T0331927

Pharmacotherapeutics
for Advanced Practice
A PRACTICAL APPROACH

FIFTH EDITION

Pharmacotherapeutics for Advanced Practice

A PRACTICAL APPROACH

FIFTH EDITION

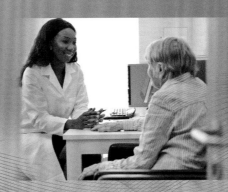
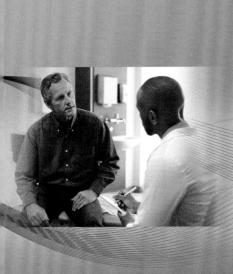
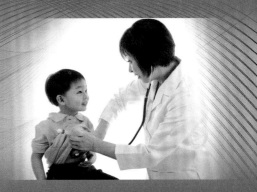

EDITORS

Virginia P. Arcangelo, PhD, NP
Family Nurse Practitioner, Retired
Canton, Georgia

Andrew M. Peterson, PharmD, PhD, FCPP
Executive Director,
Substance Use Disorders Institute
John Wyeth Dean Emeritus
Professor of Clinical Pharmacy and
Professor of Health Polity
University of the Sciences in Philadelphia
Philadelphia, Pennsylvania

**Veronica F. Wilbur, PhD, APRN-FNP, CNE,
FAANP**
Associate Professor – Graduate Nursing
Department of Nursing
West Chester University
West Chester, Pennsylvania

Tep M. Kang, PharmD, BCPS
Clinical Pharmacy Specialist,
Surgical Critical Care
Christiana Care Health Services
Adjunct Instructor, University of Delaware

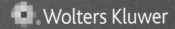
Wolters Kluwer

Philadelphia · Baltimore · New York · London
Buenos Aires · Hong Kong · Sydney · Tokyo

Not authorised for sale in United States, Canada, Australia, New Zealand, Puerto Rico, and U.S. Virgin Islands.

Acquisitions Editor: Jamie Blum
Development Editor: Maria M. McAvey
Editorial Coordinator: Julie Kostelnik
Senior Production Project Manager: Sadie Buckallew
Design Coordinator: Stephen Druding
Manufacturing Coordinator: Kathleen Brown
Marketing Manager: Linda Wetmore
Prepress Vendor: Lumina Datamatics

5th edition

Library of Congress Cataloging-in-Publication Data

ISBN-13: 978-1-9751-6059-3

Cataloging in Publication data available on request from publisher.

This book is dedicated to all of our past, current and future students who have, or will have, touched our lives so deeply. We hope that our experience in clinical practice and teaching, and that of all our contributors in this edition, will help promote excellence in patient care.

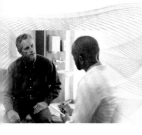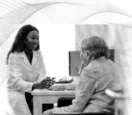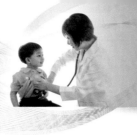
Pharmacotherapeutics for Advanced Practice originated from our combined experience in teaching nurse practitioners and practice in primary care. As a nurse practitioner and educator herself, Virginia P. Arcangelo, PhD, NP, saw a need for practical exposure to the general principles of prescribing and monitoring drug therapy, particularly in the Family Practice arena. As a PharmD, Andrew M. Peterson saw a need to be able to teach new prescribers how to think about prescribing systematically, regardless of the disease state. Veronica F. Wilbur, PhD, NP, joined the editorial team in the last edition, and her expertise as a Family Nurse Practitioner and educator added tremendous value to the staff. Joining the editorial team in the 5th edition is Dr. Tep M. Kang, a clinical pharmacist working in the acute care setting. As a past chapter author and now editor, he adds another dimension to the text.

This edition continues to build upon the foundations of the previous four editions by providing up-to-date pharmacology and disease state knowledge underscored by a process and framework through which learners can begin to think pharmacotherapeutically. While primarily geared toward the learner, this text meets both students' and practitioners' needs by providing a user-friendly, practical approach to prescribing and managing drug therapy. The book has evolved over the years, based on input from students, academicians, and practitioners. Long-standing contributors and new contributors updated their chapters to provide a combination of evidence-based medicine and practical experience. The text considers disease- and patient-specific information. With each chapter, there are tables and evidence-based algorithms that are practical and easy to read and complement the text.

This text provides a step-therapy approach that allows the learner to see select first-line, second-line, and even third-line therapy for treating the diseases. New drugs are always coming on the market; therefore, drug classes are emphasized with the focus on the application of the broader, class-specific properties of new drugs. Each chapter ends with a simple case study or series of questions designed to prompt the learner to think systematically and the teacher to ask critical questions. Each section has two cases/sets of questions—one available to the student and one available for just the faculty member/teacher. The answers to both sets of cases/questions are provided for the faculty via the online portal. There are no answers to the questions in the text since we believe the purpose of the case studies is to promote discussion. There may be more than one correct answer to each question, especially as new drugs enter the market and treatment guidelines change. We realize that there may be several answers to these questions, and we have provided just one option.

New to this edition is the provision of additional ancillary tools for students and instructors. Students have online access to Concepts in Action and current articles related to various drugs. The addition of a test bank online for instructors provides ready-made questions for each chapter to use to create examinations. As in the past, faculty can access PowerPoint slides for each chapter to prepare for classroom instruction, and acronyms are available online for students to help in their learning.

ORGANIZATION OF THE BOOK

Units 1 and 2—Principles of Therapeutics

As with previous editions, the book's Principles Unit reviews the basic therapeutics elements necessary for safe and effective prescribing. The first chapter introduces the prescribing process, including how to avoid medication errors. The following two chapters provide the foundation of therapeutics, including information on the pharmacokinetics and pharmacodynamics of drugs and drug–drug/drug–food interactions. In this edition, we've combined the pediatric and pregnancy/lactation chapters to provide a more cohesive approach to the spectrum of birth through childhood. We've kept geriatric, antimicrobial, and pharmacogenomics chapters in the foundational section and moved the Economics of Therapeutics chapter here to emphasize further the critical role this element has to play in drug therapy selection and management.

However, the reader will note we added a separate section on pain management. The book still has a chapter anchored in pain management basics, but two new chapters have been added. The first focuses on treating pain in the patient with opioid use disorder (OUD) and another on cannabis as a tool for pain management. These additions reflect the ever-changing landscape of medicine, and we hope to help introduce the student and practitioner to these—once-taboo—topics.

Units 3 through 15—Disorders

This unit of the book, consisting of 45 chapters, reviews commonly seen disorders in the primary care setting. Although not all-inclusive, the array of disorders allows the reader to gain an understanding of how to approach the pharmacotherapeutic treatment of any condition. The chapters are designed to give a brief overview of the disease process, including the causes and pathophysiology, emphasizing how drug therapy can alter the pathologic state.

We have made some significant changes to the content of these units. We have added three new chapters—liver diseases, organ transplantation, and substance use disorders. These additions reflect the clinician's expanded responsibility to have a more in-depth understanding of how these conditions affect patients' care and treatment. It is well known that liver dysfunction affects drug metabolism. Still, the clinician needs to understand liver diseases as an entity to appreciate better how to care for patients living with such disorders.

Similarly, more and more people are receiving and living with transplanted organs. The drugs and treatments required to maintain remission affect the treatment of other chronic conditions, thus obliging the practitioner to grasp these life-saving drugs. And lastly, the opioid epidemic has brought the issue of substance use disorders into the forefront of society's mind, and it is being recognized that these disorders are not limited to just prescription drugs. People are—and have been—living with substance use disorders—most notably alcohol and opioid use disorders—and the clinician must understand these conditions to treat the patient holistically.

Other text changes include combining the gastrointestinal (GI) disorders such as nausea/vomiting and diarrhea with physiologic and pathophysiologic diseases like irritable bowel and inflammatory bowel syndrome. We've also combined several skin disorders into a single chapter, thus reducing redundancy in diagnosis and treatment strategies. And to reflect the integral nature of some behavioral disorders, we have added Bipolar Disease to the Depression chapter.

Chapter Organization

This edition continues the consistent format approach throughout each disorder chapter. Each chapter begins with the background and pathophysiology of the disorder, followed by a discussion of the **Diagnostic Criteria** and **Goals of Therapy** that underlie the basic principles of treating patients with drugs.

The drug sections review the "agents" uses, mechanism of action, contraindications and drug interactions, adverse effects, and monitoring parameters. This discussion is organized primarily by drug class, with a notation to specific drugs within the text and the tables. The **Drug Overview Tables** are organized consistently, giving the reader much information on each drug, including the usual dose, contraindications, side effects, and any special considerations a prescriber should be aware of during therapy. The tables provide the reader with quick access to generic and trade names and dosages, adverse events, contraindications, and special considerations. Together, the text and tables provide the reader with sufficient information to begin to choose drug therapy.

The section on **Selecting the Most Appropriate Agent** aids the reader in deciding which drug to choose for a given patient. This section contains information on first-line, second-line, and third-line therapies, with rationales for the classification of drugs in these categories. Accompanying this section is an **algorithm** outlining the thought process by which clinicians select an initial drug therapy. Again, the text organization and the illustrative algorithms provide readers with a means of thinking by selecting drugs for patients. As with previous editions, we have kept the **Recommended Order of Treatment tables** and updated them, along with the algorithms and drug tables, to reflect current knowledge. Each chapter has been updated to reflect the most current guidelines available at the time of writing. However, medicine and pharmacotherapy are constantly changing, and it remains the clinician's responsibility to identify the most current information.

Included in each chapter is a section on **Monitoring Patient Response**. Each section encompasses clinical and laboratory parameters, times to monitor items, and actions to take the parameters that do not meet the specified therapy goals. Also, special patient populations are discussed when appropriate. These discussions include pediatric and geriatric patients but may also include ethnic- or sex-related considerations. The last item in this section consists of a discussion of patient education material relevant to the disease, and drugs are chosen. In each chapter, a patient education section includes information on complementary and alternative medicine related to that disorder and sections on external information for patients and practitioners.

A **Case Study** is provided for each disorder discussed and designed to stimulate discussion among students and instructors. In this edition, each case has been reviewed and updated with questions tailored to reinforce the process of thinking pharmacotherapeutically. As previously stated, answers to these case studies are not supplied to the student since the purpose is to promote discussion and evoke a thought process. Also, as time changes, so do therapies. The cases are short, compelling the learner to ask questions about the patient and allowing flexibility for multiple correct answers to be developed by the instructor as they work through the clinical decision-making process.

Pharmacotherapeutics for Advanced Practice continues to provide primary care students with a reasoned approach to learning pharmacotherapeutics and serves as a reference for the seasoned practitioner. Prescribing is becoming increasingly complex, and the information in this book has helped us in our own practices. As experienced educators and practitioners, we provide you with a textbook that will meet your needs.

Virginia P. Arcangelo
Andrew M. Peterson
Veronica F. Wilbur
Tep M. Kang

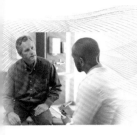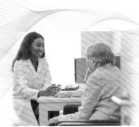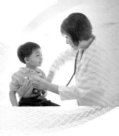

Iman I. Aberra
Clinical Pharmacist
Department of Pharmacy
ChristianaCare Health System
Newark, Delaware

Jennifer Andres, PharmD, BCPS
Clinical Pharmacist
Clinical Associate Professor of Pharmacy Practice
Temple University School of Pharmacy
Philadelphia, Pennsylvania

Virginia P. Arcangelo, PhD, NP
Family Nurse Practitioner, Retired
Canton, Georgia

Caroline Attia, PharmD, MBA, BCPS, BCGP, CPHQ
Clinical Pharmacist Specialist
Department of Pharmacy
ChristianaCare Health Services
Newark, Delaware

Kristen M. Audley, PharmD, BCCCP
Clinical Pharmacy Specialist, Neurocritical Care
Pharmacy Department
Overlook Medical Center
Atlantic Health System
Summit, New Jersey

Kelly Barranger, MSN, RN, CRNP
Certified Registered Nurse Practitioner
Department of Nursing
Veterans Affairs
Philadelphia, Pennsylvania

John Barron, PharmD
Staff Vice President and Clinical Research Advisor
HealthCore, Inc.
Wilmington, Delaware

Laura L. Bio, PharmD, BCPS
Assistant Professor
Department of Pharmacy Practice
Philadelphia College of Pharmacy
Philadelphia, Pennsylvania
Clinical Pharmacist
Department of Pharmacy
Children's Regional Hospital at Cooper University Hospital
Camden, New Jersey

Lyndsay Carlson, PharmD BCACP
Adjunct Clinical Assistant Professor
Binghamton University School of Pharmacy and
Pharmaceutical Sciences
Anticoagulation Clinical Pharmacist
UHS Wilson Medical Center
Johnson City, New York

Jesse Chen, PharmD
Clinical Pharmacist
Department of Pharmacy
ChristianaCare Health Services
Newark, Delaware

Caragh E. Clayton, PharmD
Clinical Pharmacist
Department of Pharmacy
ChristianaCare Health Services
Newark, Delaware

Lauren M. Czosnowski, PharmD, BCPS
Assistant Professor
Department of Pharmacy Practice
Butler University
Clinical Specialist
Pharmacy Department
IU Health Methodist Hospital
Indianapolis, Indiana

Quinn A. Czosnowski, PharmD
Clinical Pharmacy Specialist
Pharmacy Department
IU Health Methodist Hospital
Indianapolis, Indiana

Ryan G. D'Angelo
Advanced Practice Pharmacist
Department of Pharmacy
Thomas Jefferson University Hospital
Philadelphia, Pennsylvania

Sarah E. Diamond
Clinical Pharmacist
Department of Pharmacy
ChristianaCare Health System
Newark, Delaware

Rachel Dimeo, PharmD BCPS
Clinical Pharmacist
ChristianaCare Health System Newark, Delaware

David Dinh, PharmD, BCPS
Clinical Pharmacy Specialist, Emergency Medicine
Department of Pharmacy
Yale New Haven Hospital
New Haven, Connecticut

Amy M. Egras, PharmD, BCPS, BC-ADM
Associate Professor
Department of Pharmacy Practice
Jefferson School of Pharmacy
Clinical Pharmacist
Jefferson Family Medicine Associates
Thomas Jefferson University
Philadelphia, Pennsylvania

Tracy S. Estes, PhD, DNP, RN, FNP-BC
Family Nurse Practitioner Partner
Next Century Medical Care LLC
Wilmington, Delaware

Kelleen N. Flaherty, MS
Adjunct Assistant Professor
Department of Biomedical Writing
University of the Sciences in Philadelphia
Philadelphia, Pennsylvania

Maria C. Foy, PharmD, BCPS, CPE
Clinical Specialist, Palliative Care
Pharmacy Department
Abington Memorial Hospital
Abington, Pennsylvania

Steven P. Gelone, PharmD
Chief Development Officer
Nabriva Therapeutics
King of Prussia, Pennsylvania

Andrew J. Grimone, PharmD, BCPS-AQ ID
Assistant Professor
Department of Nursing
Clarion University of Pennsylvania
Clarion, Pennsylvania
Clinical Pharmacy Manager
Department of Pharmacy
Saint Vincent Hospital
Allegheny Health Network
Erie, Pennsylvania

Anisha B. Grover, PharmD, BCACP
Assistant Professor of Clinical Pharmacy
Department of Pharmacy Practice and Pharmacy Administration
Philadelphia College of Pharmacy
University of the Sciences
Philadelphia, Pennsylvania

Diane E. Hadley, PharmD, BCACP
Assistant Professor of Clinical Pharmacy
Department of Pharmacy Practice and Pharmacy Administration
University of the Sciences
Philadelphia, Pennsylvania

Kelsey C. Haines, PharmD, BCPS
Clinical Pharmacist
ChristianaCare Health Services
Newark, Delaware

Emily R. Hajjar, PharmD, BCPS, BCACP, CGP
Associate Professor
Department of Pharmacy Practice
Jefferson School of Pharmacy
Philadelphia, Pennsylvania

Amalia M. Issa PhD, MPH, FCP
Founding Director, Personalized Medicine & Targeted Therapeutics
Professor of Health Policy
Professor of Pharmaceutical Sciences
University of the Sciences in Philadelphia
Philadelphia, Pennsylvania

Sarah Jung, PharmD, MS, BCCCP
Clinical pharmacy specialist - Neurocritical care
Wellstar Kennestone Regional Medical Center
Atlanta, Georgia

Tep M. Kang, PharmD, BCPS
Adjunct Instructor
Department of Nursing
University of Delaware
Newark, Delaware
Wilmington University
New Castle, Delaware
Critical Care Pharmacist
Department of Pharmacy
Christiana Care Health Services
Newark, Delaware

Lauren Isaacs Karel, PharmD, BCPS
Clinical Pharmacy Specialist, Drug Information
Department of Pharmacy
Children's Hospital of Philadelphia
Philadelphia, Pennsylvania

Samantha Landolfa
Director Ambulatory & Specialty Pharmacy Services
Department of Pharmacy
ChristianaCare Health System
Newark, Delaware

Thuy Le, PharmD, BCPS
Clinical Pharmacist
Department of Pharmacy
ChristianaCare
Newark, Delaware

Jessica M. Leri, PharmD
Clinical Pharmacist
Department of Pharmacy
ChristianaCare Health Services
Newark, Delaware

Jenny R. Liu, PharmD
Clinical Pharmacist
Department of Pharmacy
Christiana Hospital
Newark, Delaware

Laura A. Mandos, BS, PharmD, BCPP
Professor of Clinical Pharmacy
Department of Pharmacy Practice and Pharmacy
Administration
Philadelphia College of Pharmacy
University of the Sciences
Philadelphia, Pennsylvania

Stephen May, PharmD
Clinical Pharmacist
Department of Pharmacy
ChristianaCare Health Services
Newark, Delaware

Lauren K. McCluggage, PharmD
Associate Professor
Lipscomb University College of Pharmacy
Clinical Pharmacist
Department of Pharmacy
St. Thomas West Hospital
Nashville, Tennessee

Karleen Melody, PharmD, BCACP
Assistant Professor of Clinical Pharmacy
Department of Pharmacy Practice and Pharmacy
Administration
Philadelphia College of Pharmacy
University of the Sciences
Philadelphia, Pennsylvania

Isabelle Mercier, PhD
Associate Professor
Pharmaceutical Sciences
University of the Sciences
Philadelphia, Pennsylvania

Lorraine Nowakowski-Grier, MSN, APRN, BC, CDE
Adjunct Faculty
Department of Nursing
College of Health Professions
Wilmington University
New Castle, Delaware
Nurse Practitioner, Diabetes Educator
Department of Nursing Education
and Development
Christiana Care Health Services
Newark, Delaware

Judith A. O'Donnell, MD
Associate Professor of Medicine
Division of Infectious Diseases
Perelman School of Medicine at the University of
Pennsylvania
Chief, Division of Infectious Diseases
Hospital Epidemiologist and Director, Infection Prevention
& Control
Penn Presbyterian Medical Center
Philadelphia, Pennsylvania

Staci Pacetti, PharmD
Assistant Professor
Department of Nursing
Rutgers University School of Nursing
Camden, New Jersey

Andrew M. Peterson, PharmD, PhD, FCPP
John Wyeth Dean
Professor of Clinical Pharmacy and Professor
of Health Policy
University of the Sciences in Philadelphia
Philadelphia, Pennsylvania

Daniel A. Peterson, PharmD
Patient Care Pharmacist
Thomas Jefferson University Hospitals
Philadelphia, Pennsylvania

Louis R. Petrone, MD
Clinical Assistant Professor
Family and Community Medicine
Sidney Kimmel Medical College
Attending Physician
Family and Community Medicine
Thomas Jefferson University Hospital
Philadelphia, Pennsylvania

Daniel Purzycki, PharmD
Clinical Pharmacist
ChristianaCare Health System
Newark, Delaware

A. Maggie Randazzo, PharmD, BCPS
Assistant Professor
Department of Physician Assistant Studies
Jefferson College of Health Professions
Thomas Jefferson University
Voorhees, New Jersey
Clinical Pharmacist
Pharmacy Department
Shore Medical Center
Somers Point, New Jersey

Jennifer A. Reinhold, BA, PharmD, BCPS, BCPP
Associate Professor of Clinical Pharmacy
Philadelphia College of Pharmacy
University of the Sciences in Philadelphia
Philadelphia, Pennsylvania

Christopher C. Roe, MSN, ACNP-BC
Nurse Practitioner Manager
Center for Heart and Vascular Health
Christiana Care Health Systems
Newark, Delaware

Jola Salavaci
Clinical Pharmacist
Department of Pharmacy
ChristianaCare Health System
Newark, Delaware

David M. Salerno, PharmD, BCPS
Clinical Pharmacy Manager, Liver Transplant
NewYork-Presbyterian Hospital,
Weill Cornell Medical Center
New York, New York

Brooke Salzman
Associate Professor
Department of Family and Community Medicine
Thomas Jefferson University
Philadelphia, Pennsylvania

Cynthia A. Sanoski, PharmD, BCPS, FCCP
Department Chair and Associate Professor
Department of Pharmacy Practice
Jefferson School of Pharmacy
Thomas Jefferson University
Philadelphia, Pennsylvania

Briana L. Santaniello, MBA, PharmD
PGY1 Managed Care Pharmacy Resident
University of Massachusetts Medical School's Clinical
Pharmacy Services
Shrewsbury, Massachusetts

Alice (Lim) Scaletta, PharmD, BCACP
Assistant Professor of Clinical Pharmacy
Department of Pharmacy Practice and Pharmacy
Administration
Philadelphia College of Pharmacy
Philadelphia, Pennsylvania

Jason J. Schafer, PharmD, MPH
Associate Professor
Department of Pharmacy Practice
Jefferson School of Pharmacy
Thomas Jefferson University
Philadelphia, Pennsylvania

Shelly R. Schneider, APN
Nurse Practitioner
Premier Dermatology
Haddon Heights, New Jersey

Jean M. Scholtz, BS, PharmD, BCPS, FASHP
Associate Professor, Vice Chair
Department of Pharmacy Practice
Philadelphia College of Pharmacy
Philadelphia, Pennsylvania

Mily Shah, PharmD
Post-Doctoral Fellow
Department of Medical Affairs
Janssen Pharmaceuticals
Voorhees, New Jersey

Pooja Shah, PharmD, BCPPS
Clinical Associate Professor
Department of Pharmacy Practice and Pharmacy
Administration
Rutgers, The State University of New Jersey
Piscataway, New Jersey
Clinical Pharmacy Specialist, Neonatal Intensive Care &
General Pediatrics
Department of Pharmacy
Hackensack University Medical Center
Hackensack, New Jersey

Priya M. Shah, PharmD
Clinical Pharmacist
Department of Pharmacy
ChristianaCare
Newark, Delaware

Anita Siu, PharmD
Clinical Professor
Department of Pharmacy Practice and Pharmacy
Administration
Rutgers, The State University of New Jersey
Piscataway, New Jersey
Neonatal/Pediatric Pharmacotherapy Specialist
Department of Pharmacy
Jersey Shore University Medical Center
Neptune, New Jersey

Sarah A. Spinler, PharmD
Professor of Clinical Pharmacy
Department of Pharmacy Practice and Pharmacy
Administration
Philadelphia College of Pharmacy
University of the Sciences
Philadelphia, Pennsylvania

Joshua J. Spooner, PharmD, MS
Associate Professor of Pharmacy
College of Pharmacy
Western New England University
Springfield, Massachusetts

Linda M. Spooner, PharmD, BCPS, FASHP
Professor of Pharmacy Practice
Department of Pharmacy Practice
MCPHS University School of Pharmacy–
Worcester/Manchester
Clinical Pharmacy Specialist in Infectious Diseases
Saint Vincent Hospital
Worcester, Massachusetts

Richard G. Stefanacci, DO, MGH, MBA, AGSF, CMD
Faculty
School of Population Health
Thomas Jefferson University
Philadelphia, Pennsylvania
Chief Medical Officer
The Access Group
Berkeley Heights, New Jersey
Senior Physician
Mercy LIFE
Trinity Health System
Philadelphia, Pennsylvania

Jeffrey Raymond F. Tagle, PharmD, BCPS
Clinical Pharmacist, Anticoagulation Center
Department of Pharmacy Services
ChristianaCare
Newark, Delaware

**Angela Thompson DNP, FNP-C, BC-ADM, CDCES,
FAANP**
Family Nurse Practitioner
Hendricks Endocrinology
Danville, Indiana
Medical Director
Diabetes Youth Foundation of Indiana
Noblesville, Indiana

Tyan F. Thomas, PharmD
Associate Professor of Clinical Pharmacy
Department of Pharmacy Practice and Pharmacy
Administration
Philadelphia College of Pharmacy at the University of the
Sciences
Clinical Pharmacy Specialist
Department of Pharmacy
Philadelphia VA Medical Center
Philadelphia, Pennsylvania

Karen J. Tietze, PharmD
Professor of Clinical Pharmacy
Philadelphia College of Pharmacy
University of the Sciences in Philadelphia
Philadelphia, Pennsylvania

Rachel Trichtinger, BCPP
Unit-Based Pharmacist- Psychiatry
Pharmacy Department
Abington Jefferson Health
Abington, Pennsylvania

Elena M. Umland, PharmD
Associate Dean, Academic Affairs
Professor, Pharmacy Practice
Jefferson School of Pharmacy
Thomas Jefferson University
Philadelphia, Pennsylvania

Sarah F. Uroza, PharmD
Assistant Professor
Department of Pharmacy Practice
Lipscomb University
Clinical Pharmacist
Faith Family Medical Clinic
Nashville, Tennessee

Michael Weissberger, MD
Fellow
Department of Family and Community Medicine
Thomas Jefferson University
Philadelphia, Pennsylvania

Veronica F. Wilbur, PhD, APRN-FNP, CNE, FAANP
Assistant Professor of Graduate Nursing
West Chester University
West Chester, Pennsylvania

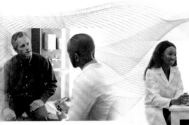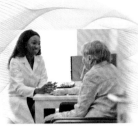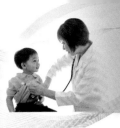

Virginia P. Arcangelo, PhD, NP

Laura Aykroyd, PharmD

Kelly Barranger, MSN, RN, CRNP

John Barron, PharmD

Laura L. Bio, PharmD, BCPS

Lauren M. Czosnowski, PharmD, BCPS

Quinn A. Czosnowski, PharmD

David Dinh, PharmD, BCPS

Amy M. Egras, PharmD, BCPS, BC-ADM

Kelleen N. Flaherty, MS

Maria C. Foy, PharmD, BCPS, CPE

Steven P. Gelone, PharmD

Andrew J. Grimone, PharmD, BCPS-AQ ID

Anisha B. Grover, PharmD, BCACP

Diane E. Hadley, PharmD, BCACP

Emily R. Hajjar, PharmD, BCPS, BCACP, CGP

Amalia M. Issa, PhD, MPH, FCPP

Tep M. Kang, PharmD, BCPS

Alice (Lim) Scaletta, PharmD, BCACP

Laura A. Mandos, BS, PharmD, BCPP

Lauren K. McCluggage, PharmD

Karleen Melody, PharmD, BCACP

Isabelle Mercier, PhD

Carol Gullo Mest, PhD, RN, ANP-BC

Samir K. Mistry, PharmD

Lorraine Nowakowski-Grier, MSN, APRN, BC, CDE

Judith A. O'Donnell, MD

Staci Pacetti, PharmD

Andrew M. Peterson, PharmD, PhD, FCPP

Louis R. Petrone, MD

Melody D. Randle, DNP, FNP-C, MSN, CCNS, CNE

Troy L. Randle, DO, FACC, FACOI

Jennifer A. Reinhold, BA, PharmD, BCPS, BCPP

Christopher C. Roe, MSN, ACNP-BC

Cynthia A. Sanoski, PharmD, BCPS, FCCP

Briana L. Santaniello, MBA, PharmD

Jason J. Schafer, PharmD, MPH

Shelly R. Schneider, APN

Jean M. Scholtz, BS, PharmD, BCPS, FASHP

Anita Siu, PharmD

Sarah A. Spinler, PharmD

Joshua J. Spooner, PharmD, MS

Linda M. Spooner, PharmD, BCPS, FASHP

Richard G. Stefanacci, DO, MGH, MBA, AGSF, CMD

James C. Thigpen Jr, PharmD, BCPS

Tyan F. Thomas, PharmD

Karen J. Tietze, PharmD

Elena M. Umland, PharmD

Sarah F. Uroza, PharmD

Craig B. Whitman, PharmD, BCPS

Veronica F. Wilbur, PhD, APRN-FNP, CNE, FAANP

Vincent J. Willey, PharmD

Eric T. Wittbrodt, PharmD, MPH

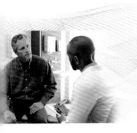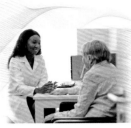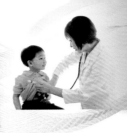

CONTENTS

Preface vii
Contributors ix
Previous Edition Contributors xv

UNIT

1 Principles of Therapeutics *1*

1 Issues for the Practitioner in Drug Therapy *3*
Veronica F. Wilbur

2 Pharmacokinetic Basis of Therapeutics and Pharmacodynamic Principles *17*
Andrew M. Peterson and A. Maggie Randazzo

3 Impact of Drug Interactions and Adverse Events on Therapeutics *33*
Tep M. Kang

4 Principles of Pharmacotherapy in Pediatrics, Pregnancy, and Lactation *55*
Pooja Shah and Anita Siu

5 Pharmacotherapy Principles in Older Adults *71*
Richard G. Stefanacci

6 Principles of Antimicrobial Therapy *93*
Steven P. Gelone, Staci Pacetti, and Judith A. O'Donnell

7 Pharmacogenomics *121*
Isabelle Mercier and Amalia M. Issa

8 The Economics of Pharmacotherapeutics *131*
Briana L. Santaniello and Joshua J. Spooner

UNIT

2 Principles of Pain Management *143*

9 Pharmacotherapy of Pain Management *145*
Maria C. Foy

10 Pain Management in Opioid Use Disorder (OUD) Patients *167*
Rachel Trichtinger and Maria C. Foy

11 Cannabis and Pain Management *179*
Andrew M. Peterson and Mily Shah

UNIT

3 Pharmacotherapy for Skin Disorders *189*

12 Contact Dermatitis *191*
Jeffrey Tagle and Virginia P. Arcangelo

13 Fungal, Viral, and Bacterial Infections of the Skin *199*
Iman I. Aberra, Virginia P. Arcangelo, and Jason J. Schafer

14 Psoriasis *229*
Shelly R. Schneider

15 Acne Vulgaris and Rosacea *241*
Shelly R. Schneider

UNIT

4 Pharmacotherapy for Eye and Ear Disorders *255*

16 Ophthalmic Disorders *257*
Joshua J. Spooner

17 Otitis Media and Otitis Externa *281*
Laura L. Bio

UNIT

5 Pharmacotherapy for Cardiovascular Disorders *293*

18 Hypertension *295*
Samantha Landolfa and Diane E. Hadley

19 Hyperlipidemia *313*
Thuy Le and John Barron

20 Chronic Stable Angina and Myocardial Infarction *329*
Lauren Isaacs Karel and Christopher C. Roe

21 Heart Failure *349*
Stephen May and Andrew M. Peterson

22 Arrhythmias *371*
Andrew M. Peterson, Daniel A. Peterson, and Cynthia A. Sanoski

UNIT

6 Pharmacotherapy for Respiratory Disorders *401*

23 Respiratory Infections *403*
Sara Jung, Karleen Melody, Anisha B. Grover, and Andrew J. Grimone

24 Asthma and Chronic Obstructive Pulmonary Disease *425*
Tracy S. Estes and Karen J. Tietze

UNIT

7 Pharmacotherapy for Gastrointestinal Disorders *449*

25 Gastric, Functional, and Inflammatory Bowel Disorders *451*
Veronica F. Wilbur

26 Gastroesophageal Reflux Disease and Peptic Ulcer Disease *523*
Alice (Lim) Scaletta

27 Liver Diseases *541*
Ryan G. D'Angelo and Jennifer Andres

UNIT

8 Pharmacotherapy for Genitourinary Tract Disorders *565*

28 Urinary Tract Infection *567*
Veronica F. Wilbur

29 Prostatic Disorders and Erectile Dysfunction *577*
Veronica F. Wilbur

30 Overactive Bladder *595*
Sarah E. Diamond

31 Sexually Transmitted Infections *615*
Caragh E. Clayton and Virginia P. Arcangelo

UNIT

9 Pharmacology for Musculoskeletal Disorders *639*

32 Osteoarthritis and Gout *641*
Rachael DiMeo, Daniel Purzycki, and Sarah F. Uroza

33 Osteoporosis *663*
Jola Salavaci and Virginia P. Arcangelo

34 Rheumatoid Arthritis *675*
Lauren K. McCluggage and Kelsey C. Haines

UNIT

10 Pharmacotherapy for Neurological Disorders *691*

35 Headaches *693*
Kelleen N. Flaherty

36 Seizure Disorders *725*
Jesse Chen and Quinn A. Czosnowski

37 Alzheimer's Disease *755*
Emily R. Hajjar, Brooke Salzman, and Michael Weisberger

38 Parkinson's Disease *765*
David Dinh, Karleen Melody, and Anisha B. Grover

UNIT

11 Pharmacotherapy for Mental Health Disorders *781*

39 Major Depressive Disorder and Bipolar Disorders *783*
Priya M. Shah

40 Anxiety Disorders *809*
Sarah Jung and Laura A. Mandos

41 Sleep Disorders *829*
Veronica F. Wilbur

42 Attention Deficit Hyperactivity Disorder *855*
Kristen M. Audley

43 Substance Use Disorders *869*
Andrew M. Peterson

UNIT

12 Pharmacotherapy for Endocrine Disorders *885*

44 Diabetes Mellitus *887*
Angela Thompson and Lorraine Nowakowski-Grier

45 Thyroid and Parathyroid Disorders *911*
Alice (Lim) Scaletta and Louis R. Petrone

UNIT

13 Pharmacotherapy for Immunology *927*

46 Allergies and Allergic Reactions *929*
Lauren M. Czosnowski

47 Human Immunodeficiency Virus *947*
Linda M. Spooner

48 Organ Transplantation *965*
David M. Salerno

UNIT

14 Pharmacotherapy for Thromboembolic Disorders *979*

49 Thromboembolic Disorders *981*
Sarah A. Spinler and Lyndsay Carlson

50 Anemias *1013*
Caroline Attia and Kelly Barranger

UNIT

15 Pharmacotherapy for Health Promotion *1031*

51 Immunizations *1033*
Jean M. Scholtz

52 Smoking Cessation *1057*
Tyan F. Thomas

53 Weight Loss *1077*
Amy M. Egras

UNIT

16 Pharmacotherapy for Women's Health *1087*

54 Contraception *1089*
Jenny R. Liu and Virginia P. Arcangelo

55 Menopause *1101*
Jessica M. Leri and Elena M. Umland

56 Vaginitis *1115*
Iman I. Aberra and Virginia P. Arcangelo

Index 1129

UNIT
1

Principles of Therapeutics

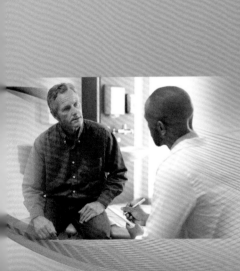
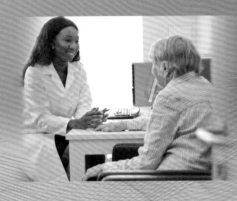
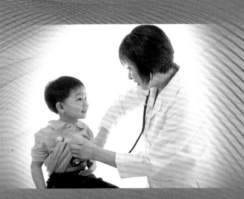

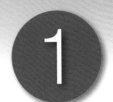

1 Issues for the Practitioner in Drug Therapy

Veronica F. Wilbur

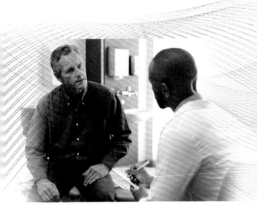
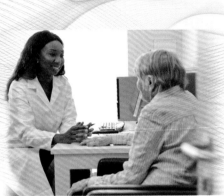
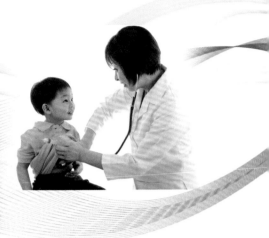

Learning Objectives

After reading this chapter, the reader will be able to:

1. Describe the approval process for prescribed drugs in the United States.
2. Analyze the practitioner's role and responsibilities in prescribing.
3. Explain the process for prescribing, whether in writing or through the electronic health record.

INTRODUCTION

Drug therapy is often the mainstay of treatment of acute and chronic diseases. An essential role of health care practitioners is to develop a treatment plan with the patient, and an integral part of the treatment plan of illness and health promotion is drug therapy. According to Center for Disease Control as reported in the Health in the United States (2018), from 2013 to 2016, among individuals aged 45 to 64, 64% of males and 73% of females used three or more prescription drugs and 13.3% used five or more during the last 30 days. Additionally, according to the National Ambulatory Medical Survey (2016), there were 2.9 billion drugs (73.9%) prescribed during office visits, 365.8 million drugs (72.5%) prescribed during visits to a hospital outpatient department, and 286.2 million drugs (81.1%) prescribed during visits to a hospital emergency department (Rui & Kang, 2017). In an analysis by the AARP Public Policy Institute, there has been a consistent increase in drug prices that is higher than inflation between 2006 and 2017 (RxPrice Watch, 2019). Even though the price of generic

drugs has dropped, the amount spent out of pocket annually for a chronic generic drug of a Medicare patient can equal $365 (Schondelmeyer & Purvis, 2018). Therefore, prescribers must have a breadth of knowledge about the principles of prescribing.

In developing a treatment plan that includes drug therapy, the prescribing practitioner considers many issues in achieving the goal of safe, appropriate, and effective treatment. Among them are drug safety and product safeguards, the practitioner's role and responsibilities, the step-by-step process of prescribing therapy and writing the prescription, and follow-up measures. Particularly noteworthy are promoting adherence to the therapeutic regimen and keeping up to date with the latest developments in drug therapy.

DRUG SAFETY AND MARKET SAFEGUARDS

Drug safety is ensured in the United States primarily by the U.S. Food and Drug Administration (FDA), which is the federal agency charged with conducting and monitoring clinical trials, approving new drugs for market and manufacture, and ensuring safe drugs for public consumption. Although the federal government supplies guidelines for a pure and safe drug product, guidelines for prescribers of drug therapy are dictated both by state and by federal governments and by licensing bodies in each state.

Clinical Trials

Various legislated mechanisms are in place to ensure pure and safe drug products. One of these mechanisms is the clinical trial process by which the FDA carefully checks new drug

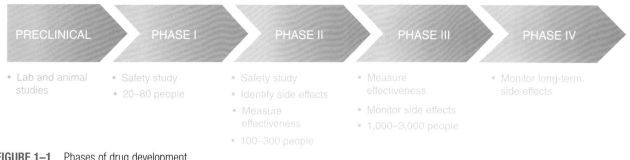

FIGURE 1–1 Phases of drug development.

development. Every new drug must successfully pass through several stages of development (see **Figure 1.1**). The first stage is preclinical trials, which involve testing in animals and monitoring efficacy, toxic effects, and untoward reactions. An application to the FDA for investigational use of a drug occurs after the preclinical trials are completed.

Clinical trials, which begin only after the FDA grants approval for investigation, consist of four phases and may last up to 9 years before the adoption of a drug for widespread use. During clinical trials, performed on informed volunteers, data are gathered about the proposed drug's purity, bioavailability, potency, efficacy, safety, and toxicity.

Phase I of clinical trials is the initial evaluation of the drug. It involves supervised studies on 20 to 100 healthy people and focuses on absorption, distribution, metabolism (sometimes interchangeable with biotransformation), and elimination of the drug. In phase I, the most effective administration routes and dosage ranges are determined. During phase II, up to several hundred patients with the disease for which the drug is intended are subjects. The testing focus is the same as in phase I, except that drug effects are monitored on people with the disease.

Phase III begins once the FDA determines that the drug causes no apparent serious adverse effects and that the dosage range is appropriate. Double-blind research methods are utilized during this phase. The investigators are blinded to who is receiving the study drug or placebo. Usually, several thousand subjects are involved in this phase, which lasts several years, and during this time, most of the risks for the drug become evident. After phase III, the FDA evaluates data presented and accepts or rejects the application for the new drug. Approval of the application means that the drug can be marketed—but only by the company seeking approval.

Once on the market, the drug enters phase IV or postmarketing surveillance. Objectives at this stage are (1) to compare the drug with others on the market, (2) to monitor for long-term effectiveness and impact on the quality of life, and (3) to analyze cost-effectiveness (Center Watch, 2015). During postmarketing surveillance, drugs can be taken off the market or restricted if additional findings emerge of the drug and side effects.

Food and Drug Administration Fast Track

In some cases, it is crucial to increase the speed of approval for drugs that treat serious diseases and meet an unmet medical need. However, *fast* does not mean the sacrifice of safety. There are four categories whereby pharmaceutical companies can request for review of their products. The first category is called the *fast track*, where the company developing the drug gets more frequent communication and has a rolling review. The second category is *breakthrough therapy*, where clinically significant surrogate endpoints are used to show effectiveness against irreversible morbidity or mortality. The third category is *accelerated approval*, and the last category is a *priority review*. Accelerated approval is another example of surrogate clinical endpoints for approval. Finally, priority review decreases the amount of time to 6 months from 10 months.

In the case of a public health emergency, the FDA can authorize a drug for use under an Emergency Use Authorization (EUA) (FDA, 2020). This is done in the public's best interest, but is in light of the fact that the FDA does not have all the evidence it would usually have to approve a drug. The EUA process was invoked to approve the drug remdesivir for the treatment of COVID-19, along with the approval of several vaccines used to combat the COVID-19 epidemic.

Prevention of Harm and Misuse

The passage of the FDA's Controlled Substances Act of 1970 established the schedule of the ranking of drugs that have the potential for abuse or misuse. The drugs on the schedule are considered controlled substances. These drugs have the potential to induce dependency and addiction, either psychologically or physiologically. **Box 1.1** defines the five categories of scheduled drugs, with Schedule 1 drugs having the most significant potential for abuse and Schedule 5 drugs the least.

Scheduled drugs can be prescribed only by a practitioner who is registered and approved by the U.S. Drug Enforcement Agency (DEA). In some states, practitioners must possess a controlled substance (CS) license as well. The DEA issues approved applicants a number, which must be written on the prescription for a CS for the prescription to be valid. The prescriber's DEA number must also appear on a prescription that was filled in another state.

The incidence of overdose emergencies and abuse of scheduled drugs continue to increase in the United States. While the overall rate of overdose deaths decreased in 2018 to 67,367, down 4.1% from its 2017 figure, there is still significant mortality in the United States (Hedegaard

---

BOX 1.1   Scheduled Drugs

Schedule 1 drugs have a high potential for abuse. There is no routine therapeutic use for these drugs, and they are not available for regular use. They may be obtained for "investigational use only" by applying to the U.S. DEA. Examples include heroin and LSD (lysergic acid diethylamide).

Schedule 2 drugs have a valid medical use but a high potential for abuse, both psychological and physiologic. In an emergency, a Schedule 2 drug may be prescribed by telephone if a written prescription cannot be provided at the time. However, a written prescription must be provided within 72 hours with the words *authorization for emergency dispensing* written on the prescription. These prescriptions cannot be refilled. A new prescription must be written each time. Examples include certain amphetamines and barbiturates.

Schedule 3 drugs have a potential for abuse, but the potential is lower than for drugs on Schedule 2. These drugs contain a combination of controlled and noncontrolled substances. Use of these drugs can cause a moderate to low physiologic dependence and a higher psychological dependence. A verbal order can be given to the pharmacy, and the prescription can be refilled up to five times within 6 months. Examples include certain narcotics (codeine) and nonbarbiturate sedatives.

Schedule 4 drugs have a low potential for abuse. They can cause psychological dependency but limited physiologic dependency. Examples include nonnarcotic analgesics and antianxiety agents, such as lorazepam (Ativan).

Schedule 5 drugs have the least potential for abuse. They contain a moderate amount of opioids and are used mainly as antitussives and antidiarrheals.

---

et al., 2020). Currently, the number of prescriptions for opioid pain medications in 2019 is 191 million and varies from state to state. In the effort to promote safe prescribing practices, many states have enacted legislation requiring the implementation of prescription drug monitoring programs (PDMPs). These programs have interconnected databases that collect a variety of information about the prescribing of substances from the DEA schedules 2 to 4. According to the National Association of State Controlled Substance Authorities (NASCSA), in 2014, 49 of 50 states had a PDMP. The program allows prescribers of a CS to look up patients for previous prescriptions of CSs, including the type of medication, amount, and name of the prescriber. The information obtained from this program helps to reveal those patients who "prescriber shop" and are receiving too many CSs. However, these programs are not without controversy, due to a lack of consensus on the scope of PDMP outcomes on patient care. Despite these concerns, the information from the PDMP helps to start a conversation with the patients, exploring their health care needs when using potentially addictive drugs.

National Provider Identifier

The Administrative Simplification provisions of the Health Insurance Portability and Accountability Act of 1996 (HIPAA) mandated the adoption of standard unique identifiers for health care providers and health plans. This identification system improves the efficiency and effectiveness of electronically transmitting health information. The National Provider Identifier (NPI) Final Rule, published on January 23, 2004, through the Centers for Medicare & Medicaid Services (CMS) developed the National Plan and Provider Enumeration System (NPPES) to assign each provider a unique NPI. Covered health care providers and all health plans and health care clearinghouses must use NPIs in the administrative and financial transactions adopted under HIPAA. The NPI is a 10-position, intelligence-free numeric identifier (10-digit number). The NPI does not carry other information about the health care provider, such as the health care provider's specialty or in which state the provider practices. Covered providers must also share their NPI with other providers, health plans, clearinghouses, and any entity that may need it for billing purposes.

The purpose of the NPI is to identify all health care providers by a unique number in standard transactions such as health care claims. NPIs may also be used to identify health care providers on prescriptions, in internal files to link proprietary provider identification numbers and other information, in the coordination of benefits between health plans, in inpatient medical record systems, in program integrity files, and in different ways. The NPI is the only health care provider identifier that can be used in standard transactions by covered entities.

Prescription versus Nonprescription Drugs

Many drugs are now available that could previously be obtained only with a prescription and at the prescription dosage. Although these drugs are accessible over the counter (OTC) without a prescription, the FDA still approves drugs with specific indications, doses, cautions, and boxed warnings. Even though these medications are within easy reach, many have the potential for interacting adversely with prescribed drugs or complicating the existing disease. The self-prescribed use of OTC drugs may delay the diagnosis and treatment of potentially serious problems. Additionally, individuals do not consider these agents to be drugs and often overuse or misuse the medication. On the other hand, the use of OTC drugs can be beneficial for the treatment of self-limiting disorders that are not serious.

Generic Drugs versus Brand Name Drugs

Substituting a generic drug for a brand name drug is a common practice, and in many states, it is required. When the patent on a brand name drug expires, other drug manufacturers can then produce the same drug formula under its generic name (the generic name and formula of a drug are always the same; only the brand names change). Due to the rising prices of brand name drugs, using generic drugs can yield savings for the consumer on the costs of medication. On average, over 2016 through 2017, the cost of generic medicines dropped by 9.3% in comparison to the inflation rate of 2.1% (Schondelmeyer & Purvis, 2018). To ensure safety, the FDA must approve generic drugs, and rigorous testing is again required to ensure that all medicines meet specifications for quality, purity, strength, and potency. Generic drugs must demonstrate therapeutic equivalence to the brand name equivalent matching the same strict standards of a branded drug. The process includes administering the generic medication in a single dose to at least 18 healthy human subjects. Next, peak serum concentration and the area under the plasma concentration curve (AUC) are measured. The values obtained for the generic drug must be within 80% to 125% of those measured for the brand name drug. Most generic drugs have a mean AUC within 3% of the brand name drug. There has been no reported therapeutic difference of a serious nature between brand name products and FDA-approved generic products. For more information, see **Table 1.1**, which presents FDA equivalency ratings for brand name and generic drugs.

Complementary and Alternative Medicine

In the United States, the use of herbal preparations as treatments for disease and disease prevention has increased tremendously. According to the National Center for Complementary and Integrative Health, the most recent survey about alternative medicines, in 2012, found that approximately 33% of adults and 11% of children use some form of complementary medication in their health care. The findings mirror results

TABLE 1.1	
Food and Drug Administration Therapeutic Equivalence Ratings	
Rating Scale	**Definition**
A	*Therapeutically Equivalent*
AA	Products in conventional dosage forms not presenting bioequivalence problems
AB	Products meeting necessary bioequivalence requirements
AN	Solutions and powders for aerosolization
AO	Injectable oil solutions
AP	Injectable aqueous solutions and, in certain instances, intravenous nonaqueous solutions
AT	Topical products
B	*Not Therapeutically Equivalent*
BB	Drug products requiring further FDA investigation and review to determine therapeutic equivalence
BC	Extended-release dosage forms (capsules, injectables, and tablets)
BD	Active ingredients and dosage forms with documented bioequivalence problems
BE	Delayed-release oral dosage forms
BN	Products in aerosol–nebulizer drug delivery systems
BP	Active ingredients and dosage forms with potential bioequivalence problems
BR	Suppositories or enemas that deliver drugs for systemic absorption
BS	Products having drug standard deficiencies
BT	Topical products with bioequivalence issues
BX	Drug products for which the data are insufficient to determine therapeutic equivalence
AB	Products for which potential equivalence problems have been resolved with adequate in vivo or in vitro evidence supporting bioequivalence

FDA, Food and Drug Administration.

U.S. Department of Health and Human Services, Food and Drug Administration, Center for Drug Evaluation and Research, Office of Pharmaceutical Science, Office of Generic Drugs. (2010). *Approved drug products with therapeutic equivalence evaluation* (30th ed.).

of similar surveys from 2007. The most popular products for adults (7.8%) and children (1.1%) are fish oils or Omega-3 fatty acids. These are followed by glucosamine with or without chondroitin (2.6%), probiotics/prebiotics (1.6%) and melatonin (1.3%) for adults, and melatonin (0.7%) for children (Clarke et al., 2015).

Historically, herbs were the first healing system used. Herbal medicines are derived from plants and thought by many to be harmless because they are products of nature. Some prescription drugs in current use, however, such as digitalis, are also "natural," which is not synonymous with "harmless." Before 1962, herbal preparations were drugs, but now they are sold as foods or supplements and therefore do not require FDA approval as drugs. Hence, there are no legislated standards on the purity or quantity of active ingredients in herbal preparations. Measurement of the value of herbal therapy relies on anecdotal reports and is not verified by research. Like synthetic products, herbal preparations may interact with other drugs and may produce undesirable side effects as well.

The Dietary Supplement Health and Education Act (1994) passed by the 103rd Congress, specific labeling is required about the effect of herbal products on the body and requires the statement that the herbal product has not been reviewed by the FDA and is not intended to be used as a drug. Complementary and alternative medicine (CAM) is discussed in within each chapter.

Foreign Medications

In today's global society, practitioners will experience encounters with patients from many countries. These individuals may request refills of drugs for treating their chronic conditions. These drugs may have unrecognizable names, different dosages/dosage forms, or different active ingredients. Additionally, patients may get their drugs from online pharmacies in other countries because they are less expensive. According to the National Association of Boards of Pharmacy (2019), there are over 35,000 active online pharmacies, and 96% violate applicable U.S. laws. According to the World Health Organization, there is a global problem with substandard and falsified medical products (2018). The U.S. FDA has many resources for the practitioner to guide patients toward sound decision-making about prescription drug acquisition.

Disposal of Medications

Many medications can be potentially harmful if taken by someone other than the person for whom they are prescribed. Improperly disposed drugs can leak into the environment, and the best disposal method is through community drug take-back programs. Almost all medicines can be safely disposed of if they are mixed with an undesirable substance, such as cat litter or coffee grounds, and placed in a closed container. Any personal information should be removed from the container by using a black marker or duct tape. Many communities have a drug take-back program for disposal, or drugs can be disposed of when the community collects hazardous material. Drugs should not be flushed down the toilet or drain unless the dispensing directions say this is allowed.

THE PRACTITIONER'S ROLE AND RESPONSIBILITIES IN PRESCRIBING

Before prescribing therapy, the practitioner has a responsibility to gather data by taking a thorough history and performing a physical examination. Once the data are collected and evaluated, one or more diagnoses are formulated and a treatment plan established. As noted, the most often-used treatment modality is drug therapy, usually with a prescription or OTC drug.

If a drug is deemed necessary for therapy, the practitioner needs to understand the responsibility involved in prescribing. The decision-making process includes the class of medication that is most appropriate for the patient. The decision is reached based on a thorough knowledge of diagnosis and treatment.

Drug Selection

Many responsibilities are inherent in prescribing medication. While determining the best therapy for the patient, the practitioner conducts a risk–benefit analysis, evaluating the therapeutic value versus the risk associated with each drug to be prescribed. The practitioner then selects from a vast number of pharmacologic agents used for treating the specific medical problem. Factors to consider when choosing the drug or drugs are the subtle or significant differences in action, side effects, interactions, convenience, storage needs, route of administration, efficacy, and cost. Another factor in the decision may involve the patient pressuring the practitioner to prescribe medication because that is the expectation of many patients at the beginning of a health care encounter.

Initial questions to ask when selecting drug therapy include "Is there a need for this drug in treating the presenting problem or disease?" and "Is this the best drug for the presenting problem or disease?" See additional questions listed in **Box 1.2**.

Concerns Related to Ethics and Practice

Specific ethical and practical issues must be considered as well. One overriding question may be the lack of a clinical indication for using medication. As mentioned, many patients visit a practitioner with the sole purpose of obtaining a prescription. In seeking medical attention, the ill patient expects the health care provider to promote relief from symptoms. In today's world, an abundance of information available in books, magazines, television, Web sites, and other media suggests that the health care provider can do this by prescribing that medication. This expectation that a magic pill or potion—the prescription—is the ticket that will relieve reflux, kill germs, end pain, and restore health puts pressure on the practitioner to prescribe for the sake of prescribing. A typical example of

BOX 1.2 Questions to Address When Prescribing a Medication

- Is there a need for the drug in treating the presenting problem?
- Is this the best drug for the presenting problem?
- Are there any contraindications to this drug with this patient?
- Is the dosage correct? Or is it too high or too low?
- Does the patient have allergies or sensitivities to the drug?
- What drug treatment modalities does the patient currently use, and will the potential new drug interact with the patient's other drugs or treatments?
- Is there a problem with storage of the drug?
- Does the dosage regimen (schedule) interfere with the patient's lifestyle? For example, if a child is in school, a drug with a once- or twice-daily dosing schedule is more realistic than one with a four-times-daily schedule.
- Is the route of administration the most appropriate one?
- Is the proposed duration of treatment too short or too long?
- Can the patient take the prescribed drug?
- Has the patient been informed of possible side effects and what to do if they occur?
- Is there a genetic component to consider?
- What is the cost of the drug?
- What, if any, prescription plan does the patient have?

this involves the patient with a cold who seeks an antibiotic, such as penicillin. In such a situation, the practitioner has a responsibility to prescribe only medications that are necessary for the well-being of the patient and that will be effective in treating the problem. In the example of the patient with an uncomplicated head cold that is viral, an antibiotic would not be useful, and the responsible practitioner must be prepared to make an ethical and prudent decision not to prescribe an antibiotic and explain it to the patient.

Patient Education

An integral part of the practitioner's role and responsibility is educating the patient about drug therapy and the intended therapeutic effect, potential side effects, and strategies for dealing with possible adverse drug reactions. These explanations include any black box warnings that involve the specific drugs. FDA black box warnings take their name from the black border around the warning information. These warnings notify the public of serious, permanent, or fatal side effects. Any instructions about the drug(s) may be explained verbally, with written instructions given when appropriate. Instructions that

are printed and handed to the patient must be readable, in a language that the patient can understand, and in the proper health literacy. If side effects are discussed in advance, the patient will know what to expect and will contact the prescriber with symptoms. When patients are well informed, they may be less likely to stop the drug before discussing it with the prescriber.

Medications can also have a placebo effect. Patients must believe that the drug will work for them to be committed to taking it as recommended. Without a belief the medication works, the drug may not be perceived as effective and may not be taken as directed.

The practitioner may want to recommend that the patient use only one pharmacy when filling prescriptions. The choice of only one pharmacy has several advantages, which include keeping a record of all medications that the patient currently receives and serving as a double-check for drug–drug interactions.

Prescriptive Authority

The prescribing practices of each practitioner are regulated by the state in which the practitioner practices. Each state determines practice parameters by statutes (laws enacted by the legislature), rules, and regulations (administrative policies determined by regulatory agencies). Each practitioner is responsible for knowing the laws and regulations in the state of practice.

Depending on the state, the State Board of Nursing can regulate prescriptive authority, sometimes in conjunction with the Board of Medicine or Board of Pharmacy, depending on the state. States vary in the level of practice authority for prescribers, allowing full practice authority, collaborative practice, supervised practice, or delegated practice. Full practice authority has no requirements for mandatory physician collaboration or supervision. Collaborative practice requires a formal agreement with a collaborating physician, ensuring a referral–consultant relationship. Supervised practice is overseen or directed by a supervisory physician. Delegated practice means that prescription writing is a delegated medical act. The Division of Professional Regulation for prescribers in each state holds the regulations.

Drug Sampling

Related to prescriptive authority issues is the issue of drug samples. Most drug companies engage in the promotional practice of distributing sample drugs to practitioners for use by patients. The Prescription Drug Marketing Act (PDMA), which was enacted in 1988 to protect the American consumer from ineffective drugs, also affects the receipt and dispensing of sample drugs. Prescription drugs can be distributed only to licensed practitioners (one authorized by the state to prescribe drugs) and health care entity pharmacies at the request of a licensed practitioner. There are penalties for violations of the act. This act affects the distribution and use of pharmaceutical samples.

The provisions of the PDMA protects the public in several ways:

- It bans foreign countries from reimporting prescription drugs and the sale, trade, and purchase of any drug samples.
- It prohibits the resale of prescription drugs from hospitals, health care entities, and charitable organizations.
- The practitioner must ask for drug samples in writing.
- It regulates the wholesale distribution of prescription drugs through the requirement of licensing in states where facilities are located.

Because these samples are freely available, some assume that all practitioners can distribute them, but this is not the case. The practitioner must be aware of the rules that govern requesting, receiving, and distributing these agents because the regulations vary from state to state.

Accepting drug samples requires specific procedures. The pharmaceutical representative's Sample Request Form must be signed. It includes the name, strength, and quantity of the sample. The sample must then be recorded on the Record of Receipt of Drug Sample sheet. The samples must be stored away from other drug inventories and where unauthorized access is not allowed or in a locked cabinet or closet in a public area. Samples are to be inspected monthly for expiration dates, proper labeling and storage, presence of intact packaging and labeling, and appropriateness for the practice. If a sample has expired, disposal occurs in a manner that prevents access to the general public; it is not disposed into the trash.

When distributing samples, each must be labeled with the patient's name, clear directions for use, and cautions. All samples are to be dispensed free of charge, along with pertinent information. The medication is then documented in the patient's chart with dose, quantity, and directions.

ADVERSE DRUG EVENTS

Prescription and nonprescription drugs have become an increasing part of life in the United States. Between 2013 and 2016, 48.4% of individuals took at least one prescription drug in the last 30 days (CDC, FastStats, 2018). Adverse drug events (ADE) have consequently become an increasing problem resulting in adverse events both in the inpatient and outpatient settings. Due to the magnitude of the problem, the Home of the Office of Disease Prevention and Health Promotion (2014) has created a National Action Plan for Adverse Drug Event Prevention (http://health.gov/hcq/ade.asp). Therefore, a prudent prescriber must always be aware of any medications when a patient is presenting for healthcare. Chapter 3 reviews the impact of ADE in depth.

Lack of Drug Knowledge

Due to the sheer number of prescription drugs, prescribers must have current knowledge. Prescribers can lack knowledge about indications and contraindications for drugs. They must understand the pharmacodynamics and pharmacokinetics of medications to order medication safely.

Dosing errors can occur, especially when prescribing for children. These errors can be attributed to the limited inclusion of pediatric patients in drug studies (Meyers et al., 2020).

Lack of knowledge about drug–drug interactions can also cause errors. For example, many drugs interfere with warfarin and cause increased bleeding if taken together. The prescriber must be aware of the potential for drug–drug interactions (see Chapter 3 for more information).

Lack of Patient Information

A standard error in prescribing is the failure to obtain an adequate history from the patient. Often, a satisfactory drug history is not obtained, and the provider does not specifically inquire about herbal preparations or OTC medications. As mentioned previously, patients do not think OTC medications are drugs and, therefore, do not include them on intake documents. Also, information on allergies to medicines is not reviewed. In addition to allergies, it is imperative to ascertain the reaction to the medication. While nausea is not considered an allergic reaction, the prescriber would not want to prescribe the drug. An allergy history should be taken and documented at each visit before a new medication is prescribed. Additionally, asking multiple times about allergies or reactions to drugs during an office visit is a safety cross-check to responsible prescribing.

Poor Communication

Poor communication among health care providers, pharmacists, and patients can be a result of poor handwriting, incorrect abbreviations, misplaced decimals, and misunderstanding of verbal prescriptions. These potential errors can be mitigated using electronic health records (EHR); however, new errors can occur if the practitioner does not click on the correct medication or enter the right directions. Additionally, there are areas in the United States where providers still handwrite prescriptions. Poor communication also results when the prescriber fails to discuss potential side effects or ask about side effects at subsequent visits.

SPECIAL POPULATION CONSIDERATIONS

Doses for children are usually based on the weight in kilograms. The prescriber has a responsibility to calculate and write the correct dose rather than relying on calculation by the pharmacist. See Chapter 4 for more information about pediatric drug dosing.

Older patients may have some difficulty hearing or reading small print. Additionally, they may be taking multiple prescription medications and OTC medications. The prescriber needs to be specific about when the patient should take each medication and if one drug cannot be administered with others. When the practitioner prescribes for older adults, he or she must consider renal function because some medicines can cause toxicity, even in small doses, with decreased renal function. Chapter 5 reviews the considerations necessary for good prescribing in older adults.

PHARMACOGENOMICS

Recently, the role of pharmacogenomics in prescribing medication is gaining more importance. Many different genes influence the way a person responds to a drug. Without knowing all the genes involved in drug response, it has not been possible to develop genetic tests that could predict a person's response to a drug. Knowing that people's genes show small variations in the DNA base makes genetic testing for predicting drug response possible. Genetic factors can account for 20% to 95% variability in the patient's reaction to a drug. When pharmacogenetic testing is available, it can enable providers to understand why patients react differently to various drugs and to make better decisions about therapy. This understanding may allow for highly individualized therapeutic regimens. This concept is discussed in detail in Chapter 7.

STEPS OF THE PRESCRIBING PROCESS

At each visit, the prescriber obtains a medication history with the name of the drug, dosage, and frequency of administration. Additionally, the information on any allergies should also be reviewed or documented. It is also helpful if the patient brings his or her actual drugs to the visit.

Multiple steps (**Figure 1.2**) are involved in prescribing drugs and evaluating their effectiveness. Again, the first step is determining an accurate diagnosis based on the patient's history, physical examination, and pertinent test findings.

Next, in selecting the best agent, the practitioner thoroughly evaluates the patient's condition, taking into consideration the effect that various medications may have on the patient and the disorder, the expected outcomes of therapy, and other variables (**Box 1.3**). To prescribe any drug therapy, the practitioner must have substantial knowledge and background in the pathophysiology of the disease, pharmacotherapeutics, pharmacokinetics, pharmacodynamics, and any interactions (see Chapter 2).

The practitioner needs to be knowledgeable about the best class of drugs for the diagnosed disorder or presenting problem, the recommended dosage, potential side effects, possible interactions with other medications, and special prescribing considerations, such as required laboratory tests, contraindications, and patient instructions.

FIGURE 1–2   Process for prescribing.

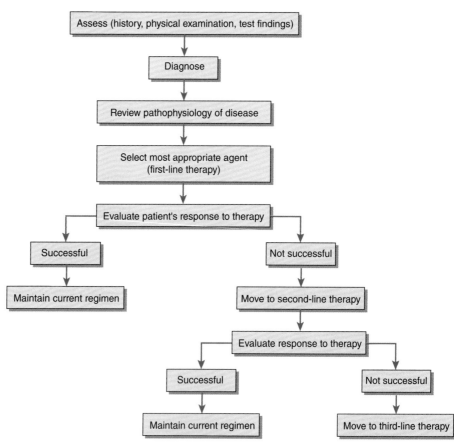

BOX 1.3   Variables to Consider in Prescribing a Medication

- Age
- Sex
- Race
- Weight
- Culture
- Allergies
- Pharmacogenomics
- Other diseases or conditions
- Other therapies
  - Prescription medications
  - Over-the-counter medicines
  - Alternative therapies
- Previous therapies
  - Effectiveness
  - Adverse effects
  - Adherence
- Socioeconomic issues
  - Insurance status
  - Income level
  - Daily schedule
  - Living environment
  - Support systems
- Health beliefs

Next, the practitioner sets goals for therapy. Goals need to be patient centered and realistic and the outcomes measurable. Evaluation of any treatment, nonpharmacologic or pharmacologic, is based on the results.

Selecting the Most Appropriate Agent

For most disease entities, there is a recommendation for first-line, second-line, and third-line therapy. Therapies are identified by evidence-based research, which shows specific agents to be more effective than others. For each recommended treatment line, the prescriber evaluates the effectiveness and potential side effects. The patient response and preferences dictate changes in the drugs. For more information, see the chapter case study outlining the prescribing process. Case studies that emphasize these processes have been provided throughout the text.

Consideration of Special Populations

Another step in prescribing drugs is considering specific concerns related to special populations, such as children, pregnant or breast-feeding women, and older adults. Cultural beliefs are also considered to ensure that the drug regimen honors individual and family customs and preferences.

Identifying Outcomes

Expected outcomes can include improvement in clinical symptoms or pathologic signs or changes in biochemistry as determined by laboratory tests. To assess whether expected results have been achieved, the practitioner reviews data collected on subsequent visits, evaluates the effectiveness of drug therapy, and investigates any adverse reactions.

The frequency of follow-up visits is determined by the disease and the patient's response to treatment. While outcomes are being assessed, the practitioner educates the patient about the results of therapy as well. Topics for discussion include drug benefits, side effects, dosage adjustments, and monitoring parameters.

An undesirable outcome can occur with any medication. Practitioners need to advise patients about the potential side effects and advise them to report issues related to the drugs. Reactions that may be expected and must be discussed include side effects, drug or food interactions, and toxicity. If a patient experiences a serious adverse drug reaction, the practitioner files a report with the FDA's MedWatch program on a special form obtainable from MedWatch (5600 Fishers Lane, Rockville, Maryland 20852-9787) or reports it online, at https://www.accessdata.fda.gov/scripts/medwatch/ (see Chapter 3 for a sample of the MedWatch form). Similarly, adverse reactions to vaccines are reported through the Vaccine Adverse Event Reporting System (VAERS) online, at http://vaers.hhs.gov/esub/index-#Online, or by mail by completing a VAERS form requested by calling 1-800-822-7967 and mailing it to VAERS, P.O. Box 1100, Rockville, Maryland 20849-1100. Adverse events are discussed in Chapter 3.

WRITING THE PRESCRIPTION

The practice of handwriting prescriptions is quickly becoming an exercise of the past; however, there are still rare instances where a practitioner needs to know the steps. A prescription is a form of communication between the practitioner and the pharmacist. It is also the basis for written directions to patients, and it is a legal document. Each prescription should be distinctly written to avoid errors of misinterpretation in filling the prescription. Although potentially serious errors occur infrequently, they are avoidable and should not occur at all.

An early step in the prescribing process involves ensuring that frequent and potentially severe errors are not made. The first step is a failure to identify a patient's allergies, particularly to a medication. In determining a drug allergy, the practitioner should also investigate the kind of reaction experienced with the medication to differentiate between a real, life-threatening drug allergy and less acute drug sensitivity. Some cross-sensitivities between categories of medication classes must also be considered. Another error is the failure to instruct the patient to stop a previously prescribed medication that treats the same condition, such as an increase in dose, and the patient does not stop the other drug. Drug–drug interactions are essential to consider when prescribing. There are now programs that can perform multiple checks for interactions. One of these is Epocrates for mobile devices and desktops.

Date, Name, Address, and Date of Birth

There are standard components of any prescription. One is the date, and another is the full name, address, and date of birth of the patient. The person's name should be the patient's given name (the one on the medical record) and not a nickname. If a different name is used each time, the patient could have multiple files in pharmacy record-keeping systems. The address should be the current home address of the patient and not a work address or a post office box.

Prescriber's Name, Address, and Phone Number

State laws mandate prescribing pads to contain the name, address, and phone number of the prescriber and, if required by state law or regulations, the collaborating physician. This information enables the pharmacist to contact the prescriber if there is a question about the prescription.

Name of Drug

Of course, the name of the drug is an essential part of the prescription. Ideally, the generic name (with the trade or brand name in parentheses) needs to be used. Legibly writing the drug name avoids errors in filling the prescription correctly. For instance, some drugs have names that are commonly confused or misread, such as Norvasc and Navane, Prilosec and Prozac, carboplatin and cisplatin, and Levoxine and Lanoxin. Severe problems may result if the wrong drug is supplied erroneously. The diagnosis may optionally be added to the prescription, which can help the pharmacist avoid misinterpreting the prescribed medication.

Dose, Dosage Regimen, and Route of Administration

The drug dose is essential because many drugs are available in various strengths. Write the dose in numerals. If the dose is a fraction of 1, it is written in decimal form with a leading zero to the left of the decimal point (e.g., 0.75). However, a whole number should not be followed by a decimal point and a trailing zero ("10.0" could be misread as "100"). The numeric dose is followed by the correct metric specification, such as milligram (mg), gram (g), milliliter (mL), or microgram (mcg). Many practitioners spell out *microgram* to avoid confusion with *milligram*. Some drugs are manufactured in units that should be specified, and the term *unit* should be written out ("insulin 10 units," not "10 U"). There are many combination drugs, and it is important to designate the strength of each medication. An example of two drugs in one tablet is losartan 25 mg/hydrochlorothiazide

12.5 mg—this drug also formulated different dose combinations without dose specificity errors in prescribing.

The prescription also mentions how frequently the drug is to be taken. A drug prescribed to be taken as needed is termed a *prn* drug. For example, dosage frequency can be written as "prn every 4 hours" (or another appropriate interval) for the problem for which the drug is prescribed (e.g., "as needed for nausea"). It is good practice to write out the number (10—ten), especially with CSs. Any special instructions, such as "after meals," "at bedtime," or "with food," also should be specified. If the dose is once a day, it is a safer practice to write out "daily" than to write "O.D." because this can be confused with every other day.

The prescription also includes the number of pills, vials, suppositories, or containers or amount in milliliters or ounces to be dispensed. Prescription reimbursement or health care insurance programs often allow for 30- or 90-day supplies to be dispensed at a time; working with the pharmacist is imperative for optimal prescribing practices. They are the best connection regarding the rules of various prescription plans. The prescription indicates whether the medicine may be refilled and the number of refills permitted.

When prescribing a new drug for a patient, the practitioner may want to consider prescribing just a few doses or a 7-day supply initially, but this could be problematic with insurance paying for additional medications in the month. In that case, another alternative, if available, is to provide samples, if allowed by law or regulations. This practice enables the prescriber to determine if the patient can tolerate the drug and if it is effective. When deciding on the number of refills, the practitioner may decide when the patient should return for a follow-up visit and allow just the number of refills that the patient should take until the next visit to ensure that the patient returns to the office. Some drug prescriptions cannot be refilled. For all Schedule 2 drugs, for example, a new prescription must be written each time.

Allowable Substitutions

There are many generic equivalents for brand name drugs. Indication of whether a substitution is allowed is a part of the prescription. Generally, on prescription pads, there is a specific line to sign for a generic replacement. As discussed earlier, a generic drug substitute must have the same chemical composition and dosage as the brand name drug initially prescribed. In many states, a generic drug will automatically be substituted for a brand name drug. If there is a medical reason to require a brand name drug (that has a generic equivalent), "Brand Medically Necessary" must be written on the prescription.

Prescriber's Signature and License Number

The signature of the prescriber is required. It should be legible and should be the person's legal signature. The state regulations

Sally Jones, FNP
111 High Street
Hometown, NH 00440
555-432-1111

Serial #00001
NPI 1234567890

Patient's Name ______________ Date ________

Patient's Address ______________________

____

Date of Birth ________

Drug ________ Dosage ________

Number ________

Directions ________

Number of refills ________

Generic substitution yes____ no____

Signature ________

License Number ________

DEA Number (if required) ________

Sally Jones, FNP
111 High Street
Hometown, NH 00440
555-432-1111

Serial #00001
NPI 1234567890

Patient's Name John Smith Date 6/29/00

Patient's Address 13 Comstock Street

Newtown, NH 33300

Date of Birth 1/2/33

Enalapril (Vasotec) 5 mg

#30

Take one daily

Number of refills 5

Substitution yes X no

Signature *Sally Jones, FNP*

License Number RN0000033

DEA Number (if required) MJ 1234563

FIGURE 1–3 Example of a blank prescription form (*left*) and a completed form (*right*).

vary regarding the inclusion of the prescriber or collaborating physician' license number on the prescription. In some instances, the NPI number of the prescriber is also required. The DEA number is required for prescribing a CS and sometimes needed when prescribing between states. **Figure 1.3** illustrates a blank prescription and a completed prescription. Each state has specific requirements for obtaining the components on a printed prescription. The practitioner must comply with state regulations and may prescribe only in the state in which he or she holds a license. Although the prescription may be filled in another state (if allowed by state regulations), a DEA number is usually required. An NPI number must be included on each prescription along with a serial number of the prescription form. If the practitioner is a federal employee, he or she may prescribe in any federal facility.

Any drug prescribed should be documented in the medical record with date of order, dosage, the amount prescribed, and the number of refills. It is helpful to have a specific area in the medical record to record all drugs taken by the patient—prescription, OTC, and CAM—for ease of audit, reference, and communication among health care professionals.

Electronic Prescriptions

Electronic prescribing has become increasingly popular and mandated by many states. Federally, CMS has mandated that all Part D prescriptions be generated electronically from January 2021 onward. The benefits of using health care technology are the reduction of medication errors with the use of drug-checking software, which checks the medication dose, potential interactions with other medications the patient may be taking, and the patient's known allergies. This drug-checking software may be part of the EHR or a freestanding e-prescribing system. Integrated EHRs can calculate dosing based on a patient's weight and carry out other contextual medication checking against a patient's laboratory results, age, and disease states. Also, computer systems provide pick lists of frequently selected medications with a precalculated dose, frequency, and route. This list reduces the opportunity for clinicians to order inappropriate amounts of medications with the wrong frequency and route of administration.

E-prescribing improves the legibility of prescriptions and the rate of completed prescriptions. There are many benefits to patients when medication is e-prescribed. Patients no longer need to carry paper copies of a prescription to a pharmacy, formulary-compliant medications are prescribed, and the order is waiting for them when they arrive at the pharmacy. Therefore, e-prescribing leads to patient convenience, shorter wait times, and increased compliance with formulary requirements. E-prescribing has yielded a 12% to 20% decrease in adverse drug reactions (Figge, 2009).

ADHERENCE ISSUES

A prescribed drug must be used correctly to produce optimal benefits. Patient nonadherence to a prescribed regimen leads to less-than-optimal outcomes, such as progression of the disease state and an increased incidence of hospitalizations. Studies demonstrate that the more complex the treatment regimen, the less likely the patient is to follow it. Benner (2009) studied 5,759 patients taking antihypertensive and lipid-lowering drugs. In patients with 0, 1, and 2 prior medications, 41%, 35%, and 30% of patients were adherent, respectively, to antihypertensive and lipid-lowering therapy. Of patients with 10 or more prior medications, 20% were adherent.

Karter (2009) found that 22% of patients had the prescription filled 0 or 1 time. The proportion of newly prescribed patients who never became ongoing users was eight times greater than the proportion who maintained ongoing use but with inadequate adherence. Four percent of those who had the prescription filled at least two times discontinued therapy during the 24-month follow-up. Nonadherence was significantly associated with high out-of-pocket costs and clinical response to therapy.

Several variables are associated with improved adherence to a drug regimen. These include variables associated with the patient's perception of the encounter and of the benefit of the treatment. If a patient is nonadherent to the prescribed regimen, it is important to document that in the chart. The risks of nonadherence are discussed, and that discussion is documented. It is essential to ask why the patient is not following the prescribed treatment, and actions to rectify the problem should be taken. All of this is documented. One issue may be that the patient is unable to swallow the pill. The medicine may be available in liquid form, or the pill may be split or crushed. The practitioner needs to review and understand the factors that affect adherence to a regimen (**Box 1.4**).

UPDATING DRUG INFORMATION

Many sources of drug information can be accessed by practitioners, who must keep current on changes in drug therapy and continually update their fund of knowledge. Resources include reference books, pharmacists (who are expertly informed about drugs, interactions, dosages, etc.), easy-to-carry drug handbooks and pocket guides for quick reference, and online databases and programs for mobile devices and desktop computers (**Tables 1.2** and **1.3**).

BOX 1.4   Factors Influencing the Patient's Adherence to a Medication Regimen

- Approachability of the health care provider
- Perception of respect with which the patient is treated by the practitioner
- Belief that the therapy is beneficial
- Belief that the benefits of therapy outweigh the risks or side effects
- Degree to which the patient participates in developing the treatment regimen
- Cost of the regimen
- Simplicity of the regimen

- Patient's understanding of the treatment regimen
- Degree to which the patient feels that expectations are being met
- Degree to which the patient perceives his or her concerns are important and being addressed
- Degree to which the practitioner motivates the patient to adhere to the regimen
- Degree to which the regimen is compatible with the patient's lifestyle

---

TABLE 1.2

Common Drug Reference Books

Reference	Features
American Hospital Formulary Service. Bethesda, MD: American Society of Health System Pharmacists.	Drug entries are indexed by generic and brand names and organized by pharmacologic–therapeutic class.
Drug Facts and Comparisons. Philadelphia, PA: Wolters Kluwer Health.	Drugs are indexed by generic and brand names and organized by major classes of drugs. Updates are issued monthly (in print and CD-ROM).
Physician's Desk Reference (PDR). Montvale, NJ: Medical Economics.	Drugs are indexed by manufacturer name, brand name, generic name, and product category. Volume contains product identification section. Information replicates the official package insert from the drug manufacturer.

TABLE 1.3		
Online Drug Reference Data		
Reference	**Address**	**Features**
AHRQ	www.ahrq.gov	Guidelines for clinical practice from the AHRQ, National Guidelines Clearinghouse, U.S. Preventive Services Task Force
Center Watch Clinical Trials	www.centerwatch.com	Lists clinical research trials and drug therapy newly approved by the U.S. FDA and the FDA New Drug Listing Service
Coreynahman	www.coreynahman.com	Pharmaceutical news and information
		Gives a choice of many sites for information
Epocrates	www.epocrates.com	Website with drug information, interactions, etc.
Mediconsult	www.mediconsult.com	Professional- and consumer-focused
		Detailed medical and drug information
Medscape	www.medscape.com	Drug search database
		Links to online journals
RxList—The Internet Drug Index	www.rxlist.com	Cross-index of U.S. prescription products

AHRQ, Agency for Healthcare Research and Quality; FDA, Food and Drug Administration.

CASE STUDY*

The first patient in the clinic today is A.J., who is a 16–year–old who has just started soccer practice at school. She complains of increased shortness of breath with exercise and describes having a hard time catching her breath when she runs, which she does five to six times a week. She does not wake up at night with a cough or shortness of breath and has no problems at any other time except in the spring when the trees start to blossom. The soccer coach advised A.J.'s mother to seek health care because A.J. had a very difficult time breathing at practice that afternoon. A.J. also has a history of eczema and seasonal allergies for which she takes an over-the-counter antihistamine when symptoms get severe.

Social history: Nonsmoker. Lives in an urban area with mother, father, and brother. Does not use street drugs.

Family history: Father has a history of asthma.
Physical examination:
    Nose: Mucosa pale and boggy bilaterally
    Lungs: Respirations 26 and shallow; diffuse expiratory wheezing; peak flow 340
Diagnosis: Mild persistent asthma

QUESTIONS

1. What is the prescriber's responsibility regarding potential drug therapy for A.J.?
2. Explain the factors that can contribute to adverse drug events for any medications prescribed for A.J.
3. Describe the factors that could improve the adherence of A.J. to your prescribed therapy.

* Answers can be found online.

Bibliography

Starred references are cited in the text.

*103rd Congress. (1994). *Dietary supplement health and education act of 1994.* National Institutes of Health. https://ods.od.nih.gov/About/DSHEA_Wording.aspx

Aseeri, M. A. (2013). The impact of pediatric antibiotic standard dosing table on dosing errors. *Journal of Pediatric Pharmacologic Therapeutics, 18*(3), 220–226. doi: 10.5863/1551-6776-18.3.220

Belle, D. G., & Singh, H. (2008). Genetic factors in drug metabolism. *American Family Physician, 77*(11), 1553–1168.

*Benner, J. S. (2009). Association between prescription burden and medication adherence in patients initiating antihypertensive and lipid-lowering therapy. *American Journal of Health System Pharmacies, 66*(16), 1471–1477.

Blaluck, D. V., Bosworth, H. B., Reeve, B. B., et al. (2019). Co-occurring reasons for medication nonadherence within subgroups of patients with hyperlipidemia. *Journal of Behavioral Medicine, 42*, 291–299. https://doi.org/10.1007/s10865-018-9954-3

Brown, M. T., & Bussell, J. K. (2011). Medication adherence: WHO cares? *Mayo Clinic Proceedings, 86*(4), 304–314. https://doi.org/10.4065/mcp.2010.0575

Centers for Disease Control and Prevention. (2014). Vital signs: Variation among states in prescribing of opioid pain relievers and benzodiazepines—United States, 2012. *Morbidity and Mortality Weekly Report, 63*(26), 563–568.

Centers for Disease Control and Prevention. (2015). Therapeutic drug use. Retrieved from www.cdc.gov/nchs/fastats/drug-use-therapeutic.htm on August 23, 2015.

*Center for Disease Control. (2018). *FastStats*. Therapeutic drug use. https://www.cdc.gov/nchs/fastats/drug-use-therapeutic.htm

*Center Watch. (2015). Overview of clinical trials: What is clinical research? Retrieved from http://www.centerwatch.com/clinical-trials/overview.aspx

*Clarke, T. C., Black Lindsey, L. I., Stussman, B. J., et al. (2015). Trends in the use of complementary health approaches among adults: United States, 2001–2012. *National Health Statistics Report, 79*, February 10. 1–16. Retrieved from http://www.cdc.gov/nchs/data/nhsr/nhsr079.pdf on August 23, 2015.

Court, M. H. (2007). A pharmacogenomics primer. *Journal of Clinical Pharmacology, 47*(9), 1087–1103.

Cusack, C. M. (2008). Electronic health records and electronic prescribing: Promise and pitfalls. *Obstetrics and Gynecology Clinics of North America, 35*(1), 63–79.

Doherty, K., Segal, A., & McKinney, P. (2004). The 10 most common prescribing errors: Tips on avoiding the pitfalls. *Consultant, 44*(2), 173–182.

Federal Drug Administration. (2020, May 13). *Black box warnings: Fast track drugs & increased use*. Drugwatch. https://www.drugwatch.com/fda/black-box-warnings/

FDA. (2014). Counterfeit drugs: Fighting illegal supply chains. Retrieved from http://www.fda.gov/NewsEvents/Testimony/ucm387449.htm

*FDA. (2020). Emergency use authorization. https://www.fda.gov/emergency-preparedness-and-response/mcm-legal-regulatory-and-policy-framework/emergency-use-authorization. Viewed January 2021.

*Figge, H. (2009). Electronic prescribing in the ambulatory care setting. *American Journal of Health System Pharmacy, 66*(1), 16–18.

Government Accounting Organization, Dicken, J., & Oliver, R. (2017, November). *Profits, research and development spending, and merger and acquisition deals* (GAO 18-40). https://www.gao.gov/products/GAO-18-40

Hampton, L. M., Ngyuen, D. B., Edwards, J. R., et al. (2013). Cough and cold medications adverse events after-market withdrawal and labeling revision. *Pediatrics, 132*(6), 1047–1054. doi: 10.1542/peds.2013-2236

Hedegaard, H., Minino, A., & Warner, M. (2020, January). *Drug overdose death in the United States 1999–2018* (No. 365). https://stacks.cdc.gov/view/cdc/84647

*Home of the Office of Disease Prevention and Health Promotion. (2014). National action plan for adverse drug event prevention. [online retrieved on August 23, 2015] http://health.gov/hcq/ade.asp#overview

Jankowska-Polanska, B., Uchmanowicz, I., Dudek, K., & Mazur, G. (2016). Relationship between patients' knowledge and medication adherence among patients with hypertension. *Patient Preference and Adherence, 10*, 2437–2447. https://doi.org/10.2147/PPA.S117269

*Karter, A. J. (2009). New prescription medication gaps: A comprehensive measure of adherence to new prescriptions. *Health Service Research, 44*(5 Pt. 1), 1640–1661.

Keohane, C. A., & Bates, D. W. (2008). Medication safety. *Obstetrics and Gynecology Clinics, 35*(1), 37–52.

Kleinsinger, F. (2018). The unmet challenge of medication nonadherence. *The Permanente Journal, 22*, 18–033. https://doi.org/10.7812/TPP/18-033

Mahoney, D. F. (2010). More than a prescriber: Gerontological nurse practitioners' perspectives on prescribing and pharmaceutical marketing. *Geriatric Nursing, 31*(1), 17–27.

Medication Errors: Technical Series on Safer Primary Care. Geneva: World Health Organization; 2016. License: CC BY-NC-SA 3.0 IGO.

*Meyers, R. S., Thackray, J., Matson, K. L., et al. (2020). Key potentially inappropriate drugs in pediatrics: The KIDs list. *The Journal of Pediatric Pharmacology and Therapeutics: JPPT: The Official Journal of PPAG, 25*(3), 175–191. https://doi.org/10.5863/1551-6776-25.3.175

Munsell, M., Frean, M., Menzin, J., et al. (2016). An evaluation of adherence in patients with multiple sclerosis newly initiating treatment with a self-injectable or an oral disease-modifying drug. *Patient Preference and Adherence, 11*, 55–62. https://doi.org/10.2147/PPA.S118107

National Association of Boards of Pharmacy. (2019, February). *Statement on precription drug importation proposals: Prescription drug importation is not a viable solution to high prescription drug costs.* NABP Pharmacy. https://nabp.pharmacy/wp-content/uploads/2019/03/NABP-Drug-Importation-Statement-2019.pdf

Neiman, A. B., Ruppar, T., Ho, M., et al. (2017). CDC grand rounds: Improving medication adherence for chronic disease management: Innovations and opportunities. *Morbidity and Mortality Weekly Report, 66*. http://dx.doi.org/10.15585/mmwr.mm6645a2external icon

Nguyen, T., Wong, E., & Ciummo, F. (2019). Polypharmacy in older adults: Practical applications alongside a patient case. *Journal of the Nurse Practitioner*. Published: January 05, 2020. https://doi.org/10.1016/j.nurpra.2019.11.01

O'Connor, N. R. (2010). FDA boxed warnings: How to prescribe drugs safely. *American Family Physician, 81*(3), 298–303.

Pollock, M., Bazaldua, O., & Dobbie, A. (2007). Appropriate prescribing of medications: An eight-step approach. *American Family Physician, 75*(2), 231–236.

Purvis, L., & Stephen, W. (2019, June). Schondelmeyer. *Rx PriceWatch Reports.* Washington, DC: AARP Public Policy Institute. https://doi.org/10.26419/ppi.00073.000

*Rui, P., & Kang, K. (2017). National Hospital Ambulatory Medical Care Survey: 2017 emergency department summary tables. National Center for Health Statistics. https://www.cdc.gov/nchs/data/nhamcs/web_tables/2017_ed_web_tables-508.pdf

*RxPrice Watch: Brand name drug prices increase more than twice as fast as inflation in 2018. (2019, November). AARP Public Policy Institute. https://doi.org/10.26419/ppi.00073.005

Sadee, W. (2008). Drug therapy and personalized health care: Pharmacogenomics in perspective. *Pharmacology Research, 25*(12), 2713–2719.

*Schondelmeyer, W., & Purvis, L. (2018, September). Trends in retail prices of brand name prescription drugs widely used by older Americans: 2017 year-end update. https://www.aarp.org/content/dam/aarp/ppi/2018/09/trends-in-retail-prices-of-brand-name-prescription-drugs-year-end-update.pdf

Villaseñor, S., & Piscotty, R. J., Jr. (2016, January). The current state of e-prescribing: Implications for advanced practice registered nurses. *Journal of the American Association of Nurse Practitioners, 28*(1), 54–61. doi: 10.1002/2327-6924.12263

Weber, W. W. (2008). Pharmacogenomics: From description to prediction. *Clinics in Laboratory Medicine, 28*(4), 499–511.

Wessell, A. M., Litvin, C., Jenkins, R. G., et al. (2010). Medication prescribing and monitoring errors in primary care: A report from the practice partner research network. *Quality Safety in Health Care, 19*, e21. doi: 10.1136/qshc.2009.034678

Wheeler, K. J., Roberts, M. E., & Neiheisel, M. (2014). Medication adherence part two: Predictors of nonadherence and adherence. *Journal of the American Association of Nurse Practitioners, 26*(4), 225–232. doi: 10.1002/2327-6924.12105

*World Health Organization. (2018, January 31). Substandard and falsified medical products. https://www.who.int/news-room/fact-sheets/detail/substandard-and-falsified-medical-products

Wysocki, K., & Seibert, D. (2019, August). Pharmacogenomics in clinical care. *Journal of the American Association of Nurse Practitioners, 31*(8), 443–446. doi: 10.1097/JXX.0000000000000254

Yeam, C. T., Chia, S., Tan, H. C. C., et al. (2018). A systematic review of factors affecting medication adherence among patients with osteoporosis. *Osteoporosis International, 29*, 2623–2637. https://doi.org/10.1007/s00198-018-4759-3.

2 Pharmacokinetic Basis of Therapeutics and Pharmacodynamic Principles

Andrew M. Peterson and A. Maggie Randazzo

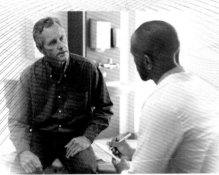 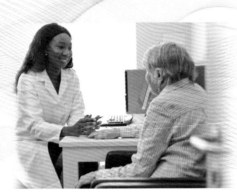 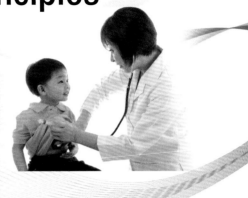

Learning Objectives

1. Describe the difference between pharmacokinetics and pharmacodynamics.
2. Discuss the impact of each of the four pharmacokinetic principles on medications administered to a patient: absorption, distribution, metabolism, and elimination.
3. Describe the concept of affinity and differentiate between an antagonist and an agonist.
4. Apply the knowledge of pharmacokinetic principles to considerations of a patient case scenario.
5. Given patient details, calculate renal function utilizing the Cockcroft-Gault formula and the Modification of Diet in Renal Disease (MDRD) equation.

INTRODUCTION

The art and science of clinical practice is based on understanding the relationship between the person and the disease and determining the most appropriate means for alleviating symptoms, curing disease, or preventing severe morbidity or even mortality. Very often, medications are prescribed to accomplish one or more of these goals.

Underpinning this treatment process is the intricate relationship between the body and the medication. Often, practitioners seek to understand the effect a drug has on the body (whether therapeutic or harmful) but neglect to consider the effect the body has on the drug—even though one cannot be understood without the other. How the body acts on a drug and how the drug acts on the body are the subjects of this chapter.

Pharmacokinetics refers to the movement of the drug through the body—in essence, how the body affects the drug. This involves how the drug is absorbed, distributed, metabolized, and eventually eliminated or excreted from the body. *Pharmacodynamics* refers to how the drug affects the body—that is, how the drug initiates its therapeutic or toxic effect, both at the cellular level and systemically. **Box 2.1** lists terms and definitions used throughout this chapter.

The purpose of pharmacokinetic processes is to get the drug to the site of action, where it can produce its pharmacodynamic effect. There is a minimum amount of drug needed at the site of action to produce the desired effect. Although the amount of drug concentrated at the site of action is difficult to measure, the amount of drug in the blood can be measured. The relationship between the concentration of drug in the blood and the concentration at the site of action (i.e., the drug receptor) is different for each drug and each person. Therefore, measuring blood concentrations is only a surrogate marker, an indication of concentration at the receptor. **Figure 2.1** shows the relationship between pharmacokinetics and pharmacodynamics.

PHARMACOKINETICS

Pharmacokinetics relates to how the drug is absorbed, distributed, metabolized, and eliminated from the body. In reality, it is the study of the fate of medications administered to a person. It is sometimes described as *what the body does to the drug*. In theory, pharmacokinetics not only deals with medications but also deals with the disposition of all substances administered externally to any living organism. Pharmacokinetic processes determine the onset and duration of a drug's action as well as

BOX 2.1 Definitions of Terms Related to Pharmacokinetics and Pharmacodynamics

Affinity: The attraction between a drug and a receptor.

Allosteric site: A binding site for substrates not active in initiating a response; a substrate that binds to an allosteric site may induce a conformational change in the structure of the active site, rendering it more or less susceptible to response from a substrate.

Bioavailability (F): The fraction or percentage of a drug that reaches the systemic circulation.

Biotransformation: Metabolism or degradation of a drug from an active form to an inactive form.

Chirality: Special configuration or shape of a drug; most drugs exist in two shapes.

Clearance: Removal of a drug from the plasma or organs.

Downregulation: Decreased availability of drug receptors.

Enantiomer (also called isomer): A mirror-image spatial arrangement, or shape, of a drug that suits it for binding with a drug receptor.

Enterohepatic recirculation: The process by which a drug excreted in the bile flows into the gastrointestinal tract, where it is reabsorbed and returned to the general circulation.

First-pass effect: The phenomenon by which a drug first passes through the liver, where it may be degraded before distribution to the tissues.

Half-life $(t_{1/2})$: The time required for half of a total drug amount to be eliminated from the body.

Hepatic extraction ratio: A comparison of the percentage of drug extracted and the percentage of drug remaining active after metabolism in the liver.

Hydrophilic (lipophobic): Molecules that do not readily cross the plasma membrane (phospholipid bilayer) because they are water soluble.

Hydrophobic (lipophilic): Molecules that easily cross the plasma membrane (phospholipid bilayer) because they are lipid soluble.

Ligand: Any chemical, endogenous or exogenous, that interacts with a receptor.

Pharmacodynamics: Processes through which drugs affect the body.

Pharmacokinetics: Processes through which the body affects drugs.

Prodrug: A drug that is transformed from an inactive parent drug into an active metabolite; in effect, a precursor to the active drug.

Receptor: The site of drug action.

Second messenger: A chemical produced intracellularly in response to a receptor signal; this second messenger initiates a change in the intracellular response.

Therapeutic window: The range of drug concentration in the blood between a minimally effective level and a toxic level.

Threshold: The level below which a drug exerts little to no therapeutic effect and above which a drug produces a therapeutic effect at the site of action.

Upregulation: Increased availability of receptors.

Volume of distribution (V_d): The extent of distribution of a drug in the body.

---

blood levels that would produce therapeutic and toxic effects. As such, one can determine the blood levels necessary to produce a desired effect. This target drug concentration is key to monitoring the effects of many medications. Assuming that the magnitude of the drug concentration at the site of action influences the drug effect, whether desired or undesired, it can be inferred that a range of drug levels produces a range of effects (**Figure 2.2**). Below a specific level, or threshold, the

drug exerts little to no therapeutic effect. Above this threshold, the concentration of drug in the blood is sufficient to produce a therapeutic effect at the site of action. However, as the drug concentration increases in the blood, so does the concentration at the site of action. Above a specific level, an increased therapeutic effect may no longer occur. Instead, an unacceptable toxicity may occur because the drug concentration is too high. Between these two levels—the minimally

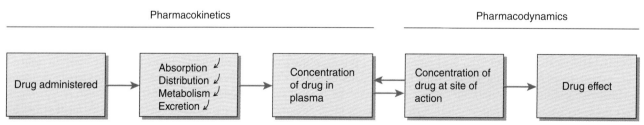

FIGURE 2–1   Relationship between pharmacokinetics and pharmacodynamics. Note the two-way relationship between the concentration of drug in the plasma and the concentration of drug at the site of action, depicting the interrelationship between pharmacokinetics and pharmacodynamics.

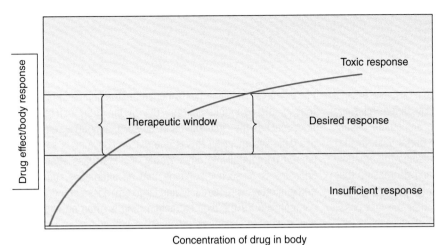

FIGURE 2–2 Therapeutic window: concentration versus response. The concentration of the drug in the body produces specific effects. A low concentration is considered subtherapeutic, producing an insufficient response. As the concentration increases, the desired effect is produced at a given drug level. A drug concentration that exceeds the upper limit of the desired response may produce a toxic reaction. The concentration range within which a desired response occurs is the therapeutic window.

effective level and the toxic level—is the *therapeutic window.* The therapeutic window is the range of blood drug concentration that yields a sufficient therapeutic response without excessively toxic reactions. This range varies based on individual differences and therefore serves only as a guide to the practitioner.

Absorption

The first phase of pharmacokinetics to consider is how drugs are administered, how they are absorbed into the body, and how they eventually reach the bloodstream. Merely introducing the drug into the body does not ensure that the compound will reach all tissues uniformly or that the drug will reach the target site at all. Commonly recognized methods of absorption include enteral absorption (after the drug is administered by the oral or rectal route) and parenteral absorption (associated with drugs administered intramuscularly [IM], subcutaneously, or topically, bypassing the gastrointestinal [GI] tract). The various administration routes are discussed in the following paragraphs and other factors affect a drug's ability to enter the bloodstream.

The extent to which the drug reaches the systemic circulation is referred to as *bioavailability,* or F, which is defined as the fraction or percentage of the drug that reaches the systemic circulation after administration. Drugs administered intravenously are 100% bioavailable because they are delivered directly to the systemic circulation. Drugs administered by other routes (e.g., oral, IM) may be 100% bioavailable, but more often, they are less than 100% bioavailable. Therefore, bioavailability depends on the route of administration and, equally important, the drug's ability to pass through membranes or barriers in the body. **Box 2.2** discusses the specific case of oral bioavailability and the first-pass effect.

Factors Affecting Absorption

A variety of factors affect absorption, such as the presence or absence of food in the stomach, blood flow to the area for absorption, and the dosage form of the drug. The following sections discuss some of the major factors affecting absorption.

Movement through Membranes and Drug Solubility

Throughout the body, biologic membranes act as barriers, blocking or permitting the passage of various substances. These membranes protect certain areas of the body from harmful chemicals and allow other areas to be accessed as needed.

Biologic membranes composed of cells serve as barriers primarily because of the structure and function of the cells that make up the membrane. Cell membranes are composed of lipids and proteins, creating a phospholipid bilayer. This bilayer acts as a barrier that is almost impermeable to water, other hydrophilic (water-loving) substances, and ionized substances. However, the bilayer does allow most hydrophobic (lipid-soluble) compounds to pass through readily. Interspersed throughout this bilayer are protein molecules and small openings, or pores. The proteins may act as carrier molecules, bringing molecules through the barrier (active transport). The pores allow hydrophilic molecules to pass through if they are small enough (passive diffusion). Therefore, drugs and other compounds that pass through membrane barriers can do so by passive or active means.

Passive diffusion. Drugs can pass through membrane barriers by diffusion. In passive diffusion, molecules move from one side of a barrier to another without expending energy. In passing, the molecules move down a concentration gradient—that is, they move from an area of higher concentration to an area of lower concentration. The rate of diffusion depends on the differences in concentrations, the relative strength of the barrier, the distance that the molecules must travel, and the size of the molecules. This relationship is known as Fick's law of diffusion. In essence, Fick's law states that the greater the distance to travel and the larger the molecule, the slower the diffusion.

Another major barrier to the absorption of a drug is its solubility. To facilitate drug absorption, the solubility of the

BOX 2.2 Oral Bioavailability and the First-Pass Effect

Drugs given orally may be subject to the first-pass effect, by which drugs are metabolized by the liver before passing into circulation. After absorption from the alimentary canal, drugs go directly to the liver through the portal vein. In the liver, hepatic enzymes act on the drug, reducing the amount of active drug reaching the bloodstream and decreasing the amount available to the body. The fraction (or percentage) of medication reaching systemic circulation after the first pass through the liver is referred to as the drug's bioavailability (F).

The first-pass effect is not the only factor contributing to the oral bioavailability of a drug. Poorly soluble drugs and drugs adversely affected by gastric pH or other presystemic factors can also have a low bioavailability.

Drugs not usually subject to the liver's first-pass effect are known as drugs with a low hepatic extraction ratio because the liver does not extract a large percentage of the drug before releasing it into the circulation. Usually, drugs with a low extraction ratio have high oral bioavailability. In contrast, drugs with a high extraction ratio have low oral bioavailability.

For example, lidocaine has a hepatic extraction ratio of 0.7; that is, the liver metabolizes 70% of the drug before the drug reaches the circulation and, as such, only 30% remains available systemically. This is one reason lidocaine is administered parenterally. In other words, the first-pass effect for lidocaine is of such magnitude that an alternative route of administration is required. Giving large oral doses of a drug to compensate for the high extraction ratio is often an alternative to parenteral administration. For example, because of the high extraction ratio of propranolol, a 1-mg dose administered intravenously is approximately equivalent to a 40-mg dose administered orally.

Examples of drugs with a high hepatic extraction ratio (70% or more) are metoprolol (Toprol XL), lidocaine (Xylocaine), and morphine; drugs with intermediate rankings are codeine, midazolam (Versed), and nifedipine (Procardia XL); and some drugs with a low extraction ratio (30% or less) are barbiturates, diazepam (Valium), theophylline (Theo-Dur), indomethacin (Indocin), and warfarin (Coumadin).

administered drug must match that of the cellular constituents of the absorption site. Lipid-soluble drugs can penetrate fatty cells; water-soluble drugs cannot. For example, a water-soluble drug such as penicillin cannot easily pass through the phospholipid bilayer between the blood and the brain, whereas a highly lipid-soluble drug such as diazepam (Valium) can. The relative strength of the barrier is important because the barrier must be permeable to the diffusing substance. Drugs diffuse more readily through the lipid bilayer if they are in their neutral, nonionized form. Most drugs are weak acids or weak bases, which have the potential for becoming positively or negatively charged. This potential is created through the pH of certain body fluids. In the plasma and in most other fluids, most drugs remain nonionized. However, in the gastric acid of the stomach, weak bases become ionized and are more difficult to absorb. As this weak base progresses through the alkaline environment of the small intestines, it becomes nonionized and therefore more easily absorbed. Similarly, weak acids remain nonionized in the stomach and become ionized in the small intestines. The result is reduced absorption by the intestines.

Active transport. In active transport, membrane proteins act as carrier molecules to transport substances across cell membranes. The role of active transport in moving drugs across cell membranes is limited. To be carried through by a protein, the exogenous drug must share molecular similarities with an endogenous substance the transport system routinely carries. Cells can accomplish this through the process of endocytosis. In this process, the cell forms a vesicle surrounding the molecule, and it is subsequently invaginated in the cell. Once inside the cell, the vesicle releases the molecule into the cytoplasm of the cell.

Pharmaceutical Preparation

Drugs are formulated and administered in such a way as to produce either local or systemic effects. Local effects (e.g., antiseptic, topical antiinflammatory, and local anesthetic effects) are confined to one area of the body. Systemic effects occur when the drug is absorbed and delivered to body tissues by way of the circulatory system.

Depending on how a drug is formulated (e.g., tablet or liquid), the means of drug delivery can target a site of action. Some drug formulations (dosage forms) deliver the drug into the GI tract quickly (immediate release), whereas others release the drug slowly. This strategy for extending the activity of drugs in the body dampens the high peaks and low troughs of drug concentrations, thereby yielding a more consistent blood level. Many medications are available in these controlled- or sustained-release dosage forms. The aim of sustained-release dosage forms is to administer them as infrequently as possible, improving patient compliance and minimizing hour-to-hour or day-to-day blood level fluctuations. The various release systems available are subject to physiologic and pathophysiologic changes in patient conditions.

Blood Flow

Blood flow ensures that the concentration across a gradient is continually in favor of passive diffusion—that is, as blood flows through an area, it continually removes the drug from the area, thereby maintaining a positive concentration gradient. Many hydrophobic–lipophilic drugs can readily pass through membranes and be absorbed. However, if the blood flow to that area is limited, the extent of absorption is limited. Because of the minimal vascularization in the subcutaneous (SC) layer compared with the greater vascularity of the musculature, drugs injected subcutaneously may undergo less absorption compared with drugs delivered by IM injection.

Gastrointestinal Motility

High-fat meals and solid foods affect GI transit time by delaying gastric emptying, which in turn delays initial drug delivery to intestinal absorption surfaces. The administration of agents that delay or slow intestinal motility (e.g., anticholinergic agents) prolongs the contact time. This increased intestinal contact time secondary to prolonged intestinal transit time may increase total drug absorption. Conversely, laxatives or diarrhea can shorten an agent's contact time with the small intestine, which may decrease drug absorption.

Enteral Absorption

Enteral absorption, with the oral route of administration being the most common and probably the most preferred, occurs anywhere throughout the GI tract by passive or active transport of the drug through the cells of the GI tract.

Following Fick's law, low molecular weight, nonionized drugs diffuse passively down a concentration gradient from the higher concentration (in the GI tract) to the lower concentration (in the blood). Active transport across the GI tract occurs more frequently with larger, usually ionized, molecules. These active mechanisms include binding of the drug to carrier molecules in the cell membrane. The molecules carry the drug across the lipid bilayer of the cells. However, most drugs are absorbed passively.

Oral Administration

The oral route of administration refers to any medication that is taken by mouth (per os or PO). The ability to swallow is implicit in oral administration; however, many practitioners consider local action, in which absorption does not occur, also to be "oral" (e.g., troches for fungal infections of the mouth). Common dosage forms administered by mouth include tablets, capsules, caplets, solutions, suspensions, troches, lozenges, and powders.

Absorption after oral administration usually occurs in the lower GI tract (small or large intestine), is slow, and depends on the patient's gastric-emptying time, the presence or absence of food, and the gastric or intestinal pH. Variations in one or more of these factors can affect the stability of the drug, the contact time with the intestinal walls, or the blood flow to the GI tract. Most of the absorption occurs in the small intestine, where the large surface area enhances and controls drug entry into the body.

Drugs administered orally must be relatively lipid soluble to cross the GI mucosa into the bloodstream. The diffusion rate, a function of the lipid solubility of a drug across the GI mucosa, is a major factor in determining the rate of absorption of a drug. The acidic pH of the stomach and the nearly neutral pH of the intestines can degrade some medications before they are absorbed. In addition, bacteria in various parts of the intestines secrete enzymes, which also can break down drugs before absorption. Many drugs are formulated to prevent the degradation of the drug before absorption.

Although the GI tract is generally resistant to a variety of noxious agents, considerable irritation and discomfort can arise from certain medications. Nausea, vomiting, diarrhea, and less often mucosal damage are common side effects of medications, and the practitioner should monitor all patients for these effects.

Sublingual Administration

Sublingual (under the tongue, SL) drug administration relies on absorption through the oral mucosa into the veins that drain those vascular beds. These veins carry the drug to the superior vena cava and eventually the heart. Drugs administered this way are not subject to the first-pass effect because they bypass the portal vein (see **Box 2.2**). This method of administration is limited by the small amount of drug that can be placed sublingually and the drug's ability to pass through the oral mucosa into the venous system. Buccal administration, in which the drug is absorbed through the mucous membranes of the mouth by putting the dosage form in the buccal/cheek area, is similar to SL administration.

Rectal Administration

Drugs administered rectally (per rectum, PR) include suppositories and enemas. Primarily used in the treatment of local conditions (e.g., hemorrhoids) and inflammatory bowel disease, this method is less effective than other enteral routes because of the erratic absorption of most agents. Bowel irritation, early evacuation, and minimal surface area contribute to erratic absorption and poor tolerability of this route. Advantages, however, include the ability to administer a medication to an unconscious or nauseated patient. Rectal administration of medications bypasses some of the first-pass effect (see **Box 2.2**).

Parenteral Absorption

All routes of administration not involving the GI tract are considered parenteral. Parenteral routes include inhalation, all forms of injection, and topical and transdermal administration.

Inhalation

Drugs that are gaseous or sprayable in small particles may be delivered by inhalation. The lungs provide a large surface area for absorption and quick entry into the bloodstream. Inhaled medications bypass the first-pass effect and therefore may have a high bioavailability. Examples of systemically active inhalants are anesthetic gases and beta-adrenergic agonists (e.g., albuterol) used in treating asthma. Conversely, agents such as inhaled corticosteroids are intended for local action in the lung tissue. Regardless of the intent of inhaled medications, the disadvantages include irritation to the alveolar space and the need for good coordination during self-administration, such as with metered-dose inhalers.

Intravenous Administration

The intravenous (IV) route provides rapid access to the circulatory system with a known quantity of drug. Bypassing the first-pass effect and any GI metabolism or degradation, drug absorption by this route is considered the gold standard with regard to bioavailability. IV bolus injections allow for large amounts of medication to be administered quickly for a high peak drug level and a rapid effect. However, adverse effects from these high levels of medications also occur with this form of administration. Repeated bolus doses of medications, at designated intervals, can produce large fluctuations in peak and trough (lowest concentration before next dose) levels. Although over time these peaks and troughs produce average desired concentrations, significant peak and trough fluctuations may not be desirable in some patients. Continuous administration via an IV infusion can minimize or eliminate these fluctuations and produce a consistent, steady-state concentration.

Like IV administration, intra-arterial administration produces a rapid effect. However, because the drug is directly instilled in an organ, this route is considered more dangerous and invasive than the IV route. Therefore, intra-arterial administration is usually reserved for a time when injection into a specific tissue is indicated (e.g., anticancer treatment for a specific tumor).

Subcutaneous Administration

Subcutaneous (SC or SQ) administration produces a slower, more prolonged release of medication into the bloodstream. Injected directly beneath the skin, a drug must diffuse through layers of fat and muscle to encounter sufficient blood vessels for entry into the systemic circulation. This route is limited by the quantity of the liquid suitable for administration (usually 2 to 3 mL). Caution must also be taken because dermal irritation, or even necrosis, may occur. More recent technological advances allow the practitioner to implant drug-releasing mechanisms under the skin, providing a reservoir of drug for long-term absorption. Etonogestrel (Nexplanon), a hormonal contraceptive, is administered in this manner.

Intramuscular Administration

Injecting medications into the highly vascularized skeletal muscle is a way of administering drugs quickly but avoiding the relatively large changes in plasma levels seen with IV administration. Local pain and muscle soreness are drawbacks to this method, as is the wide variability in the rate of absorption resulting from injections given in different muscles and in different patients. Blood flow to the area is the major factor in determining the rate of absorption. This is considered a safe way to administer irritating drugs, although not all IM injections are truly IM: In morbidly obese patients, presumed IM injections may actually be intralipomatous, which decreases the rate of absorption because of the lower vascularity of fatty tissue.

Topical Administration

Topical drug administration involves applying drugs, in various vehicles (e.g., liquids, powders), to the site of action,

primarily the skin. Topical ointments, creams, drops, and gels typically produce a local effect. Ointments are occlusive, preventing water absorption or evaporation, and therefore have a hydrating effect and typically produce greater local effects than their cream counterparts. Creams are water soluble and therefore can be washed from the skin more readily than ointments. In hairy areas, creams are preferred over ointments because creams are hydrophilic and hence easier to apply and wash off. Gels, the most water-soluble topical dosage form, allow medication to be spread more easily over a larger area.

Transdermal Administration

Transdermal (*across the skin*) administration refers to the systemic delivery of medication through the skin. Several transdermal drug delivery systems are available for a wide range of medications, including nicotine (Nicotrol) and fentanyl (Duragesic). In general, this method continuously delivers medication to achieve a constant blood level. The consistent delivery of drug throughout the dosing interval minimizes the peak-to-trough fluctuations seen with other forms of drug administration, thereby minimizing the toxicity associated with high blood levels while maintaining therapeutic concentrations.

Distribution

A discussion of the routes of administration offers the opportunity to consider the factors affecting drug absorption and bioavailability; once the medication is in the body, however, it must distribute to the site of action to be effective.

Distribution of an absorbed drug in the body depends on several factors: blood flow to an area, lipid or water solubility, and protein binding. For an absorbed drug to distribute from the blood to a specific site of action, there must be adequate blood flow to that area. In patients with compromised blood flow (e.g., from shock), relying on the blood to deliver a drug to a site of action, such as the kidney, may be risky.

In addition, drug distribution may be affected by obesity, both immediately after absorption and after achieving an equilibrium or steady state in the body. Lipid-soluble drugs readily distribute into the fatty tissues, where they may be stored and even concentrated. Water-soluble drugs, however, tend to remain in the highly vascularized spaces of the skeletal muscle. Ideal body weight is usually considered the standard for determining drug dosage, which is often adjusted for obese or cachectic patients.

Protein Binding

After absorption into the blood (and lymph), a drug may circulate throughout the body unbound (*free drug*) or bound to carrier proteins such as albumin. The extent of drug binding to carrier proteins depends on the affinity of the drug for the carrier protein and the concentrations of both the drug and the protein. Acidic drugs commonly bind to albumin and basic drugs commonly bind to alpha$_1$-acid glycoprotein or lipoproteins.

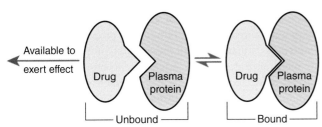

FIGURE 2–3 Relationship between bound and unbound drugs and plasma proteins.

Plasma protein binding is typically a reversible phenomenon, with binding and unbinding occurring within milliseconds. Therefore, the bound and unbound forms of the drug can be assumed to be at equilibrium at all times. As such, the degree of binding to plasma proteins can be expressed as a percentage of bound drug to total concentration (bound plus unbound). It is only the unbound or free drug that can exert a pharmacologic effect. If the drug becomes bound, it becomes inactive because it cannot leave the bloodstream or bind to an enzyme or receptor and exert its therapeutic action (**Figure 2.3**).

Once the free drug is eliminated from the bloodstream through metabolism or excretion, the bound drug can be released from the protein to become active. In essence, the bound drug may serve as a storage site or reservoir of the drug. The percentage of the free drug usually is constant for a single drug but varies among drugs. Patient-specific factors, such as nutritional status, renal function, and levels of circulating protein or albumin, can change the percentage of the free drug.

Volume of Distribution

The amount of drug in the human body can never be directly measured. Observations are made of the concentration of drug in plasma or sometimes in blood. Over time, the concentration of drug in the plasma depends on the rate and extent of drug distribution to the tissues and on how rapidly the drug is eliminated. For most drugs, distribution occurs more rapidly than elimination. The resultant plasma concentration after distribution depends on the dose and the extent of distribution into the tissues. This extent of distribution can be determined by relating the concentration obtained with a known amount of administered drug.

For example, if 100 mg of an IV drug is administered to a person and remains only in the plasma and if that person's total plasma volume measures 5 L, the resulting measured concentration of drug would be 20 mg/L (concentration = dose/volume: 100 mg/5 L). However, in reality, few drugs distribute solely in the plasma, and many bind to plasma proteins. Drugs commonly bind not only to plasma proteins but also to tissue-binding sites on fat and muscle. In addition, drugs translocate into other "compartments" or spaces throughout the body. The volume into which a drug distributes in the body at equilibrium is called the (apparent) volume of distribution (V_d). This volume does not refer to a real volume; rather, it is a mathematically calculated volume (**Box 2.3**). V_d is a direct

$$V_d = \frac{\text{Amount in body}}{\text{Plasma drug concentration}}$$

V_d is usually measured in liters (L); *amount in body* is usually measured in milligrams (mg); and *plasma drug concentration* is usually measured in milligrams per liter (mg/L).

The apparent volume of distribution is a theoretical parameter calculated by determining the amount of drug in the body (usually the dose administered) divided by the concentration of drug in the plasma taken at an appropriate time interval after administration.

measure of the extent of distribution of a drug in the body and represents the apparent volume into which a drug must distribute to contain the amount of drug homogenously.

Drugs that are highly water soluble or highly bound to plasma proteins remain in the blood compartment and do not distribute or bind to fatty tissue. These drugs have a low V_d, usually less than the volume of total body water (approximately 50 L, or 0.7 L/kg). Drugs with a low V_d usually circulate at high levels in the blood. In contrast, drugs that are not highly protein bound and are highly lipophilic have a high V_d (greater than 150 L, which is greater than the volume of total body water). These drugs distribute widely throughout the body and may even cross the blood–brain barrier.

Elimination

All drugs must eventually be eliminated from the body to terminate their effect. Drugs can be eliminated through metabolism (or biotransformation) of the drug from an active form to an inactive form. Drugs can also be eliminated by excretion from the body. Therefore, elimination is a combination of the metabolism and excretion of drugs from the body. Important concepts in understanding drug elimination are half-life, steady state, and clearance. Knowledge of these phenomena in any given patient helps practitioners understand how long a drug will last in the body and how much should be given to maintain therapeutic levels and therefore helps in determining the appropriate dose and dosing intervals.

Metabolism

Metabolism is a function of the body designed to change substances into water soluble, more readily excreted forms. The liver primarily performs the body's metabolic functions because of its high concentration of metabolic enzymes. This is why the first-pass effect is significant to the bioavailability of a drug administered orally.

Other organs, such as the kidneys and intestines, as well as circulating enzyme systems, also contribute to the metabolism

TABLE 2.1
Selected Prodrugs and Metabolites

Parent Drug (Prodrug)	Active Metabolite
Allopurinol	oxypurinol
Codeine	morphine
Enalapril	enalaprilat
Prednisone	prednisolone
Valacyclovir	acyclovir

of drugs. Metabolic processes are used to detoxify drugs and other foreign substances as well as endogenous substances. Drugs may be metabolized from active components into inactive or less active ones. Some drugs, however, may be biologically transformed from an inactive parent drug into an active metabolite. This type of drug is called a prodrug because it is a precursor to the active drug (**Table 2.1**). Not all drugs are metabolized to the same extent or by the same means. In fact, some drugs, such as the aminoglycosides (e.g., gentamicin [Garamycin]), are not metabolized at all.

Enzyme actions are the primary means for metabolizing drugs, and these actions are broadly classified as phase 1 and phase 2 enzymatic processes. Phase 1 enzymatic processes involve oxidation or reduction, by which a drug is changed to form a more polar or water-soluble compound. Phase 2 processes involve adding a conjugate (e.g., a glucuronide) to the parent drug or the phase 1–metabolized drug to further increase water solubility and enhance excretion.

The oxidative process of phase 1 metabolism is catalyzed by the flavin-containing monooxygenases (FMO), the epoxide hydrolases (EH), and the cytochrome P-450 system (CYP). The FMOs and CYP are composed of superfamilies of more than 100 enzymes each. Three families (about 15 total enzymes) of the CYP enzymes are important contributors to drug metabolism. The common feature of these enzymes is their lipid solubility. Most lipophilic drugs are substrates for one or more of the CYP enzymes (**Table 2.2**). FMOs are not considered major contributors to drug metabolism.

TABLE 2.2
Key Cytochrome P-450 Families and Isoforms in Drug Metabolism

Family	Isoform	Example of Drugs Metabolized
CYP1	CYP1A2	theophylline
CYP2	CYP2C19	omeprazole
	CYP2D6	dextromethorphan
	CYP2E1	acetaminophen
CYP3	CYP3A4	atorvastatin

CYP, cytochrome P-450.

Some drugs can induce or stimulate the production of one or more isoforms of the enzymes by a process called enzyme induction, which increases the amount of enzyme available to metabolize drugs. The result of enzyme induction is an increased metabolism of other drugs, thereby decreasing the amount of drug circulating throughout the body.

Conversely, some drugs inhibit the production of CYP enzymes and thereby decrease the metabolism of drugs and increase circulating levels. This is known as enzyme inhibition. Both enzyme induction and inhibition are the basis of metabolically mediated drug–drug interactions. See Chapter 3 for further discussion of induction and inhibition and their role in drug–drug interactions.

Although the liver is regarded as the primary site of drug metabolism, other tissues also possess the enzymes necessary for metabolism. The kidneys, for example, have several enzymes needed for drug metabolism and can serve as the site of drug inactivation. The GI tract is also known to possess several of the CYP isoforms, contributing to the extrahepatic metabolism of drugs.

The nature, function, and amount of any drug-metabolizing enzyme can be different, resulting in differing drug disposition among patients. Disease-induced changes can affect drug metabolism as well. For example, alterations in liver function induced by long-standing cirrhotic changes can reduce the production of necessary enzymes, resulting in increased concentrations of drugs typically metabolized in the liver. Also, decreased blood flow to the liver, as in the case of congestive heart failure, can decrease the delivery of drug to metabolic sites in the liver. Cigarette smoking, on the other hand, can increase the levels of enzymes responsible for drug metabolism, resulting in increased metabolic rates and the need for higher doses of drugs (e.g., theophylline) in smokers than in nonsmokers.

Drug Excretion

Metabolism eliminates a drug from the body by changing the drug molecule into something else, but drugs also can be eliminated from the body by excretion. Excretory organs include the kidneys, lower GI tract, lungs, and skin. Other structures, such as the sweat, salivary, and mammary glands, are active in excretion as well. Drugs may also be removed forcibly by dialysis.

The primary route of excretion is the kidney. After the drug is metabolized, the resultant metabolite may be filtered by the glomerulus. As the drug continues through the proximal tubule, loop of Henle, and distal tubule, several things may occur: The drug may exert action (as in the case of diuretics), be reabsorbed into the bloodstream, or remain in the nephron, eventually reaching the collecting ducts, from which it ultimately leaves the body in the patient's urine. This filtration works well for hydrophilic, ionized compounds and is a common route of elimination. Conversely, active secretion of drugs occurs in the proximal tubule. Two different systems exist, one for organic acids (e.g., uric acid) and one for organic bases (e.g., histamine). Once ionized by the acidic pH of the urine, organic bases are not reabsorbed back into the bloodstream.

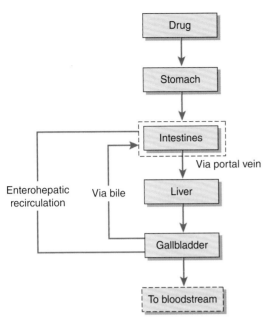

FIGURE 2–4 Enterohepatic recirculation. When a drug is absorbed from the intestine and travels to the liver and gallbladder and into the bile unchanged, it has the potential for being reintroduced into the intestine and therefore reabsorbed. This is known as enterohepatic recirculation.

If the pH of the urine rises, then more of the organic base becomes nonionized and thus more readily reabsorbed into the bloodstream. Similarly, changes in urine pH can alter the reabsorption of organic acids, increasing or decreasing the circulating levels as the pH changes. Drugs such as penicillin are excreted by the organic acid system.

Drugs are excreted by the liver into the gallbladder, resulting in biliary elimination. Biliary elimination can sometimes result in drug reabsorption. For example, if a drug is excreted in the bile, it goes into the GI tract, where it may be reabsorbed and returned to the general circulation. This is called *enterohepatic recirculation* (**Figure 2.4**). The result of significant enterohepatic recirculation is a measurable increase in the plasma concentration of a drug and a delay in its elimination from the body.

Half-Life

The time required for a drug to be eliminated from the body varies according to the drug and the individual. However, useful generalizations can be made that help practitioners estimate how long a drug will remain in the body. The first generalization has to do with the elimination half-life ($t_{1/2}$), which is the time required for half of the total drug amount to be eliminated from the body. Assuming 100% of a drug exists in the body at time X, then one half-life later, 50% of the original amount would remain in the body. An additional half-life later, 25% would remain and so on. For example, vancomycin (an IV antibiotic) has a half-life of approximately 6 hours in an adult with normal renal function. If the vancomycin concentration in a patient's body is 15 mg/L, then it would take 6 hours to decline to 7.5 mg/L, another 6 hours (12 hours total) to fall to 3.75 mg/L, and another 6 hours (18 hours total) to fall to 1.875 mg/L. The rate of elimination of a drug remains constant, but as can be seen in **Figure 2.5**, the amount of drug eliminated is proportional to the concentration of the drug—that is, the more drug there is, the faster it is eliminated. This phenomenon, known as first-order kinetics, applies to most drugs. Rate processes can also be independent of concentration, and fixed amounts of drugs, rather than a fractional proportion, are eliminated at a constant rate. This phenomenon is called zero-order kinetics. Alcohol undergoes zero-order elimination.

After five half-lives, according to first-order kinetics, approximately 97% (96.875%) of any drug is eliminated from the body. Even after three half-lives, nearly 90% (87.5%) of the drug is eliminated. In most cases, after three to five half-lives, the amount of drug remaining is too low to exert any pharmacologic effect, and the drug is considered essentially eliminated. Understanding this concept is useful for practitioners in many situations. For example, if a drug reaches a toxic level, the practitioner knows that it will take three to five half-lives for the drug to be essentially eliminated from the body. The practitioner also can estimate when the drug level will approach a minimally effective concentration and can then calculate when to administer another dose of medication to reach a therapeutic drug level.

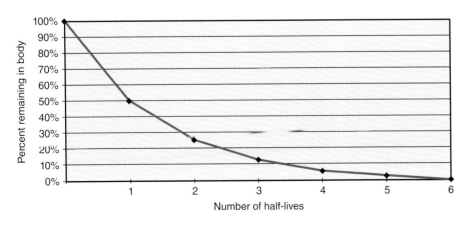

FIGURE 2–5 Drug elimination based on half-life ($t_{1/2}$).

FIGURE 2–6 Steady state achieved with regular dosing (half-life = 8 hours).

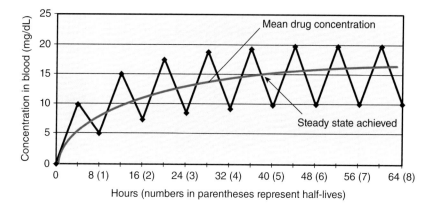

Steady State

In reality, patients take medications on a consistent basis, usually somewhere between one and four times daily. By doing so, they are absorbing and eliminating the drug throughout the day. Because the rate of elimination is proportional to the concentration, at some point, equilibrium is reached. **Figure 2.6** demonstrates how doses of a drug with a half-life of 8 hours produce this equilibrium. Note that after approximately three to five half-lives, the curve levels off. This demonstrates equilibrium between the amount of drug entering the body and the amount leaving the body. This point, which is called *steady state*, reflects a constant mean concentration of drug in the body. At steady state, even though the blood levels of a drug fluctuate above and below this mean concentration and the drug level tends to have peaks and troughs during dosing intervals, the fluctuations remain within a constant range.

For some drugs, the time required to achieve steady state may be very long. For example, digoxin (Lanoxin) has a half-life of 39 hours (1.6 days), meaning that between 4.8 and 8 days are needed to achieve steady state. Clearly, when it is imperative to gain a therapeutic level quickly, waiting this long is unacceptable. Therefore, an initial loading dose of a drug is needed to reach the desired blood concentration quickly. The loading dose is based on the volume of distribution of the drug, independent of the half-life. The maintenance dose, however, is based on the half-life of the drug. Maintenance doses of the drug are given at scheduled intervals to replace the amount of drug eliminated.

Clearance

The concept of clearance, which refers to the removal of a drug from the plasma or organ, is the final element in the process of elimination. Drugs with high clearances are removed rapidly; those with low clearances are removed slowly. Drugs can be cleared by biliary, hepatic, or renal means. The following discussion highlights renal clearance.

Clearance is related to the apparent volume of distribution and the half-life (**Box 2.4**). Clearance of a drug from the body depends directly on the apparent volume of distribution and is inversely related to the elimination half-life: The greater

BOX 2.4 Relationship among Apparent Volume of Distribution, Clearance, and Half-Life

$$\text{Clearance} = \frac{0.693 \times V_d}{t_{1/2}}$$

Clearance is usually expressed as L/hour; V_d is in L; $t_{1/2}$ is usually in hours.

Clearance of a drug is directly dependent on the apparent volume of distribution and inversely related to the elimination half-life. The larger the V_d, the faster the clearance. Also, the smaller the $t_{1/2}$, the faster the clearance.

the volume of distribution and the shorter the half-life, the faster the clearance.

Because most drugs are "cleared" through the kidney, estimating the renal elimination rate or clearance can help the practitioner to understand how fast a drug is being eliminated in an individual patient. Because directly measuring the clearance of the kidney is time intensive and often impractical, the kidney's ability to clear drugs is estimated through a surrogate substrate: creatinine. Creatinine, which is produced through the continual breakdown of muscle tissue and eliminated largely by glomerular filtration, is not significantly secreted or reabsorbed. Therefore, in estimating the creatinine clearance, the practitioner can also estimate the glomerular filtration rate (GFR). The level of creatinine is usually measured through a blood test (serum creatinine), with normal values ranging from 0.8 to 1.2 mg/dL.

In order to estimate the GFR, the practitioner generally uses one of three equations (listed in order of most accurate to least accurate): the Chronic Kidney Disease Epidemiology Collaboration (CKD-EPI) equation, the Modification of Diet in Renal Disease (MDRD) study equation, or the

TABLE 2.3

Estimating Creatinine Clearance Using Currently Accepted Formulas

Name	Equation	Value Units	Notes
CKD-EPI	$GFR = 141 \times \min(S_{Cr}/\kappa, 1)^{\alpha} \times \max(S_{Cr}/\kappa, 1)^{-1.209}$ $\times 0.993^{Age} \times 1.018$ [if female] $\times 1.159$ [if black]	mL/min/1.73 m^2	• Only for use in >18 years old and when estimated GFR is >60 mL/min/1.73 m^2 • Recommend reporting values as ≥60 mL/min/1.73 m^2 instead of an exact number
MDRD	$GFR = 175 \times (S_{Cr})^{-1.154} \times (Age)^{-0.203} \times$ (0.742 if female) $\times$ (1.212 if African American)	mL/min/1.73 m^2	• Only for use in >18 years old and when estimated GFR is <60 mL/min/1.73 m^2 • Recommend reporting values as ≥60 mL/min/1.73 m^2 instead of an exact number
CG	$C_{Cr} = \{((140\text{–}age) \times weight)/(72 \times S_{Cr})\} \times$ 0.85 (if female)	mL/min	• Should not be used for drug dosing or to estimate GFR due to possibility of significant overestimation of true GFR

CG, Cockcroft-Gault; CKD-EPI, Chronic Kidney Disease Epidemiology Collaboration; GFR, glomerular filtration rate; MDRD, Modification of Diet in Renal Disease.

Cockcroft-Gault (CG) equation. These equations consider patient demographics such as weight, gender, and race in order to *estimate* creatinine clearance and evaluate the kidney's ability to function and eliminate drugs. However, each equation will produce a different result using the same patient demographics and each has caveats (see **Table 2.3**).

For example, a 40-year-old white male who is 70 in. tall and weighs 70 kg and has a serum creatinine of 2.0 mg/dL has an estimated creatinine clearance of 41 mL/min/1.73 m^2 (CKD-EPI), 37 mL/min/1.73 m^2 (MDRD), and 49 mL/min (CG).

In any case, creatinine clearance or GFR values below 50 mL/min suggest significant impairment of renal function and thus possible impairment of renal drug elimination. This may result in administered drugs having longer half-lives and higher steady-state concentrations, which may result in toxicity if the dose is not decreased or the length of time between doses is not increased.

Not every patient needs to have creatinine clearance estimated. Two rules of thumb are useful for the practitioner: Patients older than age 65 or those with a serum creatinine value greater than 1.5 mg/dL may be at risk for accumulating drug (and therefore toxicity) because of decreased renal function. In patients with either of these characteristics, a baseline and routine evaluation of renal function (e.g., serum creatinine determination) should be performed.

PHARMACODYNAMICS

Pharmacodynamics refers to the set of processes by which drugs produce specific biochemical or physiologic changes in the body (how the drug affects the body). Most often,

pharmacodynamic effects occur because a drug interacts with a receptor. Receptors may be cell membrane proteins, extracellular enzymes, cytoplasmic enzymes, or intracellular proteins. A receptor is the component of the cell (or an enzyme) to which an endogenous substance binds, or attaches, initiating a chain of biochemical events. This chain of biochemical events culminates in a change in the physiologic function of the cell or activity of the enzyme. Like endogenous substances, drugs can initiate the biochemical chain of events. For example, a drug stimulating a receptor on the surface of an artery may ultimately cause vasoconstriction or vasodilation; or the drug's binding to a receptor may produce a change in cell wall permeability, thus allowing other substances to enter or leave a cell, as in nerve cells; or the drug attached to a receptor may initiate an increase or decrease in the production of an enzyme, thereby changing the amount of enzymatic activity for a given process.

Any chemical, endogenous or exogenous, that interacts with a receptor is called a *ligand*. Regardless of the ligand, or the actual interaction type, a substance can only alter or modify a cell or process, not impart a new function.

Drug Receptors

The capacity of a drug to bind to a receptor depends on the size and shape of the drug and the receptor. The drug acts as a "key" that fits into only a certain receptor or receptor type (**Figure 2.7**). Once the drug fits into the receptor, it may act to "unlock" the activity of the receptor, thus initiating the biochemical chain of events, much like an ignition key initiates the chain of events that starts a car.

Drug receptors are commonly classified by the effect they produce. Some drugs interact with several receptors,

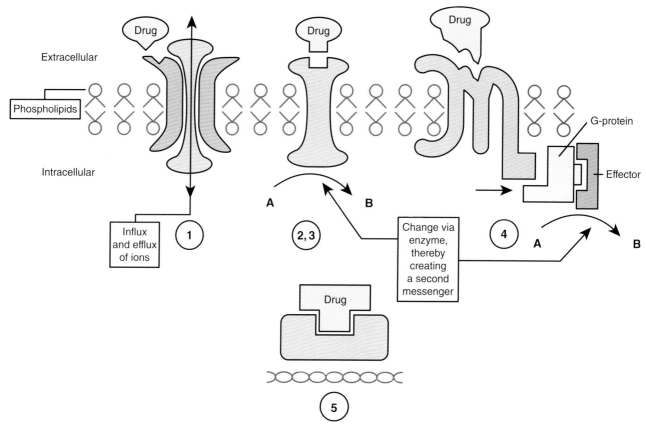

FIGURE 2–7   Drug and drug–receptor interaction and signal transduction. The five primary receptors and their mechanisms of signal transduction are (1) gated ion channels; (2 and 3) transmembranous receptors—cytoplasmic enzyme and tyrosine kinase activated; (4) G protein–coupled receptors; and (5) intracellular receptors.

causing multiple effects, whereas others interact with only a specific receptor, eliciting a single response. Epinephrine, for example, interacts with the alpha and beta receptors of the sympathetic nervous system. As a result, epinephrine produces vasoconstriction (alpha receptor action) and an increase in heart rate (beta receptor action). Various molecules or enzymes can serve as drug receptors, such as ion channels (calcium channels), enzymes (angiotensin-converting enzyme [ACE]), and even receptors that generate intracellular second messengers (substances that interact with other intracellular components).

There are four known types of receptors: gated ion channels, transmembranous receptors, G protein–coupled receptors, and intracellular receptors (see **Figure 2.7**). Understanding these receptors and the signals they generate is central to understanding the actions of many drugs.

Gated Ion Channels

The function of gated ion channel receptors is to open or close channels to allow certain ions to pass through the cell membrane. Binding of ligands to these receptors produces a conformational change that widens or narrows the channel, thereby regulating the access of soluble ions (**Figure 2.7**). The nicotinic acetylcholine receptor is a good example of a gated ion channel receptor. Its function is to translate the signal from acetylcholine into an electrical signal at the neuromuscular endplate. As such, when acetylcholine binds to this receptor, the channel opens, allowing sodium or potassium to enter the cell and cause cellular depolarization.

Other types of gated ion channel receptors are associated with the neurotransmitters. Gamma-aminobutyric acid (GABA$_A$), the primary inhibitory neurotransmitter, opens a chloride channel in the cell, which minimizes the depolarization potential. Certain drugs, such as the benzodiazepines, bind to an allosteric site and enhance the activity of GABA$_A$ by increasing the opening of the chloride channel. There is no intrinsic activity at the allosteric site, and it serves only to enhance the primary action of the endogenous ligand. Other excitatory neurotransmitters, such as L-glutamate and L-aspartate, operate by this mechanism, called signal transduction, which transfers the signal quickly.

Transmembranous Receptors: Cytoplasmic Enzyme or Tyrosine Kinase Activated

A transmembranous receptor has its ligand-binding domain, the specific region to which ligands bind, on the cell's surface. The enzymatic portion of the receptor is in the cell cytoplasm. When a ligand binds to a transmembranous receptor, several things may occur. The receptor–ligand complex produces a conformational change in the receptor and triggers a response. Alternatively, the ligand–receptor complex can pass through the cell membrane and trigger an intracellular response directly. This intracellular response often is a change in enzymatic activity. A key feature of the transmembranous receptor response is the downregulation of the receptors or a decrease in the number of receptors available for response. The opposite of this is upregulation, which does not occur as frequently. The nature of the signal depends on the specific ligand–receptor interaction, but it commonly results in the generation of second messengers. A second messenger is an intracellular chemical that interacts with other intracellular components. Ions such as calcium and potassium, along with cyclic adenosine monophosphate, are common second messengers. Hormones and other endogenous substances, such as growth factors and insulin, often operate with this signaling mechanism.

The receptor tyrosine kinase signaling pathway can bind with a polypeptide hormone or growth factor at the receptor's extracellular domain. This results in enzymatically active tyrosine kinase domains that phosphorylate each other, allowing a single receptor to activate multiple biochemical processes. For example, insulin works by stimulating the uptake of glucose as well as amino acids, resulting in changes in glycogen content within the cell. Alternatively, inhibition of tyrosine kinase processes through blockage of the external receptor can result in a decrease in stimulation of growth factors within the cell. This is particularly important in cancer treatments, when inhibiting the growth of the cell is key to treatment success.

A drawback of this system is the potential for downregulation of the receptors. Activation of these receptors leads to an endocytosis of the receptor and subsequent receptor degradation. When this activity exceeds the production of new receptors, there is a reduction in the number of receptors available for stimulation, thus resulting in a decrease in the cell's activity.

G Protein–Coupled Receptors

G protein–coupled receptors are another family of receptors that generate intracellular second messengers. These receptors also exist as transmembranous receptors composed of an extracellular protein receptor and an intracellular type G protein. The interaction of a ligand and the receptor produces a conformational change in the receptor, bringing it in contact with the G protein. This contact results in activation of an enzyme or opening of an ion channel in the cell and, in turn, increased levels of the second messenger. It is the second messenger that triggers a change in the function of the cell. Alpha- and beta-adrenergic receptors, along with several hormone receptors, use G proteins to affect cell function.

Intracellular Receptors

Lipid-soluble drugs can traverse the lipid bilayer of the cell and enter the cytoplasm. Once inside, these drugs attach to intracellular receptors and initiate direct changes in the cell by affecting DNA transcription. Glucocorticoids and sex hormones are known to act by this signaling mechanism.

Drug–Receptor Interactions

The ability of a drug to bind to any receptor is dictated by factors such as the size and shape of the drug relative to the configuration of the binding site on the receptor. The electrostatic attraction between the drug and the receptor may also be important in determining the extent to which the drug binds to the receptor.

Affinity

A drug attracted to a receptor displays an *affinity* for that receptor. This affinity, the degree to which a drug is attracted to a receptor, is related to the concentration of drug required to occupy a receptor site. Drugs displaying a high affinity for a given receptor require only a small concentration in the circulation to elicit a response, whereas those with a low affinity require higher circulating concentrations. There exists an equilibrium among the blood concentration of a drug, the concentration of drug at the site of action (i.e., near the receptor), and the amount of drug bound to a receptor. The magnitude of a drug's effect can be explained by the receptor occupancy theory—that is, a response from a cell (or group of cells) depends on the fraction of receptors occupied by a drug or endogenous substance. Therefore, one can infer a relationship between the minimally and the maximally effective concentrations needed at the site of action and the minimum and the maximum blood concentrations.

Chirality

The shape of a drug can influence its interaction with a receptor. Most drugs display chirality—that is, they exist in two forms, with mirror-image spatial arrangements called enantiomers, or isomers. Each enantiomer is distinguished from the other through its ability to rotate polarized light in pure solution to the right or left. This results in a dextrorotatory enantiomer, or D-enantiomer, and a levorotatory enantiomer, or L-companion.

A pair of enantiomers is like a left and a right hand. As such, enantiomeric pairs may not fit into a receptor equally well, just as a right hand does not fit well into a left-hand glove. This is called stereoselectivity; one enantiomer may fit better into a receptor than the other and, hence, be more active. For example, the drug dextromethorphan (the "DM" in Robitussin DM) is the D-isomer of a compound. This D-isomer is a common cough suppressant found in most over-the-counter medications. Its L-isomer counterpart, levorphanol (Levo-Dromoran), is an extremely potent narcotic analgesic. Although the L-isomer also possesses cough suppressant activity, the D-isomer is essentially devoid of analgesic activity at commonly used doses. This example illustrates the importance of isomers in pharmacodynamics.

Agonists and Antagonists

Not all drugs with an affinity for a receptor elicit a response. Drugs that display a degree of affinity for a receptor and stimulate a response are considered agonists. Others that display an affinity and do not elicit a response are called antagonists. Antagonists do not have intrinsic activity; they can only block the activity of the endogenous agonist. An antagonist may be viewed as a key that fits into the lock but, because of its different configuration, cannot be turned. Because an antagonist can occupy, or fit into, a receptor, it competes with agonists for that receptor, thereby blocking the effect of the agonist. Antagonists with a high affinity for a receptor may be able to "bump" an agonist off the receptor and reverse the agonist activity. Antagonists usually are used to block the activity of an endogenous substance, but they also can be used to block the activity of exogenously administered drugs. For example, when naloxone (Narcan) is given to a patient taking opioid drugs, the analgesic (and adverse) effects of the opioid are reversed within 1 to 2 minutes. In most cases, naloxone has a higher affinity for the opioid receptor than the opioid itself. This rough explanation of drug–receptor interactions serves only as a basis for understanding the complexity of this interplay.

Dose–Response Relationships

For many drugs, the relationship between the dose and the response is obvious: Lower doses produce smaller responses, whereas higher doses increase the response. This correlation is based on the amount of drug occupying specific receptors. As the amount of drug exceeds the number of available receptors, the response reaches a plateau, so that further increases in dose do not increase response. However, dose–response relationships such as these clearly depend on the affinity of a drug for a receptor: A drug with a high affinity for a receptor needs a significantly lower concentration to achieve the same effect compared to a drug with a lower affinity.

This difference in affinity accounts for the varying "potency" of drugs. For example, drugs such as hydromorphone (Dilaudid) and morphine produce the same effect: analgesia. However, hydromorphone is more potent than morphine and therefore requires a smaller concentration to elicit a similar level of analgesia. **Figure 2.8** demonstrates a typical dose–response relationship.

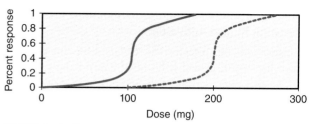

FIGURE 2–8 Two drugs with differing receptor affinities produce similar effects at different dosage ranges. The drug with the greater affinity (*solid line*) requires less drug to produce the same effect as a drug with less affinity (*dotted line*). This demonstrates the relationship between receptor affinity and drug potency.

FACTORS AFFECTING PHARMACOKINETICS AND PHARMACODYNAMICS

The goal of pharmacotherapeutics is to achieve a desired beneficial effect with minimal adverse effects. Once a medication has been selected for a patient, the practitioner must determine the dose that most closely achieves this goal. A rational approach to this objective combines the principles of pharmacokinetics with those of pharmacodynamics to clarify the dose–response relationship. Knowing the relationship between drug concentration and response allows the practitioner to take into account the various pathologic and physiologic features of a particular patient that make his or her response different from the average person's response to a drug.

Patient Variables

A host of variables affects the disposition of a drug in the body and the reaction the body has to the drug. People vary in their body type, weight, diet, ethnicity, and genetic makeup. These factors, individually and combined, contribute to significant variation in their response to drug therapy. For example, the genetic makeup of the people of Japan is known to affect the expression of certain hepatic enzymes involved in the metabolism of drugs. This suggests that, at least pharmacokinetically, some people of Japanese heritage respond differently to certain drugs. The same logic applies to people who are overweight and underweight, people of varying ages, people with various pathophysiologic problems, and even people with different diets and nutritional habits.

Pathophysiology

Structural or functional damage to an organ or tissue responsible for drug metabolism or excretion presents an obvious problem in pharmacology. Diseases that initiate changes in tissue function or blood flow to specific organs can dramatically affect the elimination of various drugs. Certain diseases may also impair the absorption and distribution of the drug, complicating the problem of individualized response. The role of disease in affecting the patient's response is crucial because the response to the medication may be affected by the same pathologic process that the drug is being used to treat. For instance, renal excretion of antibiotics, such as aminoglycosides, is altered radically in many types of bacterial infection, but these drugs are typically administered to treat the same infections that alter their own excretion. Consequently, great care must be taken to adjust the dosage accordingly when administering medications to patients with conditions in which drug elimination may be altered.

Genetics

Genetic differences are a major factor in determining the way that people metabolize specific compounds. Genetic variations may result in abnormal or absent drug-metabolizing enzymes, creating unpredictable individual responses to medication therapy despite the administration of the same drug and dose. The anomaly can be harmful or even fatal if the drug cannot be metabolized and therefore exerts a toxic effect from accumulation or prolonged pharmacologic activity. Genetic mutations may include mutations such as single nucleotide polymorphisms (SNPs), gene deletions, or gene duplications. Some people, for example, lack the enzyme that breaks down acetylcholine. In these people, a neuromuscular blocking drug such as succinylcholine (Anectine, an acetylcholine-like drug usually used to induce paralysis for procedures) is not degraded and therefore accumulates. The result is respiratory paralysis because the undegraded, accumulated succinylcholine has an increased half-life, causing it to remain active longer. Pharmacogenomics, or the study of responses of individuals to medication based on their genome, is emerging as the field of medicine dedicated to precision or personalized medicine. See Chapter 7 for more details.

Age

The influence of age on pharmacokinetics and pharmacodynamics is well known. Developmental differences in the neonate, toddler, and young child, for instance, influence how drugs are handled by the GI tract, liver, and kidneys. Of equal importance is how these children respond to drugs in light of the presence or absence of receptors at different stages of development. For example, drug-metabolizing enzymes are deficient in the fetus and premature infant. The fetus can metabolize drugs early in its development, but its expression of drug-metabolizing enzymes differs from that in the adult and is usually less efficient.

Children can metabolize many drugs more rapidly than adults, and as children approach puberty, the rate of drug metabolism approaches that of adults. Similarly, older adults undergo physiologic changes that affect the absorption, distribution, and elimination of many agents. The pharmacodynamic changes imparted by age as well as accompanying diseases pose a greater challenge for the practitioner in understanding the impact a single agent has on a patient's health and well-being. Chapter 4 discusses pediatric considerations, and Chapter 5 discusses geriatric considerations in greater detail.

Sex

The role of sex as a distinct patient variable is recognized by some but poorly understood by most. Most of the published clinical drug studies used male subjects as the primary study population, and clinicians then extrapolated the data to females. However, females in general have a higher percentage of body fat, which could ultimately alter the pharmacokinetic disposition of certain drugs. Similarly, the pharmacodynamic response of females may be different because of the presence or absence of hormones such as estrogen and testosterone. Transgender/transsexual patients present another challenge; however, current thinking suggests using their biologically assigned gender to estimate CrCl.

Ethnicity

Ethnicity is a significant factor in both the pharmacokinetic and the pharmacodynamic responses of patients. The genetic makeup of various ethnic populations governs the levels of hepatic enzymes expressed in these groups. Equally important are the habits and traditions of certain groups, such as diet or the use of home remedies.

Pharmacodynamically, ethnically based differences exist in the responses to agents. An example is the minimal response of African American patients to monotherapy with some drugs, such as ACE inhibitors. African Americans produce a low level of renin, a key component in the renin–angiotensin–aldosterone system by which the ACE inhibitors work. This low level of renin makes this system unaffected by the ACE inhibitor, thereby negating its effect.

Diet and Nutrition

Diet affects the metabolism of and response to many drugs. Animal and human studies indicate that total caloric intake and the percentage of calories obtained from different sources (carbohydrates, proteins, and fats) influence drug pharmacokinetics. Specific dietary constituents, such as cruciferous vegetables and charcoal-broiled beef, can also alter drug metabolism. Fortunately, most food–drug interactions are not serious and do not alter the clinical effects of the drug. However, a few well-known food and drug combinations should be avoided because of their potentially serious interactions. For instance, certain tyramine-containing foods, such as fermented cheese and wine, should not be ingested with drugs that inhibit the monoamine oxidase enzyme (MAO) inhibitors. Tyramine-rich foods stimulate the body to release catecholamines (norepinephrine, epinephrine). MAO-inhibiting drugs work by suppressing the destruction of catecholamines, thereby allowing higher levels of norepinephrine and epinephrine to accumulate. Consequently, when MAO inhibitors are taken with tyramine-containing foods, excessive catecholamine levels may develop and lead to a dangerous increase in blood pressure (hypertensive crisis). Practitioners should be aware of this and should be on the alert for other such interactions as new drugs arrive on the market.

CASE STUDY

J.R. is a 90-year-old Japanese male. He has been a one pack per day smoker for the past 50 years. J.R. weighs 98 kg and is 67 in. tall. He admits to eating a diet rich in processed foods and unhealthy fats. He was recently diagnosed with renal insufficiency (creatinine clearance of 32 mL/min). He comes to you because he recently started having some shortness of breath while he is resting and you are considering adding a few new medications to his regimen.

1. Which pharmacokinetic and pharmacodynamic considerations do you need to take into account in order to prescribe medicine safely to J.R., and what are the possible impacts of each of these considerations?

Bibliography

Ahmed, S., Zhou, Z., Zhou, J., et al. (2016). Pharmacogenomics of drug metabolizing enzymes and transporters: Relevance to precision medicine. *Genomics Proteonomics Bioinformatics, 14*(5), 298–313.

Bishop, B. M. (2015). Pharmacotherapy considerations in the management of transgender patients: A brief review. *Pharmacotherapy, 35*(12), 1130–1139.

Brunton, L., Brunton, L., Knollmann, B., et al. (2018). *Goodman & Gilman's the pharmacological basis of therapeutics*, 13th ed. New York: McGraw-Hill Medical.

Chudek, J., Kolonko, A., Owczarek, A., et al. (2018). Clinical factors increasing discrepancies of renal function assessment with MDRD and Cockcroft-Gault equations in old individuals. *European Geriatric Medicine, 9*, 713–720.

DiPiro, J. (2017). *Pharmacotherapy: A pathophysiologic approach,* 10th ed. New York: McGraw-Hill Education.

Katzung, B., & Katzung, B. (2018). *Basic & clinical pharmacology,* 14th ed. New York: McGraw-Hill.

Lew, A., Crass, R., & Eschenauer, G. (2020). Evolution of equations for estimating renal function and their application to the dosing of new antimicrobials. *Annals of Pharmacotherapy, 54*(5), 496–503.

National Kidney Disease Education Program. (2000–2019). Retrieved from https://www.niddk.nih.gov/health-information/professionals/clinical-tools-patient-management/kidney-disease/laboratory-evaluation/glomerular-filtration-rate-calculators. Accessed January 13, 2020.

Spruill, W., Wade, W., DiPiro, J. T., et al. (2014). *Concepts in clinical pharmacokinetics,* 6th ed. Bethesda, MD: American Society of Health-System Pharmacists.

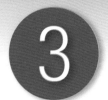

3 Impact of Drug Interactions and Adverse Events on Therapeutics

Tep M. Kang

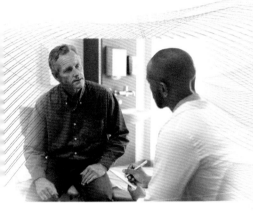
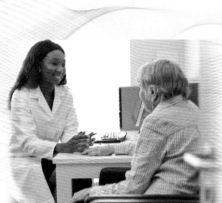
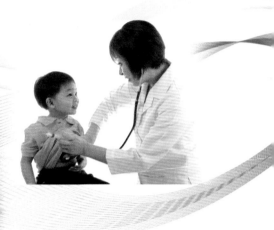

Learning Objectives

1. Able to identify factors known to cause drug–drug interactions, drug–food interactions, and drug–herb interactions.
2. Describe selected drug–drug interactions, drug–food interactions, and drug–herb interactions.
3. Recognize risk factors associated with adverse drug reactions.

INTRODUCTION

As the quantity and types of pharmacologic agents continue to expand, the likelihood of drug interactions and adverse reactions increases. Currently, more than 8,000 drugs are available to treat various conditions. Each agent is designed to alter the homeostasis of the human body to some degree, and individual responses to these agents can be unpredictable.

In a prospective study, Benard-Laribiere et al. (2014) found that 3.6% (97/2,692) of hospital admissions were due to serious adverse drug reactions (ADRs). Thirty percent of which were preventable and 16.5% of which were potentially preventable. Drug interactions caused 29.9% of ADR-related hospital admissions. According to the Institute for Safe Medicine Practices (QuarterWatch, 2014), psychiatric adverse drug events, notably suicidal behaviors, represent the major adverse effects reported in children under age 18. In a meta-analysis of observational studies, Martins et al. (2014) reported a 21.3% incidence of adverse drug events among adult inpatients. These data were captured during prospective monitoring whereby the events are detected during the hospital stay and can include interviews of the patient and/or care team and reviews of clinical and laboratory records.

ADRs present an alarming problem that warrants significant attention from health care practitioners. ADRs not only affect morbidity and mortality but also dramatically increase health care costs. In the United States, the impact of ADRs may cost up to $30.1 billion per year. Most of the cost is attributed to increased hospitalization, increased length of stay, and increased cost of performing additional tests (Sultana et al., 2013).

Similarly, drug interactions are potentially preventable ADRs posing a significant problem to the health care community. It has been reported that approximately 10% to 20% of hospital admissions are drug related and about 1% of these are secondary to drug interactions. Others have reported that drug interactions are responsible for up to 3% of hospital admissions (Bjerrum et al., 2008). In addition, the prevalence of a first dispensing of drug–drug interactions in people older than age 70 has been reported to have increased from 10.5% in 1992 to 19.2% in 2005 (Becker et al., 2008). Therefore, a thorough understanding of how drug–drug interactions occur and how they relate to ADRs should help decrease the rate of occurrence and the associated morbidity/mortality. This chapter discusses the mechanisms of drug interactions and their potential consequences. For the purpose of this chapter, these interactions are broken down into four major categories: drug–drug interactions, drug–food interactions, complementary alternative medicine (CAM) interactions, and drug–disease interactions. Each of the interaction categories can affect the drug's pharmacokinetic or pharmacodynamic profile. The definition, identification, and management of ADRs are discussed at the end of the chapter.

DRUG–DRUG INTERACTIONS

When a person takes two or more medications concomitantly, the potential exists for one or more drugs to change the effect of other drugs. The drug whose effect is altered by another drug is termed the *object* or *target* drug. Although minor interactions between drugs probably occur frequently, these interactions may not be significant enough to alter the effect of either drug. However, it is important for the practitioner to understand the mechanisms behind these interactions to predict more accurately when clinically significant (and potentially fatal) drug interactions may occur.

Pharmacokinetic Interactions

Absorption

Because most medications in the ambulatory care setting are administered orally, this route is the focus of discussion. For a drug to exert its effect, it must reach its site of action. Normally, this requires access to the bloodstream. As discussed in Chapter 2, drugs administered orally must be absorbed into the portal vein, through the intestinal wall, to reach the systemic circulation. The oral tablet must dissolve in the gastrointestinal (GI) tract before it can penetrate the intestinal wall.

Acidity (pH)

For some drugs, this process depends on the acidity in the GI tract. Therefore, if a drug that alters the gastric pH is administered concomitantly with a drug that depends on a normal gastric pH for dissolution, the absorption of the target drug will be affected. An example of this type of interaction is the concurrent administration of a histamine-2 (H_2) receptor antagonist (e.g., famotidine) and ketoconazole, an imidazole antifungal agent. Ketoconazole is the target drug that requires an acidic pH for absorption. When famotidine is administered along with ketoconazole, the increase in gastric pH hinders the dissolution of ketoconazole and therefore decreases its absorption. Similarly, this change in pH can increase the absorption of other drugs that require a more alkaline environment for absorption.

Adsorption

Another mechanism of drug–drug interactions is adsorption. Adsorption occurs when one agent binds the other to its surface to form a complex. The most common agents associated with this type of interaction are divalent and trivalent cations (Mg^{2+}, Ca^{2+}, Al^{3+}, found in antacids and some vitamin preparations) and anionic-binding resins (colestipol and cholestyramine). This type of interaction occurs when certain medications such as tetracyclines or fluoroquinolones are given with antacids. The metal ions in the antacid chelate form a complex with the antibiotic, preventing absorption of both components (ion and antibiotic). Adsorbents can interact with a variety of drugs; therefore, appropriate intervals between doses of the interacting medications are warranted. In general, with agents known to interact in this manner, the target drug should be administered at least 2 hours before or 4 to 6 hours after the interacting agent.

Gastrointestinal Motility and Rate of Absorption

Drugs that affect the motility of the GI tract produce a less common absorption-altering mechanism. These agents tend to affect the rate of absorption and not the amount of drug absorbed. Any agent—for example, metoclopramide—that stimulates peristalsis and increases gastric-emptying time can affect the rate of absorption of other medications. In most cases, an increase in the rate of absorption occurs because the target drug reaches the duodenum faster, allowing absorption to occur sooner. However, in some cases such as with metoclopramide and digoxin, a decrease in digoxin concentrations may occur (American Society of Health-System Pharmacists, 2008).

Conversely, anticholinergic agents and opiates decrease gastric motility, thereby decreasing the rate of absorption of target drugs. However, this interaction is usually clinically insignificant since the total amount of drug absorbed is not affected.

Gastrointestinal Flora and Absorption

The bacteria present in the GI tract are also responsible for a portion of the metabolism of some agents. An example of this is digoxin; concomitant administration with antibiotics (such as erythromycin or tetracycline) may alter the normal bacterial flora and reduce digoxin metabolism, thereby increasing bioavailability and serum concentrations in some patients (Susla, 2005). To the contrary, GI bacteria produce enzymes that de-conjugate inactive unabsorbable ethinyl estradiol metabolites of oral contraceptives that have been excreted into the GI tract via the bile. De-conjugation allows reabsorption of active ethinyl estradiol back into the bloodstream. By disrupting the GI flora, anti-infectives may decrease or eliminate reabsorption of active ethinyl estradiol, thereby decreasing plasma concentrations and the effectiveness of oral contraceptives (Weaver & Glasier, 1999). However, in a case-crossover study of 1,330 failure cases, Toh et al. (2011) did not find an association between concomitant antibiotic use and the risk of breakthrough pregnancy among combined oral contraceptive users.

Table 3.1 summarizes some of the major drug interactions that occur in the absorptive process.

Distribution

After drugs are absorbed into the bloodstream, most of them, to some degree, are bound to plasma protein such as albumin or α_1-acid glycoprotein. A compilation of 222 drugs for various indications showed that about 50% of them are 90% or more protein bound. As described in Chapter 2, only an unbound drug is free to interact with its target receptor site and is therefore active. The percentage of drug that binds to plasma proteins depends on the affinity of that drug for the protein-binding site. If two drugs with high affinity for circulating proteins are administered together, they may compete for a single binding site on the protein. In fact, one drug may displace the other from the binding site with the result being an increase in the unbound (free) fraction of the displaced drug. This increase in free drug may trigger an exaggerated pharmacodynamic response or toxic reaction. However, because the

TABLE 3.1

Drug Absorption Interactions

	Mechanism of Action	Target Drug	Results
Absorption Inhibitors			
Activated charcoal	Binding agent	Digoxin	Decreased absorption
Aluminum hydroxide	Unknown	Allopurinol	Decreased absorption
Antacids (Mg^{2+}, Ca^{2+}, Al^{3+})	Chelating agent	Quinolones, tetracyclines, levodopa, levothyroxine	Decreased absorption
Aluminum and Mg hydroxide	Binding agent	Digoxin	Decreased absorption
Bismuth (Pepto-Bismol)	Binding agent	Tetracycline, doxycycline	Decreased absorption
Antibiotics (i.e., erythromycin, tetracycline)	Altered GI flora	Digoxin	Increased absorption
	Altered GI flora	Oral contraceptives	Decreased reabsorption, decreased enterohepatic recycling
Anticholinergics	Decreases gastric emptying	Acetaminophen, atenolol, levodopa	Decreased absorption
Cholestyramine	Binding agent	Acetaminophen, diclofenac, digoxin, glipizide, furosemide, iron, levothyroxine, lorazepam, methotrexate, metronidazole, piroxicam	Decreased absorption
Colestipol	Binding agent	Carbamazepine, diclofenac, furosemide, tetracycline, thiazides	Decreased absorption
Desipramine	Decreases GI motility	Phenylbutazone	Decreased absorption
Didanosine	Binding agent	Ciprofloxacin	Decreased absorption
	Increases gastric pH	Imidazole, ketoconazole	Decreased absorption
Ferrous sulfate	Chelating agent	Quinolones, tetracyclines, levodopa, levothyroxine	Decreased absorption
Histamine-2 receptor antagonists/ proton pump inhibitors	Increases gastric pH	Imidazole, ketoconazole, enoxacin	Decreased absorption
Phenytoin	Unknown	Furosemide	Decreased absorption
Sucralfate	Binding agent	Quinolones, tetracyclines, phenytoin, levothyroxine	Decreased absorption
Sulfasalazine	Unknown	Digoxin	Decreased absorption
Sodium zirconium cyclosilicate	Increases gastric pH	Clopidogrel, dabigatran	Decreased absorption
Patiromer	Binding agent	Metformin, ciprofloxacin, levothyroxine	Decreased absorption
Absorption Enhancers			
Cisapride	Increases gastric emptying	Disopyramide	Increased absorption
Histamine-2 receptor antagonists	Increases gastric pH	Pravastatin, glipizide, dihydropyridine, calcium antagonists	Increased absorption
Metoclopramide	Increases gastric motility	Cyclosporine	Increased absorption
	Increases GI motility	Acetaminophen, cefprozil, ethanol	Increased absorption
Sodium zirconium cyclosilicate	Increases gastric pH	Warfarin	Increased absorption

GI, gastrointestinal.

TABLE 3.2
Protein-Bound Drug Interactions

Displacing Drug	Target Drug
Aspirin	Meclofenamate, tolmetin
Salicylates	Methotrexate
TMP-SMZ	
Sulfaphenazole	Phenytoin
Tolbutamide	
Valproic acid	
Halofenate	Sulfonylureas
Quinidine	Digoxin
Aspirin	Warfarin
Chloral hydrate	
Diazoxide	
Etodolac	
Fenoprofen	
Lovastatin	
Nalidixic acid	
Phenylbutazone	
Phenytoin	
Sulfinpyrazone	

TMP-SMZ, trimethoprim–sulfamethoxazole.

excess unbound drug is now subject to elimination processes, the increases in both free drug fraction and the effects produced are usually transient.

Clinically significant drug displacement interactions normally occur only when drugs are more than 90% protein bound and have a narrow therapeutic index. For example, warfarin is 99% protein bound, and therefore, only 1% of the drug in the bloodstream is free to induce a pharmacodynamic response (inhibition of clotting factors). If a second drug is administered that displaces even 1% of the warfarin bound to albumin, the amount of free warfarin is doubled, to 2% free. This can result in a significant increase in its pharmacodynamic action, leading to excessive bleeding. **Table 3.2** lists examples of several displacement interactions.

Metabolism

Lipophilicity (fat solubility) enables drug molecules to be absorbed and reach their site of action. However, lipophilic drugs are difficult for the body to excrete. Therefore, they must be transformed by the body to more hydrophilic (water-soluble) molecules. This is accomplished primarily through phase I, or oxidation, reactions. The main sites of metabolism in the body are the liver (hepatocytes) and small intestine (enterocytes). Other tissues, such as the kidneys, lungs, and brain, play a minor role in the metabolism of drug molecules (Michalets, 1998). These sites of metabolism contain

enzymes called cytochrome P-450 isoenzymes. This group of isoenzymes has been identified as the major catalyst of phase I metabolic reactions in humans.

The nomenclature of the cytochrome P-450 system classifies the isoenzymes (designated CYP) according to family (>36% homology in amino acid sequence), subfamily (77% homology), and individual gene (Brosen, 1990; Guengerich, 1994; Nebert et al., 1987). For example, the isoenzyme CYP3A4 belongs to family 3, subfamily A, and gene 4. As one moves down the classification system from family to gene, the structures of the isoenzymes become more similar.

This enzyme system has evolved to form new isoenzymes that metabolize foreign substrates (i.e., drugs) that are presented to the body. These enzymes are structured to recognize and bind to molecular entities on substrates. Many different substrates may have molecular structures that differ only slightly; therefore, an isoenzyme can bind to any one of these substrates. Although several different substrates may compete for the same enzyme receptor, the substrate with the highest affinity binds most often. The converse of this is also true. Two isoenzymes can bind to the same substrate (**Figure 3.1**), but the substrate binds more often to the isoenzyme to which it has the most affinity. However, not every drug molecule ("substrate") can be metabolized by every enzyme with which it binds; therefore, it is not a true substrate. These concepts form the backbone for the drug interactions that are expanded on later.

Five isoenzymes have been determined to be responsible for most metabolism-related drug interactions. They are the isoforms CYP1A2, CYP2C9, CYP2C19, CYP2D6, and CYP3A4. The CYP3A4 isoform is responsible for 40% to 45% of drug metabolism, the CYP2D6 for the next 20% to 30%, CYP2C9 about 10%, and CYP1A2 responsible for about 5% (Ingelman-Sundberg, 2004). The remaining 5% to 20% is accounted for by several lesser important isoforms. Because there are so few enzymes that transform a multitude of substrates, it is easy to see how there would be a great potential for interactions.

There are some genetic variations with respect to the distribution of the enzymes. For example, about 10% of Europeans lack the CYP2D6 enzyme and are therefore considered poor metabolizers of drugs using this pathway for biotransformation. These individuals are at greater risk for

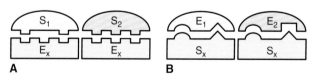

FIGURE 3–1 Substrate binding. **A,** Different substrates. Although Enzyme X (E_x) can bind to both Substrate 1 (S_1) and Substrate 2 (S_2), S_2 has greater affinity for E_x than S_1. Therefore, E_x will bind to S_2 most often. **B,** Different enzymes. Although Substrate X (S_x) can bind to both Enzyme 1 (E_1) and Enzyme 2 (E_2), E_1 has a greater affinity for S_x than E_2. Therefore, S_x will bind to E_1 most often.

ADRs related to drugs metabolized by CYP2D6. In addition, prodrugs requiring this enzyme for activation (e.g., codeine, tamoxifen) may be less effective or have no effect. In contrast, about 5% of this population are considered ultrametabolizers, have too rapid metabolism, and may show little to no response related to drugs metabolized by the CYP2D6 pathway (Ingelman-Sundberg, 2004). Similarly, there is variability within the CYP2C19 isoform, with about 14% of Chinese, 2% of Whites, and 4% of Blacks being poor metabolizers (Scott et al., 2011). The effectiveness of certain prodrugs (e.g., clopidogrel) that require metabolic activation by this enzyme system may be reduced (Holmes et al., 2010). For more information on the cytochrome P-450 enzymes, refer to Chapter 7 on Pharmacogenomics.

There has been increasing interest in genetic testing to identify strategies to reduce the risk of ADRs and to optimize therapy for individuals. Pharmacogenomic information has been incorporated into about 10% of labels for drugs approved by the U.S. Food and Drug Administration (FDA) in an effort to identify responders and nonresponders, avoid toxicity, and adjust doses of medications to optimize efficacy and ensure safety (FDA, 2015). In addition, regulatory authorities have recently recommended genetic testing to aid the clinician in determining if an agent is safe and effective in certain individuals (e.g., abacavir) (Highlights of Prescribing Information: Ziagen [abacavir sulfate] Tablets and Oral Solution accessed July 16, 2015). While commercial assays are available for genetic testing, there are some limitations. These are variable turnaround time for the results, and high cost and the reliability and reproducibility of data on the validation of techniques used are limited. Currently, there is limited evidence-based data to develop specific recommendations on the role of genetic testing in routine care (Holmes et al., 2010).

There are two types of metabolic drug interactions: drugs that inhibit the activity of an enzyme and those that induce the activity of the enzyme.

Inhibition

Inhibition of drug metabolism occurs through competitive and noncompetitive inhibition. When two drugs, administered concurrently, are metabolized by the same isoenzyme, they are defined as competitive inhibitors of each other. In essence, they compete for the same binding site on an enzyme to be metabolized.

Noncompetitive inhibition also occurs when both drugs compete for the same binding site, but one drug is metabolized by that isoenzyme and the other drug is not. The best known example of a noncompetitive inhibitor is quinidine. Quinidine is metabolized by the CYP3A4 isoenzyme but can also bind to the CYP2D6 enzyme. Therefore, although quinidine does not compete for metabolism by the CYP2D6 isoenzyme, it does compete for the CYP2D6 isoenzyme–binding site.

In both competitive and noncompetitive inhibition, the drug with the greatest affinity for the isoenzyme receptor is usually the inhibiting drug because it binds in the receptor site, preventing the other drug from being bound and metabolized

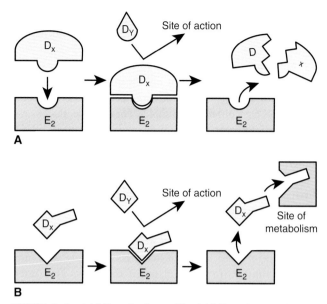

FIGURE 3–2   Inhibition. **A,** Competitive inhibition. Drug X (D_X) and Drug Y (D_Y) are both metabolized by Enzyme 2 (E_2). **B,** Noncompetitive inhibition. Although D_X and D_Y compete for the binding site on E_2, only D_Y is metabolized by E_2. Therefore, D_X noncompetitively inhibits D_Y.

(**Figure 3.2**). The significance of the drug interaction depends on several characteristics of the inhibiting drug.

Affinity.   Many drugs may inhibit the same isoenzyme but not to the same extent. The greater the affinity of an inhibiting drug for an enzyme, the more it blocks binding of other drug molecules.

Half-Life.   Along with affinity, the half-life ($t_{1/2}$) of the inhibiting drug determines the duration of the interaction. The longer the half-life of the inhibiting drug, the longer the drug interaction lasts. For example, after a regimen of ketoconazole ($t_{1/2}$ = 8 hours) is discontinued, its ability to inhibit the CYP3A4 enzyme lasts until it is eliminated, in three to five half-lives or approximately 1 day. However, the inhibiting effect of amiodarone, with a $t_{1/2}$ of approximately 53 days, lasts for weeks to months after its discontinuation.

Concentration.   The third major factor contributing to a drug's ability to inhibit hepatic enzymes is the concentration of the inhibiting drug. A threshold concentration must be reached or exceeded to inhibit an enzyme. This is similar to the threshold concentration discussed in Chapter 2 regarding minimally effective concentrations and therapeutic responses. This minimally effective threshold concentration, or concentration-dependent inhibition, is exhibited by a variety of drugs. The dose yielding this concentration-dependent inhibition varies based on volume of distribution, drug and receptor affinity, and characteristics of the individual patient. An example of a dose- or concentration-dependent inhibitor is cimetidine. In most patients, a dose of 400 mg/d results in only weak enzyme inhibition. However, at higher doses, it interacts significantly with both the CYP2D6 and CYP1A2 isoenzymes (Shinn, 1992).

Some enzyme inhibitors may affect one enzyme at a smaller concentration and more than one isoenzyme at higher concentrations. These enzyme inhibitors demonstrate that some isoenzymes have differing thresholds. For example, fluconazole at a dose of 200 mg/d significantly inhibits only the CYP2C9 isoenzyme, but as the dose increases above 400 mg/d, it also inhibits the CYP3A4 isoenzyme (Hansten & Horn, 2015).

Toxic Potential. Another consideration with regard to inhibition interactions is the toxic potential of the target drug. For example, statins like simvastatin are metabolized by the CYP3A4 isoenzyme. If a potent CYP3A4 inhibitor (e.g., ketoconazole) is administered concurrently with simvastatin, simvastatin accumulates in the body. This interaction could cause myopathy (muscle pain) as well as rare rhabdomyolysis (breakdown of skeletal muscles) leading to kidney damage. It is important to monitor for any signs of new onset muscle pain when patients are initiated on statins (Watkins et al., 2011).

Another example of toxic potential of CYP inhibition is the interaction between warfarin (Coumadin) and trimethoprim-sulfamethoxazole (TMP-SMZ). Warfarin levels are measured using a surrogate marker called international normalized ratio (INR) for therapeutic drug level monitoring on a regular bias. The CYP2C9 enzyme metabolizes warfarin but is inhibited by TMP-SMZ. This inhibition will increase the concentration of warfarin and put patients at an increased risk of bleeding due to a supratherapeutic INR (Hale & Lesar, 2014).

Efficacy. An additional consideration related to inhibition interactions is the effectiveness of the target drug. This is particularly important for prodrugs that require cytochrome P-450 metabolism to the active metabolite in order for the drug to be effective. An example of this is clopidogrel, an antiplatelet agent, which requires CYP2C19 enzymes to be metabolized to the active form. When administered with omeprazole, a CYP2C19 inhibitor, a reduction in plasma concentrations of the active metabolite of clopidogrel as well as reduced platelet function occurs (Clopidogrel [Plavix] prescribing information, 1997). In addition, tamoxifen, an agent used for breast cancer, is converted to its active metabolite by CYP2D6. Women may have a higher risk of breast cancer recurrence if they take tamoxifen in combination with CYP2D6 inhibitors such as the serotonin reuptake inhibitors paroxetine, fluoxetine, or sertraline (The Medical Letter, 2009).

Not all inhibition reactions result in harmful effects; however, some interactions may be inconsequential or even beneficial. For example, ketoconazole (a potent inhibitor of the CYP3A4 isoenzyme) can be given with cyclosporine. The consequent interaction enables practitioners to give less cyclosporine to achieve the same immunosuppressive response (Hansten & Horn, 2015).

The cytochrome P-450 system is complex, but an understanding of the basic concepts of inhibitory interactions leads to the ability to anticipate which agents are likely to interact. The affinity, half-life, and drug concentration determine the potency of the inhibiting drug. A potent enzyme inhibitor inhibits most drugs metabolized by that enzyme. A clinically significant drug interaction also depends on the toxic potential of the drug being inhibited. **Table 3.3** lists several enzymes and their inhibitors, inducers, and substrates.

Induction

Drug–drug interactions can also result from the action of one drug (inducer) stimulating the metabolism of a target drug (substrate). This enhanced metabolism is thought to be produced by an increase in hepatic blood flow or an increase in the formation of hepatic enzymes. This process, known as *enzyme induction*, increases the amount of enzymes available to metabolize drug molecules, thereby decreasing the concentration and pharmacodynamic effect of the target drug.

TABLE 3.3

Key Drug–Drug Interactions with Cytochrome P-450 Enzymes

	CYP3A4	CYP2C19	CYP2C9	CYP1A2	CYP2D6
Inhibitors*	Fluconazole, grapefruit juice, ketoconazole	Omeprazole, ritonavir	Amiodarone, fluconazole, trimethoprim/ sulfamethoxazole	Cimetidine, ciprofloxacin	Cimetidine, paroxetine, quinidine
Substrates	Carbamazepine, oral contraceptives, simvastatin	Clopidogrel, diazepam	Carvedilol, celecoxib, ibuprofen, warfarin	Clozapine, theophylline	Amitriptyline, codeine haloperidol, tamoxifen
Inducers†	Carbamazepine, rifampin, St. John's wort	Phenytoin, rifampin	Phenytoin, rifampin	Phenobarbital, rifampin	No significant inducers

* These will slow down substrate drug metabolism and increase drug effect.

† These will speed up substrate drug metabolism and decrease drug effect.

Some common CYP enzyme inducers are rifampin, phenobarbital, phenytoin, and carbamazepine. Enzyme induction, like enzyme inhibition, is substrate dependent. Therefore, any drug that is a potent inducer of a cytochrome P-450 system increases the metabolism of most drugs metabolized by that enzyme. Also, in a manner similar to that of enzyme inhibitors, inducers may affect more than one cytochrome P-450 isoform; for example, rifampin is a potent inducer of the CYP3A4, CYP1A2, and CYP2C isoforms.

Some enzyme inducers, such as carbamazepine, also increase their own metabolism. Over time, carbamazepine stimulates its own metabolism, thereby decreasing its half-life and frequently resulting in an increased dose requirement to maintain the same therapeutic drug level. This process is termed *autoinduction.*

The onset and duration/cessation of enzyme induction depend on both the half-life of the inducer and the half-life of the isoenzyme that is being stimulated. For example, rifampin ($t_{1/2}$ = 3–4 hours) results in enzyme induction within 24 hours, whereas the enzyme induction capacity of phenobarbital ($t_{1/2}$ = 53–140 hours) is not evident for approximately 7 days. The level of induction remains constant while the drugs are being administered. However, on discontinuation of the respective inducers, the inducing action of rifampin ends more rapidly because of its shorter half-life. This occurs because rifampin is removed from the body at a faster rate than phenobarbital and therefore is not available to inhibit hepatic enzymes for as long.

The initiation and duration of enzyme induction also depend on the half-life of the induced isoenzyme. It takes anywhere from 1 to 6 days for a cytochrome P-450 enzyme to be degraded or produced. Therefore, even if a drug achieves a high enough concentration to produce induction of liver enzymes, the increase in metabolism of a target drug may not be evident until more liver enzymes have formed. The effect of rifampin on warfarin metabolism is a good example of this. Although induction begins within 24 hours of rifampin administration, its effect on warfarin metabolism is not evident for approximately 4 days. On discontinuation of rifampin, the remaining drug is metabolized to negligible levels before the effect on warfarin metabolism dissipates. This occurs because the half-life of the liver enzymes is greater than the half-life of rifampin, and therefore, the enzymes remain to metabolize warfarin after rifampin is eliminated from the body.

These concepts are important to remember when monitoring laboratory values that demonstrate the effectiveness of the target medication. For example, the INR, which is a surrogate marker of warfarin levels, fluctuates significantly within a couple of days of the initiation or discontinuation of rifampin. According to a systematic review by Simmons et al., rifampin's ability to induce CYP3A4 reduces the systemic exposure of combined hormonal oral contraceptives. In theory, this could cause contraceptive failure leading to unwanted pregnancies. However, no studies have evaluated the risk of pregnancy, but the interaction is clinically relevant and warrants attention from the provider (Simmons et al., 2018). **Table 3.3** lists several enzyme inducers/inhibitors and the drugs they affect.

Excretion

Although most drugs are metabolized by the liver, the primary modes of elimination from the body are biliary and renal excretion. Drugs are removed from the bloodstream by the kidneys by filtration or by urinary secretion. However, reabsorption from the urine into the bloodstream may also occur.

Changes in these processes become important when they affect drugs that are unchanged or still active. Excretion of drug molecules can be affected in a number of ways; these include, but are not limited to, acidification or alkalinization of the urine and alteration of secretory or active transport pathways. For example, amphetamine is excreted predominantly via the urine. Thirty percent of the drug can be recovered from the urine after 24 hours of administration. Acidic urine increases while alkaline urine slows down the renal excretion of amphetamine (Jones & Karlsson, 2005). Although they are not discussed here for various reasons, there are a select number of other mechanisms of renal drug interactions.

The ionization state of drug molecules plays a key role in the excretion process. The urine pH determines the ionization state of the excreted molecule. Because lipophilic membranes are less permeable to ionized molecules (hydrophilic), ionized molecules become "trapped" in the urine and are subsequently excreted. Drugs that are nonionized in the urine may be reabsorbed and then recirculated, effectively decreasing their elimination and increasing their half-lives.

Acidic drugs remain in their nonionized state in an acidic urine and become ionized in an alkaline urine. The opposite is true for basic drug molecules, which remain nonionized in an alkaline urine and are ionized in an acidic urine. When a drug is administered that alters the urine pH, it may promote an increased reabsorption or excretion of another drug. For example, the administration of bicarbonate can potentially increase the urine pH. This leads to the increased excretion of acidic drugs (e.g., aspirin) and the increased reabsorption of basic drugs (e.g., pseudoephedrine).

Although most drugs cross the membrane of the renal tubule by simple diffusion, some drugs are also secreted into the urine through active transport pathways. These pathways, however, have a limited capacity and can accommodate only a set amount of drug molecules. Therefore, if two different drugs using the same pathway are coadministered, the transport pathway may become saturated. This causes a "traffic jam" and the excretion of one or both of the drugs is inhibited.

These interactions can be beneficial or detrimental, depending on the agents that are administered. For example, when probenecid and penicillin are given together, they compete for secretion through an organic acid pathway in the renal tubule. The probenecid blocks the secretion of the penicillin, thereby increasing the therapeutic concentration of penicillin in the bloodstream. This is a prime example of drug

TABLE 3.4

Drugs Affecting Excretion

Renal Elimination	Mechanism	Target Drug	Results
Acetazolamide	Increases urine pH	Salicylates	Increased elimination
Losartan	Unknown	Lithium	Decreased elimination
Salicylates	Unknown	Acetazolamide	Decreased elimination
Cetazolamide	Increases urine pH	Quinidine	Decreased elimination
Triamterene	Unknown	Amantadine	Decreased elimination
Amiodarone	Unknown	Digoxin	Decreased elimination
	Unknown	Procainamide	Decreased renal and hepatic elimination
Antacids	Increase urine pH	Dextroamphetamine, quinidine, pseudoephedrine	Decreased elimination
Diuretics	Inhibit sodium reabsorption with subsequent renal tubular reabsorption of lithium	Lithium	Decreased elimination
Salicylates	Inhibit renal tubular secretion of methotrexate	Methotrexate	Decreased elimination

interactions benefiting the patient. In contrast, digoxin and verapamil also share an active transport pathway. When they are administered concomitantly, their interaction leads to an increase in digoxin levels resulting in potential cardiotoxicity (e.g., arrhythmia). **Table 3.4** lists some other clinically important excretion interactions.

The other common pathway of excretion, the biliary tract, allows for the elimination of drugs and their metabolites into the feces. This route of excretion is involved in interactions with drugs that undergo enterohepatic recirculation. Drugs subject to this process are excreted into the GI tract through the biliary ducts and have the potential to be reabsorbed through the intestinal wall into the bloodstream. Some of these drugs depend on enterohepatic recirculation to achieve therapeutic concentrations. An example of a drug class that undergoes enterohepatic recirculation is the oral contraceptive. As previously described, antibiotics can adversely affect reabsorption of the estrogen components of oral contraceptives, potentially rendering them ineffective. In addition, drugs that undergo enterohepatic recirculation may also be affected by binding agents. An example of this is warfarin in combination with the bile acid sequestrants colestipol and cholestyramine. Warfarin undergoes enterohepatic recirculation. Once warfarin has been excreted in the bile, the bile acid sequestrant binds with warfarin, preventing its reabsorption and increasing its clearance, decreasing its efficacy. This has been shown to occur even when warfarin is administered intravenously (Jahnchen et al., 1978). Therefore, it is not only important to administer warfarin 2 hours before or 6 hours after cholestyramine, but consistency in the administration time of these agents is important as well (Mancano, 2005).

Pharmacokinetic interactions make up a large part of the interactions that practitioners must contend with every day.

These interactions are the most studied because they have an objective measurable outcome (e.g., drug concentrations, enzyme concentrations). However, a drug's pharmacodynamic profile must also be considered when it is administered with other agents.

P-Glycoprotein Interactions

Inhibition or induction of P-glycoprotein (P-gp), an energy-dependent efflux transporter, can result in interactions involving absorption or excretion (biliary or renal). P-gp pumps drug molecules out of cells and is found in the epithelial cells of the intestine (enterocytes), liver, and kidney. As a drug passes through the enterocyte in the intestine to be absorbed into the systemic circulation, P-gp can pick up the molecule and carry it back to the intestinal lumen, preventing absorption. P-gp in the liver and kidney acts to increase the excretion of drugs by transporting the molecules into the bile and urine, respectively (Hansten & Horn, 2015).

If P-gp is inhibited, more drugs will be absorbed through the enterocytes. This will result in an increase in plasma concentrations of the target drug. An example of this interaction is when quinidine is administered with digoxin. Quinidine inhibits intestinal P-gp, which results in increased absorption of digoxin. In addition, quinidine inhibition of renal P-gp results in reduced elimination of digoxin by the kidney. The end result is increased concentrations of serum digoxin (Horn & Hansten, 2004).

If P-gp is induced, less drug will be absorbed through the enterocytes. An example of an induction interaction of P-gp is when rifampin is given with digoxin. Rifampin induces intestinal P-gp, resulting in reduced absorption and reduced serum digoxin concentrations (Hansten & Horn, 2015).

TABLE 3.5

Examples of Substrates, Inhibitors, and Inducers of P-Glycoprotein

Substrates	Inhibitors	Inducers
Aldosterone	Amiodarone	Indinavir
Cimetidine	Atorvastatin	Morphine
Colchicine	Clarithromycin	Nelfinavir
Cyclosporine	Cyclosporine	Phenothiazine
Digoxin	Diltiazem	Rifampin
Diltiazem	Erythromycin	Ritonavir
Erythromycin	Felodipine	Saquinavir
Fexofenadine	Indinavir	St. John's wort
Indinavir	Itraconazole	
Itraconazole	Ketoconazole	
Morphine	Methadone	
Nelfinavir	Nelfinavir	
Quinidine	Nicardipine	
Ranitidine	Quinidine	
Saquinavir	Ritonavir	
Tetracycline	Sirolimus	
Verapamil	Tacrolimus	
	Verapamil	

Sources: Data from Horn, J. R., & Hansten, P. D. (2004). Drug interactions with digoxin: The role of P-glycoprotein. *Pharmacy Times* (October). Retrieved from http://www.hanstenandhorn.com/hh-article10-04.pdf; Kim, R. B. (2002). Drugs as P-glycoprotein substrates, inhibitors, and inducers. *Drug Metabolism Reviews, 34*, 47–54.

Table 3.5 provides examples of common substrates, inhibitors, and inducers of P-gp (Hansten & Horn, 2015; Kim, 2002).

Pharmacodynamic Interactions

The responses or effects produced by a drug's actions are referred to as the drug's *pharmacodynamic profile*. Although drugs are administered to elicit a specific response or change in dynamics, an agent usually causes several changes in the body. When one or more drugs are coadministered, the entire pharmacodynamic profile of each drug must be considered because of the potential for each to interact. Drugs that have a similar characteristic in their pharmacodynamic profile may produce an exaggerated response. For example, when a benzodiazepine (e.g., alprazolam) is administered with a muscle relaxant (e.g., cyclobenzaprine), the sedative effects of both drugs combine to produce excessive drowsiness. A less obvious pharmacodynamic interaction occurs with the coadministration of angiotensin-converting enzyme (ACE) inhibitors (e.g., enalapril) and potassium-sparing diuretics (e.g., triamterene). These agents individually can both produce an increase in the potassium (K^+) level. Unless the prescriber is aware of the

pharmacodynamic profile of both drugs, the potential for an excessive increase in the potassium level may go unnoticed and arrhythmia may ensue.

In contrast, drugs may also produce opposing pharmacodynamic effects. This type of interaction may cause the expected drug response to be diminished or even abolished. Unfortunately, these interactions are often overlooked. Instead of the lack of response being interpreted as a pharmacodynamic drug interaction, it is suspected to be due to an ineffective dose or drug. This often leads to an increase in the amount of drug administered and consequent unwanted side effects or interactions. This type of interaction is illustrated by the concomitant administration of an antihypertensive agent (e.g., a diuretic) and a nonsteroidal anti-inflammatory drug (NSAID). Thiazide diuretics produce their hypotensive effects by blocking sodium reabsorption in the distal tubule of the kidney, which leads to increased sodium and water excretion. If NSAIDs are administered concomitantly, the sodium and water retention effects of the NSAIDs may reduce or nullify the hypotensive action of the diuretic.

DRUG–FOOD INTERACTIONS

The interaction between food and drugs can affect both pharmacokinetic and pharmacodynamic parameters. The mechanism of these pharmacokinetic interactions is mediated by alteration of drug bioavailability, distribution, metabolism, or excretion, as seen with drug–drug interactions. The potential for pharmacodynamic drug–food interactions warrants concern about proper diet for patients on certain drugs. Although practicing clinicians often overlook drug–food interactions, these interactions can significantly affect efficacy of drug therapy. Awareness of significant drug–food interactions can reduce the incidence of these effects and optimize drug therapy.

Effect of Food on Drug Pharmacokinetics
Absorption

Food can affect the absorption of drugs in two ways: first, by altering the extent of drug absorption and second, by changing the rate of drug absorption. Usually, changes in the rate of drug absorption have less significance if only the rate of absorption is delayed without affecting bioavailability. The underlying mechanisms that mediate these interactions are highly variable and depend on both the content of food and the properties of the drug involved.

Food can either increase or decrease the amount (extent) of drug absorption, potentially altering the bioavailability of a drug. One mechanism, similar to drug–drug interactions, is adsorption. For example, tetracycline and fluoroquinolone antibiotics (e.g., ciprofloxacin, ofloxacin) can chelate with calcium cations found in milk or milk products, thus significantly limiting the drug's bioavailability.

A second type of drug–food interaction occurs when food serves as a physical barrier and prevents the absorption of orally

BOX 3.1   Drugs to Be Taken on an Empty Stomach

Azithromycin
Captopril
Erythromycin
Fluoroquinolones (e.g., ciprofloxacin, ofloxacin)
Griseofulvin
Isoniazid
Oral penicillins
Sucralfate
Tetracycline
Theophylline, timed release (e.g., Theo-Dur Sprinkle, Theo-24, Uniphyl)
Zidovudine

administered drugs. The absorptive capacity of the small intestine is related to the accessibility of a drug to the GI mucosal surfaces, the site where absorption occurs. When food is coadministered with a drug, access to the mucosa is reduced, resulting in delayed or decreased drug absorption. For example, the bioavailability of azithromycin is reduced by 43% when the drug is taken with food (Zithromax [Pfizer Pharmaceuticals], 2013). Similar types of interactions can be seen when erythromycin, isoniazid, penicillins, and zidovudine are given orally. To avoid such interactions, these drugs can be administered 2 hours apart from mealtime. **Box 3.1** identifies some commonly prescribed drugs that should be taken on an empty stomach. Note, however, if patients cannot tolerate these medications on an empty stomach (because of GI side effects like diarrhea), coadministration with food may be advisable.

In contrast, food can also decrease the absorption of some drugs. For example, phenytoin is known to bind to protein source, heavy metals such as calcium carbonate, and enteral feeding formulas (Sacks, 2004). Doses of phenytoin may have to be increased up to 1,000 mg/d compared to 300 mg/d when it is given without food. To avoid the drug–food interaction, phenytoin doses can be given 1 hour before or 2 hours after eating.

Metabolism

Food can also affect drug metabolism. Grapefruit juice, for example, can affect the metabolism of many drugs. Grapefruit juice specifically inhibits the 3A4 subset of intestinal cytochrome P-450 enzymes and thus increases the serum concentration of drugs dependent on these enzymes for metabolism (Ameer & Weintraub, 1997; Huang et al., 2004).

The extrahepatic cytochrome enzymes are found in highest concentrations in the proximal two thirds of the small intestine. These enzymes are located at the distal portion of the villi that line the small intestine and are responsible for the extrahepatic metabolism of more than 20 drugs (Ameer & Weintraub, 1997; Huang et al., 2004). The component in grapefruit juice that is responsible for this interaction remains undetermined; however, the flavonoid naringin, found in high concentrations in grapefruit juice, is suspected. Increases in the bioavailability of verapamil and dihydropyridine calcium channel blockers such as felodipine, nisoldipine, nitrendipine, nifedipine, and amlodipine have been documented with the coadministration of grapefruit juice (Bailey et al., 1991, 1992, 1993; Rashid et al., 1993). The bioavailability of carbamazepine and midazolam is markedly increased when taken with grapefruit juice (Sacks, 2004). However, unlike verapamil and dihydropyridine calcium channel blockers, diltiazem does not demonstrate an increase in bioavailability with grapefruit juice.

The amount of grapefruit juice required to increase plasma concentrations can vary between agents. A single glass of grapefruit juice can increase the area under the curve and maximum concentration (C_{max}) of felodipine by several fold (Bailey et al., 1998) while the warnings in the product labeling for some hydroxy-methylglutaryl-coenzyme A reductase inhibitors metabolized by CYP3A4 say to avoid quantities >1 quart/day (Zocor, 2015). The extent of the increase in felodipine plasma concentrations is maximal between simultaneous and 4 hours before administration of grapefruit juice. However, higher C_{max} concentrations were evident even when grapefruit juice is consumed 24 hours before felodipine. Therefore, separating doses may reduce but does not eliminate the potential for the interaction (Bailey et al., 1998). Because grapefruit juice appears to inhibit mostly intestinal CYP3A4 and not hepatic CYP3A4 enzymes, the metabolism of drugs administered intravenously is unlikely to be altered. Further, the data suggest that only those agents given at doses higher than usual or if the patients' livers are severely damaged result in the intestinal CYP3A4 as the primary metabolic pathway (Huang et al., 2004). **Box 3.2** identifies some drugs that may interact with grapefruit juice.

BOX 3.2   Drug Concentrations That Increase When Taken with Grapefruit Juice

17-beta-estradiol

Amlodipine
Benzodiazepines
Cyclosporine
Dihydropyridine calcium channel blockers
Felodipine
Lovastatin
Midazolam
Nifedipine
Nisoldipine
Nitrendipine
Simvastatin
Triazolam
Verapamil

In contrast to the ability of grapefruit juice to inhibit drug metabolism, other components of food may induce drug metabolism and therefore decrease drug efficacy. For example, in the treatment of Parkinson's disease, dopamine in the brain needs to be replenished. However, exogenous dopamine does not cross the blood–brain barrier, but its precursor, levodopa, does. Unfortunately, much of the levodopa is lost to metabolism when given orally and only approximately 1% of the administered amount enters the brain to be converted to dopamine (Trovato et al., 1991). Concomitant administration with food containing pyridoxine (or vitamin B_6) can potentially further enhance the peripheral metabolism of levodopa, thus decreasing drug efficacy (Trovato et al., 1991). Patients taking levodopa should therefore be educated about moderate intake of pyridoxine-rich foods, such as avocados, beans, bacon, beef, liver, peas, pork, sweet potatoes, and tuna. Similarly, charcoal-broiled meats can induce the activity of the CYP1A2 isoenzymes, thus increasing the metabolism of drugs such as theophylline.

Excretion

Ingestion of certain fruit juices can alter the urinary pH and affect the elimination and reabsorption of drugs such as quinidine and amphetamine. Orange, tomato, and grapefruit juices are metabolized to an alkaline residue, which can increase the urinary pH. For drugs that are weak bases, making the urine more alkaline by raising the pH increases the proportion of nonionized drug and enhances the reabsorption of the drug systemically. (Recall that the ionization of drugs helps promote water solubility and ultimately enhances drug elimination into the urine.)

Effect of Food on Pharmacodynamics

Food affects the pharmacodynamics of drugs either by opposing or potentiating a drug's pharmacologic action. For example, warfarin exerts its anticoagulant effects by inhibiting synthesis of vitamin K–dependent clotting factors. Vitamin K is required for activation by several protein factors of the clotting cascade, namely, factors II, VII, IX, and X. When foods rich in vitamin K are ingested, they can significantly oppose the anticoagulatory efficacy of warfarin. Leafy green vegetables, such as collard greens, kale, lettuce, spinach, mustard greens, and broccoli, are generally recognized to contain large quantities of vitamin K. Health care providers should educate patients who are taking warfarin about this interaction. More importantly, however, practitioners should stress maintaining a balanced diet without abruptly changing the intake of foods rich in vitamin K.

Another significant drug–food interaction occurs between monoamine oxidase (MAO) inhibitors and foods containing tyramine, an amino acid that is contained in many types of food. Tyramine can precipitate a hypertensive reaction in patients taking MAO inhibitors, such as phenelzine, tranylcypromine, or isocarboxazid. MAOs are enzymes located in the GI tract that inactivate tyramine in food. When patients are taking MAO inhibitors, the breakdown of tyramine is prevented and therefore allows for more tyramine to be

---

BOX 3.3 Foods High in Tyramine

Bean pods
Beer (draft)
Cheese (aged)
Cured meats (i.e., salami, pepperoni, sausage)
Fruits (overripe, such as figs, avocados, prunes, and raisins)
Herring (pickled)
Liver
Sauerkraut
Soy sauce
Wine

---

absorbed systemically. Because of the indirect sympathomimetic property of tyramine, this amino acid provokes the release of norepinephrine from sympathetic nerve endings and epinephrine from the adrenal glands, resulting in an excessive pressor effect. Clinically, patients may complain of diaphoresis, mydriasis, occipital or temporal headache, nuchal rigidity, palpitations, and elevated blood pressure. Examples of foods that contain tyramine are listed in **Box 3.3**.

Effect of Drugs on Food and Nutrients

Many of the aforementioned examples indicate that food can precipitate an interaction with a drug, but in some cases, a reciprocal relationship also holds true. First, some drugs can cause a depletion of nutrients or minerals found in food through various mechanisms. For example, drugs such as cholestyramine and colestipol, which were designed to bind bile acid in the GI tract, could also potentially bind to fat-soluble vitamins (i.e., vitamins A, D, E, and K) and folic acid when taken with food, resulting in the decreased absorption of these vitamins. Orlistat, an over-the-counter and prescription medication used for weight loss, reduces fat absorption. In addition to reducing fat absorption, it can also decrease the absorption of fat-soluble vitamins and beta-carotene. Similarly, the chronic use of mineral oil as a laxative reduces the absorption of fat-soluble vitamins. Careful monitoring of the INR in patients taking warfarin and drugs that affect vitamin K absorption is warranted to avoid changes in bleeding times.

Second, drug-induced malabsorption can occur in patients with preexisting poor nutritional status. For example, long-term use of isoniazid can cause pyridoxine (vitamin B_6) deficiency. Pyridoxine supplementation is recommended for patients who are malnourished or predisposed to neuropathy (e.g., patients with diabetes or alcoholism) when treated with isoniazid. Metformin is associated with vitamin B_{12} deficiency in about 7% of patients, which may lead to anemia. In general, the clinical significance of these interactions may depend on the baseline nutritional status of the patient. Patients with poor nutrition or inadequate dietary intake (e.g., older adult or alcoholic patients) are potentially at greater risk for drug-induced vitamin and mineral depletion.

Third, drugs can change nutrient excretion as well. Both thiazide and loop diuretics can enhance the excretion of potassium, possibly leading to hypokalemia. Digoxin, in the presence of diuretic-induced hypokalemia, can lead to digoxin-induced arrhythmias. Spironolactone, an aldosterone antagonist and potassium-sparing diuretic, can increase potassium levels, especially in the presence of an ACE inhibitor or angiotensin receptor blocker. Loop diuretics can increase urinary excretion of calcium, whereas thiazide diuretics can decrease it. In addition, ascorbic acid and potassium depletion can occur with high doses of long-term aspirin therapy (Trovato et al., 1991). Lithium, a drug used in the treatment of bipolar disorder, depends on renal tubular transport for clearance. Sodium can compete with this process. A diet low in sodium can enhance the renal tubular reabsorption of lithium, which could lead to lithium toxicity (Chan, 2013).

Continuous enteral feeding impairs the dissolution of levothyroxine tablets. The drug could also be bound to the enteral feeding tubes. All of which could lead to further hypothyroidism due to inadequate levothyroxine reaching the systemic circulation.

COMPLEMENTARY ALTERNATIVE MEDICINE INTERACTIONS

In today's society, the search for a "natural way" to treat and prevent diseases has become commonplace. This potentially stems from the misconception that "natural" means "safer." Among

U.S. adults aged 18 years and older, 33.2% of the population has used some form of herbal products in 2012 (Clarke et al., 2015). For the most part, these CAMs are not regulated by the FDA. In many cases, little research has been conducted to assess the efficacy and safety of these agents or the potential for pharmacokinetic or pharmacodynamic interactions. Some clinical trials have been conducted to evaluate the safety and efficacy of certain herbal medications; however, much of available data are based on animal studies, case reports, and the potential for interactions derived from what is known about the chemical characteristics and pharmacokinetic parameters of the herbs.

Pharmacokinetic Interactions
Absorption

As discussed earlier in the chapter, certain agents can interact with other medications in the GI tract to prevent absorption. Likewise, some CAMs can prevent absorption of medications and reduce the effectiveness of those medications. For example, acacia, marketed as a fiber supplement, has been shown to impair the absorption of amoxicillin. This may be secondary to the fiber content of acacia. Doses of acacia and amoxicillin should be separated by 4 hours. Dandelion has a high mineral content and has been shown to reduce the effectiveness of quinolones in animals (Ulbricht et al., 2008). **Table 3.6** summarizes some of the potential CAM interactions that can occur in the absorptive process.

Distribution

Meadowsweet and black willow contain salicylates that have the potential to displace highly protein-bound drugs. To avoid

TABLE 3.6			
Complementary Alternative Medicine Interactions Affecting Absorption			
Complementary Alternative Medication	**Mechanism of Action**	**Target Drug**	**Results**
Acacia	Fiber content may slow or reduce absorption of medications	Amoxicillin	Decreased absorption (separate doses by at least 4 h)
Carob	Decreased bowel transit time	Oral medications	Decreased absorption (separate doses by several hours)
Citrus pectin	Fiber content may slow or reduce absorption of medications	Oral medications	Take 1 h before or 2 h after intake of other oral medications
Dandelion	High mineral content (chelation)	Ciprofloxacin and potentially other medications affected by chelation	Decreased absorption; dandelion and quinolone coadministration should be avoided
Flaxseed	Fiber content may decrease absorption of oral agents	Oral agents/vitamins/minerals	Decreased absorption; oral agents should be taken 1 h before or 2 h after flaxseed
Psyllium	Fiber content may decrease absorption of oral agents	Carbamazepine, digoxin, lithium	Decreased absorption

Source: Adapted data from Ulbricht, C., Chao, W., Costa, D., et al. (2008). Clinical evidence of herb–drug interactions: A systematic review by the Natural Standard Research Collaboration. *Current Drug Metabolism, 9,* 1063–1120.

toxicity, coadministration of these products with highly protein-bound drugs with a narrow therapeutic index, such as warfarin and carbamazepine, should be avoided.

Metabolism

Certain CAMs can be inducers or inhibitors of the cytochrome P-450 enzyme system. St. John's wort, an herbal medication often used to treat depression, has consistently been shown to induce CYP3A4, CYP2E1, and CYP2C19. In addition, St. John's wort induces intestinal P-gp and has been shown to lower plasma concentrations of common P-gp substrates such as digoxin and fexofenadine. Induction of these enzymes is secondary to hyperforin, an ingredient in St. John's wort. St. John's wort has been shown to clinically interact with a number of drugs, including immunosuppressants, hypoglycemics,

anti-inflammatory agents, antimicrobial agents, antimigraine medications, oral contraceptives, cardiovascular agents, and antiretroviral and anticancer drugs as well as drugs affecting the central nervous, GI, and respiratory systems (Izzo & Ernst, 2009).

In contrast, kava, used as an anxiolytic, and garlic, used to treat dyslipidemia, have both been shown in pharmacokinetic studies to inhibit the cytochrome P-450 enzyme system, specifically CYP2E1 (Izzo & Ernst, 2009). **Table 3.7** shows some common CAM interactions affecting metabolism.

Pharmacodynamic Interactions

CAMs may contain ingredients that potentiate the pharmacodynamic effects of certain medications, which may lead to adverse effects. The causative mechanism of these effects may not be well understood in many cases.

TABLE 3.7
Complementary Alternative Medicine Metabolism Interactions

Complementary Alternative Medication	Mechanism of Action	Target Drug	Results
Garlic	Inhibitor of CYP2E1	Chlorzoxazone	Increased chlorzoxazone levels and potentially other 2E1 substrates
Ginkgo	Inducer of CYP2C19	Antiseizure medications, omeprazole	Decreased levels of valproic acid, phenytoin, and omeprazole possible
Goldenseal (berberine)	Inhibitor of CYP3A4	Cyclosporine	Increase in cyclosporine levels
Kava	Inhibitor of CYP2E1	Chlorzoxazone	Increased chlorzoxazone levels and potentially other 2E1 substrates
Licorice	Inhibitor or inducer of CYP3A4	CYP3A4 substrates	Potential increase or decrease in CYP3A4 substrate levels
Red yeast rice	CYP3A4 inhibitors can increase plasma concentrations of monacolin K	Monacolin K	Increased plasma concentrations of monacolin K can result in muscle toxicity
Scotch broom	Haloperidol (CYP2D6 inhibitor) has been shown to increase levels of sparteine	Sparteine	Increased levels of sparteine, which may be potentially cardiotoxic
St. John's wort	Inducer of CYP3A4	Alprazolam, amitriptyline, atorvastatin, erythromycin, imatinib, indinavir, irinotecan, ivabradine, methadone, midazolam, nevirapine, nifedipine, oral contraceptives, quazepam, simvastatin, tacrolimus, verapamil, warfarin	May result in decreased efficacy and/or effectiveness of the target drugs listed
	Inducer of CYP2C19	Omeprazole	Decreased levels of omeprazole possible
	Inducer of CYP2E1	Chlorzoxazone	Decreased chlorzoxazone levels and potentially other 2E1 substrates

Sources: Adapted data from Ulbricht, C., Chao, W., Costa, D., et al. (2008). Clinical evidence of herb–drug interactions: A systematic review by the Natural Standard Research Collaboration. *Current Drug Metabolism, 9,* 1063–1120; Izzo, A. A., & Ernst, E. (2009). Interactions between herbal medicines and prescribed drugs: An updated systematic review. *Drugs, 69,* 1777–1798.

Borage seed oil
Clove
Danshen
Devil's claw
Dong quai
Feverfew
Garlic
Ginger
Ginkgo
Ginseng
Goji
Omega-3 fatty acids
Papaya
Peony
Policosanol
Pycnogenol
Saw palmetto
Turmeric

Source: Adapted data from Ulbricht, C., Chao, W., Costa, D., et al. (2008a). Clinical evidence of herb–drug interactions: A systematic review by the Natural Standard Research Collaboration. *Current Drug Metabolism, 9,* 1063–1120.

Several herbal medications have been shown to inhibit platelet activity and/or have an effect on increasing the INR. Case reports of increased bleeding in patients taking certain CAMs with nonsteroidal anti-inflammatory agents, antiplatelet agents, and anticoagulants have been reported (Ulbricht et al., 2008). **Box 3.4** shows CAMs that may increase the potential for bleeding when given concomitantly with medications that inhibit platelets or alter coagulation.

Some CAMs have been shown to potentiate the central nervous system (CNS) depressant effects of some medications. Kava, lavender, and valerian may potentiate the effects of CNS depressants, such as barbiturates, benzodiazepines, and narcotics. In addition, kava may interfere with the effects of dopamine or dopamine antagonists and it is potentially hepatotoxic (Kuhn, 2002; Ulbricht et al., 2008).

Aloe has been associated with hypoglycemia in patients taking glibenclamide (glyburide). Bitter orange contains MAO inhibitor substrates such as tyramine and octopamine, and concomitant use with an MAO inhibitor may increase the potential for hypertensive effects (Ulbricht et al., 2008).

While many patients may believe CAMs are safe because they are "natural" and are available over the counter, the potential for interactions still exists. Clinicians must be aware of the potential for these interactions and encourage patients to disclose all medications they are taking, including CAMs.

DRUG–DISEASE INTERACTIONS

Certain drug–disease interactions can change drug pharmacokinetic and pharmacodynamic parameters, leading to less-than-optimal drug therapeutic outcomes and greater risk of toxicity. In addition, certain drugs can exacerbate a patient's coexisting disease.

Effect of Disease on Pharmacokinetics of Drugs

Absorption

As already discussed, the absorption of drugs may be affected by the presence of other drugs and food in the GI tract. However, drug absorption also depends on the physiologic processes that maintain normal GI function. These processes can include enzyme secretion, acidity, gastric emptying, bile production, and transit time. Thus, any disease that alters the normal physiologic function of the GI system potentially alters drug absorption.

Vitamin B_{12} deficiency is common in patients undergoing stomach surgery. Stomach acid and intrinsic factor play a critical role in the absorption of vitamin B_{12}. Without acid, vitamin B_{12} is not able to be cleaved and released from proteins in food. Vitamin B_{12} and intrinsic factor form a complex and are absorbed in the duodenum. Without intrinsic factor, vitamin B_{12} absorption is impaired (Goldenberg, 2008).

As an example, the gastric-emptying rate can be reduced in patients with duodenal or pyloric ulcers and hypothyroidism. In addition, long-term diabetes can result in diabetic gastroparesis, which delays gastric emptying. This results in later or fluctuating maximal serum concentrations and has been documented with oral hypoglycemic agents. This may become particularly important when a rapid-acting drug is required. However, drugs with longer half-lives may be less likely to be affected (Jing et al., 2009). Another example includes bowel edema and intestinal hypoperfusion from advancing heart failure, which can delay the absorption of diuretics prescribed to control edema (Hunt et al., 2009). Finally, diarrhea, a manifestation of many diseases, can pose a problem for oral absorption of drugs as well as food and nutrients.

Distribution

The distribution of drugs can be affected by certain disease states. Of significance are conditions that change plasma albumin levels and therefore can increase or decrease the concentration of drugs usually bound to albumin. Examples of conditions that may decrease plasma albumin levels include burns, bone fractures, acute infections, inflammatory disease, liver disease, malnutrition, and renal disease. Examples of conditions that may increase plasma albumin levels include benign tumors, gynecologic disorders, myalgia, and surgical procedures.

Metabolism

The metabolism of drugs can often be altered by diseases that affect the functions of the liver, such as cirrhosis. Failure of the liver (the primary organ responsible for drug metabolism) not only impairs drug metabolism but can cause a reduction in albumin synthesis. Therefore, the clinical impact of liver failure includes a strong potential for interactions with drugs. Heart failure is another disease that can cause direct reduction in the ability of the liver to metabolize drugs. In patients with heart failure, however, decreased metabolic capacity of the liver is also caused by a decrease in blood flow to the liver owing to changes in cardiac output.

In some cases, normal liver function is needed to activate a drug rather than to inactivate it. Certain drugs like enalapril are called *prodrugs*, meaning the drug needs to be converted by the liver to its active form (enalaprilat) to achieve maximal therapeutic effect. Therefore, use of a prodrug in patients with liver dysfunction can potentially reduce the efficacy of the drug.

Excretion

Renal function can influence serum drug concentrations because most drugs are eliminated by the kidneys either as unchanged drug or as metabolites. Chronic renal diseases that compromise the function of the kidney to clear drugs can result in drug accumulation. Glomerulonephritis, interstitial nephritis, long-term and uncontrolled diabetes, and hypertension are primary causes of declining renal function. In clinical practice, once the patient's estimated creatinine clearance has declined to <50 mL/min, dose adjustments usually are required for drugs that are primarily renally cleared. For example, drugs such as H_2 receptor antagonists and fluoroquinolone antibiotics commonly require dose adjustments for patients with renal insufficiency. In particular, the drug regimen of older adult patients or those with an elevated serum creatinine level above 1.5 mg/dL should be evaluated to detect any ADRs from possible drug accumulation secondary to declining renal clearance.

Effects of Drugs on Coexisting Disease

Drugs used to treat one medical condition can sometimes exacerbate the status of another comorbid disease. Practitioners, therefore, should be aware of potential drug–disease interactions. This is of particular importance in older individuals who have multiple concomitant diseases and often take multiple medications. Detected rates of drug–disease interactions range from 6% to 30% in older adults (Lindblad et al., 2006). A complete discussion of this topic is beyond the scope of this chapter. However, a consensus statement has been published from a multidisciplinary panel of health care providers whose members specialize in geriatric medicine. The statement identifies several drug–disease interactions that are common in older individuals and are considered to have a deleterious impact on coexisting disease in older individuals. **Table 3.8** lists these common and clinically significant drug–disease interactions in the older adults (American Geriatrics Society, 2012).

TABLE 3.8

Drug–Disease Interactions Common in the Older Adults

Disease/Condition	Drug/Drug Class
Benign prostatic hyperplasia	Anticholinergics
	Tricyclic antidepressants
Chronic renal failure	Nonaspirin NSAIDs
Heart failure (systolic dysfunction)	First-generation calcium channel blockers
Constipation	Anticholinergics
	Opioid analgesics
	Tricyclic antidepressants
Dementia	Anticholinergics
	Barbiturates
	Benzodiazepines
	Tricyclic antidepressants
Diabetes	Corticosteroids
Falls	Antipsychotics (thioridazine/haloperidol)
	Benzodiazepines
	Sedative hypnotics
	Tricyclic antidepressants
Heart block	Digoxin
	Tricyclic antidepressants
Narrow-angle glaucoma	Anticholinergics
Parkinson's disease	Metoclopramide
Peptic ulcer disease	Aspirin
	Nonaspirin NSAIDs
Postural hypotension	Thioridazine
	Tricyclic antidepressants
Seizures	Bupropion
Syncope	Alpha-blockers (e.g., doxazosin, terazosin, methyldopa)

Source: Data from Lindblad, C. I., Hanlon, J. T., Gross, C. R., et al. (2006). Clinically important drug–disease interactions and their prevalence in older adults. *Clinical Therapeutics, 28,* 1133–1143.
NSAID, nonsteroidal anti-inflammatory drug.

PATIENT FACTORS INFLUENCING DRUG INTERACTIONS

The outcomes of drug interactions are highly variable from one person to another. Many patient factors can influence the propensity for an interaction to occur, such as genetics, diseases, environment, smoking, diet/nutrition, and alcohol. An understanding of these factors can help to identify potential sources of drug interactions.

Heredity

As discussed previously, the cytochrome P-450 system can display genetic polymorphism. That is, the variable metabolism of drugs by cytochrome P-450 enzymes from one person to another in the population can be partly explained by genetic differences. For example, approximately 8% of Americans lack the gene to form the isoenzyme CYP2D6 and therefore are at greater risk for toxicity from psychotropic drugs and, potentially, other drugs that are metabolized by these isoenzymes. The metabolism of isoniazid also demonstrates variation among different people; some acetylate isoniazid very rapidly, whereas others acetylate it slowly.

Warfarin is a widely used oral anticoagulant. Its dose depends on age and CYP2C9 genotype. It works by depleting the supply of vitamin K. The formation of vitamin K depends on a protein known as vitamin K epoxide reductase complex subunit 1 gene. Mutations of this particular gene have been associated with a decrease in formation of clotting factors and warfarin resistance (Sconce et al., 2005).

Disease

Another important factor that influences drug interactions is the patient's existing disease state. Any disease affecting liver or kidney function can potentially predispose the patient to drug interactions and ADRs because these organs are primary sites of drug metabolism and elimination, respectively. Significant deterioration in drug metabolism or elimination can lead to increased serum drug concentrations and therefore increase the likelihood for drugs to interact. Consequently, older adult patients and those with a history of liver disease or renal insufficiency should be evaluated for dose adjustments of drugs significantly cleared by the liver and kidneys. For example, enoxaparin is a drug used to treat various clotting disorders. It is renally cleared from the body. Poor kidney function could lead to its accumulation. If the dose is not lowered in these patients, they could be exposed to too much enoxaparin resulting in excessive bleeding (Nutescu et al., 2009).

Environment

Environmental factors, such as dichlorodiphenyltrichloroethane and other pesticides, can increase the activity of liver enzymes, potentially causing an increase in drug metabolism. Although the general significance of the effect of environmental exposure on the clinical outcome of drug therapy has not been well studied, people working in occupations with prolonged exposure to toxins and chemicals should be more closely observed.

Smoking

Studies show that smoking can increase the liver's metabolism of certain drugs, including diazepam, propoxyphene, chlorpromazine, and amitriptyline. For example, the polycyclic aromatic hydrocarbons in cigarettes can induce CYP1A2 metabolism, resulting in decreased theophylline serum concentrations (Schein, 1995).

Nutrition

The nutritional status and dietary intake of the patient can influence the importance of a drug–nutrient interaction. Drugs can deplete valuable vitamins and minerals from food; however, these interactions are often difficult to recognize and may go undetected. Patients with poor baseline nutrition (e.g., alcoholics) may experience more pronounced effects mainly because of underlying nutritional deficiency. Practitioners should be aware of potential drug–nutrient interactions by identifying patients who have poor dietary intake and who concurrently take medications that can deplete vitamins and minerals.

Alcohol Intake

Alcohol can complicate drug therapy on many different levels. Alcohol has a variable effect on drug metabolism depending on acute or chronic intake. Acute alcohol ingestion can inhibit drug metabolism, thus increasing serum drug concentrations; it also can enhance the pharmacodynamic effect of drugs with properties of CNS depression. Patients concurrently taking narcotics, antihistamines, antidepressants, antipsychotics, and muscle relaxants with alcohol are at greatest risk for CNS depression and should be warned of this interaction (Trovato et al., 1991). In addition, acute ingestion of alcohol can increase the potential for hypoglycemia in diabetic patients taking insulin or insulin secretagogues (e.g., sulfonylureas). Metronidazole is an antibiotic used to treat intra-abdominal infections. When taken with alcohol, it inhibits the enzyme, aldehyde dehydrogenase, which is responsible for metabolizing alcohol. This results in an accumulation of the intermediate metabolite, acetaldehyde, causing a disulfiram-like reaction such as facial flushing, headache, nausea and vomiting, weakness, dizziness, blurred vision, confusion, and hypotension.

In contrast, chronic alcohol intake tends to increase the synthesis of drug-metabolizing enzymes, leading to induction. Enzyme induction causes decreases in serum drug levels. Enzyme induction secondary to chronic alcohol use increases conversion of acetaminophen to hepatotoxic metabolites. Chronic use of alcohol in combination with high doses of acetaminophen (often from several sources) above that recommended in the labeling may result in liver damage (Jang & Harris, 2007). In addition, chronic use of alcohol in combination with NSAIDs or aspirin increases the risk of GI bleeding. Long-term abuse of alcohol leads to liver cirrhosis, which ultimately impairs drug metabolism by destruction of functional hepatocytes.

ADVERSE DRUG REACTIONS

An ADR can be defined as an undesirable clinical manifestation that is consequent to and caused by the administration of a particular drug. ADRs are basically drug-induced toxic reactions. The World Health Organization defines an ADR as "a response to a medicine which is noxious and unintended, and which occurs at doses normally used in man" (Nebeker et al., 2004).

There are two general types to consider. The first type of ADR is an exaggeration of the principal pharmacologic action of the drug. The ADR is simply a more pronounced drug response than normal. These reactions usually are dose dependent and predictable. These are often referred to as type A reactions.

In the second type, type B reactions, the ADR is unrelated to the principal pharmacologic action of the drug itself. These reactions are precipitated by the secondary pharmacologic actions of the drug, may be unpredictable, and may or may not be dose dependent. In either type, the ADR can result from overdosage of drug or administration of therapeutic doses to a patient hyperreactive to the drug or as an indirect consequence of the primary action.

ADRs are sometimes referred to as side effects. A side effect is also recognized as an undesirable pharmacologic effect that accompanies the primary drug action and usually occurs within the therapeutic dosing range. ADRs or side effects can have varying levels of intensity. For example, the dry mouth and blurred vision that occur from drugs with anticholinergic properties are considered routine side effects of that class of medication. In contrast, drug-induced liver damage would be an uncommon and severe ADR or side effect not routinely associated with that class of medication. Patients experiencing ADRs or side effects from drugs do not necessarily require discontinuation of therapy; however, proper drug selection emphasizing agents with minimal side effect profiles may help improve patient acceptance of and compliance with the drug.

Medication Errors

Medication errors are also a potential cause of ADRs. These errors could range from switching from one dosage form to another to using foreign drugs. **Table 3.9** lists some potential causes of ADRs. Some drugs may look alike and sound alike. The Institute for Safe Medication Practices (2015) provides a list of drugs with confused drug names. For example, **Figure 3.3** shows two look-alike vials of drugs were mixed up and a patient inadvertently received phenylephrine instead of metoclopramide. Phenylephrine is a potent blood vessel vasoconstrictor often used to manage hypotension. Metoclopramide is a drug often used to treat nausea and vomiting. The event can lead to pulmonary edema and cardiac arrest.

Tracking Drug Interactions and Adverse Drug Reactions

The initial source of documented ADRs comes primarily from the experience gained while using a drug during clinical trials. Usually, the number of people taking the drug in clinical trials, on the order of hundreds to several thousands, is too few to detect all the possible adverse reactions from the drug. However, after a drug is approved by the FDA, it becomes readily available for public use in hundreds of thousands to millions of people. The potential for drug interactions and ADRs then becomes much greater than during clinical trials.

TABLE 3.9

Potential Causes of Medication Errors

Potential Causes of Medication Errors	Example
Dosage conversion	When converting from oral to IV medications and vice versa, it is often not a 1 to 1 conversion. Levothyroxine 100 mcg oral dose is equal to ~50 mcg IV dose.
Foreign drugs	Dilacor is the brand-name drug for diltiazem in the United States. In Serbia, it is the brand-name drug for digoxin.
Illegible handwriting	Isordil was mistakenly filled with Plendil.
Look alike and sound alike	Phenylephrine vial mistaken for metoclopramide vial.
Unacceptable abbreviations	Insulin 5.0 units was mistaken for 50 units.

IV, intravenous.

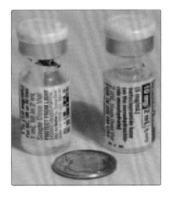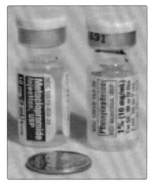

FIGURE 3–3   Look-alike drugs: Phenylephrine vial was mistaken for a metoclopramide vial.

Therefore, practitioners should have a basic understanding of drug interactions and ADRs and report these events to the FDA when they occur.

MedWatch is a medical product reporting program conducted by the FDA (**Figure 3.4**). The three ways to submit a MedWatch report are by phone (1-800-FDA-1088), by fax (1-800-FDA-0178), or online at www.fda.gov/medwatch/report.htm. The purpose of the MedWatch program is to enhance the effectiveness of surveillance of drugs and medical products after they are marketed and as they are used in clinical practice. The benefit to health care providers for reporting drug interactions and ADRs is to ensure that drug safety information is rapidly communicated to health care professionals, thus improving patient care. Health care providers should also be aware of programs in their own institutions that collect and report ADRs or drug interactions.

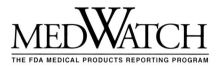

THE FDA MEDICAL PRODUCTS REPORTING PROGRAM

For **VOLUNTARY** reporting
by health professional of adverse
events and product problems

Page ____ of ____

Form Approved OMB No. 0910-0291 Expires: 12/31/94
See OMB statement on reverse
FDA Use Only **(DAVIS)**

Triage unit
sequence #

PLEASE TYPE OR USE BLACK INK

A. Patient information

1. Patient identifier

In confidence

2. Age at time of event:
or ____
Date of birth

3. Sex
☐ female
☐ male

4. Weight
____ lbs
or
____ kgs

B. Adverse event or product problem

1. ☐ **Adverse event** and/or ☐ **Product problem** (e.g., defects/malfunctions)

2. Outcomes attributed to adverse event
(check all that apply)

☐ death ____
(mo day yr)
☐ life-threatening
☐ hospitalization - initial or prolonged

☐ disability
☐ congenital anomaly
☐ required intervention to prevent
permanent impairment/damage
☐ other: ____

3. Date of event
(mo day yr)

4. Date of this report
(mo day yr)

5. Describe event or problem

6. Relevant tests/laboratory data, including dates

7. Other relevant history, including preexisting medical conditions (e.g., allergies, race, pregnancy, smoking and alcohol use, hepatic/renal dysfunction, etc.)

C. Suspect medications(s)

1. Name (give labeled strength & mfr/labeler, if known)
#1
#2

2. Dose, frequency & route used
#1
#2

3. Therapy dates (if unknown. give duration)
from to (or best estimate)
#1
#2

4. Diagnosis for use (indication)
#1
#2

5. Event abated after use stopped or dose reduced
#1 ☐ yes ☐ no ☐ doesn't apply
#2 ☐ yes ☐ no ☐ doesn't apply

6. Lot # (if known)
#1
#2

7. Exp. date (if known)
#1
#2

8. Event reappeared after reintroduction
#1 ☐ yes ☐ no ☐ doesn't apply
#2 ☐ yes ☐ no ☐ doesn't apply

9. NDC # (for product problems only)

10. Concomitant medical products and therapy dates (exclude treatment of event)

D. Suspect medical device

1. Brand name

2. Type of device

3. Manufacturer name & address

4. Operator of device
☐ health professional
☐ lay user/patient
☐ other: ____

5. Expiration date
(mo day yr)

6.
model # ____
catalog # ____
serial # ____
lot # ____
other # ____

7. If implanted, give date
(mo day yr)

8. If explanted, give date
(mo day yr)

9. Device available for evaluation? (Do not send to FDA)
☐ yes ☐ no ☐ returned to manufacturer on ____
(mo day yr)

10. Concomitant medical products and therapy dates (exclude treatment of event)

E. Reporter (see confidentiality section on back)

1. Name, address & phone #

2. Health professional?
☐ yes ☐ no

3. Occupation

4. Also reported to
☐ manufacturer
☐ user facility
☐ distributor

5. If you do NOT want your identity disclosed to the manufacturer, place an "X" in this box. ☐

FDA

Mail to: MEDWATCH
5600 Fishers Lane
Rockville, MD 20852-9787

or FAX to :
1-800-FDA-0178

FDA Form 3500 (6/93)   Submission of a report does not constitute an admission that medical personnel or the product caused or contributed to the event.

FIGURE 3–4 MedWatch form for reporting an adverse event or product problem to the U.S. FDA. (2/19) "https://www.fda.gov/safety/medical-product-safety-information/medwatch-forms-fda-safety-reporting"

CASE STUDY 1

A.C. is a 60-year-old Caucasian woman with newly diagnosed peptic ulcer disease, generalized anxiety disorder, and iron deficiency anemia. She also has a long history of asthma and depression. She is a strong believer of herbal medicine. She takes St. John's wort for her depression, iron pills for her anemia, and alprazolam (Xanax) as needed for her anxiety. During her asthma exacerbation, she is instructed to take prednisone for at least 5 days. She also takes esomeprazole (Nexium) for her peptic ulcer disease. Three months later, she experienced severe fatigue, shortness of breath, dizziness, and swelling/soreness in the tongue. Her asthma is well controlled with the occasional use of albuterol (Proventil) inhaler. During her physical exam, her physician suspected that she had bacterial vaginosis and gave her a prescription for a 1-week course of metronidazole (Flagyl). She drinks at least two to three cans of beer per day.

DIAGNOSIS: DRUG–DRUG INTERACTIONS

1. St. John's wort is known to inhibit which of her medication that is known to be metabolized by cytochrome P-450 (CYP3A4) and could potentially cause her to experience significant fatigue?
2. Which of her medication could interfere with the absorption of her iron pills?
3. Which of her medication could potentially cause her to develop vitamin B_{12} deficiency?
4. How does metronidazole interfere with alcohol?
5. If she was given a prescription for ketoconazole, which of her medication could interfere with its absorption?

Bibliography

Starred references are cited in the text.

*Ameer, B., & Weintraub, R. A. (1997). Drug interactions with grapefruit juice. *Clinical Pharmacokinetics, 33*(2), 103–121.

*American Geriatrics Society (AGS). (2012). Updated beers criteria for potentially inappropriate medication use in older adults. *Journal of the American Geriatrics Society, 60*(4), 616–631.

*American Society of Health-System Pharmacists. (2008). *AHFS drug information 2008.* (1961, 3062). Bethesda, MD: Author.

*Bailey, D. C., Arnold, J. M. O., Strong, H. A., et al. (1993). Effect of grapefruit juice and naringin on nisoldipine pharmacokinetics. *Clinical Pharmacology and Therapeutics, 54,* 589–594.

*Bailey, D. G., Malcolm, J., Arnold, O., et al. (1998). Grapefruit juice–drug interactions. *British Journal of Clinical Pharmacology, 46,* 101–110.

*Bailey, D. G., Munoz, C., Arnold, J. M. O., et al. (1992). Grapefruit juice and naringin interaction with nitrendipine [Abstract]. *Clinical Pharmacology and Therapeutics, 51,* 156.

*Bailey, D. G., Spence, J. D., Munoz, C., et al. (1991). Interaction of citrus juices with felodipine and nifedipine. *Lancet, 337,* 268–269.

*Becker, M. L., Visser, L. E., van Gelder, T., et al. (2008). Increasing exposure to drug–drug interactions between 1992 and 2005 in people aged ≥55 years. *Drugs and Aging, 25,* 145–152.

*Benard-Laribiere, A., Miremont-Salame, G., & Perault-Pochat, M. (2014). Incidence of hospital admissions due to adverse drug reactions in France: The EMIR study. *Fundamental and Clinical Pharmacology, 29,* 106–111.

*Bjerrum, L., Lopez-Valcarcel, B. G., & Petersen, G. (2008). Risk factors for potential drug interactions in general practice. *European Journal of General Practice, 14,* 23–29.

Braun, L. D. (1997). Therapeutic drug monitoring. In L. Shargel, A. H. Mutnick, P. F. Souney, et al. (Eds.). *Comprehensive pharmacy review* (3rd ed., pp. 586–597). Baltimore, MD: Lippincott Williams & Wilkins.

*Brosen, K. (1990). Recent developments in hepatic drug oxidation: Implications for clinical pharmacokinetics. *Clinical Pharmacokinetics, 18,* 220–239.

*Chan, L. (2013). Drug–nutrient interactions. *Journal of Parenteral and Enteral Nutrition, 37,* 450–459.

*Clarke, T., Black, L. I., Stussman, B. J., et al. (2015). National Health Statistics Report. Trends in the use of complementary health approaches among adults: United States, 2002–2012. *National Health Statistics, 79,* 1–15.

*Clopidogrel (Plavix®) prescribing information. Retrieved from http://products.sanofi-aventis.us/PLAVIX/PLAVIX.html on July 29, 2010.

Cupp, M., & Tracy, T. (1997). Role of the cytochrome P450 3A subfamily in drug interactions. *US Pharmacist, 22,* HS9–HS21.

Deppermann, K. M., & Lode, H. (1993). Fluoroquinolones: Interaction profile during enteral absorption. *Drugs, 45*(Suppl. 3), 65–72.

Drew, R. H., & Gallis, H. A. (1992). Azithromycin—Spectrum of activity, pharmacokinetics, and clinical applications. *Pharmacotherapy, 12,* 161–173.

FDA Drug Safety Communication. (2020). Reduced effectiveness of Plavix (clopidogrel) in patients who are poor metabolizers of the drug. Retrieved from http://www.fda.gov/Drugs/DrugSafety/PostmarketDrugSafetyInformationforPatientsandProviders/ucm203888.htm on July 16, 2015.

*FDA Table of Pharmacogenomic Biomarkers in Drug Labeling. (2020). Retrieved from http://www.fda.gov/Drugs/ScienceResearch/ResearchAreas/Pharmacogenetics/ucm083378.htm on July 16, 2015.

Fraser, A. G. (1997). Pharmacokinetic interactions between alcohol and other drugs. *Clinical Pharmacokinetics, 33*(2), 79–90.

*Goldenberg, L. (2008). Nutritional deficiencies following bariatric surgery. *Gastroenterology and Endoscopy, 65,* 31–37.

*Guengerich, F. (1994). Catalytic selectivity of human cytochrome P450 enzymes: Relevance to drug metabolism and toxicity. *Toxicology Letters, 70,* 133–138.

*Hale, S. F., & Lesar, T. S. (2014). Interaction of vitamin K antagonists and trimethoprim-sulfamethoxazole: Ignore at your patient's risk. *Drug Metabolism and Personalized Therapy, 29*(1), 53–60. doi: 10.1515/dmdi-2013-0049

Hansten, P. D. (1998). Understanding drug–drug interactions. *Science and Medicine,* (January/February), 5, 16–20.

*Hansten, P. D., & Horn, J. R. (2015). *Drug interactions: Top 100 drug interactions: A guide to patient management.* Freeland, WA: H&H Publications.

Harder, S., & Thurmann, P. (1996). Clinically important drug interactions with anticoagulants: An update. *Clinical Pharmacokinetics, 30,* 416–444.

Herb Fact Sheet. (2006). National Toxicology Program. Retrieved from http://ntp.niehs.nih.gov/ntp/Factsheets/HerbalFacts06.pdf on July 24, 2010.

*Highlights of Prescribing Information: Ziagen (abacavir sulfate) Tablets and Oral Solution. Retrieved from http://www.accessdata.fda.gov/drugsatfda_docs/label/2008/020977s019,020978s022lbl.pdf on July 27, 2010.

*Holmes, D. R., Dehmer, G. J., Kaul, S., et al. (2010). ACCF/AHA clopidogrel clinical alert: Approaches to the FDA "Boxed Warning": A report of the American College of Cardiology Foundation Task Force on Clinical Expert Consensus Documents and the American Heart Association. *Journal of the American College of Cardiology, 56,* 321–341.

*Horn, J. R., & Hansten, P. D. (2004). Drug interactions with digoxin: The role of P-glycoprotein. Pharmacy Times (October). Retrieved from http://www.hanstenandhorn.com/hh-article10-04.pdf

*Huang, S. M., Hall, S. D., Watkins, P., et al. (2004). Drug interactions with herbal products and grapefruit juice: A conference report. *Clinical Pharmacology and Therapeutics, 75,* 1–12.

*Hunt, S. A., Abraham, W. T., Chin, M. H., et al. (2009). 2009 focused update incorporated into the ACC/AHA 2005 guidelines for the diagnosis and management of heart failure in adults. *Circulation, 119,* e391–e479.

*Ingelman-Sundberg, M. (2004). Pharmacogenetics of cytochromes P450 and its applications in drug therapy; the past, present and future. *Trends in Pharmacological Sciences, 25*(4), 193–200.

*Institute for Safe Medication Practices (ISMP). (2015). ISMP's list of confused drug names. Retrieved from https://www.ismp.org/tools/confused-drugnames.pdf

*ISMP Quarter Watch. (2014). Adverse drug events in children under age 18. Retrieved from www.ismp.org/quarterwatch

*Izzo, A. A., & Ernst, E. (2009). Interactions between herbal medicines and prescribed drugs: An updated systematic review. *Drugs, 69,* 1777–1798.

*Jahnchen, E., Meinertz, T., Gilfrich, H.-J., et al. (1978). Enhanced elimination of warfarin during treatment with cholestyramine. *British Journal of Clinical Pharmacology, 5,* 437–440.

*Jang, G. R., & Harris, R. Z. (2007). Drug interactions involving ethanol and alcoholic beverages. *Expert Opinion on Drug Metabolism and Toxicology, 3,* 719–731.

*Jing, M., Rayner, C. K., Jones, K. L., et al. (2009). Diabetic gastroparesis diagnosis and management. *Drugs, 69,* 971–986.

Johnson, K. A., Strum, D. P., & Watkins, W. D. (1995). Pharmacology and the critical care patient. In P. L. Munson, R. A. Mueller, & G. R. Breese (Eds.), *Principles of pharmacology: Basic concepts and clinical application* (pp. 1673–1688). New York, NY: Chapman & Hall.

*Jones, A. W., & Karlsson, L. (2005). Relation between blood- and urine amphetamine concentrations in impaired drivers as influenced by urinary pH and creatinine. *Human and Experimental Toxicology, 24,* 615–622.

*Kim, R. B. (2002). Drugs as P-glycoprotein substrates, inhibitors, and inducers. *Drug Metabolism Reviews, 34,* 47–54.

Kirk, J. K. (1995). Significant drug–nutrient interactions. *American Family Physicians, 51*(5), 1175–1182.

Kivisto, K., Neuvonen, P., & Koltz, U. (1994). Inhibition of terfenadine metabolism: Pharmacokinetic and pharmacodynamic consequences. *Clinical Pharmacokinetics, 27,* 1–5.

*Kuhn, M. A. (2002). Herbal remedies: Drug–herb interactions. *Critical Care Nurse, 22,* 22–32.

Lazarou, J., Pomeranz, B., & Corey, P. (1998). Incidence of adverse drug reactions in hospitalized patients: A meta-analysis of prospective studies. *Journal of the American Medical Association, 279,* 1200–1205.

*Lindblad, C. I., Hanlon, J. T., Gross, C. R., et al. (2006). Clinically important drug–disease interactions and their prevalence in older adults. *Clinical Therapeutics, 28,* 1133–1143.

LOKELMA (AstraZeneca Pharmaceuticals). Package insert. (2018).

Lovastatin (Mevacor®) prescribing information. Retrieved from http://www.merck.com/product/usa/pi_circulars/m/mevacor/mevacor_pi.pdf on July 30, 2010.

Lynch, T., & Price, A. (2007). The effect of cytochrome P450 metabolism on drug response, interactions, and adverse effects. *American Family Physician, 76*(1), 391–396.

*Mancano, M. A. (2005). Clinically significant drug interactions with warfarin. *Pharmacy Times.* Retrieved from https://secure.pharmacytimes.com/lessons/200301-01.asp on July 27, 2010.

*Martins, A. C., Giordani, F., & Rozenfeld, S. (2014). Adverse events among adult patient inpatients: A meta-analysis of observational studies. *Journal of Clinical Pharmacy and Therapeutics, 39,* 609–620.

May, R. J. (1993). Adverse drug reactions and interactions. In J. T. DiPiro, R. L. Talbert, P. E. Hayes, et al. (Eds.), *Pharmacotherapy: A pathophysiologic approach* (2nd ed., pp. 71–83). East Norwalk, CT: Appleton & Lange.

*The Medical Letter. (2009). In brief: Tamoxifen and SSRI interactions. *The Medical Letter on Drugs and Therapeutics, 51,* 45.

*Michalets, E. (1998). Update: Clinically significant cytochrome P-450 drug interactions. *Annals of Pharmacotherapy, 18,* 84–112.

*Nebeker, J. R., Barach, P., & Samore, M. H. (2004). Clarifying adverse drug events: A clinician's guide to terminology, documentation, and reporting. *Annals of Internal Medicine, 140,* 795–801.

*Nebert, D., Adesnich, M., Coon, M., et al. (1987). The P450 gene superfamily: Recommended nomenclature. *DNA, 6,* 1–11.

*Nutescu, E., Spinler, S., Wittkowsky, A., et al. (2009). Low-molecular weight heparins in renal impairment and obesity: Available evidence and clinical practice recommendations across medical and surgical settings. *Annals of Pharmacotherapy, 43,* 1064–1083.

Olivier, P., Bertrand, L., Tubery, M., et al. (2009). Hospitalizations because of adverse drug reactions in elderly patients admitted through the emergency department: A prospective survey. *Drugs and Aging, 26,* 475–482.

Pharmacist's Letter. (2008). Alcohol-related drug interactions. *24,* 1–11.

Plaa, G. L., & Smith, R. P. (1995). General principles of toxicology. In P. L. Munson, R. A. Mueller, & G. R. Breese (Eds.), *Principles of pharmacology: Basic concepts and clinical application* (pp. 1537–1543). New York, NY: Chapman & Hall.

*Rashid, J., McKinstry, C., Renwick, A. G., et al. (1993). Quercetin, an in vitro inhibitor of CYP3A, does not contribute to the interaction between nifedipine and grapefruit juice. *British Journal of Clinical Pharmacology, 36,* 460–463.

*Sacks, G. (2004). Drug–nutrient considerations in patients receiving parenteral and enteral nutrition. *Practical Gastroenterology, 39,* 39–48.

*Schein, J. R. (1995). Cigarette smoking and clinically significant drug interactions. *Annals of Pharmacotherapy, 29,* 1139–1147.

*Sconce, E. A., Khan, T. I., Wynne, H. A., et al. (2005). The impact of CYP2C9 and VKORC1 genetic polymorphism and patient characteristics upon warfarin dose requirements: Proposal for a new dosing regimen. *Blood, 106*(7), 2329–2333.

*Scott, S. A., Sangkuhl, K., Gardner, E., et al. (2011). Clinical pharmacogenetics implementation consortium guidelines for cytochrome P450-2C19 genotype and clopidogrel therapy. *Clinical Pharmacology and Therapeutics, 90*(2), 328–332.

Shargel, L., & Yu, A. B. C. (1993). *Applied biopharmaceutics and pharmacokinetics* (3rd ed.). East Norwalk, CT: Appleton & Lange.

*Shinn, A. F. (1992). Clinical relevance of cimetidine drug interactions. *Drug Safety, 7,* 245–267.

*Simmons, K. B., Haddad, L. B., Nanda, K., & Curtis, K. M. (2018). Drug interactions between rifamycin antibiotics and hormonal contraception: A systematic review. *BJOG: An International Journal of Obstetrics & Gynaecology, 125*(7), 804–811. doi: 10.111/1471-0528.15027

Simvastatin (Zocor®) prescribing information. Retrieved from http://www.merck.com/product/usa/pi_circulars/z/zocor/zocor_pi.pdf on July 29, 2010.

Spinler, S., Cheng, J., Kindwall, K., et al. (1995). Possible inhibition of hepatic metabolism of quinidine by erythromycin. *Clinical Pharmacology and Therapeutics, 57,* 89–94.

*Sultana, J., Cutroneo, P., & Trifiro, G. (2013). Clinical and economic burden of adverse drug reactions. *Journal of Pharmacology and Pharmacotherapeutics, 4*(Suppl.), S73–S77.

*Susla, G. M. (2005). Miscellaneous antibiotics. In S. C. Piscitelli & K. A. Rodvold (Eds.), *Drug interactions in infectious diseases* (2nd ed., pp. 358–359). Totowa, NJ: Humana Press, Inc.

Tegretol (carbamazepine USP) Label. Retrieved from http://www.accessdata. fda.gov/drugsatfda_docs/label/2009/016608s101,018281s048lbl.pdf on July 27, 2010.

*Toh, S., Mitchell, A., Anderka, M., et al. (2011). Antibiotics and oral contraceptive failure: A case-crossover study. *Contraception*, *83*(5), 418–425.

*Trovato, A., Nuhlicek, D. N., & Midtling, J. E. (1991). Drug–nutrient interactions. *American Family Practitioner*, *44*, 1651–1658.

*Ulbricht, C., Chao, W., Costa, D., et al. (2008). Clinical evidence of herb–drug interactions: A systematic review by the Natural Standard Research Collaboration. *Current Drug Metabolism*, *9*, 1063–1120.

VELTASSA (Relypsa, Inc). (2015). Package insert. Glattbrugg, Switzerland.

*Watkins, J. L., Atkinson, B. J., & Pagliaro, L. C. (2011). Rhabdomyolysis in a prostate cancer patient taking ketoconazole and simvastatin: Case report and review of the literature. *Annals of Pharmacotherapy*, *45*(2), e9. doi: 10.1345/aph.1P433

*Weaver, K., & Glasier, A. (1999). Interaction between broad-spectrum antibiotics and the combined oral contraceptive pill: A literature review. *Contraception*, *59*, 71–78.

Zhang, F., Xue, J., Shao, J., & Jia, L. (2012). Compilation of 222 drugs' plasma protein binding data and guidance for study designs. *Drug Discovery Today*, *17*(9–10), 475–485. doi: 10.1016/j.drudis.2011.12.018

*Zithromax (Pfizer Pharmaceuticals). (2013). Package insert. New York, NY.

*Zocor (Merck & Co.). (2015). Package insert.

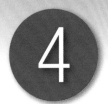

4 Principles of Pharmacotherapy in Pediatrics, Pregnancy, and Lactation

Pooja Shah and Anita Siu

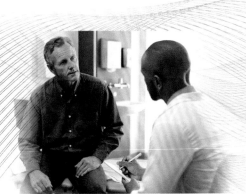
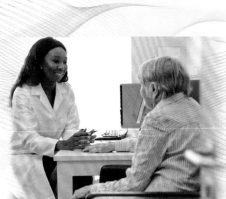
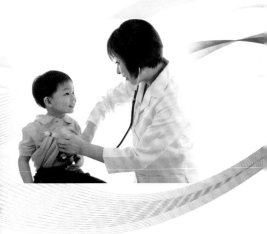

Learning Objectives

1. Describe the differences in pharmacokinetics among pregnant women, neonates, children, and adults.
2. Describe the unique challenges neonatal and pediatric patients pose to the medication system, including drug selection and dosages.
3. Explain the potential and strategies for the prevention of medication errors in neonatal and pediatric patients.
4. Identify strategies to determine safe medication use in pregnancy based on available literature.
5. Determine the drug-related factors that would help guide safe and effective medication use in breast-feeding women.

INTRODUCTION

Medication use in pediatric and pregnant patients poses a significant challenge for health care providers due to our lack of knowledge of the effects of medication on the fetus and pediatric population. Accepted terms that define the different age categories of pediatric patients are listed in **Table 4.1**. These terms should be used to ensure accuracy when describing young patients and especially when determining drug dosages. Additionally, 90% of women will use one medication during pregnancy, and about 70% will use one or more prescription medications (Mitchell et al., 2011). The rate of use of over-the-counter medications and illicit substances also continues to pose a significant challenge to understanding the risks and benefits of medication use in pregnant women and fetuses. As in the case of pediatric patients, the practitioner needs a solid

understanding of the physiologic changes that occur during pregnancy and the effects that these changes have on medication efficacy and safety. The practitioner must also balance the need to treat the mother against the potential risk of these medications to the fetus (Briggs et al., 2017).

Safe and effective drug therapy in pediatric and pregnant patients is based on a firm understanding of four concepts:

- Extent of a drug's absorption, distribution, metabolism, and excretion based on the ongoing maturation and development in pediatric patients or the altered physiologic changes in the mother. Interpatient variabilities may be attributed to physiologic changes throughout childhood or pregnancy.
- Short- and long-term effects that the prescribed drug will have on a pediatric patient's growth and development.
- The placental–fetal unit, which affects the amount of drug that crosses the placental membrane, the amount of drug metabolized by the placenta, and the distribution and elimination of the drug by the fetus.
- Effects of underlying congenital, chronic, or current diseases on the prescribed drug and vice versa.

The popular concept that the pediatric patient is merely a "little or small adult" and therefore pediatric pharmacokinetics, drug dosing, and even adverse effects can be extrapolated from the results of adult clinical drug trials is a serious misconception. Although the effects of many drugs are similar between the adult and the pediatric populations, the assumption of similarity should not be applied to all drugs. Several tragic drug misadventures in the 1960s and 1970s illustrate the invalidity of such an assumption. Extrapolated data from adult responses to chloramphenicol (Chloromycetin) led to its use in neonates in the 1960s. When given chloramphenicol, these neonates developed gray baby syndrome, hypotension,

TABLE 4.1

Age Groups of Pediatric Population

Group	Age
Preterm or premature	<36 wk gestational age
Neonate	<30 d old
Infant	Age 1 mo until 1 y
Child	Age 1 until 12 y
Adolescent	Age 12 until 18 y

and hypoxemia, leading eventually to shock and death (Haile, 1977). This occurred because neonates, unlike adults, lack the enzyme needed to metabolize chloramphenicol. Another tragedy, in the 1970s, involved the topical antimicrobial cleanser hexachlorophene. Used routinely and safely in adults, hexachlorophene caused vacuolar encephalopathy of the brain stem in premature neonates after they were repeatedly bathed in a 3% solution (Anonymous, 1972).

Pharmaceutical manufacturers face several barriers to conducting pediatric clinical trials, such as fears of unforeseen adverse events affecting growth or development or difficulties in obtaining informed consent or blood samples. In turn, the lack of clinical trials in pediatric patients prevents the U.S. Food and Drug Administration (FDA) from approving drugs for use in the pediatric population. As such, the prescribing information commonly states, "Pediatric use: Safety and effectiveness in pediatric patients has not been established."

Without FDA approval or adequate documented information, many practitioners are uncertain about the use of drugs in pediatric patients. This leaves prescribers little choice but to use drugs in pediatric patients in an off-label capacity, based on adult data, uncontrolled pediatric studies, or personal experience. In 1997, the FDA took the initiative to increase the quantity and quality of clinical drug trials in the pediatric population by proposing alternate ways to obtain FDA approval. The FDA waived the need for well-controlled clinical drug trials if drug manufacturers provided other satisfactory data for drugs already approved for the same use in adults. These data could include the results of controlled or uncontrolled pediatric studies, pharmacodynamic studies, safety reports, and premarketing or postmarketing studies. Alternatively, the drug manufacturer could provide evidence demonstrating that the disease course and drug effects are sufficiently similar in adult and pediatric patients in order to support extrapolation of data from adult clinical trials. In addition, pediatric pharmacokinetic studies are necessary to provide data for an appropriate pediatric dosage recommendation, especially age-dependent dosing. An FDA regulation issued in December 1998 required manufacturers to provide additional information about the use of their drug products in pediatric patients. The nature of the studies required to support pediatric labeling depends on the type of application, the condition being treated, and existing data about the product's safety and efficacy in pediatric patients.

Manufacturers are required to study the drug in all relevant pediatric age groups (U.S. Food and Drug Administration, 1998a). Over the years, the FDA has encouraged more well-controlled trials on drug efficacy and safety in pediatrics. The Food and Drug Administration Modernization Act of 1997 and the Best Pharmaceuticals for Children Act of 2002 offered support for the pharmaceutical industries to conduct and submit pediatric clinical trials. Companies that conduct appropriate clinical trials are eligible to receive a 6-month patent extension on their product. The Pediatric Research Equity Act of 2003 mandated that drugs used in pediatrics require literature or clinical trials supporting their use, even if the original patent did not have a pediatric indication. As a result, pediatric pharmacotherapy will evolve with additional clinical trials.

PHARMACOKINETICS IN PEDIATRICS AND PREGNANCY

Women undergo many physiologic changes during pregnancy, whereas pediatric patients differ from adults, anatomically and physiologically. For safe use of drugs in pediatrics and pregnancy, prescribers and other caregivers need to recognize the potential for very different pharmacokinetics as opposed to that for adults or nonpregnant women. In pediatrics, the differences are based on developing body tissues and organs, which affect a drug's absorption, distribution, metabolism, and excretion. In pregnancy, the differences are based on cardiovascular, gastrointestinal (GI), kidney, and hormonal changes (Pinheiro & Stika, 2020).

Changes in a pediatric patient's body proportions and composition and the relative size of the liver and kidneys can alter the pharmacokinetics of a drug. During the first several years of life, a child undergoes rapid changes in growth and development, which is most rapid during infancy. Growth is a quantitative change in the size of the body or any of its parts, and development is a qualitative change in skills or functions. Maturation, a genetically controlled development independent of the environment, is a slower process, lasting until late childhood. **Table 4.2** summarizes pharmacokinetic differences in pediatric and pregnant populations compared to adults and nonpregnant women.

By the end of the first year of life, an infant's weight triples, whereas body surface area (BSA) and length double. Accompanying these changes in growth and development are changes in body composition, intracellular and extracellular body water, fat, and protein. Approximately 75% to 80% of a full-term neonate's body weight is total body water (Friis-Hansen, 1957). By age 3 months, total body water constitutes approximately 65% of the infant's body weight. Extracellular water progressively declines and intracellular water increases faster than total body water does, exceeding extracellular water content (Friis-Hansen, 1957). The decrease in total body water as a percentage of body weight is compensated for by increased body fat during the first 5 months of life. In fact, the percentage of body weight from fat doubles in these 5 months. The protein percentage increases during the second year of life as fat is lost, primarily because of ambulation. The liver and kidney reach their maximum size

TABLE 4.2

Age- and Pregnancy-Related Pharmacokinetic Differences in Children and Women Compared with Nonpregnant Adults

	Premature Neonate	Neonate	Infant	Child	Adolescent	Pregnancy
Absorption						
Gastric acidity	↓	↓	↓	=	=	↑
Gastric emptying time	↓	↓	=	=	=	↑
GI motility	↓	↓	↓	=	=	↓
Pancreatic enzyme activity	↓↓	↓	↓	=	=	=
GI surface area	↑	↑	↑	↑	=	=
Skin permeability	↑↑	↑	=	=	=	↑
Distribution						
Blood–brain barrier	↓	↓	=	=	=	=
Plasma proteins	↓↓	↓	=	=	=	↓
Metabolism						
Liver	↓	↓	↓	=/↑	=	=/↑
Elimination						
Renal blood flow	↓	↓	↓	=	=	↑
Glomerular filtration	↓	↓	↓	=	=	↑
Tubular function	↓	↓	↓	=	=	=

GI, gastrointestinal.

relative to body weight by age 2, producing a "peak" in the child's metabolism and elimination. After age 2, the ratio of the child's liver and kidney size to body weight steadily decreases until adult liver and kidney ratios are reached by adolescence.

Oral Absorption

The extent of a drug's absorption during pregnancy may be altered and in pediatric patients can depend on a variety of factors: gastric pH, gastric and intestinal transit time, GI surface area, enzymes, microorganism flora, or any combination thereof.

Gastric pH

Basal and stimulated secretion of gastric acid controls the pH of the stomach. Pregnant women experience a reduction in gastric acid secretions (up to 40% less than in nonpregnant women) as well as an increase in gastric mucus secretion. Together, this may lead to an increase in gastric pH and a decrease in the absorption of medications that need an acidic pH for appropriate absorption.

The stomach pH is alkaline at birth (greater than 4) because of residual amniotic fluid and the immaturity of parietal cells. As gastric acid is produced, the pH falls. By the end of the first day of life, the basal and stimulated rates are equal, although lower than the rates in adults. An increased stomach pH (alkaline) adversely affects the absorption of weakly acidic drugs and improves the absorption of weakly basic drugs. This phenomenon results from increased ionization of the weakly acidic drug, producing more ionized (polar) drug, which moves poorly across the nonpolar gastric membrane, and vice versa for weakly basic drug. For example, the bioavailability of phenobarbital (a weak acid) is decreased in neonates, infants, and young children because their alkaline gastric pH produces more ionized phenobarbital, which crosses the gastric membrane poorly.

For weakly basic drugs, the alkaline stomach pH increases the nonionized form of the drug, which then easily moves across the gastric membrane. By the second year of life, the child's gastric acid output on a per kilogram body weight basis is similar to that observed in the adult (Deren, 1971). As a result, gastric pH affects the degree of drug ionization, thus changing the amount of drug absorbed.

Gastric Emptying Time and Surface Area

Pregnancy-induced maternal physiologic changes may affect GI function, and therefore, the oral absorption of some drugs may be altered. Of the many factors that can affect GI absorption of drugs, one is the decrease in GI tract motility, especially during labor. It is believed that an increase in plasma progesterone levels causes this decrease in motility, which may delay the absorption of orally administered drugs. Another reason for decreased GI absorption may be the nausea and vomiting associated with increased progesterone levels that are common during the first trimester of pregnancy. Therefore, pregnant women may be advised to take their medications at times when nausea is minimal.

Similarly, the gastric emptying time is delayed in both preterm and full-term neonates during the first 24 hours of life. No studies have been conducted beyond the immediate neonatal period. The combination of delayed gastric emptying time and gastroesophageal reflux can result in the regurgitation of orally administered drugs, producing irregular drug absorption. In general, gastric emptying is more prolonged in neonates and infants than in children.

The characteristics of a drug's movement through the intestines can drastically affect the rate and extent of drug absorption because most drugs are absorbed in the duodenum. Both neonates and infants have irregular peristalsis, which can lead to enhanced absorption. In addition, the type of feeding an infant receives can affect intestinal transit time. For instance, the gastric emptying time in breast-fed infants is faster than in formula-fed infants (Cavell, 1981).

The relative size of the absorptive surface area in the duodenum can significantly influence the rate and extent of drug absorption. In the young, the greater relative size of the duodenum compared with adults enhances drug absorption.

Gastrointestinal Enzymes and Microorganisms

The absorption of drugs that are fat soluble or carried in fat vehicles depends on lipase. Premature neonates have low lipase concentrations and no alpha amylase. The reduced activity of bile acids, lipase, alpha amylase, and protease continues until approximately age 4 months. Vitamin E absorption is decreased in neonates because of the diminished bile acid pool and biliary function; therefore, supplementation of this vitamin may be necessary.

The development of the intestinal microorganism flora depends more on diet than on age (Yaffe & Juchau, 1974), which may account for the more rapid development of flora in breast-fed infants than in formula-fed infants. The reduction of digoxin (Lanoxin) to inactive metabolites by anaerobic intestinal bacteria can be used as a marker for the development or changes in intestinal flora (Lindenbaum et al., 1981). Digoxin metabolites are not detected in children until 16 months, and an adult-like reduction of digoxin does not occur until age 9 (Linday et al., 1987).

Rectal Absorption

The rectal route of administration is seldom used; it usually is reserved for patients who cannot tolerate oral drugs or who lack intravenous access. In rectal administration, the drug is absorbed by the hemorrhoidal veins, which are not part of the portal circulation; therefore, it avoids first-pass hepatic elimination. Unfortunately, most drugs administered by this route are erratically and incompletely absorbed. Feces in the rectum, frequent bowel movements in neonates and infants, and lack of anal sphincter muscle contribute to the poor absorption profile of drugs administered rectally.

Although rectal administration may not be appropriate for routine dosing of drugs, the rectal administration of diazepam (Diastat AcuDial), valproic acid (Depakote), or midazolam (Versed) has been used to control seizures when intravenous access could not be quickly established in infants or children with status epilepticus (Brigo et al., 2015; Graves & Kriel, 1987).

Intramuscular and Subcutaneous Absorption

Both the characteristics of the patient and the properties of the drug influence the absorption of intramuscularly or subcutaneously administered drugs. Patient characteristics include blood flow to the muscle, muscle mass, tone, and activity. Important properties of the drug are its solubility, the pH of extracellular fluid, its ease in crossing capillary membranes, and the amount of drug administered at the injection site.

In pediatric patients, all the patient characteristics are highly variable. Neonates have decreased muscle mass, and their limited muscle activity decreases blood flow to and from the muscle. Collectively, these factors produce erratic and poor intramuscular drug absorption. On the contrary, infants possess a greater density of skeletal muscle capillaries than older children, allowing for more efficient drug absorption. Some drugs, such as erythromycin, can cause pain at the injection site and should not be administered intramuscularly. However, many drugs, such as the penicillins, reach concentrations in the serum with intramuscular administration that are comparable with those achieved after intravenous administration, with minimal adverse effects.

Percutaneous Absorption

An increase in the absorption of medications through the skin is evident during pregnancy. The increase in peripheral vasodilation and increase in blood flow to the skin (Kraemer, 1997) enhance this increase in absorption. Because of an increase in total body water, there is increased water content in the skin, which favors an increased rate and extent of absorption compared to water-soluble medications like lidocaine, which may be used as a topical anesthetic during pregnancy (Yankowitz & Niebyl, 2001).

The absorption of compounds is inversely related to the thickness of the stratum corneum and directly related to hydration of the skin (Morselli et al., 1980). Relative to body mass, the BSA is greatest in the infant and young child compared with older children and adults. The decreased thickness of the skin with increased skin surface hydration relative to body weight produces much greater percutaneous drug absorption in neonates than in adults. The percutaneous administration of drugs in neonates does pose some risks of toxic effects. Neonatal skin is structurally immature, resulting in less subcutaneous fat and a thinner stratum corneum and epidermis (Rutter, 1987). Adverse effects resulting from the inadvertent systemic absorption of percutaneously administered hexachlorophene emulsion, salicylic acid ointment, and hydrocortisone creams in neonates have limited the use of this route of drug administration. But since a greater skin surface area–body weight ratio is observed during the neonatal period, percutaneous drug absorption is also superior. Both the advantages and the subsequent disadvantages of enhanced percutaneous absorption disappear after infancy, however.

Mucosal Absorption

Mucosal administration of medications, whether via the nasal or the buccal route, has become a viable method for use in children. Some medications, such as nasal corticosteroids, are intended for a local effect and have almost no systemic absorption or effects. However, some medications, such as midazolam (Versed and Nayzilam) and ketamine (Ketalar), have been administered by nasal aerosolization with good absorption and systemic effect (Hosseini Jahromi et al., 2012; Klein et al., 2011). Administration by these routes avoids the trauma of placing an intravenous line and the associated costs. Also, in urgent situations, where there may be considerable difficulty placing an intravenous line (i.e., status epilepticus), nasal administration can be utilized with great effectiveness (Thakker & Shanbag, 2013).

Pulmonary Absorption

Aerosolized drug delivery to the lungs continues to be a preferred technique in many respiratory disorders, such as asthma. Factors affecting drug deposition in the lungs include particle size, lipid solubility, protein binding, drug metabolism in the lungs, and mucociliary transport (American Academy of Pediatrics, 1997). Aerosol particle size and lipid solubility are factors in determining whether the drug is deposited in the upper or lower airways; drugs with smaller particle size and lipid-soluble drugs are more likely to be absorbed and deposited in the lower airways (Bond, 1993). Besides drug considerations, physiologic changes in pregnancy favor the absorption of medications administered through the inhalation route. Both cardiac and tidal volumes are increased by approximately 50% in pregnancy, resulting in hyperventilation and increased pulmonary blood flow (Loebstein et al., 1997). These alterations aid in the transfer of medications through the alveoli into the maternal bloodstream (Loebstein et al., 1997). Because of this increased transfer into the bloodstream, it is important to consider dose reductions of certain inhaled medications such as volatile anesthetics.

Pediatric characteristics also affect aerosol drug delivery. Infants and children have lower tidal volumes and increased respiratory rates (especially while crying), reducing drug delivery and absorption in the lungs. Studies have shown that less than 2% of aerosolized drugs are deposited in young infants

and toddlers (Fok et al., 1996; Salmon et al., 1990). Therefore, adult dosing may be necessary to counteract these effects.

Distribution

Maternal blood volume increases significantly during pregnancy due to the increase in estrogen activation of the renin angiotensin–aldosterone system. The 30% to 50% increase in blood volume (Guyton & Hall, 1996; Loebstein et al., 1997) is characteristically distributed to various organ systems serving the needs of the growing fetus. The full increase in total body water during pregnancy is 8 L, with 60% distributed to the placenta, fetus, and amniotic fluid and 40% going to maternal tissues (Loebstein et al., 1997). These increases cause the volume of distribution of medications to increase, resulting in a decrease (dilutional effect) in drug concentrations. Studies show that peak and total concentrations of water-soluble drugs decrease because of the increased volume of distribution (Philipson, 1977). Conversely, drug distribution is affected by an increase in maternal fat deposits. Medications that are highly lipophilic distribute to maternal fat deposits, also resulting in decreased serum drug levels. Body fat increases during pregnancy by 3 to 4 kg and may act as a reservoir for medications that favor a fat-soluble environment (Yankowitz & Niebyl, 2001). Another factor that may affect medication distribution is the concentration of albumin in the maternal blood. The concentration of plasma albumin decreases during pregnancy. This decrease is believed to be caused by a reduction in the rate of albumin synthesis or an increase in its rate of catabolism (Fredericksen, 2001). Furthermore, there is an increase in arterial pH, which may affect drug–protein binding. Medications that are highly bound to plasma albumin (e.g., anticonvulsants) may have an increased free drug concentration due to decreased albumin binding.

Six factors affect drug distribution in the pediatric population: vascular perfusion, body composition, tissue-binding characteristics, physicochemical properties of the drug, plasma protein binding, and route of administration (Stewart & Hampton, 1987). During the neonatal period, most of these factors are significantly different from those in the adult population, while children and adolescents are very similar to or the same as adults.

Vascular Perfusion

Changes in vascular perfusion are common in neonates. For example, in neonatal respiratory distress syndrome and postasphyxia, a right-to-left vascular shunt may occur and divert blood from the lungs to the tissues and organs, potentially changing the V_d of some drugs.

Body Composition

Neonates have increased total body water (75% to 80%) with decreased fat compared with adults, resulting in a higher water–lipid ratio. After the neonatal period, fat increases and total body water decreases steadily until puberty, especially in girls. For instance, neonates and infants have increased total body and extracellular water, creating a larger volume of distribution and affecting the pharmacokinetics of some drugs, such as aminoglycosides. The larger volume, in turn, requires administering a larger milligram-per-kilogram dose of aminoglycosides to neonates and infants than to adults.

Tissue-Binding Characteristics

The mass of tissue available for binding can affect drug distribution. Drugs extensively bound to tissues exhibit increased "free" blood levels when the mass of tissue is reduced by disease or degeneration or immaturity, as in the pediatric population.

Physicochemical Properties

The physicochemical properties of a drug include lipid solubility (ionized vs. nonionized) and molecular configuration. These properties affect the ability of a drug to move across membranes into target cells or tissues. Drugs that display favorable properties for absorption may pose a greater risk for toxicity in neonates, who have enhanced percutaneous drug absorption.

Plasma Protein Binding

Preterm neonates have lower circulating amounts of alpha$_1$ acid glycoprotein, which binds alkaline drugs, than full-term neonates, who have lower alpha$_1$ acid glycoprotein levels than adults. Neonates also have a reduced amount of circulating albumin compared with adults. Albumin is responsible for binding acidic drugs, fatty acids, and bilirubin. While the affinity of drugs for either of these plasma proteins is harder to determine, theoretically a neonate's affinity for protein binding is reduced, resulting in the likelihood of displacing drugs or bilirubin bound to albumin and leading to increased serum concentrations. All these factors produce a larger volume of distribution and increased free drug concentrations (e.g., phenytoin [Dilantin]) in neonates than in adults.

Route of Administration

The route by which a drug is administered has a primary influence on the drug's distribution. If the drug is administered orally, the liver becomes the primary distribution site. However, if a drug is administered intravenously, the heart and lungs act as the primary distribution sites. This is important because when a drug passes through the liver before reaching its site of activity, it is subject to the first-pass effect of extensive hepatic metabolism, which typically reduces the amount of circulating active drug and thus limits its effects. Therefore, to achieve an equal effect, the dosage of a drug administered by the oral route usually needs to be higher than the dosage of a drug administered intravenously.

Metabolism

Clearance of many drugs is mainly reliant on hepatic metabolism. The two phases of drug metabolism in the liver are the oxidation, reduction, and hydrolysis reactions (phase I)

TABLE 4.3			
Summary of Age-Related Changes in Metabolism			
P-450 Cytochromes	**Reduced Activity versus Adults**	**Increased Activity versus Adults**	**Age at which Adult Activity Is Reached**
CYP1A2	Until age 4 mo	1–2 y	End of puberty
CYP2C9	First week of life	3–4 y	End of puberty
CYP2D6	Until age 3–5 y	3–5 y	
CYP2E1	Unknown	Unknown	Unknown
CYP3A4	First month of life	1–4 y	End of puberty

CYP, cytochrome P-450.

Based on data from Leader, J. S., & Kearns, G. L. (1997). Pharmacogenetics in pediatrics: Implications for practice. *Pediatric Clinics of North America, 44*, 55–77.

and conjugation reactions (phase II). Age-related changes in metabolism affect how drugs are broken down or transformed in pediatric patients and how certain metabolic enzymes are activated. (**Table 4.3** summarizes developmental patterns in phase I oxidation reactions.) Phase I and phase II reactions are delayed in neonates, infants, and young children, with consequential drug toxicities.

The P-450 cytochrome (CYP) is the most important component of phase I drug metabolism. Cytochromes in the CYP1, CYP2, and CYP3 families have been identified as important in human drug metabolism. Additional information suggests there is substantial genetic variability in the quantity and quality of CYP in the human body (Kearns, 1995). For example, codeine is metabolized to morphine via CYP2D6 and can result in high levels of morphine in patients who are ultrarapid metabolizers of the enzyme. Similarly, tramadol utilizes the CYP2D6 enzyme and can lead to supratherapeutic levels in patients who are ultrarapid metabolizers of this enzyme. Deaths in children who are ultrarapid metabolizers have been reported after they received codeine and tramadol. These reports led to the FDA creating a boxed warning regarding the use of codeine pain and cough medications and the use of tramadol pain medications in children less than 12 years of age with restrictions for older children (U.S. Food and Drug Administration, 2018). Additionally, breast-feeding is not recommended in mothers receiving codeine or tramadol due to the risk of adverse effects in breast-fed infants, such as sleepiness and breathing problems that could result in death.

The metabolism of caffeine and theophylline, the prototypic substrate for CYP1A2, is reduced at birth; the drug concentration increases linearly over the first year of life and exceeds adult levels in older infants and children. To maintain therapeutic serum theophylline concentrations, smaller doses are prescribed and administered less frequently in neonates than in older infants and children.

In pediatrics, phase II reactions have been less well studied than phase I reactions. In adults, acetaminophen (Tylenol), a substrate for glucuronosyltransferase 1A6 and 1A9, is metabolized by a phase II glucuronidation reaction. In neonates and infants, however, this metabolic pathway is deficient. As a result, acetaminophen metabolism is shifted to sulfate conjugation, which results in a half-life for acetaminophen that is similar to its half-life in adults.

Elimination

Almost all drugs and their metabolites are excreted through the kidneys. The kidney eliminates drugs by glomerular filtration (passive diffusion) or tubular secretion (energy-dependent channels or pumps). Hormonal changes that normally occur during pregnancy can affect the elimination of various medications. The normal increase in progesterone levels can stimulate hepatic microsomal enzyme systems, thereby increasing the elimination of some hepatically eliminated medications (e.g., phenytoin [Dilantin]). Progesterone may also decrease the elimination of some medications (e.g., theophylline [Theo-Dur]) by inhibiting specific microsomal enzyme systems. Therefore, depending on the elimination pathway of a specific medication, the elimination rate may not be predictable. The extent of these physiologic changes is difficult to quantify, and it is unknown whether changes in dosages are required.

Glomerular filtration rate (GFR) increases in pregnancy due to increase in cardiac output combined with a reduction in oncotic pressure due to decreased albumin and increased renal blood flow. With the increase in renal blood flow by 50% and increased GFR, drugs excreted primarily by the kidney show increased elimination. Cefuroxime, an antibiotic, has increased clearance and decreased half-life in pregnant women (Loebstein et al., 1997). Medications can be affected by these changes in plasma volume and increased clearance in early (12 to 15 weeks) and late pregnancy (30 to 33 weeks), as seen with enoxaparin, a low molecular weight heparin (Casele et al., 1999). The magnitude of these increases in elimination may vary depending on the medication.

The GFR increases quickly during the first 2 weeks of postnatal life and does not approach adult rates until age 2 (Rubin et al., 1949); tubular secretion and reabsorption rates do not reach adult values until age 5 to 7 months. The proximal tubules are characterized by an inability to concentrate urine or reabsorb various filtered compounds and a reduced ability to secrete organic acids. This immaturity of the renal system in neonates and infants results from restricted blood flow and a resultant decrease in cardiac output to the kidneys, combined with incomplete glomerular and tubular development. As a result, plasma clearance of many drugs via the kidneys is altered. For example, during infancy, the response to thiazide diuretics, which require a GFR greater than 30 mL/min to be effective, is diminished. Often, a larger dosage of a thiazide diuretic or substitution by a loop diuretic is required to produce adequate diuresis. Because the elimination of aminoglycosides is directly related to the GFR, aminoglycosides have a longer half-life in neonates and infants, who thus require a longer dosing interval than adults. In addition, decreased tubular secretion in neonates and infants can lengthen the elimination half-life of other antibiotics, such as the penicillins and sulfonamides. Selecting the appropriate dosing regimen based on age, weight, and kidney maturation and identifying concomitant agents renally eliminated are important factors to prevent toxicity. In general, renal excretion of many drugs is directly proportional to age.

CLINICAL IMPLICATIONS IN PREGNANCY

While multiple studies highlight pharmacokinetic changes in pregnancy, limited studies evaluate the efficacy changes of drugs and doses due to these physiologic changes. Dose changes are generally not recommended unless there are data of altered efficacy due to pharmacokinetic changes. Examples of these drugs include lamotrigine or indinavir, where dose changes are recommended. Pregnant women are often excluded from clinical trials. Therefore, there is often limited information on the effect of dose changes that would be required in pregnancy (Pinheiro & Stika, 2020).

Factors in Placental–Fetal Physiology

Until the 1960s, it was widely believed that the uterus provided a secure and protected environment for the developing fetus. Very little thought was given to the potential harm posed to the fetus from maternal drug use. After the thalidomide tragedy in the 1960s, the government required testing of drugs before human use. It is now known that by the fifth week of fetal development, virtually every drug has the ability to cross the placenta (Kraemer, 1997).

The treatment of medical conditions is complicated during pregnancy by various factors, which must be considered before initiating or continuing drug therapy. A key factor is whether the drug will cross the placenta and potentially cause fetal harm.

Placental Transfer of Medications

The following factors affect a drug's ability to cross the placenta:

- Lipid-soluble drugs can cross the placenta more freely than water-soluble drugs because the outer layers of most cell membranes are made up of lipids. Many antibiotics and opiate compounds are highly soluble in lipids and can therefore easily cross the placental membrane.
- The ionization status of the drug affects placental transfer. Drugs with high lipid solubility tend to remain in a nonionized state; therefore, placental transfer is increased. Heparin, for example, is a highly ionized drug, and therefore, it does not readily cross the placental membrane.
- The molecular weight of the drug can determine the ease of placental transfer. The lower the molecular weight or the smaller the drug molecule, the more readily the drug crosses the placenta (**Table 4.4**).

TABLE 4.4

Effect of Molecular Weight on Placental Transfer of Drugs

Molecular Weight	Drug Example	Rate of Placental Transfer
<500 g/mol	Acetaminophen, caffeine, cocaine, labetalol, morphine, penicillins, theophylline	Readily crosses the placenta
600–1,000 g/mol	Digoxin	Crosses the placenta at a slower rate
>1,000 g/mol	Heparin, insulins	Transfer across the placenta severely impeded

- Drugs that are not bound to a protein (e.g., albumin) can cross the placenta. Albumin is the most abundant protein in the human body. During pregnancy, the concentration of albumin decreases, and therefore, fewer proteins are present, allowing for more unbound or "free" drug to cross the placental membrane. Furthermore, changes in the drug–protein binding ability of albumin in pregnancy may increase the amount of "free" drug.
- Active placental transporters may also affect the concentrations of medications that cross the placenta. Specifically, P-glycoprotein (P-gp) is the most well studied and has been shown to prevent the transfer of many medications. Conversely, when mothers are administered medications that inhibit P-gp, medications that would normally be prevented from crossing the placenta are able to cross and may cause congenital abnormalities.

Placental and Fetal Metabolism

Evidence exists to support the theory that the human placenta and fetus are capable of metabolizing medications. Research findings suggest that liver enzyme systems are present in fetal livers as early as 7 to 8 weeks' gestation (Juchau & Choa, 1983). Although these enzyme systems are present, they are immature, and any drug elimination that occurs is a result of drug diffusing back into maternal blood.

Fetal Physiology

Not all drugs that cross the placental barrier cause fetal harm. Therefore, the practitioner needs to ask whether a specific drug will cross the placenta and cause fetal harm. Currently, it is not possible to directly study the effects of medications on the fetus. A single drug concentration measurement at birth from the umbilical cord is all that is available to understand the drug exposure on the fetus. Fetal factors to be considered in answering the question include the gestational age at the time of exposure to the drug, which is

important because some drugs can exert their effects on the fetus throughout gestation. On the other hand, some drugs exert their effects on the fetus at different stages of gestation. For example, angiotensin-converting enzyme inhibitors, such as captopril (Capoten), quinapril (Accupril), and enalapril (Vasotec), vary in their fetal risk during pregnancy; they pose a lesser risk in the second trimester and a higher risk in the third trimester. In other words, they become less safe as the pregnancy advances.

Within the first 14 days after conception, the embryo is protected from exogenous toxicity (Kraemer, 1997; Rayburn, 1997). The cells at this time are totipotential, meaning that if one cell is damaged or killed, another cell can perform the dead cell's function, and the embryo remains unharmed (Dicke, 1989). After this point, the developing fetus is susceptible to the effects of drugs. The first 3 months of gestation are the most crucial in terms of abnormalities and malformations, and it is estimated that approximately 70% of pregnant women take medications during the first trimester during organogenesis (Briggs et al., 2017; Mitchell et al., 2011). Medications that may be relatively safe during the middle trimester of pregnancy may not be safe in the last trimester or during delivery. For example, aspirin use late in pregnancy is associated with increased bleeding at the time of delivery. Moreover, the effect that aspirin has on prostaglandins may delay labor.

Fetal total body water and fat deposition are associated with gestational age, and they affect the absorption and distribution of drugs. As the fetus matures, total body water decreases and fat deposition increases, and the fetus is more likely to be affected by medications that are highly lipophilic (e.g., opiates) than by medications that are water soluble (e.g., ampicillin [Principen]).

Fetal circulatory patterns can alter the amount of drug distributed to the fetus. In early gestation, a disproportionately large percentage of the fetal cardiac output is presented to the brain, and consequently, the concentration of drug in the fetal circulation is increased (Kraemer, 1997).

Teratogenicity of Medications

The word *teratogenicity* is derived from the Greek root *teras*, meaning "monster." Teratogenicity is the ability of an exogenous agent to cause the dysgenesis of fetal organs as evidenced either structurally or functionally (Koren et al., 1998; Kraemer, 1997).

The risk of fetal abnormality depends on many factors, including not only the gestational age of the fetus at the time of exposure but the agent or medications the fetus is exposed to and the length of exposure. Aside from fetal malformations, fetal drug exposure may affect newborn development and function.

The health care provider must therefore balance the risk of exposing the fetus to the drug with the benefit of treatment to the mother. If it is determined that the drug is necessary, the drug with the safest profile should be used at the lowest effective dose. The practitioner should always keep in mind that the mother is not the only recipient of the drug—the fetus is as well. In addition, it is important to remember that any illnesses or chronic medical conditions that go untreated during pregnancy could potentially cause harm to the mother and fetus, even though medications to treat these illnesses may pose a risk to the fetus as well. Therefore, weighing the benefit of drug therapy to the mother against the risk of drug therapy to the fetus needs to be as balanced as possible.

In 1979, the U.S. FDA categorized drugs according to fetal risks to help practitioners guide therapy. The categories were based on animal data and the presence or absence of controlled studies in pregnant women to determine the level of fetal risk: categories A, B, C, D, and X based on level of data. Health care providers were challenged with using these oversimplified categories to assess risk–benefit ratios of medications during pregnancy due to the scarcity of controlled trials in pregnant women. This clinical dilemma prompted the new current FDA rule, entitled the Pregnancy and Lactation Labeling Rule (PLLR), which was passed in December 2014 and took effect in June 2015. The new rule includes three separate sections that are required in package labeling: pregnancy, lactation, and a new section—females and males of reproductive age.

The updated requirements for these new sections in the package labeling are summarized in **Table 4.5**. All new molecular entities coming to the market required manufacturers to include the current labeling requirements and were not assigned a pregnancy category. Pregnancy risk categories were removed from existing drugs by 2018. All drugs approved after June 2001 were required to submit new labeling information by June of 2020; however, there has a been delay in conforming to this new labeling requirement based on the initial implementation schedule. Manufacturers are also required to update labeling with new available information under the new rule. It is important to note that over-the-counter products were not affected by this new legislation. Drugs approved before 2001 must have removed pregnancy categories but are not required to conform to the new labeling requirements. The manufacturers of these drugs are encouraged to voluntarily use the new labeling sections.

DRUG THERAPY IN THE BREAST-FEEDING MOTHER

With the number of women who choose to breast-feed their infants increasing yearly, the number of questions presented to health care practitioners concerning the safety of medication use while breast-feeding is also increasing. Recommendations to discontinue or interrupt breast-feeding are often inappropriate as this cautious approach may be unnecessary for most patients. Health care practitioners are often reluctant to recommend medication use while the mother is breast-feeding because of the potential adverse effects on the infant. Most research on lactation has been conducted in small groups or on animal models. The American Academy of Pediatrics and FDA recommend that for the most up-to-date information providers use databases such as LactMed (https://www.ncbi.nlm.nih.gov/books/NBK501922/) to help guide treatment options for mothers who are breast-feeding (Sachs & Committee on Drugs, 2013). LactMed is available to all practitioners, and it has comprehensive and up-to-date information regarding the known concentrations of drug reaching the infant through breast milk, possible adverse reactions, and potential alternatives. This is an excellent resource that is powered by the National Library of Medicine. Consulting the known pharmacokinetic parameters of medications can also be helpful in prescribing medications.

Human breast milk is a complex, nutrient-enriched fluid. Containing approximately 80% water, breast milk also has immunologic properties and proteins, fats, carbohydrates, minerals, and vitamins needed for normal development. The availability of the drug to be distributed into breast milk depends on many factors. For a drug to be distributed into breast milk, it must first be absorbed into the maternal circulation. The concentration or level of the drug in the mother's plasma influences the amount and degree of drug distributed into breast milk. Once the drug is available for distribution into breast milk, several other factors need to be considered. These factors are similar to those determining whether a drug will cross the placental membrane and include the following (Dillon et al., 1997):

- Blood flow to the breast—the greater the blood flow to the breast, the greater the drug level in breast milk.
- Plasma pH (7.45) and milk pH (7.08)—the medication will stay in the maternal plasma if the medication favors a higher pH.
- Mammary tissue composition—high adipose or fat content of the breast tissue causes lipophilic medications to be distributed into the breast tissue and then into breast milk.

TABLE 4.5	
Pregnancy and Lactation Labeling Rule	
Labeling Section	**Requirements**
8.1 Pregnancy (includes labor and delivery)	Includes risk summary, clinical considerations, and data (to support the risk summary) Must include information for a pregnancy exposure registry if one is available
8.2 Lactation	Also includes risk summary, clinical consideration, and data, including the amount of drug appearing in breast milk and potential effects on the infant
8.3 Females and males of reproductive potential	Includes information about need for pregnancy testing, contraception recommendations, and infertility information when applicable

- Breast milk composition—breast milk contains proteins, fat, water, and vitamins. Any medication that has a high affinity for any of these components will have an increased distribution into breast milk.
- Physicochemical properties (i.e., lipophilicity, molecular weight, ionization of medication in plasma and breast milk) of the drug—drug characteristics that favor transfer of medication into breast milk are low molecular weight, low ionization in plasma, low protein binding, and high lipophilicity.
- Extent of drug–protein binding in plasma and breast milk—medications that are highly protein bound in the plasma are less likely to be distributed into the breast milk.
- The rate of breast milk production—the more breast milk produced, the more diluted the medication will be in the breast milk.

When considering these factors, it can easily be appreciated that different medications distribute into breast milk at different rates and to different extents. Aside from medication-specific factors, there are some general considerations for minimizing the risk of medication-related adverse effects in breast-fed infants. Medications with shorter half-lives are preferred to decrease drug accumulation in the breast milk. Similarly, sustained-release products are less preferred. Drugs with high oral bioavailability are less preferred as they are more easily absorbed. It is recommended to use the lowest effective dose and choose medications with the least serious adverse effects when possible. Dosing schedules also help in minimizing the amount of drug reaching the infant. Scheduling the mother to take the medication immediately after breast-feeding minimizes the dose to the infant by circumventing peak breast milk levels (Sachs & Committee on Drugs, 2013).

Patients with chronic conditions, such as hypertension, epilepsy, or diabetes, need to consult their health care practitioners about continuing treatment and minimizing risk to the infant. If a medication is for short-term use, the clinician can also consider if the medication could be postponed until the mother is finished breast-feeding and limiting the medication to the shortest possible duration. Without other options, patients with short-term illnesses can temporarily interrupt breast-feeding for the duration of treatment and resume breast-feeding a few days after therapy is completed if the risk of the drug to the infant is thought to outweigh the benefits. By this time, no residual drug should be concentrated in the breast milk. During the interruption, however, the mother must pump the breast and discard the milk. Doing so relieves engorgement and promotes continued milk production and flow.

DRUG SELECTION IN PEDIATRICS

Various factors are considered when prescribing a drug for a pediatric patient. Among them are the benefits of the drug in relation to the risks of administration, the long-term effects, the dosage form, and the route and frequency of administration (**Figure 4.1**).

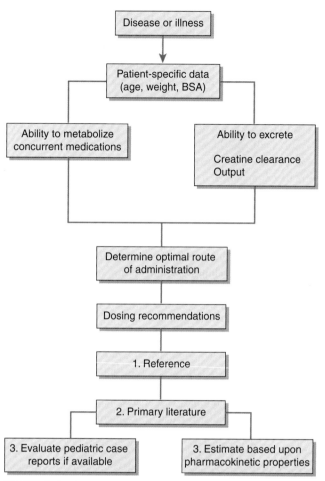

FIGURE 4–1 Approach to prescribing drug therapy for the pediatric patient.

BSA, body surface area.

Risks and Benefits

The classic medication when discussing risks and benefits in the pediatric population is ciprofloxacin (Cipro), a fluoroquinolone. Ciprofloxacin was brought to market in 1987 and carried a risk of severe degenerative arthropathy. This effect was seen in juvenile study animals during drug development. The potential for this problem led to these drugs being contraindicated in all pediatric populations. Numerous studies over the past 20 years disputing this risk have led to over 500,000 prescriptions for the drug being written annually for children younger than age 18. The American Academy of Pediatrics developed a policy statement that provides an outline for the use of fluoroquinolones in children with a clinical report update in 2016 (American Academy of Pediatrics, 2011, 2016). The use of the drug class in children is driven more by resistance patterns in pathogens covered by the class than the potential risk of arthropathy to the patient.

Cardiovascular safety and adverse psychiatric effects are a concern with the use of psychostimulants in the treatment of attention deficit hyperactivity disorder (ADHD). A very small number of case reports of sudden cardiac death have been reported in children prescribed psychostimulants for ADHD.

The risk has been found to be greater in patients with underlying cardiac structural abnormalities. However, the risk is similar to that of strenuous exercise in this population, and the use in the general population does not necessitate additional testing beyond normal screening. There is also a small risk of psychosis and mania-type reactions in children. As a result, the FDA requires the pharmaceutical industry to provide medication guides to patients and prescribers explaining the risks of ADHD drug treatments and information on their potential side effects.

Another widely used drug class with specific safety concerns in the pediatric population is antidepressants. There is a very slight increase in suicide risk in patients started on antidepressants, which likely reflects the current depressed state and other comorbidities. The FDA has included a black box warning for increased suicidality for children and adolescents initiating all classes of antidepressants. Although this is a statistically significant increased risk compared to the normal population, the risk of suicide in untreated depressed patients is much higher.

Long-Term Effects

Drugs administered to pediatric patients may take a longer time to produce adverse effects than in adults. Certain adverse effects may not be detected until decades after treatment. For example, secondary cancers, growth retardation, hypogonadism, and sterility have all been reported as late adverse effects associated with certain antineoplastic therapies. Inhaled and intranasal corticosteroids may decrease growth velocity, which is a means of comparing growth rates among children of the same age. Studies with inhaled steroids showed an approximately 1-cm/y reduction in growth velocity. The FDA suggests that the reduction is related to dose and how long the child takes the drug (U.S. Food and Drug Administration, 1998b). Lone and Pederson (2000) evaluated the long-term effect on growth of inhaled or intranasal budesonide in pediatric asthma patients. At the end of this 10-year study, the researchers concluded that normal adult height was achieved in patients receiving these corticosteroids. More recently, the Childhood Asthma Management Program (CAMP) Research Group showed a reduction of 1.2 cm in adult height in the inhaled budesonide versus placebo group (Kelly et al., 2012).

Potential long-term effects of medications used in children create a concern. The 5-year survival rates of most pediatric malignancies are exceeding 80% in most high income countries. This has led to a focus on the late effects of therapy and the quality of life in this growing population of childhood cancer survivors (Erdmann et al., 2020). Nearly two thirds of all childhood cancer survivors will experience some physical or psychologic outcome that develops or persists beyond 5 years from the initial diagnosis (Shankar et al., 2008). Other medications used in pediatrics may also carry risks for long-term effects. Unfortunately, these effects may not be seen for years after the medication is stopped, and there are likely other factors that could cause or at least contribute to the effect. Studies that evaluate the long-term effect of a medication are very difficult to perform and often yield conflicting results.

Dosage Formulation

Commercially available dosage formulations often limit the drugs that can be prescribed to children and are not always child friendly. Many drugs are available only as an oral tablet, capsule, or intravenous dilution in adult dosage strengths. Prescribing a drug as a tablet or capsule for a pediatric patient has several drawbacks. The pediatric patient may have difficulty swallowing a whole or intact tablet or capsule and attempting to break a tablet into smaller pieces or emptying part of a capsule to provide an appropriate dose leads to questionable accuracy of the administered dose. It is important to provide a dosage form that can be administered easily, accurately, and safely to a pediatric patient. A method to improve administration is via extemporaneous formulations, especially if a product is not commercially available as an elixir, solution, suspension, or syrup. However, these oral liquid formulations also have drawbacks, such as an unfavorable taste. Other alternatives to oral liquid formulations include tablet dispersion, powdered papers, and repacked capsules. Combination products are available to reduce pill burden and improve medication adherence. However, these agents contain fixed dosage forms in tablets or capsules, making it difficult for a child less than age 5 to swallow.

Ideally, a practitioner who is prescribing a dosage formulation not commercially available for a pediatric patient ought to work with a pharmacist who is willing and able to compound accurate pediatric drug dosages and formulas. Practitioners can familiarize themselves with additional drugs that can be extemporaneously compounded for use in pediatrics by a pharmacist in such publications as *Pediatric Drug Formulations* (Nahata & Pai, 2018); *Teddy Bear Book: Pediatric Injectable Drugs* (Phelps, 2018); *Pediatric Dosage Handbook* (Taketomo et al., 2019); *Extemporaneous Formulations for Pediatric, Geriatric, and Special Needs Patients* (Jew et al., 2016); or *Trissel's Stability of Compounded Formulations* (Trissel et al., 2018). A Medline search should be conducted for drugs not contained in these publications.

Dosage

In adult drug therapy, one standard dose of a drug can be used for almost all adults, but the opposite is true in pediatric drug therapy: A pediatric drug dose changes for different illnesses or as the patient grows or develops and requires age-dependent adjustments.

When writing or assessing a pediatric medication order, the following process is recommended to ensure safe and effective pharmaceutical care:

1. Determine the patient type (i.e., neonate, pediatric, adolescent).
2. Assess the appropriateness of the drug therapy selected in this patient type, patient population, and/or disease state.

3. Establish the appropriate dose, route, formulation, and frequency based on the recommended references described in the paragraph below.
4. If all resources have been exhausted or further information is needed regarding the pediatric dosage, contact a pharmacist. It is important to ensure that the dose is appropriate or reasonable based on the pharmacist's knowledge of pediatric pharmacokinetics and available resources.

Many drugs currently in use in pediatrics have established dosing recommendations based on body weight, BSA, concurrent drug therapy, and stage of development or physiologic function (age). Body weight–based dosing is the most common method for pediatric dosing. A total daily dose, milligrams per kilogram per day (mg/kg/d), is divided by the dosing interval to calculate each individual dose. Analgesics, antipyretics, and emergency drugs are often administered on a dose-by-dose method; as such, the recommended pediatric dose is reported as milligrams per kilogram per dose (mg/kg/dose). The starting or maximum doses for pediatric intravenous infusions are usually reported as micrograms per kilogram per minute (mcg/kg/min) or micrograms per kilogram per hour (mcg/kg/h). Drug dosages based on a patient's BSA are usually reserved for antineoplastic agents or critically ill patients. BSA correlates closely with many factors that influence drug elimination, including cardiac output, respiratory metabolism, blood volume, extracellular water volume, GFR, and renal blood flow. Dosages of several drugs, including docusate (Colace) and montelukast (Singulair), are based on age.

General pediatric drug references such as the *Pediatric Dosage Handbook* (Taketomo et al., 2019) and Micromedex (MICROMEDEX Solutions, 2020) provide comprehensive drug monographs, including dosage formulations, adverse events, pharmacology, and pharmacokinetics. *The Harriet Lane Handbook* (Hughes & Kahl, 2017) provides drug monographs based on the Johns Hopkins Hospital formulary and special drug topics. A specialty pediatric reference such as the *Red Book* (Kimberlin et al., 2018) covers only antimicrobial agents and vaccines; *Neofax* (Neofax, 2020) provides information about drug dosing in neonates.

Obesity

Obesity, defined in children as a body mass index (BMI) at or above the 95th percentile for age, is considered a public health crisis in the United States (Ogden et al., 2010). Nearly 1 in 5 school-age children and young people are obese in the United States (Hales et al., 2017). Children with a BMI at or above the 85th percentile are considered "at risk for overweight," and nearly 32% of U.S. children ages 2 to 19 fall into this category (Ogden et al., 2010). While it is known that there is an overall lack of information on dosages regarding most medications in children, there is far less information on proper medication dosing in the overweight child. Obesity can affect the pharmacokinetics, dosing, half-life, and metabolism of a

medication. Medications originally intended for adult use are now being utilized to treat hypertension, hyperlipidemia, and type 2 diabetes as these diseases are on the rise secondary to the increase in obesity (Kennedy et al., 2013). There is a greater risk of dosing errors in overweight children, specifically for underdosing and overdosing of antimicrobials (Matson et al., 2017). The Pediatric Pharmacy Advocacy Group recommends that weight-based dosing be utilized for all children less than age 18 and weighing less than 88 lbs (40 kg). For children who weigh over 40 kg, weight-based dosing should be used, unless the patient's dose or dose per day exceeds the recommended adult dose for the specific indication (Matson et al., 2017).

Routes of Administration

Oral

When prescribing or administering oral drugs for pediatric patients, the caregiver needs to consider not only the drug's flavor and ease of delivery but the frequency of administration, dosage form, and "inactive" ingredients, such as alcohol and sugar. A liquid dosage form is preferred for most pediatric patients.

To ensure the accuracy of each dose administered, the drug should be measured and then administered with an oral syringe or a calibrated drug cup, with the base of the meniscus viewed at eye level. If the drug is available only in tablet form and the tablet can be broken, the tablet may be crushed and mixed in compatible syrup. However, mixing a crushed or whole tablet with food should be done cautiously because many foods interfere with drug absorption.

If the patient is an infant, the head should be raised to prevent aspiration of the drug. Applying gentle downward pressure on the chin with a thumb helps open the patient's mouth. If a syringe is used, the tip of the syringe should be placed in the pocket between the patient's cheek and gum and the drug administered slowly and steadily to reduce the risk of aspiration.

For bottle-fed infants, the drug can be placed in a nipple and the infant allowed to suck the contents. However, a drug should never be mixed with the contents of a baby's bottle because the correct dose will not be received if the infant does not consume the full contents of the bottle. In addition, a drug–nutrient interaction may occur if a drug is mixed with formula feeds. A classic example of a drug–nutrient interaction is the significant reduction of oral phenytoin absorption after concurrent administration with an enteral feeding formula (Sacks & Brown, 1994).

Rectal

Toddlers being toilet trained, especially children experiencing stress or difficulty, often resist the rectal administration of drugs. Older children may perceive the procedure as an invasion of privacy and may react with embarrassment or anger and hostility. The best approach to reducing anxiety and increasing cooperation is to spend time explaining the procedure and to reassure the child that giving drugs by this route will not hurt. It may be necessary, after placing a suppository, to hold the child's buttocks together for a few minutes to prevent expulsion of the drug.

Parenteral

Establishing venous access, venipuncture for blood samples, and intramuscular injections are a great source of distress and pain for children. Several local anesthetic agents have been developed to help manage the pain and anxiety brought on by these procedures. The ideal product would have needle-free or topical administration, a rapid onset of anesthetic, and no dermal or systemic adverse effects, and the product would have no impact on the success rate of the procedure. No commercially available product has all these qualities. The three general delivery methods used to bypass the stratum corneum layer are direct injection of local anesthetics, passive diffusion from topically applied gels or creams, and several needle-free methods that hasten the rate of drug passage through the skin and speed the time to onset of action. **Table 4.6** lists the methods of drug delivery, the available agents, and the advantages and disadvantages of each (Zempsky, 2008).

Pulmonary

Nebulizers, pressurized metered-dose inhalers (pMDIs), and dry powder inhalers (DPIs) can be used to deliver bronchodilators and corticosteroids in the treatment of asthma. Nebulized drugs require connecting an air or oxygen tube to the nebulizer machine and are often used in infants and young children. pMDIs require coordination between actuation and inhalation; this is difficult in any age group, so a tube spacer is recommended for children of all ages (Global Initiative for Asthma, 2019). Spacer devices have expanded the use of metered-dose inhalers even to the neonatal population. A DPI such as budesonide powder (Pulmicort Turbuhaler) involves coordination with the patient's inspiratory flow; therefore, the delivery mechanism is not recommended in children less than age 4. **Table 4.7** summarizes the recommended population for aerosol delivery devices (Global Initiative for Asthma, 2019).

Topical

The topical delivery of medications is common in the pediatric population with diseases such as eczema and acne as well as other skin disorders that appear during childhood. Caution is

TABLE 4.6				
Topical Anesthetics				
Method	**Product(s)**	**Medication(s)**	**Onset of Topical Anesthesia**	**Adverse Reactions**
Injection of local anesthetics	Lidocaine, Lidocaine buffered with sodium bicarbonate	Lidocaine	<1 min	Pain associated with initial needlestick for injection of medication
Lidocaine needle-free injection	J-Tip®	Lidocaine	<1 min	"Popping noise" with administration (may frighten some children)
Passive diffusion with topical creams or gels	EMLA®, generic	Lidocaine, 2.5%; prilocaine, 2.5%	30 min (minimum), 60 min for more complete effect	Skin blanching, rare methemoglobinemia in infants
	LMX4®	Liposomal lidocaine, 4%	30 min	Erythema, blanching
Needle-free strategies to accelerate onset	Synera®	Lidocaine/tetracaine	10 min	Local reactions (erythema, 71%; blanching; and edema)
Lidocaine iontophoresis	Numby Stuff®	Lidocaine	10–15 min	Intolerable tingling, itching, burning sensation, discomfort, potential for burn
Lidocaine HCl monohydrate powder intradermal injection system	Zingo®	Lidocaine HCl monohydrate	1–3 min	Local reactions (erythema, 62%; petechiae, 52.8%) and edema
Vapocoolant sprays	Pain Ease®	Liquid refrigerant (ethyl chloride)	Immediate (may require two providers as effect lasts <1 min)	Some skin pigmentation changes (temporary)

J-Tip, EMLA, LMX4, Synera, Numby Stuff, Zingo, and Pain Ease

TABLE 4.7

Recommended Age Groups for Aerosol Delivery Devices

Device	Age
Nebulizer	• Any age
pMDI	• Any age (with valved spacer) • >8 y old
Breath-actuated pMDI	• >7 y old
Dry powder inhaler	• >5 y old

pMDI, pressurized metered-dose inhaler.

warranted in this population due to several factors that may lead to a higher rate of drug absorption. When compared to adults, infants and children have a higher ratio of skin surface to body weight. This increases the risk of accumulating significant serum drug levels (Metry & Herbert, 2000). It is especially true in the newborn and infant because the barrier function of their skin is immature. Parents must be cautioned to follow the directions for administration of all topical medications to prevent toxic drug levels. A fatal case of diphenhydramine toxicity has been reported in the literature, largely due to excessive application following a bath in a child with eczema (Turner, 2009).

MEDICATION SAFETY

Ensuring effective and safe delivery of drugs to fetuses and pediatric patients involves understanding the physiologic changes that occur throughout childhood and pregnancy. Since the start of the Institute for Safe Medication Practices in 1994, pediatric medication safety movements have progressed over time. In 2004, the Institute of Healthcare Improvement (IHI) introduced

the 100,000 Lives Campaign to protect patients from medical harm. Two years later, the IHI launched the 5 Million Lives Campaign with a pediatric initiative to reduce adverse drug events and decrease harm from high-alert medications (i.e., anticoagulants, sedatives, opioids, insulin) (Institute of Healthcare Improvement, 2006). The Joint Commission Sentinel Event Alert stated that harm caused by medication errors is three times greater in pediatric patients than adults (The Joint Commission, 2008). As a result, The Joint Commission Issue 39 recommends initiatives to prevent medication errors and suggests risk reduction strategies. **Box 4.1** gives some recommendations to assist health care professionals in reducing medication errors (American Academy of Pediatrics, 2003; The Joint Commission, 2008). In the future, pediatric pharmacotherapy will evolve with additional legislation and safety movements.

CONCLUSION

In summary, pediatric, pregnancy, and lactation pharmacotherapy poses a unique challenge. The lack of medications approved by the FDA, insufficient literature resources, pharmacokinetic parameters compared to adults and nonpregnant women, individual drug dosing calculations, lack of dosage forms, and inappropriate drug delivery systems are a few examples (Levine et al., 2001). Although the health benefits of breast-feeding are established, there remain a few medications that are unsafe to use during breast-feeding. As with medication use during pregnancy, the risk–benefit ratio needs to be assessed. Choice of the best medication to treat the maternal condition needs to be balanced against the risk of adverse effects to the infant. Furthermore, ensuring medication safety practices and legislations will allow for safe and effective medication therapy to this vulnerable medical population.

BOX 4.1   Preventing Pediatric Medication Errors

American Academy of Pediatrics

- Maintain an up-to-date patient allergy profile.
- Confirm the validity of a patient's weight for medications that are dosed by body weight (or BSA for medications dosed by BSA).
- State specific dosage strengths or formulation.
- Do not use abbreviations for drug names or patient instructions.
- Avoid using abbreviations for dosage units.
- Use a zero before a decimal point.
- Avoid a zero after a decimal point.

BSA, body surface area.

The Joint Commission

- Standardize concentrations of high-alert medications (i.e., heparin, insulin, or narcotics).
- Utilize oral syringes to administer liquid formulations.
- Create drug order pathways for protocols.
- Collaborate and educate all health care members involved with the patients' care.
- Use technology such as automated dispensing cabinets, smart infusion pumps, bar coding.

CASE STUDY 1

M.T. is an 18-month-old, 20-kg male who presents to the emergency department in status epilepticus, which has continued for approximately 20 minutes. He was brought to the emergency department from a small community via a family vehicle. He has not received any care at this point. The nursing staffs have attempted several intravenous line insertions but were unable to gain access. M.T. continues to convulse without interruption (Learning Objective 1).

1. Discuss the advantages and disadvantages of the different routes of administrations of medications available to treat M.T.

2. You prescribe a rescue medication for M.T.'s mom to use at home in the event M.T. has another seizure. Discuss some advantages of utilizing the mucosal route of administration for at home administration.

3. During the follow-up clinic visit after his hospital admission, Mom explains that M.T. has been having rashes all over his body. You evaluate the rash and determine that it is eczema and want to prescribe a topical steroid. Discuss some considerations regarding the absorption of topical medications in pediatric patients.

Bibliography

Starred references are cited in the text.

*American Academy of Pediatrics. (1997). Alternative routes of drug administration—Advantages and disadvantages (subject review). *Pediatrics*, *100*, 143–152.

*American Academy of Pediatrics. (2003). Prevention of medication errors in the pediatric inpatient setting. *Pediatrics*, *112*, 431–436.

*American Academy of Pediatrics. (2011). The use of systemic and topical fluoroquinolones. *Pediatrics*, *128*, e1034–e1045.

*American Academy of Pediatrics. (2016). The use of systemic and topical fluoroquinolones. *Pediatrics*, *138*, e20162706.

*Anonymous. (1972). American Academy of Pediatrics committee on fetus and newborn: Hexachlorophene and skin care of newborn infants. *Pediatrics*, *49*, 625–626.

*Bond, J. A. (1993). Metabolism and elimination of inhaled drugs and airborne chemicals from the lungs. *Pharmacology and Toxicology*, *72*, 23–47.

*Briggs, C. G., Freeman, R. K., Tovers, C. V., et al. (2017). *Drugs in pregnancy and lactation: A reference guide to fetal and neonatal risk* (11th ed.). Philadelphia, PA: Wolters Kluwer.

*Brigo, F., Nardone, R., Tezzon, F., et al. (2015). Nonintravenous midazolam versus intravenous or rectal diazepam for the treatment of early status epilepticus: A systemic review with meta-analysis. *Epilepsy and Behavior*, *25*, pii: S1525-5050(15)00090-6.

*Casele, H. L., Laifer, S. A., Woelkers, D. A., et al. (1999). Changes in the pharmacokinetics of the low-molecular-weight heparin enoxaparin sodium during pregnancy. *American Journal of Obstetrics and Gynecology*, *181*, 1113–1117.

*Cavell, B. (1981). Gastric emptying in infants fed human milk or infant formula. *Acta Paediatrica Scandinavica*, *70*, 639–641.

Centers for Disease Control and Prevention. (2014). Treating for two: Data and statistics. Updated: February 3, 2020. Retrieved from https://www.cdc.gov/pregnancy/meds/treatingfortwo/index.html on February 14, 2020.

Department of Health and Human Services. Food and Drug Administration. 21 CFR Part 201. Content and Format of Labeling Human Prescription Drug and Biological Products: Requirements for Pregnancy and Lactation Labeling. Published December 4, 2014. Retrieved from https://www.govinfo.gov/content/pkg/FR-2014-12-04/pdf/2014-28241.pdf on July 20, 2015.

*Deren, J. S. (1971). Development of structure and function of the fetal and newborn stomach. *American Journal of Clinical Nutrition*, *24*, 144–159.

*Dicke, J. M. (1989). Teratology: Principles and practice. *Medical Clinics of North America*, *73*, 567–582.

*Dillon, A. E., Wagner, C. L., Wiest, D., et al. (1997). Drug therapy in the nursing mother. *Obstetrics and Gynecology Clinics of North America*, *24*, 676–697.

Erdmann, F., Frederiksen, L.E., Bonaventure, A., et al. (2020). Childhood cancer: Survival, treatment modalities, late effects and improvements over time. *Cancer Epidemiol*. Epub ahead of print. PMID: 32461035.

*Fok, T. F., Monkman, S., Dolovich, M., et al. (1996). Efficacy of aerosol medication delivery from a metered-dose inhaler versus jet nebulizer in infants with bronchopulmonary dysphasia. *Pediatric Pulmonology*, *21*, 301–309.

*Fredericksen, M. C. (2001). Physiologic changes in pregnancy and their effect on drug disposition. *Seminars in Perinatology*, *25*(3), 120–123.

*Friis-Hansen, B. (1957). Changes in body water compartment during growth. *Acta Paediatrica*, *46*(Suppl. 110), 1–68.

*Global Initiative for Asthma. (2019). Global strategy for asthma management and prevention. Retrieved from https://ginasthma.org/wp-content/uploads/2019/07/GINA-2019-Appendix-wms.pdf on February 14, 2020.

*Graves, N. M., & Kriel, R. L. (1987). Rectal administration of antiepileptic drugs in children. *Pediatric Neurology*, *3*, 321–326.

Guyton, A. C., & Hall, J. C. (1996). *Human Physiology and Mechanisms of Disease* (6th ed.). Philadelphia, PA: Saunders.

*Haile, C. A. (1977). Chloramphenicol toxicity. *Southern Medical Journal*, *70*, 479–480.

Hales, C.M., Carroll, M.D., Fryar, C.D., et al. (2017). Prevalence of obesity among adults and youth: United States, 2015–2016. NCHS Data Brief. 288, 1–8.

*Hosseini Jahromi, S. A., Hosseini Valami, S. M., Adeli, N., et al. (2012). Comparison of the effects of intranasal midazolam versus different doses of intranasal ketamine on reducing preoperative pediatric anxiety: A prospective randomized clinical trial. *Journal of Anesthesia*, *26*, 878–882.

*Hughes, H. L., & Kahl, L. K. (2017). *The Harriet Lane handbook* (21st ed.). San Francisco, CA: Elsevier.

*Institute of Healthcare Improvement. (2006). Protecting 5 million lives from harm. Retrieved from http://www.ihi.org/IHI/Programs/Campaign/Campaign.htm?TabId=1 on August 16, 2010.

*Jew, R. K., Soo-Hoo, W., Erush, S. C., et al. (2016). *Extemporaneous formulations for pediatric, geriatric, and special needs patients* (3rd ed.). Bethesda, MD: American Society of Hospital Pharmacists.

*Juchau, M. R., & Choa, S. T. (1983). Drug metabolism by the human fetus. In M. Gibaldi & L. Prescott (Eds.), *Handbook of clinical pharmacokinetics* (pp. 58–78). New York, NY: Adis.

*Kearns, G. L. (1995). Pharmacogenetics and development: Are infants and children at increased risk for adverse outcomes? *Current Opinion in Pediatrics*, *7*, 220–233.

*Kelly, H. W., Sternberg, A. L., Lescher, R., et al. (2012). Effect of inhaled glucocorticoids in childhood on adult height. *New England Journal of Medicine*, *367*, 904–912.

*Kennedy, M. J., Jellerson, K. D., Smow, M. Z., et al. (2013). Challenges in the pharmacological management of obesity and secondary dyslipidemia in children and adolescents. *Pediatric Drugs*, *15*, 335–342.

*Kimberlin, D. W., Brady, M. T., Jackson, M. A., et al. (2018). *Red book: 2018 report of the committee on infectious diseases* (31st ed.). Elk Grove Village, IL: American Academy of Pediatrics.

*Klein, E. J., Brown, J. C., Kobayashi, A., et al. (2011). A randomized clinical trial comparing oral, aerosolized intranasal, and aerosolized buccal midazolam. *Annals of Emergency Medicine*, 58, 323–329.

*Koren, G., Pastuszak, A., & Ito, S. (1998). Drugs in pregnancy. *New England Journal of Medicine*, 338, 1128–1137.

*Kraemer, K., (1997). Placental transfer of drugs. *Neonatal Network*, 16(2), 65–67.

*Levine, S. R., Cohen, M. R., Blanchard, N. R., et al. (2001). Guidelines for preventing medication errors in pediatrics. *Journal of Pediatric Pharmacologic Therapies*, 6, 426–442.

*Linday, L., Dobkin, J. F., Wang, T. C., et al. (1987). Digoxin inactivation by the gut flora in infancy and childhood. *Pediatrics*, 79, 544–548.

*Lindenbaum, J., Rund, D. G., Butler, V. P., et al. (1981). Inactivation of digoxin by gut flora; reversal by antibiotic therapy. *New England Journal of Medicine*, 305, 789–794.

*Loebstein, R., Lalkin, A., & Koren, G. (1997). Pharmacokinetic changes during pregnancy and their clinical relevance. *Clinical Pharmacokinetics*, 33, 328–343.

*Lone, A., & Pederson, S. (2000). Effect of long-term treatment with inhaled budesonide on adult height in children with asthma. *New England Journal of Medicine*, 343, 1064–1069.

*Matson, K. L., Horton, E. R., & Capino, A. C. (2017). Medication dosage in overweight and obese children. *Journal of Pediatric Pharmacology and Therapeutics*, 22(1), 81–83.

*Metry, D. W., & Herbert, A. A. (2000). Topical therapies and medications in the pediatric patient. *Pediatric Clinics of North America*, 47, 867–876.

*MICROMEDEX® Solutions (electronic version). (2020). Truven Health Analytics, Greenwood Village, Colorado. Retrieved from http://www.micromedexsolutions.com/home/dispatch on February 14, 2020.

*Mitchell, A. A., Gilboa, S. M., Werler, M. M., et al. (2011). Medication use during pregnancy, with particular focus on prescription drugs: 1976–2008. *American Journal of Obstetrics and Gynecology*, 205(51), e1–8.

*Morselli, P. L., Franco-Morselli, R., & Bossi, L. (1980). Clinical pharmacokinetics in newborns and infants: Age-related differences and therapeutic implications. *Clinical Pharmacokinetics*, 5, 485–527.

*Nahata, M. C., & Pai, V. B. (2018). *Pediatric drug formulations* (7th ed.). Cincinnati, OH: Harvey Whitney.

*Neofax® (electronic version). (2020). Truven Health Analytics, Greenwood Village, Colorado. Retrieved from http://neofax.micromedexsolutions.com/neofax/neofax.php on February 13, 2020.

*Ogden, C. L., Carroll, M. D., Curtin, L. R., et al. (2010). Prevalence of high body mass index in U.S. children and adolescents, 2007–2008. *Journal of the American Medical Association*, 303, 242–249.

Pernia, S., & DeMaagd, G. (2016). The new pregnancy and lactation labeling rule. *Pharmacy and Therapeutics*, 41(11), 713–715.

*Phelps, S. J. (2018). *Teddy bear book: Pediatric injectable drugs* (11th ed.). Bethesda, MD: American Society of Hospital Pharmacists.

*Philipson, A. (1977). Pharmacokinetics of ampicillin during pregnancy. *Journal of Infectious Diseases*, 136, 370–376.

*Pinheiro, E. A., & Stika, C. S. (2020). Drugs in pregnancy: Pharmacologic and physiologic changes that affect clinical care. *Seminars in Perinatology*. https://doi.org/10.1016/j.semperi.2020.151221

*Rayburn, W. F. (1997). Chronic medical disorders during pregnancy. *Journal of Reproductive Medicine*, 42, 1–24.

*Rubin, M. I., Bruck, E., & Rapoport, M. J. (1949). Maturation of renal function in childhood: Clearance studies. *Journal of Clinical Investigation*, 28, 1144–1162.

*Rutter, N. (1987). Percutaneous drug absorption in the newborn: Hazards and uses. *Clinical Perinatology*, 14, 911–930.

*Sachs, H., & Committee on Drugs. (2013). The transfer of drugs and therapeutics into human breast milk: An update on selected topics. *Pediatrics*, 132, e796–e809.

*Sacks, G. S., & Brown, R. O. (1994). Drug-nutrient interactions in patients receiving nutritional support. *Drug Therapy*, 24, 35–42.

*Salmon, B., Wilson, N. M., & Silverman, M. (1990). How much aerosol reaches the lungs of wheezy infants and toddlers? *Archives of Disease in Childhood*, 65, 401–404.

*Shankar, S. M., Marina, N., Hudson, M. M., et al. (2008). Monitoring for cardiovascular disease in survivors of childhood cancer: Report from the cardiovascular disease task force of the children's oncology group. *Pediatrics*, 121, 387–396.

*Stewart, C. F., & Hampton, E. M. (1987). Effect of maturation on drug disposition in pediatric patients. *Clinical Pharmacy*, 6, 548–564.

*Taketomo, C. K., Hodding, J. H., & Kraus, D. M. (2019). *Pediatric dosage handbook* (26th ed.). Hudson, OH: Lexi-Comp.

*Thakker, A., & Shanbag, P. (2013). A randomized controlled trial of intranasal-midazolam versus intravenous-diazepam for acute childhood seizures. *Journal of Neurology*, 260, 470–474.

*The Joint Commission. (2008). Preventing pediatric medication errors. Retrieved from http://www.jointcommission.org/sentinelevents/sentinelevalert/sea_39.htm on February 13, 2020.

*Trissel, L., Ashworth, L. D., & Ashworth, J. (2018). *Trissel's stability of compounded formulations* (6th ed.). Washington, DC: American Pharmacist Association.

*Turner, J. W. (2009). Death of a child from topical diphenhydramine. *American Journal of Forensic Medical Pathology*, 30, 380–381.

*U.S. Food and Drug Administration. (1998a). Rules and regulations. *Federal Register*, 63(231), 66631–66672.

*U.S. Food and Drug Administration. (1998b). *FDA talk paper*. Rockville, MD: Author.

*U.S. Food and Drug Administration. (2018). FDA Drug Safety Communication: FDA restricts use of prescription codeine pain and cough medicines and tramadol pain medicines in children; recommends against use in breast-feeding women. Retrieved from https://www.fda.gov/drugs/drug-safety-and-availability/fda-drug-safety-communication-fda-restricts-use-prescription-codeine-pain-and-cough-medicines-and on February 13, 2020.

van Donge, T., Evers, K., Koch, G., van den Anker, J., & Pfister, M. (2019). Clinical pharmacology and pharmacometrics to better understand physiological changes during pregnancy and neonatal life. In W. Kiess, M. Schwab, & van den Anker J. (Eds.), *Handbook of experimental pharmacology*. Berlin, Heidelberg: Springer.

*Yaffe, S. J., & Juchau, M. R. (1974). Perinatal pharmacology. *Annual Review of Pharmacology*, 14, 219–238.

*Yankowitz, J., & Niebyl, J. R. (2001). *Drug therapy in pregnancy* (3rd ed.). Philadelphia, PA: Lippincott Williams & Wilkins.

*Zempsky, W. T. (2008). Pharmacologic approaches for reducing venous access pain in children. *Pediatrics*, 122, S140–S153.

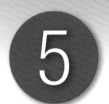

5 Pharmacotherapy Principles in Older Adults

Richard G. Stefanacci

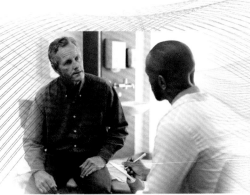
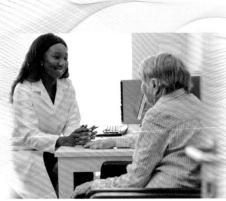
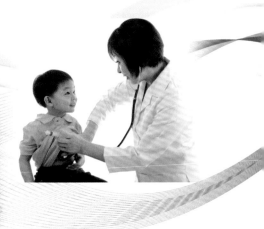

Learning Objectives

1. Describe the various physiological changes that occur in the older adult that affect pharmacokinetic and pharmacodynamics responses.
2. Identify at least four drugs that are problematic to use in the older adult.
3. Discuss safe prescribing practices for the older adult.
4. Describe the behavioral and psychological symptoms of dementia.

INTRODUCTION

While the science governing pharmacotherapy in older adults has largely remained the same for the past several years, what has significantly changed is the complexity of the environment. Today, the number and frailty of the older adult population is far "more" in every sense than ever before. The delivery system has changed, with providers now being placed at risk for clinical and financial outcomes, as well as new emerging technologies that are impacting the delivery of care, for example, the analysis of big data from electronic medical records, claims, and other data sources. Technology has also brought forward new therapies, especially for rare diseases as well as the ability to more accurately diagnose and stage patients. A strong appreciation of these environmental changes is critical to producing positive outcomes from pharmacotherapy (**Box 5.1**).

Older adults are the most pharmacotherapeutically challenging population because of the requirement to take into consideration their unique physiology and other factors in the face of the need to treat multiple chronic comorbid conditions

as well as managing within the current complex environment previously mentioned. This warrants an understanding of aging and its effects on the body. Some of the other factors impacting this population include changes such as cognitive and social issues affecting proper adherence, resulting in suboptimal outcomes. In addition, part of this challenge is the fact that many pharmaceuticals have not been tested in this population. As a result, practitioners need to rely on their knowledge of basic principles of pharmacotherapy and monitor on an individual patient basis.

This expertise of managing pharmacotherapy in the older adults is crucial given that the older population is the fastest growing of any age group. The 2016 American Community Survey (ACS) estimated the number of people in the United States aged 65 and over to be 49.2 million. Of them, more than half (28.75 million or 58%) were aged 65 to 74. The 75-to-84 age group share of the older population was around 14.3 million or 29%—more than double the number and proportion (6.3 million or 13%) for those 85 and older. There were more females than males among the older population (ACS, 2018). The latest numbers available from the Centers for Disease Control and Prevention (CDC) can be obtained through the CDC Wide-ranging ONline Data for Epidemiologic Research (CDC WONDER). This application makes many health-related data sets, such as demographic information, available to CDC staff, public health departments, researchers, and others. The data are meant to help with public health research, decision-making, priority setting, program evaluation, and resource allocation (**Table 5.1**).

A report from the National Center for Health Statistics, Division of Vital Statistics, at the CDC finds that after a slight increase in overall life expectancy from 78.7 years in 2011 to 78.8 years in 2012, life expectancy is back to 78.7 years.

Demographics
- Increasing number of older adults
- Increasing frailty through improved management of previously terminal conditions such as HIV, CHF, cancers

Health Systems
- More physicians employed by health systems
- Health systems and providers at risk for clinical and financial outcomes

Technology
- Analytic capacity of big data
- Use of electronic medical records
- Use of telemedicine and consultative services
- Genomics and advanced diagnostics

CHF, congestive heart failure. HIV, human immunodeficiency virus.

The difference in life expectancy between the white and black populations was 3.5 years in 2017 (Arias & Xu, 2019). While decreasing in frequency, cancer, heart disease, and stroke remain significant health issues for older adults, which is a concern given the rise in obesity.

The consequences of longevity are evidenced by the rising number of older adults living with multiple chronic diseases, contributing to disability, frailty, and decline in function and presenting significant challenges for medical management (Norris et al., 2008). According to a recent report, nearly 80% of Medicare beneficiaries have at least two chronic conditions and more than 60% have at least three chronic conditions (DuGoff et al., 2014). Experts have estimated that 26% of the U.S. population will be living with multiple chronic conditions by 2030 (Anderson, 2010). Although multimorbidity is not limited to older adults, its prevalence increases substantially with age. In a cross-sectional study that included 1.7 million patients in Scotland, Barnett and colleagues found that 30.4% of the population aged 45 to 64 years, 64.9% of people aged 65 to 84 years, and 81.5% of people aged 85 years or older reported at least two chronic conditions. This has led to an increased use of health care utilization.

Treating multiple problems with prescription as well as over-the-counter (OTC) medications can result in adverse drug reactions (ADRs) and interactions related to changes produced by aging. Problems of polypharmacy (the use of an inappropriate amount and combination of medications to treat a host of medical conditions), improper dosing for an older adult, and a lack of understanding by adults about medications can lead to significant but preventable adverse effects, such as falls, fractures, and delirium. This chapter discusses basic physiologic changes of aging, proper prescribing principles, and social concepts pertaining to safe medication use for the older adult.

BODY CHANGES AND AGING

Everybody is affected by the aging process, although homeostasis is often maintained despite less-than-optimal functioning of organ systems. Certain systems are more vitally affected by aging and play significant roles in the pharmacokinetic and pharmacodynamic changes in drug effects. **Box 5.2** summarizes the impact of aging on the pharmacokinetics of drugs.

Absorption

Older individuals frequently have oropharyngeal muscle dysmotility and altered swallowing of food. Reductions in esophageal peristalsis and lower esophageal sphincter (LES) pressures are also more common in the aged. Delayed motility and gastric emptying have been reported in some cases; as well, the propulsive motility of the colon is decreased, which may impact absorption. Decreased gastric secretions (acid, pepsin) and impairment of the mucous–bicarbonate barrier are frequently described in the older population and may impact absorption. The prolonged transit time in the gastrointestinal (GI) tract still allows for adequate drug absorption.

Distribution

Muscle that makes up lean body tissue decreases in the older adult, shifting to increased fat stores, and body water content decreases by 10% to 15% by age 80. Aging results in some reduction in serum albumin (by approximately 20%), leading to an increase in free drug concentration of drugs such as warfarin (Coumadin) and phenytoin (Dilantin).

There are two important plasma-binding proteins in drug metabolism: albumin and alpha$_1$-acid glycoprotein. Albumin has an affinity for acid compounds or drugs such as warfarin, whereas alpha$_1$-acid glycoprotein binds more readily with lipophilic and alkaline drugs such as propranolol (Inderal). The effects of chronic disease, nutritional deficits, immobility, and age-related liver changes contribute to the changes in serum proteins. The significance of decreased serum proteins is realized when highly protein-bound drugs compete for decreased protein-binding sites. The result can be greater levels of free or unbound circulating drug and, therefore, potential toxicity.

Body mass changes may lead to changes in total body content of drugs in older adults. A water-soluble drug (low volume of distribution [V_d]) is taken up more readily by lean tissue or muscle and attains higher serum concentrations in adults with less body water or lean tissue. Conversely, a lipid-soluble drug is retained in body fat, resulting in a higher V_d for some drugs. Coupled with a decrease or no change in total body clearance, this increase in V_d can lead to increased half-lives and drug accumulation in older adults. For example, diazepam (Valium) has a half-life ($t_{1/2}$) of approximately 20 hours in a young adult, but its $t_{1/2}$ can exceed 70 hours in the older adult. In addition, some drugs, such as tricyclic antidepressants (TCAs) and long-acting benzodiazepines, pass more readily through the blood–brain barrier, causing more pronounced central nervous

TABLE 5.1

Population by Age and Sex: 2012

Age	Both Sexes		Male		Female	
	Number	Percent	Number	Percent	Number	Percent
All ages	3,24,356	100.0	1,59,028	100.0	1,65,328	100.0
Under 55 years	2,29,813	70.9	1,15,239	72.5	1,14,573	69.3
55–59 years	21,163	6.5	10,046	6.3	11,117	6.7
60–64 years	20,592	6.3	9,819	6.2	10,773	6.5
65–69 years	17,356	5.4	8,198	5.2	9,158	5.5
70–74 years	14,131	4.4	6,691	4.2	7,440	4.5
75–79 years	9,357	2.9	4,233	2.7	5,124	3.1
80–84 years	6,050	1.9	2,519	1.6	3,532	2.1
85 years and over	5,893	1.8	2,282	1.4	3,611	2.2
Under 55 years	2,29,813	70.9	1,15,239	72.5	1,14,573	69.3
55 years and over	94,543	29.1	43,789	27.5	50,755	30.7
Under 60 years	2,50,976	77.4	1,25,286	78.8	1,25,690	76.0
60 years and over	73,380	22.6	33,742	21.2	39,638	24.0
Under 62 years	2,59,319	79.9	1,29,278	81.3	1,30,041	78.7
62 years and over	65,037	20.1	29,749	18.7	35,287	21.3
Under 65 years	2,71,568	83.7	1,35,105	85.0	1,36,463	82.5
65 years and over	52,788	16.3	23,923	15.0	28,865	17.5
Under 75 years	3,03,055	93.4	1,49,994	94.3	1,53,061	92.6
75 years and over	21,301	6.6	9,034	5.7	12,267	7.4

Note: Details may not sum to totals because of rounding.

The U.S. Census Bureau reviewed this data product for unauthorized disclosure of confidential information and approved the disclosure avoidance practices applied to this release. CBDRB-FY20-027.

Numbers in thousands. Civilian noninstitutionalized population. Plus armed forces living off post or with their families on post.

Source: U.S. Census Bureau, Current Population Survey, Annual Social and Economic Supplement, 2019. Internet release date: April 2020.

system (CNS) effects. Older adults who are treated for depression and anxiety may experience fatigue and confusion from drug therapy because antidepressant and antianxiety agents more readily cross their blood–brain barrier.

Elimination

The liver is the major organ of drug metabolism in the body. With aging comes a decrease in blood flow and liver size. However, in the absence of disease, function is maintained. Decreased size and hepatic blood flow may slow the clearance of certain drugs, and reduced dosages may be required (**Box 5.3**). This is particularly important for drugs with high hepatic extraction ratios. Phase I metabolism, particularly oxidation, is affected by aging. The result is decreased oxidation of drugs, which in turn results in a decreased total body clearance. Phase II metabolism of drugs by conjugation, which promotes drug elimination by breaking the drug into water-soluble components, is not affected by age.

After the liver, the kidneys are the most important organs for drug metabolism and excretion. After age 40, renal blood flow declines and the glomerular filtration rate (GFR) drops approximately 1% a year and accelerates with advancing age. Function is usually maintained despite decreased filtration unless illness or disease overstresses the kidney (Kelleher & Lindeman, 2003). In older adults, drugs excreted primarily by the kidney are given in smaller doses, or the time between doses is extended.

BOX 5.2 Summary of Pharmacokinetic Changes Caused by Aging

Absorptive Changes
Decreased blood flow
Increased gastric pH
Delayed gastric emptying
Distribution Changes
Decreased albumin
Decreased lean body mass
Increased total body fat
Decreased total body water
Metabolic Changes
Decreased liver blood flow
Decreased liver mass
Decreased enzymatic activity
Excretion Changes
Decreased glomerular filtration
Decreased secretion

BOX 5.3 Drugs with Reduced Hepatic Metabolism in Older Adults

Amlodipine	Nifedipine
Codeine	Phenytoin
Diltiazem	Propranolol
Ibuprofen	Quinidine
Meperidine	Theophylline
Morphine	Verapamil
Naproxen	

A serum creatinine level alone cannot be used to estimate renal function in the aging person because reductions in lean body mass result in decreased rates of creatinine formation. This, coupled with the decreased GFR, makes the serum creatinine appear normal. It cannot be assumed that the GFR is normal from a normal serum creatinine value. The most accurate means of measuring renal function is a 24-hour urine test for creatinine clearance; however, this is not standard procedure before ordering a medication. When there is a need to determine a drug choice in the setting of a potential reduction in creatinine clearance, the Cockcroft-Gault or the Modification of Diet in Renal Disease (MDR) equation (see Chapter 2) is used, which provides an estimate based on age, weight, and serum creatinine level with an adjustment for sex. **Table 5.2** lists drugs eliminated by the kidney and recommended dosage adjustments based on estimated creatinine clearance.

PHARMACODYNAMIC CHANGES IN THE OLDER ADULT

Many of the changes that occur due to aging affect major organ systems and therefore affect the pharmacokinetic disposition of the drug. However, the clinician also must consider the impact drugs have on the aging body: the pharmacodynamic effect. Although few pieces of data are available regarding age-related pharmacodynamic changes in older adults, it is known that the older adult may be more sensitive to drug–receptor interactions, because of either increased sensitivity of the receptor to the drug or decreased capacity to respond to drug-induced innervation of receptors. In addition, the number or affinity of receptors may be reduced. Nevertheless, it is commonly accepted that the CNS effects of drugs appear to be exaggerated in the older patient. Particularly egregious are the agents with anticholinergic effects, such as the TCAs, antihistamines, and antispasmodics. The anticholinergic effect induced by these agents can lead to excessive dry mouth, blurred vision, constipation, and even an exacerbation of benign prostatic hyperplasia in men. Caution should be used if these agents are prescribed at all.

Similarly, the sedative effects of agents may be intensified in older adults. The benzodiazepines and potent analgesic agents are examples of drugs to which older adults are particularly susceptible. Overprescribing, or typical prescribing without considering the potential for exaggerated effect, can lead to oversedation and a greater risk of falls and fractures.

The cardiovascular system also can be affected by changes due to aging. Orthostatic hypotension is more common in the older adult because of a loss of the baroreceptor reflex and changes in cerebral blood flow. Moreover, drugs that lower blood pressure or decrease cardiac output put the older patient at risk for a syncopal episode.

POLYPHARMACY

Polypharmacy is a significant factor in the morbidity and mortality of older adults. Increasing age puts the person at risk for multiple chronic illnesses, many of which require drug therapy For example, osteoarthritis (OA) is the most common joint disorder in the United States. Symptomatic knee OA occurs in 10% of men and 13% of women aged 60 years or older. The costs in terms of morbidity are staggering (Zhang & Jordan, 2010). Chronic stiffness and pain from arthritis have an impact on function, prompting the routine use of nonsteroidal antiinflammatory drugs (NSAIDs) and aspirin products. Long-term use of NSAIDs lowers the prostaglandin level in the GI tract, which may result in esophagitis, peptic ulcerations, GI hemorrhage, and GI perforation. In an older adult, treatment with histamine-2 blockers or proton pump inhibitors to relieve the side effects of aspirin or other NSAIDs may cause additional side effects, such as confusion and mental status changes, which in turn require more treatment. This demonstrates how easily

TABLE 5.2

Examples of Dose Adjustments Based on Estimated Creatinine Clearance

Drug	Usual Oral Dose (Nonrenally Impaired)	Dose Based on Estimated CrCl*		
		CrCl >50 mL/min	CrCl 10–50 mL/min	CrCL <10 mL/min
Amantadine	100 mg q12h	Usual dose	Increase interval to q24–72h	Increase interval to q7d
Amoxicillin	250–500 mg q8h	Usual dose	Increase interval to q12h	Increase interval to q24h
Cefaclor	250 mg TID	Usual dose	Decrease dose to 50%–100% of usual	Decrease dose to 50% of usual
Ciprofloxacin	250–750 mg q12h	Usual dose	Reduce dose to 50% of usual	Reduce dose to 33% of usual or extend to q24h
Codeine	30–60 mg q4–6h	Usual dose	Reduce dose to 75% of usual	Reduce dose to 50% of usual
Digoxin[†]	0.125–0.5 mg q24h	Usual dose	Reduce dose to 25%–75% of usual *or* increase interval to q48h	Reduce dose to 10%–25% of usual
Enalapril, gabapentin[†]	5–10 mg q12h 400 mg TID (for CrCl >60)	Usual dose 300 mg BID (for CrCl 30–60 mL/min)	Reduce dose to 75% of usual 300 mg daily (for CrCl 15–30 mL/min)	Reduce dose to 50% of usual 300 mg every other day (for CrCl 15 mL/min)
Nadolol	80–120 mg/d	Usual dose	Reduce dose to 50% of usual	Reduce dose to 25% of usual
Procainamide[‡]	350–400 mg q3–4h	Usual dose	Increase interval to q6–12h	Increase interval to q8–24h
Ranitidine	150 mg q12h or 300 mg qhs	Usual dose	Decrease dose to 50% of usual *or* increase interval to q24h	Decrease dose to 25% of usual *or* increase interval to q48h

* Dose adjustments based on actual creatinine clearance or creatinine clearance estimated by the Cockcroft-Gault formula (see Chapter 2).

† These drugs are best monitored using actual drug levels, and dose adjustments should be made based on these results.

‡ Based on manufacturer's information.

adverse events occur and snowball in an older patient. ADRs account for 30% of hospital admissions for persons older than age 65; approximately 106,000 deaths are attributed to medication problems. Sadly, 15% to 65% of these events are preventable (Nair et al., 2016; Shiyanbola & Farris, 2010) by avoiding potentially inappropriate medications, effective communication, and patient education.

Several factors contribute to polypharmacy. Among them are the varied symptoms and complaints associated with multiple chronic illnesses. In addition, adults often believe that a "pill will fix what ails them," and the health care provider feels pressured to "prescribe something" to satisfy the patient's expectations of a prescription for medication. When a particular medication regimen is unsuccessful, the health care provider typically prescribes another drug; this is referred to as the prescribing cascade. Dr. Jerry Gurwitz, a noted geriatrician, has warned that "any symptom in an elderly patient should be considered a drug side effect until proved otherwise," although his wife, Leslie Fine, a pharmacist, is actually believed to have first described this approach (Smith, 2013).

Polypharmacy is also the effect from many older adults stockpiling their discontinued medications in case they may be needed again—primarily because of the cost of prescription drugs. Many providers who visit older adults in their homes have seen evidence of stockpiled medications. Some older adults keep a drawer or cabinet full of old prescription drug bottles. Some contain the same medication, differing only in brand name. Some adults may place a current medication (prescription or OTC) in a labeled prescription bottle that was used for another drug. In addition, the stockpile may reveal prescription bottles for other family members. Adults may be sharing medications or may have received medications from others who believed that the drug that helped them would help the patient.

Other sources of polypharmacy are "polyproviders." Many older adults see multiple specialists for various chronic diseases. Medications prescribed without the provider carefully reviewing the patient's other medications can lead to drug overuse and complications. Without a primary care provider overseeing the care of the older adult seeing multiple specialists, ADRs are sure to occur.

The health care provider sometimes creates a polypharmacy situation because multiple drugs are used to treat several chronic illnesses. The provider who is not astute in the principles of safe geriatric prescribing practices may create avoidable side effects and complications. In addition, the patient, who may be a great consumer of OTC medications or home remedies, often self-prescribes without knowing the consequences of mixing these treatments with current prescription drugs.

Drug Interactions in the Older Adult

Because of normal, age-related physiologic changes, the older adult is at greater risk for complications from medications. Complications related to drug–disease, drug–drug, and drug–food interaction are all commonly encountered. (For more information on drug–drug interactions, see Chapter 3.)

Adverse Drug Reactions

ADRs often result in significant negative health outcomes, such as falls and fractures, costing billions of dollars in hospital and nursing home care (Shiyanbola & Farris, 2010). Although age itself creates a risk for ADRs, polypharmacy and the multiplicity of drugs taken by older adults present the greater risk. The older adult with multiple chronic illnesses and medications must be identified as a potential candidate for ADRs (Fick et al., 2003; Nair et al., 2016). Older women in particular are at great risk for ADRs because they often receive more prescription drugs and have a more significant loss of muscle mass than older men.

There is a paucity of information on safety and efficacy of drugs for the older patient. Most research and clinical trials are performed with younger subjects. It often is difficult or impossible to predict the consequences of a medication for its intended use on an older adult because few pieces of data may be available that specifically apply to the older population. In an effort to better understand the effects of drugs on older adults, the U.S. Food and Drug Administration (FDA) published guidelines in 1997 recommending that older adults be included in clinical trials of drugs specifically being developed to treat prevalent diseases affecting older adults (Murray & Callahan, 2003).

Contributing Lifestyle Factors

Preventing adverse events or failed treatments begins with being aware of potential drug interactions resulting from older adults commonly taking OTC medications and prescription drugs without alerting their health care providers. Additional combinations of foods or nutritional supplements can slow absorption, prolonging the time for medications to reach peak levels (see Chapter 3). Fatty foods, in particular, can increase intestinal drug absorption because of the longer time required to digest a fatty meal. This, in turn, potentially leads to increased drug levels or toxicity.

Alcohol and Other Drugs

The ingestion of alcohol and other drugs can alter the metabolism of many medications in older adults. The combination of comorbid conditions, physiological changes with age, and concomitant medications is often potentiated with alcohol usage. CNS effects such as lethargy and confusion occur, as

does hypotension, when alcohol is combined with nitrates and some cardiovascular drugs. Alcohol can be found in many OTC products such as cough and cold syrups and mouthwashes.

Alcohol use disorder may be overlooked as a potential problem in the older adult, but abuse among community-dwelling (noninstitutionalized) people aged 65 and older has a prevalence of 14% for men and 1.5% for women. High numbers of older alcoholics are treated in emergency departments and medical offices or are hospitalized for medical or psychiatric admissions. Depression, which is more prevalent in the older adult, often coexists with alcohol misuse. Moderate to heavy drinkers older than 65 are 16 times more likely to die of suicide. Practitioners need to be more aware of the potential for alcohol misuse in older adults. Although alcohol use and abuse decline with age, approximately 40% of older adults use alcohol, with between 2% and 4% meeting the criteria for alcohol use disorder. The use of alcohol is anticipated to increase as baby boomers age. The baby boomer cohort has a history of greater alcohol, tobacco, and nonmedical substance usage than previous generations. Life stressors such as retirement, loss of loved ones, dependency, and chronic illness are contributors to potential alcohol misuse. As well, with 11 states legalizing the recreational use of marijuana, it should be expected that older adults will also be among the users. So the inclusion of this potential drug–drug interaction needs to be taken into account as well.

Caffeine and Nicotine Use

Caffeine and nicotine are among some of the most commonly used products that have the potential to interact with certain drugs, thereby altering efficacy and therapeutic drug levels. Besides its presence in coffee, tea, and some sodas, caffeine is found in many OTC drug products. The interaction of caffeine and certain medications may alter drug absorption, cause CNS effects, or decrease drug effectiveness. **Table 5.3** summarizes selected caffeine–medication interactions.

Many older adults have lifelong smoking addictions and are unsuccessful in stopping them. Adults and providers alike are frequently unaware of the effects of nicotine and medications. Nicotine alters the metabolism of many drugs, causes CNS effects, and interferes with platelet activity. **Table 5.4** reviews nicotine medication effects and interactions.

ADHERENCE ISSUES

One reason older adults, similar to all patients, do not achieve the optimum outcome from their treatments is their failure to adhere to the medication regimen. In many cases, prescription drugs are not taken as prescribed: Up to 40% of older adults take their medications improperly. More than 40% of ambulatory adults aged 65 and older take at least 5 medications per week, with 12% taking at least 10 per week. Studies have shown that as the complexity of the medication regime increases, improper drug usage rises proportionately. In some cases, they may not take enough of the medication, either because they think that they will save money by making the prescription last longer

TABLE 5.3

Medication–Caffeine Interactions

Type of Interaction	Example of Interaction Effect
Caffeine-induced increase in gastric acid secretion	Decreased absorption of iron
Caffeine-induced gastrointestinal irritation	Decreased effectiveness of cimetidine; increased gastrointestinal irritation from corticosteroids, alcohol, and analgesics
Altered caffeine metabolism	Prolonged effect of caffeine when combined with ciprofloxacin, estrogen, or cimetidine
Caffeine-induced cardiac arrhythmic effect	Decreased effectiveness of antiarrhythmic medications
Caffeine-induced hypokalemia	Exacerbated hypokalemic effect of diuretics
Caffeine-induced stimulation of CNS	Increased stimulation effects from amantadine, decongestants, fluoxetine, and theophylline
Caffeine-induced increase in excretion of lithium	Decreased effectiveness of lithium

CNS, central nervous system.

TABLE 5.4

Medication–Nicotine Interactions

Type of Interaction	Example of Interaction Effect
Nicotine-induced alteration in metabolism	Decreased efficacy of analgesics, lorazepam, theophylline, aminophylline, beta blockers, and calcium channel blockers
Nicotine-induced vasoconstriction	Increased peripheral ischemic effect of beta blockers
Nicotine-induced CNS stimulation	Decreased drowsiness from benzodiazepines and phenothiazines
Nicotine-induced stimulation of antidiuretic hormone secretion	Fluid retention and decreased effectiveness of diuretics
Nicotine-induced increase in platelet activity	Decreased anticoagulant effectiveness (heparin, warfarin); increased risk of thrombosis with estrogen use
Nicotine-induced increase in gastric acid	Decreased or negated effects of H_2 antagonists (cimetidine, famotidine, nizatidine, ranitidine)

CNS, central nervous system.

or because they believe that the medicine is not needed at the prescribed dose. In other situations, a medication may not be taken if it interferes with the patient's lifestyle, for example, not taking a diuretic for fear of incontinence on certain days.

Cost Factors

Cost is actually becoming less of an issue for some of the more commonly used medications while it is still an issue for this population, especially for older adults requiring innovative biologics. For the more commonly used medications today, many are available in a generic formulation, such as those needed for hypertension, diabetes, and hypercholesterolemia. The addition of the Medicare Part D prescription drug benefit provides older adults drug coverage. When this Medicare benefit was introduced in 2006, there was a coverage gap—more commonly referred to as "the doughnut hole." During the period of this gap in the Medicare Part D benefit, beneficiaries were responsible for 100% of the cost of their medication. As a result of this sudden increase in cost from 25% during the initial benefit period to 100%, many older adults abandoned their medication at the pharmacy counter (Tseng et al., 2009). Follow-on legislation has moved to close the coverage gap, so today it no longer exists: Older adults continue to only be responsible for a maximum of 25% through their benefit until they reach the catastrophic period, where they are only responsible for 5% of the cost of their medication (Stefanacci & Spivack, 2010). The savings on prescription drugs are even greater for older adults with low income who qualify for extra help. These individuals only pay a little over $2 per prescription for generic medications and $6 for branded products. This exact copayment is adjusted annually.

Side Effects

Other reasons for nonadherence to drug treatments include the unpleasant or inconvenient side effects accompanying some medications. Dry mouth, change in taste sensations, fatigue, or frequent urination are reported as reasons for stopping a medication. The form of the medication and ease of administration are reasons as well. Large tablets and capsules may be difficult to swallow. Swallowing problems may be compounded by insufficient fluid being taken with medications. Taking several oral medications at one dosing time with too little fluid may result in the medications "getting stuck," leading to chronic esophageal irritation. Presbyesophagus (the slowing of esophageal motility with advancing age) makes it difficult and frustrating to swallow multiple medications, and it can also lead to choking or aspiration.

Many times, perceived side effects are not truly related to the medications, resulting in an inappropriate discontinuation of a needed therapy. Critical to the management of side effects are education and communication. Education requires that health care providers inform patients of the expected side effects of their medications. Communication is required to assure that patients openly describe their concerns regarding any and all real and perceived side effects. It is only through effective education and communication that side effects are appropriately managed.

Physical and Mental Changes

Functional deficits, especially those affecting the senses, can also challenge adherence to the medication regimen. Poor vision leads to difficulty reading labels and consequently taking the wrong pills or too many of the same pills. Arthritic hands and safety caps can make opening prescription bottles difficult and frustrating for an older adult.

The prevalence of dementia, which manifests in symptoms of cognitive impairment and poor short-term memory and recall, slowly progresses with age, affecting a substantial percentage of those residing in the community. The condition may be unrecognized by the family because the patient may remain seemingly independent and functional despite mental deficits. The family may be fooled into believing the loved one is fine until the condition affects the person's ability to manage basic, daily routines. Unfortunately, the affected older adult is often responsible for taking his or her own medications. Poor memory results in not taking medication properly, forgetting doses, or taking too many doses of the same drug. Approximately 30% of hospital admissions among the older adults are attributed to toxicity from medications or ADRs. Of prescription medications, almost one third are for those aged 65 and older. While technology, including personal mechanical medication management systems, is providing a wide range of solutions to assist in overcoming these challenges, having engaged caregivers is often required to overcome these issues in assuring adherence to therapy.

Self-Medication Issues

The use of OTC drugs and home remedies is another significant issue. Among community dwelling older adults, about as many take nonprescription drugs as take prescription drugs. A review of US data indicates that the average number of OTC drugs taken daily is around 1.8 (Hanlon, 2001). Of more concern is the fact that of patients who reported using an OTC medication 58% did not tell their physicians (Sleath, 2001). NSAIDs for example are one of the most commonly used OTC accounting for a significant number of ADRs (Brahma, 2013). Many OTC medications are taken without the medical provider's awareness in order to treat symptoms patients do not want to report. Family members and friends often borrow medications believed to treat a particular ailment, again without consultation with their medical provider.

The use of herbal preparations contributes to ADRs, especially when taken with prescription medications. Of those over age 65 taking herbal preparations, 49% do not divulge this information to their medical providers, compounding the risk for drug interactions and toxicity.

Many OTC medications are products that were once available only by prescription. Now, despite their decreased strength, the use of these medications, which once required medical supervision and monitoring, presents a potential hazard for side effects.

The most common OTC medications used by the older adult are analgesics, vitamins and minerals, antacids, and laxatives. Cough and cold products and sleeping aids such as Tylenol PM are frequently used by older adults. Combining these products may result in confusion, change in mental status, fluid and electrolyte imbalances, dysrhythmias, and nervousness. Cold medications may worsen hypertension without the patient's knowledge or worsen glucose control in a patient with diabetes.

The older adult must be educated to use OTC drugs safely and to do so only after consulting with the health care provider. If an alternative to drug use is feasible, such as initiating sleep hygiene practices versus taking a sleeping pill, the patient should be encouraged to try these measures first because of their limited negative side effects.

LIFE EXPECTANCY AND GOALS OF CARE

Appreciating an older adult's life expectancy and goals of care is critical for determination of when discontinuation of treatments would be appropriate. To aid in the determination of prognosis, there is a calculator available to health care providers, at www.ePrognosis.org.

The information on ePrognosis is intended as a rough guide to inform health care providers about possible mortality outcomes. This information can assist in making a determination when a medication such as a statin may no longer be appropriate because of a limited life expectancy. This situation is unique to older adults, for in the care of younger adults, discontinuation because of limited effectiveness secondary to a shortened life expectancy is typically not an issue. Understanding this dynamic such that recommendations can be made for discontinuation is essential to prevent unnecessary adverse events from occurring as well as a waste of health care resources.

SPECIAL CONSIDERATIONS IN LONG-TERM CARE

Advanced age and years of multiple illnesses and mental decline result in frailty and disability. Transitioning to a long-term care (LTC) facility occurs when an older adult requires assistance with functions of daily living, such as bathing and dressing, shows cognitive impairment, or has a significant nursing need such as wound care. The national percentage of older adults in nursing homes is about 5%, which rises to 20% for age 85 and older. With a wide array of physical, psychiatric, neurologic, and behavioral problems, the LTC resident is the most complex of all older adults. Consequently, the complexity of prescribing medications for the nursing home resident can be challenging. As a result, there is a federal requirement that all residents of skilled nursing facilities (SNFs) receive a drug regimen review by a consultant pharmacist on a monthly basis. All of these practices described for older adult residents of SNFs apply to those living in the community as well. This is especially true given that LTC needs are increasingly being served in the community. Programs such as the Program of All-Inclusive Care for the Elderly (PACE) service nursing home–eligible older adults in the community. Additionally, states are using home and community waivers to provide LTC services outside of the nursing home. This has forced clinicians to apply LTC practices outside of the nursing home to serve this increasingly community-based frail older adult population.

Falls and Medication

One of the most serious problems in LTC facilities are traumatic falls. Approximately half of nursing home residents fall annually, sustaining fractures and soft tissue and other injuries. Among the multiple causes of falls are medications, in particular psychotropic agents (e.g., sedatives, hypnotics, antidepressants, and neuroleptics). These medications are useful for treating the depression, anxiety, and behavioral problems that are not unusual in the LTC resident. However, their use presents an ongoing treatment challenge. Medication-related falls are often caused by orthostatic hypotension, sedation, extrapyramidal side effects (EPSs), myopathy, and pupil constriction. **Table 5.5** lists drug classes that lead to instability (Hile & Studenski, 2007).

Antipsychotics

Antipsychotics are an ongoing major concern for the Centers for Medicare & Medicaid Services (CMS), to improve the quality of care for SNF residents, especially when it comes to restraints and what they consider inappropriate medications. Again, because of this continuous ongoing concern due to the overuse of psychotropic medications to manage agitation and other behavioral problems associated with dementia—which

goes contrary to the U.S. FDA black box warning—CMS has been propelled to expand oversight on their use. CMS has made several initiatives to decrease the use of antipsychotic medications, including state survey application of unnecessary medication F-tags and quality measures specific to this effort, which have had success. But in an effort to decrease any medication that they consider to be a chemical restraint, CMS is looking to expand regulation in this area. As a result, effective November 28, 2017, CMS announced several regulatory changes for SNFs, including an expanded definition of psychotropic medications and new limitations on the use of as-needed (PRN) psychotropic medications within SNFs.

The definition of a psychotropic medication now includes "any drug that affects brain activities associated with mental processes and behavior" (Centers for Medicare & Medicaid Services, 2017a). These drugs include, but are not limited to, the following drug categories: antipsychotic, antidepressant, antianxiety, hypnotic, as well as medication classes that may affect brain activity. This expanded list of psychotropic medications includes CNS agents, mood stabilizers, anticonvulsants, muscle relaxants, anticholinergic medications, antihistamines, N-methyl-D-aspartate receptor modulators, and OTC natural or herbal products.

For the expanded list of psychotropic medications, CMS has placed 14-day limits on their duration of use when prescribed with PRN orders. Extension of use beyond 14 days can occur if the prescribing practitioner (a) believes it is appropriate to extend the order, (b) documents the clinical rationale for the extension, and (c) includes a specific duration of use. As detailed as these rules are for psychotropic medications, the rules regarding PRN antipsychotics specifically are even more explicit.

For antipsychotics, a 14-day limitation is applied to all PRN orders; as a result, these orders may not be extended beyond the 14-day limit. To continue their use, a new order for the PRN antipsychotic may be written if the prescribing practitioner directly examines and assesses the resident and documents the clinical rationale. This clinical rationale must include the benefit of the medication for that resident. This documentation is required every 14 days for a resident receiving a PRN antipsychotic without exception, including hospice patients. As per section F757 in the Manual (Centers for Medicare & Medicaid Services, 2017b), the continued use of these medications is permitted as long as prescribers heed the following guidance:

> When a resident is experiencing an acute medical problem or psychiatric emergency (e.g., the resident's expression or action poses an immediate risk to the resident or others), medications may be required, as delirium induced psychosis. As always, medications should only be initiated/used in the presence of active clinical symptoms and after nonpharmacological interventions and least restrictive measures have been attempted.

As a result of these expanded rules, many SNFs will likely try to discontinue orders for standing PRN antipsychotic medications. An alternative approach is to assure appropriate use,

TABLE 5.5

Medications That Contribute to Falls

Mechanism	Classes of Medications
Orthostatic hypotension	Antihypertensives, antianginals, Parkinsonian drugs, TCAs, and antipsychotics
Sedation, decreased attention	Benzodiazepines, sedating antihistamines, narcotic analgesics, TCAs, SSRIs, antipsychotics, anticonvulsants, and ethanol
Extrapyramidal side effects	Antipsychotics, metoclopramide, phenothiazines for nausea such as prochlorperazine, and SSRIs
Myopathy	Corticosteroids; colchicine; high-dose statins, especially in combination with fibrates; ethanol; and interferon
Miosis (pupil constriction)	Glaucoma medications, especially pilocarpine

SSRIs, selective serotonin reuptake inhibitors; TCAs, tricyclic antidepressants.

in which the consultant pharmacist can play a lead role with the SNF team taking the following steps:

1. Prevent initiation of inappropriate use of psychotropic medications in residents.
2. Taper and discontinue inappropriate psychotropic medications, to ensure that use of the medications is appropriate and that monitoring and documentation are properly conducted.
3. Improve disruptive behaviors while limiting/diminishing the use of psychotropic medications, by educating and encouraging prescribers and nursing facility staff to adopt a more structured and broader approach to the management of behavioral symptoms.

The team approach to management of older adults with disruptive behaviors should emphasize certain key principles:

- Individuals who exhibit disruptive behaviors should be thoroughly assessed by a qualified health professional.
- The assessment should seek to identify possible underlying causes that may contribute to disruptive behaviors, so that treatment can target the underlying cause.
- Disruptive behaviors should be objectively and quantitatively monitored by caregivers or facility staff and documented on an ongoing basis.
- If the behaviors do not present an immediate and serious threat to the patient or others, the initial approach to management should focus on environmental modifications, behavioral interventions, psychotherapy, or other nonpharmacologic interventions.
- When medicationls are indicated, an appropriate agent should be selected only after consideration of the underlying diagnosis or condition, effectiveness of the medication, and risk of side effects.

Although developed for antipsychotic medications, these practices should be applied to all classes of medications when managing pharmacotherapy in older adults. With all of these changes, it is important that SNFs utilize resources such as consultant pharmacists and medical and nursing directors to develop and implement a process to make sure patients have access to appropriate medications, especially those with less potential for adverse events. The Beers Criteria, a consensus-based document listing potentially inappropriate medications for use in older adults and guidelines for safe prescribing practices, can be used as a guide to assist with this selection process.

Anxiolytics

Anxiety is a problem frequently confronted in the nursing home setting. It may be precipitated by physical causes such as pain, infection, or chronic illness. Other stressors that contribute to anxiety include fatigue or change, such as a change in a daily routine or change of caregiver. An overly stimulating environment or expectations of staff members hurrying the older resident through daily routines may evoke anxiety. Initially, nonpharmacologic measures should be used to assess and ameliorate anxiety; prescribing a medication to relieve anxiety should be a last choice.

Several nonpharmacologic antianxiety treatments may be beneficial. They include establishing daily routines in a structured environment, consistently providing the same caregiver for bathing and hygiene assistance, avoiding overstimulation from activities, limiting social visits, and scheduling quiet time with rest or naps.

When anxiolytic drugs are prescribed, the benzodiazepines are often chosen for adults aged 65 and older. Unfortunately, side effects are prevalent, among which are the discomforts of discontinuing the therapy. Benzodiazepines can impact cognitive function and psychomotor performance in older adults. The patient may experience increased agitation, anxiety, and insomnia. More serious symptoms include tremors, tachycardia, diaphoresis, nausea, vomiting, and alterations in perception, anterograde amnesia, and seizures. The benzodiazepines have a propensity for dependence by accumulating in the older body. For this reason, they should be prescribed for short courses of up to 2 weeks at most.

The older patient receiving benzodiazepine therapy often experiences significant daytime sedation, dizziness, and subsequent falls. Studies indicate that the "oldest old," those older than age 85, have a greater risk for falls with benzodiazepine use (Hartikainen et al., 2007). When a benzodiazepine with a long half-life is prescribed, the fall rate is 10-fold greater than when a benzodiazepine with a short to moderate half-life is prescribed. Benzodiazepines with a long half-life include diazepam and flurazepam (Dalmane); benzodiazepines with a shorter half-life include lorazepam (Ativan), alprazolam (Xanax), and oxazepam (Serax). When a benzodiazepine is prescribed, it should have a short half-life, be for short-term use, and be given in the lowest dose possible.

The selective serotonin reuptake inhibitors (SSRIs), which treat depression, general anxiety, and panic and obsessive–compulsive disorders, are now considered the better choice for treating anxiety in the frail older adult due to their favorable side effect profile (Sheikh & Cassidy, 2003). There is often comorbid depression with anxiety, so an SSRI may treat both conditions, such as sertraline (Zoloft) for panic and depression.

An alternative anxiolytic is buspirone (BuSpar). It is nonsedating and has minimal drug interactions and a slow onset of action, of 2 to 3 weeks. For that reason, it is not indicated for acute anxiety but works well as an add-on drug. Caution must be used with buspirone in adults with Parkinson's disease because EPS can occur. For anxiety with underlying depression and insomnia, trazodone (Desyrel) is an alternative. Because of its sedating properties, it promotes sleep and treats underlying depression that may exacerbate anxiety.

Antidepressants

The prevalence of depression increases with age, as evidenced by 25% of those with chronic illness and a 15% to 25% rate of depression among nursing home residents (Bergman et al., 2009). Older adults with late life depression exhibit more psychotic symptoms, delusions, insomnia, and somatic complaints. In such settings, older adults with depression should be treated because antidepressant treatment usually improves nutrition and function and decreases symptoms of pain and insomnia. Better choices for antidepressants are the SSRIs (e.g., paroxetine, fluoxetine [Prozac], sertraline [Zoloft], citalopram [Celexa], and escitalopram [Lexapro]). SSRIs have the advantage of daily dosing and fewer side effects than TCAs, which were used frequently before the advent of SSRIs. Although the TCAs are still used, they are associated with many side effects that can lead to cognitive impairment and falls. Cardiovascular effects include hypotension, arrhythmias, and sudden death. Other troublesome side effects include sedation, dry mouth, urinary retention, and dizziness from anticholinergic properties.

Significant drug interactions and toxicity may occur with SSRI use because these drugs inhibit oxidative metabolism. Drugs that may be affected by SSRIs include warfarin, phenytoin, and class 1C antiarrhythmics. Studies indicate that older adults taking SSRIs have a greater risk for falls than older adults not taking antidepressants (Leipzig et al., 1999) and suggest that higher doses of combined CNS medications, such as SSRIs, benzodiazepines, and antipsychotics, can lead to cognitive decline in older adults (Wright et al., 2009). Common side effects of SSRIs in the older adult include headache, nausea, dry mouth, dizziness, constipation, dyspepsia, diarrhea, asthenia, insomnia, decreased appetite, tachycardia, and abnormal taste. Hyponatremia has been increasingly noted to occur in older adults on SSRIs. On withdrawal of the SSRI, sodium levels return to normal within days to weeks (Kirby & Ames, 2001). The prescriber needs to be aware of early signs of hyponatremia: lethargy, fatigue, muscle cramps, anorexia, and nausea.

Marijuana

An analysis from data gathered in the National Survey on Drug Use and Health (NSDUH) from 2015 and 2016 showed that about 9% of U.S. adults between ages 50 and 64 used marijuana in the previous year and about 3% of people over 65 used the drug in that time period (Han & Palamar, 2018; NPR, 2018).

There is increasing interest in the use of cannabinoids for disease and symptom management, but limited information is available regarding their pharmacokinetics and pharmacodynamics to guide prescribers. Cannabis medicines contain a wide variety of chemical compounds, including the cannabinoids delta-9-tetrahydrocannabinol (THC), which is psychoactive, and the nonpsychoactive cannabidiol (CBD). Cannabis use is associated with both pathological and behavioral toxicity and, accordingly, is contraindicated in the context of significant psychiatric, cardiovascular, renal, or hepatic illness. The pharmacokinetics of cannabinoids and the effects observed depend on the formulation and route of administration, which should be tailored to individual patient requirements. As both THC and CBD are hepatically metabolized, the potential exists for pharmacokinetic drug interactions via inhibition or induction of enzymes or transporters. An important example is the CBD-mediated inhibition of clobazam metabolism. Pharmacodynamic interactions may occur if cannabis is administered with other CNS-depressant drugs, and cardiac toxicity may occur via additive hypertension and tachycardia with sympathomimetic agents. More vulnerable populations, such as older patients, may benefit from the potential symptomatic and palliative benefits of cannabinoids but are at increased risk for adverse effects. The limited availability of applicable pharmacokinetic and pharmacodynamic information highlights the need to initiate prescribing cannabis medicines using an "start low and go slow" approach, carefully observing the patient for desired and adverse effects. Further clinical studies in the actual patient populations for whom prescribing may be considered are needed, to derive a better understanding of these drugs and enhance safe and optimal prescribing.

There are two unique aspects in the management of marijuana that are untrue for any other drug. These involve management of prescribed medical use and self-directed recreational use. One major difference is that in the case of self-directed use, information on the use and its quantity and frequency, which is often not regular, need to be obtained from the patient as opposed to medical claims or prescription data.

Other Disorders and Drug Therapies

Studies have shown that, in general, older adults are more vulnerable to severe or persistent pain and that the inability to tolerate severe pain increases with age. Further, older adults are far more likely to experience pain associated with surgical procedures, such as knee and hip replacements, arthritis, cancer, and end-of-life symptoms. Compounding the problem of pain in the older adult is the well-documented fact that pain in the institutionalized older adult population, particularly among minorities and those with dementia, is far more likely to be undertreated. According to the 2011 Institute of Medicine (IOM) report, "a study of more than 13,000 people with cancer aged 65 and older discharged from the hospital to nursing homes found that, among the 4,000 who were in daily pain, those aged 85 and older were more than 1.5 times as likely to receive no analgesia than those aged 65 to 74; only 13 percent of those aged 85 and older received opioid medications, compared with 38 percent of those aged 65 to 74" (IOM, 2011).

While many drug precautions have been in effect since the passage of the Comprehensive Drug Abuse Prevention and Control Act of 1970, they have now taken the form of forced restrictions. Some of these new restrictions are resulting in issues in managing pain for SNF residents. For example, in 2011, the U.S. FDA asked drug manufacturers to limit the strength of acetaminophen in combination prescription drugs to 325 mg per tablet by January 2014, in an attempt to reduce incidences of potentially fatal liver damage. Even though acetaminophen has been commercially available since 1953, it was not until 2009 that the FDA required manufacturers of the OTC drug Tylenol and its generic equivalents to post a black box warning for liver damage, due in large part to deaths attributable to acetaminophen use and heavy alcohol consumption. According to the FDA, more than half of manufacturers have voluntarily complied with this request. However, some prescription combination drug products containing more than 325 mg of acetaminophen per dosage unit remain available, prompting the FDA to eventually withdraw approval of any prescription combination drug products containing more than 325 mg of acetaminophen that remain on the market. The result of all of this focus is a limitation on access of higher-dose acetaminophen preparations, and as a result, appropriate adjustments for patients receiving these treatments may need to occur. To avoid hepatotoxicity, caution should be taken not to exceed 4,000 mg in 24 hours, especially in patients with known liver disease, alcoholism, or malnutrition.

The chronic pain of degenerative joint disease unrelieved by acetaminophen can be treated with an NSAID. Long-term treatment with NSAIDs, however, can result in GI bleeding, anemia, and renal insufficiency. Caution should be taken when on highly bound drugs, such as warfarin, digoxin, and anticonvulsants, because increased bioavailability occurs due to NSAIDs being highly protein bound. The cyclooxygenase 2 (COX-2) inhibitor celecoxib (Celebrex) is a nontraditional antiinflammatory drug developed to prevent GI bleeding by not affecting platelet aggregation and bleeding. Although the risk of bleeding with COX-2 inhibitors may be lower than that with traditional NSAIDs, such as naproxen or ibuprofen, it can still occur. Cardiovascular safety issues led to the withdrawal of rofecoxib and valdecoxib from the market in the United States.

Neuropathic pain from postherpetic neuralgia or diabetic neuropathy can be treated with mixed serotonin and norepinephrine uptake inhibitors, such as duloxetine (Cymbalta) and venlafaxine (Effexor), with a better side effect profile than older TCAs. The anticonvulsant agents gabapentin (Neurontin) and carbamazepine (Tegretol) are also effective in treating neuropathic pain. Pregabalin (Lyrica) is indicated for diabetic peripheral neuropathy; however, it can cause somnolence and dizziness.

Topical analgesics can be effective in pain management in the LTC setting. The 5% lidocaine patch may help with neuralgia pain, although it is often used off label for localized back pain or arthritis. The topical NSAID diclofenac (Flector) is indicated for chronic pain management with less systemic absorption than oral NSAIDs (American Geriatrics Society [AGS] Panel on Pharmacological Management of Persistent Pain in Older Persons, 2009).

Other commonly encountered drug-related problems in LTC are urinary incontinence and recurrent urinary tract infections (UTIs), evidenced by confusion and mental status changes. Respiratory infections such as bronchitis and pneumonia quickly spread through a facility because of the compromised immune state of frail residents. Thus, antibiotic use is called on more frequently than for the community-residing adult. The frail older patient with pneumonia may not have typical signs of illness. For example, the patient may not have a cough or fever. Moreover, the frail older patient becomes ill more quickly and decompensates rapidly if untreated. Dehydration, sepsis, or even death may result.

Constipation is another concern, and sometimes an obsession, of older adults. In many instances, they think they need medications to promote bowel movements. However, alternate methods of treating this problem may be judicious, including increasing physical activity and consumption of fluids, fiber, and fruit. One or two tablespoons of a mixture of prune juice, unprocessed bran, and applesauce taken daily is an alternative to stool softeners and laxatives. When assessing constipation, a review of current medications may yield clues to drug use that contributes to the constipation. For example, anticholinergics, such as oxybutynin (Ditropan), used for urinary incontinence; antidepressants, such as the TCAs; and calcium channel blockers may all cause constipation in the frail older patient.

In summary, the older resident in LTC is usually the frailest and at greatest risk for complications related to improper drug administration. The health care provider should attempt to keep medications at a minimum with the lowest dosage possible. A monthly or bimonthly review of all medications should be done to review medical necessity. A pharmacist from within the facility or from the company supplying the facility with medications should routinely review charts and write recommendations to decrease or stop medications. The suggestions should be evaluated by the health care provider and acted on if appropriate to reduce polypharmacy, side effects, and costs for the resident.

GUIDELINES FOR SAFE PRESCRIBING

Guidelines for safe prescribing apply not only to residents of LTC facilities but to all older adults. The goal of prescribing for adults in LTC should be to prevent adverse events, falls, and injuries that will further degrade the patient's function, both physical and mental. The provider must prescribe cautiously and keep the patient's safety in mind while promoting his or her comfort and dignity (**Box 5.4**). Providers in LTC need to familiarize themselves with the Beers Criteria. This extensive list of medication guidelines was created by a consensus panel of nationally recognized experts in geriatrics and updated in 2019 (AGS, 2019).

In addition to the Beers Criteria, an opportunity to improve outcomes comes from the Choosing Wisely initiative. In response to the challenge of improving health care, national organizations representing medical specialists have asked their members to *choose wisely* through the identification of tests or procedures commonly used in their field, whose necessity should be questioned and discussed. The resulting list, Five Things Providers and Patients Should Question, is meant to encourage discussion of the need—or lack thereof—for many frequently ordered tests or treatments.

The AMDA–The Society for Post-Acute and LTC Medicine developed 5 things to question, while the AGS developed 10. Considering these 15 things, one can identify 5 common themes upon which clinicians should focus their

INITIATION OF THERAPY

- Review the risks and benefits of adding a medication. Explore nonpharmacologic options first.
- If possible, choose one medication that treats two coexisting problems.
- Always start with the lowest dose possible and titrate up slowly. "Start low, go slow but get there."
- Choose a drug with the fewest daily required doses (i.e., daily or twice daily).
- Remember to consider the cost of the brand name drug and consider generic equivalents if cost issues will deter compliance.

ONGOING PHARMACOTHERAPY ASSESSMENT

- Schedule routine follow-up examinations for the patient who has multiple chronic illnesses and who takes multiple medications.
- Reduce dosages or discontinue medications if possible to avoid polypharmacy.
- Advise patients to bring all medications (prescription or OTC) to each office visit for review.
- Document accurately all current medications and dosages.

- Review medications added by other practitioners and specialists. Inform these professionals of changes made by the primary health care provider.
- Schedule blood tests regularly to monitor levels of such medications as diuretics, ACE inhibitors, antiseizure medications, anticoagulants, antiarrhythmics, and digitalis.

PATIENT SUPPORT

- Give a written list and instructions to the patient after each office visit of the medications to be taken.
- Provide the written medication instructions and changes in large print in terms easily understood by older adults.
- Explain and document both the generic and the brand name of the prescribed drug to avoid confusing the patient; also explain and document the important reason for each medication.
- Review medications and changes in the regimen with family/caregivers, especially for those caring for loved ones with cognitive impairments.
- Recommend or provide medication planners or weekly/daily dosage containers to improve compliance and promote safe medication administration.

ACE, angiotensin-converting enzyme; OTC, over-the-counter.

---

attention. These five center on the following critical areas for management of pharmacotherapy in older adults:

1. Dementia and behavioral and psychological symptoms of dementia (BPSD)
2. Screening and medication management
3. Antibiotic use
4. Diabetes management
5. Nutritional management

These five areas come from extensive work done by both AMDA and AGS and are refined here with a special focus toward the care of older adults. The result is five Choosing Wisely initiatives that when followed will serve clinicians caring for older adults well. Choosing wisely starts and often ends with a *wise* clinician, one who understands that these five initiatives are a step in that direction.

Dementia and Behavioral and Psychological Symptoms of Dementia

A starting point is the management of dementia and BPSD, for perhaps nothing is more critical given the increasing prevalence of dementia. Several of the AMDA and AGS Choosing Wisely directives are focused in this area. These include

appropriate management of dementia through not prescribing cholinesterase inhibitors for dementia without periodic assessment for perceived cognitive benefits and adverse gastrointestinal effects. The impact of cholinesterase inhibitors on institutionalization, quality of life, and caregiver burden is NOT well established. Clinicians, caregivers, and patients should discuss cognitive, functional, and behavioral goals of treatment prior to beginning a trial of cholinesterase inhibitors. Advance care planning, patient and caregiver education about dementia, diet and exercise, and nonpharmacologic approaches to behavioral issues are integral to the care of patients with dementia and should be included in the treatment plan in addition to any consideration of a trial of cholinesterase inhibitors. If goals of treatment are not attained after a reasonable trial (e.g., 12 weeks), then discontinuing the medication should be considered. Benefits beyond a year have not been investigated and the risks and benefits of long-term therapy have not been well established, resulting in a need for ongoing assessment.

Regarding other treatments for agitation and delirium, two items were raised regarding the use of chemical and physical restraints. Both the AGS and AMDA called out the use of antipsychotic medications because of their adverse effects and consideration as chemical restraints; they specifically recommended not to use antipsychotic medications for BPSD in individuals with dementia as first choice or without an assessment for an underlying cause of the behavior. People with dementia often exhibit aggression, resistance to care, and other challenging or disruptive behaviors. In such instances, antipsychotic medicines are often prescribed, but they often provide limited benefit and can cause serious harm, including stroke and premature death. Use of these drugs should be limited to cases where nonpharmacologic measures have failed and patients pose an imminent threat to themselves or others. Identifying and addressing causes of behavior change can make drug treatment unnecessary.

Careful differentiation of cause of the symptoms (physical or neurological vs. psychiatric or psychological) may help better define appropriate treatment options. The therapeutic goal of the use of antipsychotic medications is to treat patients who present an imminent threat of harm to self or others or are in extreme distress—not to treat non-specific agitation or other forms of lesser distress. Treatment of BPSD in association with the likelihood of imminent harm to self or others includes assessing for and identifying and treating underlying causes (including pain, constipation, and environmental factors such as noise and being too cold or warm), ensuring safety, reducing distress, and supporting the patient's functioning. If treatment of other potential causes of the BPSD is unsuccessful, antipsychotic medications can be considered, taking into account their significant risks compared to potential benefits. When an antipsychotic is used for BPSD, it is advisable to obtain informed consent.

Also regarding chemical restraints in older adults, using benzodiazepines or other sedative–hypnotics as the first choice for insomnia, agitation, or delirium is discouraged. Large-scale studies consistently show that the risk for falls and hip fractures leading to hospitalization and death can more than double in older adults taking benzodiazepines and other sedative–hypnotics. Older patients, their caregivers, and their providers should recognize these potential harms when considering treatment strategies for insomnia, agitation, or delirium. Use of benzodiazepines should be reserved for alcohol withdrawal symptoms/delirium tremens or severe generalized anxiety disorder unresponsive to other therapies.

And lastly, avoiding physical restraints to manage behavioral symptoms of hospitalized older adults with delirium was called out. Persons with delirium may display behaviors that risk injury or interfere with treatment. There is little evidence to support the effectiveness of physical restraints in these situations. Physical restraints can lead to serious injury or death and may worsen agitation and delirium. Effective alternatives include strategies to prevent and treat delirium, identification and management of conditions causing patient discomfort, environmental modifications to promote orientation and effective sleep–wake cycles, frequent family contact, and supportive interaction with staff. Educational initiatives and innovative models of practice have been shown to be effective in implementing a restraint-free approach to patients with delirium. This approach includes continuous observation; trying reorientation once and if not effective not continuing; observing behavior to obtain clues about patients' needs; discontinuing and/or hiding unnecessary medical monitoring devices or intravenous (IV) devices; and avoiding short-term memory questions to limit patient agitation. Pharmacologic interventions are occasionally utilized after evaluation by a medical provider at the bedside, if a patient presents harm to himself or herself or others. Physical restraints should only be used as a very last resort and should be discontinued at the earliest possible time.

Screening and Medication Management

Consider the true benefits for each and every individual resident before recommending a screening test or medication. All too often, treatments are ordered based on an overestimate of the benefits and undervaluation of the risks. This includes such actions as not recommending screening for breast or colorectal cancer or prostate cancer (with the PSA test) without considering life expectancy and the risks of testing, overdiagnosis, and overtreatment. Cancer screening is associated with short-term risks, including complications from testing, overdiagnosis, and treatment of tumors that would not have led to symptoms. For prostate cancer (Choosing Wisely, 2013), 1,055 men would need to be screened and 37 would need to be treated to avoid 1 death in 11 years. For breast and colorectal cancer, 1,000 patients would need to be screened to prevent 1 death in 10 years. For patients with a life expectancy under 10 years, screening for these three cancers exposes them to immediate harms with little chance of benefit.

In addition, a resident's life expectancy should be taken into account such that there is no routine use of lipid-lowering medications in individuals with a limited life expectancy. There is no evidence that hypercholesterolemia, or low HDL-C, is an important risk factor for all-cause mortality, coronary heart disease mortality, or hospitalization for myocardial infarction or unstable angina in persons older than 70 years. In fact, studies show that older patients with the lowest cholesterol have the highest mortality after adjusting for other risk factors. In addition, a less favorable risk–benefit ratio may be seen for patients older than 85, where benefits may be more diminished and risks from statin drugs more increased (cognitive impairment, falls, neuropathy, and muscle damage).

Drug regimen reviews are done monthly by a consultant pharmacist within the nursing home, and these assessments are critical to assuring appropriate medication use. Older patients disproportionately use more prescription and nonprescription drugs than other populations, increasing the risk for side effects and inappropriate prescribing. Polypharmacy may lead to diminished adherence, ADRs, and increased risk of cognitive impairment, falls, and functional decline. Medication review identifies high-risk medications, drug interactions, and medications continued beyond their indication. Additionally, medication review elucidates unnecessary medications and underuse of medications and may reduce medication burden.

Antibiotic Use

The CDC and other organizations are increasingly sensitive to the overuse of antibiotics. This overuse has led to dangerous drug-resistant organisms. As a result, both the AGS and AMDA have made recommendations to not use antimicrobials to treat bacteriuria in older adults unless specific urinary tract symptoms are present. Cohort studies have found no adverse outcomes for older men or women associated with asymptomatic bacteriuria. Antimicrobial treatment studies for asymptomatic bacteriuria in older adults demonstrate no benefits and show increased adverse antimicrobial effects. Consensus criteria have been developed to characterize the specific clinical symptoms that, when associated with bacteriuria, define UTI.

The inappropriate treatment of positive urine cultures starts with an inappropriate urine analysis; as such, it is recommended not to obtain a urine culture unless there are clear signs and symptoms that localize to the urinary tract. Chronic asymptomatic bacteriuria is frequent in the LTC setting, with prevalence as high as 50%. A positive urine culture in the absence of localized UTI symptoms (i.e., dysuria, frequency, urgency) is of limited value in identifying whether a patient's symptoms are caused by a UTI. Colonization (a positive bacterial culture without signs or symptoms of a localized UTI) is a common problem in LTC facilities, which contributes to the overuse of antibiotic therapy, leading to an increased risk for diarrhea, resistant organisms, and infection due to *Clostridium difficile*. An additional concern is that the finding of asymptomatic bacteriuria may lead to an erroneous assumption that a UTI is the cause of an acute change of status, which leads to failure in detecting or a delay in the detection of a patient's possibly more serious underlying problem. A patient with advanced dementia may be unable to report urinary symptoms. In this situation, it is reasonable to obtain a urine culture if there are signs of systemic infection such as fever (an increase in temperature of equal to or greater than 2°F [1.1°C] from baseline), leukocytosis, or a left shift or chills in the absence of additional symptoms (e.g., new cough) to suggest an alternative source of infection. Remember, it often starts with clinicians believing a patient's change in condition and requesting a urine analysis despite there not being any signs of a urinary infection. Thoughtful recommendations in this area can go a long way in assuring appropriate antibiotic use.

Diabetes Management

Diabetes management was another area where both the AGS and AMDA found common ground. The inappropriate treatment of residents with diabetes can result in falls from hypoglycemia as well as painful frequent fingersticks and injections from the overuse of sliding scale insulin (SSI). As a result, it is recommended to avoid using medications to achieve hemoglobin A1c less than 7.5% in most adults aged 65 and older; moderate control is generally better. There is no evidence that using medications to achieve tight glycemic control in older adults with type 2 diabetes is beneficial. Among non-older adults, except for long-term reductions in myocardial infarction and mortality with metformin, using medications to

achieve glycated hemoglobin levels less than 7% is associated with harms, including higher mortality rates. Tight control has been consistently shown to produce higher rates of hypoglycemia in older adults. Given the long time frame to achieve theorized microvascular benefits of tight control, glycemic targets should reflect patient goals, health status, and life expectancy. Reasonable glycemic targets would be 7% to 7.5% in healthy older adults with long life expectancy, 7.5% to 8% in those with moderate comorbidity and a life expectancy less than 10 years, and 8% to 9% in those with multiple morbidities and shorter life expectancy.

SSI was called out as a term to be avoided for long-term diabetes management for individuals residing in the nursing home. SSI is a reactive way of treating hyperglycemia after it has occurred rather than preventing it. Good evidence exists that neither is SSI effective in meeting the body's insulin needs nor is it efficient in the LTC setting. Use of SSI leads to greater patient discomfort and increased nursing time because patients' blood glucose levels are usually monitored more frequently than may be necessary and more insulin injections may be given. With SSI regimens, patients may be at risk from prolonged periods of hyperglycemia. In addition, the risk of hypoglycemia is a significant concern because insulin may be administered without regard to meal intake. Basal insulin, or basal plus rapid-acting insulin with one or more meals (often called basal/bolus insulin therapy), most closely mimics normal physiologic insulin production and controls blood glucose more effectively. Clinicians can raise awareness of inappropriate SSI with recommendations for changes to scheduled dosing or oral or insulin treatments.

Nutritional Support

Lastly, appropriate nutritional support is often critical at the end of life. This involves avoiding inappropriate nutritional interventions. One such intervention is percutaneous feeding tubes. As such, it is recommended not to use percutaneous feeding tubes in individuals with advanced dementia. Instead, oral-assisted feedings may be offered. Strong evidence exists that artificial nutrition does not prolong life or improve quality of life in patients with advanced dementia. Substantial functional decline and recurrent or progressive medical illnesses may indicate that a patient who is not eating is unlikely to obtain any significant or long-term benefit from artificial nutrition. Feeding tubes are often placed after hospitalization, frequently with concerns for aspirations and for those who are not eating. Contrary to what many people think, tube feeding does not ensure the patient's comfort or reduce suffering; it may cause fluid overload, diarrhea, abdominal pain, local complications, and less human interaction and may increase the risk for aspiration. Assistance with oral feeding is an evidence-based approach to provide nutrition for patients with advanced dementia and feeding problems.

Careful hand-feeding for patients with severe dementia is at least as good as tube feeding for improving the outcomes of death, aspiration pneumonia, functional status, and patient comfort. Food is the preferred nutrient. Tube feeding is associated with agitation, increased use of physical and chemical restraints, and worsening pressure ulcers.

Also called out regarding nutritional support was avoiding the use of prescription appetite stimulants or high-calorie supplements for treatment of anorexia or cachexia in older adults; instead, social supports may be optimized, feeding assistance provided, and patient goals and expectations clarified. Unintentional weight loss is a common problem for medically ill or frail older adults. Although high-calorie supplements increase weight in older people, there is no evidence that they affect other important clinical outcomes, such as quality of life, mood, functional status, or survival. Use of megestrol acetate results in minimal improvements in appetite and weight gain, no improvement in quality of life or survival, and increased risk for thrombotic events, fluid retention, and death. In patients who take megestrol acetate, 1 in 12 will have an increase in weight and 1 in 23 will die. The AGS Beers Criteria lists megestrol acetate and cyproheptadine as medications to avoid in older adults (AGS, 2019). Systematic reviews of cannabinoids, dietary polyunsaturated fatty acids (DHA) and eicosapentaenoic acid (EPA), thalidomide, and anabolic steroids have not identified adequate evidence for the efficacy and safety of these agents for weight gain. Mirtazapine is likely to cause weight gain or increased appetite when used to treat depression, but there is little evidence to support its use to promote appetite and weight gain in the absence of depression. In the end, clinicians can assist by increasing family involvement in feeding and promoting this oral feeding activity to prevent the potential inappropriate use of pharmacotherapy.

Executing on These Five

These five areas—dementia and BPSD management, screening and medication management, antibiotic use, diabetes management, and nutritional management—are critical to improving outcomes for nursing home residents. A common thread running through these Choosing Wisely initiatives is that the prudent use of services involves a patient centered approach, taking into account the benefits and risks. This requires thoughtful assessments to assure that interventions are not encouraged that are truly not of benefit for that particular patient. In the end, all clinicians can play a key role in assuring that each resident receives appropriate care. And it is this care that will assist in improving the quality of life and death for older adults (**Box 5.5**).

Exploring Alternatives to Medication

The health care provider must evaluate new problems and determine if a medication is necessary as part of the treatment plan. If there are alternatives to medications, such as diet, exercise, and weight loss for borderline hypertension or antiembolism stockings instead of a diuretic for pedal edema, these options should be explored first. Only after nonpharmacologic treatments fail should a medication be initiated. In

---

BOX 5.5 | **Guidelines for Safe Prescribing in Dementia and Behavioral and Psychological Symptoms of Dementia**

1. Assure that dementia and BPSD are properly managed through use of physical and chemical restraints such as antipsychotics and benzodiazepines as well as cholinesterase inhibitors.
2. Assist in the reduction of inappropriate screening and medications that are not beneficial because of limited effectiveness and dangerous adverse effects.
3. Do not request a urine analysis or order for an antibiotic unless there is clear indication of a bacterial infection.
4. Assure appropriate diabetes management through a reasonable hemoglobin A1c target and use of regularly scheduled antidiabetic medications, thus avoiding SSI.
5. Assist in the promotion of oral feeding such that percutaneous feeding tube and appetite stimulants are only used in rare situations.

BPSD, behavioral and psychological symptoms of dementia; SSI, sliding scale insulin.

---

knowing the patient's overall situation—physically, mentally, and socially—the provider has a baseline from which to consider the risks and benefits of medication therapy. **Table 5.6** lists 20 medications that should not be prescribed to any older patients. All of the drugs in this table are also present in the 2019 Beers Criteria.

When deciding on a medication for an older adult, assisting with that decision, or evaluating a selection, a drug that treats two coexisting conditions should be considered. For example, a calcium channel blocker might be selected for the patient with angina and hypertension. An older man with hyperplasia of the prostate and hypertension may benefit from an alpha-adrenergic blocking agent such as terazosin (Hytrin). Treating two conditions with one medication reduces cost, cuts down on dosing schedules, and improves adherence and patient satisfaction.

Simplifying the Regimen

Simplifying the medication plan is a key to therapeutic adherence and safety. Drugs are started at the lowest dose possible and the dosage increased as needed. Lower doses are often effective and reduce the risk of toxicity. Dosing schedules must be easy to follow and remember. If two drugs are equally suitable to treat the same condition, it is desirable to prescribe the one that requires the less frequent dosing.

Another important concern is the cost of the drug, especially if the drug is for long-term use. Many older adults are on fixed incomes and find the cost of prescription drugs

TABLE 5.6

Twenty Drugs to Avoid in Older Adults

Prescription Drug	Use	Reason for Avoiding
Amitriptyline	To treat depression	Other antidepressant medications cause fewer side effects.
Carisoprodol	To relieve severe pain caused by sprains and back pain	Minimally effective while causing toxicity. Potential for toxic reaction is greater than potential benefit.
Chlordiazepoxide	To tranquilize or to relieve anxiety	Shorter-acting benzodiazepines are safer alternatives.
Chlorpropamide	To treat diabetes	Other oral hypoglycemic medications have shorter half-lives and do not cause inappropriate antidiuretic hormone secretion.
Cyclandelate	To improve blood circulation	Effectiveness is in doubt. This drug is no longer available in the United States.
Cyclobenzaprine	To relieve severe pain caused by sprains and back pain	Minimally effective while causing toxicity. Potential for toxic reaction is greater than potential benefit.
Diazepam	To tranquilize or to relieve anxiety	Shorter-acting benzodiazepines are safer alternatives.
Dipyridamole	To reduce blood clot formation	Effectiveness at low dosage is in doubt. Toxic reaction is high at higher dosages. Safer alternatives exist.
Flurazepam	To induce sleep	Shorter-acting benzodiazepines are safer alternatives.
Indomethacin	To relieve the pain and inflammation of rheumatoid arthritis	Other NSAIDs cause fewer toxic reactions.
Isoxsuprine	To improve blood circulation	Effectiveness is in doubt.
Meprobamate	To tranquilize	Shorter-acting benzodiazepines are safer alternatives.
Methocarbamol	To relieve severe pain caused by sprains and back pain	Minimally effective while causing toxicity. Potential for toxic reaction is greater than potential benefit.
Orphenadrine	To relieve severe pain caused by sprains and back pain	Minimally effective while causing toxicity. Potential for toxic reaction is greater than potential benefit.
Pentazocine	To relieve moderate to severe pain	Other narcotic medications are safer and more effective.
Pentobarbital	To induce sleep and reduce anxiety	Safer sedative–hypnotics are available.
Phenylbutazone	To relieve the pain and inflammation of rheumatoid arthritis	Other NSAIDs cause fewer toxic reactions.
Propoxyphene	To relieve mild to moderate pain	This drug is no longer available in the United States.
Secobarbital	To induce sleep and reduce anxiety	Safer sedative–hypnotics are available.
Trimethobenzamide	To relieve nausea and vomiting	Least effective of the available antiemetics

NSAIDs, nonsteroidal anti-inflammatory drugs.

unaffordable. If the most suitable medication for the condition is expensive, this is explained to the patient before purchase to prevent "sticker shock," or the embarrassment of not having enough money to pay for the prescription. Understanding the impact of a patient's out-of-pocket expenses on adherence is important. As Dr. C. Everett Koop, former U.S. surgeon general, has been quoted, "A medication only works if the patient takes it."

Educating Adults and Caregivers

Potential side effects need to be discussed in a nonthreatening way to prevent needless fear or anticipation when starting a

new medication. Many older adults forgo starting a medication for fear of potential side effects that may occur. The media are powerful in alarming adults about potentially undesirable or dangerous adverse effects, proven or not. Many older adults stop taking essential medications after reading or hearing something in the media pertaining to that particular drug.

Reviewing Medications

The provider working with a geriatric patient should have the patient bring in all of his or her medications to each office visit or review a current medication card if the patient carries one.

The current medications taken by the patient are recorded at each office visit as part of the progress note. This review alerts the provider to improper dosing and drug administration, misunderstanding of medications, and changes made by specialists and other professionals. The specialist is not always aware of all the medications or OTC drugs the patient takes and may prescribe a drug that places the patient at risk for interactions. As part of the review, the health care provider should ask about topical creams, vitamins, eye drops, and OTC products that may interact with prescription drugs. Adults do not always view these products as medications.

The provider should review all drugs periodically to determine if the dosage can be reduced or the drug discontinued. The goal should always be to use as little medication as possible to treat the multiple illnesses that challenge the older adult.

At the end of each office visit, the provider needs to give the medication list to the patient. Doses and times to take the medications and any special instructions need to be clearly stated and communicated in writing as appropriate. New medications should be listed by brand and generic name so there is no confusion. Clear writing with large lettering should be used, particularly if the patient has common vision impairments, such as cataracts, glaucoma, or macular degeneration.

The caps of the medication bottles that the patient brings to the office can be labeled with the reason for the drug (e.g., "blood pressure," "water pill," or "diabetes"). This helps to ensure that the patient has a basic understanding of the importance of each drug. If the caregiver of an older patient is available, the provider should explain any new medication changes or special instructions, especially for the patient with cognitive impairment or other changes in mental status.

THERAPEUTIC MONITORING

When memory problems are an issue, a medication planner helps. Labeled with the days of the week and four dosing times per day, the planner is a useful device for preparing medications for a week. A patient who fails to take the medications despite visual cues and careful labeling may be sending a signal that the family or other responsible caregivers need to investigate additional interventions, home care services, or future placement in assisted living or LTC facilities.

It is important routinely to schedule and monitor the results of laboratory tests when the patient is taking medications that may result in fluctuating drug blood levels. For example, older adults taking such drugs as warfarin, theophylline (Theo-Dur), digoxin, and quinidine (Quinaglute) need careful monitoring, as do adults taking anticonvulsant medications, such as phenytoin, carbamazepine (Tegretol), and valproic acid (Depakote), for seizure disorders.

Adults taking diuretics or angiotensin-converting enzyme (ACE) inhibitors require periodic evaluation with a renal profile to detect electrolyte imbalances, as well as renal insufficiency (as evidenced by rising blood urea nitrogen

[BUN] and creatinine levels). Adults starting ACE inhibitor therapy should have a baseline BUN/creatinine level documented with a follow-up test in 2 weeks to alert for renal artery stenosis (evidenced by a rise in the BUN/creatinine levels). Because of the potential for elevations in serum potassium concentration with ACE inhibitor therapy, the older adult needs routine renal profiles to detect such changes, especially when drug therapy also includes diuretics and digoxin (Lanoxin). (**Box 5.4** presents guidelines for prescribing drugs safely for older adults.)

SUMMARY

Three quotes that summarize best practices in pharmacotherapy principles in older adults follow:

1. "Any symptom in an elderly patient should be considered a drug side effect until proved otherwise."
2. "Start low, go slow but get there (the therapeutic dose)."
3. "A medication only works if the patient takes it."

It begins with determination of the right treatment in the face of new symptoms or issues. This may not always mean beginning a new medication but rather may mean instead reducing a dose of a current medication, discontinuing a therapy, or starting a nonpharmacologic treatment. The quote from Leslie Fine should be remembered and practiced, that "any symptom in an elderly patient should be considered a drug side effect until proved otherwise." This is important to prevent polypharmacy issues in older adults. Also, when determining if a new medication should be started, careful assessment of the benefits versus the costs should be undertaken such that only those treatments that offer benefits over costs should be started. Assessing costs includes not only financial costs but also potential side effects, while benefits analyses need to take into account benefits given the life expectancy and other concerns in the older adult.

The second quote deals with starting a new medication. It begins with a standard geriatric quote but with a new addition. The quote is that medications in older adults should "start low and go slow" but, to be complete, should include "but get there." This translates to initiating medications at a low starting dose and titrating slowly but getting to the therapeutic dose. This is not only to prevent adverse events from too quick a titration at too high a dose but also to caution against therapies that are not being used at a therapeutic level.

The final quote comes from C. Everett Koop describing the importance of adherence—"A medication only works if the patient takes it": for after a careful determination and initiation of the "right" medication, at the right dose for the right duration, has been made, assurance of adherence is the final step in producing optimum outcomes. Of course, there is no final step; pharmacotherapy management, especially in older adults, requires educated clinicians' ongoing evaluation and support to assure optimum outcomes.

CASE STUDY[*]

R.S. is an 85-year-old female who has congestive heart failure. Over the past 3 months, she has had four hospitalizations. Like many older adults, R.S. is experiencing difficulty swallowing and psychologic changes affecting her medication absorption.

1. Which of the following would be an appropriate starting point for identifying causes for R.S.'s frequency of hospitalizations?
   a. Simply ask if she is taking her medications as directed.
   b. Assume that her frequent hospitalizations are secondary to expected changes, which are normal features of aging.
   c. Examine all of R.S.'s medication vials to complete an assessment including pill count for adherence.
   d. Assume that her frequent hospitalizations are the result of undertreating her conditions.
2. In determining the most appropriate course of treatment for R.S., assessing her life expectancy should never be taken into account. Rather, the same course of treatment should be pursued without regard for life expectancy or her unique goals of care.
   a. True
   b. False
3. Which of the following best describes a concern that R.S. is taking nonprescribed drugs, which may impact her cardiac function?
   a. Assume that although R.S. likely has not discussed her taking nonprescribed drugs with her health care providers that this is most likely not an issue.
   b. Assume because older adults typically do not take nonprescribed drugs that this is not an issue with R.S.
   c. Because older adults take a significant number of nonprescribed drugs without knowledge of their physicians, R.S.'s use is best assessed through a home visit and the asking of open-ended questions.

[*] Answers can be found online.

Bibliography

Starred references are cited in the text.

*AGS Beers Criteria 2019. https://onlinelibrary.wiley.com/doi/abs/10.1111/jgs.15767

*AMDA action for improving dementia care in nursing homes. American Medical Directors Association. http://www.amda.com/advocacy/dementiacare.cfm. Accessed January 6, 2014.

*American Community Survey Reports (ACS). (2018). The population 65 years and older in the United States: 2016. https://www.census.gov/content/dam/Census/library/publications/2018/acs/ACS-38.pdf

American Geriatric Society & American Association for Geriatric Psychiatry. (2003). Consensus statement on improving the quality of mental health care in U.S. nursing homes: Management of depression and behavioral symptoms associated with dementia. *Journal of the American Geriatric Society, 51*(9), 1287–1298.

*American Geriatrics Society Panel on Pharmacological Management of Persistent Pain in Older Persons (2009). Pharmacological management of persistent pain in older persons. (2009). *Journal of the American Geriatrics Society, 57*(8), 1331–1346. https://doi.org/10.1111/j.1532-5415.2009.02376.x

*Anderson, G. (2010). *Chronic care: Making the case for ongoing care.* Princeton, NJ: Robert Wood Johnson Foundation, p. 43.

Arias, E., & Xu, J. Q. (2019). United States life tables, 2017. National Vital Statistics Reports, 68(7). Hyattsville, MD: National Center for Health Statistics.

Barnett, K., Mercer, S. W., Norbury, M., et al. (2012). Epidemiology of multimorbidity and implications for health care, research, and medical education: A cross-sectional study. *Lancet, 380,* 37–43.

*Bergman, S., Ronald, K., Gonzales, M., et al. (2009). Pharmacotherapy update 2009. Part 1. Cardiology, neurology, and psychiatry. *Annals of Long-Term Care, 17*(12), 30–34.

*Brahma, D. K., Wahlang, J. B., Marak, M. D., & Ch Sangma, M. (2013). Adverse drug reactions in the elderly. *Journal of Pharmacology & Pharmacotherapeutics, 4*(2), 91–94. https://doi.org/10.4103/0976-500X.110872

Brooks, B. R., Crumpacker, D., Fellus, J., et al. (2013). PRISM: A novel research tool to assess the prevalence of pseudobulbar affect symptoms across neurological conditions. *PLoS One, 8*(8), e72232.

Burdick, K., & Goldberg, J. (2002). Cognitive advantages of new anticonvulsants in treating a geriatric population. *Clinical Geriatrics, 10*(10), 25–36.

Caracci, G. (2003). The use of opioid analgesics in the older. *Clinical Geriatrics, 11*(11), 18–21.

*Centers for Disease Control and Prevention (CDC) (2012). Wide-ranging Online Data for Epidemiologic Research (WONDER). https://healthdata.gov/dataset/wide-ranging-online-data-epidemiologic-research-wonder. Accessed January 11, 2021.

Centers for Medicare & Medicaid Services. (2017a). State Operations Manual, §483.45(c)(3). https://healthdata.gov/dataset/wide-ranging-online-data-epidemiologic-research-wonder

Centers for Medicare & Medicaid Services. (2017b). State Operations Manual, Sec F757. https://www.cms.gov/Regulations-and-Guidance/Guidance/Manuals/downloads/som107ap_pp_guidelines_ltcf.pdf.

Choosing Wisely. (2013). American Geriatrics Society. Wide-ranging Online Data for Epidemiologic Research (WONDER). https://www.choosingwisely.org/societies/american-geriatrics-society/

Christian, R., Saavedra, L., Gaynes, B. N., et al. (2012, February). Future research needs for first- and second-generation antipsychotics for children and young adults. Future Research Needs Paper No. 13. (Prepared by the RTI-UNC Evidence-based Practice Center under Contract No. 290 2007 10056 I.) Rockville, MD: Agency for Healthcare Research and Quality. http://www.effectivehealthcare.ahrq.gov/ehc/products/419/967/FRN13_Antipsychotics_FinalReport_20120427.pdf. Accessed February 10, 2014

CMS. Freedom of Information Act (FOIA) Service Center: Contacts by region. http://www.cms.gov/center/freedom-of-information-act/regional-contacts.html. Accessed February 4, 2014.

CMS. MDS 3.0 for Nursing Homes and Swing Bed Providers. Retrieved from https://www.cms.gov/Medicare/Quality-Initiatives-Patient-Assessment-Instruments/NursingHomeQualityInits/NHQIMDS30.html on February 27, 2016.

CMS. MDS 3.0 history. http://www.cms.gov/Medicare/Quality-Initiatives-Patient-Assessment-Instruments/NursingHomeQualityInits/NHQIMDS30.html. Accessed February 10, 2014.

CMS. (2016). Medicare prescription drug benefit manual, Chapter 6. https://www.cms.gov/Medicare/Prescription-Drug-Coverage/PrescriptionDrugCovContra/Downloads/Part-D-Benefits-Manual-Chapter-6.pdf. Updated January 15, 2016. Accessed November 15, 2017.

CMS. National Partnership to Improve Dementia Care in Nursing Homes. Retrieved from https://www.cms.gov/Medicare/Provider-Enrollment-and-Certification/SurveyCertificationGenInfo/National-Partnership-to-Improve-Dementia-Care-in-Nursing-Homes.html on February 27, 2016.

CMS. (2013). New data show antipsychotic drug use is down in nursing homes nationwide [news release]. https://ltc.health.mo.gov/archives/6037. Accessed January 11, 2021.

CMS. Quality measures. http://www.cms.gov/Medicare/Quality-Initiatives-Patient-Assessment-Instruments/NursingHomeQualityInits/NHQIQuality Measures.html. Accessed January 13, 2014.

CMS. (2017). Revision to State Operations Manual (SOM) appendix PP for phase 2, F-tag revisions, and related issues, Section F757. https://www.cms.gov/Medicare/Provider-Enrollment-and-Certification/GuidanceforLawsAndRegulations/Downloads/Advance-Appendix-PP-Including-Phase-2-.pdf. Accessed November 10, 2017.

Cooke, C., & Proveaux, W. (2003). A retrospective review of the effect of COX-2 inhibitors on blood pressure change. *American Journal of Therapeutics*, *10*(5), 311–317.

Drug Effectiveness Review Project. (2010, July). Drug class review: Atypical antipsychotics drugs. Final update3 report. https://www.ncbi.nlm.nih.gov/books/NBK50583/pdf/TOC.pdf. Accessed January 17, 2014.

DuGoff, E. H., Canudas-Romo, V., Buttorff, C., et al. (2014). Multiple chronic conditions and life expectancy: A life table analysis. *Medical Care*, *52*, 688–694.

Espinoza, R., & Eslami, M. (2004). Update on treatment for Alzheimer's disease—Part II: Management of noncognitive, psychiatric, and behavioral complications. *Clinical Geriatrics*, *12*(1), 45–53.

FDA requests boxed warnings on older class of antipsychotic drugs [news release]. (2008). https://www.fdanews.com/articles/107752-fda-expands-mortality-warnings-on-antipsychotic-drugs. Accessed February 10, 2014.

*Fick, D., Cooper, J., Wade, W., et al. (2003). Updating the Beers criteria for potentially inappropriate medication use in older adults. *Archives of Internal Medicine*, *163*, 2716–2724.

Guralnik, J., & Havlik, R. (2000). Demographics. In M. Beers & R. Berkow (Eds.), *The Merck manual of geriatrics* (3rd ed., pp. 9–21). Whitehouse Station, NJ: Merck Research Laboratories.

*Han, B. H., & Palamar, J. J. (2018). Marijuana use by middle-aged and older adults in the United States, 2015–2016. *Drug and Alcohol Dependence*, *191*, 374–381.

*Hanlon, J. T., Fillenbaum, G. G., Ruby, C. M., Gray, S., & Bohannon, A. (2001). Epidemiology of over-the-counter drug use in community dwelling elderly: United States perspective. *Drugs Aging*, *18*(2),123-31. doi: 10.2165/00002512-200118020-00005. PMID: 11346126.

*Hartikainen, S., Lönnroos, E., & Louhivuori, K. (2007). Medication as a risk factor for falls: Critical systematic review. *The Journals of Gerontology: Series A*, *62*(10), 1172–1181. http://consultgerirn.org/uploads/File/trythis/try_this_d2.pdf

Hayes, B., Klein-Schwartz, W., & Barrueto, F. (2007). Polypharmacy and the older adult. *Clinics in Geriatric Medicine*, *23*(2), 371–390.

Horgas, A. L. (2018). Assessing pain in older adults with dementia. *Try this:*® *Best practices in nursing care to older adults with dementia*. ConsultGeriRN: http://consultgerirn.org/uploads/File/trythis/try_this_d2.pdf. Accessed January 6, 2014.

Hospital Elder Life Program (HELP). Hospital Elder Life Program (HELP) for Prevention of Delirium. http://www.hospitalelderlifeprogram.org/public/public-main.php. Accessed January 6, 2014.

Herr, K., Bjoro, K., & Decker, S. (2006). Tools for assessment of pain in nonverbal older adults with dementia: A state-of-the-science review. *Journal of Pain and Symptom Management*, *31*(2), 170–192.

*Hile, E., & Studenski, S. (2007). Instability and falls. In E. Duthie, P. Katz, & M. Malone (Eds.), *Practice of geriatrics* (4th ed.). Philadelphia, PA: Saunders.

Horowitz, M. (2000). Aging and the gastrointestinal tract. In M. Beers & R. Berkow (Eds.), *The Merck manual of geriatrics* (3rd ed., pp. 1000–1052). Whitehouse Station, NJ: Merck Research Laboratories.

Improving Dementia Care Treatment for Older Adults Act of 2012, S 3604, 112th Cong, 2nd Sess. (2012). http://www.gpo.gov/fdsys/pkg/BILLS-112s3604is/pdf/BILLS-112s3604is.pdf. Accessed January 6, 2014.

Institute of Medicine (US) Committee on Advancing Pain Research, Care, and Education. (2011). Relieving Pain in America: A Blueprint for Transforming Prevention, Care, Education, and Research. National Academies Press (US).

Juurlink, D., Mamdani, M., Kopp, A., et al. (2003). Drug–drug interactions among older adults hospitalized for drug toxicity. *Journal of the American Medical Association*, *289*(13), 1652–1658.

*Kelleher, C., & Lindeman, R. (2003). Renal diseases and disorders. In E. Flaherty, T. Fulmer, & M. Mezey (Eds.), *Geriatric nursing review syllabus* (pp. 357–365). New York, NY: American Geriatric Society.

*Kirby, D., & Ames, D. (2001). Hyponatremia and selective serotonin re-uptake inhibitors in older adults. *International Journal of Geriatric Psychiatry*, *16*(5), 484–493.

Leading Age. http://www.leadingage.org/. Accessed January 17, 2014.

*Leipzig, R., Cumming, R., & Tinetti, M. (1999). Drugs and falls in older people: A systematic review and meta-analysis: Psychotropic drugs. *Journal of the American Geriatric Society*, *47*(1), 30–39.

Lester, P., Kohen, I., Stefanacci, R. G., et al. (2011). Antipsychotic drug use since the FDA black box warning: Survey of nursing home policies. *Journal of the American Medical Directors Association*, *12*(8), 573–577.

Moore, A., Karno, M., Grella, C., et al. (2009). Alcohol, tobacco, and non-medical drug use in older U.S. adults: Data from the 2001/02 national epidemiologic survey of alcohol and related conditions. *Journal of the American Geriatric Society*, *57*(12), 2275–2281.

*Murray, M., & Callahan, C. (2003). Improving medication use for older adults: An integrated research agenda. *Annals of Internal Medicine*, *139*(5), 425–428.

*Nair, N. P., Chalmers, L., & Bereznicki, L. R. (2016). Hospitalization in older patients due to adverse drug reactions – the need for a prediction tool. *Clinical Interventions in Aging*, *11*, 497–505. https://www.ncbi.nlm.nih.gov/pmc/articles/PMC4859526/

*Norris, S., High, K., Gill, T., et al. (2008). Health care for older Americans with multiple chronic conditions: A research agenda. *Journal of American Geriatric Society*, *56*(1), 149–159.

*NPR. (2018). More older Americans are turning to marijuana. Retrieved from https://www.npr.org/sections/health-shots/2018/09/12/646423762/more-older-americans-are-turning-to-marijuana on November 11, 2020.

Mitka, M. (2012). Overprescribing antipsychotics. *JAMA*, *308*(18), 1849. doi:10.1001/jama.2012.33462

Pain Assessment in Advanced Dementia Scale (PAINAD). Iowa Geriatric Education Center. https://geriatricpain.org/assessment/cognitively-impaired/pain-assessment-advanced-dementia-painad-instructions. Accessed January 6, 2014.

*Sheikh, J., & Cassidy, E. (2003). Anxiety disorders. In E. Flaherty, T. Fulmer, & M. Mezey (Eds.), *Geriatric nursing review syllabus* (pp. 220–223). New York, NY: American Geriatric Society.

*Shiyanbola, O., & Farris, K. (2010). Concerns and beliefs about medicines and inappropriate medications: An internet-based survey on risk factors for self-reported adverse drug events among older adults. *American Journal of Geriatric Pharmacotherapy*, *8*(3), 245–257.

*Smith, M. (2013). *Pharmacy and the US healthcare system* (4th ed.). London, UK: Pharmaceutical Press.

*Sleath, B., Rubin, R. H., Campbell, W., Gwyther, L., & Clark, T. (2001). Physician-patient communication about over-the-counter medications. *Social Science & Medicine* (1982), *53*(3), 357–369. https://doi.org/10.1016/s0277-9536(00)00341-5

Stefanacci, R. G. (2017). New CMS rules on psychotropic medications in SNFs. *Annals of Long-Term Care*, *25*(6), 19–20.

*Stefanacci, R., & Spivack, B. (2010). Impact of healthcare reform on today's Medicare beneficiaries—and on those who care for them. *Clinical Geriatrics*, *18*(6), 42–48.

*Tseng, C., Dudley, R., Brook, R., et al. (2009). Older adults' knowledge of drug benefit caps and communication with providers about exceeding caps. *Journal of the American Geriatric Society, 57*(5), 848–854.

Warden, V., Hurley, A. C., & Volicer, L. (2003). Development and psychometric evaluation of the Pain Assessment in Advanced Dementia (PAINAD) scale. *Journal of the American Medical Directors Associations, 4*(1), 9–15.

*Wright, R., Roumani, Y., Boudreau, R., et al. (2009). Effect of central nervous system medication use on decline in cognition in community-dwelling older adults: Findings from the health, aging and body composition study. *Journal of the American Geriatric Society, 57*(2), 243–250.

Zarowitz, B. J., & O'Shea, T. (2013). Clinical, behavioral, and treatment differences in nursing facility residents with dementia, with and without pseudobulbar affect symptomatology. *Consultant Pharmacyst, 28*(11), 713–722.

*Zhang, Y., Jordan, J. M, (2010). Epidemiology of osteoarthritis. *Clinics in Geriatric Medicine, 26*(3), 355–369. https://doi.org/10.1016/j.cger.2010.03.001

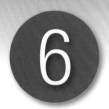

6 Principles of Antimicrobial Therapy

Steven P. Gelone, Staci Pacetti, and Judith A. O'Donnell

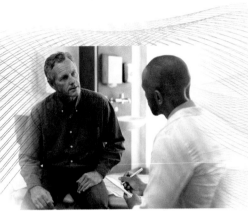
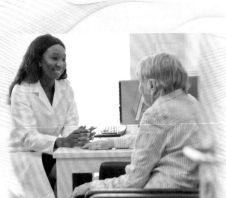
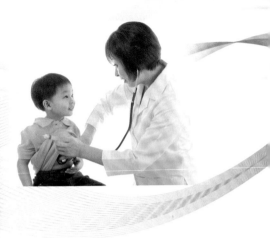

Learning Objectives

1. Discuss factors that may influence the selection of an appropriate antimicrobial regimen.
2. Given a clinical scenario, recommend a safe, effective and patient-specific antimicrobial treatment option.
3. Identify common mechanisms of antimicrobial resistance and the antimicrobial stewardship strategies that may be utilized.

INTRODUCTION

The selection of an appropriate antimicrobial agent to treat an infection is guided by a number of factors. Typically, empiric antimicrobial therapy is based on the epidemiology of the suspected infection, with therapy directed toward the most likely organisms. Laboratory studies, including Gram stain as well as culture and sensitivity testing, help to identify the pathogen and its susceptibility to a variety of antimicrobials. Although there may be several options, efficacy, toxicity, pharmacokinetic profile, and cost ultimately determine the agent of choice. The optimal dose and duration of the antimicrobial therapy are then determined by patient factors such as age, weight, and concurrent disease states as well as the site and severity of infection.

FACTORS INVOLVED IN SELECTING AN ANTIMICROBIAL REGIMEN

Before initiating antibiotic therapy, a systematic approach to identify the source and site of infection must be undertaken. A complete medical history and physical examination should be conducted to identify signs and symptoms consistent with the presence of infection. Identifying underlying medical or social conditions such as diabetes, immunosuppression (cancer, human immunodeficiency virus [HIV] infection), past medications, or intravenous (IV) drug use may help in identifying a predisposition toward infection or the most likely pathogen causing disease. In addition, determining where the infection was acquired (in the community vs. a nursing home or hospital setting) may also help to limit the list of most likely pathogens. Health care–acquired pathogens may necessitate broad-spectrum empiric therapy to cover multidrug-resistant (MDR) pathogens.

Identifying the causative pathogen is the ultimate goal because it allows for optimal antibiotic selection and patient outcome. Updated recommendations from the Infectious Diseases Society of America (IDSA) and the American Society of Microbiology on the appropriate utilization of microbiologic laboratory testing may guide health care providers in their diagnostic approach. Specimens from the most likely body sites should be properly collected and sent to the microbiology laboratory. Depending on the body site involved, specimens will be stained (e.g., Gram stain) to determine morphology and cell wall structure (cocci vs. bacilli and gram-positive vs. gram-negative) and analyzed to detect white blood cells (which indicate inflammation and infection). The gold standard of diagnosis in infectious diseases is to be able to grow the causative organism in culture and perform antibiotic susceptibility testing to determine which agents are most likely to be effective in eradicating the pathogen. Susceptibility results often take 48 to 72 hours after cultures are obtained. Newer methods of testing can help identify specific pathogens (such as methicillin-resistant *Staphylococcus aureus* [MRSA] and *Candida*) more quickly.

TABLE 6.1

Infection and Most Likely Infecting Organism

Body Site (Infection)	Most Likely Organism
Heart (Endocarditis)	
Subacute	*Streptococcus viridans*
Acute	*Staphylococcus aureus*
Injection drug user	*Staphylococcus aureus*, gram-negative aerobic bacilli, *Enterococcus* spp.
Prosthetic valve	*Staphylococcus epidermidis*
Intra-abdominal tissues	*Escherichia coli, Enterococcus* spp., anaerobes (especially *Bacteroides fragilis*), other gram-negative aerobic bacilli
Brain (Meningitis)	
Children < age 2 mo	*E. coli*, group B streptococci, *Listeria monocytogenes*
Children age 2 mo to 12 y	*Streptococcus pneumoniae, Neisseria meningitidis, Haemophilus influenzae*
Adults (community acquired)	*S. pneumoniae, N. meningitidis*
Adults (hospital acquired)	*S. pneumoniae, N. meningitidis*, gram-negative aerobic bacilli
HIV coinfected	*Cryptococcus neoformans, S. pneumoniae*
Respiratory Tract	
Upper tract, community acquired	*S. pneumoniae, H. influenzae, Moraxella catarrhalis*, group A streptococci
Lower tract, community acquired	*S. pneumoniae, H. influenzae, M. catarrhalis, Klebsiella pneumoniae, Mycoplasma pneumoniae, C. pneumoniae*, viruses
Aspiration pneumonia	Mouth flora (anaerobic and aerobic)
Lower tract, hospital acquired	*S. aureus (including MRSA), P. aeruginosa*, other gram-negative aerobic bacilli
HIV coinfected	*Pneumocystis jiroveci, S. pneumoniae*
Skin and Soft Tissue	
Diabetic ulcer	*Staphylococcus* spp., *Streptococcus* spp., gram-negative aerobic bacilli, anaerobes
Urinary Tract	
Community acquired	*E. coli*, other gram-negative aerobic bacilli, *Enterococcus* spp., *Staphylococcus saprophyticus*
Hospital acquired	*E. coli*, other gram-negative aerobic bacilli, *Enterococcus* spp.

HIV, human immunodeficiency virus; MRSA, methicillin-resistant *S. aureus*.

Often, antibiotic therapy is initiated before culture and sensitivity testing is complete. Empiric antibiotic therapy is based on the premise of providing coverage for the most likely pathogens (**Table 6.1**). In general, the most likely organism is based on the suspected site of the infection. **Table 6.2** outlines key pathogens and spectra of activity for the most commonly prescribed antibiotics.

In most patients treated initially with a parenteral antibiotic who are clinically improving, therapy should be switched to the oral route. This may not apply to certain infections, such as osteomyelitis and endocarditis, in which parenteral antibiotics are often continued to ensure adequate concentrations at the infection site. This oral conversion should be based on the following criteria:

- The patient is responding to therapy, as evidenced by a return to normal or a trend toward normal values in the patient's temperature and white blood cell count.

- The patient can take oral medications and absorb them adequately.
- An oral equivalent to the parenteral regimen exists. Not all parenteral agents are available orally. In choosing the oral equivalent, the goal is to select an agent (or agents) that provides a similar spectrum of antimicrobial activity and possesses good oral bioavailability. This may necessitate the use of oral agents that are from a different class from the parenteral agent.

The patient's response to therapy should be monitored regularly. This includes monitoring both efficacy and toxicity. If the patient responds to the prescribed antibiotic regimen, the presenting signs and symptoms of the infection should resolve. Parameters to be considered for response regardless of the site of infection include vital signs, white blood cell count, and, if the culture proved positive for bacteria, subsequent negative cultures as clinically indicated. Other signs and symptoms

TABLE 6.2

Sensitivity of Organisms to Specific Agents

Agent	Streptococci	Enterococcus	MSSA	MRSA	Gram-Negative Aerobes (e.g., E. coli, K. pneumoniae)	Pseudomonas	Gram-Negative Anaerobes (e.g., Bacteroides fragilis)	Chlamydia pneumoniae, Legionella pneumophila, M. pneumoniae
Penicillins								
Amoxicillin	+++	+++	+	−	+/++	−	−	−
Ampicillin	+++	+++	+	−	+/++	−	−	−
Dicloxacillin	+++	−	+++	−	−	−	−	−
Nafcillin	+++	−	+++	−	−	−	−	−
Penicillin G	+++	++	+	−	+	−	−	−
Penicillin V	+++	++	+	−	+	−	−	−
Piperacillin	+++	+++	++	−	++	+++	++	−
Beta-Lactam/Beta-Lactamase Inhibitors								
Amoxicillin–clavulanic acid	+++	+++	+++	−	++	−	+++	−
Ampicillin–sulbactam	+++	+++	+++	−	++	−	+++	−
Ceftazidime–avibactam	+++	+++	+++	−	+++	+++	+++	−
Ceftolozane–tazobactam	+++	+++	+++	−	+++	+++	+++	−
Piperacillin–tazobactam	+++	+++	+++	−	+++	+++	+++	−
Meropenem–vaborbactam	+++	−	+++	−	+++	++	+++	−
Imipenem–cilastatin–relebactam	++	+	+++	−	+++	++	+++	−
First-Generation Cephalosporins								
Cefadroxil	+++	−	+++	−	++	−	−	−
Cefazolin	+++	−	+++	−	++	−	−	−
Cephalexin	+++	−	+++	−	++	−	−	−
Second-Generation Cephalosporins								
Cefotetan	++	−	+	−	++/+++	−	++	−
Cefoxitin	++	−	++	−	++	−	++/+++	−
Cefuroxime	+++	−	+++	−	++	−	−	−

(Continued)

TABLE 6.2

Sensitivity of Organisms to Specific Agents (*Continued*)

Agent	Streptococci	Enterococcus	MSSA	MRSA	Gram-Negative Aerobes (e.g., E. coli, K. pneumoniae)	Pseudomonas	Gram-Negative Anaerobes (e.g., Bacteroides fragilis)	Chlamydia pneumoniae, Legionella pneumophila, M. pneumoniae
Third-Generation Cephalosporins								
Cefotaxime	+++	–	++	–	+++	+	+/++	–
Ceftazidime	++	–	+	–	+++	+++	++	–
Ceftriaxone	+++	–	++	–	+++	+	+	–
Fourth-Generation Cephalosporins								
Cefepime	+++	–	++	–	+++	++/+++	–	–
Ceftaroline	+++	–	++	–	+++	–	–	–
Siderophore Cephalosporins								
Cefiderocol	+++	–	++	–	+++	+++	–	–
Monobactams								
Aztreonam	–	–	–	–	++/+++	++/+++	–	–
Carbapenems								
Doripenem	+++	++	+++	–	+++	+++	+++	–
Ertapenem	+++	++	+++	–	+++	–	+++	–
Imipenem	+++	++	+++	+/++	+++	++/+++	+++	–
Meropenem	+++	+	+++	–	+++	++/+++	+++	–
Fluoroquinolones								
Ciprofloxacin	+/++	+	++	–	+++	++	–	++
Delafloxacin	+++	++	+++	++	+++	+++	–	++
Gemifloxacin	++/+++	+	++	+/++	++	–	–	+++
Levofloxacin	++/+++	+	++	–	+++	+	+	+++
Moxifloxacin	++/+++	+	++	+/++	+++	–	+/++	+++
Norfloxacin†	++	+	++	–	+++	–	–	–

Macrolides							
Azithromycin	++/+++	—	—	++	—	+	—
Clarithromycin	++/+++	—	—	++	—	+	—
Erythromycin	++/+++	—	—	+/++	—	++	—
Aminoglycosides							
Amikacin*	++	—	+++	++	—	++	—
Gentamicin*	++	—	++	++	—	++	‡
Tobramycin*	++	—	+++	++	—	++	—
Tetracyclines							
Doxycycline	++/+++	++	—	+/++	+/++	++	+
Minocycline	+++	++	—	+/++	+/+++	+/+++	+
Tetracycline	++/+++	+	—	+	+/++	++	+
Tigecycline	+++	++	—	++	++	+++	++
Omadacycline	+++	+/++	—	++	++	+++	‡
Eravacycline	++	+++	—	++	++	+++	++
Sulfonamides							
Trimethoprim–sulfamethoxazole	++	—	—	+/+++	+	++	—
Glycopeptides							
Dalbavancin	+++	—	—	—	++	+++	+++
Oritavancin	+++	—	—	—	+++	+++	+++
Telavancin	+++	—	—	—	+++	+++	+++
Vancomycin	++	—	—	—	+++	+++	+++

(Continued)

TABLE 6.2
Sensitivity of Organisms to Specific Agents (Continued)

Agent	Streptococci	Enterococcus	MSSA	MRSA	Gram-Negative Aerobes (e.g., E. coli, K. pneumoniae)	Pseudomonas	Gram-Negative Anaerobes (e.g., Bacteroides fragilis)	Chlamydia pneumoniae, Legionella pneumophila, M. pneumoniae
Oxazolidinones								
Linezolid	+++	+++	+++	+++	–	–	–	+
Tedizolid	+++	+++	+++	+++	–	–	–	–
Lipopeptides								
Daptomycin	+++	+++	+++	+++	–	–	–	–
Streptogramins								
Quinupristin–dalfopristin	+++	++	+++	+++	+	–	–	+
Pleuromutilins								
Lefamulin	+++	++	+++	+++	+/++	–	–	+++
Antianaerobic Agents								
Clindamycin	+++	–	+++	+/++	–	–	+++	–
Metronidazole	–	–	–	–	–	–	+++	–
Miscellaneous Agents								
Chloramphenicol	+/++	++	–	–	++	–	+++	+
Nitrofurantoin†	+++	+++	++	–	+++	–	–	–
Rifampin	++/+++	–	+++	++	–	+	–	++

*Provides synergistic activity against gram-positive organisms when combined with a cell wall-active agent.

†Applicable only to organisms isolated in the urine.

– = No activity or no information available.

+ = Poor to moderate activity; use only when known to be susceptible.

++ = Good activity; resistance in some strains and geographical location may limit use.

+++ = Excellent activity; generally reliable coverage for empiric therapy.

The symbol next to nitrofurantoin - Applicable only to organisms isolated in the urine.

MRSA, methicillin-resistant S. aureus; MSSA, methicillin-sensitive S. aureus.

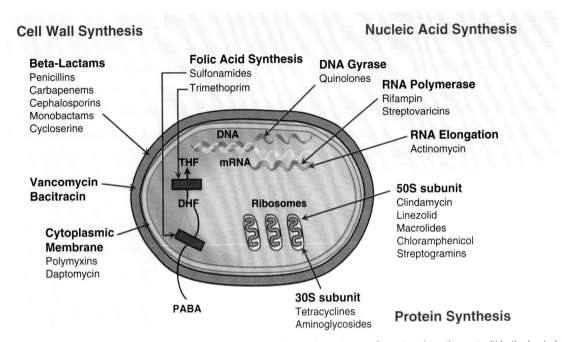

FIGURE 6–1 Antibiotic Sites and Mechanism of Action. This figure identifies various classes of agents, where they act within the bacterial cell and the specific bacterial function they inhibit. Used with permission from Tornetta, P., Ricci, W., Court-Brown, C. M., McQueen, M. M., & McKee, M. (2019). *Rockwood and Green's fractures in adults* (9th ed.). Wolters Kluwer.

DHF, dihydrofolic acid; DNA, deoxyribonucleic acid; mRNA, messenger RNA; PABA, para-aminobenzoic acid; RNA, ribonucleic acid; THF, tetrahydrofolic acid.

are specific to the body site involved. Monitoring for adverse events is specific to the agents prescribed. All patients should be taught how to recognize the most common adverse events, and they should be advised to notify their health care provider if an adverse reaction occurs. The following sections highlight antimicrobials used in practice and include pharmacokinetics, pharmacodynamics, mechanism of action (see **Figure 6.1**), spectrum of activity, common clinical uses, adverse events, drug interactions, and antimicrobial resistance.

PENICILLINS

First isolated in 1928, the penicillins were used successfully to treat streptococcal and staphylococcal infections. Since then, many synthetic penicillins have been developed to address the emerging problem of resistance. Despite resistance, the penicillins remain an important class of antimicrobials. They are classified based on their spectra of activity.

Pharmacokinetics and Pharmacodynamics

Most of the penicillins are unstable in the acid environment of the stomach and must be administered parenterally. Those that are acid stable are given orally. They are widely distributed in the body and penetrate the cerebrospinal fluid (CSF) in the presence of inflammation. Most penicillins are excreted by the kidneys, and renal impairment necessitates dosage adjustment. The half-life of the penicillins in adults with normal renal function is 30 to 90 minutes. The penicillins are removed by hemodialysis, with

the exception of nafcillin and oxacillin. The penicillins exhibit time-dependent bactericidal activity and a postantibiotic effect (PAE) against most gram-positive organisms. See **Box 6.1** for information on PAE. Also, see **Table 6.3** for dosing information.

Mechanism of Action and Spectrum of Activity

The mechanism of action of the penicillins is the inhibition of bacterial cell growth by interference with cell wall synthesis. Penicillins bind to and inactivate the penicillin-binding proteins (PBPs).

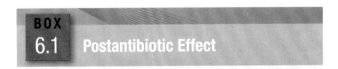

BOX 6.1 Postantibiotic Effect

The PAE is defined as "persistent suppression of bacterial growth after a brief exposure (1 or 2 hours) of bacteria to an antibiotic even in the absence of host defense mechanisms" (Craig & Vogelman, 1987, pp. 900–902). This delayed growth of bacteria results in an increased efficacy of the drugs and allows for less frequent dosing of medications, potentially lowering toxicity and improving compliance. The duration of the PAE is affected by the class of antibiotic, the relevant exposure time, and the specific bacterial species. Bacteriostatic agents, such as macrolides, clindamycin, streptogramins, tetracyclines, and linezolid, have long PAEs, whereas drugs with relatively slow bactericidal action (e.g., penicillins) have moderate PAE.

TABLE 6.3

Penicillin Dosages

Drug	Adult Dosages	Pediatric Dosages
Natural		
Penicillin G	2–4 million units IV q4–6h	100,000–400,000 units/kg/d IV divided q4–6h
Penicillin G benzathine	1.2–2.4 million units IM at specified intervals	300,000–2.4 million units IM at specified intervals
Penicillin G procaine	0.6–4.8 million units IM in divided doses q12–24h at specified intervals	25,000–50,000 units/kg/d IM divided 1–2 times/d
Penicillin VK	250–500 mg PO q6h	25–50 mg/kg/d PO divided q6–8h
Aminopenicillins		
Ampicillin	1–2 g IV q4–6h	100–400 mg/kg/d IV divided 4–6h
Amoxicillin–ampicillin	250–500 mg PO q8h or 875–1,000 mg PO q12h	400–100 mg/kg/d PO divided q6–12h
Penicillinase Resistant		
Cloxacillin	250–500 mg PO q6h	50–100 mg/kg/d PO divided q6h
Dicloxacillin	250–500 mg PO q6h	12.5–100 mg/kg/d PO divided q6h
Nafcillin	500 mg–1 g IV q4–6h	50–200 mg/kg/d IV divided q4–6h
Oxacillin	500–2 g IV q4–6h	100–200 mg/kg/d IV divided q4–6h
Ureidopenicillins		
Piperacillin	3–4 g IV q4–6h	200–300 mg/kg/d IV divided q4–6h

Note: Dosage adjustment of all drugs required in patients with impaired renal function, with the exception of penicillinase-resistant penicillins.

IM, intramuscular; IV, intravenous.

Clinical Uses

Although the use of penicillin itself is limited due to widespread resistance, the penicillin class is effective in treating many infections, including those of the upper and lower respiratory tract, urinary tract, and central nervous system (CNS) as well as sexually transmitted diseases. They are the agents of choice for treating gram-positive infections such as endocarditis caused by susceptible organisms. The ureidopenicillins may be used to treat infections caused by *Pseudomonas aeruginosa*.

Adverse Events

There is a low incidence of adverse reactions with penicillin administration. Hypersensitivity reactions characterized by maculopapular rash and urticaria are most common. Gastrointestinal (GI) side effects are most common with oral administration. In the presence of severe renal dysfunction, high-dose penicillins have been associated with seizures and encephalopathy. Thrombophlebitis has occurred with IV administration. The Jarisch-Herxheimer reaction, characterized by fever, chills, sweating, and flushing, may occur when penicillin is used in treating spirochetes, in particular syphilis. Release of toxic particles from the organism precipitates the reaction. In rare cases, leukopenia, thrombocytopenia, and hemolytic anemia can occur with penicillins.

Drug Interactions

Drug interactions involving penicillins are rare. Probenecid has been shown to increase the half-life of the penicillins by inhibiting renal tubular secretion. The ureidopenicillins have been shown to inactivate the aminoglycosides, and these agents should not be mixed in the same IV solution.

BETA-LACTAM/BETA-LACTAMASE INHIBITOR COMBINATIONS

Resistance to beta-lactams develops when the drug is inactivated by the enzymes known as penicillinases or beta-lactamases produced by bacteria. After several attempts over the years to prevent penicillin degradation by this enzyme, clavulanic acid became the first beta-lactamase inhibitor introduced and combined with a beta-lactam. Other beta-lactamase inhibitors, avibactam, relebactam, sulbactam, tazobactam, and vaborbactam, are also available in combination with ampicillin, ceftazidime, ceftolozane, piperacillin, and the carbapenems imipenem and meropenem. The role of the beta-lactamase inhibitor is to prevent the breakdown of the beta-lactam by organisms that produce the enzyme, thereby enhancing antibacterial activity. These combinations are suitable alternatives for infections caused

TABLE 6.4

Beta-Lactam/Beta-Lactamase Inhibitor Dosages

Drug	Adult Dosages	Pediatric Dosages
Amoxicillin–clavulanic acid (Augmentin)	250–500 mg PO q8h or	20–40 mg/kg/d PO divided q8–12h
	500–875 mg PO q12h or	
	2 g PO q12h*	80–90 mg/kg/d PO divided q12h[†]
Ampicillin–sulbactam (Unasyn)	1.5–3 g IV q6h	100–400 mg/kg/d IV divided q6h
Piperacillin–tazobactam (Zosyn)	4.5 g IV q6–8h or 3.375 g IV q6h	240–300 mg/kg/d IV divided q8h
Ceftazidime–avibactam (Avycaz)	2.5 g IV q8h	—
Ceftolozane–tazobactam (Zerbaxa)	750 mg IV q8h	—
Meropenem-vaborbactam (Vabomere)	4 g IV q8h	—
Imipenem-cilastatin-relebactam (Recarbrio)	1.25 g IV q6h	—

Note: Dosage adjustment required for all drugs administered to patients with renal impairment.

*Amoxicillin–clavulanic acid (Augmentin XR) extended-release formulation.

[†] Amoxicillin/clavulanic acid (Augmentin ES-600) formulation.

IV, intravenous.

by beta-lactamase-producing organisms such as *S. aureus*, *Haemophilus influenzae*, and *Bacteroides fragilis*.

Pharmacokinetics and Pharmacodynamics

The beta-lactam/beta-lactamase inhibitors diffuse into most body tissues, with the exception of the brain and CSF. The half-life of both components in each combination is approximately 1 hour. Because these drugs are eliminated by glomerular filtration, renal dysfunction necessitates dosage changes (**Table 6.4**). The compounds are removed by hemodialysis and peritoneal dialysis.

Mechanism of Action and Spectrum of Activity

The beta-lactam components of the combinations are cell wall–active agents. They interfere with bacterial cell wall synthesis by binding to and inactivating PBPs. The beta-lactamase inhibitors irreversibly bind to most beta-lactamase enzymes, protecting the beta-lactam from degradation and improving their antibacterial activity. The beta-lactamase inhibitors by themselves lack significant antibacterial activity. The spectrum of activity is similar to that of the beta-lactam derivative, with broader coverage against beta-lactamase-producing organisms.

Clinical Uses

Based on their broad spectrum of activity, the beta-lactam/beta-lactamase inhibitors are frequently used in treating polymicrobial infections. They are used extensively to treat intra-abdominal and gynecologic infections and skin and soft tissue infections, including human and animal bites, as well as foot infections in diabetic patients. Respiratory tract infections,

including aspiration pneumonia, sinusitis, and lung abscesses, have been successfully treated with these combinations.

Adverse Events

The addition of the beta-lactamase inhibitor to the various beta-lactams has not resulted in any new or major adverse events. The major effects associated with the beta-lactam/beta-lactamase inhibitor combinations are hypersensitivity reactions and GI side effects such as nausea and diarrhea associated with oral administration. Elevated aminotransferase levels have been documented for all agents.

Drug Interactions

Some of the combinations are physically incompatible with parenteral aminoglycosides. Each of the penicillins in the combinations has been associated with the inactivation of aminoglycosides in vitro. The clinical significance of this interaction is unknown.

CEPHALOSPORINS

The cephalosporins, a beta-lactam group, are structurally similar to the penicillins. Substitutions on the parent compound, 7-aminocephalosporanic acid, produce compounds with different pharmacokinetic properties and spectra of activity. The cephalosporins are divided into *generations* based on their antimicrobial spectrum of activity. The progression from first to fourth generation in general reflects an increase in gram-negative coverage and a loss of gram-positive activity. The fifth generation cephalosporins are considered MRSA-active agents. The siderophore cephalosporins represent a novel class of cephalosporins with activity against drug-resistant gram-negative organisms.

Pharmacokinetics and Pharmacodynamics

The cephalosporins are well absorbed from the GI tract. In some cases, food enhances absorption. They penetrate well into tissues and body fluids and achieve high concentrations in the urinary tract. Noncephamycin second-generation agents and all third- and fourth-generation agents penetrate the CSF and play a role in treating bacterial meningitis. Most of the oral and parenteral cephalosporins are excreted by the kidney, with the exception of ceftriaxone (Rocephin) and cefoperazone (not available in the United States), which are eliminated by the liver. The cephalosporins exhibit a time-dependent bactericidal effect and a prolonged PAE against staphylococci. **Table 6.5** provides dosing information.

Mechanism of Action and Spectrum of Activity

Like other beta-lactams, the cephalosporins interfere with bacterial cell wall synthesis by binding to and inactivating the PBPs. The siderophore cephalosporins utilize the siderophore–iron complex pathway to penetrate the outer membrane of gram-negative organisms in addition to normal passive diffusion through membrane porins.

Clinical Uses

The cephalosporins are used in treating many infections. In general, the first-generation cephalosporins are used in

TABLE 6.5

Cephalosporin Dosages

Drug	Adult Dosages	Pediatric Dosages
First Generation		
Cefazolin	500 mg–1 g IV q8h	50–100 mg/kg/d IV divided q8h
Cephalexin	250–1,000 mg PO q6h	25–100 mg/kg/d PO divided q6h
Cefadroxil	500 mg–1 g PO q12h	30 mg/kg/d PO divided q12h
Second Generation		
Cefotetan	1–2 g IV q12h	40–80 mg/kg/d IV divided q12h
Cefoxitin	1–2 g IV q6–8h	80–160 mg/kg/d IV divided q4–8h
Cefuroxime	750–1.5 g IV q8h	75–150 mg/kg/d IV divided q8h
Cefuroxime axetil	250–500 mg PO q12h	20–30 mg/kg/d PO divided q12h
Cefaclor	250–500 mg PO q8h	20–40 mg/kg/d PO divided q8–12h
Third Generation		
Cefotaxime	1–2 g IV q8h	100–300 mg/kg/d IV divided q6–8h
Ceftazidime	1–2 g IV q8h	90–150 mg/kg/d IV divided q8h
Ceftriaxone*	1–2 g IV q12–24h	50–100 mg/kg/d IV divided q12–24h
Ceftibuten	400 mg PO q24h	9 mg/kg/d PO divided q24h
Cefpodoxime proxetil	100–400 mg PO q12h	10 mg/kg/d PO divided q12h
Cefprozil	250–500 mg PO q12h	15–30 mg/kg/d PO divided q12h
Cefdinir	300 mg PO q12h or 600 mg PO q24h	7–14 mg/kg/d PO divided q12–24h
Fourth Generation		
Cefepime	1–2 g IV q8–12h	50 mg/kg/d IV divided q8h
Ceftaroline	600 mg IV q8h	—
Siderophore Cephalosporins		
Cefiderocol	2 g IV q8h	—

Note: Dosage adjustment necessary for all agents in patients with renal impairment except ceftriaxone.

*Dosage adjustment necessary in patients with liver dysfunction.

IV, intravenous.

treating gram-positive skin infections, pneumococcal respiratory infections, and urinary tract infections and for surgical prophylaxis. The second-generation cephalosporins are used in treating community-acquired pneumonia, other respiratory tract infections, and skin infections. Mixed aerobic and anaerobic infections may be treated with the second-generation cephamycins (cefotetan and cefoxitin). In addition, treating community-acquired bacterial meningitis typically includes a third-generation cephalosporin such as ceftriaxone or cefotaxime (Claforan). Nosocomial infections are commonly treated with ceftazidime (Fortaz) or cefepime (Maxipime), whose broad spectrum of activity includes gram-negative organisms, especially *P. aeruginosa*. Ceftaroline fosamil (Teflaro), a new IV cephalosporin, has activity similar to ceftriaxone but is the only cephalosporin that covers MRSA. The spectrum of activity of cefiderocol (Fetroja), the novel siderophore cephalosporin, encompasses both lactose-fermenting and non-lactose-fermenting gram-negative pathogens, including carbapenem-resistant Enterobacterales.

Adverse Events

The cephalosporins are a safe class of antimicrobials with a favorable toxicity profile. With a few exceptions, the adverse events are similar across the generations. Hypersensitivity reactions, not unlike those with the penicillins, are characterized by maculopapular rash and urticaria. The cross-reactivity between penicillins and cephalosporins is 3% to 10%. Patients who experience allergic reactions to penicillins (other than a type 1 allergy [see Chapter 46]) can often tolerate a cephalosporin. The most common side effects with oral administration are nausea, vomiting, and diarrhea. GI effects are usually transient. Less common reactions include a positive Coombs test and rarely hemolytic reactions.

Drug Interactions

Drug interactions involving cephalosporins are rare. Probenecid has been shown to increase the half-life of some cephalosporins by inhibiting the renal tubular secretion.

MONOBACTAMS

The monobactams are a unique class of beta-lactams with a four-membered ring but lacking a fifth or sixth member, like other beta-lactams. Because aztreonam (Azactam) is the only agent of its class commercially available, most of the information relates specifically to that agent. With primary activity against gram-negative organisms, including *Pseudomonas*, aztreonam is considered a safer alternative to the aminoglycosides, with a similar spectrum of activity.

Pharmacokinetics and Pharmacodynamics

Aztreonam distributes well into most tissues, with a volume of distribution of 0.16 L/kg. Penetration into the CSF is

TABLE 6.6		
Aztreonam Dosages		
Monobactams		
Drug	**Adult Dosages**	**Pediatric Dosages**
Aztreonam	1–2 g IV q6–12h	90–120 mg/kg/d IV divided q6–8h

Note: Dosage adjustment required in patients with impaired renal function.

IV, intravenous.

increased in the presence of inflamed meninges. Aztreonam is not extensively bound to proteins. The approximate half-life is 2 hours, and dosages are typically calculated according to the severity of disease (**Table 6.6**). Aztreonam is excreted primarily unchanged by glomerular filtration, so dosage adjustments are necessary in patients with renal insufficiency. Aztreonam is cleared by hemodialysis and peritoneal dialysis.

Mechanism of Action and Spectrum of Activity

Aztreonam, like other beta-lactams, interferes with bacterial cell wall synthesis by binding to and inactivating PBPs. The principal activity of aztreonam is against most aerobic gram-negative organisms, including *P. aeruginosa*, *Serratia marcescens*, and *Citrobacter* species. It has virtually no activity against gram-positive organisms. Its gram-negative coverage is similar to that of the aminoglycosides and the third-generation cephalosporin ceftazidime. Aztreonam is not active against anaerobic organisms.

Clinical Uses

Aztreonam is commonly used in treating complicated and uncomplicated urinary tract and respiratory tract infections such as pneumonia and bronchitis when aerobic gram-negative coverage is necessary. To broaden coverage, it is usually used in combination with an agent exhibiting gram-positive activity. It is a reasonable substitute for the aminoglycosides in treating gram-negative infections in patients at high risk for toxicity.

Adverse Events

Aztreonam has a relatively safe toxicity profile. Most of the adverse events associated with aztreonam are local reactions and GI symptoms. Elevated aminotransferase levels have also been documented. Patients allergic to penicillins and cephalosporins usually do not manifest an allergic reaction to aztreonam, despite its beta-lactam structure. A cross-allergy specifically with ceftazidime has been reported and linked to an identical side chain on both compounds.

Drug Interactions

No clinically significant drug interactions have been documented with aztreonam.

CARBAPENEMS

The carbapenems, ertapenem (Invanz), doripenem (Doribax), imipenem (Primaxin), and meropenem (Merrem), are bicyclical beta-lactams with a common carbapenem nucleus (**Table 6.7**). Imipenem is extensively metabolized by renal dehydropeptidases, yielding only limited activity in the urine. Cilastatin, a competitive inhibitor of the dehydropeptidases, was introduced to overcome imipenem degradation and is commercially available in combination with imipenem in a one-to-one ratio. Subsequently, ertapenem, meropenem, and doripenem were developed; they maintain stability against dehydropeptidase metabolism without the addition of a cilastatin-like agent. Imipenem-cilastatin-relebactam (Recarbrio) is the first of a new triple combination that includes a beta-lactamase inhibitor to assist in the treatment of complicated gram-negative infections of the urinary and abdominal tracts. The carbapenems are the most broad-spectrum agents commercially available.

Pharmacokinetics and Pharmacodynamics

Carbapenems are not absorbed after oral administration. They exhibit linear pharmacokinetics; thus, peak serum levels increase proportionally as the dose is increased. They are widely distributed into most tissues, with an approximate volume of distribution of 0.25 L/kg. With the exception of ertapenem, they are minimally bound to plasma proteins. Penetration into the CSF varies and depends on the degree of meningeal inflammation. The half-life of the carbapenems is approximately 1 hour. They are primarily eliminated by urinary excretion of unchanged drug. Imipenem, meropenem, and doripenem are removed by hemodialysis and hemofiltration.

The carbapenems, like other beta-lactams, exhibit time-dependent bactericidal effects. Unlike other beta-lactams, they exhibit a PAE against gram-negative aerobes lasting at least 1 to 2 hours.

TABLE 6.7

Carbapenem Dosages

Drug	Adult Dosages	Pediatric Dosages
Ertapenem	1 g IV/IM daily	30 mg/kg/d IV divided q12h
Doripenem	500 mg IV q8h	Not recommended
Imipenem	250–1,000 mg IV q6h	25–100 mg/kg/d IV divided q6h
Meropenem	500–1,000 mg IV q8h	30–120 mg/kg/d IV divided q8h

Note: Dosage adjustment required for all above drugs administered to patients with renal impairment.

IM, intramuscular; IV, intravenous.

Mechanism of Action and Spectrum of Activity

Similar to the penicillins and cephalosporins, the carbapenems bind to several PBPs on the cell wall and interfere with bacterial cell wall synthesis.

Imipenem, meropenem, and doripenem possess the broadest spectrum of activity of any of the beta-lactam compounds. They have excellent activity against aerobic gram-positive organisms, including staphylococci and streptococci, and gram-negative organisms such as Enterobacteriaceae, *P. aeruginosa*, and *Acinetobacter* species. They are also active against most gram-negative anaerobic organisms, including *B. fragilis*. Ertapenem has a similar spectrum of activity as the other carbapenems, with the noted exceptions of *P. aeruginosa* and *Acinetobacter* species, for which ertapenem has no clinically significant activity.

Clinical Uses

Their broad spectrum of activity and stability to many beta-lactamases make the carbapenems useful as single agents in treating polymicrobial infections. They have been used extensively in treating skin and soft tissue, bone and joint, intra-abdominal, and lower respiratory tract infections. In addition, meropenem is used in treating CNS infections because it has a lower risk than imipenem of causing seizures.

Adverse Events

Neurotoxicity, a well-known effect of the carbapenems, is characterized by seizure activity. Imipenem has been reported to lower the seizure threshold more frequently than meropenem and doripenem. Risk factors for seizures include impaired renal function, improper dosing, age, previous CNS disorder, and concomitant agents that lower the seizure threshold. Meropenem and more recently doripenem are the carbapenems of choice in patients with a seizure disorder or underlying risk factors. Such GI side effects as nausea, vomiting, and diarrhea have also been reported. Decreasing the infusion rate may lessen their severity.

Drug Interactions

Concomitant administration of probenecid and meropenem or doripenem results in decreased clearance of these agents and a substantial increase in half-life; therefore, the concurrent administration of meropenem or doripenem with probenecid is not recommended. A similar interaction with imipenem occurs but to a lesser degree.

FLUOROQUINOLONES

Since 1990, the fluoroquinolones (FQs) have become a dominant class of antimicrobial agents. No other class of antimicrobial agents has grown so rapidly or been developed with such interest by pharmaceutical research companies. Although

TABLE 6.8	
Fluoroquinolone Dosages	
Drug	**Adult Dosages**
Ciprofloxacin	250–750 mg PO q12h; 200–400 mg IV q12h; 400 mg IV q8h (severe infections)
Delafloxacin	300 mg IV q12h or 450 mg PO q12h
Gemifloxacin	320 mg PO daily
Levofloxacin	250–750 mg PO/IV daily
Moxifloxacin	400 mg PO/IV daily
Norfloxacin	400 mg PO q12h
Ofloxacin	200–400 mg PO q12h

Note: With the exception of ciprofloxacin for the treatment of urinary tract infections and anthrax, these drugs are not recommended for use in children younger than age 18. Dosage adjustment is required for all drugs (except moxifloxacin) administered to patients with renal impairment.

IV, intravenous.

multiple medications in this class have been approved by the U.S. Food and Drug Administration (FDA), several FQs have been removed from the U.S. market due to the identification of postmarketing adverse events. This emphasizes the importance of postmarketing research and adverse-event reporting. In 2016, the FDA issued a warning stating that adverse effects associated with FQs outweigh the benefits in certain infections (FDA, 2016). Today, the routine use of FQs to treat various types of uncomplicated infections is no longer recommended. **Table 6.8** lists the available FQs. Ciprofloxacin, levofloxacin, and moxifloxacin are most commonly prescribed.

Pharmacokinetics and Pharmacodynamics

The FQs are bactericidal antibiotics. Delafloxacin is unique in that it is an anionic FQ, whereas other FQs are zwitterionic. This basically means that delafloxacin has increased accumulation in bacteria, allowing for enhanced bactericidal activity.

The FQs display a concentration-dependent killing effect. All FQs have excellent bioavailability, making it easy to transition from an IV to an oral formulation. They have a volume of distribution ranging from 1.5 to 6.1 L/kg and distribute well into most tissues and fluids except the CNS. The half-life for the FQs ranges from 4 to 12 hours, with levofloxacin, gemifloxacin, and moxifloxacin having the longest half-lives. These three agents are dosed once daily. All FQs undergo renal elimination with the exception of moxifloxacin. The FQs are removed by hemodialysis and peritoneal dialysis, with percentages varying between products. All FQs also exhibit a PAE, which also appears to be a concentration-dependent parameter. The newer compounds have been reported to have PAEs of 1 to 6 hours, depending on the pathogen and drug.

Mechanism of Action and Spectrum of Activity

The quinolone antibiotics are strong inhibitors of deoxyribonucleic acid (DNA) gyrase and topoisomerase IV. These enzymes are critical to the process of supercoiling DNA. Without such enzymatic activity, bacterial DNA cannot replicate.

All FQs possess activity against aerobic gram-negative organisms. Ciprofloxacin and levofloxacin have activity against *P. aeruginosa*, representing the oral antibiotics commonly used to treat this pathogen. However, widespread use of the FQs since the late 1990s have led to increased resistance against gram-negative pathogens and limited use in some parts of the United States. Newer FQs, such as levofloxacin, moxifloxacin, and gemifloxacin, have activity against gram-positive organisms including *Streptococcus* species. These agents are sometimes referred to as the *anti-pneumococcal* or *respiratory* FQs given their activity against *Streptococcus pneumoniae* and usefulness in treating community-acquired pneumonia. Moxifloxacin (Avelox) has some activity against anaerobic bacteria. Delafloxacin (Baxdela) possesses in vitro activity against MRSA, *P. aeruginosa*, and certain anaerobic bacteria including *B. fragilis*.

Clinical Uses

The FQs have been shown to be effective in treating many infections, including urinary tract infections, pneumonia, sexually transmitted diseases, skin and soft tissue infections, GI infections (in combination with an agent for anaerobic coverage), traveler's diarrhea, and osteomyelitis. For hospital-acquired infections such as nosocomial pneumonia, ciprofloxacin (Cipro) or levofloxacin (Levaquin) is the preferred agent, as part of a drug combination, because these agents have the best activity against *P. aeruginosa*. Ciprofloxacin is also recommended for meningococcal prophylaxis as a single 500-mg oral dose.

Adverse Events

The most common side effects include nausea, diarrhea, dizziness, and confusion. QTc interval prolongation remains a potentially serious effect as well. Enhanced warnings include disabling and potentially permanent side effects involving tendons, muscles, joints, nerves, and the CNS.

Drug Interactions

The FQs have several significant drug–drug interactions. Ciprofloxacin is a potent inhibitor of the cytochrome P-450 (CYP) 1A2 isoenzyme and may increase the effect of other medications, including theophylline, warfarin (Coumadin), tizanidine, and propranolol. Antacids, sucralfate, and magnesium, calcium, or iron salts will decrease the absorption of the FQs if given concomitantly. These agents should be separated when administered orally. Due to the risk of QTc prolongation and torsades de pointes, medications that prolong the QTc interval should be used cautiously with the FQs. Prolonged administration of FQs in combination with corticosteroids increases the risk of tendonitis and tendon rupture. Hyperglycemic and hypoglycemic events have been reported with FQs when administered with insulin or other antidiabetic agents.

MACROLIDES

Erythromycin (E-Mycin), the prototypical macrolide, has been used in treating many infections over the years. However, its use has been diminished by its GI side effects. This toxicity has even been used as a means of treating patients with diabetic gastroparesis. Newer agents (clarithromycin and azithromycin) have been developed with improved GI tolerance and longer half-lives. Telithromycin (Ketek), a related ketolide with a similar mechanism of action and antibacterial coverage, was withdrawn from the market due to safety concerns of acute hepatic failure. Fidaxomicin (Dificid) is the first macrolide antibiotic with a narrow spectrum of activity targeted against *Clostridium difficile*.

Pharmacokinetics and Pharmacodynamics

The macrolides are usually administered orally and are absorbed from the GI tract if not inactivated by gastric acid. Fidaxomicin is not systemically absorbed and acts locally in the colon. The macrolides have good tissue penetration, achieve high intracellular concentrations, and exhibit minimal protein binding. The macrolides are metabolized via the liver and excreted in the urine. Half-lives vary throughout the class, from 2 hours for erythromycin, 4 to 5 hours for clarithromycin (Biaxin), and 50 to 60 hours for azithromycin (Zithromax). The long half-life and high intracellular concentrations of azithromycin permit once-daily dosing and short courses. Dosage adjustment in patients with renal failure is necessary with clarithromycin (Biaxin) and erythromycin (**Table 6.9**). The macrolides are minimally cleared via hemodialysis and peritoneal dialysis.

Mechanism of Action and Spectrum of Activity

The mechanism of action of the macrolides is inhibition of bacterial protein synthesis by binding to the 50S ribosomal subunit. The spectrum of activity of the macrolides includes gram-positive and gram-negative aerobes and atypical organisms, including chlamydia, mycoplasma, legionella, rickettsia, mycobacteria, and spirochetes.

Clinical Uses

The macrolides are used in several settings. Their broad spectrum of activity makes them useful in treating respiratory tract, skin, and soft tissue infections, sexually transmitted diseases, HIV-related *Mycobacterium avium–Mycobacterium intracellulare* complex infection, and other infections caused by atypical organisms such as chlamydia, rickettsia, and legionella. Fidaxomicin is solely used to treat both severe and non-severe cases of *C. difficile* infection.

Adverse Events

The macrolides are in general considered safe agents. Particularly with erythromycin, GI effects such as abdominal pain, nausea, and vomiting are most common. The newer macrolides cause fewer GI effects. Hepatotoxicity related to the macrolides is rare but serious; it also is less frequent with the newer agents. Extremely high doses of IV erythromycin and oral clarithromycin have been associated with ototoxicity. Phlebitis may occur with IV erythromycin administration.

Drug Interactions

Among the macrolides, erythromycin and clarithromycin are potent inhibitors of the CYP3A4 isoenzyme. When administered concomitantly, they have been shown to prolong the half-life of an extensive list of agents, including cyclosporine, tacrolimus, carbamazepine, theophylline, warfarin, and most statins. Azithromycin does not undergo significant cytochrome P-450 metabolism, so the possibility of similar interactions is low. Macrolides have the potential to increase the QTc interval, so caution should be used in patients receiving concomitant medications that can also prolong the QTc interval.

TABLE 6.9		
Macrolide/Ketolide Antibiotic Dosages		
Drug	**Adult Dosages**	**Pediatric Dosages**
Azithromycin	250–500 mg IV/PO daily or 2,000 mg (ER) PO single dose	5–12 mg/kg IV/PO daily or 30 mg/kg PO single dose
Clarithromycin*	250–500 mg PO q12h or 1,000 mg (ER) PO daily	15 mg/kg/d PO divided q12h
Erythromycin base*	250 mg–1 g PO q6h	30–50 mg/kg/d PO divided q6–8h
Erythromycin ethyl succinate	400–800 mg PO q6–12h	30–50 mg/kg/d PO divided q6–8h
Erythromycin injection	500–1,000 mg IV q6–8h	15–50 mg/kg/d IV divided q6h

*Dosage adjustment necessary in patients with renal impairment.

ER, extended-release product; IV, intravenous.

AMINOGLYCOSIDES

Despite the advent of many new antibiotics over the past several decades, the aminoglycosides remain an important therapeutic drug class. Their major drawback has been their potential for drug-related toxicities (nephrotoxicity and ototoxicity). Because of these, their use or the length of therapy has been restricted. The introduction of a modified dosing regimen that uses once-daily (or extended-interval) dosing of these agents for several infections has provided a way of maximizing their therapeutic effects while minimizing the risk of toxicity.

Pharmacokinetics and Pharmacodynamics

The aminoglycosides are poorly absorbed from the GI tract, and parenteral administration is necessary to treat systemic infections. They are weakly bound to serum proteins (10%) and freely distribute into the extracellular fluid. The approximate volume of distribution is 0.25 L/kg, which may be significantly affected in intensive care patients and in disease states such as malnutrition, obesity, and ascites. The aminoglycosides are excreted unchanged via glomerular filtration. The half-life of aminoglycosides in an adult with normal renal function is approximately 1 to 3 hours. Dosage adjustments are necessary in patients with renal impairment because substantial increases in the half-life are seen. Aminoglycosides can be removed by hemodialysis, peritoneal dialysis, and continuous hemofiltration/dialysis.

Because of a narrow range between efficacy and toxicity, renal function and serum levels are used to monitor therapy with aminoglycosides. **Table 6.10** gives dosage guidelines.

Pharmacodynamically, the bactericidal effect of the aminoglycosides depends on drug concentration. The number of organisms decreases more rapidly when a higher peak concentration is achieved. In addition, the aminoglycosides exhibit a PAE for both gram-positive and gram-negative organisms.

Mechanism of Action and Spectrum of Activity

The aminoglycosides are actively taken up by bacteria and subsequently bind to the smaller 30S subunit of the bacterial ribosome, thus inhibiting bacterial protein synthesis.

The principal activity of the aminoglycosides is against aerobic gram-negative bacilli such as *Escherichia coli*, *Klebsiella* species, *Proteus mirabilis*, *Enterobacter* species, *Acinetobacter* species, and *P. aeruginosa*. They are also generally active against gram-positive cocci, particularly *Staphylococcus*, *Enterococcus*, and *Streptococcus* species, but they must be used in combination (for synergy) with a cell wall–active agent such as ampicillin, nafcillin, or vancomycin. Streptomycin is also active against *Francisella tularensis* and *Mycobacterium tuberculosis*. Plazomicin (Zemdri) is a novel aminoglycoside that has been modified to maintain stability against common mechanisms of *Enterobacteriaecae* resistance.

Clinical Uses

The aminoglycosides are primarily used in treating gram-negative infections. They have long been used in the empiric treatment of neutropenic fever and nosocomial infections because of their broad coverage of *P. aeruginosa* and Enterobacteriaceae. They are also frequently used with cell wall–active agents such as penicillins, cephalosporins, and vancomycin to achieve synergy in treating gram-positive infections, including

TABLE 6.10

Aminoglycoside Dosages

Aminoglycoside	Adult Dosages	Pediatric Dosages
Multiple Daily Dosing		
Gentamicin, tobramycin	1–1.7 mg/kg IV q8h	6–7.5 mg/kg/d IV divided q8h
Netilmicin*	1.7–2 mg/kg IV q8h	
Amikacin, kanamycin*	5 mg/kg IV q8h or 7.5 mg/kg IV q12h	15–22.5 mg/kg/d IV divided q8h
Streptomycin	0.5–2 g IV q24h	20–40 mg/kg/d IV divided q6–12h
Once-Daily Dosing†		
Gentamicin, tobramycin	5–7 mg/kg IV q24h	5–7.5 mg/kg IV q24h
Netilmicin*	4–6 mg/kg IV q24h	
Amikacin	15–20 mg/kg IV q24h	20 mg/kg IV q24h
Plazomicin	15 mg/kg IV q24h	

Note: Dosage adjustment required for all drugs administered to patients with renal impairment.

* Not routinely available for use in the United States.

† Once-daily dosing of aminoglycosides is not recommended for enterococcal infections, during pregnancy, in instances of gram-positive synergy, or for endocarditis, meningitis, or ascites.

IV, intravenous.

staphylococcal and enterococcal infections. They are routinely used in combination with other agents in treating pneumonia, bacteremia, and intra-abdominal and skin and soft tissue infections. Monotherapy usually is not recommended, with the noted exception of patients with urinary tract infections. The aminoglycosides have been used in treating tuberculosis, with streptomycin having the greatest activity against *M. tuberculosis*. Streptomycin is also the treatment of choice for tularemia, a potential agent of bioterrorism.

Adverse Events

In general, the aminoglycosides have been associated with a variety of adverse events (GI and CNS), most of which are mild and transient. They rarely produce hypersensitivity reactions and are well tolerated at the sites of administration. Nephrotoxicity and ototoxicity are also associated with aminoglycoside use.

Nephrotoxicity results from accumulation of the drug in the proximal tubule cells of the kidney, causing nonoliguric renal failure. This renal failure is usually mild and reversible and rarely progresses to the need for dialysis. Factors that increase the risk of toxicity to the kidney include increased age, renal disease, increased trough levels, dehydration, and concomitant administration of nephrotoxic agents such as amphotericin B, cyclosporine, and vancomycin. Blood urea nitrogen and serum creatinine values are monitored in addition to serum levels to ensure safe and effective therapy. **Table 6.11** provides optimal serum concentrations for aminoglycosides.

Two forms of ototoxicity—auditory and vestibular—may occur alone or simultaneously. Auditory toxicity presents as

hearing loss and tinnitus; vestibular toxicity is manifested by nausea, vomiting, and vertigo. Ototoxicity may be irreversible and has been associated with high serum trough levels. The risk of ototoxicity increases when the aminoglycosides are administered in combination with high-dose loop diuretics, high-dose macrolide antibiotics, or vancomycin. Long courses of aminoglycosides warrant baseline and periodic auditory monitoring.

Drug Interactions

The aminoglycosides have the potential to cause or prolong neuromuscular blockade, although this is uncommon. It is recommended that parenteral aminoglycosides be administered over a 30-minute interval. The risk of neuromuscular blockade increases in patients receiving concurrent neuromuscular blockers, general anesthetics, or calcium channel blockers and in those with myasthenia gravis. Administration of calcium gluconate usually reverses the neuromuscular blockade.

TETRACYCLINES

The tetracyclines possess activity against gram-positive, gram-negative, and atypical organisms, including rickettsia, chlamydia, mycobacteria, and spirochetes. The classic tetracyclines are separated into short-, intermediate-, and long-acting agents (such as doxycycline and minocycline). The tetracyclines became the first class of antimicrobials to be labeled *broad spectrum*, and they remain a frequently used class of antimicrobials. Alterations to the tetracycline structure have also yielded a newer generation of agents. Tigecycline (Tygacil), eravacycline (Xerava), and omadacycline (Nuzyra) have recently been added to the tetracycline armamentarium.

Pharmacokinetics and Pharmacodynamics

Absorption from the GI tract along with protein binding varies among agents. The long-acting agents have the highest absorption and are protein bound to the greatest extent. With the exception of the long-acting agents, absorption is improved with administration on an empty stomach. The tetracyclines have excellent tissue distribution. The primary route of elimination is through the kidney by glomerular filtration, with the exception of doxycycline and the newer generation agents. In general, the short-acting agents have a half-life of 8 hours and the long-acting agents 16 to 18 hours. The tetracyclines are removed to a small degree by hemodialysis. **Table 6.12** provides dosing information.

Mechanism of Action and Spectrum of Activity

The tetracyclines inhibit bacterial protein synthesis by binding to the 30S subunit of the ribosome and are typically bacteriostatic. The tetracyclines are active against gram-positive and gram-negative bacteria and atypical organisms, including spirochetes, rickettsia, chlamydia, mycoplasma, and legionella. The newer generation agents possess enhanced activity

TABLE 6.11		
Aminoglycoside Concentration Monitoring		
Aminoglycoside	**Target Peak**	**Target Trough**
*Multiple Daily Dosing**		
Gentamicin, tobramycin	4–10 mcg/mL	<2 mcg/mL
Netilmicin	4–10 mcg/mL	<2 mcg/mL
Amikacin, kanamycin	20–30 mcg/mL	<8 mcg/mL
Streptomycin	20–30 mcg/mL	<8 mcg/mL
Once-Daily Dosing†		
Gentamicin, tobramycin	>15 mcg/mL	<1 mcg/mL
Netilmicin	>15 mcg/mL	<1 mcg/mL
Amikacin	>50 mcg/mL	<5 mcg/mL
Plazomicin		<3 ug/mL

*Serum concentrations based upon steady state for multiple daily dosing. Peak concentrations should be obtained 30–60 minutes after infusion and trough concentrations 30 minutes before next infusion.

† Random concentrations routinely measured for once-daily dosing in lieu of peak and trough serum concentrations and dosage adjustments based upon dosing nomograms.

TABLE 6.12
Tetracycline Dosages

Drug	Adult Dosages
Doxycycline (Vibramycin)	100 mg IV or PO q12h
Eravacycline (Xerava)	1 mg/kg IV q12h
Minocycline (Minocin)	100–200 mg PO q12h
Tetracycline (Sumycin)	250–500 mg PO q6h
Omadacycline (Nuzyra)	200 mg IV on day 1, then 100 mg IV q24h or 450 mg PO daily on days 1–2, then 300 mg PO daily
Tigecycline (Tygacil)	50 mg IV q12h

Note: Dosage adjustment necessary for demeclocycline, minocycline, and tetracycline in patients with renal impairment. The tetracyclines are not recommended for use in children less than age 8 or during pregnancy and breast-feeding.

IV, intravenous.

against MRSA, vancomycin-resistant enterococci (VRE), and extended-spectrum beta-lactamase-producing organisms.

Clinical Uses

Because of their broad spectrum of activity, the tetracyclines are used extensively in many settings. They are typically used as alternatives when beta-lactams are not an option. They are frequently used in treating rickettsial, chlamydial, and gram-negative infections, in addition to acne vulgaris and pelvic inflammatory disease (PID). Doxycycline is the drug of choice for the treatment of early Lyme disease and is used in treating community-acquired pneumonia. Doxycycline and minocycline are used as sclerosing agents for pleurodesis. Additionally, minocycline and doxycycline have gained popularity as a treatment for community-acquired MRSA infections. Though a tetracycline, demeclocycline (Declomycin) is primarily used to treat the syndrome of inappropriate antidiuretic hormone and not as an antibiotic. The newer generation agents may be used to treat complicated skin and skin structure infections and intra-abdominal infections and may prove useful in the treatment of tetracycline-resistant organisms. Given their spectrum of activity, they may also be used for gram-negative organisms resistant to alternative agents.

Adverse Events

The most frequent side effects associated with the tetracyclines are anorexia, nausea, vomiting, and epigastric distress. These are typically lessened if the agents are administered with food. Thrombophlebitis is associated with IV administration, and it is recommended that doxycycline be administered in a large volume and infused slowly. Hepatotoxicity is a rare but potentially fatal toxicity. The risk of hepatotoxicity increases if the patient is concurrently receiving other hepatotoxic agents. Gray-brown discoloration of the teeth can be a permanent effect of the tetracyclines. It results from stable tetracycline–calcium complexes in bone and teeth and is related to dose and duration of therapy. Therefore, children younger than age 8 should not receive tetracyclines. Patients receiving tetracyclines are more sensitive to the effects of the sun because of accumulation of the drug in the skin. Minocycline has been associated with dose-related vertigo. Tigecycline has been reported to cause asymptomatic hyperbilirubinemia.

Drug Interactions

There are multiple drug interactions involving the tetracyclines. The absorption of the tetracyclines is affected by several agents. Tetracyclines form chelating complexes with divalent and trivalent cations, decreasing tetracycline absorption. It is recommended that the administration of tetracyclines and antacids, iron, cholestyramine, and sucralfate be separated by at least 1 hour. Likewise, food decreases the absorption of most tetracyclines, with the exception of doxycycline. Milk and dairy products also impair their absorption. Phenytoin and carbamazepine, CYP (cytochrome P-450) enzyme inducers, decrease the half-life of doxycycline. Concomitant administration of the tetracyclines and oral contraceptives results in decreased levels of the oral contraceptive, so an additional form of contraception is recommended. The tetracyclines also potentiate the effect of warfarin by impairing vitamin K production by intestinal flora.

SULFONAMIDES

In 1932, the dye prontosil rubrum was found to be effective in treating streptococcal infections. Subsequently, it was determined that one of the by-products was sulfanilimide. Manipulation of this by-product created the class of antimicrobials known as the sulfonamides.

Pharmacokinetics and Pharmacodynamics

Oral sulfonamides are readily absorbed from the GI tract. They are distributed through all body tissues and enter the CSF, pleural fluid, and synovial fluid. They are eliminated from the body by glomerular filtration and hepatic metabolism. The half-lives of the sulfonamides vary from hours to days; sulfadoxine (Fansidar) (no longer available in the United States), at 5 to 10 days, has the longest half-life. **Table 6.13** gives dosing information.

Mechanism of Action and Spectrum of Activity

The sulfonamides work by inhibiting the incorporation of para-aminobenzoic acid, the basic building block used by bacteria to synthesize dihydrofolic acid. Making dihydrofolic acid is the first step leading to folic acid synthesis, which is required for bacterial cell growth. Sulfamethoxazole (SMX) competitively inhibits the bacterial enzyme dihydropteroate synthetase.

Trimethoprim (TMP), combined with SMX, inhibits the enzyme dihydrofolate reductase, synergistically inhibiting

TABLE 6.13
Sulfonamide Dosages

Drug	Adult Dosages	Pediatric Dosages
Sulfadiazine	4–8 g PO in divided doses q6–12h	100–150 mg/kg/d PO divided q6h
Sulfisoxazole	4–8 g PO in divided doses q4–6h	120–150 mg/kg/d PO divided q4–6h
Trimethoprim	100 mg PO q12h or 200 mg PO q24h	4–6 mg/kg/d PO divided q12h
Trimethoprim–sulfamethoxazole*	160/800 mg PO q12h or 10–20 mg/kg/d IV in divided doses	6–20 mg/kg/d PO/IV divided q6–12h

Note: Dosage adjustment necessary in patients with renal impairment.

* Dosing recommendations are based on the trimethoprim component.

IV, intravenous.

folic acid formation at another step in the pathway. Because bacterial dihydrofolate reductase is inhibited much more than the mammalian enzyme and because humans obtain exogenous dietary folate, inhibition of folate synthesis by SMX–TMP in humans is not a major problem.

The sulfonamides are active against a wide range of gram-positive and gram-negative organisms, with the exception of *Pseudomonas* species and group A streptococci. In combination with other folate antagonists, they also demonstrate activity against *P. jiroveci* and *Toxoplasma gondii.*

Clinical Uses

The sulfonamides are frequently used in treating many infections. Sulfasalazine (Azulfidine), a sulfonamide derivative lacking significant antimicrobial activity, is poorly absorbed and is used in the management of ulcerative colitis. Because of their limited spectrum of activity and increasing resistance, the sulfonamides are typically used in combination with other agents to increase efficacy or expand coverage. TMP–SMX (Bactrim) is the combination of choice in treating urinary tract infections, *P. jiroveci* pneumonia (PCP), toxoplasmosis, and some resistant gram-negative infections. Mafenide (Sulfamylon) and silver sulfadiazine (Silvadene) are topical agents frequently used in treating burns.

Adverse Events

Several side effects are reported for sulfonamides. The most common are rash, fever, and GI side effects. The rash occurs within 1 to 2 weeks of initiating therapy. Severe dermatologic reactions, such as Stevens-Johnson syndrome and vasculitis, are uncommon and associated more with longer-acting preparations.

Hemolytic anemia can occur in patients with glucose-6-phosphate dehydrogenase deficiency.

Drug Interactions

The sulfonamides potentiate the effects of warfarin, phenytoin, hypoglycemic agents, and methotrexate as a result of drug displacement or decreased liver metabolism.

GLYCOPEPTIDES

Vancomycin, a glycopeptide antibiotic, was introduced in 1958. Shortly after its introduction, vancomycin became known as *Mississippi Mud* because of the color and impurities in the manufacturing process. The clinical use of vancomycin was initially limited due to its potential for drug-related toxicities, alternative available agents, and concern for the development of resistance. However, since the early 1980s, vancomycin has been an important agent in treating gram-positive infections. More recent additions to this class include dalbavancin (Dalvance), oritavancin (Orbactiv), and telavancin (Vibativ). All of these agents have a narrow spectrum of activity directed toward gram-positive organisms. The newest agents, dalbavancin and oritavancin, have prolonged half-lives that allow for much less frequent dosing.

Pharmacokinetics and Pharmacodynamics

Vancomycin is poorly absorbed from the GI tract. Because of its poor bioavailability, oral administration of vancomycin provides concentrations in the stool sufficient to treat *Clostridium difficile* colitis. The volume of distribution for vancomycin and telavancin, respectively, is 0.6 to 0.9 L/kg and 0.1 L/kg. Vancomycin is minimally bound to proteins; however, telavancin is highly bound to proteins (greater than 90%). They have relatively good penetration into most body fluids and tissues. Unpredictable levels are attained in the CSF and bone. Telavancin is dosed 10 mg/kg IV once daily. Vancomycin is dosed 15 to 20 mg/kg IV with the interval based on kidney function. **Table 6.14** provides an example of a vancomycin-dosing nomogram, and **Table 6.15** provides the dosing of dalbavancin, oritavancin, and telavancin. Monitoring renal function is important in determining proper dosing because dosage adjustments are necessary in patients with renal insufficiency. Both vancomycin and telavancin are renally excreted, primarily as unchanged drug. Vancomycin's half-life in adults with normal renal function is 5 to 11 hours. The half-life of telavancin is approximately 8 hours. Neither telavancin nor vancomycin is cleared to a significant extent by hemodialysis or peritoneal dialysis.

Serum drug monitoring has been used for vancomycin in patients with unpredictable kidney function or severe infections or those receiving therapy for more than 3 to 5 days. In general, the target trough concentration ranges from 15 to 20 mg/mL for pneumonia, osteomyelitis, meningitis, and endocarditis and from 10 to 15 mg/mL for other infections.

TABLE 6.14

Vancomycin Dosages

Dosing Interval

Estimated Creatinine Clearance (mL/min)	40–55 kg, 500 mg*	55–75 kg, 750 mg*	75–100 kg, 1,000 mg*
>80	q8h	q12h	q12h
54–80	q12h	q18h	q18h
40–53	q18h	q24h	q24h
27–39	q24h	q36h	q36h
21–26	q36h	q48h	q48h
16–20	q48h		

Note: These recommendations represent one of several nomograms used in the empiric dosing of vancomycin. Some prescribers use pharmacokinetic calculations and monitor serum trough levels to evaluate the efficacy and toxicity of a particular regimen. Therapeutic trough levels are typically maintained between 10 and 20 mcg/mL.

* Patient's body weight and IV dose of vancomycin.

TABLE 6.15

Glycopeptide Dosages

Drug	Adult Dosages	Pediatric Dosages
Dalbavancin (Dalvance)	1,000 mg IV followed by 500 mg IV 1 wk later	—
Oritavancin (Orbactiv)	1,200 mg IV as a single injection	—
Telavancin (Vibativ)	10 mg/kg IV q24h	—

IV, intravenous.

However, recent evidence suggests that trough levels may not correlate well to area under the concentration (AUC) values. An updated consensus guideline on the therapeutic monitoring of vancomycin was recently published and now recommends AUC-based dosing that includes both peak and trough levels. Serum monitoring is not required for dalbavancin, oritavancin, or telavancin. All of these agents exhibit bactericidal activity and a PAE of 1 to 4 hours.

Mechanism of Action and Spectrum of Activity

Glycopeptides are cell wall–active agents. They work by inhibiting the binding of the D-alanyl-D-alanine portion of the cell wall precursor or by interfering with the polymerization and cross-linking of peptidoglycan. The newer agents have more rapid bactericidal activity than vancomycin.

The principal activity of the glycopeptides is limited to gram-positive aerobic and anaerobic bacteria such as methicillin-sensitive and methicillin-resistant staphylococci, streptococci, enterococci, and *Clostridium* species.

Clinical Uses

Vancomycin is used to treat many infections. It is frequently used to treat serious gram-positive infections in patients allergic to or unable to tolerate beta-lactam antibiotics, and it is the drug of choice for MRSA and other resistant gram-positive infections. Neutropenic fever, endocarditis, and meningitis are commonly treated with vancomycin. Oral vancomycin is now recommended as a first-line treatment of both severe and non-severe cases of *C. difficile* colitis. The newer agents are currently indicated only for the treatment of skin and skin structure infections.

Adverse Events

The most common side effects associated with vancomycin administration are fever and chills, phlebitis, and *red man* syndrome, a histamine-mediated phenomenon associated with the rate of vancomycin infusion. The typical syndrome consists of pruritus; flushing of the head, neck, and face; and hypotension. It usually resolves when the drug is discontinued. This reaction can also occur with telavancin. Vancomycin and telavancin should be infused over at least 1 hour.

Nephrotoxicity as a result of vancomycin alone is uncommon. Typically, a combination of variables and risk factors precipitates renal insufficiency. Risk factors include age, preexisting renal disease, and the use of other nephrotoxic agents such as aminoglycosides, amphotericin B, acyclovir, and cyclosporine. In clinical trials evaluating telavancin and vancomycin, an increase in serum creatinine was more common with telavancin. Vancomycin has been classified as an ototoxic agent. Although rare, ototoxicity has occurred in patients receiving high-dose therapy or concurrent ototoxic agents (e.g., aminoglycosides). Hematologic effects from vancomycin such as thrombocytopenia and neutropenia are rare. The most commonly reported adverse effects of telavancin are taste disturbances, nausea, vomiting, and foamy urine. Due to the risk to the fetus, telavancin is contraindicated during pregnancy.

Drug Interactions

Since the glycopeptides do not undergo significant hepatic metabolism, drug–drug interactions with these agents are unlikely.

OXAZOLIDINONES

The oxazolidinones are a totally synthetic antibiotic class first investigated in the late 1980s as antidepressant agents. Serendipitously, these agents were discovered to have excellent antibacterial activity. The main reason for their clinical development has been the emergence and spread of resistance in gram-positive pathogens. Linezolid (Zyvox) and tedizolid (Sivextro) are the only agents available in this class.

Pharmacokinetics and Pharmacodynamics

Linezolid and tedizolid are well absorbed from the GI tract. Peak levels are achieved within 1 to 2 hours, and levels increase linearly as the dose is increased. The absolute bioavailability of these agents is greater than 90%. The oral formulation may be administered without regard to meals. Oxazolidinones are predominantly eliminated by nonrenal mechanisms, and their metabolism does not involve the CYP enzyme system. Linezolid is removed by hemodialysis and should be dosed following hemodialysis sessions, while tedizolid is not significantly affected. **Table 6.16** provides dosing information.

Oxazolidinones are considered bacteriostatic agents. Oxazolidinones exhibit a modest to prolonged PAE against staphylococci and enterococci.

Mechanism of Action and Spectrum of Activity

Oxazolidinones bind to the 50S ribosome at a unique binding site and disrupt bacterial protein synthesis. Antagonism has been described with chloramphenicol and clindamycin.

The principal activity of the oxazolidinones is against gram-positive aerobic organisms, including staphylococci, streptococci, and enterococci. In particular, activity against resistant pathogens, including MRSA, penicillin-resistant streptococci, and VRE, is excellent.

Clinical Uses

Linezolid has FDA approval for the treatment of community and nosocomial pneumonia, skin and skin structure infections, and vancomycin-resistant *Enterococcus faecium*, while tedizolid is only approved for the treatment of skin and skin structure infections.

Adverse Events

In general, oxazolidinones are well tolerated when used for short-course therapy. The most common adverse events include diarrhea, nausea, taste perversion, and vomiting. Thrombocytopenia has been reported on average in 3% to 4% of patients in studies of linezolid. Additionally, anemia, leukopenia, and pancytopenia have been reported. A complete blood count should be monitored in patients, especially if receiving linezolid for longer than 2 weeks.

Drug Interactions

As mentioned earlier, this class of agents was initially investigated for its antidepressant activity and as such linezolid and tedizolid possess weak monoamine oxidase inhibitory activity. There is a potential for drug interactions with sympathomimetic agents, such as pseudoephedrine, selective serotonin reuptake inhibitor antidepressants like citalopram, some herbal products, and foods rich in tyramine.

LIPOPEPTIDES

Daptomycin is an antibacterial agent belonging to the class known as the lipopeptides. This class of agents has been studied for its antibacterial activity for several decades; however, daptomycin is the only agent available. Daptomycin (Cubicin) is a natural product developed for the treatment of MDR gram-positive pathogens.

Pharmacokinetics and Pharmacodynamics

Daptomycin's pharmacokinetics are nearly linear and time independent at doses of up to 6 mg/kg administered once daily for 7 days. Its half-life is approximately 8 hours. The apparent volume of distribution in healthy adults is approximately 0.1 L/kg. Daptomycin reversibly binds human plasma proteins, primarily to serum albumin, with a mean serum protein binding of 90%. Because renal excretion is the primary route of elimination, dosage adjustments are necessary in patients with severe renal insufficiency (creatinine clearance less than 30 mL/min). The dose for patients with normal renal function is 4 to 6 mg/kg IV administered daily (**Table 6.17**). There is very limited information to support the use of daptomycin in pediatric patients. Daptomycin exhibits rapid, concentration-dependent bactericidal activity against gram-positive organisms.

TABLE 6.16
Oxazolidinone Dosages

Drug	Adult Dosages	Pediatric Dosages
Linezolid (Zyvox)	400–600 mg PO/IV q12h	20 mg/kg/d PO/IV divided q12h or 30 mg/kg/d PO/IV divided q8h
Tedizolid (Sivextro)	200 mg PO/IV daily	–

IV, intravenous.

TABLE 6.17
Lipopeptide Dosages

Drug	Adult Dosages	Pediatric Dosages
Daptomycin (Cubicin)	4–6 mg/kg IV q24h	

Note: Dosage adjustment necessary for CrCl < 30 mL/min.

IV, intravenous.

Mechanism of Action and Spectrum of Activity

The mechanism of action of daptomycin is distinct from that of any other antibiotic. It binds to bacterial membranes and causes a rapid depolarization of membrane potential. The loss of membrane potential leads to bacterial cell death.

Daptomycin covers most gram-positive pathogens such as *S. aureus* (including methicillin-resistant strains), streptococcus, and enterococcus. It is active against MRSA and VRE.

Clinical Uses

Daptomycin is indicated for the treatment of complicated skin and skin structure infections and *S. aureus* bloodstream infections (bacteremia), including those with right-sided infective endocarditis, caused by methicillin-susceptible and methicillin-resistant isolates. Daptomycin is a useful alternative to other agents (linezolid, quinupristin/dalfopristin) for treating infections caused by resistant gram-positive pathogens because there are few options at present for treating these infections. For complicated skin and skin structure infections, combination therapy may be clinically indicated if the documented or presumed pathogens include gram-negative or anaerobic organisms. Daptomycin is not indicated for the treatment of pneumonia.

Adverse Events

Daptomycin may cause GI reactions such as constipation, nausea, diarrhea, and vomiting. Injection site reactions and headache may occur. Skeletal muscle toxicity manifested as muscle pain has been reported with daptomycin. This is accompanied by an increase in creatinine phosphokinase (CPK) levels.

Drug Interactions

CPK monitoring should be done at least weekly for patients concomitantly receiving a statin and/or those with renal insufficiency. Otherwise, daptomycin does not have any significant drug–drug interactions.

STREPTOGRAMINS

The streptogramin antibiotics are naturally occurring products that have been used clinically in Europe for more than 40 years. The semisynthetic derivative quinupristin/dalfopristin (Synercid) is the only streptogramin antibiotic available in the United States. It is a combination of two antibiotics.

Pharmacokinetics and Pharmacodynamics

Quinupristin/dalfopristin is not absorbed from the GI tract. After IV administration, both quinupristin and dalfopristin have a serum half-life of approximately 1 hour. Each drug is moderately protein bound; the volume of distribution is 0.45 and 0.24 L/kg for quinupristin and dalfopristin, respectively.

TABLE 6.18

Streptogramin Dosages

Drug	Adult Dosages	Pediatric Dosages
Quinupristin-dalfopristin (Synercid)	7.5 mg/kg IV q8–12h	7.5 mg/kg IV q8–12h

IV, intravenous.

Metabolism of both agents is through the liver. The drug is primarily excreted in the feces.

Quinupristin/dalfopristin is a bactericidal agent against most organisms, with the noted exception of vancomycin-resistant *E. faecium*. Quinupristin/dalfopristin possesses a PAE ranging from 8 to 18 hours. The dosage for adults and children is 7.5 mg/kg every 8 to 12 hours (**Table 6.18**). It is not significantly removed by hemodialysis or peritoneal dialysis.

Mechanism of Action and Spectrum of Activity

The streptogramins inhibit protein synthesis by binding to the 50S ribosome. The interaction of quinupristin and dalfopristin is synergistic. Either compound alone is bacteriostatic, whereas the combination results in a bactericidal effect.

The principal activity of quinupristin/dalfopristin is against gram-positive aerobic organisms, including staphylococci, streptococci, and enterococci. In particular, its activity against resistant pathogens, including methicillin-resistant staphylococci, penicillin-resistant streptococci, and vancomycin-resistant *E. faecium*, is excellent. Quinupristin/dalfopristin is not active against *Enterococcus faecalis*.

Clinical Uses

Quinupristin/dalfopristin is approved by the FDA for treating skin and skin structure infections and vancomycin-resistant *E. faecium* infections. The use of this agent is limited due to adverse effects and the need for administration through a central venous line. It can be used to treat gram-positive infections caused by methicillin-resistant staphylococci, penicillin-resistant *S. pneumoniae*, and vancomycin-resistant *E. faecium* when alternative agents are contraindicated.

Adverse Events

The most common adverse reactions are infusion related. Infusion site reactions, including pain, inflammation, edema, and thrombophlebitis, have been reported in as many as 75% of patients receiving quinupristin/dalfopristin through a peripheral IV catheter. Arthralgias and myalgias have also been reported. They may be severe and result in discontinuation of therapy. They usually occur after several days of therapy. After discontinuation of therapy, these reactions are uniformly reversible. The most common laboratory abnormality is an increased level of conjugated bilirubin.

Drug Interactions

The CYP3A4 isoenzyme (responsible for the metabolism of many drugs) is significantly inhibited by quinupristin/dalfopristin. Close clinical or serum level monitoring of known substrates of the CYP3A4 enzyme is recommended.

PLEUROMUTILINS

Lefamulin (Xenleta) belongs to a new class of agents known as the pleuromutilins. This class is structurally unrelated to other anti-infective agents and is derived from the naturally occurring tricyclic pleuromutilin, which received its name from the edible mushroom, *Pleurotus mutilus* (now called *Clitophilus scyphoides*). Lefamulin is a semisynthetic compound with a modification at the C-14 side chain, which is largely responsible for its excellent pharmacokinetics and tissue distribution profile, enhanced antimicrobial spectrum, and the availability of both IV and oral formulations.

Pharmacokinetics and Pharmacodynamics

Following IV and oral administration, lefamulin has a half-life of approximately 8 hours in patients with community-acquired bacterial pneumonia (CABP). It is 95% bound to plasma proteins and has a volume of distribution of 1.25 L/kg. **Table 6.19** provides dosing information for lefamulin. The dose in adults is 150 mg IV or 600 mg orally every 12 hours. Lefamulin is not extensively metabolized in the liver and does not require adjustments for renal insufficiency or those with mild to moderate hepatic insufficiency. No data are available for patients with severe liver disease. Lefamulin is not removed by hemodialysis.

Lefamulin is bactericidal against *S. pneumoniae*, *H. influenzae*, *Neisseria gonorrhoeae*, and *Mycoplasma genitalium* and bacteriostatic against *S. aureus*.

Mechanism of Action and Spectrum of Activity

Lefamulin inhibits bacterial protein synthesis by binding to the peptidyltransferase center of the 50S ribosomal subunit with high affinity and specificity at a unique binding site that is different than other antimicrobial classes. Lefamulin is active against many gram-positive, fastidious gram-negative, and some anaerobic organisms and spirochetes. It is noteworthy that lefamulin activity possesses against MRSA and VRE, as well as multidrug resistant strains of *S. pneumoniae*, *N. gonorrhoeae*, and *M. genitalium*.

TABLE 6.19
Pleuromutilin Dosages

Drug	Adult Dosages	Pediatric Dosages
Lefamulin (Xenleta)	150 mg IV q12h or 600 mg PO q12h	—

Clinical Uses

Lefamulin is approved by the FDA for treating CABP in adults.

Adverse Events

Lefamulin is generally well tolerated, with nausea and abdominal upset being the most common adverse effects reported after oral administration and local infusion reactions most commonly reported after IV administration. Lefamulin can produce a concentration-dependent prolongation in the QTc interval; this is more pronounced (~10 ms increase on average) after IV administration.

Drug Interactions

Lefamulin tablets are contraindicated with sensitive CYP3A4 substrates that prolong the QT interval (e.g., pimozide) as this may result in increased plasma concentrations of these drugs, leading to QT prolongation.

Concomitant use of lefamulin IV or oral tablets with strong and moderate CYP3A4 inducers or P-gp inducers should be avoided unless the benefit outweighs the risks. In addition, concomitant use of lefamulin tablets should be avoided with strong CYP3A inhibitors or P-gp inhibitors. Concomitant use of sensitive CYP3A substrates with lefamulin tablets requires close monitoring for adverse effects of these drugs (e.g., alprazolam, diltiazem, verapamil, simvastatin, vardenafil).

ANTIANAEROBIC AGENTS

Clindamycin

Clindamycin (Cleocin) has been used extensively in treating gram-positive and anaerobic bacterial infections. It was first used orally to treat streptococcal and staphylococcal infections, but it soon became the drug of choice for anaerobic infections. The combination of clindamycin and gentamicin (Garamycin) is still frequently used in treating mixed aerobic and anaerobic infections.

Pharmacokinetics and Pharmacodynamics

Both the hydrochloride and palmitate hydrochloride salts of clindamycin are well absorbed and converted to active forms in the blood. Clindamycin reaches most tissues and bone, but its distribution into CSF is limited. It is 93% bound to proteins. The half-life is approximately 3 hours. Clindamycin is metabolized by the liver, necessitating dosage adjustment in patients with liver impairment (**Table 6.20**). Hemodialysis and peritoneal dialysis do not remove clindamycin to a significant extent.

Mechanism of Action and Spectrum of Activity

Clindamycin binds to the 50S subunit of the bacterial ribosome and inhibits protein synthesis. It acts at the same site as chloramphenicol and the macrolides.

TABLE 6.20
Antianaerobic Agents: Dosages

Drug	Adult Dosages	Pediatric Dosages
Clindamycin	150–450 mg PO q6–8h or 600 mg IV q8h	10–30 mg/kg/d PO divided q6–8h 25–40 mg/kg/d IV divided q6–8h
Metronidazole	250–500 mg PO q6–8h or 500 mg IV q6–12h	15–35 mg/kg/d PO/IV divided q6h

Note: Dosage adjustment recommended for patients with liver dysfunction.

IV, intravenous.

Clinical Uses

Clindamycin is typically included in regimens for its anaerobic coverage in mixed infections and may also be used in treating gram-positive infections, toxoplasmosis, and PCP or in combination with other agents to treat PID. In addition, it is frequently used to inhibit toxin production as part of the treatment for staphylococcal or streptococcal toxic shock.

Adverse Events

The major side effect associated with clindamycin is diarrhea and associated *C. difficile* colitis. This adverse event is unrelated to dose and may range from acute, self-limiting symptoms to life-threatening toxic megacolon. Pain at the site of IV administration may occur.

Drug Interactions

In rare cases, clindamycin use in combination with skeletal muscle relaxants has been reported to potentiate neuromuscular blockade.

Metronidazole

Metronidazole (Flagyl) was first recognized for its antiprotozoal activity in treating *Trichomonas vaginalis* infections. Subsequently, its utility as an antianaerobic agent was used in treating *B. fragilis* infections. Metronidazole has become a treatment of choice for anaerobic infections and is part of a number of regimens to eradicate *Helicobacter pylori*–associated duodenal ulcers. Metronidazole is no longer a first-line treatment option for adults with *C. difficile* colitis.

Pharmacokinetics and Pharmacodynamics

Metronidazole is completely absorbed from the GI tract after oral administration. It penetrates well into most tissues, with an apparent volume of distribution of 0.3 to 0.9 L/kg. Its binding to plasma protein is minimal. The liver metabolizes metronidazole, and dosage adjustments are necessary in patients with hepatic impairment (**Table 6.20**). The half-life is approximately 6 to 9 hours. Metronidazole is removed by hemodialysis and peritoneal dialysis.

Mechanism of Action and Spectrum of Activity

Metronidazole is reduced to a toxic product that interacts with DNA, causing strand breakage and resulting in protein synthesis inhibition. Metronidazole has excellent activity against gram-positive and gram-negative anaerobes, *H. pylori*, and protozoa such as *T. vaginalis*.

Clinical Uses

Metronidazole is typically included in regimens for its anaerobic coverage in mixed infections. In addition, metronidazole is the treatment of choice for bacterial vaginosis and trichomoniasis and may be used to treat *C. difficile* diarrhea in patients who cannot tolerate or do not have access to vancomycin or fidaxomicin.

Adverse Events

Metronidazole is usually safe and well tolerated. GI side effects such as nausea, vomiting, abdominal pain, and a metallic taste are most common. More serious but rare effects include seizures, peripheral neuropathy, and pancreatitis. Seizures have been associated with high doses, whereas peripheral neuropathy has been documented in patients receiving prolonged courses of metronidazole.

Drug Interactions

Metronidazole enhances the anticoagulant effect of warfarin, resulting in a prolonged half-life of warfarin. A disulfiram-like reaction characterized by flushing, palpitations, nausea, and vomiting may occur when alcohol is consumed during metronidazole therapy. Metronidazole is an inhibitor of the CYP3A4 isoenzyme. It has the potential to interact with multiple medications. Additionally, phenobarbital, phenytoin, and rifampin increase the metabolism of metronidazole, which may result in treatment failure. A careful review of a patient's medication list for drug interactions should be done before initiating metronidazole.

MISCELLANEOUS ANTIMICROBIAL AGENTS

Chloramphenicol

Chloramphenicol has a wide spectrum of activity against gram-positive, gram-negative, and anaerobic organisms. However, its use has been limited by its toxicity profile, which includes *gray baby syndrome*, optic neuritis, and fatal aplastic anemia. Nonetheless, in selected situations, chloramphenicol remains an important agent.

Pharmacokinetics and Pharmacodynamics

Chloramphenicol is available as an IV succinate ester. The dose is based on age and indication (**Table 6.21**). The ester formulation is hydrolyzed in the body to the active drug. Chloramphenicol penetrates well into most tissues and bodily

TABLE 6.21		
Miscellaneous Agents: Dosages		
Drug	**Adult Dosages**	**Pediatric Dosages**
Chloramphenicol	Older children and adults: 50–100 mg/kg/d IV divided q6h (max 4,000 mg daily)	—
	Older children and adults with meningitis: 75–100 mg/kg/d IV divided q6h	—
Nitrofurantoin	50 mg PO q6h (macrocrystal) or	5–7 mg/kg/d PO divided q6h
	100 mg PO q12h (macrocrystal monohydrate)	
Rifampin	600 mg PO once daily or	10–20 mg/kg IV generally once daily
	10–20 mg/kg IV daily	

Notes: Chloramphenicol should be used with caution in patients with renal impairment, and serum concentrations should be monitored to guide dosing and prevent toxicity.

Dosage adjustment for rifampin is recommended for patients with liver dysfunction.

Nitrofurantoin is contraindicated in patients with a creatinine clearance of <60 mL/min.

IV, intravenous.

fluids, including the CSF. Chloramphenicol readily crosses the placenta in pregnant females. It is conjugated in the liver and excreted by the kidney in an inactive, nontoxic form. The serum half-life is 3 to 4 hours. Chloramphenicol is 25% to 50% bound to protein.

Serum levels are frequently monitored in high-risk patients. The therapeutic range of chloramphenicol is 5 to 20 mg/dL. Dose-related myelosuppression typically occurs at serum levels exceeding 25 mg/dL.

Mechanism of Action and Spectrum of Activity

Chloramphenicol reversibly binds to the larger 50S subunit of the ribosome, thereby inhibiting bacterial protein synthesis. It is variably bactericidal.

Chloramphenicol is active against gram-positive and gram-negative aerobes and anaerobes as well as atypical organisms, including mycoplasma, chlamydia, and rickettsia. Its gram-negative activity includes *E. coli*, *Proteus* species, and *Salmonella* species but not *P. aeruginosa*.

Clinical Uses

Newer agents have reduced the need to use chloramphenicol in treating infection. However, it can be used as an alternative in treating bacterial meningitis when a patient has a life-threatening penicillin allergy. It is also useful in treating rickettsial diseases such as Rocky Mountain spotted fever and typhus fever in patients allergic to tetracyclines or in pregnant women. Chloramphenicol may be used in treating VRE infections as well.

Adverse Events

The major adverse events associated with chloramphenicol are gray baby syndrome, blood dyscrasias, and optic neuritis. Gray baby syndrome typically occurs in neonates and is manifested by vomiting, lethargy, respiratory collapse, and death. It results from drug accumulation because neonates cannot conjugate chloramphenicol. Two forms of hematologic toxicity may occur with chloramphenicol administration. Dose-related

bone marrow suppression has occurred in patients receiving doses exceeding 4 g/d and at serum levels exceeding 25 mg/dL. It may present as a combination of anemia, leukopenia, and thrombocytopenia. Aplastic anemia is an idiosyncratic effect independent of dose and may occur weeks after therapy with chloramphenicol. It is associated with a greater than 50% mortality rate and often necessitates bone marrow transplantation. Optic neuritis is a major neurologic complication and is associated with long courses of chloramphenicol. The toxicity involves red-green color changes and loss of vision. It may be reversible or permanent. GI side effects have been associated with high doses of chloramphenicol.

Drug Interactions

Chloramphenicol is metabolized by the liver and is an inhibitor of the CYP2C19 and CYP3A4 enzymes. It prolongs the half-life of warfarin, phenytoin, and cyclosporine.

Rifampin

Rifampin is a macrocyclic antibiotic used in a variety of settings, and it is a first-line agent in treating tuberculosis. It is typically combined with other antibiotics such as vancomycin in treating MRSA infections.

Pharmacokinetics and Pharmacodynamics

Rifampin is completely absorbed after oral administration. It distributes into most tissues and fluids, including the CSF. The half-life of rifampin is approximately 3 hours. It is metabolized by the liver and is not removed by hemodialysis or peritoneal dialysis. **Table 6.21** provides dosing information.

Mechanism of Action and Spectrum of Activity

Rifampin suppresses initiation of chain formation for ribonucleic acid (RNA) synthesis in susceptible bacteria by inhibiting DNA-dependent RNA polymerase. The beta-subunit of the enzyme appears to be the site of action.

Rifampin is extremely active against gram-positive cocci. It has moderate activity against aerobic gram-negative bacilli.

Neisseria meningitidis, Neisseria gonorrhoeae, and *H. influenzae* are the most sensitive gram-negative organisms. Rifampin maintains activity against *M. tuberculosis.*

Clinical Uses

Rifampin is commonly used in combination with a cell wall–active agent to treat serious, gram-positive infections that fail to respond to other courses of therapy. This combination is used for synergistic activity and prevents rapid resistance development. It is the drug of choice for postexposure meningitis prophylaxis against *N. meningitidis* and *H. influenzae* type B. Rifampin is a first-line agent in the treatment of *M. tuberculosis* infection, and it is used to treat nontuberculous mycobacterial infections as well.

Adverse Events

The most common side effects associated with rifampin are GI distress (nausea, vomiting, and diarrhea), headache, and fever. Rifampin changes bodily fluids such as sweat, saliva, and tears to a red-orange color. Hepatotoxicity is rare, but the risk increases when it is administered in combination with isoniazid. Liver function should be monitored while patients receive rifampin. Anemia or thrombocytopenia also has been reported.

Drug Interactions

Rifampin is a potent inducer of hepatic CYP drug metabolism and precipitates many drug interactions. Rifampin increases the clearance of agents such as antiarrhythmics, azole antifungals, clarithromycin, estrogens, most statins, warfarin, and many HIV medications. A careful review of the patient's medication list for drug interactions should be done before initiating rifampin.

Nitrofurantoin

Nitrofurantoin is an antimicrobial agent used only for treating and preventing urinary tract infections. Nitrofurantoin has been used in the United States since 1953 and still remains very effective. It is a synthetic nitrofuran-compound derivative, a class that also includes furazolidone, available in Europe.

Pharmacokinetics and Pharmacodynamics

Following oral administration, nitrofurantoin is rapidly absorbed. The bioavailability of nitrofurantoin is approximately 40% to 50%. Absorption can be enhanced with food. Nitrofurantoin serum concentrations are low, with a serum half-life of less than 30 minutes. For this reason, nitrofurantoin should not be used for complicated urinary tract infections or in patients for whom a concern of bacteremia exists. Nitrofurantoin undergoes renal elimination. Inadequate urinary concentrations are achieved in patients with renal insufficiency; thus, the drug is ineffective. It is contraindicated in patients with a creatinine clearance of less than 60 mL/min. **Table 6.21** provides dosing information.

Mechanism of Action and Spectrum of Activity

The exact mechanism of nitrofurantoin is poorly understood. The drug does inhibit several bacterial enzymes, which results in impaired bacterial cell wall synthesis.

Nitrofurantoin has adequate antimicrobial coverage against common organisms that cause urinary tract infections such as *E. coli, Citrobacter* species, *Staphylococcus saprophyticus, E. faecalis,* and *E. faecium.* Nitrofurantoin frequently covers strains of VRE. Resistance has increased against some types of bacteria, such as *Enterobacter* and *Klebsiella* species.

Clinical Uses

Nitrofurantoin is only used for the treatment and prophylaxis of uncomplicated urinary tract infections. As mentioned earlier, it should not be used for complicated urinary tract infections such as pyelonephritis.

Adverse Events

The most common side effects of nitrofurantoin include nausea and vomiting. Nitrofurantoin may cause a harmless yellow-brown discoloration of urine. Allergic reactions are rare. Pulmonary reactions (pulmonary infiltrates, pneumonitis, pulmonary fibrosis) and hepatic effects (hepatitis, hepatic necrosis) have been reported in rare cases, usually associated with long-term use. Additionally, peripheral neuropathy has been associated with long-term use in patients with renal failure.

Drug Interactions

Nitrofurantoin is not associated with significant drug interactions.

ANTIMICROBIAL RESISTANCE

There are multiple mechanisms by which bacteria form or acquire antibiotic resistance. Some types of resistance occur naturally, while others are acquired from another strain of bacteria. Additionally, resistance can sometimes be induced during antibiotic treatment. **Table 6.22** summarizes the most common resistance mechanisms.

1. The most common type of resistance is bacterial enzyme production. For example, bacteria frequently produce enzymes that disrupt beta-lactam antibiotics, altering the structure so they cannot bind to the PBPs. There are hundreds of different types of these enzymes known as *beta-lactamases.* Some enzymes have activity only against penicillins (penicillinases), whereas others, such as extended-spectrum beta-lactamases, can render almost all beta-lactam antibiotics ineffective. Separate from beta-lactamases, bacteria also produce enzymes that can alter the chemical structure or inactivate the drug. This can occur with aminoglycosides, chloramphenicol, macrolides, streptogramins, and tetracyclines.
2. Resistance can occur as the bacteria alter their own cell membranes, not permitting antibiotics to enter the bacteria.

TABLE 6.22

Antimicrobial Resistance

Antibiotic/Antibiotic Class	Bacterial Enzyme Production	Decreased Membrane Permeability	Promotion of Antibiotic Efflux	Altered Target Sites/Protection of Target Site	Altered Target Enzymes	Overproduction of Target
Penicillins	✓	✓	✓		✓	
Cephalosporins	✓	✓	✓		✓	
Monobactams	✓	✓				
Carbapenems	✓	✓	✓			
Fluoroquinolones		✓	✓	✓	✓	
Macrolides	✓		✓	✓		
Aminoglycosides	✓			✓		
Tetracyclines	✓		✓	✓		
Sulfamethoxazole/trimethoprim					✓	✓
Glycopeptides				✓		
Oxazolidinones				✓		
Streptogramins	✓		✓	✓		
Clindamycin	✓			✓		
Metronidazole		✓			✓	
Chloramphenicol	✓	✓				
Rifampin				✓		
Nitrofurantoin					✓	
Lefamulin			✓	✓		

An example of this is loss of porins on the gram-negative bacterial cell outer membrane. Specifically, with beta-lactam antibiotics, loss of these porins alters the ability of the antimicrobial agent to enter the cell.

3. A third, common mechanism of resistance is the activation of efflux pumps that expel antibiotics out of the intracellular space back across the cell membrane. This prevents antibiotics from acting at their intracellular target site. This is a common mechanism of resistance with classes such as tetracyclines and macrolides.

4. A fourth type of resistance is alteration of the antibiotic's target site of action. This occurs with macrolides, among other classes, when mutations alter the ribosomal binding site. The antibiotic does not bind as well or at all to the ribosome anymore. Similarly, VRE is a result of altered cell wall precursors. Plasmid-mediated resistance results in a modified peptidoglycan precursor that binds vancomycin, preventing it from binding to its intended target site.

5. A fifth type of resistance is alteration of target enzymes. For example, the FQs work by inhibiting the enzymes DNA gyrase and topoisomerase IV. Mutations to a variety of different chromosomes on these enzymes can reduce the efficacy of the FQs.

6. Last, overproduction of target enzymes can result in resistance. The best example of this is with sulfonamides and

TMP. SMX–TMP works by inhibiting folic acid synthesis by inhibiting the dihydropteroate synthetase and dihydrofolate reductase enzymes, respectively. These enzymes are required for bacterial folic acid synthesis. Excess production of these two enzymes in some strains of bacteria can render the antibiotic ineffective.

A specific area of interest in antimicrobial development is targeting the prevention of or overcoming drug resistance.

ANTIMICROBIAL STEWARDSHIP

Overuse of antibiotics is well documented and has led to increased resistance to various strains of bacteria worldwide. Some examples of drug-resistant bacteria include extended-spectrum beta-lactamases against *E. coli* and *Klebsiella*, carbapenem-resistant *Klebsiella*, FQ-resistant gonococcus, MRSA, and vancomycin-intermediate *S. aureus*. The IDSA and Centers for Diseases Control and Prevention have developed core principles for the implementation of antimicrobial stewardship programs for both the inpatient and the outpatient settings. These guidelines stress the importance of a multidisciplinary team approach to improving antibiotic use, with a focus on ensuring that the best drug, at the best dose and duration, is prescribed to patients.

CASE STUDY[*]

J.G., a 55-year-old man, is started on daptomycin for methicillin-resistant *Staphylococcus aureus* (MRSA) bacteremia and presumptive endocarditis. His medications include rivaroxaban, atorvastatin, and lorazepam.

1. Which of the following is true for daptomycin?
   a. It is effective against MRSA and vancomycin-resistant enterococci (VRE).
   b. It works by disrupting bacterial cell wall synthesis.
   c. He can be converted to oral treatment as soon as his white blood cell count decreases.
   d. Thrombocytopenia occurs in a small percentage of patients.

2. About 1 week later, J.G. complains of lower extremity muscle aches and pains. Which of the following is a probable reason for these signs/symptoms?
   a. Daptomycin is known for causing flu-like symptoms.
   b. Daptomycin is interacting with the rivaroxaban, leading to a deep vein thrombosis.
   c. J.G.'s infection is getting worse and vancomycin needs to be added to the regimen.
   d. Atorvastatin is interacting with the daptomycin, creating a rhabdomyolysis-like syndrome.

[*] Answers can be found online.

A few examples of ways to improve antibiotic use include infectious disease specialist oversight of the use of specific antimicrobials, the use of rapid diagnostics and evidence-based prescribing, the use of pharmacokinetic-pharmacodyamic-guided dose optimization, antibiotic streamlining, and de-escalation and the use of vaccines and other infection prevention principles.

Bibliography

Starred references are cited in the text.

Aloisamy, S., Abdul-Mutakabbir, J. C., Kebriaci, R., et al. (2020). Evaluation of eravacycline: A novel fluorocycline. *Pharmacotherapy*, *40*(3), 221–238.

Barber, K., Bell, A. M., Wingler, M. J. B., et al. (2018). Omadacycline enters the ring: A new antimicrobial contender. *Pharmacotherapy*, *38*(12), 1194–1204.

Barlam, T. F., Cosgrove, S. F., Abbo, L. M., et al. (2016). Implementing an antibiotic stewardship program: Guidelines by the Infectious Diseases Society of America and the Society for Healthcare Epidemiology of America. *Clinical Infectious Diseases*, *62*(10), e51–e77.

Bonomo, R. A. (2019). Cefiderocol: A novel siderophore cephalosporin defeating carbapenem-resistant pathogens. *Clinical Infectious Diseases*, *69*(7), S519–S520.

Burdette, S. D., & Trotman, R. (2015). Tedizolid: The first once-daily oxazolidinone class antibiotic. *Clinical Infectious Diseases*, *61*(8), 1315–1321.

CDC. (2019). Core Elements of Hospital Antibiotic Stewardship Programs. Atlanta, GA: US Department of Health and Human Services, CDC. Available at https://www.cdc.gov/antibiotic-use/core-elements/hospital.html

Cho, J. C., Crotty, M. P., White, B. P., et al. (2018). What is old is new again: Delafloxacin, a modern fluoroquinolone. *Pharmacotherapy*, *8*(1), 108–121.

Coggins, M. D. (2019). Fluoroquinolone antibiotic risks. *Today's Geriatric Medicine*, *9*(5), 6.

*Craig, W. A., & Vogelman, B. (1987). The postantibiotic effect. *Annals of internal medicine,* *106*, 900–902.

Doi, Y. (2019a). Ertapenem, imipenem, meropenem, doripenem and aztreonam. In G. L. Mandell, J. E. Bennett, R. Dolin, & M. J. Blaser (Eds.), *Principles and practice of infectious diseases* (9th ed.). Philadelphia, PA: Elsevier.

Doi, Y. (2019b). Penicillins. In G. L. Mandell, J. E. Bennett, R. Dolin, & M. J. Blaser (Eds.), *Principles and practice of infectious diseases* (9th ed.). Philadelphia, PA: Elsevier.

*FDA drug safety communication: FDA advises restricting fluoroquinolone antibiotic use for certain uncomplicated infections; warns about disabling side effects that can occur together. US Food and Drug Administration. http://www.fda.gov/Drugs/DrugSafety/ucm500143.htm. Updated June 7, 2016. Accessed May 25, 2020.

Hooper, D. C., & Strahilevitz, J. (2019). Quinolones. In G. L. Mandell, J. E. Bennett, R. Dolin, & M. J. Blaser (Eds.), *Principles and practice of infectious diseases* (9th ed.). Philadelphia, PA: Elsevier.

Huckell, V. F. (2018). Infective endocarditis. In R. S. Porter & J. L. Kaplan (Eds.), *The Merck manual of diagnosis and therapy* (20th ed.). Whitehouse Station, NJ: Merck Sharpe & Dohme Corp.

Lepak, A. J., & Andes, D. R. (2019). Cephalosporins. In G. L. Mandell, J. E. Bennett, R. Dolin, & M. J. Blaser (Eds.), *Principles and practice of infectious diseases* (9th ed.). Philadelphia, PA: Elsevier.

Levison, M. E. (2004). Pharmacodynamics of antimicrobial drugs. *Infectious Disease Clinics of North America*, *184*, 51–65.

Maslow, M. J., & Portal-Celhay, C. (2019). Rifamycins. In G. L. Mandell, J. E. Bennett, R. Dolin, & M. J. Blaser (Eds.), *Principles and practice of infectious diseases* (9th ed.). Philadelphia, PA: Elsevier.

Miller, J. M., Binnicker, M. J., Campbell, S., et al. (2018). A guide to utilization of the microbiology laboratory diagnosis of infectious diseases: 2018 update by the Infectious Diseases Society of America and the American Society for Microbiology. *Clinical Infectious Diseases*, *67*(6), e1–e94.

Moffa, M., & Brook, I. (2019). Tetracyclines, glycylcyclines and chloramphenicol. In G. L. Mandell, J. E. Bennett, R. Dolin, & M. J. Blaser (Eds.), *Principles and practice of infectious diseases* (9th ed.). Philadelphia, PA: Elsevier.

Mounsey, A., Lacy Smith, K., Reddy, V. C., et al. (2020). Clostridium difficile infection: Update on management. *American Family Physician*, *101*(3), 168–175.

Nagel, J. L., & Aronoff, D. M. (2019). Metronidazole. In G. L. Mandell, J. E. Bennett, R. Dolin, & M. J. Blaser (Eds.), *Principles and practice of infectious diseases* (9th ed.). Philadelphia, PA: Elsevier.

Nesbitt, W. J., & Aronoff, D. M. (2019). Macrolides and clindamycin. In G. L. Mandell, J. E. Bennett, R. Dolin, & M. J. Blaser (Eds.), *Principles and practice of infectious diseases* (9th ed.). Philadelphia, PA: Elsevier.

Opal, S. M., & Pop-Vicas, A. (2019). Molecular mechanisms of antibiotic resistance in bacteria. In G. L. Mandell, J. E. Bennett, R. Dolin, & M. J. Blaser (Eds.), *Principles and practice of infectious diseases* (9th ed.). Philadelphia, PA: Elsevier.

Rice, L. B. (2009). The clinical consequences of antimicrobial resistance. *Current Opinion in Microbiology*, *12*(5), 476–481.

Rybak, M. J., Le, J., Lodise, T. P., et al. (2020). Therapeutic monitoring of vancomycin for serious methicillin-resistant *S. aureus* infections:

A revised consensus guideline and review by the American Society of Health-System Pharmacists, the Infectious Diseases Society of America, the Pediatric Infectious Diseases Society, and the Society of Infectious Diseases Pharmacists. *American Journal of Health-System Pharmacy*, *77*(11), 835–864.

Saravolatz, L. D., & Stein, G. E. (2019). Plazomicin: A new aminoglycoside. *Clinical Infectious Diseases*, *70*(4), 704–709.

Smith, J. R., Rybak, M. J., & Claeys, K. C. (2020). Imipenem-cilastatin-relebactam: A novel β-lactam-β-lactamase inhibitor combination for the treatment of multidrug-resistant gram-negative infections. *Pharmacotherapy*, *40*(4), 343–356.

Society for Healthcare Epidemiology of America; Infectious Diseases Society of America; Pediatric Infectious Diseases Society. (2012). Policy statement on antimicrobial stewardship by the Society for Healthcare Epidemiology of America (SHEA), the Infectious Diseases Society of America (IDSA), and the Pediatric Infectious Diseases Society (PIDS). *Infection Control and Hospital Epidemiology*, *33*(4, Special Topic Issue: Antimicrobial Stewardship (April 2012)), 322–327.

Stahlmann, R., & Lode, H. (2010). Safety considerations of fluoroquinolones in the elderly. *Drugs and Aging*, *27*(3), 193–209.

Veve, M. P., & Wagner, J. L. (2018). Lefamulin: Review of a promising novel pleuromutilin antibiotic. *Pharmacotherapy*, *38*(9), 935–946.

Wu, J. Y., Srinivas, P., & Pogue, J. M. (2020). Cefiderocol: A novel agent for the management of multidrug-resistant gram-negative organisms. *Infectious Diseases Therapy*, *9*(1), 17–40.

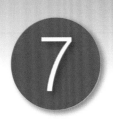

7 Pharmacogenomics

Isabelle Mercier and Amalia M. Issa

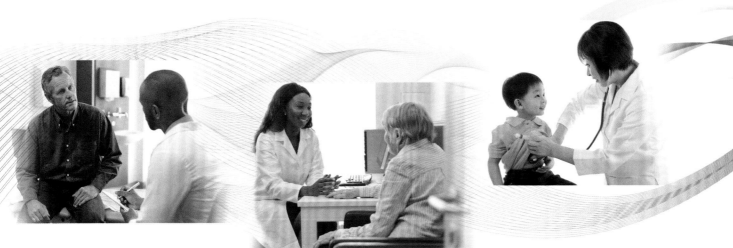

Learning Objectives

1. Explain the basic concepts of pharmacogenomics and be familiar with its terminology.
2. Discuss how genetics affect the activity of drug-metabolizing enzymes.
3. Consider how pharmacogenomics may play a role in drug therapy selection given a specific case.

INTRODUCTION

Pharmacogenomics and Precision Medicine

Interpatient variability in drug therapy response is a well-known pharmacotherapeutic concept. Indeed, as far back as 1892, William Osler is reputed to have said, "If it were not for the great variability among individuals, medicine might be a science and not an art" (Golden, 2004). In addition to factors such as age, sex, drug–drug interactions, and comorbidities, genetics also is known to play a role in interpatient variability of drug response.

The ability of genetic variability (inherited differences) to influence therapeutic drug response is the basis of pharmacogenetics and pharmacogenomics. Generally, *pharmacogenetics* refers to single or a few gene variations (called polymorphisms), whereas *pharmacogenomics* refers more broadly to the genome-wide (or an individual's entire deoxyribonucleic acid [DNA] sequence) effects on drug therapy. *Precision medicine* is a more recently coined term that includes pharmacogenetics/pharmacogenomics and refers to "an emerging approach for disease treatment and prevention that takes into account individual variability in genes, environment, and lifestyle for each person" (National Library of Medicine (2020).

We can think of pharmacogenomics as the basic science of precision medicine, and indeed, much of the progress that has been made in the field of precision medicine to date has been largely focused on pharmacogenomics.

This chapter is geared toward future clinicians, particularly nurse practitioners and physician assistants, to provide them with an overview of pharmacogenomics, the current state of the science, including some pertinent examples, some relevant applications, and promises, pitfalls and policy implications.

BASIC CONCEPTS

Because pharmacogenomics is rooted in genetics, it is helpful to review some basic genetic concepts. Several of the definitions of key terms that are associated with genetics and pharmacogenomics can be found in **Box 7.1**.

The human genome is the underpinning of every human's individuality. With the exception of identical twins, the genome is different for every individual, although in the grand scheme of things, there are only small differences among people's DNA that make us unique. The human genome consists of approximately three billion base pairs, 99.9% of which are the same among all humans, with only 0.1% variation among individuals. The variations that occur with DNA (*polymorphisms*), along with environmental and dietary factors, create a patient's individuality, susceptibility to disease, and response to treatments. Included in this individuality is a person's ability to absorb, distribute, metabolize, and excrete drugs. Understanding the

BOX 7.1   Definitions

Adenine (A)—One of the four nucleotide bases. Pairs with thymine.

Alleles—Multiple versions of a gene. Each person typically inherits two alleles of each gene, one from the mother and one from the father.

Autosomal—Pertains to any chromosome that is not a sex chromosome. Humans have 22 autosomal pairs (i.e., 44 autosomes) in each cell.

Biomarkers—Molecules that indicate the status of a biological process.

Chromosome—The organized structure of DNA and proteins, the *double-helix*. It contains genes and nucleotide sequences.

Cytosine (C)—One of the four nucleotide bases. Pairs with guanine.

DNA—Deoxyribonucleic acid, a nucleic acid that contains genetic information and/or instructions used in the function of living organisms.

Exon—The portion of a gene that codes for amino acids.

Gene—A sequence of DNA that codes for a type of protein or RNA, serving a particular function in a cell.

Genome—All of the genetic material in chromosomes of an organism.

Guanine (G)—One of the four nucleotide bases. Pairs with cytosine.

Haplotype—A combination of alleles. A haplotype may be a single locus of alleles, multiple loci, or even an entire chromosome.

Nucleotide—Molecules that make up the structural units of DNA and RNA. The four DNA nucleotides are adenine, cytosine, guanine, and thymine. For RNA, uracil is substituted for thymine.

Precision medicine—A more recently coined term that includes pharmacogenetics/pharmacogenomics and refers to "an emerging approach for disease treatment and prevention that takes into account individual variability in genes, environment, and lifestyle for each person" (National Library of Medicine, 2020).

Pharmacogenetics—Refers to the study of inherited differences in single gene variations (called polymorphisms) or a few genes, in drug metabolism and response.

Pharmacogenomics—Refers to the effects of genome-wide sequence (or an individual's entire DNA sequence) on drug therapy.

Polymorphism—DNA sequence variation.

RNA—Ribonucleic acid, a nucleic acid that carries genetic information and produces proteins used in the function of living organisms.

SNP—Single-nucleotide polymorphism, a DNA sequence variation occurring when a single nucleotide differs among members of a species.

Thymine (T)—One of the four nucleotide bases. Pairs with adenine.

Wild-type—The normal, as opposed to the mutant, gene or allele.

---

genetic components affecting these pharmacokinetic processes can help the clinician tailor treatment for a patient.

Each human has 23 pairs of *chromosomes*—22 are autosomal and look the same in males and females, and 1 pair is the sex chromosome, in which females have two X chromosomes and males have an X and a Y chromosome. These chromosomes reside in the nucleus of a cell (**Figure 7.1**). Each chromosome is composed of DNA, which carries the genetic information for the individual. Each chromosome can have hundreds or thousands of genes; it is estimated that there are more than 25,000 genes on the human genome. However, genes only make up about 1% of the total DNA found in humans.

Genes function to produce proteins involved in the millions of biological processes that support the function of the body every day. Genes that mutate or malfunction can have profound effects on the body. In the case in which a single gene mutates or malfunctions, the result is a monogenic disease, such as sickle cell anemia or cystic fibrosis. In most cases, however, there are multiple genes involved in the disease process. These are referred to as polygenic disorders.

Polygenic disorders may appear as a single clinical disorder but at the molecular level have multiple *biomarkers*. Biomarkers are molecules that indicate the status of a biological process. Examples of biomarkers include prostate-specific antigen for prostate cancer or hemoglobin A1c (HbA1c), now considered more reliable than glucose tests as a marker of hyperglycemia. HbA1c has been added as standard of care according to the recommendations of the American Diabetes Association not only to detect diabetes but also to inform about the prediabetic status, which is a powerful predictive tool to manage this disease in high-risk patients (Lyons & Basu, 2012). Genetic biomarkers, specific DNA sequences, are also being discovered.

The building blocks of DNA are the four *nucleotide* bases, including the two purines—*adenine* (A) and *guanine* (G)—and the two pyrimidines—*thymine* (T) and *cytosine* (C). DNA strands are linked through base pairing of the pyrimidines with the purines (A with T; G with C), conceptually forming the well-known double helix (See **Figure 7.1**). The arrangement of these base pairs along each chromosome is called the *DNA sequence*. Variations in the base pairings range from *single*

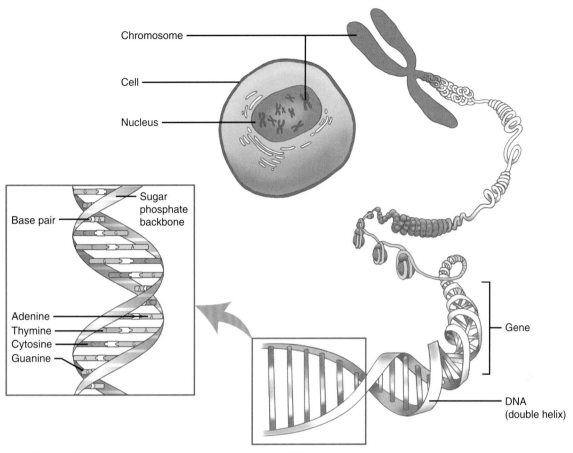

FIGURE 7–1   Relationship among human cell, chromosome, genes, and DNA.

DNA, deoxyribonucleic acid.

nucleotide polymorphisms (SNPs), insertions, or deletions of a nucleotide base to changes in the number of copies of genes. These variations can alter the production or function of proteins, thus creating the variation in the expression of a disease or the response to drug therapy.

Single Nucleotide Polymorphisms

A SNP is a variation in the DNA sequence that differs among members of a species or paired chromosomes in an individual. For example, the following are two sequenced DNA fragments from different individuals: AAGCTA and AAGTTA. Note that the only difference between these sequences is the substitution of thymidine (T) for cytosine (C). In this case, there are two versions (or *alleles*) of this gene. Each person typically inherits two alleles of each gene: one from the mother and one from the father. There can be up to 10 million SNPs in humans, but only those SNPs on coding regions of the gene or the area of the DNA responsible for turning genes on or off have an effect on humans. This concept of SNPs and differing alleles is important in the study of pharmacogenomics, as many of the genes responsible for drug activity and metabolism (e.g., cytochrome P450 [CYP]) have different alleles on the same gene, producing different metabolic effects.

CLINICAL APPLICATIONS OF PHARMACOGENOMICS

A major current issue in medical care is that many therapies given to patients to treat their diseases (e.g., cardiovascular, cancer, diabetes) are misaligned with the patient's genetic makeup. There are two main consequences that directly result from this lack of molecular knowledge at the time of drug treatment: (1) Patients can be given a therapy that inefficiently treats the underlying cause of the disease (lack of therapeutic effect) and (2) patients can be given a medication that can lead to adverse drug reactions (ADRs) that can be harmful or even fatal due to a difference in their genetic makeup. Clinicians and health care professionals must understand and acknowledge that some patients could be genetically predisposed to respond differently to a given drug. This genetic information should then be utilized to assure tailored therapy and safety.

The main organ involved in detoxification/metabolism of drugs is the liver. The CYP superfamily of liver enzymes is a key player in drug metabolism as these enzymes are directly involved in the modification and processing of approximately 75% of all medications taken (Di, 2014; Tornio & Backman, 2018). The impact of genetic modifications in these

CYP enzymes has therefore an important impact on patient treatment. The following examples are focused on genetic alterations in these CYP enzymes and their clinical implications focused on commonly used cardiovascular medications as well as a specific class of commonly used antibiotics.

Clopidogrel: Metabolism and Polymorphism

The P450 2C19 (CYP2C19) liver enzyme is one of the best characterized P450 isoenzymes with clinical implications linked to this genetic polymorphism. The *CYP2C19* gene has 9 *exons* and is situated on chromosome 10. To date, more than 30 different SNPs have been identified for this gene. Interestingly, several years ago, reports emerged that not all patients metabolized clopidogrel in a similar manner, regardless of their age or weight, suggesting that additional components might be involved.

Clopidogrel is a very common medication that is prescribed to patients undergoing acute coronary syndrome (ACS). When patients arrive at the hospital with a partial coronary obstruction, antiplatelet agents are the gold standard in preventing irreversible cardiac ischemia. Clopidogrel is given as an inactive prodrug that is rapidly converted to its active metabolite via hepatic bioactivation through CYP2C19 enzymes (see Chapters 2 and 3 for a review of prodrugs and biotransformation). Clopidogrel inhibits ADP-mediated platelet activation and aggregation by irreversibly binding to the platelet purinergic receptor P2RY12. About 15% of clopidogrel is modified into an active compound and 85% is hydrolyzed to inactive forms to be excreted.

Due to its potent nature, a timely intervention with this pharmacologic agent is essential to preventing further blockage and death, making dosage key to attaining efficacious and safe treatment. The metabolism of clopidogrel to its active metabolite is critical to successful treatment, and thus inherited genetic polymorphisms associated with *CYP2C19* have a high impact on the physiological responses to clopidogrel in patients. Genetic variants of the *CYP2C19* gene result in normal, reduced, or absent enzyme activity or can directly lead to an overactive enzyme. As summarized in **Figure 7.2**, different mutations are responsible for these levels of enzymatic activity. In pharmacogenomics, genetic variants are identified using a special nomenclature (see **Box 7.2**). While CYP2C19*1 is the *wild-type* allele resulting in normal enzyme activity, the most common loss-of-function variant is referred to as CYP2C19*2 (681G>A) (Schuldiner et al., 2009). The CYP2C19*2 allele is inherited as an autosomal codominant trait that co-segregates mostly to the Asian population and is less common in Caucasian and Africans (Scott et al., 2011). A much less common variant associated with a reduced or absent function of this enzyme is referred to as CYP2C19*3 (636G>A), which is detected only in less than 10% of the Asian population. The distribution of these mutations in patients dictates how patients metabolize clopidogrel. Around 2% to 15% of patients carry loss-of-function mutations (*2/*2,*2/*3,*3/*3) on both alleles, resulting in significantly reduced or lack of CYP2C19 activity, and these patients are referred to as poor metabolizers (PMs).

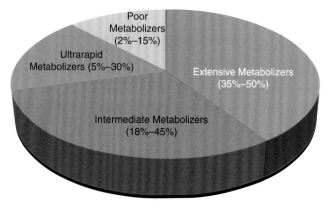

- ◼ Normal Enzyme Activity: *1/*1 (wild-type alleles), no detected mutations
- ◼ Intermediate Enzyme Activity: *1/*2 or *1/*3 one wild-type allele (*1) paired with an allele with decreased activity *2 (681G>A) or *3 (636G>A)
- ◼ Normal or Increased Enzyme Activity: *1/*17 or *17/*17 enhanced activity allele *17 (–806C>T) with or without a wild-type allele (*1)
- ◻ Low or Absent Enzyme Activity: Combination of mutated alleles *2/*2, *2/*3, or *3/*3 resulting in a poor metabolizer phenotype

FIGURE 7–2   Clopidogrel therapy and CYP2C19.

CYP, cytochrome P450.

Other individuals carry a gain-of-function mutation, which makes CYP2C19 more active (*1/*17,*17/*17); these patients are referred to as ultrarapid metabolizers (URMs) and comprise about 5% to 30% of patient populations. Most patients, however, have a normal *CYP2C19* gene (*1/*1) without any mutations, who are called extensive metabolizers (EMs), or with only one loss-of-function allele (*1/*2,*1/*3), who are referred to as intermediate metabolizers (IMs). EMs and IMs comprise 35% to 50% and 18% to 45% of a given population, respectively.

Warfarin: Metabolism and Polymorphism

Warfarin is a commonly prescribed blood thinner used to prevent atrial fibrillation–induced strokes, as well as permanent damage following the onset of venous thromboembolism or pulmonary embolism. Warfarin exists as a racemic mixture of R-warfarin and S-warfarin (Qayyum et al., 2015). S-warfarin possesses the most anticoagulant properties through its action as a vitamin K antagonist. Vitamin K plays a crucial role in the coagulation cascade as its reduced form acts as a cofactor of gamma-glutamyl carboxylase, an important enzyme that renders the coagulation factors II, VII, IX, and X functional through post-ribosomal synthesis (**Figure 7.3**). Importantly, in order for the coagulation cascade to be fully active, vitamin K needs to be in its reduced form. This is accomplished by an upstream enzyme called the vitamin K epoxide reductase complex, subunit 1 (VKORC1). VKORC1 is the therapeutic target of warfarin, and its inhibition results in decreased amounts of vitamin K, preventing coagulation factors from being activated (**Figure 7.3**; Pan et al., 2015). Once its therapeutic window is achieved, S-warfarin is rapidly metabolized

Pharmacogenomics uses a special nomenclature to identify alleles rather than by their cDNA or genomic positions (as in other areas of genetics). For pharmacogenomics, variants are identified using a simple system of numbers and letters divided by a star. Consider the following as an example: CYP3A5*2. This common example is pronounced or spoken as "sip-3-A-5-star-2." It refers to the allele or variant in the *CYP3A5* gene located at position g.27289C>A, which leads to the substitution in the amino acid p.T398N. The star nomenclature was first used to identify variations in the *CYP450* genes and then was adopted for use in other pharmacogenomic genes.

From a clinical perspective, the CYP450 genetic variations are particularly interesting as they signify four different phenotypic states of drug metabolism:

- An URM
- An EM
- An IM
- A PM

Individuals with two standard copies of the normally functioning allele are called *extensive drug metabolizers*. Using the star nomenclature, this wild-type allele corresponds to *1. An individual with double or multiple copies of an allele, called an *ultrarapid metabolizer*, typically has increased functionality. On the other hand, persons considered *intermediate or poor drug metabolizers* have one or more alleles harboring reduced functionality. The star nomenclature *2, *3, *4, and so on is used to denote alleles with altered functionality (i.e., increased or reduced drug metabolism).

CYP, cytochrome P450; DNA, deoxyribonucleic acid; EM, extensive metabolizer; IM, intermediate metabolizer; PM, poor metabolizer; URM, ultra rapid metabolizer.

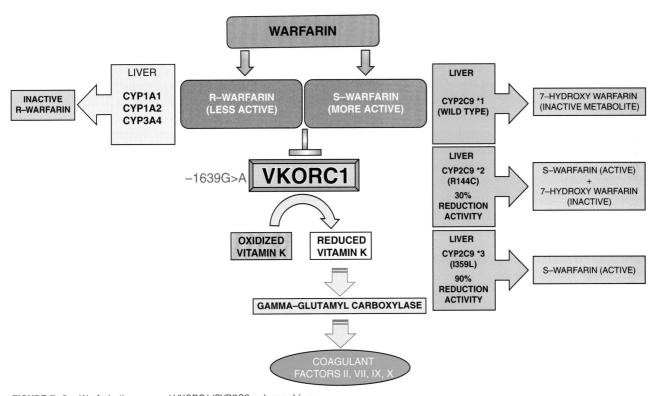

FIGURE 7–3   Warfarin therapy and VKORC1/CYP2C9 polymorphism.

CYP, cytochrome P450; VKORC1, vitamin K epoxide reductase complex, subunit 1.

through the P450 liver enzyme CYP2C9 to its inactive oxidized form (7-hydroxy warfarin). The rate at which S-warfarin is metabolized is highly dependent on the enzymatic activity of CYP2C9. As one might expect, a less efficient metabolism and clearance of warfarin could lead to accumulation of its active form systemically leading to sustained anticoagulation effects. Indeed, several incidents have been reported where accidental deaths have occurred due to excessive bleeding following warfarin treatment. It was later discovered that some patients do not have a fully functional CYP2C9 enzyme due to alleles containing mutations, preventing the proper inactivation of the potent active S-warfarin. There are two main CYP2C9 SNPs found in patients, *2 (R144C) and *3 (I359L); *1 is referred to as the wild-type allele without mutations. The CYP2C9*1 individuals possess normal enzyme activity while CYP2C9*2 carriers exhibit a 30% decrease in activity and CYP2C9*3 patients have as much as a 90% decrease in their enzymatic activity. Patients can express a functional CYP2C9 enzyme by carrying two normal copies of the gene *1/*1, a normal copy and a polymorphic *1/*2, or could have both copies with polymorphism *2/*3. Clinical implication will be discussed in the following. The target enzyme VKORC1 has also shown the presence of inactivating mutation, the most common being −1639G>A.

Mitochondrial Mutation Linked to Antibiotics-Induced Ototoxicity

Aminoglycosides are a class of antibiotics that are still currently used to treat gram-negative infections. Antibiotics within this class are associated with increased risk of both nephrotoxicity and ototoxicity in both young and adult patients. Damage to the ear ranges from tinnitus to irreversible hearing loss, which has been linked both in animal models and in human studies to doses, frequency, and length of treatment (Bitner-Glindzicz & Rahman, 2007; Hutchin et al., 1993). However, there seems to be a segregation of mitochondrial mutations that have been identified that correlate with hypersensitivity of aminoglycosides-induced ototoxicity in patients (Bitner-Glindzicz & Rahman, 2007; Hutchin et al., 1993). At the molecular level, aminoglycosides are designed to bind bacterial ribosomes to halt protein synthesis. However, an inherited mutation in the mitochondrial DNA (transferred maternally) increases the affinity by which aminoglycosides bind to mitochondrial ribosomes, resulting in an increased half-life of these antibiotics in the hair cells of the inner ear (Bitner-Glindzicz & Rahman, 2007). This increased presence of aminoglycoside-binding affinity in the ear of genetically predisposed individuals is specifically thought to affect mitochondrial protein synthesis and disrupt adenosine triphosphate production and ion gradients in the ear, leading to hearing impairment (Hutchin et al., 1993).

Genetic Testing to Predict Drug Efficacy and Adverse Response

The active metabolite of clopidogrel dictates its therapeutic efficacy. Therefore, the degree to which patients are capable of effectively producing these active metabolites through their liver CYP2C19 enzymes is directly linked to their treatment success and recovery from an ACS. In the case of clopidogrel, the PMs are those who could benefit the most from genetic testing prior to therapy, as stated on package inserts and as suggested by the U.S. Food and Drug Administration (FDA). These PMs are incapable of producing the active metabolite of clopidogrel, due to inactivating mutations in CYP2C19 liver enzyme responsible to convert clopidogrel to its active metabolite. If a PM patient suddenly suffers a coronary blockage and is administered clopidogrel, this would result in an unsuccessful treatment of the patient's coronary blockage. The Clinical Pharmacogenetics Implementation Consortium also recommends that special attention be given to URMs and that alternative therapies be used in PMs to treat their coronary obstruction (Scott et al., 2011). In addition, IMs are also challenging to treat with clopidogrel, as these patients have a higher number of residual platelets, which could lead to adverse cardiovascular outcomes (Shirasaka et al., 2015), and might also benefit from other forms of therapy.

For patients receiving warfarin treatment, genetic testing is recommended in order to predict which patients are carrying these mutations who would be at higher risk for bleeding (Maluso, 2015). For example, those who carry the VKORC1 mutation −1639 G>A produce less VKORC1 (referred to as A haplotype) than those with the regular G allele (G haplotype). Consequently, the A haplotype individual would require less warfarin to inhibit VKORC1 to produce similar anticoagulant effects. The same is true for patients who carry CYP2C9 *2 and *3, where the active form of warfarin does not go through clearance normally, leading to immediate excessive bleeding. As a consequence, the therapeutic index of this blood thinner is extremely narrow and needs to be carefully assessed. Genetic testing is thus highly suggested to assess those patients who are genetically predisposed to metabolize clopidogrel and warfarin differently. Genetic testing offers knowledge of this genetic information ahead of time to predict the efficacy of these lifesaving drugs and guide the therapeutic window toward more successful therapy.

In theory, hearing loss associated with possible mitochondrial mutations inherited by the mother following aminoglycoside treatment could be a preventable adverse event. The extensive rehabilitation required for children affected by this irreversible hearing loss should motivate genetic screening prior to aminoglycoside therapy. Such genetic testing would identify early on which patients should not be receiving this antibiotic or provide information about dosage.

PROMISES, PITFALLS, AND POLICY IMPLICATIONS

In addition to pharmacogenomics, progress is being made with newer technologies such as next generation sequencing, including whole genome sequencing (WGS), exome sequencing, and targeted ribonucleic acid (RNA) sequencing, as well as CRISPR-Cas9 genome editing. One new trend that is increasing within the pharmaceutical industry is to use pharmacogenomics for drug re-purposing and re-positioning (Ferrero & Agarwal, 2018). Collectively, the rapid scientific developments are leading to a number of implications for policy, including both opportunities and challenges (Issa, 2015; Issa et al., 2019; Joly et al., 2020).

Pharmacogenomics and personalized medicine provide both economic opportunities and challenges. The cost of different pharmacogenomic tests continues to decline, and there is increasing evidence for the cost-effectiveness of pharmacogenomics as well as its potential to reduce ADRs. It is also important to consider how pharmacogenomics might increase costs, including the storage of genetic samples, resources for computational analysis, and interpretation of the findings. While electronic health records (EHRs) and clinical decision support (CDS) systems are getting better and more user-friendly, they are generally not yet well equipped for the large amount of data that is being generated by the increasing amount of genomic information, particularly from WGS. In order for EHR and CDS systems to become more useful for the greater implementation of pharmacogenomics and personalized medicine, a substantive investment in computational and clinical laboratory infrastructure has to be made at a national level.

Biobanks and handling of DNA samples present both scientific opportunities and policy challenges for regulatory agencies worldwide. Efforts to establish best practices and address the regulation of processing, storage, and uses of samples are being undertaken by a number of national and international regulatory agencies, including the U.S. FDA, the European Medicines Agency, Japan's Pharmaceuticals and Medical Devices Agency, and Health Canada. One promising opportunity is that these agencies are working toward global harmonization of standards for the use of pharmacogenomic tests and targeted therapeutics.

Another area that is broadly presenting policy challenges involves ethical, legal, and social issues (ELSIs), such as patient privacy and protection of data and genetic samples, return of results obtained within the context of research studies to patients, decisions related to the use of genomic information and insurance coverage, and more recently the open science movement (Granados Moreno et al., 2019). Aimed at protecting Americans from future genetic discrimination, the *Genetic Information Nondiscrimination Act* (GINA) was passed in 2008 (GINA, 2008). However, a number of ELSIs related to privacy and protection of genetic data remain to be addressed by legislators and policy makers (Joly et al., 2020). Issues surrounding the education of health care providers and other stakeholders are also increasingly presenting barriers and challenges to the full implementation of pharmacogenomics. A number of studies have concluded that there remains a serious lack of knowledge of genetics and genomics on the part of clinicians Squassina et al. (2010). Steps are increasingly being taken to address the educational needs of current and future health care providers. Pharmacogenomics is being incorporated in the curricula of medical and pharmacy schools.

Keeping Up with Clinical Pharmacogenomics Science

This discussion of the educational needs of future clinicians, including nurse practitioners and physician assistants, brings us to a discussion of how nurse practitioner or physician assistant (PA) students can keep up with the state of science and clinical practice in pharmacogenomics. Although this is a rapidly evolving and fast-moving field, there are some resources that students (Rackover et al., 2007) and clinicians should be aware of and consult on a regular basis. Currently, there are over 260 U.S. FDA–approved drugs that incorporate pharmacogenomic information in the label (https://www.fda.gov/drugs/science-and-research-drugs/table-pharmacogenomic-biomarkers-drug-labeling). In addition to the FDA Web site and the FDA's Table of Pharmacogenomic Biomarkers in Drug Labeling, there are other useful Web sites. For example, the DailyMed project (http://dailymed.nlm.nih.gov/dailymed/), administered by the U.S. National Library of Medicine of the National Institutes of Health (NIH), provides detailed information about package inserts of many prescription drugs, including pharmacogenomic information. The DailyMed Web site is user-friendly and has a powerful search engine, making it easy to navigate.

There are also several organizations with online resources related to pharmacogenomics and its implementation in clinical practice, such as the Clinical Pharmacogenomics Implementation Consortium (Relling & Klein, 2011) and the Dutch Pharmacogenomics Working Group (Swen et al., 2011). In particular, these organizations provide guidelines and recommendations for the clinical use of pharmacogenomics. As they continually update their resources, their Web sites are worth checking routinely (**Box 7.3**).

The CDC's Office of Public Health Genomics tracks and provides evidence related to various genomic tests from research to clinical and public health application. The NIH also maintains the clinicaltrials.gov Web site, which is a mandatory listing of all clinical trials being conducted; this Web site includes information on the purpose of the clinical trial, the study's eligibility requirements, sites where the clinical study is being conducted, the status of patient recruitment and enrollment, and contact information for the investigators. Although clinicaltrials.gov is not restricted to pharmacogenomics and includes all ongoing trials, it is possible to search for pharmacogenomics studies, thereby providing clinicians opportunities to learn more about the latest in clinical pharmacogenomics research and possibly provide their patients with opportunities to enroll in specific trials.

There are also an increasing number of resources that are specifically targeted toward equipping specific health care professionals with knowledge and information about pharmacogenomics and how to use it in clinical settings, such as the Community Pharmacist Pharmacogenetics Network (https://rxpgx.wordpress.com).

BOX 7.3   Selected Pharmacogenomics Information Resources for Clinicians

CDC Office of Public Health Genomics: https://www.cdc.gov/genomics/default.htm

Clinical Pharmacogenomics Implementation Consortium: https://cpicpgx.org/guidelines/

Community Pharmacist Pharmacogenetics Network: https://rxpgx.wordpress.com

Dutch Pharmacogenomics Working Group Guidelines: https://www.knmp.nl/patientenzorg/medicatiebewaking/farmacogenetica/pharmacogenetics-1/pharmacogenetics

FDA Table of Pharmacogenomic Biomarkers in Drug Labeling: https://www.fda.gov/drugs/science-and-research-drugs/table-pharmacogenomic-biomarkers-drug-labeling

National Library of Medicine DailyMed Project: https://dailymed.nlm.nih.gov/dailymed/

Pharmacogenomics Knowledge Base, PharmGKB: www.Pharmgkb.org

Ubiquitous Pharmacogenomics (U-PGx): http://upgx.eu

CASE STUDY 1

J.T. suffers from an irregular heartbeat called atrial fibrillation. On a Sunday afternoon, his wife noticed as J.T. was watching a football game on television that his face started to droop and his speech seemed abnormal. She asked him to smile and his smile was all of sudden very uneven. After he arrives at the hospital, it is determined he is having a stroke as a consequence of his newly diagnosed atrial fibrillation.

1. The therapy of choice for J.T. in this particular case is warfarin. However, following a few hours of warfarin therapy, J.T.'s wife notice excessive nose bleeds and bruising appearing under his skin that seemed to be coming out of nowhere. From the following options given and from a genetic standpoint, what could be happening to J.T.?
   a. He could have a mutation in his liver CYP2C19 enzyme, causing a 90% decrease in warfarin clearance, leaving more S-warfarin in his blood, causing excessive bleeding.
   b. He could have a mutation in his liver CYP2C9 enzyme, causing a 90% decrease in warfarin clearance, leaving more S-warfarin in his blood, causing excessive bleeding.
   c. He could have a mutation in his liver CYP2C9 enzyme, causing a 90% decrease in warfarin clearance, leaving more R-warfarin in his blood, causing excessive bleeding.
   d. He could have a mutation in his liver CYP1A1 enzyme, causing a 90% decrease in warfarin clearance, leaving more S-warfarin in his blood, causing excessive bleeding.

2. Surprisingly, following genetic testing, it was discovered that J.T. can metabolize warfarin perfectly through his liver as all of his CYP enzymes came back normal (no mutations). Which of the following options could thus explain his excessive bleeding?
   a. J.T. is A haplotype for VKORC1.
   b. J.T. is G haplotype for VKORC1.
   c. J.T. is T haplotype for VKORC1.
   d. J.T. is C haplotype for VKORC1.

3. Knowing J.T.'s genetic testing results, what should be done concerning the dose of warfarin?
   a. A lower dose should be given.
   b. A higher dose should be given.
   c. No change in the dosage is necessary.
   d. No warfarin should be given to J.T. in the first place.

CONCLUSION

In summary, among the most promising applications of pharmacogenomics is the potential to minimize or prevent ADRs. Progress has been made in the clinical implementation of pharmacogenomics, with several molecular companion diagnostics paired with targeted therapeutics. Many other biomarkers are currently being tested to predict response to therapies. However, to date, the implementation of pharmacogenomics in clinical practice has presented various ELSI and policy challenges.

Bibliography

Starred references are cited in the text.

*Bitner-Glindzicz, M., & Rahman, S. (2007). Ototoxicity caused by aminoglycosides in severe and permanent in genetically susceptible people. *British Medical Journal, 335*, 784–785.

*ClinicalTrials.gov. Bethesda (MD): National Library of Medicine (US). 2000–. Available from: clinicaltrials.gov. Accessed March 11, 2020.

*Di, L. (2014). The role of Drug Metabolism Enzymes in Clearance. *Expert Opinion on Drug Metabolism & Toxicology, 10*(3), 379–393.

*Ferrero, E., & Agarwal, P. (2018). Connecting genetics and gene expression data for target prioritisation and drug repositioning. *BioData Mining, 11*, 7. Published May 31, 2018. doi: 10.1186/s13040-018-0171-y

*Genetic Information Nondiscrimination Act of 2008, Public Law 110–233, Stat. 122 (2008).

*Golden, R. (2004). A history of William Osler's The principles and practice of medicine. Osler Library studies in the history of medicine No. 8. Montreal, McGill University.

*Granados Moreno, P., Ali-Khan, S., Capps, B., et al. (2019). Open-science precision medicine in Canada: Points to consider, *FACETS, 4*, 1–19.

*Hutchin, T., Haworth, I., Higashi, K., et al. (1993). A molecular basis for human hypersensitivity of aminoglyscoside antibiotics. *Nucleic Acids Research, 21*, 4174–4179.

*Issa, A. M. (2015). Ten years of personalizing medicine: How the incorporation of genomic information is changing practice and policy. *Personalized Medicine, 12*(1), 1–3.

*Issa, A. M., Thorogood, A., Joly, Y., et al. (2019). Accelerating evidence gathering and approval of precision medicine therapies: The FDA takes aim at rare mutations. *Genetics in Medicine, 21*, 542–544.

*Joly, Y., Dupras, C., Pinkesz, M., et al. (2020). Looking beyond GINA: Policy approaches to address genetic discrimination [published online ahead of print, January 21, 2020]. *Annual Review of Genomics and Human Genetics*. doi: 10.1146/annurev-genom-111119-011436

*Lyons, T., & Basu, A. (2012). Biomarkers in diabetes: Hemoglobin A1c, vascular and tissue marker. *Translational Research, 159*(4), 303–312.

*Maluso, A. (2015). Pharmacogenomic testing and Warfarin Management. *Oncology Nursing Forum, 42*(5), 563–565.

*National Library of Medicine (US). Daily Med project. https://dailymed.nlm.nih.gov/dailymed/index.cfm. Accessed March 10, 2020.

*National Library of Medicine (US). Genetics Home Reference Bethesda (MD): The Library. https://ghr.nlm.nih.gov/primer/precisionmedicine/definition. Accessed February 10, 2020.

*Pan, Y., Cheng, R., Li, Z, et al. (2015). PGWD: Integrating personal genome for warfarin dosing. *Interdisciplinary Sciences, Computational Life Sciences, 8*, 23–27.

*Qayyum, A., Najmi, M. H., Khan, A. M., et al. (2015). Determination of S- and R-warfarin enantiomers by using modified HPLC method. *Pakistan Journal of Pharmaceutical Sciences, 28*(4), 1315–1321.

*Rackover, M., Goldgar, C., Wolpert, C., et al. (2007). Establishing essential physician assistant clinical competencies guidelines for genetics and genomics. *The Journal of Physician Assistant Education, 18*(2), 47–48.

*Relling, M. V., & Klein, T. E. (2011). CPIC: Clinical Pharmacogenetics Implementation Consortium of the pharmacogenomics research network. *Clinical Pharmacology & Therapeutics, 89*, 464–467.

*Scott, S. A., Sangkuhl, K., Gardner, E. E., et al. (2011). Clinical pharmacogenetics implementation consortium guidelines for cytochrome P450-2C19 (CYP2C19) genotype and clopidogrel therapy. *Clinical Pharmacology & Therapeutics, 90*(2), 328–332. doi: 10.1038/clpt.2011.132. Epub 2011.

*Shirasaka, Y., Chaudhry, A. S., McDonald, M., et al. (2015). Interindividual variability of CYP2C19-catalyzed drug metabolism due to differences in gene diplotypes and cytochrome P450 oxidoreductase content. *The Pharmacogenomics Journal*. doi: 10.1038/tpj.2015.58. [Epub ahead of print]

*Shuldiner, A. R., O'Connell, J. R., Bliden, K. P., et al. (2009). Association of cytochrome P450 2C19 genotype with the antiplatelet effect and clinical efficacy of clopidogrel therapy. *JAMA, 302*(8), 849–857. doi: 10.1001/jama.2009.1232

Squassina, A., Manchia, M., Manolopoulos, V. G., et al. (2010). Realities and expectations of pharmacogenomics and personalized medicine: Impact of translating genetic knowledge into clinical practice. *Pharmacogenomics, 11*(8), 1149–1167. doi: 10.2217/pgs.10.97

*Swen, J. J., Nijenhuis, M., deBoer A., et al. (2011). Pharmacogenetics: From bench to byte–an update of guidelines. *Clinical Pharmacology & Therapeutics, 89*, 662–673.

*Tornio, A., & Backman, J. T. (2018). Cytochrome P450 in Pharmacogenetics: An update. *Adv Pharmacol, 83*, 3–32.

*U.S. Food and Drug Administration Table of Pharmacogenomic Biomarkers in Drug Labels. https://www.fda.gov/drugs/science-and-research-drugs/table-pharmacogenomic-biomarkers-drug-labeling. Accessed March 11, 2020.

8

The Economics of Pharmacotherapeutics

Briana L. Santaniello and Joshua J. Spooner

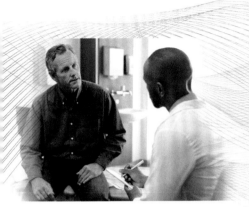
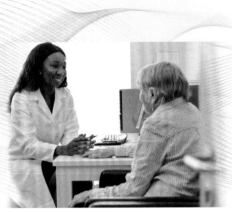
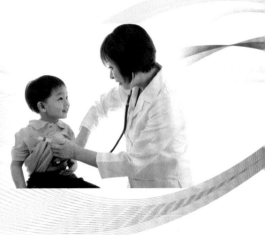

Learning Objectives

1. Describe the historical origins and evolution of health insurance and managed care organizations in the United States.
2. Compare and contrast the common types of prescription drug formularies and corresponding prescription copayment strategies.
3. Explain the responsibilities of a pharmacy and therapeutics (P&T) committee and describe the factors that P&T committees consider in their decision-making processes.
4. Discuss how formulary management tools (generic substitution, therapeutic interchange, prior authorization, and step therapy programs) can influence prescribing patterns.
5. Explain how emerging health technologies (electronic prescribing, electronic medical records, and telehealth) have influenced the delivery of care.

INTRODUCTION

As few as 100 years ago, health insurance in the United States was a scarce commodity. Although President George Washington had signed a law establishing prepaid health care in 1798, health insurance plans were slow to develop. Traditionally, patients in the United States paid health care providers and hospitals directly for their services out of their own pocket on a fee-for-service basis. This system worked well for patients in times of good health; however, a serious injury or illness could place the patient in severe financial peril.

The goal of this chapter is to provide a fundamental understanding of the principles used by managed care organizations (MCOs) and pharmacy benefit managers (PBMs) to manage pharmacy costs while providing access to appropriate patient care. This chapter provides a brief review of pharmacoeconomic principles, educates the reader about the strategies used by MCOs and PBMs to manage health care expenditures, explains how these strategies are developed and implemented, and reviews how MCOs evaluate the performance of contracted providers. Through a better understanding of the practices, benefits, and challenges of MCOs and PBMs, practitioners can better prescribe appropriate and cost-effective medications for their patients.

ORIGINS OF MANAGED CARE

The origins of modern health insurance can be traced to 1929, when the Baylor University Hospital in Dallas, Texas, began to offer school teachers up to 21 days of hospital care a year for an annual payment (premium) of $6 per person (Starr, 1982). Other groups also entered into agreements to prepay for Baylor's services. Shortly thereafter, several other Dallas-area hospitals followed suit and offered similar plans. Other early health insurance plans included the Kaiser Health Plans (early to mid-1930s) and the Group Health Association in Washington, DC (1937). As the country slid into the depression and hospital revenues plummeted by 75% per patient, hospitals began to rely on insurance payments for a greater proportion of their operating budget (Starr, 1982).

Most health plans offered indemnity insurance (also known as *fee-for-service insurance*), in which patients paid for health care expenses out of their own pockets and then requested reimbursement from the insurer (often receiving reimbursement for 80% of incurred expenses). However, indemnity insurance did little to control health care expenditures because physicians and hospitals received payments proportional to the volume of services they provided. Concerned with the rising cost of providing health care, insurance providers sought ways to slow the increases in health care expenditures. After extensive lobbying and negotiations in Congress, President Richard Nixon signed the federal Health Maintenance Organization (HMO) Act into law in 1973. This act encouraged the growth of managed care by providing grants and loans to develop HMOs, overturned restrictive state laws regulating health providers, defined a basic package of services that HMOs were required to offer, and established procedures by which HMOs could become federally qualified.

Because HMOs could deliver cost-effective health care benefits while maintaining a reasonable quality of care, they were viewed as an attractive health insurance alternative for employers. The rate of enrollment in HMOs grew rapidly during the 1980s and 1990s, growing to rival preferred provider organizations (PPOs) as the leading source of employer-sponsored health insurance in the United States in the late 1990s. The federal government also encouraged the use of HMOs to manage the health care costs of Medicare-eligible beneficiaries; HMOs were reimbursed on a prospective basis by the government. The states soon followed suit, offering HMO-based options to Medicaid recipients. Of late, there has been a significant decline in employer-sponsored HMO enrollment, with a shift in favor of PPOs and high-deductible health plans (Kaiser Family Foundation, 2019).

OVERVIEW OF PHARMACOECONOMICS

When MCOs make decisions related to what medications are covered and placed on formularies, those decisions could impact hundreds of thousands of members. Applying economic principles to analyze the impact of a medication on the MCO's overall health care cost and disease management of the patient population is essential to appropriate decision making. *Pharmacoeconomic* research assesses the "overall value" of medications in the treatment or prevention of the disease(s) they are intended to treat (Navarro et al., 2009). Because they evaluate both cost and human data, studies on pharmacoeconomics are important tools for MCOs in making drug therapy decisions. To provide an overview, some different pharmacoeconomic study designs are described in the following sections.

Cost–Benefit Analysis

A cost–benefit analysis is used to determine the overall cost of a particular intervention or protocol by evaluating all pertinent data and converting the data to a monetary endpoint (e.g., U.S. dollars or EU Euros). Most often, this type of analysis is used to compare two different programs that also have different units for endpoints because the data can then be converted to one common monetary unit. The limitation to this analysis involves the evaluation of "intangible" endpoints, or data that cannot be equated to a monetary value.

Cost Minimization Analysis

A cost minimization analysis evaluates the cost of two or more interventions with equivalent components or endpoints and determines which intervention is least costly. The most appropriate use for such analyses involves situations in which every aspect of compared interventions is identical except the cost of the intervention. Because efficacy and safety are identical, the cost of each intervention becomes the differential outcome. The outcomes of these analyses are also expressed in a monetary endpoint.

Cost-Effectiveness Analysis

A cost-effectiveness analysis may help determine the best program or intervention, where the desired outcome is a combination of both a monetary endpoint and a nonmonetary endpoint relative to an improvement in health (e.g., life expectancy, blood glucose measurements). An example of this would be dollars spent per life-year saved.

Cost–Utility Analysis

A cost–utility analysis, which is closely related to a cost-effectiveness analysis, measures data in terms of quality of life. Quality of life is an assessment of a patient's well-being and social functioning, which can assist practitioners in determining a patient's response to drug therapy (Hunter et al., 2015). Along with traditional clinical results (e.g., laboratory values, blood pressure, serum glucose level), a cost–utility analysis provides a more complete evaluation of a patient's progress and compares the cost of an intervention or program in terms of more intangible endpoints, rather than dollars. These analyses predominantly use quality-adjusted life-years (QALYs) gained as a major outcome. The QALY is symbolic of healthy years of life and is the unit of measurement that encompasses outcomes (e.g., morbidity and mortality) in preferential sequence. This method has been very successful in evaluating various procedures compared with drug therapy in which a patient's quality of life is the chosen outcome (Hunter et al., 2015). The Institute for Clinical and Economic Review, a non-partisan research organization that objectively evaluates the value of health care, has identified the QALY as the gold standard for measuring how well a medical treatment improves and lengthens patients' lives (Institute for Clinical and Economic Review, 2018).

Pharmacoeconomic research compares cost and consequence with respect to pharmaceutical products and their impact on individuals, the health care system, and society. Such parameters are seldom analyzed in most studies.

FORMULARIES AND PHARMACY AND THERAPEUTICS COMMITTEES

An evaluation of American health expenditures identified $3.6 trillion in total health care spending in 2018 (Centers for Medicare & Medicaid Services [CMS], 2019a), which accounted for 17.7% of the national gross domestic product (GDP). Of this $3.6 trillion in health expenditures, $335 billion (9.9%) was spent on prescription drugs. Although this represents a minor portion of overall health care expenditures, it remains a target for intervention by MCOs due to large annual increases in prescription drug spending. Prescription drug spending in the United States tripled during the 1980s, tripled again during the 1990s, and doubled during the first decade of the 21st century (CMS, 2019b).

Formularies

One of the most effective methods by which an MCO can improve the quality of care provided to patients and mitigate the increasing costs of providing a prescription benefit is by implementing a formulary. Also known as a *preferred drug list*, a medication formulary is a list of preferred medications approved for use within an HMO, a third-party payer, or a PBM (Navarro et al., 2009). Formularies are usually organized by therapeutic area and medication class, with the formulary status and reimbursement category listed for each medication.

Formularies encourage the use of medications considered to be safer, more clinically effective, or more cost-effective than other medications within the same therapeutic category. When an MCO wants to limit the use of a drug for a specific reason (safety, efficacy, or cost), the formulary allows the flexibility to implement restrictions or limitations on utilization. Examples of such restrictions include prior authorizations, step therapies, quantity limitations, and tiered copayments.

Evolution of Formularies

The use of formularies can be traced back to 1925, when the physicians and pharmacists of Syracuse University Hospital collaborated to establish a formulary system to monitor drug use and reduce therapeutic duplication (the unnecessary use of two or more medications to treat the same condition) in their drug therapy program (Sonnedecker, 1976). By the 1960s, formularies were being implemented in hospitals throughout the country with the guidance of the *American Hospital Formulary Service*, a prominent set of formulary development materials published by the American Society of Hospital Pharmacists. Following the HMO Act of 1973, many HMOs adopted the hospital formulary to monitor medication use. Formularies were initially used by MCOs as an inventory control mechanism for staff model HMOs (Navarro et al., 2009), but they have evolved into effective tools for monitoring and regulating medication utilization for all types of MCOs.

Structure of Formularies

Although formats may differ among plans, a formulary usually contains the same fundamental information. Formularies usually begin with a basic plan summary and detailed key points of reference and then proceed to the list of drugs. The drugs are most often categorized within their respective therapeutic classes, with the therapeutic classes listed in alphabetic order. The order of the drugs within each therapeutic class can vary, but the drugs are often listed alphabetically, either in complete alphabetical order (generic and brand drugs intermixed) or as generic drugs listed before brand-name drugs. Additional information usually detailed for each drug includes the brand/generic status; the drug's relative cost (often symbolized by dollar signs, with one $ representing the lowest cost medication and additional $s representing increasingly costly medications); copay tier; and any potential utilization management programs. An example of a formulary is shown in **Table 8.1**. A *formulary medication* is a drug that is covered (reimbursed) by the health plan; formulary medications can be subdivided into different groups such as preferred and nonpreferred agents. *Preferred* agents are drugs that the health plan would prefer that the practitioner prescribe, due to safety, efficacy, and/or relative cost. *Nonpreferred* drugs are not the preferred drugs of the health plan but will nonetheless be covered by the plan at a higher out-of-pocket cost to the patient. Most formularies have different tiered copays for preferred and nonpreferred drugs, in which preferred drugs have a lower-cost tiered copay than the nonpreferred drugs. *Nonformulary medications* are drugs that are excluded from the formulary; health plans generally do not publish the nonformulary medications on their formularies. Prescribers must usually provide justification for a patient to receive reimbursement for a nonformulary medication.

Formularies can be grouped into three different categories: closed, open, and tiered formularies. Closed formularies limit clinicians to prescribing from a limited list of preferred agents (Edlin, 2015). Open formularies usually do not involve

TABLE 8.1

Example of a Formulary

Drug Name	Brand or Generic	Relative Cost	Tier	Edits
Drug A	Generic	$	Tier 1	
Drug B	Generic	$	Tier 1	QL
Drug C	Brand	$$	Tier 2	QL, ST
Drug D	Brand	$$	Tier 2	
Drug E	Brand	$$$	Tier 3	ST
Drug F	Brand	$$$$	Tier 3	PA
Drug G (specialty injectable)	Brand	$$$$$$	Tier 4	QL, ST

PA, prior authorization; QL, quantity limits; ST, step therapy; Tier 1, generic; Tier 2, preferred brand drug; Tier 3, nonpreferred brand drug; Tier 4, specialty injectable.

a preferred group of agents; instead, they allow the prescriber to select any covered medication. Tiered formularies are essentially the compromise between closed and open formularies. Tiered formularies are open formularies that set different copay tiers for generic, preferred, and nonpreferred medications (Edlin, 2015).

Impact of Formularies on Patients

The price that consumers pay for prescription medications varies from plan to plan. Patients are commonly required to pay a portion of the cost of the prescription, also known as the *copayment*, or *copay*. Copay amounts can differ from plan to plan and by geographic region. Closed and open formularies usually only have two copays: one for generic drugs and one for brand drugs. Tiered formularies have more than two copays, and each tier is associated with a different copay amount.

Most copays are set to cover up to a 1-month supply of medication (28–31 days of therapy, depending on the health plan). Thus, a patient who received a prescription for a 7-day course of therapy of prednisone for an acute allergic reaction would likely have the same copayment as a patient who received a prescription for a 30-day course of therapy of prednisone for chronic use.

Some plans may allow patients who are receiving a stable dose of a maintenance medication (medications used for chronic conditions) to receive more than 1 month of medication at a time. For these maintenance medications, many health plans allow patients to receive a 90-day supply of medication. Health plans usually charge patients three copays for a 90-day supply (three 1-month supply copays). For example, if a patient paid a $10 copay for a 1-month supply, then the 90-day supply would cost $30. Health plans can offer reduced copayments as an enticement for patients to order their maintenance medications from a mail-order pharmacy service; a 90-day supply of medication might only cost the patient the equivalent of two copayments instead of three.

In the rigid formulary systems utilized in the 1990s, a two-tiered prescription copayment system was used by most health plans and pharmacy benefits managers (PBM); the lower copayment tier was used for generic medications, whereas the higher copayment tier was used for formulary brand-name medications. Nonformulary medications were rarely covered by health plans or PBMs without prior approval; if granted, the prescription would fall into the higher copayment tier. Nonformulary medications that were not approved by the health plan were not covered; either patients paid the full retail price for the prescription out of their own pocket or the prescription was switched to a formulary agent by the prescriber.

Fueled by unsustainable prescription cost increases, MCOs abandoned the two-tiered formulary system in favor of higher-tiered formulary designs, ranging from three-tiered systems up to the more recently adopted four- or higher-tiered systems. Within three-tiered formulary systems, the first two tiers are set up the same as the previous two-tiered system, with the first (lowest) tier copayment reserved for generic products and the second-tier copayment reserved for preferred brand-name products. Agents in the third tier are the nonpreferred brand-name products; the copayment is substantially higher than the second-tier copayment. Plans are increasingly adding fourth or fifth tiers to their formulary, which include high-cost specialty medications (with the highest prescription copayments). Among employer-sponsored prescription drug benefit plans, 39% operate formularies with three copayment tiers and 45% have four or more copayment tiers (Kaiser Family Foundation, 2019). Three- and four-tiered formularies have introduced value considerations to patients: Do they value a specific third-tier or fourth-tier product enough to pay the higher copayment or will a first-tier or second-tier product (with a lower copayment) be suitable for their needs? The multiple-tiered copayment has been proven to successfully move patients to products in the first and second tiers of the formulary without restricting access to prescription products (Edlin, 2015).

Functions of Formularies

Formularies have been used to promote the prescribing of safe, efficacious, and cost-effective medications. Formularies' main functions are to promote the use of less costly and equally efficacious medications (which are most often generic medications). For brand-name medications, formularies financially incentivize the use of preferred brand drugs over nonpreferred brand drugs or place barriers that prevent nonpreferred branded medications from being covered by the MCO. MCOs also implement policies or programs with their formularies to promote appropriate drug utilization and the use of generic drugs and preferred brand drugs prior to the use of nonpreferred and nonformulary drugs. Examples of such policies or programs include generic substitution, therapeutic interchange, prior authorization, step therapy, medical necessity, and dispensing limitations around quantity, duration of therapy, age and gender.

Generic Substitution

A highly effective method of reducing the cost of the pharmacy benefit is generic substitution. Generic substitution is the process of dispensing an appropriate generic equivalent of a prescribed brand-name drug. Prescribing generic products can reduce the cost of providing prescription medications for patients; generic-medication use resulted in 10-year savings of nearly $2 trillion from 2009 to 2018 (Association for Accessible Medicines, 2019). Generic substitution has been supported by cost minimization analyses; as the brand and generic agents are considered identical in composition and activity, cost becomes the contributing factor for an agent's selection.

A generic medication is considered equal, or bioequivalent, to its parent brand-name medication, must undergo stringent safety and equivalency testing, and comply with specific criteria established by the U.S. Food and Drug Administration (FDA). The FDA has set certain therapeutic equivalence evaluation codes to show the relative bioequivalence of generic agents to their corresponding brand-name drugs (Food and Drug Administration, 2018). There are two basic rating codes: A and B. The "A" rating indicates that the drug is considered therapeutically equivalent to other pharmaceutically equivalent products. The "B" rating indicates that the agent is not therapeutically equivalent to other pharmaceutically equivalent agents. Both A- and B-rated drugs are further differentiated based on dosage form. An "AB" rating states that the product's bioequivalence problems have been resolved, and evidence exists supporting the bioequivalence to pharmaceutically equivalent agents.

An example of generic substitution is dispensing pregabalin when the prescriber writes the prescription for Lyrica and the prescriber has not indicated that the brand-name product is medically necessary. In such a situation, the pharmacist is filling the prescription with an FDA-approved, bioequivalent form of the brand-name drug. Some insurance plans may allow the patient or prescriber to request the brand-name agent, but this often results in a higher copayment for the patient (Navarro et al., 2009). The increase in copayment may be as large as the difference in cost to the health plan between the brand and the generic agents.

To maximize generic substitution, plans may use restrictive strategies such as *dispense as written* (DAW) blocks. A DAW code describes the rationale for the drug's selection and is entered into the prescription claim by the pharmacist before it is transmitted to the health plan for adjudication. There are DAW codes for *substitution permissible* (DAW 0), *dispense as written* (DAW 1), *patient requests brand* (DAW 2), and other choices to provide a rationale for the chosen agent. A health plan can require that the patient receive an acceptable generic substitution for a brand-name product unless a suitable DAW code has been entered. A DAW code of 7 is used for products with a narrow therapeutic index. Due to the risk of disrupting the level of drug in the patient's blood, drugs with a narrow therapeutic index may not have to be automatically substituted for an equivalent generic agent. A DAW code of 7 informs the health plan that the physician, pharmacist, or patient has elected to continue use of the brand-name product. Drugs in this category include warfarin (Coumadin) and levothyroxine (Synthroid).

Therapeutic Interchange

Therapeutic interchange is defined as the procedure of dispensing prescribed medications that are chemically different but deemed therapeutically similar to the medication prescribed (Holmes et al., 2011). In general, therapeutic interchange involves the substitution of drugs that are different chemical compounds but are considered to exert the same therapeutic effect and have similar toxicity and side effect profiles (e.g., HMG-CoA reductase inhibitors: substitution of generic atorvastatin [Lipitor] for Crestor). The use of therapeutic interchange has increased significantly because of a large influx of new medications that do not offer any therapeutic advantages over existing therapies but are priced much higher than the established products. These medications are commonly known as *me too drugs*. Some popular examples of therapeutic

categories that contain me too drugs include proton pump inhibitors (PPIs), HMG-CoA reductase inhibitors (statins), angiotensin receptor blockers, and bisphosphonates.

Pharmaceutical manufacturers offer rebates to health plans to compete for preferred status on formularies, which lowers the prescription benefit cost. Controversies tend to arise when discounts are used to exchange one drug over another when the drugs are in different classes. If a therapeutic interchange involves two drugs of the same therapeutic class, it can be considered an example of therapeutic minimization because the only difference between the two agents is cost (assuming that the relative safety/efficacy data for the two agents are similar).

Therapeutic interchange is used for reasons other than controlling costs, including promoting the use of agents associated with fewer drug–drug interactions (e.g., substitution of fluconazole for ketoconazole) or of agents with a more convenient dosing schedule (e.g., once-daily enalapril instead of two- to three-times daily captopril). These interventions may prevent unnecessary drug–drug interactions or enhance medication compliance, which could, in turn, improve care and decrease overall health care costs.

In the outpatient pharmacy setting, therapeutic interchange must be verified and accepted by the prescribing practitioner. In the institutional setting, therapeutic interchange does not necessarily require a prescriber's approval if the institution's pharmacy and therapeutics (P&T) committee approves the specific interchange protocol. The American Medical Association (AMA) endorses the practice of therapeutic interchange in settings that have an organized medical staff and a functioning P&T committee (American Medical Association [AMA], 1994).

Drug-Dispensing Limitations

Limitations regarding dispensing drugs are developed and implemented to promote appropriate prescribing of medications and are often structured around FDA-approved labeling and evidence-based medical data. Examples of drug limitations include drug quantity limits, duration of therapy limits, age limits, and gender limits. Drug quantity limitations are used to promote the appropriate quantity of medication that should be prescribed. There are two main types of quantity limits: quantity per filled prescription and quantity per days. Limits on quantity per filled prescription are implemented for drugs that are prescribed for short-term use, such as analgesics and antibiotics. An example of such a quantity limit would be limiting the prescribing of addictive, high-potency narcotic analgesics indicated for acute pain to 10 tablets per prescription. Limits on quantity per days are utilized for chronically used (maintenance) medications. An example of this type of quantity limit would be limiting the prescribing of simvastatin to 1 tablet per day. Limits on duration of therapy are implemented to manage how long a drug should be used, especially for medications that are not considered maintenance medications. An example of a such a limit would be a 3-week duration-of-therapy limit for the prescribing of muscle relaxants (e.g., cyclobenzaprine). Age limitations prevent the use of medications either above or below what is recommended by the FDA. An example of an age limit would be to prevent the use of barbiturates in members greater than 65 years of age. Gender limits prevent the use of medications for a gender when prescribing would not be safe and/or appropriate; an example of this type of limits would be prevention of prescriptions of oral contraceptives for males.

Prior Authorization and Step Therapy Programs

Prior authorization refers to the approval process that health plans may require for certain medications before they will be covered. The primary purpose of a prior authorization process is to control the use of and prevent the overuse of nonformulary, hazardous, or inappropriately prescribed medications. More recently, health plans have begun to move toward increasingly open formularies with three and four tiers of copayments. Further, health plans are requiring prior authorizations for most nonformulary drugs, expensive drugs, newly approved drugs, and drugs with less expensive alternatives (Navarro et al., 2009). Ninety-four percent of employers offering health insurance used prior authorization programs in 2018 (Takeda Pharmaceuticals, 2018), and prior authorizations are used by a majority of the states in their Medicaid programs (National Conference of State Legislatures, 2018).

The criteria for approval of each drug undergoing the prior approval process will depend on the drug, the patient, the disease state involved, and the prescribing practitioner. Some prior authorizations may require a diagnosis along with pertinent laboratory values, whereas others may require a patient to fail therapy with certain drugs that are indicated to treat the same disease as the restricted agent. Other criteria may include patient demographics, such as age or gender limits, or prescriber limits, where only specific specialty types are allowed to prescribe for certain medications (e.g., only allowing dermatologists to prescribe isotretinoin).

The usual chain of events involving prior authorization starts with a patient presenting a pharmacist with a prescription for a newly prescribed medication. The pharmacist, after submitting a claim and having it rejected, learns that the medication requires prior authorization (often from a message sent with the rejected claim). The pharmacist or patient then contacts the prescriber, tells the prescriber that the medication requires prior authorization, and requests that the prescriber contact the MCO to explain why the patient requires that medication. Either prescribers can decide to contact the MCO and pursue prior authorization or they may choose not to pursue prior authorization and select an alternative agent. MCOs often accept prior authorization requests from practitioners by mail, fax, telephone, or Internet. Completing the prior authorization process may result in the drug's approval for use in that patient, or the MCO may again reject the claim and offer a list of alternative medications that are covered by the plan.

If the prescriber knows that the drug requires prior authorization, the necessary paperwork can be completed to have the drug approved for the patient before the patient enters the pharmacy. Problems arise when the patient and prescriber are unaware of which agents on the MCO's formulary require prior authorization. This confuses many patients, possibly leading them to think that the prescriber ordered the wrong medication or the pharmacist made an error in filling the prescription (Bendix, 2013).

Step therapy programs are utilization management programs that are a version of prior authorization, in which they promote the use of one drug before another (Navarro et al., 2009). There are two main types of step therapy programs: those driven by cost-effectiveness and those that promote more clinically effective medications before less effective medications. The cost-effectiveness step therapy programs promote the use of cost-effective generic medication before the use of an expensive branded medication. They can be implemented using drugs within the same therapeutic class or different categories. An example of a step therapy within a therapeutic class would be to require the use of a generic atypical antipsychotic, such as aripiprazole for the adjunctive treatment of major depressive disorder, before the approval of a branded atypical antipsychotic like Rexulti. An example of a step therapy using different categories would be to require the use of metformin before the approval of dipeptidyl peptidase-4 (DPP4) inhibitors like sitagliptin and saxagliptin. Step therapy programs implemented for the purpose of promoting clinical effectiveness are usually based on practice guidelines or evidence-based medical data. An example of this type of program would be to require the use of nasal corticosteroids or non-sedating antihistamines before the approval of leukotriene inhibitors for the treatment of allergic rhinitis.

MCOs have increased their efforts to prospectively review prescriptions requiring prior authorization during the claim adjudication process. When a pharmacy sends a claim for a prior authorization drug to the PBM for adjudication, the PBM can review the patient's prescription claim history and the claim itself to determine if the prior authorization criteria have been met. This step can decrease the number of rejected prescription claims and minimize the time and efforts of prescribers, pharmacists, and patients in obtaining prior authorizations. When initiated effectively by informing practitioners of the drug's status and the preapproval process, prior authorization can become a very efficient mechanism for controlling costs and drug use.

Medical Necessity

Some MCOs use the term *medical necessity* interchangeably with *prior authorization*. In most settings, a medication listed as a medical necessity is a nonformulary drug that is often extremely expensive and usually has less expensive generic alternatives and/or less expensive brand name alternatives, or is considered a relatively unsafe medication compared to available alternatives (Navarro et al., 2009). Some MCOs make medical necessity drugs available only after failure of drug therapy with a drug requiring prior authorization. MCOs carefully evaluate drugs before classifying them as medical necessity drugs, knowing that the drugs will be restricted if they are covered. Like the criteria for medications requiring prior authorization, the criteria for coverage vary from drug to drug.

PHARMACY AND THERAPEUTICS COMMITTEE

Structure and Function

A P&T committee is a group that meets periodically to review and revise the organization's formulary. The committee is composed primarily of physicians and pharmacists and may also include nurses, nurse practitioners, physicians' assistants, patient care advocates, and members of the organization's administration. The physicians on the committee often comprise a diverse group from various fields of practice, with general practitioners and multiple specialists represented. The committee should be a well-balanced mix of practitioners who can view health care policies from different perspectives and provide sound recommendations.

Formulary Management

The main responsibilities of a P&T committee are to develop and revise the formulary, create and implement medication use policies, and provide education for practitioners. Formulary reviews include evaluating new medications for formulary consideration, periodic drug class reviews, and utilization analyses. A major goal of the P&T committee is to provide cost-effective, clinically safe, and effective therapy. Frequent formulary revisions are needed for several reasons: the introduction of new products into the marketplace, modifications to a product's labeling to include new treatment indications, emerging research indicating a previously unknown benefit or risk of therapy, changes in consensus disease treatment guidelines, and changes in the brand/generic status of a product or other pricing concerns.

The inclusion and exclusion of agents are a time-intensive process for P&T committees. As such, many P&T committees elect to delay their consideration of a new product until it has a sufficient body of evidence to perform a review and/or it has been on the market for a sufficient length of time (e.g., 1 year), which provides an opportunity for any adverse events undetected in clinical trials to be noted. P&T committees may consider a wide variety of information when evaluating a new product, including peer-reviewed clinical trials, adverse event/safety data, patient-oriented health outcomes (e.g., the ability of an antihypertensive to reduce the risk of myocardial infarctions, not merely to lower blood pressure), the FDA-approved product labeling for the new agent, quality-of-life research, and pharmacoeconomic data (**Box 8.1**). The committee must consider the issue of bias when evaluating results of clinical or health outcomes research, data analyses, or pharmacoeconomic modeling sponsored by the pharmaceutical manufacturer. Publications that include data comparing the new agent with an agent currently used to treat the same disorder are prized by P&T committees for their utility in comparing one drug with another. If the new agent offers a clinical, safety, or economic advantage over existing formulary agents, the P&T committee may place the agent on the formulary and can do

---

BOX 8.1 Information Considered by a Pharmacy and Therapeutics Committee When Reviewing a Product for the Formulary

1. FDA-approved indications
2. Pharmacology/mechanism of action
3. Pharmacokinetic/pharmacodynamic data
4. Dosing and administration, including special monitoring or drug administration requirements
5. Adverse effect profile, warnings, precautions, contraindications, and black box warnings
6. Drug interactions (with other drugs, foods, or medical conditions)
7. Clinical evidence: clinical trials, health outcomes research, retrospective database analyses, quality-of-life research
8. Risks versus benefits regarding clinical efficacy and safety of a particular drug relative to other drugs with the same indication
9. Pharmacoeconomic data and modeling
10. Off-label uses and utilization rates for off-label uses
11. Cost comparisons against other drugs available to treat the same medical condition(s)
12. Source of supply and reliability of manufacturer and distributor

---

so by adding the new product; this may be accompanied by removing or not removing an existing product or products from the formulary. Further, committees can add the drug to the formulary unconditionally or may recommend implementation of certain restrictions on the coverage (prior authorization, quantity limitations, step therapy) of the new agent to allow its inclusion in the formulary.

Because of the increase in prescription drug spending by health plans, cost now plays a more significant role in the formulary decision-making process and formulary tier placement, although many organizations claim that cost is considered only after safety and efficacy data have been evaluated. Pharmacoeconomic modeling allows an organization to estimate the impact of a formulary change on both the health outcomes experienced by their members and the total prescription drug and health care spending. To improve the likelihood of a drug's addition to a formulary, pharmaceutical manufacturers may offer prescription volume-dependent rebates to MCOs as incentives.

Development of Disease Management Programs and Treatment Protocols

Another responsibility of a P&T committee is to develop or approve disease management programs or treatment protocols for the organization. These programs and protocols provide useful recommendations for practitioners treating various diseases.

They may be based on current consensus practice guidelines, or they may be developed by the P&T committee using current clinical data. A main purpose of guidelines or algorithms is to minimize treatment variations and improve patient outcomes while minimizing costs (Navarro et al., 2009).

ENSURING FORMULARY AND PRACTICE GUIDELINE COMPLIANCE

One of the primary reasons that MCOs develop formularies and practice guidelines is to minimize the cost of the prescription drug benefit. Unfortunately, merely printing and distributing formularies and algorithms often are not enough to alter prescribing practices. Patients and pharmacists may also be wary of the formulary system, failing to understand both its necessity and its utility. While educational programs (including seminars, newsletters, provider peer-to-peer communications, and one-on-one meetings) are useful, these tools alone do not ensure improved formulary compliance. MCOs have developed a variety of payment and reimbursement strategies to improve formulary compliance. The following sections describe the ways that MCOs evaluate formulary and treatment guideline compliance and how they use different levels of payments to improve compliance.

Prescriber Incentives for Compliance

MCOs can monitor compliance to the formulary and treatment protocols with a variety of tools. Many MCOs use the level of peer compliance to determine the amount of a prescriber's or practice's year-end incentives. Prescribers can be eligible for financial incentives if their compliance to the formulary or treatment protocols meets the threshold established by the MCO (Navarro et al., 2009).

Some MCOs may tie a portion of a provider's compensation to their level of compliance. If a practitioner fails to follow treatment protocols closely and inexplicably high prescription costs result, an MCO may withhold a portion of the provider's compensation. In a capitated plan, the provider receives a fixed, predetermined, per-member payment by the MCO to provide services for members, regardless of how much or how frequently a member uses the service. Providers can reap financial reward if they can provide services at a cost lower than their level of payment but are responsible for all costs if expenses should rise above their level of payment. While capitation remains a frequently utilized tool by MCOs to manage medical costs and encourages providers to focus on efficiency and cost control (Hodgin, 2018), few (if any) health plans utilize a capitated pharmacy benefit.

Evaluating Compliance: Percentage Formulary Compliance

The simplest way for an MCO to evaluate formulary compliance is to determine the prescriber's percentage of prescriptions for generic and preferred branded formulary products.

Although this method is useful for determining formulary compliance (e.g., the use of generic and branded formulary angiotensin receptor blockers [ARBs] compared with nonformulary-branded ARBs), it does not evaluate the quality of prescribing; just because a formulary agent is prescribed does not make the prescription appropriate. It may be more useful to determine if the prescriber is following consensus disease treatment guidelines. A prescriber who prescribes a formulary agent but is not following treatment guidelines may have the same percentage formulary compliance as a prescriber who uses a different and potentially less expensive or more appropriate formulary medication by following treatment guidelines. Also, prescribers who use medically necessary or appropriate nonformulary drugs are penalized in this system. Many MCOs have initiated programs to evaluate the quality of the prescriber by implementing practitioner profiling programs, where MCO clinicians evaluate questionable prescribing with the provider.

Because of these limitations with percentage formulary compliance, MCOs also use another tool to evaluate compliance: per-member–per-month (PMPM) reports.

Health Care Trend Reporting

When analyzing health care trends for an MCO, many variables are reviewed and factored in to evaluate and justify the trends during any particular year. PMPM reports are a unit of measure related to each enrollee for each month. When used to evaluate prescribing practices, average PMPM prescription costs are determined for each provider. Theoretically, prescribers who adhere to formulary and practice guidelines will achieve lower PMPM prescription costs than their peers who do not. This is not a foolproof method to evaluate compliance because a small number of patients requiring expensive therapy (e.g., chemotherapy, antipsychotics) can substantially increase a prescriber's PMPM amount. More frequently, MCOs use PMPM reports to evaluate prescription costs for a specific disease. An example of a disease-specific PMPM report appears in **Table 8.2**. Although prescriber A is responsible for the highest

TABLE 8.2			
Per-Member–Per-Month Prescription Costs for Patients Receiving Antihyperlipidemic Therapy			
Prescriber	**Number of Member Months**	**Lipid Prescription Costs ($)**	**PMPM Prescription Costs ($)**
A	561	67,622	120.54
B	240	26,462	110.26
C	285	36,759	128.98
D	496	53,464	107.79
E	357	43,568	122.04
F	489	56,978	116.52
All prescribers	2,428	284,853	117.32

PMPM, per-member–per-month.

dollar expenditure on antihyperlipidemics, their PMPM prescription cost is close to the average of the prescriber's peers. On the other hand, despite prescriber C's low overall dollar expenditure on lipid agents, their PMPM prescription cost is the highest.

Another factor that is considered in evaluating health care trends is drug cost. Monitoring the rate of increase in drug cost has become a significant factor in overall health care spending. As the prices of prescription medications increase, MCOs are adjusting their overall plan designs to compensate for that increase. These adjustments may include changes in product status on drug formularies, implementation of prior authorization and step therapy programs for expensive products, increases in member copayments, or increases in member premiums.

Improving Formulary Compliance

In addition to prescribers, MCOs have an opportunity to improve formulary and practice guideline compliance by providing financial incentives or disincentives to the prescription dispenser (pharmacist) and the prescription recipient (patient). These financial incentives include bonuses, differential reimbursement rates, and different levels of prescription copayment.

Pharmacist Reimbursement

An MCO can influence pharmacists as a secondary step in limiting the use of nonformulary medications. As a part of the contracting process, MCOs impose requirements on pharmacies if the pharmacy wishes to serve members of the plan. MCOs can require that pharmacies dispense generic products when available, unless the prescriber requires the prescription to be DAW or the medication has a narrow therapeutic index (e.g., phenytoin [Dilantin], warfarin). Many states already require automatic generic substitution when applicable. To reduce wasted or unused medication, MCOs often impose a limit on the amount of medication that a community pharmacist can dispense—usually no more than 30 days' worth at a time. Once a patient is stabilized on a maintenance dose for medications used to treat chronic illnesses (e.g., hypertension, diabetes), MCOs may require that patients receive a 3-month supply of medication from a mail-order pharmacy; this can be done at a lower expense to the MCO.

Pharmacies that are successful in increasing formulary compliance or reducing member pharmacy costs may be eligible for bonuses or they may receive a higher reimbursement rate. Alternatively, pharmacies that fail to meet the requirements of the contract may receive a lower reimbursement rate or have their contract terminated altogether. MCOs frequently audit the claims of pharmacies with a higher-than-average number of DAW orders to ensure that the prescriber does in fact require that the brand-name drug be dispensed to the patient.

Patient Prescription Copayment

The impact of prescription copayment on patients was reviewed earlier in this chapter. In summary, as formularies have progressively become more open, health plans have responded by using differential copayments with significant price differentials between tiers in an effort to encourage patients to use lower-cost generic or preferred brand medications. Patients who are hesitant to pay a high prescription copayment when lower-priced alternatives are available frequently ask their provider to prescribe the product with the lower copayment; the provider will often comply with the patient's request if they believe the change can be made without adversely affecting the expected outcomes of care.

ELECTRONIC PRESCRIBING AND ELECTRONIC HEALTH RECORDS

Before the introduction of electronic prescribing, practitioners were faced with a variety of options by which they could prescribe medications: written orders on prescription pads, typed orders sent via fax, or verbal orders communicated through telephone calls. These prescribing options leave room for error, as there is the potential for illegible handwriting, poorly scanned images, and inaudible messages. Furthermore, these options are not exempt from tampering or fraud, as individuals can alter handwritten prescriptions, send falsified prescriptions via fax, or call in fake prescriptions over the phone. With the advent of electronic prescribing, practitioners were presented with an additional option that has the potential to save time and money, as well as reduce medication errors and fraud. The SUPPORT for Patients and Communities Act requires the use of electronic prescribing for all controlled substances covered under Medicare Part D beginning January 1, 2021 (Uhrig, 2019). Due to the COVID-19 pandemic, a compliance date of January 1, 2022 was set to allow healthcare providers additional time to implement electronic prescribing without penalty (CMA, 2020).

Electronic prescribing, or e-prescribing, is the process whereby a prescriber orders and submits a prescription through an application that electronically transmits the prescription to a pharmacy in real time (CMS, 2014). A variety of e-prescribing software programs exist, and thus, there may be differences in functionality among the e-prescribing software programs available to clinicians. Ideally, the software programs should allow the prescribers to view a patient's current medication list, medication history, available pharmacy, and prescription insurance plan (Health Resources and Services Administration [HRSA], 2015).

E-prescribing software requires a user (the prescriber or an authorized representative) to log in to a secure system and verify his or her identity using a username and password combination. After authentication, the prescriber can search for and select a patient record within the e-prescribing system using patient-specific information (i.e., first name, last name, date of birth, etc.). The prescriber can then choose to review the patient's records and begin to enter and edit a prescription (HRSA, 2015).

After entering the intended prescription information, the prescriber can send the order to the transaction hub, which links the prescriber to both the pharmacy and the PBM. This interoperability allows for the verification of patient eligibility for prescription coverage by submitting the prescription information to the PBM before the e-prescription arrives at the pharmacy. Once the information has been submitted, the PBM determines if the drug is a covered benefit for the member. The prescriber then receives a message regarding the drug's coverage status. If the drug is covered, the prescriber may choose to send the prescription to the pharmacy for it to be filled. On the other hand, if the drug is not covered, the prescriber has the option of ordering a different medication or contacting the PBM for prior authorization of the drug (HRSA, 2015).

The ability of prescribers to directly transmit prescriptions from the office to the pharmacy eliminates the need for the patient to take it to the pharmacy to be filled. Since patients are not required to take electronically transmitted prescriptions to the pharmacy, there are increased chances that the prescriptions actually arrive at the pharmacy.

E-prescribing has also been shown to reduce prescribing errors. Researchers at Weill Cornell Medical College found 37 errors for every 100 prescriptions written by hand but only 7 errors for every 100 prescriptions ordered via e-prescribing software (Kaushal et al., 2010). These benefits, along with the potential for time and cost savings, explain the rationale behind the *meaningful use* incentive payments program offered by the Centers for Medicare & Medicaid Services (CMS), which began in 2009 and ended in 2013 (CMS, 2019c).

E-prescribing represents only one part of a greater change to the health care system: electronic health records (EHRs). EHRs are digital versions of patient-centered medical records, which can be updated in real time (HealthIT, 2019). In 2009, the American Recovery and Reinvestment Act (ARRA) authorized CMS to offer financial incentives to providers and hospitals that exhibit *meaningful use* of EHR technology (AMA, 2015). With the recent advances in technology, many providers have already adopted the software necessary to maintain EHRs. However, these systems can impart challenges to smaller practices because of the significant cost to upgrade technology and the operational changes needed to use the system. Aside from the large costs associated with the purchase of EHR software, the universal implementation of EHR represents an opportunity for enhanced interoperability, improved continuity of care, and medical error reduction.

The terms *telemedicine* and *telehealth* are sometimes used interchangeably; however, the term *telehealth* refers to a broader variety of digital health services than *telemedicine* (NEJM Catalyst, 2018). Telemedicine is the delivery of remote clinical services, which may include the remote diagnosis, treatment, and monitoring of patients through telecommunication (Center for Connected Health Policy, 2019; NEJM Catalyst, 2018). The term *telehealth* refers to the delivery and facilitation of health care (including diagnosis and management of conditions), education, information, and related services through digital communication technologies (Center for Connected Health Policy, 2019; NEJM Catalyst, 2018). Many MCOs are beginning to adopt and encourage the use of telehealth as it has the potential to reduce costs and wait times, improve access to care, and enhance overall health care delivery. For example, some health plans encourage members to utilize telehealth services for their non-life-threatening urgent care needs. By seeking care through the telehealth system, patients may be able to skip the visit to the urgent care office or the unnecessary and costly emergency department visit, which can help save time and money for both the patient and the health plan. Telehealth services can also improve patients' access to a broader network of specialists. In a traditional health care setting, patients are sometimes required to visit their primary care provider in order to receive a referral to a specialist. With telehealth, patients may be able to be seen by the specialist through a virtual visit, during which their health records, including test results and images, are reviewed and an evaluation, diagnosis, and treatment plan can be made.

CURRENT ISSUES IN MANAGED CARE

In March 2010, the U.S. Congress passed the Affordable Care Act, commonly known as either the Healthcare Reform Bill or Obamacare. The objective for the act was to ensure accountability of MCOs, lower health care costs, improve quality of care, and provide improved consumer choice for health care services (U.S. Department of Health & Human Services, 2010). Components of the Affordable Care Act include provisions requiring insurers to provide coverage for individuals with preexisting conditions, provisions allowing individuals under the age of 26 years to remain on a parent's insurance plan, an elimination of lifetime and annual dollar limits for essential health benefits, and requirements for specific preventive services (e.g., colorectal cancer screening for adults over 50, breast cancer mammography screening for women over 40, vision screening for children) without having to pay a copayment or coinsurance when delivered by a network provider (U.S. Department of Health & Human Services, 2019). A mandate written into the act requires individuals not covered by an employer-sponsored health plan or a public insurance plan to obtain an approved private insurance policy or pay a penalty. This individual mandate provision of the act was upheld by the U.S. Supreme Court in June 2012 as a constitutional action under Congress's taxation powers (*National Federation of Independent Businesses vs. Sebelius*, 2012). In 2018, a tax bill that repealed the Affordable Care Act's tax penalty was signed, and the federal individual mandate penalty was eliminated in most states in 2019; however, the penalty still exists in some state tax codes such as Massachusetts's (Norris, 2019). While the Affordable Care Act has increased consumer choice and improved quality of care, it has not been as effective in lowering health care costs, as evidenced by the continued increases to the cost of insurance premiums. The average family's annual premium costs were nearly $20,600 in 2019, with covered workers paying 29% of the premium (Kaiser Family Foundation, 2019).

The act continues to face legal and legislative challenges in its funding and implementation, and the regulations and provisions noted here may be modified or eliminated in the future.

Due to the escalation in prescription copayment expenses that consumers are expected to pay, some pharmaceutical manufacturers have begun to issue copayment cards, which are designed to reduce or eliminate a customer's out-of-pocket spending for prescriptions. These *copay cards* are available to individuals with commercial or private health insurance; copay cards cannot be utilized for prescriptions paid for (in part or in whole) by Medicare or Medicaid. Consumers apply for copay cards through patient assistance programs (PAPs) operated by manufacturers; these PAPs are often need based and place household income caps (often set at 400% of the federal poverty limit) on enrollees. If approved for a copay card, the card is valid for prescriptions covered by the PAP, with benefits often limited to a single medication or line of products from the manufacturer sponsoring the PAP. Consumers redeem these copay cards at the prescription point of sale; the pharmacy would then receive the copay directly from the PAP and not the consumer. Copay cards are thought to improve patient adherence and persistence with prescription therapy, as lower copayment levels are associated with higher rates of prescription adherence and improved health outcomes (Amin et al., 2017; Gourzoulidis et al., 2017). MCOs generally oppose PAPs because they undermine prescription cost-sharing requirements and benefit designs that incentivize cost-effective prescribing practices (Linehan, 2019). MCOs have responded by implementing copay accumulator programs. Under a copay accumulator program, the health plan does not count PAP payments toward the customer's annual deductible or annual out-of-pocket maximum, which may result in a patient being unable to continue to afford the prescription if the copay card has been exhausted of value. Despite criticism from patients, prescribers, and consumer advocates that copay accumulator programs are harmful to public health, these programs are being adopted by an increasing number of MCOs to shift upfront costs to consumers (Silverman, 2018).

Despite its critics and shortcomings, managed care is likely to remain the leading manner of financing and delivering health care in the United States. Through more effective communication and cooperation, practitioners and MCOs may someday resolve their conflicting issues. It is imperative for practitioners and MCOs to understand each other's role in health care. Although practitioners and MCOs have quite different responsibilities in health care, both groups share a common goal: the delivery of high-quality care to patients.

Bibliography

Starred references are cited in the text.

Academy of Managed Care Pharmacy. (2019). AMCP format for formulary submissions, version 4.1. Alexandria, VA: Author.

Agarwal, R., Mazurenko, O., & Menachemi, N. (2017). High-deductible health plans reduce health care cost and utilization, including use of needed preventive services. *Health Affairs, 36*(10), 1762–1768.

Agency for Healthcare Research and Quality. (2019). Electronic health records. Retrieved from http://psnet.ahrq.gov/primer/electronic-health-records on March 11, 2020.

American Academy of Family Physicians. (2020). What's the difference between telemedicine and telehealth? Retrieved from http://www.aafp.org/media-center/kits/telemedicine-and-telehealth.html on March 11, 2020.

American Academy of Pediatrics. (2020). What is telehealth? Retrieved from http://www.aap.org/en-us/professional-resources/practice-transformation/telehealth/Pages/What-is-Telehealth.aspx on March 11, 2020.

*American Medical Association. (1994). AMA policy on drug formularies and therapeutic interchange in inpatient and ambulatory patient care settings. *American Journal of Hospital Pharmacy, 51*, 1808–1810.

*American Medical Association. (2015). Meaningful use: Electronic health record (EHR) incentive programs. Retrieved from https://www.ama-assn.org/practice-management/medicare/meaningful-use-electronic-health-record-ehr-incentive-programs on February 10, 2020.

*Amin, K., Farley, J. F., Maciejewski, M. L., et al. (2017). Effect of Medicaid policy changes on medication adherence: Differences by baseline adherence. *Journal of Managed Care and Specialty Pharmacy, 23*(3), 337–345.

*Association for Accessible Medicines. (2019). The case for competition: 2019 generic drug & biosimilars access & savings in the U.S. report. Retrieved from http://accessiblemeds.org/sites/default/files/2019-09/AAM-2019-Generic-Biosimilars-Access-and-Savings-US-Report-WEB.pdf on February 9, 2020.

*Bendix, J. (2013). Curing the prior authorization headache. *Medical Economics*. Retrieved from http://medicaleconomics.modernmedicine.com/medical-economics/content/tags/americas-health-insurance-plans/curing-prior-authorization-headache?page=full on May 10, 2015.

*California Medical Association. (2020). CMS delays enforcement of e-prescribing requirement for controlled substances. Retrieved from http://www.cmadocs.org/newsroom/news/view/ArticleId/49150/CMS-delays-enforcement-of-e-prescribing-requirement-for-controlled-substances on January 14, 2021.

*The Center for Connected Health Policy. (2019). About telehealth. Retrieved from http://www.cchpca.org/about/about-telehealth on January 29, 2020.

*Centers for Medicare & Medicaid Services. (2014). Electronic prescribing (eRx) incentive program. Baltimore, MD: Author. Retrieved from https://www.cms.gov/Medicare/Quality-Initiatives-Patient-Assessment-Instruments/ERxIncentive/index.html on February 10, 2020.

*Centers for Medicare & Medicaid Services. (2019a). Office of the Actuary, National Health Statistics Group. National health expenditures fact sheet. Washington, DC: Author.

*Centers for Medicare & Medicaid Services. (2019b). Office of the Actuary, National Health Statistics Group. National health expenditures accounts: historical data [Table 16] Washington, DC: Author.

*Centers for Medicare & Medicaid Services. (2019c). E-prescribing. Baltimore, MD: Author. Retrieved from https://www.cms.gov/Medicare/E-Health/Eprescribing/index.html?redirect=/eprescribing on February 10, 2020.

Cohen, J. P., El Khoury, C., Milne, C., et al. (2018). Rising drug cost drives the growth of pharmacy benefit managers exclusion lists: Are exclusion decisions value-based? *Health Services Research, 53*(S1), 2758–2769.

*Edlin, M. (2015). Closed formularies hold the line on costs: One of a number of strategies in use. *Managed Healthcare Executive, 25*(3), 48.

Enthoven, A. C., & Baker, L. C. (2018). With roots in California, managed competition still aims to reform health care. *Health Affairs, 37*(9), 1425–1430.

*Food and Drug Administration. (2018). Electronic Orange Book preface 39th edition. http://www.fda.gov/Drugs/DevelopmentApprovalProcess/ucm079068.htm. Accessed February 10, 2020.

Fullerton, D. S., & Atherly, D. S. (2004). Formularies, therapeutics, and outcomes. New opportunities. *Medical Care, 42*(4 Suppl.), 39–44.

*Gourzoulidis, G., Kourlaba, G., Stafylas, P., et al. (2017). Association between copayment, medication adherence, and outcomes in the management of patients with diabetes and heart failure. *Health Policy, 121*(4), 363–377.

*Health Resources and Services Administration. (2015). How does e-prescribing work? http://www.hrsa.gov/healthit/toolbox/HealthITadoptiontoolbox/ElectronicPrescribing/epreswork.html. Accessed May 30, 2015.

*HealthIT.gov. (2019). What is an electronic health record (EHR)? https://www.healthit.gov/faq/what-electronic-health-record-ehr. Accessed January 12, 2020.

*Hodgin, S. (2018). Capitation vs. fee for service. http://www.insight-txcin.org/post/capitation-vs-fee-for-service. Accessed January 14, 2020.

*Holmes, D. R., Becker, J. A., Granger, C. B., et al. (2011). ACCF/AHA 2011 health policy statement on therapeutic interchange and substitution. *Circulation, 124*, 1290–1310.

Howard, J. N., Harris, I., Frank, G., et al. (2018). Influencers of generic drug utilization: A systematic review. *Research in Social and Administrative Pharmacy, 14*(7), 619–627.

*Hunter, R. M., Baio, G., Butt, S., et al. (2015). An educational review of the statistical issues in analysing utility data for cost utility analysis. *Pharmacoeconomics, 33*, 355–366.

*Institute for Clinical and Economic Review. (2018). The QALY: Rewarding the care that most improves patients' lives. White Paper. Boston, MA: Author.

James, B. C., & Poulsen, G. P. (2016). The case for capitation. *Harvard Business Review*, July/August, *61*, 87–94.

Johnson, T. L., Rinehart, D. J., Durfee, J., et al. (2015). For many patients who use large amounts of health care services, the need is intense yet temporary. *Health Affairs, 34*(8), 1312–1319.

*Kaiser Family Foundation and Health Research Educational Trust. (2019). Employer health benefits 2019 annual survey. San Francisco, CA: Author.

Kaufman, B. G., Spivack, B. S., Stearns, S. C., et al. (2019). Impact of accountable care organizations on utilization, care, and outcomes: A systematic review. *Medical Care Research and Review, 76*(3), 255–290.

*Kaushal, R., Kern, L. M., Barron, Y., et al. (2010). Electronic prescribing improves medication safety in community-based office practices. *Journal of General Internal Medicine, 6*, 530–536.

*Linehan, J. S. (2019). Assessing the legal and practical implications of copay accumulator and maximizer programs. *Managed Care, 28*(2), 42–44.

*National Conference of State Legislatures. (2018). State Pharmaceutical Assistance Programs 2010. Retrieved from http://www.ncsl.org/default.aspx?tabid=14334. Denver, CO: Author.

National Federation of Independent Businesses vs. Sebelius, 567.U.S. 2012, 132 S. Ct 2566. June 28, 2012.

*Navarro, R. P., Dillon, M. J., & Grzegorczyk, J. E. (2009). Role of drug formularies in managed care organizations. In R. P. Navarro (Ed.), *Managed care pharmacy practice* (2nd ed., pp. 233–252). Sudbury, MA: Jones and Bartlett Publishers.

*NEJM Catalyst. (2018). What is telehealth? Retrieved from http://catalyst.nejm.org/doi/full/10.1056/CAT.18.0268 on January 29, 2020.

*Norris, L. (2019). Chapter Six: What is the Obamacare penalty? Retrieved from http://www.healthinsurance.org/obamacare-enrollment-guide/what-is-the-obamacare-penalty/ on February 9, 2020.

Penna, P. M. (2002). AMCP format for formulary submissions: Who is using them, who will be evaluating them, and what regulatory concerns do they raise? International Society for Pharmacoeconomics and Outcomes Research Seventh International Meeting, Arlington, VA.

Seeley, E., & Kesselheim, A. S. (2019). Pharmacy benefit managers: Practices, controversies, and what lies ahead. Commonwealth Fund [issue brief], March, pp. 1–11.

*Silverman, E. (2018). Backlash against copay accumulators. *Managed Care, 27*(9), 15.

*Sonnedecker, G. (1976). *Kremer's and Urdang's history of pharmacy*. Madison, WI: American Institute of the History of Pharmacy.

*Starr, P. (1982). *The social transformation of American medicine*. New York: Basic Books.

Sweet, B. T., Wilson, M. W., Waugh, W. J., et al. (2002). Building the outcomes-based formulary. *Disease Management and Health Outcomes, 10*, 525–530.

*Takeda Pharmaceuticals. (2018). 2018 Trends in drug benefit design report. Plano, TX: Pharmacy Benefit Management Institute.

*Uhrig, P. (2019). It's official: Half of all states will soon require E-prescribing to combat the opioid epidemic. Retrieved from http://surescripts.com/news-center/intelligence-in-action/opioids/it-s-official-half-of-all-states-will-soon-require-e-prescribing-to-combat-the-opioid-epidemic/ on February 9, 2020.

*U.S. Department of Health & Human Services. (2010). Understanding the affordable care act: About the law. Retrieved from http://www.hhs.gov/healthcare/rights/index.html on April 27, 2015.

*U.S. Department of Health & Human Services. (2019). About the Affordable Care Act. Retrieved from https://www.hhs.gov/healthcare/about-the-aca/index.html on February 10, 2020.

U.S. Food & Drug Administration. (2018). FYs 2013-2017 Regulatory Science Report: Analysis of Generic Drug Utilization and Substitution. Retrieved from http://www.fda.gov/drugs/generic-drugs/fys-2013-2017-regulatory-science-report-analysis-of-generic-drug-utilization-and-substitution on March 11, 2020.

Principles of Pain Management

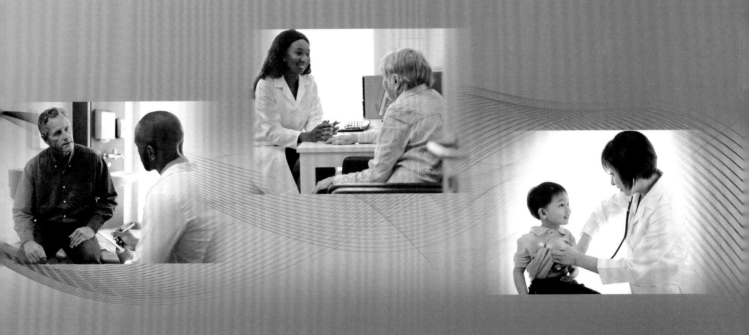

9 Pharmacotherapy of Pain Management

Maria C. Foy

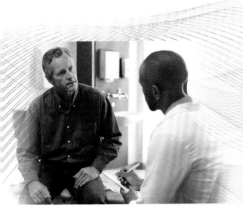
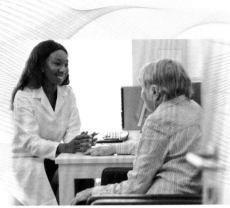
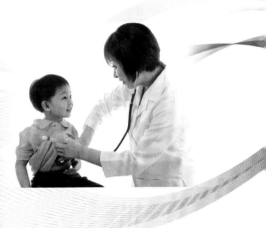

Learning Objectives

1. Explain pain pathophysiology and the neurotransmitters involved in the facilitation of pain.
2. Classify pain based on source and chronicity.
3. Select first-line treatments for a patient with acute or chronic pain.
4. Compare and contrast the current medication options for the treatment of acute and chronic pain.

INTRODUCTION

One of the most widely encountered clinical situations is a patient in pain. Treatment of pain is one of the most difficult aspects of patient care. Pain is defined by the International Association for the Study of Pain as "an unpleasant sensory and emotional experience associated with actual or potential tissue damage, or described in terms of such damage" (Merskey & Bogduk, 2012, p. 210). Pain is subjective, and its intensity varies from patient to patient, day to day. The clinician has a large array of medications available with which to assist patients in relieving their pain. The principles of managing the various types of pain are described in this chapter, which introduces the practicing nurse to the many types and classes of drugs available for therapeutic management.

Analgesics represent one of the most frequently prescribed and administered classes of medications used in pain management. Managing pain in the acutely or chronically ill patient requires both a sound comprehension of the clinical pharmacology of analgesics and a clear understanding of how pain is perceived. Clinicians caring for chronically ill patients not only find themselves assisting the patient in dealing with the physical component of pain but often are confronted by the patient's psychological, spiritual, and social perceptions of pain and pain medications.

In 2000, in an effort to deal with the inadequate treatment of pain, The Joint Commission developed a standard recommendation that pain be considered "the Fifth Vital Sign" (Phillips, 2000). However, education on the appropriate assessment and treatment of various conditions did not follow and prescribers were pressured to utilize opioids as their main analgesic option. Unfortunately, overprescribing occurred when the main focus on pain control moved away from a multidisciplinary approach to aggressive treatment with opioids. Prior to the release of the standards in 2001, opioid prescribing patterns were on the rise, but a more rapid escalation occurred after 2001, with prescriptions peaking around 2011. Subsequently, unintended residual harm occurred with an increase in opioid overdoses and related deaths. Despite efforts to control overprescribing, deaths continued to rise. When the opioid "supply" was taken away, sometimes inappropriately, many would obtain opioids from the streets.

Prior to starting opioid therapy, a patient's risk for opioid abuse or misuse must be assessed. Various assessment tools are available to determine the risk of opioid use disorder (OUD) which are discussed in Chapter 10.

Additional assessments are needed in order to determine the most appropriate approach to pain management. Renal and liver dysfunction will affect the choice and dosing of analgesic agents. Respiratory comorbidities can increase the risk of opioid-induced respiratory depression. Age is another major consideration in assessing pain and appropriate therapies. In general, older patients are less likely to complain about pain, are more sensitive to medications, and request fewer analgesics to alleviate pain, often secondary to incorrect beliefs and biases. A corollary exists in pediatric patients, whose inability to adequately express suffering leads some clinicians to believe that children cannot feel pain, which we know now is untrue. Because of the identified communication barrier, clinicians need to evaluate a child by utilizing special pain assessment tools developed for children. Similar assessment tools are utilized for adults who may not be able to verbally communicate their pain.

TYPES OF PAIN

Pain can be categorized as nociceptive, neuropathic, or "other" based on the presumed underlying cause. Nociceptive pain occurs as a result of nerve receptor stimulation following a mechanical, thermal, or chemical insult. Nociceptive pain is purposeful, because the pain tells you to stop doing whatever is causing discomfort. Nociceptive pain can be further classified as somatic or visceral. Somatic pain associated with muscle, skin, or bone injury is often well localized. Pain affecting internal organs is referred to as visceral pain. Inflammatory pain is another subtype of nociceptive pain, which results from the release of proinflammatory cytokines at the site of tissue injury. Inflammatory pain may be present in acute pain from bruises or infection and chronically from rheumatoid arthritis or osteoarthritis.

Neuropathic pain is caused by abnormal signal processes in the central nervous system (CNS). Pain can be peripheral or central in origin and is no longer protective in nature. Peripheral neuropathies include pain from diabetes and postherpetic neuralgia. Examples of central neuropathic pain syndromes include pain from multiple sclerosis, spinal cord injuries, migraine, and poststroke syndrome. Descriptors of neuropathic pain, such as electric-like, burning, tingling, stabbing, or shooting pain, can differentiate nerve pain from nociceptive pain and help determine appropriate treatment.

More than one type of pain may occur simultaneously. Failed back surgery syndrome, cancer pain, and chronic regional pain syndrome (CRPS) may have characteristics of a mixed nociceptive–neuropathic picture.

New evidence is now directed toward the consideration that many chronic pain conditions should be viewed as a biopsychosocial disease with pain facilitated by the combination of biological, psychological, and environmental factors. Noxious pain precipitants are no longer present and no pathology exists that would explain the symptomology. This other pain category is often referred to as dysfunctional pain, caused by changes in the analgesic pathway. Structural changes consist of increases in nerve endings and receptive fields and a decreased threshold for nerve activation. Sensitized pain resulting from nervous system changes and cortical reorganization is referred to as neuroplasticity. Patients with psychological comorbidities, such as anxiety, depression, poor sleep patterns, and a history of both physical and psychological trauma, are predisposed to the development of chronic sensitized pain

conditions (Ru-Rong et al., 2018). The fear and the lack of the ability to cope can be underlying factors in the development of chronic sensitized pain. Some examples of sensitized conditions include CRPS, fibromyalgia, and migraines (Ru-Rong et al., 2018).

CLASSIFICATION OF PAIN

Pain can be classified into two categories—acute and chronic—which help identify the derivation of the pain and provide a framework for treatment. Pain can subsequently be categorized and treated based on the expected chronicity of the pain and on whether it is nociceptive, neuropathic, or mixed in origin.

Acute Pain

Acute pain has a sudden onset, usually subsides quickly, and is characterized by sharp, localized sensations with an identifiable cause. Acute pain is a natural physiologic response to injury, useful in warning individuals of disease or harmful situations. Inflammation seen in acute pain influences pain perception and provides a protective role by removing the painful stimuli, restoring tissue health and facilitating healing. This process is often seen as a signal that the body is invoking critical immunologic and physiologic responses to cellular or tissue damage. Concomitant physiologic responses include excessive sympathetic nervous system activity, such as tachycardia, diaphoresis, and increased blood pressure and respiratory rate. Acute pain is somewhat instructive and purposeful by signaling danger. Pain is usually brief and resolves within a few months of onset. Surgical intervention and trauma are common sources of acute pain.

When acute pain responses become unremitting, constant, or undertreated, the biologic responses outlive their usefulness and can lead to chronic pain. Patients with chronic pain become tolerant to the physiologic response seen in acute pain. In addition, these patients often do not appear to be suffering. The body becomes tolerant to the autonomic indicators, where heart rate, blood pressure, and respiratory rate normalize as pain persists. Undesired consequences, such as anxiety and depression, are often associated with constant, long-term pain. The goal of acute pain management is to avoid progression to a chronic pain state. Early pain control will often prevent the development of chronic pain.

Chronic Pain

Chronic pain is defined by the Institute of Clinical Systems Improvement as "pain without biological value that has persisted beyond the normal time and despite the usual customary efforts to diagnose and treat the original condition and injury" (Hooten et al., 2013, p. 7). Chronic pain may be nociceptive, neuropathic, or mixed in origin. Pain can be either the main complaint, where no evidence of structural or nerve damage is present to explain the discomfort, or secondary to an underlying disease. Some conditions may have a verifiable source, as in patients with arthritis, diabetic peripheral neuropathy, or postherpetic neuralgia. In some patients, however, pain can be referred to as *chronic primary pain*, when no apparent evidence of structural or nerve damage exists (Treed et al., 2019). In these patients, the pain is most likely from neuroplastic changes resulting in peripheral and central sensitization of the nociceptive pathways, explained later in this chapter.

Identifying and differentiating pain through careful examination of the history, location, quality, chronicity, and presence of psychological comorbidities is important because treatment choices are dictated by the cause and type of pain. Patients with pain as the main complaint are especially difficult to treat, and a multimodal approach to treatment is needed. Cognitive factors such as pain catastrophizing and anxiety have a strong correlation to pain and disability. The current biomedical approach focusing only on tissue and tissue injury as the cause has often been ineffective in people with sensitized pain. Cases are often complicated, and patients need an individualized approach to therapy.

Pain may respond to most traditional analgesic approaches, including opioid therapy. However, higher doses of opioids may be required to control chronic and sensitized pain. Over time, opioid therapy often becomes less effective and fails to improve function, especially when it's the only modality of analgesia offered to the patient. With chronic pain, the goals of therapy are to decrease the pain to a tolerable level and improve function using a combination of various types of therapies to ultimately enhance quality of life. The patient must have realistic expectations and agree that the goal of pain control is to reduce discomfort to a tolerable level and that the pain may never totally resolve. Active versus passive patient involvement is necessary. Examples of types of chronic pain are shown in **Box 9.1**.

Opioid Use in Chronic Pain

Opioid use for chronic pain is controversial. In an effort to address the "pain crisis" due to reports of a substantial number of patients suffering from pain, a focus was placed on treatment based on subjective patient self-reports alone. In the late 1990s, opioids were advocated as a safe and effective analgesic with minimal risk of abuse when used in persistent noncancer pain, leading to an increase in prescribing by health care providers. In addition, providers were not given adequate training in the appropriate assessment and management of pain and regarding where opioids fit in the treatment plan. By 2012, enough prescriptions were written to give virtually every American a bottle of opioid medications (Paulozzi et al., 2014). A marked increase in opioid-related SUD and deaths resulted. Between 1999 and 2014, more than 165,000 deaths due to opioids were reported (Centers for Disease Control and Prevention [CDC], 2014).

Overprescribing of opioids with subsequent increases in opioid-related morbidity and mortality has led to the development of guidelines in 2016 by the CDC. The guidelines provide recommendations for the use of opioids in the treatment of chronic noncancer pain (CNCP), focusing on multiple analgesic options. Guidance to primary care physicians on when to initiate or continue opioids, choice/duration of treatment, and risk assessment of harm and SUD in patients prescribed opioids for chronic pain is provided. However, methods on how to accomplish the recommendations are not outlined within the guidelines. In the subsequent years since implementation, various challenges have been identified that can potentially cause residual harm to patients. In a report in *Pain Medicine* in 2019, a multidisciplinary CDC panel highlighted several issues, which included inflexible application of recommendations, abrupt discontinuation of long-term opioid

---

BOX 9.1   Classification of Chronic Pain

NOCICEPTIVE PAIN

Arthropathies (e.g., rheumatoid arthritis, osteoarthritis, gout)
Ischemic disorders
Mechanical low back pain
Myalgia (e.g., myofascial pain syndromes)
Nonarticular inflammatory disorders (e.g., polymyalgia rheumatica)
Postoperative pain
Skin and mucosal ulcerations
Superficial pain (sunburn, thermal burns, skin cuts)
Visceral pain (appendicitis, pancreatitis)

NEUROPATHIC PAIN

Alcoholic neuropathy
Cancer-related pain and some cancer treatments

Chronic regional pain syndrome
Diabetic peripheral neuropathy
Human immunodeficiency virus (HIV)–related pain and some HIV treatments
Multiple sclerosis–related pain
Phantom limb pain
Postherpetic neuralgia
Poststroke pain
Trigeminal neuralgia
Vitamin B_{12} deficiency

MIXED OR UNDETERMINED PATHOPHYSIOLOGY

Carpal tunnel syndrome
Chronic recurrent headaches
Low back pain with radiculopathy
Painful vasculitis

therapies without proper tapering, failure to involve patients in decisions regarding their opioid therapy, lack of access to pain specialists, and barriers to provision for treatment of opioid use disorder (OUD) (Kroenke et al., 2019). Lack of insurance coverage for analgesic alternatives remains a significant barrier to recommended treatment options. Some patients, who have had abrupt tapering or discontinuation of opioids, have turned to the streets for supply in order to treat pain and/or prevent withdrawal from established tolerance to opioid therapy. In fact, despite leveling off of opioid prescriptions, deaths continue to rise at an alarming rate due to increase in the use of heroin and illicit fentanyl. A balance between appropriate and safe options for pain control and risks and harms from opioid therapy is needed. Clinicians must provide individualized treatment plans based on patient-specific factors, and risks and policies should allow flexibility in individualization with coverage available for options besides medications. Education is needed on various pain management modalities and assessment of a patient's risk of abuse before initiating opioid therapies. In addition, we now know that titration to high-dose opioid therapy is no longer recommended, especially when improvement of function is not seen.

Cancer-Related Pain

Cancer-related pain is associated with malignancy and can result from the disease itself, disease treatments, or damage to secondary tissue. Disease-induced pain may be secondary to direct tumor involvement of bone, nerves, viscera, or soft tissue. In addition, muscle spasm, muscle imbalance, and other body structure/function changes secondary to the tumor are considered disease induced. Pain may be associated with treatment of the disease and may be seen with biopsies, surgeries, and/or chemotherapy and radiation treatments. Pain may be present in sites where cancer has metastasized (i.e., bone pain). Cancer treatment interventions may activate peripheral nociceptors, causing somatic and visceral nociceptive pain. Neuropathic pain involving the sympathetic nervous system may also be seen. In metastatic cancer, opioids are the mainstay of treatment for severe pain. Nonsteroidal agents or steroids may be an additional option for pain control, especially when bony metastasis are present.

Breakthrough Pain

Breakthrough pain (BTP) is defined as a transitory discomfort often seen in conjunction with cancer-related pain, where moderate to severe pain occurs in patients with an otherwise well-controlled analgesic baseline. True BTP is characterized as brief, lasting minutes to hours, and can interfere with functioning and quality of life. True BTP has historically been associated with a cancer diagnosis but may also be seen in other chronic pain conditions, such as neuropathic pain and chronic lower back pain.

Other types of BTP include pain caused by certain activities (incident pain) or when the duration of analgesia is less than the dosing interval (end-of-dose failure). Giving an analgesic prior to the event known to cause pain will often allow the activity to be performed with minimal discomfort to the patient. Shortening the dosing interval is recommended in patients with end-of-dose failure.

PAIN PATHOPHYSIOLOGY

Several theories exist as to how information resulting from tissue damage is perceived by the brain as pain. Noxious stimuli from the point of the initial injury move through specialized nerve fibers within the CNS, where the signal reaches the brain and is interpreted as pain. This transmission through the CNS is termed *nociception*. Free nerve endings of small myelinated A-delta fibers and larger unmyelinated C fibers are called nociceptors and are responsible for delivering signals to the brain. In the past, the *gate control theory* proposed that the "closing of the gate" to pain signals was accomplished primarily through stopping the transmission of the pain signal to the brain. However, recent studies theorize that changes in the brain and the CNS have a much larger role in the facilitation and perception of pain (Woo et al., 2015). Anxiety, fear, depression, and previous pain experiences may influence an individual's perception of pain, especially when pain becomes chronic.

A description of nociception can be divided into four main categories: transduction, transmission, perception, and modulation (**Figure 9.1**).

Transduction

Transduction refers to a process of nociceptor activation due to mechanical, thermal, or chemical injury. Nerve endings are activated through the release of various excitatory chemical neurotransmitters, such as proinflammatory cytokines, prostaglandins (PGs), substance P, histamine, bradykinin, and serotonin.

Transmission

Transduction results in an action potential transmitted via the myelinated A-delta and unmyelinated C fibers, by way of the dorsal root ganglia, synapsing in the dorsal horn of the spinal cord. Second-order neurons are then activated and convey pain signals to the higher centers of the CNS. Neurotransmitters in the dorsal horn directly or indirectly depolarize the second-order neurons, facilitating transmission of information to the brain, leading to the perception of pain. Inhibitory substances are also released in the dorsal horn (see the section titled Modulation that follows) and may decrease the number of signals reaching the brain, thereby lessening transmission.

Perception

Nociceptive information travels through different areas of the CNS to the brain, where the pain is perceived. Perception is the end result of the nociceptive transmission to the brain; at this point, we become consciously aware of discomfort. Pain

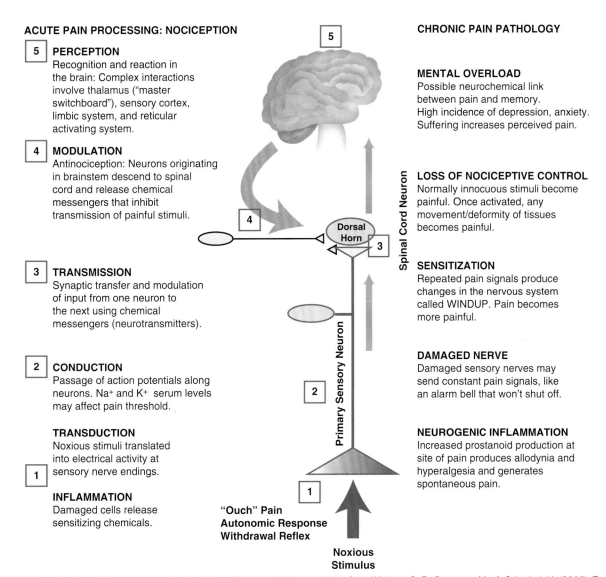

ACUTE PAIN PROCESSING: NOCICEPTION

5 PERCEPTION
Recognition and reaction in the brain: Complex interactions involve thalamus ("master switchboard"), sensory cortex, limbic system, and reticular activating system.

4 MODULATION
Antinociception: Neurons originating in brainstem descend to spinal cord and release chemical messengers that inhibit transmission of painful stimuli.

3 TRANSMISSION
Synaptic transfer and modulation of input from one neuron to the next using chemical messengers (neurotransmitters).

2 CONDUCTION
Passage of action potentials along neurons. Na+ and K+ serum levels may affect pain threshold.

TRANSDUCTION
Noxious stimuli translated into electrical activity at sensory nerve endings.

1 INFLAMMATION
Damaged cells release sensitizing chemicals.

Dorsal Horn

Spinal Cord Neuron

Primary Sensory Neuron

**"Ouch" Pain
Autonomic Response
Withdrawal Reflex**

**Noxious
Stimulus**

CHRONIC PAIN PATHOLOGY

MENTAL OVERLOAD
Possible neurochemical link between pain and memory. High incidence of depression, anxiety. Suffering increases perceived pain.

LOSS OF NOCICEPTIVE CONTROL
Normally innocuous stimuli become painful. Once activated, any movement/deformity of tissues becomes painful.

SENSITIZATION
Repeated pain signals produce changes in the nervous system called WINDUP. Pain becomes more painful.

DAMAGED NERVE
Damaged sensory nerves may send constant pain signals, like an alarm bell that won't shut off.

NEUROGENIC INFLAMMATION
Increased prostanoid production at site of pain produces allodynia and hyperalgesia and generates spontaneous pain.

FIGURE 9–1 Acute and chronic pain pathophysiology. Reprinted with permission from Whitten, C. E., Donovan, M., & Cristobal, K. (2005). Treating chronic pain: New knowledge, more choices. *The Permanente Journal, 9*(4), 9–18. Retrieved from http://www.thepermanentejournal.org. Copyright 2005 The Permanente Journal.

perception is not just a manifestation of physical injury but is affected by psychosocial factors and previous painful experiences. In a chronic pain state, the perception of pain is no longer influenced by the initial noxious stimuli. The presence of psychologic comorbidities in many patients with chronic pain may result in fear of the pain and pain catastrophizing, thereby increasing its perception.

Modulation

Pain modulation occurs at various levels of the CNS. Endogenous opioids work through binding to opioid receptors in both the peripheral and CNS. The main central inhibitory neurotransmitters involved in modulation are serotonin and norepinephrine. These neurotransmitters fight pain by increasing their concentration in the spinal cord and brainstem.

Pain-Modulating Receptors

Historically, pain modulation was thought to be primarily due to descending inhibitory information from the brain. Experts now theorize that both descending inhibitory pain pathways and inhibitory neurotransmitters decrease the perception of pain. Inhibitory substances, such as endogenous opioids, norepinephrine, and serotonin are released in various areas of the CNS and attenuate the transmission of pain by modulating the signals in the dorsal horn (Pasero & McCaffrey, 2011). Endogenous opioid substances, primarily beta endorphins, stimulate inhibitory neuronal receptors known as the opioid receptors. Stimulation of these receptors, particularly the *mu* opioid receptor, inhibits the transmission of pain signals to and from the higher brain centers. These receptors are stimulated by morphine-like drugs (opioids) and account for a great deal of the pain relief associated with this class of analgesics.

In contrast, neuropathic pain syndromes do not respond as well to conventional analgesic therapy. Neuropathic pain is often the result of peripheral and central sensitization or from actual nerve damage. Sensitization of the *N*-methyl-D-aspartic acid (NMDA) receptors by various mechanisms is primarily responsible for this type of pain. Use of coanalgesic agents, such as antidepressants, anticonvulsants, and antiarrhythmic agents, is recommended for treatment. Details on the use of coanalgesics are found later in this chapter.

More information is being assimilated on the endocannabinoid system and pain control. Cannabinoid receptor activation may facilitate analgesia by inhibition of excitatory neurotransmitters in a retrograde fashion, thereby attenuating the hyperalgesic and inflammatory components of pain. See Chapter 11, on cannabinoids and pain, for more information.

CHEMICAL MEDIATORS

Coupled with the neuronal component of pain is the release of chemical mediators initiating or continuing the stimulation of pain-conducting fibers. Peripheral chemical mediators include the neurotransmitters norepinephrine, serotonin, and histamine and polypeptides such as bradykinin, PGs, and substance P. Neurotransmitters may be both excitatory and inhibitory, depending on the site of activity in the CNS. The role of excitatory neurotransmitters in the pain pathway is activating and sensitizing nociceptors and increasing neuronal activity. Blocking the production of these mediators, particularly inhibiting the production of PGs with antiinflammatory medications or similar compounds, minimizes nociceptor activation and neuronal firing, thereby lessening the transmission of pain through the CNS. Because of their role in initiating the pain pathway, these chemicals are targets for many of the medications currently available to treat pain.

Both excitatory and inhibitory neurotransmitters can be found in the dorsal horn of the spinal cord. Excitatory amino acids, glutamate and aspartate, along with substance P facilitate activation of second-order neurons in the dorsal horn primarily through activation of the NMDA receptors.

Natural endocannabinoids may also play a role in inhibition of pain. Anandamide and 2-arachidonoylglycerol are the main natural endocannabinoids that elicit analgesia through modulation of pain signaling, perception, and mood (see also Chapter 11).

PERIPHERAL AND CENTRAL SENSITIZATION

Often, pain persists despite healing, and no biomedical explanation can be found. Pain pathways become "broken," and pain is experienced without an obvious cause. Modifications occurring in the nociceptive conduction pathways of the peripheral nervous system and CNS, where hypersensitivity to a stimulus and neuronal structural changes result in chronic pain syndromes, are referred to as *peripheral sensitization* and *central sensitization*.

Peripheral Sensitization

When pain receptors in the periphery are continually stimulated (i.e., untreated acute pain), the threshold for stimulation becomes lowered and increased nerve firing occurs. Nociceptive neurons become hypersensitized through activation of various protein kinases and modulation of ion channels. Increased frequency of nerve impulses result in more pain signals reaching the dorsal horn of the spinal cord. Release of excitatory neurotransmitters is also increased, producing neuronal hyperexitabiltiy that contributes to the development of central sensitization.

Central Sensitization

Central sensitization is defined as "an amplification of neural signaling within the CNS that elicits pain hypersensitivity" (Woolf, 2011, p. 4). When nociceptive information repeatedly stimulates nerve fibers, increased dorsal horn neuronal activity is seen. With actual or potential nerve damage, as seen in many cases of uncontrolled pain, the increase in firing leads to an increased excitability and responsiveness, termed *central sensitization*. Neuroinflammation of the peripheral nervous system and the CNS is now thought to play a major role in the transition from acute to chronic pain. Characteristics of neuroinflammation include production of inflammatory cytokines, infiltration of leukocytes into the CNS, and activation of various protein kinases and glial cells. The end result is a decrease of central pain inhibition, increased spontaneous neuronal activity in the dorsal horn, a decreased threshold for neuronal firing, and spread of pain sensitivity in areas not affected by the initial insult. Sensitization of the NMDA receptor in the area of the dorsal horn also contributes to central sensitization. Allodynia (pain response to something painless), hyperalgesia (increased response to pain), persistent pain, or referred pain may result.

Central sensitization can occur in many chronic pain states, especially when associated with nerve injury or dysfunction. Factors associated with the development of sensitized pain include inadequate treatment of acute pain, concomitant psychological comorbidities, and poor coping skills, leading to the development of chronic pain through the sensitization of the CNS. Evidence is accumulating on the role of neuroinflammation in patients with *chronic overlapping pain conditions*, caused by dysregulation of sensory, inflammatory, and psychological pathways. Examples include but are not limited to patients suffering with fibromyalgia, headache, and irritable bowel syndrome, where multiple factors contribute to the chronicity of pain (Ru-Rong et al., 2018). Pain associated with central sensitization often responds poorly to traditional therapies. The addition of coanalgesics, reviewed later in this chapter, should be considered for the treatment of chronic pain associated with central sensitization.

GENERAL PRINCIPLES OF PAIN MANAGEMENT

Treatment of pain in today's society rests on three major principles: appropriate assessment of the severity and intensity of the pain, selection of the most appropriate agent to relieve pain with minimal side effects, and assessment for risks of misuse or abuse. Pain relief, especially with chronic pain, often requires a multimodal approach, using multiple agents that target different receptors and neurotransmitters in the CNS. Non-opioid-based pain modalities should be utilized initially for treatment. Additional mind–body approaches such as cognitive–behavioral therapy, massage, acupuncture, and mindful meditation are often recommended to be used in addition to pharmacologic therapy in patients suffering from chronic nonmalignant pain. Prior to initiation of opioid therapy, assessment for risk of abuse/misuse and appropriate monitoring should be established.

Pain Assessment

The individual assessment of pain is extremely important for determining proper treatments as well as monitoring effectiveness over time. According to the National Institutes of Health (NIH), self-reporting by patients is "the most reliable indicator of the existence and intensity of pain" (Hooten et al., 2013, p. 14). Along with self-reporting, involving the caregiver's assessment, especially in the very young or noncommunicating older patient, may be helpful. The self-report should include a description of the pain, location, intensity/severity, aggravating and relieving factors, and effect of pain on quality of life. Assessment tools are recommended to be brief and easy to use in order to reliably document pain intensity and pain relief. Various tools, especially those used in chronic pain, will also evaluate other factors that may facilitate pain perception, such as the presence of psychological comorbidities. One routine clinical approach to pain assessment and management is summarized by the mnemonic PQRSTU (**Box 9.2**). Assessment tools should be used initially to obtain a baseline level of pain and impaired function. Follow-up assessments should be performed to measure the progress toward acceptable pain relief based on the individual functional goals of the patient.

Because pain is subjective and is not easily quantifiable, several tools are available to determine the quantity and quality of a patient's pain. The various pain scales can be classified as single or multidimensional and self-report or observational. Common single-dimensional tools include the visual analog scale (VAS), numerical rating scale (NRS), and verbal description scale (**Figure 9.2**). The single-dimensional scales evaluate pain intensity. However, single-dimensional scales do not take into account function, which may be a more reliable indicator of pain control. Multidimensional scales consider location, pattern, and affective responses in addition to a severity score alone. Examples of multidimensional scales include the Brief Pain Inventory and the Initial Pain Assessment Tool (Pasero & McCaffrey, 2011).

The information obtained, particularly from the NRS and VAS, is helpful in determining appropriate treatment and drug selection. The Institute for Clinical Systems Improvement (ICSI), the NIH, and the CDC have published guidelines on the appropriate evaluation and treatment of acute and chronic pain. Acute pain is recommended to be assessed with a 0-to-10 scale to determine a patient's current level of discomfort. Zero defines a pain-free state, and a 10 describes the most severe pain imaginable by the patient. Pain rated at 1 to 3 is classified as mild; 4 to 6 is classified as moderate; and 7 to 10 is classified as severe (Jensen et al., 2001). Other validated scales are available for use in special populations, such as in children and adults unable to self-report.

> **BOX 9.2 — PQRSTU Mnemonic for Assessing Pain**
>
> **P**—Presenting, precipitating, palliating. When and how did the pain start? What makes the pain better? What have you used for pain in the past that wasn't effective?
> **Q**—Quality of the pain. What does the pain feel like? (descriptors such as sharp, stabbing, burning)
> **R**—Region, radiation. Where is the pain? Does the pain stay in one location or does the pain radiate?
> **S**—Severity. On a scale of 0 to 10, 0 being no pain, 10 being the worst pain imaginable, what is your pain now? In the last 24 hours? After a pain medication?
> **T**—Temporal pattern. Is the pain constant, intermittent, associated with movement?
> **U**—How does the pain affect *you*? Quality-of-life indicator.

Do you have

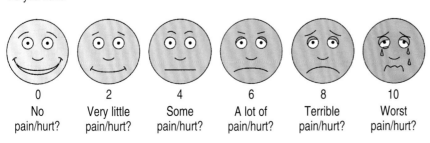

0	2	4	6	8	10
No pain/hurt?	Very little pain/hurt?	Some pain/hurt?	A lot of pain/hurt?	Terrible pain/hurt?	Worst pain/hurt?

FIGURE 9–2 Visual analog scale used for ranking pain. Used with permission from Wong-Baker FACES Foundation (2019).

New assessment scales are being evaluated for assessment of chronic pain. Acute pain is easier to assess via available validated tools. Chronic pain is often driven by maladaptive thought processes in patients with comorbid anxiety and depression. Functional capacity is often limited; therefore, in a patient with chronic pain, functional improvement is a better indicator of successful treatment than a score from a single-dimensional tool. Anxiety and depression are often present in patients with chronic pain and may limit their ability to cope with pain, thereby further affecting function. The Indiana Polyclinic Combined Pain Scale, developed in 2005, is a four-part assessment tool that takes into account pain score, function, depression, and anxiety when evaluating chronic pain (Arbuck & Fleming, 2019). Each of the four scales offer both descriptions and associated numeric ratings for the area of evaluation and may be of value for use in patients with chronic pain to better determine a successful treatment regimen. Further study is needed to validate the scale when compared to currently utilized assessment tools. Subsequent monitoring should evaluate the effectiveness of the treatment plan. If pain remains uncontrolled, determine if the reason for increased pain is related to the progression of disease, disease treatments, or a new cause, as in cancer that has metastasized. Unrelieved pain may also be due to the development of opioid tolerance, where the same amount of pain requires increasing doses of opioids in order to provide relief. In chronic pain, untreated psychological comorbidities and unrealistic expectations are often the cause of poor pain control and should be addressed in conjunction with medication management. The assessment of the patient's pain and the efficacy of the treatment plan should be ongoing, and the pain reports should be documented. Continued use of the same pain scale is crucial to the continued assessment of treatment progress and communication between health care providers.

Pain Management

Treatment options for pain control include nonpharmacologic and pharmacologic therapies. **Box 9.3** lists treatments that complement medication management of pain. Often, a multimodal, multidisciplinary approach using a combination of both pharmacologic and nonpharmacologic treatments is necessary to reduce pain to an acceptable level and provide an improvement in function, especially when opioid therapies are used. Maximizing the patient's quality of life and function, while minimizing the adverse effects of treatments, is the goal of the treatment plan. Individualization of drug regimens according to the type and severity of pain is essential when using medications to manage both acute and chronic pain states.

For mild to moderate pain, acetaminophen, nonsteroidal antiinflammatory agents (NSAIDs), and/or topical analgesics are recommended for initial therapy. Acetaminophen is used for mild pain across all age groups, mainly due to its favorable side effect profile. NSAIDs are very effective in pain associated with inflammation. However, patients may be at risk for gastrointestinal (GI), cardiac, or renal toxicities. Discussion of risk versus benefits of NSAID therapies are discussed later in this chapter.

For pain assessed as moderate to severe, opioid agonists either alone or in combination with acetaminophen or ibuprofen can be used. Around the clock (ATC) acetaminophen and NSAIDs can provide non-opioid choices for persistent pain in conjunction with as-needed opioid therapy and may reduce the need for opioids as the main treatment option when pain is moderate to severe. Combination opioids, such as oxycodone or hydrocodone in conjunction with acetaminophen or ibuprofen, can also be used in patients where pain is intermittent.

Morphine, hydromorphone, oxycodone, oxymorphone, and fentanyl are examples of pure *mu* opioid agonists. Moderate to severe pain can be treated with low-dose opioids when a patient has contraindications to NSAIDs or acetaminophen or when these agents are being used around the clock. Opioids may be combined with other coanalgesic medications based on severity, description, and type of pain. The combination of an opioid and non-opioid and/or coanalgesic medications may provide more pain control than utilizing a single modality agent for analgesia.

When developing a treatment plan, members of the health care team should take into account the preferences and needs of patients whose education or cultural traditions may impede effective treatment. Certain cultures have strong beliefs about pain and its management. Members of these cultures may hesitate to report unrelieved pain or may have alternative methods of treatment. Clinicians should be aware of the unique needs and circumstances of patients from different age groups or various ethnic and cultural backgrounds. In addition, the current environment of the opioid crisis has increased fear and stigma surrounding opioid use for persistent pain, especially when not related to cancer. Patient and provider education may be effective in addressing cultural concerns and alleviating biases associated with opioid therapies.

Pharmacologic treatment is the most common modality in pain control. However, nonpharmacologic options and therapies have been shown to be effective, especially in patients with chronic pain. Nonpharmacologic approaches include the use of therapies such as heat, cold, exercise, and physical therapy. Transcutaneous electrical nerve stimulation therapy and implantable spinal cord stimulators are recommended to

---

BOX 9.3   Adjunctive Pain Control Options

Acupuncture
Cognitive–behavioral therapy
Coping skills training
Massage
Mindful meditation
Patient education (therapeutic neuroscience education)
Physical methods (stretching, exercise, gait training, immobilization, hot or cold applications)
Transcutaneous electrical nerve stimulation

be used for treatment of certain types of nerve-related pain. Complementary therapies such as acupuncture and massage may also be effective.

More data are emerging on how CNCP needs to be seen more as a biopsychosocial phenomenon and not as a purely biological condition, especially when no obvious cause is present. Realistic expectations need to be established with the patient early in the treatment plan. Fear of any discomfort and catastrophizing behaviors are often the main drivers of pain and must be addressed before treatment strategies can be effective. Behavioral therapies, including systematic coping approaches and relaxation strategies, have been shown to be essential in these patients in order to improve function and quality of life. Cognitive–behavioral therapy, acceptance therapy, and meditation are active treatment strategies that can help overcome psychological issues central to adequate pain control. Treatment of difficult pain conditions that cannot be managed by noninvasive and/or pharmacologic treatments may require a consultation with a pain specialist or a pain psychologist to evaluate other options or interventions.

Drug Therapy by Type of Pain

The assessment of the source of pain and intensity is important when determining initial analgesic therapies. Mild to moderate pain can be treated with lower-potency medications such as acetaminophen and NSAIDs. These agents can also be part of a multimodal therapy plan in combination with opioids for severe pain. Historically, aspirin had been used as a pain modality for short-term pain treatment. However, increased adverse effects have limited its chronic use. Aspirin is mostly used today to prevent cardiac events and is not routinely used as part of first-line pain management therapy.

Combination opioids, ketorolac, and tramadol are commonly used to treat moderate pain. Combination opioids contain the addition of a "nonopioid," such as acetaminophen or ibuprofen, creating a treatment ceiling dose (maximum dose). Low doses of strong opioids may also be utilized for moderate pain in patients who have contraindications to NSAIDs, acetaminophen, or tramadol.

Opioids are the most common therapy recommended for severe pain. Morphine is the gold standard and the most studied opioid. When used in equivalent doses, most pure opioids (*mu* receptor agonists) are equally effective in controlling pain, but individual variation may exist among patients. Morphine, oxycodone, hydromorphone, oxymorphone, and fentanyl are pure *mu* opioid agonists indicated for the treatment of severe pain. Morphine is considered the opioid of first choice unless a contraindication exists or the patient has failed prior morphine therapy. Meperidine is another opioid that has historically been utilized for the treatment of severe pain. Use of this agent is no longer recommended due to neurotoxicity associated with accumulation of the active metabolite with routine use or in patients with renal insufficiency.

In most cases involving persistent cancer pain, analgesics should be administered ATC, with as-needed medications used to treat BTP. This recommendation is based on the finding that regularly scheduled medications maintain a constant baseline level of drug in the body and help prevent a recurrence of pain. BTP medications are indicated when intermittent pain occurs despite ATC therapy.

An essential principle in using medications to manage pain is to individualize medication regimens according to severity (**Table 9.1**). For mild to moderate pain, acetaminophen or an NSAID is usually considered initial therapy. Management of moderate to severe pain may require low dose opioids, a

---

TABLE 9.1
Treatment Strategy Based on Initial Pain Assessment

Pain Rating	Classification	NSAID/APAP	Opioids	Coanalgesics
1–3	Mild	✓	Sometimes	✓
4–6	Moderate	✓	Usually	✓
7–10	Severe	✓	Usually	✓

Supplement each level with nonpharmacologic therapy: *psychological*, cognitive–behavioral therapy, biofeedback, relaxation, imagery, psychotherapy; *physical rehabilitation/alternative therapy*, stretching, exercise, reconditioning, thermotherapy, massage, acupuncture.

Pain Assessment Tools

Single Dimensional	Multidimensional
NRS	McGill Pain Questionnaire
VAS	Brief Pain Inventory
Thermometer Pain Scale	Behavioral Pain Scales
Faces Pain Scale	Pain/comfort Journals
Painad Scale	Multidimensional Pain Inventory
FLACC Scale	Pain Disability Index

APAP, acetaminophen; FLACC, faces, legs, activity, cry, consolability; NRS, numerical rating scale; NSAIDs, nonsteroidal antiinflammatory agents; VAS, visual analog scale.

combination opioid, or tramadol. Severe pain is treated with higher-potency and doses of opioids, such as morphine, hydromorphone, or oxycodone. Various classes of coanalgesics, such as anticonvulsants and antidepressants, can also be utilized in combination with the opioids.

Acute Pain

Acute pain is often a response to tissue injury or trauma and is usually nociceptive in nature. Treatment includes nonopioids such as NSAIDs and acetaminophen for mild to moderate pain and opioid medications for moderate to severe pain. As acute pain increases and persists, it becomes more difficult to manage. Therefore, it is important to treat acute pain promptly and effectively. Also, untreated acute pain is often the catalyst in the development of chronic pain conditions in which pain persists despite healing of the original injury.

Acetaminophen is the drug of choice for treating minor, noninflammatory pain, especially in patients at risk for GI damage. NSAIDs are also effective as monotherapy in the treatment of mild to moderate pain. Both acetaminophen and NSAIDs are available in combination with opioids for moderate pain. Pure or multiple-mechanism opioids are used when pain is severe. The opioids, as a class, generally exhibit equal analgesic effects when given at equipotent doses (adjusted for route of administration and duration of action).

Various strategies are currently implemented in the control of pain. Postoperative pain is often treated with multimodal therapies including non-opioid analgesics, opioid medications, and various adjunctive therapies. The use of preemptive analgesia, defined as the administration of various analgesics prior to procedures, is often part of a multimodal treatment plan using two or more medications with different mechanisms of action. Intra-operative ketamine and lidocaine may be utilized, especially in surgeries performed on opioid-tolerant patients (use of 60 mg or more oral morphine or equivalent over a minimum of the previous 7 days). Postoperative ATC non-opioid medications will minimize the need for opioids for pain control. Central regional and local anesthetic blocks have also been shown to provide additional analgesia when added to opioid therapy. Choice of medications, doses, and use of local interventional techniques should be individualized to suit the patient (**Box 9.4**).

Chronic Pain

Noncancer Pain

NSAIDs and salicylates are effective for chronic inflammatory conditions, such as arthritis and musculoskeletal disorders. The efficacy of NSAID treatment varies greatly among patients. Those who do not respond to an NSAID in one class may respond to an NSAID from the same or a different class. Opioids may be considered as an alternative or in addition to NSAID therapy if pain is moderate to severe in appropriately assessed CNCP. Administration of a

---

BOX 9.4 Interventional Techniques for Chronic Pain

Injections
- Epidural steroid injection
- Facet joint injections
- Nerve blocks
- Nerve root blocks
- Sacroiliac joint injection

Kyphoplasty

Neuromodulatory therapy
- Intrathecal pump implants
- Spinal cord stimulants

Percutaneous disc decompression

Radiofrequency rhizotomy

Spinal fusion

Vertebroplasty

---

lower-potency opioid in conjunction with a coanalgesic may be indicated if treatment failure with NSAIDs or acetaminophen occurs. NSAIDs may not provide analgesic benefit in neuropathic pain conditions.

The long-term use of opioids for CNCP in patients with psychological comorbidities or risk for misuse and/or SUD may not provide long-term benefits and increase in functionality (Franklin, 2014). Overprescribing of opioids over the past 20 years has resulted in a staggering increase in opioid-related deaths. Historically, opioids were thought to have no ceiling effect, be effective for long-term use in CNCP, and be nonaddictive when used for analgesia. Today, opioid prescribing must be initiated with caution, especially when used for CNCP. Opioid monotherapy in high-risk patients may increase the incidence of development of OUD without improvement in function or quality of life. Proper patient selection and continual monitoring is vital when evaluating the appropriateness of opioid therapy.

Buprenorphine, a partial agonist to the *mu* receptor, is mainly used for SUD therapy but is increasingly being utilized as a pain treatment modality. Due to its better safety profile, less chance of developing OUD, and its efficacy in chronic pain, buprenorphine may be a valuable option for pain control for CNCP, especially in patients with comorbid substance abuse (see Chapter 10 for more information).

Despite risks, physical dependence and fear of addiction should not be the overriding considerations when choosing a pain modality for patients but must be taken into consideration. A balance of the individual treatment benefits versus risk of therapy is recommended when opioid therapy is being considered for severe pain. Appropriate assessment tools may provide guidance on which patients may or may not benefit from opioid therapy. A multidisciplinary approach using medications, physical therapy, massage, acupuncture, meditation, and cognitive–behavioral therapy is indicated in patients with chronic pain, especially if medications alone have not provided benefit in function. Often, patients expect pain to be totally eliminated, which is usually not possible. Multimodal therapy with various pharmacologic and nonpharmacologic approaches along with a motivated patient with realistic expectations provides the best hope to bring chronic pain to a tolerable level.

Cancer Pain

The National Comprehensive Cancer Network (NCCN) has released guidelines for the management of cancer pain. In the past, the World Health Organization utilized a three-step analgesic ladder, where therapy is started with mild analgesics, moving to stronger therapies when the current treatment fails (Reidenberg, 1996). We now know that cancer pain is much more complex and needs to be individualized for the patient based on type of pain, degree of pain, and comorbidities that may affect pain and suffering. The NCCN provides an algorithm for a treatment approach with recommendations for therapy (Swarm et al., 2019). Opioids are the mainstay of cancer pain management. The addition of nonopioids and coanalgesics is advocated as part of a multimodal approach to treatment. The goal of therapy is to safely use medications in order to improve function and quality of life.

Morphine, oxycodone, oxymorphone, hydromorphone, and fentanyl are the commonly used opioids in the management of severe pain. Methadone is a long-acting opioid with multiple mechanisms of action, working by activating opioid receptors, by inhibiting norepinephrine reuptake, and as an NMDA receptor antagonist. These actions help to modulate and inhibit pain. Methadone can be difficult to dose and has many drug–drug interactions and adverse reactions. Therefore, for safety reasons, methadone should be reserved for treatment failure with other opioids. Referral to a pain professional trained in the safe dosing of methadone is recommended.

MEDICATIONS USED IN PAIN MANAGEMENT

The current pharmacotherapeutic options for pain management include nonopioid and opioid agents. Coanalgesic therapies, such as antidepressants, anticonvulsants, local anesthetics, and topical treatments are often added, especially in chronic, neuropathic, and/or mixed persistent pain conditions. Selection of the appropriate agent rests on an assessment of the patient's type and source of pain as well as the intensity level of the pain.

Nonopioid Analgesics

The nonopioid analgesics utilized for mild to moderate pain can be found in **Table 9.2**. Pain is reduced, and beneficial antiinflammatory action may also be seen with some agents in this class. Onset of analgesia occurs within 1 hour of oral administration, and drug effects last anywhere from 4 to 12 hours.

The agents can be classified by their mechanism of action, chemical class, and antiinflammatory activity. When choosing a nonopioid, the lowest effective dose should be used to minimize possible adverse reactions.

Acetaminophen

Acetaminophen is one of the most commonly prescribed analgesic–antipyretic medications.

The mechanism of analgesic activity is unknown, but it is postulated that pain may be mediated through PG inhibition in the CNS as a cyclooxygenase-3 (COX-3) inhibitor. Lack of peripheral PG inhibition makes acetaminophen a weak antiinflammatory agent and therefore is not considered useful in treating inflammatory disorders such as rheumatoid arthritis. Acetaminophen does not adversely affect platelet aggregation or the gastric mucosa and is generally well tolerated.

Acetaminophen is almost completely absorbed from the GI tract and has a quick onset of action, with a time-to-peak effect of 1 to 3 hours. Extensive liver metabolism to inactive substances makes acetaminophen a relatively nontoxic agent. However, a small portion (4%) of the drug is converted to a toxic metabolite, normally inactivated by glutathione pathways. Once glutathione stores are depleted, as seen in cases of chronic ingestion or acute overdosage, the toxic metabolite can cause potentially fatal liver necrosis.

Acetaminophen is being increasingly used as an ATC agent in postoperative pain management and chronic pain conditions. Generally, the maximum daily dose of acetaminophen should not exceed 4,000 mg. Lower maximum doses (2,000 mg) are recommended when two or more alcoholic drinks per day are ingested or if liver disease is present. In older adults, some experts are recommending reducing the maximum dose to 3,000 mg/d to reduce risk of overdose and to minimize adverse effects (Byrd, 2013).

Nonsteroidal Antiinflammatory Drugs

NSAIDs as a class have antiinflammatory, analgesic, and antipyretic activity. Cyclooxygenase, consisting of the isoforms COX-1 and COX-2, is the enzyme involved in the formation of PGs. Aspirin causes irreversible inactivation of COX-1 and COX-2, where nonaspirin NSAIDs cause reversible inactivation. The COX-1 isoform produces PGs that regulate blood flow to the kidneys and GI tract and decrease platelet aggregation. The COX-2 isoenzyme is usually expressed as a result of tissue injury and is the source of inflammatory pain. First-generation NSAIDs inhibit both isoenzymes, thereby reducing inflammation but also decreasing the gastroprotective effects of COX-1. Pain is decreased but gastroprotection is lost from damage to the GI mucosa, increasing the risk of GI bleeding. COX-2 inhibitors were developed in hopes of relieving pain while reducing the chance for GI toxicities. Unfortunately, a subsequent increase in cardiovascular events was seen. All NSAIDs have some degree of COX-2 inhibition. Those that have a greater proportion of COX-2 versus COX-1 inhibition may have a higher risk for thrombus, heart attack, and stroke.

TABLE 9.2

Pharmacokinetic and Pharmacodynamic Properties of Nonopioid Analgesics

Generic Name	Trade Name	Dosage Forms	Half-Life (h)	Onset (h)	Duration (h)	Route	Usual Starting Dosage	Maximum Dosage (24 h)
Acetaminophen	Tylenol, others	Tablet	2–7	0.5–0.75	4–6	PO	650 mg q4–6h	4,000 mg
		Suspension				PR		
		Suppository						
		Intravenous		5–10 min	4–6	IV	1 g q6h	
Diclofenac	Voltaren	Tablets	2	0.5	8–12	PO	25 mg q12h	200 mg
		Gel	1–2			Topical		
Diclofenac epolamine	Flector	Topical patch	12	1	12	Topical	1 patch q12h	2 patches
Diflunisal	Dolobid	Tablet	8–12	1	8–12	*PO*	1 g × 1, then 500 mg q8–12h	1,500 mg
Ibuprofen	Motrin, Advil	Tablets	1.8–2.4	0.5–1	6–8	PO	200–400 mg q4–6h	3,200 mg
	Caldolor	Suspension						
		Injection				IV	400–800 mg q6h	
Ketorolac	Toradol	Tablets	5.5–7	0.5–1	4–6	PO	10 mg q6h	120 mg
		Injection		0.5	4–6	IV, IM	15–30 mg IV q6h	40 mg
Naproxen	Naprosyn	Tablets						
		Suspension	12–17	0.5–1	8–12	PO	500 mg × 1, then 250 mg q8h	1,250 mg
Naproxen sodium	Aleve	Tablets	12–17	0.5–1	8–12	PO	550 mg × 1, then 275 mg q12h	1,375 mg

IM, intramuscular; IV, intravenous.

Some NSAIDs, including aspirin, ketoprofen, and indomethacin, inhibit both COX-1 and COX-2 enzymes but are more selective for inhibiting COX-1. Diflunisal and diclofenac may be more selective for COX-2 inhibition and therefore may be less likely to cause GI toxicity. Only one COX-2 inhibitor, celecoxib (Celebrex), has benefits that outweigh its risks and remains on the market today.

The analgesic effect of NSAIDs is achieved within 1 hour of administration, with maximal effects within 2 or 3 hours. Antiinflammatory effect has a longer onset, with maximal effects seen in 7 to 10 days. Decreased pain due to reduced tissue swelling is an indirect response to NSAIDs. In general, NSAIDs should be avoided in the older adult population. If clinically indicated, lower doses of nonsteroidal therapies for the shortest duration possible should be used.

Long-term use of NSAIDs at high doses (antiinflammatory doses) can increase the risk for serious adverse effects. Indomethacin (Indocin) is associated with more CNS and ocular adverse effects than other NSAIDs. In patients at risk for a GI bleed or who are taking concomitant aspirin and NSAID therapy, addition of acid suppression therapy preferably with a proton pump inhibitor is recommended. Misoprostol, a synthetic PG, is also effective for the prevention of bleeding, but GI adverse reactions (nausea, abdominal cramps, and diarrhea) limit its use.

A black box warning on cardiovascular toxicities has been added to all NSAID products. Unlike NSAIDs, acetaminophen and salicylates have minimal GI toxicity and no effect on platelet aggregation at usual doses. See Chapters 32 and 34 for more discussion of NSAIDs and acetaminophen.

Opioids

Receptors in the CNS (*mu* [μ], *kappa* [κ], or *delta* [δ]) bind with opioids exerting their analgesic effect primarily with *mu* receptor binding. Full *mu* opioid agonists include codeine, morphine, hydrocodone, oxycodone, hydromorphone, oxymorphone, fentanyl, and meperidine. Meperidine is associated with significant adverse effects and is no longer recommended as first-line therapy. Meperidine's active metabolite, normeperidine, can accumulate and induce seizures with high doses following extended use or use in patients with decreased renal function.

Activation of the *mu* opioid receptor produces effective analgesia as well as undesired adverse effects, including respiratory depression, sedation, confusion, nausea/vomiting, pruritus, miosis, constipation, and urinary retention. With the exception of constipation and possibly pruritus, tolerance to adverse effects develops over time. Morphine and other *mu* opioid receptor agonists provide pain relief over a broad dosage range. Multiple *mu* receptor subtypes exist, which may explain why opioids do not have the same outcomes for everyone. Opioid effects may also differ due to individual differences in hepatic metabolism and genetic factors. For example, codeine is a pro-drug, and conversion to morphine is facilitated by hepatic CYP2D6 enzyme action. The CYP2D6 genotype is associated with polymorphism, causing variability of CYP2D6 activity effecting the amount of morphine converted from codeine. See **Box 9.5** for an explanation of genotype versus phenotype effects of CYP metabolism (Eckhardt et al., 1998).

Opioids vary in onset, duration, and half-life (**Table 9.3**). At equianalgesic doses and appropriate dosing intervals, there is no appreciable difference in potency among opioid agents (McPherson, 2010). The described potency is a reflection of the dose needed to achieve a desired level of analgesia. In general, more potent agents will provide equivalent pain control at lower doses (**Table 9.4**).

Opioids are primarily metabolized by the liver to active and inactive metabolites. The metabolites of morphine and hydromorphone are eliminated by the kidneys. In renal failure, morphine's active metabolites may accumulate and cause neurotoxicity, such as hyperalgesia, myoclonus, confusion, and coma. Death may result if this accumulation is not identified.

Hydromorphone has historically been thought to be safe in renal disease. Data are emerging that hydromorphone metabolites may also accumulate, causing neurotoxicity. The metabolites of morphine and hydromorphone differ in that hydromorphone's metabolites are eliminated by dialysis and morphine metabolites are not dialyzable. Hydromorphone is recommended to be used cautiously in patients with renal failure, especially if renal failure is acute or if the patient is not currently receiving dialysis (Arnold et al., 2007).

Metabolites of oxycodone are inactive, making this a good option in patients with renal failure. Lower initial doses should be started and titrated with caution as increased sensitivity to opioids is seen in general in this patient population. Sustained-release [SR] formulations should also be used with caution in end-stage renal and liver disease. Fentanyl and methadone do not have active metabolites and are considered the drugs of choice in the treatment of chronic pain in patients with renal failure. Fentanyl is the drug of choice in patients with liver failure.

The onset of the analgesic effects of oral opioids is 30 to 60 minutes, and the peak effect is seen within 1 to 2 hours. Fentanyl has a quicker onset and shorter duration of action. Moderate-acting opioids, with duration of action between 4 and 6 hours, include morphine, codeine, hydromorphone, oxycodone, and oxymorphone. Methadone, a dual-mechanism, long-acting opioid, has a variable duration of action and half-life of approximately 24 to 36 hours. Steady state may take 5 to 7 days to be reached; therefore, upward titration should not occur for at least 5 days after therapy initiation.

Morphine and Congeners

Morphine is a low-cost, readily available agent with well-characterized pharmacokinetic and pharmacodynamic properties. Other opioids are compared to morphine due to the extensive clinical experience of practitioners and literature available supporting its use. Morphine is absorbed erratically from the GI tract and undergoes significant first-pass hepatic metabolism when given by the oral route. Morphine is distributed throughout the body with sufficient amounts crossing the blood–brain barrier, which accounts for most of its pharmacologic effects. Morphine has a plasma half-life of approximately 3 hours, which is due mainly to its nearly complete metabolism in the liver. Morphine crosses the placental barrier and is excreted in maternal milk.

BOX 9.5   Pharmacogenomic Considerations

The metabolism of codeine to its active metabolite, morphine, is pharmacogenetically determined. Individuals with more than one copy of the "normal" gene producing the cytochrome P450 enzyme 2D6 (CYP2D6) will be *ultrarapid metabolizers*, and in the case of codeine, will produce more morphine than expected; this will have a much greater effect on the patient. In contrast, those patients with variations in the gene producing CYP2D6 will have less metabolism. If the patient does not have the normal gene present, the patient will be considered a *poor metabolizer*. See Chapter 7 for more information on the effects of genetic variations on drug metabolism.

Genotype/Phenotype	Drug Effect
Genotype: Normal (2 pairs of genes) Phenotype: Ultrarapid metabolizer	Decreased efficacy of active drug—inactivated quickly Increased efficacy of prodrug—activated quickly
Genotype: Normal (single pair of normal alleles) Phenotype: Extensive metabolizer	Usual expected activity
Genotype: Normal and variant pair of alleles Phenotype: Intermediate metabolizer	Usual expected activity
Genotype: Variant (single pair of variant alleles) Phenotype: Poor metabolizer	Increased efficacy of active drug—remains in system longer Decreased efficacy of prodrug—activated slowly

TABLE 9.3

Pharmacokinetic and Pharmacodynamic Properties of Opioid Analgesics

Generic Name	Trade Name(s)	Route	Onset (min)	Half-Life (h)	Duration (h)	Usual Starting Dose
Fentanyl	Duragesic	Transdermal patch	12–16	1.5–6	48–72	Individualize dose
		IV	0–5	2–4	30–60 min	
	Actiq, Fentora	Transmucosal	5–15	17	4–8	*
Hydrocodone combination	Vicodin, Lortab, Lorcet, generic	PO	10–20	3.3–4.5	4–8	1 tablet (5 mg hydrocodone) q4h
Hydrocodone	Zohydro ER, Hysingla ER			8	24	Individualize
Hydromorphone	Dilaudid,	PO	15–30	1–3	3–13	2 mg q4h
	Exalgo		360	11		Individualize dose
		IV, SC	5–10	2–3	4–5	0.5 mg q4h
Morphine, immediate release	Various, generic	PO	30–60	2–4	3–6	5–15 mg q3–4h
Sustained release	MS Contin, Kadian, Avinza	PO	30–60	15	8–12 (formulation dependent)	Individualize dosing
Injection	Various, generic	IV, SC	5–10	2–4	2–4	2–5 mg q3–4h
Oxycodone combination	Percocet, Percodan, generic	PO	15	2–3	4–5	1 tablet (5 mg oxycodone) q4h
Oxycodone-immediate release	Oxy IR, Roxicodone	PO	15–60	2–3	3–4	5 mg q3–4h
Sustained release	Oxycontin	PO	50–60	5	8–12	Individualize dose
Oxymorphone	Opana	PO	30	7–9	4–6	5 mg q4–6h
	Opana ER	PO	3	10	12	Individualize dosage
Combination Mechanism						
Methadone	Dolophine, others	PO	15–60	8–59	2–10 (acute) >12 (chronic)	2.5–5 mg q8–12h
		IV	10–20	8–59	>8 (chronic)	1–2 mg q8h
Tapentadol	Nucynta	PO	30–45	4	4–6	50 mg q4–6h
Tramadol	Ultram	PO	60	6–7	4–6	50 mg q6h

Opioid Pearls

1. Use lower initial opioid doses in older adults and in patients with respiratory comorbidities.
2. *Hydrocodone* for pain is available in combination with acetaminophen or ibuprofen. A long-acting formulation for chronic pain is also available.
3. *Oxycodone* is available in combination with acetaminophen, aspirin, and ibuprofen or available as a single analgesic agent.
4. *Morphine* is the opioid of choice unless contraindications exist. Morphine is relatively contraindicated in renal failure.
5. *Hydromorphone* is approximately five times the potency of morphine.
6. *Fentanyl* patch is contraindicated for acute pain and/or opioid naive patients.
   - Fentanyl patch may not be appropriate for patients with fever, diaphoresis, cachexia, morbid obesity, and ascites, all of which affect absorption and clinical effectiveness.
   - Patch may be appropriate for patients who cannot take long-acting oral opioids.
   - Onset of action is 12–16 hours after application. Utilize BTP medications for pain control until onset of analgesia. Full effect takes 72 hours.
   - Application of external heat sources will increase the release of fentanyl from the transdermal system.
   - Titration of the patch should not occur before 3 days after the initial dose or no more frequent than every 7 days thereafter.
7. Due to the long half-life of methadone, full analgesic effects may not be seen until steady state is reached (5–7 days on average after initiation), making the drug difficult to dose.
   - Conservative dose conversions with careful titration are recommended. Use a higher conversion ratio in patients currently on high-dose opioids.
   - Steady state is not reached for at least 5–7 days.[†] Use BTP medications early in the titration, as analgesic effects are shorter than the half-life of the drug. Observe for accumulation-related side effects during titration (>2 days treatment).
   - Consult a pain management specialist for dosing.

* Cancer-related BTP only.

[†] Not initial therapy for opioid-naive patients.

BTP, breakthrough pain; IM, intramuscular; IV, intravenous; SC, subcutaneous.

TABLE 9.4
Basic Opioid Conversion Table

Opioid	Oral	Parenteral
Morphine	30 mg	10 mg
Oxycodone	20 mg	—
Hydrocodone	30 mg	—
Hydromorphone	7.5 mg	1.5 mg
Oxymorphone	10 mg	1 mg
Codeine	200 mg	120 mg
Fentanyl	—	0.1 mg
Tramadol	300 mg	—
Tapentadol	150 mg	
Methadone	Refer to a pain management specialist for methadone dosing	2:1 oral to IV

Source: Institute for Clinical Systems Improvement (ICSI). (2017). Pain: Assessment, Non-Opioid Treatment Approaches and Opioid Management. www.icsi.org. Accessed February 21, 2020.

IV, intravenous.

Morphine may be administered by multiple routes. Oral, injectable, rectal, intrathecal, and epidural formulations are available. Dosage forms include immediate-release [IR] and SR tablets and capsules. Liquid formulations are also available. With chronic dosing, the potency of the intravenous dose is three times that of the equivalent oral dose.

Morphine effectively relieves severe pain, particularly nociceptive pain, regardless of its cause or anatomic source. Analgesia is due to the drug's binding to *mu* receptors in the CNS. Opioids can cause respiratory depression due to both the drug's actions on the brain's medullary respiratory control center and the drug's ability to suppress the medulla's response to blood carbon dioxide levels. Respiratory depression is seen mainly in opioid-naive patients or with upward dose titration in both acute and chronic pain. Tolerance develops relatively quickly to respiratory depressive effects. A person in whom tolerance has developed may experience only moderate respiratory effects when receiving doses that could cause serious or fatal respiratory depression in a non-tolerant person.

Opioids also increase smooth muscle tone in various parts of the GI tract. *Mu* receptors are located throughout the GI tract, where receptor binding results in reduced peristalsis and increased tone of the rectal sphincter. The overall resultant effect is constipation. Prophylactic bowel regimens consisting of a stimulant laxative or osmotic diuretic plus/minus a stool softener is recommended with initiation of opioid therapy. See the section titled Bowel Regimen for the Prevention of Constipation later in the chapter.

Hydromorphone is considered more potent and more soluble than morphine with a similar pharmacologic profile. Hydromorphone is available as an oral IR tablet, a suppository,

and an injectable formulation. A long-acting formulation of hydromorphone is also available on the U.S. market.

Oxycodone is slightly more potent than morphine. This agent may be used as monotherapy or in combination with nonopioid analgesics, such as ibuprofen or acetaminophen. Oxycodone is available as an IR tablet, an oral liquid formulation, and a SR tablet. No injectable form of oxycodone is currently available.

Hydrocodone is available in combination with nonopioid analgesics and is equipotent to morphine on a milligram-to-milligram basis. Hydrocodone is available in combination with acetaminophen or ibuprofen and is used for moderate to severe pain. Long-acting formulations indicated for severe pain are also available. The Drug Enforcement Agency reclassified hydrocodone from Schedule 3 to Schedule 2 in 2014.

Oxymorphone, the metabolite of oxycodone, is used to treat moderate to severe pain. Previously, oxymorphone was available as an injectable (Numorphan) but currently is only available as IR and SR tablets. Oxymorphone is approximately twice as strong as oxycodone, with 10 mg of oxymorphone equivalent to 20 mg of oxycodone. Adverse effects and mechanisms of action are similar to those of other opioids.

Codeine is usually administered orally either alone or in combination with nonopioid analgesics, such as acetaminophen, for moderate pain. If the patient is a poor metabolizer or if CYP2D6 enzyme is not available to convert codeine to the active ingredient, morphine, pain control will not be achieved. To the opposite extreme, rapid metabolizers of codeine may convert a higher amount to morphine, increasing overdose risk. See **Box 9.5** for more information on the effect of metabolic enzymes on drug activity. In addition, their use has fallen out of favor due to increased adverse effects when compared to other opioids. Other more potent and better-tolerated pain management modalities are available. At equianalgesic doses, codeine induces greater histamine release than do other opioids. This increases the risk of hypotension, cutaneous vasodilation, urticaria, and bronchoconstriction. Currently, codeine is primarily used as an antitussive agent.

Fentanyl and Congeners

Fentanyl is an alternative to morphine and its congeners, with low to no cross-allergenicity in patients with true hypersensitivity to morphine-like drugs. Fentanyl is available for acute pain as injectable and buccal formulations. The long-acting transdermal patch is available for stable chronic pain and is only to be used in opioid-tolerant patients with a chronic pain process. Patients are required to have taken oral morphine 60 mg/day, oxycodone 30 mg/day, or hydromorphone 8 mg/day for the previous 7 days or longer to be considered opioid tolerant (Janssen Pharmaceuticals, 2006). Transdermal fentanyl has an onset of effect of approximately 12 hours after patch placement. Peak systemic concentrations occur between 24 and 72 hours after initial patch application. The duration of effect is approximately 72 hours. However, some patients may require patch changes after 48 hours. Use of the buccal transmucosal formulation is limited to severe

BTP associated with cancer. A recent study demonstrated that transmucosal fentanyl formulations have better efficacy in cancer BTP when compared to oral short-acting morphine (Maroo et al., 2014). Onset of action is 15 minutes versus 45 to 60 minutes with oral formulations. Practitioners are required to become certified prior to being able to prescribe transmucosal fentanyl as part of a Risk Evaluation Mitigation Strategy requirement for safe use.

Other agents, such as sufentanil (Sufenta) and alfentanil (Alfenta), also fall in this class but are used primarily for perioperative and postoperative pain relief and are available only in an injectable formulation.

Meperidine is a synthetic analgesic that binds strongly to both *mu* and *kappa* receptors. Potency is less than that of morphine. Most of the pharmacologic effects of this drug are similar to those of morphine; however, adverse effects limit its use. Prolonged use of meperidine may cause CNS excitation characterized by tremors and seizures due to the accumulation of its active metabolite, normeperidine. The half-life of normeperidine ranges between 15 and 20 hours, and it is almost completely renally eliminated. The possibility of accumulation of this metabolite leading to detrimental CNS effects has limited the use of meperidine in the treatment of pain. Meperidine is still used for treatment of rigors and in procedural sedation.

Multiple-Mechanism Analgesics

Tramadol is a centrally acting weak *mu* receptor agonist. Pain is also modulated by norepinephrine reuptake inhibition and serotonin release. Tramadol is used to treat moderate to severe pain and is available alone or in combination with acetaminophen. Tramadol may be useful for pain management in patients where a pure *mu* opioid is not an option and an NSAID may introduce undue risk (e.g., GI bleeding). Patients with a true allergy to morphine and other structurally similar opioids can use tramadol for pain relief. In addition, there may be a place for it in neuropathic pain management due to the additional norepinephrine reuptake inhibition. Maximum dose of tramadol is 400 mg/d. Dosing should be initiated slowly and titrated to an effective dose. Tramadol may have less abuse potential when compared to other opioids but misuse has been reported. In addition, consideration of increased seizure potential and drug–drug interactions must be assessed prior to initiation. Tramadol is rapidly absorbed, with peak serum levels obtained within 2 hours. A 4-to-6-hour duration of effect is seen. Tramadol is metabolized in the liver by the CYP2D enzyme system to an active metabolite (*O*-dimethyl tramadol), similar to codeine. Drug–drug interactions are common. Decreased maximum doses are recommended in older adults and in patients with renal impairment. Increased seizure risk is seen with high doses or in patients with a history of seizure disorders.

Tapentadol is a combination opioid that works on opioid receptors in addition to working as a specific norepinephrine reuptake inhibitor. This medication has been shown to be effective in various pain conditions, such as osteoarthritis and postoperative pain. Tapentadol has less affinity for the *mu* receptor than morphine, but the analgesic effect is augmented due to norepinephrine reuptake inhibition. Fewer incidences of GI adverse effects (nausea, vomiting, constipation) are seen when compared with other opioids due to less effect on the *mu* receptor. Tapentadol is another agent that can be used in patients with allergy to morphine-like drugs.

Methadone hydrochloride is an effective analgesic alternative when other opioid therapies have failed. Due to its different chemical structure, methadone can also be used as an analgesic alternative in patients with a true allergy to morphine-like compounds (anaphylaxis, hives). Methadone is effective both orally and parenterally and has an average oral bioavailability of 80%. It is more than 90% bound to plasma tissue proteins and is extensively metabolized by the CYP-450 enzyme system. Methadone is known to cause cardiac toxicity. Patients may be at risk for ventricular arrhythmias (QTc prolongation and torsades de pointes) especially when methadone is given with other medications that also prolong the QTc. Methadone is most often associated with the treatment of opioid substance abuse but is being used more frequently in the treatment of chronic severe pain. Methadone works as both a *mu* receptor agonist and an NMDA receptor antagonist, making it effective for the treatment of severe neuropathic pain and mixed pain syndromes. The lack of active metabolites makes methadone a viable choice in patients with renal failure. The drug has a long half-life of approximately 24 hours (range between 10 and 60 hours), with an analgesic effect of approximately 4 to 8 hours. Early in methadone titration, pain control may be inadequate until steady state is reached. Aggressive BTP therapies may be required during the first 3 to 5 days of therapy. A tendency to dose methadone aggressively early in titration can lead to serious adverse effects, including fatal respiratory depression. Patients should be monitored carefully for signs of drug accumulation and toxicity. The long biologic half-life also accounts for the mild, but prolonged, withdrawal syndrome if use is stopped abruptly. Due to a rise in methadone-associated deaths, the *Journal of Pain* released guidelines on methadone safety (Chou et al., 2014). These guidelines provide direction on the appropriate use of methadone for chronic pain and OUD based on the available evidence. Information on dosing, titration, and ECG monitoring are areas covered in the guidelines.

Opioid Antagonist: Naloxone

Naloxone is a pure opioid antagonist that competitively binds to opioid receptors without producing an analgesic response. Naloxone is inactivated when given orally and therefore is given mainly by injection. Naloxone is indicated for treating opioid-induced respiratory depression. Efforts are being made to make naloxone readily available as a response to the increasing opioid-related deaths. Many states have a "standing order" giving pharmacists the freedom to sell naloxone to patients at a risk of an overdose. An intra-nasal dosage form is approved for outpatient use.

The duration of naloxone's drug action is approximately 45 minutes. In most cases, this duration is shorter than that of the offending opioid, and the overdose effect from the opioid may return, requiring readministration of naloxone. Care must be taken to avoid precipitation of withdrawal in opioid-tolerant patients when administering naloxone. Rare adverse effects of naloxone include tachycardia, ventricular fibrillation, and cardiac arrest due to the release of neurotransmitters when naloxone is administered. Opioid withdrawal syndrome may occur in opioid-tolerant patients when excessive or rapid reversal is used.

Safety of Opioids

Side effects common to all opioids include sedation, confusion, respiratory depression, itching, nausea/vomiting, and constipation. Opioid-induced bowel dysfunction develops due to reduced movement through the lower GI tract due to reduction of bowel tone and motility, increased anal sphincter tone, and increased absorption of fluids. Although considered the most dangerous side effect, severe respiratory depression is seen not only in overdose situations but also in patients who are opioid naive. Patients who are at risk for respiratory depression include older adults, patients who have respiratory comorbidities such as obstructive sleep apnea, and patients with kidney/liver failure. Patients with chronic pain on opioids usually develop tolerance to the respiratory depression effects. However, if substantial opioid doses are used in addition to chronic therapy, as in the case of a postoperative opioid-tolerant patient, risk for respiratory depression is increased. In patients with closed head injury or recent brain surgery, opioids should be used with caution because hemodynamic effects (e.g., hypotension, orthostasis) may be exaggerated.

Care should be taken when administering opioids to older adults or in patients with renal failure, liver failure, and respiratory diseases. In patients with renal failure, morphine should be used with caution due to accumulation of neurotoxic metabolites. Opioid-induced hyperalgesia can result, a phenomenon where rapid upward titration of opioid doses or metabolite accumulation can cause pain to escalate. Myoclonus can be the initial telltale sign that hyperalgesia is present. In patients with end-stage liver disease, lower doses and extended dosing intervals are recommended due to decreases in opioid metabolism. Lower doses should be initiated in these patients and titrated slowly based on response. Utilizing coanalgesics as monotherapy or in combination with opioids may be effective in chronic pain treatment and may decrease opioid requirements.

Bowel Regimen for the Prevention of Constipation

Tolerance usually develops within a few days to most of the adverse reactions associated with opioids, except for constipation. Constipation prevention is needed in patients receiving opioids. The general approach for patients on opioid therapy is to institute a prophylactic bowel regimen consisting of a mild stimulant or osmotic agent plus/minus a stool softener. The dose of the stimulant can be titrated based on patient response. Initial dosing would consist of senna 2 tablets daily or twice daily. Polyethylene glycol (PEG) powder packets used daily is another effective alternative. PEG is usually dosed initially at

1 packet (17 g) daily. Up to 4 packets per dose daily can be utilized. Docusate sodium 100 mg twice daily is often used when stool softening is needed. However, a 2013 study comparing senna alone to senna/docusate showed no difference in the efficacy of docusate versus placebo when added to senna (Tarumi et al., 2013). If there is no bowel movement produced in 48 hours, consider using an additional agent (e.g., bisacodyl suppository, lactulose, sorbitol, additional PEG) to stimulate peristalsis. If interventions continue to be ineffective, assess for impaction. If no impaction is present, utilizing an additional method (e.g., enema) is recommended. Once the patient has a bowel movement, titrate the dosage of the current regimen to an effective dose. (Up to 8 tablets senna per day or the liquid equivalent has been used in the hospice and palliative care population.) Docusate sodium should not be titrated aggressively because sodium salt may affect sodium levels.

Use of bulk-forming laxatives in patients receiving opioids is not recommended. Due to slower peristalsis in patients receiving opioids and potential inadequate fluid intake, the medication may lodge in the colon, causing bowel obstruction.

New novel agents are now available to treat refractory constipation due to opioids by specifically targeting the *mu* receptors in the gut. These medications were developed by altering the structure of naltrexone and naloxone, making them unable to cross the blood–brain barrier, thereby preventing reversal of analgesia. Methylnaltrexone is available as an injectable and oral formulation with effect seen within minutes to a few hours with the injectable product. Naloxegol is an oral agent with a time to effect of approximately 12 hours.

Opioid Tolerance, Dependence, Pseudo-Addiction, and Addiction

Opioid tolerance develops when chronic use of opioids causes the need for upward dose titration to maintain analgesia. Opioid dependence is defined as an emergence of withdrawal symptoms when the drug is abruptly discontinued or when the dose is rapidly decreased. Tolerance and physical dependence of opioids can develop quickly. Apparent dependence and/or tolerance in a patient with chronic pain should not impede titration of therapy to an effective dose. However, if no pain control is seen with increasing doses, an alternate opioid should be considered.

Patients taking opioids for as briefly as 2 or 3 days may become dependent and can experience withdrawal symptoms upon discontinuation. Withdrawal symptoms range from mild tremors to sweating and fever and mimic flu-like symptoms. Severe withdrawal symptoms in opioid-dependent patients may consist of increased respiratory rate, perspiration, lacrimation, mydriasis, hot and cold flashes, and anorexia.

Patients with pain may demonstrate signs of maladaptive behavior, which may be a result of undertreated pain or worsening pain due to disease progression, rather than active SUD. Pseudo-addiction, defined as drug-seeking behaviors due to inadequate pain management, can be differentiated from true addiction because "pseudo-addictive" behaviors will resolve once adequate pain management is achieved.

Addiction is defined as "a treatable, chronic medical disease involving complex interactions among brain circuits, genetics, the environment, and an individual's life experiences. People with addiction use substances or engage in behaviors that become compulsive and often continue despite harmful consequences" (American Society of Addiction Medicine [ASAM] 2019). The term *addiction* has been replaced by the term *SUD* due to the negative connotations associated with the former. Severe SUD is characterized by behaviors that include 6 of 11 criteria set by the American Psychiatric Association. Criteria include impaired control over drug use, compulsive use, continued use despite harm, and cravings. In 2016, an estimated 2.1 million Americans were reported to be suffering from an opioid use disorder (Substance Abuse and Mental Health Services Administration [SAMHSA] 2017). Opioid abuse has been reported in patients with chronic pain with psychological comorbidities who use opioids to treat pain resulting from depression or anxiety. The concept of substance abuse with respect to opioids is an important consideration in patients presenting with uncontrolled pain but is beyond the scope of this chapter. For further information, see Chapters 10 and 43.

Co-analgesics

Several medications have been evaluated for use either alone or in conjunction with other analgesics to treat many persistent pain conditions. The most benefit is seen in chronic pain, neuropathic pain, and sensitized pain syndromes.

Antidepressants

Antidepressants, including tricyclic antidepressants (TCAs) and selective norepinephrine reuptake inhibitors (SNRIs), exhibit analgesic effects by primarily blocking the reuptake of norepinephrine, thereby increasing pain-modulating pathway activity. TCAs also block peripheral sodium channels, which may also help reduce pain. TCAs and SNRIs have been useful in neuropathic pain resulting from cancer or cancer therapies and chronic noncancer, neuropathic pain syndromes (i.e., diabetic or postherpetic neuropathy, chronic low back pain, and fibromyalgia). Several TCAs have beneficial effects in neuropathic pain, including amitriptyline, desipramine, and nortriptyline. Common adverse reactions include dry mouth, weight gain, dizziness, urinary retention, confusion, and sedation. Dosing of TCAs is initiated at 10 to 25 mg nightly and titrated weekly to an effective dose of 75 to 100 mg each evening. Therapy with TCAs should be initiated with caution in older adults due to an increased incidence of confusion and sedation due to anticholinergic activity, which may lead to falls. TCAs should not be used as a first-line agent and should be reserved for treatment failures to other agents in the older adult population. Amitriptyline is the most studied TCA. The second-generation agents nortriptyline and desipramine may be better tolerated than amitriptyline because of less cholinergic and sedative effects.

The SNRIs duloxetine and venlafaxine may be safer alternatives for the treatment of neuropathic pain conditions. Duloxetine dosing is initiated at 20 to 30 mg/d to a target dose of 60 mg/d. Dosing can be titrated to 120 mg/d if indicated. Venlafaxine dose is initiated at 75 mg/d and titrated to a maximum dose of 225 mg/d either once daily or divided twice daily based on dosage form (SR vs. IR) These medications are better tolerated than the TCAs because no cholinergic side effects are seen. GI disturbances, sedation, insomnia, sweating, and confusion may be seen with SNRI use. Venlafaxine has also been associated with increases in blood pressure.

Abrupt discontinuation of TCAs and SNRIs may precipitate withdrawal symptoms. Patients can experience flu-like symptoms, insomnia, nausea, and anxiety. The phenomenon is seen more when short-acting agents are stopped without an appropriate taper. Symptoms are generally not serious but can be severe in some patients. Restarting the medications, transitioning to a long-acting antidepressant prior to decreasing the dose, or slowing the taper can help with reducing the symptoms of withdrawal.

Anticonvulsants

Another group of agents commonly prescribed for neuropathic pain conditions are the anticonvulsants. The most common agents used in this class are the gabapentinoids, which include gabapentin and pregabalin. The anticonvulsants carbamazepine and oxcarbazepine are specifically used for pain due to trigeminal neuralgia. Gabapentin has historically been the first-line anticonvulsant agent recommended for pain treatment. Pregabalin is structurally similar to gabapentin and has the same mechanism of action. The mechanism of action is not totally understood, but it is postulated to be due to the effects of binding to the alpha-2-delta subunit of voltage-dependent calcium channels, resulting in a reduction of the influx of calcium into the dorsal horn. This results in a decreased release of glutamate, causing lower activation of the second-order neurons responsible for transmission of the pain signal to the brain. Gabapentin and pregabalin are generally well tolerated. Most common side effects include nausea, sedation, dizziness, weight gain, and ataxia. Peripheral edema has been associated with pregabalin use. Gabapentinoids have been shown to be effective for many neuropathic pain conditions, including diabetic neuropathy, trigeminal neuralgia, restless leg syndrome, phantom limb pain, and pain after a stroke. Generally, gabapentin doses are started at 100 to 300 mg daily and titrated up to 1,800 to 3,600 mg daily in three to four divided daily doses. A SR formulation is also available with a lower maximum dose of 1,800 mg/d. The SR and IR products are not interchangeable.

Pregabalin is better absorbed than gabapentin, and efficacy is seen in approximately 1 week, compared to 4 to 6 weeks with gabapentin. The dose should be started low and titrated. Initial doses are 50 mg two to three times daily, titrated to an effective dose. The maximum dose of pregabalin is 600 mg/d. A generic formulation of pregabalin has recently been released. Side effects are similar to those of gabapentin. Dosing of gabapentin and pregabalin should be reduced in patients with renal impairment.

Carbamazepine and oxcarbazepine are considered the drugs of choice for trigeminal neuralgia. Other anticonvulsants including topiramate, lamotrigine, and divalproex may be tried for neuropathic pain treatment if other modalities have failed.

Sodium Channel Blockers (Local Anesthetics)

This class of medications exerts its analgesic effects by blocking sodium channels, thereby slowing pain transmission and increasing the firing threshold of the second-order neurons. Several routes of administration exist and are chosen based on the indication for use. Topical applications help control localized neuropathic pain with minimal absorption. Lidocaine patches and EMLA(R) cream (mixture of lidocaine and prilocaine) are available for topical use. Lidocaine patches are indicated for postherpetic neuralgia, but efficacy is reported in painful conditions such as diabetic peripheral neuropathy and osteoarthritis. Patches may be cut, and up to three patches may be used. Application is usually 12 hours on and 12 hours off daily. Systemic absorption is minimal. The safety and tolerability of 24-hour administration were demonstrated in a study published in the *Annals of Pharmacotherapy* in 2002, which compared safety of 24-hour administration to the recommended 12-hour application (Gammaitoni & Alvarez, 2002). Pharmacokinetic data on 24-hour administration reported in the study showed systemic absorption markedly below the level needed for toxicity and was well tolerated. Lidocaine patches are now available over the counter.

Local injections of anesthetics can be utilized as regional anesthesia, injected into tissue or the epidural space. Epidural analgesia is commonly utilized in managing obstetric or postoperative pain. Rarely, lidocaine has been administered intravenously to control refractory pain conditions in subanesthetic dosages. Intravenous infusions must be administered in a monitored setting because of the potential for severe adverse drug reactions with possible exceptions in the end-of-life population. Evidence has shown that the use of lidocaine as a palliative measure for refractory pain may be efficacious when other methods have failed.

N-*Methyl-D-Aspartate Receptor Antagonists*

Evidence is emerging in the use of the NMDA antagonists, specifically ketamine, for both acute and chronic pain. Ketamine, an anesthetic agent, is used as a bolus dose or an intravenous infusion for treatment of a variety of pain conditions, such as postoperative pain, chronic refractory pain, and acute pain in the emergency department. Doses for analgesia are lower than doses used for anesthesia. Cancer and noncancer pain refractory to other treatments may benefit from the addition of ketamine to opioid therapy. Better pain control and an opioid-sparing effect have been demonstrated in studies using this combination. Ketamine reduces firing of the NMDA receptor, thereby decreasing sensitivity to pain impulses. Ketamine, by the oral and topical routes, also shows promise for the treatment of

pain. Adverse effects are dose related and increased in patients who have a history of psychiatric comorbidities. The most common side effects with ketamine are vivid dreams and sedation. Delirium, dysphoria, hallucinations, hypotension, hypertension, and increased intracranial pressure have also been associated with its use. Other NMDA antagonists, such as dextromethorphan, memantine, amantadine, and magnesium, have not shown promise for pain reduction in studies related to use as analgesics.

An upsurge of ketamine usage for a variety of conditions has prompted the release of guidelines for both acute (Schwenk et al., 2018) and chronic (Cohen et al., 2018) pain management. The consensus guidelines were developed by three pain organizations to address the use of ketamine for acute and chronic pain. For acute pain, the guidelines provide recommendations on indications, contraindications, use as an adjunctive agent to opioids, use of non-parenteral dosage forms, and the appropriate analgesic dosing range. Chronic pain guidelines suggest possible efficacy for use in CRPS for up to 12 weeks (moderate evidence) and possible short-term improvement of spinal cord injury pain (weak evidence). Contraindications include pregnancy, active psychosis, uncontrolled cardiovascular disease, severe hepatic disease and elevated intracranial/intraocular pressure. Ketamine should be administered by health care personnel certified in advanced life support with clinical experience and training in administration of moderate sedation to ensure patient safety.

Skeletal Muscle Relaxants

In the past, skeletal muscle relaxants were one of the most extensively prescribed agents for treatment of musculoskeletal disorders, such as low back pain, muscle sprains, or athletic injury. Currently, muscle relaxants are recommended for the short-term treatment of acute musculoskeletal conditions. Long-term use is not recommended. Two categories of skeletal muscle relaxants exist: antispasmodic agents used for musculoskeletal conditions and antispastic agents for central spasticity in conditions such as multiple sclerosis and cerebral palsy.

Antispasmodic Skeletal Muscle Relaxants

Skeletal muscle relaxants are often used in the treatment of acute low back pain. The most benefit is usually demonstrated within the first few days of treatment. Adverse effects such as drowsiness and dizziness are commonly seen, and some agents in this class have potential for abuse. If a muscle relaxant is indicated, choice should be based on adverse effect profile, drug interaction potential, and identified risk of abuse.

Cyclobenzaprine has been the most studied skeletal muscle relaxant. The manufacturer's recommended dose of cyclobenzaprine is 10 mg. However, a 5-mg dose has been shown to be effective with less toxicity. Its anticholinergic properties must be taken into account if used in older adults. Tizanidine (Zanaflex) is a centrally acting, alpha$_2$-adrenergic agonist, reducing spasticity by increasing presynaptic inhibition of motor neuron excitation. Tizanidine is very sedating and a useful adjunct in patients with sleep disturbances as a result of musculoskeletal pain. Benzodiazepines, such as diazepam, may be effective for acute pain associated with muscle spasms. The predominance of adverse reactions, especially sedation and risk of abuse, limit benzodiazepine use for this indication.

Antispastic Agents

Limited evidence exists for using antispastic agents to treat musculoskeletal conditions. Baclofen is the most utilized agent in this class. Baclofen is indicated for managing signs and symptoms of spasticity resulting from multiple sclerosis and spinal cord injuries. Some anecdotal evidence exists for the use of baclofen in persistent neuropathic states and is used off label for hiccups. Available formulations include an oral tablet and an injectable formulation for intrathecal administration. Common side effects of the oral form include drowsiness, hypotension, weakness, nausea/vomiting, and headache. Intrathecal administration results in hypotension, somnolence, dizziness, constipation, and headache. Respiratory depression and difficulty with concentration or coordination are also seen with intrathecal administration. Due to the possible precipitation of withdrawal symptoms with abrupt discontinuation, tapering baclofen is recommended when discontinuing the drug, especially with the intrathecal formulation or prolonged oral use. Seizures and delirium may occur and can progress to rhabdomyolysis, disseminated intravascular coagulation, and hepatic/renal failure with abrupt discontinuation.

Cannabis

Cannabis is being used more often as a method for pain control, but its use is controversial. Cannabis may provide analgesia through anti-nociceptive and anti-hyperalgesic properties and may be synergistic with exogenous and endogenous opioids. Preclinical evidence has shown that cannabis may be beneficial in the treatment of chronic cancer and neuropathic pain, with minimal efficacy when used for acute pain. Cannabis is considered Schedule 1 at the federal level; however, more and more states are approving cannabis for medical use. Evidence is lacking, however; more quality studies need to be conducted to determine the place of cannabis in pain control. However, research on cannabis is difficult due to the variability of strains and terpine profiles in individual strains. Please see Chapter 11, "Cannabis and Pain Management," for more information.

CONCLUSION

Pain is difficult to manage and often needs a multidisciplinary approach to therapy. Treatment needs to be individualized for each patient, especially when a chronic pain condition exists. A proper assessment must be performed in order to differentiate the type and chronicity of pain. Once the type of pain is determined, patient-specific factors should be evaluated in order to choose the appropriate analgesic for pain treatment. A combination of therapies is often needed to provide a pain management goal of an acceptable level of pain and improvement in function. By utilizing the information provided in this chapter, the nursing practitioner will obtain the knowledge and the tools to effectively assess, treat, and monitor pain. The subsequent development of the individualized treatment plan will then provide improvement in the quality of life of the patient suffering in pain.

CASE STUDY 1

J.T. is a 65-year-old male admitted to the hospital with a history of chronic cancer pain using morphine sustained-release (SR) 60 mg orally every 8 hour. On admission, morphine 2 mg IV every 4 hour was ordered. The patient reports that his pain went from a 9 to an 8 only after the morphine dose and is asking for more pain medication. The staff begin to question the motivation of the patient and if addiction is present. The resident decides to start patient controlled analgesia (PCA). (A PCA device is a delivery system that allows the patient to self-administer analgesic medication at a specific dose and time interval). In a few hours, the patient is comfortable, resting in bed.

1. J.T.'s behavior is best described as
   a. Tolerance
   b. Addiction
   c. Pseudo-addiction
   d. Dependence

2. During his hospital stay, J.T. went into acute renal failure. He is increasingly lethargic and is experiencing confusion and some hallucinations. The physician believes that the morphine metabolites may be responsible and would like to convert to an alternative regimen. What would be your recommendation?
   a. Decrease morphine SR dose to 60 mg orally every 8 hour.
   b. Switch to hydromorphone 8 mg orally every 4 hour as needed.
   c. Add haloperidol 1 mg orally every 6 hour.
   d. Switch to a fentanyl patch 75 mcg every 3 days.

3. Tolerance will not develop to which adverse opioid effect?
   a. Respiratory depression
   b. Sedation
   c. Constipation
   d. Nausea

Bibliography

Starred references are cited in the text.

*American Society of Addiction Medicine. (2019). Definition of Addiction. www.asam.org. Accessed March 1, 2020.

*Arbuck, D. M., & Fleming, A. (2019). Pain assessment: Review of current tools. Practical Pain Management. practicalpainmanagement.com. Accessed January 5, 2020.

*Arnold, R. M., Verrico, P., & Davison, S. N. (2007). Opioid use in renal failure 161. *Journal of Palliative Medicine, 10*(6), 1403–1404.

*Byrd, L. (2013). Managing chronic pain in older adults: A long-term care perspective. Retrieved from http://www.annalsoflongtermcare.com/article/managing-chronic-pain-older-adult-long-term-care on April 20, 2015.

*Centers for Disease Control and Prevention. (2014). National Vital Statistics System mortality data. www.cdc.gov. Accessed January, 2020.

*Centers for Disease Control and Prevention. (2016). CDC Guideline for Prescribing Opioids for Chronic Pain—United States. *MMWR, 265*, 1–50.

*Chou, R., Cruciani, R., Fiellin, D., et al. (2014). Methadone safety: A clinical practice guideline from the American Pain Society and College on problems of drug dependence, in Collaboration with the Heart Rhythm Society. *The Journal of Pain, 15*(4), 321–337.

*Cohen, S. P., Bhatia, A., Buvanendran, A., et al. (2018). Consensus Guidelines on the Use of Intravenous Ketamine Infusions for Chronic Pain From the American Society of Regional Anesthesia and Pain Medicine (ASRA), the American Academy of Pain Medicine (AAPM), and the American Society of Anesthesiologists (ASA). *Regional Anesthesia and Pain Medicine, 43*, 521–546.

*Eckhardt, K., Li, S., Ammon, S., et al. (1998). Same incidence of adverse drug events after codeine administration irrespective of the genetically determined differences in morphine formation. *Pain, 76*(1–2), 27–33.

*Franklin, G. (2014). Opioids for chronic noncancer pain: A position paper of the American Academy of Neurology. *Neurology, 83*, 1277–1284.

*Gammaitoni, A. R., & Davis, M. W. (2002). Pharmacokinetics and tolerability of lidocaine patch 5% with extended dosing. *Annals of Pharmacotherapy, 36*(2), 236–240. doi: 10.1345/aph.1A185. PMID: 11847940.

Henry, D. E., Chiodo, A. E., & Yang, W. (2011). Central nervous system reorganization in a variety of chronic pain states: A review. *American Academy of Physical Medicine and Rehabilitation, 3*(12), 1116–1125.

*Herr, K., & Garand, L. (2001). Assessment and measurement of pain in older adults. *Clinics in Geriatric Medicine, 17*, 457–478.

*Hooten, W. M., Timming, R., Belgrade, M., et al. (2013). Assessment and management of chronic pain. Retrieved from www.icsi.org/_asset/bw798b/ChronicPain.pdf on April 15, 2015.

*Institute for Clinical Systems Improvement (ICSI). (2017). Pain: Assessment, Non-opioid Treatment Approaches and Opioid Management. www.icsi.org. Accessed February 21, 2020.

*Janssen Pharmaceuticals. (2006). Product Information DURAGESIC® (Fentanyl Transdermal Patch).

*Jensen, M. P., Smith, D. G., & Ehde, D. M. (2001). Pain site and the effects of amputation pain: Further clarification of the meaning of mild, moderate, and severe pain. *Pain, 91*(3), 317–322.

Kim, H., & Nelson, L. S. (2015). Reducing the harm of opioid overdose with the safe use of naloxone: A pharmacologic review. *Expert Opinion Drug Safety, 14*(7), 1137–1146.

*Kroenke, K., Alford, D. P., Argoff, C., et al. (2019). Challenges with implementing the Centers for Disease Control and Prevention opioid guideline: A consensus panel report. *Pain Medicine, 20*(4), 724–735.

Manchikanti, L., Falco, F., Singh, V., et al. (2013). An update of comprehensive evidence-based guidelines for interventional techniques in chronic spinal pain. *Pain Physician, 16*, S1–S48.

*Maroo, S., Patel, K., Bhatnagar, S., et al. (2014). Safety and efficacy of oral transmucosal fentanyl citrate compared to morphine sulphate immediate release tablet in management of breakthrough cancer pain. *Indian Journal of Palliative Care, 20*, 182–187.

*McPherson, M. (2010). *Demystifying opioid conversion calculations: A guide for effective dosing*. Bethesda, MD: American Society of Health-System Pharmacists.

*Merskey, H., & Bogduk, N. (2012). In Part III: Pain terms: A current list with definitions and notes on usage. Classification of chronic pain (2nd ed., pp. 209–214). Seattle, WA: IASP Task Force on Taxonomy.

The NSDUH Report: Substance use and mental health estimates from the 2013 National Survey on Drug Use and Health: Overview of findings. (2014). Retrieved from http://www.samhsa.gov/data/sites/default/files/NSDUHresultsPDFWHTML2013/Web/NSDUHresults2013.pdf on April 20, 2015.

*Pasero, C., & McCaffery, M. (2011). *Pain assessment and pharmacologic management*. St. Louis, MO: Elsevier/Mosby.

*Paulozzi, L. J., Mack, K. A., & Hockenberry, J. M. (2012). Vital signs: Variation among states in prescribing of opioid pain relievers and benzodiazepines—United States. *Morbidity and Mortality Weekly Report, 63*, 563–568.

*Phillips, D. M. (2000). JCAHO pain management standards are unveiled: Joint Commission on Accreditation of Healthcare Organizations. *JAMA, 284*(4), 428–429.

*Reidenberg, M. M. (1996). Assessment of patients' pain. *The New England Journal of Medicine, 334*, 59.

*Ru-Rong, J., Nackley, A., Huh, Y., et al. (2018). Neuroinflammation and central sensitization in chronic and widespread pain. *Anesthesiology, 129*, 343–366.

Savage, S., Joranson, D., Covington, E., et al. (2003). Definitions related to the medical use of opioids: Evolution towards universal agreement. *Journal of Pain and Symptom Management, 26*(1), 655–667.

*Schwenk, E. S., Viscusi, E. R., Buvanendran, A., et al. (2018). Consensus guidelines on the use of intravenous ketamine infusions for acute pain management from the American Society of Regional Anesthesia and Pain Medicine (ASRA), the American Academy of Pain Medicine (AAPM) and the American Society of Anesthesiologists (ASA). *Regional Anesthesia and Pain Medicine, 43*(5), 456–466.

Substance Abuse and Mental Health Services Administration (SAMHSA). (2017). Key substance use and mental health indicators in the United States: Results from the 2016 National Survey on Drug Use and Health. Rockville, MD: Center for Behavioral Health Statistics and Quality, Substance Abuse and Mental Health Services Administration. Retrieved from https://www.samhsa.gov/data/. Accessed January 5, 2020.

*Swarm, R. A., Paice, J. A., & Anghelescu, D. L. (2019). Adult Cancer Pain, Version 3. 2019, NCCN clinical practice guidelines in oncology. *Journal of the National Comprehensive Cancer Network, 17*(8), 977–1007.

*Tarumi, Y., Wilson, M. P., Szafran, O., et al. (2013). Randomized, double-blind, placebo-controlled trial of oral docusate in the management of constipation in hospice patients. *Journal of Pain and Symptom Management, 45*(1), 2–13.

*Treed, R., Rief, W., Barke, A., et al. (2019). Chronic pain as a symptom or a disease: The IASP Classification of Chronic Pain for the *International Classification of Diseases* (ICD-11). *PAIN, 160*(1), 19–27.

Ventafridda, V., & Stjernsward, J. (1996). Pain control and the World Health Organization analgesic ladder. *The Journal of the American Medical Association, 275*, 835–836.

Wilcock, A., & Twycross, R. (2011). Therapeutic reviews: Ketamine. *Journal of Pain and Symptom Management, 41*(3), 640–648.

*Woo, C. W., Roy, M., Buhle, J. T., et al. (2015). Distinct brain systems mediate the effects of nociceptive input and self-regulation on pain. Retrieved from http://wagerlab.colorado.edu/files/papers/Woo_PLOS.pdf on April 15, 2015.

*Woolf, C. (2011). Central sensitization: Implications for the diagnosis and treatment of pain. *Pain, 152*(Suppl. 3), S2–S15.

10 Pain Management in Opioid Use Disorder (OUD) Patients

Rachel Trichtinger and Maria C. Foy

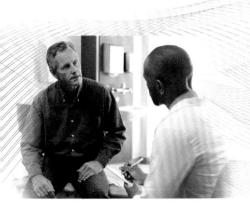
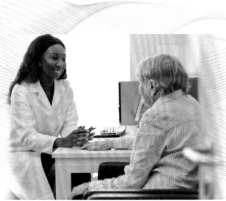
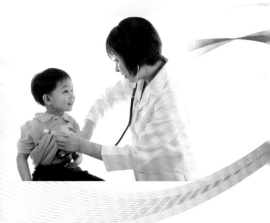

Learning Objectives

1. Screen and assess pain in patients with opioid use disorder (OUD).
2. Develop treatment plans to both alleviate pain and prevent relapse when on medication-assisted treatment.
3. Monitor the safety and efficacy of pharmacotherapy for pain in OUD.

INTRODUCTION

In 2017, the U.S. Department of Health and Human Services declared the opioid crisis a "public health emergency" (U.S. Department of Health and Human Services, 2019). Approximately 2 million people were diagnosed with an opioid use disorder (OUD) in 2018 (U.S. Department of Health and Human Services, 2019). The course of this disorder is both chronic and relapsing. Currently only 20% of diagnosed patients are receiving substance abuse treatment, leaving a large portion of patients untreated. Addressing the crisis involves not only supporting the treatment of OUD but also confronting the underlying issues that may have precipitated the addiction in the first place, with one of these issues being undertreated pain. Relief of pain is the most frequent reason that opioids are abused. Historically, opioids have been effective in managing acute pain; however, there is less evidence supporting the use of this class of medication in long-term treatment of chronic noncancer pain. Conversely, there is evidence that long-term opioid use leads to an increased risk of OUD and other adverse outcomes. In patients with current or remitted OUD who are experiencing pain, the appropriate management of the pain

will help prevent inappropriate use of opioids often obtained from nonmedical sources.

Managing pain in patients with OUD is challenging and complex, and treatment relies on assessing risk versus benefit and applying the ultimate goal of *do no harm*. Practitioners should be mindful to not stigmatize a patient diagnosed with OUD as this can interfere with effectively managing pain. Another barrier to treating this population is that patients diagnosed with OUD generally have a higher tolerance to opioids and an increased pain sensitivity, making their pain even more difficult to treat. Two of the most common medications used for both prevention of withdrawal symptoms and maintenance treatment of OUD that can proficiently manage pain are buprenorphine and methadone; these two medications are first-line treatment options for medication-assisted treatment (MAT) in OUD. Both medications have effects at the *mu* opioid receptor, alleviating pain while also reducing cravings. In patients in need of pharmacotherapy for pain management with a history of substance abuse not responding to non-opioid interventions, methadone or buprenorphine may be beneficial. Also, in patients with OUD already being treated with methadone or buprenorphine, the dosing can be adjusted to maximize their analgesic effect.

PATHOPHYSIOLOGY BETWEEN PAIN AND ADDICTION

Refer to Chapter 9 and Chapter 44 for the individual pathophysiology of pain and OUD.

The experience of pain occurs via nociception, defined as the transmission of pain signaling through the central nervous system (CNS). Chronic use of opioids, whether prescribed or misused, alters the processing of pain stimuli, which leads to

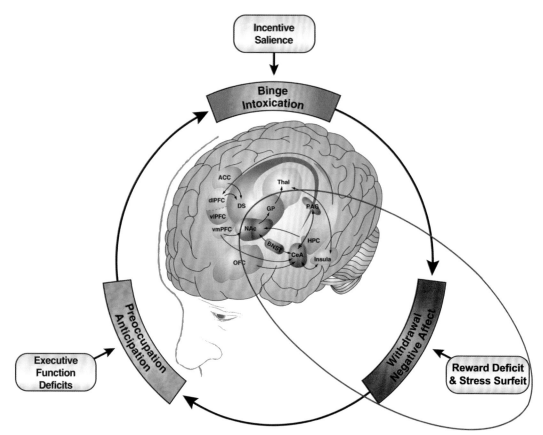

FIGURE 10–1   Reward and intoxication cycle in the brain. (From Koob, G. F. (2020). Neurobiology of opioid addiction: Opponent process, hyperkatifeia, and negative reinforcement. *Biological Psychiatry*, *87*(1), 44–53. doi: 10.1016/j.biopsych.2019.05.023.)

ACC, anterior cingulate cortex; BNST, bed nucleus of the stria terminalis; dlPFC, dorsolateral prefrontal cortex; DS, dorsal striatum; GP, globus pallidus; HPC, hippocampus; NAc, nucleus accumbens; OFC, orbitofrontal cortex; PAG, periaqueductal gray; vlPFC, ventrolateral prefrontal cortex; vmPFC, ventromedial prefrontal cortex.

increased pain sensitivity and the occurrence of opioid tolerance. In patients with OUD, the mesolimbic pathway (reward pathway) facilitated by the actions of *mu* opioid agonists also plays a major role in the reinforcing effect leading to its addictive properties.

Pain provides both a positive and negative reinforcement of opioid use. Opioids produce feelings of pleasure primarily due to activation of the ventral tegmental area and subsequent release of dopamine from the nucleus accumbens. Continued misuse of opioids leads to dysregulation of the neurochemical system causing severe distress and discomfort when opioids are withdrawn or absent. This dysphoria, which may be further exacerbated by concomitant pain, correlates to negative reinforcement motivating continued opioid use. The positive and negative reinforcement of opioids is decreased in chronic pain resulting in the need for higher and more frequent doses (**Figure 10.1**).

classification of pain) using subjective information offered by the patient. In addition, clinical examination and testing (e.g., magnetic resonance imaging, X-ray, etc.) can be performed when applicable. The patient's ability to function is critical in the evaluation. After completion of a detailed workup of the patient's pain complaints, collateral information should be obtained. The patient's concomitant diseases, especially any psychological comorbidities, must be taken into consideration when developing a treatment and monitoring plan. Review all medications (including over-the-counter and herbal medicine) for the presence of drug interactions and potential side effects. If the patient has been diagnosed with OUD, determination of current or past MAT must be reviewed. It is also important to be aware of responses to any previous pain management treatments. Lastly, identify and confirm a strong support system before interventions are initiated.

SCREENING AND ASSESSMENT FOR PAIN

When assessing pain, patients with OUD should be treated like any other patient. A thorough assessment should be conducted with type and class of pain identified (refer to Chapter 9 for

SCREENING AND ASSESSMENT OF OPIOID USE DISORDER

While all patients should be screened routinely for OUD (and other substance use disorders), it is essential to perform this assessment before initiating opioid analgesics. Continuously assessing for potential opioid misuse, as well as monitoring for worsening or continued pain, is recommended. Differentiate OUD diagnosis from "pseudo-addictive" behavior (refer to Chapter 9 for definition). Nonjudgmental and open communication should be applied when assessing the patient. Patients are often reluctant to divulge a present or past history of opioid misuse. Some patients may not be ready to disclose when they struggle with opioid use due to concern of their pain being left untreated or fear of withdrawal. Other patients may not realize that overutilization of opioid dosing reflects tolerance and/or addiction. Evaluation and diagnosis of a substance use disorder can be based on the *Diagnostic and Statistical Manual of Mental Disorders, Fifth Edition* criteria (refer to Chapter 44 on substance use disorder).

Urine drug screens may also assist in the assessment; however, false-positive or -negative results can and do occur. Both quantitative and qualitative tests are available to assess for illicit substances in the urine. Immunoassays used for screening are quick and inexpensive but may produce false positives and negative results. For example, patients taking an antipsychotic medication may produce a false-positive result for fentanyl on a urine drug screen assay (Wang et al., 2014). If an immunoassay returns an unanticipated positive or negative finding, a more precise gas chromatography-mass spectrometry is advised for confirmation. Gas chromatography-mass spectrometry is more sensitive and tests for specific medications (Standridge et al., 2010).

Referencing a prescription drug monitoring program (PDMP), an electronic database that relays information on filled prescriptions for controlled substances, can assist in identifying opioid misuse in an individual patient. This database displays the medication, date, and quantity/day supplied as well as the name of the prescribing physician and dispensing pharmacy. Early fills, large quantities, and multiple pharmacies and providers on a patient's PDMP profile alert a provider to potential misuse.

If opioid misuse is suspected or confirmed, referral for treatment should be offered. A tool that can be used to help guide a practitioner on whether or not an opioid may be safely prescribed is the Opioid Risk Tool (Webster & Webster, 2005). This tool is used on patients with chronic pain and is based on risk factors for OUD including family history of substance abuse, personal history of substance abuse, age, history of preadolescent sexual abuse, and psychological diseases. The Screener and Opioid Assessment for Patients with Pain-Revised (SOAPP®-R) is an alternative or adjunctive tool a prescriber can use to help further evaluate risk for misuse with prescribed opioids (Butler et al., 2008). See **Box 10.1** for a list of risk assessment tools.

When a patient is on buprenorphine or methadone for treatment of OUD, doses should be confirmed before starting any new medications. Buprenorphine dosing can be confirmed by referencing a PDMP and clarifying with pharmacy or provider. Methadone dosing will need to be verified by patient's methadone clinic.

BOX 10.1 Risk Assessment and Monitoring Tools for Opioid Use Disorder

OPIOID RISK ASSESSMENTS

Screening

- ORT (Opioid Risk Tool)
- SOAPP®-R (Screener and Opioid Assessment for Patients with Pain-Revised)
- SISAD (Screening Instrument for Substance Abuse Potential)

Monitoring

- PDUQ (Prescription Drug Use Questionnaire)
- COMM (Current Opioid Misuse Measure)
- PMQ (Patient Medication Questionnaire)
- PADT (Patient Assessment and Documentation Tool)
- ABC (Addiction Behavior Checklist)

INITIATING DRUG THERAPY

Goals of Drug Therapy

The goals of treating pain in patients with OUD include (1) reducing or eliminating pain and treating underlying injury/disease, (2) reducing or eliminating cravings, (3) preventing relapse, (4) minimizing or managing side effects, and (5) improving quality of life. Medications used in OUD include buprenorphine, methadone, and naltrexone. Naltrexone, an opioid antagonist, is not routinely used in the management of chronic pain (**Table 10.1**).

Buprenorphine and Buprenorphine/Naloxone

Buprenorphine is a partial *mu* opioid receptor agonist providing analgesic effects similar to full *mu* opioid receptor agonists (opioids). The partial agonism feature creates a ceiling effect, which lessens both its euphoria and its risk of causing respiratory depression. Partial agonist properties are reflected in the dose response, which plateaus as the dose is increased. Therefore, higher doses of buprenorphine do not produce greater euphoric or respiratory depressive outcomes. The analgesic impact of buprenorphine does not seem to be limited by this ceiling effect.

Antinociception and anti-hyperalgesia may also be seen through agonizing the opioid receptor like-1, making buprenorphine an option for the treatment of neuropathic pain (Marquez et al., 2008). Buprenorphine has additional benefits over other *mu* agonists. Buprenorphine does not cause spasm of the sphincter of Oddi and therefore induces less constipation. Cognitive dysfunction may be lessened, making a safe and effective therapeutic option for older patients when compared to full *mu* opioid agonists.

Buprenorphine has high binding affinity to the *mu* opioid receptor. When given to a patient with recent opioid

TABLE 10.1

Drugs Used in the Treatment of Opioid Use Disorder and Pain

Generic Name and Dosage	Selected Adverse Effects	Contraindications	Special Considerations
Methadone			

Opioid Use Disorder:
Oral:
  Initial: 20–30 mg (as a single dose)
  Maximum initial dose: 30 mg. Lower doses (5–10 mg) and much slower titration should be considered in patients with no or low tolerance at initiation. Patients should be monitored for oversedation and withdrawal symptoms for 2–4 hours after initial dose. An additional 5–10 mg may be provided if withdrawal symptoms have not been suppressed or if symptoms reappear after 2–4 hours. Total daily dose on the first day should not exceed 40 mg.
  Maintenance: Titrate to a dosage that prevents opioid withdrawal symptoms for 24 hours, prevents craving, attenuates euphoric effect of self-administered opioids, and reduces tolerance to sedative effects of methadone. Usual range: 80–120 mg/d (titration should occur cautiously).
Pain Management:
Oral:
Initial: 2.5 mg q8–12h
IM, IV, SQ:
Initial: 2.5–10 mg q8–12h
	Hypotension
	EKG changes
	Torsades de pointes
	Syncope
	Tachycardia
	Sedation
	Nausea
	Respiratory depression
	Constipation
		Hypersensitivity to methadone or any component	Older patients: Decrease initial dose and monitor closely when initiating and titrating. Monitor closely due to an increased potential for risks, including certain risks such as falls/fracture, cognitive impairment, and constipation. Clearance may also be reduced in older adults, increasing the risk for respiratory depression or overdose.
			Neonatal opioid withdrawal syndrome is an expected and treatable outcome of use of methadone during pregnancy. Neonatal opioid withdrawal syndrome may be life threatening if not recognized and treated in the neonate. Signs and symptoms include irritability, hyperactivity and abnormal sleep pattern, high-pitched cry, tremor, vomiting, diarrhea, and failure to gain weight. Onset, duration, and severity depend on the drug used, duration of use, maternal dose, and rate of drug elimination by the newborn.
			Incomplete cross-tolerance: Use caution in converting patients from other opioids to methadone. Follow appropriate conversion recommendations. Patients tolerant to other *mu* opioid agonists may not be tolerant to methadone and may be at risk for severe respiratory depression when converted to methadone.
			Opioid use disorder: When switching patients from methadone to buprenorphine, patients should preferably be on low doses of oral methadone (<30–40 mg/d) prior to the switch to lessen discomfort. Patients switching from methadone to naltrexone (oral or extended-release IM) require complete withdrawal from methadone or other opioids before naltrexone initiation (typically achieved in 7 days but up to 14 days may be necessary).

Buprenorphine			
Opioid Use Disorder: Sublingual tablet average daily dose: 16 mg/d; (max daily dose: 32 mg but doses over 24 mg do not seem to provide a clinical advantage)	Hypertension Fatigue Headache Dizziness Opioid withdrawal syndrome	Hypersensitivity (e.g., anaphylaxis) to buprenorphine or any component of the formulation	Discontinuation of therapy: When discontinuing sublingual buprenorphine for long-term treatment of opioid use disorder, use a gradual taper to prevent withdrawal; do not abruptly discontinue.

TABLE 10.1			
Drugs Used in the Treatment of Opioid Use Disorder and Pain (*Continued*)			
Generic Name and Dosage	**Selected Adverse Effects**	**Contraindications**	**Special Considerations**
Sublingual tablet/film (with naloxone) average daily dose: 11.4/2.9 mg or 16/4 mg/d depending on product (max daily dose: 17.2/4.2 mg or 24/6 mg depending on product) Buccal tablet (with naloxone) average daily dose: 8.4/1.4 mg/d (max daily dose: 12.6/2.1 mg) Extended-release subcutaneous injection average dose: 100 mg monthly; (max monthly dose: 300 mg) Subdermal implant: 4 implants are inserted for 6-month duration; each implant contains 74.2 mg of buprenorphine, equivalent to 80 mg of buprenorphine hydrochloride.	Anemia Constipation Skin rashes Specific to implant: Local pruritus, local edema, local hemorrhage Injection: pain at injection site, bruising at injection site, induration at injection site, swelling at injection site, erythema at injection site	Significant respiratory depression GI obstruction Extended-release injection is not recommended in patients with moderate to severe hepatic impairment.	Prescribing for opioid dependence is limited to physicians who have met the qualification criteria and have received a DEA number specific to prescribing this product. Older patients are more sensitive to the CNS depressant effects of opioid analgesic; therefore, use agents with caution. Monitor older patients for sedation and respiratory depression, particularly when initiating therapy. Extended-release injection: indicated for the treatment of moderate to severe opioid use disorder in patients who have initiated treatment with a transmucosal buprenorphine-containing product, followed by dose adjustment for a minimum of 7 days Subdermal implant: indicated for maintenance treatment of opioid dependence in patients who have achieved and sustained prolonged clinical stability on low to moderate doses of a transmucosal buprenorphine- containing product (i.e., doses of no more than 8 mg per day of Subutex® or Suboxone® sublingual tablet or generic equivalent) Neonatal abstinence syndrome is an expected and treatable outcome of use of buprenorphine during pregnancy. Neonatal abstinence syndrome may be life-threatening if not recognized and treated in the neonate.

CNS, central nervous system; DEA, Drug Enforcement Agency; EKG, electrocardiography; GI, gastrointestinal; IM, intramuscular; IV, intravenous.

Source: Lexicomp Online. (2021). Lexicomp: Evidence-based drug referential solutions. Retrieved from http://www.wolterskluwercdi.com/lexicomp-online/ on December 27, 2019.

use, buprenorphine will displace the previous opioids from the receptors and precipitate a very substantial and exaggerated withdrawal. To avoid this, patients with recent opioid use should not have buprenorphine initiated until objective symptoms of withdrawal are seen. Withdrawal symptoms can be assessed using the Clinical Opiate Withdrawal Scale (Wesson & Ling, 2003).

Buprenorphine is highly protein bound and has a large volume of distribution. The drug is a substrate of cytochrome P450 3A4 (CYP3A4); therefore, CYP3A4 inducers and inhibitors will decrease or increase buprenorphine concentrations, respectively. Also, decreased doses should be used in patients identified as poor metabolizers of CYP3A4. Adverse effects of buprenorphine include precipitated withdrawal (when given concurrently or after recent opioid use) with subsequent nausea/vomiting and tremors. Other common side effects include headache, insomnia, and peripheral edema. While buprenorphine has a dose-ceiling effect on respiratory depression, risk increases when used with other CNS depressants such as benzodiazepines.

The dosing of buprenorphine for OUD is generally once a day. Because the analgesic effect of buprenorphine is shorter (6–8 hours) than its properties related to treatment of OUD, the drug should be dosed twice to thrice daily to optimize the analgesic effect when used for pain management (in contrast to the once-a-day dosing used in OUD). While buccal and sublingual formulations of buprenorphine are the most commonly used formulations for OUD, a long-acting implant and extended-release subcutaneous injection are available for use in patients who have been maintained on transmucosal buprenorphine. These formulations are long-acting and consequently less beneficial in treating pain. Various formulations of buprenorphine (such as Suboxone®) may contain naloxone, a *mu* opioid reversal agent. The purpose of the addition of naloxone is to deter abuse. When taken buccally or sublingually, the absorption of the naloxone is very poor, rendering it ineffective. However, when injected, the naloxone will antagonize the opioid receptors, thereby lessening the euphoric effects. The formulation of buprenorphine with naloxone can be very beneficial in the outpatient setting.

While buprenorphine formulations approved for OUD can be used off-label to treat pain, formulations of buprenorphine approved by the Food and Drug Administration (FDA) are available specifically for the treatment of pain. The analgesic effects of buprenorphine are seen at lower doses than what is used for OUD. Since higher doses are needed to prevent opioid cravings, many of the buprenorphine formulations indicated for the treatment of pain are not as efficacious for concomitantly treating OUD. When both pain control and OUD treatments are needed, increased analgesic benefit may be obtained by dividing the dose of formulations indicated for OUD. Formulations are not interchangeable and no current dosing equivalents among agents are available. Bioavailability of the products must be assessed in order to determine safe interchange among products (**Table 10.2**).

Buprenorphine is a Schedule 3–controlled medication requiring a Drug Enforcement Agency (DEA) number for its prescribing. In order to prescribe buprenorphine for OUD, the Drug Addiction Treatment Act (DATA) requires prescribers to request a waiver and complete specific requirements of the Center for Substance Abuse Treatment. Restrictions on the number of patients a prescriber can treat at any given time are also included in the DATA prescribing information. However, any prescriber can write buprenorphine when used as an analgesic (**Table 10.3**).

Patients should be educated on how to properly administer buprenorphine. The sublingual or buccal tablet/film should be placed under the tongue or placed inside the cheek, respectively, until completely dissolved. The long-acting implant and extended-release subcutaneous injection formulation require

TABLE 10.2
Bioavailability of Buprenorphine Formulations

Formulation	Average Bioavailability (%)*
Buccal formulation (Belbuca®)	55
Transdermal patch (Butrans®)	15
Sublingual—Zubsolv®	25
Sublingual—Suboxone®	35
Sublingual—Bunavail®	50

*Information obtained from respective package inserts.

TABLE 10.3
Drug Addiction Treatment Act Prescribing Information

Brand Name	Generic Name	Formulation	Indication
Belbuca®	Buprenorphine	Buccal film	Pain
Bunavail®	Buprenorphine/naloxone	Buccal film	Opioid dependence
Buprenex®	Buprenorphine	Solution for injection (IV/IM)	Pain
Butrans®	Buprenorphine	Transdermal patch	Pain
Probuphine®	Buprenorphine	Intradermal implant	Opioid dependence
Sublocadelate	Buprenorphine	Solution for injection (SQ) or (SC)	Opioid dependence
Suboxone®	Buprenorphine/naloxone	Sublingual film/tablet	Opioid dependence
Subutex®	Buprenorphine	Sublingual tablet	Opioid dependence
Zubsolv®	Buprenorphine/naloxone	Sublingual tablet	Opioid dependence

IV, intravenous; IM, intramuscular.

administration by a trained health care provider and are not available in retail pharmacies. Buprenorphine should be used cautiously in patients with respiratory depression as well as pre-existing hepatic impairment. Patients should have liver function tests assessed at baseline, 6 months, and then annually.

Methadone

Methadone is effective in treating OUD due to its very long half-life, which reduces cravings and dulls the euphoric effects of other opioid agonists. Because of its full *mu* opioid agonist properties, methadone is also efficacious in pain control and is thought to be less likely to produce tolerance due to its antagonistic effects at the N-methyl-D-aspartate receptor. Methadone is a Schedule 2–controlled substance. When being used for pain, prescriptions can be filled at a retail pharmacy, usually dispensed in tablet formulation. When being used for OUD, dosing is usually once a day, and the medication is only available through federally regulated opioid treatment programs often referred to as *methadone clinics*. At these facilities, the liquid formulation is usually dispensed, and doses are provided daily by the clinic directly to the patient. Methadone that is provided to patients from a clinic may not display in the PDMP report.

Similar to buprenorphine, methadone is primarily metabolized by CYP3A4 (also by CYP2B6 and CYP2D6). Drug interactions should be analyzed and used cautiously in patients who are poor metabolizers of these enzymes. Pharmacokinetics of methadone are widely variable. Methadone's half-life can range between 8 and 59 hours with a duration of effect lasting approximately 30 hours. Unlike buprenorphine, there is no ceiling effect and therefore carries a greater risk of respiratory depression if dosed inappropriately.

The FDA black box warnings associated with methadone use emphasize dangerous adverse effects such as respiratory depression and risk of abuse/dependence. Respiratory rate should be monitored during initiation and titration of methadone doses. When taken with other medications that cause CNS depression, the incidence of respiratory depression increases. Also, methadone is associated with an increased risk of torsades de pointes by prolonging the QTc interval. Electrocardiography (EKG) should be done prior to treatment initiation, within 30 days of starting, and then once a year. Electrolytes such as potassium and magnesium need to be in normal range to prevent risk of arrhythmias. If the QTc interval exceeds 500 ms, stopping or reducing methadone is recommended, and an alternative medication should be considered. Risk is increased when methadone is given with other medications that also prolong the QTc interval (e.g., antipsychotics, antiarrhythmics). Common side effects are similar to other opioids and can include nausea/vomiting, sedation, and hypotension.

Unfortunately, methadone has incomplete cross-tolerance with other opioids, and conversions are not bidirectional. When converting from high-dose opioids to methadone, a higher conversion factor is used as opposed to switching off methadone. Tolerance will not generally develop to methadone as is seen with other opioids such as morphine. Therefore, when converting between methadone and other opioids, no standard equivalent analgesic dose recommendations are available. Dosing recommendations suggest starting low and titrating up gradually. In the past, increases in deaths were seen when methadone was initiated for pain without a thorough understanding of the properties of the medication. This prompted development of guidelines for methadone use in pain, providing direction for initial dosing in both opioid-naive and -tolerant patients (Chou et al., 2014). While methadone is usually dosed once a day for OUD, more frequent dosing is necessary when being used for pain. In general, higher once-daily doses for methadone are recommended for OUD compared to lower doses given multiple times a day for pain management. When both acute pain and OUD are present, the methadone dose can be divided three to four times daily in order to provide analgesic treatment.

Non-opioid and Multimodal Analgesia

Non-opioid analgesics are first line for mild to moderate pain. Examples of non-opioid analgesics are acetaminophen and nonsteroidal anti-inflammatory drugs. These medications do not have an effect on the opioid receptors that may lead to abuse and therefore are good analgesic options for patients with OUD, especially for acute pain treatment. Also, the use of coanalgesics, either alone or as adjunct treatment, can also be used in patients with OUD, particularly if pain is chronic. Classes of adjunctive pain modalities include antidepressants, anticonvulsants, cannabinoids, sodium channel blockers, antispasmodic skeletal muscle relaxers, and antispastic agents. While tramadol is technically not an opioid, its weak *mu* receptor properties may elicit cravings. Therefore, tramadol is generally not recommended in patients with OUD due to misuse potential (but can be considered in certain situations). Refer to Chapter 9 for additional information on each class of non-opioid agents indicated for pain.

Opioids

Opioids are not generally recommended for pain in patients with diagnosed or suspected OUD. There *may* be a place for opioids in acute pain or cancer-related pain when used in controlled settings after the potential risks and benefits of treatment have been weighed and other options have been exhausted. If indicated, opioids with less rewarding properties should be selected and titrated up slowly to an effective dose (avoid supratherapeutic doses). Recently, some opioids have been reformulated to deter abuse by making the medication more arduous to tamper with once manipulated.

Dosing is more complicated because of existing tolerance. If opioids must be used in patients with OUD, active substance abuse should not be present. If an opioid is added to a patient already stabilized on MAT, higher doses may be required with shorter intervals due to increased pain sensitivity and opioid tolerance. Patients will require close monitoring, and only limited quantities should be dispensed at a time. Urine drug screens can be utilized, but unexpected results should be confirmed due to a high frequency of false positives/negatives. Refer to Chapter 9 for more information on opioid pharmacotherapy.

Selecting the Most Appropriate Therapy

Non-opioid medications are recommended for use in patients with OUD. If a patient is receiving MAT, the dosing interval can be adjusted to allow full analgesic potential. Single daily doses of methadone and buprenorphine for OUD are not adequate in controlling pain due to the shorter-acting analgesic effects of both medications compared to long half-lives. For example, methadone's analgesic effects last about 6 hours although its half-life can be up to 59 hours in some patients.

A recommended outpatient option for treating pain in a patient established on buprenorphine therapy is dividing the total daily dose and administering every 6 to 8 hours. Non-opioid medications dosed continuously or "as needed" can also be added to the regimen.

Currently there are no established perioperative or postoperative guidelines for patients on buprenorphine. Limited literature offers suggestions on treatment methods, but often decisions are made based on patient- and institution-specific factors. For patients on buprenorphine in need of inpatient analgesic treatment, there are a few options (Alford et al., 2006):

1. Continue buprenorphine once-daily maintenance and titrate a short-acting opioid to effect. Due to increased pain sensitivity and the mechanism of action of buprenorphine, higher doses of the opioid will need to be administered to treat pain. An opioid with a high affinity to the *mu* receptor, such as hydromorphone or fentanyl, would be needed to overcome the strong receptor binding of buprenorphine.
2. Divide total daily dose of buprenorphine and administer every 6 to 8 hours. Low-dose buprenorphine can be considered as needed for additional acute pain control.
3. For anticipated acute pain from scheduled surgery, buprenorphine can be discontinued or dosage can be reduced while full opioid agonists are initiated (including methadone) for the treatment of anticipated postoperative pain. Initially, higher doses of opioids will be needed to overcome the high affinity of buprenorphine to the *mu* receptor. Patients should be monitored for possible respiratory depression that may occur once the buprenorphine is no longer in the system, that is, if buprenorphine is stopped when acute pain treatments are initiated.
4. When acute pain is resolved and opioids discontinued, the buprenorphine can be restarted after the patient is in confirmed withdrawal.

No consensus exists on the proper method of switching to buprenorphine from a full opioid agonist. Level of dependence, type of opioid used (long acting vs. short acting), and time since last dose of opioid taken should be determined prior to switching to buprenorphine. One method of transition recommends discontinuing the opioid (by tapering, if high dose-opioid use) and waiting for the patient to experience objective symptoms of withdrawal. Once the patient is in withdrawal, low-dose buprenorphine (2 mg) with available redosing every 1 to 2 hours as needed for signs of withdrawal and cravings can be prescribed. Each subsequent day, the dose can be adjusted to the previous day's total dose with breakthrough doses accessible until effective dose is established. The buprenorphine/naloxone (Suboxone®) package insert recommends that when switching from short-acting opioids or heroin, buprenorphine should be given at least 6 to 12 hours after last use of a short-acting opioid, at least 24 to 96 hours after long-acting opioid, and/or preferably when moderate objective signs of opioid withdrawal are observed. Therapy should be titrated to clinical effectiveness as quickly as possible.

Induction in the package insert is as follows (Indivior, Inc., 2019):

On Day 1, an induction dosage of up to 8 mg/2 mg SUBOXONE sublingual film is recommended. Clinicians should start with an initial dose of 2 mg/0.5 mg or 4 mg/1 mg buprenorphine/naloxone and may titrate upwards in 2 or 4 mg increments of buprenorphine, at approximately 2-hour intervals, under supervision, to 8 mg/2 mg buprenorphine/naloxone

based on the control of acute withdrawal symptoms. On Day 2, a single daily dose of up to 16 mg/4 mg SUBOXONE sublingual film is recommended.

When switching from long-acting opioids (such as methadone) to buprenorphine/naloxone, withdrawal symptoms may be more likely to occur. Also, the naloxone component may be minimally absorbed, potentially worsening withdrawal. For this reason, buprenorphine monotherapy is recommended with an eventual switch to combination formulation when converting from long-acting formulations.

For treatment of acute pain for patients on methadone that have failed non-opioid adjuncts, the total daily dose of methadone can be divided every 6 to 8 hours. If unable to partition methadone dosing (only some methadone clinics will offer split dosing), opioids (not including mixed agonist/antagonist opioids) may need to be prescribed under close monitoring.

When a patient is diagnosed with OUD and not receiving medication and/or therapy for OUD, referral should be made for treatment. If the patient is currently on prescribed or recreational opioids, consider a switch to methadone or buprenorphine. Buprenorphine with naloxone may be considered a safer option due to its ceiling effect and presence of an opioid reversal agent that minimizes abuse potential.

Special Considerations

Pediatric

The safety of buprenorphine when used for OUD has not been established in patients less than 16 years old, and the safety and effectiveness of methadone have not been established in patients less than 18 years old.

The American Academy of Pediatrics recommends the consideration of MAT in adolescents with severe OUD ("Medication-Assisted Treatment," 2016). Generally, at least two documented attempts at psychosocial treatment within 12 months before being considered for methadone maintenance are recommended (Feder et al., 2017).

Geriatric

Methadone and buprenorphine need to be used cautiously in older patients due to decreases in hepatic, renal, and cardiac function; and alterations in absorption, distribution, metabolism, and excretion of medications. Recommendations are to start at lower doses and gradually titrate up to efficacy. This patient population may also be on multiple medications, thereby increasing the risk of drug-drug interactions. Monitor closely for signs and symptoms of overdose or toxicity.

Women

Methadone historically has been considered the standard of care for treating pregnant patients with OUD; however, both methadone and buprenorphine (without naloxone) are considered safe and effective for use in pregnancy. Data on buprenorphine with naloxone are currently limited and therefore buprenorphine monotherapy is preferred. Prolonged exposure to opioids in utero can result in neonatal abstinence syndrome (NAS). Buprenorphine and methadone both cross the placenta and can result in withdrawal of a neonate in the first week after birth. NAS can occur with either treatment option although some studies have shown that buprenorphine may be associated with reduced severity of NAS as well as improved fetal growth outcomes when compared to methadone (Krsak et al., 2017). However, there is also evidence that methadone maintenance in opioid-dependent women may also improve maternal and newborn outcomes (Kumar, 2020). It is undetermined whether or not intrauterine exposure to methadone or buprenorphine leads to developmental issues in infants, but there is also no current evidence showing that either results in birth defects (Kumar, 2020). Overall, the risk of using MAT during pregnancy is commonly preferred to the risk of overdose or withdrawal. Pregnant women who are on MAT are generally encouraged to continue on buprenorphine or methadone throughout pregnancy. Transmucosal buprenorphine is the preferred formulation for pregnant women (Lexicomp, 2019). The pharmacokinetics of buprenorphine and methadone change as pregnancy progresses, and therefore, higher doses or more frequent dosing may be needed. After childbirth, the doses can be gradually tapered back down to prepregnancy doses.

Buprenorphine and its metabolite norbuprenorphine have been detected in low levels in breast milk although available data have not yet shown adverse events in infants who were breast-fed (possibly due to low oral bioavailability). Methadone is also excreted into breast milk with incidences of infant respiratory depression and sedation. Weaning breast-fed infants gradually to prevent withdrawal may be necessary (Bostwick et al., 2019). Infants of patients receiving buprenorphine or methadone should be monitored for breathing difficulties and respiratory depression.

Nonpharmacologic

Nonpharmacologic treatments are recommended for the treatment of pain in conjunction with both non-opioid medications and MAT (see **Box 10.2**).

Cognitive behavioral therapy (CBT) is a psychotherapy that helps patients change negative and maladaptive thoughts about pain with the goal of reducing and gaining better functioning and coping skills. It involves multiple intensive sessions and has been found to be efficacious in patients with chronic pain. During CBT, patients are able to learn techniques to transition their thoughts away from pain and lessen the exacerbation of symptoms that they may be experiencing through pain-related coping mechanisms (Lemmon & Hampton, 2018).

Examples of exercise-based therapy include tai chi, yoga, and therapeutic exercise. Each of these therapies has evidence to support the treatment of common causations of pain such as knee osteoarthritis, chronic lower back pain, and fibromyalgia. As with medications, different nonpharmacologic treatment options have greater efficacy for different conditions. For example, tai chi, with its low impact and flowing movements, was found to be an effective treatment of knee osteoarthritis, but lower-quality evidence of improvement in the chronic low back pain and fibromyalgia (Lemmon, 2018). Complementary modalities include treatment options such as spinal manipulative therapy, massage therapy, and acupuncture. One of the most important things to remember when considering nonpharmacologic options is to use a combination of alternative treatments.

MONITORING PATIENT RESPONSE

Self-reported pain and utilization of "as needed" medications for treatment should be reassessed at all subsequent visits. Discuss and manage any side effects that the patient may be experiencing. Patient's quality of life should also be considered. The 5 A's of analgesia can be applied to assess pain as well as response to treatment (see **Box 10.3**). In patients with OUD, it is important to evaluate for cravings and/or for the need to use more medication than prescribed. Verifying pharmacy fills through a PDMP may be helpful in monitoring adherence in some cases, although methadone obtained from a clinic will not be documented in this system. Random urine drug screens

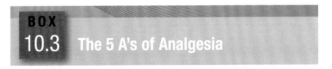

BOX 10.2 Nonpharmacologic Treatment Options for Pain

Other Nonpharmacologic Treatment Options for Pain

- Acupuncture
- Hypnosis
- Massage Therapy
- Meditation
- Transcutaneous Electrical Nerve Stimulation
- Mindfulness

BOX 10.3 The 5 A's of Analgesia

- Analgesia
  - How well is therapy working? How much pain relief is achieved with current dosing?
- Adverse Reactions
  - Constipation, nausea, dizziness, drowsiness, confusion
- Aberrant Behaviors
  - Are medications being taken as prescribed? Have there been lost prescriptions and early refills requested?
- Activity of Daily Living
  - Has the patient's function improved on therapy?
- Affect
  - Is pain impacting mood? Is there concurrent depression/anxiety?

can be conducted using immunoassays. Confirmatory testing will need to be completed for unexpected results.

PATIENT EDUCATION

Patients must be educated on proper administration of their pain medication. Common side effects should be discussed with patients and follow-up appointments established. Encourage patients to report increased or recurring pain at their follow-up appointments. Patients can also be educated on drug take-back programs (DEA, 2020). These programs help reduce the quantity of circulating opioids by promoting and making accessible the return of unused prescriptions. Resources on pain management and OUD should be provided to patient. Instruct patients to keep an opioid reversal agent such as naloxone (Narcan®) in the household. Educate on the proper administration of this medication to the patient and their family members.

APPENDIX 10-1

Bibliography

Starred references are cited in the text.

*Alford, D. P., Compton, P., & Samet, J. H. (2006). Acute pain management for patients receiving maintenance methadone or buprenorphine therapy. *Annals of Internal Medicine, 144*(2), 127. doi: 10.7326/0003-4819-144-2-200601170-00010

Bonnie, R. J., Ford, M. A., & Phillips, J. K. (2017). Pain management and the opioid epidemic: Balancing societal and individual benefits and risks of prescription opioid use. Consensus Study Report. National Academies of Sciences, Engineering, and Medicine. doi: 10.17226/24781

*Bostwick, J., Carnahan, R., Cole, T., et al. (2019). *2020–2021 Psychiatric pharmacotherapy review.* Lincoln, NE: College of Psychiatric and Neurologic Pharmacists.

*Butler, S. F., Fernandez, K., Benoit, C., et al. (2008). Validation of the revised screener and opioid assessment for patients with pain (SOAPP-R). *The Journal of Pain, 9*(4), 360–372. doi: 10.1016/j.jpain.2007.11.014

Centers for Disease Control and Prevention. (2017). What states need to know about PDMPs. https://www.cdc.gov/drugoverdose/pdmp/states.html

Cheattle, M. D. (2019). Risk assessment: Safe opioid prescribing tools. Retrieved from https://www.practicalpainmanagement.com/resource-centers/opioid-prescribing-monitoing/risk-assessment-safe-opioid-prescribing-tools on March 10, 2020.

*Chou, R., Cruciani, R. A., Fiellin, D. A., et al. (2014). Methadone safety: A clinical practice guideline from the American pain society and college on problems of drug dependence, in collaboration with the heart rhythm society. *The Journal of Pain, 15*(4), 321–337. doi: 10.1016/j.jpain.2014.01.494

Cosio, D., & Lin, E. H. (2020). Behavioral medicine: How to incorporate into pain management. Retrieved from https://www.practicalpainmanagement.com/treatments/psychological/cognitive-behavioral-therapy/behavioral-medicine-how-incorporate-pain

Davis, M. P. (2012). Twelve reasons for considering buprenorphine as a frontline analgesic in the management of pain. *The Journal of Supportive Oncology, 10*(6), 209–219. doi: 10.1016/j.suponc.2012.05.002

*DEA National RXTake Back Day. (2020). Retrieved from https://takeback-day.dea.gov/ on March 18, 2020.

Dowell, D., Haegerich, T. M., & Chou, R. (2016). CDC guideline for prescribing opioids for chronic pain—United States, 2016. *MMWR Recommendations and Reports, 65*(1), 1–49. doi: 10.15585/mmwr.rr6501e1

*Feder, K. A., Krawczyk, N., & Saloner, B. (2017). Medication-assisted treatment for adolescents in specialty treatment for opioid use disorder. *Journal of Adolescent Health, 60*(6), 747–750. doi: 10.1016/j.jadohealth.2016.12.023

*Indivior Inc. (2019). *Suboxone (buprenorphine and naloxone): Highlights of prescribing information.* Warren, NJ: Author.

Kampman, K., & Jarvis, M. (2015). American Society of Addiction Medicine (ASAM) National Practice Guideline for the use of medications in the treatment of addiction involving opioid use. *Journal of Addiction Medicine, 9*(5), 358–367. doi: 10.1097//adm.0000000000000166

*Koob, G. F. (2020). Neurobiology of opioid addiction: Opponent process, hyperkatifeia, and negative reinforcement. *Biological Psychiatry, 87*(1), 44–53. doi: 10.1016/j.biopsych.2019.05.023

*Krsak, M., Trowbridge, P., Regan, N., et al. (2017). Buprenorphine with, or without, Naloxone for pregnant women? Review of current evidence and practice in Massachusetts. *Journal of Alcoholism and Drug Dependence, 5*(3), 1–5, doi: 10.4172/2329-6488.1000269

*Kumar, R. (2020, February 27). Buprenorphine. Retrieved from https://www.ncbi.nlm.nih.gov/books/NBK459126/#_article-18708_s10_ on March 17, 2020.

*Lemmon, R., & Hampton, A. (2018). Nonpharmacologic treatment of chronic pain: What works? *The Journal of Family Practice, 67*(8), 474–477, 480–483.

*Lexicomp Online. (2021). Lexicomp: Evidence-based drug referential solutions. Retrieved from http://www.wolterskluwercdi.com/lexicomp-online/ on December 27, 2019.

Lingford-Hughes, A., Welch, S., Peters, L., et al. (2012). BAP updated guidelines: Evidence-based guidelines for the pharmacological management of substance abuse, harmful use, addiction and comorbidity—Recommendation from BAP. *Journal of Psychopharmacology, 26*(7), 899–952.

Macintyre, P. E., Russell, R. A., Usher, K. A. N., et al. (2013). Pain relief and opioid requirements in the first 24 hours after surgery in patients taking buprenorphine and methadone opioid substitution therapy. *Anaesthesia and Intensive Care, 41*(2), 222–230. doi: 10.1177/0310057x1304100212

Malinoff, H. L., Barkin, R. L., & Wilson, G. (2005). Sublingual buprenorphine is effective in the treatment of chronic pain syndrome. *American Journal of Therapeutics, 12*(5), 379–384. doi: 10.1097/01.mjt.0000160935. 62883.ff

*Marquez, P., Borse, J., Nguyen, A., et al. (2008). The role of the opioid receptor-like (ORL1) receptor in motor stimulatory and rewarding actions of buprenorphine and morphine. *Neuroscience, 155*(3), 597–602. doi: 10.1016/j.neuroscience.2008.06.027

Mitra, S., & Sinatra, R. S. (2004). Perioperative management of acute pain in the opioid-dependent patient. *Anesthesiology, 101*(1), 212–227. doi: 10.1097/00000542-200407000-00032

National Institute on Drug Abuse. (2017, July 31). Pain relief most reported reason for misuse of opioid pain relievers. Retrieved from https://www.drugabuse.gov/news-events/news-releases/2017/07/pain-relief-most-reported-reason-misuse-opioid-pain-relievers on December 20, 2019.

Norton, M. (2018). *The pharmacists guide to opioid use disorder.* Bethesda, MD: American Society of Health-System Pharmacists.

Rosen, K., Gutierrez, A., Haller, D., et al. (2014). Sublingual buprenorphine for chronic pain: A survey of clinician prescribing practices. *The Clinical Journal of Pain, 30*(4), 295–300.

Rosenblum, A., Cruciani, R., & Strain, E. (2012). Sublingual buprenorphine/naloxone for chronic pain in at-risk patients: Development and pilot test of a clinical protocol. *Journal of Opioid Management, 8*(6), 369–382. doi: 10.5055/jom.2012.0137

Roux, P., Sullivan, M. A., Cohen, J., et al. (2013). Buprenorphine/naloxone as a promising therapeutic option for opioid abusing patients with chronic pain: Reduction of pain, opioid withdrawal symptoms, and abuse liability of oral oxycodone. *Pain, 154*(8), 1442–1448.

*Standridge, J. B., Adams, S. M., & Zotos, A. P. (2010, March 1). Urine drug screening: A valuable office procedure. Retrieved from https://www.aafp.org/afp/2010/0301/p635.html

Substance Abuse and Mental Health Services Administration. (2019). *2018 National Survey on Drug Use and Health: Methodological summary and definitions.* Rockville, MD: Center for Behavioral Health Statistics and

Quality, Substance Abuse and Mental Health Services Administration. Retrieved from https://www.samhsa.gov/data/

TIP 63 Part 3: Pharmacotherapy for Opioid Use Disorder. (2018). Medications for opioid use disorder. Retrieved from https://store.samhsa.gov/system/files/sma18-5063pt3.pdf on December 20, 2019.

*U.S. Department of Health and Human Services. (2019). *What is the U.S. opioid epidemic?* Retrieved from https://www.hhs.gov/opioids/about-the-epidemic/index.html

U.S. Department of Health and Human Services, Substance Abuse and Mental Health Services Administration, Center for Substance Abuse Treatment. (2011). *Managing chronic pain in adults with or in recovery from substance use disorders.* Rockville, MD.

*Wang, B.-T., Colby, J. M., Wu, A. H., et al. (2014). Cross-reactivity of acetylfentanyl and risperidone with a fentanyl immunoassay. *Journal of Analytical Toxicology, 38*(9), 672–675. doi: 10.1093/jat/bku103

*Webster, L. R., & Webster, R. M. (2005). Predicting aberrant behaviors in opioid-treated patients: Preliminary validation of the opioid risk tool. *Pain Medicine, 6*(6), 432–442. doi: 10.1111/j.1526-4637.2005.00072.x

*Wesson, D. R., & Ling, W. (2003). The clinical opiate withdrawal scale (COWS). *Journal of Psychoactive Drugs, 35*(2), 253–259. doi: 10.1080/02791072.2003.10400007

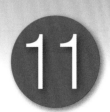

11 Cannabis and Pain Management

Andrew M. Peterson and Mily Shah

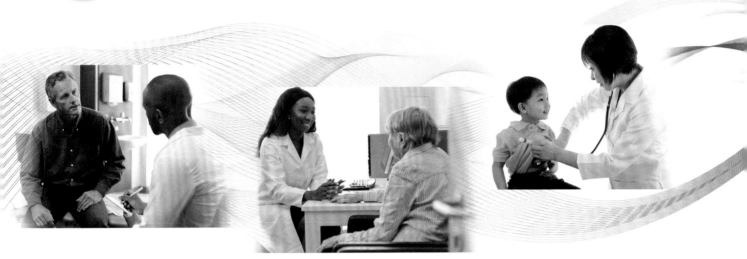

INTRODUCTION

Cannabis, more commonly known as marijuana, has a history that dates back more than 12,000 years. Throughout mankind's history, humans have cultivated cannabis for longer than any other plant. There is a common misconception of cannabis as a harmful substance of abuse, but in reality, it can be both good and bad. Cannabis can be used medicinally but can also cause harm if not used with the right knowledge. There are hundreds of chemicals in the cannabis plant, many of which act in the body by mimicking regulatory molecules that contribute to physiologic processes. Cannabis acts on the endocannabinoid system (ECS), a complex regulatory system with a broad function in the human body, which regulates pain, appetite, immunity, and other physiologic processes (Backes, 2014). This chapter reviews the basics of cannabis pharmacology and discusses the currently approved drugs derived from or mimicking chemicals in the cannabis plant.

CANNABIS

Cannabis as a Plant

The cannabis plant is comprised of many different structures (see **Figure 11.1**). Cannabis plants can be male, female, or both depending on the reproductive organs, but female plants produce the potent flowers that patients consume. Cannabis plants stem off a long branch called the node, and the male and the female both contain a cola. The cola is a cluster of buds that grow closely together, and the main cola grows at the top of the plant. The pistil of the plant contains the reproductive parts of the flower, and the hair-like strands that stem off from the pistil are known as the stigmas. Stigmas are found only on female plants and are used to collect the pollen from the male plants. The bract of the female plant is essential because it is covered in the resin glands. The resin glands produce the highest concentration of cannabinoids. On the cannabis bud, there is a layer of crystal resin; when it is dry, the resin is known as kief. The calyx is the layer over the ovule at the flower's base. The last part of the cannabis plant is the trichome. Trichomes were developed to protect the plant against the environment and predators; this resin creates an ooze, which is known as terpenes. The ooze also contains cannabinoids such as tetrahydrocannabinol (THC) and cannabidiol (CBD).

There are over 100 cannabinoids in the cannabis plant, and THC and CBD are currently the most studied compounds in health care. THC is the compound that produces the psychoactive effects, whereas CBD contains no psychoactive effects. There are currently three species identified: *Cannabis sativa*, *Cannabis indica*, and *Cannabis ruderalis*. *C. sativa* contains

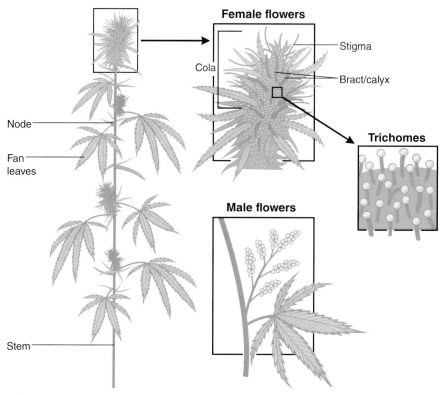

FIGURE 11–1   Structure of the cannabis plant.

higher levels of THC than CBD, whereas *C. indica* contains more CBD than THC.

Cannabis as Medicine

Cannabis and cannabinoids have been used to alleviate numerous symptoms and treat diseases. Cannabinoids have been studied in the treatment of chronic pain in patients with neuropathic pain, fibromyalgia, rheumatoid arthritis, and mixed chronic pain. Current evidence suggests that cannabinoids are safe, with minimal side effects, and are effective in the treatment of neuropathic pain, specifically fibromyalgia and rheumatoid arthritis.

Cannabinoids have also been studied as agents in alleviating chemotherapy-related nausea. A THC-based agent such as dronabinol has been approved for use as an antiemetic. Along with alleviating nausea, cannabis-based medicine has been used for treating epilepsy, multiple sclerosis (MS), Huntington's disease, and Tourette's. Medical cannabis has been used for a variety of conditions, including Alzheimer's disease, human immunodeficiency virus (HIV)/acquired immunodeficiency syndrome (AIDS), amyotrophic lateral sclerosis, cancer, inflammatory bowel disease, glaucoma, autoimmune disorders, Parkinson's disease, posttraumatic stress disorder (PTSD), autism, cachexia, chronic pain, migraine headaches, nausea and vomiting, seizure disorders, and muscle spasticity.

Cannabis's Legal Status

Between the 1800s and the 1900s, cannabis was widely used across multiple countries, including the United States. In 1850, cannabis was included in the U.S. pharmacopeia and was used to treat a wide variety of conditions ranging from chronic cough to gonorrhea. However, in the later 1800s, attitude toward the medical use of marijuana shifted, with the growth of opium and morphine abuse. While it did not specifically address marijuana, the enactment of the 1906 Pure Food and Drug Act took its toll on all mind-altering substances. Subsequently, in 1914 the Harrison Act made drug consumption a crime and by 1937, 23 states had outlawed the use of marijuana. Following this, the federal government passed the Marijuana Tax Act of 1937, which made nonmedical use of marijuana a crime. After World War II, the Boggs Act (1951) and Narcotics Control Act (1956) were passed, which introduced compulsory sentences for drug offenders. While there was a general relaxation in marijuana laws during the 1960s, largely associated with changing public perception, President Nixon introduced the Controlled Substances Act (CSA) in 1970, which classified marijuana as a Schedule 1 drug, deeming it to have a high potential for abuse and no accepted medical use. Today, the U.S. Drug Enforcement Agency (DEA) still considers marijuana a Schedule 1 drug under the CSA.

Prior to 2018, marijuana and hemp were often considered the same, as they both are under the cannabis umbrella. In 2018, Congress passed the Agricultural Improvement Act, also known as the 2018 Farm Bill, which separated, legally, marijuana and hemp. In this bill, any part or derivative of the *C. sativa* plant that contains less than 0.3% THC is considered hemp; anything over this is considered marijuana. Further, this bill amended the CSA, legalizing hemp and thus removing it from the DEA Schedule 1 classification.

As of January 2020, cannabis is legal for adult use in 11 states and the District of Columbia: Alaska, California, Colorado, Illinois, Maine, Massachusetts, Michigan, Nevada, Oregon, Vermont, and Washington. There are currently 33 states where medical marijuana is legal. This requires patients to sign up through the state, which allows them to purchase medical marijuana at an approved retail location. Due to regulatory implications, physicians are unable to legally prescribe medicinal marijuana due to its Schedule 1 classification. In accordance with the state law, physicians are only able to certify or recommend patients for medical marijuana treatment. As of July 2020, there were four states where marijuana remains completely illegal: Idaho, Kansas, Nebraska, and South Dakota.

PATHOPHYSIOLOGY

Refresher on the Pathophysiology of Pain

Pain itself is the end result of the central nervous system's processing stimuli. Pain can be classified as either nociceptive or neuropathic. Nociceptive pain is the pain secondary to an insult (chemical, thermal, or mechanical) to the body, resulting in nerve receptor stimulation. This can be either somatic or visceral, depending on the pain's origin. Inflammatory pain, another nociceptive subtype, is a result of cytokine release secondary to tissue injury and is often seen in chronic pain syndromes such as rheumatoid arthritis. Neuropathic pain, either peripheral or central, is caused by damage to the somatosensory nervous system. The abnormal pain signaling occurring due to the damaged nerves either increases the excitatory action or decreases the inhibitory action, and this leads to variation in the way pain messages are modulated in the central nervous system.

The molecular and biochemical processes involved in the transmission of pain signals to and from the central nervous system are often the target of drug therapy, since many drugs can enhance inhibitory pain signals or block excitatory pain signals. For more information, please see Chapter 9, "Principles of Pharmacology in Pain Management."

The Endocannabinoid System and Its Relationship to Pain

The ECS is a biological system recently discovered (in the early 1990s) and is composed of lipid-based endogenous neurotransmitters. Two such transmitters, anandamide and 2-arachidonoylglycerol (2-AG), have been fairly well characterized. These neurotransmitters act in a retrograde fashion; they are created in the postsynaptic neuron and bind to receptors on the presynaptic neuron. This mechanism creates a feedback loop to the sending neuron, thus regulating the release of neurotransmitters from the presynaptic neuron. The endocannabinoids are created "on demand"—that is, they are created in response to a need and then destroyed in the synapse once the need for them is abated. The ECS is found throughout the central and peripheral nervous systems, is found in most vertebrates, and is involved in maintaining homeostasis. Alterations in the ECS have been implicated in a variety of disease states, from immune-regulated diseases (e.g., rheumatoid arthritis) to neurological disorders such as epilepsy and MS.

Within the ECS are cannabinoid (CB) receptors located throughout the body. The two receptors most characterized are the CB1 and CB2 receptors. These receptors receive signals from the endocannabinoids and in turn transmit messages to the presynaptic neuron, regulating the release of other neurotransmitters. These receptors are of the G-coupled protein type and are the most commonly found receptors in the human body. The CB1 receptors are primarily located in the central nervous system, while the CB2 receptors are primarily located in the periphery, especially in the immune cells (**Figure 11.2**).

Activation of the CB1 receptor is linked to a decrease in the release of glutamate (an excitatory neurotransmitter) or a decrease in gamma-aminobutyric acid (GABA), an inhibitory neurotransmitter. The overall net effect is typically a reduction in the excitation of the postsynaptic neuron. Activation of the CB1 receptor has been associated with changes in pain perception, appetite stimulation, and memory/cognition changes. Anandamide appears to be the primary endogenous agonist of CB1 receptors. The exogenous cannabinoid THC interacts with the CB1 receptor but has a much lower affinity for the receptor than anandamide. In this respect, THC may be considered a *partial* agonist of the CB1 receptor. CBD has a low affinity for this receptor and may even act as an *antagonist*. Thus, THC may decrease the release of neurotransmitters presynaptically while CBD may increase them. The specific neurotransmitter is location and function dependent.

CB2 receptors are found more in the peripheral nervous system than in the central nervous system but have similar pharmacologic properties as the CB1 receptors. That is, they too are G-coupled receptors and regulate the release of neurotransmitters from presynaptic neurons. Activation of the CB2 receptors, depending on the peripheral organ, can have positive effects on pain, the immune system, and neurological disorders such as epilepsy. Anandamide has a high affinity for the CB2 receptor, but the endocannabinoid 2-AG has a higher affinity and these endogenous ligands serve as agonists

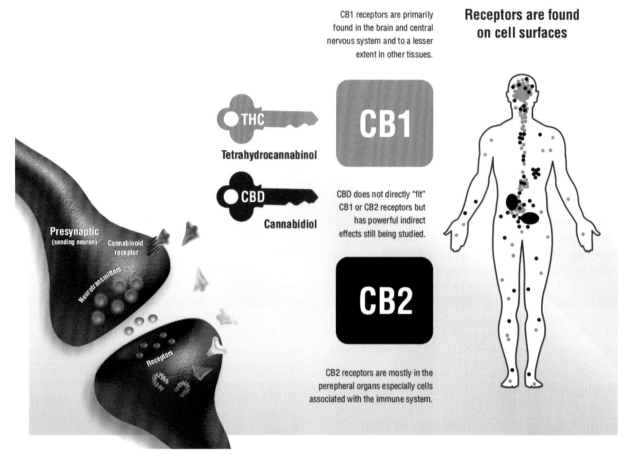

FIGURE 11–2 Structure and function of the endocannabinoid system.

CB1, cannabinoid 1; CB2, cannabinoid 2; CBD, cannabidiol.

at this receptor. Similar to the CB1 receptor, THC acts as a partial agonist to the CB2 receptor and CBD acts as an antagonist.

The components of the ECS can be found all along the pain pathway, from periphery to the brain. The ECS receptors are involved in the modulation of pain thresholds through inhibition or release of neurotransmitters involved in pain.

DIAGNOSTIC CRITERIA

As noted in Chapter 9, the diagnosis and assessment of pain is a complex process. Once the pain has been classified as nociceptive or neuropathic, the treatment modality can be better selected.

Discussion of Disease States Where Cannabis May Be Effective

Cannabis and cannabinoid derivatives are becoming more accepted in the treatment of disease or alleviation of symptoms. However, the data supporting their efficacy for specific

indications are not well established. In 2011, Lynch and Campbell published a systematic review of 18 randomized, controlled trials investigating the use of cannabinoids in the treatment of noncancer chronic pain such as neuropathic pain, fibromyalgia, and rheumatoid arthritis (Lynch & Campbell, 2011). The cannabinoids included smoked cannabis, oral cannabis-based medicine, nabilone, dronabinol, and a THC analogue, ajulemic acid. Fifteen of the 18 included trials demonstrated a significant analgesic effect of cannabinoids compared with the placebo. Cannabinoid use was generally well tolerated; adverse effects most commonly reported were mild to moderate in severity.

The National Academies of Sciences, Engineering and Medicine (NASEM) conducted a review of the literature surrounding the use of cannabis (NASEM, 2017). The NASEM report concluded that there is substantial or conclusive evidence regarding the efficacy of cannabis or cannabinoids in the treatment of chronic pain in adults, chemotherapy-induced nausea and/or vomiting, and spasticity symptoms in patients with MS. The report further asserted that there is moderate evidence that these agents are effective for short-term sleep disturbances in patients with fibromyalgia, sleep apnea syndrome, chronic pain, and MS. There was limited evidence reported or none reported on the efficacy of cannabis or cannabinoids in the treatment of all other diseases.

INITIATING DRUG THERAPY

Since marijuana/cannabis is a Schedule 1 drug, the focus of the rest of this chapter will be on the Food and Drug Administration (FDA)–approved cannabinoids. **Table 11.1** shows the FDA-approved cannabis products.

One of the key *mantras* used when treating patients with cannabis products is "start low, go slow." Depending on the product and the dose, the adverse effects of too high a dose may deter the user from adhering to treatment.

Goals of Drug Therapy

Given the focus of this chapter is on pain management using cannabinoids, it must be mentioned that the goals of drug therapy using these agents are the same as those of any other agent used to treat pain. With chronic pain, the goals of therapy are to decrease the pain to a tolerable level and improve

---

TABLE 11.1

Overview of Cannabis Drugs Approved by the U.S. Food and Drug Administration

Generic (Trade) Name and Adult Dosage	Selected Adverse Effects	Contraindications	Special Considerations
Cannabidiol (Epidiolex): The initial dose for the treatment of LGS or DS in patients ≥2 years of age is 2.5 mg/kg BID. May be increased to 5 mg/kg after 1 week, up to a maximum of 10 mg/kg BID.	Drowsiness, sedation, fatigue, sleep disturbances, including insomnia. GI disturbances, such as diarrhea and loss of appetite may occur.	Hypersensitivity to cannabidiol, sesame oil, or dehydrated alcohol. Individuals with severe liver disease may also be at risk for adverse effects.	Hepatic injury may occur (increased ALT/AST ~10%), typically in the first 2 months but has been seen in patients 18 months after initiation of treatment. Treatment should be discontinued if transaminase levels exceed 3 times the upper limit of normal or bilirubin levels are 2 times greater than normal
Dronabinol (Marinol): 2.5 mg before lunch and 2.5 mg before supper; chemotherapy-induced nausea and vomiting; an initial dose of Marinol is 5 mg/m^2 1–3 hours prior to the administration of chemotherapy. Syndros: 2.1 mg before lunch and dinner; chemotherapy-induced nausea and vomiting; 4.2 mg/m^2, 1 to 3 hours prior to the administration of chemotherapy.	Most common adverse reactions (≥3%) are abdominal pain, dizziness, euphoria, nausea, paranoid reaction, somnolence, thinking abnormal, and vomiting.	Contraindicated in any patient with a hypersensitivity to the active ingredient or any cannabinoid. For Marinol, patients with sensitivity to sesame oil and patients with a hypersensitivity to alcohol or taking disulfiram or metronidazole should not take Syndros because alcohol is used in its formulation.	Patients should be instructed not to crush, break, or chew the Marinol capsule.
Nabilone (Cesamet): Usual starting dose is 1–2 mg BID and can be increased to 2 mg TID, with a maximum dose of 6 mg daily (2 mg TID).	Euphoria, hypotension impaired cognition. Delayed adverse reactions include depression and ataxia. Less severe adverse reactions include drowsiness, headache, vertigo/dizziness, insomnia and/or fatigue, asthenia, and dry mouth.	Contraindicated in any patient with a cannabinoid hypersensitivity. Patients with psychiatric conditions (e.g., bipolar disorder, schizophrenia) should not receive this agent unless necessary because of the risk for exacerbating the psychotic disorder.	Caution in patients with cardiac conditions due to the tachycardia and orthostatic hypotension.

ALT, alanine aminotransferase; AST, aspartate aminotransferase; DS, Dravet syndrome; GI, gastrointestinal; LGS, Lennox-Gastaut syndrome.

function using a combination of various types of therapies to ultimately enhance quality of life.

Dronabinol

Dronabinol (Marinol, Syndros) is a synthetic THC product that is indicated for the treatment of anorexia associated with weight loss in patients with AIDS and for the treatment of chemotherapy-induced nausea and vomiting.

Mechanism of Action

Dronabinol, as a synthetic version of THC, has complex effects on the central nervous system, which may include partial agonism of the CB1 and CB2 receptors.

Dosage

Marinol is available in 2.5-mg, 5-mg, and 10-mg capsules. These capsules contain sesame oil as part of the formulation. Syndros is formulated as a 5-mg/mL oral solution, with 50% dehydrated alcohol.

For appetite stimulation and antiemetic effects, dosing of Marinol starts at 2.5 mg before lunch and 2.5 mg before supper. Syndros is administered at 2.1 mg before lunch and dinner. The maximum recommended dose of Syndros is 8.4 mg twice daily.

For treatment of chemotherapy-induced nausea and vomiting, the initial dose of Marinol is 5 mg/m^2 and that of Syndros is 4.2 mg/m^2, 1 to 3 hours prior to the administration of chemotherapy, then every 2 to 4 hours after chemotherapy. In both cases, the dose may be increased or decreased depending on the desired effect or undesired side effects, respectively.

Patients should be instructed not to crush, break, or chew the Marinol capsule.

Time Frame for Response

Dronabinol has an onset of action of 0.5 to 1 hour with a peak effect occurring at 2 to 4 hours. The appetite stimulation effect may continue for 24 hours after administration while the psychoactive effect lasts only about 4 to 6 hours.

Contraindications

Marinol is contraindicated in any patient with a hypersensitivity to the active ingredient, any cannabinoid, or sesame oil, which is used in the product's formulation. Patients with a hypersensitivity to alcohol, or taking disulfiram or metronidazole, should not take Syndros because alcohol is used in its formulation.

Patients taking dronabinol should be warned not to drive or operate machinery until they are able to tolerate the drug and to perform such tasks safely.

Adverse Events

Most common adverse reactions ($\geq 3\%$) are abdominal pain, dizziness, euphoria, nausea, paranoid reaction, somnolence, thinking abnormally, and vomiting.

Interactions

Dronabinol is primarily metabolized by the CYP2C9 and 3A4 systems, and thus one could presume drug–drug interactions with agents using one or more of these metabolic pathways. Thus, inhibitors or inducers of these enzymes can alter the systemic concentration of dronabinol, and caution must be taken when used concomitantly. However, dronabinol is not currently considered an inhibitor or inducer of either of these enzyme systems.

The Syndros formulation contains 50% (w/w) alcohol, and this formulation should be avoided in patients taking disulfiram (Antabuse) or metronidazole (Flagyl) since these agents inhibit the aldehyde dehydrogenase enzyme and can cause severe reactions (disulfiram-like reactions—cramps, nausea/vomiting, flushing).

Nabilone

Nabilone (Cesamet) is a synthetic derivative of THC, approved by the FDA for the treatment of nausea and vomiting associated with cancer chemotherapy in patients who have failed to respond adequately to conventional antiemetic treatments. Similar to dronabinol, nabilone has psychotomimetic reactions that are not normally observed with other antiemetic agents.

Mechanism of Action

As a synthetic analogue to THC, nabilone exerts its effects on the CB1 and CB2 receptors similarly. It acts as a partial agonist of the CB1 and CB2 receptors and thus would have similar effects.

Dosage

Nabilone is available orally as a 1-mg capsule. The usual starting dose is 1 to 2 mg twice daily, which can be increased to 2 mg thrice daily, with a maximum dose of 6 mg daily (2 mg thrice daily). For children under 18 kg, the dose is 0.5 mg twice daily and for children 18 to 30 kg, the dose is 1 mg twice daily. For those over 30 kg, the dose would be 1 mg thrice daily. The manufacturer does not report any adjustment for older adults or patients renally or hepatically impaired.

Time Frame for Response

After oral administration, the peak plasma level occurs in about 2 hours. The parent compound has a half-life of about 2 hours, while the half-life of the metabolites is about 35 hours. The activity of the metabolites has not been completely established, but it is speculated that they may play a role in the long duration of action of the agent.

Contraindications

Nabilone is contraindicated in any patient with a cannabinoid hypersensitivity. Further, it should be used with caution in patients with cardiac conditions because of tachycardia and the adverse effects of orthostatic hypotension associated with its use. In addition, patients with psychiatric conditions (e.g., bipolar disorder, schizophrenia) should not receive this agent unless necessary because of the risk of exacerbating the psychotic disorder.

Adverse Events

Early in treatment, euphoria and hypotension may occur, as well as impaired cognition. Delayed adverse reactions include depression, ataxia, and orthostatic hypotension. Less severe adverse reactions include drowsiness, headache, vertigo/dizziness, insomnia and/or fatigue, asthenia, and dry mouth.

Interactions

Nabilone is similar to THC; thus, the mechanism of metabolism is similar to that of THC and other cannabinoids. The nabilone prescribing information states that nabilone is extensively metabolized by multiple cytochrome P450 enzymes, including CYP3A4, CYP2E1, CYP2C9.

Cannabidiol (Epidiolex)

Cannabidiol (Epidiolex) is a 98% pure plant-derived oral CBD solution with an FDA-approved indication for the treatment of seizures associated with Lennox-Gastaut syndrome (LGS) or Dravet syndrome (DS) in pediatric patients 2 years of age and older. It is the first plant-derived cannabis product approved by the FDA and is considered a non-psychoactive cannabinoid.

Although it has not been evaluated in depth for the treatment of pain (as monotherapy), its antiinflammatory, anti-spasmodic benefits and good safety profile suggest that it could be an effective and safe analgesic. Due to the farm bill

of 2018, the over-the-counter market for CBD has exploded. See **Box 11.1** for more information.

Mechanism of Action

CBD is thought to have significant analgesic, antiinflammatory, anti-convulsant, and anxiolytic activities without the psychoactive effect of THC. CBD has very little affinity for the CB1 and CB2 receptors as an agonist but may serve as an antagonist, particularly in the presence of THC. CBD is thought to regulate the perception of pain by affecting the activity of other target receptors found in the ECS.

Dosage

Epidiolex comes in a 105-mL bottle of a 100-mg/mL solution. The initial dose for the treatment of LGS or DS in patients ≥2 years of age is 2.5 mg/kg twice daily. This dose may be increased to 5 mg/kg after 1 week, up to a maximum of 10 mg/kg twice daily. There are no dose adjustments for patients with renal or mild hepatic impairment. However, for those patients with moderate to severe hepatic impairment (Child-Pugh classification of B or C), the dose is adjusted to 1.25 mg/kg and 0.5 mg/kg twice daily, respectively.

Time Frame for Response

An oral dose peaks in 2.5 to 5 hours and the drug has a half-life of approximately 56 to 61 hours. Full response for treating LGS or DS is approximately 4 weeks. However, for the relief of pain, little clinical data is available. Animal models suggest that pain relief occurs after repeated dosing, and one expert suggests a time frame of up to a week before a response is seen (McNamara, 2018).

BOX 11.1   Caution Using Unregulated Cannabidiol

The 2018 farm bill is the first piece of federal legislation legalizing hemp and removing its DEA Schedule 1 controlled substance designation. However, the FDA notes that although hemp and products derived from hemp are no longer illegal substances under federal law, it remains a regulated product under the Food, Drug, and Cosmetic Act (FD&C Act). The agency bases their authority on the fact that CBD is an active ingredient in FDA-approved drugs and is subject to the FD&C Act. Therefore, any marketed cannabis product, including CBD derived from hemp, with a claim of therapeutic benefit must be approved by the FDA before it can be sold legally.

The FDA also states that adding CBD to food products or dietary supplements would be unlawful.

Despite these restrictions, many CBD products are being sold online and in pharmacies, food stores, health stores, and specialty cannabis shops. Because there are so many CBD products being produced and sold throughout the United

States, and none of them are federally regulated by the FDA, some of these products may be of questionable quality and safety. Further, there may be variability between products and batches with respect to quantity of active ingredient. Bonn-Miller and colleagues (2017) examined 84 CBD products from 31 companies. They found that nearly 43% contained 10% or more CBD than labeled (under-labeled), 31% were accurately labeled, and 26% were over-labeled. Therefore, the clinician must advise a patient using CBD from these sources that he or she cannot know for sure that the product purchased has the active ingredients as listed on the label and must advise that the product may contain other, in some cases, unknown elements.

Further, the clinician should inquire with the patient regarding his or her use of CBD products. Untold drug interactions and adverse effects may occur in the patient using these products without supervision and guidance.

CBD, cannabidiol; DEA, drug enforcement agency; FDA, Food and Drug Administration.

Contraindications

Epidiolex is contraindicated in patients with hypersensitivity to CBD or any of the inactive ingredients (sesame oil, dehydrated alcohol). Hypersensitivity reactions, including angioedema, erythema, and pruritus requiring antihistamines, have been reported. Individuals with severe liver disease may also be at risk for adverse effects.

Adverse Events

Drowsiness, sedation, fatigue, and lethargy are common in patients taking CBD. Other sleep disturbances, including insomnia, may occur. Gastrointestinal (GI) disturbances, such as diarrhea and loss of appetite, may occur. Hepatic injury may occur (increased alanine aminotransferase [ALT]/aspartate aminotransferase [AST] ~10%), typically in the first 2 months but has been seen in patients 18 months after initiation of treatment. Treatment should be discontinued if transaminase levels exceed 3 times the upper limit of normal or if bilirubin levels are 2 times greater than normal.

Interactions

CBD is metabolized by the CYP2C9, CYP2C19, CYP2D6, and CYP3A4 enzyme systems. CBD can inhibit the metabolism of medications metabolized by these systems and thus may increase the risk for adverse events. A reduction in the dose of medications metabolized by these systems should be considered when used concomitantly. Similarly, drugs inhibiting or inducing these enzymes may increase or decrease the level of CBD in the body, and thus dosage adjustments for CBD may be necessary.

Combination Treatment of Tetrahydrocannabinol and Cannabidiol (Sativex [Nabiximols])

Sativex, nabiximols, is available as a 1:1 combination of THC and CBD. It is a plant-derived oral mucosal spray formulation not yet available in the United States. Outside of the United States, nabiximols is indicated for the "symptom improvement in adult patients with moderate to severe spasticity due to multiple sclerosis (MS) who have not responded adequately to other anti-spasticity medication" (Sativex Prescribing Info, 2010).

Terpenes and Other Chemicals in Pain Management

Terpenes are the main constituents of essential oils and are commonly found in cannabis plants. Essential oils extracted from plants are the compounds that typically produce the plant's fragrance. The oil can come from any part of the plant, and sometimes different oils come from the same plant, just from different parts. Terpenes are the volatile hydrocarbons found in these oils and are the actual molecular compounds that give the plant its characteristic odor. For example, menthol is a terpene from the peppermint plant, and limonene can be found in orange peel and other citrus fruits.

Cannabis contains a variety of terpenes that contribute to the naming vernacular commonly referred to as *strain* names. Strains of cannabis often relate to the fragrance conferred by terpenes. However, the growing conditions and large genetic variability among strains thwart the creation of an accurate and reproducible chemotaxic classification based on terpene content. Nonetheless, many practitioners and patients rely on the terpene content of cannabis to confer the desired therapeutic effect.

The FDA has noted that many terpenes are generally recognized as safe (Smith et al., 2005). Terpenes can be pharmacologically active. They are lipophilic and interact with many different parts of a cell. Terpenes interact with cell membranes, neuronal and muscle ion channels, G-protein-coupled receptors, neurotransmitter receptors, and secondary messenger systems and enzymes (Russo, 2019). These terpenes include, but are not limited to, limonene, pinene, and myrcene. Cannabis products containing terpenes in concentrations above 0.05% are considered of pharmacological interest (Russo, 2011). **Box 11.2** lists the most common terpenes found in cannabis plants at pharmacologically relevant concentrations. When seen in these concentrations, terpenes can have anxiolytic, antiinflammatory, analgesic, and sedative effects. Terpenes are thought to have a synergistic effect with THC and/or CBD. This synergistic effect is often referred to as the *entourage effect* (Russo, 2011). The theory is supported by the evidence that isolated, non-plant-derived THC-based products (e.g., dronabinol or nabilone) may not have the same effects as the full plant (Russo, 2019).

Selecting the Most Appropriate Drug

As of the year 2020, use of marijuana—or any cannabis plant containing more than 0.3% THC—is illegal in the United States per federal law. While more than 50% of the states have some form of medical marijuana law allowing patients access to it, primary care practitioners should consider cannabis-based pain treatment only after sufficient trials of approved, proven treatments have been tried. And once that point has arrived, the patient needs to be certified by a medical practitioner (in most states, it is a physician) that the patient has an underlying condition that is on the state's list of approved conditions

BOX 11.2 Common Pharmacologically Active Terpenes Found in Cannabis Plants

Alpha-pinene
Beta-caryophyllene
Beta-myrcene
Limonene
Linalool

for medical marijuana use. After that certification, a patient may access a product by going to a dispensary.

The product selected clearly depends on the condition and the theoretical need for CBD, THC, and/or terpenes. In all cases, the mantra *start low, go slow* should always be kept in mind.

Special Considerations

Pediatric

CBD is used in pediatric patients 2 years or older. It is FDA approved for the treatment of seizures associated with LGS and DS. The most common adverse reactions are infection, somnolence, decreased appetite, diarrhea, fatigue, and elevated transaminases. Serum transaminases (ALT and AST) and total bilirubin levels should be monitored in all pediatric patients.

Geriatric

Medical marijuana should be used cautiously in geriatric populations due to the sedative properties of certain marijuana strains and should be initiated at the lower end of the dosing range.

Women

Although there is limited evidence regarding the use of marijuana during pregnancy, it is strongly recommended that women avoid its use while pregnant. Infants who are born from mothers who have been exposed to cannabis during pregnancy tend to have lower birth weight.

Ethnic

Cannabis dependence was found to be the greatest among blacks, mixed-race adults, and Native Americans (Wu et al., 2016).

Genomics

Minimal evidence has been published regarding pharmacogenomics and the association with cannabis. The opioid receptor mu 1 (*OPRM1*) gene encodes opioid receptors in humans and is associated with marijuana dependency. Patients with the AA genotype may be at an increased risk for developing dependence when compared to patients with the GG or AG genotype of the *OPRM1* gene (PharmGKB, 2016).

MONITORING PATIENT RESPONSE

There are various dosage forms of cannabis; inhalation results in the fastest onset of action (5–10 minutes) and the shortest duration of action (2–4 hours). There is difficulty in finding the safe therapeutic dose for each patient; therefore, it is recommended that prescribers start low and go slow when titrating

to ensure that the dose given is safe. It is recommended that physicians follow up with patients every 3 months to monitor for any complications or risks of abuse, diversion, or misuse.

PATIENT EDUCATION

Drug Information

Cannabis is a drug that affects most body systems. It produces anxiolytic, sedative, psychedelic, and analgesic properties and is also known to stimulate appetite in patients. Although it has a wide panel of effects, the side effects profile is mild.

Common adverse effects of cannabis include dizziness, reddened eyes, dry mouth, dysphoria, ataxia, sedation, changed visual perceptions, altered sense of time, and bronchitis.

The biggest effect of cannabis is the psychological effect that comes from THC. THC is the compound that produces the "high," which can ease anxiety and pain and produce the psychedelic feeling. The high can cause perceptual changes that may make colors seem brighter and music seem louder, and hallucinations can occur with higher doses of cannabis. The effects of cannabis on a patient's cognition is similar to the effects of alcohol and benzodiazepines. It can cause a slowing of reaction time, defects in short-term memory, motor incoordination, and a loss of attention. Patients should not operate a vehicle when under the influence of cannabis.

Tolerance has been studied in patients and has been shown to develop to the high as well as other effects that cannabis causes in a patient. Increase in tolerance can cause patients to increase the dosage. Cannabis use disorder (CUD) can occur and is diagnosed as other use disorders per the *Diagnostic and Statistical Manual of Mental Disorders, Fifth Edition* (*DSM-5*) criteria (Patel & Marwaha, 2020). The prevalence of dependence peaks in the age group of 20 to 24 and decreases with age. Withdrawal symptoms of cannabis are similar to those of alcohol and benzodiazepine and can include insomnia, anxiety, restlessness, and increased aggression.

Patient-Oriented Information Sources

Most states with approved medical marijuana programs have a Web site dedicated to providing additional information for the patient. Major reputable health Web sites also include patient information regarding medical cannabis. One such example is Americans for Safe Access (see https://www.safeaccessnow.org/resources_for_patients).

Nutrition or Lifestyle Changes

Cannabis use can lead to increased appetite and increased somnolence and fatigue. *C. indica* is known to stimulate appetite and promote relaxation and sleep. *C. sativa* is known to promote a more euphoric and uplifting experience and also increase energy in the user. Dronabinol (Marinol) is an oral form of THC that is clinically used for the treatment of anorexia and weight loss in patients with HIV infection.

CASE STUDY 1

H.P. is a 67-year-old female with a history of hypertension, high cholesterol, and chronic neuropathic pain. She currently takes the following:
– Atenolol 50 mg daily
– Simvastatin 40 mg daily
– Tramadol 100 mg extended-release twice daily

She receives dronabinol (off-label use) for chronic neuropathic pain at a dose of 5 mg in the morning and 2.5 mg at lunch.

1. What concerns do you have?
2. What are the potential drug interactions?
3. H.P. calls 4 days later and tells you she is experiencing dry mouth, dysphoria, ataxia, sedation, changed visual perceptions, and an altered sense of time. What do you do?

Bibliography

Starred references are cited in the text.

Andreae, M. H., Carter, G. M., Shaparin, N., et al. (2015). Inhaled cannabis for chronic neuropathic pain: A meta-analysis of individual patient data. *Journal of Pain, 16*(12), 1121–1232.

Backes, M. (2014). *Cannabis Pharmacy: The Practical Guide to Medical Marijuana.* New York: Black Dog & Leventhal Publishers.

Berry, E. M., & Mechoulam, R. (2002). Tetrahydrocannabinol and endocannabinoids in feeding and appetite. *Pharmacology & Therapeutics, 95,* 185–190.

*Bonn-Miller, M. O., Loflin, M. J. E., Thomas, B. F., et al. (2017). Labeling accuracy of cannabidiol extracts sold online. *JAMA, 318,* 1708–1709.

Fitzcharles, M. A., Ste-Marie, P. A., Hauser, W., et al. (2016). Efficacy, tolerability, and safety of cannabinoid treatments in the rheumatic diseases: A systematic review of randomized controlled trials. *Arthritis Care and Research, 68*(5), 681–688.

Goncalves, J., Rosado, T., Soares, S., et al. (2019). Cannabis and its secondary metabolites: Their use as therapeutic drugs, toxicological aspects and analytical determination. *Medicines (Basel), 6*(1), 31.

Leafly Cannabis Anatomy. https://www.leafly.com/news/cannabis-101/cannabis-anatomy-the-parts-of-the-plant. Accessed on June 13, 2020.

Leafly Where Is Cannabis Legal? https://www.leafly.com/news/cannabis-101/where-is-cannabis-legal. Accessed on June 13, 2020.

*Lynch, M. E., & Campbell, F. (2011). Cannabinoids for treatment of chronic noncancer pain: A systematic review of randomized trials. *British Journal of Clinical Pharmacology, 72,* 735–744.

*McNamara, D. (2018). Repeated CBD doses required for effective pain relief. Medscape. https://www.medscape.com/viewarticle/904290

Mouhamed, Y., Vishnyakov, A., Qorri, B., et al. (2018). Therapeutic potential of medicinal marijuana: An educational primer for health care professionals. *Drug, Healthcare and Patient Safety, 10,* 45–66.

*National Academies of Sciences, Engineering, and Medicine (NASEM). (2017). *The health effects of Cannabis and Cannabinoids: The current state of evidence and recommendations for research.* Washington, DC: The National Academies Press. https://doi.org/10.17226/24625

*Patel, J., & Marwaha, R. (2020). *Cannabis use disorder.* [Updated June 24, 2020]. In StatPearls [Internet]. Treasure Island (FL): StatPearls Publishing; 2020 Jan-. https://www.ncbi.nlm.nih.gov/books/NBK538131/

*PharmGKB. (2016). Clinical Annotation for rs1799971 (OPRM1); cannabinoids; Marijuana Abuse (level 4 Toxicity/ADR). https://www.pharmgkb.org/disease/PA443602/clinicalAnnotation/1450823791. Accessed on June 5, 2020.

Richards, B. L., Whittle, S. L., Van Der Heijde, D. M., et al. (2012). Efficacy and safety of neuromodulators in inflammatory arthritis: A Cochrane systematic review. *Journal of Rheumatology, 39*(Suppl 90), 28–33.

*Russo, E. B. (2011). Taming THC: Potential cannabis synergy and phytocannabinoid-terpenoid entourage effects. *British Journal of Pharmacology, 163,* 1344–1364.

*Russo, E. B. (2019). The case for the entourage effect and conventional breeding of clinical cannabis: No "strain," no gain. *Frontiers in Plant Science, 9,* 1969–1976.

Safe Access Now. Resources for patients. https://www.safeaccessnow.org/resources_for_patients. Accessed on June 5, 2020.

*Sativex. UK Prescribing info. (2010). GW Pharma Ltd. https://www.medicines.org.uk/emc/product/602/smpc

Smith, R.L., Cohen, S.M., Doull, J., et al. (2005). GRAS Flavoring Substances 22. *Food Technology, 59*(8), 24-62.

Snedecor, S. J., Sudharshan, L., Cappelleri, J. C., et al. (2013). Systematic review and comparison of pharmacologic therapies for neuropathic pain associated with spinal cord injury. *Journal of Pain Research, 6,* 539–547.

Whiting, P. F., Wolff, R. F., Deshpande, S., et al. (2015). Cannabinoids for medical use: A systematic review and meta-analysis. *JAMA, 313*(24), 2456–2473.

*Wu, L. T., Zhu, H., & Swartz, M. S. (2016). Trends in cannabis use disorders among racial/ethnic population groups in the United States. *Drug and Alcohol Dependence, 165,* 181–190.

UNIT

3

Pharmacotherapy for Skin Disorders

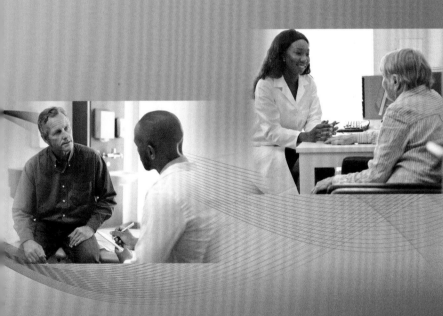
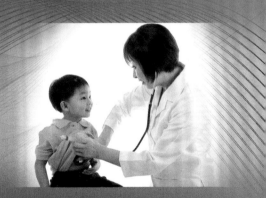

12 Contact Dermatitis

Jeffrey Tagle and Virginia P. Arcangelo

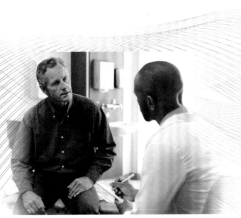
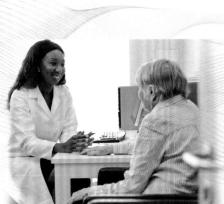
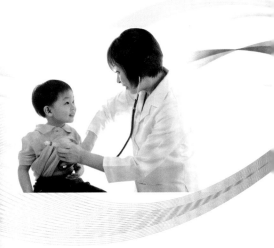

Learning Objectives

1. Identify the differences in the causes and the patho-physiology of contact dermatitis and atopic dermatitis.
2. Differentiate the symptoms of each disease state to appropriately diagnose a patient.
3. Compare available treatment options to treat dermatitis.
4. Formulate a treatment plan for a patient who presents with symptoms of dermatitis.

INTRODUCTION

Contact dermatitis (CD) is defined as any skin disorder caused by exposure to a substance that elicits an allergic or irritant response. This inflammatory reaction can occur after a single exposure or multiple exposures to an agent or in response to an allergen. According to the American Academy of Dermatology, CD is a common problem and results in approximately 5.7 million visits to health care providers each year. CD is also prevalent in occupational settings and can be a significant cause of workplace disability. CD is divided into irritant contact dermatitis (ICD) and allergic contact dermatitis (ACD). ICD is more common, especially in the occupational setting. About 80% of cases of occupational dermatitis are attributed to ICD. ACD is also prevalent, affecting about 20% of the general adult population.

Atopic dermatitis (AD), also known as eczema, is a form of allergic dermatitis characterized as a pruritic, chronic inflammatory condition. AD affects about 12% of children and 7% of adults.

CAUSES

As previously mentioned, CD occurs after exposure to an offending agent. ICD results from exposure to chemical stimuli that has a toxic effect on the skin. Examples of offending agents include hand soap and hydrofluoric acid from chemical plants. ACD results from exposure to an antigen that causes an immunologic response. A prime example of ACD is a reaction from exposure to poison ivy.

Many factors play a role in AD, including generic, immunologic, and environmental factors, which all lead to dysfunctional skin barrier and dysregulation of the immune system.

PATHOPHYSIOLOGY

In ICD, exposure to the offending agent results in release of proinflammatory cytokines from the keratinocytes. This leads to skin barrier disruption and epidermal cellular changes, causing damage to the water–protein–lipid matrix of the outer layer of skin.

ACD is T-cell mediated and requires initial activation of the innate immune system. This reaction occurs in two phases: the sensitization phase and the elicitation phase. During the sensitization phase, first contact of the antigen with the skin leads to activation of skin cells, most importantly the epidermal Langerhans cells and dermal dendritic cells. These cells migrate to local lymph nodes and present the antigens to naïve T-cells. This leads to proliferation of contact-allergen-specific T-cells and differentiation into effector T-cells, which further distribute throughout the blood. During the elicitation phase, repeated skin exposure to the antigen induces inflammation, and these effector T-cells are recruited to the site of inflammation, which leads to the clinical symptoms of ACD.

The complex pathogenesis of AD involves genetic factors, skin barrier defects, and immune dysregulation. The filaggrin gene is responsible for encoding FLG (fillagrin protein), which is a structural protein in the stratum corneum. Mutations in this gene impair skin barrier function, leading to an increased risk for AD. This disruption in the epidermis and environmental triggers lead to stimulation of keratinocytes, which release cytokines (interleukins, chemokines, and lymphopoietins), which in turn activate dendritic and Langerhans cells. In the acute phase, these play a role in suppression of antimicrobial peptide (AMP) production and itching. In the chronic stages of AD, other T-helper cells release certain cytokines that result in epidermal thickening and abnormal keratinocyte proliferation.

PHARMACOGENOMICS

There is ongoing research looking into gene expression and proteomics that will assist in the identification of biomarkers to help improve diagnosis and treatment of dermatitis, namely in ACD and AD. Clinical appearance of ACD can be similar for different allergens, but the underlying immune responses can be different. Inflammation and skin barrier–related genes and proteins are differentially regulated in all studies, but the challenge is to identify biomarkers that allow for the differentiation among ACD, ICD, and other forms of dermatitis.

Various risk factors have been identified in AD, but only family history of atopy and loss-of-function mutations in the FLG gene have been strongly associated with the development of AD. Allergen-specific serum immunoglobulin E (IgE) levels are nonspecific, since they are found in 55% of the U.S. population and may also be elevated in other nonatopic conditions. There is ongoing research looking into different T-lymphocyte subsets, chemokines, and cytokines as reliable biomarkers. Once novel biomarkers are identified, this may lead to identification of targeted drug therapy.

DIAGNOSTIC CRITERIA

The typical symptoms of ICD include burning, itching, stinging, soreness, and pain on presentation. In contrast, pruritus is more commonly associated with ACD. In both types of CD, there are three phases of morphological patterns during which the patient may present: acute, subacute, and chronic. In the acute phase, erythema, edema, oozing, crusting, tenderness, vesicles, or pustules are common. In the subacute phase, crusts, scales, and hyperpigmentation are often present. In the chronic phase, lichenification is most common. Visual symptoms are mostly scattered in appearance or present on the hands or face. It is important to obtain a complete history regarding the patient's occupation, hobbies, and any topicals or oral medications that the patient takes or uses, including any cosmetics and jewelry the patient wears. This may help identify any possible allergens or irritants that contribute to the patient's symptoms. Patch testing is the gold standard to confirm a diagnosis of

ACD, where the allergens are placed on the patient's back and the results are interpreted after 48 to 72 hours. The local allergic reaction is graded from negative to extreme reaction.

Features typically present in AD include pruritus and eczema and are commonly seen at an early age, although patients may develop symptoms later on in life. Dry skin (xerosis) is also fairly common. Nonspecific symptoms include atypical vascular responses (facial pallor, delayed blanch response), ocular changes, and lichenification. In infants and children, symptoms are common in the face, neck, and extensor areas. In adolescents and adulthood, symptoms appear in the flexural areas.

Other skin conditions, such as scabies, cutaneous T-cell lymphoma, psoriasis, immune deficiency diseases, and photosensitivity dermatoses, should be excluded from the differential diagnosis.

INITIATING DRUG THERAPY

The most effective form of treatment is prevention. Once the allergen or irritant has been identified, the patient must become aware of the causes or triggers and either avoid the allergen and/or irritant or use appropriate skin protection. The use of personal protective equipment such as gloves, goggles, or uniforms in the occupational setting is helpful.

Cool compresses may offer relief from itching. Colloidal oatmeal baths, calamine lotion, and Burow solution are effective for drying the vesicles and bullae that may be associated with CD. If these treatments fail or if the dermatitis is more extensive, drug therapy is initiated.

Before initiating drug therapy, delivery of the drug to the skin, protection/barrier function, and cosmetic acceptability must be considered. Ointment and gels offer the best delivery and protection barrier. Creams are less greasy but less effective. Lotions are dilute creams. Solutions are alcohol-based liquids and are useful for treating the scalp because they do not coat the hair.

Lipid-rich moisturizers increase skin hydration and help protect the barrier function of the skin.

Barrier creams containing dimethicone or perfluoropolyethers, cotton liners, and softened fabrics also help to protect the skin from irritants.

Goals of Drug Therapy

The goals of drug therapy for dermatitis are as follows:

- Restoration of a normal epidermal barrier
- Treatment of inflammation of skin
- Control of itching

Topical agents are the mainstay of AD, although they may be considered for off-label use in CD as well. Therefore, many therapeutic options for AD and CD overlap. Topical corticosteroids (TCSs) are used as first-line therapy in AD and are also used in the treatment of acute and chronic CD. Topical calcineurin inhibitors (TCI), such as tacrolimus or pimecrolimus, are immunosuppressants and are mostly used for AD. Systemic therapy is recommended for widespread symptoms, although it should not be used long term due to adverse effects. Antihistamines are used for relieving intense pruritus.

Nonpharmacologic Therapy

Moisturizers are recommended to prevent xerosis (dry skin) and transepidermal water loss. Emollients, occlusive agents, and humectants are ingredients in moisturizers that provide benefits. Emollients help lubricate and soften the skin, occlusive agents prevent evaporation of water, and humectants attract and retain water. Moisturizers should be helpful in patients with mild dermatitis but should also be considered as adjunct therapy in patients with moderate and severe dermatitis. They also should be used as maintenance therapy and to prevent flare-ups in AD. Bathing may be helpful, although no specific bathing practice has been shown to be beneficial. Limited use of neutral-low pH, hypoallergenic, and fragrance-free cleansers is also recommended. The patient should be instructed to use moisturizers after bathing to prevent water loss.

Wet-wrap therapy (WWT) involves using a topical agent that is covered by an initial wet layer, consisting of either gauze or bandages, and a secondary dry layer. This may help increase penetration of the topical agent and also provides protection to the skin. Phototherapy can be considered as an option for treatment in AD after the use of moisturizers, TCSs, and TCIs.

Topical Corticosteroids

TCSs act on immune cells to interfere with antigen processing and suppress the release of cytokines, thereby reducing inflammation. TCSs are the first-line topical agents in AD and may be considered in patients with localized lesions in CD. They may also be used to prevent flares in AD. Patients with more localized disease and failure to respond to adequate skin care and use of moisturizers may benefit from the addition of TCSs. The selection of TCSs is generally based on age, area of the body that is affected, patient preference in the type of vehicle, and cost.

Dosage

TCSs are classified according to potency (**Table 12.1**), from very low to very high potency. There is no recommended dosing strategy to use. Some practitioners utilize a short burst of high-potency TCSs, followed by a quick taper in potency. Others utilize low-potency TCSs titrated upward based on response to therapy. Low-potency TCSs should be used in the facial and intertriginous regions because medium- and high-potency corticosteroids applied to the face may cause atrophy of the tissue or trigger steroidal rosacea. Higher-potency steroids should be reserved for the extremities and torso. TCSs may be applied once or twice daily to the affected area of dermatitis.

In CD, TCSs should be used for the shortest possible duration. Prolonged periods of their use in the treatment of CD should be avoided. For acute flares in AD, TCSs are recommended every day until lesions have improved. To prevent further flares, TCSs once or twice a week can reduce the rate of flares.

Preparations

TCSs are available in creams, ointments, lotions, gels, solutions, or sprays. Creams are the most desirable because they are

TABLE 12.1
Classification of Topical Corticosteroids by Potency

Low Potency	Medium Potency	High Potency	Very High Potency
Alclometasone dipropionate 0.05% (c, o)	Betamethasone valerate 0.1% (c, f, l, o)	Amcinonide 0.1% (c, l, o)	Betamethasone dipropionate augmented 0.05% (o)
Desonide 0.05% (c, g, f, o)	Clocortolone pivalate 0.1% (c)	Betamethasone dipropionate augmented 0.05% (c)	Clobetasol propionate 0.05% (c, f, o)
Dexamethasone 0.1% (c)	Desoximetasone 0.05% (c)	Desoximetasone 0.05% (g), 0.25% (c, o)	Diflorasone diacetate 0.05% (o)
Fluocinolone acetonide 0.01% (c, s)	Fluocinolone acetonide 0.025% (c, o)	Diflorasone diacetate 0.05% (c)	Halobetasol propionate 0.05% (c, o)
Hydrocortisone 0.25%, 0.5%, 1% (c, l, o, s)	Flurandrenolide 0.05% (c, o)	Fluocinonide 0.05% (c, g, o, s)	
Hydrocortisone acetate 0.5%–1% (c, o)	Fluticasone propionate 0.05% (c), 0.005% (o)	Halcinonide 0.1% (c, o)	
	Mometasone furoate 0.1% (c)	Mometasone furoate 0.1% (o)	
	Triamcinolone acetonide 0.1% (c, o)	Triamcinolone acetonide 0.5% (c, o)	
	Lower-Medium Potency		
	Hydrocortisone butyrate 0.1% (c, o, s)		
	Hydrocortisone probutate 0.1% (c)		
	Hydrocortisone valerate 0.2% (c, o)		
	Prednicarbate 0.1% (c)		

c, cream; f, foam; g, gel; l, lotion; o, ointment; s, solution.

Used with permission from "Guidelines of care for the management of atopic dermatitis: Management and treatment of atopic dermatitis with topical therapies," by Eichenfield, L. F., Tom, W. L., Berger, T. G., et al. (2014a). *Journal of the American Academy of Dermatology, 71*(1), 116–132. Copyright 2014 by Elsevier Inc.

not as obvious when applied. They are, however, water based, which causes more skin drying. Ointments and gels are the most potent and the most lubricating, and they have occlusive properties. In areas with large amounts of hair or widespread dermatitis, lotions, gels, spray products, and solutions are easiest to apply. Occlusion by a dressing of an area of a TCS application increases hydration and hence penetration, thereby enhancing efficacy.

Application

There is no standard amount of TCS that should be applied, but the amount should be individualized to the patient. In general, an amount equal to the length from the fingertip to the distal interphalangeal joint is sufficient. Penetration of a TCS is enhanced when the skin is hydrated. This can be accomplished by moistening the skin before application or by using an occlusive dressing constructed from a material such as a plastic shower cap (for the scalp), gloves (for hands), or a plastic wrap or a sock (on other extremities).

Adverse Events

TCSs are generally safer than systemic corticosteroids, although some adverse events may occur. Adverse effects on the skin include purpura, telangiectasia, striae, focal hypertrichosis, and rosacea-like effects. Skin atrophy can occur in older patients, through use of TCSs on thin skin or use of higher-potency TCSs.

Although TCSs are applied to the skin, systemic effects may occur, especially with the use of high- and very high-potency agents for a prolonged period of time. The main adverse effect is hypothalamic–pituitary–adrenal axis suppression.

TCSs, or ingredients in their formulation, may also be a suspected allergen in CD and should be considered as a source of contact sensitization if lesions fail to respond or worsen despite therapy.

Topical Calcineurin Inhibitors

TCIs inhibit calcineurin-dependent T-cell activation, which prevents production of cytokines and other mediators that play a role in inflammation. They also play a role in mast cell activation. TCIs are typically used as second-line treatment in AD and may be used in immunocompetent patients with AD who cannot tolerate TCSs and are not responsive to other treatments or used when there is a concern for topical steroid–induced atrophy. Because they do not cause skin atrophy, these medications are especially useful for the treatment of AD involving the face, including the periocular and perioral areas. Use of TCSs and TCIs together to treat AD may also be considered. Efficacy in ACD and ICD has not been established yet.

Tacrolimus and pimecrolimus are the two preparations currently available. Tacrolimus is approved for use in moderate to severe AD, and pimecrolimus is approved for mild to moderate AD.

Dosage

Tacrolimus comes in ointments of 0.03% and 0.1% concentrations, whereas pimecrolimus comes in a 1% cream only. They are applied twice daily until the lesions and inflammation resolve. Prophylactic application 2 to 3 times a week to areas of recurrent disease may also be considered to prevent relapse. The skin is dried before application, but TCIs should not be used with occlusive dressings.

Contraindications

If patients experience hypersensitivity to TCIs, the agent should be discontinued. Caution is needed with use during acute infection, since these agents are immunosuppressants.

Adverse Effects

TCIs can cause transient burning and pruritus, which disappear with continued use or with short-term application of TCSs prior to use. More severe adverse effects include immunosuppression and, in rare cases, malignancy. Due to concerns of malignancy, the patient should limit sun exposure and use of sun protection is recommended.

Crisaborole

Crisaborole is a topical phosphodiesterase-4 (PDE-4) inhibitor that may be used in the treatment of mild to moderate AD. Through the inhibition of PDE-4, intracellular levels of cAMP are elevated and this plays a role in reducing inflammation. The place in therapy is not well known since this medication is still fairly new, having been approved in 2016. It's available as a 2% cream that can be applied twice daily to the affected area. The most common side effects include application site reactions, nasopharyngitis, and upper respiratory tract infections.

Topical Antimicrobials and Antiseptics

Patients with AD are susceptible to skin infections due to a compromised skin barrier. The prominent colonizer of the skin is *Staphylococcus aureus*. Despite this risk factor, there is no recommendation for the use of anti-staphylococcal treatment in patients with AD. If secondary infection is suspected, bleach baths and intranasal mupirocin may help reduce the severity of disease.

Antihistamines

Antihistamines are used to relieve pruritus associated with CD, especially allergic CD. Topical antihistamines have not been shown to help with AD. Antihistamines come in oral and topical preparations. The best time to use them is before bed to promote sleep because the main side effect is drowsiness. Antihistamines are discussed further in Chapter 46.

Systemic Corticosteroids

If the dermatitis is widespread or refractory to treatment with TCSs, TCIs, or phototherapy, oral systemic therapy may be used.

The first oral therapy option is corticosteroids, which should be reserved for refractory CD. Oral corticosteroids inhibit cytokine and mediator release, attenuate mucus secretion, upregulate beta-adrenergic receptors, inhibit IgE synthesis, decrease microvascular permeability, and suppress the influx of inflammatory cells and the inflammatory process.

Dosing

Corticosteroids should be prescribed at an initial dose of 1 mg/kg/d equivalent to prednisone and tapered down. The entire dose can be taken at the same time in the morning to minimize sleep disturbances. Taking corticosteroids for less than 2 weeks may cause rebound dermatitis, especially with poison ivy. If dermatitis flares up during the tapering, the dosage can be increased and tapered down again.

Contraindications

Because they suppress the immune response, systemic corticosteroids are contraindicated in patients with systemic fungal infections and in patients receiving a live or live attenuated vaccination. These drugs should also be used cautiously in people with tuberculosis, hypothyroidism, cirrhosis, renal insufficiency, hypertension, osteoporosis, and diabetes mellitus.

Adverse Effects

Systemic corticosteroids mask infection. In short-term use, they may cause gastrointestinal upset. Mood changes (hyperactivity, anxiety, depression) may be evident, and sleep disturbances may occur. The effects of systemic corticosteroids may be decreased if they are administered with barbiturates, hydantoins, or rifampin. For more information about systemic corticosteroids, refer to Chapter 25.

Other Systemic Therapy Options

Examples of other oral therapy options include cyclosporine, azathioprine, methotrexate, and mycophenolate. These four agents may be considered in refractory AD.

Cyclosporine is a calcineurin inhibitor. It inhibits production and release of interleukin II, which prevents activation of T-cells. Dosing is 150 to 300 mg daily in adults and 3 to 6 mg/kg/d in children. Adverse effects include renal impairment, hypertension, and infection. This agent should not be used in patients with active malignancy or impaired renal function.

Azathioprine is an immunosuppressant that produces metabolites that incorporate into deoxyribonucleic acid (DNA) and prevent replication. It also plays a role in inhibiting purine synthesis. Dosing is 1 to 3 mg/kg/d in adults and 1 to 4 mg/kg/d in children. If the patient is pregnant, this medication should only be used if the benefit outweighs the risk.

Methotrexate is a folate antimetabolite that binds to dihydrofolate reductase and thymidylate synthetase, which play a role in DNA synthesis, repair, and cell replication. The mechanism in skin disease is unknown, but it is thought to affect proliferation of epithelial cells. Dosing is 7.5 to 25 mg a week in adults and 0.2 to 0.7 mg/kg/wk in children. A test dose of 1.25 to 5 mg should be considered to assess if the patient can tolerate the medication. Many adverse effects are associated with methotrexate, including pulmonary fibrosis, cytopenia, and ulcerative stomatitis. This drug should not be used in pregnant patients or patients with liver disease.

Mycophenolate is an immunosuppressant that inhibits guanosine nucleotide synthesis, which affects the proliferation of T- and B-cells. Dosing is 1 to 1.5 g twice daily in adults and 1,200 mg/m^2 daily (~30–50 mg/kg/d) in children. Gastrointestinal upset is most commonly seen with this agent. Use caution in patients who are pregnant and in patients receiving a live vaccine.

Selecting the Most Appropriate Agent

The recommended treatment order is listed in **Tables 12.2** and **12.3**.

First-Line Therapy

Nonpharmacologic options should first be considered in both CD and AD. This includes avoidance of the offending agent, use of skin protection, and use of moisturizers to maintain the skin barrier. If these approaches do not help, pharmacologic therapy can be considered.

TCSs are the first-line topical medication for use in CD and AD. If improvement does not occur, a higher-potency TCS may be considered. TCSs can be applied for both treatment and prevention of future flares of AD.

Oral antihistamines are used to relieve pruritus and should only be considered in CD.

Second-Line Therapy

If the patient does not respond to TCS or if the use of a steroid-sparing agent is warranted, a TCI can be considered

TABLE 12.2

Recommended Order of Treatment for Contact Dermatitis

Order	Intervention	Comments
First line	Prevention and avoidance of offending agent May consider use of TCS Oral antihistamine for relief of pruritus	Occlusive dressing is helpful Apply to moist skin surface
Second line	Increased potency of topical corticosteroid	Avoid using moderate- or high-potency topical corticosteroid on face or intertriginous areas
Third line	Oral corticosteroids	Common dosage: 1 mg/kg and tapered down Consider increasing dose if CD persists

TCS, topical corticosteroids.

TABLE 12.3

Recommended Order of Treatment for Atopic Dermatitis

Order	Intervention	Comments
First line	Nonpharmacologic approaches; may consider TCS in treatment and prevention of flares	Nonpharmacologic therapy includes the use of moisturizers, bathing, and WWT
Second line	TCI, crisaborole, or phototherapy	May consider TCI as a steroid-sparing agent or use in conjunction with TCS Phototherapy can be considered if patient does not respond to topical therapy
Third line	Oral systemic therapy	Reserved for refractory AD

AD, atopic dermatitis; TCI, topical calcineurin inhibitors; TCS, topical corticosteroids; WWT, wet-wrap therapy.

as second-line therapy in AD. The use of both a TCS and a TCI can be considered. One common strategy is the use of a TCS during an acute flare of AD and the use of a TCI to prevent future flares as a steroid-sparing option. Crisaborole can also be considered as an alternative to TCSs and TCIs. Phototherapy may also be considered if topical agents do not resolve the patient's condition.

Third-Line Therapy

Systemic therapy may be considered if the patient does not respond to topical therapy and phototherapy. Unfortunately, the adverse effect profiles of available systemic options are vast, and monitoring of these adverse effects is warranted.

A proposed treatment algorithm is provided in **Figures 12.1** and **12.2**.

Special Populations

Pediatric

Since children have greater body surface area–weight ratio, they can absorb more of a TCS than adults. Therefore, the least potent TCS should be used to minimize adverse effects when used for long-term disease.

Tacrolimus 0.03% and pimecrolimus 1% are approved for use in patients who are 2 years old or older, and tacrolimus 1% is only approved for patients who are 15 years old or older. Despite this, the use of tacrolimus 0.03% or pimecrolimus 1% may be considered in patients who are less than 2 years old.

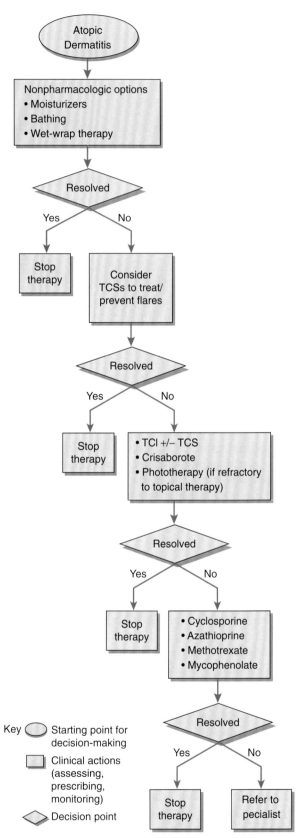

FIGURE 12–1   Proposed treatment algorithm for a topic dermatitis.

TCIs, topical calcineurin inhibitors; TCSs, topical corticosteroids.

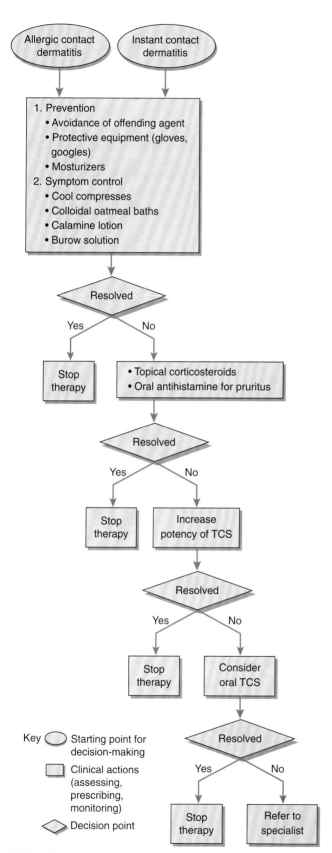

FIGURE 12–2 Proposed treatment algorithm for contact dermatitis.

TCSs, topical corticosteroids.

Geriatric

The most common causes of CD in older patients are topical medications (e.g., neomycin [Myciguent]) and the bases of other topical medications. The adhesives on adhesive patches may also cause CD. The rash of CD does not present in a classic pattern in the older adult. Instead of vesicles or inflammation, the area exposed to the irritant may simply become scaly. TCSs can cause atrophy of the skin in older adults, which is a problem because their skin is already friable.

Women

Apply caution when using various systemic therapy options in women who are pregnant. Most systemic therapy options pose a risk to the fetus, and the risks oftentimes outweigh the benefits. The one medication to avoid in pregnancy is methotrexate.

MONITORING PATIENT RESPONSE

The response to therapy is monitored by visual examination of the affected parts of the anatomy and the reported resolution of symptoms. The patient should return for follow-up evaluation within 2 or 3 days of initiation of therapy. If a bacterial infection recurs secondary to CD, it may be treated as discussed in Chapter 13, "Bacterial, Fungal, and Viral Infections of the Skin."

PATIENT EDUCATION

Education includes teaching patients to avoid the causative substance. Using mild soaps without perfume is an important preventive measure. As appropriate, the practitioner can demonstrate how to apply topical preparations to moist skin and apply an occlusive dressing to increase the efficacy of TCSs. Penetration of TCSs is enhanced 10- to 100-fold by hydrating (moistening) the area before applying the medication. An easy-to-make occlusive dressing consists of plastic wrap applied over the medicated area and held in place by a sock or tape. On the hands, a glove can act as an occlusive dressing. On the head area, a shower cap can be used. Occlusive dressings should not be used with topical immunosuppressants. The patient should avoid alcohol and should use sunscreen.

The practitioner should also address any fears or misconceptions about the use of TCSs since patients may have a fear of adverse effects from TCSs. This may lead to incorrect usage or noncompliance to the TCSs. In general, TCSs are well tolerated as long as they are being applied appropriately.

Most patients with AD require hydration through the liberal use of bland emollients, which serve to hydrate the stratum corneum and maintain the lipid barrier. Sufficient emollients applied liberally several times a day may be enough to significantly reduce the disease activity of AD. Parents of infants and toddlers should apply a bland emollient to the entire body with each diaper change. Older children should apply bland emollients in the morning, after school, and at bedtime. Bathing should be limited to brief, cool showers once daily. Soap, which dries and irritates the skin, should be avoided, but gentle lipid-free cleansers are beneficial.

Skin hydration is best accomplished through daily soaking baths for 10 to 20 minutes. It is important to remind patients and caregivers to apply a topical medication or moisturizer immediately after bathing. This is to seal in the water that has been absorbed into the skin and to prevent evaporation, which can lead to further drying of the skin.

For additional information that is patient friendly, the practitioner may refer the patient to the Web site of the American Academy of Dermatology (aad.org) and the National Eczema Association (nationaleczema.org).

Some adjunctive and complementary interventions are thought to be helpful in AD, although there is limited or no evidence to show benefit. Food allergies may coexist with AD, but the frequency of that food allergy causing a flare is probably low. Vitamin D and E supplementation may have a mild benefit. Overall, these strategies and other alternative therapies should not be routinely recommended.

CASE STUDY 1

J.F., a 15-year-old boy who weighs 110 pounds, is seeking treatment for a very itchy rash consisting of linear streaks of papules, vesicles, and blisters on his arms, legs, and face. He tells you he was hiking in the woods 2 days ago along trails lined with patches of shiny weeds with three leaves. He tried using calamine lotion and over-the-counter diphenhydramine cream but the itching still persists (Learning Objectives 1 and 3).

1. What condition does J.F. present with? What symptoms does J.F. present with and what is the most likely offending agent that suggests this condition?
2. What would be the first-line option for drug therapy?
3. What would be the best choice for second-line therapy?
4. What lifestyle changes would you recommend to J.F.?

Bibliography

Edwards, T., Patel, N. U., Blake, A., et al. (2018). Insights into future therapeutics for atopic dermatitis. *Expert Opinion on Pharmacotherapy, 19*(3), 265–278.

Eichenfield, L. F., Tom, W. L., Berger, T. G., et al. (2014a). Guidelines of care for the management of atopic dermatitis: Management and treatment of atopic dermatitis with topical therapies. *Journal of the American Academy of Dermatology, 71*(1), 116–132.

Eichenfield, L. F., Tom, W. L., Chamlin, S. L., et al. (2014b). Guidelines of care for the management of atopic dermatitis: Diagnosis and assessment of atopic dermatitis. *Journal of the American Academy of Dermatology, 70*(2), 338–351.

Fonacier, L., Bernstein, D. I., Pacheco, K., et al. (2015). Contact dermatitis: A practice parameter-update 2015. *The Journal of Allergy and Clinical Immunology: In Practice, 3*(3), S1–S39.

Kim, J., Kim, B. E., & Leung, D. Y. M. (2019). Pathophysiology of atopic dermatitis: Clinical implications. *Allergy and Asthma Proceedings, 40*(2), 84–92.

Kostner, L., Anzengruber, F., Guillod, C., et al. (2017). Allergic contact dermatitis. *Immunology and Allergy Clinics of North America, 37*(1), 141–152.

LEO Pharma Inc. (2019). *PROTOPIC- tacrolimus ointment.* Madison, NJ: Author.

Litchman, G., Nair, P. A., Atwater, A. R., et al. (2019). Contact dermatitis, *StatPearls.* (pp. 1–8). Treasure Island, FL: StatPearls Publishing.

Sidbury, R., Davis, D. M., Cohen, D. E., et al. (2014a). Guidelines of care for the management of atopic dermatitis: Management and treatment with phototherapy and systemic agents. *Journal of the American Academy of Dermatology, 71*(2), 327–349.

Sidbury, R., Tom, W. L., Bergman, J. N., et al. (2014b). Guidelines of care for the management of atopic dermatitis: Prevention of disease flares and use of adjunctive therapies and approaches. *Journal of the American Academy of Dermatology, 71*(6), 1218–1233.

Souto, E. B., Dias-Ferreira, J., Oliviera, J., et al. (2019). Trends in atopic dermatitis-from standard pharmacotherapy to novel drug delivery systems. *International Journal of Molecular Sciences, 20*(22), 5659.

13 Fungal, Viral, and Bacterial Infections of the Skin

Iman I. Aberra, Virginia P. Arcangelo, and Jason J. Schafer

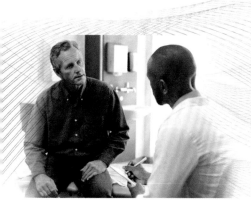
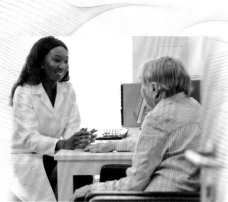
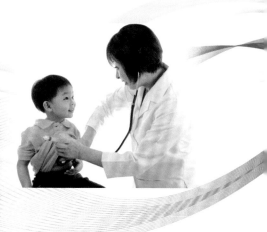

Learning Objectives

1. Recognize signs, symptoms, and presentation of various types of bacterial, fungal, and viral skin infections.
2. Identify the causes and risk factors for different types of skin infections.
3. Create a treatment plan including pharmacologic, nonpharmacologic, and preventive measures for skin infections.

INTRODUCTION

Skin infections are common problems that will cause patients to seek medical attention. Bacterial skin infections can become a life-threatening infection if not promptly and appropriately treated. Viral and fungal infections can be contagious, and patients should be counseled on appropriate preventive measures to reduce transmission to others.

BACTERIAL SKIN INFECTIONS

Introduction

Bacterial skin infections range from those that are minor and heal without consequence to those that are more severe and may be disfiguring or even life threatening. Minor infections are quite common and are often self-treated by patients without formal medical care. The majority of wounds seen in health care practice are easily managed with appropriate wound care and antibiotic therapy, if indicated.

Common primary skin infections resulting from bacteria include impetigo, bullous impetigo, folliculitis, felons, paronychias, and cellulitis. (See **Box 13.1** for information about associated problems.) These are discussed in this chapter, along with the less common infections erysipelas, ecthyma, furuncles, and carbuncles. This chapter also contains a brief discussion of necrotizing fasciitis, a very serious infection treated in an inpatient setting by specialists.

Causes

Bacteria most commonly responsible for causing skin infections are *Staphylococcus aureus* and beta-hemolytic streptococci such as *Streptococcus pyogenes* (group A *Streptococcus*, or GAS) and *Streptococcus agalactiae* (group B *Streptococcus*, or GBS) (**Tables 13.1** and **13.2**).

Impetigo and Ecthyma

Impetigo is a common superficial skin infection characterized by scattered vesicular lesions due to *S. aureus*, GAS, or both. Bullous impetigo, a variation of impetigo where blisters or bullae form, is caused primarily by *S. aureus*. Ecthyma is a chronic form of impetigo that affects deeper layers of the skin. Ecthyma can develop from minor wounds, scabies, insect bites, or any condition that causes itching, scratching, and excoriation.

Impetigo is more common in children but can also be seen in adults. Hot and humid weather promotes growth of bacteria on the skin and can result in these infections. Both impetigo and ecthyma are communicable and can be transmitted through person-to-person contact, often in schools or day care centers. Poor hygiene and crowded living conditions are other factors that can contribute to the development of these infections.

BOX 13.1   Danger: Bites and Other Puncture Wounds

Human and animal bites and puncture wounds of other sorts are infections waiting to develop. Because these wounds are associated with such a high risk for infection, antibiotic prophylaxis with broad-spectrum penicillin usually begins with the patient's request for health care. Tetanus is also an important consideration in puncture wounds and bites, and patients should be immunized as appropriate. If patients are unsure of when their last tetanus vaccine was done, it is best to err on the side of caution and give the tetanus vaccine.

If the wound was created by a clean object and is in an area that is well vascularized, treatment may consist simply of washing thoroughly; soaking in warm, soapy water several times a day; and observing the site for a few days.

If the wound was made by an object contaminated with fecal material, soil, or other debris, or if the patient is diabetic or has a compromised circulation, antibiotics should be initiated based on the probable causative organism. These patients may need close observation to ensure that they do not develop a systemic infection.

Care for bite wounds depends on several factors, including whether the bite was from a human or an animal, the location of the wound, and whether the wound is primarily a puncture or a laceration. All bite wounds should be cleaned thoroughly with soap and water. Puncture bites should be irrigated with normal saline solution. Extensive wounds may require surgical debridement, tendon repair, or suturing. If the bite is located on an extremity, elevation of the extremity will help prevent swelling.

All human bites that break the skin should be treated with antibiotics. Appropriate choices include oral amoxicillin–clavulanate or ampicillin–sulbactam for IV treatment. Oral or IV doxycycline can be used for patients who are allergic to penicillin. Treatment should be given for 3 to 5 days.

Minor animal bites may not require antibiotic therapy unless the wound is on the hand, foot, or face. Patients who are immunocompromised should be treated with antibiotics. The possibility of rabies must also be addressed, and local health officials may need to be contacted to determine the need to administer post-exposure rabies vaccination to the patient. The same agents used for human bites are also appropriate for animal bites.

Although most puncture wounds heal without incident, patients should be instructed to observe for signs of infection, including inflammation, persistent pain, swelling, or purulent drainage. If a puncture wound becomes infected, further systemic antibiotic therapy is required and should be based on Gram stain and culture results. A follow-up visit should be scheduled within days to ensure that the wound is healing without further infection.

Source: Stevens, D. L., Bisno, A. L., Chambers, H. F., et al. (2014). Practice guidelines for the diagnosis and management of skin and soft tissue infections:2014 update by the Infectious Diseases Society of America. *Clinical Infectious Diseases: An Official Publication of the Infectious Diseases Society of America, 59*(2), e10–e52.

TABLE 13.1

Selected Organisms That Cause Skin Infections

	Impetigo and Ecthyma	Bullous Impetigo	Erysipelas	Folliculitis, Furuncles, and Carbuncles	Paronychias
Gram-Positive Organisms					
Staphylococcus aureus	X	X	X (very few)	X	X
Group A *Streptococcus*	X		X		X
Group B *Streptococcus*	X (newborn impetigo)		X (newborn)		

Cellulitis and Erysipelas

Cellulitis is an infection involving the subcutaneous tissue. It has the potential to spread systemically and cause serious illness. It can develop from any type of skin breakage including those that are not visibly noticeable. Examples of conditions that may cause skin breakage include venous insufficiency, edema, and obesity. In intravenous (IV) drug users, cellulitis typically develops at injection sites, and patients are at risk for deep-seeded infection. The characteristics of infection depend on many factors, including the type of wound, the organisms involved, and the patient.

Most cases of non-purulent cellulitis are caused by GAS. Patients with certain predisposing factors, however, may be at risk for infections caused by other organisms. *Pasteurella multocida* is the primary cause of cellulitis from animal bites and scratches. **Table 13.2** lists additional causes.

Methicillin-resistant *S. aureus* (MRSA) infections can be particularly challenging to manage because commonly used

TABLE 13.2

Bacteria That Can Cause Cellulitis Under Certain Conditions

Organism	Condition
Staphylococcus aureus	Common
Group A *Streptococcus*	Common
Haemophilus influenzae B	Children (periorbital cellulitis*)
Group B *Streptococcus*	Newborns
Escherichia coli	Opportunistic in compromised patients
Pseudomonas aeruginosa	Folliculitis from under-chlorinated hot tubs Burns
Klebsiella species	Opportunistic in compromised patients
Enterobacter species	Opportunistic in compromised patients
Pasteurella multocida	Animal bites and scratches
Anaerobic organisms	Diabetes, ulcers, trauma, crush wounds
Aeromonas hydrophila	Freshwater-related injury, immunosuppressed patients
Vibrio species	Seawater-related injuries, wound contact with raw or undercooked seafood

*Uncommon now because of the use of the HIB vaccine.

antibiotics such as penicillins and cephalosporins are inactive against MRSA. Those at risk for MRSA infections are those with penetrating trauma, other active MRSA infection, positive MRSA nasal swab, IV drug use, purulent drainage, or septic (severe non-purulent infection).

Erysipelas, predominantly caused by *S. pyogenes*, occurs in the superficial epidermis and is seen more often in children, especially infants, and older adults.

Purulent Skin Infections

Pustular infections include abscesses, folliculitis, furunculosis, and carbunculosis and are commonly caused by *S. aureus*. Abscesses are sometimes polymicrobial depending where on the body it forms. A majority of cases are due to MRSA.

Folliculitis is a superficial infection of the hair follicle. *Pseudomonas aeruginosa* can also cause folliculitis, particularly in those who frequently use hot tubs, as a result of inadequate chlorination. Furunculosis (furuncles) and carbunculosis (carbuncles) involve deeper areas of the skin and can develop from unresolved cases of folliculitis.

Irritation from shaving, plucking, and waxing of hair may contribute to folliculitis. Other predisposing factors include humid conditions, tight clothing, diabetes, occlusion of the

hair follicles from cosmetics or sunscreens, poor hygiene, and occupational exposure to heavy grease or solvents.

Other common skin infections, such as acute paronychia (an infection in at least one nail fold of the fingers or toes) and a felon (a finger infection on the palm side), are usually caused by *S. aureus*, *S. pyogenes*, or *Pseudomonas* species and occasionally other gram-negative bacilli. Women are at more risk for these types of skin infections perhaps because of their more frequent utilization of nail services.

Diabetic Foot Infection

Diabetes can cause many microvascular and macrovascular complications. The best way to mitigate the risk for developing these complications is to maintain good glycemic control. A microvascular complication that can be a devastating and recurring problem is diabetic foot infection (DFI).

It is estimated that 25% of people with diabetes will develop a DFI at least once in their lifetime (Barwell et al., 2017). DFIs increase the likelihood of needing an amputation and therefore affecting quality of life. It is associated with prolonged hospital stay and both physical and psychological morbidity (Barwell et al., 2017). Risk factors in patients with diabetes include neuropathy, foot deformities, peripheral artery disease (PAD), increased age and duration of diabetes, ethnic minority, ill-fitting shoes, other microvascular complications including renal dysfunction, and past foot ulcerations (Boulton et al., 2018).

Necrotizing Fasciitis

Necrotizing fasciitis is an extremely serious infection of the subcutaneous tissues between the skin and the underlying muscle. It can be life threatening if not diagnosed early and treated appropriately. Management requires emergent surgical interventions to remove infected tissue in combination with antibiotic therapy. Risk factors for developing necrotizing fasciitis include alcohol abuse, diabetes, severe debilitation, and trauma. Mortality is high, especially if surgical debridement is delayed or incomplete.

Necrotizing fasciitis type 1 is a polymicrobial infection typically including many aerobic and anaerobic organisms. It is commonly associated with perianal abscesses, penetrating trauma, complicated bowel procedures, decubitus ulcers, Bartholin abscess, and episiotomy wounds.

Necrotizing fasciitis type 2 is monomicrobial, most commonly involving GAS, although *S. aureus*, and anaerobic bacteria such as *Peptostreptococcus*, can also be the cause. In some cases, GAS and *S. aureus* can cause necrotizing fasciitis alone as a monomicrobial infection. Varicella infection is considered a risk factor for invasive skin infections, including necrotizing fasciitis caused by GAS and rarely MRSA.

Necrotizing fasciitis type 3, or *gas gangrene*, is often caused by *Clostridium perfringens*, an anaerobic bacterium commonly found in soil. This can occur following deep penetrating trauma injuries.

Pathophysiology

The skin is composed of three layers. The outer layer is the epidermis, the first line of defense against infection. Nail tissue is part of the epidermis. Underneath is the dermis, which contains connective tissue, blood vessels, nerves, hair follicles, sweat glands, and sebaceous glands. The innermost layer, hypodermis, is composed of subcutaneous tissue. Skin infections may be classified according to the depth of penetration and the layer and skin structure affected.

Under normal circumstances, bacteria present on the skin as normal flora cause no harm. However, a break in the skin can allow these organisms to penetrate and proliferate, resulting in a skin infection. Some people are persistent carriers of *S. aureus* in the nasal, perineal, or axillary areas. These individuals may be more prone to developing skin infections and more likely to experience recurrences.

Patients with predisposing medical conditions (**Box 13.2**), such as diabetes, immune system disorders, and malnutrition from alcoholism or other causes, are more prone to skin infection because of poor wound healing. Also at a higher risk for skin infection are those with circulatory compromise of the arterial, venous, or lymphatic systems. Wound infections in patients with these conditions have the potential to become more serious and invasive, requiring IV antibiotic therapy, hospitalization, or referral to a specialist. Wound infections can also become more serious when treatment is delayed. The practitioner must be alert for these situations and act promptly.

In addition, many organisms aside from GAS and *S. aureus* may cause skin infections in patients with chronic conditions like diabetes. These organisms include *Escherichia coli (E. coli)*, *Klebsiella* species, and *P. aeruginosa*. Infections in these patients are often more difficult to manage clinically and have the tendency to become chronic. Infections that do resolve with appropriate therapy have a high risk of recurrence. A common example of this scenario is a DFI.

BOX 13.2   Predisposing Factors in Skin Infections

Chronic carriers of *Staphylococcus aureus*
Diabetes mellitus
Debilitation
Peripheral vascular disease
Venous stasis
Alcoholism (malnutrition)
Immune deficiency
Corticosteroid therapy
Obesity
Trauma or burns
Poor hygiene
Warm, humid conditions
Topical irritants
Tight clothing

Diagnostic Criteria

Impetigo and Ecthyma

Impetigo, a highly contagious, common primary skin infection in children, is most frequently found on the face, scalp, or extremities. It begins as scattered, discrete macules that itch and are spread by scratching. These macules then develop into vesicles and pustules on an erythematous base that eventually rupture, oozing a purulent liquid. Once dried, the lesions appear thick, with a characteristic honey-colored crust on the surface. Once healed, scarring is rare. Regional lymphadenopathy may be present, and lesions may itch; however, fever or other systemic complaints are uncommon. The infection is diagnosed clinically by the appearance of hallmark honey-colored crusts. Although not commonly done in practice due to time restrictions, gram stain and culture of the pus or exudates to identify if the cause is from *S. aureus* or GAS are recommend by the Infectious Diseases Society of America (IDSA). It is acceptable, however, to proceed with treatment without these tests.

Impetigo may also present with bullous lesions and can be referred to as bullous impetigo. Found on the face, scalp, extremities, trunk, and intertriginous areas, it affects primarily newborns and children under the age of 2. Bullous impetigo is characterized by the formation of superficial, flaccid bullae on the skin. The brownish-gray lesions are sometimes crusted or have an erythematous halo. They also appear to be smooth and shiny.

Both treated and untreated impetigo caused by nephrogenic GAS can develop into poststreptococcal glomerulonephritis. It presents as acute kidney injury, usually 2 to 6 weeks after the occurrence of impetigo.

Ecthyma occurs when a case of impetigo worsens and spreads deeply to the dermis. Much less common than impetigo, ecthyma usually affects the lower extremities of debilitated individuals and older adults. It begins with the formation of vesicles that then develop into shallow ulcerations. The ulcerations enlarge over several days and are surrounded by an erythematous halo. Because the infection affects the deeper layers of the skin, scarring is often seen after ulcerations heal. Lesions are usually painful and may persist for weeks to months.

Cellulitis and Erysipelas

Cellulitis is a potentially serious infection involving the skin and subcutaneous tissue. The disease can spread through the superficial layers of skin and cause painful erythema, with the affected area warm and tender to the touch. Pitting edema can also be present, and the skin may be pink, shiny, and resemble the surface of an "orange peel." The margins of cellulitis are diffuse, not sharply demarcated, and the affected area is flat and usually edematous. In open wounds, purulent drainage and necrosis may be present. Red streaks may develop proximal to the area of infection, indicating lymphatic spread or lymphangitis. Systemic symptoms of fever, chills, and malaise and regional adenitis are also common and can indicate bacteremia, in which case, blood cultures should be obtained.

Blood cultures should also be obtained in those who are immunocompromised, are neutropenic, or have immersion injuries or animal bites. Cultures of aspirates, biopsies, or swabs may be considered in this population. In all other cases of cellulitis, these studies are not routinely recommended.

Erysipelas is most commonly found on the lower extremities but can also be present on the face and scalp. Erysipelas begins as an area of sharply demarcated erythema that spreads rapidly over a period of minutes to hours. The affected area is raised, red, firm, warm, and tender to the touch. Erythema spreads along local lymphatic channels, which gives the skin a typical "orange peel" appearance due to lymphatic obstruction.

Common systemic symptoms include pain, malaise, chills, and fever. Erysipelas occurring on the face often follows a streptococcal sore throat infection. The face is usually so inflamed that the eyes are swollen shut.

Purulent Skin Infections

Abscesses are localized collections of pus located deep within the dermis. They are tender to the touch, often accompanied with painful erythematous swelling. The swelling is usually firm at first but then becomes fluctuant.

Folliculitis is superficial and occurs on the hairy areas of the skin, especially the bearded parts of the face and the intertriginous areas. Early lesions appear as clusters of small, erythematous, pruritic papules that may quickly turn into pustules. Each papule or pustule contains a single hair follicle in its center.

A furuncle or boil, which develops from folliculitis, is a painful, pus-filled nodule that encircles a hair follicle. Common sites are the neck, face, axillae, forearms, upper back, groin, buttocks, and thighs. A carbuncle is a confluence of several furuncles that form deep within the dermis. They are bigger and form deeper in the skin. Common sites of infection are the upper back, neck, or lateral thigh. Systemic manifestations are not usually seen with furuncles, but carbuncles are frequently accompanied by systemic signs such as fever, malaise, and headache. Cultures of the pus from carbuncles and abscesses are recommended for severe cases, although treatment should not be delayed if obtaining the specimens is not feasible.

A paronychia is an infection of the tissue surrounding a nail bed. It is associated with nail biting, hangnails, or finger sucking; it may occur in people who have their hands in water frequently. Diabetic patients are also at a higher risk. A paronychia involving the toenail most often results from an ingrown nail. The infected area appears red and swollen and is painful. Pus, which may accumulate, may sometimes be expressed with gentle pressure; this usually relieves the discomfort. Systemic symptoms are uncommon.

A felon, which may follow a fingertip wound, is an infection that involves the pulp space in the tip of a digit. It is potentially more serious than a paronychia because it is confined in a closed space. The affected digit is erythematous, edematous, and exquisitely tender. The edema has the potential to compromise the arterial supply of the digit. If left untreated,

abscess and tissue necrosis can occur. An additional danger is the possibility of bony or joint involvement, which can lead to loss of function.

Diabetic Foot Infection

It is important to realize that not all diabetic foot ulcers are infected. It is essential to make this distinction as giving antibiotics unnecessarily can harbor resistant organisms that make future infections difficult to treat. Ulcers that show purulence or at least two signs of inflammation are deemed infectious. Signs of inflammation include erythema, warmth, tenderness, pain, and induration. Other signs can include non-purulent secretions, discolored granulation tissue, and foul odor (Lipsky et al., 2012). A validated classification system should be used to classify the severity of infection, which will aid in treatment. An example of a validated classification system is the one developed by the IDSA (**Table 13.3**). All other causes of inflammation of the skin should be ruled out, such as gout, distal venous thrombosis, and venous stasis. PAD should be evaluated and for severe infections vascular surgery may need to be consulted to evaluate for limb ischemia.

Tissue culture should be obtained from infectious wounds after debridement and cleansing and prior to initiating antibiotics if possible. Purulent secretions should be aspirated if possible and sent for culture. Wound swabs should be avoided as they can be contaminated with normal skin flora and will be less accurate in identifying the pathogenic organism. Mild DFIs in patients who have not recently received

TABLE 13.3	
Infectious Diseases Society of America Classification of Diabetic Foot Infection	
Classification	**Manifestation**
Noninfectious	No signs or symptoms of infection.
Mild	Local infection without involvement of deeper tissues. If erythema is present, it should be >0.5 cm to ≤2 cm around the ulcer.
Moderate	Local infection with erythema >2 cm or involving structures deeper than skin and subcutaneous tissues.
Severe	Local infection (as described previously) with the signs of SIRS, as manifested by ≥2 of the following: • Temperature >38°C or <36°C • Heart rate >90 bpm • Respiratory rate >20 breaths/min or PaCO₂ <32 mm Hg • White blood cell count >12,000 or <4,000 cells/mcL or ≥10% immature (band) forms

SIRS, systemic inflammatory response syndrome.

Adapted from the Infectious Diseases Society of America Diabetic Foot Infection Guidelines, 2012.

antibiotics do not need culture. In severe infections, cultures can be taken in the operating room if there is need for extensive debridement.

Patients presenting with a DFI should have radiographs taken to rule out osteomyelitis, gas formation, or any other abnormalities on the foot. If X-ray imaging cannot rule out osteomyelitis, additional imaging with magnetic resonance imaging (MRI) needs to be performed to rule out bone involvement as that will affect the duration and dosing of antimicrobials.

Necrotizing Fasciitis

Patients with necrotizing fasciitis are extremely ill, requiring intensive care and emergent surgical debridement. The infection may initially appear similar to cellulitis, although excruciating pain, erythema, and edema are commonly present. Necrotizing fasciitis may be differentiated from cellulitis by its rapid spread, tissue destruction, and lack of response to usual antibiotic therapy. The subcutaneous tissue will have a wooden-hard feel, as compared to cellulitis and erysipelas, where this tissue is usually yielding and can be palpated. As this infection progresses and tissue destruction spreads, pain may be replaced by anesthesia due to necrotized superficial nerve endings, and patients may show signs of sepsis, including hemodynamic instability and multiorgan dysfunction. There may also be crepitus, bullous lesions, and ecchymoses.

MRI can be done to look for edema along the fascia, although this should not delay treatment. Diagnosis is made by clinical judgment. Diagnosis is confirmed during surgical exploration of the site. The fascia will appear swollen and gray with areas of string-like necrosis. Cultures of the deep tissue should be obtained while in surgery. It is important not to take superficial skin cultures as the organisms that grow will not be truly reflective of the organism(s) in the deep tissue.

Initiating Drug Therapy

An increasing challenge in treating skin infections is the problem of antibiotic-resistant organisms. Choosing the appropriate agent is not as simple as it once was, and prescribers must be aware of resistance, as well as regional variations in the prevalence and susceptibility of infecting organisms.

Because warm, humid conditions and poor hygiene may play a role in skin infections, especially impetigo, treatment begins with good hygiene (**Box 13.3**), avoidance of irritants, and meticulous wound care as appropriate. For some very minor infections, these measures along with a topical agent may be sufficient. Adjunctive treatment for most skin infections (e.g., bullous impetigo and erysipelas) includes warm soaks and elevation of the affected area if the infection involves an extremity. However, most bacterial skin infections require treatment with systemic antibiotics.

The majority of infections are treated in the outpatient setting with oral antibiotic agents. Patients with more serious infections, however, may require hospitalization, IV antibiotics, and consultation with an infectious diseases specialist. Treatment decisions are based on the practitioner's knowledge

---

BOX 13.3   Strategies to Prevent Skin Infections

Wash hands frequently with soap and water or an alcohol-based hand gel, especially after touching infected skin to prevent spread of infecting organisms.
Bathe regularly.
Avoid scratching.
Avoid irritants, including tight clothing and occlusive cosmetics and deodorants.
Avoid reusing or sharing personal items such as disposable razors, towels, and bedsheets.
Disinfect commonly touched surfaces such as door knobs, counters, and toilet seats.

Lipsky, B. A., Berendt, A. R., Cornia, P. B., et al. 2012 Infectious Diseases Society of America clinical practice guideline for the diagnosis and treatment of diabetic foot infections. *Clinical Infectious Diseases: An Official Publication of the Infectious Diseases Society of America, 54*(12), e132–e173.

---

of the patient's predisposing conditions and presentation and the type and stage of the infection.

In many cases, systemic antibiotic therapy (**Table 13.4**) is prescribed empirically based on knowledge of the organisms commonly responsible for specific skin infections, such as *S. aureus* and GAS. Therapy is then narrowed once culture results, if collected.

In the case of puncture or bite wounds that are not initially infected, antibiotics are prescribed as prophylaxis in immunocompromised individuals because of the high risk of infection associated with these wounds (**Box 13.1**).

Topical medications, such as mupirocin (Bactroban) ointment, can be occasionally used as primary therapy for minor infections (e.g., impetigo) or alternatively used in combination with systemic agents for more serious infections. In some patients thought to be chronic carriers of *S. aureus*, infections may be recurrent.

Several other adjunctive measures may also be used in combination with drug therapy. Bedside warm soaks and incision and drainage procedures may help resolve pustular lesions. Patients with a paronychia may need to have the nail bed decompressed to relieve the pressure, and deeper and more invasive infections almost always require incision and drainage.

Goals of Drug Therapy

The goals in treating bacterial skin infections are to cure the infection, prevent worsening, minimize scarring, and prevent recurrence. Many minor infections resolve within 10 to 14 days. If resolution does not occur, alternative agents may be prescribed. The prescriber must decide when it is appropriate to initiate treatment with an alternative agent or whether a referral to a specialist for more definitive diagnosis and treatment is indicated.

TABLE 13.4

Overview of Selected Antibiotics for Skin Infections

Generic (Trade) Name and Dosage	Selected Adverse Events	Contraindications	Special Considerations
Broad-Spectrum Penicillins			
Amoxicillin–clavulanate (Augmentin) Adults: 500–875 mg q12h Children: weight-based dosing based on the formulation	Nausea, vomiting, diarrhea, rash, allergic reactions, fungal infection **Serious:** Pseudomembranous colitis, seizures (high doses)	Allergy to penicillin Use with caution in severe renal disease, less severe allergy to cephalosporins.	Food may decrease GI symptoms Renal adjustments: Comes in suspension for children Interactions: warfarin (may increase INR), oral contraceptives (decrease effectiveness of contraceptive)
Dicloxacillin (Dynapen) Adults: 125–250 mg PO q6h Children: 6.25–12.5 mg/kg PO q6h	Same as amoxicillin–clavulanate	Penicillin allergy Use with caution in severe renal dysfunction	Take on empty stomach for best absorption Interactions: warfarin (Decreases INR)
First-Generation Cephalosporins			
Cephalexin (Keflex) Adults: 500 mg PO q6h Children: 25–50 mg/kg/d divided in 3–4 doses	Nausea, vomiting, diarrhea, rash, allergic reactions, fungal infections **Serious:** Pseudomembranous colitis, seizures (high doses)	Serious penicillin allergy, allergy to cephalosporins Use with caution in renal disease	Food may decrease GI symptoms. Renal adjustments
Cefazolin (Ancef) Adults: 1 g IV q8h Children: 50 mg/kg/d IV divided into 3 doses	Same as cephalexin	Same as cephalexin	Same as cephalexin
Second-Generation Cephalosporins			
Cefaclor (Ceclor) Adults: Immediate release: 250–500 mg PO q8h Extended release: 500 mg PO q12h Children: 20–40 mg/kg/d q8h not to exceed 1 g/d	Same as cephalexin	Same as cephalexin	Same as cephalexin
Cefprozil (Cefzil) Adults: 250–500 mg PO q12h or 500 mg PO q24h Children: 20 mg/kg q24h	Same as cephalexin	Same as cephalexin	Same as cephalexin
Cefuroxime (Ceftin, Zinacef) Adults: 500 mg PO q12h Children: 15 mg/kg PO q12h	Same as cephalexin	Same as cephalexin	Same as cephalexin; swallow whole because of bitter taste
Third-Generation Cephalosporins			
Cefpodoxime (Vantin) Adults: 400 mg q12h PO	Same as cephalexin	Same as cephalexin	Same as cephalexin Not recommended for children <12 years
Ceftriaxone (Rocephin) Adults: 0.5–1.0 g q12h IM or IV or 1–2 g q24h IM or IV Children: 50–75 mg/kg q24h IM or IV	Same as cephalexin and also pseudolithiasis	Same as cephalexin	IM: Dilute with lidocaine to reduce pain at injection site No renal dose adjustments needed

(Continued)

TABLE 13.4

Overview of Selected Antibiotics for Skin Infections (*Continued*)

Generic (Trade) Name and Dosage	Selected Adverse Events	Contraindications	Special Considerations
Fluoroquinolones			
Ciprofloxacin (Cipro) Adults: 500–750 mg PO q12h Levofloxacin (Levaquin) Adults: 750 mg PO/IV q24h Moxifloxacin (Avelox) Adults: 400 mg PO/IV q24h	Nausea, diarrhea, altered taste, dizziness, drowsiness, headache, insomnia, agitation, confusion, hypoglycemia **Serious:** Pseudomembranous colitis, Stevens-Johnson syndrome	Allergy to fluoroquinolone. Myasthenia gravis Children younger than age 18, pregnancy Use with caution in renal and hepatic disease, central nervous system disease, older adults, lactation (safety not established)	Black box warning about serious adverse effects associated with fluoroquinolones: Tendinitis and tendon rupture, peripheral neuropathy, central nervous system effects, and aortic ruptures or tears Food slows absorption. Interactions: antacids, zinc, sucralfate, iron, theophylline, warfarin, probenecid, foscarnet, glucocorticoids, didanosine Renal adjustments QTc prolongation
Miscellaneous			
Clindamycin (Cleocin) Adults: 300–450 mg PO q6h Children: 20–40 mg/kg/d divided into 3–4 doses	Nausea, vomiting, diarrhea, rash, allergic reaction, fungal infections **Serious:** Pseudomembranous colitis	Allergy clindamycin or lincomycin	Take with or without food with full glass of water to avoid esophageal irritation Check antibiogram for local susceptibility rates for MRSA
Daptomycin (Cubicin) Adults: 4 mg/kg IV daily Children: not approved	CPK elevation with or without myopathy (reversible)	Allergy to daptomycin, children younger than age 18	Monitor for CPK elevations, especially in patients receiving HMG-CoAreductase inhibitors
Doxycycline (Doxy 100) Adults: 100 mg PO q12h Children: not approved	Photosensitivity, diarrhea, upper abdominal pain	Pregnancy Children <8 years	No renal dose adjustments Unreliable streptococcus coverage: check local antibiogram
Linezolid (Zyvox) Adults: 600 mg IV or PO q12h Children: 10 mg/kg q8h	Bone marrow suppression, rare optic neuritis, or peripheral neuropathy with use >2 weeks	Allergy, uncontrolled hypertension, and concurrent use of MAO inhibitors	Interaction with selective serotonin reuptake inhibitors and MAO inhibitors
Tigecycline (Tygacil) Adults: 100 mg × 1 dose, then 50 mg q12h Children: not approved	Nausea, vomiting, diarrhea, headache, hepatic dysfunction	Allergy to tigecycline; also use caution in patients with allergies to tetracyclines	Dosage adjustment is necessary for severe hepatic impairment Reserved for very resistant cases
Sulfamethoxazole–trimethoprim (Bactrim) Adults: 1–2 double-strength tablets q12h Children: 8 mg/kg trimethoprim component/day PO divided q12h	Bone marrow suppression, rash, nausea, and vomiting, hyperkalemia, renal dysfunction	Allergy to sulfonamides or trimethoprim, pregnant patients, nursing mothers, folate deficiency, or those who have developed severe thrombocytopenia from prior therapy	Poor coverage against GAS Requires renal dose adjustments Monitor potassium and serum creatinine Administer with a full glass of water Renal adjustments
Vancomycin (Vancocin) Adults: 15 mg/kg IV q12h Children: 10 mg/kg IV q6h	Infusion-related reactions (red man syndrome) phlebitis, renal injury	Allergy to vancomycin.	Monitor levels or consult pharmacy to dose Rate of infusion can be slowed if red man syndrome occurs

CPK, creatine phosphokinase; GAS, *Group A streptococcus*; GI, gastrointestinal; IM, intramuscular; INR, international normalized ratio; IV, intravenous; MAO, monoamine oxidase; MRSA, methicillin-resistant *S. aureus*; QTc, corrected Q-T interval.

Antibiotics

Several classes of antibiotics are useful for treating bacterial skin infections. For information on specific agents, refer to **Table 13.4**. In certain circumstances, a combination of antibiotics may be necessary to treat an infection because of multiple pathogens (i.e., a polymicrobial infection). Agents may be administered topically, orally, intramuscularly, or intravenously, depending on the specific infection and the condition of the patient.

The most common adverse effects occurring with most antibiotics are nausea, vomiting, diarrhea, rashes, allergic reactions, and urticaria. Patients taking antibiotic therapy, especially for a prolonged duration, can develop fungal infections such as vaginal candidiasis or thrush.

A less common but potentially life-threatening adverse effect of antibiotic therapy is pseudomembranous colitis. This causes severe diarrhea and is the result of overgrowth of the bacterium *Clostridium difficile*. Anaphylaxis and seizures (especially when high doses of beta-lactam antibiotics are used) may also occur. To minimize the risk of these events, a thorough patient history is essential before prescribing these drugs. There are also potentially many interactions between antibiotics and other medications a patient might be taking. Since antibiotics are not without risk, it is important to limit duration to the shortest effective course. Antibiotic therapy should be narrowed to cover the pathogenic organism when possible to limit adverse effects, save costs, and reduce development of resistance organisms.

Broad-Spectrum Penicillins

Most skin infections are caused by GAS and *S. aureus*. In the past, therapy with penicillin was usually effective in treating these infections. With the growing problem of antibiotic resistance, however, it is now necessary to choose a broad-spectrum agent. For example, many strains of *S. aureus* produce the enzyme penicillinase, which can inactivate penicillin. In this case, the provider should choose an agent that is penicillinase resistant. Useful agents in this class for treating specific skin infections include amoxicillin–clavulanate (Augmentin) or dicloxacillin (Dynapen). Penicillin usually still has good coverage of GAS, but local resistance patterns should be checked to show susceptibility.

Amoxicillin–clavulanate has bactericidal action against many organisms, including beta-hemolytic streptococci, *S. aureus*, *E. coli*, and *Proteus mirabilis (P. mirabilis)*. The clavulanate portion of the drug is a beta-lactamase inhibitor that allows amoxicillin to remain active in the presence of certain beta-lactamase enzymes such as the penicillinase produced by *S. aureus*. Amoxicillin–clavulanate is well absorbed orally and is more resistant to acid inactivation than other penicillins.

Common side effects are nausea, vomiting, diarrhea, rash, and urticaria. Patients who are allergic to penicillin should not be given this agent, and it needs dose adjustments when used in patients with renal dysfunction.

Dicloxacillin has bactericidal activity against penicillinase-producing strains of *S. aureus*. It is administered orally, and the adverse effect profile is similar to that of amoxicillin–clavulanate. It is dosed four times daily, which may be more difficult to comply with than amoxicillin–clavulanate, which is dosed twice daily (see **Table 13.4**).

First-Generation Cephalosporins

In this class, commonly used drugs for treating skin infections are cephalexin (Keflex) and cefazolin (Ancef). These agents have bactericidal activity against many organisms, including GAS and penicillinase-producing *S. aureus*. They also have activity against *Klebsiella pneumoniae (K. pneumoniae)*, *P. mira bilis*, and *E. coli*.

Cephalexin is administered orally and has excellent bioavailability, while cefazolin is administered intravenously. Their adverse effect profiles are similar to those of the broad-spectrum penicillins. These drugs should not be used in patients with a severe penicillin or cephalosporin allergy, and dosage adjustments are necessary in patients with renal insufficiency (see **Table 13.4**).

Second-Generation Cephalosporins

Second-generation cephalosporins that are useful for skin infections include cefaclor (Ceclor), cefuroxime (Ceftin, Zinacef), and cefprozil (Cefzil). They are effective against the same organisms as first-generation cephalosporins but have additional activity against certain gram-negative organisms, including *Haemophilus influenzae (H. influenzae)*, *E. coli*, *K. pneumoniae*, and *Proteus* organisms. These agents are all well absorbed orally and their adverse effect profiles are similar to those of the first-generation cephalosporins. They should not be given to patients who have a severe allergy to penicillin or an allergy to other cephalosporins. Dosage adjustments are necessary in patients with renal insufficiency (see **Table 13.4**).

Third-Generation Cephalosporins

Useful third-generation cephalosporins for treating skin infections include cefpodoxime (Vantin), ceftriaxone (Rocephin), and ceftazidime (Fortaz). These drugs are usually reserved for more serious infections and are not typically chosen as first-line agents. In addition, ceftriaxone and ceftazidime are not available as oral agents. Cefpodoxime is available only as an oral agent.

The spectrum of antibacterial activity for these agents is similar to that of the second-generation cephalosporins. However, they are less effective against *S. aureus* and more effective against certain gram-negative organisms, including *Enterobacter*, *H. influenzae*, *E. coli*, *K. pneumoniae*, and *Proteus* species. Ceftazidime is the only agent in this group that can be recommended for infections caused by *P. aeruginosa*. Ceftriaxone is absorbed intramuscularly, but this route of administration may be painful. Cefpodoxime is well absorbed orally when taken with food, although absorption is less than that of oral first-generation cephalosporins.

The adverse effect profile for these agents is similar to that of the other cephalosporins and broad-spectrum penicillins.

These antibiotics need to be renally adjusted in patients with renal dysfunction, with the exception for ceftriaxone. Caution should be used before administering these medications to patients with severe penicillin or cephalosporin allergies and generally should be avoided. Rarely, ceftriaxone may cause pseudolithiasis (see **Table 13.4**).

Clindamycin

Clindamycin (Cleocin) is an alternative agent that can be considered for treating bacterial skin infections due to *S. aureus* and GAS when patients are allergic to penicillins and cephalosporins. Susceptibility to *S. aureus* including MRSA may be low, and the clinician should check this with the local antibiogram, if available. In addition, clindamycin may be considered when gram-positive anaerobic bacterial coverage is necessary for polymicrobial infections.

Clindamycin is available for oral or IV administration and is generally well tolerated. Common side effects include diarrhea, nausea, and abdominal pain. Also, this agent has been more commonly associated with *C. difficile*–associated pseudomembranous colitis.

Fluoroquinolones

Levofloxacin (Levaquin), moxifloxacin (Avelox), and ciprofloxacin (Cipro) are the fluoroquinolone antibiotics used in the treatment of skin and skin structure infections. They are useful for serious infections in patients with penicillin allergies that have infections caused by gram-negative organisms. Their spectrum of activity includes many gram-negative bacteria, such as *E. coli, Klebsiella,* and *Enterobacter* species. In addition, levofloxacin and ciprofloxacin are active against *P. aeruginosa.* Each fluoroquinolone agent is available IV and orally and each has excellent bioavailability.

Common adverse effects are diarrhea, nausea, abdominal pain, dizziness, drowsiness, headache, and insomnia. Uncommon but severe events include Stevens-Johnson syndrome, seizures, Achilles tendon rupture, and pseudomembranous colitis. In addition, there have been several black box warnings issued by the Food and Drug Administration (FDA) regarding serious adverse effects such as tendinitis, tendon rupture, peripheral neuropathy, central nervous system (CNS) effects, and aortic ruptures or tears. These agents should be used as last-line therapy. Fluroquinolones also have several drug interactions (see **Table 13.4**).

Fluoroquinolone antibiotics are not recommended in children younger than age 18 or during pregnancy and lactation. They are also contraindicated in patients allergic to other fluoroquinolones. These medications should be used cautiously in older adults and patients with CNS diseases, seizure disorders, or renal impairment.

Additional Antimicrobial Agents

Vancomycin, daptomycin, telavancin, dalbavancin, oritavancin, linezolid, tedizolid, and tigecycline have antibacterial activity against drug-resistant, gram-positive pathogens including MRSA. Vancomycin remains the drug of choice for bacterial skin infections due to MRSA when parenteral therapy is necessary; however, daptomycin, telavancin, dalbavancin, oritavancin, linezolid, tedizolid, and tigecycline are also effective but are more expensive options. Dalbavancin and oritavancin are unique due to their very long half-lives. As a result, treatment with dalbavancin requires only two doses given 1 week apart, while oritavancin is indicated to treat bacterial skin infections using only a single IV dose. Linezolid and tedizolid are the only agents in this group that are available orally, which provides an option for clinicians to switch from IV to oral therapy when patients are clinically stable but require additional treatment. Linezolid should not be continued for more than 14 days due to the increased incidence of developing serious adverse effects. Tedizolid is often used for 6 days maximum for a skin and soft tissue infection, but it is very expensive and often reserved for special cases needing infectious diseases consultation.

Despite their activity against MRSA, each agent has significant side effects, and the potential for drug–drug interactions should be considered prior to initiating therapy.

Sulfamethoxazole–Trimethoprim

Sulfamethoxazole–trimethoprim (SMX–TMP) is another useful agent for the treatment of MRSA infections that can be managed with oral therapy. It is important, however, to remember that this agent does not have reliable activity for infections caused by GAS. Therefore, the diagnosis of MRSA should be made prior to treatment.

Adverse effects associated with SMX–TMP include gastrointestinal (GI) intolerance, rash, pruritus, and hyperkalemia. In addition, this agent may cause photosensitivity, and patients should be counseled to wear sun protection during therapy.

Topical Agents

Topical agents may be used as first-line treatment or adjunctively in bacterial skin infections. Mupirocin ointment is effective against *S. aureus* and some streptococcal infections.

Mupirocin ointment is minimally absorbed systemically. It is metabolized by the skin and usually well tolerated. Adverse effects are few but include headache, cough, rhinitis, pharyngitis, upper respiratory tract congestion, and taste perversion with nasal use. Burning, stinging, rash, erythema, or itching can occur when applied topically. Mupirocin should not be used in patients with an allergy to the drug and should not be used with other nasal products.

The topical preparation of gentamicin is available in a cream or an ointment. It is a powerful topical agent and is effective against many organisms, including GAS, *S. aureus*, and *Pseudomonas* species. Topical gentamicin can be used for a variety of primary and secondary skin infections. It is usually well tolerated, although irritation may occur. Occasionally, fungal infection or overgrowth of non-susceptible bacteria may occur at the site of use.

Selecting the Most Appropriate Agent

Practice guidelines are available to assist clinicians in the management of skin infections including the selection of appropriate antimicrobial therapy (Stevens et al., 2014). Most bacterial skin conditions are treated empirically based on the prescriber's knowledge of the organisms most likely to cause a particular infection (**Table 13.5**). When the organism is not known, the potential for serious infection is present, or if the patient is already extremely ill, the prescriber needs to confirm the diagnosis and organism either by skin biopsy or by wound culture. In such cases, empiric treatment begins with a broad-spectrum agent until organism susceptibility is available and a diagnosis is made.

Other important factors in choosing an antibiotic agent include patient allergies, pregnancy status, renal and hepatic function, and age. Practical concerns that affect compliance include the taste of the medication (especially in treating children), its adverse effect profile, how frequently it must be taken, and how much it costs. An antibiotic agent may be changed if the condition does not improve or if intolerable effects impede compliance or pose a danger to the patient. **Figure 13.1** gives an overview of the drug selection process.

First-Line Therapy: Impetigo and Ecthyma

For minor cases of bullous and non-bullous impetigo, topical mupirocin ointment applied twice daily for 5 days is recommended. For other cases of impetigo and ecthyma, an oral antibiotic with *S. aureus* coverage is prescribed for 7 days. A broad-spectrum penicillin (e.g., amoxicillin–clavulanate or dicloxacillin) or a first-generation cephalosporin (e.g., cephalexin) is a good first choice. In cases where cultures are taken and grow GAS only, penicillin is recommended. If MRSA is suspected or confirmed or in those with a penicillin allergy, doxycycline, clindamycin, or SMX–TMP may be used. In many communities, *S. aureus* has become resistant to clindamycin. Clinicians need to check with their local antibiogram if available. Because of the depth of ulceration and chronic nature of ecthyma, healing takes weeks to months, and scarring is likely. Debridement is painful and not recommended and unnecessary. When there are outbreaks of streptococcal glomerulonephritis, IV penicillin should be used to help control and eliminate nephritogenic GAS.

First-Line Therapy: Cellulitis and Erysipelas

Treatment for mild non-purulent cellulitis and erysipelas should begin promptly and usually on an outpatient basis with oral antibiotic therapy. Antibiotics should cover GAS. Penicillin VK, amoxicillin–clavulanate, a cephalosporin such as cephalexin, clindamycin, or dicloxacillin would be acceptable options. Clindamycin should be reserved for those with a penicillin allergy. For those with mild infections caused by MRSA, oral options include SMX–TMP, a tetracycline such as doxycycline or minocycline, or linezolid (Sartelli et al., 2018). Treatment duration is typically for 5 days, which may be extended if there is no improvement.

Those with moderate cellulitis require parenteral therapy with penicillin, cefazolin, ceftriaxone, or clindamycin. For infections caused by MRSA, IV vancomycin, daptomycin, linezolid, ceftaroline, or dalbavancin can be used. Most commonly, IV vancomycin is used and these other agents are often reserved for infectious diseases specialists for special and complicated cases. Severe infections require emergency surgical inspection to rule out necrotizing infection. Broad-spectrum empiric antibiotic treatment should be initiated with vancomycin and piperacillin–tazobactam. Improvement usually occurs rapidly within the first 48 hours.

Second-Line Therapy: Cellulitis and Erysipelas

If the infection does not respond to the initial course of treatment, patients should be promptly referred or admitted for IV therapy. Wounds that become secondarily infected may require debridement, with frequent cleansing and dressing changes. Surgical debridement may be necessary.

First-Line Therapy: Purulent Skin Infections

In all cases of purulent skin infections such as abscesses, furuncles, and carbuncles, incision and drainage are indicated. In mild cases, antibiotics are usually not needed since source control has been obtained and no systemic signs of infection are present. In moderate cases, systemic signs are present and empiric therapy with SMX–TMP or doxycycline should be started. If treatment fails, it is then considered a severe infection. Additionally, patients who present with fever, tachycardia, tachypnea, leukopenia, or leukocytosis or

TABLE 13.5		
Recommended Order of Treatment for Bacterial Skin Infections		
Infection	**First-Line Therapy**	**Second-Line Therapy**
Minor bullous and nonbullous impetigo	Topical mupirocin BID × 5 days	Oral antibiotic × 7 days or refer to an infectious diseases specialist
Impetigo and ecthyma	Oral antibiotic × 7 days	Admit for IV antibiotic treatment or refer
Cellulitis and erysipelas	Oral antibiotic × 5 days	Admit for IV antibiotic treatment or refer
Furuncles and carbuncles	Incision and drainage. Oral antibiotic × 7 days if infectious symptoms noted	Alternate oral antibiotic or refer

IV, intravenous.

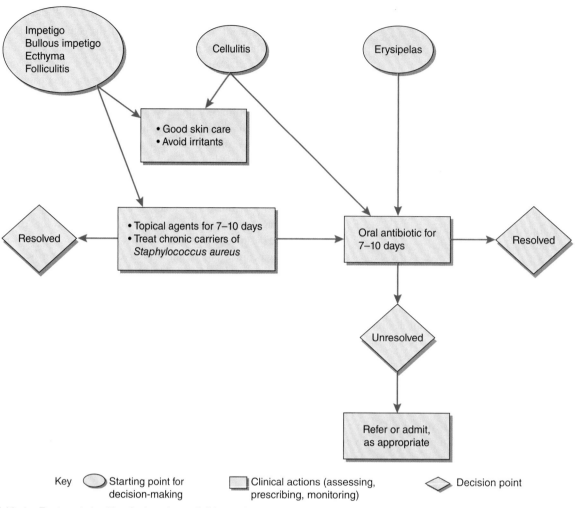

FIGURE 13–1   Treatment algorithm for impetigo, cellulitis, erysipelas, and other bacterial skin infections.

Note: If the patient has necrotizing fasciitis, admit to hospital and refer to specialist.

are immunocompromised should be treated as patients with severe infection. IV antibiotics with MRSA coverage such as vancomycin, daptomycin, linezolid, telavancin, or ceftaroline should be started. Pus obtained from incision and drainage in moderate to severe infections should be cultured. Once the culture speciates and sensitivities are available, antibiotic therapy should be narrowed as appropriate. In moderate infections, oral therapy with SMX–TMP for MRSA, or cephalexin or dicloxacillin for methicillin-susceptible *Staphylococcus aureus* (MSSA), may be used. In severe infections, de-escalation to cefazolin, nafcillin, or oxacillin may be done if MSSA is cultured. Antibiotics should be given for 7 to 14 days for severe infections.

Systemic therapy is not needed for folliculitis, and it often heals without treatment in 7 to 10 days. Topical mupirocin or clindamycin may be used in cases of widespread disease. Moist heat applications can help drain the pus in folliculitis and mild furunculosis.

For patients with paronychia, soaking the finger or toe in warm water helps with spontaneous drainage. For paronychias

with abscesses or felons, incision and drainage is recommended. Antibiotics are not recommended if no system signs of infection are present.

Second-Line Therapy: Purulent Skin Tissue Infections

For skin infections that fail oral therapy, IV therapy should be considered. Additionally, recurrence of a pustular infection in the same location should prompt a workup for a differential diagnosis such as a pilonidal cyst or other dermatologic disease.

First-Line Therapy: Diabetic Foot Infections

For ulcers that are not infected, antibiotics are not recommended. For mild to moderate DFIs, patients can be treated in the outpatient setting with oral antibiotics covering *S. aureus* and *Streptococcus* if they have not recently received antibiotics, in the past month. Such antibiotics include cephalexin and amoxicillin–clavulanate. Patients with severe DFIs will require inpatient admission and initiation of broad-spectrum parenteral antibiotics. Some patients with moderate infections but with certain risk factors like PAD may be initially treated as those with severe infections. Additionally, patients who fail outpatient therapy may need to be admitted to a hospital for parenteral antibiotics and further workup.

Empiric antibiotic coverage for pseudomonas is often unnecessary unless there are risk factors for pseudomonas infection, such as warm climate, high local prevalence, or walking barefoot in bodies of water (Lipsky et al., 2012). Empiric coverage for MRSA should be initiated in patients with severe-appearing infection or prior history of MRSA infection or in areas where prevalence of MRSA colonization or infection is high. Patients who have received antibiotics in the past month should receive antibiotic coverage against gram-negative bacilli. Coverage of anaerobic bacteria may be needed in cases of severe DFIs.

Antibiotic therapy should be narrowed once cultures result and susceptibilities are available. For mild and moderate DFIs, 1 to 2 weeks of therapy is typically sufficient and can be stopped once clinical signs of infection are resolved. For patients who have bone involvement, a 4-to-6-week course of antibiotics is recommended (Boulton et al., 2018). Antibiotic therapy without appropriate wound care is insufficient. Wound care specialists should be consulted if needed and available. For any DFI with necrotic tissue, debridement should be performed.

First-Line Therapy: Necrotizing Fasciitis

Surgical debridement is needed emergently for the treatment of necrotizing fasciitis. Additional debridement is usually required to fully remove all necrotic tissue. Broad-spectrum empiric antibiotic therapy should be started. An example of an empiric antibiotic regimen for necrotizing fasciitis includes piperacillin–tazobactam, clindamycin, or vancomycin. Clindamycin is primarily used for its toxin and cytokine-suppressing properties. Once culture results are available, antibiotic therapy can be tailored appropriately. Antibiotics are continued for 48 to 72 hours after clinical stability and when no further procedures are needed.

Special Considerations

When choosing topical or systemic therapy in a pregnant patient, a drug in category B should be chosen over a drug in category C whenever possible. Following is a list of commonly used medications for skin and skin structure infections and their associated categories. Of particular note, tigecycline, a derivative of tetracycline, is a category D medication and should be avoided during pregnancy. In general, beta-lactams are considered safe in pregnancy.

Amoxicillin–clavulanate: category B
Cephalexin and other cephalosporins: category B
Clindamycin: category B
Daptomycin: category B
Dicloxacillin: category B

Fluoroquinolones: category C
Vancomycin: category C
Linezolid: category C
Tigecycline: category D
SMX–TMP: category D

Monitoring Patient Response

The therapy for bacterial skin conditions is monitored by follow-up visits (see **Figure 13.1**). Most cases of impetigo heal rapidly without scarring or other adverse effects. These patients may not need to be seen again unless the condition does not resolve. However, untreated lesions may last for weeks and develop into ecthyma, which is the more chronic and severe form of impetigo. These patients should continue to be followed. Folliculitis, although not serious, is often recurrent or chronic. Emphasis should be placed on controlling aggravating factors and promoting good hygiene measures. Follow-up or referral is required if the condition spreads or does not resolve.

Patients with cellulitis and erysipelas should be followed closely because of the potential for a serious systemic infection. It is sometimes necessary to change antibiotic agents or increase the duration of treatment if the patient fails to improve. Follow-up or referral may be necessary for paronychia, which often recurs.

Patient Education
Drug Information

Patients treated with systemic antibiotic therapy must be taught to take their medication around the clock to sustain the proper blood level. They also must understand the importance of taking the medication for the prescribed length of time and not to discontinue their medication even if they feel their infection is resolved.

There are common side effects with most antibiotics, such as nausea, vomiting, diarrhea, and rash. Some medications must be taken with or without food. These instructions should be emphasized to the patient. Some medications may cause dizziness, drowsiness, or photosensitivity, and patients should be advised accordingly.

Antibiotics can predispose a patient to fungal infections such as vaginal candidiasis or oral thrush. Patients should be told to report these symptoms so that appropriate treatment can be implemented. Some antibiotics may cause a decreased effectiveness of oral contraceptives, so patients should be told to use an alternate form of contraception while on their medication until their next menstrual cycle.

Patients should be told to report signs of allergic reaction, fever, or severe diarrhea, especially if it contains blood, mucus, or pus. Unusual bleeding or bruising should also be reported. These adverse effects may be signs of a serious medication reaction.

Most topical medications are relatively well tolerated. However, some are in an alcohol base and are flammable. Patients should avoid smoking while on and shortly after applying their medication.

Nutrition and Lifestyle Changes

Patients need to learn proper methods of hygiene (**Box 13.3**) to prevent the spread of infection, secondary infection, or recurrence. Patients with paronychia must be instructed to keep their hands dry as much as possible.

In cases where there are open wounds, proper wound care instruction is essential. Some infections, such as impetigo, present a risk to others. Patients with impetigo should avoid contact with infants, small children, older adults, or those who are debilitated due to the highly contagious nature of the illness.

Although most bacterial skin infections are self-limiting and resolve quickly with treatment, some have the potential to become much more serious. Patients should be taught to report symptoms such as fever, increased erythema or streaking, chills, or malaise that may indicate a worsening of their condition. Also, the chronic nature of some skin infections, such as folliculitis, should be emphasized so that patients understand that treatment may be long term and recurrent.

It is important that patients with diabetes wear proper-fitting shoes to prevent ulceration and therefore prevent subsequent infection. A referral to establish care with a podiatrist should be made as a podiatrist can measure a patient's feet for custom-made shoes and insoles and assist in foot care. Patients should be counseled to avoid walking barefoot as that makes the foot more susceptible to injury. Additionally, patients with diabetes should have yearly foot exams and should be encouraged to self-monitor their feet at home with a mirror. This is especially important for patients with diabetic neuropathy, who may have decreased sensation on the bottom of their feet, making it difficult to feel an injury. A multidisciplinary team with vascular surgeons, podiatrists, and wound care specialists is helpful in reducing the risk of developing infectious wounds that could result in amputation (Lipsky et al., 2012).

Complementary and Alternative Medicine

Tea tree oil can have some activity against MRSA, although one study found it to be significantly less effective than topical mupirocin in clearing nasal colonization of MRSA (Dryden et al., 2004). A Cochrane review on Chinese herbal medicine in the treatment of skin and soft tissue infections found that there is not enough evidence to support its use (Wang et al., 2014).

Topical trypsin is possibly effective for wound cleansing and wound healing. Trypsin is contained in some U.S. FDA–approved products for wound debridement, such as Granulex and Dermaspray. Pain and burning may occur with their use.

FUNGAL INFECTIONS

Introduction

Fungi live in the dead, horny outer layer of the skin. The organisms penetrate only the stratum corneum—the surface layer of the skin—and infect the skin, hair, and nails. They cause tinea, tinea versicolor, and candidiasis.

Causes

Tinea

Dermatophytes are a group of fungi that infect nonviable keratinized cutaneous tissues. Dermatophytosis, more commonly called tinea, is a condition caused by dermatophytes. Tinea is further classified by the location of the infection (**Box 13.4**).

Tinea capitis primarily affects children of ages 3 to 9. This age group may also be infected with tinea corporis. Tinea pedis most commonly affects the adolescent population and young adults. Immunocompromised patients have an increased incidence and more intractable dermatophytosis.

General factors that predispose an individual to a fungal infection include warm, moist, occluded environments; family history; and a compromised immune system. Infection is spread from people, inanimate objects, and animals, especially cats and dogs. Different types of dermatophytes cause infection on specific sites of the body. These common site-specific dermatophytes differ by geographic location. For example, a dermatophyte causing the majority of cases of tinea capitis in Canada will not necessarily be the same dermatophyte causing the majority of tinea capitis infections in Italy.

Tinea Versicolor

Tinea versicolor, also called pityriasis versicolor, is a superficial fungal skin infection. It is a chronic, asymptomatic infection characterized by well-demarcated, scaling patches of varied coloration, from whitish to pink, tan, or brown.

An overgrowth of the hyphal form of *Malassezia*, a lipophilic fungus part of normal skin flora, causes tinea versicolor. *Malassezia* is typically found on sebaceous areas of the skin, where lipid-rich sebum is found. It causes hyper or hypopigmentation, when certain triggers cause it to convert to its pathogenic hyphal form. Tinea versicolor is most common in teenagers and young adults. It occurs mostly in subtropical and tropical areas. In temperate zones, it is more common in the summer months but is seen in physically active people year-round. Other risk factors include excessive perspiration, diabetes, poor nutrition, and possibly genetics. The infection

---

BOX 13.4   Varieties of Tinea Infections

Tinea infections are identified by their location on the body as follows:

- *Head:* tinea capitis
- *Body:* tinea corporis
- *Hand:* tinea manus
- *Foot:* tinea pedis
- *Groin:* tinea cruris
- *Nails:* tinea unguium (onychomycosis)

rarely causes symptoms other than discoloration, and patients usually seek treatment for cosmetic purposes.

Candidiasis

Cutaneous candidiasis is a superficial fungal infection of the skin and mucous membranes. It is commonly found in the diaper area, oral cavity, intertriginous areas, nails, vagina, and male genitalia. It can occur at any age and in both sexes. It is classified by its location on the body (**Box 13.5**).

Cutaneous candidiasis, which is caused by *Candida albicans*, a yeast-like fungus, occurs on moist cutaneous sites. It thrives in occluded sites. Predisposing factors include infection, diabetes, use of systemic and topical corticosteroids, and immunosuppression.

Pathophysiology

Tinea

Dermatophytes grow only on or within keratinized structures. Most infections result from three genera of fungi: *Trichophyton*, *Microsporum*, and *Epidermophyton*. These can be found on humans, on animals, and in the soil. They produce keratinases, an enzyme that digests keratin, causing epidermal scale, thickened nails, and hair loss.

Tinea Versicolor

Malassezia has an enzyme that oxidizes fatty acids in the skin surface lipids, forming dicarboxylic acids, which inhibit tyrosinase in epidermal melanocytes and cause hypomelanosis (loss of pigmentation).

Candidiasis

Normally found on the skin and mucous membranes, *C. albicans* invades the epidermis when warm, moist conditions prevail or when there is a break in the skin that allows overgrowth.

BOX 13.5   Varieties of Candidiasis

Candidal infections are identified by their location on the body as follows:

- *Axillae, under pendulous breasts, groin, intergluteal folds:* intertrigo
- *Glans penis:* balanitis
- *Follicular pustules:* candidal folliculitis
- *Nail folds:* candidal paronychia
- *Mouth and tongue:* oral candidiasis (thrush)
- *Area included under diaper:* diaper dermatitis

Diagnostic Criteria

Tinea

General symptoms of cutaneous fungal infections include pruritus, burning, and stinging of the scalp or skin. An inflammatory dermal reaction may cause erythema and vesicles. Diagnosis is confirmed by several mechanisms. One mechanism is microscopic evaluation of the stratum corneum. Fungi appear as rod-shaped filaments with branching.

Another mechanism for diagnosis is fungal culture, which can take 7 to 14 days for fungus to grow. This may not be feasible for use if prompt treatment is needed. However, given the severity of adverse effects associated with the use of oral antifungals, culture is often recommended to select appropriate antifungal therapy if treatment can be deferred without harm to the patient.

A third diagnostic method involves using a Wood lamp, which produces a bright green fluorescence in the presence of a tinea infection caused by *Microsporum* species. A major disadvantage of this test is that other fungal infections may be undiagnosed because the Wood lamp test identifies only *Microsporum*. Another limitation to this test is that it needs to be performed by a trained technician.

Tinea Capitis

Presentation of tinea capitis varies widely. There may be generalized, diffuse seborrheic dermatitis-like scalp scaling, although more common signs and symptoms include patches of alopecia with or without scaly patches or black dots. Kerion, a severe form of tinea capitis, can be recognized by impetigo-like lesions with crusting and redness, areas of tender plaque, and possibly inflammatory nodules. Cervical lymphadenopathy can be suggestive of tinea capitis. Most cases of tinea capitis are found in pre-pubertal children, with a disproportionate number of African Americans. It is very contagious. If left untreated, it can cause permanent alopecia and scarring.

Most cases (90%) in the United States are caused by *Trichophyton tonsurans (T. tonsurans)*. *Microsporum canis* is the most common cause of tinea capitis in most parts of Europe, and *Trichophyton violaceum (T. violaceum)* is a common cause in Africa and the Middle East.

Tinea capitis presents in several ways:

- Inflamed, scaly, alopecic patches, especially in infants
- Diffuse scaling with multiple round areas with alopecia secondary to broken hair shafts, leaving residual black dots
- *Gray patch* type with round, scaly plaques of alopecia, in which the hair shaft is broken off close to the surface

Tinea Corporis

Tinea corporis is called *ringworm* and affects the face, limbs, or trunk but not the groin, hands, or feet. The typical presentation of tinea corporis is a ring-shaped lesion with well-demarcated margins, central clearing, and a scaly, erythematous border. It is transmitted by contact with infected animals, humans, and objects such as infected mats in wrestling. Transmission via humans is low, estimated to be around 10% (Woo et al., 2019).

The organisms most commonly responsible are *Trichophyton rubrum (T. rubrum)*, and *Trichophyton mentagrophytes (T. mentagrophytes)*. This is commonly seen in children and young adults.

Tinea Cruris

Tinea cruris is often referred to as *jock itch*. It is a fungal infection of the groin and inguinal folds and sometimes can spread to the upper inner thighs. The most common causes are *T. rubrum* and *E. floccosum*. Typically, the lesion borders are well demarcated and peripherally spreading. The lesions are large, erythematous, and macular, with a central clearing. A hallmark of tinea cruris is pruritus and a burning sensation. There is often an accompanying fungal infection of the feet.

Tinea Pedis

Interdigital tinea pedis, commonly called *athlete's foot*, is characterized by scaling and itching in the web spaces between the toes and sometimes by maceration of the skin. It is the most common type of tinea pedis. Another variation is inflammatory tinea pedis, which presents with vesicles involving the mid-anterior plantar surface of the foot. A third variety is the moccasin style, which presents with chronic noninflammatory scaling and thickness and cracking of the epidermis on the sole, heel, and often up the side of the foot. The fourth variation is the ulcerative type. It presents with vesicles, pustules, and ulcers on the foot. It is most common in those with diabetes or an immunocompromising condition. Most cases of tinea pedis are caused by *T. rubrum*, which evokes a minimal inflammatory response. *T. mentagrophytes* organism produces vesicles and bullae. *T. interdigitale* and *E. floccosum* are also common causes of tinea pedis. All types of tinea pedis present with itching and burning sensation.

Tinea Manuum

Tinea manuum is a dermatophyte infection of the hand. The lesions are marked by mild, diffuse scaling of the palmar skin, and vesicles may be grouped on the palms or fingernails involved. It can cause itching and a burning sensation.

Tinea Unguium

Tinea unguium, also called onychomycosis, is a fungal infection of the nail common in older adults. Typically affected are the toenails, which become thick and scaly with subungual debris. Onycholysis, a separation of the nail from the nail bed, may be seen. The infection usually begins distally at the tip of the toe and moves proximally and through the nail plate, producing a yellowish discoloration and striations in the actual nail. Under the nail, a hyperkeratotic substance accumulates that lifts the nail up. If untreated, the nail thickens and turns yellowish brown. Onychomycosis is usually asymptomatic but may be painful when wearing occlusive footwear. In immunocompromised patients, tinea unguium can act as a portal of entry for a more serious infection.

Organisms causing onychomycosis include *T. interdigitale*, *T. rubrum*, *T. mentagrophytes*, and sometimes *C. albicans*. Some health insurance plans refuse to reimburse for drug therapy without confirmation of the diagnosis. Tests that verify the diagnosis include the potassium hydroxide (KOH) test and culture.

Tinea Versicolor

Skin lesions of tinea versicolor are well-defined, round or oval macules with an overlay of scales that may coalesce to form larger patches. They most often form on the trunk, upper arms, and neck. There may be mild itching. The diagnosis is confirmed by positive KOH test findings, which reveal budding yeast and hyphae.

Candidiasis

Candidiasis has several classifications. Intertrigo presents as red, moist papules or pustules. It is found in the axillae, inframammary areas, groin, and skin folds and between fingers and toes.

Diaper dermatitis presents as erythema and edema with papular and pustular lesions, erosion, and oozing. Scaling may be evident at the margin of the lesions.

Interdigital candidiasis is an erythematous eroded area with surrounding maceration between the fingers and toes, whereas balanitis presents as multiple discrete pustules on the glans penis and preputial sac. Balanitis that involves the scrotum can be painful. It is most common in uncircumcised men.

Paronychia and onychia present as redness and swelling of the nail folds. Swelling lifts the wall from the nail plate, causing purulent infection.

Initiating Drug Therapy

Drug therapy should be initiated when the diagnosis is confirmed. For indications that require oral antifungal therapy, it is often recommended to obtain culture to ensure that the selected antifungal will be active against the cultured dermatophyte. This is so that the patient will not be exposed to avoidable potential harm since oral antifungals are not without risk. There is a black box warning issued by the FDA recommending against the use of oral ketoconazole for the treatment of onychomycosis or cutaneous dermatophyte infections due to risk of hepatotoxicity. A discussion of oral ketoconazole is beyond the scope of this chapter.

Topical agents for treating tinea versicolor include selenium sulfide, sulfur plus salicylic acid, ketoconazole, or zinc pyrithione shampoos, and azole creams. For widespread or stubborn disease, systemic itraconazole for 5 days or once-weekly fluconazole for 2 weeks may be prescribed.

Candidiasis can be prevented by keeping intertriginous areas dry when possible. Therapy should be initiated when clear signs and symptoms are present and a clinical diagnosis is made.

Goals of Drug Therapy

Pharmacologic therapy is directed against the offending fungus and the site of infection. Therapy is topical or systemic, depending on the location of the lesion. Topical therapy is used for most skin infections. The exceptions are tinea capitis and tinea unguium.

The goal of therapy for tinea versicolor is resolution of lesions. Because the lesions are likely to recur in warm weather, prophylaxis consists of applying selenium sulfide shampoo twice a month for 6 months.

Topical Azole Antifungals

Topical azoles (**Table 13.6**) impair the synthesis of ergosterol, the main sterol of fungal cell membranes. This allows for increased permeability and leakage of cellular components, ultimately resulting in cell death. Topical azoles are fungicides that are effective against tinea corporis, tinea cruris, and tinea pedis as well as cutaneous candidiasis. They should be applied once or twice a day for 2 to 4 weeks. Therapy should continue for 1 week after the lesions clear. Adverse effects include pruritus, irritation, and stinging.

Topical Allylamine Antifungals

These agents are effective against dermatophyte infections but have limited effectiveness against yeast such as *candida*. Patients treated with these agents may undergo a shorter treatment period with less likelihood of relapse. Topical allylamines are applied twice daily and include terbinafine, naftifine, and tolnaftate. Potential side effects include burning and irritation.

Griseofulvin
Mechanism of Action

Griseofulvin is a fungistatic that deposits in keratin precursor cells, increasing new keratin resistance to fungal invasion.

Adverse Events

Adverse effects include nausea, vomiting, diarrhea, headache, insomnia, and photosensitivity. It is contraindicated in hepatic impairment and can cause hematologic abnormalities. This drug may aggravate lupus erythematosus.

Interactions

Griseofulvin decreases levels of warfarin (Coumadin), cyclosporine (Sandimmune), and oral contraceptives. It is important for

TABLE 13.6			
Overview of Antifungal Medications			
Generic (Trade) Name and Dosage	**Selected Adverse Events**	**Contraindications**	**Special Considerations**
Topical Agents			
Clotrimazole (Lotrimin) ointment, powder, cream, solution. Gently massage ointment, cream, or solution into affected and surrounding skin areas BID for 2–4 weeks.	Erythema, irritation, stinging, pruritus	Hypersensitivity to clotrimazole or any component of the formulation	Available OTC
Miconazole (Micatin, Monistat Derm) ointment, powder, cream, solution. Cover affected areas with BID for 2–4 weeks.	Allergic contact dermatitis, burning sensation, maceration	Hypersensitivity to miconazole or any component of the formulation	Available OTC
Ketoconazole (Nizoral) cream. Apply to affected and surrounding areas once daily for 2–4 weeks.	Irritation, stinging, pruritus	Hypersensitivity to ketoconazole or any component of the formulation.	RX only
Oxiconazole (Oxistat) cream, lotion. Apply to affected and surrounding areas once or twice daily for 2–4 weeks.	Pruritus, burning	Hypersensitivity to oxiconazole or any component of the formulation	Available OTC
Sulconazole (Exelderm) cream. Apply to affected and surrounding areas BID for 3–4 weeks.	Pruritus, burning sensation, erythema	Hypersensitivity to sulconazole or any component of the formulation	Not recommended in children Avoid contact with eyes RX only
Ciclopirox (Loprox cream, Penlac lacquer). Cream—apply to affected area BID for 4 weeks Lacquer—apply to affected nails and adjacent skin daily. Remove with alcohol weekly	Burning sensation	Hypersensitivity to ciclopirox or any component of the formulation	Not recommended in children younger than age 10 Not studied in immunocompromised patients Avoid occlusive dressing RX only

(Continued)

TABLE 13.6

Overview of Antifungal Medications (*Continued*)

Generic (Trade) Name and Dosage	Selected Adverse Events	Contraindications	Special Considerations
Naftifine (Naftin) cream. Apply to affected area once daily for 2–4 weeks.	Burning, stinging, dryness, erythema, itching	Hypersensitivity to naftifine or any component of the formulation	Not recommended in children ≤2 years Avoid occlusive dressings Avoid contact with mucous membranes RX only
Terbinafine (Lamisil) cream, spray, gel. Apply to affected area one to twice daily for 1–2 weeks. Spray, gel—apply once daily for 1 week	Burning, irritation, skin exfoliation, dryness		Not recommended in children ≤12 years Avoid occlusive dressings. Avoid contact with mucous membranes Available OTC
Tolnaftate (Tinactin) cream. Apply small amount BID for 4 weeks	Stinging, burning, irritation		Not recommended in children ≤2 years Available OTC
Selenium sulfide (Selsun) lotion, shampoo. Massage into affected area, rest 10 min and rinse thoroughly	Irritation, hair loss	Hypersensitivity to selenium sulfide or any component of the formulation	Available OTC
Nystatin (Mycostatin) 100,000 units/mL Oral candidiasis dosing: Infants: 2–4 mL PO QID each side of mouth Adults: 4–6 mL PO QID (swish and swallow)	GI upset, oral irritation	Hypersensitivity to nystatin or any component of the formulation	Continue use for at least 48 hours after clinical cure. Keep in mouth as long as possible (minutes) before swallowing
Oral Agents			
Griseofulvin (Gris-PEG) Microsize: Adult: 500–1,000 mg PO in one or divided doses Child: 20–25 mg/kg/d in single daily dose or in 2 divided doses (maximum 1,000 mg/d) Ultramicrosize: Adult: 375–750 mg PO in divided doses Child: 10–15 mg/kg/d (maximum 750 mg/d)	Headaches, nausea, vomiting, diarrhea, photosensitivity, insomnia, weakness, liver dysfunction, severe skin reactions	Pregnancy, patients with porphyria or hepatic failure	Ultramicrosize formulation has better absorption than microsize formulation Prescribe with caution to patients who are sensitive to penicillin Drug is most effective when taken with a high-fat meal Monitor complete blood count and LFT with long-term use. Drug use may aggravate lupus erythematosus Use with alcohol produces antabuse-like effects Drug interactions: decreases effect of oral contraceptives and warfarin and barbiturates may decrease effectiveness of friseofulvin
Itraconazole (Sporanox) Adult: 100-200 mg PO once or twice daily Child: 5 mg/kg/dose (max 100 mg) PO daily	GI upset, rash, fatigue, headache, dizziness, edema, heart failure exacerbation, QTc prolongation	Many drug interactions through inhibition CYP3A4 Concomitant use with ticagrelor, ivabradine, dofetilide, dronedarone, eplerenone, methadone Pregnancy	Limited data in children Ingestion of food increases absorption of capsules/tablets and should be taken with food Oral solution should be taken on an empty stomach Capsules are not bioequivalent to solution formulation

TABLE 13.6

Overview of Antifungal Medications (*Continued*)

Generic (Trade) Name and Dosage	Selected Adverse Events	Contraindications	Special Considerations
Terbinafine (Lamisil) 250 mg PO daily Child: <25 kg: 125 mg once daily for 6 weeks 25–35 kg: 187.5 mg once daily for 6 weeks >35 kg: 250 mg once daily for 6 weeks	Depression, taste disturbances including loss of taste, LFT abnormalities, pruritus, headache, thrombotic microangiopathy	CrCl <50 mL/min Liver disease	Granules for suspension are not available in the United States. Only comes in 250 mg tablet dosage form. Pulse dosing is less effective but may reduce AEs. Only approved for children ≥4 years for tinea capitis. Taste disturbances may be permanent. Confirmatory culture testing recommended prior to initiating therapy due to potential toxicity.
Fluconazole (Diflucan) Adults: 150–300 mg PO once weekly for 2–6 weeks	GI disturbance, headache, rash, hepatotoxicity	QTc prolonging medications: use with caution	Decrease dose if CrCl <50 mL/min CYP3A4 inhibitor may increase the concentration of substrates Drug interactions: potentiates warfarin, theophylline. May increase serum levels of phenytoin, cyclosporine

AEs, adverse events; CrCl, creatinine clearance; CYP3A, cytochrome P-450 enzyme 3A; GI, gastrointestinal; LFT, liver function tests; OTC, over the counter; QTc, corrected QT-interval; RX, prescription.

females of reproductive age to be placed on effective contraceptive while on therapy as griseofulvin is pregnancy category X. A disulfiram-like reaction may occur when taken with alcohol. Patients should be advised not to drink alcoholic beverages while taking this drug.

Systemic Allylamine Antifungals

Terbinafine (Lamisil) is a synthetic allylamine derivative that inhibits squalene epoxidase, a key enzyme in fungal biosynthesis. This causes a deficiency of ergosterol, causing fungal cell death. It is used in the treatment of onychomycosis and can be used in other tinea infections.

Dosage

The dose for onychomycosis treatment is 250 mg by mouth daily for 6 weeks if on the fingernail and 12 weeks if on the toenail. Various pulse-dosing regimens exist and may be used to improve compliance and reduce cost and risk for adverse events (AEs); although pulse-dosing may result in treatment failure. Clearance is reduced by about 50% when creatinine clearance is less than 50 mL/min.

Adverse Events

AEs include diarrhea, dyspepsia, rash, increase in liver enzymes, and headache. Evaluation of alanine aminotransferase and

aspartate aminotransferase levels is recommended before starting therapy and at 6 to 8 weeks into therapy if it is long term because it can cause liver failure, although this is rare. Terbinafine may permanently alter ability to taste and smell. Therapy should be discontinued if the patient reports taste or smell disturbances. Depression has also been reported, and it is important to counsel patients on this adverse effect and to report it immediately.

Interactions

Terbinafine may increase the serum concentration of clozapine, amitriptyline, and imipramine. Terbinafine may decrease the serum concentration of tamoxifen and tramadol.

Systemic Azole Antifungals

Systemic azoles inhibit cytochrome P-450 (CYP) enzymes and fungal 14-alpha-demethylase, inhibiting synthesis of ergosterol. Systemic therapy is required for tinea capitis and tinea unguium. Itraconazole (Sporanox), a systemic azole, has a high affinity for keratin and is lipophilic, which causes high levels to accumulate in the hair and nail. It has a long half-life, so pulse dosing, in which periods of drug therapy are alternated with periods without therapy, is feasible. The capsule requires gastric acidity to aid in absorption and therefore should be taken with food. Itraconazole suspension should be taken on an empty stomach to increase absorption. These two formulations are not interchangeable.

Dosage

The dose of itraconazole is 200 mg once daily for 12 weeks for toe onychomycosis. For fingernail onychomycosis, the dose is 200 mg twice daily for 1 week, then 3 weeks off, and repeat dosing with 200 mg twice daily for 1 week. This pulse regimen may also be done for toe onychomycosis, but the repeat dosing is done for two more times after the initial week. Itraconazole is not recommended for children, and ingestion of food increases absorption.

Various regimens of fluconazole have been studied for the treatment of tinea infections. One such is 150 mg once weekly for 2 to 6 weeks for the treatment of tinea pedis. For tinea corporis or cruris, the treatment duration is usually 2 to 4 weeks. Fluconazole has not been extensively studied in pediatrics for the treatment of tinea infections.

Contraindications

All systemic azoles can prolong corrected QT-interval (QTc) interval. Caution should be used when using other drugs that can also prolong QTc interval, especially drugs that are metabolized by CYP3A4, such as erythromycin and quinidine, as their use with azoles is contraindicated. Azole antifungals inhibit CYP3A4. Systemic azole antifungals should be avoided in pregnancy. Itraconazole has many contraindications. It should not be used for skin infections in patients with ventricular dysfunction such as heart failure and women who are planning to become pregnant.

Adverse Events

Adverse effects associated with systemic azole therapy include GI upset, rash, fatigue, hepatic dysfunction, edema (with itraconazole), and hypokalemia.

Interactions

Concomitant use with QTc-prolonging drugs should be avoided. Itraconazole capsules should not be taken with antacids as it needs an acidic environment for absorption. Itraconazole should not be used in patients taking ticagrelor, rivaroxaban, ivabradine, or dofetilide.

Selenium Sulfide

Selenium sulfide has antifungal properties. It is applied once a day to the affected skin for 10 minutes and then rinsed off daily for 1 week. It should be used with caution in instances of acute inflammation or exudation. Skin folds and genitalia are carefully rinsed. Selenium sulfide must be kept away from eyes. Potential adverse effects include irritation and hair loss.

Nystatin

Nystatin (Mycostatin) is a fungicide that binds to sterols in the cell membrane of the fungus, causing a change in the membrane's permeability. This allows intracellular components to leak, thereby causing cell death. Nystatin cream is preferred over ointment for treatment in intertriginous areas. Moist areas are better treated with nystatin powder.

Selecting the Most Appropriate Agent

Topical agents work well for most tineas but not for tinea capitis and tinea unguium. To be effective, all therapy must be adequate in dose and duration. If a pet carries the fungus, the pet must be treated.

When selecting an oral agent to treat onychomycosis, consideration must be given to the cost of the agent, patient motivation and compliance, the age and health of the patient, and drug interactions and side effect profile of the medications.

First-Line Therapy: Tinea

Topical therapy is recommended for cases of tinea corporis, pedis, cruris, or manuum when the infection affects a limited area. The topical antifungal is applied 3 cm beyond the margin of the lesion. Therapy should continue for at least 2 weeks and for 1 week after the lesion clears.

Tinea capitis can only be cured with oral therapy since topical therapies cannot adequately penetrate the hair follicles. Therapy for tinea capitis caused by *Microsporum* is microsize griseofulvin administered with milk or food to promote absorption. Treatment is for 6 weeks. The adult dose is 500 mg daily, and the pediatric dose is 10 mg/kg/d. For infections caused by *T. tonsurans*, terbinafine 250 mg orally daily should be used for 4 weeks in children at least 4 years of age and greater than 35 kg. Children who weigh less than 25 kg are dosed with 125 mg and those who weigh between 25 and 35 kg are dosed with 187.5 mg daily. Children may attend school during therapy.

First-line therapy for tinea unguium consists of systemic terbinafine based on a Cochrane review that showed that both terbinafine and azole antifungals are better than placebo at achieving clinical and mycological cure, but terbinafine is probably better than azole antifungals at achieving clinical cure rates with no significant difference in AE rates (Kreijkamp-Kaspers et al., 2017). Dosing for adults is 250 mg orally daily for at least 6 weeks for fingernails and 12 weeks for toenails. Treatment success rates vary between 51% and 71%. Use of terbinafine may be limited due to its adverse effect profile, especially in older adults, who may be more vulnerable to its effects. Topical preparations are not effective because they penetrate the nails poorly.

Second-Line Therapy: Tinea

Topical therapies are often successful for tinea corporis, pedis, cruris, and manuum, although second-line therapy is needed if the infection fails to respond to topical therapy or if there is extensive and chronic disease. Second-line therapy consists of terbinafine 250 mg orally daily for 1 to 3 weeks or itraconazole 100 to 200 mg orally daily for 1 to 4 weeks.

Second-line therapy for tinea capitis involves using an alternate antifungal such as itraconazole, terbinafine, fluconazole, or griseofulvin.

Second-line therapy for tinea unguium includes systemic azole antifungals and topical nail solutions. Itraconazole is given by pulse dosing, 200 mg twice daily with a full meal for 7 consecutive days per month. Treatment for fingernails lasts 2 months and for toenails 3 months. Also effective for toenails is 200 mg itraconazole per day for 12 weeks. Pulse dosing has less impact on the liver and is more popular than continuous dosing due to fewer side effects, easier patient compliance, and decreased cost. Fluconazole can be given at a dose of 150 to 300 mg once weekly for 12 to 24 weeks for fingernails and 24 to 52 weeks for toenails. When systemic therapy with terbinafine and azoles is contraindicated, topical nail treatments can be used. Available agents are efinaconazole (Jublia) 10% solution, tavaborole (Kerydin) 5% solution, and ciclopirox (Ciclodan) 8% solution. Therapy lasts for 48 weeks, although mycologic and clinical cure rates are low. It is important to keep in mind that these topical nail solutions can be expensive but may be the only option for those who cannot or are unable to tolerate systemic therapy. In clinical practice, patients are seldom placed on systemic therapy due to risks associated with their use.

First-Line Therapy: Tinea Versicolor

Selenium sulfide 2.5% solution is applied once a day for 7 days. Pyrithione zinc (Head & Shoulders shampoo) may also be used. An antifungal topical agent can also be used, such as terbinafine, ketoconazole, or sulconazole nitrate creams twice daily for 2 weeks.

Lesions may reappear because the infection is a result of microorganisms that normally inhabit the skin, so twice-monthly application of selenium sulfide is suggested as prophylaxis for 6 months following initial treatment.

Second-Line Therapy: Tinea Versicolor

For resistant or widespread tinea versicolor, systemic therapy with itraconazole 200 mg orally for 5 days or fluconazole 300 mg orally once weekly for 2 weeks may be prescribed. If infection reoccurs in warm weather, it is appropriate to repeat the previously effective regimen.

First-Line Therapy: Candidiasis

For cutaneous candidiasis, topical treatment with nystatin, clotrimazole, ketoconazole, oxiconazole, or econazole should be applied twice daily until infection clears. For diaper dermatitis caused by candida, nystatin ointment or cream can be applied two to four times daily.

Second-Line Therapy: Candidiasis

For failure to respond to treatment, once weekly oral fluconazole 150 mg for 4 weeks may be prescribed to adults for intertrigo.

Monitoring Patient Response

When patients use terbinafine, fluconazole, or itraconazole, liver function tests should be monitored at 6 to 8 weeks. Follow-up evaluations need to monitor both the effectiveness of the therapy and labs to evaluate liver, kidney, and hematopoietic function. If tests disclose elevated liver function or if there is an acute change in renal function, drug therapy should be discontinued. For itraconazole, patients should be monitored for signs and symptoms of heart failure.

For cutaneous candidiasis, response to therapy should be evaluated in 2 weeks. Human immunodeficiency virus infection and diabetes mellitus should be ruled out in patients who have recurring problems with candidiasis.

Patient Education

An important role of the practitioner is teaching the patient about hygiene and ways to avoid transferring fungal infection to others. Patients should be instructed to complete the full course of treatment and not to stop treatment when symptoms subside. Parents and other caregivers also need to know that children can attend school while being treated.

It is important to inform patients with tinea versicolor that it may take several months for the discoloration to disappear. Prophylactic application of selenium sulfide shampoo twice a month can prevent recurrence.

Complementary and Alternative Medicine

Tea tree oil has natural antifungal compounds that help kill the fungi that cause fungal infections, particularly in interdigital tinea pedis (Satchell et al., 2002). Data on this are sparse, and this should only be used if patients are resistant to recommended therapy.

VIRAL SKIN INFECTIONS

Introduction

Viruses producing skin lesions may be categorized into three groups: herpes viruses, papillomaviruses, and pox viruses. Viruses' genetic material can be made of ribonucleic acid (RNA) or deoxyribonucleic acid (DNA). Herpes viruses, papillomaviruses, and pox viruses are all DNA viruses.

Viruses are obligate small parasites that consist of a nucleic acid core surrounded by one or more proteins. A host cell is required for viral replication. Several mechanisms exist for viral replication, and different DNA viruses replicate by their own specific mechanism. Pox viruses replicate entirely in the cytoplasm. Herpes viruses and papillomaviruses replicate in the nucleus of the host cell. Pox viruses are not discussed in this chapter, since they are very rare. An example of a pox virus is smallpox, which has been eradicated from the world by widespread use of the smallpox vaccine.

Causes

Herpes Virus Infections

Nine types of herpes viruses are associated with human illness: herpes simplex virus type 1 (HSV-1), herpes simplex virus type 2 (HSV-2), varicella-zoster virus (VZV), Epstein-Barr virus, cytomegalovirus, human herpes virus type 6 (HHV-6) types A and B, and Kaposi sarcoma-associated herpesvirus (HHV-8).

HSV-1 infection usually involves the face, mostly mouth and eyes, and skin above the waist. It is most often the cause of cold sores, or herpes simplex labialis, and herpetic whitlow, an infectious blister on the digits. Whitlow infection commonly is the cause of HSV-1 spread to the digits from thumb-sucking in children or to health care professionals who acquire HSV-1 infection while working without gloves. HSV-2 is most commonly associated with the genitalia and the skin below the waist, although HSV-1 can also infect those areas. A life-threatening neonatal infection is associated with HSV-2 in a baby whose mother is infected with the virus; the infection is typically transmitted during vaginal birth.

Herpes zoster (shingles) and varicella (chickenpox) are the result of VZV reactivation and infection, respectively. The incidence of herpes zoster increases with age and is most common in older adults and immunocompromised individuals. Varicella infection occurs mostly in children, although with vaccination, active infection is uncommon. Risk factors for herpes zoster include age more than 50 years, female gender, white race, immunodeficiency, solid organ transplant, and hematologic malignancy. Infectious mononucleosis is a result of Epstein-Barr virus infection. HHV-6 is associated with a mild childhood illness called roseola. HHV-8 is associated with Kaposi sarcoma, especially in patients with HIV infection. HSV-1 and VZV are discussed in this chapter; HSV-2 is discussed in Chapter 35.

Warts (Verrucae)

Verrucae, or warts, are caused by the human papillomavirus (HPV). There are more than 100 types of HPV. They are transferred by skin-to-skin contact. The common viruses can be classified as those causing anogenital infections and non-anogenital infections. Anogenital infections are discussed in Chapter 35. Non-anogenital HPV infections typically present as warts. They are very common, especially in children. At some time in their life, approximately 20% of school-age children have one or more warts, which usually regress spontaneously (Becker & Childress (2018)).

It is thought that microtraumas on the skin provide an entry way for the virus. The virus then causes keratinocyte proliferation, which results in the formation of a wart on the surface of the epidermis. In immunocompromised individuals, this is a benign infection and is self-limiting. HPV is transmitted by direct contact with an object or someone shedding the virus.

Factors that predispose individuals to HPV include the following:

- Immunosuppression
- Walking barefoot
- Use of communal showers
- Handling raw meat, fish, or other animal matter

Pathophysiology

Herpes Virus Infections

Herpes viruses replicate their own polymerase along with several of their own enzymes. HSV-1 and VZV are highly contagious, especially when lesions are in the vesicular phase. The virus is spread by direct contact with wet vesicles on skin or mucous membranes. The individual is no longer contagious once lesions have crusted over.

After primary infection with HSV-1 or varicella, most often in childhood, the virus retreats to the ganglia, where it remains latent until it is reactivated. The virus can be latent for years. For HSV-1, triggers such as stress, extremes in temperature, sun exposure, and weakened immune system can reactivate the latent infection. For herpes zoster, the virus typically stays dormant for many years and is reactivated with no apparent direct cause. Either active infection with varicella or immunization with the varicella vaccine as a child causes latent disease, although those who are vaccinated are less likely to have activation of herpes zoster. Because of these viruses' ability to stay dormant in the ganglia, they are never fully eradicated. Recurrent infection is common for HSV-1, and although recurrent infection with herpes zoster is possible, it is not common in immunocompetent individuals. Additionally, due to the location of the latent virus, reactivation can cause neuropathic pain, a common complication in herpes zoster. In HSV-1, a tingly and burning sensation can be felt at the site of infection.

Warts (Verrucae)

HPV proteins contribute to the initiation of DNA replication. The virus enters through skin abrasions and infects the cells of the basal layers of the skin. Viral replication is slow, with an incubation period of 4 to 6 months. Once viral replication in the basal layers of the skin produces enough keratin, a wart is produced on the superficial layer of the skin.

Diagnostic Criteria

Herpes Virus Infections

Infection with HSV-1 causes vesicular eruptions that are painful and often recurrent. Prodromal symptoms can occur with recurrent infections and include burning, tingling, or itching. Within hours, the lesion presents as a single vesicle or group of vesicles that overlie an erythematous base. They become pustules and become crusted or erode. Lesions commonly recur at the primary site innervated by the ganglion inhabited by the virus. The diagnosis is typically made from clinical presentation and history. Objective tools such as viral culture, serology, direct fluorescent antibody testing, polymerase chain reaction

(PCR), and Tzanck test can be used to confirm diagnosis. The sensitivity of viral culture decreases with more time lapsed from the first appearance of symptoms, and it is best to collect the specimen within 24 to 28 hours. Viral cultures can take up to 7 days to yield a positive result. Serology is not recommended because of its poor specificity for active disease since it cannot differentiate new from old infection. Serology, however, can be used for detecting HSV-1 exposure. Direct fluorescent antibody testing has low sensitivity. PCR is the most sensitive and specific test for detecting HSV-1 and yields results quickly (Miller et al., 2018). It is recommended to swab and test un-crusted lesions to get an accurate result. The Tzanck test cannot differentiate between HSV-1 and HSV-2 and requires skilled personnel to collect and examine the specimen under microscope (Usatine & Tinitigan, 2010). It is not recommended due to low sensitivity.

The two different diseases caused by varicella (chickenpox and shingles) have similar symptoms. After an incubation period of 10 to 20 days, chickenpox (primary varicella) manifests with fever and malaise followed by the outbreak of itchy, vesicular lesions on an erythematous base. The outbreak usually begins on the trunk and progresses to the extremities and face. Primary varicella occurs most often in children. Adults infected with primary varicella tend to have more systemic effects, especially if they are immunocompromised.

A reactivation of varicella in the dorsal root ganglion is referred to as herpes zoster, or shingles. The infection characteristically begins with neuralgia in the affected dermatome, followed by an outbreak of grouped vesicles on an erythematous base, clustered in a unilateral pattern of the dermatome. In two thirds of infections, the lesions are on the trunk. Additional symptoms include fever, myalgia, and increasing localized pain. The most common presentation of herpes virus infection in older adults is VZV in the form of herpes zoster. A significant complication of herpes zoster is postherpetic neuralgia, which is defined as pain in the dermatome site that lasts longer than 6 weeks after resolution of the infection.

VZV can be diagnosed objectively similarly to HSV-1. The most sensitive and specific method is PCR. The test is quick and has become a standard approach to testing. Serology, direct fluorescent antibody testing, and culture are less sensitive than PCR and not commonly performed if PCR is available.

Warts (Verrucae)

Warts are papillomatous, corrugated, hyperkeratotic growths found only on the epidermis, especially in areas subjected to repeated trauma. They can be solitary, multiple, or clustered. Warts are named based on their clinical appearance or location. Diagnosis is made based on clinical appearance. Lab tests are rarely needed to make a diagnosis.

Plantar warts (verruca plantaris) commonly occur on the heels, toes, soles of the feet, and the palms of the hands. Verruca vulgaris, common warts, presents on the hands, fingers, knees, elbows, or toes or at sites of trauma. They are flesh-colored-to-brown, hyperkeratotic papules and have an asymmetric distribution. Flat warts (verruca plana) are located on the face, neck,

and chest or flexor regions of the forearms and legs. They are flat and well defined and may be flesh colored or darker brown. Flat warts can be spread by shaving and are found in the beard area in men and on the legs in women. Filiform warts (verruca filiformis) are found primarily on the face and neck and present as tan, finger-like projections.

Initiating Drug Therapy

Herpes labialis is usually self-limiting, lasting approximately 7 to 10 days without scarring. Initial infection is usually the most severe, and recurrent infections are milder and shorter in duration. It typically does not require treatment, although it can be bothersome and visually unappealing, encouraging the affected individual to seek treatment. Topical antivirals can be used, although they are marginally efficacious. Systemic therapy with oral antivirals may shorten the duration of pain and infection.

For primary VZV infections that manifest as chickenpox, systemic therapy is used only in special cases, and is not recommended for uncomplicated disease that is self-limiting. If treatment is initiated, it should be initiated within 24 hours from the first varicella rash for treatment to be effective. For VZV infections that manifest as herpes zoster, antiviral agents may help relieve symptoms. Patients should be treated if the rash has been present for fewer than 72 hours or if new lesions are still developing. If therapy starts within 72 hours of the appearance of the lesion, systemic therapy decreases the duration of the rash and the acute pain associated with herpes zoster. In addition, any patient who is immunocompromised should be considered for treatment with IV antivirals and inpatient observation. Antiviral agents used are acyclovir, famciclovir, and valacyclovir. All antiviral agents have been shown to shorten the duration of herpes zoster infection and the severity of acute pain, but none prevent postherpetic neuralgia.

The natural history of cutaneous HPV infection is spontaneous resolution in months or a few years. Therapy is not needed unless the patient reports pain or requests removal for cosmetic purposes. Warts on the face need to be removed by a dermatologist, usually with liquid nitrogen cryotherapy. Topical treatment with salicylic acid (DuoFilm) is usually the starting point for all other warts. It is easier to treat small verrucae rather than waiting until they are large.

Goals of Drug Therapy

In herpes virus infections, the goal of therapy is to reduce the duration of symptoms, suppress pain, and stop viral shedding. It is important to know that herpes infections are never cured since the virus retreats into the ganglia and may be reactivated.

The goal of therapy for warts is eradication of the lesion safely and effectively while also keeping in mind the cost of therapy. There is no way to actually kill HPV.

Topical Antiviral Agents

Acyclovir 5% (Zovirax) and penciclovir (Denavir) are available to treat herpes labialis. These agents work by inhibiting viral DNA synthesis (**Table 13.7**). They may decrease time to

TABLE 13.7

Overview of Antiviral Agents for Herpes Virus Infections

Generic (Trade) Name and Dosage*	Selected Adverse Events	Contraindications	Special Considerations
Topical Therapy			
Acyclovir 5% (Zovirax) Apply five times daily for 4 days	Local pain and transient stinging	Hypersensitivity to drug or its components	Not studied in children younger than 12 years of age
Penciclovir 1% (Denavir) Apply q2h while awake for 4 days	Erythema		Begin using at first sign or symptom of cold sore
Docosanol 10% (Abreva) Apply five times daily until healed for up to 10 days	N/A		Docosanol is available OTC
Systemic Therapy			
Acyclovir (Zovirax) For HSV-1: 400 mg TID for 5–10 days HSV-1 suppression: 400 mg BID For VZV infection: Chickenpox, pediatric: 20 mg/kg QID for 5 days Herpes zoster: 800 mg 5X a day for 7 days	Malaise, nausea, vomiting, headache, renal dysfunction	Hypersensitivity to drug or its components	Poor oral bioavailability Frequent dosing may be difficult for compliance Relatively inexpensive Encourage hydration while on therapy to protect kidneys Renal dose adjustments needed
Famciclovir (Famvir) For HSV-1: 1,500 mg PO once For VZV infection: 500 mg TID for 7 days	Headache, nausea, fatigue, paresthesias	Hypersensitivity to drug or its components	Initiate therapy as soon as symptoms develop Renal dose adjustments needed Limited data on the use in children
Valacyclovir (Valtrex) For HSV-1: 2 g BID for 1 day Suppression: 500–1,000 mg daily For VZV infection: 1 g TID for 7 days	Nausea, headache, fatigue, abdominal pain, LFT elevations, nasopharyngitis	Hypersensitivity to drug or its components	Use caution in older adults as it can cause CNS effects Renal dose adjustments needed Limited data in severely immunosuppressed patients

*Dosing in chart is for the immunocompetent patient. Refer to text for dosing in the immunocompromised patient.

CNS, central nervous system; HSV, herpes simplex virus; LFT, liver function test; OTC, over the counter; VZV, varicella-zoster virus.

heal, although clinical significance is marginal (Spruance et al., 1997; Worrall, 2009). Patients should apply topical acyclovir five times daily for 4 days. Penciclovir is applied every 2 hours during waking hours for 4 days. Adverse effects include mild skin irritation and pruritus.

Docosanol cream (Abreva) is a saturated aliphatic alcohol with antiviral properties marketed for the treatment of cold sores, although its clinical significance in reducing healing time and duration of symptoms is minimal (Usatine & Tinitigen, 2010). It is available over the counter. It is essential to inform patients they should apply topical treatments with a glove or an applicator so that they do not infect other areas of the body with the virus.

Systemic Antiviral Agents

Systemic antivirals used for herpes virus include acyclovir (Zovirax), famciclovir (Famvir), and valacyclovir (Valtrex). Famciclovir and valacyclovir have higher oral bioavailability than acyclovir. Systemic antivirals are highly effective against herpes virus. In general, antiviral therapy is recommended for adolescents, adults, and high-risk patients but not usually for healthy children younger than age 12 (see **Table 13.7**).

Contraindications

Caution should be used in patients with renal disease because antivirals are excreted renally. Creatinine clearance should be calculated and used to renally adjust antiviral therapy.

Adverse Events

Adverse effects include headaches, depression, and increased liver enzymes. Patients may also experience GI symptoms and rashes.

Interactions

The effect of acyclovir and valacyclovir is increased in patients taking foscarnet. Acyclovir and valacyclovir may increase the concentrations of tizanidine, clozapine, and zidovudine. Famciclovir does not have any significant drug interactions. Patients on antiviral therapy should not receive the live attenuated zoster vaccine (Zostavax) or varicella virus vaccine. Patients should be off antiviral therapy for greater than 24 hours prior to receiving those vaccines and should not receive antiviral therapy within 14 days of receiving the vaccine. This is because antivirals will decrease the efficacy of the vaccine.

Acyclovir

The prototypical antiviral agent acyclovir acts by inhibiting viral DNA replication. The drug works only in cells infected by HSV. A disadvantage of oral acyclovir is its low bioavailability of 10% to 20% and need for frequent dosing.

The recommended acyclovir dosage for an initial and recurrent HSV-1 orolabial disease in both immunocompetent and immunocompromised patients is 400 mg orally thrice daily for 5 to 10 days (see **Table 13.7**). Immunocompromised patients should continue therapy until complete resolution of lesions has occurred. Suppressive therapy may be initiated for patients with severe or frequent recurrent infections, although benefit is minimal (Chi et al., 2015). The regimen for prophylaxis is acyclovir 400 mg orally twice daily. The need for prophylaxis should be regularly assessed. Pediatric dosing of acyclovir in HIV-exposed or-positive patients is 20 mg/kg four times daily, with a maximum dose of 400 mg, four times daily for 5 days. For immunocompetent pediatric patients requiring chronic suppressive therapy for severe and frequent recurrences, the dose of acyclovir should be 10 mg/kg thrice daily, with a maximum daily dose of 1 g/d. This should be reevaluated annually.

The recommended dosage for treating VZV infections in immunocompetent children is 20 mg/kg orally four times daily for 5 days, with a maximum daily dose of 3.2 g. For pediatric patients exposed to HIV or who are HIV positive, it is recommended to extend treatment duration to 7 to 10 days and until 48 hours after the last new lesion forms. Adult dosing is 800 mg orally five times daily for 5 to 7 days and until all lesions have dried. For complicated cases requiring hospitalization, IV therapy is warranted.

Famciclovir

Famciclovir is a pro-drug that is metabolized to its active form, penciclovir. The dose of famciclovir for herpes labialis is 1,500 mg once for immunocompetent patients. It is best to start therapy within 1 hour of the first sign of infection if the patient has prodromal symptoms. In patients with HIV, the recommended dose of famciclovir is 500 mg by mouth twice daily for 5 to 10 days.

In uncomplicated varicella infection (chickenpox), the regimen is famciclovir 500 mg by mouth thrice daily for 5 to 7 days in a HIV-infected patient. For herpes zoster, the dose is 500 mg by mouth thrice daily for 7 days. For patients with HIV, this regimen can be extended to 10 days or longer if lesions have not completely healed.

Valacyclovir

Valacyclovir is a pro-drug of acyclovir and is converted rapidly. First-pass metabolism converts valacyclovir to acyclovir, with approximately 55% bioavailability. For herpes labialis, the recommended dose in immunocompetent patients is 2 g by mouth twice daily for 1 day. For severe and frequently recurring infections, suppressive therapy with valacyclovir 500 mg to 1 g by mouth daily can be initiated and periodically reassessed. In immunocompromised patients, the recommended dose is 1 g by mouth twice daily for 5 to 10 days and until lesions are completely healed. Suppressive therapy can be initiated in case of severe and frequent recurrences. The dose is 500 mg by mouth twice daily.

For uncomplicated and mild varicella (chickenpox) infection, the recommended dose is 1 g by mouth thrice daily for 5 to 7 days and until lesions have completely crusted over. The recommended regimen for herpes zoster infection is valacyclovir 1 g by mouth thrice daily for 7 days. In immunocompromised patients, treatment duration can be extended to 10 days or longer if there is slow resolution of lesions.

Salicylic Acid

Salicylic acid is a keratolytic agent that may be used for common and plantar warts. It is available over the counter and in a variety of strengths for specific types or sites of verrucae. It comes in various dosage forms including plaster, collodion-like vehicle, and karaya gum-glycol plaster vehicle. Usually, 17% salicylic acid is used to treat small lesions. A patch product that is 40% salicylic acid plaster is useful for large lesions and can be cut to fit the wart. Compared to no treatment, salicylic acid cures warts faster (Loo & Tang, 2014).

Dosage

For salicylic acid that comes in a collodion-like vehicle, a drop should be applied on the wart and allowed to dry. When using the karaya gum-glycol plaster vehicle preparation, the wart should be initially flattened gently with a pumice stone. A drop of warm water should then be applied to the wart, and the plaster should be applied at bedtime and kept on for at least 8 hours. It should be removed when awake; this process can continue nightly until the wart is removed for up to 12 weeks. Salicylic acid patches come in plaster strengths ranging from 12% to 40%. The plaster should be cut to fit the wart and left on for 48 hours. This can be repeated until the wart is removed for up to 12 weeks. There are various over-the-counter products with salicylic acid, and patients should be counseled on reading and following the directions of use on the package.

Contraindications

Topical therapy is contraindicated in patients with diabetes mellitus or impaired circulation and on moles, birthmarks, or unusual warts with hair growth. Some systemic absorption can occur, and therapy should be avoided in patients with salicylate hypersensitivity, including those with an aspirin allergy. The most common adverse effect is skin irritation, which can be severe enough to discontinue treatment.

Selecting the Most Appropriate Agent

When selecting an agent, it is necessary to consider ease of compliance, cost, and efficacy profile of medication. For warts, most patients will seek treatment for cosmetic purposes, and treatment with salicylic acid will work for most common and plantar warts. Warts located on the face or neck, such as filiform or flat warts, may need to be removed by a dermatologist. This procedure is commonly done in the office. Most warts cure themselves over time, especially in the immunocompetent host.

First-Line Therapy: Herpes Simplex Virus Type 1

Herpes labialis is typically self-limiting without treatment. For patients with recurrent or severe herpes labialis, oral antiviral therapy with acyclovir, famciclovir, or valacyclovir should be initiated. Topical antiviral therapy may be prescribed for mild cases in immunocompetent patients, although symptoms may only be reduced by a day, which may not be worth the expense of the treatment. Immunocompromised patients should be treated with oral antiviral therapy. Cost is typically a deciding factor in which agent to select. Most insurances will cover valacyclovir or acyclovir, but most topical antiviral preparations are not covered and expensive.

Evidence for suppressive therapy suggests that topical antiviral preparations are ineffective in preventing recurrences and should not be used for that purpose. Oral antiviral suppressive therapy can prevent recurrences, although the benefit is minimal (Chi et al., 2015).

First-Line Therapy: Varicella-Zoster Virus

Systemic therapy is used only in patients with complicated disease, children with chronic pulmonary or cutaneous disease or taking inhaled corticosteroids or long-term salicylate therapy, or anyone healthy above the age of 12 years. It is prescribed only if the rash has been present for less than 24 hours, as that is when it will work best.

First-Line Therapy: Herpes Zoster

Systemic antiviral therapy can be started if the herpes zoster outbreak is less than 72 hours in duration or longer than 72 hours but with new lesions appearing, the patient being older than age 50, or the patient being immunosuppressed. Therapy consists of systemic therapy with acyclovir, famciclovir, or valacyclovir. Most often, valacyclovir is prescribed to patients with insurance coverage as it is typically covered and has a less frequent dosing schedule (**Figure 13.2**). For patients without insurance or with insurance that does not cover valacyclovir, acyclovir would be a cheaper alternative. Patients who have received a stem cell transplant or any transplant on anti-rejection medication or those who are showing signs of extracutaneous infection should be hospitalized and managed with IV acyclovir. They can finish the recommended 14-day course of antiviral therapy with oral acyclovir, famciclovir, or valacyclovir.

Oral analgesics, such as acetaminophen, aspirin, and nonsteroidal antiinflammatory drugs, are helpful in pain control. Patients with neuropathic pain, commonly associated with shingles, may need medication targeting neuralgia prescribed, such as gabapentin or lidocaine patches.

First-Line Therapy: Verrucae

For common warts, topical salicylic acid in a 17% concentration is used; it is applied at bedtime for approximately 8 to 12 weeks or until the wart has healed. For plantar warts, a 40% salicylic acid preparation is used in plaster or patch form that is cut to the size of the wart and applied at bedtime.

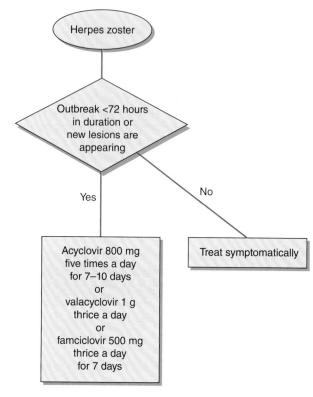

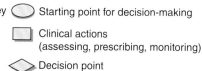

FIGURE 13–2 Treatment algorithm for the Herpes zoster virus infection manifested as shingles.

The preparation remains in place for 24 to 48 hours. When removed, the area is rubbed with a pumice stone to remove dead white keratin. This can be repeated for up to 12 weeks or until the wart is gone (**Figure 13.3** and **Table 13.8**).

Second-Line Therapy: Verrucae

If patient-applied therapy fails, cryotherapy, carbon dioxide laser therapy, or pulsed dye laser therapy can be performed. Pulsed dye laser therapy seems to have the least adverse effects associated with it when compared with other laser therapies (Nguyen et al., 2016).

Monitoring Patient Response

Follow-up evaluation of HSV infection is not required if the symptoms resolve. For patients with herpes zoster, follow-up is recommended if pain or symptoms have not resolved.

In non-anogenital HPV infections, multiple treatments may be necessary. Patients should understand the importance of follow-up beyond the initial wart removal, because the virus may remain. Patients may need weekly treatment until the wart is eradicated.

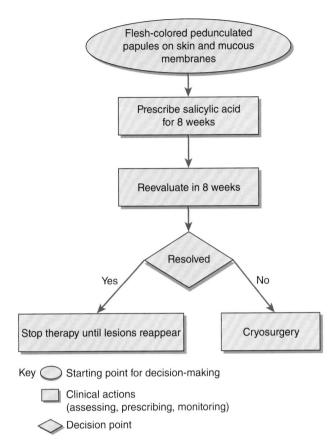

FIGURE 13–3   Treatment algorithm for common warts.

TABLE 13.8

Recommended Order of Treatment for Non-anogenital Infection with Human Papillomavirus

Order	Agent	Comments
First line	Salicylic acid	Used as first-line agent to treat any wart not on face Available OTC
Second line	Cryotherapy or laser treatment	Refer patient to specialist

OTC, over the counter.

Patient Education

Lifestyle Changes

Educating the patient about hygiene, precipitating factors, and prevention is imperative. Viral infections are spread by skin contact, so patients need to recognize the importance of wearing gloves when applying medications and of thorough hand washing. Skin-to-skin contact should be avoided. Patients with warts should be informed that they may recur.

Complementary and Alternative Medicine

Capsaicin cream can be used for pain control in herpes zoster, although data on its efficacy are insufficient. Tea tree and eucalyptus oil have been reported to have activity against herpes simplex. Use of alternative medications have very limited data and should not be routinely recommended.

Special Populations

VZV infections during pregnancy are extremely rare and can cause fetal abnormalities. If a pregnant woman is infected, varicella zoster immunoglobulin and antiviral drugs should be considered.

Prevention

There are no vaccinations for the prevention of HSV-1 infections. Patients should be counseled on preventing transmission to other people by not sharing drinks and avoiding kissing with active herpes labialis lesions.

Vaccination reduces the incidence of VZV infections. The varicella vaccine is a two-dose series that can be given after 12 months of birth. There has been significant decline in the incidence of chickenpox since the varicella vaccination program per the Centers for Disease Control and Prevention. There are two different vaccinations for the prevention of herpes zoster and postherpetic neuralgia in adults. Live zoster vaccine (Zostavax) is a subcutaneous one-time injection given to adults over the age of 60 years, and since it is a live attenuated vaccine, it cannot be given to immunocompromised individuals. Recombinant zoster vaccine (Shingrix) is the preferred shingles vaccine due to its better efficacy and longer-lasting effect (Dooling et al., 2018). The vaccine is given as two doses 2 to 6 months apart intramuscularly in adults older than the age of 50 years.

CASE STUDY 1

B.H. is a 72-year-old man who presents for evaluation of several painful red bumps on his left side. The pain radiates around to his chest. The rash resembles blisters that are just forming. He noticed them yesterday, and more are forming. His laboratory results are all normal, and his creatinine is 0.8 mg/dL. He has prescription insurance (Learning Objectives 2 and 3).

DIAGNOSIS: HERPES ZOSTER

1. What, if any, risk factors does this patient have for developing herpes zoster?
2. What, if any, drug therapy would you prescribe? Why?
3. Discuss patient education and preventive measures based on his history and the therapy.

Bibliography

Starred references are cited in the text.

Ahn, K. H., Park, Y. J., Hong, S. C., et al. (2016). Congenital varicella syndrome: A systematic review. *Journal of Obstetrics and Gynaecology: The Journal of the Institute of Obstetrics and Gynaecology, 36*(5), 563–566.

American Academy of Pediatrics Committee on Infectious Diseases. (1993). The use of oral acyclovir in otherwise healthy children with varicella. *Pediatrics, 91*(3), 674–676.

Ashbee, H. R., & Evans, E. G. (2002). Immunology of diseases associated with Malassezia species. *Clinical Microbiology Reviews, 15*(1), 21–57.

*Barwell, N. D., Devers, M. C., Kennon, B., et al. (2017). Diabetic foot infection: Antibiotic therapy and good practice recommendations. *International Journal of Clinical Practice, 71*(10). doi:10.1111/ijcp.13006

*Boulton, A., Armstrong, D. G., Kirsner, R. S., et al. (2018). Diagnosis and management of diabetic foot complications. American Diabetes Association.

*Becker, B. A., & Childress, M. A. (2018). Common foot problems: Over-the-counter treatments and home care. *American Family Physician, 98*(5), 298–303.

Burnham, J. P., Kirby, J. P., & Kollef, M. H. (2016). Diagnosis and management of skin and soft tissue infections in the intensive care unit: A review. *Intensive Care Medicine, 42*(12), 1899–1911.

Burnham, J. P., & Kollef, M. H. (2018). Treatment of severe skin and soft tissue infections: A review. *Current Opinion in Infectious Diseases, 31*(2), 113–119.

*Chi, C. C., Wang, S. H., Delamere, F. M., et al. (2015). Interventions for prevention of herpes simplex labialis (cold sores on the lips). *The Cochrane Database of Systematic Reviews, 2015*(8), CD010095.

Chussil, J. T. (2015). Superficial fungal infections. In M. Bobonich & M. Nolen (Eds.), *Dermatology for advanced practice clinicians* (pp. 181–195). Philadelphia, PA: Wolters Kluwer.

*Dooling, K. L., Guo, A., Patel, M., et al. (2018). Recommendations of the advisory committee on immunization practices for use of herpes zoster vaccines. *Morbidity and Mortality Weekly Report, 67*(3), 103–108.

*Dryden, M. S., Dailly, S., & Crouch, M. (2004). A randomized, controlled trial of tea tree topical preparations versus a standard topical regimen for the clearance of MRSA colonization. *The Journal of Hospital Infection, 56*(4), 283–286.

Everett, E., & Mathioudakis, N. (2018). Update on management of diabetic foot ulcers. *Annals of the New York Academy of Sciences, 1411*(1), 153–165.

Gupta, A. K., & Foley, K. A. (2015). Antifungal treatment for pityriasis versicolor. *Journal of Fungi (Basel, Switzerland), 1*(1), 13–29.

Hay, R. J. (2017). Tinea capitis: Current status. *Mycopathologia, 182*(1–2), 87–93.

Hudson, A., Carroll, B., & Kim, S. J. (2017). Folliculocentric tinea versicolor. *Dermatology Online Journal, 23*(2). Retrieved from https://escholarship.org/uc/item/5kj574bd

John, A. R., & Canaday, D. H. (2017). Herpes zoster in the older adult. *Infectious Disease Clinics of North America, 31*(4), 811–826.

Kalra, M. G., Higgins, K. E., & Kinney, B. S. (2014). Intertrigo and secondary skin infections. *American Family Physician, 89*(7), 569–573.

Kovitwanichkanont, T., & Chong, A. H. (2019). Superficial fungal infections. *Australian Journal of General Practice, 48*(10), 706–711. https://doi.org/10.31128/AJGP-05-19-4930

*Kreijkamp-Kaspers, S., Hawke, K., Guo, L., et al. (2017). Oral antifungal medication for toenail onychomycosis. *The Cochrane Database of Systematic Reviews, 7*(7), CD010031.

Kukhanova, M. K., Korovina, A. N., & Kochetkov, S. N. (2014). Human herpes simplex virus: Life cycle and development of inhibitors. *Biochemistry. Biokhimiia, 79*(13), 1635–1652.

Laureano, A. C., Schwartz, R. A., & Cohen, P. J. (2014). Facial bacterial infections: folliculitis. *Clinics in Dermatology, 32*(6), 711–714.

Leggit, J. C. (2017). Acute and chronic paronychia. *American Family Physician, 96*(1), 44–51.

*Lipsky, B. A., Berendt, A. R., Cornia, P. B., et al. (2012). 2012 Infectious Diseases Society of America clinical practice guideline for the diagnosis and treatment of diabetic foot infections. *Clinical Infectious Diseases: An Official Publication of the Infectious Diseases Society of America, 54*(12), e132–e173.

*Loo, S. K., & Tang, W. Y. (2014). Warts (non-genital). *BMJ Clinical Evidence, 2014*, 1710.

Melancon, J. M. (2014a). Herpes simplex. In K. A. Arndt, T. S. Hsu, M. Alam, et al. (Eds.), *Manual of dermatologic therapeutics* (8th ed., pp. 150–160). Philadelphia, PA: Wolters Kluwer.

Melancon, J. M. (2014b). Herpes zoster and varicella. In K. A. Arndt, T. S. Hsu, M. Alam, et al. (Eds.), *Manual of dermatologic therapeutics* (8th ed., pp. 161–172). Philadelphia, PA: Wolters Kluwer.

*Miller, J. M., Binnicker, M. J., Campbell, S., et al. (2018). A guide to utilization of the microbiology laboratory for diagnosis of infectious diseases: 2018 update by the Infectious Diseases Society of America and the American Society for Microbiology. *Clinical Infectious Diseases: An Official Publication of the Infectious Diseases Society of America, 67*(6), e1–e94.

Mulhem, E., & Pinelis, S. (2011). Treatment of nongenital cutaneous warts. *American Family Physician, 84*(3), 288–293.

Nardi, N. M., & Schaefer, T. J. (2020). Impetigo. In *StatPearls*. StatPearls Publishing.

*Nguyen, J., Korta, D. Z., Chapman, L. W., et al. (2016). Laser treatment of nongenital verrucae: A systematic review. *JAMA Dermatology, 152*(9), 1025–1034.

Noska, K. (2015). Viral infections. In M. Bobonich & M. Nolen (Eds.), *Dermatology for advanced practice clinicians* (pp. 147–164). Philadelphia, PA: Wolters Kluwer.

Pappas, P. G., Kauffman, C. A., Andes, D. R., et al. (2016). Clinical practice guideline for the management of candidiasis: 2016 update by the Infectious Diseases Society of America. *Clinical Infectious Diseases: An Official Publication of the Infectious Diseases Society of America, 62*(4), e1–e50.

Ramakrishnan, K., Salinas, R. C., & Agudelo Higuita, N. I. (2015). Skin and soft tissue infections. *American Family Physician, 92*(6), 474–483.

Rawla, P., & Ludhwani, D. (2020). Poststreptococcal Glomerulonephritis. In StatPearls [Internet]. Treasure Island (FL): StatPearls Publishing; 2020 Jan–. https://www.ncbi.nlm.nih.gov/books/NBK538255/

Renati, S., Cukras, A., & Bigby, M. (2015). Pityriasis versicolor. *BMJ (Clinical research ed.), 350*, h1394.

Saguil, A., Kane, S., Mercado, M., et al. (2017). Herpes zoster and postherpetic neuralgia: Prevention and management. *American Family Physician, 96*(10), 656–663.

Sahoo, A. K., & Mahajan, R. (2016). Management of tinea corporis, tinea cruris, and tinea pedis: A comprehensive review. *Indian Dermatology Online Journal, 7*(2), 77–86.

*Sartelli, M., Guirao, X., Hardcastle, T. C., et al. (2018). 2018 WSES/SIS-E consensus conference: Recommendations for the management of skin and soft-tissue infections. *World Journal of Emergency Surgery, 13*, 58.

*Satchell, A. C., Saurajen, A., Bell, C., et al. (2002). Treatment of interdigital tinea pedis with 25% and 50% tea tree oil solution: A randomized, placebo-controlled, blinded study. *Australasian Journal of Dermatology, 43*, 175–178.

Schnitzler, P., Schön, K., & Reichling, J. (2001). Antiviral activity of Australian tea tree oil and eucalyptus oil against herpes simplex virus in cell culture. *Die Pharmazie, 56*(4), 343–347.

Spruance, S. L., Nett, R., Marbury, T., et al. (2002). Acyclovir cream for treatment of herpes simplex labialis: Results of two randomized, double-blind, vehicle-controlled, multicenter clinical trials. *Antimicrobial Agents and Chemotherapy, 46*(7), 2238–2243.

*Spruance, S. L., Rea, T. L., Thoming, C., et al. (1997). Penciclovir cream for the treatment of herpes simplex labialis. A randomized, multicenter, double-blind, placebo-controlled trial. Topical Penciclovir Collaborative Study Group. *JAMA, 277*(17), 1374–1379.

*Stevens, D. L., Bisno, A. L., Chambers, H. F., et al. (2014). Practice guidelines for the diagnosis and management of skin and soft tissue infections: 2014 update by the Infectious Diseases Society of America. *Clinical Infectious Diseases: An Official Publication of the Infectious Diseases Society of America, 59*(2), e10–e52.

Stevens, D. L., & Bryant, A. E. (2016). Impetigo, Erysipelas and Cellulitis. In J. J. Ferretti et al. (Eds.), *Streptococcus pyogenes: Basic biology to clinical manifestations*. University of Oklahoma Health Sciences Center.

*Usatine, R. P., & Tinitigan, R. (2010). Nongenital herpes simplex virus. *American Family Physician, 82*(9), 1075–1082.

*Wang, Y. F., Que, H. F., Wang, Y. J., & Cui, X. J. (2014). Chinese herbal medicines for treating skin and soft-tissue infections. *The Cochrane Database of Systematic Reviews, 7*, CD010619.

Winters, R. D., & Mitchell, M. Folliculitis. (2019). In: StatPearls [Internet]. Treasure Island (FL): StatPearls Publishing; 2020 Jan-. https://www.ncbi.nlm.nih.gov/books/NBK547754/

*Woo, T. E., Somayaji, R., Haber, R. M., et al. (2019). Diagnosis and management of cutaneous tinea infections. *Advances in Skin & Wound Care, 32*(8), 350–357.

*Worrall, G. (2009). Herpes labialis. *BMJ Clinical Evidence, 2009*, 1704.

14 Psoriasis

Shelly R. Schneider

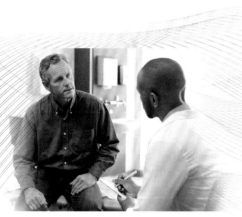
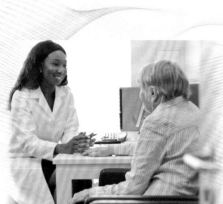
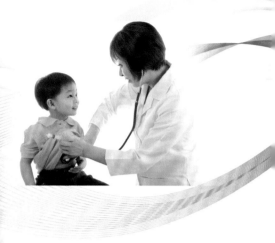

Learning Objectives

1. The learner will discuss treatment options that include topical, oral, and injectable pharmacologic agents.
2. The learner will distinguish between first-, second-, and third-line agents with regard to severity of disease, side effects, and risk–benefit.
3. The learner will be able to recognize factors in choosing biologic agents to treat psoriasis for preventing systemic complications, as well as treat local lesions.

INTRODUCTION

Psoriasis is a chronic debilitating disease characterized by recurrent exacerbations and remissions. It affects between 2% and 3% of the U.S. population, with a higher incidence in whites and an equal distribution between the genders. Approximately 36% of patients with psoriasis have a positive family history. The cost of outpatient treatment for psoriasis averages $1.6 to $3.2 billion annually. There appear to be two peak ages of onset: between ages 16 and 22 and between ages 57 and 60.

Psoriatic lesions are associated with physical discomfort including pain, itching, stinging, cracking, and bleeding. In approximately 10% of patients with psoriasis, the disease develops into psoriatic arthritis. Psoriasis affects almost all aspects of life, including sexual relationships and emotional well-being. In addition, patients with psoriasis spend one or more hours a day caring for their skin. Of a survey group of patients with psoriasis, up to 25%, at some point in their life, felt that they would rather be dead than alive with psoriasis.

Psoriasis affects approximately 2.5% of whites and 1.3% of blacks in the United States, with approximately 150,000 newly diagnosed cases every year. The incidence of psoriasis is somewhat lower in Asians (0.4%). Generally, it is more common in individuals living at higher latitudes or in colder locales and less common in individuals who have greater sun exposure.

There seems to be a genetic factor associated with psoriasis. Based on population studies, the risk of psoriasis in children is estimated to be 41% if both parents are affected, 14% if one parent is affected, and 6% if one sibling is affected, and a family history can be found in 5% to 10% of patients who have psoriasis.

CAUSES

A definitive cause for psoriasis is unknown, although there are several possible etiologic factors: abnormal epidermal cell cycle, hereditary factors, and triggers, including trauma, infection, endocrine imbalance, climate, and emotional stress. Physical trauma, such as rubbing, scratching, or sunburn, is a major exacerbating factor in psoriasis, which results in a reaction known as *Koebner phenomenon*. Stress plays a role in as many as 40% of psoriasis flares in adults and children. Exacerbations of psoriasis may develop from the use of certain drugs (**Box 14.1**).

PATHOPHYSIOLOGY

Psoriasis is a T cell–mediated disease involving a dysregulation of the inflammatory process, as well as skin barrier dysfunction. Believed to be multifaceted, insults to the body

Systemic corticosteroids (when dose is decreased or
    stopped)
Lithium carbonate
Antimalarials
Beta blockers
Systemic interferon
Alcohol

due to genetic influences in addition to stress, infection, or drugs can elicit the altered and disruptive inflammatory process exhibited in the skin as plaques. Any immunologic or environmental trauma may trigger an abnormal immune response, resulting in a cascade of events, not fully understood. Hallmarks of the condition include hyper-proliferation and abnormal differentiation of epidermal keratinocytes with infiltrative T lymphocytes. Epidermal thickening and remodeling occurs externally while pro inflammatory substances are released into systemic circulation. This may account for chronic health issues and joint involvement later in the disease process.

Research shows an association with epidermal defense genes, six of which are located on chromosome 8p23. Tumor necrosis factor alpha (TNF-alpha), interleukin (IL)-23, and IL-17 have been shown to be elevated in patients with psoriasis. These cytokines act to attract and activate neutrophils which are responsible for much of the inflammation seen in the skin. In addition, IL-17 A downregulates the expression of filaggrin which binds to keratin fibers in epithelial cells causing disruption in the skin barrier. Intercellular adhesion molecule is altered along with TNF-alpha and lymphocytic antigen cells, which initiate inflammatory cytokines IL-7 and IL-6 and pro-inflammatory transcription factor. High levels of IL-6 suppress T regulatory activity, which results in unopposed activity of pathogenic T cells. Increased IL-22 leads to epidermal acanthuses and abnormal differentiation of keratinocytes. Activation of these cells can occur through specific interactions with antigen-presenting cells (APCs) or via nonspecific super antigen reaction (i.e., guttate psoriasis is triggered by streptococcal antigens). This becomes a continuous feedback loop of inflammation.

Activation of these T cells can occur through specific interactions with APCs or via nonspecific super antigen interactions (i.e., guttate psoriasis is triggered by streptococcal antigens). APC activation requires co-stimulatory signals. Three main pathways, TNF-alpha, IL-23, and IL-17, have been shown to affect those with psoriasis. These cytokines act to attract and activate neutrophils which are responsible for much of the inflammation seen in psoriasis.

DIAGNOSTIC CRITERIA

Clinical presentation of the plaque type of psoriasis consists of sharp, well-demarcated, erythematous papules or plaques surrounded by silvery-white scales. The lesions are symmetric, and many are found on the extensor surfaces—elbows and knees. Other common areas affected include scalp, nails, anogenital, intertriginous (inverse psoriasis), trunk, and ears. The plaque type is the most common form. Other forms of psoriatic disease include guttate, erythrodermic, and pustular. The guttate type is characterized by small, scattered, teardrop-shaped papules and plaques. In many cases psoriasis begins as the guttate form and may evolve into any of its other forms. The erythrodermic form is characterized by generalized erythema and shedding with scales.

Individuals are extremely ill and should be treated similar to burn victims. Finally, the pustular type has three additional forms: generalized, localized, and palmo-plantar. All these forms share a similar characteristic: 2- to 3-mm sterile pustules on specific body regions.

Bleeding may follow removal of the scales (Auspitz sign). Pitting and discoloration of the nails are also some of the characteristics of psoriasis. In some cases, the nail may separate from the nail bed—referred to as onycholysis.

INITIATING DRUG THERAPY

Before beginning drug therapy, the patient is usually counseled to avoid precipitating factors. Cigarette smoking is discouraged since this can exacerbate the condition.

There are three treatment modalities available: topical, phototherapy, and systemic agents. To select the most appropriate treatment, one must determine whether the patient has localized or generalized psoriasis. Patients with 10% or less of body involvement can usually be successfully treated in a primary care setting with topical agents, whereas those with greater body surface area (BSA) involvement usually require treatment by a dermatologist with phototherapy or systemic therapy. In estimating BSA involvement, the prescriber keeps in mind that the palm represents 1% BSA; this can be used as a tool to estimate total BSA involvement.

Goals of Drug Therapy

The goals of therapy are the following:

- Decrease the size and thickness of the plaques.
- Decrease pruritus.
- Improve emotional well-being and quality of life.
- Put the patient in remission.
- Ensure minimal side effects from treatment.

It is imperative to use a management strategy with the least possible toxicity deemed acceptable to the patient. **Table 14.1** identifies topical and systemic preparations used in psoriasis treatment.

TABLE 14.1

Overview of Selected Agents for Psoriasis

Generic (Trade) Name and Dosage	Selected Adverse Events	Contraindications	Special Considerations
Topical Agents			
Emollients (Eucerin, Lubriderm, Moisturel, CeraVe, Cetaphil). Apply to affected skin TID or QID	Folliculitis, maceration, miliaria	Sensitivity	Avoid applying near eyes
Tar Preparations			
Coal tar Apply at bedtime and allow to remain on skin. Emulsion: 15–25 mL dissolved in bath water Shampoo	Irritation, photoreactions, unpleasant odor, folliculitis	Open or infected lesions	Preparation may stain skin and clothing. With emulsion, immerse affected area for 10–20 minutes 3 to 7 times a week. Shampoo should be massaged into wet scalp and rinsed, then applied a second time and left on for 5 minutes
Antipsoriatics			
Anthralin (Drithocreme, Micanol) Apply for 30–60 minutes, and then remove.	Irritation	Renal disease, acute psoriasis	Preparation may stain skin, towels, sinks, and tubs. Avoid applying near eyes and mucous membranes. Irritation can be avoided by applying emollients to unaffected skin
Vitamin D Analogs			
Calcipotriene (Dovonex) Apply BID.	Burning and stinging, skin peeling, rash	Hypercalcemia, vitamin D toxicity	Avoid use on face
Vitamin A Derivatives			
Tazarotene (Tazorac) Once a day at bedtime	Pruritus, erythema	Pregnancy	Avoid vitamin A.
Topical Corticosteroids			
Hydrocortisone (Cortisporin)	Burning, folliculitis, hypothalamic–pituitary–adrenal axis suppression Local irritation	Primary bacterial infections or fungal infections	Use lowest effective dose. Avoid prolonged use. Use occlusive dressing.
Combination Products			
Betamethasone and calcipotriene (Enstillar foam, Taclonex scalp solution, ointment)	Hypopigmentation, irritation, stinging, burning	Infection	Once daily convenience
Halobetasol proprionate and Tazarotene lotion (Duobrii)	Same as above	Infection	Once daily dosing
Systemic Agents			
Apremilast (Otezla)	GI upset, diarrhea	Known hypersensitivity	Starter kit to minimize side effects
Cyclosporine (Cyclosporine A, Sandimmune) Maximum dose 2–5 mg/kg/d	Tremor, gingival hyperplasia, GI upset, hypertension, renal dysfunction, acne	Pregnancy and lactation; caution in impaired renal and hepatic function	Increased risk of digoxin toxicity. Interacts with lovastatin, diltiazem, ketoconazole. Decreased therapeutic effect with use of hydantoins, rifampin, sulfonamides

(Continued)

TABLE 14.1

Overview of Selected Agents for Psoriasis (*Continued*)

Generic (Trade) Name and Dosage	Selected Adverse Events	Contraindications	Special Considerations
Etretinate (Acitretin) 25–50 mg daily	Elevation in lipid levels, abnormal liver function, alopecia, rash, dry skin, pruritus	Alcohol use, pregnancy, and lactation	Perform pretreatment lipid and liver function tests. Advise female patients not to become pregnant while taking this medication. Take with meals
Methotrexate (MTX, Rheumatrex) 7.5–25 mg/kg/wk	Headache, blurred vision, fatigue, malaise, GI distress, gingivitis, hepatotoxicity, chills, bone marrow depression, rash alopecia, fever	Pregnancy and lactation; caution in patients with renal and hepatic compromise, leukopenia	Drug decreases the level of digoxin. Increased risk of toxicity with salicylates, phenytoin, and sulfonamides. Take folic acid 1 mg on nontreatment days
Biologics			
Adalimumab (Humira) 80 mg subcutaneously initially then 40 mg every other week	Headache, nausea, rash, reaction at injection site	Concurrent live vaccine, active infection; caution in pregnancy	Used for psoriatic arthritis. May benefit Crohns, IBS
Etanercept (Enbrel) 50 mg twice a week for 3 months, then 50 mg weekly by subcutaneous injection	Infection, injection site pain, localized erythema, rash, upper respiratory infection, abdominal pain, vomiting	Concurrent live vaccine, active infection; caution in pregnancy, impaired renal function, asthma, blood dyscrasia, central nervous system demyelinating disease, history of recurrent infections	A maximum of 25 mg can be given in each site, requiring two injections. It is given subcutaneously
Infliximab (Remicade) IV 5 mg/kg	GI upset, headache, fatigue, cough, congestive heart failure Nasopharyngitis, upper respiratory infection, cellulitis	Severe congestive heart failure Infection Malignancy, infection Infections Inflammatory bowel	Intravenous infusion Monitor for tuberculosis
Secukinumab (Cosentyx) 150–300 mg	Local injection site reaction	Malignancy, infection	Monitor for tuberculosis Avoid with IBS
Ustekinumab (Stelara)	Same, cellulitis	Malignancy, infection	Monitor for tuberculosis
Certikuzumab (Cimzia) 200 mg	Same as above	Malignancy, infection	Monitor for tuberculosis
Tildrakizumab (Ilumya)	Same as above	Same for all biologics	Monitor for tuberculosis
Abatacept (Orenzia)	Same as above	Same for all biologics	Monitor for tuberculosis
Brodalumab (Siliq)	Same as above	Same for all biologics	Monitor for tuberculosis, for depression
Golimumab (Simponi)	Same as above	Same for all biologics	Monitor for tuberculosis
Risarkizymab (Skyrizi)	Same as above	Same for all biologics	Monitor for tuberculosis
Ixekizumab (Taltz)	Same as above	Same for all biologics	Monitor for tuberculosis, avoid with IBS
Guselkumab (Tremfya)	Same as above	Same for all biologics	Monitor for tuberculosis
Tofacitnib (Xeljannz)	Same as above	Same for all biologics	Monitor for tuberculosis

GI, gastrointestinal; IBS, irritable bowel syndrome.

Emollients

Emollients are useful for all cases of psoriasis as an adjunct therapy. These agents hydrate the stratum corneum, decrease water evaporation, and soften the scales of the plaques. Multiple products are available commercially in lotions, creams, and ointments. The thicker the preparation, the more effective it is. In addition to preserving moisture, emollients have a mild antipruritic effect. Gentle cleansers are encouraged.

Topical Corticosteroids

The foundation of topical treatment is topical corticosteroids. They play an important role in treating psoriasis by decreasing erythema, pruritus, and scaling. They promote vasoconstriction. They are fast acting but not intended for long-term use. Topical corticosteroids are classified into several categories based on potency and vasoconstrictive properties. Low-potency corticosteroids are safer for long-term use and for use at thin-skinned sites such as the face and groin. The most effective topical treatment is a medium- or high-potency agent used for a limited time, followed by a less potent agent for maintenance. Occlusion of the area where the topical steroid is applied is recommended. Saran wrap can be used; Cordran tape is also effective but quite expensive.

This method increases the absorption (hence the potency) of the topical preparation. Topical corticosteroids may be used twice daily for 2 weeks and then decreased to alternating days. Topical corticosteroids have a rapid onset of action giving quick relief. For more information on topical corticosteroids, see Chapter 12. Intralesional steroid use may also be helpful for individual plaques.

Coal Tars

Coal tar (Cutar) contains polycyclic hydrocarbon compounds formed from bituminous coal. It depresses deoxyribonucleic acid (DNA) synthesis and has antiinflammatory and antipruritic properties. Several preparations are available over the counter (OTC), including ointments, gels, bath preparations, and shampoos. Coal tar can be used as an initial therapy, usually with adjunct topical corticosteroids. The emulsion is dissolved in bath water (15–25 mL), and the patient immerses the affected area in the water for 10 to 20 minutes. It is used for 30 to 45 days, 3 to 7 times a week. The shampoo preparation is massaged into a wet scalp and rinsed. It is applied a second time and left on the scalp for 5 minutes. Disadvantages of coal tar include the unpleasant odor; staining of clothes, skin, and fiberglass tubs or sinks (even with the clear preparation); and photosensitivity. These disadvantages tend to lead to poor compliance.

Anthralin

Anthralin (Drithocreme, Micanol) is another topical treatment for psoriasis. Similar to cutar, this is a coal tar derivative.

Mechanism of Action

There are two possible mechanisms of action: inhibition of DNA synthesis and a decrease in epidermal proliferation. Anthralin is a good alternative therapy if the patient has a limited number of lesions, because its use is time consuming.

Dosage

Anthralin is applied for 30 minutes to 1 hour and then removed. It should be applied only to the lesions. Treatment starts with a low strength that is gradually increased. Staining of the psoriasis plaques signifies that treatment is decreasing cellular proliferation. Treatment is time consuming but short term.

Time Frame for Response

There is a slow onset of action, and response is slow as well.

Contraindications

Anthralin therapy is contraindicated in acute psoriasis and inflammation.

Adverse Events

Anthralin therapy may be limited by irritation of the unaffected skin. The medication stains clothing a brownish purple and permanently stains towels, tubs, and sinks.

Vitamin D Analogs

Calcipotriene (Dovonex) and Calcipotriol are vitamin D analogs for treating mild to moderate psoriasis. They are supplied in creams, ointments, and topical foams.

Mechanism of Action

Its mechanism of action is a reduction of cell proliferation by binding to receptors in epidermal keratinocytes. The drug is also thought to have an antiinflammatory effect. It is effective for long-term use and maintenance therapy and is often used as rotational therapy with topical corticosteroids.

Dosage

A thin layer is applied twice daily to affected skin for 6 to 8 weeks. It may be used as rotational therapy or by pulse dosing (off-and-on therapy) in which the patient follows the therapeutic regimen for 2 weeks, followed by 1 week off. Use with a potent topical corticosteroid is most effective.

Time Frame for Response

Some improvement is usually seen in 2 to 4 weeks, although therapy is recommended for 6 to 8 weeks. An advantage of calcipotriene is its efficacy similar to that of medium- to high-potency topical corticosteroids. Unlike corticosteroids, however, calcipotriene does not cause skin atrophy or hypothalamus–pituitary–adrenal axis suppression. However, it is an irritant and should not be used on the face.

Contraindications

It is contraindicated in patients with hypercalcemia and vitamin D toxicity.

Adverse Events

The most common adverse effects of calcipotriene are mild and include dry skin, peeling, and rash. Hypercalcemia may be caused by vitamin D ingestion but is rare if the patient uses less than 100 g of calcipotriene per week.

Retinoid (Vitamin A Derivative)

Tazarotene (Tazorac) is a topical retinoid used for mild to moderate psoriasis.

Mechanism of Action

This drug normalizes epidermal differentiation, decreases hyperproliferation, and diminishes inflammation of the cells in the skin. Use of tazarotene promotes longer remission of psoriasis.

Dosage

It comes in a clear, nonstaining gel, in cream (0.05% and 0.1%), and in foam (Fabior) preparations and is applied in a thin layer once a day at bedtime. Skin must be air dried and the area left un-occluded. The preparation can be used for the body, scalp, hairline, and face but not on the genitalia, on the intertriginous areas, or around the eyes.

Time Frame for Response

After 1 week of therapy, diminished scaling is noted. Clearing is seen in approximately 8 weeks.

Contraindications

Tazarotene can cause fetal harm, so it is started in women during the menstrual cycle. Women using this agent should ensure that they do not get pregnant during therapy.

Adverse Events

Adverse effects of tazarotene include pruritus, erythema, and mild to moderate burning. The use of topical corticosteroids counteracts these effects. The patient must be warned that the psoriasis may get worse before it improves.

Interactions

Vitamin A ingestion is to be avoided, and tazarotene is to be used with caution with other photosensitizers such as tetracyclines and with other topical irritants such as abrasives, depilatories, or permanent wave solutions.

Combination Products

Newer therapies include topical steroids in combination with keratolytic agents: betamethasone 0.064% and calcipotriene 0.005% gel and ointment (Taclonex), foam (Enstilar), halobetasol propriante 0.01%, and tazaratene 0.045% lotion (Duobrii).

Mechanism of Action

The mechanism is same as that described previously for individual products.

Dosage

The dosage is same as that described previously for individual products.

Contraindications

The contraindications are same as those described previously for individual products.

Adverse Events

Combination products may reduce the irritating side effects due to decreased dosage of each product while maximizing results.

Interactions

The interactions are the same as those described previously for individual products.

Systemic Retinoids

Acitretin (Soriatane) is a systemic retinoid used for long-term psoriasis therapy.

Mechanism of Action

Acitretin normalizes epidermal differentiation and diminishes hyperproliferation and inflammation of cells in the skin. Prior to initiation of drug therapy, complete blood count (CBC) with differential diagnosis, comprehensive metabolic panel (CMP), and lipid profile should be obtained.

Dosage

Initially, acitretin 10 mg once daily and then up to 50 mg once daily must be taken with the main meal until the lesions clear, which occurs gradually.

Contraindications

Acitretin is contraindicated in pregnancy and lactation and with the use of alcohol. It cannot be used in patients with severe renal impairment and increased lipid levels. The patient cannot donate blood for three years after therapy. Caution is exercised if the patient has a history of depression, obesity, or alcohol abuse.

Adverse Events

Adverse effects include lipid elevations, abnormal liver function, alopecia, skin peeling, pruritus, dry skin, dry mouth, epistaxis, paresthesia, paronychia, and pseudotumor cerebri.

Interactions

Drug interactions occur with methotrexate (MTX, Rheumatrex), alcohol, and progestin-only contraceptives. Women must not ingest alcohol during therapy or for 2 months afterward because alcohol prolongs the teratogenic potential of the drug.

Methotrexate

MTX is used to treat generalized psoriasis.

Mechanism of Action

MTX inhibits folic acid reductase, resulting in the inhibition of cellular replication and selection of the most rapidly dividing cells.

Dosage

The initial dose is 7.5 mg a week administered in three doses over a 24-hour period. It is then titrated to a dose of 12.5 to 25 mg a week. With improvement in the disease, the dose is reduced and other agents are used. Folic acid, 1 mg daily, should be taken on nontreatment days.

Contraindications

MTX is contraindicated in pregnancy and lactation, and the drug is used with caution in patients with renal, hepatic disorders and leukopenia.

Adverse Events

Common adverse effects include headache, blurred vision, fatigue, malaise, gastrointestinal (GI) distress, gingivitis, hepatic toxicity, bone marrow depression, rashes, alopecia, and chills and fever.

Interactions

There is an increased risk of toxicity if the patient is taking other medications, such as salicylates, phenytoin (Dilantin), and sulfonamides. Use of MTX also decreases the serum level of digoxin (Lanoxin).

Cyclosporine

Mechanism of Action

Cyclosporine suppresses cell-mediated immune reactions and humoral immunity. It inhibits the production of IL-2, which is responsible for producing T cell proliferation. Cyclosporine promotes rapid remission in severe psoriasis flares. It is usually used for short-term treatment (3–6 months) for severe exacerbations due to toxicity.

Dosage

The maximum dose for use in psoriasis is 2 to 5 mg/kg/d. Maintenance therapy is at lower doses. It is supplied in 100-mg tablets and dosed twice daily.

Contraindications

Cyclosporine is contraindicated in pregnancy and lactation and must be used with caution in patients with impaired renal function and malabsorption.

Adverse Events

Adverse effects include hypertension and nephrotoxicity, as well as tremor, gingival hyperplasia, GI upset, hirsutism, and acne. Lesions can recur within days to weeks after treatment ends, and rebounds with worse symptoms are not uncommon.

Interactions

Cyclosporine use increases the risk for nephrotoxicity if the patient uses other nephrotoxic agents, and it also increases the risk for digoxin toxicity. Cyclosporine interacts with lovastatin, diltiazem, and ketoconazole, and its therapeutic effect is decreased with concomitant hydantoin (Dilantin), rifampin, and sulfonamide use. Patients must avoid grapefruit products.

PHOSPHODIESTERASE 4 INHIBITORS

Apremilast (Otezla)

Mechanism of Action

Apremilast, an oral agent, is a small molecule specific to cyclic adenosine monophosphate. The underlying mechanism is not well understood. No prior lab studies are required prior to initiating therapy, unlike the requirement with most other agents.

Dosage

A starter pack is designed to allow for titration to maintenance dose 30 mg twice daily.

Contraindications

Patients with a known hypersensitivity to apremilast and its ingredients.

Adverse Events

The most common adverse event is GI distress and diarrhea which for some may be self-limiting. Weight loss may also occur as a side effect. Caution is needed with use in patients with a history of depression, as this drug may exacerbate symptoms.

Interactions

Apremilast activity is decreased when coadministered with strong cytochrome P-450 inducers (i.e., rifampin), and may decrease efficacy.

BIOLOGICS

The biologics interact with specific targets in the T cell–mediated inflammatory process. They have an antiinflammatory effect through the inhibition of cytokine release, prevention of T cell activation, depletion of pathologic T cells, and blocking of the interactions that lead to T cell activation or migration into the tissue. They also alter the balance of the T cell types and inhibit key inflammatory cytokines, such as TNF-alpha inhibitors (Enbrel and Humira), IL-17 blockage (Taltz Cosentyx and Siliq), IL-12/23 blockade (Stelara), and IL-23 antagonists (Tremfya, Ilumya, Skyrizi). Testing for tuberculosis (TB) prior to drug initiation is recommended by placing purified protein derivative (PPD) intradermal or Quantiferon Gold via blood samples for all agents. For individuals who have received the Bacillus Calmette-Guerin (BCG) vaccine, a chest X-ray is recommended. If tested positive, a consult to the infectious disease department is recommended for treatment prior to biologic use. Due to the immune-suppressive nature of these drugs, other laboratory studies recommended include CBC, CMP, lipid panel, hepatitis B (must treat prior to biologic use), and hepatitis C.

TNF-alpha inhibitors were the first biologics used to treat moderate to severe plaque psoriasis. The following are currently approved drugs in this class:

Etanercept (Enbrel)
Infliximab (Remicade)
Adalimumab (Humira)
Certolizumab pegol (Cimzia)

Mechanism of Action

Binds and inhibits TNF, the cytokine that helps regulate the body's immune response to inflammation. It is used to treat moderate to severe psoriasis.

Dosage

Etanercept (Enbrel) in psoriasis is dosed at 50 mg subcutaneously twice a week initially for 3 months. The maintenance dose is 50 mg subcutaneously weekly, with a maximum of 25 mg given at one site. It requires two injections in separate sites. Infliximab (Remicade) is given by intravenous infusion over at least 2 hours. The dose is 5 mg/kg at week 0, week 2, and week 6 and then once every 8 weeks. Adalimumab (Humira) is administered subcutaneously initially 80 mg followed by 40 mg every other week starting the week after the initial dose. Certolizumab (Cimzia) is dosed at 400 mg subcutaneously initially and then every other week.

Contraindications

Contraindications include live vaccines, malignancy, and/or active infection. Caution is exercised in females of reproductive age. It is not recommended for patients in pregnancy or those with impaired renal function, asthma, history of blood dyscrasias, demyelinating disease, that is, multiple sclerosis, history of chronic recurrent infections, and/or malignancy. Infliximab is contraindicated in patients with moderate to severe congestive heart failure.

Adverse Events

Adverse events include infection, injection site reaction, localized erythema, rash, upper respiratory infections, abdominal pain, and vomiting.

Interactions

There is an increased chance of infection with those individuals who are immunocompromised. Live vaccines should be given prior to initiation of therapy or dosage should be withheld for 2 weeks before and then 1 month after administration of the vaccine to ensure adequate immune response. Similar discontinuation used for voluntary surgical procedures.

Ustekinumab

Mechanism of Action

Ustekinumab (Stelara) is a human IL-12 and IL-23 antagonist.

Dosage

Administered subcutaneously, it is available in two weight-based doses: Patients weighing less than 100 kg (220 lbs) receive a 45-mg dose and those weighing greater than 100 kg (220 lbs) receive 90 mg four times a year.

Contraindications

Ustekinumab is not recommended for patients with sensitivity to any of the excipients.

Adverse Events

May include nasopharyngitis and upper respiratory tract infections. Serious infections and malignancies may occur.

Interactions

Live vaccines should not be given to patients taking ustekinumab.

Interleukin-17 Inhibitors

Mechanism of Action

Secukinumab (Cosentyx), Ixekizumab (Taltz), and Brodalumab (Siliq) are monoclonal antibodies that bind to IL-17, blocking the ability of the cytokine to interact with its receptor.

Dosing

The following are the dosages:

Secukinumab—300 mg administered subcutaneously (in divided doses of 150 each) every week for 5 weeks and then once every month

Ixekizumab—80 mg administered every 2 weeks for 3 months and then once every 4 weeks

Brodalumab—210 mg administered at weeks 0, 1, and 2 and then once every 2 weeks.

Contraindications

Similar to all other biologic agents.

Adverse Events

Adverse events are similar to those of all other biologic agents.

Contraindications

No live vaccines.

Interleukin-23 inhibitors

Mechanism of Action

Guzelkumab (Tremfya), Tildrakizumab (Ilumya), and risanki-zumab (Skyrizi) block IL-23. Inhibition of IL-23 cytokine prevents the cascade of inflammatory cells. By blocking the IL 23 pathway, it activates and maintains the T helper 17 pathway.

Dosing

Guselkumab 100 mg subcutaneously at weeks 0, 4, and then every 8 weeks. Tildrakizumab 100 mg subcutaneously at weeks 0, 4, and then every 12 weeks.

Contraindications

Similar to all other biologic agents.

Adverse Events

Similar to all other biologic agents.

Contraindications

No live vaccines.

Biosimilars are also now available for some of these agents.

Selecting the Most Appropriate Agent

Selection of therapy depends on the patient's age, type of lesion, involvement, and previous treatments. Mild to relatively moderate psoriasis (less than 10% BSA) can be treated by a primary care provider. Topical treatment of psoriasis is the first step and is usually effective for mild disease. Patients with more generalized disease are referred to a dermatologist

for treatment and phototherapy, and systemic agents are used (**Table 14.2** and **Figure 14.1**).

It appears that combination therapy with systemic agents and other modalities have synergistic value. In combination therapy, the dose can often be reduced, causing less toxicity from higher dose individual drugs. Systemic therapy with phototherapy is also effective, but time constraints of biweekly therapy hinder use.

First-Line Therapy

First-line therapy includes moisturizers and topical steroids. For 2 weeks, a high-potency or very high–potency topical steroid is applied twice daily and covered by an occlusive dressing of plastic wrap. A low-potency preparation is used on the face and intertriginous areas. An ointment is recommended because it provides the most moisture. An emollient is also used to keep the skin hydrated.

Second-Line Therapy

If the patient's response to first-line therapy is not optimal, several second-line choices are available. If the patient shows a good response, therapy may consist of a week's rest from the topical corticosteroids. Another option is the use of corticosteroids twice daily weekends and vitamin D analog twice daily weekdays. Limiting the use of high-potency topical corticosteroids to once or twice a week and adding a lower-strength or a vitamin D analog twice daily to the regimen are other options. This produces a better result than either drug used alone. The topical corticosteroid helps clear the plaques and reduces irritation from the vitamin D preparation.

Third-Line Therapy

If first- and second-line treatments fail, a patient is referred to a dermatologist, who may use ultraviolet (UV) B light treatments, antimetabolites, biologic agents, or psoralens plus UVA = PUVA.

TABLE 14.2		
Recommended Order of Treatment for Psoriasis		
Order	**Therapy**	**Comments**
First line	High-potency topical corticosteroids applied to moist skin and use of occlusive dressing twice daily for 2 weeks. Use emollients as adjunct therapy	Use when <10% of body surface area is affected
Second line	If the patient responded well to first-line therapy, provide a 1-week rest from the topical corticosteroids and initiate another 2 weeks of therapy with the same agent for two more times OR Taper the high-potency topical corticosteroid use to once or twice a week and add a vitamin D analog twice daily	If there is remission, applying the topical steroids once or twice a week may maintain remission
Third line	Refer to dermatologist for systemic therapy	For use with >20% body surface area, UVB is used with coal tar or anthralin; PUVA is used with psoralens

PUVA, Psoralen and ultraviolet A therapy; UVB, ultraviolet B treatments.

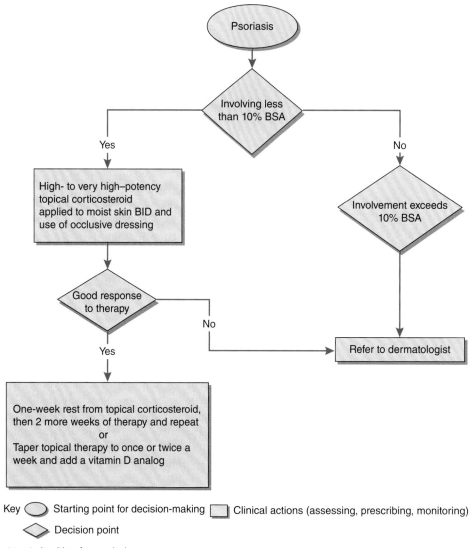

FIGURE 14–1 Treatment algorithm for psoriasis.

BSA, body surface area.

MONITORING PATIENT RESPONSE

The goal of chronic topical corticosteroid therapy is to use the lowest effective potency to control symptoms. Initially, follow-up may have to be done monthly and then may progress to every 2 to 3 months.

PATIENT EDUCATION

Drug Information

In patients with psoriasis, education regarding stress reduction and symptom control is important to prevent progression of disease and reach therapy goals. The population should understand that psoriasis is not contagious. In addition, referral for counseling may help with related emotional issues.

Psychosocial concerns should be addressed since this condition can affect self-esteem and social interactions with others. Patients may also benefit from information and support from groups such as the National Psoriasis Foundation (1-800-723-9166, www.psoriasis.org).

Demonstration for proper application of topical steroids is an important aspect of care. The medications are to be used twice daily and applied lightly on moist skin for maximum benefit.

Lifestyle Changes

Symptom control, rather than cure, is the goal of therapy. Patients may help control symptoms by exposing their skin to the sun. This should be accomplished by gradually increasing the length of exposure. Emphasis should be placed on the importance of using sunscreen and avoiding sunburn.

To prevent infection, patients must take care to not cut the lesions when shaving (if there are lesions in the area). Psoriasis can be triggered by infections, stress, and changes in climate that can dry skin. These should be avoided when possible.

Complementary and Alternative Medicine

Fish oil is thought to alter the immune response and in small quantities can relieve itching and scaling. It has an effect on chronic plaque psoriasis in doses of 6 to 15 g daily. An alternative is to eat fish thrice a week. Aloe vera was shown to be effective in treatment of psoriasis. In a 16-week study, there was an 82.8% clearing of psoriatic plaque by use of 0.5% hydrophilic aloe vera cream thrice daily. Glucosamine has been shown to relieve some of the pain of arthritis from psoriasis. Dietary changes to avoid inflammatory substances are encouraged.

CASE STUDY 1

P.B. is a 58-year-old woman with a history of hypertension. She seeks treatment for scattered plaques with a silvery-white scale on her elbows, forearms, and knees. The body surface area affected is approximately 8%. She is very self-conscious about the lesions: "I just want them to go away." Her medications include propranolol 40 mg thrice daily and furosemide 40 mg daily. She has a positive family history of psoriasis and reports high levels of stress in her job and life. She smokes a pack of cigarettes per day.

DIAGNOSIS: PSORIASIS

1. List specific goals for treatment for P.B.
2. What drug therapy would you prescribe? Why?
3. What are the parameters for monitoring the success of the therapy?
4. Discuss specific patient education based on the prescribed therapy.
5. List one or two adverse reactions for the selected agent that would cause you to change therapy.
6. What would be the choice for second-line therapy?
7. What over-the-counter or alternative medications would be appropriate for P.B.?
8. What lifestyle changes would you recommend to P.B.?
9. Describe one or two drug–drug or drug–food interactions for the selected agent.

Bibliography

Busard, C., Zweegers, J., Limpens, J., et al. (2014). Combined use of systemic agents for psoriasis: A systematic review. *JAMA Dermatology, 150*(11), 1213–1220.

Egeberg, A., Byrd, L., & Skov, L. (2019). Drug survival of Secukinumab and Ixekizumab for moderate to severe plaque psoriasis. *Journal of American Academy of Dermatology, 81*(1), 173–178.

Elmets, C., Lim, H., et al. (2019). Joint academy of dermatology-national psoriasis foundation guidelines of care for the management and treatment of psoriasis with phototherapy. *Journal of American Academy of Dermatology, 81*(3), 778–804.

Feldman, S. (2014). Five factors for choosing the right biologic treatment. *The Dermatologist, 22*(9), 26–29.

Fu, Y., Lee, C. et al. (2018). Association of psoriasis with inflammatory bowel disease: A systemic review and meta-analysis. *JAMA Dermatology, 154*(12), 1417–1423.

Green, L., Yamauchi, P., & Kircik, L. (2019). Comparison of the safety and efficacy of tumor necrosis factor inhibitors and interleukin-17 inhibitors in patients with psoriasis. *Journal of Drugs in Dermatology, 18*(8), 776–789.

Habif, T., Diunlos, J., Chapman, M.S. et al. (2018). *Skin disease: Diagnosis and treatment.* New York: Elsevier.

Han, G. (2019). What's new in topical treatments for psoriasis. *Cutis, 103*(2), 65–66.

Lebwohl, M., Sugarman, J., et al. (2018). Long term safety results from a phase 3 open-label study of a fixed combination halobetasol propronate 0.01% and tazarotene 0.045% lotion in moderate to severe plaque psoriasis. *Journal of American Academy of Dermatology, 80*(1), 282–285.

Menter, A., Korman, N., Elmets, C., et al. (2010). Guidelines of care for management of psoriasis and psoriatic arthritis. *Journal of the American Academy of Dermatology, 62*(1), 114–135.

Murphy, E., Nussbaum, D., et al. (2019). Use of complementary and alternative medicine by patients with psoriasis. *Journal of American Academy of Dermatology, 81*(1), 281–283.

Stein-Gold, L., Lain, E., et al. (2019). Halobetasol 0.01%/ tazarotene 0.045% lotion for moderate-to-severe plaque psoriasis: Maintenance of therapeutic effect after cessation of therapy. *Journal of Drugs in Dermatology, 18*(8), 815–820.

Yamauchi, P. S., & Bagel, J. (2015). Next generation biologics in the management of plaque psoriasis: A literature review of IL-17 inhibition. *Journal of Drugs in Dermatology, 14*(3), 244–250.

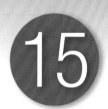

15 Acne Vulgaris and Rosacea

Shelly R. Schneider

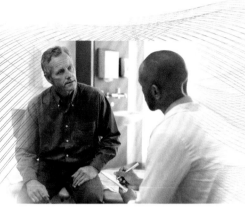
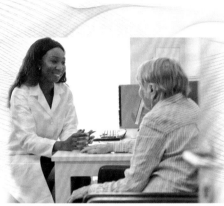
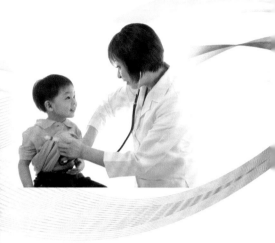

Learning Objectives

1. The learner will identify agents used to treat mild to moderate acne lesions.
2. The learner will distinguish the need for topical therapy, understand when to add oral agents if appropriate, and understand when to refer to dermatology.
3. The learner will discuss the varied topical agents available to treat both telangectatic and papulopustular rosacea.

ACNE VULGARIS

Acne vulgaris is viewed by some as a rite of passage during the adolescent years. Up to 90% of all teenagers report having some form of acne. Adults suffer from the effects of acne as well: between 30% and 50% of adult women report experiencing acne. Consumers spend millions of dollars annually on prescription and over-the-counter (OTC) acne preparations. The psychosocial costs of acne are high. Adolescents are particularly affected by physical defects, no matter how minor they appear to others. The health care practitioner must be particularly sensitive to the perceived seriousness of the acne in addition to the clinical picture. What may seem inconsequential to the practitioner may be devastating to the patient. No matter how minor the acne may appear to the provider, it is important to ask patients if they are concerned about their acne and whether they would like treatment.

CAUSES

Historically, numerous theories of the cause of acne vulgaris have been proposed, yet the exact cause remains unknown. Foods, stress, and hormones, although not causative, may exacerbate existing acne, which is why it is important to obtain a complete health history to ascertain precipitating factors. For example, a variety of drugs, topical agents, and medical conditions may exacerbate acne. Certain drugs used to treat tuberculosis, seizure disorders, chronic illness, or depression and steroid dependency may be the cause of drug-induced acneiform rash (**Table 15.1**). Drug-induced acne should be suspected when all lesions are in the same stage (e.g., the lesions are uniformly all pustules or all open comedones), covering the face, chest, trunk, arms, and legs.

Acne may be exacerbated in teenagers and adults whose skin is exposed to oily agents, such as makeup, oil-based sunscreen, and oil-based hair products that come in contact with the forehead and temporal regions of the face (referred to as *pomade acne*). Friction acne from tight-fitting clothes (sports bras in females), football helmets (chin straps), and hatbands may be found over the skin rubbed by the clothes. Exposure to animal vegetable and petroleum-based oils used in workplaces such as fast-food restaurants and automotive garages may also exacerbate acne. Emotional stress may contribute to acne exacerbations in persons prone to breakouts, but studies have not consistently proven this correlation. Women with a history of menstrual irregularities, hirsutism, and treatment-resistant acne should be evaluated for androgen excess associated with polycystic ovarian syndrome.

TABLE 15.1

Medications That Cause Acneiform Rash

Medication	Underlying Condition
Corticosteroids	Chronic inflammatory conditions
Isoniazid	Tuberculosis
Lithium	Depression
Phenytoin	Seizure disorder
Trimethadione	Seizure disorder

PATHOPHYSIOLOGY

Acne usually begins 1 to 2 years before the onset of puberty, when androgen production increases. Excess androgen causes increased sebum production. For unknown reasons, abnormal keratinization causes retention of sebum in the pilosebaceous follicle. This produces open comedones (blackheads) and closed comedones (whiteheads). When closed comedones continue to produce keratin and sebum, the pilosebaceous follicle ruptures and inflames the surrounding tissue. If the inflammation is close to the surface, a papule forms. If it is deeper in the dermis, a larger papule or nodule forms. These deeper, nodular acne cysts can cause permanent scars.

Although *Cutibacterium acnes* (*C. acnes*) formerly known as *Propionibacterium acnes*, an anaerobic gram-positive bacterium, is present as normal flora in the pilosebaceous follicle, acne is not an infectious entity. Rather, it is believed that *C. acnes* produces lipolytic enzymes that in turn produce biologically active extracellular products. These in turn attract polymorphonuclear leukocytes and monocytes, which increase inflammation.

DIAGNOSTIC CRITERIA

Acne vulgaris is diagnosed from the clinical presentation of the patient's skin. It is classified and subsequently treated depending on its severity. The mildest form of acne is comedonal. Both open and closed comedones may be present. Mild inflammatory acne is manifested by papules. Moderate inflammatory acne consists of pustules and some cysts. Severe cystic acne consists of cysts, nodules, and scarring (**Table 15.2**).

TABLE 15.2

Classification of Acne Vulgaris

Classification	Physical Findings
Comedonal acne	Open comedones (blackheads), closed comedones (whiteheads)
Mild inflammatory acne	Papules
Moderate inflammatory acne	Pustules, cysts
Severe cystic acne	Cysts, nodules, "ice-pick" scarring

INITIATING DRUG THERAPY

Skin care is the most important nonpharmacologic tool in the management of acne vulgaris. The patient should be instructed to wash the face gently twice a day with a mild agent. A cleanser is less drying and harsh than soap, and multiple preparations are available OTC. Washing should be gentle because scrubbing the skin may exacerbate the acne. Comedonal removal, although therapeutic, should be undertaken only by someone skilled in the proper technique. Picking or popping pimples may increase tissue damage, leading to scarring and infection. The health care provider should advise the patient to avoid manipulating the acne with the fingers.

In general, moisturizers and cosmetics should be water based, non-comedogenic, and fragrance free. If hair preparations are used, they should also be water based. The patient should be instructed to apply hair products so that they avoid contact with sides of face, shoulders, and trunk.

The practitioner also needs to stress that ingestion of specific foods, such as sugar and dairy, may contribute to inflammatory factors that predispose one to acne. Heredity may also be a precipitating a factor for severe scarring acne.

Goals of Drug Therapy

The goal of pharmacotherapy is to minimize the number and severity of new lesions, prevent scarring, and improve the patient's appearance. The patient must be counseled that improvement of acne vulgaris takes time—usually 4 to 6 weeks. Some form of therapy will probably need to be continued throughout adolescence and even into young adulthood.

Pharmacotherapy choices are based on the severity of the acne. Currently, successful therapy usually relies on a combination of medications. The synergistic effect of two or more drugs from different classes produces the best results. See **Table 15.3** for a summary of acne medications.

Comedolytics

Tretinoin

Mechanism of Action

When applied topically, retinoic acid (Retin A, Retin A Micro, Altreno) acts on the epidermis with little systemic absorption to decrease cohesion between epidermal cells and increase epidermal cell turnover. The result is expulsion of open comedones and the conversion of closed comedones to open ones.

Dosage

Retinoic acid is available in creams (0.025%, 0.05%, 0.06%, 0.08%, and 0.1%), gels (0.01%, 0.025%, and 0.05%), and microsphere (0.04% and 0.1%) formulations. The microsphere formulation encapsulates the active ingredient in microspheres, which act as a reservoir that slowly releases the retinoic acid into the skin.

TABLE 15.3			
Overview of Topical and Oral Acne Preparations			
Generic (Trade) Name and Dosage	**Selected Adverse Events**	**Contraindications**	**Special Considerations**
Topical Medications			
Tretinoin (Retin-A, Retina A Micro, Renova, Altreno) 0.025%, 0.05% cream, gel 0.04%, 0.06%, 0.08%, 0.1% microspheres Apply once daily; increase strength as tolerated	Erythema, local skin irritation, photosensitivity	Eczema, sunburn	Apply to dry skin for short periods or on alternate nights until better tolerated. Avoid products with high concentrations of alcohol, astringents, spices
Benzoyl peroxide (many) 2.5%–5.0% once daily; increase to BID/TID	Irritation	Sunscreens containing PABA may cause transient skin discoloration	Product may bleach fabrics. Apply at different time from other topical medications
Azelaic acid (Azelex) 20% cream Apply twice daily	Pruritus, irritation		Darker-pigmented people may have hypopigmentation. Exacerbation of asthma
Clindamycin (Clindagel) 1% Apply to skin twice daily	Burning; stinging of eyes, possibly pseudomembranous colitis		Discontinue use if diarrhea develops. Pseudomembranous colitis may develop. Drug may potentiate neuromuscular blocking agents
Erythromycin (many) 2%–3% topical Apply twice daily	Irritation	Allergy to erythromycin	None
Dapsone (Aczone) 5% and 7.5%	Local irritation	Sensitivity to G6P deficiency, glaucoma	May leave brownish discoloration if used in combination with BPO
Combination Topicals			
Clindamycin/Tretinoin (Veltin, Ziana) 1.2%/0.025%	Same as for each individual	Pregnancy	Same as above
Adapalene/BPO (Epiduo, Epiduo Forte) 0.03%/2.5% and 0.1%/2.5%	Same as for each individual	Pregnancy	Same as above
Oral Medications			
Tetracycline (many) 500–1,000 mg daily divided BID/QID Taper to 250 mg/d after improvement; attempt to discontinue after 4–6 months of therapy	Photosensitivity, gastric irritation, decreased effectiveness of oral contraceptives	Age younger than 8 years	Drug may increase serum digoxin levels. Drug absorption is reduced if taken with antacids, iron, zinc, dairy products. Drug use may increase blood urea nitrogen values if renal system is impaired
Erythromycin (many) 250, 333, 500–1,000 mg/d divided	Nausea, vomiting, diarrhea, rash, allergic reactions, fungal infection, hepatitis, ototoxicity	Allergy to erythromycin or macrolide Not recommended for children younger than age 2 months	Take on an empty stomach for better absorption 1 hour before or 2 hours after a meal. Enteric-coated form can be taken with or without food. Interactions: warfarin, theophylline, cisapride, digoxin, and others
Sarecycline (Seysara) 60, 100, and 150 mg	Nausea	Hypersensitive to tetracycline	Once daily with or without food

(Continued)

TABLE 15.3

Overview of Topical and Oral Acne Preparations (*Continued*)

Generic (Trade) Name and Dosage	Selected Adverse Events	Contraindications	Special Considerations
Isotretinoin (Absorica) generic options: Amnesteem, Claravis, Myorisan 0.5–1.0 mg/kg BID	Increased cholesterol and triglyceride levels; dry skin and mucous membranes; depression; aggressive, violent behaviors; back pain; arthralgias in pediatric patients	Adolescents before cessation of growth Pregnancy	Prescriber must be registered in iPledge program. Female patients of childbearing age must test negative for two pregnancy tests prior to therapy initiation, with monthly pregnancy tests while on therapy. Monitor cholesterol and triglyceride levels, CBC, liver function tests before therapy, at 4 weeks, and as indicated
Ethinyl estradiol with norgestimate (Ortho Tri-Cyclen, Tri-Sprintec) 1 tablet daily		Pre-menarchial girls, male patients	Women who smoke should avoid use of oral contraceptives
Aldactone (Spironolactone) 25–200 mg	Rarely hyperkalemia	Pregnancy	Avoid hyperkalemia

BPO, benzyl peroxide; CBC, complete blood count; PABA, para-aminobenzoic acid.

Contraindications

All retinoids are considered teratogenic, and women should ensure that they do not become pregnant while using these agents.

Side Effects

Erythema, dryness, and peeling of the skin may result if overused. Some patients cannot tolerate daily use or prolonged contact at the initiation of therapy.

Special Considerations

Fair-skinned and sensitive patients should be advised to start out using the product every other day. Alternatively, the patient may be instructed to apply retinoic acid to the face for 15 to 30 minutes each night and then wash off the medication. Gradually, the length of time the medication remains on the face is increased until it can be tolerated overnight. It is best to apply the medication on clean, thoroughly dry skin to avoid excessive irritation. Patients should be advised to avoid prolonged exposure to the sun or to wear a non-comedogenic sunscreen formulated specifically for use on the face.

Informing individuals to stop the topical preparation for at least 3 days before facial waxing is recommended due to sensitivity and sloughing. In addition, avoidance of corners of eyes, nose, and mouth due to increased sensitivity and irritation in such sensitive areas is recommended.

Adapalene

Mechanism of Action

Adapalene (Differin) 0.1% and 0.3% gel, a topical medication for treating noninflammatory acne, is a derivative of naphthoic acid, which binds to retinoid receptors.

Dosage

It is applied once daily in evening to avoid sun sensitivity.

Contraindications

The drug is considered teratogenic, so females of childbearing potential should be cautioned to avoid pregnancy while using these agents.

Side Effects

Erythema, dryness, and peeling of the skin may result if overused. Some patients cannot tolerate daily use or prolonged contact at the initiation of therapy.

Special Considerations

It is considered less irritating than retinoic acid. Up to 40% of patients report irritation, but it subsides during the first month of treatment. Adapalene is applied in the same way as retinoic acid. The lower dose is now available OTC.

Tazarotene

Mechanism of Action

A retinoid prodrug, tazarotene (Tazorac) 0.05% gel, 0.1% gel, cream, and foam preparation is effective against both comedonal and inflammatory acne.

Dosage

It is applied once daily in evening. The user may alternate every other day when first introduced.

Contraindications

All retinoids are considered teratogenic, and women should be cautioned to use contraception and/or prevent pregnancy.

Side Effects

Redness, dryness, burning, and peeling of the skin may result when initiating therapy. Some patients tolerate alternate daily use or less prolonged contact at the initiation of therapy.

Special Considerations

Alternating days of application, as well as using a pea-sized dose for the entire face, can reduce irritation. Use of a moisturizer prior to application is helpful. Address the use of a gentle cleanser if dryness continues or seek a less potent form of therapy.

Comedolytic Bactericidals

Benzyl Peroxide

Method of Action

Benzyl peroxide (BPO) is both comedolytic and bactericidal to *C. acnes*. It has a role in inflammatory acne because of its antibacterial qualities. Decreasing *C. acnes* levels decreases the inflammation caused by leukocytic and monocytic attraction to the pilosebaceous follicle. The major side effect of BPO is irritation.

Dosage

BPO is available in various strengths and forms in OTC preparations. Gel formulations are considered more effective, but all are available in many different strengths. It is also available as washes or leave-on lotion and creams. This product can be used once or twice daily, in addition to use on alternate days.

Contraindications

Hypersensitivity reactions may occur in those with more sensitive skin types.

Side Effects

Irritation, erythema, and dryness may all be experienced with the use of BPO products.

Special Considerations

Similar to all comedolytics, BPO is applied initially in a low-percentage formulation in a nonirritating base. The patient increases the dosage strength and frequency as tolerated. Since BPO may bleach colored items, the patient should be instructed to not let the product come in contact with brightly colored towels, pillowcases, or clothing.

Azelaic Acid

Mechanism of Action

Azelaic acid (Azelex) 20% cream is believed to interfere with the deoxyribonucleic acid synthesis of acne-causing bacteria. Used to treat mild to moderate acne, the drug is also available in 15% gel and foam formulations for use in rosacea.

Dosage

Azelaic acid is applied once daily to clean skin initially; dosing may be increased to twice daily.

Side Effects

Irritation, erythema, and dryness initially can occur with first time use. Alternating days when initiating therapy can be recommended.

Special Considerations

This agent is a milder, less irritating topical than most BPO preparations. Its use along with a moisturizer prior to application prevents overdrying and irritation.

Dapsone

Mechanism of Action

Drug properties of dapsone (Aczone) include both antiinflammatory and antibacterial activity, although the exact mechanism of action is not well understood.

Dosage

Dapsone is applied once daily with other acne agents or twice daily as a single agent. It is administrated to both adolescents and middle-aged females.

Contraindications

Hypersensitivity to any ingredients has been noted.

Side Effects

A rare but potentially lethal side effect is methemogloinemia. This condition results in an abnormal production of red blood cell protein, which delivers oxygen throughout the body.

Special Considerations

Caution must be exercised when using dapsone with topical BPO products due to the formation of an orange-brown discoloration. This is easily wiped away but may be concerning initially. Oral dapsone has been indicated in dose-related hemolysis in patients with a glucose-6-phosphate dehydrogenase deficiency.

Topical Antibiotics

Topical antibiotics may be prescribed when comedolytic antibacterials are either not effective or not tolerated and systemic antibiotics are not desired. Topical antibiotics inhibit the growth of *C. acnes* and decrease the number of comedones, papules, and pustules. Clindamycin 1% (Clindagel) is supplied in solutions, saturated pads, lotions, and gels. Rarely, topical clindamycin has been implicated in pseudomembranous colitis and regional enteritis. The practitioner should advise patients to discontinue therapy if diarrhea develops. To avoid resistance and to improve results, the practitioner may suggest washing with BPO and then applying clindamycin. The combination of BPO and clindamycin used together has been shown to prevent drug resistance and improve results. Now a novel topical foam minocycline 4% (Amzeeq) formulation is available by prescription and applied once daily.

Oral Antibiotics

Mechanism of Action

When improvement cannot be achieved with topical therapy, oral antibiotics may be considered. Oral antibiotics are indicated for inflammatory acne because they suppress *C. acnes*, as well as inhibit bacterial lipases, neutrophil chemotaxis, and follicular plugging.

Tetracycline

Although tetracycline is rarely used first line due to gastrointestinal (GI) upset, its derivatives doxycyline and minocycline are used for treating inflammatory acne. Newer weight-based once-daily formulations minocycline (Ximino) are available, as well as a small-to-swallow doxycycline (Targadox), providing a wide range of options.

Dosage

Doxycycline and minocyline doses are administered at 50, 75, 100, and 200 mg/d and are tapered to 100 mg/d after improvement occurs. Clinical improvement takes at least 3 to 4 weeks. Ximino, brand minocycline, is available as 45, 90, and 135 mg tablets taken once daily as weight-based options. Targadox is available in 50-mg tablets.

Contraindications

The contraindication noted is hypersensitivity to products containing tetracycline and its by-products.

Side Effects

The side effects of the tetracycline class include photosensitivity, gastric irritation, blood dyscrasias, and pseudotumor cerebri (benign intracranial hypertension). Caution should be exercised in treating patients who have renal failure or who are concurrently taking digoxin because tetracycline may increase serum digoxin levels.

Special Considerations

Tetracycline permanently stains the teeth in children, so it should not be prescribed for patients younger than 12 years of age. Moreover, the drug is a teratogen. It may also decrease the effectiveness of oral contraceptives. Therefore, caution should be exercised when prescribing it for sexually active female patients. Patient education should include directions to avoid concurrent ingestion of dairy products, iron preparations, and antacids which decrease absorption. Ideally, the medication should be taken on an empty stomach.

Sun protection should be encouraged due to sun sensitivity. Long-term use of these agents is not recommended due to drug resistance. Change of therapy to oral isotretinoin if not improved after three months of oral antibiotic therapy should be considered. Difficult-to-treat acne may also respond to other less often used antibiotics including but not limited to cephalexin (Keflex) or sulfamethoxazole/trimethoprim (Bactrim DS) when other agents have not demonstrated improvement.

Trimethoprim/Sulfamethoxazole

Trimethoprim/sulfamethoxazole has been used successfully in patients with acne refractory to other antibiotics and in gram-negative acne.

Other Systemic Drugs

Sarecycline (Seysara)
Dosage
Sarecycline (Seysara) was approved in 2018 and is available as 50-mg tablets. This tertracycline-derived antibiotic is effective for moderate to severe acne vulgaris.

Erythromycin

Erythromycin and its derivatives are alternatives when tetracycline fails or is not tolerated. They can also be used when the patient is younger than age 12. A common side effect is GI upset. There are drug interactions with digoxin, theophylline, and cyclosporine.

Dosage

Available in doses of 250, 333, 500, and 1,000 mg/d, erythromycin can be as effective as tetracycline. It is helpful in treating those individuals with tetracycline allergy.

Other Systemic Drugs

Retinoic Acid Derivatives: Isotretinoin
Mechanism of Action
Isotretinoin (formerly Accutane, now Absorica) has changed the management of acne therapy. It is reserved for patients with severe nodulocystic acne when other treatments have failed. Isotretinoin is a retinoic acid derivative. Although the exact mechanism is unknown, it decreases sebum production, follicular obstruction, and the number of skin bacteria. It also has an antiinflammatory action.

Dosage
Isotretinoin is given at a dose of 0.5 to 1 mg/kg/d. Therapy continues for 20 to 24 weeks. If therapy needs to be repeated, 6 months should elapse before restarting the drug. Isotretinoin is available in 10-, 20-, and 40-mg capsules usually twice daily.

Contraindications
Because isotretinoin is associated with serious birth defects, only prescribers registered in the iPledge program may prescribe the drug. This program was established to prevent pregnancy for the course of therapy and 1 month after. Female patients are required to consent to pregnancy prevention and/or contraception while on drug therapy.

Adverse Events

The most significant adverse effect of isotretinoin is teratogenicity. A 25-fold increase in fetal abnormalities has been documented. Even without external abnormalities, approximately 50% of children exposed to isotretinoin in utero had subnormal intelligence. Approximately 25% of patients experience cholesterol and triglyceride elevations.

Special Considerations

It is recommended that this drug be prescribed by a dermatologist. Two negative pregnancy tests 1 month apart prior to initiation of the drug are required. Registration with the iPledge program is mandatory, and monthly pregnancy screening should be performed while on this drug. Obtaining monthly pregnancy tests during therapy is mandatory for all female patients of childbearing potential.

Before initiating therapy, baseline CBC, chemistry profile, fasting triglyceride, and cholesterol levels should be obtained. In addition, a repeat CBC and a chemistry profile should then be obtained 1 month after the start of therapy and after each dosage adjustment. Pregnancy should be avoided at least 1 month after therapy is discontinued. Pseudotumor cerebri has been reported when isotretinoin therapy is combined with oral antibiotics, that is, tetracycline. Almost all patients report dry skin and mucous membranes, including cheilitis, severe dry skin, and difficulty wearing contact lenses. Other side effects include musculoskeletal aches and corneal opacities. Therapy should not be initiated in adolescents who have not completed growing due to concern regarding premature closure of the epiphyses.

A black box warning was added in 2002, warning of an increase in aggressive or violent behaviors in patients; consent is required through the iPledge agreement for all patients (male and female) regarding depressive symptoms.

Other Medications

Topical Combinations

Marketed as Benzamycin, the combination of erythromycin 3% and benzoyl peroxide 5% in gel base may increase compliance when a topical antibiotic is needed in addition to one or more other topical medications. The gel is applied once or twice daily. Although the product requires refrigeration, small quantities may be transferred to another container for up to 10 days, which tends to promote therapeutic adherence.

Similarly, a combination of clindamycin 1% and BPO 5% gel (BenzaClin Gel, Duac Gel) is available. Unlike Benzamycin, these products have a shelf life of 3 months at room temperature and do not require refrigeration. Additionally, newer topical agents are available with varying percentages of each active agent. This allows for increased use in different skin types, especially those with more sensitive complexion. Clindamycin 1.2%/Tretinoin 0.25% (Veltin, Ziana), Adapalene 0.1%/BPO 2.5% (Epiduo), and Adapalene 0.3%/BPO 2.5% (Epiduo forte) are just a few of the options now available. Other benefits to using combination products include reducing side effects and preventing drug resistance with the individual products.

Hormonal Therapy

Oral contraceptives can be used in women when conventional topical and systemic therapies have failed. This will be discussed in Chapter 55. Oral contraceptives that contain ethinylestradiol, levonorgestrel, and norgestimate or drospirenone are effective in the treatment of acne. Some other oral contraceptives may exacerbate acne. Relative to other therapies, oral contraceptives are inexpensive. They reduce both comedonal and inflammatory acnes and are worth considering for women who are already taking or considering taking systemic contraceptives.

Spironolactone

Mechanism of Action

Originally marketed to treat hypertension, spironolactone (Aldactone) is a potassium-sparing weak diuretic and androgen blocker. It is a reliable option for treatment in adult women with cyclic painful hormonal acne, particularly at the jawline. Long-term effectiveness and tolerability have proven this agent to be a reliable and safe option. Although no longer required, annual laboratory monitoring for potassium levels may be performed. Education regarding concerns for hyperkalemia should be discussed prior to therapy. Pregnancy prevention is important while using this drug therapy. Usually, improvement is evident within 3 months of use.

Dosage

Starting dosage can be 25 to 50 mg and then can be increased if necessary to maximum 200 mg/d. Long-term use has proven effective in managing adult female acne.

Side Effects

GI upset may be experienced in addition to dry mouth and dizziness. Gynecomastia and irregular menses have also been reported as possible side effects.

Selecting the Most Appropriate Agent

The most important consideration in selecting a therapeutic regimen is matching the severity of the acne to the appropriate pharmacologic agent (**Figure 15.1** and **Table 15.4**).

First-Line Therapy

The first line of therapy for comedonal acne is topical medication. Topical comedolytics encourage faster turnover of the surface skin. The addition of bacteriocidal or topical antibiotics enhances results for patients with closed comedones and pustules.

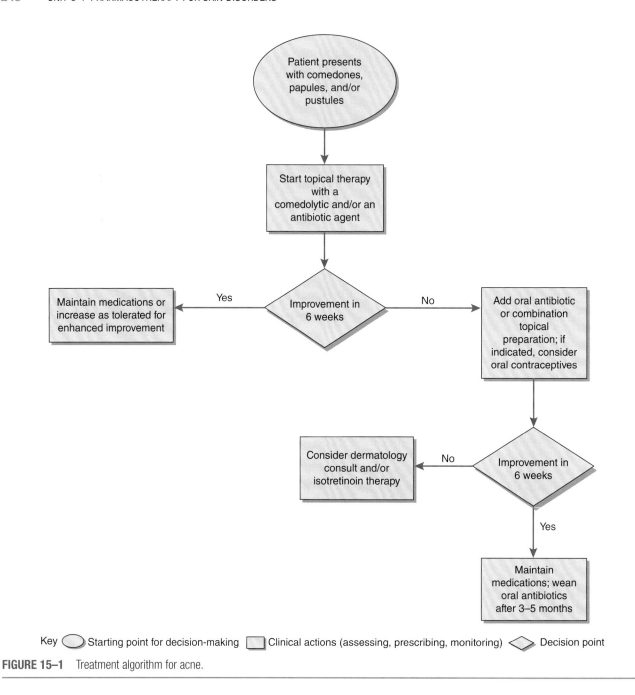

FIGURE 15–1   Treatment algorithm for acne.

TABLE 15.4		
Recommended Order of Treatment for Acne		
Order	**Agent**	**Comments**
First line	Topical therapy	Improvement takes ~6 weeks.
Second line	Oral medications	Monitor in 6 weeks
Third line	Isotretinoin or refer to dermatologist	Prescribe with caution to women of childbearing age

Second-Line Therapy

Patients whose acne does not respond to topical therapy may need oral medications. The practitioner may initiate treatment with oral antibiotics in addition to topical medications for more severe papulocystic acne. Oral contraceptives are a useful and cost-effective alternative for sexually active women.

Third-Line Therapy

Isotretinoin is reserved for the most severe forms of nodulocystic acne. Special care must be taken when prescribing this agent for women who can become pregnant. Practitioners who are not registered in the iPledge program or who cannot comply with the necessary monitoring and follow-up may feel more comfortable referring the patient to an individual who is, for evaluation and treatment.

SPECIAL POPULATION CONSIDERATIONS

Pediatric

Because of the risk of dental enamel defects and bone growth retardation, the use of tetracycline is contraindicated in children younger than age 12. Growth retardation in children who have not reached adult height is associated with isotretinoin use. Children may also experience increased arthralgias and back pain with the use of isotretinoin.

Women of Childbearing Age

Women of childbearing age who are using isotretinoin or tazarotene gel must not become pregnant because of the teratogenicity of both products. Practitioners may suggest that a long-acting contraceptive, such as Depo-Provera, be used. If pregnancy occurs, the patient must be counseled accordingly. Tetracycline, also considered teratogenic, may decrease the effectiveness of oral contraceptives. Women taking this antibiotic should rely on a long-acting contraceptive or a barrier method to prevent pregnancy. Topical retinoic acid is not recommended for use in pregnant women or nursing mothers.

Ethnic

Azelaic acid may cause hypopigmentation in patients with dark skin.

MONITORING PATIENT RESPONSE

Follow-up should be scheduled monthly to monitor the patient's response to therapy, provide reassurance, and encourage adherence to therapy. Monthly visits provide the opportunity to adjust medications and dosages as the patient's acne responds to treatment. The ideal management is long-term topical therapy. If isotretinoin is prescribed, laboratory tests should be obtained before therapy and 1 month into therapy, as described previously.

PATIENT EDUCATION

Drug Information

The practitioner may show the patient how to apply topical preparations correctly to prevent excessive irritation (**Box 15.1**). An important consideration in prescribing topical

---

> **BOX 15.1   General Principles for Applying Topical Acne Preparations**
>
> - Initiate therapy with a lower concentration of active ingredient and then work up to a higher concentration as tolerated.
> - Choose a product with a lower percentage of alcohol for people with sensitive skin.
> - Apply the product to clean, dry skin. Allow at least 20 minutes to elapse between washing the face and applying the medication.
> - Use the smallest amount of medication necessary for coverage.
> - Apply in "dots" over the desired area and then gently massage into skin.
> - Apply one drying agent in the morning and another in the evening to avoid excessive irritation.

---

therapy is that many gels and solutions contain significant amounts of alcohol. If a patient is sensitive to alcohol-based preparations or is experiencing significant dryness despite low concentrations of active ingredients, the practitioner may consider switching to a preparation that does not contain alcohol, such as a cream or aqueous gel or lotion.

Nutritional factors may play an important role in the pathogenesis of acne. A diet with a low glycemic load, higher in protein than carbohydrates and fats, can decrease lesion counts in acne vulgaris. A low glycemic–load diet has also been associated with a reduction in calorie intake, body mass index, and insulin resistance. Improved insulin sensitivity leads to a decrease in androgen production and a concordant improvement in the symptoms of acne vulgaris.

Patients should be cautioned to avoid using excessive amounts of topical medications in the hope that it will speed improvement. Instead, irritation will most likely be the result, and that may discourage continuation of therapy.

Patience is the key to resolution of acne. Adolescents looking for a quick cure may be disappointed, so the practitioner should discuss realistic expectations for improvement with the patient. All forms of acne therapy require a minimum of 4 to 6 weeks before results are seen. It is important to provide appropriate follow-up and encouragement and to have the patient return for evaluation and refinement of the treatment program.

Patient-Oriented Information Sources

The Web sites www.acne.org and www.nih.gov/medlineplus/acne.html (a site from the National Institutes of Health) provide information about acne and treatment.

COMPLEMENTARY AND ALTERNATIVE MEDICINE

Zinc is involved in the maintenance of skin health and immune function, local hormone activation, and production of retinol-binding protein. It has shown some bacteriostatic action against *C. acnes* and inhibitory action on the production of retinol-binding protein.

Another product that has been shown to improve acne severity is tea tree oil. It has less skin irritation than benzoyl peroxide. A solution of 5% to 15% is applied once daily.

Witch hazel is inexpensive and less drying than alcohol and can be used as a toner for those individuals with oily skin. Nicotinamide is a member of the vitamin B group. More specifically, a form of B$_3$ complex is available in a 4% topical cream or an oral dietary supplement. Nicomide is a generic vitamin that includes zinc, copper, and folic acid taken once or twice daily. It is believed to decrease inflammation in the skin which subsequently reduces acne lesions.

ROSACEA

Occasionally mistaken for acne vulgaris, rosacea is an acneiform disorder that begins in midlife (ages 30–50). It is estimated that rosacea affects over 16 million people by the National Rosacea Society. The rash is symmetric and limited to the central part of the face. Fair-skinned people with a tendency to blush are more often affected. Although rosacea is more likely to develop in women, men who are affected may have a more severe form of the disorder. Rosacea is not frequently seen in skin of color but does occur.

CAUSES

Rosacea does not have a clear cause. Various theories suggest bacterial infection, fungal infection, mite (*Demodex folliculorum*) infestation, menopausal changes, and more recently *Helicobacter pylori* infection. Sun exposure, heat, excessive washing, and irritating cosmetics may exacerbate rosacea along with other triggers such as alcohol, hormones, stress, and spicy foods.

PATHOPHYSIOLOGY

Early vascular rosacea consists of simple erythema in response to cold exposure. Extravascular fluid accumulates. As a result, blood flow to the superficial dermis increases. Persistent telangiectasia occurs late in the vascular stage of the disorder. During this period, ocular involvement may develop, consisting of mild conjunctivitis, dry eyes, burning, blepharitis, and occasionally keratitis and corneal ulceration. The second stage of rosacea represents lymphatic failure. It results in epidermal epithelial hyperplasia and pilosebaceous gland hyperplasia with fibrosis, inflammation, and telangiectasia. Clinical changes include persistent erythema, telangectasia, papules, and pustules. Rhinophyma, the characteristic deep inflammation and connective tissue hypertrophy of the nose, may begin to develop during this stage. Rhinophyma is almost exclusively seen in men older than age 40 and is treatable only by laser or surgery. Late-stage rosacea is recognized by persistent deep erythema, dense telangiectases, papules, pustules, nodules, and persistent edema of the central part of the face.

DIAGNOSTIC CRITERIA

The diagnosis of rosacea is based on the history and clinical presentation. Fixed telangiectasia is the hallmark of this disorder. In patients younger than age 30, acne should be ruled out. In patients with systemic symptoms, systemic lupus erythematosus should be considered. Bacterial cultures should be performed to rule out *Staphylococcus aureus* and gram-negative folliculitis. Patients who do not respond to systemic antibiotics should be evaluated for *Demodex folliculorum* infestation. Approximately 50% of patients report ocular involvement, so any ocular symptoms should be investigated.

Referral to an ophthalmologist should be considered if the practitioner suspects corneal ulceration or keratitis.

INITIATING DRUG THERAPY

The goal of therapy is to minimize the disfiguring effects of rosacea and prevent further tissue damage. As with acne, the patient's concerns with regard to appearance must be considered. Patients with rosacea may feel stigmatized. Treatment during the early phase (vasodilation) is easier to treat with the addition of topical therapies with vasoconstrictive properties, discussed later in the chapter.

Topical Antibacterials

Metronidazole

Mechanism of Action
Topical metronidazole (MetroGel, Noritate) has anti-inflammatory properties (**Table 15.5**). It is available in 0.75% and 1% strengths and is applied once or twice daily in a thin layer on the face, avoiding the eyes.

Dosage
Metronidazole is available in forms of cream, gel, and lotion. Initial results should be seen in approximately 3 weeks and the full effect in approximately 9 weeks. Patients are then maintained on the agent indefinitely with drug holidays as appropriate. Patients who receive concurrent anticoagulant therapy should be monitored closely for an enhanced anticoagulation effect.

TABLE 15.5

Overview of Topical Agents for Rosacea

Generic (Trade) Name and Dosage	Selected Adverse Events	Contraindications	Special Considerations
Metronidazole 0.75% gel, cream, lotion (MetroGel, etc.) 1.0% cream (Noritate)	Burning sensation, irritation, erythema (transient), mild dryness, pruritus	Children Breastfeeding mothers	Avoid eyes. With anticoagulant therapy, monitor closely for enhanced anticoagulation
Sodium sulfacetamide 10% with sulfa 5%, (Sulfacet) sodium sulfacetamide 10% with sulfa 5% and urea 10% (Rosula), one to thrice daily in thin layer	Local irritation, allergic dermatitis	Kidney disease Breastfeeding mothers Sulfa allergy	Avoid eyes and denuded skin
Azelaic acid 15% (Finacea) gel, foam Apply thin film BID	Burning, stinging, pruritus	Allergy Not for internal use	Hypopigmentation in patients with dark complexions
Oxymetazoline HCl 1% (Rhofade) gel	Local irritation	Not for internal use Not for use in pregnancy	Not for internal use. Child-proof cap available. Helps reduce persistent erythema
Brimonidine gel 0.33% (Mirvaso)	Local irritation	Not for internal use Not for use in pregnancy	Not for internal use childproof cap
Ivermectin gel 1% (Soolontra)	Local irritation	Not for internal use Not for use in pregnancy	For use with papules

Contraindications

There are no contraindications.

Side Effects

Adverse events include burning, skin irritation, transient erythema, mild dryness, and pruritus.

Special Considerations

Least expensive generic options for those without insurance or those with coverage limitations may be recommended.

Combination Medications

Sodium sulfacetamide 10% with sulfur 5% (Sulfacet-R, Clenia, Plexion) also has anti-inflammatory properties when used to treat rosacea.

Dosage

It is applied one to thrice daily as needed for flares.

Contraindications

It is contraindicated in patients with kidney disease, and caution should be exercised in those sensitive to sulfa drugs. Application to eyes and areas of denuded skin is to be avoided.

Side Effects

Adverse events include local irritation and allergic dermatitis.

Special Considerations

Rosula is a branded combination of sulfacetamide 10%, sulfur 5%, and urea 10%. Addition of urea helps to soothe and relieve redness and inflammation.

Azelaic Acid

Azelaic acid 15% (Finacea) is indicated for the topical application for mild to moderate rosacea.

Dosage

Supplied as gel or foam formulation applied once or twice daily. For more information regarding azelaic acid, see acne section earlier in this chapter.

Antiparasitic

Ivermectin

Mechanism of Action

Ivermectin 1% (Soolontra) is a macrocyclic lactone working as a topical anti-infective. The mechanism of action is unknown. It is used alone or in combination with other agents.

Dosage

It is applied once daily on clean dry face.

Side Effects

As with any of the topical agents on sensitive skin, local irritation, peeling, and redness may result.

Decongestants and Vasoconstrictors

Oxyometazoline HCl Cream 1% (Rhofade), Brimonidine 0.33% Gel (Mirvaso)

Mechanism of Action

Both are alpha-adrenergic agonists that work through decongestion and vasoconstriction. This provides temporary external constriction to surface vessels.

Dosage

Apply pea-sized amounts once daily in the morning to fore-head, cheeks, nose, and chin. This drug shows benefit and may be effective for up to 8 to 12 hours. It is helpful in preventing the severe forms of this condition.

Contraindications

These products are not for internal consumption and for top-ical use only. A safety cap is provided to prevent accidental internal consumption. Caution should be exercised in use with individuals with glaucoma due to increased incidence risk for angle closure glaucoma.

Side Effects

Side effects include erythema, flushing, and burning sensations.

Oral Antibiotics

When topical agents have not improved the patient's condi-tion, oral anti-infective agents may be considered.

Mechanism of Action

Antibiotics are used for their antiinflammatory effect in lower doses as opposed to higher doses in acne for antimi-crobial properties. Oral antibiotics are indicated for patients with ocular symptoms and when topical agents alone are ineffective.

Dosage

Doxycycline (Vibramycin, Monodox, Doryx, Oracea) is the antibiotic of choice for treating rosacea. It is prescribed in doses of 20 mg twice daily, 50 mg once daily, or 40 mg slow-release preparations. After 3 to 5 months, the practitioner may consider discontinuing oral agent while continuing topi-cal therapy. Patients should be cautioned to avoid sun exposure while taking doxycycline as discussed earlier.

Erythromycin (E-mycin, Ery-Tab) 250 and 500 mg is a useful agent when tetracycline is contraindicated. Dosages and tapering regimens are identical to those used for tetracycline and are discussed earlier in chapter.

Isotretinoin

Isotretinoin may be prescribed for patients who do not respond to oral and topical agents. The drug is prescribed in doses of 0.5 to 1.0 mg/kg/d for up to 8 months. Precautions and labo-ratory follow-up as described earlier in this chapter.

Selecting the Most Appropriate Agent

Initial drug therapy choices should include a topical agent. Cases that involve ocular symptoms should be treated with oral antibiotics initially.

TABLE 15.6

Recommended Order of Treatment for Rosacea

Order	Agent	Comments
First line	Topical medication	Improvement takes 6 weeks
Second line	Oral antibiotics	Improvement takes 6 weeks
Third line	Oral isotretinoin; consider referral to dermatologist	Teratogenic

First-Line Therapy

The first-line treatment of rosacea consists of topical therapy. If no improvement is seen after 6 weeks, second-line therapy begins.

Second-Line Therapy

Second-line treatment consists of adding an oral antibiotic. After 2 weeks, the dose is reduced by 50%, and then, after 6 weeks, the oral antibiotic is discontinued altogether and the topical treatment continues indefinitely.

Third-Line Therapy

Third-line treatment consists of oral isotretinoin or referral to a dermatologist. **Table 15.6** lists the lines of therapy for rosa-cea, and **Figure 15.2** outlines rosacea treatment.

MONITORING PATIENT RESPONSE

As discussed throughout this chapter, the patient's response is monitored regularly by observation and follow-up visits to adjust medications and provide support and encouragement during therapy.

PATIENT EDUCATION

Patients with rosacea need to recognize what triggers their con-dition. The goal of management is to avoid flare-ups. Although each patient responds differently to triggers, common triggers are sun exposure, strong winds, cold weather, warm environ-ment, strenuous exercise, alcoholic beverages, spicy foods, hot foods and beverages, and stress.

It is important that a broad-spectrum ultraviolet A (UVA)/ ultraviolet B (UVB) sunscreen be used and applied routinely.

Patients may be advised to avoid harsh cleansers and avoid skin irritants. Cosmetic foundations with a green tint may camouflage redness. Additional information and consumer education may be obtained through the National Rosacea Society (1-888-NO BLUSH, http://www.rosacea.org).

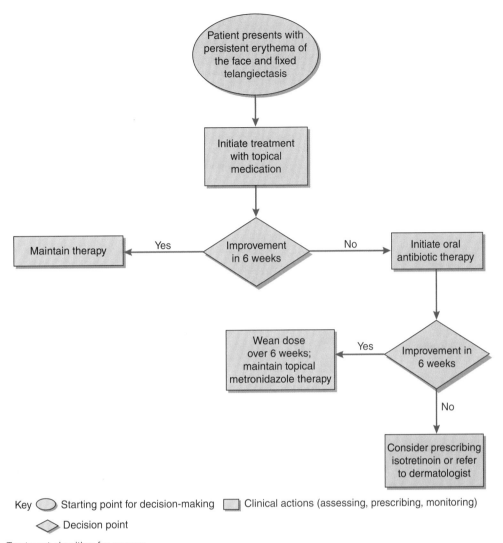

FIGURE 15–2   Treatment algorithm for rosacea.

CASE STUDY 1*

J.S. age 16, comes to your office for a routine physical examination. You notice that she has facial acne that she is hiding with heavy makeup. She has tried Clearasil inconsistently without relief. She works at a fast-food restaurant as a cook after school and on the weekends. Her mother has made her stop eating chocolates and greasy foods, but that has not seemed to help her. She is concerned because her prom is in 6 weeks and she wants her face clear. On physical examination, there are open and closed comedones, as well as papules, on her face and back. No scarring is evident. J.S. confides that she has recently become sexually active.

DIAGNOSIS: ACNE VULGARIS

1. List specific treatment goals for J.S.
2. What drug therapy would you prescribe? Why?

3. What are the parameters for monitoring the success of the therapy?
4. Describe specific patient education based on the prescribed therapy.
5. List one or two adverse reactions for the selected agent that would cause you to change therapy.
6. What would be the choice for second-line therapy?
7. What over-the-counter or dietary supplement would you recommend to J.S.?
8. What dietary and lifestyle changes should be recommended for J.S.?
9. Describe one or two drug–drug or drug–food interactions for the selected agent.

*Answers can be found online.

Bibliography

Barbier, J., Chol, J., et al. (2019). Real world drug usage of surveillance of spironolactone vs oral antibiotic for the management of female patients with acne. *Journal of American Academy of Dermatology, 81*(3), 848–851.

Bobonich, M., & Nolen, M. (2015). *Dermatology for advanced practice clinicians*. Philadelphia, PA: Wolters Kluwer.

Burris, J., Rietkerk, W., & Woolf, K. (2013). Acne: The role of medical nutrition therapy. *Journal of the Academy of Nutrition and Dietetics, 113*(3), 416–430.

Friedman, A. (2015). Spironolactone for adult female Acne. *Cutis, 96*(4), 216–217.

Grove, G., Zerweck, C., & Gwazdauskas, J. (2013). Tolerability and irritation potential of four topical acne regimens in healthy subjects. *Journal of Drugs in Dermatology, 12*(6), 644–649.

Habif, T., Dinulos, J., Chapman, M. S., & Zug, K. A. (2018). *Skin disease: Diagnosis and treatment*. New York: Elsevier.

Leyden, J., Berk, D., et al. (2017). Efficacy to safety of oral sarecycline for the treatment of moderate to severe facial acne. *Journal of American Academy of Dermatology, 6*(6), AB113.

Maloney, M., & Stone, S. (2011). Isotretinoin and IPledge: A view of results. *Journal of American Academy of Dermatology, 65*(2), 418–419.

Saint-Jean, M., et al. (2019). Adult acne in women is not associated with a specific type of *Cutibacterium acnes*. *Journal of American Academy of Dermatology, 81*(3), 851–852.

Snyder, S., Crandell, I., Davis, S. A., et al. (2014). Medical adherence to acne therapy: A systematic review. *American Journal of Clinical Dermatology, 15*(2), 87–94.

Thiboutot, D., et al. (2016). Once daily topical dapsone gel 7.5% for Acne Vulgaris. *Journal of American Academy of Dermatology, 74*(5), AB7.

Zaenglein, A., Pathy, A., et al. (2016). Guidelines of care for the management of acne vulgaris. *Journal of American Academy of Dermatology, 74*(5), 945–973.

Pharmacotherapy for Eye and Ear Disorders

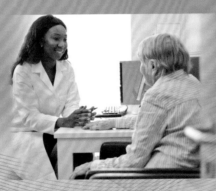

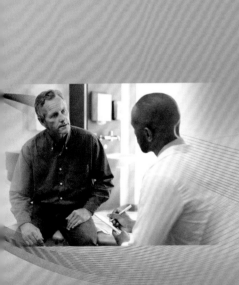

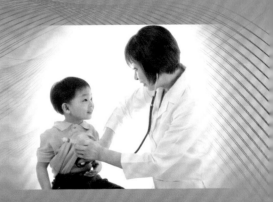

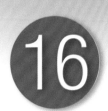

16 Ophthalmic Disorders

Joshua J. Spooner

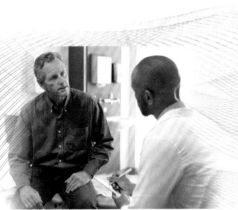
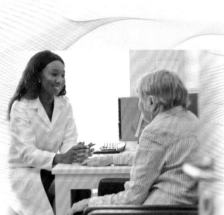
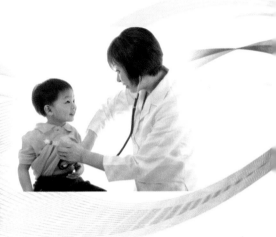

Learning Objectives

1. Describe the pathophysiology of common ophthalmic disorders routinely presenting in primary care practice.
2. Evaluate signs and symptoms of these common ophthalmic disorders and interpret these signs and symptoms in order to diagnose subtypes of blepharitis and conjunctivitis.
3. Present nonpharmacologic and first- and second-line treatment options for these common ophthalmic disorders.
4. Discuss key patient counseling points for ophthalmic disorder and treatment options.

INTRODUCTION

There are many conditions and disorders of the eye, but only a few, such as blepharitis and conjunctivitis, should be diagnosed and treated by a primary care provider. The remaining ocular conditions are usually treated by eye care specialists. Nonetheless, prescribers should be familiar with drug therapy for the more common ophthalmic conditions (glaucoma, dry eye disease [DED]), as they are likely to encounter patients being treated for these disorders.

EYELID MARGIN INFECTIONS: BLEPHARITIS

The eye is well protected externally by the eyebrow, eyelashes, and eyelids. If these protective mechanisms are compromised, the eye becomes predisposed to disease. Externally, the eyelid structures are composed of skin with a high degree of elasticity, muscles that elevate the upper eyelid and close the eyelids, and the tarsal plate, which contains the meibomian glands. Through frequent blinking, the eyelids maintain an even flow of tears over the cornea. Internally, the eyelid structure is lined by the palpebral conjunctiva, which folds upon itself and then covers the sclera of the eyeball up to the corneoscleral junction. Located at the lid margins are the openings to the long sebaceous meibomian glands; these glands secrete the oily film that prevents tears from evaporating. At the base of the eyelash are the superficial modified sebaceous glands of Zeis and the sweat glands of Moll. Any of these glands may become functionally disrupted.

Blepharitis is an inflammation of the eyelid margin. Although it is a common eye disorder in the United States, epidemiologic information on its incidence or prevalence is not robust.

Causes

Blepharitis can be caused by a bacterial infection (staphylococcal blepharitis), inflammation or hypersecretion of the sebaceous glands (seborrheic blepharitis), meibomian gland dysfunction (MGD blepharitis), or a combination of these (American Academy of Ophthalmology [AAO], 2018a). Staphylococcal and seborrheic blepharitis primarily involve the anterior eyelid; both have also been referred to as *anterior blepharitis*.

Pathophysiology

Although the gram-positive organism *Staphylococcus aureus* and coagulase-negative species such as *Staphylococcus epidermidis* are found on the eyelids of a high proportion of healthy subjects, *S. aureus* is observed more frequently among patients with staphylococcal blepharitis. While *S. epidermidis* and *S. aureus* are thought to play a role in the development of staphylococcal blepharitis, their role in disease production remains unclear. Toxin production, immunologic mechanisms, *Demodex folliculorum* mite infestation, and antigen-induced inflammatory reactions have all been reported with blepharitis (AAO, 2018a; Fromstein et al., 2018). Isotretinoin use is also associated with an increase in *S. aureus* conjunctival colonization and blepharitis.

Seborrheic blepharitis typically occurs as part of the more comprehensive condition of seborrheic dermatitis, with dandruff of the scalp, eyebrows, eyelashes, nasolabial folds, and external ears. Seborrheic blepharitis is more commonly found in the geriatric population because of its association with rosacea.

Manifestations of MGD blepharitis include thickening of the eyelid margin, plugging of the meibomian orifices, prominent blood vessels crossing the mucocutaneous junction, and formation of chalazia (painless firm lumps on the eyelid). These changes may lead to atrophy of the meibomian glands (AAO, 2018a). Compared to healthy patients, meibomian gland secretions are more turbid among patients with MGD blepharitis. These secretions block the gland orifices and become a growth medium for bacteria. Patients with MGD blepharitis frequently have coexisting rosacea or seborrheic dermatitis.

Diagnostic Criteria

There are no specific diagnostic tests for blepharitis; the diagnosis is often based upon patient history and characteristic symptoms. Patients with blepharitis frequently present with irritated red eyes and report a burning sensation. Increases in tearing, blinking, and photophobia are frequently reported, as are eyelid sticking and contact lens intolerance. Symptoms are typically worse in the morning (worsening symptoms later in the day are more indicative of keratoconjunctivitis sicca). Upon close inspection, the eyelid margins appear red, greasy, and crusted, with eyelid deposits that cling to the eyelashes. The eyelid margins may be ulcerated and thickened, and eyelashes may be missing.

Although the clinical features of staphylococcal, seborrheic, and MGD blepharitis are similar, there are differences that can aid in the differential diagnosis of these conditions. Eyelash loss and eyelash misdirection frequently occur in staphylococcal blepharitis but are rare in seborrheic blepharitis. The eyelid deposits are matted and scaly in staphylococcal blepharitis, oily or greasy in seborrheic blepharitis, and fatty and foamy in MGD blepharitis. Chalazia are most likely to occur in MGD blepharitis.

Initiating Drug Therapy

The underlying cause of the blepharitis must be treated, particularly if it is due to seborrheic dermatitis or rosacea. Treatment for all types of blepharitis includes strict eyelid hygiene and warm compresses. The use of warm compresses with a clean washcloth can soften adherent encrustations; once-daily use of compresses is generally sufficient (AAO, 2018a). Patients with MGD blepharitis often benefit from eyelid massage following warm compress use to remove excess oil. Following warm compress use, eyelid cleaning is performed by having the patient rub the base of the eyelashes with a commercially available eyelid cleaner (EyeScrub, OCuSOFT) or a diluted mixture of baby shampoo (e.g., Johnson & Johnson) and water on a cotton swab, cotton ball, or gauze pad. Performing eyelid hygiene daily or several times a week often blunts the symptoms of chronic blepharitis (Duncan & Jeng, 2017). Patients should be advised that warm compresses and eyelid cleansing may be required for life because symptoms frequently recur if eyelid hygiene is discontinued.

Patients suspected of having a new case of seborrheic or MGD blepharitis should be referred to an eye care specialist for a workup. Patients with staphylococcal blepharitis need a topical antibiotic.

Goals of Drug Therapy

The goals of drug therapy are to eradicate the pathogens causing the staphylococcal blepharitis and to reduce the signs and symptoms of blepharitis.

Topical Ophthalmic Antimicrobials

Topical ophthalmic antimicrobials are used for the treatment of and prophylaxis against external bacterial infections (**Table 16.1**). They kill the offending pathogen and other susceptible organisms.

Selecting the Most Appropriate Agent

Topical antimicrobials that are effective against staphylococci are listed in **Table 16.2**.

First-Line Therapy

Topical antibiotics such as bacitracin ointment or erythromycin 0.5% ophthalmic ointment are used first line for staphylococcal blepharitis and should be applied to the eyelid margins one or more times daily or at bedtime for a few weeks. Therapy selection is based on allergies and patient preference for ointment or solution (drops). Ointments tend to cause a greater degree of blurry vision than the solutions; if a patient prefers a solution, azithromycin or a fluoroquinolone (besifloxacin, gatifloxacin, levofloxacin, or moxifloxacin) would be suitable. The AAO (2018a) recommends that the frequency and duration of treatment should be guided by the severity of the condition and the response to treatment.

Second-Line Therapy

If the blepharitis fails to respond to the first-line therapy after several weeks or the condition appears to worsen at any time (including any vision loss or corneal involvement), the patient should be referred to an ophthalmologist for a complete evaluation.

TABLE 16.1

Overview of Antimicrobial Ophthalmic Agents

Generic (Trade) Name and Dosage	Selected Adverse Events	Contraindications	Special Considerations
Single-Agent Products			
Sulfacetamide sodium 10% solution (Bleph-10) Dosing Solution: 1–2 drops q2–3h initially according to the severity of infection Dosing may be tapered as the condition responds. Usual duration of therapy is 7–10 d.	Local irritation, itching, stinging, burning, periorbital edema	Allergy to sulfa drugs Do not use in infants less than age 2 mo.	A significant percentage of *Staphylococcus* species are completely resistant to sulfa drugs.
Bacitracin 500 units/g ointment Dosing: apply BID and HS	Blurred vision, redness, burning, eyelid edema		Ointments may blur vision and retard corneal wound healing.
Erythromycin 0.5% ointment Dosing: apply up to 1 cm to the affected eye(s) up to six times daily	Redness, ocular irritation		Ointments may blur vision and retard corneal wound healing.
Gentamicin sulfate 0.3% solution or ointment (Gentak) Dosing Solution: 1–2 drops in the affected eye(s) q4h Ointment: 0.5 inch to the affected eye(s) BID or TID	Ocular burning and irritation, nonspecific conjunctivitis, conjunctival epithelial defects, conjunctival hyperemia, bacterial and fungal corneal ulcers		In severe infections, dosage of the solution may be increased to as much as 2 drops every hour. Ointments may blur vision and retard corneal wound healing.
Tobramycin 0.3% solution or ointment (Tobrex) Dosing Solution: 1–2 drops into the infected eye q4h Ointment: 0.5 inch BID or TID	Lid itching, lid swelling, conjunctival hyperemia, nonspecific conjunctivitis, bacterial and fungal corneal ulcers		Ointments may blur vision and retard corneal wound healing. For more severe infections, the initial dose may be increased to 2 drops q60min (solution) or 0.5 inch q3–4h (ointment).
Besifloxacin 0.6% suspension (Besivance) Dosing: 1 drop in the affected eye(s) TID for 7 d	Conjunctival redness, blurred vision, eye irritation, eye pain, pruritus		
Ciprofloxacin 0.3% solution or ointment (Ciloxan) Dosing Solution: 1–2 drops q2h while awake for 2 d and then 1–2 drops q4h while awake for 5 d Ointment: 0.5 inch TID for 2 d and then 0.5 inch BID for 5 d	Local burning and discomfort, white crystalline precipitate formation, conjunctival hyperemia, altered taste		Ointments may blur vision and retard corneal wound healing. This is the only ophthalmic fluoroquinolone available as an ointment.
Gatifloxacin 0.3% solution (Zymaxid) Dosing: 1 drop in the affected eye(s) q2h while awake for 1 d (up to 8 times daily) and then 1 drop in the affected eye(s) up to QID while awake for 6 d	Conjunctival irritation, tearing, papillary conjunctivitis, eyelid edema, ocular itching, dry eye		

(Continued)

TABLE 16.1

Overview of Antimicrobial Ophthalmic Agents (*Continued*)

Generic (Trade) Name and Dosage	Selected Adverse Events	Contraindications	Special Considerations
Levofloxacin 0.5% solution (Quixin) Dosing: 1 drop in the affected eye(s) q2h while awake for 2 d (up to 8 times daily) and then 1 drop in the affected eye(s) up to QID while awake for 5 d	Temporarily decreased or blurred vision, eye irritation, itching, dry eye		
Moxifloxacin 0.5% solution (Moxeza, Vigamox) Dosing: Moxeza: 1 drop in the affected eye(s) BID for 7 d Vigamox: 1 drop in the affected eye(s) TID for 7 d	Decreased visual acuity, dry eye, ocular itching and discomfort, ocular hyperemia		
Ofloxacin 0.3% solution (Ocuflox) Dosing: 1–2 drops in the affected eye(s) q2–4h for 2 d and then 1–2 drops QID for 5 d	Ocular burning and stinging, itching, redness, edema, blurred vision, photophobia		Rare reports of dizziness and nausea with use
Azithromycin 1% solution (AzaSite, Klarity-A) Dosing: 1 drop in affected eye(s) BID for 2 d and then 1 drop once daily for 5 d	Eye irritation, dry eye, ocular discharge		Refrigerate bottle; once opened, discard after 14 d.
Combination Products			
Polymyxin B sulfate, bacitracin ointment (AK-Poly-Bac) Dosing: apply q3–4h for 7–10 d, depending upon the severity of infection.	Local irritation (burning, stinging, itching, redness), lid edema, tearing, rash		Ointments may blur vision and retard corneal wound healing.
Polymyxin B sulfate, trimethoprim sulfate solution (Polytrim) Dosing: 1 drop in the affected eye(s) q3h (maximum six doses daily) for 7–10 d	Local irritation (burning, stinging, itching, redness), lid edema, tearing, rash		
Polymyxin B sulfate, gramicidin, neomycin solution (Neosporin) Dosing: 1–2 drops into the affected eye(s) q4h for 7–10 d	Itching, swelling, conjunctival erythema, local irritation		Dosage of the solution may be increased to as much as 2 drops every hour for severe infections.
Polymyxin B sulfate, bacitracin zinc, and neomycin ointment (Neo-Polycin) Dosage: apply q3–4h for 7–10 d, depending upon the severity of infection.	Itching, swelling, conjunctival erythema, local irritation		Ointments may blur vision and retard corneal wound healing.

Patient Education

Patients should be educated about the chronic nature of blepharitis. While chronic blepharitis is rarely cured, improved eyelid hygiene, warm massages, and occasional antibiotic use (for staphylococcal blepharitis) can improve symptoms. Counsel contact lens wearers to refrain from wearing contact lenses during an acute case of blepharitis, especially if antibiotic therapy has been initiated. Contact lens wearers with chronic blepharitis should consult with their eye care professional to determine whether contact lens use is safe.

TABLE 16.2

Recommended Order of Treatment for Blepharitis

Order	Agent	Comments
First line	Erythromycin 0.5% ophthalmic ointment *or* Bacitracin 500 units/g ointment *or* Azithromycin 1% solution *or* An ophthalmic fluoroquinolone solution (besifloxacin, gatifloxacin, levofloxacin, or moxifloxacin)	Ointments tend to cause a greater degree of blurry vision than solutions. Erythromycin and bacitracin are available as inexpensive generic products. The remaining ophthalmic fluoroquinolones do not provide good staphylococcal coverage.
Second line	Referral to an ophthalmologist	

EXTERNAL SURFACE OCULAR INFECTIONS: CONJUNCTIVITIS

Conjunctivitis is the most common cause of a painful red eye in the United States (Horton, 2015). Conjunctivitis is an inflammation of the bulbar conjunctiva (the clear membrane that covers the white part of the eye) or the palpebral conjunctiva (the lining of the inner surfaces of the eyelids). Conjunctivitis is commonly referred to as *pink eye*.

Causes

The most common organisms seen in acute bacterial conjunctivitis are the gram-positive *Staphylococcus* and *Streptococcus* species and the gram-negative *Moraxella* and *Haemophilus* species; less common organisms include *Neisseria gonorrhoeae* and *Chlamydia trachomatis* (Centers for Disease Control and Prevention [CDC], 2020). In children, up to 50% of conjunctivitis cases are of bacterial origin. The most common pathogens in neonates are *N. gonorrhoeae* and *C. trachomatis*, while *S. aureus, Haemophilus influenzae, Streptococcus pneumoniae*, and *Pseudomonas aeruginosa* are the most commonly isolated organisms in children with bacterial conjunctivitis, with *H. influenzae* most frequently found in children below 7 years of age and *S. aureus* most frequently found in children 7 years of age and older (Chen et al., 2018; Sethuraman & Kamat, 2009).

Viruses account for the majority of conjunctivitis cases in adults. The most common viral etiology is adenovirus infection (Horton, 2015); conjunctivitis due to an adenovirus is highly contagious. Other viruses associated with conjunctivitis include the herpes simplex virus, the varicella-zoster virus, and molluscum contagiosum (AAO, 2018b).

Allergic conjunctivitis is fairly common and is frequently mistaken for bacterial conjunctivitis. There are three common types of allergic conjunctivitis: seasonal/perennial (hay fever) conjunctivitis, due to seasonal release of plant allergens, outdoor air pollution, and exposure to pets and farm animals; vernal conjunctivitis, which is of unknown origin but is thought to be due to hot, dry environments and airborne environmental antigens; and atopic conjunctivitis, which occurs in people with atopic dermatitis or asthma.

Conjunctivitis can also be caused by mechanical or chemical irritants. A foreign body on the eye (typically a contact lens) can lead to giant papillary conjunctivitis.

Pathophysiology

General mechanisms of infection are at work in bacterial and viral conjunctivitis. In bacterial conjunctivitis, the infecting organism is obtained via contact with an infected individual and transmitted to the eye by fingertips. Neonates with conjunctivitis may have become inoculated during childbirth by their infected mother. Transmission of viral conjunctivitis is usually through direct contact with infected persons, contaminated surfaces, or contaminated swimming pool water (Fredrick, 2018). In both bacterial and viral conjunctivitis, the infectious agent causes the inflammation of the conjunctiva. Mechanical and chemical irritants that cause conjunctivitis operate in the same manner.

In allergic conjunctivitis, symptoms are caused by the immunoglobulin (Ig) E–mediated release of mast cells in the conjunctiva (Leonardi et al., 2017).

Diagnostic Criteria

In addition to the hallmark red or pink eye, classic patient complaints that occur in conjunctivitis include itching or burning sensations of the eyes, ocular discharge ("leaky eye"), eyelids that are stuck together in the morning, and a sensation that a foreign body is lodged in the eye. Patients may also report a feeling of fullness around the eye. Moderate to severe pain and light sensitivity are not typical features of a primary conjunctival inflammatory process (Azari & Barney, 2013; Narayana & McGee, 2015). If these symptoms are present, or if the patient reports blurred vision that does not improve with blinking, the patient should be referred to an eye care professional as a more serious ocular disease process (such as a corneal abrasion or keratoconjunctivitis) may be occurring. Neonates with signs of conjunctivitis should be referred to an eye care professional for immediate examination as bacterial conjunctivitis due to *C. trachomatis* or *N. gonorrhoeae* can lead to serious eye damage.

Although many symptoms of conjunctivitis are nonspecific (tearing, irritation, stinging, burning, and conjunctival swelling), inspection and patient history can help determine the cause of illness. Patients who report that their eyelids were stuck together upon awakening most likely have bacterial conjunctivitis (Garcia-Ferrer et al., 2018); this sticking is caused by a purulent ocular discharge. Because gonococcal conjunctivitis produces a copiously purulent discharge, the cause of any copiously purulent conjunctivitis should be suspected as *N. gonorrhoeae* until Gram stain testing proves otherwise.

Bacterial conjunctivitis usually starts in one eye and can become bilateral a few days later.

Viral conjunctivitis produces a profuse watery discharge. Similar to bacterial conjunctivitis, viral conjunctivitis usually starts in one eye and can become bilateral within a few days. While unlikely, photophobia and a foreign body sensation may be reported. Examination may reveal a tender preauricular node. A rapid, in-office immunodiagnostic test with high specificity for adenovirus is available (Holtz et al., 2017; Kam et al., 2015).

In allergic conjunctivitis, itching is the hallmark symptom; it can be mild to severe and may manifest as excessive blinking. A history of recurrent itching or a personal or family history of hay fever, asthma, atopic dermatitis, or allergic rhinitis is suggestive of allergic conjunctivitis. In general, a patient with conjunctivitis who does not report an itchy eye does not have allergic conjunctivitis. Unlike bacterial or viral conjunctivitis, allergic conjunctivitis usually presents with bilateral symptoms. An ocular discharge may or may not be present; if present, it may be watery or mucoid. Aggressive forms of allergic conjunctivitis are vernal conjunctivitis in children and atopic conjunctivitis in adults. Atopic and vernal conjunctivitis are associated with shield corneal ulcers and perilimbal accumulation of eosinophils (Garcia-Ferrer et al., 2018). Atopic conjunctivitis is associated with eyelid thickening, conjunctival scarring, blepharitis, and corneal scarring (AAO, 2018b).

Giant papillary conjunctivitis occurs mainly in contact lens wearers. These patients report excessive itching, mucus production and discharge, and increasing intolerance to contact lens use—symptoms resemble those of vernal conjunctivitis. Upon examination, the upper tarsal conjunctiva may show inflammation and papillae greater than 1 mm (Ackerman et al., 2016). Ptosis may occur in severe cases (AAO, 2018b).

Initiating Drug Therapy

Before drug therapy is prescribed, both the patient and the practitioner should be aware that bacterial and viral conjunctivitis are highly contagious and are spread by contact. Therefore, good handwashing and instrument-cleansing techniques are imperative. The etiology of illness should be determined as treatment is different for bacterial, viral, and allergic conjunctivitis.

Goals of Drug Therapy

The goals of drug therapy are to eradicate the offending organism (for bacterial conjunctivitis), to relieve symptoms, and to quicken the resolution of the disease. A patient with bacterial conjunctivitis should experience improvement in symptoms a few days after the start of antibiotic therapy; the organisms remain active (and contagious) for 24 to 48 hours after therapy begins. With viral conjunctivitis, the disease is contagious for at least 7 days after symptoms appear; it may be contagious for up to 14 days.

Antibiotics

Although bacterial conjunctivitis caused by typical pathogens (*Staphylococcus*, *Streptococcus*, *Pneumococcus*, *Moraxella*, and *Haemophilus* species) is usually self-limiting, antibiotic therapy is justified because it can shorten the course of the disease, which reduces person-to-person spread and lowers the risk of sight-threatening complications. The choice of antibiotic is usually empirical; clinical evidence indicating the superiority of any particular antibiotic is lacking (AAO, 2018b). Five to 7 days of therapy with agents such as erythromycin ointment or bacitracin–polymyxin B ointment is usually effective. While well tolerated, sulfacetamide has weak to moderate activity against many organisms. The aminoglycosides have good gram-negative coverage but incomplete coverage of *Streptococcus* and *Staphylococcus* species and a relatively high incidence of corneal toxicity. The fluoroquinolones also have good gram-negative coverage; the older fluoroquinolones (ciprofloxacin, norfloxacin, and ofloxacin) have poor coverage of *Streptococcus* species, while the newer fluoroquinolones (besifloxacin, gatifloxacin, levofloxacin, and moxifloxacin) offer improved gram-positive coverage and are available in a solution.

Because gonococcal infection is serious, immediate treatment of conjunctivitis due to *N. gonorrhoeae* with a 250-mg intramuscular (IM) injection of ceftriaxone (Rocephin) plus a single 1-g dose of oral azithromycin is recommended for adults and children who weigh at least 45 kg. Children who weigh less than 45 kg should receive a single 125-mg IM injection of ceftriaxone, while 25 to 50 mg/kg of ceftriaxone intravenous or IM (not to exceed 125 mg) is the appropriate dose for neonates. Cephalosporin-allergic patients should be referred to an infectious disease specialist. Topical antibiotic therapy is not necessary but is often initiated to prevent secondary infection (AAO, 2018b).

As *C. trachomatis* is now the most common cause of conjunctivitis in neonates in the United States, the long-time standard prophylactic agent for neonates, topical 1% silver nitrate solution, is no longer recommended (nor commercially available) in the United States. Topical treatment of neonatal chlamydial conjunctivitis is ineffective and unnecessary (American Academy of Pediatrics, 2015). In adults and children at least 8 years old, *C. trachomatis* infection is treated with a single 1-g dose of azithromycin or 7 days of therapy with doxycycline 100 mg twice daily. Children who weigh at least 45 kg but are less than 8 years old should receive the single dose of azithromycin 1 g. Neonates and children who weigh less than 45 kg should receive 50 mg/kg/d of erythromycin base or erythromycin ethylsuccinate, divided into four doses a day for 14 days (AAO, 2018b). Identification of either *Chlamydia* or *N. gonorrhoeae* conjunctivitis requires that the patient's sexual partner also be treated.

Antihistamines

The ophthalmic antihistamines alcaftadine and emedastine prevent the histamine response in blood vessels by preventing histamine from binding with its receptor site and are useful in reducing the symptoms of allergic conjunctivitis. Ocular adverse events with these agents include transient stinging or burning upon instillation, dry eyes, red eyes, and blurred vision. Oral antihistamines can also help to relieve symptoms in patients with vernal/atopic conjunctivitis (see **Table 16.3**).

TABLE 16.3

Overview of Antiallergy Ophthalmic Agents

Generic (Trade) Name and Dosage	Selected Adverse Events	Contraindications	Special Considerations
Antihistamines			
Alcaftadine 0.25% solution (Lastacaft) Dosing: 1 drop in the affected eye(s) once daily	Eye irritation, burning and stinging, itching		Labeling: wait 10 min following administration before inserting contact lenses.
Emedastine 0.05% solution (Emadine) Dosing: 1 drop in the affected eye(s) up to QID	Blurred vision, burning and stinging, dry eyes, foreign body sensation, hyperemia, itching		Labeling: wait 10 min following administration before inserting contact lenses.
Mast Cell Stabilizers			
Bepotastine 1.5% solution (Bepreve) Dosing: 1 drop into the affected eye(s) BID	Mild taste following instillation, eye irritation		Labeling: wait 10 min following administration before inserting contact lenses.
Cromolyn 4% solution (Crolom) Dosing: 1–2 drops in each eye four to six times daily at regular intervals	Burning and stinging, conjunctival injection, watery eyes, itching, dry eye, styes		Labeling: refrain from contact lens use while under treatment.
Lodoxamide 0.1% solution (Alomide) Dosing: 1–2 drops in each eye QID	Burning and stinging, ocular itching, blurred vision, dry eye, tearing, hyperemia, foreign body sensation		Labeling: refrain from contact lens use while under treatment.
Nedocromil 2% solution (Alocril) Dosing: 1–2 drops in each eye BID	Ocular burning and stinging, unpleasant taste, redness, photophobia		Labeling: refrain from contact lens use while exhibiting the signs and symptoms of allergic conjunctivitis.
Antihistamine/Mast Cell Stabilizer			
Azelastine 0.05% solution (Optivar) Dosing: 1 drop into each affected eye BID	Ocular burning and stinging, headache, bitter taste, eye pain, blurred vision		Labeling: wait 10 min following administration before inserting contact lenses.
Epinastine 0.05% solution (Elestat) Dosing: 1 drop in each eye BID	Burning sensation, folliculosis (hair follicle inflammation), hyperemia, itching		Labeling: wait 10 min following administration before inserting contact lenses.
Ketotifen 0.025% solution (Alaway, Claritin Eye, Zaditor, Thera Tears Allergy) Dosing: 1 drop in the affected eye(s) q8–12h, once daily or BID	Headache, conjunctival injection, burning and stinging, conjunctivitis, dry eye, itching, photophobia		Labeling: wait 10 min following administration before inserting contact lenses.
Olopatadine 0.1% (Patanol), 0.2% (Pataday), or 0.7% (Pazeo) solution Dosing 0.1%: 1 drop in each affected eye BID at an interval of 6–8 h 0.2%, 0.7%: 1 drop in the affected eye(s) once daily	Ocular burning and stinging, dry eye, headache, foreign body sensation, hyperemia, lid edema, itching		Labeling: wait 5–10 min following administration before inserting contact lenses.
Nonsteroidal Antiinflammatory Drugs			
Ketorolac 0.5% solution (Acular) Dosing: 1 drop QID	Stinging and burning, corneal edema, iritis, ocular irritation or inflammation		Use with caution in patients with aspirin sensitivities and patients with bleeding disorders or those receiving anticoagulant therapy. Labeling: do not administer while wearing contact lenses.

(Continued)

TABLE 16.3

Overview of Antiallergy Ophthalmic Agents (*Continued*)

Generic (Trade) Name and Dosage	Selected Adverse Events	Contraindications	Special Considerations
Vasoconstrictors (Decongestants)			
Naphazoline 0.0125% or 0.03% solutions (Clear Eyes) and 0.1% solution (AK-Con) Dosing: 1–2 drops in the affected eye(s), up to QID	Stinging, blurred vision, mydriasis, redness, punctate keratitis, increased IOP	Narrow-angle glaucoma Narrow-angle without glaucoma	Use should be limited to 72 h. Contains benzalkonium chloride; use with contact lenses not addressed in labeling. 0.1% solution requires a prescription.
Tetrahydrozoline 0.05% solution (Visine Advanced Relief, Murine for Red Eyes, Clear Eyes Triple Action, GoodSense, Opti-Clear) Dosing: 1–2 drops up to QID	Stinging, blurred vision, mydriasis, redness, punctate keratitis, increased IOP	Narrow-angle glaucoma Narrow-angle without glaucoma	Use should be limited to 72 h. Contains benzalkonium chloride; use with contact lenses not addressed in labeling
Topical Corticosteroids			
Dexamethasone 0.1% solution (AK-Dex, Decadron) or 0.1% suspension (Maxidex) Dosing Solution: 1–2 drops every hour during the day and q2h at night initially, reduced to 1 drop q4h with favorable response Suspension: 1–2 drops less than four to six times a day in mild disease; hourly in severe disease	IOP elevation, loss of visual acuity, cataract formation, secondary ocular infection, globe perforation, stinging and burning	Dendritic keratitis Fungal disease Viral disease of the cornea and conjunctiva Mycobacterial eye infection	Labeling: wait 15 min following administration before inserting contact lenses.
Fluorometholone 0.1% ointment or suspension (FML, Flarex) or 0.25% suspension (FML Forte) Dosing Ointment: 0.5 inch ribbon one to TID; during initial 24–48 h, dosing may be increased to q4h. Suspension: 1 drop BID to QID; during initial 24–48 h, dosing may be increased to q4h.	IOP elevation, glaucoma, posterior subcapsular cataract formation, delayed wound healing	Dendritic keratitis Vaccinia and varicella Fungal disease Viral disease of the cornea and conjunctiva Mycobacterial eye infection	
Loteprednol 0.2% or 0.5% suspension (Alrex, Lotemax) Dosing 0.2% solution: 1 drop in the affected eye(s) QID 0.5% solution: 1–2 drops in the affected eye(s) QID	IOP elevation, loss of visual acuity, cataract formation, secondary ocular infection, globe perforation, stinging and burning, dry eye, itching, photophobia	Dendritic keratitis Fungal disease Viral disease of the cornea and conjunctiva Mycobacterial eye infection	If needed, dosing of the 0.5% solution can be increased to 1 drop every hour during the first week of therapy. Labeling: wait 15 min following administration before inserting contact lenses.
Prednisolone 0.12% or 1% suspension (Pred Mild, Omnipred, Pred Forte) or 1% solution Dosing Solution: 2 drops QID Suspension: 1–2 drops BID to QID; dose may be increased during the initial 24–48 h.	IOP elevation, cataract formation, delayed wound healing, secondary ocular infection, acute uveitis, globe perforation, stinging and burning, conjunctivitis	Dendritic keratitis Fungal disease Viral disease of the cornea and conjunctiva Mycobacterial eye infection Acute, purulent, untreated eye infections	Labeling: wait 15 min following administration before inserting contact lenses.

IOP, increased intraocular pressure.

Mast Cell Stabilizers

The mast cell stabilizers (bepotastine, cromolyn, lodoxamide, and nedocromil) inhibit hypersensitivity reactions and prevent the increase in cutaneous vascular permeability that accompanies allergic reactions. These agents may be helpful for patients with allergic conjunctivitis. Ocular adverse events include transient burning, stinging or discomfort, pruritus, blurred vision, dry eyes, taste alteration, and foreign body sensation (see **Table 16.3**).

Antihistamine/Mast Cell Stabilizer

Several products (azelastine, epinastine, ketotifen, and olopatadine) have the combined properties of an antihistamine and a mast cell stabilizer, providing immediate relief of itching and long-term suppression of histamine release. Ketotifen is available without a prescription. These agents are given once or twice a day and have an adverse effect profile similar to the antihistamines and mast cell stabilizers (see **Table 16.3**).

Nonsteroidal Antiinflammatory Ophthalmic Drugs

The ophthalmic nonsteroidal antiinflammatory drug (NSAID) ketorolac may be useful for treating the itch associated with allergic conjunctivitis. The NSAIDs inhibit the biosynthesis of prostaglandin by decreasing the activity of the enzyme cyclooxygenase. Ketorolac is administered 1 drop four times a day into the affected eye. It should be used with caution in patients with aspirin sensitivities and patients who have bleeding disorders or are receiving anticoagulant therapy because ophthalmic NSAIDs are absorbed systemically. Adverse events include transient stinging and burning, irritation and inflammation, corneal edema, and iritis (see **Table 16.3**).

Vasoconstrictors (Decongestants)

Vasoconstrictor eye drops (naphazoline and tetrahydrozoline) may offer relief to patients with allergic conjunctivitis. With the exception of the higher-strength (0.1%) naphazoline solution, these agents are available without a prescription. Adverse effects include stinging, blurred vision, mydriasis, and increased redness; punctate keratitis and increased intraocular pressure (IOP) may also occur. These agents are contraindicated in patients with narrow-angle glaucoma or a narrow angle without glaucoma. Rebound congestion may occur with extended use of these agents; use should be limited to a maximum of 72 hours (see **Table 16.3**).

Topical Corticosteroids

Topical corticosteroids have been shown to reduce inflammation in allergic conjunctivitis. Low-dose corticosteroid therapy can be used at infrequent intervals for short-term periods (1–2 weeks) (AAO, 2018b). Long-term use of topical corticosteroids is associated with severe adverse effects including ocular infection, cataract formation, and glaucoma (Oray et al., 2016) (see **Table 16.3**).

Selecting the Most Appropriate Agent

Treatment of bacterial conjunctivitis is aimed at eradicating the offending organism. Cultures are not indicated unless the infection does not resolve with first-line therapy (**Table 16.4** and **Figure 16.1**).

There is conflicting information about the use of soft contact lenses while taking ophthalmic medications that contain the preservative benzalkonium chloride. This preservative, which is in many of the ophthalmic antihistamines, mast cell stabilizers, NSAIDs, vasoconstrictors, and topical steroids reviewed in this section, may be absorbed by contact lenses. While no products identify contact lens use as an absolute contraindication to therapy, some (e.g., cromolyn, lodoxamide, and nedocromil) have warnings advising against the use of contact lenses during therapy; others advise patients to wait 10 to 15 minutes after administering the medication before reinserting contact lenses (see **Table 16.3**). Regardless of the etiology, contact lens wearers should refrain from wearing contact lenses during an acute case of conjunctivitis.

Bacterial Conjunctivitis

The treatment of bacterial conjunctivitis is aimed at the organisms *S. aureus*, *S. pneumoniae*, and *H. influenzae*. First-line treatments include 5 to 7 days of therapy with erythromycin ointment (twice or three times daily) or polymyxin B–trimethoprim solution (1 drop every 3–4 hours). Therapy selection can be based on patient preference for ointment or solution. If bacterial conjunctivitis does not resolve with first-line therapy, the patient should be referred to an eye care professional so that cultures may be taken to rule out *C. trachomatis*. The ophthalmic fluoroquinolones with improved gram-positive organism coverage (besifloxacin, gatifloxacin, levofloxacin, or moxifloxacin) can be used as second-line therapy.

Gonococcal infection requires immediate treatment. Ceftriaxone plus azithromycin is recommended for adults and children who weigh at least 45 kg; children who weigh less than 45 kg and neonates should receive a reduced dose of ceftriaxone. In adults and children at least 8 years old, *C. trachomatis* infection is treated with azithromycin or doxycycline. Azithromycin should be used in children who weigh at least 45 kg but are less than 8 years old, while neonates and children who weigh less than 45 kg should receive erythromycin base or erythromycin ethylsuccinate.

Seasonal (Hay Fever) Conjunctivitis

Steps should be taken to minimize exposure to the offending allergen. The ophthalmic antihistamines alcaftadine or emedastine can be used as first-line therapy for mild seasonal conjunctivitis. If symptom control is inadequate, a brief course (1–2 weeks) of a low-potency topical corticosteroid can be added to the regimen. If the condition is persistent, a mast cell stabilizer or, preferably, an agent with antihistamine and mast cell stabilizer properties (azelastine, epinastine, ketotifen, or olopatadine) can be used. The ophthalmic NSAID ketorolac should be reserved for third-line therapy, as it is generally less

TABLE 16.4

Recommended Order of Treatment for Conjunctivitis

Order	Agent	Comments
Bacterial Conjunctivitis (nongonococcal, nonchlamydial)		
First line	Erythromycin ointment *or* Bacitracin–polymyxin B ointment	Ointments tend to cause a greater degree of blurry vision than solutions.
Second line	Ophthalmic fluoroquinolone (besifloxacin, gatifloxacin, levofloxacin, or moxifloxacin) solution	The remaining ophthalmic fluoroquinolones do not provide good staphylococcal coverage.
Seasonal (Hay Fever) Conjunctivitis		
First line	Topical antihistamine (alcaftadine or emedastine)	Minimization of exposure to the offending allergen, cool compresses, and artificial tears may also be helpful.
Second line	Addition of a brief course of low-potency topical corticosteroid to the first-line agent *or* For recurrent or persistent disease: a product with antihistamine/ mast cell stabilizer properties (azelastine, epinastine, ketotifen, or olopatadine)	Use of the topical corticosteroids should not exceed 2 wk.
Third line	Ophthalmic ketorolac	
Vernal/Atopic Conjunctivitis		
First line	Topical antihistamine or oral antihistamine or mast cell stabilizer	Minimization of exposure to the offending allergen, cool compresses, and artificial tears may also be helpful.
Second line	For acute exacerbations: addition of a brief course of low-potency topical corticosteroid to the first-line agent	
Viral Conjunctivitis		
First line	Topical antihistamines *or* Artificial tears *or* Cold compresses	There is no effective treatment for viral conjunctivitis; treatment is for symptom mitigation.
Second line	In severe cases: a low-potency topical corticosteroid	Use of the topical corticosteroids should not exceed 2 wk.
Giant Papillary Conjunctivitis		
Mild disease	One or more of the following: replace contact lenses more frequently, decrease contact lens wearing time, increase the frequency of enzyme treatment, use preservative-free lens care systems, switch to disposable lenses, administer mast cell stabilizer, change the contact lens polymer	
Moderate or severe disease	Same as mild disease *and* Discontinuation of contact lens wear for several weeks or a brief course of topical corticosteroid treatment	

effective than the ophthalmic antihistamines (Abelson et al., 2015). Many of these agents can be stored in the refrigerator and provide a cooling sensation and symptomatic relief upon instillation. Patients may also benefit from the use of cool compresses and artificial tears (which dilute allergens and help manage coexisting tear deficiency).

Vernal/Atopic Conjunctivitis

Similar to seasonal conjunctivitis, general treatment measures for vernal/atopic conjunctivitis include minimizing exposure to the offending allergen and use of cool compresses and artificial tears. The topical antihistamines (alcaftadine or emedastine), oral antihistamines, or mast cell stabilizers (bepotastine,

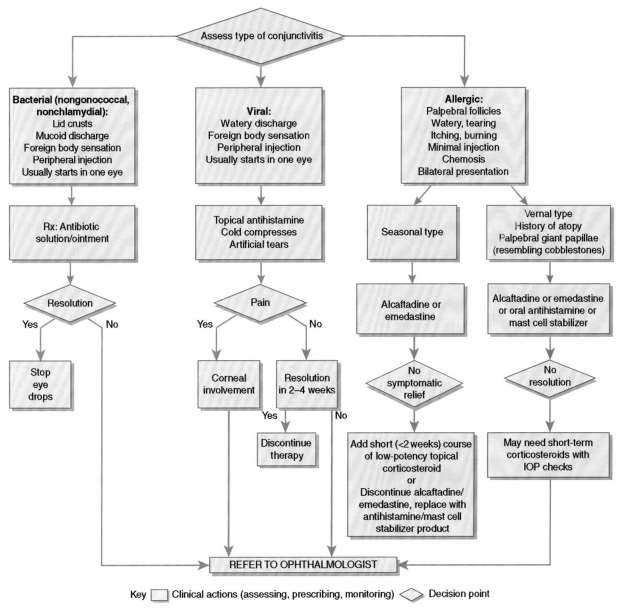

FIGURE 16–1   Treatment algorithm for conjunctivitis.

IOP, increased intraocular pressure.

cromolyn, lodoxamide, or nedocromil) can be used as first-line agents for the treatment of vernal or atopic conjunctivitis. For patients with acute exacerbations, a topical corticosteroid can be added to the first-line agent for control of severe symptoms.

Viral Conjunctivitis

There is no effective treatment for viral conjunctivitis; patients should be informed of the risk of spreading the infection to the other eye (in unilateral infection) or to other people. Topical antihistamines, artificial tears, or cool compresses can be used to relieve symptoms. In severe cases of adenoviral keratoconjunctivitis with marked chemosis or lid swelling, epithelial sloughing, or membranous conjunctivitis, topical corticosteroids can be helpful in reducing symptoms and preventing scarring.

Giant Papillary Conjunctivitis

Management of giant papillary conjunctivitis centers around identifying and modifying the causative entity. Treatment of mild giant papillary conjunctivitis due to contact lens use can consist of one or more of the following: more frequent replacement of contact lenses, reduction in contact lens wearing time, increase in the frequency of enzyme treatment, use of preservative-free lens care systems, switching to disposable daily-wear lenses, administration of a mast cell stabilizer, and change of the contact lens polymer (AAO, 2018b). In moderate or severe giant papillary conjunctivitis due to contact lens use, discontinuation of contact lens use for several weeks or a brief course of topical corticosteroid therapy may be necessary.

Monitoring Patient Response

If symptoms begin to improve within 48 hours, no follow-up is needed. If there is no improvement, the patient should be referred to an eye care professional for evaluation.

Patient Education

It is important to instruct patients with bacterial or viral conjunctivitis to wash their hands carefully to prevent spreading infection. Organisms in bacterial conjunctivitis remain active (and contagious) for 24 to 48 hours after therapy begins, while patients with viral conjunctivitis can remain contagious for up to 14 days. Patients should be taught how to apply the medication in the inner aspect of the lower eyelid. The tip of the container should not touch the eyelashes, as it may contaminate the medication and result in therapy failure or reinfection. Patients should not share eye medications because this can spread the infection. To improve the effectiveness of an ophthalmic antibiotic, crusted eyelids should be gently cleansed before instilling medication. Regardless of the etiology, contact lens wearers should refrain from wearing contact lenses during an acute case of conjunctivitis.

DRY EYE DISEASE: KERATOCONJUNCTIVITIS SICCA

Keratoconjunctivitis sicca, commonly referred to as dry eye disease (DED) or *dry eye syndrome*, is a common ophthalmologic abnormality involving bilateral disruption of tear film on the ocular surface. Estimates of the prevalence of dry eye in the United States range from 10% to 20%, with the prevalence markedly higher for individuals over the age of 80 years compared to those younger than 60 years of age (19.0% vs. 8.4%) (Moss et al., 2000). DED can occur intermittently or as a chronic condition that becomes a self-perpetuating syndrome. While the majority of patients with DED experience non-sight-threatening ocular irritation and intermittently blurred vision, patients with severe DED are at risk for severe vision loss due to ocular surface keratinization, corneal scarring, and corneal ulceration (AAO, 2018c).

Causes

DED is a multifactorial disease. It can be the result of decreased tear production, increased tear evaporation, or a combination of these factors (Craig et al., 2017). In addition, decreased tear secretion and clearance initiate an inflammatory response on the ocular surface, and research suggests that this inflammation plays a role in the pathogenesis of DED (Lee et al., 2018).

Risk factors for DED include advanced age, female gender, and a history of laser-assisted in situ keratomileusis surgery. Individuals with concomitant inflammatory conditions (rosacea, lupus, sarcoidosis, or rheumatoid arthritis), systemic viral infections (hepatitis C, human immunodeficiency virus/ acquired immunodeficiency syndrome, or Epstein-Barr virus), or conditions such as MGD blepharitis, Sjögren syndrome, Parkinson's disease, and Bell palsy are also at increased risk for DED. Symptoms caused by dry eye may be exacerbated by environmental factors such as wind, reduced humidity, cigarette smoke, and heating and air-conditioning (Calogne et al., 2017). Systemic medications such as antihistamines, diuretics, anticholinergics, antidepressants, beta blockers, antipsychotics, menopausal hormone therapy, oral contraceptives, and isotretinoin can also exacerbate dry eye symptoms (AAO, 2018c; Clayton, 2018).

Pathophysiology

Tears are composed of three layers: a mucus layer produced by goblet cells, which coats the cornea, allowing the tear to adhere to the eye; a middle aqueous layer produced by the lacrimal glands, which provides moisture and supplies oxygen and nutrients to the cornea; and an outer lipid film layer produced by the meibomian glands, which seals the tear film on the eye and prevents evaporation. The outer lipid film layer is replenished by eyelid blinking, which relubricates and redistributes the lipid layer across the ocular surface. The ocular surface and tear-secreting glands function as an integrated unit to maintain the tear supply and to clear used tears. Aging, ocular surface diseases (such as herpes simplex virus keratitis), surgeries that disrupt the trigeminal afferent sensory nerves, systemic inflammatory diseases, and systemic diseases and medications that disrupt the efferent cholinergic nerves that stimulate tear secretion can disrupt this functional unit and result in an unstable and poorly maintained tear film (AAO, 2018c; Pfulgfelder & de Paiva, 2017). Decreased tear secretion and clearance leads to an inflammatory response on the ocular surface, which is also believed to play a role in DED.

Diagnostic Criteria

Family practitioners should always refer patients reporting dry eye to an ophthalmologist if there is moderate to severe pain, vision loss, corneal infiltration or ulceration, or no response to therapy (AAO, 2018c). Making the diagnosis of DED, particularly the mild form, can be difficult because of the unpredictable correlation between reported symptoms and clinical signs and the relatively poor sensitivity/specificity of existing diagnostic tests (AAO, 2018c). Because most dry eye conditions are chronic, repeat observation will allow a more accurate clinical diagnosis of DED.

Signs and symptoms of DED include a dry eye sensation, ocular irritation, redness, burning, stinging, a foreign body or gritty sensation, blurred vision, photophobia, contact lens intolerance, an increased frequency of blinking, and, paradoxically, increased tearing (AAO, 2018c; National Eye Institute [NEI], 2019). DED symptoms tend to worsen in dry climates, in the wind, during air travel, with prolonged visual efforts (e.g., reading or computer use), and toward the end of the day (AAO, 2018c).

A physical examination (including a test of visual acuity, an external examination, and slit-lamp biomicroscopy) should be performed to document the signs of DED; to assess the quality, quantity, and stability of the tear film; and to rule out other causes of ocular irritation (AAO, 2018c). Evaluative tools (the Dry Eye Questionnaire 5 or Ocular Surface Disease Index) can be utilized to screen for DED; positive symptom scores should trigger a more detailed examination, which may include fluorescein tear break-up time, tear osmolarity testing, or ocular surface staining (Craig et al., 2017). Individuals with moderate to severe dry eye who have a family history of autoimmune disorders and/or signs and symptoms of an autoimmune disorder should be evaluated for an underlying autoimmune disorder.

Initiating Drug Therapy

Before starting drug therapy, the patient should try nonpharmacologic interventions such as environmental control (increasing air humidity, avoiding drafts and cigarette smoke) and scheduling regular breaks during computer use and reading. Unfortunately, these interventions result in limited effectiveness and produce few lasting improvements in DED symptoms. Exogenous medical factors that can cause DED (i.e., blepharitis, meibomianitis) should be addressed, and prescription medications that can exacerbate DED symptoms should be discontinued when possible.

If the nonpharmacologic interventions fail to eliminate DED symptoms, drug therapy is appropriate. **Table 16.5** gives information about the drugs used to treat DED.

Goals of Drug Therapy

The goals of therapy in DED are to relieve discomfort, maintain and improve visual function, and reduce or prevent structural damage (AAO, 2018c). Therapy should attempt to normalize tear volume and composition so that the eye tissues are properly lubricated, nourished, and protected, resulting in improved patient satisfaction and clinical outcomes.

Artificial Tears and Lubricants

Artificial tears and lubricants can be used as palliative therapies to relieve DED symptoms. Designed to mimic the composition of natural tears, artificial tears contain lipids, water with dissolved salts and proteins, and mucin. Artificial tears and lubricants are over-the-counter products, available in a variety of formulations (emulsions, gels, ointments). Ointments and gels may make the eyelids sticky and blur vision and are often used only at bedtime.

For patients with mild DED, use of artificial tears four times daily plus a lubricating ointment at bedtime may be useful. As the severity of dry eye increases, administration of artificial tears can increase to hourly. Preservative-free preparations should be used if the patient applies tears more than four times a day (AAO, 2018c).

Cholinergic Agonists

The cholinergic agonists pilocarpine and cevimeline are indicated for the treatment of dry mouth in patients with Sjögren syndrome. These agents bind to muscarinic receptors, stimulating secretion of the salivary and sweat glands and improving tear function. However, these agents are more effective for

treating dry mouth compared to dry eye. The main adverse event with these agents is excessive sweating, reported in 18% to 40% of patients. The use of these agents is contraindicated in patients with uncontrolled asthma and when miosis is undesirable (acute iritis, narrow-angle glaucoma).

Fatty Acid Supplements

Supplementation with n-3 fatty acids has been reported to provide benefits in DED due to their antiinflammatory activity and has been recommended by clinicians (Serhan et al., 2008). However, there is no definitive evidence supporting fatty acid supplementation in the management of DED, and a large, multicenter, double-blind clinical trial failed to demonstrate the effectiveness of n-3 fatty acid supplementation in patients with moderate to severe DED (Asbell et al., 2018).

Topical Cyclosporine

Cyclosporine ophthalmic emulsion has been reported to increase aqueous tear production and decrease ocular irritation symptoms in patients with DED. It prevents T cells from activating and releasing cytokines that incite the inflammatory component of dry eye. Adverse effects include ocular burning, conjunctival hyperemia, discharge, itching, and blurred vision.

Lifitegrast

Lifitegrast is a lymphocyte function-associated antigen-1 (LFA-1) antagonist. The exact mechanism of action of lifitegrast in DED is not known, though lifitegrast blocks the interaction of cell surface proteins LFA-1 and intercellular adhesion molecule-1 and may inhibit T cell–related inflammation in DED. Adverse effects include taste alteration and decreased visual acuity.

Topical Corticosteroids

Topical corticosteroids have been shown to reduce inflammation in DED by reducing cytokine levels in the conjunctival epithelium. Low-dose corticosteroid therapy can be used at infrequent intervals for short-term (2 weeks) suppression of irritation secondary to inflammation (AAO, 2018c). Long-term use of topical corticosteroids is associated with severe adverse effects, including ocular infection, cataract formation, and glaucoma (Cutolo et al., 2019).

Selecting the Most Appropriate Agent

Agent selection is determined by the severity of DED and the underlying pathophysiology (**Table 16.6**).

First-Line Therapy

For patients with mild DED, the use of a tear substitute four times a day is appropriate. For moderate or severe DED, artificial tears can be used as often as hourly, although administration that frequently may be cumbersome. Preservative-free preparations should be used if the patient uses tears more than four times a day. A lubricating ointment applied at bedtime may also be useful.

A patient with DED and underlying Sjögren syndrome may benefit from therapy with oral pilocarpine 5 mg four times daily or oral cevimeline 30 mg three times daily.

TABLE 16.5

Overview of Dry Eye Disease Agents

Generic (Trade) Name and Dosage	Selected Adverse Events	Contraindications	Special Considerations
Artificial Tear Substitutes			
Solutions containing preservatives: Dakrina, Dwelle, Fresh Kote, GenTeal Tears, GoodSense, GoodSense Ultra, Natural Balance Tears, Nutra Tear, Soothe XP, Systane Contacts, Systane Complete, Tears Again, Tears Again Advanced Eyelid	Stinging, blurred vision		Should not be used more than four to six times per day (except in severe disease); if use in excess of QID is necessary, use a preservative-free preparation.
Preservative-free solutions: Bion Tears PF, FreshKote PF, GenTeal Tears PF, GenTeal Tears Moderate PF, Optics Mini Drops, Refresh, Systane PF, Systane PF Ultra, Tears Naturale Free	Stinging, blurred vision		
Ocular Lubricants			
Ointments containing preservatives: Refresh Lacri-Lube, Refresh PM	Blurred vision		
Gels containing preservatives: Systane	Blurred vision		
Preservative-free ointments: GenTeal Tears Night-Time, HypoTears, LubriFresh PM, Puralube, Refresh PM, Systane Nighttime, Tears Again, Tears Naturale PM, Ultra Fresh PM	Blurred vision		
Preservative-free gels: GoodSense	Blurred vision		
Cholinergic			
Cevimeline 30-mg tablets (Evoxac) Dosing: 1 tablet TID	Excessive sweating, nausea, rhinitis, excessive salivation, asthenia	Uncontrolled asthma Acute iritis Narrow-angle glaucoma	Dehydration may develop from excessive sweating. Visual disturbances may impair the ability to drive, especially at night.
Pilocarpine 5-mg tablets (Salagen) Dosing: 1 tablet QID	Excessive sweating, headache, urinary frequency, nausea, flushing, dyspepsia, rhinitis, dizziness	Uncontrolled asthma Acute iritis Narrow-angle glaucoma	Dehydration may develop from excessive sweating.
Antiinflammatory			
Cyclosporine 0.05%, 0.09%, or 0.1% emulsion (Restasis, Restasis Multidose, Cequa, Klarity) Dosing: 1 drop in each eye BID, approximately 12 h apart	Ocular burning, blurred vision, conjunctival hyperemia, discharge, eye pain, foreign body sensation, pruritus, stinging		For the single-use vials (Restasis, Cequa): use immediately after opening; discard the remaining contents.
Lifitegrast 5% solution (Xiidra) Dosing: 1 drop in each eye q12h	Taste alteration, decreased visual acuity		Use the single-use vials immediately after opening; discard the remaining contents. Labeling: wait 15 min following administration before inserting contact lenses.

TABLE 16.6

Recommended Order of Treatment for Dry Eye Disease

Order	Agent	Comments
First line	Mild DES: artificial tear substitute QID *or* Moderate to severe DES: preservative-free artificial tear substitute, administered up to hourly	If the patient has underlying Sjögren syndrome, administer pilocarpine tablets 5 mg QID or cevimeline tablets 30 mg TID.
Second line	Cyclosporine 0.05% ophthalmic emulsion BID *or* Lifitegrast 5% solution q12h	Ophthalmic corticosteroid therapy may be useful for the short-term (2-wk) suppression of irritation secondary to inflammation.

DES, dry eye syndrome.

Second-Line Therapy

Patients with moderate to severe DED who fail to experience any improvement in symptoms with artificial tears may benefit from therapy with 0.05% cyclosporine ophthalmic emulsion 1 drop in each eye twice daily or lifitegrast 5% ophthalmic solution 1 drop in each eye every 12 hours. Due to the adverse effect profile, corticosteroid therapy is limited to second-line therapy for short-term (2 weeks) suppression of irritation secondary to inflammation.

Third-Line Therapy

Patients with severe DED that fails to respond to drug therapy are candidates for permanent punctal occlusion or tarsorrhaphy.

Monitoring Patient Response

The frequency and extent of follow-up will depend upon the severity of DED and the therapeutic approach selected. Patients with mild DED can be seen once or twice per year for follow-up if symptoms are controlled by therapy. Patients with sterile corneal ulceration associated with DED require careful, sometimes daily, monitoring (AAO, 2018c).

Patient Education

Patients with DED should be educated about the chronic nature of the disease and given specific instructions about their therapeutic regimens. Patients with moderate to severe DED are at an elevated risk for contact lens intolerance.

GLAUCOMA: PRIMARY OPEN-ANGLE GLAUCOMA

Glaucoma is a group of eye diseases involving optic neuropathy characterized by irreversible damage to the optic nerve and retinal ganglion cells (**Figure 16.2**). Over time, this deterioration

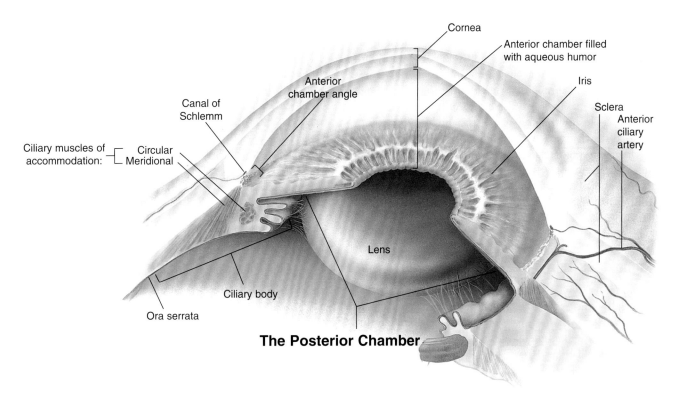

FIGURE 16–2   Anatomy of the eye.

results in the loss of visual sensitivity and field, which frequently goes unnoticed until a significant amount of damage has occurred. Glaucoma is the leading cause of irreversible blindness in the world (Bourne et al., 2017). There are numerous types of glaucoma, including primary open-angle glaucoma (POAG), acute closed-angle glaucoma, and narrow-angle glaucoma. POAG accounts for up to 80% of glaucoma cases in the United States and afflicts 2.7 million Americans (Liu & Tanna, 2016; Weinrab et al., 2014); as such, this section will specifically review POAG.

Causes

Several studies have shown that the prevalence of POAG increases with increasing IOP (Gordon et al., 2002; Leske et al., 2003). The median IOP in large populations is 15.5 ± 2.5 mm Hg. Previously, it was thought that increased IOP was the sole cause of POAG, but it is now recognized that IOP is one of several factors associated with the development of POAG, and an increased IOP is not required for the diagnosis of POAG.

Additional risk factors for the development of POAG include increasing age, black race (three times greater than whites), a family history of glaucoma, a thin central cornea, and type 2 diabetes mellitus (AAO, 2020; Kapetenakis et al., 2016).

Pathophysiology

The pathophysiology of glaucoma-induced vision loss is not well understood. Aqueous humor is produced by the ciliary body and secreted into the posterior chamber of the eye. A pressure gradient in the posterior chamber forces the aqueous humor between the iris and lens and through the pupil into the anterior chamber. Aqueous humor in the anterior chamber leaves the eye through two methods: filtration through the trabecular meshwork to Schlemm canal (80%–85%) or traversal of the anterior face of the iris and absorption into iris blood vessels (uveoscleral outflow). In POAG, degenerative changes in the trabecular meshwork and Schlemm canal result in a decrease in the outflow of the aqueous humor, resulting in IOP elevation and compression of the optic nerve resulting in damage and optic neuropathy (Marshall et al., 2018).

Diagnostic Criteria

Symptoms of POAG do not manifest until substantial damage has already occurred. The diagnosis of any glaucoma should be made by an eye care professional. Any patients reporting visual field loss should be referred to an eye care professional for prompt evaluation.

During the physical examination, IOP is measured in each eye, preferably with a Goldmann-type applanation tonometer, before gonioscopy or dilation of the pupil (AAO, 2020). Unfortunately, the measurement of IOP is not an effective method for screening populations for glaucoma. At an IOP cutoff of 21 mm Hg, the sensitivity for the diagnosis of POAG by tonometry was 47.1% (Tielsch et al., 1991), and half of all individuals with POAG are measured with an IOP of less than 22 mm Hg at a single screening (Leske et al., 2003). As such, the AAO recommends, in addition to the measurement of IOP, that a physical examination include the following elements: patient history, test of pupil reactivity, slit-lamp biomicroscopy of the anterior segment, determination of central corneal thickness, gonioscopy, evaluation of the optic nerve head and retinal nerve fiber layer, documentation of the optic nerve head appearance, evaluation of the fundus, and evaluation of the visual field (AAO, 2020).

Initiating Drug Therapy

The goals of therapy for POAG are to control IOP, to stabilize the status of the optic nerve and retinal fiber layer, and to stabilize the visual field (AAO, 2020). Most cases of glaucoma can be controlled and vision loss prevented with early detection and treatment. Treatment of POAG entails decreasing aqueous humor production, increasing aqueous outflow, or a combination of both.

Over the past 30 years, glaucoma management has changed significantly, primarily due to the introduction of pharmaceutical agents that have shown clinical effectiveness (**Table 16.7**). These agents have been associated with a significant reduction in surgery rates among glaucoma patients (Conlon et al., 2017).

Once a target IOP has been determined, treatment may include drug therapy, laser therapy, or surgery. Topical medication is, in most cases, indicated as first-line therapy. Several trials have clearly shown that reducing IOP by treatment with ocular hypotensive medication can prevent or reduce the risk of progression of glaucoma. Furthermore, the more IOP is reduced, the more the risk of glaucomatous eye damage decreases.

Goals of Drug Therapy

The goals of drug therapy for POAG are to reduce IOP to a target level and to prevent or slow the progression of vision loss. In patients with POAG, the initial IOP target should be 20% to 30% lower than baseline. Additional IOP lowering may be justified, based upon the severity of the existing optic nerve damage, the speed at which the damage occurred, and the presence of other risk factors such as family history, age, or disc hemorrhage. (AAO, 2020). Visual fields and optic nerve status should be monitored for signs of change; if progression is detected, the IOP target should be lowered.

Beta Blockers

Beta blockers are the benchmark against which other IOP-lowering medications are measured. Beta blockers reduce adenylyl cyclase activity, which in turn reduces the production of aqueous humor in the ciliary body. Beta blockers lower IOP

TABLE 16.7

Overview of Glaucoma Agents

Generic (Trade) Name and Dosage	Selected Adverse Events	Contraindications	Special Considerations
Beta Blockers			
Betaxolol 0.5% solution or 0.25% suspension (Betoptic S) Dosing: 1–2 drops in the affected eye(s) BID	Discomfort on instillation, tearing, decreased corneal sensitivity, edema, bradycardia, hypotension, dizziness, photophobia	Cardiogenic shock Second- or third-degree AV block Sinus bradycardia Overt cardiac failure	A cardioselective (beta-1) blocker; it has fewer effects on pulmonary and cardiovascular parameters.
Carteolol 1% solution Dosing: 1 drop in the affected eye(s) BID	Transient eye irritation, burning, tearing, conjunctival hyper-emia, edema, bradycardia, hypotension, arrhythmia, palpitations, photophopia	Bronchial asthma or severe COPD Sinus bradycardia Second- or third-degree AV block Overt cardiac failure Cardiogenic shock	May be absorbed systemically; the same adverse reactions seen with oral beta blockers may occur. May mask the symptoms of acute hypoglycemia or hyperthyroidism
Levobunolol 0.5% solution (Betagan) Dosing: 1–2 drops in the affected eye(s) once daily; dose can be increased to 1 drop BID in severe glaucoma.	Burning and stinging, blepharoconjunctivitis, urticaria, ataxia, bradycardia, arrhythmia, hypotension, syncope, heart block, bronchospasm	Bronchial asthma or severe COPD Sinus bradycardia Second- or third-degree AV block Overt cardiac failure Cardiogenic shock	May be absorbed systemically; the same adverse reactions seen with oral beta blockers may occur. May mask the symptoms of acute hypoglycemia or hyperthyroidism
Metipranolol 0.3% solution Dosing: 1 drop in the affected eye(s) BID	Transient local discomfort, con-junctivitis, eyelid dermatitis, blepharitis, blurred vision, photophobia, headache, asthenia, angina, palpitation, bradycardia	Bronchial asthma or severe COPD Symptomatic sinus bradycardia Second- or third-degree AV block Overt cardiac failure Cardiogenic shock	May be absorbed systemically; the same adverse reactions seen with oral beta blockers may occur. May mask the symptoms of acute hypoglycemia or hyperthyroidism
Timolol 0.25% or 0.5% solution (Timoptic, Timoptic Ocudose, Betimol, Istalol) or gel-forming solution (Timoptic-XE) Dosing: Solution: 1 drop in the affected eye(s) BID; Islatol: 1 drop in the affected eye(s) once daily AM Gel-forming solution: 1 drop in the affected eye(s) once daily	Ocular irritation, decreased corneal sensitivity, visual disturbances, conjunctivitis, tearing, headache, dizziness, bradycardia, arrhythmia, angina, bronchospasm	Bronchial asthma or severe COPD Sinus bradycardia Second- or third-degree AV block Overt cardiac failure Cardiogenic shock	May be absorbed systemically; the same adverse reactions seen with oral beta blockers may occur. May mask the symptoms of acute hypoglycemia or hyperthyroidism. Other ophthalmic medications should be administered 10 min before the gel-forming solution.
Carbonic Anhydrase Inhibitors			
Brinzolamide 1% suspension (Azopt) Dosing: 1 drop in the affected eye(s) TID	Blurred vision, bitter taste, blepharitis, dermatitis, dry eye, headache, hyperemia ocular pain, pruritus		Use with caution in patients with renal impairment, hepatic impairment, or sulfonamides hypersensitivity.
Dorzolamide 2% solution (Trusopt) Dosing: 1 drop in the affected eye(s) TID	Ocular burning and stinging, bitter taste, keratitis, ocular allergy, blurred vision, tearing, photophobia	Sulfa allergy	Use with caution in patients with renal impairment, hepatic impairment, or sulfonamides hypersensitivity.

(Continued)

TABLE 16.7

Overview of Glaucoma Agents (*Continued*)

Generic (Trade) Name and Dosage	Selected Adverse Events	Contraindications	Special Considerations
Prostaglandin Analogs			
Bimatoprost 0.03% solution (Lumigan) Dosing: 1 drop in the affected eye(s) once daily PM	Conjunctival hyperemia, growth of eyelashes, ocular pruritus, dry eye, iris discoloration, visual disturbance, eye pain, pigmentation of the periocular skin, foreign body sensation		Iris discoloration is irreversible; incidence less than with latanoprost
Latanoprost 0.005% solution (Xalatan) Dosing: 1 drop in the affected eye(s) once daily PM	Iris discoloration, blurred vision, burning and stinging, conjunctival hyperemia, itching, eyelash changes, eyelid skin darkening		Iris discoloration is irreversible. Requires refrigeration until dispensed
Tafluprost 0.0015% solution (Zioptan) Dosing: 1 drop in the affected eye(s) once daily PM	Conjunctival hyperemia, ocular stinging, headache, ocular pruritus, dry eye, growth of eyelashes, iris discoloration, pigmentation of the periocular skin		Iris discoloration is irreversible.
Travoprost 0.004% solution (Travatan Z) Dosing: 1 drop in the affected eye(s) once daily PM	Ocular hyperemia, decreased visual acuity, eye discomfort, foreign body sensation, eye pain, pruritus		Iris discoloration is irreversible. May interfere in pregnancy; should not be used during pregnancy or by those attempting to become pregnant
Nitric Oxide Donating Prostaglandin Analogs			
Latanoprostene bunod 0.024% solution (Vyzulta) Dosing: 1 drop in the affected eye(s) once daily PM	Same as latanoprost		Same as latanoprost
Adrenergic Agonists			
Apraclonidine 0.5% solution (Iopidine) Dosing: 1–2 drops in the affected eye(s) TID	Hyperemia, tearing, pruritus, lid edema, dry mouth, foreign body sensation, eyelid retraction	Hypersensitivity to clonidine Patients receiving MAO inhibitors	For short-term use only as an adjunct therapy A 1% solution is available for prevention of postsurgical elevations in IOP.
Brimonidine 0.1%, 0.15%, or 0.2% solution (Alphagan P) Dosing: 1 drop in the affected eye(s) TID, approximately 8 h apart	Ocular hyperemia, ocular pruritus, visual disturbance, allergic conjunctivitis somnolence, headache, hypertension, fatigue, drowsiness, dry mouth	Patients receiving MAO inhibitors	Not recommended in children less than age 2
Cholinergic Agonists			
Pilocarpine 1%, 2%, or 4% solution (Isopto Carpine) Dosing: 1–2 drops TID or QID	Stinging and burning, tearing, ciliary spasm, blurred vision, brow ache, hypertension, tachycardia, bronchospasm, salivation	Acute iritis or other conditions where papillary constriction is undesirable	

TABLE 16.7

Overview of Glaucoma Agents (*Continued*)

Generic (Trade) Name and Dosage	Selected Adverse Events	Contraindications	Special Considerations
Rho Kinase Inhibitors			
Netarsudil 0.02% solution (Rhopressa) Dosing: 1 drop in the affected eye(s) once daily	Conjunctival hyperemia, corneal verticillata, stinging and burning, conjunctival hemorrhage, blurred vision, decreased visual acuity		Labeling: wait 15 min following administration before inserting contact lenses.
Combination Products			
Brimonidine and timolol 0.2%–0.5% solution (Combigan) Dosing: 1 drop in the affected eye(s) q12h	See individual components.	See individual components.	Combined effect results in greater IOP lowering than either agent alone, but not as great as brimonidine TID and timolol BID administered concomitantly.
Dorzolamide and timolol 2%–0.5% solution (Cosopt) Dosing: 1 drop into the affected eye(s) BID	See individual components.	See individual components.	Combined effect results in greater IOP lowering than either agent alone, but not as great as dorzolamide TID and timolol BID administered concomitantly.
Brinzolamide and brimonidine 1%–0.2% solution (Simbrinza) Dosing: 1 drop into the affected eye(s) TID	See individual components.	See individual components.	
Netarsudil and latanoprost 0.02%–0.005% solution (Rocklatan) Dosing: 1 drop into the affected eye(s) once daily PM	See individual components	See individual components	

AV, atrioventricular mode; COPD, chronic obstructive pulmonary disease; IOP, increased intraocular pressure; MAO, monoamine oxidase.

by an average of 20% to 25%. There are five ophthalmic beta blockers available in the United States: timolol, levobunolol, carteolol, and metipranolol are nonselective beta blockers, while betaxolol is a beta$_1$-selective agent. Although nonselective beta blockers may be more efficacious in lowering IOP, selective beta blockers appear to be better tolerated systemically, particularly in patients with chronic obstructive pulmonary disease.

The ophthalmic beta blockers are typically applied twice daily. Timolol is available in a solution that forms a gel upon application, allowing once-daily dosing. Adverse effects include stinging, burning, dry eye, and blurred vision. Topical beta blockers can be absorbed systemically and may cause bradycardia, reduced blood pressure, aggravation of congestive heart failure, heart block, bronchospasm in asthma patients, and central nervous system (CNS) side effects such as hallucinations and depression. Betaxolol is less

likely to cause these systemic side effects, but a risk remains. All of the ophthalmic beta blockers are contraindicated in patients with sinus bradycardia, second- or third-degree atrioventricular node block, overt cardiac failure, and cardiogenic shock, and all except betaxolol are contraindicated in patients with bronchial asthma or severe chronic obstructive pulmonary disease.

Prostaglandin Analogs

The prostaglandin F$_{2\alpha}$ analogs such as bimatoprost, latanoprost, tafluprost, and travoprost reduce IOP by improving the uveoscleral outflow of aqueous humor. Given once daily, the prostaglandin F$_{2\alpha}$ analogs reduce IOP by 25% to 33%. Studies of bimatoprost, latanoprost, and travoprost found no statistical difference in IOP lowering among agents (Li et al., 2006).

These agents are more effective when given at bedtime rather than in the morning. Latanoprost requires refrigeration until dispensed; latanoprost and travoprost should be discarded within 6 weeks of the time the package is opened. Tafluprost is supplied in single-use containers packaged within a foil pouch; unused single-use containers should be discarded 28 days after opening the pouch. Adverse effects of the prostaglandins include ocular hyperemia, blurred vision, pruritus, dry eye, lengthening and thickening of the eyelashes, and conjunctival hyperemia. These agents are also associated with irreversible iris discoloration, most often affecting patients with mixed-color irises. Iris discoloration is reported by 7% to 12% of latanoprost users, with discoloration starting between 18 and 26 weeks after commencement of therapy. Compared to latanoprost, the incidence of iris discoloration is lower for bimatoprost and travoprost. In addition, darkening of the eyelid skin (periocular hyperpigmentation) can occur with these agents; therapy discontinuation often results in reversal of periocular hyperpigmentation 3 to 6 months after therapy discontinuation.

Nitric Oxide Donating Prostaglandin Analogs

Latanoprostene bunod is a molecule that is metabolized on the ocular surface to latanoprostic acid (the active form of latanoprost) and butanediol monohydrate, which itself is further metabolized to form nitric oxide and an inactive metabolite. In addition to the role of latanoprost in improving uveoscleral outflow of aqueous humor (described previously), the nitric oxide acts to reduce cellular contractility and volume, which facilitates outflow of aqueous humor through the trabecular meshwork and Schlemm's canal (Hoy, 2018; Marshall et al., 2018). Latanoprostene bunod reduces IOP by 26% to 34% and provides a greater degree of IOP lowering than latanoprost or timolol monotherapy. The adverse effect profile of latanoprostene bunod is similar to latanoprost.

Carbonic Anhydrase Inhibitors

The topical carbonic anhydrase inhibitors (CAIs) brinzolamide and dorzolamide work through the reversible and competitive binding of carbonic anhydrase. Carbonic anhydrase acts as a catalyst for the reversible hydration of carbonic acid, which plays a role in fluid transport in various cell systems. By decreasing bicarbonate formation, the movement of bicarbonate, sodium, and fluid into the posterior chamber of the eye declines, and less aqueous fluid is generated, reducing IOP (Abel & Sorensen, 2018). While the topical CAIs reduce IOP to a lesser extent (15%–26%) than beta blockers, prostaglandins, or systemic CAIs, they are rarely associated with systemic adverse effects.

The topical CAIs are given three times daily. Adverse effects include ocular burning and stinging, bitter taste, blurred vision, itching, tearing, and keratitis. The topical CAIs are not recommended for use in patients with severe renal impairment, respiratory acidosis, and electrolyte disorders and should be used with caution in patients with hypersensitivity to sulfonamides.

The systemic CAIs (acetazolamide, methazolamide, and dichlorphenamide) are the most potent agents for reducing IOP, producing a 25% to 40% decrease in IOP. However, these agents produce severe adverse effects such as paresthesias, gastrointestinal disturbances (anorexia, nausea, and weight loss), metallic taste, CNS effects (lethargy, malaise, and depression), electrolyte disturbances, and renal calculi, which limit their use in the older population (Swenson, 2014).

Adrenergic Agonists

The adrenergic agonists apraclonidine and brimonidine activate the presynaptic alpha-2 receptors, inhibiting the release of norepinephrine. As less norepinephrine is available for activation of postsynaptic beta receptors on the ciliary epithelium, the formation of aqueous humor is reduced.

Apraclonidine and brimonidine reduce IOP by 18% to 27%. Brimonidine is a highly selective alpha-2 agonist, causing little or no alpha-1 activity. In addition to decreasing aqueous humor, it increases uveoscleral outflow. Adverse effects include dry mouth, fatigue, ocular hyperemia, somnolence, and headache. Apraclonidine is a relatively selective alpha-2 agonist; it is associated with some alpha-1 activity, which can lead to mydriasis, conjunctival bleeding, and eyelid retraction. Apraclonidine is primarily indicated for short-term adjunctive therapy, as the efficacy of apraclonidine diminishes over time; the benefit for most patients lasts less than 1 to 2 months. Both agents are contraindicated in patients taking monoamine oxidase inhibitors. In addition, brimonidine has been associated with respiratory and cardiac depression in infants and should be used with caution in children under age 2.

The nonselective ophthalmic adrenergic agonists epinephrine and dipivefrin (epinephrine prodrug) are no longer available in the United States. These agents provided lackluster IOP control and were associated with adverse reactions such as stinging and tearing, brow ache, and the formation of black conjunctival spots and conjunctival deposits.

Cholinergic Agonists

Pilocarpine is a direct-acting cholinergic agonist. Pilocarpine stimulates the parasympathetic muscarinic receptor site to increase aqueous outflow through the trabecular meshwork. While effective in lowering IOP by 20% to 30%, pilocarpine usually needs to be given four times a day. Adverse effects include eye pain, brow ache, blurred vision, and accommodative spasms. It can also provoke miotic responses such as papillary constriction, which can decrease night vision. The intense dosing regimen and the adverse effect profile make adherence difficult.

Rho Kinase Inhibitors

The rho kinase inhibitor netarsudil increases aqueous humor outflow by relaxing the cells that line Schlemm's canal, reducing the resistance to the flow of aqueous humor (Tanna & Johnson, 2018). Netarsudil reduces IOP by 14% to 22%; head-to-head clinical trials found that netarsudil produced lesser IOP lowering compared to latanoprost and timolol. Netarsudil is likely most effective when used as an adjunctive therapy for patients utilizing other classes of IOP-lowering agents (Schehlein & Robin, 2019).

Netarsudil is dosed once daily. Adverse effects associated with netarsudil include conjunctival hyperemia, stinging and burning, blurred vision, and decreased visual acuity. Conjunctival hemorrhage and corneal verticillata (corneal deposits that form a faint brown whorl pattern) were observed in approximately 20% of patients receiving netarsudil in clinical trials; the verticillata did not alter visual function, and most dissipated upon discontinuation of treatment.

Combination Products

Combination products simplify administration and can promote adherence to therapy. Solutions of timolol 0.5% in combination with dorzolamide 2% or brimonidine 0.2% are available, as are combinations of brimonidine 0.2% and brinzolamide 1% as well as netarsudil 0.02% and latanoprost 0.005%. The combined effect results in additional IOP reduction compared to either agent alone, but the result is often less than each agent administered separately.

Selecting the Most Appropriate Agent

The AAO does not recommend a specific agent as first-line therapy. When the first-line agent drug fails to reduce IOP, the AAO recommends that it be discontinued in favor of another therapy before the original agent is supplanted by other medications. If a first-line agent lowers IOP but fails to lower IOP to the target level, combination therapy and discontinuation of therapy in favor of another agent are appropriate options. When selecting the first-line therapy for glaucoma, factors such as efficacy, adverse effects, cost, and dosing frequency should all be considered. **Table 16.8** lists the recommended order of treatment for these agents.

First-Line Therapy

The prostaglandins are often utilized as first-line therapy for POAG because they possess the best balance among efficacy, safety, cost, and ease of dosing regimen.

Second-Line Therapy

If the prostaglandin fails to decrease IOP to a significant extent, the patient should be switched to a different class of medicine. Beta blockers are recommended because of their efficacy, tolerability, and ease of dosing. If the IOP decreases with a prostaglandin but fails to reach the target IOP, an additional medication from a different class (such as a beta blocker) should be added.

TABLE 16.8

Recommended Order of Treatment for Glaucoma

Order	Agent	Comments
First line	Prostaglandin ophthalmic solution (bimatoprost, latanoprost, tafluprost, or travoprost)	
Second line	Substitution of an ophthalmic beta blocker (if failure to decrease IOP to a significant extent)	
	or	
	Addition of an ophthalmic beta blocker (if IOP is significantly decreased but not to goal)	
Third line	Addition of an ophthalmic carbonic anhydrase inhibitor *or* addition of brimonidine	Dorzolamide is available in a combination product with timolol.

IOP, increased intraocular pressure.

Third-Line Therapy

If a patient fails to reach the target IOP with the first-line and second-line therapies, a topical CAI (usually the fixed combination of timolol and dorzolamide to keep the dosing regimen simple) can be added. If this fails, dorzolamide should be discontinued in favor of brimonidine.

Monitoring Patient Response

Patients with POAG should receive follow-up evaluations and care from their eye care professional to determine the effectiveness of therapy. In addition to a recent history, a physical examination including a slit-lamp biomicroscopy and tests of visual acuity and IOP in each eye should be performed (AAO, 2020). The practitioner must distinguish between the impact of a prescribed agent on IOP and ordinary background fluctuations of IOP.

Patient Education

Patients should wash their hands before administering glaucoma medications. Patients should be taught how to apply the medication in the inner aspect of the lower eyelid. The tip of the container should not touch the eyelashes or any part of the eye because this may contaminate the medication. Contact lenses should be removed prior to administration, and patients should separate administration of different glaucoma medications by at least 10 minutes.

CASE STUDY 1

V.S. is a 15-year-old white female who presents with a feeling that there is sand in her eye. She had a cold one week ago, which recently resolved. Her mother reports that V.S. woke up this morning with her left eyelid crusted with yellowish drainage. On physical examination, V.S. has swollen conjunctiva on her left side, no adenopathy, and no vision changes. Her vision is corrected to 20/20 with contact lenses, but she was unable to insert them this morning and is wearing glasses instead. Fluorescein staining reveals no abrasion. She is afebrile. She is allergic to sulfonamides (Learning Objective 2).

1. What is the most likely diagnosis for V.S.?
2. List specific goals of treatment for V.S.
3. What drug therapy would you prescribe? Why?
4. Discuss the education you would give to V.S.'s parents regarding treating this condition.

Bibliography

Starred references are cited in the text.

*Abel, S. R., & Sorensen, S. J. (2018). Eye disorders. In C. S. Zeind, et al. (Eds.), *Applied therapeutics: The clinical use of drugs* (11th ed., pp. 1148–1169). Philadelphia, PA: Wolters Kluwer.

*Abelson, M. B., Shetty, S., Korchak, M. et al. (2015). Advances in pharmacotherapy for allergic conjunctivitis. *Expert Opinion on Pharmacotherapy, 16*(8), 1219–1231.

*Ackerman, S., Smith, L. M., & Gomes, P. J. (2016). Ocular itch associated with allergic conjunctivitis: Latest evidence and clinical management. *Therapeutic Advances in Chronic Disease, 7*(1), 52–67.

*American Academy of Ophthalmology Cornea/External Disease Panel, Preferred Practice Guidelines Committee. (2020). *Primary open-angle glaucoma.* San Francisco, CA: AAO.

*American Academy of Ophthalmology Cornea/External Disease Panel, Preferred Practice Guidelines Committee. (2018a). *Blepharitis.* San Francisco, CA: AAO.

*American Academy of Ophthalmology Cornea/External Disease Panel, Preferred Practice Guidelines Committee. (2018b). *Conjunctivitis.* San Francisco, CA: AAO.

*American Academy of Ophthalmology Cornea/External Disease Panel, Preferred Practice Guidelines Committee. (2018c). *Dry eye syndrome.* San Francisco, CA: AAO.

*American Academy of Pediatrics. (2015). Chlamydia trachomatis. In D. W. Kimberlin (Ed.), *Red book: Report of the committee on infectious diseases* (30th ed., pp. 288–293). Elk Grove Village, IL: American Academy of Pediatrics.

Andalibi, S., Haidara, M., Bor, N., et al. (2015). An update on neonatal and pediatric conjunctivitis. *Current Ophthalmology Reports, 3*, 158–169.

*Asbell, P. A., Maguire, M. G., Pistilli, M., et al. (2018). n-3 fatty acid supplementation for the treatment of dry eye disease. *New England Journal of Medicine, 378*, 1681–1690.

*Azari, A. A., & Barney, N. P. (2013). Conjunctivitis: A systematic review of diagnosis and treatment. *Journal of the American Medical Association, 310*(16), 1721–1729.

Bielory, B. P., Shah, S. P., O'Brien, T. P., et al. (2016). Emerging therapeutics for ocular surface diseases. *Current Opinion in Allergy & Clinical Immunology, 16*(5), 477–486.

*Bourne, R. R. A., Flaxman, S. R., Braithwaite, T., et al. (2017). Magnitude, temporal trends, and projections of the global prevalence of blindness and distance and near vision impairment: A systematic review and meta-analysis. *Lancet Global Health, 5*, e888–e897.

*Calogne, M., Pinto-Fraga, J., Gonzalez-Garcia, M. J., et al. (2017). Effects of the external environment on dry eye disease. *International Ophthalmology Clinics, 57*(2), 23–40.

*Centers for Disease Control and Prevention. (2020). *Conjunctivitis (pink eye) for clinicians.* Atlanta, GA: National Center for Immunization and Respiratory Diseases.

*Chen, F. V., Chang, T. C., & Cavuoto, K. M. (2018). Patient demographic and microbiology trends in bacterial conjunctivitis in children. *Journal for the American Association for Pediatric Ophthalmology and Strabismus, 22*(1), 66–67.

*Clayton, J. A. (2018). Dry eye. *New England Journal of Medicine, 378*, 2212–2223.

*Conlon, R., Saheb, H., & Ahmed, I. I. K. (2017). Glaucoma treatment trends: A review. *Canadian Journal of Ophthalmology, 52*(1), 114–124.

*Craig, J. P., Nelson, J. D., Azar, D. T., et al. (2017). TFOS DEWS II report executive summary. *Ocular Surface, 15*(4), 802–812.

*Cutolo, C. A., Barbarino, S., Bonzano, C., et al. (2019). The use of topical corticosteroids for treatment of dry eye syndrome. *Ocular Immunology and Inflammation, 27*(2), 266–275.

De Paiva, C. S., Pflugfelder, S. C., Ng, S. M., et al. (2019). Topical cyclosporine A therapy for dry eye syndrome. *Cochrane Database of Systematic Reviews,* CD010051.

Donnenfeld, E. D., Perry, H. D., Nattis, A. S., et al. (2017). Lifitegrast for the treatment of dry eye disease in adults. *Expert Opinion in Pharmacotherapy, 18*(14), 1517–1524.

Downie, L. E., & Keller, P. R. (2015). A pragmatic approach to the management of dry eye disease: Evidence into practice. *Optometry and Vision Science, 92*(9), 957–966.

*Duncan, K., & Jeng, B. H. (2017). Medical management of blepharitis. *Current Opinion in Ophthalmology, 26*(4), 289–294.

*Fredrick, D. R. (2018). Conjunctivitis beyond the neonatal period. In S. S. Long, C. G. Prober, M. Fischer (Eds.), *Principles and practice of pediatric infectious diseases* (5th ed., pp. 501–505). Philadelphia, PA: Elsevier, Inc.

*Fromstein, S. R., Harthan, J. S., Patel, J. P., et al. (2018). Demodex blepharitis: Clinical perspectives. *Clinical Optometry, 10*, 57–63.

*Garcia-Ferrer, F. J., Augsburger, J. J., & Correa, Z. M. (2018). Conjunctiva and tears. In P. Riordan-Eva, et al. (Eds.), *Vaughan & Asbury's general ophthalmology* (19th ed.). New York, NY: McGraw-Hill.

*Gordon, M. O., Beiser, J. A., Brandt, J. D., et al. (2002). The ocular hypertension treatment study: Baseline factors that predict the onset of primary open-angle glaucoma. *Archives of Ophthalmology, 120*, 714–720.

Gupta, D., & Chen, P. P. (2016). Glaucoma. *American Family Physician, 93*(8), 668–674.

Gupta, P., Zhao, D., Guallar, E., et al. (2016). Prevalence of glaucoma in the United States: The 2005–2008 National Health and Nutrition Examination Survey. *Investigative Ophthalmology & Visual Science, 57*, 2905–2913.

*Holtz, K. K., Townsend, K. R., Furst, J. W., et al. (2017). An assessment of the AdenoPlus point-of-care test for diagnosing adenoviral conjunctivitis and its effect on antibiotic stewardship. *Mayo Clinic Proceedings: Innovation, Quality, and Outcomes, 1*(2), 170–175.

*Horton, J. C. (2015). Disorders of the eye. In D. L. Kasper et al. (Ed.), *Harrison's principles of internal medicine* (19th ed.). New York, NY: McGraw-Hill.

Hoy, S. M. (2018). Latanoprostene bunod ophthalmic solution 0.024%: A review in open angle glaucoma and ocular hypertension. *Drugs, 78,* 773–780.

Jhanji, V., Chan, T. C. Y., Li, E. Y. M., et al. (2015). Adenoviral keratoconjunctivits. *Survey of Ophthalmology, 60*(5), 435–443.

Jonas, J. B., Aung, T., Bourne, R. R., et al. (2017). Glaucoma. *Lancet, 390,* 2083–2093.

Jones, L., Downie, L. E., Korb, D., et al. (2017). TFOS DEWS II management and therapy report. *Ocular Surface, 15,* 575–628.

*Kam, K. Y. R., Ong, H. S., Bunce, C., et al. (2015). Sensitivity and specificity of the AdenoPlus point-of-care system in detecting adenovirus in conjunctivitis patients at an ophthalmic emergency department: A diagnostic accuracy study. *British Journal of Ophthalmology, 99,* 1186–1189.

*Kapetenakis, V. V., Chan, M. P. Y., Foster, P. J., et al. (2016). Global variations and time trends in the prevalence of primary open-angle glaucoma (POAG): A systematic review and meta-analysis. *British Journal of Ophthalmology, 100,* 86–93.

Keen, M., & Thompson, M. (2017). Treatment of acute conjunctivitis in the United States and evidence of antibiotic overuse: Isolated issue or a systematic problem? *Ophthalmology, 124*(8), 1096–1098.

Kuklinski, E., & Asbell, P. A. (2017). Sjogren's syndrome from the perspective of ophthalmology. *Clinical Immunology, 182*(9), 55–61.

*Leonardi, A., Doan, S., Fauquert, J. L., et al. (2017). Diagnostic tools in ocular allergy. *Allergy, 72,* 1485–1498.

*Leske, M. C., Heijl, A., Hussein, M., et al. (2003). Factors for glaucoma progression and the effect of treatment: The early manifest glaucoma trial. *Archives of Ophthalmology, 121,* 48–56.

*Li, N., Chen, X. M., Zhou, Y., et al. (2006). Travoprost compared to other prostaglandin analogues or timolol in patients with open angle glaucoma or ocular hypertension: Meta-analysis of randomized, controlled trials. *Clinical and Experimental Ophthalmology, 34,* 755–764.

Li, F., Huang, W., & Zhang, X. (2018). Efficacy and safety of different regimens for primary open-angle glaucoma or ocular hypertension: A systematic review and network meta-analysis. *Acta Ophthalmologica, 96,* e277–e284.

*Liu, D., & Tanna, A. P. (2016). Glaucoma's rising prevalence in the US. *Ophthamology Management, 20,* 38–40.

Lusthaus, J., & Goldberg, I. (2019). Current management of glaucoma. *Medical Journal of Australia, 210*(4), 180–187.

*Marshall, L. L., Hayslett, R. L., & Stevens, G. A. (2018). Therapy for open-angle glaucoma. *Consultant Pharmacist, 33,* 432–445.

Milner, M. S., Beckman, K. A., & Luchs, J. I. (2017). Dysfunctional tear syndrome: Dry eye disease and associated tear film disorders—new strategies for diagnosis and treatment. *Current Opinion in Ophthalmology, 28* (Suppl 1), 3–47.

*Moss, S. E., Klein, R., & Klein, B. E. (2000). Prevalence and risk factors for dry eye syndrome. *Archives of Ophthalmology, 118,* 1264–1268.

Mounsey, A. L., & Gray, R. E. (2016). Topical antihistamines and mast cell stabilizers for treating allergic conjunctivitis. *American Family Physician, 93*(11), 915–916.

Murphy, C., Ogston, S., Cobb, C., et al. (2015). Recent trends in glaucoma surgery in Scotland, England, and Wales. *British Journal of Ophthalmology, 99,* 308–312.

*Narayana, S., & McGee, S. (2015). Bedside diagnosis of the 'red eye': A systematic review. *The American Journal of Medicine, 128*(11), 1220–1224.

*National Eye Institute. (2019). *At a glance: Dry eye.* Bethesda, MD: Author.

*Oray, M., Samra, K. W., Ebrahimiadib, N., et al. (2016). Long-term side effects of glucocorticoids. *Expert Opinion on Drug Safety, 15*(4), 457–465.

Patel, D. S., Arunakirinathan, M., Stuart, A., & Angunawela, R. (2017). Allergic eye disease. *British Medical Journal, 359,* j4706.

Pelletier, A. L., Rojas-Roldan, L., & Coffin, J. (2016). Vision loss in older adults. *American Family Physician, 94*(3), 219–226.

*Pfulgfelder, S. C., & de Paiva, C. S. (2017). The pathophysiology of dry eye disease: What we know and future directions for research. *Ophthalmology, 124*(11 Suppl), S4–S13.

Sambursky, R., Tauber, S., Schirra, F., et al. (2013). Sensitivity and specificity of the AdenoPlus test for diagnosing adenoviral conjunctivitis. *JAMA Ophthalmology, 131,* 17–21.

Schehlein, E. M., Novack, G., & Robin, A. L. (2016). New pharmacotherapy for the treatment of glaucoma. *Expert Opinion on Pharmacotherapy, 18,* 1939–1946.

*Schehlein, E. M., & Robin, A. L. (2019). Rho-associated kinase inhibitors: Evolving strategies in glaucoma treatment. *Drugs, 79,* 1031–1036.

*Serhan, C. N., Chaing, N., & Van Dyke, T. E. (2008). Resolving inflammation: Dual anti-inflammatory and pro-resolution lipid mediators. *Nature Reviews Immunology, 8*(3), 349–361.

*Sethuraman, U., & Kamat, D. (2009). The red eye: Evaluation and management. *Clinical Pediatrics, 48,* 588–600.

Shekwahat, N. S., Shtein, R. M., Blachley, T. S., et al. (2017). Antibiotic prescription fills for acute conjunctivitis among enrollees in a large United States managed care network. *Ophthalmology, 124*(8), 1099–1107.

*Swenson, E. R. (2014). Safety of carbonic anhydrase inhibitors. *Expert Opinion on Drug Safety, 13,* 459–472.

*Tanna, A. P., & Johnson, M. (2018). Rho kinase inhibitors as a novel treatment for glaucoma and ocular hypertension. *Ophthalmology, 125,* 1741–1756.

Tanna, A. P., & Lin, A. B. (2015). Medical therapy: What to add after a prostaglandin analog? *Current Opinion in Ophthalmology, 26,* 116–120.

Tarff, A., & Behrens, A. (2017). Ocular emergencies: Red eye. *Medical Clinics of North America, 101*(3), 615–639.

*Tielsch, J. M., Katz, J., Singh, K., et al. (1991). A population-based evaluation of glaucoma screening: The Baltimore eye survey. *American Journal of Epidemiology, 134,* 1102–1110.

Vivino, F. B., Al-Hashima, I., Khan, Z., et al. (1999). Pilocarpine tablets for the treatment of dry mouth and dry eye symptoms in patients with Sjögren syndrome. *Archives of Internal Medicine, 159,* 174–181.

*Weinrab, R. N., Aung, T., & Medeiros, F. A. (2014). The pathophysiology and treatment of glaucoma: A review. *Journal of the American Medical Association, 311,* 1901–1911.

World Health Organization. (2019). Blindness and vision impairment. Fact Sheet 282.

Yadav, K. S., Rajpurohit, R., & Sharma, S. (2019). Glaucoma: Current treatment and impact of advanced drug delivery systems. *Life Sciences, 221,* 362–376.

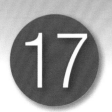

17 Otitis Media and Otitis Externa

Laura L. Bio

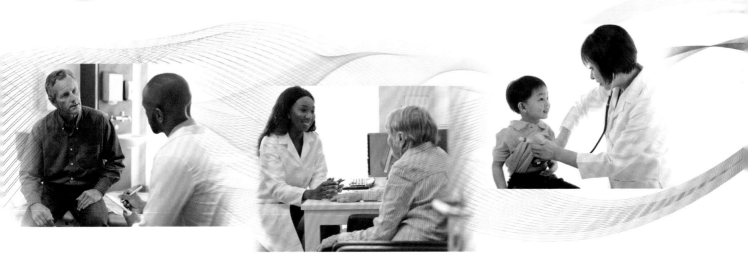

Learning Objectives

1. Compare and contrast the clinical presentations of acute otitis media (AOM) and otitis externa (OE).
2. Ascertain the necessity for antibiotic therapy based on the presentation of a patient with AOM.
3. Determine appropriate management strategies for AOM and OE.

INTRODUCTION

Infections of the ear are a common problem in children due to anatomical predisposition, but adults are susceptible to ear infections as well. The most common infections or inflammatory conditions of the ear include acute otitis media (AOM), otitis media with effusion (OME), and otitis externa (OE; also known as *swimmer's ear* or *tropical ear*). Although antibiotics and vaccination programs have decreased the frequency of these types of infections, identification, diagnosis, and management of these infections are essential to prevent complications such as permanent hearing loss, chronic or recurrent ear infections, mastoiditis, meningitis, and speech or language delay.

OTITIS MEDIA AND OTITIS EXTERNA

Otitis media (OM) continues to impact antibiotic expenditures as the most common infection for which antibiotics are prescribed in children. However, not all cases of OM require antibiotic treatment as it depends on the presentation as AOM or chronic OME (Lieberthal et al., 2013). Despite the stringent 2013 American Academy of Pediatrics (AAP) AOM guidelines, the rate of antibiotic prescribing for AOM has remained constant; however, a downward trend in the rates of AOM episodes has been observed, resulting in reduced direct medical expenditures for AOM (Suaya et al., 2018). Judicious antibiotic prescribing for upper respiratory infections (URIs), including OM, is required to reduce the risk of antibiotic resistance and adverse effects.

AOM is defined as an acute onset of signs and symptoms of a middle ear infection and inflammation, such as middle ear effusion (MEE) and erythema, respectively (**Table 17.1**). AOM is the most common bacterial URI in children and predominantly affects infants and children aged 6 months to 2 years. AOM poses a major social and economic burden, occurring at an alarming rate of 709 million cases worldwide each year, with 51% of these occurring in children under 5 years of age (Monasta et al., 2012). In contrast, OME is characterized by MEE without fever or otalgia and typically is not caused by bacterial infection (Pelton, 2012). OME typically precedes or follows AOM.

OE is defined as an inflammation of the outer ear and ear canal, and may present in acute and chronic forms. While AOM primarily affects children, OE occurs with similar frequency in children and adults. Acute OE roughly affects 1 in 123 persons in the United States based on the 2.4 million visits to ambulatory care centers and emergency departments in 2007 (Centers for Disease Control and Prevention, 2011). Half of the visits occurred among adults aged more than or equal to 20 years compared to children 5 to 14 years of age, accounting for approximately 34% of all visits. OE is most often associated with swimming, local trauma, use of

TABLE 17.1
Comparing Types of Otitis

Type of Otitis	Etiology	Symptoms	Clinical Findings
AOM	*Streptococcus pneumoniae* *Haemophilus influenzae* nontypable *Moraxella catarrhalis*	Otalgia Ear pulling Upper respiratory infection symptoms	Diffuse erythema and bulging of the TM Decreased mobility of the TM
OME	Eustachian tube obstruction causing sterile effusion in the middle ear	Hearing loss that may be manifested by delayed language development in young children or decreased school performance in older children Feeling of ear fullness Popping sensation with swallowing, yawning, or blowing the nose	Clear, yellowish, or bluish-gray fluid behind the TM, with or without air bubbles TM may be retracted with decreased movement
OE	*Pseudomonas aeruginosa,* *Staphylococcus aureus,* *Streptococcus* species	Erythema and swelling of the external canal with otalgia and itching, muffled hearing, watery or thick discharge from the ear	Pain with movement of tragus, raised area of induration on the tragus, swollen external auditory canal, red pustular lesions
Necrotizing (malignant) OE	*P. aeruginosa*	Persistent foul-smelling discharge, deep otalgia	Progressive cranial nerve palsies, granulations in the external ear canal

AOM, acute otitis media; OE, otitis externa; OME, otitis media with effusion; TM, tympanic membrane.

hearing aids, and high, humid temperatures (**Table 17.1**). Unlike AOM, in which the mainstay of treatment is systemic antibiotics, topical antibiotic therapy is usually adequate for the treatment of OE.

CAUSES

Acute Otitis Media and Otitis Media with Effusion

The most frequently isolated bacteria from middle ear fluid during AOM are *Streptococcus pneumoniae*, nontypable *Haemophilus influenzae*, and *Moraxella catarrhalis*, followed by the less common *Streptococcus pyogenes* and *Staphylococcus aureus*. The precise frequency for each AOM pathogen has changed over time due to changes in vaccination coverage. Historically, *S. pneumoniae* dominated AOM etiology, but after implementation of the 13-serotype pneumococcal conjugate vaccine (PCV), beta-lactamase producing *H. influenzae* and *M. catarrhalis* has emerged as more common (Kaur et al., 2017).

Although many cases are caused by bacterial pathogens, viruses play a significant role in the pathogenesis and treatment decisions. Viral pathogens, such as respiratory syncytial virus (RSV), influenza A and B, parainfluenza, enterovirus, and rhinovirus, have been studied extensively and implicated with AOM (Marom et al., 2012). Inflammatory changes in the upper airways caused by viral URI facilitate bacterial AOM by impairing local host defenses, enhancing the bacteria's ability to ascend the nasopharynx, and infecting the middle ear. For example, RSV has been recovered from 2% to 20% of AOM tympanocenteses.

Otitis Externa

Ninety-eight percent of OE cases in the United States are caused by bacteria, most commonly *Pseudomonas aeruginosa* and *S. aureus* (Rosenfeld et al., 2014). The etiology of OE is different than that of OM because the flora of the external auditory canal is similar to that of the skin including *Staphylococcus epidermidis*, *S. aureus*, *Corynebacteria* species, and *Propionibacterium acnes*. Fungal OE, otomycosis, predominantly *Aspergillus* and *Candida* species, cause less than 5% of OE in the United States (Boyce & Balakrishnan, 2018) and may be associated with prolonged use of topical antibiotics. Chronic OE may be noninfectious but caused by inflammatory skin disorders and allergic reactions. Necrotizing (malignant) OE results from invasive infection of the external ear canal and is predominantly caused by *P. aeruginosa*.

PATHOPHYSIOLOGY

Otitis Media

AOM frequently follows a URI (usually of viral etiology) in which the eustachian tube is obstructed secondary to inflamed mucous membranes (Marom et al., 2012). The pathophysiology of AOM is multifactorial but is mainly the result of eustachian tube dysfunction. The eustachian tube protects the middle ear from nasopharyngeal secretions, provides drainage of secretions produced in the middle ear into the nasopharynx, and permits equilibration of air pressure to atmospheric pressure in the middle ear. The structure of a child's eustachian tube differs from that of an adult's. The adult eustachian tube lies at 45 degrees to the horizontal plane and allows for secretions to drain from the middle ear to the nasopharynx. The child's eustachian tube, however, is short and horizontal. When a child develops mild inflammation or edema of the eustachian tube, the ear has difficulty clearing secretions due to the almost horizontal placement of the eustachian tube. Persistent secretions, incomplete drainage, and the absence of aeration promote an environment for bacterial growth within the middle ear, resulting in AOM (Marom et al., 2012). The incidence of AOM peaks during 6 to 12 months of age and in the winter months due to high correlation with URIs. Risk factors for AOM include day care attendance, family history of AOM, male sex (only in the first year of life), non-Hispanic white race, and children who attend day care or are relatives of children in day care (Kaur et al., 2017). Exposure to second-hand smoke has also been associated, however inconsistently, with an increased risk of AOM.

OME occurs when fluid builds up in the middle ear which may occur after AOM or during URI due to eustachian tube dysfunction, and can be associated with conductive hearing loss (Rosenfeld et al., 2016). The major difference between OME and AOM is that in OME the fluid is not actively infectious and pain may be absent or minimal.

Otitis Externa

OE is cellulitis of the ear canal skin and subdermis, which is typically unilateral and associated with head immersion in water, especially freshwater or hot tubs (Rosenfeld et al., 2014). Persons of all ages are at risk for developing this infection. The common predisposing factor is swimming. Additional risk factors for OE include eczema or seborrhea, resulting in excessive scratching, trauma from cerumen removal, use of hearing aids, and immunocompromised states such as diabetes (Boyce & Balakrishnan, 2018). Disruption of the ear canal homeostasis from prolonged periods of water exposure, loss of the protective cerumen barrier, and disruption of the epithelium all result in varied pH and compromised local immune defenses, which allows bacteria and other pathogens to produce infection.

Resistance

The increasing rates of antimicrobial resistance are a major concern worldwide and warrants the judicious use of antibiotics. Common bacterial mechanisms of resistance associated with AOM include production of antibiotic-inactivating enzymes, such as beta-lactamases, and alteration of drug-binding sites, such as mutations in the penicillin-binding protein. Beta-lactamase production is the mechanism by which bacteria such as *H. influenzae* and *M. catarrhalis* develop resistance, with a prevalence of 45% and 100% in tympanocentesis specimens, respectively (Kaur et al., 2017). Production of these enzymes renders many beta-lactam antibiotics useless. Beta-lactamase inhibitors in combination with beta-lactam therapy, such as amoxicillin–clavulanic acid or beta-lactamase stable cephalosporins (i.e., cefixime, cefpodoxime), can overcome this mechanism of resistance. Therefore, these agents should

be recommended for treatment if these bacteria are suspected, specifically in the setting of treatment failure or recurrent infection. A detailed discussion of treatment options is presented in the Initiating Drug Therapy section of this chapter.

Historically, penicillin had been the mainstay of treatment against *S. pneumoniae*, but increasing prevalence of penicillin-intermediate and penicillin-resistant strains has discouraged the use of penicillin and its derivatives. The mechanism of resistance is alteration of the penicillin-binding site, resulting in elevated minimum inhibitory concentration. Drug-resistant *S. pneumoniae* (DRSP) remains a threat in the treatment of AOM. However, following the introduction of the PCV with 7 serotypes (PCV-7) in 2000 and subsequent 13-serotype vaccine (PCV-13) in 2010, not only have the number of pneumococcal isolates decreased but the incidence of DRSP strains isolated from cultures of children with OM has also decreased, including serotype 19A (Kaplan et al., 2015).

DIAGNOSTIC CRITERIA AND CLINICAL PRESENTATION

Acute Otitis Media

The differentiation between AOM and OME is dependent on an accurate and consistent OM diagnosis, as emphasized in the 2013 AAP guidelines. However, difficulties remain, and AOM diagnoses unsubstantiated by physical examination findings result in inappropriate and overprescribing of antibiotics. For example, cerumen or debris may impede otoscopic examination of the ear canal and tympanic membrane (TM), and may require removal for visualization. Therefore, novel noninvasive technologies are highly desirable and could improve the diagnosis of OM, such as optical coherence tomography (Shirai & Preciado, 2019). However, the validity and reliability of new methods must be proven prior to adoption; a thorough patient history and physical examination remain the standard of care.

AOM presents abruptly with symptoms such as fever, otalgia, and irritability. The averbal infant may express otalgia and irritability by tugging, rubbing, or holding the affected ear, and excessive crying, or changes in sleep or behavior pattern. Visualization of the TM via otoscope reveals a bulging and erythematous TM that is immobile to pneumatic otoscopy indicating MEE. Tips for pneumatic otoscopy can be found in the "Otitis Media with Effusion: Clinical Practice Guideline" (Rosenfeld et al., 2016). The diagnosis of AOM requires abrupt onset of symptoms (less than 48 hours), presence of MEE, and signs or symptoms of middle ear inflammation (e.g., otalgia, erythema of the TM, hearing loss) (Lieberthal et al., 2013). Otorrhea may also be present and a sign of TM perforation which will greatly impact the decision to treat with antibiotics (Table 17.2).

The differentiation between AOM and OME is imperative since OME should not be treated with antibiotics due to noninfectious etiology. The absence of acute inflammatory signs and symptoms presumes a diagnosis of OME. Patients with OME

TABLE 17.2

Diagnostic Criteria for Acute Otitis Media

1. History of acute onset of signs/symptoms
2. Presence of middle ear effusion (indicated by one of the following):
   a. Bulging of TM
   b. Limited or absent TM mobility
   c. Otorrhea
   d. Air–fluid interface behind TM
3. Signs and symptoms of middle ear inflammation
   a. Erythema of TM
   b. Otalgia

TM, tympanic membrane.

are usually asymptomatic but may complain of ear fullness and hearing loss. Upon otoscopic examination, the TM may appear normal or with an air-fluid level behind the TM with no signs or symptoms of middle ear inflammation; the only sign of effusion is reduced mobility (Rosenfeld et al., 2016). Tympanometry is an objective tool for the diagnosis of OME as a confirmatory measure or alternative to pneumatic otoscopy by assessing TM mobility. When the diagnosis of OME is uncertain after pneumatic otoscopy is used or attempted, tympanometry is recommended in specific situations, for example, child intolerance to otoscopy, unreliable equipment, TM obstruction.

INITIATING DRUG THERAPY

Goals of Drug Therapy

The goals of therapy for AOM include symptomatic pain relief, appropriate use of antibiotics to prevent complications, and judicious use of antibiotics to prevent future antimicrobial resistance. Symptomatic pain relief can be achieved with over-the-counter analgesics such as acetaminophen or a nonsteroidal antiinflammatory drug (NSAID) such as ibuprofen, and should be offered regardless of antibiotic use, unless hypersensitivity exists. Local topical anesthetics containing benzocaine or procaine should be reserved for children over 5 years of age and may provide brief additional pain relief. Antibiotics are utilized to eradicate the infecting organism and prevent complications such as mastoiditis and hearing impairment. However, due to concerns of microbial resistance and adverse effects, clinicians should avoid unnecessary use of antibiotics.

Observational Therapy versus Antibiotic Therapy

The decision to manage AOM with antibiotics is based on patient-specific characteristics such as age, bilateral involvement, presence of otorrhea, and severity of illness (Lieberthal et al., 2013). All patients with suspected AOM who are younger than ages 6 months should receive antibiotics due to diagnostic difficulties and high risk of complications. For patients with non-severe, unilateral AOM without otorrhea who are older than age

6 months, the role of antibiotics is unclear, and the decision to provide symptomatic relief with close observation can be made. The decision to observe and withhold antibiotics is based on the high rate of spontaneous resolution (approximately 80%) and overlap of nonspecific AOM symptoms with viral URIs (Hersh et al., 2013). Observation therapy requires implementation of follow-up within 48 to 72 hours to ensure antibiotics can be initiated if the child's condition worsens or fails to improve. The technique for observational therapy is controversial: observe with or without a prescription with instructions to fill after 2 to 3 days if symptoms persist (Chao et al., 2008). This decision should be based on the prescriber's discussion with the caregiver and assessment of likelihood to adhere to the plan.

Patients with otorrhea or severe symptoms (i.e., toxic-appearing child, persistent otalgia more than 48 hours, temperature more than or equal to 102.2°F in the past 48 hours, or uncertain access to follow up) require antibiotic therapy regardless of age. If AOM is identified bilaterally, the decision to treat is based on the patient's age: AOM requires antibiotic therapy only if the patient is less than 2 years of age. Patients 2 years old or greater with bilateral AOM without otorrhea or severe symptoms may initially be managed with observation therapy after a discussion with the child's family to understand the decision.

Penicillins

First-line therapy for AOM is high-dose amoxicillin for adequate middle ear penetration and to overcome intermediate-resistant *S. pneumoniae* (Lieberthal et al., 2013; **Figure 17.1**; **Table 17.3**). If the child has received amoxicillin in the past 30 days or has concurrent purulent conjunctivitis or allergy to penicillin, amoxicillin may not be appropriate. Recent receipt of amoxicillin or failure to improve while on amoxicillin raises concern of resistant organisms causing the infection, such as *M. catarrhalis* and *H. influenzae*. Therefore, the addition of beta-lactamase inhibitor to a beta-lactam or use of a beta-lactam stable cephalosporin (see Cephalosporins section following) is necessary. Amoxicillin–clavulanate is a combination product commercially available in the United States in various concentrations of the oral suspension, chewables, tablets, and extended-release tablets. The major difference among these formulations is the ratio of clavulanate to amoxicillin and therefore may not be interchanged. The most common adverse effect of antibiotics is diarrhea, which is even more so with amoxicillin–clavulanate when the dosage of clavulanate is too high (Hoberman et al., 2017). Since high-dose amoxicillin is recommended for AOM treatment, use of amoxicillin–clavulanate standard ratio (clavulanate to amoxicillin, 1:7) would result in excess exposure of clavulanate and diarrhea. Therefore, the ES oral suspension formulation (ratio 1:14) or XR formulation for tablets (ratio 1:16) should be recommended to limit excessive exposure to clavulanate and therefore reduce the incidence of diarrhea.

Cephalosporins

If the presence of a penicillin allergy is elicited from the patient or caregiver, the type of reaction should be assessed.

AOM Treatment Algorithm

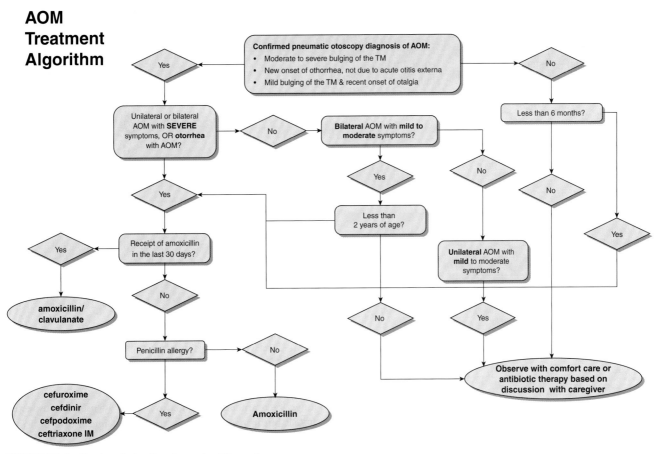

FIGURE 17–1   Treatment algorithm for acute otitis media.

AOM, acute otitis media; IM, intramuscular; TM, tympanic membrane.

TABLE 17.3

Overview of Antibiotics for Acute Otitis Media

Generic (Trade) Name	Usual Pediatric Daily Dose	Usual Adult Daily Dose	Adverse Effects	Dosage Formulations
Amoxicillin (various)	80–90 mg/kg/d PO divided into 2 doses per day	2–3 g/d PO divided into 2 to 3 doses per day	Abnormal taste, diarrhea, headache, skin rash	Suspension, PO: 125 mg/5 mL, 250 mg/5 mL, 400 mg/mL Chewable, PO: 125 mg, 200 mg, 250 mg, 400 mg Tablet, PO: 500 mg, 875 mg Capsule: 250 mg, 500 mg
Amoxicillin–clavulanate (Augmentin)	80–90 mg/kg/d based on amoxicillin component PO divided into 2 doses per day	250–500 mg PO q8h; or 875–1000 mg PO q12h	Abnormal taste, diarrhea, headache	Suspension, PO: amoxicillin* 200 mg/5 mL, 400 mg/5 mL; Augmentin ES-600†: 600 mg/5 mL Chewable, PO:* amoxicillin 200 mg, 400 mg Tablet, PO:‡ 500 mg, 875 mg Augmentin XR§ 1,000 mg
Ceftriaxone (Rocephin)	50 mg/kg/d IM once daily for 1 or 3 days	1 g IM once daily for 1 or 3 days	Skin rash, injection site reactions	IM: 250–350 mg/mL with lidocaine
Cefdinir (Omnicef)	14 mg/kg/d PO divided into 2 doses per day	300 mg PO BID	Skin rash and GI upset but otherwise generally well tolerated	Suspension, PO: 125 mg/5 mL, 250 mg/5 mL Capsule, PO: 300 mg

(Continued)

TABLE 17.3

Overview of Antibiotics for Acute Otitis Media (*Continued*)

Generic (Trade) Name	Usual Pediatric Daily Dose	Usual Adult Daily Dose	Adverse Effects	Dosage Formulations
Cefpodoxime (Vantin)	10 mg/kg/d PO once daily	200 mg PO BID	Skin rash and GI upset but otherwise generally well tolerated	Suspension, PO: 50 mg/5 mL, 100 mg/5 mL Tablet, PO: 100 mg, 200 mg
Cefuroxime (Ceftin)	30 mg/kg/d PO divided into 2 doses per day	250–500 mg PO BID	Skin rash and GI upset but otherwise generally well tolerated	Suspension, PO: 125 mg/5 mL, 250 mg/5 mL Tablet, PO: 250 mg, 500 mg
Clindamycin (various)	30 mg/kg/d PO divided into 3 doses per day	300–450 mg PO q6–8h	Diarrhea, *C. difficile–*associated diarrhea, rash	Suspension, PO: 75 mg/5 mL Capsule, PO: 75 mg, 150 mg, 300 mg

*Standard ratio of clavulanate to amoxicillin of 1:7.

†ES ratio of clavulanate to amoxicillin of 1:14.

‡Standard 125 mg of clavulanate per tablet.

§XR ratio of clavulanate to amoxicillin of 1:16.

ES, extra strength; GI, gastrointestinal; IM, intramuscular; TM, tympanic membrane; XR, extended release.

Fortunately, the cross-reactivity between penicillins and most second-generation and third-generation cephalosporins is low due to distinct chemical structures (Norton et al., 2018). Therefore, oral formulations of cefdinir and cefpodoxime, which are third-generation cephalosporins, and cefuroxime, which is a second-generation cephalosporin, are recommended for penicillin-allergic patients, regardless of reaction type (both anaphylactic and urticarial reaction) (**Table 17.3**).

For patients who are persistently vomiting or cannot tolerate oral medication for other reasons, ceftriaxone, a third-generation cephalosporin, administered as an intramuscular (IM) injection, is an option as a single dose for initial treatment or daily dosing for a total of three for repeat antibiotic treatment due to treatment failure.

Macrolides

Historically, macrolides including azithromycin and erythromycin were recommended for patients with a history of anaphylactic reaction to penicillins. Due to limited macrolide efficacy against both *S. pneumoniae* and *H. influenzae* and realized lower rate of cross-sensitivity to cephalosporins among penicillin-allergic patients than previously reported, macrolides are no longer recommended by the AAP for AOM (Lieberthal et al., 2013).

Clindamycin

Similar to macrolides, clindamycin historically was an option for patients who had an anaphylactic to penicillin. But again, due to concerns of clindamycin's lack of activity against gram-negative bacteria, such as *H. influenzae* or *M. catarrhalis*, it is no

longer recommended. Clindamycin may be used for suspected DRSP, but it may not be effective against multi–drug-resistant strains, such as serotype 19A (Kaplan et al., 2015).

Selecting the Most Appropriate Agent

Figure 17.1 outlines the process for selecting the most appropriate agent.

First-Line Antibiotic Therapy

Once the decision to initiate antibiotics is made, regardless of whether an observation period has passed or not, the same antibiotic decision algorithm applies (**Figure 17.1**). Amoxicillin is considered the first-line treatment for AOM in patients who show severe symptoms and who did not have a course of amoxicillin in the past 30 days or are not allergic to penicillin. For those patients who had a course of amoxicillin in the recent past, treatment with the combination amoxicillin–clavulanate is indicated. In patients with penicillin allergy, one of the cephalosporins is indicated as the first-line treatment.

Second-Line Antibiotic Therapy

Patients who receive antibiotics for more than 72 hours with persistent, severe symptoms are deemed treatment failure. This may be due to the presence of a resistant organism, a viral infection which would be unresponsive to antibiotic therapy, inadequate concentration of antibiotic in the middle ear, or noncompliance with the prescribed regimen. Treatment failure requires escalation to the next step in management and is highly dependent on the initial therapy. If the patient's condition does not improve with high-dose amoxicillin treatment, therapy should be switched to amoxicillin–clavulanate. For patients who fail either amoxicillin–clavulanate or an oral cephalosporin (i.e., cefpodoxime, cefuroxime, cefdinir), escalation to ceftriaxone as a single daily IM or intravenous injection for a 3-day course is recommended (Leibovitz et al., 2000). Tympanocentesis for bacteriologic diagnosis is an option for patients who have repeatedly failed therapy. The effusion is sent for Gram stain, culture, and antibiotic susceptibility testing to tailor therapy to the causative organism.

Monitoring Patient Response

The duration of antibiotic therapy is dependent on the severity and age of the patient: severe AOM or patients younger than age 2 years should receive a 10-day course, patients of age 2 years or older should be treated with a 7-day course, and those of age 6 years and older may benefit from a shorter, 5-day course of therapy (Lieberthal et al., 2013). Reduced duration of 5 days was compared to a 10-day duration of amoxicillin/clavulanate in children of age 6 to 23 months with AOM; this was associated with significantly worse outcomes (Hoberman et al., 2016). Symptom resolution should occur within 2 to 3 days, and the patient should achieve complete resolution of AOM symptoms after 7 days; however, asymptomatic MEE may persist if inspected by pneumatic otoscope. The patient or caregiver must be counseled to continue antibiotic therapy even if symptoms resolve before completion of the entire therapy course to prevent recurrence.

RECURRENT ACUTE OTITIS MEDIA

Recurrent AOM is defined as more than 3 episodes within 6 months or 4 episodes within 12 months, with 1 episode in the preceding 6 months. Recurrence is most commonly due to relapse (infection with the same organism) or reinfection (infection with a different organism). Management of recurrent AOM remains controversial, but may include episodic antibiotic treatment, adenoidectomy, or tympanostomy tube insertion. However, the effect of these interventions on OM recurrence is inconsistent, and evidence is contradictory. The American Academy of Otolaryngology: Head and Neck Surgery Foundation published guidelines stating tympanostomy tube insertion should be offered to children with bilateral OME and documented hearing difficulties for 3 months or longer (Rosenfeld et al., 2013). An additional indication is for children at increased risk of speech, language, or learning problems from OME due to baseline sensory, physical, cognitive, or behavioral factors. Myringotomy and insertion of tympanostomy tubes improve AOM symptoms by allowing drainage of the effusion; however, reduction in OME recurrence is not consistent. Complications of tube placement include otorrhea, myringosclerosis, perforation, and tissue granulation as seen on otoscopic examination.

Prophylaxis and/or Prevention

Use of antibiotic prophylaxis for recurrent AOM is controversial due to lack of supporting evidence. Cost, adverse effects, and contribution to bacterial resistance emergence do not outweigh the small reduction in frequency of AOM with long-term antibiotic prophylaxis. Therefore, antibiotic prophylaxis is no longer recommended for children with recurrent AOM.

The Centers for Disease Control and Prevention's (CDC) childhood vaccination schedule should be followed to reduce preventable diseases. The vaccines pertinent to the prevention of AOM are the pneumococcal, *H. influenzae* type B (HiB), and influenza vaccine. Please refer to the prevention section of this chapter for a detailed discussion on targeted vaccine groups and current recommendations.

OTITIS EXTERNA

Diagnostic Criteria and Clinical Presentation

OE diagnosis requires all three criteria: symptoms of ear canal inflammation such as otalgia (often severe), itching, or fullness; signs of ear canal inflammation such as tenderness of tragus and/or pinna; and an erythematous ear canal with occasional otorrhea (Rosenfeld et al., 2014). Hearing is usually unaffected unless pressure and fullness in the ear exist, producing occasional conductive or sensorineural hearing loss. Jaw pain may also be present. Acute OE diagnosis requires rapid onset of signs and symptoms within 48 hours in the past 3 weeks. Differentiation from other possible causes of otalgia, otorrhea, and inflammation of the ear canal, such as AOM, is important due to overlapping pathologies that require different treatment management.

Patient evaluation should include history of symptoms, water exposure, local trauma, past medical history of inflammatory skin disorders or diabetes, and history of ear surgeries or local radiotherapy. As mentioned in the Diagnostic Criteria and Clinical Presentation section, otoscopic examination may require cerumen or debris removal. If the TM is bulging or erythematous, the patient should be worked up for OM. Examination of pinna and adjacent skin for regional lymphadenitis and cellulitis is included as well. Otomycosis, that is, fungal OE, presents with intense pruritus, aural fullness, clear otorrhea, and fluffy, cotton-like debris in the external ear canal upon examination (Kesser, 2011). Necrotizing OE diagnosis is confirmed with an elevated erythrocyte sedimentation rate and abnormal computed tomography or magnetic resonance imaging scan to detect a skull base osteomyelitis (Rosenfeld et al., 2014).

INITIATING DRUG THERAPY

Goals of Drug Therapy

The goals of OE treatment are similar to those of OM: decreasing the accompanying pain and eradicating the causative organisms.

This can be accomplished with systemic analgesic and/or antiinflammatory drugs and direct ototopical application of antimicrobial agents, respectively.

Pain relief can be achieved with orally administered acetaminophen or NSAIDs given alone or in combination with an opioid for mild to moderate pain (Rosenfeld et al., 2014). Topical anesthetic drops, such as benzocaine otic solution, are not recommended due to potential masking of underlying disease states and lack of Food and Drug Administration (FDA) approval for OE indication.

Management of OE begins with clearing any obstructing debris or excess cerumen from the canal (i.e., aural toilet) and checking the integrity of the TM to determine if extension beyond the ear canal is present. Topical therapy is the mainstay of OE treatment (i.e., antibiotics, steroids, or combination treatments). Topical antimicrobials are preferred over systemic administration to achieve high concentration at the site of infection while reducing systemic adverse effects to the patient. Selection of the appropriate product must include evaluation of the patient's infection, predisposing factors, adherence, and medication costs (Boyce & Balakrishnan, 2018). The duration of ototopical antibiotic treatment is 7 to 10 days.

Oral antibiotics may be recommended for patients with acute OE infections extending outside the ear canal or certain host factors such as diabetes, immune deficiency, or inability to effectively deliver topic therapy. Systemic antibiotics should also be considered for patients with recurrent episodes of OE or clinical signs of necrotizing (i.e., malignant) OE, which is a serious and potentially life-threatening complication of the infection extending to the mastoid or temporal bone. Immunocompromised patients, including the elderly with diabetes and human immunodeficiency virus, are at the highest risk of necrotizing OE. Chronic OE is a single episode lasting longer than 3 months or 4 or more episodes in 1 year; it is often the result of allergies, chronic dermatologic conditions, or inadequately treated acute OE (Rosenfeld et al., 2014; Schaefer & Baugh, 2012).

Antibiotic Therapy

If edema prevents application of the drops, a compressed cellulose ear wick can be placed into the ear to facilitate drug delivery. The medication should be applied to the wick until inflammation subsides and the wick falls out or is removed as instructed by a clinician (usually within 24–48 hours). Ototopical antimicrobials for OE include aminoglycosides, polymyxin B, and quinolones. Ototopical selection is based on several factors including TM condition (e.g., perforation, tympanostomy tubes), risk of adverse effect, adherence issues, cost, patient preference, and physician experience/preference (**Table 17.4**). Systemic antimicrobials are not recommended for uncomplicated, acute OE, but they are recommended for infections extending beyond the ear canal or when certain factors are present, such as uncontrolled diabetes, immunocompromised status, history of radiotherapy, or inability to deliver topical antibiotics. Otomycosis requires debridement and topical antifungal therapy, such as a powdered mixture of chloromycetin, sulfanilamide, amphotericin, and hydrocortisone (Kesser, 2011). Necrotizing OE is managed with surgical debridement and systemic, prolonged antipseudomonal and antistaphylococcal antibiotics.

Fluoroquinolones

The fluoroquinolone antibiotics, that is, ciprofloxacin and ofloxacin, are often used to treat infections associated with OE, due to its ideal antipseudomonal activity. Higher bacteriologic and clinical cure rates have been observed with quinolone-containing otic drops than with non-quinolone therapy (Mösges et al., 2011). In addition, these agents may be more tolerable than neomycin–polymyxin B due to infrequent administration, less adverse effects (e.g., stinging), and lower risk of hypersensitivity. This information must be balanced with the high cost of quinolone otic preparations. Ciprofloxacin 0.3%–dexamethasone 0.1% (Ciprodex) and ofloxacin (Floxin Otic) are commercially available fluoroquinolone otic formulations. (See **Table 17.4** for dosage and adverse effect information.) However, the addition of

TABLE 17.4

Overview of Treatment for Otitis Externa

Generic (Trade) Name and Dosage	Selected Adverse Events	Contraindications	Special Considerations
Polymyxin B sulfate, neomycin, and hydrocortisone Children: 3 drops into ear canal TID–QID for maximum of 10 days Adults: 4 drops into ear canal TID–QID for maximum of 10 days	Superinfection, contact dermatitis, ototoxicity with prolonged use	Herpes simplex, fungal, tubercular, or viral otic infections Perforated eardrum Prescribe with caution in pregnancy (category C drug) and in breast-feeding patients	Use otic drops for a maximum of 10 days
Ofloxacin (Floxin) Children 6 months–12 years: 5 drops into ear canal once daily for 10 days Children >12 years and adults: 10 drops once daily for 10 days	Pruritus, site reaction, dizziness, earache, vertigo, taste perversion, paresthesia, rash	Perforated eardrum Prescribe with caution in pregnancy (category C drug) and in breast-feeding patients	Use otic drops for a maximum of 10 days

a corticosteroid to the antibiotic formulation is controversial. The antiinflammatory effects of corticosteroids potentially include reduced pain, swelling, and itching. Ciprofloxacin otic solution was found to be non-inferior to the corticosteroid plus antibiotic otic combination solution, polymixin B–neomycin–hydrocortisone based on clinical cure (Drehobl et al., 2008). The risk of local immunosuppression and potential hypersensitivity reactions should be studied before recommending corticosteroid–fluoroquinolone antibiotic combination otic solutions first line. Of note, the Floxin Otic preparation does not contain a corticosteroid.

Aminoglycoside Antibiotics

The combination product neomycin sulfate–polymyxin B–hydrocortisone acetate (Cortisporin) has historically been used for OE. The combination of the gram-positive coverage of the aminoglycoside neomycin and the antipseudomonal activity of polymyxin has made this combination the gold standard of treatment in the past. As stated in the Fluoroquinolones section, the addition of a corticosteroid with this combination remains controversial. Concerns associated with the side effect profile, particularly the hypersensitivity reactions related to neomycin (and possibly the preservative), and frequency of dose administration must be weighed against the low cost for this generic product. Furthermore, ototoxicity with neomycin has been reported, although the number of reports is low and the data are speculative. Due to concerns of ototoxicity, aminoglycosides should not be used if the TM is not intact since the risk of injury outweighs the benefit and efficacious, non-ototoxic antibiotics are available (i.e., quinolones).

Selecting the Most Appropriate Agent

First-Line Therapy

OE with intact or non-intact TM is treated initially with a fluoroquinolone antibiotic. The selection of ciprofloxacin versus ofloxacin depends on the formulary status of the agents, as well as the clinician's experience with added corticosteroids (**Table 17.5**).

Second-Line Therapy

Neomycin-polymyxin B combinations are considered second-line agents, primarily due to their side effect profile and precaution against use for nonintact TM OE. The lower cost of these agents, however, warrants consideration, particularly in patients without insurance or other means of paying for the more expensive fluoroquinolones.

Third-Line Therapy

Antifungals can be considered if a patient fails to respond to initial topical antibiotic therapy (e.g., clotrimazole, miconazole, bifonazole, ciclopirox olamine, tolnaftate) (Vennewald et al., 2010). Systemic antibiotic therapy with *P. aeruginosa* and *S. aureus* coverage is recommended if ear canal obstruction cannot be relieved or if infection extends beyond the ear canal.

TABLE 17.5

Recommended Order of Treatment for Otitis Externa

Order	Agents	Comments
First line	Fluoroquinolone drops	Floxin is not recommended for patients <6 months. Use all otic drops for a maximum of 10 days
Second line	Combination neomycin-polymyxin B drops	All drops are contraindicated in cases of perforated eardrum
Third line	Antifungal drops Systemic antipseudomonal or antistaphylococcal agent	Consider if a patient fails to respond to initial topical antibiotic therapy. Consider if ear canal obstruction cannot be relieved or if infection extends beyond the ear canal

Special Population Considerations

Children with tympanostomy tubes placed within 1 year of an acute OE episode are assumed to have nonintact TM and therefore should not receive an ototoxic antibiotic. Historical concerns of fluoroquinolone use in children are not relevant due to the minimal systemic absorption and small dose administered ototopically.

MONITORING PATIENT RESPONSE

Symptom improvement should occur within 48 to 72 hours after appropriate treatment initiation, but complete symptom resolution may take up to 2 weeks. Reassessment of patients who fail initial therapy may include addressing patient adherence with therapy, re-examination of the ear canal and TM, a culture of the ear canal to identify causes of infection and target therapy, and consideration of underlying dermatologic disorders.

PREVENTION

Prevention is the key and plays a significant role in reducing the overall burden of illness (e.g., office visits, antibiotic expenditures, severity of illness). Vaccination programs have been shown to have a favorable outcome on decreasing the overall incidence of the AOM, namely, those caused by *S. pneumoniae*, *H. influenzae*, and influenza virus.

The introduction of the heptavalent pneumococcal polysaccharide conjugate vaccine (PCV-7, Prevnar-7; serotypes 4, 6B, 9V, 14, 18C, 19F, and 23F) decreased the overall incidence of invasive pneumococcal disease by 69% in children younger than age 2 from 1998 to 1999 and 2001 (Pichichero & Casey, 2007). Specifically, reductions in OM office visits and severity of illness have been observed since the introduction of the vaccine (Black et al., 2000). When the 7-valent vaccine was brought to the market in 2000, the serotypes represented approximately 70% of the serotypes found in AOM. Unfortunately, after the introduction of PCV-7, otopathogenic *S. pneumoniae* serotype 19A has been identified as being resistant to all FDA-approved antibiotics for children with AOM (Pichichero & Casey, 2007). A 13-valent pneumococcal conjugate vaccine (PCV-13, Prevnar-13) was approved by the U.S. FDA in 2010 to contain the 6 serotypes responsible for 63% of invasive pneumococcal disease (serotypes 1, 3, 5, 6A, 7F, and 19A, in addition to the 7 serotypes of PCV-7). PCV-13 has replaced PCV-7 in the childhood vaccination schedule (Centers for Disease Control and Prevention, 2020).

In addition to the routine pneumococcal vaccination with PCV, the polysaccharide (PPSV) is recommended for children older than age 2 years with comorbidities. It is not indicated in infants younger than age 2 years due to poor immunogenicity to PPSV. PPSV contains 23 pneumococcal serotypes and is indicated for children with chronic diseases such as chronic lung disease or congenital heart disease, cochlear implant, and more. Check the most up-to-date recommendations from the Advisory Committee on Immunization Practices (ACIP).

The HiB and influenza vaccines are also routinely recommended in the childhood immunization schedule. The HiB vaccine is a polysaccharide, conjugated protein carrier indicated for infants of age 6 weeks and older. The influenza vaccine is recommended for all persons over 6 months of age, but the selection of the correct formulation is dependent on the age of the patient. Influenza vaccine is available as a trivalent or quadrivalent inactivated influenza vaccine (IIV) for IM injection, and live attenuated vaccine (LAIV) as an intranasal administration. The IIV requires two doses during a single flu season for children of age 6 months through 8 years if it's their first vaccinated season, depending on the current ACIP. The minimum age to receive the LAIV is age 2 years. In addition, the LAIV should not be given to individuals who are not immunocompromised or pregnant. Current restrictions on LAIV use must be checked before recommending (Centers for Disease Control and Prevention, 2020).

For up-to-date ACIP vaccine administration schedules, check the CDC Web site at www.cdc.gov/vaccines (Centers for Disease Control and Prevention, 2020).

PATIENT EDUCATION

Drug Information

Administration of ototopical products requires patient education and potentially an assistant to administer the drops for them as self-administration may be difficult. Ototopicals should be warmed to body temperature before instillation to avoid dizziness. To warm the otic solution, the patient should hold or roll the bottle in the hand for 1 to 2 minutes. To instill drops, the patient should lie with the affected ear upward, administer enough drops to fill the ear canal (or saturate the ear wick if in place), gently tug the auricle to help expel trapped air and assist drug delivery, and remain in this position for about 5 minutes to help the solution penetrate into the ear canal.

Nutrition/Lifestyle Changes

The use of hypoallergenic ear canal molds when swimming or showering is controversial for the prevention of OE. Drying the ears with a cool hair dryer to aid removal of fluid after swimming may be beneficial. The patient should avoid trying to remove ear wax mechanically with cotton-tipped swabs to prevent trauma. It is important for the patient to avoid water in the ear until the infection clears (usually 5–7 days) and for 4 to 6 weeks afterward. To accomplish this, hair can be washed in a sink instead of a shower or tub, and the patient can use a shower cap when bathing.

Complementary and Alternative Medications

"Home remedies" of a 1:1 solution of white vinegar and rubbing alcohol have never been evaluated or substantiated and therefore are not recommended for OE. In addition, ear candles are not efficacious and may be harmful (e.g., hearing loss).

CASE STUDY 1

C.J., age 17, is on his high school swim team. He presents with sudden onset of right ear pain that worsens at night. He says that the pain intensifies when he touches his ear and that he has a feeling of fullness in the ear. On examination of his right ear, the auditory canal is edematous and erythematous, with yellow crusting. His temperature is 97.8°F, and his tympanic membrane (TM) is pearly gray with landmarks intact. His left ear exam is within normal limits (Learning Objectives 1 and 3).

DIAGNOSIS: OTITIS EXTERNA

1. What drug therapy would you prescribe for C.J.? Why?
2. What are the parameters for monitoring success of the therapy?
3. What lifestyle changes would you recommend to C.J.?

Bibliography

Starred references are cited in the text.

*Black, S. L., Shinefield, H., Fireman, B., et al. (2000). Efficacy, safety and immunogenicity of heptavalent pneumococcal conjugate vaccine in children. Northern California Kaiser Permanente Vaccine Study Center Group. *Pediatric Infectious Disease Journal, 19*(3), 187–195.

*Boyce, T. G., & Balakrishnan, K. (2018). Otitis externa and necrotizing otitis externa. In S. Long (Ed.), *Principles and practices of pediatric infectious diseases* (5th ed.). Edinburgh, UK: Saunders.

*Centers for Disease Control and Prevention. (2011). Estimated burden of acute otitis externa—United States, 2003–2007. *MMWR Morbidity and Mortality Weekly Report, 60,* 605–609.

*Centers for Disease Control and Prevention. (2020). Immunization schedules. Retrieved from http://www.cdc.gov/vaccines/schedules/

*Chao, J. H., Kunkov, S., Reyes, L. B., et al. (2008). Comparison of two approaches to observation therapy for acute otitis media in the emergency department. *Pediatrics, 121*(5), e1352–e1356.

*Drehobl, M., Guerrero, J. L., Lacarte, P. R., et al. (2008). Comparison of efficacy and safety of ciprofloxacin otic solution 0.2% versus polymyxin B-neomycin-hydrocortisone in the treatment of acute diffuse otitis externa. *Current Medical Research Opinion, 24,* 3531–3542.

*Hersh, A. L., Jackson, M. A., Hicks, L. A., et al. (2013). Principles of judicious antibiotic prescribing for bacterial upper respiratory tract infections in pediatrics, *Pediatrics, 132,* 1146–1154.

*Hoberman, A., Paradise, J. L., Rockette, H. E., et al. (2016). Shortened antimicrobial treatment for acute otitis media in young children. *New England Journal of Medicine, 375*(25), 2446–2456.

*Hoberman, A., Paradise, J. L., Rockette, H. E., et al. (2017). Reduced-concentration clavulanate for young children with acute otitis media. *Antimicrobial Agents and Chemotherapy, 61*(7), e00238–e00217.

*Kaplan, S. L., Center, K. J., Barson, W. J., et al. (2015). Multicenter surveillance of *Streptococcus pneumoniae* isolates from middle ear and mastoid cultures in the 13-valent pneumococcal conjugate vaccine era. *Clinical Infectious Diseases, 60*(9), 1339–1345.

*Kaur, R., Morris, M., & Pichichero, M. E. (2017). Epidemiology of acute otitis media in the postpneumococcal conjugate vaccine era. *Pediatrics, 140*(3), e20170181.

*Kesser, B. W. (2011). Assessment and management of chronic otitis media. *Current Opinion in Otolaryngology & Head and Neck Surgery, 19,* 341–347.

Leach, A. J., & Morris, P. S. (2006). Antibiotics for the prevention of acute and chronic suppurative otitis media in children. *Cochrane Database of Systematic Reviews, 4,* CD004401.

*Leibovitz, E., Piglansky, L., Raiz, S., et al. (2000). Bacteriologic and clinical efficacy of one day vs. three day intramuscular ceftriaxone for treatment of nonresponsive acute otitis media in children. *The Pediatric Infectious Diseases Journal, 19*(11), 1040–1045.

*Lieberthal, A. S., Carroll, A. E., Chonmaitree, T., et al. (2013). The diagnosis and management of acute otitis media: Clinical practice guideline. *Pediatrics, 113,* e964–e999.

*Marom, T., Nokso-Koivisto, J., & Chonmaitree, T. (2012). Viral-bacterial interactions in acute otitis media. *Current Allergy and Asthma Reports, 12*(6), 551–558.

McDonald, S., Langton Hewer, C. D., & Nunez, D. A. (2008). Grommets (ventilation tubes) for recurrent acute otitis media in children. *Cochrane Database of Systematic Reviews, 4,* CD004741.

*Monasta, L., Ronfani, L., Marchetti, F., et al. (2012). Burden of disease caused by otitis media: Systematic review and global estimates. *PLoS One, 7*(4), e36226.

*Mösges, R., Nematian-Samani, M., Hellmich, M., et al. (2011). A meta-analysis of the efficacy of quinolone containing otics in comparison to antibiotic-steroid combination drugs in the local treatment of otitis externa. *Current Medical Research and Opinion, 27*(10), 2053–2060.

*Norton, A. E., Konvinse, K., Phillips, E. J., et al. (2018). Antibiotic allergy in pediatrics. *Pediatrics, 141*(5), e20172497.

*Pelton, S. (2012). Otitis media. In S. Long (Ed.), *Principles and practices of pediatric infectious diseases* (4th ed.). Edinburgh, UK: Saunders.

Pichichero, M. E. (2013). Otitis media. *Pediatric Clinics of North America, 60,* 391–407.

*Pichichero, M. E., & Casey, J. R. (2007). Emergence of a multiresistant serotype 19a pneumococcal strain not included in the 7-valent conjugate vaccine as an otopathogen in children. *Journal of the American Medical Association, 298*(15), 1772–1778.

Prevnar. (2011). *Pneumococcal 13-valent Conjugate Vaccine package insert.* Philadelphia, PA: Wyeth Pharmaceuticals.

*Rosenfeld, R. M., Schwartz, S. R., Cannon, C. R., et al. (2014). Clinical practice guideline: Acute otitis externa. *Otolaryngology—Head and Neck Surgery, 150*(1S), S1–S24.

*Rosenfeld, R. M., Schwartz, S. R., Pynnonen, M. A., et al. (2013). Clinical practice guideline: Tympanostomy tubes in children. *Otolaryngology—Head and Neck Surgery, 149,* S1–S35.

*Rosenfeld, R. M., Shin, J. J., Schwartz, S. R., et al. (2016). Clinical practice guideline: Otitis media with effusion. *Otolaryngology—Head and Neck Surgery, 154*(1S), S1–S41.

*Schaefer, P., & Baugh, R. F. (2012). Acute otitis externa: An update. *American Family Physician, 86*(11), 1055–1061.

Seely, D. R., Quigley, S. M., & Langman, A. W. (1996). Ear candles—efficacy and safety. *Laryngoscope, 106*(10), 1226–1229.

*Shirai, N., & Preciado, D. (2019). Otitis media: What is new? *Current Opinion in Otolaryngology & Head and Neck Surgery, 27,* 495–498.

Soni, A. (2008). Ear infections (otitis media) in children (0–17): Use and expenditures. Statistical Brief No. 228. Agency for Healthcare Research and Quality. Retrieved from http://www.meps.ahrq.gov/mepsweb/data_files/publications/st228/stat228.pdf on June 28, 2015.

*Suaya, J. A., Gessner, B. D., Fung, S., et al. (2018). Acute otitis media, antimicrobial prescriptions, and medical expenses among children in the United States during 2011–2016. *Vaccine, 36*(49), 7479–7486.

*Vennewald, I., Nat, D. R., & Klemm, E. (2010). Otomycosis: Diagnosis and treatment. *Clinics in Dermatology, 28,* 202–211.

Pharmacotherapy for Cardiovascular Disorders

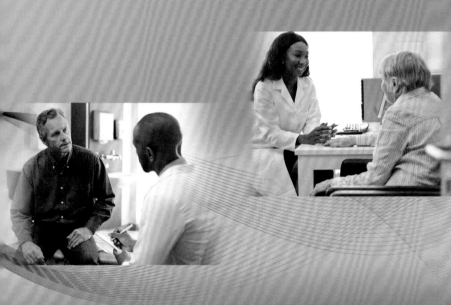

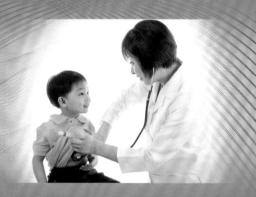

18 Hypertension

Samantha Landolfa and Diane E. Hadley

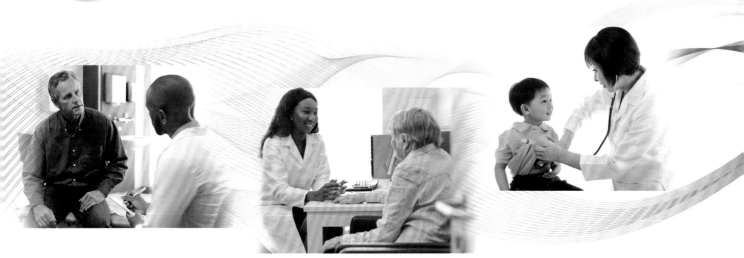

Learning Objectives

1. Diagnose and classify patients with hypertension.
2. Determine appropriate blood pressure goals for specific patient populations.
3. Develop an appropriate patient-specific treatment regimen.
4. Educate patients on nonpharmacologic interventions to treat hypertension.

INTRODUCTION

Hypertension (HTN) or high blood pressure (BP) is one of the most common chronic conditions managed by primary care providers and other health practitioners. It increases the risk for cardiovascular disease (CVD) and chronic kidney disease (CKD). Approximately 45.6% of adults in the United States have HTN. The average annual estimated direct and indirect costs of HTN from 2014 to 2015 was $55.9 billion (Virani et al., 2020). Heart disease is a widely prevalent cause of death in the United States, thus making management of a patient's BP crucial. The death rate attributable to HTN increased 25.7% from 2007 to 2017, causing more than 90,000 deaths in 2017. Despite these alarming numbers, 35.3% of U.S. adults with HTN are not aware they have HTN because the disease can be asymptomatic; therefore, the disease is appropriately nicknamed "the silent killer."

The prevalence of HTN continues to grow due to the increasing age of our population, obesity, and high dietary salt intake (Beckett et al., 2008). The prevalence of obesity was 38.3% among adults aged 20 years and older, according to

data from the 2013 to 2016 National Health and Nutrition Examination Survey. Obesity, impaired renal function, and diabetes mellitus are all associated with resistant HTN (Vongpatanasin, 2014).

HTN increases with age and affects all ethnic groups. However, blacks suffer disproportionately from HTN and its effects, leading to high rates of cardiovascular morbidity and mortality. HTN in blacks occurs at an earlier age, is more severe, and results in organ damage such as coronary heart disease, stroke, and end-stage renal disease more often than it does in whites. HTN also disproportionately affects people with lower socioeconomic status.

CAUSES

HTN is classified as primary (essential), secondary, or idiopathic when there is no identifiable cause for elevated BP. Approximately 95% of adults with HTN have primary or essential HTN, and the exact cause of primary HTN is not known. Environmental factors (excess salt, obesity, and sedentary lifestyle) and genetic factors (inappropriately high activity of the renin–angiotensin–aldosterone system [RAAS] and the sympathetic nervous system) are hypothesized contributing factors and are being studied. An additional cause of HTN is stiffening of the aorta artery, secondary to increasing age. This is referred to as isolated or predominant systolic HTN. It is characterized by high systolic blood pressure (SBP) with normal diastolic blood pressure (DBP) and is found primarily in older adults.

Secondary HTN, where the cause can be identified, accounts for 5% of all cases of HTN. The main causes of secondary HTN are CKD (anemia, low glomerular filtration rate, small kidney), renovascular HTN (abdominal bruit, elevated plasma renin activity, >30% elevation of serum creatinine [SCr] upon initiation of BP-lowering agents), hypothyroidism (elevated thyroid-stimulating hormone), hyperparathyroidism (elevated calcium), pheochromocytoma, sleep apnea, and primary aldosteronism (hypokalemia, ratio serum aldosterone/plasma renin activity >25:30).

Furthermore, medications can serve as a factor that may increase BP. Examples include oral contraceptives, nicotine, steroids, appetite suppressants, tricyclic antidepressants, venlafaxine (Effexor), cyclosporine (Sandimmune), nonsteroidal antiinflammatory drugs (NSAIDs), and some nasal decongestants (which include over-the-counter preparations). Herbal products that affect BP include capsicum, goldenseal, licorice root, ma huang (Ephedra), Scotch broom, witch hazel, and yohimbine.

PATHOPHYSIOLOGY

Role of the Nervous System

The central and autonomic nervous systems play a key dual role in regulating BP. Centrally located presynaptic beta receptors stimulate the release of norepinephrine, while alpha-2 receptors inhibit norepinephrine release. Receptors located in the periphery also regulate BP. These receptors are located on effector cells that are innervated by sympathetic neurons. Stimulation of alpha-1 receptors located on arterioles and venules causes vasoconstriction, while activation of the beta-2 receptors on these vessels produces vasodilation. Beta-1 receptors, which are located in the heart and kidneys, regulate heart rate and contractility, which ultimately impacts cardiac output. Because BP is the product of cardiac output and peripheral resistance, any reduction in cardiac output results in a decrease in BP. Therefore, blockade of beta-1 receptors decreases cardiac output, peripheral resistance, and BP.

Baroreceptors, which are nerve endings located in large arteries such as the aortic arch and carotids, additionally play a significant role in regulating BP. These receptors are sensitive to changes in BP. When BP drops drastically, the baroreceptors send an impulse to the brain stem, which results in vasoconstriction and increased heart rate and contractility. In contrast, elevation in BP increases baroreceptor activity, which results in vasodilation and decreased heart rate and contractility.

Peripheral autoregulatory components also play a role in controlling BP. Normally, rises in BP result in sodium and water elimination by the kidney. In turn, plasma volume, cardiac output, and BP decrease. Dysfunction of this mechanism can raise plasma volume and BP.

Role of the Renal System

RAAS regulates sodium, potassium, and fluid balance in the body. Renin, an enzyme secreted by the juxtaglomerular cells on the afferent arterioles of the kidney, is released in response to changes in BP caused by reduced renal perfusion, decreased intravascular volume, or increased circulation of catecholamines. Renin catalyzes the conversion of angiotensinogen to angiotensin I. Angiotensin I is converted to the potent vasoconstrictor angiotensin II by angiotensin-converting enzyme (ACE). Angiotensin II causes direct vasoconstriction and stimulation of the sympathetic nervous system. Angiotensin II also stimulates release of aldosterone from the adrenal gland, which results in the retention of sodium and water. In normal physiology, angiotensin II directly inhibits further release of renin through a negative feedback system. If the negative feedback system fails, BP rises. Hyperinsulinemia is another contributing factor to HTN, by causing sodium retention and stimulating the sympathetic nervous system.

DIAGNOSTIC CRITERIA

HTN is defined as an elevation in SBP and/or DBP. HTN is not diagnosed on an initial reading; rather, it is confirmed after at least 2 readings at least 1 week apart. BP measurements should be obtained after the patient has had time to relax for at least 5 minutes. Patients should be seated in a chair, back supported (rather than on an examination table), with feet on the floor, legs uncrossed, and arm supported at heart level. Patients should avoid smoking cigarettes 30 minutes before the reading, should not exercise heavily immediately before the reading, should not drink caffeine during the hour preceding the reading, and should avoid adrenergic stimulants, such as phenylephrine. For an accurate reading, the appropriate size sphygmomanometer cuff should be used. The cuff should encompass 80% of the arm, and the width of the cuff should be at least 40% of the length of the upper arm (U.S. Preventive Services Task Force, 2007). At the initial evaluation, BP should be measured in both arms. If the readings are different, the arm with the higher reading should be used for measurements thereafter. It is preferable to take two readings, 1 to 2 minutes apart, and use the average of these measurements. In older people, it is useful to obtain standing BP, after 1 minute and again after 3 minutes, to check for postural effects.

Ambulatory BP monitoring (ABPM) is recommended for patients with suspected variable BP. Contributing factors can include "white coat hypertension," episodic HTN, HTN resistant to increasing medication regimens, hypotensive symptoms while taking antihypertensive medications, and autonomic dysfunction. Patients with white coat hypertension have a persistently elevated BP in the doctor's office but a persistently normal BP at other times. ABPM readings correlate better with target organ damage than clinical measurements. ABPM also identifies patients in whom BP does not drop significantly during sleep. More aggressive treatment may be necessary for these patients, who are known to be at higher cardiovascular risk. An elevated systolic BP is a more potent cardiovascular risk factor than an elevated diastolic BP.

In 2014, the Eighth Report of the Joint National Committee (JNC 8) was published. The updated guidelines established new definitions for HTN and removed the classifications that had existed in JNC 7 (**Table 18.1**).

TABLE 18.1

Definition of Hypertension of the Eighth Report of the Joint National Committee

Patient Population	BP (mm Hg)
<60 years old	≥140/90
≥60 years old	≥150/90
≥18 years old with CKD or diabetes	≥140/90

BP, blood pressure; CKD, chronic kidney disease.

Two studies within the primary literature, systolic hypertension in the elderly program (SHEP) and systolic hypertension in Europe, used placebo-controlled approaches to evaluate people over the age of 60 with systolic HTN, and the Hypertension in the Very Elderly Trial (HYVET) evaluated patients over the age of 80. The JNC 8 panel could not recommend a lower threshold value for those over 60 since no evidence existed that a systolic BP less than 140 mm Hg was better than a systolic BP less than 150 mm Hg for protecting patients from harm.

In 2017, the American College of Cardiology (ACC) and American Heart Association (AHA) published a Guideline for the Prevention, Detection, Evaluation, and Management of Blood Pressure in Adults. This guideline recommends categorizing BP into four stages to reflect data suggesting a gradient in CVD risk as the BP increases. Notably, the BP categories that had been specified by JNC 7 (and since removed by JNC 8) differ significantly from those in the most recent ACC/AHA guidelines (**Table 18.2**).

The diagnosis of HTN should be confirmed at an additional patient visit, usually 1 to 4 weeks after the first measurement. On both occasions, the SBP and DBP should be higher than recommendations listed previously per age. The U.S. Preventive Services Task Force recommends BP monitoring in adult patients over the age of 18. If the BP is very high (SBP >180 mm Hg), initiation of the appropriate triage and treatment should occur. If available resources are not adequate to permit a convenient second visit, the initial diagnosis can be made and treatment can be started.

TABLE 18.2

2017 American College of Cardiology/American Heart Association Classification of Blood Pressure

Classification	Systolic BP (mm Hg)	Diastolic BP (mm Hg)
Normal	<120	<80
Elevated	120–129	<80
Stage 1 HTN	130–139	80–89
Stage 2 HTN	≥140	≥90

BP, blood pressure; HTN, hypertension.

Physical Examination

A thorough examination should be performed, including a personal history, first-degree family history of CVD, dietary habits, and a history of prescription and over-the-counter medications, smoking/tobacco product use, caffeine intake, alcohol consumption, and herbal products. For patients with documented HTN, evaluate lifestyle and other cardiovascular risk factors or concomitant disorders to determine the extent of target organ damage and to assess the patient's overall cardiovascular risk status. Most prevalent target damage concern is concentrated on the cardiovascular, cerebral, and renal tissues.

Physical examination includes two or more measured, seated BP readings with verification in the contralateral arm; weight and height; body mass index (BMI); waist circumference; muscle strength; funduscopy exam; auscultation for carotid, abdominal, and femoral bruits; palpation of the thyroid gland; thorough examination of the heart and lungs; examination of the abdomen for enlarged kidneys, enlarged liver, masses, and abnormal aortic pulsation; palpation of the lower extremities for edema and pulses; and neurologic assessment for sign of previous stroke.

Diagnostic Tests

The following laboratory tests should be routinely performed: electrocardiogram, hemoglobin, hematocrit, complete urinalysis, and complete chemistry panel (which includes serum potassium, SCr, blood glucose, and liver function tests), calcium and magnesium, glycosylated hemoglobin (hemoglobin A1c), and fasting lipid panel (9- to 12-hour fast), which includes total cholesterol, low-density lipoprotein cholesterol, high-density lipoprotein cholesterol, and triglycerides. Further testing should be performed based on clinical findings.

INITIATING DRUG THERAPY

Goals of Drug Therapy

The goal of antihypertensive therapy is to manage HTN, reduce cardiovascular complications (including lipid disorders, glucose intolerance or diabetes, obesity, and smoking), and prevent renal disease. Treating HTN can decrease the risk of stroke by 40%, myocardial infarction (MI) by 25%, and heart failure by 50%. It is important to inform patients that the treatment of HTN is usually expected to be a lifelong commitment and that it can be dangerous for them to terminate without first consulting their provider (Whelton et al., 2018).

Treatment guidelines are cumbersome due to the different classifications of hypertensive patients with or without comorbidities of diabetes and/or CKD, and elderly versus nonelderly patients. BP goals specified in national guidelines are summarized in **Table 18.3**.

In the past, guidelines have recommended treatment values of less than 130/80 mm Hg for patients with diabetes, CKD, or coronary artery disease. However, evidence to support

TABLE 18.3
Blood Pressure Goals

Patient Population	BP Goal (mm Hg)
2014 Eighth Joint National Committee	
≥60 years old	<150/90
<60 years old	<140/90
≥18 years old with diabetes or CKD	<140/90
2020 American Diabetes Association	
Diabetes and 10-year ASCVD risk <15%	<140/90
Diabetes and existing ASCVD or 10-year ASCVD risk ≥15%	<130/80
Diabetes and pregnancy	≤135/85
2017 American College of Cardiology/American Heart Association	
Stage 1 HTN and existing ASCVD or 10-year ASCVD risk ≥10%	<130/80
Stage 2 HTN	<130/80
≥65 years old	<130/NA
Comorbidities (diabetes, CKD, stable ischemic heart disease, heart failure, PAD, secondary stroke prevention)	<130/80
2012 Kidney Disease Improving Global Outcomes	
Urine albumin excretion <30 mg/24 hours	<140/90
Urine albumin excretion ≥30 mg/24 hours	<130/80

ASCVD, atherosclerotic cardiovascular disease; BP, blood pressure; CKD, chronic kidney disease; HTN, hypertension; PAD.

this lower target is lacking and newer guidelines have increased the BP goal. For instance, the ACCORD trial demonstrated that aggressive reduction of the BP target (<120/80 mm Hg) in patients with type 2 diabetes did not reduce combined cardiovascular and renal outcomes compared with usual care (target BP <140/90 mm Hg) (Cushman et al., 2010). Among secondary outcomes, strokes were reduced by the lower BP goals, but at the expense of twice as many serious side effects. Several meta-analyses have demonstrated that lowering SBP to below 130 mm Hg does not reduce mortality rates or most cardiovascular outcomes (Mancia et al., 2013).

In adult patients with HTN and diabetes, treatment should be initiated when BP is 140/90 mm Hg or higher, regardless of age, per the JNC 8 guidelines. The guidelines of the American Diabetes Association 2020 Standards of Medical Care in Diabetes recommend different BP targets based on cardiovascular risk. In contrast, the ACC/AHA 2017 guidelines recommend a goal of less than 130/80 mm Hg for all patients with diabetes.

Diuretics

There are five classes of diuretics: carbonic anhydrase inhibitors, thiazides, thiazide-like diuretics, loop diuretics, and potassium-sparing diuretics. Carbonic anhydrase inhibitors are not used for HTN because of their weak antihypertensive effects; therefore, they will not be discussed in this chapter. Diuretics decrease BP by causing diuresis, which results in decreased plasma volume, stroke volume, and cardiac output. During chronic therapy, their major hemodynamic effect is reduction of peripheral vascular resistance. As a result of drug-induced diuresis, adverse effects of hypokalemia and hypomagnesemia may lead to cardiac arrhythmias. Patients at greatest risk are those receiving digitalis therapy, those with left ventricular hypertrophy (LVH), and those with ischemic heart disease (**Table 18.4**).

Thiazide Diuretics
Mechanism of Action
Thiazide diuretics work by increasing the urinary excretion of sodium and chloride in equal amounts. They inhibit the reabsorption of sodium and chloride in the thick ascending limb of the loop of Henle and the early distal tubules. The antihypertensive action requires several days to produce effects.

TABLE 18.4
Thiazides and Thiazide-like Diuretics

Agent	Initial Dose	Maximum Total Daily Dose	Clinical Pearls
Chlorothiazide (Diuril)	500 mg PO daily or BID	2,000 mg	
Hydrochlorothiazide (often abbreviated as HCTZ)	12.5–25 mg PO daily	50 mg	Doses above 25 mg often result in increased adverse effects with minimal added benefit
Chlorthalidone	12.5–25 mg PO daily	100 mg	
Indapamide	1.25 mg PO daily	5 mg	Titrate every 4 weeks; Give with food or milk to decrease GI side effects
Metolazone	2.5 mg daily	20 mg	Other thiazides are usually preferred; May be added to loop diuretics in hospitalized patients to augment effect

GI, gastrointestinal.

The duration of action of the thiazides requires a single daily dose to control BP. Thiazide diuretics cause increased potassium and bicarbonate excretion and decreased calcium excretion. They may be helpful in patients with osteoporosis as they can slow demineralization. Additionally, they cause uric acid retention, so caution should be used in patients with a history of gout.

Contraindications

Thiazide diuretics are contraindicated in those who are anuric or are hypersensitive to thiazides or sulfonamides. They are not recommended in patients with a creatinine clearance (CrCl) of less than 30 mL/min because they are ineffective.

Adverse Events

Side effects include hypokalemia, hypomagnesemia, hypercalcemia, hyperuricemia, and hyperglycemia. As a result of drug-induced diuresis, hypokalemia occurs in 15% to 20% of patients taking low-dose thiazide diuretics; therefore, potassium supplements can be utilized by some patients. Combination therapy with thiazide and potassium-sparing diuretics (e.g., hydrochlorothiazide and triamterene) may be prudent when the potassium level is less than 4.0 mEq/L and the patient is taking a thiazide diuretic or when a low potassium level may potentiate drug toxicity, as in patients concurrently taking digoxin. Monitor the SCr, sodium, and potassium within 7 to 10 days after initiation or dose titration.

Other side effects include tinnitus, paresthesia, abdominal cramps, nausea, vomiting, diarrhea, muscle cramps, weakness, and sexual dysfunction. Thiazides can also worsen gout due to an increase in serum uric acid. Diuretic-induced hyperuricemia may produce gouty arthritis or uric acid stones. There is also a greater risk of developing diabetes with thiazides than with ACE inhibitors (ACEIs), angiotensin II receptor blockers (ARBs), or calcium channel blockers (CCBs) (**Table 18.5**).

Loop Diuretics

Mechanism of Action

Loop diuretics are indicated in the presence of edema associated with congestive heart failure, hepatic cirrhosis, and renal disease. This drug class is useful when greater diuresis is desired compared with thiazide diuretics. In general, loop diuretics should be reserved for hypertensive patients with chronic renal insufficiency and/or the need for more severe diuresis.

Furosemide and ethacrynic acid inhibit the reabsorption of sodium and chloride, not only in proximal and distal tubules but also in the loop of Henle. In contrast, bumetanide is more chloruretic than natriuretic and may have an additional action in the proximal tubule.

Loop diuretics are especially useful in patients with heart failure and CKD using twice daily dosing.

Contraindications

Loop diuretics are contraindicated in patients who are anuric and in patients with hepatic coma or in states of severe electrolyte depletion. Ethacrynic acid is contraindicated in infants. Furosemide, bumetanide, and torsemide are sulfonamide-based loop diuretics that should not be used in patients with hypersensitivity to sulfonylureas; ethacrynic acid is generally reserved for this patient population as it does not contain a sulfa moiety.

Adverse Events

Loop diuretics may cause the same side effects as thiazides, although the effects on serum lipids and glucose are not as significant, and hypocalcemia may occur instead. The metabolic abnormalities, such as hyperlipidemia and hyperglycemia, usually occur with high doses of diuretics and can be avoided by using low doses of the drug.

Loop diuretics may lead to electrolyte and volume depletion more readily than thiazides; they have a short duration of

| **TABLE 18.5** | | | |
| **Loop Diuretics** | | | |
Agent	Initial Dose	Maximum Total Daily Dose	Clinical Pearls
Bumetanide (Bumex)	0.5–1 mg PO daily	10 mg	If initial dose does not result in diuresis, double the single dose (instead of increasing frequency) until diuresis occurs and then administer that dose 1–3 times daily.
Furosemide (Lasix)	20–40 mg PO daily	600 mg	If initial dose does not result in diuresis, double the single dose (instead of increasing frequency) until diuresis occurs and then administer that dose 1–2 times daily; Tablets may be administered sublingually.
Torsemide	5 mg PO daily	200 mg	Titrate after 4–6 weeks; Antihypertensive effect may take up to 12 weeks.
Ethacrynic acid (Edecrin)	50 mg PO daily	400 mg	Reserved for patients with hypersensitivity to sulfonamide-based loop diuretics; Titrate by 25–50 mg in at least 24-hour intervals; Dose may be divided BID.

Equivalent doses in patients with normal renal function: bumetanide 1 mg = furosemide 40 mg = torsemide 10–20 mg = ethacrynic acid 50 mg.

TABLE 18.6

Potassium-Sparing Diuretics and Aldosterone Receptor Antagonists

Agent	Initial Dose	Maximum Daily Dose	Clinical Pearls
Amiloride (Midamor)	5 mg PO daily	10 mg	Minimal effect as monotherapy, so it is typically added to thiazide diuretics.
Eplerenone (Inspra)	50 mg PO daily	100 mg	Titrate after 4 weeks.
Spironolactone (Aldactone)	12.5–25 mg PO daily	100 mg	Preferred in patients with congestive heart failure.
Triamterene (Dyrenium)	50–100 mg PO daily or divided BID	300 mg	Minimal effect as monotherapy, so it is typically added to thiazide diuretics.

action, but the thiazide diuretics are more effective than loop diuretics in reducing BP in patients with normal renal function. Therefore, loop diuretics should be reserved for hypertensive patients with renal dysfunction (SCr >2.5 mg/dL). Monitor SCr, sodium, and potassium within 7 to 10 days after initiation or dose titration.

Loop diuretics may also cause ototoxicity. This is more likely to occur with high doses, during rapid IV administration, or with severe renal impairment. It is more common with ethacrynic acid (**Table 18.6**).

Potassium-Sparing Diuretics and Aldosterone Receptor Antagonists

Mechanism of Action

In the kidney, potassium is filtered at the glomerulus and then absorbed parallel to sodium throughout the proximal tubule and the thick ascending limb of the loop of Henle, so that only minor amounts reach the distal convoluted tubule. As a result, potassium appearing in urine is secreted at the distal tubule and collecting duct. The potassium-sparing diuretics interfere with sodium reabsorption at the distal tubule, thus decreasing potassium secretion. These drugs can be used as a possible agent for HTN; however, their true benefit is in patients with heart failure. In the Randomized Spironolactone Evaluation Study, low-dose spironolactone was shown to improve morbidity and mortality rates in patients with severe heart failure (Pitt et al., 1999).

Aldosterone receptor antagonists inhibit the effect of aldosterone by competitively binding to aldosterone receptors in the cortical collecting duct. This results in decreased reabsorption of sodium and water, while decreasing potassium secretion. They are typically used in patients with refractory HTN.

These diuretics have the potential for causing hyperkalemia and hyponatremia, in particular, in patients with renal insufficiency or diabetes and in patients receiving concurrent treatment with an ACEI inhibitor, NSAIDs, or potassium supplements.

Contraindications

Potassium-sparing diuretics are contraindicated in patients with hyperkalemia, Addison disease, anuria, or patients taking eplerenone.

Adverse Events

Side effects include gynecomastia, hirsutism, and menstrual irregularities. Asymptomatic hyperuricemia may occur, and gout may be precipitated. Potassium-sparing diuretics should be avoided in patients with CrCl below 10 mL/min, and aldosterone antagonists should not be used in patients with CrCl below 30 mL/min. Monitor SCr and potassium within 7 to 10 days after initiation or titration of potassium-sparing diuretics. SCr and potassium should be monitored in 3 days and in 7 days and monthly for 3 months after initiation or titration of aldosterone antagonists (**Table 18.7**).

Beta-Adrenergic Blockers

Mechanism of Action

Beta-1 receptors, located predominantly in the heart and kidney, regulate heart rate, renin release, and cardiac contractility. Beta-2 receptors, located in the lungs, liver, pancreas, and arteriolar smooth muscle, regulate bronchodilation and vasodilation. Beta blockers reduce BP by blocking central and peripheral beta receptors, which results in decreased cardiac output and sympathetic outflow.

Beta blockers have been included in clinical guidelines since the 1980s and remain a mainstay of HTN treatment. Despite several pharmacologic differences in the available beta blockers, they are all effective in treating HTN. Beta blockers that mostly bind to beta-1 receptors are referred to as *cardioselective* because they do not significantly block beta-2 receptors and are typically used for treating HTN. These agents include metoprolol tartrate, metoprolol succinate, atenolol, nebivolol, and bisoprolol. These may be safer than nonselective beta blockers for patients with asthma, chronic obstructive pulmonary disease, and peripheral vascular disease. At higher doses, however, selective beta blockers lose cardioselectivity and may aggravate a preexisting condition.

Drugs with beta-1 and alpha-1 receptor blockade are more effective in lowering blood pressure compared to drugs with single receptor blockade. Agents with dual receptor blockade include carvedilol and labetalol.

Some beta blockers possess intrinsic sympathomimetic activity (ISA); these agents are partial beta-receptor agonists

TABLE 18.7

Beta-Adrenergic Blockers

Agent	Initial Dose	Maximum Daily Dose	Clinical Pearls
Atenolol (Tenormin)	50 mg PO daily	100 mg	Beta-1 selective, except at high doses; Titrate every 1–2 weeks; Doses above 100 mg are unlikely to produce further benefit.
Bisoprolol	2.5–5 mg PO daily	10 mg	Beta-1 selective
Carvedilol immediate release (Coreg)	6.25 mg PO BID	50 mg	Nonselective—has alpha-blocking activity; Titrate in intervals of at least 1 week; Give with food to reduce risk of orthostatic hypotension.
Carvedilol extended release (Coreg CR)	20 mg PO daily	80 mg	
Labetalol	100 mg PO BID	800 mg	Nonselective—blocks beta-1, beta-2, and alpha-1; Can be titrated by 100 mg BID every 2–3 days; Can be increased to 2,400 mg/day, but it is usually preferred to use a combination of agents once dose reaches 800 mg/day; Bioavailability is increased when given with food.
Metoprolol succinate (Toprol XL)	25–100 mg PO daily	400 mg	Beta-1 selective; Titrate in intervals of at least 1 week; Tablets may be divided but not crushed or chewed.
Metoprolol tartrate (Lopressor)	50 mg PO BID	400 mg	Beta-1 selective; Titrate in intervals of at least 1 week; Should be given with or immediately after meals.
Nebivolol (Bystolic)	5 mg PO daily	40 mg	Highly beta-1 selective; Titrate every 2 weeks.

that reduce heart rate and contractility during excessive sympathetic outflow. In resting states, heart rate and contractility are maintained. Typical medications include pindolol and acebutolol.

Studies suggest that beta blockers may decrease sympathetic activity involved with the progression of heart failure (see Chapter 21, "Heart Failure"). For example, carvedilol and metoprolol succinate decreased mortality rates in patients with heart failure and decreased ventricular remodeling (which results in LVH). Beta blockers should be used only in patients with stable congestive heart failure and be temporarily discontinued if the patient has an acute decompensation. Practitioners should refer any patient with heart failure to a cardiologist for evaluation of therapy.

Patients should be cautioned not to discontinue therapy abruptly. The dose of beta blockers should be tapered gradually over 14 days to prevent withdrawal symptoms, which include unstable angina, MI, or even death in patients with underlying CVD. Patients without coronary artery disease may experience sinus tachycardia, palpitations, increased sweating, and fatigue.

Contraindications

Beta blockers are contraindicated in patients with sinoatrial or atrioventricular (AV) node dysfunction, decompensated heart failure, and severe bronchospastic disease. They should be used with caution, especially at higher doses, in patients with asthma or chronic obstructive pulmonary disease due to blockade of pulmonary beta receptors. Beta blockers should be avoided in patients who have sinus bradycardia, second- or third-degree heart block, or overt cardiac failure.

Non-ISA beta blockers are the preferred agents for treating HTN in patient with coexisting coronary artery disease and especially in patients after MI.

Beta blockers should be used cautiously, but not avoided, in patients with resting ischemia or severe claudication secondary to peripheral vascular disease, reactive airway disease, systolic congestive heart failure, diabetes mellitus, or depression.

Adverse Events

The most common side effects of beta blockers are fatigue, drowsiness, dizziness, bronchospasm, nausea, and vomiting. Serious side effects include bradycardia, AV conduction abnormalities, and the development of congestive heart failure. The dose should be adjusted in patients who develop symptomatic bradycardia or greater than first-degree heart block.

In patients with diabetes, beta blockers can mask all symptoms of hypoglycemia, except for sweating. Beta blockers may also cause depression. Similar to the thiazides, there is a higher risk of developing diabetes with beta blockers than with ACEIs, ARBs, or CCBs.

Some of these adverse effects can be beneficial for certain patients. For example, beta blockers may be favorable

TABLE 18.8

Angiotensin-Converting Enzyme Inhibitors

Agent	Initial Dose	Maximum Daily Dose	Clinical Pearls
Captopril	12.5–25 mg PO BID or TID	150 mg	Titrate every 1–2 weeks; Give at least 1 hour before meals.
Enalapril (Epaned, Vasotec)	5 mg PO daily or 2.5 mg PO BID	40 mg	Titrate every 4–6 weeks by doubling the dose.
Lisinopril (Prinvil, Zestril)	5–10 mg PO daily	40 mg	
Ramipril (Altace)	2.5 mg PO daily	20 mg	Titrate every 2–4 weeks.

in treating patients with atrial fibrillation, tachyarrhythmias, angina, migraines, and essential tremor (**Table 18.8**).

Angiotensin-Converting Enzyme Inhibitors

Mechanism of Action

ACEIs, such as lisinopril, enalapril, captopril, ramipril, and trandolapril (see **Table 18.5**), exert an antihypertensive effect by preventing the conversion of angiotensin I to angiotensin II, which is a potent vasoconstrictor. ACEIs also inhibit the degradation of bradykinin and increase the synthesis of vasodilating prostaglandins. ACEIs decrease morbidity and mortality in patients with congestive heart failure, post-MI, and systolic dysfunction.

Contraindications

ACEIs are contraindicated in patients with bilateral renal artery stenosis because of the risk of acute renal failure. They are also contraindicated in pregnancy due to their teratogenic effects, so consider avoiding their use in women of child-bearing age. Additionally, ACEIs are contraindicated in patients with a history of angioedema.

Adverse Events

The most common side effects associated with ACEIs include chronic dry cough, rashes (most common with captopril), and dizziness. Hyperkalemia can occur but is a higher risk in patients with renal disease, with diabetes, or taking concomitant potassium-sparing drugs or potassium supplements. Angioedema is a rare but dangerous side effect that occurs 2 to 4 times more frequently in African Americans; it is reversible upon discontinuation of the agent. Laryngeal edema, another rare adverse effect, is life threatening and requires immediate medical attention. ACEIs can also cause a rise in SCr; a modest rise of up to 30% from baseline is acceptable and should be considered the new baseline.

ACEIs are not recommended to be used in combination with an ARB or a renin inhibitor because all of these agents affect the RAAS system, thereby increasing the incidence of side effects. When initiating or titrating the dose of an ACEI, the potassium and SCr should be checked within 1 to 2 weeks (**Table 18.9**).

TABLE 18.9

Angiotensin Receptor Blockers

Agent	Initial Dose	Maximum Daily Dose	Clinical Pearls
Candesartan (Atacand)	8 mg PO daily	32 mg	Titrate every 4–6 weeks.
Losartan (Cozaar)	25–50 mg PO daily	100 mg	
Valsartan (Diovan)	80–160 mg PO daily	320 mg	

Angiotensin II Receptor Blockers

Mechanism of Action

ARBs block the vasoconstriction and aldosterone-secreting effects of angiotensin II by selectively blocking the binding of angiotensin II to the angiotensin II receptor found in many tissues (see **Table 18.6**). This reduces end organ responses to angiotensin II and results in decreased afterload and preload. They are indicated for patients with HTN, nephropathy in type 2 diabetes, and heart failure and those who cannot tolerate the side effects associated with ACEIs.

The results of the Losartan Intervention for Endpoint Reduction in HTN study suggest that losartan is more effective than atenolol in reducing cardiovascular morbidity and mortality in patients who have diabetes, HTN, and LVH (Dahlöf et al., 2002). The incidence of cough and hyperkalemia associated with this class of drugs is lower than with ACEIs but may still occur.

Contraindications

Like the ACEIs, ARBs are contraindicated in patients with bilateral renal artery stenosis and pregnancy. Angioedema can be seen with ARB therapy but with much less frequency than with ACEIs. There should be some justification (heart failure or proteinuric nephropathy) for the use of ARBs in patients having experienced ACEI-related angioedema. Combination with ACEI and/or renin inhibitors is not recommended. Caution should be used in patients with renal and hepatic function impairment.

TABLE 18.10
Renin Inhibitor

Agent	Initial Dose	Maximum Daily Dose	Clinical Pearls
Aliskiren	150 mg PO daily	300 mg	High-fat meals significantly decrease absorption.

Adverse Events

Adverse reactions include dizziness, upper respiratory tract infections, viral infection, fatigue, diarrhea, pain, sinusitis, pharyngitis, and rhinitis. Like ACEIs, there is a risk of hyperkalemia in patients taking another potassium-sparing medication or potassium supplements. ARBs can also elevate the SCr; like ACEIs, a modest rise of 30% above baseline is acceptable and should be considered the new baseline. When initiating or titrating the dose of an ARB, the potassium and SCr should be checked within 7 to 10 days (**Table 18.10**).

Renin Inhibitors

Mechanism of Action

Renin inhibitors block the conversion of angiotensinogen to angiotensin I. Angiotensin I suppression decreases the formation of angiotensin II. Angiotensin II functions within the RAAS as a negative inhibitory feedback mediator within the renal parenchyma to suppress the further release of renin. The reduction in angiotensin II levels suppresses this feedback loop, leading to further increased plasma renin concentrations and subsequent low plasma renin activity. Aliskiren is the first renin inhibitor approved by the U.S. Food and Drug Administration, in March 2007. It is currently the only renin inhibitor on the market in the United States. Aliskiren lowers BP by a degree comparable to most other agents. There are no clinical trial data of aliskiren monotherapy on outcomes in HTN. The Aliskiren Trial in Type 2 Diabetes Using Cardiovascular and Renal Disease Endpoints, which compared aliskiren added to an ACEI or ARB with placebo, was terminated early due to an increase in adverse events and lack of apparent benefit. It is also important to note that patients with renal insufficiency were excluded from clinical trials.

Contraindications

This drug is not recommended in combination with ACEI and ARB therapy due to similar mechanisms of action. It is contraindicated for use with an ACEI or ARB in patients with diabetes. Aliskiren is contraindicated during pregnancy because it directly acts on the renin–angiotensin system and can cause fetal and neonatal morbidity.

Adverse Events

Significant adverse events include dose-related diarrhea, hyperkalemia when used with an ACEI, and angioedema (rare) (**Table 18.11**).

Calcium Channel Blockers

Mechanism of Action

CCBs share the ability to inhibit the movement of calcium ions across the cell membrane. The effect on the cardiovascular system is muscle relaxation and vasodilation. Non-dihydropyridines,

TABLE 18.11
Calcium Channel Blockers

Agent	Initial Dose	Maximum Daily Dose	Clinical Pearls
Non-dihydropyridines			
Diltiazem 12-hour (Cardizem)	60–120 mg PO BID	360 mg	Titrate every 1–2 weeks.
Diltiazem 24-hour (Cardizem LA, Cardizem CD, Cartia XT)	120–240 mg PO daily		
Verapamil immediate release (Calan)	40–80 mg PO TID	480 mg	Titrate weekly.
Verapamil extended release (Calan SR, Verelan)	120–180 mg PO daily		
Verapamil extended release, delayed onset (Verelan PM)	100 or 200 mg PO QHS	400 mg	
Dihydropyridines			
Amlodipine (Norvasc)	2.5–5 mg PO daily	10 mg	Titrate every 1–2 weeks.
Felodipine (Plendil)	2.5–5 mg PO daily	10 mg	Titrate every 1–2 weeks.
Isradipine (Dynacirc)	2.5 mg PO BID	10 mg	Titrate every 2–4 weeks.
Nifedipine (Procardia XL)	30–60 mg PO daily	90 mg	Titrate every 1–2 weeks.
Nicardipine (Procardia)	20 mg PO TID	120 mg	Titrate in intervals of at least 3 days.

such as verapamil and diltiazem, decrease heart rate and slow cardiac conduction at the AV node. The dihydropyridines (amlodipine, felodipine, nifedipine, nicardipine, nisoldipine, and isradipine) are potent vasodilators. CCBs are effective as monotherapy and are especially effective in black patients. CCBs are similar in antihypertensive effectiveness but differ in other pharmacodynamic effects. The non-dihydropyridines are typically used in patients with atrial fibrillation or stable angina.

Contraindications

The non-dihydropyridines (verapamil and diltiazem) are contraindicated in patients with heart block or sick sinus syndrome. They may accelerate the progression of congestive heart failure in a patient with cardiac dysfunction; therefore, these agents are not first line. Diltiazem and verapamil should also be avoided in patients with left ventricular (systolic) dysfunction when the ejection fraction measures less than 40%.

Short-acting nifedipine should not be used for treating essential HTN or hypertensive emergencies because of its association with causing inconsistent fluctuations in BP and reflex tachycardia.

Adverse Events

Diltiazem and verapamil can cause gastrointestinal (GI) upset, peripheral edema, and hypotension. Rare side effects include bradycardia, AV block, and congestive heart failure. Verapamil can cause constipation in older adults. These medications are also potent CYP450 inhibitors; therefore, they have the potential for severe drug–drug interactions. They should also be used with caution in patients also taking a beta blocker.

The dihydropyridine agents (nifedipine, nicardipine, isradipine, felodipine, nisoldipine, and amlodipine) produce symptoms of vasodilation, such as headache, flushing, palpations, and peripheral edema. Other side effects of nifedipine include dizziness, gingival hyperplasia, mood changes, and various GI complaints. Nifedipine may cause reflex tachycardia as a result of stimulating the baroreceptors in response to an acute drop in BP (**Table 18.12**).

Peripheral Alpha-1 Receptor Blockers

Mechanism of Action

Doxazosin, prazosin, and terazosin are selective alpha-1 receptor blockers that are effective in patients with benign prostatic hypertrophy and are not usually prescribed solely for HTN treatment. Peripheral alpha-1 receptor blockers act by inhibiting the action of adrenaline on smooth muscle in blood vessel walls, dilating both arterioles and veins, causing relaxation of smooth muscle.

In the presence of CVD, alpha-1 receptor blockers should be avoided, as the Antihypertensive and Lipid-Lowering Treatment to Prevent Heart Attack (ALLHAT) study showed that these patients had an increase in mortality (Papademetriou et al., 2003). Alpha-1 blockers are generally viewed as fourth- or fifth-line agents. These drugs are typically reserved for male patients with benign prostatic hyperplasia.

Contraindications

The use of tadalafil, sildenafil, and vardenafil is not recommended with alpha-1 receptor blockers due to an increased risk of symptomatic hypotension. If both agents are prescribed, a washout window of at least 4 to 6 hours is recommended.

Adverse Events

The most common side effect associated with this class of antihypertensive medications is the first-dose phenomenon, which consists of dizziness or faintness, palpitations, or syncope. Orthostatic hypotension may also occur. These agents should be administered initially at bedtime, and the dosage should be adjusted slowly. With chronic administration, even at low doses, fluid and sodium accumulate, requiring concurrent diuretic therapy. Other side effects include vivid dreams and depression (**Table 18.13**).

Central Alpha-2 Receptor Agonists

Mechanism of Action

Central alpha-2 agonists stimulate alpha-2 adrenergic receptors in the brain, resulting in decreased sympathetic outflow, cardiac output, and peripheral resistance. These agents may cause fluid retention, and in most cases, combination with a diuretic can be considered. Clonidine, methyldopa, and guanfacine should not be used as initial monotherapy. Abrupt cessation of alpha-2 agonist therapy may result in a compensatory increase in the norepinephrine level, thereby increasing BP.

TABLE 18.12			
Peripheral Alpha-1 Receptor Blockers			
Agent	**Initial Dose**	**Maximum Daily Dose**	**Clinical Pearls**
Doxazosin (Cardura)	1 mg PO QHS	16 mg	If discontinued for several days, restart titration at 1 mg.
Prazosin (Minipress)	1 mg PO BID or TID	40 mg	If adding another antihypertensive, decrease prazosin to 1–2 mg TID and retitrate.
Terazosin	1 mg PO QHS	20 mg	If discontinued for several days, restart titration at 1 mg.

TABLE 18.13

Central Alpha-2 Receptor Antagonists

Agent	Initial Dose	Maximum Daily Dose	Clinical Pearls
Clonidine (Catapres)	0.1 mg PO BID 0.1 mg/24-hour patch every 7 days	2.4 mg	Titrate by 0.1 mg every week; Doses above 0.6 mg are generally not used; Onset of patch is 2–3 days after application.
Methyldopa	250 mg PO BID or TID	3,000	Titrate every 2 days; Initial dose should be limited to 500 mg/day when used with antihypertensives other than a thiazide.
Guanfacine (Intuniv)	0.5–1 mg PO QHS	2 mg	Titrate after 3–4 weeks; Adverse reactions significantly increase at doses above 3 mg/day; Given at bedtime to decrease somnolence.

Contraindications

Central agonists should be used cautiously in patients with severe coronary insufficiency, conduction disturbances, recent MI, cerebrovascular disease, and renal failure.

Adverse Events

These agents may cause fluid retention, sedation, and dry mouth. They should be avoided in patients with heart failure. The first-dose effect of dizziness and syncope is possible. Abrupt cessation should be avoided due to the risk for rebound HTN, which is higher in patients also taking a beta blocker (**Table 18.14**).

Direct Vasodilators

Mechanism of Action

The direct vasodilators hydralazine and minoxidil cause arteriolar smooth muscle relaxation, resulting in BP reduction. Direct vasodilators should be reserved for patients with essential or severe HTN. Both hydralazine and minoxidil may cause fluid retention and reflex tachycardia, which can be treated with a concurrent diuretic and a beta blocker or another agent (clonidine, diltiazem, or verapamil) that slows the heart rate.

Contraindications

Hydralazine should be used with caution in patients with coronary artery disease and mitral valvular rheumatic heart disease.

Minoxidil is contraindicated in patients with pheochromocytoma, acute MI, and dissecting aortic aneurysm.

Adverse Events

Hydralazine is associated with drug-induced lupus-like syndrome that is dose related at dosages greater than 200 mg/day. It can also cause tachycardia when used in combination with a beta blocker. Other adverse reactions include dermatitis, drug fever, and peripheral neuropathy. Minoxidil may cause drug-induced hirsutism and pericardial effusion. Both medications can cause fluid retention, so concomitant diuretic use should be considered.

Selecting the Most Appropriate Agent

First-Line Therapy

First-line therapy should be influenced by the age, ethnicity/race, and presence of comorbidities (diabetes, coronary disease, etc.). Long-acting drugs that can be taken once daily are preferred to shorter-acting drugs because this will improve medication adherence. Most patients will require at least two antihypertensive mediations to control BP, especially those with diabetes. Patients with CKD often need three or more agents. In patients with BP more than 20/10 mm Hg above goal, initiating two agents simultaneously should be considered.

TABLE 18.14

Direct Vasodilators

Agent	Initial Dose	Maximum Daily Dose	Clinical Pearls
Hydralazine	10 mg PO QID for 2–4 days, then 25 mg PO QID for the rest of the first week	300 mg	Doses above 200 mg/day are avoided due to the risk of drug-induced lupus-like syndrome.
Minoxidil	5 mg PO daily	100 mg	Titrate at intervals of at least 3 days; May be administered in divided doses 1–3 times daily; Boxed warning: maximum doses of a diuretic and 2 other medications should be used before adding minoxidil.

For this reason, when more than one drug is prescribed, combination products can simplify treatment and reduce pill burden. However, combination products can be more expensive.

According to the JNC 8 guidelines, for black patients with HTN, with or without diabetes, CCBs or thiazide diuretics are recommended. For all other ethnicities, initial treatment options include ACEIs or ARBs, thiazide diuretics, or CCBs. Additionally, all adult patients with CKD, regardless of age, race, or the presence of diabetes, should be on an ACEI or an ARB to improve renal outcomes. The 2017 ACC/AHA guidelines recommend initial treatment with two agents that have complementary mechanisms of action, especially in black patients or those with stage 2 HTN. These guidelines are summarized in **Table 18.15**.

If a diuretic is chosen, the longer-acting and more potent agent chlorthalidone should be considered as first-line treatment given that it has the highest level of clinical trial evidence supporting its use. Data support the view that monotherapy with a beta blocker (in particular atenolol because of excess risks of strokes) or an alpha blocker (caused by excess risks of CHF events by doxazosin in the ALLHAT study) should be discouraged because they are less effective than most other agents (Law et al., 2009). Meta-analyses also suggest that beta blockers are inferior in the prevention of strokes (Bangalore

TABLE 18.15
Initial Treatment Recommendations

Patient Population	First-Line Treatment
JNC 8	
Nonblack patients	Thiazide diuretic, CCB, ACEI, or ARB
Black patients	Thiazide diuretic or CCB
All patients with CKD	ACEI or ARB
ACC/AHA	
Stage 1 HTN	Thiazide diuretic, CCB, ACEI, or ARB
Stage 2 HTN	2 drugs from different classes (thiazide diuretic, CCB, ACEI, or ARB)
Black patients without HF or CKD	Thiazide diuretic or CCB, in combination with another agent
ADA	
Diabetes	Thiazide diuretic, CCB, ACEI, or ARB
KDIGO	
CKD	No evidence to support preference of any agent
CKD with high levels of urinary albumin or protein excretion	ACEI or ARB

ACC, American College of Cardiology; ACEI, angiotensin-converting enzyme inhibitors; AHA, American Heart Association; ARB, angiotensin II receptor blocker; CCB, calcium channel blockers; CKD, chronic kidney disease; HF, heart failure; HTN, hypertension; JNC, Joint National Committee.

et al., 2007). However, beta blockers might be effective in the secondary prevention of ischemic heart disease.

Studies have shown that isolated systolic HTN (SBP >160 mm Hg with DBP <90 mm Hg) is a potent risk factor for stroke and CVD. Among patients older than 50 years, SBP levels are more strongly related to CVD and renal disease than DBP. Treatment of isolated systolic HTN leads to improved CVD outcomes regardless of achieved DBP. Although there have been long-standing concern and debate about the risks of the J-curve, whereby excessive reductions in DBP may lead to increased risk for CHD events, the overall evidence supports the view that this effect is limited to high-risk patients with established CAD. Treatment-induced reduction in SBP to less than 140 mm Hg provides a greater overall event reduction and is offset by any adverse effects of excessive lowering of DBP (Mancia et al., 2013). Nevertheless, careful monitoring of certain individuals in this scenario is warranted, including those older than 80 years, patients with active angina worsened by BP lowering, and people with excessively low DBP (<65 mm Hg) or orthostatic hypotension.

Additionally, the Avoiding Cardiovascular Events through Combination Therapy in Patients Living with Systolic Hypertension trial demonstrated a significant reduction (20%) in combined cardiovascular events in patients treated with a combination of an ACEI plus CCB (benazepril + amlodipine) compared with patients treated with an ACEI plus a thiazide diuretic (benazepril + hydrochlorothiazide) (Jamerson et al., 2008). Furthermore, the Ongoing Telmisartan Alone and in Combination with Ramipril Global Endpoint Trial study demonstrated that combined ACEI and ARB therapy did not prevent cardiovascular events more than monotherapy. In fact, it showed that renal outcomes were worsened by this combination and higher risk of adverse events (Yusuf et al., 2008). Therefore, ACEIs and ARBs should not be used in combination.

Second-Line Therapy

There are several different strategies for intensifying pharmacologic therapy. **Figure 18.1** summarizes a few of these strategies. Data are lacking to support a preference of one strategy over another. Therefore, the selected strategy may be tailored to the patient based on drug tolerability, cost, pill burden, and adherence. It is important to consider that many of these patients have comorbidities that may also require the use of several drugs. Fortunately, most HTN medications are available as a generic drug and have been on the market for quite some time, which helps with affordability. Antihypertensive medications that are prescribed once daily or that are available as combination products are particularly helpful in patients requiring multiple medications.

Third-Line Therapy

Should the patient still not be at goal, providers should question patient adherence, request BP readings from home, or

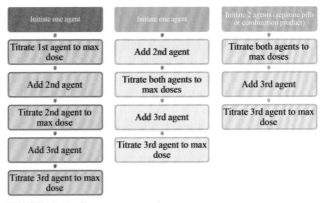

FIGURE 18-1 Treatment strategies.

consider secondary causes of HTN. It may be necessary to add an agent from a drug class not listed in **Table 18.15**. An HTN specialist should be considered if the patient still fails to achieve the goal BP after being on multiple medications, since the patient may have resistant HTN.

For select individuals, it was concluded that some alternative treatments, notably resistance and isometric exercise, device-guided slow breathing, and certain meditation techniques, can serve as effective and helpful adjuvants to lower BP. Whether or not patients are able to adhere to these nonpharmacologic lifestyle treatments to control BP over several years remains uncertain.

Special Considerations

Pediatric Patients

HTN diagnosis and treatment guidelines in pediatric patients are published by the American Academy of Pediatrics. The most recent guidelines were published in 2017. This guideline highlights diagnosis based on the child's age, and goal ranges of the SBP and/or DBP are determined by height and weight percentiles. In general, BP should be treated to below the 90th percentile in patients under age 13, or less than 130/80 mm Hg in patients 13 years and older. Initial treatment is recommended with an ACEI, ARB, long-acting CCB, or thiazide diuretic. It is important to note that recommended dosing for children is different than that for adults and may vary based on age due to differences in renal and hepatic function (Beckett et al., 2008).

Geriatric Patients

Approximately two thirds of patients over age 65 have HTN. The Trial of Nonpharmacological Interventions in the Elderly showed that in older patients with HTN, BP can be reduced by low-sodium diets and weight loss. In some instances, patients could discontinue their antihypertensive medications or reduce the number of medications required to remain normotensive (Sander, 2002). The HYVET demonstrated that a goal BP of less than 150/80 mm Hg in patients over age 80 significantly decreases the risk of stroke and all-cause mortality.

Older adults are very sensitive to medications that cause sympathetic inhibition and are at greater risk of becoming

volume depleted than younger patients. Decreased renal and hepatic function complicates HTN treatment and increases the risk of adverse events in this population. Antihypertensive medications should be started at lower initial doses and titrated slowly, even though standard doses and multiple agents are usually required to achieve BP control. If choosing to use beta blockers in older adults, it is prudent to use the newer beta blockers such as nebivolol and carvedilol as they may provide a better safety profile and better morbidity and mortality outcome (Kaiser et al., 2014). According to the SHEP trial, patients with isolated systolic HTN should start hypertensive therapy with a diuretic due to decrease in stroke incidence unless there is a compelling reason to avoid its use. The long-acting dihydropyridine CCBs are also effective and are an alternative in these patients. Clinical trials have demonstrated that in older patients with isolated systolic HTN, low diastolic BP was associated with a higher mortality rate for any given level of systolic BP. Postural hypotension should also be closely monitored in this population.

Female Patients

There are no significant differences in BP response between genders. Women taking oral contraceptives may have an increase in BP, and the risk of HTN may increase with the duration of oral contraceptive use. If HTN develops as a result of oral contraceptive use, an alternate contraception method should be used. Because of the risk of stroke associated with oral contraceptive use and cigarette smoking, women taking oral contraceptives should be encouraged not to smoke cigarettes, and women older than age 35 should not take oral contraceptives if they continue to smoke.

Women diagnosed with HTN before pregnancy should continue taking antihypertensive agents throughout pregnancy. Few are safe for use, however, during pregnancy. ACEIs, renin inhibitors, and ARBs should be avoided during pregnancy because they are teratogenic. Beta blockers should also be avoided during early pregnancy because of the risk of fetal growth retardation. However, labetalol is preferred later in pregnancy. Methyldopa is recommended for women who are diagnosed with HTN during pregnancy. Consultation with an obstetrician-gynecologists specialist regarding an antihypertensive recommendation should occur in all cases.

African-American Patients

The incidence of HTN and HTN-related complications is believed to be higher in blacks than in any other ethnic group. Some blacks experience HTN before age 10, which is attributed to two major risk factors: obesity and inactivity. Other risk factors include a diet high in sodium and low in potassium. This has resulted in the greatest incidence of stroke, end-stage renal disease, CVD, and death in this population. Blacks who are diagnosed and treated have a lower incidence of complications.

Blacks also have physiologic characteristics that contribute to this risk, including low circulating renin levels with excessive levels of angiotensin II, endothelial dysfunction as a result of reduced bradykinin and nitric oxide, abnormal sympathetic nervous system activation, and higher levels of intracellular calcium stores. As a result, they are less responsive to certain drug classes, such as beta blockers, ACEIs, and ARBs. Blacks are more responsive to monotherapy with diuretics. Results from ALLHAT found that chlorthalidone and amlodipine were superior to ACEIs in treating blacks, and alpha blockers should not be used as initial monotherapy (Papademetriou et al., 2003). ACEIs may induce angioedema, which occurs two to four times more frequently in blacks.

Patients with Diabetes

The coexistence of HTN and diabetes mellitus is very common. HTN increases cardiovascular risks in patients with diabetes. Current guideline recommendations for patients with diabetes have been discussed earlier in this chapter.

All patients should be encouraged to make lifestyle modifications: limit sodium intake, lose weight, and exercise for 150 minutes per week. All major antihypertensive drug classes, RAAS blockers, beta blockers, diuretics, and calcium blockers are useful in diabetic patients. ACEIs and ARBs are considered the cornerstone of therapy. Studies have shown these classes to be beneficial in reducing overall cardiovascular risk, nephropathy, renal failure, and retinopathy. Combination therapy consisting of two RAAS blockers or the use of ACEI and an ARB in combination is not recommended because of the risk of causing renal impairment, hypotension, and hyperkalemia.

HYPERTENSIVE EMERGENCY/ HYPERTENSIVE URGENCY

Hypertensive crisis or malignant HTN is defined as an extremely high SBP and/or DBP according to JNC 7. Hypertensive emergency was not addressed by JNC 8 guidelines. Hypertensive crisis is further divided into two categories based upon evidence of target organ damage. Hypertensive crisis without evidence of organ damage is classified as hypertensive urgency and can be treated in the ambulatory setting. Most of these patients present as a result of nonadherence or inadequate treatment. If end organ damage is present, the condition is classified as hypertensive emergency and typically requires hospitalization.

In hypertensive emergencies, the therapeutic goal is to protect remaining end organ function, reduce risk of complications, and improve outcomes. BP reduction should be made in a controlled fashion and not aimed at normalizing the BP quickly, as this can exacerbate target organ damage. The BP itself may not be as important as the rate of elevation. Patients with a history of chronic HTN can tolerate higher levels than those normotensive patient can tolerate.

Presenting symptoms may include chest pain, dyspnea, and neurologic deficits. The physical examination must include serial BP measurements in both arms, lung and heart auscultation, renal artery auscultation, neurologic evaluation, and funduscopic evaluation. Imaging studies should be obtained if the patient presents with chest or back pain and unequal pulses in the upper extremities. Electrocardiogram and cardiac enzymes are part of the initial workup for shortness of breath or chest pain, and echocardiogram is useful if heart failure is suspected.

Immediate treatment with an intravenous (IV) antihypertensive agent(s) is needed to salvage viable tissue. The marked elevation in BP results in arteriolar fibrinoid necrosis, endothelial damage, platelet and fibrin deposition in the media of smooth muscle, and loss of autoregulatory function. This results in end organ ischemia such as encephalopathy, MI, unstable angina, pulmonary edema, eclampsia, stroke, intracranial hemorrhage, life-threatening arterial bleeding, or aortic dissection.

The drug of choice to treat hypertensive emergencies depends on the clinical situation. BP control can be achieved over several hours (24–48 hours) with either IV or oral medications depending on the urgency of the situation. Commonly used medications include direct vasodilators (hydralazine), nitrates (sodium nitroprusside, nitroglycerin), CCBs (nicardipine, clevidipine), sympathoplegic agents (labetalol, esmolol), alpha-1 blockers (phentolamine), and ACEIs (enalaprilat). After the BP is lowered, the patient's drug regimen should be assessed to determine possible causes of the hypertensive emergency/urgency such as medication nonadherence, adverse effects that interfere with the patient's lifestyle, and/or a complex medication regimen that could be simplified. Patients should have follow-up within several days.

MONITORING PATIENT RESPONSE

Follow-Up and Monitoring

BP should be measured at every routine visit. The patient's efforts and lifestyle modifications should be discussed at each visit. Patients should be evaluated monthly until the goal BP is achieved. More frequent evaluation may be necessary in patients with stage 2 HTN or multiple comorbidities. Referral to a HTN specialist may be indicated if the BP goal is not achieved despite several medications, if resistant HTN is suspected, or if clinical consultation is needed for more complicated patients. When initially adding medication or increasing doses of drugs that have electrolyte abnormalities as an adverse effect, frequent monitoring is warranted. SCr and potassium levels should be monitored once or twice a year in patients taking antihypertensive medications once the levels have proven to be stable.

The importance of adhering to the drug regimen cannot be overemphasized. It is extremely important to ask open-ended questions. The practitioner needs to be alert for signs of nonadherence and should ask patients about their experiences or problems with adhering to the drug regimen. Side effects should be discussed, and changes in medications may or may not be considered at each visit.

PATIENT EDUCATION

Patient education is a vital component of HTN treatment. Because most patients are free of symptoms, they must be educated about the disease, the importance of adhering to therapy, and the consequences of uncontrolled HTN. Patient education booklets are available from most national organizations such as the AHA, which may be used to reinforce the information provided by the practitioner.

Because each antihypertensive medication has some side effects, the patient needs to be informed about what they are, what actions can be taken to relieve minor side effects, and what to do about intolerable or dangerous side effects. Adherence to the antihypertensive medication regimen should be assessed at each office encounter. Since the objective of drug therapy is to lower BP without intolerable effects, the patient needs to know which adverse reactions should be reported to the practitioner and which ones may be relieved by switching to an alternative drug in a different class. The patient also needs to know that several different agents may be tried before finding the one that best controls the patient's BP with minimal or no side effects. Providing information about lifestyle changes is also important.

Nutrition/Lifestyle Changes

As described previously, it is important to remind patients about the key role of lifestyle in BP. Patients should follow a healthy diet, restrict sodium, quit smoking (if applicable), and limit alcohol consumption. Patients should also be reminded to maintain a healthy weight and get regular exercise for better control of BP. Lifestyle changes and nonpharmacologic treatment are an important aspect of HTN treatment and should always be emphasized, even in patients on antihypertensive medications. In some cases, it is possible to reduce or eliminate medications altogether in patients who make significant lifestyle changes.

All patients diagnosed with HTN should be counseled about the benefits of and how to implement a combination of dietary and lifestyle modifications for BP reduction. Patients are encouraged to maintain appropriate body weight (BMI of 19.5–24.9). A reduction in SBP of 5 to 20 mm Hg occurs per 10 kg weight loss. Patients should also adopt a healthy diet, such as the Dietary Approaches to Stop Hypertension diet, U.S. Department of Agriculture Food Pattern diet, or the AHA diet. These diets focus on a high quantity of fruits, vegetables, and low-fat dairy products. They specifically focus on reduction of intake of saturated and total fat. A healthy diet can decrease the SBP by 11 mm Hg. Other recommended lifestyle modifications include restriction of dietary sodium to less than 2.4 g daily, encouragement of physical activity (at least 120 minutes per week of aerobic activity), and reduction in alcohol consumption (Eckel & Cornier, 2014). All patients diagnosed with HTN should be utilizing lifestyle modifications as a backbone to treatment.

Complementary and Alternative Medications

To date, there is no evidence that alternative medications reduce BP.

CASE STUDY 1

Robert is a 65-year-old African-American man who was referred to the hypertension clinic for evaluation of high blood pressure (BP) noted on an initial screening. On physical exam, his BP readings are 145/90 mm Hg and 141/96 mm Hg. He was diagnosed with diabetes 10 years ago, has a history of gout, and currently smokes 2 packs of cigarettes per day. His current medications include metformin 1,000 mg twice daily, aspirin 81 mg daily, allopurinol 300 mg daily, and rosuvastatin 20 mg daily (Learning Objectives 1–3).

Laboratory findings
    Total cholesterol: 201 mg/dL
    High-density lipoprotein cholesterol: 30 mg/dL
    Low-density lipoprotein cholesterol: 142 mg/dL
    Triglycerides: 167 mg/dL

1. Based on the patient's blood pressure readings, Robert is best classified as having what stage of hypertension?
2. According to JNC 8, his blood pressure goal is:
3. Which antihypertensive drug class is preferred for Robert based on his comorbid conditions and ethnicity?

Bibliography

Starred references are cited in the text.

*American Diabetes Association. (2020). Standards of medical care in diabetes—2020. *Diabetes Care, 43* (Supplement 1), S1–S2.

*Bangalore, S., Parkar, S., Grossman, E., et al. (2007). A meta-analysis of 94,492 patients with hypertension treated with beta blockers to determine the risk of new onset diabetes mellitus. *American Journal of Cardiology, 100*, 1254–1262.

Basile, J. (2010). One size does not fit all: The role of vasodilating β-blockers in controlling hypertension as a means of reducing cardiovascular and stroke risk. *The American Journal of Medicine, 123*, S9–S15.

*Beckett, N., Peters, R., Fletcher, A., et al. (2008). Treatment of hypertension in patients 80 years of age or older. *New England Journal of Medicine, 358*(18), 1887–1898.

Bloch, M. J. (2003). The diagnosis and management of renovascular disease: A primary care perspective. *Journal of Clinical Hypertension, 5*, 210–218.

Brown, N. J., Ray, W. A., Snowden, M., et al. (1996). Black Americans have an increased rate of angiotensin-converting enzyme inhibition associated angioedema. *Clinical Pharmacology and Therapeutics, 60*, 8–13.

Burkhart, G. A., Brown, N. J., Griffin, M. R., et al. (1996). Angiotensin-converting enzyme inhibitor-associated angioedema: Higher risk in blacks than whites. *Pharmacoepidemiology and Drug Safety, 5*, 149–154.

CAPRICORN Investigators. (2001). Effects of carvedilol on outcome after myocardial infarction in patients with left-ventricular dysfunction: The CAPRICORN randomised trial. *Lancet, 357*, 1385–1390.

Chobanian, A. (2008). Does it matter how hypertension is controlled? *New England Journal of Medicine, 359*, 2485–2488.

*Cushman, W., Evans, G., Byington, R., et al. (2010). Effects of intensive blood-pressure control in type 2 diabetes mellitus. *New England Journal of Medicine, 362*, 1575–1585.

*Dahlöf, B., Devereux, R., Kjeldsen, S., et al. (2002). Cardiovascular morbidity and mortality in the Losartan Intervention For Endpoint reduction in hypertension study (LIFE): A randomised trial against atenolol. *Lancet, 359*, 995–1003.

Eckel, R. H., & Cornier, M. A. (2014). Update on the NCEP ATP-III emerging cardiometabolic risk factors. *BMC Medicine, 12*, 115. https://doi.org/10.1186/1741-7015-12-115

Eknoyan, G., Lameire, N., Eckardt, K.-U., et al. (2012). KDIGO clinical practice guideline for the management of blood pressure in chronic kidney disease. *Kidney International Supplements, 2*, 341–342.

Escobar, C., & Barrios, V. (2009). Combined therapy in the treatment of hypertension. *Fundamental & Clinical Pharmacology, 24*, 3–8.

*Flynn, J., Kaelber, D., Baker-Smith, C., et al. (2017). Clinical practice guideline for screening and management of high blood pressure in children and adolescents. *Pediatrics, 140*(3), e20171904.

Forman, J., & Brenner, B. (2006). Hypertension and microalbuminuria: The bell tolls for thee. *Kidney International, 69*, 22–28.

Garcia-Donaire, J., & Ruilope, L. (2009). Multiple action fixed combinations. Present or future? *Fundamental & Clinical Pharmacology, 24*, 37–42.

Go, A., Bauman, M., Coleman, S., et al. (2014). An effective approach to high blood pressure control. *Hypertension, 63*, 878–885.

Go, A., Mozaffarian, D., Roger, V., et al. (2014). Heart disease and stroke statistics—2014 update: A report from the American Heart Association. *Circulation, 129*(3), e28–e292. doi: 10.1161/01.cir.0000441139.02102.80

Grossman, Y., Shlomai, G., & Grossman, E. (2014). Treating hypertension in type 2 diabetes. *Expert Opinion on Pharmacotherapy, 15*, 2131–2140.

He, J., Klag, M. J., Appek, L. J., et al. (1999). The renin–angiotensin system and BP: Differences between blacks and whites. *American Journal of Hypertension, 12*(6), 555–562.

Head, G. (2014). Ambulatory blood pressure monitoring is ready to replace clinic blood pressure in the diagnosis of hypertension. Pro side of the argument. *Hypertension, 64*, 1175–1181.

*Jamerson, K., Weber, M., Bakris, G., et al. (2008). Benazepril plus amlodipine or hydrochlorothiazide for hypertension in high-risk patients (ACCOMPLISH). *New England Journal of Medicine, 359*(23), 2417–2428.

*James, P., Oparil, S., Carter, B., et al. (2014). 2014 evidence-based guideline for the management of high blood pressure in adults: Report from the panel members appointed to the eighth Joint National Committee (JNC 8). *Journal of the American Medical Association, 311*, 507–520.

Joint National Committee on Prevention, Detection, Evaluation, and Treatment of High BP. (2003). Seventh report of the joint national committee on prevention, detection, evaluation, and treatment of high BP (JNC VII). *Journal of the American Medical Association, 289*, 2560–2572.

Jordan, J., & Grassi, G. (2010). Belly fat and resistant hypertension. *Journal of Hypertension, 28*, 1131–1133.

*Kaiser, E., Lotze, U., & Schafer, H. (2014). Increasing complexity: Which drug class to choose for treatment of hypertension in the elderly? *Clinical Interventions in Aging, 9*, 459–475.

*Law, M., Morris, J., & Wald, N. (2009). Use of blood pressure lowering drugs in the prevention of cardiovascular disease: Meta-analysis of 147 randomised trials in the context of expectation from perspective epidemiological studies. *British Medical Journal, 338*, b1665.

Lee, M. (2014). Erectile dysfunction. In J. T. DiPiro, R. L. Talbert, G. C. Yee, et al. (Eds.), *Pharmacotherapy: A pathophysiologic approach* (9th ed., p. 1349). New York, NY: McGraw-Hill.

Mancia, G., De Backer, G., Dominiczak, A., et al. (2007). 2007 guidelines for the management of arterial hypertension: The task force for the management of arterial hypertension of the European Society of Hypertension (ESH) and of the European Society of Cardiology (ESC). *Journal of Hypertension, 25*, 1105–1187.

*Mancia, G., Fagard, R., Narkiewicz, K., et al. (2013). 2013 ESH/ESC guidelines for the management of arterial hypertension: The task force for the management of arterial hypertension of the European Society of Hypertension (ESH) and of the European Society of Cardiology (ESC). *Journal of Hypertension, 31*, 1281–1357.

Messerli, F., & Panjrath, G. (2009). The J-curve between blood pressure and coronary artery disease or essential hypertension: Exactly how essential? *Journal of the American College of Cardiology, 20*, 1827–1834.

*Papademetriou, V., Piller, L., Ford, C., et al. (2003). Characteristics and lipid distribution of a large, high-risk, hypertension population: The lipid-lowering component of the antihypertensive and lipid-lowering treatment to prevent heart attack trail (ALLHAT). *Journal of Clinical Hypertension, 5*, 377–385.

Parving, H., Brenner, B., McMurray, J., et al. (2012). Cardiorenal End Points in a Trial of Aliskiren for Type 2 Diabetes (ALTITUDE). *New England Journal of Medicine, 367*(23), 2204–2213.

Piper, M. A., Evans, C. V., Burda, B. U., et al. (2014). Screening for high blood pressure in adults: A systematic evidence review for the U.S. Preventive Services Task Force. Evidence Synthesis No. 121. AHRQ Publication No. 13-05194-EF-1. Rockville, MD: Agency for Healthcare Research and Quality.

*Pitt, B., Remme, W., Cody, R., et al. (1999). The effect of spironolactone on morbidity and mortality in patients with severe health failure (RALES). *New England Journal of Medicine, 341*(10), 709–717.

Poole-Wilson, P., Swedberg, K., Cleland, J., et al. (2003). Comparison of carvedilol and metoprolol on clinical outcomes in patients with chronic heart failure in the Carvedilol Or Metoprolol European Trial (COMET): Randomised controlled trial. *Lancet, 362*, 7–13.

Rakel, R., & Rakel, D. (2013). *Textbook of family medicine. Cardiovascular disease* (9th ed.). Philadelphia, PA: Elsevier.

Ramos, A., & Varon, J. (2014). Current and newer agents for hypertensive emergencies. *Current Hypertension Reports, 16*, 450.

Redon, J., & Lurbe, E. (2014). Ambulatory blood pressure monitoring is ready to replace clinic blood pressure in diagnosis of hypertension. Con side of the argument. *Hypertension, 64*, 1169–1174.

*Sander, G. (2002). High blood pressure in the geriatric population: Treatment considerations. *American Journal of Geriatric Cardiology, 11*, 223–232.

Saseen J. J., & MacLaughlin E. J. (2014). Hypertension. In: J. T. DiPiro, R. L. Talbert, G. C. Yee, et al. (Eds.), *Pharmacotherapy: A pathophysiologic approach* (9th ed., pp. 49–84). New York, NY: McGraw-Hill.

SHEP Cooperative Research Group. (1991). Prevention of stroke by antihypertensive drug treatment in older persons with isolated systolic hypertension. *Journal of the American Medical Association, 265*, 3255–3264.

Sica, D. (2002). ACE inhibitors and stroke: New considerations. *Journal of Clinical Hypertension, 4*, 126–129.

Sica, D., & Black, H. (2002). ACE inhibitor-related angioedema: Can angiotensin-receptor blockers be safely used? *Journal of Clinical Hypertension, 4*(5), 375–380.

*Taler, S., Agarwal, R., Bakris, G., et al. (2013). KDOQI US Commentary on the 2012 KDIGO clinical practice guideline for management of blood pressure in CKD. *American Journal of Kidney Diseases, 62*, 201–213.

Taylor, A., & Bakris, G. (2010). The role of vasodilating B-blockers in patients with hypertension and the cardiometabolic syndrome. *The American Journal of Medicine, 123*, S21–S26.

Tierney, L., McPhee, S., & Papadakis, M. (2004). *Current medical diagnosis and treatment*. New York, NY: McGraw-Hill.

Ungar, A., Pepe, G., Lambertucci, L., et al. (2009). Low diastolic ambulatory blood pressure is associated with greater all-cause mortality in older patients with hypertension. *Journal of the American Geriatrics Society, 57*, 291–296.

*U.S. Preventive Services Task Force. (2007). Screening for high blood pressure: U.S. Preventive Services Task Force reaffirmation recommendation statement. *Annals of Internal Medicine, 147*, 783–787.

*Virani, S. S., Alonso, A., Benjamin, E. J., et al. (2020). Heart disease and stroke statistics—2020 update. *Circulation, 141*(9), e139–e596.

*Vongpatanasin, W. (2014). Resistant hypertension: A review of diagnosis and management. *Journal of the American Medical Association, 311*, 2216–2224.

*Whelton, P., Carey, R., Aronow, W., et al. (2018). 2017 ACC/AHA/AAPA/ABC/ACPM/AGS/APhA/ASH/ASPC/NMA/PCNA guideline for the prevention, detection, evaluation, and management of high blood pressure in adults: A report of the American College of Cardiology/American Heart Association Task Force on Clinical Practice Guidelines. *Journal of the American College of Cardiology, 71*(19), e127–e248.

Wright, J., Jamerson, K., & Ferdinand, K. (2007). The management of hypertension in African Americans. *Journal of Clinical Hypertension, 9*, 468–475.

Yancy, C., Fowler, M., Colucci, W., et al. (2001). Race and the response to adrenergic blockade with carvedilol in patients with chronic heart failure. *New England Journal of Medicine, 344*, 1358–1365.

*Yusuf, S., Teo, K., Pogue, J., et al. (2008). Telmisartan, ramipril, or both in patients at high risk for vascular events. *New England Journal of Medicine, 358*, 1547–1559.

19 Hyperlipidemia

Thuy Le and John Barron

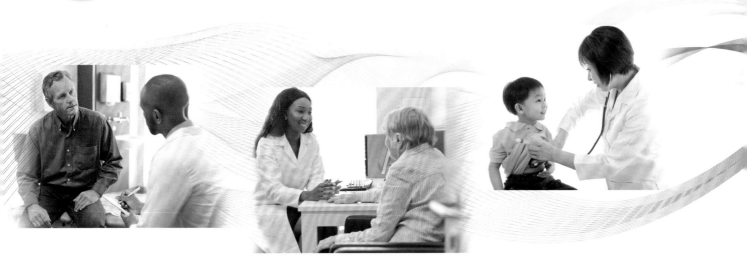

Learning Objectives

1. Evaluate risk factors for the development of atherosclerotic cardiovascular disease and identify when pharmacologic treatment may be indicated for hyperlipidemia.
2. Design a hyperlipidemia pharmacologic plan of care using evidence-based guidelines.
3. Describe the monitoring parameters for drug efficacy, side effects, and contraindications of cholesterol-lowering medications.

INTRODUCTION

Hyperlipidemia is a blood disorder characterized by elevations in blood cholesterol levels. The term is often used synonymously with *dyslipidemia* and *hypercholesterolemia*. Hyperlipidemia is one of the major contributing risk factors in the development of coronary heart disease (CHD). It is estimated that approximately 15.5 million people in the United States have CHD, with approximately 375,000 deaths each year (American Heart Association, 2015). In addition, approximately $215 billion is spent each year on direct and indirect costs from CHD.

Informed estimates indicate that approximately more than 100 million adults aged 20 and older had total cholesterol levels above 200 mg/dL, using data from 2009 to 2012, representing approximately 47% of adults in the United States (American Heart Association, 2015). However, data from the National Health and Nutrition Examination Survey suggest that the percentage of patients with elevated cholesterol may be decreasing.

Numerous large studies have shown that reducing elevated cholesterol levels reduces morbidity and mortality rates in patients with and without existing CHD (Downs et al., 1998; Frick et al., 1987; Heart Protection Study Collaborative Group, 2002; Lewis et al., 1998; Long-Term Intervention with Pravastatin in Ischaemic Disease [LIPID] Study Group, 1998; Ridker et al., 2008; Scandinavian Simvastatin Survival Study Group, 1994; Shepherd et al., 1995). Specifically, the lowering of low-density lipoprotein cholesterol (LDL-C), or "bad" cholesterol, is associated with significant risk reduction of atherosclerotic cardiovascular disease (ASCVD). Although these and other trials have clearly shown the benefits of treating high cholesterol levels and other preventive measures, including the use of aspirin, beta blockers, and angiotensin-converting enzyme inhibitors, in the management of patients with coronary artery disease, long-term use of statin medications across the population is still suboptimal, particularly in high-risk populations, minorities, women, and the uninsured (Salami et al., 2017).

CAUSES

In hyperlipidemia, serum cholesterol levels may be elevated as a result of an increased level of any of the lipoproteins. (See the section titled Lipoproteins and Lipid Metabolism.) The mechanisms for hyperlipidemia appear to be genetic (primary) and environmental (secondary). In fact, the most common cause of hyperlipidemia (95% of all those with hyperlipidemia) is a combination of genetic and environmental factors.

Disease States	Drugs
Acute hepatitis	Alcohol
Diabetes mellitus	Beta blockers
Hypothyroidism	Glucocorticoids
Nephrotic syndrome	Oral contraceptives
Primary biliary cirrhosis	Progestins
Systemic lupus erythematosus	Thiazide diuretics
Uremia	

Some individuals are genetically predisposed to elevated cholesterol levels. They may inherit defective genes that lead to abnormalities in the synthesis or breakdown of cholesterol. These may include abnormalities in LDL receptors (LDLR) and mutations in apolipoproteins that lead to increased production of cholesterol or decreased clearance of cholesterol from the bloodstream. (See the section titled Lipoproteins and Lipid Metabolism.)

Secondary factors may include medications (e.g., beta blockers and oral contraceptives), concomitant disease states or other conditions (e.g., diabetes mellitus and pregnancy), diets high in fat and cholesterol, lack of exercise, obesity, and smoking (**Box 19.1**).

PATHOPHYSIOLOGY

The major plasma lipids are cholesterol, triglycerides (TGs), and phospholipids. Cholesterol is a naturally occurring substance that is required by the body to synthesize bile acids and steroid hormones and to maintain the integrity of cell membranes. Although cholesterol is found predominantly in the cells, approximately 7% circulates in the serum. It is this serum cholesterol that is implicated in atherosclerosis. TGs are made up of free fatty acids and glycerol and serve as an important source of stored energy. Phospholipids are essential for cell function and lipid transport. Because these lipids are insoluble in plasma, they are surrounded by special fat-carrying proteins, called *lipoproteins*, for transport in the blood.

Lipoproteins are produced in the liver and intestines, but endogenous production of lipoproteins occurs primarily in the liver. Lipoproteins consist of a hydrophobic (water-insoluble) inner core made of cholesterol and TGs and a hydrophilic (water-soluble) outer surface composed of apolipoproteins and phospholipids. Apolipoproteins are specialized proteins that identify specific receptors to which the lipoprotein will bind. They are thought to play a role in the development or prevention of hyperlipidemia because they control the interaction and metabolism of the lipoproteins.

Lipoproteins and Lipid Metabolism

The major lipoproteins are named according to their density. They include chylomicrons, very-low-density lipoproteins (VLDLs), intermediate-density lipoproteins (IDLs), LDLs, and high-density lipoproteins (HDLs).

Chylomicrons

Chylomicrons, the largest lipoproteins, are composed primarily of TGs. Chylomicrons are produced in the gut from dietary fat and cholesterol that has been solubilized by bile acids (exogenous pathway). Chylomicrons normally are not present in the blood after a 12- to 14-hour fast.

Very-Low-Density Lipoproteins

VLDLs are primarily composed of cholesterol and TGs and are the major carrier of endogenous TGs. On secretion into the bloodstream, lipoprotein lipase and hepatic lipase hydrolyze the TG core by a mechanism similar to that which occurs with chylomicrons. As the TG content decreases, the lipoprotein becomes progressively smaller with a higher percentage of cholesterol; it is now referred to as an *IDL*. IDL is a short-lived lipoprotein that is converted to LDL or is taken up by LDLR on the liver. LDL, the final product of the metabolism of VLDL, contains the most cholesterol by weight of all the lipoproteins. It is estimated that 60% to 75% of the total cholesterol is contained in LDLs (Talbert, 1997).

Approximately 50% of LDL is taken up by the liver, and the remaining 50% is taken up by peripheral cells. Increased levels of LDL cholesterol are directly related to the probability that atherosclerosis will develop. Thus, LDL cholesterol is usually referred to as *bad* cholesterol.

High-Density Lipoproteins

HDL particles are produced in the liver and intestine. The primary function of HDL cholesterol is to remove LDL cholesterol from the peripheral cells and to remove TGs that result from the degradation of chylomicrons and VLDL particles. The HDL then transports these particles to the liver for metabolism. This process is termed *reverse cholesterol transport*. For this reason, HDL is often referred to as *good* cholesterol.

Pathogenesis of Atherosclerosis

Atherosclerosis is characterized by the development of lesions resulting from accumulations of cholesterol in the blood vessel wall, leading to an increased risk of ASCVD. Atherosclerosis primarily affects the larger arteries, including the coronary arteries.

The atherogenic process begins with the accumulation of LDL cholesterol under the endothelial lining of the innermost arterial layer, the intima. As LDLs accumulate, circulating monocytes attach to the endothelial lining and penetrate between the endothelial cells into the subendothelial space. On entry into the subendothelial space, the monocytes form into macrophages, which then ingest the LDLs. Macrophages, in particular, have a high affinity for modified (oxidized) LDL. As the macrophages ingest the modified LDL, they are converted into foam cells and form the *fatty streak*, which is the initial lesion in the atherogenic process. These lesions commonly affect the coronary arteries. Formation begins in the mid-teens, and the lesions grow as the person ages.

Once the fatty streak forms, the oxidized LDL and macrophages act in other ways that promote the progression of the atherogenic lesion. Oxidized LDL appears to act as a chemotactic agent, recruiting other circulating monocytes and preventing macrophages from leaving the subendothelial space. Macrophages also produce chemotactic factors and growth factors. The growth factors cause proliferation of smooth muscle cells from the media into the fatty streak, leading to the formation of a fibrous plaque (Ross & Glomset, 1976). Fibrous plaques are usually raised and protrude into the lumen of the artery, thereby compromising blood flow.

As the foam cells grow, the endothelium stretches and may become damaged. This leads to platelet aggregation and clot formation. In many instances, these fissures heal and incorporate the thrombi inside the plaque. This process may occur dozens of times and eventually may produce a complicated lesion. The formation of complicated lesions is the major cause of acute cardiovascular (CV) events. However, in some instances, rupture of a small, unstable plaque may also cause the formation of a single large clot that totally occludes the vessel. The fibrous plaques that are most likely to rupture are those that have large lipid cores and a thin fibrous cap, a layer of smooth muscle cells directly over the lipid core. Large plaques with a strong fibrous cap may be more stable and less likely to rupture (Cooke & Bhatnagar, 1997; McKenney & Hawkins, 1995).

The primary symptom associated with atherosclerosis is chest pain known as *angina*. Symptoms occur when the lesion compromises blood flow in the vessel lumen. A lesion that occludes approximately 50% of the lumen usually causes symptoms when more blood flow is required (i.e., exercise-induced angina). As the lesions grow and occlude more than 70% of the vessel, anginal symptoms may occur even when the person is resting (Cooke & Bhatnagar, 1997).

RISK ASSESSMENT

In 2018, the American College of Cardiology (ACC) and the American Heart Association (AHA) released updated guidelines on the management of blood cholesterol. The previous 2013 guidelines echoed a framework that the intensity of an intervention should be proportional to the individual's absolute risk for having a future ASCVD event (**Box 19.2**). Health care practitioners can then utilize this framework by assessing a patient's ASCVD risk, discussing benefits and risks associated with potential therapies, and reviewing the patient's goals and preferences for treatment.

Similar to the previous guidelines, the 2018 ACC/AHA guidelines recommend assessment of traditional ASCVD risk

BOX 19.2 Atherosclerotic Vascular Disease

Acute coronary syndrome
History of myocardial infarction
Stable or unstable angina
History of arterial revascularization (coronary artery bypass graft, coronary angioplasty)
Peripheral arterial disease (including aortic aneurysm of atherosclerotic origin)
Thrombotic stroke
Transient ischemic attack

factors in patients aged 20 to 79 without a history of CVD every 4 to 6 years. In addition to lipid levels, these traditional risk factors include age, gender, systolic blood pressure, antihypertensive therapy use, presence of diabetes, and smoking status. While for the estimation of 10-year risk for ASCVD, only total and HDL cholesterol levels are required, a full lipid panel, which also contains LDL cholesterol and TGs, should be obtained to fully evaluate a patient's ASCVD risk. A past medical history should also be obtained to determine if the patient has already had an ASCVD event such as a myocardial infarction (MI) or thromboembolic stroke. Those patients with a past medical history of ASCVD, labeled as *secondary prevention patients*, are at a higher risk for a future ASCVD event than those without a history of ASCVD, labeled as *primary prevention patients*.

To quantify the ASCVD risk in a primary prevention patient, the ACC/AHA guidelines recommend the use of the pooled cohort equations (PCE) that are race and gender specific. The PCE calculator can be assessed online through the ACC or AHA Web site. This risk assessment tool estimates the 10-year ASCVD risk for patients 40 to 79 years of age and the lifetime ASCVD risk for patients 20 to 59 years of age. The PCE are based on multiple studies beyond the original Framingham study and were hoped to be an improvement on the Framingham risk calculator because the equations were developed in a broader population, including African-Americans, and a fuller definition of ASCVD was utilized (CHD death, nonfatal MI, and fatal/nonfatal stroke). While the PCE calculator is a robust tool for predicting population risk, limitations exist for predicting individual risk that can potentially underestimate or overestimate risk for ASCVD in individual patients. In order to improve the ASCVD risk assessment in patients with borderline risk based on the traditional risk factors and help inform treatment decisions, the 2018 ACC/AHA cholesterol guidelines introduced risk-enhancing factors (**Table 19.1**), which help clinicians quantify a patient's overall risk to further confirm whether statin therapy should be initiated when risk is borderline. Furthermore, the ACC/AHA guidelines recommend the utilization of coronary artery calcium (CAC) score to further explore the decision of

TABLE 19.1

Atherosclerotic Cardiovascular Disease Risk-Enhancing Factors

ASCVD Risk Enhancers

Chronic kidney disease

Family history of premature ASCVD

Inflammatory diseases (psoriasis, rheumatoid arthritis, HIV)

Metabolic syndrome

Persistently elevated cholesterol (LDL-C $\geq$160 mg/dL, non-HDL-C 190–219 mg/dL)

Persistently elevated cholesterol (LDL-C $\geq$160 mg/dL, non-HDL-C 190–219 mg/dL)

South Asian ancestry

Preeclampsia or premature menopause (before age 40 year old)

Elevated biomarkers:
Hs-CRP $\geq$2 mg/L; Lp (a) levels $\geq$50 mg/dL or >15 nmol/L; ABI <0.9

ABI, ankle-brachial index; ASCVD, atherosclerotic cardiovascular disease; HDL-C, high-density lipoprotein cholesterol; HIV, human immunodeficiency virus; Hs-CRP, high-sensitivity C-reactive protein; LDL-C, low-density lipoprotein cholesterol; Lp(a), lipoprotein (a).

TABLE 19.2

Clinical Application Using Coronary Artery Calcium Score

10-Year ASCVD Risk	CAC Score	Statin Recommendation
<5%	Any value	Not recommended
5%–7%	0	Not recommended
	>1	Consider statin therapy
7.6%–20%	0	Not recommended
	>0	Statin recommended
>20	Any value	Statin recommended

ASCVD, atherosclerotic cardiovascular disease; CAC, coronary artery calcium.

statin initiation in these patients. Other risk markers include family history of CVD, high-sensitivity C-reactive protein (hs-CRP), and ankle–brachial index. hs-CRP is a marker for inflammation, and levels 2 mg/L or higher have been associated with an increased risk of ASCVD.

Coronary Artery Calcium

A CAC scan is a noninvasive procedure that detects atherosclerotic plaque burden (total plaque area and density). The result of the CAC scan is characterized by the Agatston score. The CAC score can assist clinicians and patients to further determine the ASCVD risk of an individual for future CV events and also to determine whether statin therapy should be initiated or delayed. Subset of patients who may benefit from knowing their CAC score includes patients who have borderline risk (i.e., ASCVD risk of 5%–7.4%) or patients who are reluctant or curious to start statin therapy and require more objective data to better understand their condition.

A CAC score can range from 0 to over 400. A score of zero categorizes a patient at a lower ASCVD risk level for the next 10 years. In other words, statin therapy may be delayed in these patients. Experts recommend that a CAC be repeated in 5 to 10 years in this case. On the contrary, the following high-risk conditions favor statin initiation regardless of CAC score: diabetes mellitus, active smoking, and premature or a strong family history of ASCVD or chronic inflammatory conditions. A CAC score of 1 to 99 favors initiation of statin in adults aged more than 55 years. A CAC score of 100 or more correlates to an ASCVD score of 7.5% or more and favors the initiation of statin therapy (**Table 19.2**). It is important to note that a CAC score is only useful in patients who are not actively on statin therapy, and it currently has no clinical utility in those patients already on a statin.

Lifestyle Modification

In 2013, the ACC and the AHA released guidelines on lifestyle management to reduce CV risk (2013 ACC/AHA lifestyle guidelines). These guidelines focused primarily on dietary therapy, exercise, weight loss, moderation of alcohol intake, and smoking cessation.

Diet

The guidelines recommend a diet that is high in fruits, vegetables, whole grains, low-fat dairy products, poultry, fish, legumes, nontropical vegetable oils, and nuts. It also recommends limiting sweets, sugar-sweetened beverages, and red meats. Individuals should try to limit caloric intake of saturated fat to no more than 5% to 6% of total calories. Additionally, it is recommended to limit intake of trans fats. Diets that are recommended include the Dietary Approaches to Stop Hypertension dietary pattern, the U.S. Department of Agriculture Food Pattern, or the AHA Diet. Strict adherence to a healthy diet can reduce LDL-C levels by 10% to more than 15%.

In addition, overweight patients should attempt to lose weight. The ability to lose weight depends on the amount of calories consumed and the amount of calories burned. The goal for overweight patients should be a realistic, gradual, and steady loss of weight. Once an ideal weight is achieved, caloric intake is adjusted to maintain that weight.

Exercise

Regular physical exercise may provide several benefits in patients with hyperlipidemia.

The guidelines encourage individuals to participate in aerobic physical activity three to four times a week, with each session averaging about 40 minutes. As mentioned, it should be used along with dietary therapy to promote weight loss. Exercise may benefit the lipid profile by reducing TGs and raising HDL levels. Exercise may also improve control of diabetes and coronary blood flow.

Moderation of Alcohol Intake and Smoking Cessation

Excessive alcohol intake may elevate serum lipid levels, specifically TG levels, but in moderation (no more than one drink per day for women and two drinks per day for men), alcohol may improve HDL levels and has been associated with lower ASCVD rates (Brien et al., 2011). Despite these benefits, alcohol should not be recommended for ASCVD prevention because the consequences associated with excessive alcohol use outweigh any benefits.

Cigarette smoking is an independent risk factor in the development of ASCVD (Huxley & Woodward, 2011). Although smoking minimally affects cholesterol levels, it contributes to the development of ASCVD by damaging the vascular endothelium and promoting platelet aggregation, which results in increased risk of clot formation. Smoking cessation can reduce this risk and should be encouraged by all health care professionals. The risk of developing ASCVD decreases by approximately 50% within 1 to 2 years of smoking cessation.

STATIN BENEFIT GROUPS

The ACC/AHA cholesterol guidelines recommend use of beta-hydroxy-beta-methylglutaryl coenzyme A (HMG-CoA) reductase inhibitors (statins) for ASCVD prevention in four groups of patients, termed *statin benefit groups*. The statin benefit groups include individuals who (1) have clinical ASCVD (highest-risk group), (2) do not have ASCVD but have severe hyperlipidemia defined as LDL-C 190 or more and are 20 to 75 years of age (high-risk group), (3) are 40 to 75 years old with type 1 or type 2 diabetes mellitus and have LDL-C values of 70 to 189 mg/dL, or (4) are 40 to 75 years old with LDL-C values of 70 to 189 mg/dL and have a 10-year risk of ASCVD of 7.5% or more.

The recommended statin and dose to use are based upon the expected reduction in LDL-C levels. High-intensity statins are those that can lower LDL-C by 50% or more, on average. Moderate-intensity statins reduce LDL-C by about 30% to 49%, and low-intensity statins typically reduce LDL-C by less than 30%. Specific medications and doses for each category are listed in **Table 19.3**.

In individuals with clinical ASCVD, a high-intensity statin is recommended in those 75 years or less of age, unless contraindicated (known hypersensitivity, active liver disease, women who are pregnant or may become pregnant, or nursing mothers) or unable to tolerate dose, in which a moderate-intensity statin should be used. For individuals with ASCVD who are more than 75 years of age, a moderate-dose statin is recommended.

Individuals who do not have ASCVD but whose LDL-C is 190 mg/dL or more should receive high-intensity statin, unless contraindicated or unable to tolerate high-intensity statin.

A moderate-intensity statin is recommended for individuals aged 40 to 75 years old who have diabetes mellitus and have LDL-C between 70 and 189 mg/dL. High-intensity statin is recommended for patients meeting these criteria whose 10-year ASCVD risk is 20% or more. For diabetic patients aged less than 40 or more than 75 years old, it is recommended

TABLE 19.3			
Statin Dose Intensity (Daily Dose)			
Generic Name (Trade Name)	**High Intensity (mg)**	**Moderate Intensity (mg)**	**Low Intensity (mg)**
Atorvastatin (Lipitor)	40–80	10–20	NA
Rosuvastatin (Crestor)	20–40	5–10	NA
Simvastatin (Zocor)	NA	20–40	10
Lovastatin (Mevacor)	NA	40–80	20
Pravastatin (Pravachol)	NA	40–80	10–20
Fluvastatin (Lescol)	NA	80	20–40
Pitavastatin (Livalo)	NA	1–4	NA

to evaluate 10-year ASCVD risk to determine whether or not statin therapy should be considered.

For patients aged 40 to 75 years old without ASCVD, without diabetes mellitus, and whose LDL-C is between 70 and 189 mg/dL, treatment with a moderate-intensity statin is indicated when 10-year ASCVD risk is 7.5% or more or a high-intensity statin if ASCVD risk is 20% or more.

Goals of Statin Therapy and Monitoring

Studies have found a direct relationship between reduction of LDL cholesterol and reduction in risk of major ASCVD events. Generally speaking, for every 1% of LDL-C reduction, there is approximately a 1% reduction in risk of ASCVD. Patients with higher baseline LDL-C may potentially see greater benefits. The measure of efficacy is hence measured by percentage reduction in LDL-C from baseline in addition to monitoring for patient medication adherence.

A baseline cholesterol panel is recommended prior to initiating therapy. In most cases, cholesterol blood levels can be obtained without regard to fasting due to the relatively minimal difference in LDL-C levels under normal food intake. However, if the patient has a TG of 400 mg/dL or more, has a family history of premature ASCVD, or has familial hyperlipidemia, then a fasting cholesterol is preferred.

Cholesterol levels should be repeated within 1 to 3 months after initiating treatment. For individuals whose response is less than expected, providers should assess reasons such as nonadherence, including intolerance to the statin or affordability. Lifestyle modifications should also be reemphasized. Inadequate response would include an LDL-C reduction of less than 50% in those on high-intensity statin and less than 30% LDL-C reduction in those on moderate-intensity statin. If response continues to be lower than expected, addition of a non-statin may be considered for patients who are adherent but still not meeting the LDL-C reduction desired. Threshold LDL-C for adding a second agent can be found in **Figure 19.1**. Individuals who do have the expected response should be monitored every 3 to 12 months for continued assessment. See **Box 19.3** for a step-wise approach to hyperlipidemia treatment.

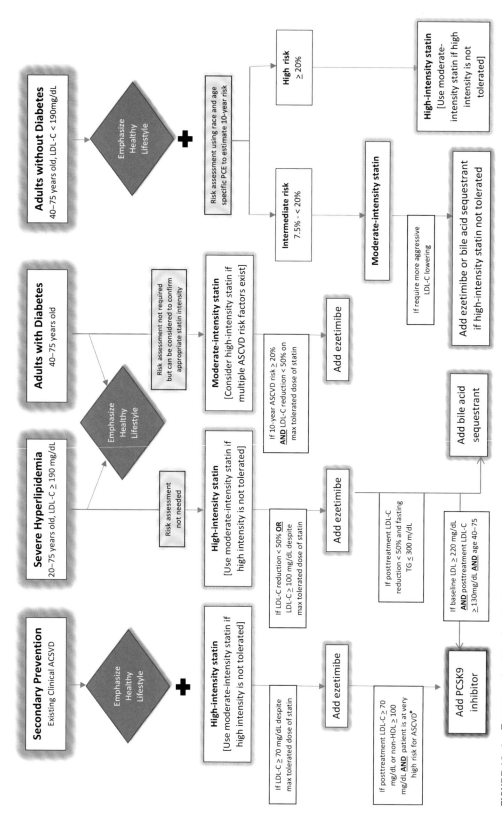

FIGURE 19–1   Treatment algorithm for initiating cholesterol-lowering therapy.

*Very high risk for ASCVD: (1) One major ASCVD event and several high-risk conditions or (2) history of multiple major ASCVD events (see **Box 19.2** for clinical ASCVD conditions).
ASCVD, atherosclerotic cardiovascular disease; LDL-C, low-density lipoprotein cholesterol; PCE, pooled cohort equations; PCSK9 inhibitor, proprotein convertase subtilisin/kexin type 9 inhibitor; TG, triglyceride.

BOX 19.3 Approach to Hyperlipidemia Treatment in Adult Patients

1. Obtain baseline lipid panel.
2. Evaluate and categorize patients in statin benefit group based on risks.
3. Emphasize healthy lifestyle in all patients.
4. Calculate ASCVD 10-year risk (40–75 year old) or lifetime risk (20–39 year old):
   a. Use risk enhancers to quantify overall risk.
   b. Obtain other markers to confirm if necessary (e.g., CAC score).
5. Initiate statin therapy if criteria are met and patient is agreeable.
6. Recheck lipid panel in 1 to 3 months.
7. Assess response:
   a. **LDL-C not at goal:** Evaluate and reinforce medication compliance and lifestyle changes. Consider adding non-statin if still not at goal after intervention.
   b. **LDL-C at goal:** Monitor lipid panel every 3 to 12 months.

Statin Intolerance

The statins are well tolerated by most patients, and long-term therapy does not appear to have any serious risks. The most common complaint with statin use is muscle-related symptoms, including pain, tenderness, weakness, and fatigue. These symptoms combined with a creatine phosphokinase level 10 times above the upper normal limits are consistent with a diagnosis of myopathy. If severe symptoms occur, the patient should be evaluated for rhabdomyolysis, a severe breakdown of muscle cells that leak into the urine and can result in renal failure. If suspected, the statin should be discontinued, and creatinine kinase, serum creatinine, and urinalysis should be performed.

If individuals develop mild to moderate muscle-related symptoms, it is reasonable to discontinue the statin and see if the symptoms resolve. If symptoms resolve after discontinuation, and the patient has no other contraindications, it is recommended to restart the same statin at a lower dose or start a different statin at a lower-intensity dose. If the patient is able to tolerate the lower-dose statin, the dose can gradually be increased to the recommended dose as tolerated. Individuals who are unable to achieve recommended statin dose or tolerate statins all together should consider use of non-statin medications.

Beta-Hydroxy-Beta-Methylglutaryl Coenzyme A Reductase Inhibitors (Statins)

Statins primarily block the conversion of HMG-CoA to mevalonate, which is the rate-limiting step in the production of cholesterol in the liver. Blocking the production of cholesterol in the liver leads to an increase in the number of LDL cholesterol receptors on the liver. As a result, a larger amount of LDL cholesterol is taken up by the liver, thereby decreasing the amount of LDL cholesterol in the bloodstream (**Figure 19.2**).

LDLR are also involved with the uptake of VLDL and IDL, thus leading to a decrease in TG levels. In addition, modest increases in HDL tend to occur. Despite having the same mechanism of action, there are differences between the agents, including the magnitude of their cholesterol lowering (**Table 19.3**). For example, fluvastatin (Lescol) can lower LDL cholesterol levels up to approximately 36% with the maximum dose, whereas atorvastatin (Lipitor) and rosuvastatin (Crestor) can lower LDL cholesterol levels up to 60% at maximum doses.

Maximum effects usually are seen after 4 to 6 weeks of therapy. For this reason, dosage adjustments should not be made more frequently than every 4 weeks.

Contraindications

There are several instances when statins are contraindicated or should be used with caution. Although no studies have been conducted in pregnant women, lovastatin causes skeletal malformations in rats, so statins are contraindicated during pregnancy. These agents should be used with extreme caution in women who are breast-feeding because they may be excreted in breast milk.

Statins are also contraindicated in patients with active liver disease or with unexplained elevated aminotransferase levels. They should be used with caution in patients who consume large amounts of alcohol or have a history of liver disease.

Adverse Events

The statins are well tolerated by most patients, and long-term therapy does not appear to have any serious risks, although statin intolerance is still an important issue. As mentioned previously, the most common cause of statin intolerance is due to myopathies. Gastrointestinal (GI) complaints and headache are typically among the most commonly reported adverse events, but they are usually mild and transient. Asymptomatic elevations in liver function test (LFT) values may also occur. Traditionally, LFTs were recommended to be monitored at baseline (before starting therapy), at 6 and 12 weeks after starting or titrating therapy, and periodically thereafter.

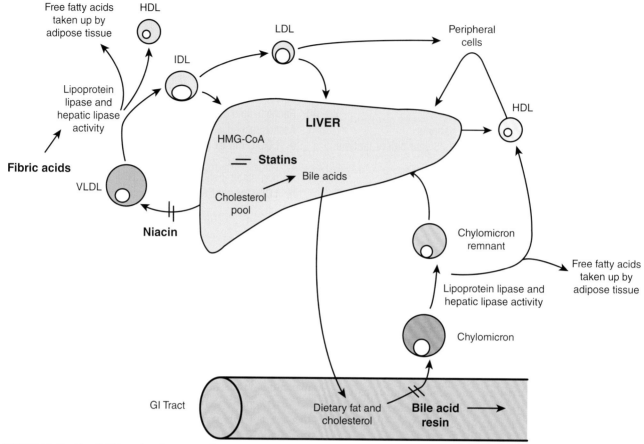

FIGURE 19–2   How lipid-lowering drugs work. The statins work in the liver by blocking the conversion of beta-hydroxy-beta-methylglutaryl coenzyme A to mevalonate, which is involved in producing cholesterol. The bile acid resins bind bile acid in the intestines for excretion in the feces so that lipids are not absorbed by the intestinal tract and returned to the liver. Niacin works to decrease circulating TG and low-density lipoprotein cholesterol, and fibric acid derivatives appear to lower TG levels and stimulate lipoprotein lipase, which enhances the breakdown of very-low-density lipoprotein to low-density lipoprotein cholesterol.

GI, gastrointestinal; HDL, high-density lipoprotein; IDL, intermediate-density lipoprotein; LDL, low-density lipoprotein; VLDL, very-low-density lipoprotein.

However, after decades of use and data from numerous clinical trials, these monitoring parameters have been relaxed. The 2018 guidelines recommend that a creatine kinase level and liver transaminases including aspartate aminotransferase and alanine aminotransferase levels should be performed during therapy only as clinically indicated if hepatotoxic symptoms present. In patients with chronic but stable liver disease who require statin therapy, baseline labs should be obtained and periodically monitored for safety.

Interactions

The risk of myopathy is most common when using statins at high doses or in combination with drugs that can also cause myopathy (including other lipid-lowering agents) or that can affect the metabolism of the statins (e.g., cyclosporine, erythromycin, azole antifungals). Moreover, myopathy may occur at any time during therapy. Patients should be instructed to report any unusual muscle pain or weakness during therapy.

The practitioner should encourage the patient to take the statins in the evening or at bedtime because a significant amount of cholesterol production seems to occur during sleep. By taking the medication before bedtime, peak concentrations of medication occur during sleep. Exceptions are lovastatin, which has an increased bioavailability when taken with food and is usually taken with the evening meal, and atorvastatin and rosuvastatin, which can be taken at any time during the day because of their long half-lives.

NON-STATIN CHOLESTEROL-LOWERING MEDICATIONS

The role of non-statin cholesterol-lowering drugs is limited to add-on therapy. Of the non-statin drug group, only cholesterol absorption inhibitors and proprotein convertase subtilisin/kexin type 9 (PCSK9) inhibitors are recommended in the 2018 ACC/AHA guidelines. Other classes of non-statin cholesterol-lowering medications currently have a limited role in clinical practice due to their lack of evidence in reducing ASCVD risks.

Cholesterol Absorption Inhibitors

Currently, there is only one cholesterol absorption inhibitor on the market: ezetimibe (Zetia). Ezetimibe appears to act at the brush border of the small intestine and inhibits the absorption of cholesterol, leading to a decrease in the delivery of intestinal cholesterol to the liver. This causes a reduction of hepatic cholesterol stores and an increase in clearance of cholesterol from the blood; this distinct mechanism is complementary to that of HMG-CoA reductase inhibitors.

Zetia, introduced in April 2003, is indicated for use as monotherapy or as combination therapy with a statin. LDL cholesterol levels are reduced by up to 18% with monotherapy and up to an additional 25% when added to ongoing statin therapy. Together with a statin, LDL cholesterol reductions of more than 50% have been noted. The recommended dosage of ezetimibe is 10 mg daily. If taken with a bile acid sequestrant, ezetimibe should be taken 2 hours before or 4 hours after the bile acid (**Table 19.4**).

The Ezetimibe and Simvastatin Hypercholesterolemia Enhances Atherosclerosis Regression trial, which evaluated the impact of adding ezetimibe to simvastatin, found no significant change in carotid artery intima–media thickness (a marker for atherosclerosis progression) despite significant decreases in LDL cholesterol and CRP levels (Kastelein et al., 2008). However, the more recent Improved Reduction in Outcomes: Vytorin Efficacy International Trial showed that the addition of ezetimibe 10 mg to simvastatin 40 mg reduced CV events compared to simvastatin alone. While the magnitude of the results was not large (5.8% relative risk reduction, 2.0% absolute risk reduction—both statistically significant), they were very important in that it was the first trial to demonstrate incremental benefit in ASCVD event reduction with a non-statin added to a statin compared to the statin alone.

TABLE 19.4
Doses and Lipid-Lowering Ability of Other Available Agents

Class	Generic Name (Trade Name)	Usual Daily Dose	LDL*	HDL*	Triglycerides*
Bile acid resins	Cholestyramine (Questran, Questran Light, Prevalite)	4–16 g	↓13%–32%	↑3%–5%	↑0%–15%
	Colesevelam (Welchol)	3.75 g	↓15%–18%	↑3%	↑9%–10%
Cholesterol absorption inhibitors	Ezetimibe (Zetia)[†]	10 mg	↓16%–19% ↓33%–60%	↑3%–4% ↑8%–11%	↓5% ↓19%–40%
PCSK9 inhibitors	Alirocumab (Praluent) Evolocumab (Repatha)	75–300 mg 140–420 mg	↓43%–64%	↑8%–10%	↓8–10%
Niacin[‡]	Niacin (various)	1.5–3.0 g	↓12%–21%	↑18%–30%	↓15%–44%
Fibric acid derivatives	Gemfibrozil (Lopid)	600 mg BID	0	↑6%	↓31%
	Fenofibrate (various)	48–200 mg daily	↓20%	↑11%	↓38%
ACL inhibitors[§]	Bempedoic acid	180 mg	↓18%	↓6%	↑3% ↓2%
Combination products	Lovastatin/niacin	20/500–40/2,000 mg	↓30%–42%	↑20%–30%	↓32%–44%
	Simvastatin/ezetimibe	10/10–80/10 mg	↓45%–60%	↑6%–10%	↓23%–31%
	Bempedoic acid/ezetimibe	180/10 mg	↓38%	↓5%	↓11%

*Effects on lipid levels are dose dependent.

[†]Results in first line are those seen when used as monotherapy (Adapted from Bays, H. E., Moore, P. B., Drehobl, M. A., et al. [2001]. Effectiveness and tolerability of ezetimibe in patients with primary hypercholesterolemia: Pooled analysis of two phase II studies. *Clinical Therapeutics, 23*[8], 1209–1230). Second results are those seen when used with statin therapy (Adapted from Kerzner, B., Corbelli, J., Sharp, S., et al. [2003]. Efficacy and safety of ezetimibe coadministered with lovastatin in primary hypercholesterolemia. *American Journal of Cardiology, 91*[4], 418–424) (lovastatin); (Adapted from Davidson, M. H., McGarry, T., Bettis, R., et al. [2002]. Ezetimibe coadministered with simvastatin in patients with primary hypercholesterolemia. *Journal of the American College of Cardiology, 40*[12], 2125–2134) (simvastatin); (Adapted from Ballantyne, C. M., Houri, J., Notarbartolo, A., et al. [2003]. Effect of ezetimibe coadministered with atorvastatin in 628 patients with primary hypercholesterolemia: A prospective, randomized, double-blind trial. *Circulation, 107*[19], 2409–2415) (atorvastatin).

[‡]Dose must be titrated slowly (usually weekly) to avoid side effects.

[§]Results in first line are those seen in the CLEAR Harmony trial. (Adapted from Ray, K. K., Bays, H. E., Catapano, A. L, et al. [2019]. Safety and efficacy of bempedoic acid to reduce LDL cholesterol. *The New England Journal of Medicine, 380*[11], 1022–1032. doi: 10.1056/NEJMoa1803917). Second results are those seen in the CLEAR Wisdom trial (Adapted from Goldberg, A. C., Leiter, L. A., Stroes, E., et al. [2019]. Effect of bempedoic acid vs placebo added to maximally tolerated statins on low-density lipoprotein cholesterol in patients at high risk for cardiovascular disease: The CLEAR wisdom randomized clinical trial. *JAMA, 322*[18], 1780–1788. doi: 10.1001/jama.2019.16585).

ACL, adenosine triphosphate-citrate lyase; HDL, high-density lipoprotein; LDL, low-density lipoprotein; PCSK9, proprotein convertase subtilisin/kexin type 9.

Contraindications

Ezetimibe is contraindicated in patients who have a hypersensitivity to any component of the medication. The combination of ezetimibe with an HMG-CoA reductase inhibitor is contraindicated in patients with active liver disease or unexplained persistent elevations in serum transaminases. There are no adequate, controlled studies of ezetimibe in pregnant women, so use during pregnancy is indicated only if the potential benefit outweighs any potential risk to the fetus.

Adverse Events

Adverse events with ezetimibe are minimal. Adverse events noted in clinical trials include headache, diarrhea, and abdominal pain. In addition, myopathy and rhabdomyolysis have been noted when given in combination with statins. The incidence of elevated liver enzymes was similar to placebo.

Proprotein Convertase Subtilisin/Kexin Type 9 Inhibitors

PCSK9 inhibitors are a novel class of monoclonal antibodies for LDL cholesterol lowering. LDLR on the surface of hepatocytes play an important role in clearing LDL in the circulation. PCSK9 regulates LDLR by binding to LDLR, promoting its degradation and reducing the number of LDLR available, hence, increasing circulating LDL cholesterol. By inhibiting PCSK9, LDL cholesterol can significantly be lowered.

Two medications in this class, evolocumab (Repatha) and alirocumab (Praluent), were approved by the Food and Drug Administration (FDA) in late 2015. These agents, which are injectables, provide LDL cholesterol lowering of up to 60% or more when used alone or when added on to statin therapy. PCSK9 inhibitors are FDA approved as add-on therapy to maximally tolerated statin therapy in adults with familial hypercholesterolemia (FH) or clinical ASCVD.

Studies showed evolocumab and alirocumab to be effective in significantly reducing CV events including CV death, MI, and stroke in patients who are on maximally tolerated statin (Sabatine et al., 2017; Schwartz et al, 2018).

Contraindications

PCSK9 inhibitors are contraindicated in patients who have a hypersensitivity to PCSK9 inhibitors in the past.

Adverse Effects

Long-term safety data for PCSK9 inhibitors are still lacking due to their relatively new status on the market. The most common adverse effects reported in patients on PCSK9 inhibitors have been nasopharyngitis and local injection-site reaction. No drug interactions have been reported to date. In patients who develop LDL cholesterol less than 25 mg/dL for two consecutive readings while on a PCSK9 inhibitor, deintensification of lipid-lowering therapy is recommended due to lack of safety data.

Bile Acid Resins

The agents in this class are cholestyramine (Questran, Questran Light, Prevalite), colestipol (Colestid), and colesevelam (Welchol). Bile acid resins decrease cholesterol absorption through the exogenous pathway. These agents are not absorbed from the GI tract. They act to bind bile acids in the intestines, forming an insoluble complex that is excreted in the feces. This decreases the return of cholesterol to the liver. The body responds to this by increasing LDLR on the liver, which in turn increases the amount of LDL cholesterol taken up by the liver and thus decreases LDL cholesterol levels in the bloodstream (see **Figure 19.2**). Unfortunately, this process also leads to increased production of VLDL particles. As a result, TG levels rise, especially in patients with elevated baseline TG levels. Bile acid resins can decrease LDL cholesterol levels by 15% to 30%, increase HDL levels by approximately 3%, and increase TG levels by up to 15% (**Table 19.4**). As with the statins, these effects are related.

Maximum effects of cholesterol lowering are seen in approximately 3 weeks. Although there is a weak level of evidence, bile acid resins may be considered as adjunct therapy in select patients who do not respond to maximally tolerated statin and ezetimibe therapy. Because of their safety with long-term use, they may be useful in young adult men and premenopausal women who are at relatively low CV risk.

Contraindications

Bile acid resins should not be used in patients whose fasting TG levels are 300 mg/dL or more, as it may lead to a severe increase in TG levels. They can be used with caution in patients whose baseline TGs are between 250 and 299 mg/dL, with monitoring every 4 to 6 weeks. These agents are contraindicated in patients with biliary obstruction or chronic constipation.

Adverse Events

Bile acid resins are not absorbed, and therefore, systemic adverse events are minimal. Monitoring for abnormal LFT values is not required. The most common adverse events are GI related and include flatulence, bloating, abdominal pain, heartburn, and constipation. For these reasons, some patients, such as older patients, may not be good candidates for bile acid resins. Colesevelam is least likely to cause GI-related adverse effects and is better tolerated compared to cholestyramine and colestipol.

Interactions

Because bile acid resins block the absorption of cholesterol from the GI tract, they should be taken with meals to maximize effectiveness. These agents are usually administered once or twice daily but can be taken up to four times a day. If taken once a day, a bile acid resin should be taken with the largest meal.

Cholestyramine is available as a powder, colestipol is available as granules or tablets, and colesevelam is available in both powder and tablet forms. The powder and granules should be mixed with water, noncarbonated beverages, soups, or pulpy fruits such as applesauce. The tablets should be swallowed whole with water or other fluids. These agents should not be taken dry because they can cause esophageal distress. Patients should avoid taking these agents with carbonated beverages because it may result in increased GI discomfort. Medications taken concomitantly, such as thyroid hormones, antibiotics, and fat-soluble vitamins, should be taken at least 1 hour before or 4 hours after the bile acid resin because of their potential to bind to other medications and decrease their bioavailability.

Niacin

Niacin (nicotinic acid) is a naturally occurring B vitamin that can improve cholesterol levels when used at doses 100 to 300 times the recommended daily allowance as a vitamin. Niacin's mechanism of action is uncertain, but the substance appears to decrease VLDL synthesis in the liver, inhibit lipolysis in adipose tissue, and increase lipoprotein lipase activity. This results in decreased TG and LDL cholesterol levels in the bloodstream (see **Figure 19.2**). LDL cholesterol levels can be decreased by 15% to 25% and TGs by up to 50%, whereas HDL cholesterol levels may be increased by up to 35% (see **Table 19.4**). Although niacin is one of the most effective agents in improving cholesterol levels, most patients cannot tolerate the adverse events associated with its use (see Adverse Events). Additionally, there is very little evidence to suggest that it can reduce ASCVD events further when added to statin therapy.

Dosage

Niacin immediate release products are at least 1.5 g niacin daily are usually required to achieve beneficial effects on lipid levels. However, to minimize adverse events, dosages need to be titrated gradually. The usual starting dose for immediate release products is 50 to 100 mg twice or thrice daily. The dose can be increased every 1 to 2 weeks until a dosage of 1.0 to 1.5 g daily is reached; this should take approximately 4 to 5 weeks. This dosage range provides significant increases (15%–30%) in HDL cholesterol levels and decreases (20%–30%) in TG levels. However, for maximal LDL cholesterol lowering, dosages of 3 g/d or more may be necessary. Niacin is available in both immediate-release and sustained-release formulations. Maximum effects usually are seen after 4 to 6 weeks of therapy on the aforementioned dosages.

Contraindications

Niacin is contraindicated in patients with hepatic dysfunction, severe hypotension, persistent hyperglycemia, acute gout, new-onset atrial fibrillation, or active peptic ulcers. In addition, niacin can elevate uric acid levels and worsen glucose control. Therefore, niacin is not a first-line treatment agent in patients with gout or diabetes mellitus, and it should be used cautiously in these populations.

Adverse Events

Niacin use has been limited primarily because of its extensive adverse events. Although it is one of the most effective agents for improving lipid profiles, many patients cannot tolerate the adverse events. The most common adverse events are attributed to an increase in prostaglandin activity and include pruritus and flushing of the face and neck. A dose of aspirin, 325 mg, taken 30 minutes before the niacin dose may decrease the severity. As mentioned earlier, niacin can also increase uric acid levels and worsen glucose control and should be used cautiously, if at all, in patients with a history of gout or diabetes mellitus. Baseline glucose and uric acid levels should be checked in all patients starting niacin therapy.

Other adverse events include GI side effects (it is contraindicated in patients with an active peptic ulcer), rash, hepatotoxicity, and, rarely, acanthosis nigricans (hyperpigmentation of the skin, usually in the axilla, neck, or groin). Unlike statins, LFTs are still recommended to be monitored at 6 and 12 weeks after initiating or titrating therapy and periodically thereafter.

Fibric Acid Derivatives

Fibric acid derivatives class of lipid-lowering drugs mainly affects TG and HDL cholesterol levels. The exact mechanism of action of fibric acid derivatives is unclear, but the principal effect of TG lowering appears to result from the stimulation of lipoprotein lipase, which enhances the breakdown of VLDL to LDL cholesterol (see **Figure 19.2**).

These agents may also inhibit hepatic VLDL production, and they lower TG levels up to 60% and increase HDL cholesterol by up to 30%. Although gemfibrozil and clofibrate (Atromid-S) have minimal effects on LDL cholesterol lowering, fenofibrate (TriCor) has been shown to decrease LDL cholesterol by up to 20%. Fibric acid derivatives are primarily indicated in patients who have severely elevated TG levels (≥500 mg/dL) and who have not responded to dietary therapy (see **Table 19.4**).

Gemfibrozil and fenofibrate are the currently available fibric acid derivatives.

Dosage

Gemfibrozil is given in 600-mg doses twice daily with breakfast and dinner. No titration of dose is necessary, although some patients may respond at lower doses. Fenofibrate therapy is initiated at 43 to 67 mg/d (depending upon formulation). The dosage can be increased to a maximum of 200 mg/d. Because its absorption is increased when taken with food, fenofibrate should be taken with meals.

Contraindications

Fibric acid derivatives are contraindicated in patients with a history of gallstones and in those with severe hepatic or renal dysfunction. No studies have been conducted in pregnant women, so, these agents should be used only if the benefits clearly outweigh any risks to the fetus.

Adverse Events

The fibric acid derivatives usually are well tolerated. The most common adverse events are GI related and include epigastric pain, nausea and vomiting, dyspepsia, flatulence, and constipation. Myopathy may occur, and the incidence is increased when fibric acid derivatives are used with lovastatin and simvastatin and, to a lesser degree, other statins and niacin. As with the other systemic lipid-lowering agents, hepatotoxicity can occur, and LFTs should be monitored at 6 and 12 weeks and periodically thereafter. If LFT values increase to more than three times the upper normal limits, the fibric acid derivative should be discontinued. Other adverse events include rhabdomyolysis, cholestatic jaundice, gallstones, and, rarely, leukopenia, anemia, and thrombocytopenia.

Interactions

As mentioned previously, the incidence of myopathy is increased when fibric acids, especially gemfibrozil, are used in combination with lovastatin and simvastatin and, to a lesser degree, other statins and niacin. In fact, the combination of gemfibrozil and simvastatin is contraindicated. Fenofibrate should be used with caution in patients taking anticoagulant therapy because it can increase the effects of the anticoagulant. Doses of the anticoagulant should be lowered and levels monitored closely if fenofibrate therapy is initiated.

Omega-3 Fatty Acids

Similar to fibric acids, omega-3 fatty acids are not considered a major class of lipid-lowering drugs due to a lack of LDL cholesterol lowering. In some cases, omega-3 fatty acids may increase LDL cholesterol levels. Additionally, there have been no studies showing reduced CV morbidity and mortality. There are numerous over-the-counter dietary supplements that contain omega-3 fatty acids, as well as omega-3 acid ethyl esters by prescription. These agents are all indicated as an adjunct to diet for the treatment of severe hypertriglyceridemia. Patients should be on a lipid-lowering diet before treatment with any omega-3 fatty acids or omega-3 acid ethyl esters is initiated.

Dosage

All prescription drugs of omega-3 products are given as a once- or twice-daily dose. Patients can take either 4 g (four capsules) daily or 2 g (two capsules) twice daily. There is no dose titration.

Contraindications

Any omega-3 fatty acid is contraindicated in patients with a known hypersensitivity to the drug. To date, there is no evidence to suggest that patients who have fish allergies are at an increased risk for an allergic reaction with these agents. There are no studies that have included pregnant women, so it should only be used if the benefits outweigh any potential risks to the fetus.

Adverse Events

Omega-3 fatty acids are generally well tolerated. Some of the side effects noted in clinical trials include flu-like symptoms, belching, taste changes, upset stomach, and back pain.

Interactions

There has been some evidence to suggest that omega-3 fatty acids prolong bleeding time, but no studies have been performed to determine if there is an interaction with concomitant use of anticoagulants.

Adenosine Triphosphate-Citrate Lyase Inhibitors

ACL inhibitors are the newest class of LDL cholesterol-lowering medication on the market. ACL is an enzyme upstream of HMG-CoA reductase in the cholesterol synthesis pathway. Inhibition of ACL reduces cholesterol biosynthesis in the liver and subsequently decreases LDL cholesterol by up-regulation of LDLR.

Approved by the FDA in 2020, bempedoic acid (Nexletol) is the first and only medication of this class. Shortly after its approval, bempedoic acid/ezetimibe combination tablet was approved. Bempedoic acid is indicated as an adjunct therapy for the treatment of hyperlipemia in patients with a history of heterozygous familial hypercholesteremia or established ASCVD who require additional lowering of LDL cholesterol despite maximally tolerated statin. Bempedoic acid reduces LDL cholesterol by approximately 18% when used with a statin, and bempedoic acid/ezetimibe decreases LDL cholesterol by about 38% when used with maximally tolerated statin therapy (see **Table 19.4**).

Due to its recent introduction to the market, the effects of bempedoic acid on CV morbidity and mortality have not been determined. The results of the Cholesterol Lowering via Bempedoic acid, an ACL-Inhibiting Regimen (CLEAR) Outcomes trial should provide better insight as to whether bempedoic acid has an effect on CV outcomes. The study is expected to be completed by 2022 (https://clinicaltrials.gov/ct2/show/NCT02993406).

Dosage

Bempedoic acid is available as 180 mg tablets, dosed once daily and can be taken without regard to meals. There is a combination pill available formulated with bempedoic acid and ezetimibe (Nexlizet) in a single tablet. This combination pill comes in the standard dose of 180 mg of bempedoic acid and 10 mg of ezetimibe and is also dosed once daily.

Contraindication

No contraindications have been identified by the manufacturer for bempedoic acid. There is currently no data available for pregnant women. Unless the potential benefit outweighs any potential risk to the fetus, bempedoic acid should be discontinued at the time when pregnancy is known.

Adverse Effects

Side effects of bempedoic acid include upper respiratory tract infection, bronchitis, muscle spasms, back pain, abdominal pain or discomfort, extremity pain, anemia, and elevated liver enzymes.

Two rare but notable adverse effects reported in the clinical trials are tendon rupture or injury and hyperuricemia (increased uric acid blood level), which can lead to gout. Uric acid elevation usually occurs within the first 4 weeks of initiating bempedoic acid. For this reason, uric acid blood levels should be monitored periodically throughout the course of therapy. In clinical trials, tendon rupture occurred in a small number (0.5%) of patients while taking bempedoic acid. Tendon rupture or injury can occur within weeks or months after starting therapy. Risk factors include age 60 years or older, a history of tendon disorders, renal failure, or concomitant use of fluoroquinolone antibiotics or corticosteroids.

Interactions

When given concomitantly with simvastatin or pravastatin, bempedoic acid may increase the concentration of these specific statins, thereby increasing the risk of myopathy. To ameliorate this drug interaction, bempedoic acid should not be given with simvastatin dose of more than 20 mg or pravastatin dose of more than 40 mg.

Medications for Homozygous Familial Hypercholesterolemia

Homozygous FH is a rare genetic disorder characterized by dysfunctional LDL cholesterol receptors on the liver, which leads to severely elevated cholesterol levels (LDL cholesterol levels >600 mg/dL) and ASCVD at an early age. Due to the lack of function of the LDL cholesterol receptors, many lipid-modifying agents including statins show significantly reduced effects on LDL cholesterol reduction in this clinical setting. In 2013, mipomersen and lomitapide were approved in the United States for the treatment of FH. Mipomersen (Kynamro) and lomitapide (Juxtapid) have been shown to reduce LDL cholesterol levels by 25% and 40%, respectively, on top of what had been achieved with maximum tolerated statin doses. Due to the extremely small overall patient population affected by FH, ASVCD event reduction studies will not be possible. Severe liver toxicity is associated with these agents. Due to this, specific FDA-mandated training is required before prescribing these medications, which should only be used in patients with FH.

PCSK9 inhibitors can also be considered in the treatment of FH as adjunct treatment to maximally tolerated lipid-lowering therapy (statin and ezetimibe) in adults with homozygous FH and heterozygous FH.

Combination Therapy

In the past, it was thought that it would be beneficial for patients to be prescribed combination lipid-lowering therapy to achieve desired cholesterol levels, particularly for those with severe hypertriglyceridemia or severely elevated LDL cholesterol levels who do not respond adequately to a statin alone or are intolerant to statin doses needed to attain desired LDL-C reduction. Statin/niacin and statin/gemfibrozil have been used together for patients with severely elevated LDL cholesterol, low HDL cholesterol, and hypertriglyceridemia. Currently, there are two products available that include a statin and niacin in a single formulation: lovastatin/niacin (Advicor) and simvastatin/niacin (Simcor). However, to date, there have been no studies showing an increased benefit in reducing CV morbidity and mortality from either of these combinations. Combining statins with a cholesterol absorption inhibitor has shown added benefits in reducing both LDL cholesterol and ASCVD event rates. As previously mentioned, this is the only lipid medication combined with a statin to show incremental benefits in ASCVD event rates. Bile acid resins can be used safely and effectively with statins, niacin, and fibric acid derivatives to enhance LDL cholesterol lowering. The only concern with using bile acid resins in combination is ensuring that the concomitant medications are taken at least 1 hour before or 4 hours after the resin to ensure adequate GI absorption.

Special Population Considerations

Pediatric

Pharmacologic therapy with a statin may be considered in children older than age 10 if lifestyle modifications cannot adequately lower cholesterol levels. Use in children younger than age 10 usually is not recommended because atherosclerotic lesions are not thought to develop before this age. A consultation with a lipid specialist is recommended for any child with elevated cholesterol levels.

Young Adults (20–39 Years of Age)

Due to the limited available data in young adults with moderately elevated LDL-C (20–39 years of age with LDL-C 160–189 mg/dL), the latest guidelines recommend screening patients for risk enhancers and carefully weighing the risks versus benefits of statin therapy. Note that there are no randomized controlled trials available to support the long-term use of statins in patients in this group.

Geriatric (>75 Years of Age)

Literature to support statin use in older adults are limited and conflicting, particularly in adults more than 80 years of age. For patients 75 years of age and older with LDL-C level of 70 to 189 mg/dL, it may be reasonable to initiate a moderate intensity for primary prevention. However, due to the collective risks associated with statin therapy in this patient population, the potential risks may outweigh the benefits. Clinicians may even consider deprescribing statin therapy in patients with limited life expectancy or other factors that may limit the benefits of long-term statin therapy (e.g., physical or cognitive decline, frailty, multiple comorbidities).

Women

Statins are classified as category X by the U.S. FDA and should not be used by pregnant women because of the potential for fetal abnormalities. Most other agents are classified as category C, meaning that tests have not been performed in humans.

PATIENT EDUCATION

Patient education consists of a thorough explanation of the value of modifying habits and making lifestyle changes (diet, exercise) to avoid or enhance drug therapy in reducing lipid levels. Equally important is thorough teaching about the need for regular laboratory tests to evaluate the effect of drug therapy on body systems and organs, such as the liver. Such education will encourage the patient to cooperate with the therapeutic plan.

Two Web sites that provide useful information for patients are www.americanheart.org (American Heart Association)

and www.nhlbi.nih.gov (Department of Health and Human Services, National Institutes of Health, National Heart, Lung, and Blood Institute). On the latter site, the patient can calculate his or her 10-year risk of having a heart attack.

Cholesterol screening should begin at age 20 and should be done every 5 years if it is normal unless there has been a significant lifestyle change, such as significant weight gain. Children should be screened if their parents have a cholesterol level more than 240 mg/dL or they have grandparents aged 55 or younger with overt ASCVD.

CASE STUDY 1

J.J., a 55-year-old white male, has come in for his annual physical. He has hypertension and type 2 diabetes mellitus (type 2 DM). His blood pressure (BP) is controlled with lisinopril 20 mg daily and amlodipine 5 mg daily (BP 132/82 mm Hg). His most recent hemoglobin A1c was 7.2% while taking metformin. His father died at age 55 of a myocardial infarction, and his brother, age 57, just underwent angioplasty. J.J. eats fast food at least five times a week because of his work schedule. He weighs 245 lb and stands 5 feet 11 inches. His total cholesterol is 237 (low-density lipoprotein [LDL], 190; high-density lipoprotein [HDL], 35; triglycerides, 200).

1. Does J.J. fall into any of the statin risk categories? If so, which one?
2. What drug therapy and dose would you prescribe, and why?
3. What are the parameters for monitoring the success of the therapy?
4. List one or two adverse reactions for the drug therapy that you have prescribed for J.J. that would cause you to change therapy.
5. When rechecked, J.J.'s total cholesterol is 174 (LDL, 100; HDL, 38), but he is complaining of muscle pain. How would you manage J.J.'s treatment?

BIBLIOGRAPHY

Starred references are cited in the text.

*American Heart Association. (2015). Heart disease and stroke statistics. Retrieved from www.americanheart.org

*Ballantyne, C. M., Houri, J., Notarbartolo, A., et al. (2003). Effect of ezetimibe coadministered with atorvastatin in 628 patients with primary hypercholesterolemia: A prospective, randomized, double-blind trial. *Circulation, 107*(19), 2409–2415.

Ballantyne, C. M., Laufs, U., Ray, K. K., et al. (2020). Bempedoic acid plus ezetimibe fixed-dose combination in patients with hypercholesterolemia and high CVD risk treated with maximally tolerated statin therapy. *European Journal of Preventive Cardiology, 27*(6), 593–603. doi: 10.1177/2047487319864671

*Bays, H. E., Moore, P. B., Drehobl, M. A., et al. (2001). Effectiveness and tolerability of ezetimibe in patients with primary hypercholesterolemia: Pooled analysis of two phase II studies. *Clinical Therapeutics, 23*(8), 1209–1230.

Boekholdt, S. M., Hovingh, G. K., Mora, S., et al. (2014). Very low levels of atherogenic lipoproteins and the risk for cardiovascular events: A meta-analysis of statin trials. *Journal of the American College of Cardiology, 64*(5), 485–494. doi: 10.1016/j.jacc.2014.02.615

*Brien, S. E., Ronksley, P. E., Turner, B. J., et al. (2011). Effect of alcohol consumption on biological markers associated with risk of coronary heart disease: Systematic review and meta-analysis of interventional studies. *British Medical Journal, 342*, d636. doi: 10.1136/bmj.d636

Cannon, C. P. (2014). IMPROVE-IT trial: A comparison of ezetimibe/simvastatin versus simvastatin monotherapy on cardiovascular outcomes after acute coronary syndromes. American Heart Association 2014 Scientific Sessions, November 17, 2014. Chicago, IL.

*ClinicalTrials.gov. National Library of Medicine (U.S.). (2016, November 18). Evaluation of major cardiovascular events in patients with, or at high risk for, cardiovascular disease who are statin intolerant treated with bempedoic acid (ETC-1002) or placebo (CLEAR Outcomes). Identifier NCT02993406. Retrieved from https://clinicaltrials.gov/ct2/show/NCT02993406 on November 25, 2020.

Cholesterol Treatment Trialists' (CTT) Collaboration, Baigent, C., Blackwell, L., et al. (2010). Efficacy and safety of more intensive lowering of LDL cholesterol: A meta-analysis of data from 170,000 participants in 26 randomised trials. *Lancet (London, England), 376*(9753), 1670–1681. doi: 10.1016/S0140-6736(10)61350-5

*Cooke, J. P., & Bhatnagar, R. (1997). Pathophysiology of atherosclerotic vascular disease. *Disease Management and Health Outcomes, 2*(Suppl. 1), 1–8.

*Davidson, M. H., McGarry, T., Bettis, R., et al. (2002). Ezetimibe coadministered with simvastatin in patients with primary hypercholesterolemia. *Journal of the American College of Cardiology, 40*(12), 2125–2134.

*Downs, J. R., Clearfield, M., Weis, S., et al. (1998). Primary prevention of acute coronary events with lovastatin in men and women with average cholesterol levels: Results of AFCAPS/TexCAPS. *Journal of the American Medical Association, 279*, 1615–1622.

Eckel, R. H., Jakicic, J. M., Ard, J. D., et al. (2014). 2013 AHA/ACC guideline on lifestyle management to reduce cardiovascular risk: A report of the American College of Cardiology/American Heart Association Task Force on Practice Guidelines. *Circulation, 129*(25 Suppl 2), S76–S99. doi: 10.1161/01.cir.0000437740.48606.d1

Expert Panel, National Cholesterol Education Program. (2001). Executive summary of the third report of the National Cholesterol Education Program (NCEP) Expert Panel on Detection, Evaluation and Treatment of High Blood Cholesterol in Adults (Adult Treatment Panel III). *Journal of the American Medical Association, 285*, 2486–2497.

Filippatos, T. D., Kei, A., Rizos, C. V., et al. (2018). Effects of PCSK9 inhibitors on other than low-density lipoprotein cholesterol lipid variables. *Journal of Cardiovascular Pharmacology and Therapeutics, 23*(1), 3–12. doi: 10.1177/1074248417724868

*Frick, H., Elo, O., Kaapa, K., et al. (1987). Helsinki Heart Study: Primary prevention trial with gemfibrozil in middle-aged men with dyslipidemia. *New England Journal of Medicine, 257*, 3233–3240.

Genest, J., McPherson, R., Frohlich, J., et al. (2009). Canadian Cardiovascular Society/Canadian guidelines for the diagnosis and treatment of dyslipidemia and prevention of cardiovascular disease in the adult—2009 recommendations. *Canadian Journal of Cardiology, 25*, 567–579.

*Goldberg, A. C., Leiter, L. A., Stroes, E., et al. (2019). Effect of bempedoic acid vs placebo added to maximally tolerated statins on low-density lipoprotein cholesterol in patients at high risk for cardiovascular disease: The CLEAR wisdom randomized clinical trial. *JAMA, 322*(18), 1780–1788. doi: 10.1001/jama.2019.16585

Grundy, S. M., Stone, N. J., Bailey, A. L., et al. (2019). 2018 AHA/ACC/AACVPR/AAPA/ABC/ACPM/ADA/AGS/APhA/ASPC/NLA/PCNA Guideline on the management of blood cholesterol: A report of the American College of Cardiology/American Heart Association task force on clinical practice guidelines. *Journal of the American College of Cardiology, 73*(24), e285–e350. doi: 10.1016/j.jacc.2018.11.003

Guyton, J., Bays, H., Grundy, S., et al. (2014). An assessment by the Statin Intolerance Panel: 2014 update. *Journal of Clinical Lipidology, 8*(3), S72–S81. doi: 10.1016/j.jacl.2014.03.002

*Heart Protection Study Collaborative Group. (2002). MRC/BHF Heart Protection Study of cholesterol lowering with simvastatin in 20,536 high-risk individuals: A randomised placebo-controlled trial. *Lancet, 360*, 7–22.

*Huxley, R., & Woodward, M. (2011). Cigarette smoking as a risk factor for coronary heart disease in women compared with men: A systematic review and meta-analysis of prospective cohort studies. *Lancet, 378*(9799), 1297–1305.

*Kastelein, J. J., Akdim, F., Stroes, E. S., et al.; For the ENHANCE Investigators. (2008). Simvastatin with or without ezetimibe in familial hypercholesterolemia. *New England Journal of Medicine, 358*, 1431–1443.

*Kerzner, B., Corbelli, J., Sharp, S., et al. (2003). Efficacy and safety of ezetimibe coadministered with lovastatin in primary hypercholesterolemia. *American Journal of Cardiology, 91*(4), 418–424.

*Lewis, S. J., Moye, L. A., Sacks, F. M., et al. (1998). Effect of pravastatin on cardiovascular events in older patients with myocardial infarction and cholesterol levels in the average range: Results of the Cholesterol and Recurrent Events (CARE) Trial. *Annals of Internal Medicine, 129*, 681–689.

*Long-Term Intervention with Pravastatin in Ischaemic Disease (LIPID) Study Group. (1998). Prevention of cardiovascular events and death with pravastatin in patients with coronary heart disease and a broad range of initial cholesterol levels. *New England Journal of Medicine, 339*, 1349–1357.

Malguria, N., Zimmerman, S., & Fishman, E. K. (2018). Coronary artery calcium scoring: Current status and review of literature. *Journal of Computer Assisted Tomography, 42*(6), 887–897. doi: 10.1097/RCT.0000000000000825

*McKenney, J. M., & Hawkins, D. W. (1995). *Handbook on the management of lipid disorders*. Springfield, NJ: National Pharmacy Cholesterol Council/Scientific Therapeutics Information, Inc.

McKenney, J. M., Jones, P. H., Adamczyk, M. A., et al. (2003). Comparison of efficacy of rosuvastatin vs. atorvastatin, simvastatin and pravastatin in achieving lipid goals. Results from STELLAR trial. *Current Medical Research and Opinion, 19*(8), 689–698.

Mozaffarian, D., Benjamin, E., Go, A., et al. (2015). Executive summary: Heart disease and stroke statistics—2015 update. A report from the American Heart Association. *Circulation, 131*, 434–441. doi: 10.1161/CIR.0000000000000157

National Heart, Lung and Blood Institute. (2002). *Morbidity and mortality: 2002 chartbook on cardiovascular, lung and blood disease*. Bethesda, MD: U.S. Department of Health and Human Services, Public Health Service.

*Newby, L. K., LaPointe, N. M., Chen, A. Y., et al. (2006). Long-term adherence to evidence-base secondary prevention therapies in coronary artery disease. *Circulation, 113*, 203–212.

Pearson, T. A., Mensah, G. A., Alexander, R. W., et al. (2003). Markers of inflammation and cardiovascular disease: Application to clinical and public health practice—A statement for healthcare professionals from the centers for disease control and prevention and the American Heart Association. *Circulation, 107*, 499–511.

Pokhrel, B., Yuet, W. C., & Levine, S. N. (2020). PCSK9 inhibitors. In *StatPearls [Internet]*. Treasure Island (FL): StatPearls Publishing; 2020 Jan-. Available from: https://www.ncbi.nlm.nih.gov/books/NBK448100/.

*Ray, K. K., Bays, H. E., Catapano, A. L., et al. (2019). Safety and efficacy of bempedoic acid to reduce LDL cholesterol. *The New England Journal of Medicine, 380*(11), 1022–1032. doi: 10.1056/NEJMoa1803917

*Ridker, P. M., Danielson, E., Fonseca, F. A., et al. (2008). Rosuvastatin to prevent vascular events in men and women with elevated C-reactive protein. *New England Journal of Medicine, 359*, 2195–2207.

Ridker, P. M., Hennekens, C. H., Buring, J. E., et al. (2000). C-reactive protein and other markers of inflammation in the prediction of cardiovascular disease in women. *New England Journal of Medicine, 342*, 836–884.

*Ross, R., & Glomset, J. A. (1976). The pathogenesis of atherosclerosis (first of two parts). *New England Journal of Medicine, 295*, 369–377.

Rubins, H. B., Robins, S. J., Collins, D., et al. (1999). Gemfibrozil for the secondary prevention of coronary heart disease in men with low levels of high-density lipoprotein cholesterol. *New England Journal of Medicine, 341*, 410–418.

*Sabatine, M. S., Giugliano, R. P., Keech, A. C., et al. (2017). Evolocumab and clinical outcomes in patients with cardiovascular disease. *The New England Journal of Medicine, 376*(18), 1713–1722. doi: 10.1056/NEJMoa1615664

Sacks, F. M., Pfeffer, M. A., Moye, L. A., et al. (1996). The effect of pravastatin on coronary events after myocardial infarction in patients with average cholesterol levels: The Cholesterol and Recurrent Events Trial. *New England Journal of Medicine, 335*, 1001–1009.

*Salami, J. A., Warraich, H., Valero-Elizondo, J., et al. (2017). National trends in statin use and expenditures in the US adult population from 2002 to 2013: Insights from the medical expenditure panel survey. *JAMA Cardiology, 2*(1), 56–65. doi: 10.1001/jamacardio.2016.4700

*Scandinavian Simvastatin Survival Study Group. (1994). Randomized trial of cholesterol lowering in 4,444 patients with coronary heart disease: The Scandinavian Simvastatin Survival Study (4S). *Lancet, 344*, 1383–1389.

*Schwartz, G. G., Steg, P. G., Szarek, M., et al. (2018). Alirocumab and cardiovascular outcomes after acute coronary syndrome. *The New England Journal of Medicine, 379*(22), 2097–2107. doi: 10.1056/NEJMoa1801174

*Shepherd, J., Cobb, S. M., Ford, I., et al. (1995). Prevention of coronary heart disease with pravastatin in men with hypercholesterolemia: The West of Scotland Coronary Prevention Study. *New England Journal of Medicine, 333*, 1301–1307.

Silverman, M. G., Ference, B. A., Im, K., et al. (2016). Association between lowering LDL-C and cardiovascular risk reduction among different therapeutic interventions: A systematic review and meta-analysis. *JAMA, 316*(12), 1289–1297. doi: 10.1001/jama.2016.13985

Spence, J. D., & Dresser, G. K. (2016). Overcoming challenges with statin therapy. *Journal of the American Heart Association, 5*(1), e002497. doi: 10.1161/JAHA.115.002497

Stone, N. J., Robinson, J. G., Lichtenstein, A. H., et al. (2014). 2013 ACC/AHA guideline on the treatment of blood cholesterol to reduce atherosclerotic cardiovascular risk in adults: A report of the American College of Cardiology/American Heart Association Task Force on Practice Guidelines. *Circulation, 129*(25 Suppl 2), S1–S45. doi: 10.1161/01.cir.0000437738.63853.7a

*Talbert, R. L. (1997). Hyperlipidemia. In J. T. Dipiro, R. L. Talbert, G. C. Yee, G. R. Matzke, B. G. Wells, & L. M. Posey (Eds.), *Pharmacotherapy: A pathophysiologic approach* (3rd ed., pp. 459–489). Stamford, CT: Appleton & Lange.

*Wei, M., Ito, M., Cohen, J., et al. (2013). Predictors of statin adherence, switching, and discontinuation in the USAGE survey: Understanding the use of statins in America and gaps in patient education. *Journal of Clinical Lipidology, 7*(5), 472–483. doi: 10.1016/j.jacl.2013.03.001

Weinberger, Y., & Han, B. (2015). Statin treatment for older adults: The impact of the 2013 ACC/AHA cholesterol guidelines. *Drugs and Aging, 32*, 87–93. doi: 10.1007/s40266-014-0238-5

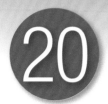

20 Chronic Stable Angina and Myocardial Infarction

Lauren Isaacs Karel and Christopher C. Roe

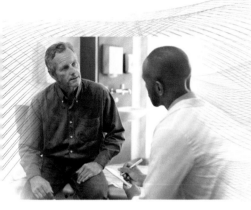
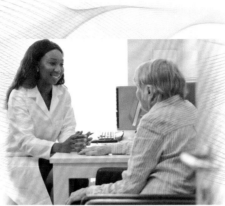
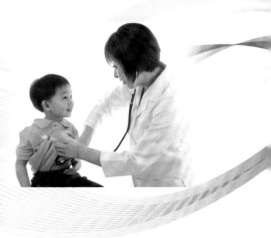

Learning Objectives

1. Identify risk factors for chronic stable angina and myocardial infarction.
2. Understand the pathophysiology of coronary heart disease and its relation to the medical therapies utilized in chronic stable angina and myocardial infarction.
3. Recognize contraindications to use, adverse reactions, and significant drug interactions for medications utilized in the management of chronic stable angina and myocardial infarction.
4. Recommend evidence-based treatment and monitoring strategies for chronic stable angina and myocardial infarction.

INTRODUCTION

Cardiovascular disease, which includes coronary heart disease (CHD), heart failure, stroke, and hypertension, continues to affect millions of Americans each year. The cost of cardiovascular disease in the United States was estimated to be nearly $351.2 billion in 2014 (Benjamin et al., 2019). Angina is a clinical syndrome caused by CHD that affects nearly 9.4 million Americans. CHD accounted for 43.2% of all cardiovascular disease–related death in the United States in 2016 (Benjamin et al., 2019).

Fortunately, the overall mortality rate due to CHD has been declining. The reason for this decline is the improved treatments for cardiovascular disease, including angina. Despite this hopeful note, angina remains a significant challenge for primary care management. Successful management depends on an in-depth understanding of the pathologic process, diagnosis, and treatment of this symptom complex.

Angina is a syndrome—a constellation of symptoms—that results from myocardial oxygen demand being greater than the oxygen supply (myocardial ischemia). By definition, angina is associated with reversible ischemia, so it does not result in permanent myocardial damage. Myocardial infarction (MI), a type of acute coronary syndrome, is the result of irreversible ischemia from an abrupt change in coronary blood flow that causes permanent damage to myocardial tissue.

Patients with angina may report left-sided chest pain, discomfort, heaviness, or pressure, and the sensation may radiate to the back, neck, jaw, and throat or arms. Usually, these sensations last 1 to 15 minutes. Patients may also experience shortness of breath or fatigue. It is important to note, however, that not all patients present with "angina" in a typical fashion. For example, dyspnea on exertion may be the only presenting symptom. If a patient presents with unique symptoms, his or her group of symptoms associated with identified ischemia is called that patient's *anginal equivalent*. **Box 20.1** lists common and unique terms used to describe angina.

Angina is called *stable* when the paroxysmal chest pain or discomfort is provoked by physical exertion or emotional stress and is relieved by rest and/or nitroglycerin (NTG). Stable angina exists when the stimulating factors or activities and the degree and duration of discomfort have not changed for the past 60 days.

Anginal episodes that increase in frequency, duration, or severity are referred to as *unstable*. Unstable angina is experienced when the patient is at rest or if the episode is prolonged or progressive. Unstable angina has also been called *preinfarction angina*, *crescendo angina*, or *intermittent coronary syndrome*. It is differentiated from stable angina by the fact that symptoms may be triggered by minimal physical exertion or may be present at rest. Patients who experience unstable angina are at high risk for developing an MI.

Other types of angina include variant (or Prinzmetal) angina, nocturnal angina, angina decubitus, and postinfarction angina. Stable angina is frequently managed in the primary care setting, while acute coronary syndromes such as MI are considered medical emergencies. Chronic stable angina and MI will be the focus of this chapter.

CAUSES

The development of angina is directly related to the risk factors that have been identified for CHD. Nonmodifiable risk factors for CHD cannot be altered or improved by the patient; they include age, family history, and gender. Modifiable risk factors may be controlled or treated by lifestyle modifications or pharmacologic therapy to reduce the risk of morbidity or mortality from CHD. Modifiable risk factors include cigarette smoking, hypertension, dyslipidemia, diabetes, obesity, and physical inactivity. **Box 20.2** lists the risk factors for chronic stable angina.

**BOX
20.2 Risk Factors for Chronic Stable Angina**

NONMODIFIABLE RISK FACTORS

Age
Heredity
Gender

MODIFIABLE RISK FACTORS

Cigarette smoking
Hypertension
Dyslipidemia
Diabetes
Obesity
Physical inactivity

Nonmodifiable Risk Factors

Age

It is uncommon for men younger than age 40 and premenopausal women to have symptomatic CHD, but the incidence increases with age and is increased in women after menopause. The average age at which a patient experiences a first MI is 65.6 years for males and 72 years for females (Benjamin et al., 2019). Moreover, the incidence of death within 5 years following a first MI rises with increasing age (Benjamin et al., 2019). This increasing incidence of CHD with age is likely linked to age-related changes in the vasculature and the higher prevalence of other CHD risk factors among older persons.

Heredity

A family history of premature CHD in a first-degree relative (i.e., mother, father, sister, or brother) is a strong predictor for CHD in an individual. Premature CHD is defined as occurring in a man younger than age 55 or in a woman younger than age 65. The strong association between family history and the development of CHD has been consistently demonstrated in several studies. Furthermore, race has been shown to be a factor. Data show that the prevalence of high blood pressure is higher in blacks than in whites, contributing to higher risk of a cardiovascular event (Benjamin et al., 2019). Therefore, individuals with a family history of CHD should be carefully screened for other CHD risk factors and managed appropriately.

Gender

In general, the risk of CHD is higher for men than women. Male gender is considered a nonmodifiable risk factor for CHD. While prevalence of CHD is higher in men, women may be more likely present with atypical symptoms and may be more likely to experience adverse outcomes including higher rate of death following a coronary event (Khamis et al., 2016). This is an area that requires further research, but highlights the importance of prompt evaluation and treatment when CHD is suspected in female patients.

Modifiable Risk Factors

Cigarette Smoking

Cigarette smoking increases the risk of CHD by at least twofold to threefold. Smoking increases the incidence of atherosclerosis by a mechanism that is not clearly understood. It is thought to increase the release of catecholamines, which leads to elevated blood pressure due to an increased workload of the heart caused by an increase in the heart rate and peripheral vascular constriction. Catecholamines also increase the release of free fatty acids, which increases the amount of lipids in the blood. Smoking lowers high-density lipoprotein (HDL) levels and increases low-density lipoprotein (LDL) levels and is thought to promote platelet activation, which increases the risk of clot formation in the arteries. All patients with CHD risk factors or established disease should be instructed to stop smoking. See Chapter 53 for a more detailed discussion of smoking cessation.

Hypertension

It is estimated that 116.4 million Americans have elevated blood pressure (Benjamin et al., 2019). Hypertension is a major risk factor for CHD and can lead to vascular complications that increase morbidity and mortality. Additionally, the higher the blood pressure, the higher the risk of MI and other cardiovascular events.

Atherosclerotic changes in the vasculature are exacerbated by increased pressure. Increased blood pressure alone also causes injury to the inner lining of the arteries, resulting in atherosclerotic changes and thrombus formation. As the arteries become stiff and narrow, the blood flow that normally increases during physical activity is restricted to a greater degree, resulting in ischemic symptoms. Chapter 18 provides further discussion of drug therapy for hypertension.

Dyslipidemia

Nearly half of the American population has high cholesterol (American Heart Association, 2010; Benjamin et al., 2019). Cholesterol plays a substantial role in the pathophysiology of atherosclerosis and CHD. High levels of LDL cholesterol and low levels of HDL cholesterol are associated with an increased risk of cardiovascular disease and occurrence of MI or other poor cardiovascular outcomes. Treatment of dyslipidemia in patients with CHD using pharmacologic and non-pharmacologic means has been shown in multiple large-scale studies to reduce the risk of cardiovascular death. In 2018, a new guideline was developed outlining the diagnosis and treatment of dyslipidemia in adults (Grundy et al., 2019). See Chapter 19 for more detailed information on the treatment of dyslipidemia.

Diabetes

Cardiovascular disease is the most common cause of death in patients with diabetes. In fact, patients with diabetes have the same risk of having an MI as a patient who already has a history of an MI. Although data have not shown a clear or conclusive link between glucose control and cardiovascular risk reduction, an effort should be made to prevent or treat diabetes in these patients. For a complete discussion of diabetes treatment, see Chapter 45.

Obesity

In the United States, 69.4% of the adult population is considered overweight or obese (Benjamin et al., 2019). The increasing incidence of obesity has been attributed to poorer nutrition and a more sedentary lifestyle.

Obesity is a risk factor for CHD in both men and women. Hypertension, dyslipidemia, and diabetes are more common in patients who are obese, but obesity also increases cardiovascular risk independent of these other risk factors by a mechanism that is not well understood. Even modest weight loss can improve blood pressure, hypertension, and insulin resistance and reduce cardiovascular risk. Weight loss is discussed in Chapter 53.

Physical Inactivity

A sedentary lifestyle predisposes patients to CHD. Regular physical exercise reduces blood pressure, maintains a healthy weight, and improves dyslipidemia, but it also reduces the risk of CHD independent of these changes. Patients should be carefully screened and counseled before beginning an exercise program. Exercise may include walking, running, cycling, or formalized aerobic exercise routines. It is recommended that patients get 30 to 60 minutes of aerobic exercise every day, at least 5 days per week. Resistance training on 2 days per week may also be of benefit.

PATHOPHYSIOLOGY

Angina is a symptomatic manifestation of reversible myocardial ischemia, which occurs when demand for oxygen in the myocardium exceeds available supply. This imbalance between oxygen supply and demand is caused by limited blood supply due to narrowing of the blood vessels that supply the heart muscle. The most common cause of this narrowing of the coronary arteries is atherosclerotic disease. Rarely, vasospasm of the coronary arteries narrows the arteries, thereby limiting the blood supply to the heart muscle. Other even more uncommon sources of anginal symptoms are thrombosis, aortic stenosis, primary pulmonary hypertension, and severe hypertension.

Atherosclerotic Disease

The pathophysiology of angina involves atherosclerosis, a disorder of lipid metabolism resulting in the deposit of cholesterol in the blood vessel. Over time, this causes a reactive endothelial injury that eventually results in a narrowing of the vessels by episodes of acute thrombosis. The narrow arteries impair the ability of oxygen and nutrients to reach the myocardium. This reduction in blood supply, or ischemia, impairs myocardial metabolism. The myocardial cells remain alive but cannot function normally. Once the blood supply is restored, cardiac function returns to normal. If the ischemia is caused by complete occlusion of the coronary artery, an MI (cell death) occurs.

Regardless of the risk factors that cause the development of atherosclerosis and resulting restriction of coronary blood supply, the pathophysiologic process is essentially the same. The three layers of the arterial wall—intima, media, and adventitia—are affected by structural changes that lead to CHD. The intima is a single layer of endothelial cells, constituting the innermost surface of the artery. It is impermeable to the substances in the blood. The media is the middle layer of the artery and is made up almost entirely of smooth muscle. The outer layer, or adventitia, consists mainly of smooth muscle cells, fibroblasts (which are normally only in this layer), and loose connective tissue. Atherosclerotic changes in the artery occur in stages. Normally, the intima is thin and contains only an occasional muscle cell. As a person ages, the intima slowly increases in thickness and muscle cells proliferate.

Atherosclerosis primarily affects the intima of the arterial wall. It normally takes years to develop, and clinical manifestations do not occur until the disorder is well advanced. CHD progresses through three developments—the fatty streak, the fibrous plaque, and the complicated lesion.

The Fatty Streak

Thought to begin in childhood, the fatty streak is caused by the development of fatty, lipid-rich lesions that result from macrophages adhering to the intact endothelial surface. The macrophages take in lipids, which leads to a thickening of the intimal layer. Smooth muscle cells migrate to the intima and become lipid laden. The lesions at this stage do not obstruct the artery. However, on examination, fatty streaks appear in the coronary arteries as early as age 15. They continue to enlarge through the third decade of life and appear to be a precursor to plaque formation, although the process is not clearly understood.

The Fibrous Plaque

The raised fibrous plaque is a white, elevated area on the surface of the artery. It signals the beginning of progressive changes in the arterial wall, including protrusion of the lesion into the lumen of the artery. These more advanced lesions begin to develop at approximately age 30 in most patients. The major change in the arterial intima during this phase is the migration and proliferation of smooth muscle cells and the formation of a fibrous cap over a deeper deposit of extracellular lipid and cell debris. The lipid accumulation directly or indirectly reduces the blood supply. The decrease in blood supply is permanent and results in cell necrosis and cell debris.

The Complicated Lesion

A complicated lesion contains a fibrous plaque, calcium deposits, and a thrombus formed by hemorrhage into the plaque. The complicated lesion results from continuing cell degeneration. As the complicated lesion, with its lipid, necrotic center, becomes larger, it calcifies. The intimal surface may develop open or ruptured areas that degenerate into an ulcer. The damage is most likely to occur in areas where blood flow creates the greatest amount of stress in the vessel, such as at branches and bifurcations. The damaged surface allows blood from the artery lumen to enter the lipid core. Then, platelets adhere and thrombus formation begins. The thrombus expands and distorts the plaque, which becomes larger and begins to block the lumen of the artery. The blockage impedes the blood flow needed to supply extra oxygen and nutrients to meet the increased workload of the heart. The result is cardiac ischemia and anginal symptoms. These symptoms are relieved when either the workload of the heart is decreased or administration of vasodilating drugs increases blood flow to the myocardium. Complete blockage from the arterial thrombus can cause permanent myocardial death because the cells are entirely deprived of oxygen, and blood flow cannot be restored in time to revive the cardiac cells, resulting in an MI.

Coronary Artery Vasospasm

A less common cause of restricted coronary blood supply may be coronary vasospasm, a narrowing of the coronary artery lumen. This narrowing is produced by an arterial muscle spasm and limits the blood supply to the myocardium. The exact cause is unknown, but it is thought to occur when the smooth muscles of the coronary arteries contract in response to neurogenic stimulation. Cigarette smoking and hyperlipidemia appear to play a role in this type of angina because they interfere with normal neurogenic control of the arterial intima.

Spasm is suspected of playing a role in acute MI, as well as in triggering anginal episodes. Coronary artery spasm also can occur with abrupt nitrate withdrawal, cocaine use, and direct mechanical irritation from cardiac catheterization. However, the exact mechanisms leading to spasm are still unclear.

Activation of Ischemic Episodes

Regardless of the existing pathophysiologic process, ischemic episodes that result in anginal pain are usually activated by two situations occurring simultaneously or independently: (1) ambient factors that increase myocardial oxygen demand and (2) circumstances that decrease oxygen supply. For example, suppose that the person with atherosclerosis (noncompliant arteries) climbs a flight of stairs. The activity increases the workload of the heart, and the myocardium needs more oxygen. The damaged arteries are unable to meet this demand. In some situations, the arteries may be so constricted that they are unable to deliver an adequate amount of oxygen even if the person is in a resting state. Therapy to address angina symptoms is directed at resolution or control of these situations so that the heart can receive the oxygen it needs to meet the physical demands of the body. In acute MI with complete obstruction by an arterial thrombus, therapy is aimed at breaking up the formed thrombus to restore blood flow to cardiac tissue.

DIAGNOSTIC CRITERIA

Health History

The health history is an important part of the diagnosis and management of angina and MI. The chief complaint for most patients with angina is usually chest pain or discomfort, but other symptoms may predominate, such as neck or jaw pain or shortness of breath. The patient should be asked to describe the duration, quality, location, severity, and radiation of the pain. Additionally, the practitioner should inquire about potential triggers of the pain and any accompanying symptoms, such as dyspnea, diaphoresis, nausea, or palpitations. The practitioner also should explore what interventions relieved the patient's pain or symptoms, such as rest or NTG. Patients presenting with continuing chest pain lasting for 10 minutes or longer, severe dyspnea, syncope, or palpitations should immediately be referred and/or transported to the emergency department for evaluation of an acute coronary syndrome.

For all patients with angina, and/or following an acute MI, an assessment of CHD risk factors should be performed to determine an individual patient's risk for CHD and to better target pharmacologic and nonpharmacologic management. Practitioners should ask patients about both nonmodifiable and modifiable risk factors, including family history, cigarette smoking, hypertension, dyslipidemia, diabetes, and physical inactivity. A past history of cerebrovascular disease or the presence of peripheral vascular disease also increases a patient's risk of CHD.

Physical Findings

Most commonly, practitioners will not have the opportunity to examine a patient during an acute anginal episode. In that case, the physical examination should focus on the assessment of risk factors and the cardiovascular system as a whole. For example, the practitioner should assess a patient for obesity during the physical examination. Additionally, the vasculature may be evaluated by looking for funduscopic changes or decreased peripheral pulses. Hypertension may be evident from taking the patient's blood pressure, and clinical signs and symptoms of heart failure may include murmurs, gallops, changes in the heart sounds, edema, rales, or organomegaly. Patients with dyslipidemia may exhibit xanthomas or cholesterol nodules.

If a physical exam is performed during an episode of anginal pain, a variety of findings may be present. These may include extra heart sounds, mild hypertension, tachycardia, or tachypnea. A paradoxical split of S2 may indicate altered left ventricular (LV) heart function associated with the ischemic discomfort. This finding may also be present during physical exam in acute coronary syndromes.

A physical exam is also crucial in the differential diagnosis of acute MI versus other conditions associated with chest pain. The practitioner should assess pain on palpation that may be indicative of musculoskeletal disease or inflammation. Patients reporting back pain should have blood pressure evaluated in both arms as a large difference in systolic blood pressure between right and left sides may be concerning for aortic dissection.

Diagnostic Tests

Before therapy for angina can be properly prescribed, diagnostic testing is necessary to identify a cardiac cause of the patient's chest pain. Diagnostic testing includes electrocardiography, echocardiography, exercise tolerance testing, radioisotope imaging, and coronary artery angiography.

Patients with new, current, or recent chest pain should have an electrocardiogram (ECG) to detect signs of cardiac ischemia. During an acute anginal episode, ST segment depressions with or without symmetric T-wave inversions may be noted in the leads that correspond to the myocardium affected. During pain-free intervals, however, the ECG reverts to baseline. ECG changes that may be present in the patient with chronic CHD include evidence of a prior MI, LV hypertrophy, and repolarization abnormalities.

Echocardiography is recommended if valvular disease or heart failure is suspected, if the patient has a history of MI, or if the patient experiences ventricular arrhythmias. Most patients with intermittent episodes of chest pain should undergo an exercise tolerance test with ECG monitoring (also called a *stress test*) to evaluate the risk of future cardiac events. Those suspected of having coronary ischemia based on the presence of anginal symptoms should undergo testing within 72 hours of symptoms (Fihn et al., 2012). One notable exception would be patients with a high probability of CHD, such as a patient with known coronary disease and classical angina symptoms; these patients should be referred to a specialist for potential advanced interventional therapies. Further testing with radioisotope perfusion testing or coronary artery angiography may be indicated for subgroups of patients. If diagnostic testing confirms cardiac ischemia as the cause of anginal symptoms, drug therapy is warranted.

In the patient presenting with an acute coronary syndrome, an ECG should be performed within 10 minutes of arrival to emergency services. An ECG showing ST segment elevation or new left bundle branch block is referred to as *ST elevation MI* (STEMI) and warrants urgent coronary angiography. No ST elevation noted on ECG is indicative of non-ST elevation MI (NSTEMI). Similar to ECG findings in an acute anginal episode, ST segment depression with or without T-wave inversion may be seen in the patient presenting with NSTEMI.

Laboratory biomarkers are also utilized in the diagnosis of acute MI. With myocardial injury, cardiac troponin levels rise shortly after symptom onset and remain elevated for several days to weeks. In the patient presenting with acute chest pain, a lack of elevated cardiac troponins may suggest an alternative cause of the patient's symptoms.

INITIATING DRUG THERAPY

Goals of Drug Therapy

The treatment goals for the management of angina include relieving the acute anginal episode, preventing additional anginal episodes, preventing progression of CHD, reducing the risk of MI, improving functional capacity, and prolonging survival. These goals should be accomplished while maintaining the patient's quality of life and avoiding adverse events associated with therapy.

The immediate goal for an acute coronary syndrome is restoring coronary blood flow to reduce the extent of myocardial injury. For the patient diagnosed with STEMI, reperfusion therapy should occur within 12 hours of symptom onset. Percutaneous coronary intervention (PCI) is the preferred method of reperfusion therapy; however, if not available, fibrinolytic therapy should be initiated barring contraindications to treatment (O'Gara, et al., 2013).

For the patient with NSTEMI, the practitioner should assess the risk for mortality and major adverse cardiac events

Age 65 years or more
Presence of 3 or more risk factors for coronary artery disease
Prior coronary stenosis 50% or more
ST deviation on ECG
Two or more anginal events in prior 24 hours
Use of aspirin in previous 7 days
Elevated cardiac biomarkers

to guide further management. Risk assessment is conducted using the thrombolysis in myocardial infarction (TIMI) risk score, in which one point each is given for the presence of up to seven variables as listed in **Box 20.3**. The total number of points is then used to determine prognosis and inform treatment decisions. The patient with higher TIMI risk scores (at least three points) may be more likely to benefit from treatment with additional antiplatelet therapy and invasive management strategies (Amsterdam et al., 2014).

Nonpharmacologic therapy is the cornerstone of treatment for patients with angina and following acute MI. The practitioner must assess the patient's modifiable risk factors and work with him or her to reduce the risk for or progression of CHD. Practitioners should counsel patients on smoking cessation at each clinic visit and provide support and access to pharmacologic treatment if necessary. Patients should be instructed to maintain a normal weight by consuming a low-fat, low-cholesterol diet, and practitioners should provide dietary counseling and refer interested patients to dietitians for further support. Finally, practitioners should encourage patients to engage in regular aerobic exercise. Further details on these lifestyle modifications are provided in Chapters 18, 19, 52, and 53.

The practitioner should emphasize to the patient that nonpharmacologic therapy and lifestyle modifications supplement drug therapy and should continue indefinitely.

After the patient has been properly instructed on nonpharmacologic therapy for angina, appropriate drug therapy may be initiated. A summary of selected agents is provided in **Table 20.1**. Several classes of medications are used to treat angina, including angiotensin-converting enzyme (ACE) inhibitors, nitrates, beta blockers, calcium channel blockers, and antiplatelet agents. Additional medications that are used in the treatment of acute MI include morphine, anticoagulants, fibrinolytics, and aldosterone antagonists. Supplemental oxygen should also be offered for arterial oxygen saturation less than 90%, cyanosis, or difficulty breathing.

Angiotensin-Converting Enzyme Inhibitors, Angiotensin Receptor Blockers, and Aldosterone Antagonists

The 2012 Guideline for the Diagnosis and Management of Patients with Stable Ischemic Heart Disease and 2014 Guideline for the Management of Patients with Non-ST-Elevation Acute Coronary Syndromes recommend that patients with ejection fractions of less than 40% or those with hypertension, diabetes, or kidney disease be placed on an ACE inhibitor unless contraindicated (Amsterdam et al., 2014; Fihn et al., 2012). When patients cannot take an ACE inhibitor, an angiotensin receptor blocker (ARB) may be used (Amsterdam et al., 2014; Fihn et al., 2012). Guideline recommendations for NSTEMI also recommend an aldosterone antagonist for patients with ejection fraction of less than 40%, diabetes, or heart failure who are already receiving ACE inhibitor and beta-blocker therapy and who have adequate kidney function and normal potassium levels (Amsterdam et al., 2014). ACE inhibitors include captopril (Capoten), ramipril (Altace), enalapril (Vasotec), quinapril (Accupril), benazepril (Lotensin), perindopril (Aceon), and lisinopril (Prinivil, Zestril). ARBs include losartan (Cozaar), valsartan (Diovan), candesartan (Atacand), telmisartan (Micardis), eprosartan (Teveten), olmesartan (Benicar), and irbesartan (Avapro). Aldosterone antagonists include spironolactone (Aldactone) and eplerenone (Inspra).

Mechanism of Action

ACE inhibitors affect the enzyme responsible for the conversion of angiotensin I to angiotensin II. ARBs block the vasoconstriction and aldosterone-secreting effects of angiotensin II by selectively blocking angiotensin II from binding to angiotensin II receptors found in many tissues. Angiotensin II is a potent vasoconstrictor and also stimulates aldosterone secretion. Aldosterone binding to mineralocorticoid receptors in the kidney increases sodium and water reabsorption. Blocking the production and downstream effects of angiotensin II results in reduced vasoconstriction and sodium and water retention, thus reducing preload, afterload, and ejection fraction. These benefits are helpful in chronic stable angina, heart failure, and hypertension.

Dosage

ACE inhibitors, ARBs, and aldosterone antagonists should be initiated at low doses and followed by gradual dosage increases if the lower doses are well tolerated. Renal function and serum potassium should be assessed within 1 to 2 weeks of starting therapy and periodically thereafter, especially in patients with preexisting diabetes or those receiving potassium supplementation. **Table 20.1** shows the doses of some common ACE inhibitors, ARBs, and aldosterone antagonists when used to treat chronic stable angina and following acute MI.

Contraindications

ACE inhibitors are contraindicated in pregnancy and should be avoided in patients with bilateral renal artery stenosis or unilateral stenosis. Aldosterone antagonists are contraindicated in patients with hyperkalemia.

TABLE 20.1			
Overview of Agents Used to Treat Chronic Stable Angina and Myocardial Infarction			
Generic (Trade) Name and Dosage	**Selected Adverse Events**	**Contraindications**	**Special Considerations**
Selected Angiotensin-Converting Enzyme Inhibitors			
Captopril (Capoten) Start: 6.25 mg or 12.5 mg TID Therapeutic range: 25–50 mg TID	Common: cough; hypotension, particularly with a diuretic or volume depletion; hyperkalemia, loss of taste, and leukopenia; angioedema, neutropenia, and agranulocytosis in <1% of patients; rash in >10% of patients	Contraindicated in pregnancy; avoid in patients with bilateral renal artery stenosis or unilateral stenosis.	Renal impairment related to ACE inhibitors is seen as an increase in serum creatinine and azotemia, usually in the beginning of therapy. Monitor BUN, creatinine, and K levels when starting.
Enalapril (Vasotec) Start: 2.5 mg daily or BID Range: 5–20 mg daily or BID	Same as for captopril	Same as for captopril	Same as for captopril Use only 2.5 mg/d in patient with impaired renal function or hyponatremia.
Fosinopril (Monopril) Start: 10 mg daily Range: 10–40 mg daily	Same as for captopril	Same as for captopril	Same as for captopril Use only 5 mg/d in patient with impaired renal function or hyponatremia.
Lisinopril (Zestril, Prinivil) Start: 5 mg daily Range: 5–40 mg daily	Same as for captopril	Same as for captopril	Same as for captopril Use only 2.5 mg/d in patient with impaired renal function or hyponatremia.
Quinapril (Accupril) Start: 5 mg BID Range: 20–40 BID	Same as for captopril	Same as for captopril	Same as for captopril Use only 2.5 mg/d in patient with impaired renal function or hyponatremia.
Ramipril (Altace) Start: 1.25 mg BID Range: 1.25–5 mg BID	Same as for captopril	Same as for captopril	Same as for captopril
Selected Angiotensin Receptor Blockers			
Losartan (Cozaar) Start: 12.5 mg/d Range: 50–100 mg/d	Dyspnea, hypotension, hyperkalemia	Angioedema secondary to ACE inhibition	May be used in patients experiencing cough due to ACE inhibitor
Valsartan (Diovan) Start: 80 mg/d Range: 80–160 mg BID	Same as for losartan	Same as for losartan	Same as for losartan
Aldosterone Antagonists			
Spironolactone (Aldactone) Start: 25 mg/d Range: 25–50 mg/d	Hyperkalemia, hypotension, gynecomastia	Hyperkalemia, Addison's disease, combination with eplerenone	Dose may be reduced to 25 mg QOD due to hyperkalemia.
Eplerenone (Inspra) Start: 25 mg/d Range: 25–50 mg/d	Hyperkalemia	Hyperkalemia, kidney failure, combination with strong CYP3A inhibitors	Dose may be reduced to 25 mg QOD due to hyperkalemia.

(Continued)

TABLE 20.1

Overview of Agents Used to Treat Chronic Stable Angina (Continued)

Generic (Trade) Name and Dosage	Selected Adverse Events	Contraindications	Special Considerations
Short-Acting Nitrates			
Nitroglycerin (Nitrostat, NitroQuick) 0.4 mg SL PRN	Headache, dizziness, tachycardia, hypotension, edema	Combination with phosphodiesterase-5 inhibitors (e.g., sildenafil, vardenafil, and tadalafil)	For acute treatment of anginal episodes
ISDN; Isordil, Sorbitrate, 5 mg SL PRN	Same as for nitroglycerin	Same as for nitroglycerin	Same as for nitroglycerin
Long-Acting Nitrates			
Nitroglycerin	Previous notes also apply.	Previous notes also apply.	For chronic prevention of anginal episodes
Topical ointment (Nitro-Bid) ½–1 inch BID–TID	Local irritation and erythema with topical application		Use nitrate-free interval to reduce risk of nitrate tolerance.
Transdermal patch (Minitran, Nitro-Dur, Nitrol, Transderm-Nitro) 0.2–0.8 mg/h			Potential hypotensive effect with vasodilators Tapering is recommended after long-term use. Onset of action with transdermal application is ~60 min.
Isosorbide mononitrate	Previous notes also apply.	Previous notes also apply.	Previous notes also apply.
Immediate release (Ismo, Monoket) 5–20 mg BID Extended release (Imdur) 30–120 mg daily			Extended-release formulations should be swallowed whole.
Beta Blockers			
Propranolol Immediate release (Inderal) 40–160 mg BID Extended release (Inderal LA) 80–240 mg daily	Fatigue, dizziness, decreased exercise tolerance, bradycardia, hypotension, dyspnea	Use with caution in patients with reactive airway disease. Bradycardia (heart rate <45 beats per minute) Acutely decompensated heart failure	Abrupt cessation of beta-blocker therapy should be avoided. Extended-release formulations should be swallowed whole.
Atenolol (Tenormin) 25–100 mg daily	Same as for propranolol	Same as for propranolol	Previous notes also apply. Dose adjustment needed in chronic kidney disease
Metoprolol Immediate release (metoprolol tartrate, Lopressor) 25–200 mg BID Extended release (metoprolol succinate, Toprol-XL) 50–400 mg daily	Same as for propranolol	Same as for propranolol	Toprol-XL tablets may be split but should not be chewed or crushed.
Calcium Channel Blockers			
Amlodipine (Norvasc) 2.5–10 mg daily	Headache, dizziness, flushing, edema, gingival hyperplasia	Severe conduction abnormalities Use with caution in patients with preexisting bradycardia or CHF.	Useful for patients with isolated systolic hypertension
Nifedipine (extended release, Adalat CC, Procardia XL) 30–60 mg daily	Same as for amlodipine	Same as for amlodipine	Should be swallowed whole

TABLE 20.1

Overview of Agents Used to Treat Chronic Stable Angina (*Continued*)

Generic (Trade) Name and Dosage	Selected Adverse Events	Contraindications	Special Considerations
Diltiazem (extended release, Cardizem CD, Dilacor XR, Tiazac) 180–360 mg daily	Headache, nausea, conduction abnormalities, gingival hyperplasia	Same as for amlodipine	Should be swallowed whole
Verapamil Immediate release (Calan, Isoptin) 80–160 mg TID Extended release (Calan SR, Isoptin SR) 120–480 mg daily	Same as for amlodipine Constipation	Same as for amlodipine	Extended-release formulations should be swallowed whole.
Selected Antiplatelet Agents			
Aspirin 81–325 mg daily	Bleeding, bruising, nausea, dyspepsia	Allergy to aspirin Bleeding disorders Allergy to clopidogrel	For primary and secondary prevention of cardiovascular events
Clopidogrel (Plavix) Load (acute MI): 300 mg Maintenance: 75 mg daily	Bleeding, bruising, nausea	Bleeding disorders	Alternative antiplatelet agent for aspirin-intolerant or aspirin-allergic patients
Prasugrel (Effient) Load (acute MI): 60 mg Maintenance: 10 mg daily	Same as for clopidogrel	Bleeding disorders Prior stroke	Same as for clopidogrel
Ticagrelor (Brilinta) Load (acute MI): 180 mg Maintenance: 60–90 mg BID	Same as for clopidogrel	Bleeding disorders Prior intracranial hemorrhage	Same as for clopidogrel Preferred to clopidogrel during the first 12 months of therapy following acute MI
Selected Anticoagulant Agents			
Unfractionated heparin Load: 60 IU/kg (maximum 4,000 IU) Maintenance infusion: 12 IU/kg/hour (maximum 1,000 IU/hour)	Bleeding, bruising, HIT	Uncontrolled active bleeding, history of HIT, hypersensitivity to pork products	Infusion rate adjusted per aPTT
Enoxaparin (Lovenox) 1 mg/kg SubQ q12h	Same as for unfractionated heparin	Same as for unfractionated heparin	Reduce dose to 1 mg/kg SubQ once daily if CrCl <30 mL/min.
Bivalirudin (Angiomax) Load: 0.75 mg/kg Maintenance infusion: 1.75 mg/kg/h	Bleeding, bruising	Active major bleeding	Additional 0.3 mg/kg bolus dose may be given per ACT level. Reduce infusion rate to 1 mg/kg/h if CrCl <30 mL/min.
Ranolazine			
Ranolazine (Ranexa) 500–1,000 mg BID	Dizziness, nausea, constipation	Patients taking strong inhibitors of CYP3A4 and/or severe hepatic impairment	Should be swallowed whole

ACE, angiotensin-converting enzyme; ACT, activated clotting time; aPTT, activated partial thromboplastin time; BUN, blood urea nitrogen; CHF, congestive heart failure; HIT, heparin-induced thrombocytopenia; ISDN, isosorbide dinitrate; ISMN, isosorbide mononitrate; MI, myocardial infarction; SL, sublingual.

Adverse Effects

Side effects of ACE inhibitors are uncommon but may include an irritating cough and excessive drops in blood pressure, particularly in hypovolemic patients or those already on diuretics. Hyperkalemia may also occur; however, the incidence is less with ARBs than with ACE inhibitors. A serious adverse effect with ACE inhibitors is angioedema, which usually occurs early in treatment. Angioedema secondary to an ACE inhibitor is a contraindication to further ACE inhibitor use, but an ARB may be used cautiously in its place. Other adverse effects include rash, loss of taste, neutropenia, and agranulocytosis. Hyperkalemia is a serious adverse effect with aldosterone antagonists, and risk may be increased in patients with kidney dysfunction, with potassium supplementation, or with concomitant use of ACE inhibitor or ARB therapy. Spironolactone specifically may also cause gynecomastia, which is usually reversible after therapy is stopped.

Interactions

Due to the effects on angiotensin II and aldosterone, ACE inhibitors, ARBs, and aldosterone antagonists contribute to potassium retention as sodium is preferentially excreted. This raises the possibility of a hyperkalemia state for the patient and must be monitored routinely. Similarly, patients taking lithium are at increased risk for lithium toxicity due to its decreased renal excretion. Other important ACE inhibitor interactions can be found in Chapter 18, **Table 18.3**.

Nitrates

The nitrates are one of the original medications used for controlling angina, and they are still commonly used to halt an acute anginal attack, to prevent predictable episodes, and for chronic treatment to prevent anginal episodes. Nitrates are also used to treat ischemic pain with acute MI.

Mechanism of Action

Nitrates and their analogs are potent agents and have profound effects on vascular smooth muscle. The nitrates cause dilation throughout the vasculature—in the peripheral arteries and veins as well as the coronary arteries. When dilated, the veins return less blood to the heart, thereby reducing LV filling volume and pressure (preload). This decreases the workload of the heart. Another primary effect of the nitrates is coronary arterial dilation, which results in increased blood flow and oxygen supply to the myocardium. Nitrates do not directly influence the chronotropic or inotropic actions of the heart, so their administration does not affect or alter cardiac function but rather decreases the work of the heart and increases myocardial oxygenation. Nitrates are moderately effective in lessening coronary vasospasm.

Rapid-Acting Nitrates

The sublingual forms of NTG are rapid acting (see **Table 20.1**). These medications are used for acute attacks of angina. Short-acting nitrates are also used for prophylaxis of angina in situations when an anginal episode can be reasonably predicted by the patient, such as during walking, climbing stairs, or sexual activity. To be effective, NTG must be administered sublingually to avoid hepatic first-pass metabolism, which would inactivate the medication.

Sublingual NTG (Nitrol, Isordil, others) remains a first-line therapy for managing acute angina episodes and NSTEMI. NTG may be adequate treatment for patients who experience angina no more frequently than once a week. NTG usually relieves anginal symptoms within 1 to 5 minutes and provides short-term (up to 30 minutes) relief. NTG tablets or spray (0.3–0.6 mg) is used sublingually for immediate symptomatic treatment of anginal episodes. The practitioner instructs the patient to rest at the time of pain, take a single dose, repeat the dose if the pain does not resolve within 5 minutes, and call emergency medical services if the pain is not relieved with three doses. In the patient with NSTEMI, intravenous NTG may be considered for continued ischemic pain, heart failure, or hypertension.

Patients should be instructed to mark the date they open a bottle of NTG tablets or first use an NTG spray canister. Tablets in an opened glass bottle of NTG retain efficacy for only 1 year and should be discarded after that time period. NTG canisters retain their efficacy for up to 3 years.

The main advantage of rapid-acting nitrates is their ability to halt an episode of angina once it has begun. Generally, the adverse effects of short-acting nitrates are related to their vasodilatory effects; however, patients may also experience burning under the tongue with sublingual preparations.

Long-Acting Nitrates

Due to their short duration of action, short-acting nitrates such as sublingual NTG are not suitable for maintenance therapy; long-acting nitrates must be used for chronic prophylaxis of anginal episodes. Long-acting nitrates act to maintain vasodilation, thereby continuously decreasing the workload of the heart and maintaining blood flow to the heart. The most prescribed long-acting nitrates are isosorbide dinitrate (ISDN; oral [Cedocard SR, Isordil, others]), isosorbide mononitrate (ISMN; oral [Imdur, Ismo, Monoket, others]), and long-acting transdermal NTG preparations (transdermal [Minitran, Nitro-Dur, Transderm-Nitro, others], topical [Nitro-Bid, others]).

Isosorbide Dinitrate (Oral)

Single oral doses of 20 to 40 mg significantly improve hemodynamic parameters and exercise tolerance, and the effect continues for several hours. The starting dose should be low (e.g., ISDN 5 mg thrice daily), and the dosage should be advanced slowly in small increments every 1 to 2 weeks to minimize side effects. The dose is increased until control is obtained, side effects become intolerable, systolic blood pressure falls to 100 mm Hg or below, resting heart rate increases more than 10 beats per minute, or postural hypotension occurs.

Intestinal absorption with ISDN is unpredictable, especially when taken with food, so oral nitrates should be taken on an empty stomach, 1 hour before or 2 hours after food intake. A drawback to ISDN products is the short half-life (~2–4 hours) and duration of action, which necessitates multiple doses during the day.

Isosorbide Mononitrate (Oral)

ISMN is a long-acting metabolite derivative of ISDN. Formulated in extended-release tablets, ISMN can be administered in fewer doses (Imdur, once daily; other products, twice daily). A common twice-daily starting regimen is 20 mg (immediate release) orally at 7 a.m. and 3 p.m., allowing for a nitrate-free period to reduce the risk of nitrate tolerance. A starting dose using extended-release ISMN (Imdur) is 30 to 60 mg orally in the morning. Like ISDN, ISMN should also be taken on an empty stomach. Extended-release formulations of ISMN must be taken whole, without crushing or chewing the tablet.

Nitroglycerin (Transdermal)

Transdermal NTG is long acting and effective for treating and preventing anginal pain. Two percent (2%) NTG ointment may be applied to the skin as an adjunct to isosorbide therapy for nocturnal pain or, with repeated daily dosing, used alone for anginal treatment. One half to one inch of the ointment is applied to a clean, hairless area of the torso before bed. Alternatively, the ointment may be applied every 4 to 6 hours while awake, allowing for an 8- to 12-hour nitrate-free interval. Measurement guides are provided with the product to assist in dosing. The dose is increased by a half inch at a time until pain relief is achieved.

Transdermal NTG patches may also be used as a long-acting nitrate. Therapy is typically initiated with a 5-mg (0.2 mg/h) or 10-mg (0.4 mg/h) patch, which should be left in place for 12 to 14 hours and then removed to prevent nitrate tolerance. Nitrate patches should be applied to the torso intact, since cutting a patch destroys the drug delivery system. Care should be taken to ensure that a previously applied patch is removed before applying a new patch.

Nitrate Tolerance

A drawback to the use of nitrates to treat angina is the potential for the development of nitrate tolerance. Nitrate tolerance refers to the loss of ability of the smooth muscles to respond to the action of the nitrates. Tolerance develops to both the peripheral and coronary vasodilator effects of nitrates. This phenomenon occurs with continuous nitrate use over prolonged periods. Tolerance is both dose and time dependent. Nitrate tolerance can be seen after as few as 7 to 10 days of continuous administration. Nitrate tolerance may also develop with frequent sublingual administration of nitrates, if the oral tablets are given four times daily in evenly spaced intervals or if the transdermal patches are left on the skin for 24-hour periods.

Prevention of nitrate tolerance is based on a treatment plan that provides for rapid changes in blood nitrate levels over a given time, usually 24 hours. To prevent nitrate tolerance, one 10- to 12-hour nitrate-free interval per day is necessary. In this manner, the intervals between doses need not be equal. For example, the patch can be applied in the morning and removed in the evening. The same schedule can be developed for patients taking oral medications. The medication is given three times during the day when the patient is awake. The patient does not receive any medication during the night to minimize the risk of nitrate tolerance. Combination antianginal therapy (e.g., a beta blocker plus a long-acting nitrate) should be used for patients whose anginal symptoms are not controlled during the nitrate-free interval.

Adverse Events

The common side effects of the nitrates are related to their vasodilatory effects: headache, flushing, dizziness, weakness, and orthostatic hypotension. Additionally, since all segments of the vascular system relax in response to nitrates, reflex tachycardia often results as the heart compensates for the blood pressure drop to maintain cardiac output. Transdermal nitrate products may also cause irritation of the skin at the site of application.

Most of the side effects associated with nitrates abate or disappear with continuation of therapy. By starting therapy at a low dose and slowing titrating the dose upward, side effects are minimized and may not present at all. However, starting with a high dose can produce severe side effects (especially headache), and if side effects are intolerable, the patient may self-discontinue the medication.

If a patient has been receiving nitrate therapy long term, it should not be abruptly discontinued because of the risk of rebound hypertension and angina. If discontinuation of nitrate therapy is required, it should be done by tapering the dose over a period of time.

Caution should be exercised when using nitrates in combination with vasodilators due to additive hypotensive effects. Concurrent use of nitrates and phosphodiesterase-5 inhibitors such as sildenafil (Viagra), vardenafil (Levitra), or tadalafil (Cialis) is contraindicated due to the potential for severe hypotension.

Beta Blockers

Beta blockers are very effective in managing angina. They reduce the workload of the heart and decrease overall myocardial oxygen demand and consumption through antagonism of adrenergic receptors. This is accomplished by a reduction in the heart rate and myocardial contractility, both at rest and during periods of normal exercise. As such, they are particularly beneficial for treating exertional angina. In the management of NSTEMI, beta blockers should be started within the first 24 hours after symptom onset unless contraindicated (Amsterdam et al., 2014).

Nitrates and beta blockers have complementary effects on myocardial oxygen supply and demand and therefore are often used together. Because beta blockers reduce the heart rate, they can be used to control the reflex tachycardia that sometimes occurs with the administration of nitrates. This reduction in heart rate also allows more time for coronary artery filling and therefore myocardial perfusion during diastole.

Mechanism of Action

Beta blockers can be categorized according to their cardioselectivity, that is, the degree of preferential affinity for beta-1 receptors, which predominate in the heart and are the principal target of these medications. Beta antagonists that block only beta-1 receptors are considered cardioselective beta blockers. Those that block both beta-1 and beta-2 receptors are nonselective. There are many beta blockers available, all of which block beta-1 receptors. However, many agents also block beta-2 receptors, which predominate in the lungs.

Beta-1-receptor blockade is desirable in a patient with angina because it causes a slowing of the heart rate and a reduction in myocardial contractility. These effects reduce myocardial oxygen demand and therefore improve and prevent anginal symptoms.

Blockage of beta-2 receptors can lead to bronchoconstriction; therefore, nonselective beta blockers should be used with caution in patients with uncontrolled or unstable reactive airway disease. At low to intermediate doses, cardioselectivity is demonstrated by atenolol (Tenormin) and metoprolol (Lopressor). Propranolol (Inderal) is an example of a nonselective beta blocker. However, even cardioselective beta blockers show nonselective action at high doses.

Propranolol is a nonselective beta blocker with a short half-life (4–6 hours). Immediate-release formulations of propranolol must be dosed multiple times per day, but sustained-release preparations for once-daily dosing are also available. Other nonselective beta blockers include nadolol and timolol.

Atenolol and metoprolol are selective beta-1 antagonists. These drugs, which preferentially block beta-1 receptors, were developed to eliminate the unwanted bronchoconstriction effect of the agents that also block beta-2 receptors. These agents may be a better choice for patients with severe or uncontrolled asthma or chronic obstructive pulmonary disease (COPD). However, when these agents are prescribed at high-dosage levels, they lose their cardioselective properties. Atenolol has a long duration of action and therefore may be dosed once daily. Atenolol is renally cleared; therefore, dose adjustments must be made based on the patient's estimated glomerular filtration rate. Immediate-release metoprolol tartrate (Lopressor) must be given twice to thrice daily, but extended-release metoprolol succinate (Toprol-XL) is given only once daily. Both atenolol and metoprolol tartrate are available in generic forms and are relatively inexpensive. A generic form of metoprolol succinate is now available; however, it remains expensive when compared to the immediate-release preparation.

Pindolol and acebutolol are beta blockers that also possess some agonist activity. They are not completely blockers in that they also have the ability to stimulate weakly both beta-1 and beta-2 receptors, possessing so-called *intrinsic sympathomimetic activity* (ISA). Drugs possessing ISA can stimulate the beta receptor to which they are bound, yet, as antagonists, they block the activation of the receptor by the more potent endogenous catecholamines, epinephrine and norepinephrine. Because of the agonist action, there is a diminished effect on cardiac rate and cardiac output. Patients who cannot tolerate the other beta blockers because of preexisting bradycardia or heart block may tolerate these agents.

Three beta blockers have proven to reduce mortality in patients with heart failure: extended-release metoprolol succinate, carvedilol, and bisoprolol. The patient with concomitant heart failure should receive beta blocker therapy with one of these three agents.

Contraindications

Beta blockers are relatively contraindicated and therefore should be used cautiously in patients with preexisting bradycardia because beta blockade may lower the heart rate further. Additionally, beta blockers should not be used if a patient is experiencing an acute episode of decompensated heart failure. The addition of a beta blocker in this situation has the potential to negatively impact the patient by further reducing heart rate and contractility. Finally, as discussed earlier, beta blockers should be used with caution in patients with reactive airway disease. In patients with stable or controlled asthma or COPD, a selective beta blocker may be a better choice to minimize the risk of bronchospasm.

Adverse Events

Beta blockers have the potential to adversely affect cardiac function. These effects include slowing the sinoatrial node and atrioventricular (AV) conduction, leading to symptomatic bradycardia and heart block. Sinus arrest is possible. If the patient has preexisting cardiac conduction system disease, a preparation with some intrinsic beta-agonist activity may be chosen to minimize these adverse events. These patients require close and frequent monitoring to ensure that early conduction system disease is managed promptly. Beta blockers should not be given to patients with a slow heart rate at baseline due to the potential for severe bradycardia.

Since beta blockers attenuate the "fight or flight" response, the clinical manifestations of hypoglycemia may be masked. Therefore, patients with diabetes should be instructed to more closely monitor their serum glucose to avoid severe hypoglycemic reactions. Typical symptoms of hypoglycemia, including tachycardia, tremor, or sweating, may be decreased or absent when these patients are taking a beta blocker.

Abrupt withdrawal of beta blockers can precipitate an acute withdrawal syndrome that may be manifested by tachycardia, hypertensive crises, angina exacerbation, acute coronary insufficiency, or even MI (Antman & Sabatine, 2013). For this reason, beta-blocker therapy should always be tapered. Withdrawal is of particular concern in the anginal patient on large doses of beta blockers who is faced with an emergency situation that makes it impossible to continue taking the prescribed beta blocker for more than 48 hours.

Beta blockers may also cause adverse central nervous system effects, including drowsiness and depression. These effects may occur more frequently in older patients or in patients with preexisting depression or psychiatric disorders. In these patients, careful monitoring of mood, sleep pattern, and sexual and cognitive functioning is necessary.

Calcium Channel Blockers

Calcium channel blockers are effective in managing angina because they exert vasodilatory effects on the coronary and peripheral vessels. Depending on the specific agent, they have the potential to depress cardiac contractility, heart rate, and conduction, which may mediate their antianginal effects. These drugs are effective in relieving coronary constriction associated with vasospastic angina. Nondihydropyridine calcium channel blockers are used in the initial management for NSTEMI in patients who have a contraindication or intolerance to beta blockers (Amsterdam et al., 2014).

Mechanism of Action

Calcium plays a major role in the electrical excitation and contraction of cardiac and vascular smooth muscle cells. The calcium channel blockers inhibit the entrance of calcium into smooth muscle cells of the coronary and systemic arterial vessels, which inhibits muscular contraction and therefore causes vasodilation. These vasodilatory effects are more pronounced on arteries than veins because of the relatively large amount of smooth muscle found in the arteries. Because calcium channel blockers do not cause substantial venous dilation, they do not reduce preload. Nondihydropyridine calcium channel blockers reduce heart rate by slowing conduction through the sinoatrial and AV nodes, and they depress cardiac contractility.

Two major groups of calcium channel blockers are available: the dihydropyridines and the nondihydropyridines.

Dihydropyridines

The dihydropyridine calcium channel blockers are potent dilators of the coronary and peripheral arteries. Due to the vasodilatory effect of these agents, they may cause reflex tachycardia due to a reduction in systemic blood pressure. Since dihydropyridines do not alter conduction, they do not slow the sinus rate.

There are many dihydropyridine calcium channel blockers available. Nifedipine is an example of a first-generation dihydropyridine; nicardipine, felodipine, isradipine, and amlodipine are second-generation dihydropyridines. In general, the second-generation agents are better tolerated than the first-generation agents.

All of these agents are administered orally, and they have relatively short half-lives. Doses should be titrated upward slowly to minimize orthostasis or other adverse events. Several dihydropyridines (e.g., nifedipine, nicardipine) must be administered as multiple daily doses unless the sustained formulations are used. Amlodipine is administered once daily.

Nondihydropyridines

Although diltiazem and verapamil are both nondihydropyridine calcium channel blockers, they display different effects on the cardiovascular system. Verapamil has a pronounced effect on cardiac conduction, reducing the rate of electrical conduction through the AV node. Verapamil also exerts negative inotropic and chronotropic effects, suppressing contractility, reducing heart rate, and therefore causing a reduction in oxygen demand. However, due to this effect, verapamil should be used with caution in those patients with depressed cardiac function or AV conduction abnormalities. Immediate-release formulations of verapamil must be administered as divided doses, but sustained-release products are administered once daily.

Like verapamil, diltiazem reduces the heart rate but to a lesser extent. Diltiazem also has a less potent effect than verapamil on conduction and contractility, but it is a more potent vasodilator. Diltiazem has immediate- and sustained-release formulations. The immediate-release formulation usually is taken four times daily before meals; the sustained-release formulation is taken daily on an empty stomach.

Contraindications

Before a calcium channel blocker can be selected for treating angina, a careful assessment must be done to determine a patient's LV and conduction system function. Nondihydropyridine calcium channel blockers with negative inotropic properties may worsen preexisting LV dysfunction. Patients with conduction system disease are poor candidates for nondihydropyridine calcium channel blocker therapy because of the risk of bradyarrhythmias.

The nondihydropyridine calcium channel blockers are contraindicated in patients with heart block because of the significant depression of AV node conduction. Additionally, calcium channel blockers should be used with caution in patients with sick sinus syndrome and hypotension.

Adverse Events

In general, adverse events accompanying the dihydropyridine calcium channel blockers are more common with the first-generation than the second-generation agents. Leg edema, a common problem, results from vasodilation, which causes fluid to pool in the legs. In some cases, the edema may be so severe that new-onset heart failure may be suspected. In this situation, dosage reduction or drug discontinuation may be considered. Other common side effects of the calcium channel blockers include fatigue, dizziness, headache, flushing, and gingival hyperplasia. Verapamil is associated with constipation much more often than the other calcium channel blockers.

Antiplatelet Therapy

In patients with stable angina, the risk of MI can be lowered with daily aspirin therapy. Current angina recommendations suggest that all patients with acute or chronic ischemic heart disease receive aspirin 75 to 162 mg daily as primary or secondary prevention of cardiovascular disease (Fihn et al., 2012). Doses of aspirin greater than 162 mg have been shown to increase the risk of adverse events without any enhanced benefit.

All patients with acute MI should receive non-enteric-coated aspirin 162 to 325 mg as soon as possible following symptom onset, unless contraindicated for use (Amsterdam et al., 2014). Thereafter, daily aspirin should be continued indefinitely.

P2Y12 inhibitors, which include clopidogrel, prasugrel, ticagrelor, and cangrelor, reduce adenosine diphosphate (ADP)–induced platelet activation. Clopidogrel is recommended for prevention of MI in angina patients who have contraindications to aspirin. Like aspirin, clopidogrel has been shown to reduce the incidence of morbidity and mortality in patients with established cardiovascular disease.

P2Y12 inhibitor loading and maintenance doses should be administered to patients with acute MI. Dual antiplatelet treatment with both aspirin and an oral P2Y12 inhibitor should be continued for 6 to 12 months, utilizing lower maintenance doses of aspirin (75–100 mg daily) to reduce the risk of bleeding (Amsterdam et al., 2014; Levine et al., 2016). Cangrelor is the only P2Y12 inhibitor for intravenous administration that may be considered in patients unable to tolerate oral therapy upon presentation with acute MI. Following the loading dose and maintenance infusion, patients should be transitioned to an oral P2Y12 inhibitor for continuation of antiplatelet therapy. Cangrelor has not been studied in patients receiving glycoprotein IIb/IIIa (GPIIb/IIIa) inhibitors, which are parenteral antiplatelet agents used in the management of high-risk patients with acute MI. GPIIb/IIIa inhibitors include tirofiban, eptifibatide, and abciximab.

Mechanism of Action

Antiplatelet drugs inhibit platelet aggregation through a variety of mechanisms. Aspirin acts by irreversibly blocking prostaglandin synthesis, which prevents formation of the platelet-aggregating substance thromboxane A2. The P2Y12 inhibitors reduce ADP-induced platelet activation by antagonizing the platelet ADP receptors. Lastly, the GPIIb/IIIa inhibitors prevent binding of fibrinogen to the GPIIb/IIIa on platelets, which further halts platelet aggregation. Aggregation is a normal process that causes disease when the platelets adhere to vessel walls, causing thrombus formation. Antiplatelet therapy limits the formation of the thrombus, thereby decreasing the risk of progressive CHD. When antiplatelet medications are used to treat patients with angina, the chances of having an MI are reduced.

Contraindications

Aspirin is contraindicated in patients with a known aspirin hypersensitivity. P2Y12 inhibitors should not be used in patients with known bleeding disorders. GPIIb/IIIa inhibitors should be avoided in patients with active bleeding or recent major surgery or trauma. Additional agent-specific contraindications are listed in **Table 20.1**.

Adverse Events

Adverse events associated with aspirin use include dyspepsia, bruising, and bleeding. Enteric-coated aspirin may be prescribed to minimize gastrointestinal symptoms. Bleeding events associated with P2Y12 inhibitors are similar to aspirin, although they typically exhibit better gastrointestinal tolerance. In addition to bleeding risk, GPIIb/IIIa inhibitors are also associated with allergic reactions that could range from urticaria to severe anaphylaxis.

Interactions

Clopidogrel is metabolized to its active component, in part by the CYP2C19 system, which may be affected by medications that induce or inhibit CYP2C19. Certain patients also show significant genetic variation in the activity of this enzyme. Data have shown that this genetic variation may play a role in the effectiveness of clopidogrel, particularly in those who have a slow metabolism. For further discussion of antiplatelet agents, refer to Chapter 50.

Anticoagulant and Fibrinolytic Therapy

Anticoagulant therapy is recommended for all patients undergoing PCI in the management of acute MI (Amsterdam et al., 2014; O'Gara et al., 2013). Anticoagulant agents slow down the clotting cascade, reduce fibrin clumping within the developing thrombus, and prevent further clot formation. Although effective as antithrombotic therapy, it is important to note that use of anticoagulants confers further bleeding risk in addition to the risk of bleeding from antiplatelet therapy. Anticoagulant therapies utilized in the management of acute MI include unfractionated heparin, low molecular weight heparin (enoxaparin), fondaparinux, bivalrudin, and argatroban.

Fibrinolytic therapy should only be utilized in the management of STEMI, as this class of medications has no role in the treatment of NSTEMI. These agents are only used in the patient who is unable to receive PCI as reperfusion therapy. Fibrinolytics are effective in reperfusion because they directly break apart the existing thrombus, allowing blood supply to return to myocardial tissue. Fibrinolytic agents include tenecteplase, reteplase, and alteplase.

Mechanism of Action

Anticoagulant agents exert their antithrombotic effect in a variety of mechanisms. Unfractionated heparin binds to and activates the antithrombin III enzyme. Antithrombin III is a naturally occurring anticoagulant that balances prothrombotic activity through two mechanisms: inhibiting the ability of factor Xa to convert prothrombin to thrombin (factor IIa) and inhibiting the ability of thrombin to convert fibrinogen to fibrin. In the presence of heparin, more antithrombin III is in the active state, thereby limiting further fibrin formation and thrombus development. Low molecular weight heparins, as the name suggests, are approximately one-third the molecular weight of heparin and have higher antifactor Xa activity compared to unfractionated heparin. Fondaparinux is a synthetic pentasaccharide that specifically promotes antithrombin III–mediated inhibition of factor Xa. Bivalrudin and argatroban directly bind and inhibit thrombin. While anticoagulant agents halt further thrombus development, fibrinolytic medications break apart existing clots by converting plasminogen to plasmin, a naturally occurring protein that degrades fibrin.

Contraindications

Anticoagulants should not be used in the patient with active uncontrolled major bleeding. Heparin treatment may cause an immune-mediated thrombocytopenia, and future use of heparin would be contraindicated if this condition were to occur. Certain anticoagulants, such as fondaparinux, should be used with caution or avoided depending on the degree of a patient's kidney dysfunction. Argatraban should be avoided in the patient with severe liver impairment.

Since fibrinolytic activation of plasmin leads to nonspecific fibrin degradation, use is contraindicated in the patient with active internal bleeding, history of stroke or recent (within 3 months) neurosurgery or head trauma, or severe uncontrolled hypertension as use in these settings could increase the risk of a life-threatening bleeding event.

Adverse Events

As an extension of their pharmacologic activity, anticoagulants and fibrinolytics increase the risk for bleeding events. During therapy, the practitioner should closely monitor for signs and symptoms of major bleeding, which include decreased hemoglobin levels, changes in hemodynamic stability, altered mental status, or the presence of blood in stool. To reduce the risk of major bleeding while ensuring adequate anticoagulation, some agents have specific laboratory monitoring recommendations to adjust dosing based on the patient's coagulant test results. Heparin dosing is titrated to maintain a goal-activated partial thromboplastin time, and the practitioner should refer to institution-specific protocols to guide dose adjustments.

Platelet counts should be monitored in the patient receiving heparin therapy to identify the occurrence of heparin-induced thrombocytopenia (Linkins et al., 2012). Also referred to as *heparin-induced thrombocytopenia* (HIT), this disorder is a serious immune-mediated adverse reaction that places the patient in a paradoxical hypercoagulable state, increasing the risk of thrombosis. Onset of HIT is typically five to ten days following initial heparin exposure and is managed with non-heparin anticoagulant therapy such as argatroban.

Other Agents

Ranolazine

Ranolazine (Ranexa) is a unique antianginal agent that can be used alone or in combination with nitrates, beta blockers, calcium channel blockers, or ACE inhibitors. Currently, its primary role is as an adjunctive agent for patients who are not achieving adequate symptom relief with other agents.

Mechanism of Action

The mechanism of action of ranolazine is not well understood, but it is thought to block late-phase sodium channels, which often remain open during hypoxic or ischemic events. An increase in intracellular sodium during late phase affects sodium-dependent calcium channels, thus increasing the amount of calcium entering the cell and causing a calcium overload. This overload can lead to further or continued contraction of the myocardium, increasing oxygen demand. By blocking late-phase sodium channels, ranolazine decreases calcium overload and breaks the cycle of ischemia.

Dosage

Ranolazine is taken orally at 500 mg twice daily and can be titrated up to a maximum of 1,000 mg twice daily. Ranexa tablets should be swallowed whole, not crushed or split. There may need to be a dose reduction in patients taking CYP3A4 inhibitors, such as diltiazem and verapamil.

Contraindications

Ranolazine is contraindicated in patients taking ketoconazole, itraconazole, clarithromycin, and other strong CYP3A4 inhibitors.

Adverse Events

Ranolazine prolongs the QTc interval in a dose-related manner; however, in long-term studies, there has been no association with an increased risk of proarrhythmia or sudden death. Regardless, caution should still be used because there is little experience with doses greater than 1,000 mg twice daily. Dose-related dizziness, headache, constipation, and nausea are common adverse effects. Other adverse events include palpitations, vertigo, dry mouth, peripheral edema, hypotension, and, less commonly, angioedema and renal failure.

Interactions

As noted earlier, patients taking potent CYP3A4 inhibitors should not take ranolazine, and less-potent inhibitors warrant monitoring. Conversely, agents that induce the CYP3A4 system, such as rifampin, carbamazepine, phenytoin, and St. John's wort, may decrease plasma concentrations of ranolazine. Ranolazine, through the P-glycoprotein system, may increase digoxin levels.

Selecting the Most Appropriate Antianginal Therapy

Choosing the appropriate medications for treating a patient with angina can be challenging. The primary goal is to design a regimen that will reduce the frequency and severity of anginal episodes. Subsequent adjustments are made empirically based on the patient's response to treatment, disease progression, risk factor modification, and patient satisfaction and adherence (**Figure 20.1**).

Acute Treatment of Anginal Episodes

All patients with angina should be provided a short-acting nitrate for acute treatment of anginal episodes. Additionally,

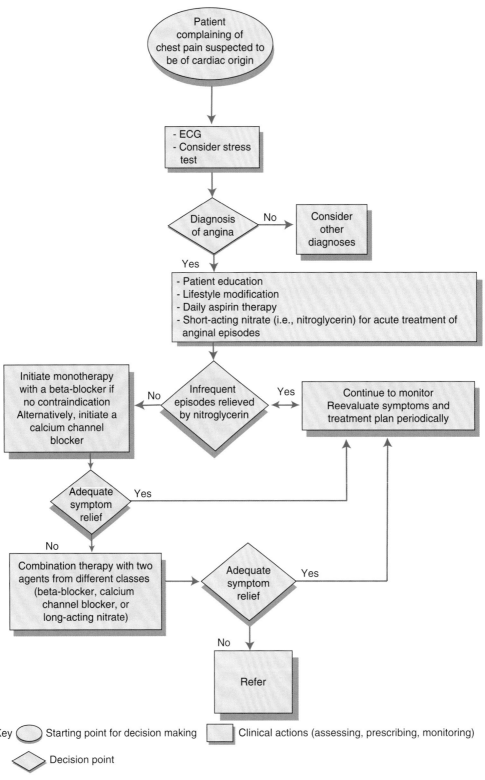

FIGURE 20–1 Treatment algorithm for angina.

ECG, electrocardiogram.

patients with infrequent episodes of angina can be managed effectively with short-acting nitrates alone. They are a good choice for the patient who has infrequent attacks or predictable pain on exertion.

Chronic Prevention of Anginal Episodes

Patients with repeated episodes of angina should receive long-acting therapy for chronic prophylaxis. All patients should be receiving aspirin. In addition, there are three classes of agents that may be used for chronic antianginal therapy: beta blockers, calcium channel blockers, and long-acting nitrates. The initial choice of an antianginal agent should be based on the patient's specific characteristics, such as physical exam findings and coexisting medical conditions. Treatment with a single agent is generally used for initial antianginal therapy, whereas combination therapy is instituted for patients who fail monotherapy.

First-Line Therapy

In the absence of contraindications, beta blockers are the agents of choice for prevention of acute anginal episodes in patients with or without a history of MI. Beta blockers reduce the frequency and likelihood of anginal episodes and reduce CHD-related morbidity and mortality. Additionally, beta blockers are useful as antihypertensive and antiarrhythmic agents. Beta blockers are particularly useful in patients whose anginal symptoms are related to physical exertion.

For patients whose anginal symptoms have been linked to coronary vasospasm, a calcium channel blocker may be considered for initial treatment. See **Table 20.2** for more information.

Second-Line Therapy

For patients who do not respond sufficiently to therapy with a single antianginal agent, combination therapy should be attempted. When initial treatment with a beta blocker is not successful, either a calcium channel blocker or a long-acting nitrate may be added to beta blocker therapy.

A long-acting nitrate/beta blocker regimen is safe, effective, and low in cost. Nitrates and beta blockers are well tolerated, and their effects are complementary. Reflex tachycardia caused by nitrates is blunted by a beta blocker. The control of reflex tachycardia is beneficial because a decrease in heart rate lowers myocardial oxygen demand. The combination of nitrates and beta blockers is an accepted treatment of angina, and they are often used together.

A beta blocker plus a calcium channel blocker is another typical combination. Patients who have anginal symptoms that cannot be controlled by either beta blocker or calcium channel blocker monotherapy often respond to a combination of the two. However, a beta blocker plus non-dihydropyridine calcium channel blocker combination should be used with caution. When drugs from these two classes are given together, the additive effect is potent suppression of AV conduction, which may be problematic in patients with preexisting cardiac conduction abnormalities. It is best to start with low doses of each drug and monitor each dosage increase so that side effects can be identified early.

Nitrates are often combined with a nondihydropyridine calcium channel blocker, such as diltiazem or verapamil, or a second-generation dihydropyridine calcium channel blocker, such as amlodipine. Since nitrates and first-generation dihydropyridine calcium channel blockers are potent vasodilators, they should be used together with extreme caution and only if no other treatment option is available.

Third-Line Therapy

In patients who are refractory to a two-drug regimen, a three-drug regimen of a calcium channel blocker, beta blocker, and a long-acting nitrate may be used. In general, patients whose

---

TABLE 20.2
Recommended Order of Treatment for Angina

Order	Agents	Comments
For all patients	Short-acting nitrate	For acute treatment of anginal episodes
	Aspirin (if not contraindicated)	May be used to prevent predictable episodes
		May be used alone in patients with infrequent episodes
Chronic Prevention of Anginal Episodes		
First line	Beta blocker	Reduces workload of heart by decreasing overall myocardial oxygen consumption
	Calcium channel blocker	Useful for patients who cannot tolerate a beta blocker
Second line	Combination therapy	If monotherapy fails, add another agent from a different class: beta blocker, calcium channel blocker, long-acting nitrate (e.g., beta blocker and long-acting nitrate)

TABLE 20.3

Recommended Treatment Options for Acute Myocardial Infarction

Phase of Care	Agents	Comments
Acute phase	Aspirin	Give as soon as possible
	Nitrates	Give sublingual nitroglycerin as initial treatment; may consider intravenous nitroglycerin if needed Reduces left ventricular preload and increases coronary blood flow
	Oxygen	May consider if oxygen saturation <90% or respiratory distress
	Morphine	May consider if ischemic pain persists despite nitroglycerin
Intervention phase	P2Y$_{12}$ inhibitor	Recommended for all patients
	GPIIa/IIIb inhibitor	Recommended in high-risk patients, such as those with positive cardiac troponin levels
	Anticoagulant agent	Recommended for all patients
	Fibrinolytic agent	Only considered in management of ST elevation myocardial infarction in patients unable to receive PCI
Maintenance phase	Dual antiplatelet therapy	P2Y$_{12}$ inhibitor with aspirin for up to 12 months if medically treated or for at least 12 months if treated with coronary stent; aspirin continued indefinitely
	Beta blocker	Initiate within 24 hours of care.
	Calcium channel blocker	Useful for patients who cannot tolerate a beta blocker
	ACE inhibitor	Recommended for patients with LVEF<40%, hypertension, diabetes mellitus, or stable CKD

ACE, angiotensin-converting enzyme; CKD, chronic kidney disease; LVEF, left ventricular ejection fraction; PCI, percutaneous coronary intervention; ST, step therapy.

anginal symptoms do not respond to two antianginal agents should be referred to a specialist's care.

Treatment Selection in Acute Coronary Syndromes

The American College of Cardiology and American Heart Association provide evidence-based recommendations for the management of NSTEMI and STEMI (Amsterdam et al., 2014; O'Gara et al., 2013). In the immediate treatment of acute MI, the goals of therapy are to provide symptom relief, prevent or limit the extent of myocardial injury, and improve patient outcomes. A summary of guideline recommendations can be found in **Table 20.3**.

Acute Treatment of Myocardial Infarction

In the absence of contraindications, patients presenting with acute MI should be given non-enteric-coated chewable aspirin (162–325 mg) as soon as possible after symptom onset as clinical trials have shown this treatment to reduce the risk of recurrent MI and death. Additional medications for acute symptom management include sublingual NTG (0.3–0.4 mg) administered every five minutes for up to three doses, oxygen for patients with respiratory distress, and morphine for patients with persistent ischemic pain. Caution is advised for routine use of oxygen and morphine therapies, as observational studies have associated these treatments with poor outcomes (McCarthy et al., 2017).

After initial stabilization, patients may either go to coronary angiography for PCI or be managed with medical therapy (Amsterdam et al., 2014; O'Gara et al., 2013). In either treatment strategy, a P2Y12 inhibitor is initiated in conjunction with daily aspirin. Certain high-risk patients, such as those with elevated cardiac troponins, may also receive additional antiplatelet therapy with a GPIIb/IIIa inhibitor until PCI. All patients should also receive anticoagulation. If a patient is diagnosed with STEMI and PCI is not available, fibrinolytic therapy may be initiated as reperfusion therapy.

Maintenance Therapy

Following acute MI, patients will be continued on lifelong aspirin therapy. Dual antiplatelet therapy with a P2Y12 inhibitor is continued for up to 12 months if the patient was managed with medical therapy alone or continued for at least 12 months if the patient received PCI. A beta blocker should be initiated within the first 24 hours of therapy. Additional maintenance treatments include ACE inhibitor or ARB therapy, aldosterone, and cholesterol management therapies.

MONITORING PATIENT RESPONSE

In patients with CHD, monitoring is important to evaluate for progression or stability of the disease, response to therapy, and presence or absence of adverse events.

Patient monitoring begins when a stress test is performed to confirm the diagnosis of angina. Once the diagnosis is made, stress tests may be repeated if there is a change in the pattern of anginal symptoms. Additionally, patients with stable angina should have an ECG if the history or physical examination changes or if the practitioner suspects new myocardial ischemia or development of a conduction abnormality (Fihn et al., 2012).

Routine follow-up for CHD depends on the frequency and severity of the patient's complaints. Stable patients should be seen every 2 to 6 months, but visits should be more frequent if the patient's symptoms change or become more severe or more frequent. Medication initiation and adjustment also require more office visits. At each office visit, vital signs should be taken and a complete physical examination performed. The patient should be questioned about anginal pain and associated symptoms and side effects of the drug regimen. Additional monitoring parameters should be determined by the specific drug regimen. Ideally, a patient's antianginal regimen should make him or her symptom-free.

PATIENT EDUCATION

For optimal control of anginal symptoms, the patient should be educated on his or her disease and medications. Patients should be informed of the seriousness of coronary artery disease and the potential consequences of leaving their angina untreated. Education about lifestyle modification strategies should be provided to all patients as often as possible. Additionally, patients need to know how to recognize worsening or escalating symptoms so they know when to seek emergency care.

Drug Information

There are many sources of information relating to the treatment of angina and acute MI. Several therapeutic guidelines are available to the practitioner, including those from the American College of Cardiology and American Heart Association, the American College of Chest Physicians, the European Society of Cardiology, and many other organizations. Specific questions relating to pharmacologic agents used in the treatment of angina may be addressed using the Physician's Desk Reference, Drug Facts and Comparisons,

Epocrates, or another drug reference. Finally, information regarding ongoing clinical trials for angina, MI, and other conditions may be obtained from a Web site provided by the National Institutes of Health (www.clinicaltrials.gov).

Patient-Oriented Information Sources

Practitioners may provide disease- and treatment-related information to patients from a variety of sources. The Web site for the American Heart Association (www.americanheart.org) has many resources available to explain cardiovascular disease and angina in a fashion that patients will understand. Also, the American Academy of Family Physicians (www.familydoctor.org) provides on its Web site a variety of resources under the heading "Patient Ed." Finally, the National Heart, Lung, and Blood Institute describes for patients angina, its causes, and appropriate treatments under "Diseases and Conditions Index" (http://www.nhlbi.nih.gov/health/dci/Diseases/Angina/Angina_WhatIs.html).

Complementary and Alternative Medications

Although there are a variety of complementary medications, such as Coenzyme Q10 and vitamin E, that allege to provide symptom relief for patients with angina, no herbal or supplement medication has been shown to have efficacy similar to that of the traditional agents described previously. Chelation therapy also has anecdotal reports of anginal symptom improvement, but there are no randomized controlled trials that support its use (Fihn et al., 2012). If at all possible, practitioners should counsel patients to adhere to treatment regimens that have shown efficacy in the treatment of angina.

Patients should be educated on each of the medications they are provided. They should know the importance of taking their medications as prescribed. They should be informed of each medication's indication and possible side effects, and what to do if they miss one or more doses of a scheduled medication, such as a long-acting nitrate. Additionally, practitioners should educate patients about the proper storage of all medications.

CASE STUDY 1

E.H. is a 45-year-old African-American man who has recently moved to the community from another state. He requests renewal of a prescription for a calcium channel blocker, prescribed by a physician in the former state. He is unemployed and lives with a woman, their son, and the woman's two children. His past medical history is remarkable for asthma and six "heart attacks," which he claims occurred because of a 25-year history of drug use

(primarily cocaine). He states that he has used drugs as recently as 2 weeks ago. He does not have any prior medical records with him. He claims that he has been having occasional periods of chest pain. He is unable to report the duration or pattern of the pain.

Before proceeding, explore the following questions: What further information would you need to diagnose angina (substantiate your answer)? What is the connection between cocaine use and angina? Identify at least three tests that you would order to diagnose angina.

DIAGNOSIS: ANGINA

1. List specific goals of treatment for E.H.
2. What dietary and lifestyle changes should be recommended for this patient?
3. What drug therapy would you prescribe for E.H. and why?
4. How would you monitor for success in E.H.?
5. Describe one or two drug–drug or drug–food interactions for the selected agent.
6. List one or two adverse reactions for the selected agent that would cause you to change therapy.
7. What would be the choice for the second-line therapy?
8. Discuss specific patient education based on the prescribed first-line therapy.
9. What over-the-counter and/or alternative medications would be appropriate for E.H.?

Bibliography

Starred references are cited in the text.

Alaeddini, J. (2015). Angina pectoris. Retrieved from http://emedicine.medscape.com/article/150215-overview on August 20, 2015.

*Antman, E., & Sabatine, M. (2013). *Cardiovascular therapeutics: A companion to Braunwald's heart disease.* New York, NY: Elsevier Health Sciences.

*Amsterdam, E. A., Wenger, N. K., Brindis, R. G., et al. (2014). 2014 AHA/ACC guideline for the management of patients with non-ST-elevation acute coronary syndromes: A report of the American College of Cardiology/American Heart Association Task Force on Practice Guidelines. *Journal of the American College of Cardiology, 64*(24), e139–e228. doi: 10.1016/j.jacc.2014.09.017.

*Benjamin, E. K., Muntner, P., Alonso, A., et al. (2019). Heart disease and stroke statistics-2019 update: A report from the American Heart Association. *Circulation, 139*, e56–e528.

*Fihn, S. D., Gardin, J. M., Abrams, J., et al. (2012). 2012 ACCF, AHA, ACP, AATS, PCNA, SCAI, STS guideline for the diagnosis and management of stable ischemic heart disease. *Journal of the American College of Cardiology, 60*, e44–e164.

Franchi, F., Rollini, F., & Angiolillo, D. J. (2017). Antithrombotic therapy for patients with STEMI undergoing primary PCI. *Nature Reviews Cardiology, 14*(6), 361–379. doi: 10.1038/nrcardio.2017.18

*Grundy, S. M., Stone, N. J., Bailey, A. L., et al. (2019). 2018 AHA/ACC/AACVPR/AAPA/ABC/ACPM/ADA/AGS/APhA/ASPC/NLA/PCNA guideline on the management of blood cholesterol: A report of the American College of Cardiology/American Heart Association Task Force on Clinical Practice Guidelines. *Journal of the American College of Cardiology, 73*(24), e285–e350. doi: 10.1016/j.jacc.2018.11.003

Hirsh, J. (2008). Antithrombotic therapy. Retrieved from https://www.hematology.org/About/History/50-Years/1523.aspx on February 11, 2020.

Jneid, H., Anderson, J. L., Wright, R., et al. (2012). 2012 ACCF/AHA focused update of the guideline for the management of patients with unstable angina/NSTEMI (updating the 2007 guideline and replacing the 2011 focused update): A report of the American College of Cardiology Foundation/American Heart Association Task Force on practice guidelines. *Journal of the American College of Cardiology, 60*(7), 645–681. doi: 10.1016/j.jacc.2012.06.004

Katzung, B., & Chatterjee, M. (1998). Vasodilators and the treatment of angina pectoris. In B. Katzung (Ed.), *Basic and clinical pharmacology* (7th ed.). Stamford, CT: Appleton & Lange.

Khamis, R. Y., Ammari, T., & Mikhail, G. W. (2016). Gender differences in coronary heart disease. *Heart, 102*, 1142–1149.

Kones, R. (2010). Recent advances in the management of chronic stable angina I: Approach to the patient, diagnosis, pathophysiology, risk stratification, and gender disparities. *Vascular Health and Risk Management, 6*, 635–656.

Lanza, G. A., Careri, G., & Crea, F. (2012). Contemporary reviews in cardiovascular medicine: Mechanisms of coronary artery spasm. *Circulation, 124*, 1774–1782. doi: 10.1161/Circulationsaha.222.037283

*Levine, G. N., Bates, E. R., Bittl, J. A., et al. (2016). 2016 ACC/AHA guideline focused update on duration of dual antiplatelet therapy in patients with coronary artery disease: A report of the American College of Cardiology/American Heart Association Task Force on Clinical Practice Guidelines. *Journal of the American College of Cardiology, 68*(10), 1082–1115. doi: 10.1016/j.jacc.2016.03.513

Libby, P., Ridken, P., & Hansson, G. (2011). Progress and challenges in translating the biology of atherosclerosis. *Nature, 473*, 317–325. doi: 10.1038/nature10146

*Linkins, L. A., Dans, A. L., Moores, L. K., et al. (2012). Treatment and prevention of heparin-induced thrombocytopenia: Antithrombotic Therapy and Prevention of Thrombosis, 9th ed: American College of Chest Physicians Evidence-Based Clinical Practice Guidelines. *Chest, 141*(2 Suppl), e495S–e530s. doi: 10.1378/chest.11-2303

Maron, D. J., Grundy, S. M., Ridler, P. M., et al. (2004). Dyslipidemia, other risk factors, and the prevention of coronary heart disease. In V. Fuster, R. W. Alexander, & R. A. O'Rourke (Eds.), *Hurst's the heart* (11th ed., pp. 1093–1122). New York, NY: McGraw-Hill.

*McCarthy, C. P., Donnellan, E., Wasfy, J. H., Bhatt, D. L., & McEvoy, J. W. (2017). Time-honored treatments for the initial management of acute coronary syndromes: Challenging the status quo. *Trends in Cardiovascular Medicine, 27*(7), 483–491. doi: 10.1016/j.tcm.2017.05.001

*O'Gara, P. T., Kushner, F. G., Ascheim, D. D., et al. (2013). 2013 ACCF/AHA guideline for the management of ST-elevation myocardial infarction: A report of the American College of Cardiology Foundation/American Heart Association Task Force on Practice Guidelines. *Journal of the American College of Cardiology, 61*(4), e78–e140. doi: 10.1016/j.jacc.2012.11.019

O'Rourke, R. A., O'Gara, P., & Douglas, J. S. (2004). Diagnosis and management of patients with chronic ischemic heart disease. In V. Fuster, R. W. Alexander, & R. A. O'Rourke (Eds.), *Hurst's the heart* (11th ed., pp. 1465–1494). New York, NY: McGraw-Hill.

Palaniswamy, C., & Aronow, W. (2011). Treatment of stable angina pectoris. *American Journal of Therapeutics, 18*(5), e138–e152. doi: 10.1097/MJT.0b013e3181f2ab9d

Patrano, C., Coller, B., FitzGerald, G. A., et al. (2004). Platelet-active drugs: The relationships among dose, effectiveness, and side effects: The seventh ACCP conference on antithrombotic and thrombolytic therapy. *Chest, 126*(3, Suppl.), 234S–264S.

Ross, R. (1998). Factors influencing atherogenesis. In R. W. Alexander, R. Schant, & V. Fuster (Eds.), *Hurst's the heart* (9th ed., pp. 1139–1160). New York, NY: McGraw-Hill.

Sitia, S., Tomasoni, L., Atzeni, F., et al. (2010). From endothelial dysfunction to atherosclerosis. *Autoimmunity Reviews, 9*(12), 830–834. doi: 10.1016/j.autrev.2010.07.016

Tarkin, J., & Kaski, J. (2013). Pharmacological treatment of chronic stable angina pectoris. *Clinical Medicine, 13*(1), 63–70.

Undas, A., & Zabczyk, M. (2018). Antithrombotic medications and their impact on fibrin clot structure and function. *Journal of Physiology and Pharmacology, 69*(4). doi: 10.26402/jpp.2018.4.02

Walker, B. F. (2004). Nonatherosclerotic coronary heart disease. In V. Fuster, R. W. Alexander, & R. A. O'Rourke (Eds.), *Hurst's the heart* (11th ed., pp. 1173–1214). New York, NY: McGraw-Hill.

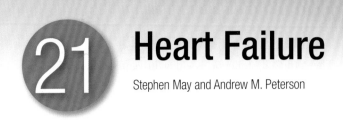

21 Heart Failure

Stephen May and Andrew M. Peterson

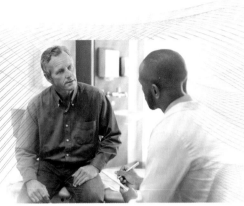
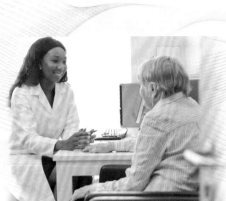
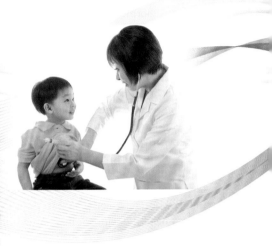

Learning Objectives

1. Describe the goals of therapy for heart failure (HF).
2. Recognize medications that are used to treat HF and discuss the mechanism of action, therapeutic effects, monitoring, contraindications, and adverse effects.
3. Identify appropriate therapies for patients with HF.

INTRODUCTION

Heart failure (HF), one of the most serious consequences of cardiovascular disease, has rapidly become one of the most important health problems in cardiovascular medicine. More than 6 million Americans have HF today, with an incidence approaching 21 per 1,000 among persons older than age 65 (Benjamin et al., 2019). At age 45 years through age 95 years, the estimated lifetime risk of developing HF is notably high, between 20% and 45%. The incidence of HF increases with age (Benjamin et al., 2019). HF is more common in men than in women, due to the higher incidence of ischemic heart disease in men. As the population is aging, the number of people with HF will significantly increase in the future. In people diagnosed with HF, the mortality rates remain approximately 50% within 5 years of diagnosis (Benjamin et al., 2019). Health care disparities place African-Americans at highest risk for HF (Bahrami et al., 2008).

In the United States, HF incidence has largely remained stable over the past several decades, with more than 650,000 new HF cases diagnosed annually. HF incidence increases with age, rising from approximately 20 per 1,000 individuals 65 to 69 years of age to greater than 80 per 1,000 individuals aged 85 or older. Approximately 5.1 million persons in the United States have clinically manifest HF, and the prevalence continues to rise, and 7% of all cardiac deaths are due to HF.

The economic impact of HF is also significant. The large number and often high complexity of hospitalizations for HF make this diagnosis very costly. The total cost of HF hospitalizations in the United States has been estimated at $8 billion (Go et al., 2013). After hypertension, HF is the second most common indication for physician office visits. The estimated direct and indirect cost of HF in the United States for 2012 was $30.7 billion (Benjamin et al., 2019). Consequently, improved quality of life is considered a worthy health care goal, and the therapeutic approach to HF is directed toward increasing the patient's ability to maintain a positive quality of life with symptom-free activity and to enhance survival. Vasodilator therapy, especially with the angiotensin-converting enzyme (ACE) inhibitors, has made significant contributions toward achieving this goal.

CAUSES OF HEART FAILURE

The development of HF may be related to many etiologic variables. Coronary artery disease, hypertension, and idiopathic cardiomyopathy are the most frequently cited risk factors for HF. Acute conditions that may result in HF include acute myocardial infarction (MI), arrhythmias, pulmonary embolism, sepsis, and acute myocardial ischemia. Gradual development of HF may be caused by liver or renal disease, primary cardiomyopathy, cardiac valve disease, anemia, bacterial endocarditis, viral myocarditis, thyrotoxicosis, chemotherapy, excessive dietary sodium intake, and ethanol abuse.

Drugs can also worsen HF. Drugs that may cause fluid retention, such as nonsteroidal antiinflammatory drugs (NSAIDs), steroids, hormones, antihypertensives (e.g., hydralazine [HYD] [Apresoline], nifedipine [Procardia XL]), sodium-containing drugs (e.g., carbenicillin disodium [Geopen]), and lithium (Eskalith, others), may cause congestion. Beta blockers, antiarrhythmics (e.g., disopyramide [Norpace], flecainide [Tambocor], amiodarone [Cordarone], sotalol [Betapace]), tricyclic antidepressants, and certain calcium channel blockers (e.g., diltiazem [Cardizem], nifedipine, verapamil [Calan]) have negative inotropic effects and further decrease contractility in an already depressed heart. Direct cardiac toxins (e.g., amphetamines, cocaine, daunorubicin [DaunoXome], doxorubicin [Adriamycin], and ethanol) can also worsen or induce HF. The American Heart Association (AHA) also provides a helpful document describing drugs that may cause or exacerbate HF (Pagell et al., 2016).

PATHOPHYSIOLOGY

HF is a pathophysiologic state in which abnormal myocardial function inhibits the ventricles from delivering adequate quantities of blood to metabolizing tissues at rest or during activity. It results not only from a decrease in intrinsic systolic contractility of the myocardium but also from alterations in the pulmonary and peripheral circulations (Braunwald, 2015).

The cardiac dysfunction is either in ventricular contraction/ejection (systolic) or ventricular filling/relaxation (diastolic).

HF resulting from systolic dysfunction may be referred to as *systolic HF* or *HF with reduced ejection fraction* (HFrEF). HF resulting from diastolic dysfunction may be referred to as *diastolic HF* or *HF with preserved ejection fraction* (HFpEF).

When the heart fails as a pump and cardiac output (the volume of blood pumped out of the ventricle per unit of time) decreases, a complex scheme of compensatory mechanisms to raise and maintain cardiac output occurs. These compensatory mechanisms include increased preload (volume and pressure or myocardial fiber length of the ventricle prior to contraction [end of diastole]), increased afterload (vascular resistance), ventricular hypertrophy (increased muscle mass), and dilatation, activation of the sympathetic nervous system (SNS), and activation of the renin–angiotensin–aldosterone system (RAAS).

Although initially beneficial for increasing cardiac output, these compensatory mechanisms are ultimately associated with further pump dysfunction. In effect, the consequence of activating the compensatory systems is worsening HF. This is often referred to as the *vicious cycle of HF* (**Figure 21.1**). Without therapeutic intervention, some of the compensatory mechanisms continue to be activated, ultimately resulting in a reduced cardiac output and a worsening of the patient's symptoms. An understanding of the compensatory mechanisms makes it clear why one goal in treating HF is to interrupt this vicious cycle and why various drugs are used in managing patients with HF.

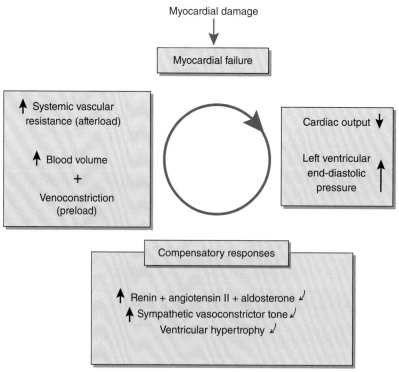

FIGURE 21–1 Vicious circle of heart failure.

DIAGNOSTIC CRITERIA

The signs and symptoms of HF are useful in diagnosing and assessing a patient's clinical response to therapy. The clinical manifestations of HF are in part due to pulmonary or systemic venous congestion and edema. When the left ventricle malfunctions, congestion initially occurs proximally in the lungs. When the right ventricle functions inadequately, congestion in the supplying systemic venous circulation results in peripheral edema, liver congestion, and other indicators of right HF (**Box 21.1**). Both pulmonary and systemic congestion eventually develop in most patients with left HF. In fact, the chief cause of right HF is left HF.

Depressed ventricular function may be confirmed by echocardiography, radionuclide ventriculography, magnetic resonance imaging, or cardiac catheterization. Abnormalities in the electrocardiogram (ECG) are common and include arrhythmias, conduction delays, left ventricular (LV) hypertrophy, and nonspecific ST segment and T-wave changes, which typically reflect the underlying etiology. Laboratory findings from liver function or other tests disclose such abnormalities as elevated blood urea nitrogen (BUN) and creatinine levels, hyponatremia, and elevated serum enzymes of hepatic origin. The circumstances in which the symptoms of HF occur are also particularly important in determining the severity of disease in a particular patient.

The New York Heart Association (NYHA) classifies the functional incapacity of patients with cardiac disease into four levels, depending on the degree of effort needed to elicit symptoms (**Table 21.1**):

- *Class I:* Patients may have symptoms of HF only at levels that would produce symptoms in normal people.
- *Class II:* Patients may have symptoms of HF on ordinary exertion.
- *Class III:* Patients may have symptoms of HF on less-than-ordinary exertion.
- *Class IV:* Patients may have symptoms of HF at rest.

BOX 21.1 Clinical Manifestations of Heart Failure

Left Ventricular Failure—Pulmonary Congestion
Symptoms: Cough, dyspnea, dyspnea on exertion, orthopnea, paroxysmal nocturnal dyspnea, nocturia
Signs: Cardiomegaly, S_3 heart sound, bibasilar rales, signs of pulmonary edema, tachycardia, increased respiratory rate

Right Ventricular Failure—Systemic Congestion
Symptoms: Peripheral pitting edema, abdominal pain, anorexia, bloating, constipation, nausea, vomiting
Signs: Hepatomegaly, distention of the jugular veins, hepatojugular reflex, signs of portal hypertension, ascites, splenomegaly

Decreased Cardiac Output
Peripheral cyanosis, fatigue, decreased tissue perfusion, decrease in metabolism and renal elimination of drugs, decreased appetite, angina, increased risk for thromboembolism

---

The American College of Cardiology (ACC)/AHA has developed a classification system that categorizes the progression of HF and is intended to complement the NYHA classification (**Table 21.1**):

- *Stage A:* Patients who are at high risk for developing HF but have no structural heart disease
- *Stage B:* Patients with structural heart disease who have never had symptoms of HF
- *Stage C:* Patients with past or current symptoms of HF associated with underlying structural heart disease

---

TABLE 21.1

New York Heart Association Functional Classification/American College of Cardiology Foundation/American Heart Association Stages of Heart Failure

Class	Definition	Stage	Definition
None		A	At high risk for HF without structural heart disease or symptoms of HF
I	No limitation of physical activity. Ordinary physical activity does not cause undue fatigue or dyspnea.	B	Structural heart disease but without signs or symptoms of HF
II	Slight limitation of physical activity. Comfortable at rest, but ordinary physical activity results in fatigue or dyspnea.	C	Structural heart disease with prior or current symptoms of HF
III	Marked limitation of physical activity. Comfortable at rest, but less-than-ordinary activity causes fatigue or dyspnea.		
IV	Unable to carry on any physical activity without symptoms. Symptoms are present even at rest. If any physical activity is undertaken, symptoms are increased.	D	Refractory HF requiring specialized interventions

HF, heart failure.

- *Stage D:* Patients with end-stage disease who require specialized treatment strategies, such as mechanical circulatory support, continuous intravenous (IV) inotrope infusions, cardiac transplantation, or hospice care.

INITIATING DRUG THERAPY

In the past, digitalis, glycosides, and diuretics were the mainstays of therapy for HF. However, the concept of HF has changed dramatically from a narrow focus on the weakened heart to a broadened view of the systemic pathophysiologic state, with peripheral and myocardial factors playing important roles. Individualization of pharmacologic therapy is a cornerstone of care and now based on the stage of HF. The goals of therapy are to improve the quality of life, decrease mortality, and reduce the compensatory mechanisms causing the symptoms. Three general approaches are used:

1. An underlying cause of HF is treated if possible (e.g., surgical correction of structural abnormalities/valvular heart disease or medical treatment of conditions such as hypertension, diabetes mellitus, or dyslipidemia).
2. Precipitating factors that produce or worsen HF are identified and minimized (e.g., fever, anemia, arrhythmias, medication noncompliance, or drugs).
3. After these two steps, drug therapy to control the HF and improve survival becomes important.

Nonpharmacologic management techniques should be used along with pharmacologic therapy in patients with HF. In the past, reduced activities and bed rest were considered a standard part of the care of patients with HF. However, it has been determined that short periods of bed rest result in reduced exercise tolerance and aerobic capacity. There is insufficient evidence to recommend a specific type of training program or the routine use of supervised rehabilitation programs. Although most patients should not participate in heavy labor or exhausting sports, aerobic activity should be encouraged (except during periods of acute decompensation). For example, according to the Agency for Healthcare Research and Quality (AHRQ), regular exercise (e.g., walking or cycling) is recommended for patients with stable class I to III disease. The introduction of a new agent, an angiotensin receptor-neprilysin inhibitor (ARNI), and its role in therapy is also discussed later.

Goals of Drug Therapy

Pharmacologic management of patients with HF is critical in reducing symptoms and decreasing mortality. In most cases, drug therapy is long term and consists of ACE inhibitors (ACE-I) and beta blockers for class I indications. Diuretics, aldosterone antagonists, HYD, nitrates, digoxin (Lanoxin), and others medications are also used. **Table 21.2** provides an overview of drugs used to treat HF.

In patients with a history of HF with reduced ejection fraction (EF), ACE-I, angiotensin receptor blockers (ARBs),

or ARNI should be used to reduce morbidity and mortality. In patients with an MI and reduced EF, beta blockers should be used to prevent HF, and a statin should also be given.

Angiotensin-Converting Enzyme Inhibitors

Patients who have HF resulting from LV systolic dysfunction and who have an LV EF less than 35% to 40% should be given a trial of ACE-I, unless they cannot tolerate treatment with these drugs. The ACE-I may be considered therapy in the subset of patients who present with fatigue or mild dyspnea on exertion and who do not have any other signs or symptoms of volume overload. In patients with evidence for, or a prior history of, fluid retention, ACE-I are usually used together with diuretics (see section titled Selecting the Most Appropriate Agent). ACE-I are also recommended for use in patients with LV systolic dysfunction who have no symptoms of HF. The clinical and mortality benefits of the ACE-I have been shown in numerous uncontrolled and controlled, randomized clinical trials.

ACE-I have a positive effect on cardiac function (i.e., reduced preload and afterload, increased cardiac index, and EF) and the signs and symptoms of HF (e.g., dyspnea, fatigue, orthopnea, and peripheral edema). As a result, exercise capacity is increased, NYHA functional classification is significantly improved, and morbidity and mortality rates in patients with HF, including those who have suffered an MI, are reduced because these drugs can attenuate ventricular dilation and remodeling.

Captopril (Capoten), enalapril (Vasotec), fosinopril (Monopril), lisinopril (Zestril), quinapril (Accupril), trandolapril (Mavik), ramipril (Altace), and perindopril (Aceon) are the ACE-I currently indicated for treating HF (see **Table 21.2**). The ACE-I that are approved for use in patients with LV dysfunction, and have been shown to prolong survival, are enalapril, captopril, and lisinopril. Quinapril and fosinopril are labeled for symptom reduction in HF, but data are lacking as to their effect on mortality rates.

American College of Cardiology Foundation (ACCF)/AHA HF guidelines recommend that in all patients with a recent or remote history of MI or acute coronary syndrome (ACS) and reduced EF, ACE-I should be used to prevent symptomatic HF and reduce mortality. The guidelines also comment that, in patients intolerant of ACE-I, ARBs are appropriate unless contraindicated. They also recommend that ACE-I should be used in all patients with a reduced EF to prevent symptomatic HF, even if they do not have a history of MI. In regard to patients with HF stage C, the guidelines recommend ACE-I for patients with HFrEF and current or prior symptoms, unless contraindicated, to reduce morbidity and mortality (Yancy et al., 2013). The role of ARNI in this patient population is discussed in a corresponding section later.

Mechanism of Action

"Balanced" vasodilators, including the ACE-I and angiotensin II receptor blockers, cause vasodilation on both the venous and arterial sides of the heart and therefore provide

TABLE 21.2

Overview of Selected Agents Used to Treat Heart Failure

Generic (Trade) Name and Dosage	Selected Adverse Events	Contraindications	Special Considerations
Selected Angiotensin-Converting Enzyme Inhibitors			
Captopril (Capoten) Start: 6.25 mg or 12.5 mg TID Therapeutic range: 25–100 mg TID	Common: cough; hypotension, particularly with a diuretic or volume depletion; hyperkalemia, loss of taste, leukopenia; angioedema, neutropenia, and agranulocytosis in <1% of patients; rash in >10% of patients	Contraindicated in pregnancy Avoid in patients with bilateral renal artery stenosis or unilateral stenosis.	Renal impairment related to ACE-I is seen as an increase in serum creatinine and azotemia, usually in the beginning of therapy. Monitor BUN, creatinine, and K levels when starting.
Enalapril (Vasotec) Start: 2.5 mg daily or BID Range: 5–20 mg daily or BID	Same as captopril	Same as captopril	Same as captopril Use only 2.5 mg/d in patient with impaired renal function or hyponatremia.
Fosinopril (Monopril) Start: 10 mg daily Range: 10–40 mg daily	Same as captopril	Same as captopril	Same as captopril Use only 5 mg/d in patient with impaired renal function or hyponatremia.
Lisinopril (Zestril, Prinivil) Start: 5 mg daily Range: 5–20 mg daily	Same as captopril	Same as captopril	Same as captopril Use only 2.5 mg/d in patient with impaired renal function or hyponatremia.
Quinapril (Accupril) Start: 5 mg BID Range: 20–40 BID	Same as captopril	Same as captopril	Same as captopril Use only 2.5 mg/d in patient with impaired renal function or hyponatremia.
Ramipril (Altace) Start: 1.25 mg BID Range: 1.25–5 mg BID	Same as captopril	Same as captopril	Same as captopril
Trandolapril (Mavik) Start: 0.5–1 mg daily Target dose: 4 mg	Same as captopril	Same as captopril	Same as captopril
Selected Thiazide and Thiazide-Like Diuretics			
Chlorthalidone (Hygroton) 12.5–50 mg daily	Hyperuricemia, hypokalemia, hypomagnesemia, hyperglycemia, hyponatremia, hypercalcemia, hypercholesterolemia, hypertriglyceridemia, pancreatitis, rashes and other allergic reactions	High doses are relatively contraindicated in patients with hyperlipidemia, gout, and diabetes.	Thiazide diuretics preferred in patients with CrCl >30 mL/min
Hydrochlorothiazide (HydroDIURIL, Microzide) 12.5–50 mg daily	Same as chlorthalidone	Same as chlorthalidone	Same as chlorthalidone
Metolazone (Zaroxolyn) 2.5–10 mg daily	Less or no hypercholesterolemia	Same as chlorthalidone	Same as chlorthalidone

(Continued)

TABLE 21.2

Overview of Selected Agents Used to Treat Heart Failure (*Continued*)

Generic (Trade) Name and Dosage	Selected Adverse Events	Contraindications	Special Considerations
Loop Diuretics			
Bumetanide (Bumex) 0.5–5 mg daily–BID	Dehydration, circulatory collapse, hypokalemia, hyponatremia, hypomagnesemia, hyperglycemia, metabolic alkalosis, hyperuricemia (short duration of action, no hypercalcemia)	High doses are relatively contraindicated in patients with hyperlipidemia, gout, and diabetes.	Effective in patients with CrCl <30 mL/min Monitor BUN, creatinine, and K levels when starting and with dosage changes.
Ethacrynic acid (Edecrin) 25–100 mg BID–TID	Same as bumetanide (only nonsulfonamide diuretic, ototoxicity)	Same as bumetanide	Same as bumetanide
Furosemide (Lasix) 20–320 mg BID–TID	Same as bumetanide	Same as bumetanide	Same as bumetanide
Torsemide (Demadex) 5–20 mg daily–BID	Short duration of action, no hypercalcemia	Same as bumetanide	Same as bumetanide
Potassium-sparing Diuretics			
Amiloride (Midamor) 5–20 mg daily–BID	Hyperkalemia, GI disturbances, rash	High doses are relatively contraindicated in patients with hyperlipidemia, gout, and diabetes.	Same as bumetanide
Spironolactone (Aldactone) 12.5–100 mg daily–BID	Hyperkalemia, GI disturbances, rash, gynecomastia	Same as amiloride	Spironolactone ideal in patients with heart failure
Triamterene (Dyrenium) 50–150 mg daily–BID	Hyperkalemia, GI disturbances, nephrolithiasis	Same as amiloride	Same as bumetanide
Selected Angiotensin Receptor Blockers			
Losartan (Cozaar) Start: 12.5 mg/d Range: 50–100 mg/d	Dyspnea, hypotension, hyperkalemia	Angioedema secondary to ACE inhibition	May be used in patients experiencing cough due to ACE-I
Valsartan (Diovan) Start: 80 mg/d Range: 80–160 mg BID	Same as losartan	Same as losartan	Same as losartan
Angiotensin Receptor-Neprylisin Inhibitor			
Sacubatril/valsartan (Entresto) Start: 24 mg/26 mg or 49 mg/51 mg BID Target: 97 mg/103 mg BID	Hypotension, hyperkalemia, cough, serum creatinine increase, and angioedema	History of angioedema related to previous ACE-I or ARB therapy, concomitant use or use within 36 hours of ACE-Is, concomitant use of aliskiren in patients with diabetes, pregnancy	36-hour washout period of ACE-I is required prior to initiation of ARNI
Beta Blockers			
Bisoprolol (Zebeta) Start: 5 mg daily Range: 5–20 mg daily	Bradycardia, congestive heart failure, atrioventricular block, postural hypotension, vertigo, fatigue, depression, bronchospasm, impotence, insomnia, decreased exercise tolerance, impaired peripheral circulation, generalized edema, sinusitis	Sinus bradycardia, second- or third-degree heart block, asthma, liver abnormalities	Advise patient to avoid abrupt cessation of therapy. Observe for signs of dizziness for 1 h when dose is increased.

TABLE 21.2

Overview of Selected Agents Used to Treat Heart Failure (*Continued*)

Generic (Trade) Name and Dosage	Selected Adverse Events	Contraindications	Special Considerations
Carvedilol (Coreg) 3.125–50 mg BID	Same as bisoprolol	Same as bisoprolol	Same as bisoprolol
Metoprolol Start: 6.25 mg BID–TID Range: 50–100 mg BID–TID	Same as bisoprolol	Same as bisoprolol	Same as bisoprolol
Hydralazine/Isosorbide Dinitrate			
Hydralazine (Apresoline) 25–75 mg TID	Postural hypotension, tachycardia	Coronary artery disease, aortic stenosis	Advise patient to avoid rapid changes in position. Patient can be started on 10 mg TID if older, with severe heart failure, or hypotensive.
ISDN (Isordil) 10–40 mg TID	Headache, dizziness, tachycardia, retrosternal discomfort, blurred vision, rash, flushing	Hypersensitivity to nitrates, closed-angle glaucoma, early MI, head trauma, pregnancy (category C)	Advise patient to avoid rapid changes in position.
Hydralazine/ISDN Initial: 1 tab TID Goal: 2 tab TID	Same as individual agents	Same as individual agents	Each tablet contains 37.5 mg of hydralazine and 20 mg of ISDN
Other Agents			
Digitalis/digoxin (Lanoxin) 0.25 mg daily	Ventricular tachycardia, paroxysmal atrial tachycardia, fatigue, anorexia, nausea	Allergy, ventricular tachycardia, ventricular fibrillation, heart block, sick sinus syndrome, idiopathic hypertrophic subaortic stenosis, acute MI, renal insufficiency, electrolyte abnormalities Use with caution in pregnancy and lactation.	Check potassium levels before starting. Check serum levels once a year.
Dobutamine (Dobutrex) 2–5 mcg/kg/min intravenously	Elevated blood pressure, increased heart rate, angina, hypotension	Idiopathic hypertrophic subaortic stenosis	May increase insulin requirements
Ivabradine (Corlanor) 2.5–7.5 mg BID	Bradycardia, HTN, atrial fibrillation, visual disturbances	Severe hepatic impairment, sick sinus syndrome, SA block without pacemaker, resting HR <60, atrial fibrillation, BP <90/50	Avoid grapefruit.

ACE, angiotensin-converting enzyme; ACE-I, ACE inhibitors; ARB, angiotensin receptor blocker; ARNI, angiotensin receptor-neprilysin inhibitor; BP, blood pressure; BUN, blood urea nitrogen; GI, gastrointestinal; HR, heart rate; HTN, hypertension; ISDN, isosorbide dinitrate; MI, myocardial infarction; SA, sinoatrial.

the hemodynamic and clinical benefits of both preload and afterload reduction.

Activation of the RAAS is an important compensatory mechanism in HF (**Figure 21.2**). ACE catalyzes the conversion of angiotensin I to angiotensin II, a potent vasoconstrictor and stimulant of aldosterone secretion. ACE-I are uniquely effective in managing HF by interrupting stimulation of the RAAS, inhibiting the contributions of this system

to the downward spiral of HF. The pharmacodynamic properties of ACE-I involve specific competitive binding to the active site of ACE.

Angiotensin II interacts with at least two known membrane receptors, type 1 and type 2 (AT_1 and AT_2). By blocking formation of angiotensin II, ACE-I indirectly produce vasodilation and a decrease in systemic vascular resistance (LV afterload). In addition, because angiotensin II stimulates

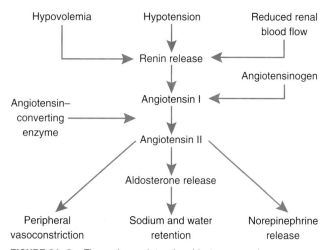

FIGURE 21–2   The renin–angiotensin–aldosterone syndrome.

aldosterone secretion by the adrenal cortex and provides negative feedback for plasma renin, inhibition of angiotensin II may lead to decreased aldosterone and increased renin activity. This prevents aldosterone-mediated sodium and water retention and may produce a small increase in serum potassium levels. The reduction in volume expansion due to ACE inhibition decreases ventricular end-diastolic volume (i.e., preload). Because ACE (kininase II) is involved in the breakdown of bradykinin, a vasodilator, a decrease in kininase II activity by an ACE-I could increase bradykinin and prostaglandin production, either of which can lead to vasodilation.

ACE-I produce vasodilation, inhibit fluid accumulation, and increase blood flow to vital organs, such as the brain, kidney, and heart, without precipitating reflex tachycardia. The hemodynamic effects of ACE-I in HF include decreased preload, afterload, and mean arterial pressure, as well as increased cardiac output. EF is also improved. Clinical benefits to patients with HF include improvement in exercise duration, NYHA functional class, dyspnea/fatigue focal index, and signs and symptoms of HF, as well as increased survival.

Dosage

ACE-I should be initiated at low doses followed by gradual dosage increases if the lower doses have been well tolerated. Renal function and serum potassium should be assessed within 1 to 2 weeks of starting therapy and periodically thereafter, especially in patients with preexisting hypotension, hyponatremia, diabetes, or azotemia, or if they are receiving potassium supplementation. Doses should be titrated as tolerated by the patient to the target doses shown in clinical trials to decrease morbidity and mortality (e.g., 150 mg/d in divided doses of captopril; 20 mg/d of enalapril or lisinopril). The doses of ACE-I can be increased to these effective doses unless the patient cannot tolerate high doses.

The practitioner should provide the following information to patients taking ACE-I:

- Adverse effects may occur early in therapy but do not usually prevent long-term use of the drug.
- Symptomatic improvement may not be seen for several weeks or months.
- ACE-I may reduce the risk of disease progression even if the patient's symptoms have not responded favorably to treatment (Savarese et al., 2013).

Captopril, lisinopril, ramipril, and trandolapril have been shown to reduce mortality rates in patients who have had an MI and who have HF symptoms. The indications for these ACE-I in this population vary slightly, and the dosing for patients after MI differs from the dosing for patients with chronic HF. Captopril is indicated to improve survival after MI in clinically stable patients with LV dysfunction manifested as an EF of 40% or less and to reduce the incidence of overt HF and subsequent hospitalizations for HF. Captopril may be initiated with a single dose of 6.25 mg. If the patient tolerates this dose, the dose should be titrated in increments to a maximum of 50 mg thrice daily as long as tolerated (systolic blood pressure >100 mm Hg). Other post-MI therapies (e.g., thrombolytics, aspirin, and beta blockers) may be used concurrently.

Lisinopril has been shown to decrease mortality rates in both acute and post-MI patients. It also is indicated for treating hemodynamically stable patients within 24 hours of an acute MI to improve survival. Patients should receive, as appropriate, the standard recommended treatments such as thrombolytics, aspirin, and beta blockers. The first 2.5-mg dose of lisinopril may be given to hemodynamically stable patients within 24 hours of the onset of symptoms of acute MI. The dose of lisinopril should be titrated as tolerated to a dose of 10 mg daily. Dosing should be continued for 6 weeks. At that time, the patient should be assessed for signs and symptoms of HF, and therapy should be continued if necessary. The dose should be decreased to 2.5 mg in patients with a low systolic blood pressure (below 120 mm Hg) when treatment is started or during the first 3 days after the MI. If hypotension occurs (systolic blood pressure below 100 mm Hg), a daily maintenance dose of 5 mg may be given with temporary reductions to 2.5 mg if needed. If prolonged hypotension occurs (systolic blood pressure below 90 mm Hg for at least 1 hour), lisinopril therapy should be discontinued. Patients who develop symptoms of HF should receive the usual effective dose of lisinopril for HF, with a goal of 20 mg/d.

Ramipril has also been approved for stable patients who have shown clinical signs of HF within the first few days after an acute MI. It is used to decrease the risk of death (principally cardiovascular death) and to decrease the risks of HF-related hospitalization and progression to severe or resistant HF. The starting dose is 2.5 mg twice daily. A patient who becomes hypotensive at this dose may be switched to 1.25 mg twice daily, but all dosages should then be titrated, as tolerated, toward a target dose of 5 mg twice daily. In patients with a creatinine clearance less than 40 mL/min/1.73 m^2 (serum creatinine level of <2.5 mg/dL), the dose should be decreased to 1.25 mg once daily. The dosage may be increased to 1.25 mg twice daily up to a maximum dose of 2.5 mg twice daily, depending on clinical response and tolerability.

Trandolapril is also approved for use in stable patients who have evidence of LV systolic dysfunction (identified by wall motion abnormalities) or who have symptoms of HF within the first few days after an acute MI. This drug has proved beneficial for the treatment of LV dysfunction after MI and has been found considerably important in treatment of patients with comorbid diabetes. It also reduces the progression to proteinuria in high-risk patients (Diaz & Ducharme, 2008). The recommended starting dose is 1 mg once daily. Dosages should be titrated, as tolerated, toward a target dose of 4 mg/d. If the 4-mg dose is not tolerated, patients can continue therapy with the highest tolerated dose.

Contraindications

Patients should not receive an ACE-I if they have experienced life-threatening adverse effects (e.g., angioedema or anuric renal failure) during previous exposure or if they are pregnant. Angioedema is a potentially fatal allergic reaction that may cause sudden difficulty in breathing, speaking, and swallowing accompanied by obvious swelling of the lips, face, and neck. Patients should receive an ACE-I with caution if they have any of the following:

- Very low systemic blood pressure (systolic blood pressure <80 mm Hg)
- Markedly increased serum creatinine levels (above 3 mg/dL)
- Bilateral renal artery stenosis (previously considered a contraindication)
- Elevated serum potassium levels (above 5.5 mmol/L)

In addition, ACE-I should not be given to hypotensive patients who are at immediate risk for cardiogenic shock and who require IV pressor support (e.g., dobutamine [Dobutrex] or epinephrine [Adrenalin, others]). These patients should receive treatment for their pump failure first; then, once they are stabilized, the HF should be reevaluated.

When taken by pregnant women during the second and third trimesters, ACE-I can cause injury and even death to the fetus. When pregnancy is detected, the ACE-I should be discontinued immediately due to the teratogenic effects.

Adverse Events

The most common adverse reactions of ACE-I are dizziness, headache, fatigue, diarrhea, cough, and hypotension. Angioedema of the face, extremities, lips, tongue, glottis, or larynx has also been reported in patients treated with ACE-I. Angioedema associated with throat or laryngeal edema may be fatal because of airway blockage, which causes suffocation. Patients should be advised about this possible adverse effect and told to go to an emergency department immediately if they experience any of the symptoms suggesting angioedema.

Hypotension may occur with any of the ACE-I and is usually observed after the first dose. It is more common in patients who are sodium or volume depleted, such as those treated vigorously with diuretics or those on dialysis, and in patients with severe HF. Hypotension can be minimized by starting with a very low dose and then increasing it slowly (usually every 3–7 days based on response) to the highest clinically effective level that does not produce hypotension. The diuretic dose may also need to be decreased or discontinued before starting the ACE-I. Blood pressure should be followed closely after the first dose (until the blood pressure is stabilized), for the first 2 weeks of therapy, and whenever the dose of the ACE-I or diuretic is increased. Hypotension, an anticipated problem among older patients with HF because of blunted baroreceptor reflexes, is no more common in older patients than in other age groups.

Changes in renal function may occur in susceptible patients (i.e., patients with hyponatremia; those taking high doses of diuretics; those with low cardiac output, diabetes mellitus, severe HF, or preexisting renal impairment) because of inhibition of the RAAS. Patients with bilateral or unilateral renal artery stenosis should receive ACE-I with extreme caution and should be monitored closely because renal failure may occur. The increases in serum creatinine and BUN that may occur are usually reversible by adjusting the dose of the ACE-I, diuretic, or both. Furthermore, an increase in serum creatinine not exceeding 30% of the basal value is now being viewed as an indicator that the drug is working (i.e., there is adequate ACE inhibition) and that it has not caused renal failure and the drug may be continued in these patients. However, the initial dose of an ACE-I should be reduced with increasing severity of HF, and the titration period should be monitored carefully. Age-related declines in renal function may slow the elimination of ACE-I and thus may increase the level and duration of their effects. Therefore, it may be necessary to reduce the initial dose of ACE-I in older patients or in patients with a serum creatinine level of 2.5 mg/dL or more. These patients may not tolerate as high a dose as other patients with HF but should be titrated to the highest possible dose.

Diuretic-induced potassium loss (hypokalemia) may be reduced when an ACE-I is used in combination with a diuretic. However, hyperkalemia may occur in patients with renal impairment or in those receiving a potassium-sparing diuretic, a potassium supplement, or potassium-containing salt substitutes. ACE-I should be administered cautiously if hypokalemia exists and discontinued if hyperkalemia exists. Frequent monitoring of serum potassium levels should be performed.

A cough is a common adverse event associated with ACE-I therapy, occurring in 5% to 20% of patients. It is thought to be due to increased production of bradykinins or substance P, both of which lower the cough reflex. The cough is described as an annoying, ticklish, dry cough that is reversible on discontinuation of the ACE-I. In patients with HF, cough is rarely severe enough to require discontinuation of therapy. Patients who experience cough should be questioned to determine whether this symptom is due to the ACE-I or pulmonary edema.

The ACE-I should be implicated only after other causes have been excluded. In most cases, the patient and family can be advised that if the cough is bothersome but not intolerable, the benefits of ACE-I therapy outweigh this adverse effect. However, if the cough is persistent and troublesome, the clinician can suggest withdrawing the ACE-I and trying alternative medications (e.g., an ARB or a combination of HYD and isosorbide dinitrate [ISDN]).

Because HF is common among older patients and increases in prevalence with age, safety and efficacy in this population are important. When ACE-I first became available, many experts believed that because older patients tend to have low plasma renin activity, these agents would be relatively ineffective. Furthermore, the physiologic consequences of aging may alter the absorption, distribution, and elimination of drugs, as well as the sensitivity of the patient to drugs. Thus, it was recognized that safety and efficacy studies should be conducted in this important patient population. A number of studies have been completed, and they document that ACE-I are well tolerated and effective for older patients with HF. Studies have not yet identified differences in response between older and younger patients. However, greater sensitivity of some older patients cannot be ruled out. Older patients receiving ACE-I do not experience more adverse effects than do younger patients (Masoudi et al., 2004).

Interactions

The ACE-I have been associated with very few significant drug–drug interactions. One or all of the ACE-I have been used in combination with digoxin, methyldopa (Aldomet), prazosin (Minipress), HYD, beta blockers, nitrates, and calcium channel blockers. The drug interactions that should be kept in mind are listed in **Table 21.3**.

Diuretics

During initial evaluation, the clinician should determine whether the patient manifests symptoms (e.g., orthopnea, paroxysmal nocturnal dyspnea, or dyspnea on exertion) or signs (e.g., pulmonary rales, a third heart sound, or jugular venous distention) of volume overload. Patients with HF and significant volume overload should be started immediately on a diuretic in conjunction with an ACE-I and a beta blocker (see **Table 21.2**).

ACCF/AHA HF guidelines recommend diuretics in patients with HFrEF who have evidence of fluid retention, unless contraindicated, to improve symptoms. These guidelines also provide specific recommendation for aldosterone receptor antagonists. The guidelines recommend aldosterone receptor antagonists (or mineralocorticoid receptor antagonists) in patients with NYHA class II–IV HF and who have left ventricular ejection fraction (LVEF) of 35% or less, unless contraindicated, to reduce morbidity and mortality. It is recommended that patients with NYHA class II HF should have a history of prior cardiovascular hospitalization or elevated plasma natriuretic peptide levels to be considered for

aldosterone receptor antagonists. The guidelines also recommend that creatinine should be 2.5 mg/dL or less in men or 2.0 mg/dL or less in women (or estimated glomerular filtration rate >30 mL/min/1.73 m^2), and potassium should be less than 5.0 mEq/L. It is suggested that careful monitoring of potassium, renal function, and diuretic dosing should be performed at initiation and closely followed thereafter to minimize risk of hyperkalemia and renal insufficiency. The guidelines also recommend use of aldosterone receptor antagonists to reduce morbidity and mortality following an acute MI in patients who have LVEF of 40% or less, who develop symptoms of HF, or who have a history of diabetes mellitus, unless contraindicated (Yancy et al., 2013).

Mechanism of Action

Diuretics cause an increase in sodium and water excretion by the kidney by inhibiting the reabsorption of sodium or chloride. Thiazide diuretics work at the distal tubule of the kidney. Loop diuretics (bumetanide, furosemide, or torsemide) exert their effect at the loop of Henle as well as the

TABLE 21.3

Drug Interactions Associated with the Angiotensin-Converting Enzyme Inhibitors

Interacting Agent	Potential Effect
Antacids	Decrease the bioavailability of captopril; therefore, separate administration times by 2 h.
Aspirin	Decreases hemodynamic response of ACE-I
Capsaicin	Triggers or exacerbates the coughing that is associated with ACE-I treatment
Lithium	In combination with ACE-I, causes increased serum lithium levels and symptoms of lithium toxicity
Nonsteroidal antiinflammatory drugs	In combination with ACE-I, promotes sodium and water retention and diminishes control of hypertension and heart failure
Potassium supplements/ potassium-sparing diuretics/salt substitutes	In combination with ACE-I, increases risk of hyperkalemia
Rifampin	Reduces the pharmacologic effects of enalapril
Tetracycline	In combination with quinapril, tetracycline undergoes decreased absorption (28%–37%), possibly from the high magnesium content in quinapril

ACE, angiotensin-converting enzyme; ACE-I, ACE inhibitors.

proximal and distal tubules. Thus, loop diuretics are more potent in inhibiting sodium, chloride, and water excretion. Diuretics decrease preload by reducing the volume overload. An immediate effect (extrarenal) is an increase in venous capacity with resultant redistribution of venous blood away from the lungs toward the periphery, which results in a decrease in pulmonary capillary pressure.

Dosage

Therapy is commonly initiated with low doses of a diuretic (e.g., furosemide [Lasix] 20–40 mg/d), and the dose is increased until urine output increases and weight decreases, usually by 0.5 to 1.0 kg daily. Increases in the dose of the diuretic may be required to sustain the loss of weight. The goal is to reduce symptoms as well as eliminate physical signs of fluid retention by restoring jugular venous pressures toward normal, by eliminating edema, or by both. Patients with persistent volume overload despite initial medical management may require one of the following:

- More aggressive administration of the current diuretic (e.g., IV administration)
- A combination of diuretics (e.g., loop diuretic and metolazone [Zaroxolyn])
- Short-term use of drugs that increase renal blood flow (e.g., dopamine [Intropin])

Although patients are commonly prescribed a fixed dose of diuretic, the dose of these drugs should be adjusted ideally on a daily basis. This can be accomplished in most cases by having the patient record his or her weight daily and allowing the patient or an appropriately trained health professional to adjust the dosage if the weight increases or decreases beyond a specified range for that patient. Thus, the most useful approach for practitioners to select the dose of, and monitor the response to, diuretic therapy is by measuring body weight, preferably on a daily basis. Practitioners should educate patients on the importance of weighing themselves and contacting a health care professional when weight increases or symptoms return. This may help to avoid hospitalization of the patient with HF.

Patients with pulmonary edema or marked volume overload should be given an IV loop diuretic initially. Diuretics should then be titrated to achieve resolution or improvement of signs and symptoms of volume overload. There is no standard target dose. Excessive diuresis should be avoided before starting an ACE-I. Volume depletion may lead to hypotension or renal insufficiency when ACE-I are started.

Spironolactone (Aldactone) has taken a larger, but controversial, role in the treatment of HF. In the Randomized Aldactone Evaluation Study (RALES), study of spironolactone use in HF revealed a decrease in morbidity and mortality (Pitt et al., 1999). A more recent global study of spironolactone did not support the findings of RALES (Pitt et al., 2014). Spironolactone lacked efficacy within patient subgroups who also had comorbid problems of blood pressure and diabetes. The researchers speculated this variance could be explained

by different treatments around the world. However, in the absence of any other similar drug, cardiology experts still support the use of spironolactone. Spironolactone acts to competitively bind at the aldosterone receptor site of the distal convoluted renal tubules, which causes increased amounts of water and sodium to be excreted. Spironolactone may be initiated at a dose of 12.5 to 25 mg daily, and creatinine should be 2.5 mg/dL or less in men or 2.0 mg/dL or less in women (or estimated glomerular filtration rate >30 mL/min/1.73 m^2) prior to initiation. Close monitoring of potassium, renal function and diuretic dosing, should be conducted at agent initiation and closely thereafter as discussed previously.

Adverse Events

Potassium depletion commonly occurs when patients are treated chronically with diuretics, except with the use of spironolactone. However, ACE-I decrease renal potassium losses and raise serum potassium levels, so many patients with HF who are treated with both agents may not have potassium depletion. Concomitant administration of ACE-I alone or in combination with potassium-sparing agents (e.g., spironolactone) can prevent electrolyte depletion in most patients with HF. Diuretics may also cause magnesium depletion, which often accompanies potassium depletion. If high doses of diuretics are used, magnesium levels should be followed and oral supplementation given when needed (Mg 1.5 mEq/L).

Interactions

NSAIDs (including aspirin) may blunt the natriuretic effect of diuretics. Therefore, patients receiving daily therapy with NSAIDs may need an increase in the dose of the diuretic to compensate for fluid retention. Diuretics may decrease lithium clearance, which may raise lithium levels into the toxic range. Lithium levels should be monitored in patients receiving both drugs. Patients may be at an increased risk of ototoxicity when high doses of loop diuretics and other ototoxic drugs (e.g., aminoglycosides) are used concomitantly.

Angiotensin II Type 1 Receptor Blockers

These antagonists were developed to offer the advantages of increased selectivity and specificity and to maintain blockade of the circulating and tissue RAAS at the AT$_1$ receptor level without the adverse reactions associated with ACE-I. ARBs do not block the degradation of vasoactive substances (e.g., bradykinin, enkephalins, and substance P) and may not cause the adverse effects, such as cough, related to ACE-I–induced bradykinin accumulation.

Of the currently approved ARBs, losartan (Cozaar) has been the most extensively studied in patients with HF. Losartan lowers blood pressure, systemic vascular resistance, pulmonary capillary wedge pressure, and heart rate and raises the cardiac index. Dyspnea on exertion and HF exacerbation decrease with losartan. Compared with the ACE-I enalapril, losartan shows no significant difference in terms of altered exercise capacity (6-minute walk test), clinical status (dyspnea–fatigue index), neurohumoral activation (norepinephrine, N-terminal atrial natriuretic factor), laboratory evaluation, or incidence of adverse effects. Comparisons with another ACE-I, captopril, show that losartan has the same incidence of persistent renal dysfunction and no difference in the incidence of death or HF hospital admissions. Further studies with other ACE-I in various patient populations are needed to determine whether losartan reduces morbidity and mortality to a greater degree than the ACE-I. The initial studies of losartan for treating HF seem promising. In addition, studies of the combination of ARBs and ACE-I are also being conducted. Although combination therapy with an ACE-I and ARB has been shown to be of benefit in the Valsartan Heart Failure Trial (Val-HeFT) and Candesartan in Heart Failure Assessment of Reduction in Mortality and Morbidity trial, there is hesitancy in clinical practice due to effects on renal function. It is reasonable to prescribe ARBs instead of ACE-I only in patients who cannot tolerate ACE-I because of angioedema or intractable cough. Even though the pathways are different, ARBs should be used cautiously (if at all) in patients who developed angioedema with ACE-I.

ACCF/AHA HF guidelines recommend that in all patients with a recent or remote history of MI or ACS and reduced EF, ACE-I should be used to prevent symptomatic HF and reduce mortality. The guidelines also recommend that ACE-I should be used in all patients with a reduced EF to prevent symptomatic HF, even if they do not have a history of MI. They also recommend that in patients intolerant of ACE-I, ARBs are appropriate unless contraindicated. With regard to HF patients with stage C HF, the guidelines recommend ARBs for patients with HFrEF with current or prior symptoms and who are ACE-I intolerant, unless contraindicated, to reduce morbidity and mortality. These guidelines recommend that ARBs are reasonable to reduce morbidity and mortality as alternatives to ACE-I as first-line therapy for patients with HFrEF, especially for patients already taking ARBs for other indications, unless contraindicated (Yancy et al., 2013). The role of ARNI in this patient population is discussed in a corresponding section given later.

Mechanism of Action

ARBs block the physiologic effects of angiotensin II by inhibiting receptor stimulation. The currently marketed ARBs—candesartan (Atacand), eprosartan (Teveten), losartan (Cozaar), olmesartan (Benicar), telmisartan (Micardis), valsartan (Diovan), and irbesartan (Avapro)—are approved by the U.S. Food and Drug Administration (FDA) for the management of hypertension. These antagonists were developed to offer the advantages of increased selectivity and specificity and to maintain blockade of the circulating and tissue RAAS at the AT_1 receptor level without the adverse reactions associated with ACE-I. ARBs do not block the degradation of vasoactive substances (e.g., bradykinin, enkephalins, and substance P) and may not cause the adverse effects, such as cough, related to ACE-I–induced bradykinin accumulation.

When ARBs were introduced into practice, there was a theoretical consideration that reducing the production of angiotensin II with an ACE-I and blocking the remaining angiotensin II with an ARB would be better than either therapy alone. However, the Val-HeFT study showed that adding an ARB to ACE-I therapy is not beneficial.

Dosage

The doses of these agents vary. **Table 21.2** lists selected ARBs and their doses. Regardless of which agent is selected, the practitioner should monitor the patient's renal function and blood pressure.

Adverse Events

ARB therapy may be associated with hypotension. This usually occurs with the first dose but may also occur during upward titration or when clinical status worsens. This situation is most common among patients with hyponatremia, hypovolemia, low baseline blood pressure, renal impairment, and high baseline levels of renin or aldosterone. Potentiation of the vasodilator effects of bradykinin and prostaglandins appears to contribute to this hypotension. Theoretically, ARBs, which do not interfere with the degradation of these peptides, should result in fewer episodes of first-dose hypotension. However, this beneficial effect remains to be proven in clinical trials. In addition, specific ARBs could block the deleterious effects of angiotensin II produced by non-ACE-dependent pathways that are not blocked by ACE-I.

The most common adverse events with losartan include dyspnea, worsening of HF, hypotension, dizziness, cough, and upper respiratory tract infection. The ARBs appear as likely as the ACE-I to produce hypotension, worsening renal function, and hyperkalemia. Also, like ACE-I, these agents are contraindicated in pregnancy, especially during the second and third trimesters.

Angiotensin Receptor-Neprilysin Inhibitor

The emergence of a new class of medication, ARNI, has changed treatment recommendations within the latest updates to HF guidelines (mentioned earlier in both the Angiotensin-Coverting Enzyme Inhibitors and the Angiotensin II Type 1 Receptor Blockers sections). Sacubitril/valsartan (Entresto) was approved by the FDA in 2015. The medication is a combination of valsartan, an ARB that has been well studied, and sacubitril, which is a neprylisin inhibitor (described further in the section titled Mechanism of Action).

The landmark Prospective Comparison of ARNI with ACEI to Determine Impact on Global Mortality and Morbidity in Heart Failure trial study was published in 2014 and was a multicenter, prospective, randomized controlled trial, which aimed to evaluate sacubitril/valsartan versus an active treatment control group receiving enalapril. The primary outcome of the study was a composite outcome of cardiovascular mortality or HF hospitalization. The study found that treatment with ARNI provided a statistically significant improvement over comparator group with regard to the composite outcome of cardiovascular mortality or HF hospitalization, as well as each individual outcome of cardiovascular mortality and HF hospitalization when evaluated individually. Adverse effects of ARNI were evaluated and appeared to be relatively well tolerated overall; side effects similar to ACE-I and ARBs were observed, including hypotension, hyperkalemia, cough, serum creatinine increase, and angioedema (McMurray et al., 2014).

The ACC/AHA/ Heart Failure Society of America (HFSA) HF guideline updates in 2016 and 2017 provided new recommendations for pharmacological treatment for patients of stage C HF with reduced EF. Relevant guideline recommendations are included in their entirety later in this chapter. The guidelines comment that the clinical strategy of inhibition of the renin–angiotensin system with ACE-I, *or* ARBs, *or* ARNI, in conjunction with evidence-based beta blockers and aldosterone antagonists in selected patients, is recommended for patients with chronic HFrEF to reduce morbidity and mortality. The use of ACE-I is beneficial for patients with prior or current symptoms of chronic HFrEF to reduce morbidity and mortality. The use of ARBs to reduce morbidity and mortality is recommended in patients with prior or current symptoms of chronic HFrEF who are intolerant to ACE-I because of cough or angioedema. In patients with chronic, symptomatic HFrEF NYHA class II or III who tolerate an ACE-I or ARB, replacement by an ARNI is recommended to further reduce morbidity and mortality. ARNI should not be administered concomitantly with ACE-I or within 36 hours of the last dose of an ACE-I. ARNI should not be administered to patients with a history of angioedema (Yancy et al., 2017).

There are currently large-scale randomized clinical trials seeking further information on a potential role of sacubatril/valsartan in patients with HFpEF (Solomon et al., 2019), as well as a potential role in patients with acute decompensated HF (Velazquez et al., 2019).

Mechanism of Action

Valsartan, the ARB component of the ARNI, functions by blocking the physiologic effects of angiotensin II by inhibiting receptor stimulation. The mechanism of ARBs was previously discussed; refer to the preceding section for further information.

Notably, there are various endogenous vasoactive peptides that are degraded to inactive metabolites via neprylisin, a neutral endopeptidase. These endogenous vasoactive peptides (including natriuretic peptides, bradykinin, adrenomedullin, substance P and calcitonin gene-related peptides) provide beneficial physiologic functionality, serving to reduce vascular tone, neurohormonal activation, sodium retention, as well as cardiac fibrosis and hypertrophy. Inhibiting neprilysin with sacubitril functions to antagonize endogenous vasoactive peptide degradation and maintains beneficial effect of these peptides within the RAAS system (McMurray et al., 2014).

Dosage

When transitioning from an ACE-I to ARNI, a 36-hour washout period is recommended.

In patients previously taking a moderate- to high-dose ACE-I (>10 mg/day of enalapril or equivalent) or ARB (>160 mg/day of

valsartan or equivalent), treatment may be initiated with sacubitril 49 mg/valsartan 51 mg twice daily. The dose may be doubled as tolerated after 2 to 4 weeks to target maintenance dose of sacubitril 97 mg/valsartan 103 mg twice daily.

In patients not previously on an ACE-I or an ARB or who were previously taking a low-dose ACE-I (≤10 mg/day of enalapril or equivalent) or ARB (≤160 mg/day of valsartan or equivalent), treatment may be initiated with sacubitril 24 mg/valsartan 26 mg twice daily. The dose may be doubled as tolerated every 2 to 4 weeks to target maintenance dose of sacubitril 97 mg/valsartan 103 mg twice daily. This lower initial dose may also be utilized for patients with estimated glomerular filtration rate less than 30 mL/min/1.73 m^2 or moderate hepatic impairment.

Similar to ACE-I and ARBs, serum electrolytes, renal function, and blood pressure should be monitored closely when sacubatril/valsartan is initiated, upon dose adjustment of sacubatril/valsartan or other interacting medications, and periodically thereafter.

The valsartan salt formulation utilized in sacubatril/valsartan (Entresto) is more bioavailable than valsartan in other market formulations; thus valsartan 26, 51, and 103 mg in sacubatril/valsartan (Entresto) is equivalent to valsartan 40, 80, and 160 mg in other marketed tablet formulations, respectively.

Adverse Events

The most common adverse events with sacubatril/valsartan include side effects similar to ACE-I and ARBs, such as hypotension, hyperkalemia, cough, serum creatinine increase, and angioedema.

Contraindications

As described previously, use of sacubatril/valsartan is contraindicated in patients with history of angioedema related to previous ACE-I or ARB therapy. Use of sacubatril/valsartan is also contraindicated with concomitant use or use within 36 hours of ACE-I. Use of sacubatril/valsartan is also contraindicated with concomitant use of aliskiren in patients with diabetes. Also, like ACE-I and ARBs, ARNIs are contraindicated in pregnancy, especially during the second and third trimesters. The U.S. boxed warning for this agent comments that drugs that act directly on the RAAS system can cause injury and death to the developing fetus. When pregnancy is detected, discontinue sacubatril/valsartan as soon as possible.

Interactions

Sacubatril/valsartan has been associated with interactions similar to those expected of ACE-I or ARBs. As discussed earlier, concomitant use of ACE-I may increase the adverse/toxic effect profile of sacubatril/valsartan; specifically, the risk of angioedema may be increased within this combination, resulting in labeled contraindication. Concomitant use of aliskiren may increase the adverse/toxic effect profile of sacubatril/valsartan; specifically, the risk of hyperkalemia, hypotension, and nephrotoxicity may be increased within this combination, resulting in labeled contraindication for concomitant use in patients with diabetes.

Beta Blockers

Historically, beta blockers have been contraindicated for treating HF. The negative inotropic effect, bradycardic effect, and peripheral constriction of the beta blockers can all exacerbate HF. However, observations from experimental studies and controlled clinical trials indicate that prolonged activation of the SNS can accelerate the progression of HF. The studies also determined that the risks of such progression can be substantially decreased through the use of pharmacologic agents that interfere with the actions of the SNS on the heart and peripheral blood vessels. Thus, the use of beta blockers is gaining acceptance as a treatment for HF.

The new recommendations strongly advocate using beta blockers for treating patients with HF. As stated previously, the recommendations state that all patients with stable NYHA class II to class IV HF due to LV systolic dysfunction should receive a beta blocker unless they have a contraindication to its use or have shown to be unable to tolerate treatment with the drug. Beta blockers should not be used in unstable patients or in acutely ill patients ("rescue" therapy), including those who are in the intensive care unit with refractory HF requiring IV support. Beta blockers can be initiated once patients are clinically compensated. Also, if a patient is already on a beta blocker, it can be continued as long as the patient is hemodynamically stable. Beta blockers are recommended to improve symptoms and clinical status and to decrease the risk of death and hospitalization in patients with mild to moderate (NYHA class II) or moderate to severe (NYHA class III) HF and in those who have an LV EF of less than 35% to 40%. Beta blockers should be added to preexisting treatment with diuretics and an ACE-I and may be used together with digitalis or vasodilators.

Carvedilol, a nonselective beta adrenergic receptor blocker with vasodilating action (through alpha-adrenergic blocking action) previously approved for the management of essential hypertension, has become the first beta blocker approved in the United States for treating HF. It is intended to reduce the progression of disease as evidenced by cardiovascular death, cardiovascular hospitalization, or the need to adjust other HF medications. Similarly, the extended-release formulation of metoprolol, metoprolol succinate, was shown to be superior to placebo in decreasing mortality in HF patients. Bisoprolol (Zebeta) is also a beta blocker used in the treatment of HF that decreases mortality.

ACCF/AHA HF guidelines recommend that in all patients with a recent or remote history of MI or ACS and reduced EF, evidence-based beta blockers should be used to reduce mortality. The guidelines also recommend that beta blockers be used in all patients with a reduced EF to prevent symptomatic HF, even if they do not have a history of MI. They also recommend use of one of the three beta blockers proven to reduce mortality (e.g., bisoprolol, carvedilol, and sustained-release metoprolol succinate) for all patients with current or prior symptoms of HFrEF, unless contraindicated, to reduce morbidity and mortality (Yancy et al., 2013).

Mechanism of Action

Catecholamines can cause peripheral vasoconstriction that can exacerbate loading conditions in the failing heart and may precipitate myocardial ischemia and ventricular arrhythmias. In addition, activation of the SNS can increase heart rate, which may adversely affect the relation between myocardial supply and demand and more importantly may exacerbate the abnormal force–frequency relation that exists in HF. In addition, catecholamines activate cellular pathways that can lead to the loss of myocardial cells by a process of programmed cell death (apoptosis), which has been implicated in the progression of HF.

In experimental models of HF, pharmacologic interference with the SNS can favorably alter the natural history of the disease, similar to the manner in which antagonism of the RAAS by ACE-I can modify the course of HF. Extensive research implicating the target mechanism, increased adrenergic drive, as being unfavorable to the natural history of systolic dysfunction, and the HF clinical syndrome has been done. This has led to the conclusion that the primary mechanism of action of beta blockers in chronic HF is to prevent and reverse adrenergically mediated intrinsic myocardial dysfunction and remodeling. This occurs through a time-dependent, biologic effect involving inhibition of beta-adrenergic mechanisms directly or indirectly responsible for the development of cellular contractile dysfunction and remodeling (Doughty et al., 2004). In addition, one of the beta blockers used in patients with HF, carvedilol, has direct antioxidant effects that may decrease the role played by apoptosis in the progression of HF (Dandona et al., 2007).

Studies have shown that carvedilol and metoprolol improve LV function, hemodynamic parameters, and various symptoms of HF. Carvedilol also improves submaximal exercise tolerance and NYHA classification. In multicenter clinical trials, carvedilol was associated with a highly significant 65% reduction in the risk of death versus placebo (all patients received conventional therapy in addition to carvedilol or placebo). This was due to a decrease in death due to both pump failure and sudden death. In addition, carvedilol decreases the risk of hospitalization for cardiovascular causes and the combined risk of all-cause mortality and cardiovascular hospitalization (Pasternak et al., 2014).

Dosage

Adverse effects with carvedilol usually occur early in therapy and are more frequent and severe with higher doses. Because of this, the starting dose of carvedilol is 3.125 mg twice daily, and each dose titration should be done slowly over a 2-week period, doubling the dose each time. At initiation of each new dosage, the patient should be observed for 1 hour for signs of dizziness or light-headedness. In addition, blood pressure should be monitored. The maximum recommended dosage is 25 mg twice daily in patients weighing less than 85 kg and 50 mg twice daily in patients weighing 85 kg or greater. In addition, patients should be seen in the office during titration and evaluated for symptoms of worsening HF, vasodilation (i.e., dizziness, light-headedness, and symptomatic hypotension), or bradycardia to determine their tolerance for carvedilol. Treatment with metoprolol starts at 6.25 mg twice or thrice daily, and the dose is titrated slowly up to a target of 100 mg twice or thrice daily.

Initiation of therapy with a beta blocker may produce fluid retention, which may be severe enough to cause pulmonary or peripheral congestion and worsening symptoms of HF. Increases in body weight may occur after 3 to 5 days of starting treatment and, if untreated, may lead to worsening symptoms within 1 to 2 weeks. For this reason, practitioners should ask patients to weigh themselves daily. The amount of weight gain then guides the practitioner in prescribing an increase in the diuretic dosage until the patient's weight is restored to pretreatment levels. The dose of carvedilol may also have to be decreased; occasionally, the drug must be temporarily discontinued.

Excessive vasodilation may occur with initiation of therapy. It is usually asymptomatic but may be accompanied by dizziness, light-headedness, or blurred vision. Vasodilatory adverse effects are usually seen within 24 to 48 hours of the first dose or increments in dose but usually subside with repeated dosing without any change in the dose of carvedilol or other medications. The risk of hypotension may be minimized by taking the beta blocker, ACE-I, or vasodilator (if used) at different times during the day. Practitioners can work with patients to develop a regimen that is convenient and minimizes adverse effects. The practitioner may need to reduce the dose of the ACE-I or vasodilator if hypotension is excessive. If the patient's heart rate decreases to less than 50 beats per minute or if second- or third-degree heart block occurs, the patient should contact the practitioner, who may then decrease the dose of the beta blocker. Practitioners should evaluate the patient's concomitant medications for drug interactions that may also decrease heart rate or cause heart block (e.g., diltiazem or flecainide).

Contraindications

Beta blockers should not be used in patients with bronchospastic disease, symptomatic bradycardia, or advanced heart block (unless treated with a pacemaker). Patients should receive a beta blocker with caution if they have asymptomatic bradycardia (heart rate below 60 beats per minute). Despite concerns that beta blockade may mask some of the signs of hypoglycemia, patients with diabetes mellitus may be particularly likely to experience a reduction in morbidity and mortality with beta blocker therapy. The Glycemic Effects in Diabetes Mellitus: Carvedilol-Metoprolol Comparison in Hypertensives Study (GEMINI) trial showed that carvedilol improved insulin resistance, maintained glycemic control, and reduced progression to microalbuminuria.

Adverse Events

The adverse effect profile of beta blockers in patients with HF is consistent with the pharmacology of the drug and the health status of the patient. The most common adverse effects are dizziness,

fatigue, and worsening of HF. Other adverse reactions that occur less frequently include bradycardia, hypotension, generalized edema, dependent edema, sinusitis, and bronchitis. Rare cases of liver function abnormalities have been reported in patients receiving carvedilol, but no deaths due to these abnormalities have been reported. Mild hepatic injury related to carvedilol has been reversible and has occurred after short- and long-term therapy. Carvedilol should be discontinued if a patient has laboratory evidence of liver function abnormalities or jaundice.

Practitioners should advise patients receiving therapy with carvedilol or other beta blockers about the following:

- Adverse effects may occur early in therapy but usually do not prevent long-term use of the drug.
- Symptomatic improvement may not be seen for 2 to 3 months.
- Beta blockade may reduce the risk of disease progression even if the patient's symptoms have not responded favorably to treatment.

Digoxin

Digoxin can prevent clinical deterioration in patients with HF due to LV systolic dysfunction and can improve these patients' symptoms. However, it does not decrease the mortality rate. The latest large trial, the Digitalis Investigation Group study, showed that survival was not changed by use of digoxin (0.125–0.5 mg) in NYHA class II and III patients with HF who were taking diuretics and ACE-I. However, digoxin significantly decreased the number of hospitalizations compared with placebo. This effect seemed to be more pronounced in patients with the lowest EFs and the most enlarged hearts. However, digoxin increased the risk of non-HF causes of cardiac death from presumed arrhythmia or MI (Digitalis Investigation Group, 1997).

The ACTION HF organization recommends digoxin to improve the clinical status of patients with HF due to LV systolic dysfunction and recommends that it should be used in conjunction with diuretics, an ACE-I, and a beta blocker. In addition, digoxin is recommended in patients with HF who have rapid atrial fibrillation, even though beta blockers may be more effective in controlling the ventricular response during exercise. If a patient is receiving digoxin but not an ACE-I or a beta blocker, treatment with digoxin should not be withdrawn, but appropriate therapy with the neurohormonal antagonists should be instituted. Patients should not receive digoxin if they have significant sinus or atrioventricular (AV) block, unless the block has been treated with a permanent pacemaker. Digoxin should be used cautiously in patients receiving other drugs that can depress sinus or AV nodal function (e.g., amiodarone or a beta blocker), although these patients usually tolerate digoxin without difficulty. In addition, digoxin is not indicated for the stabilization of patients with acutely decompensated HF (unless they have rapid atrial fibrillation). There are no data to recommend using digoxin in patients with asymptomatic LV dysfunction (NYHA class I).

ACCF/AHA guidelines recommend that digoxin can be beneficial in patients with HFrEF, unless contraindicated, to decrease hospitalizations for HF (Yancy et al., 2013).

Mechanism of Action

Digoxin produces a mild inotropic effect by inhibiting cell membrane sodium–potassium adenosine triphosphatase activity and thereby enhancing calcium entry into the cell. Calcium enhances contractile protein activity, allowing for a greater force and velocity of contraction.

Dosage

Loading doses of digoxin usually are not needed in patients with HF. The typical dosage of 0.25 mg daily may be initiated if there is no evidence of renal dysfunction. Patients who have reduced renal function, who have baseline conduction abnormality, or who have low body weight or older should be started on 0.125 mg daily or lower (such as every other day). The ACCF/AHA HF guidelines suggest that digoxin levels of 0.5 to 0.9 ng/mL are considered therapeutic for HF patients and that higher level were not associated with better outcomes (Yancy et al., 2013). A recent study, which evaluated patients with atrial fibrillation taking digoxin, found that the risk of death was independently related to serum digoxin concentration and was highest in patients with concentrations 1.2 ng/mL or more; this was true both in patients with and without HF (Lopes et al., 2018). Although it has been suggested that serum levels may be used to guide the selection of an appropriate dose of digoxin, there is no evidence to support this approach (Packer & Cohn, 1999).

Steady state is reached in approximately 1 week in patients with normal renal function, although 2 to 3 weeks may be required in patients with renal impairment. When steady state is achieved, the patient should be evaluated for symptoms of toxicity. In addition, an ECG, serum digoxin level, serum electrolytes, BUN, and creatinine should be obtained. It is not clear whether regular serum digoxin monitoring is necessary, but levels should be checked once a year after a steady state is achieved. In addition, levels should be checked if HF status worsens, renal function deteriorates, signs of toxicity develop (e.g., confusion, nausea, anorexia, visual disturbances, arrhythmias), or additional medications are added, which could affect the digoxin level.

Adverse Events

Signs of digoxin toxicity develop in approximately 20% of patients, and up to 18% of digoxin-toxic patients die from the arrhythmias that occur. Noncardiac symptoms are related to the central nervous system (CNS) and gastrointestinal (GI) tract. Anorexia is often an early manifestation, with nausea and vomiting following. The CNS adverse effects include headache, fatigue, malaise, disorientation, confusion, delirium, seizures, and visual disturbances. The noncardiac symptoms do not always precede the cardiac symptoms. Cardiac toxicity manifested by arrhythmias can take the form of almost every known rhythm disturbance (e.g., ectopic and reentrant cardiac rhythms and heart block).

Digoxin should be discontinued (often with consideration of reinstitution at a lower dose after 2–3 days if the patient is benefiting from therapy) if any of the following is noted:

- Elevated digoxin level
- Substantial reduction in renal function
- Symptoms of toxicity
- Significant conduction abnormality (e.g., symptomatic bradycardia due to second- or third-degree AV block or high-degree AV block in atrial fibrillation)
- An increase in ventricular arrhythmias

Practitioners should counsel patients about the potential adverse effects of digoxin. They also should stress the importance of taking digoxin exactly as it is prescribed to avoid toxicity or a subtherapeutic effect.

Interactions

The medications that most often cause an increase in digoxin levels are quinidine (Cardioquin, others), amiodarone, flecainide, propafenone (Rythmol), spironolactone, and verapamil. It may be necessary to decrease the dose of digoxin when treatment with these drugs is initiated. Antibiotics may decrease gut flora and prevent bacterial inactivation of digoxin, and anticholinergic agents may decrease intestinal motility. Both of these drug classes may also increase digoxin levels. Antacids, cholestyramine (Questran), neomycin (Mycifradin Sulfate), and kaolin–pectin (Kaopectate) may inhibit the absorption of digoxin and decrease digoxin levels. Patients should be advised to take digoxin at least 2 hours before these medications. Diuretics can enhance digoxin toxicity by decreasing renal clearance of digoxin and by causing electrolyte changes, including hypokalemia, hypomagnesemia, and hypercalcemia (thiazides). Before any new medications are added to a patient's regimen, the prescriber should determine whether the medication interacts with digoxin.

Hydralazine/Isosorbide Dinitrate

The HYD/ISDN combination of vasodilators is an appropriate alternative in African-American patients with contraindications to, or intolerance of, ACE-I. The combination should not be used for treating HF in patients who have not tried ACE-I and should not be substituted for ACE-I in patients who are tolerating ACE-I without difficulty. No studies have specifically addressed the use of HYD/ISDN for patients who cannot take or tolerate ACE-I, and the FDA has not approved HYD/ISDN for use in patients with HF. Isosorbide mononitrate is also not approved for HF and has not been studied for treating HF. HYD/ISDN is not as beneficial as the ACE-I enalapril in reducing mortality rates during the first 2 years of treatment. However, this combination has been shown to achieve an absolute reduction in mortality rates compared with placebo during the first 3 years of treatment. The combination increases exercise capacity as much as enalapril, but adverse effects are a significant problem.

ACCF/AHA guidelines recommend the combination of HYD and ISDN to reduce morbidity and mortality for patients self-described as African-Americans with NYHA classes III–IV HFrEF receiving optimal therapy with ACE-I and beta blockers, unless contraindicated. The guidelines also recommend that a combination of HYD and ISDN can be useful to reduce morbidity or mortality in patients with current or prior symptomatic HFrEF and in those who cannot be given an ACE-I or ARB because of drug intolerance, hypotension, or renal insufficiency, unless contraindicated (Yancy et al., 2013).

Mechanism of Action

Vasodilators may be classified by their mechanism of action or their site of action (venodilators, arteriolar dilators, or "balanced" vasodilators). ISDN is a venodilator that redistributes blood volume to the venous side of the heart to the systemic circulation, away from the lungs, which decreases the ventricular blood volume (preload). HYD, along with prazosin and minoxidil (Loniten), which are not used for treating HF, is an arteriolar dilator. HYD decreases the resistance the heart encounters during contraction (afterload), which allows for increased stroke volume (volume of blood leaving the heart) and increased cardiac output. Balanced vasodilators, including the ACE-I and ARBs, cause vasodilation on both the venous and arterial sides of the heart and therefore provide the hemodynamic and clinical benefits of both preload and afterload reduction (as discussed in other sections).

Dosage

There is now a fixed-dose combination of the two agents commonly available. The guidelines recommend that the initial dose should be one tablet (containing 37.5 mg of HYD hydrochloride and 20 mg of ISDN) thrice daily. They also recommend that the dose can be increased to two tablets thrice daily for a total daily dose of 225 mg of HYD hydrochloride and 120 mg of ISDN (Yancy et al., 2013).

If the fixed-dose combination is not available, or if the two drugs are being used separately, both pills should be administered at least thrice daily. Doses may be initiated at HYD 25 to 50 mg, three or four times daily (maximum 300 mg daily in divided doses) and ISDN 20 to 30 mg three or four times daily (maximum 120 mg daily in divided doses). The guidelines state that initial low doses of the drugs given separately may be progressively increased to a goal similar to that achieved in the fixed-dose combination trial (Yancy et al., 2013).

Adverse Events

Adverse events include reflex tachycardia, headache, flushing, nausea, dizziness, syncope, nitrate tolerance, and sodium and water retention. Nitrate tolerance can be avoided by providing a nitrate-free period of 10 to 14 hours.

Interactions

Other drugs that lower blood pressure, including diuretics, may cause additive hypotension, and blood pressure should be monitored.

Ivabradine (Corlanor)

Ivabradine is a relatively new drug in the treatment of HF to reduce the risk of hospitalization. It is indicated for patients with stable, symptomatic, chronic HF with LVEF 35% or less and in sinus rhythm with resting heart rate greater than or equal to 70 bpm, for those taking beta blockers at the highest dose they can tolerate or those who are not taking beta blockers because there is a medical reason to avoid the use of beta blockers.

The ACC/AHA/HFSA HF guideline updates recommend that ivabradine can be beneficial to reduce HF hospitalization for patients with symptomatic (NYHA classes II and III), stable, chronic HFrEF (LVEF ≤35%) who are receiving guideline-directed management and therapy, including a beta blocker at maximum tolerated dose, and who are in sinus rhythm with a heart rate of 70 bpm or greater at rest (Yancy et al., 2017).

Mechanism of Action

Ivabradine (Corlanor) is a hyperpolarization-activated cyclic nucleotide-gated channel blocker that reduces the spontaneous pacemaker activity of the cardiac sinus node by selectively inhibiting the I_f current (I_f), resulting in heart rate reduction with no effects on ventricular repolarization and no effects on myocardial contractility.

Dosage

The initial dose is 5 mg orally twice daily with meals, and the maximum dose is 7.5 mg orally twice daily. Dosing is adjusted based on keeping the heart rate between 50 and 60 bpm and the overall tolerability of the drug. In patients who have a resting heart rate greater than 60 bpm, dosing should be increased by 2.5 mg up to the maximum of 7.5 mg twice daily. For patients with resting heart rate between 50 and 60 bpm, the dose should be maintained. Finally, if the resting heart rate is less than 50 bpm, the dose should be decreased by 2.5 mg and tolerability reassessed. If the dose is already 2.5 mg twice daily, then discontinue the drug.

Interaction

Because ivabradine is metabolized by the CYP3A4 pathway of the P450 concomitant, use of CYP3A4 inhibitors will increase the concentration of ivabradine and use of CYP3A4 inducers will decrease the concentration. With increased plasma concentrations, bradycardia and conduction disturbance may be exacerbated. Examples of strong CYPA4 inhibitors include azole antifungals (e.g., ketoconazole, itraconazole), macrolide antibiotics (e.g., clarithromycin), and HIV protease inhibitors. Examples of moderate CYPA4 inhibitors include diltiazem, verapamil, and grape juice. Finally, examples of strong CYPA4 inducers include St. John's wort, rifampicin, barbiturates, and phenytoin.

Contraindications

Ivabradine is contraindicated in sick sinus syndrome or AV block (unless a pacemaker is inserted), severe liver disease, worsened HF symptoms, resting heart rate of less than 60, and blood pressure less than 90/50. Ivabradine is also contraindicated in chronic obstructive pulmonary disease, hypotension, or asthma and concomitant use of strong cytochrome P450 3A4 (CYP3A4) inhibitors.

Adverse Events

The most common adverse events in ivabradine are bradycardia, hypertension, atrial fibrillation and phosphenes, and visual brightness. Postmarketing reports of additional reactions include hypotension, angioedema, rash, pruritus, urticaria, vertigo, and diplopia.

Other Agents

Amiodarone

Amiodarone (Cordarone) is approved in the United States for treating refractory life-threatening ventricular arrhythmias. Amiodarone has been studied in patients with HF with ventricular arrhythmias to assess whether it reduces mortality rates. Some studies demonstrated that low-dose amiodarone (300 mg/d) reduced mortality rates, whereas others found no improvement (Doval et al., 1994; Singh et al., 1995). A meta-analysis of 13 randomized controlled trials of prophylactic amiodarone in patients with recent MI (8 trials) or HF (5 trials) found that amiodarone reduced the rate of arrhythmic/sudden death in high-risk patients with recent MI or HF (Amiodarone Trials Meta-Analysis Investigators, 1997).

The FDA has not approved amiodarone for treating HF. According to the most recent HF guidelines (Yancy et al., 2013), amiodarone is the only antiarrhythmic to have neutral effects on mortality from HF. Further studies are needed to determine whether it is useful for routine prophylactic treatment of patients with ventricular arrhythmias and non-ischemic HF. It may be beneficial in patients at high risk for arrhythmic/sudden death, patients with primary cardiomyopathy, or patients with both (Amiodarone Trials Meta-Analysis Investigators, 1997; Gheorghiade et al., 1998). The recommendations suggest that some class III antiarrhythmic agents (e.g., amiodarone) do not appear to increase the risk of death in patients with chronic HF. Such drugs are preferred to class I agents when used for treating atrial fibrillation in patients with LV systolic dysfunction. Because of its known toxicity and equivocal evidence for efficacy, amiodarone is not recommended for general use to prevent death (or sudden death) in patients with HF already treated with drugs that reduce mortality rates (e.g., ACE-I or beta blockers).

Mechanism of Action

Amiodarone is classified as a Vaughn-Williams class III (potassium channel blocking) antiarrhythmic drug, but it also possesses class I (sodium blocking), class II (beta blocking), and class IV (calcium channel blocking) antiarrhythmic effects. It also has vasodilatory properties. The therapeutic benefit of amiodarone may be due to its beta-blocking effects and not due to an antiarrhythmic effect.

Dosage

Before treatment with amiodarone starts, the practitioner should make sure the patient does not have hyperthyroidism or advanced liver disease. In addition, pulmonary function tests, chest radiography, ophthalmologic examination, and neurologic assessment are recommended before initiating therapy. The maintenance dosage should be 200 to 300 mg/d. High doses of amiodarone may cause initial cardiac decompensation with abnormal hemodynamics; therefore, use of high loading doses in patients with very severe forms of HF should be avoided.

Interactions

Amiodarone interacts with warfarin (Coumadin; increases the international normalized ratio) and digoxin (increases digoxin levels).

Selecting the Most Appropriate Agent

The 2013 ACCF/AHA clinical practice guidelines changed the approach to the management of patients with HF. Updated guidelines were published by the ACC/AHA/HFSA in 2016 and 2017 with the introduction of ARNI as a treatment option for patients with stage C HFrEF as well as guidance for the use of ivabradine. **Table 21.4** and **Figure 21.3** summarize therapeutic regimens. Note that **Figure 21.3** does not include the updates regarding the place of ARNI or ivabradine in treatment. In patients with a history and HF with reduced EF, ACE-I, ARBs, or ARNI should be used to reduce morbidity and mortality. In patients with an MI and reduced EF, beta blockers should be used to prevent HF, and a statin should also be given.

TABLE 21.4		
Recommended Order of Treatment for Heart Failure		
Order	**Agents**	**Comments**
First line	ACE-I or ARB or ARNI with or without a diuretic (depends on fluid retention)	Monitor patient's response carefully.
Second line	ACE-I or ARB or ARNI and beta blocker with a diuretic	In patient with mild heart failure, use a potassium-sparing diuretic when serum potassium level is <4.0 mEq/L.
Third line	ARB, beta blocker, aldosterone agonist, diuretic, and digoxin	Hydralazine/Isosorbide dinitrate or ivabradine may be considered for indicated patient populations.

ACE-I, ACE inhibitors; ARB, angiotensin receptor blocker; ARNI, angiotensin receptor-neprilysin inhibitor.

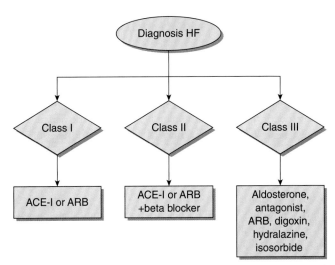

FIGURE 21–3 Treatment algorithm for chronic heart failure. (Adapted with permission from Yancy, C. W., Jessup, M., Bozkurt, B., et al. [2013]. 2013 ACCF/AHA guideline for the management of heart failure. *Journal of the American College of Cardiology, 62*(16), e147–e239. Copyright © 2013 American College of Cardiology Foundation and the American Heart Association, Inc. Published by Elsevier Inc. All rights reserved.)

ACE-I, angiotensin-converting enzyme inhibitor; ARB, angiotensin receptor blocker; HF, heart failure.

First-Line Therapy

The ACE-I are considered the first-line choice for routine use in patients with HF. ACE-I may also be considered for treatment of those who are stage A as classified by the ACC/AHA (Yancy et al., 2013). According to the clinical practice guidelines, patients with systolic dysfunction should receive a trial of an ACE-I unless contraindications are present (see discussion of Angiotensin-Converting Enzyme Inhibitors). The ACE-I may be considered sole therapy in HF patients who have fatigue or mild dyspnea on exertion and who do not have any other signs or symptoms of volume overload. However, if these symptoms persist after the target dose of the ACE-I is reached, a diuretic should be added (see Second-Line Therapy). Thus, ACE-I therapy is appropriate for patients in NYHA class I as a means of preventing HF and for patients in NYHA class II to IV with symptoms to decrease mortality rates (see discussion of Angiotensin-Converting Enzyme Inhibitors). They may be used in conjunction with beta blockers, which are also considered first-line therapy.

If the patient is unable to tolerate an ACE-I, an ARB can be used.

The 2016 and 2017 updates to guidelines highlighted the place of ARNI in patients with stage C HF with reduced EF. The guideline commented that the clinical strategy of inhibition of the renin–angiotensin system with ACE-I, *or* ARBs, *or* ARNI, in conjunction with evidence-based beta blockers and aldosterone antagonists in selected patients, is recommended for patients with chronic HFrEF, to reduce morbidity and mortality. In patients with chronic, symptomatic HFrEF NYHA class II or III, who tolerate an ACE-I or ARB, replacement by

an ARNI is recommended to further reduce morbidity and mortality (Yancy et al., 2017).

Beta blockers with vasodilating action have been approved for treating HF (see discussion in Beta Blocker section). Beta blockers are initial therapy.

The recommendations state that all patients with stable NYHA class II or III HF due to LV systolic dysfunction should receive a beta blocker unless the drug is contraindicated or cannot be tolerated. Beta blockers should be used with diuretics and ACE-I. Beta blockers should not be used in unstable patients or in acutely ill patients (rescue therapy), including those who are in the intensive care unit with refractory HF requiring IV support. Studies of beta-blocker therapy in various types of patients with HF are continuing to define their role.

Second-Line Therapy

Diuretics are used to increase sodium and water excretion, correct volume overload (which manifests as dyspnea on exertion), and maintain sodium and water balance. Patients with HF and signs of significant volume overload should be started immediately on a diuretic in addition to an ACE-I. Patients with mild HF or concomitant hypertension may be managed adequately on thiazide diuretics. However, a loop diuretic is preferred in most patients, particularly those with renal impairment or marked fluid retention. A potassium-sparing diuretic or potassium supplement should be used for patients with serum potassium concentrations less than 4.0 mEq/L. Patients with persistent volume overload despite initial medical management may require more aggressive administration of the current diuretic (e.g., IV administration), more potent diuretics, or a combination of diuretics (e.g., furosemide and metolazone, or furosemide and spironolactone).

Third-Line Therapy

The AHRQ clinical practice guidelines state that digoxin should be used in patients with severe HF and should be added to the medical regimen of patients with mild or moderate failure and those who remain symptomatic after optimal management with ACE-I and diuretics. The ACTION HF recommendations state that digoxin is recommended to improve the clinical status of patients with HF due to LV systolic dysfunction and should be used with diuretics, an ACE-I, and a beta blocker. Both groups suggest that digoxin may be beneficial in patients with HF when there is a second indication for digoxin therapy (e.g., a supraventricular arrhythmia for which digoxin is specifically indicated). However, there remains a question of whether the benefits of digoxin therapy outweigh its risks.

Fourth-Line Therapy

Fourth-line therapy consists of ARBs, such as losartan, the HYD/ISDN combination of vasodilators, or an aldosterone antagonist, such as spironolactone. A newer medication, ivabradine, can be added to the regimen for specific patients.

According to the AHRQ guidelines and the ACTION HF recommendations, the HYD/ISDN combination is an appropriate alternative in African-American patients with contraindications to, or intolerance of, ACE-I, although some practitioners continue to use it in all patient populations. There is little evidence to support using nitrates alone or HYD alone in treating HF. Spironolactone at a low dosage of 12.5 to 25 mg once daily should be considered for patients who are receiving standard therapy and who have severe HF (with recent or current NYHA class IV standing) caused by LV systolic dysfunction. Patients should have a normal serum potassium level (5.0 mmol/L) and adequate renal function (serum creatinine 2.5 mg/dL).

Special Populations

Pediatric

Children with HF usually have maturational differences in contractile function or congenital, structural, or genetic heart dysfunction. Drug data for children with HF are not well established. In general, treatment for class I acute HF includes IV inotropes (excluding digoxin) and IV diuretics. For class II failure, digoxin may be added, and for class III, oxygen may be administered. Drug therapy in children is highly individualized according to the child's condition and setting and is usually managed by a specialist in pediatric cardiology.

Geriatric

Because of age-related reductions in renal function, older patients may be particularly susceptible to drug-induced decreases in blood pressure, making careful monitoring essential not only at baseline but also when dosage or drug adjustments are instituted. Blood pressure, renal function, and potassium levels should be monitored regularly. Changes in renal function may also affect the elimination of digoxin, and patients should be monitored for digoxin toxicity and educated to recognize its signs and symptoms.

An important issue in drug therapy for older patients with HF is therapeutic compliance. In one study, investigators identified the primary reason for hospitalization of older patients with HF as noncompliance with diet and medication therapy; moreover, the investigators concluded that up to 40% of readmissions could be prevented by therapeutic compliance and appropriate discharge planning, follow-up, and adequate patient and caregiver education (SOLVD Investigators, 1991).

Women

In pregnant women, ACE-I therapy may pose the risk of congenital birth defects. The same is true for ARB and ARNI therapies. Ivabradine (Corlanor) has also potential for fetal toxicity, and appropriate birth control is necessary. For ACE-I, ARBs, ARNI, and ivabradine if a woman becomes pregnant, the drug should be stopped immediately.

MONITORING PATIENT RESPONSE

A careful history and a physical examination guide outcomes and direct therapy. The patient's symptoms and activities should be explored; any worsening symptom suggests the need to adjust therapy. Although ECG exercise testing is not recommended, repeated testing may be ordered if the patient has a new heart murmur or a new MI or suddenly deteriorates despite compliance with the medication regimen. Serum electrolyte levels, renal function, blood pressure, and diuretic use should be monitored regularly, particularly in patients taking ACE-I. Within 2 weeks of initial ACE-I therapy, serum potassium, creatinine, and BUN measurements should be repeated. If values are stable, monitoring can occur at 3-month intervals or within 1 week of a change in dosage of the ACE-I or diuretic drug.

Response to initial ACE-I therapy should be monitored by blood pressure measurements at 1 to 2 hours (captopril) and 4 to 6 hours for long-acting drugs (enalapril or lisinopril). Blood pressure and heart rate should be monitored for 1 hour after initiating carvedilol to assess tolerance to the drug; clinical reevaluation should occur at each increase in dose and with any worsening of symptoms (increasing fatigue, decreased exercise tolerance, weight gain).

Patients taking spironolactone should have their serum potassium level measured after the first week of therapy, at regular intervals thereafter, and after any change in dose or concomitant medications that may affect potassium balance.

PATIENT EDUCATION

Practitioners must take an active role in patient education to enhance compliance and help prevent medication errors and adverse effects. Patients taking ACE-I, such as captopril and moexipril (Univasc), should take them at least 1 hour before meals. They should also be advised of potential adverse effects, particularly the effects that signal a dangerous reaction: sore throat, fever, swelling of hands or feet, irregular heartbeat, chest pains, and signs of angioedema (swelling of the face, eyes, lips, or tongue; difficulty swallowing or breathing; hoarseness). If these occur, the patient should notify the health care professional at once.

Patients taking diuretics need to know that they can take the medication with food or milk to prevent GI upset, and they can schedule administration so that the need to urinate does not interrupt sleep. Because some diuretics cause photosensitivity, patients should use sunblock or avoid extensive exposure to sunlight. The practitioner can show the patient how to rise slowly from a lying or sitting position to avoid orthostatic hypotension.

Patients need to understand how to monitor their symptoms and weight fluctuations, restrict their sodium intake, take their medications as prescribed, and stay physically active.

Patients taking digoxin should understand that discontinuing the medication can be dangerous and that they should consult their health care provider before doing so. They should avoid taking over-the-counter medications such as antacids, cold and allergy products, and diet drugs. Reportable signs and symptoms are loss of appetite, lower abdominal pain, nausea, vomiting, diarrhea, unusual fatigue or weakness, headache, blurred or yellow vision, rash or hives, or mental depression.

Women of childbearing age need to know that ACE-I and ARBs should be avoided if pregnancy is a possibility. Patients taking spironolactone should know the signs and symptoms to report (muscle weakness or cramps and fatigue).

Nutrition/Lifestyle Changes

Dietary sodium intake should be limited to 2 or 3 g daily. Although a 2-g daily sodium intake is preferred, patient compliance may be poor because most patients find such a diet unpalatable. Patients with mild or moderate (NYHA class II or III) HF may tolerate 3 g daily. Alcohol decreases myocardial contractility, and therefore, consumption of alcoholic beverages should be discouraged or limited to one drink (i.e., a glass of beer or wine or a cocktail containing 1 ounce or less of alcohol) per day. Patients with HF should avoid excessive fluid intake, but fluid restriction is not advisable unless hyponatremia develops.

Patients should stop smoking because cigarettes cause cardiac injury. In addition to pharmacology therapy and lifestyle, revascularization may be necessitated. Some patients with HF experience severe limitation or repeated hospitalizations despite aggressive drug therapy and intervention; thereby, cardiac transplantation may be a reasonable option.

CASE STUDY 1

I.W., aged 62, is a male who is new to your practice. He is reporting shortness of breath on exertion, especially after climbing two to three flights of stairs or walking three to four blocks. His symptoms clear with rest. He also has difficulty sleeping at night (he tells you he needs two pillows to be comfortable).

He tells you that 2 years ago, he suddenly became short of breath after hurrying for an airplane. He was admitted to a hospital and treated for acute pulmonary edema. Three days before the episode of pulmonary edema, he had an upper respiratory tract infection with fever and mild cough. After the episode of pulmonary edema, his blood pressure has been consistently elevated. His previous physician started him on a sustained-release preparation of diltiazem 180 mg/d. His medical history includes moderate prostatic hypertrophy for 5 years, adult-onset diabetes mellitus for 10 years, hypertension for 10 years, and degenerative joint disease for 5 years. His medication history includes hydrochlorothiazide (HydroDIURIL) 50 mg orally daily, carvedilol (Coreg) 25 mg immediate-release orally twice daily, controlled-delivery diltiazem 180 mg orally daily, glyburide (DiaBeta) 5 mg orally daily, and indomethacin (Indocin) 25 to 50 mg orally thrice daily as needed for pain. While reviewing his medical records, you see that his last physical examination revealed a blood pressure of 160/95 mm Hg, a pulse of 95 bpm, a respiratory rate of 18, normal peripheral pulses, mild edema bilaterally in his feet, a prominent S3 and S4, neck vein distention, and an enlarged liver (Learning Objectives 1–3).

DIAGNOSIS: HEART FAILURE CLASS II

1. List specific goals of treatment for I.W.
2. What drug(s) would you prescribe? Why?
3. What are the parameters for monitoring the success of your selected therapy?
4. Discuss specific patient education based on the prescribed therapy.
5. Describe one or two drug–drug or drug–food interactions for the selected agent(s).
6. List one or two adverse reactions for the selected agent(s) that would cause you to change therapy.
7. What would be the choice for the second-line therapy?
8. What over-the-counter (OTC) or alternative medications would be appropriate for this patient?
9. What dietary and lifestyle changes should be recommended for I.W.?

Bibliography

Starred references are cited in the text.

Ahmed, A., & Dell'Italia, L. J. (2004). Use of beta-blockers in older adults with chronic heart failure. *American Journal of the Medical Sciences, 328*(2), 100–111.

*Amiodarone Trials Meta-Analysis Investigators. (1997). Effect of prophylactic amiodarone on mortality after acute myocardial infarction and in congestive heart failure: Meta-analysis of individual data from 6500 patients in randomized trials. *Lancet, 350,* 1417–1424.

Anderson, J., Jacobs, A., Albert, N., et al. (2013). 2013 ACCF/AHA guideline for the management of heart failure. *Journal of the American College of Cardiology, 62*(16), 147–239. doi: 10.1016/j.jacc.2013.05.019

*Bahrami, H., Kronmal, R., Bluemke, D. A., et al. (2008). Differences in the incidence of congestive heart failure by ethnicity: The multi-ethnic study of atherosclerosis. *Archives of Internal Medicine, 168*(19), 2138–2145. doi: 10.1001/archinte.168.19.2138

*Benjamin, E. J., Munter, P., Alonso, A., et al. (2019). Heart disease and stroke statistics—2019 update: A report from the American Heart Association. *Circulation, 139,* e56–e528.

*Braunwald, E. (2015). Clinical manifestations of heart failure. In E. Braunwald (Ed.), *Heart disease* (pp. 471–484). Philadelphia, PA: W.B. Saunders.

*Dandona, P., Ghanim, H., & Brooks, D. P. (2007). Antioxidant activity of carvedilol in cardiovascular disease. *Journal of Hypertension, 25*, 731–741.

*Diaz, A., & Ducharme, A. (2008). Update on the use of trandolapril in the management of cardiovascular disorders. *Vascular Health and Risk Management, 4*(6), 1147–1158.

*Digitalis Investigation Group. (1997). The effect of digoxin on mortality and morbidity in patients with heart failure. *New England Journal of Medicine, 336*, 525–533.

*Doughty, R. N., Whalley, G. A., Walsh, H. A., et al. (2004). CAPRICORN Echo Substudy Investigators. Effects of carvedilol on left ventricular remodeling after acute myocardial infarction: The CAPRICORN Echo Substudy. *Circulation, 109*, 201–206.

*Doval, H. C., Nul, D. R., Grancelli, H. O., et al. (1994). Randomized trial of low-dose amiodarone in severe congestive heart failure. *Lancet, 344*, 493–498.

*Gheorghiade, M., Cody, R. J., Francis, G. S., et al. (1998). Current medical therapy for advanced heart failure. *American Heart Journal, 135*, S2231–S2248.

*Go, A. S., Mozaffarian, D., Roger, V. L., et al. (2013). Heart disease and stroke statistics—2013 update: A report from the American Heart Association. *Circulation, 127*(1), e6–e245.

Gottlieb, S. S., Dickstein, K., Fleck, E., et al. (1993). Hemodynamic and neurohormonal effects of the angiotensin II antagonist losartan in patients with congestive heart failure. *Circulation, 88*, 1602–1609.

Kober, L., Torp-Pedersen, C., Carlsen, J. E., et al. (1995). A clinical trial of the angiotensin-converting-enzyme inhibitor trandolapril in patients with left ventricular dysfunction after myocardial infarction. *New England Journal of Medicine, 333*, 1670–1676.

Konstam, M. A., Neaton, J. D., Dickstein, K., et al. (2009). Effects of high-dose versus low-dose losartan on clinical outcomes in patients with heart failure (HEAAL study): A randomised, double-blind trial. *Lancet, 374*, 1840–1848.

Krum, H., & Teerlink, J. (2011). Heart failure 2: Medical therapy for chronic heart failure. *Lancet, 378*, 713–721.

*Lopes, R. D., Rordorf, R., De Ferrari, G. M., et al. (2018). Digoxin and mortality in patients with atrial fibrillation. *Journal of the American College of Cardiology, 71*(10), 1063–1074.

Margo, K., Luttermoser, G., & Shaugnessy, A. (2001). Spironolactone in left-sided heart failure: How does it fit in? *American Family Physician, 64*(8), 1393–1398, 1399.

*Masoudi, F., Rathore, S., Wang, Y., et al. (2004). National patterns of use and effectiveness of angiotensin-converting enzyme inhibitors in older patients with heart failure and left ventricular systolic dysfunction. *Circulation, 110*, 724–731. doi: 10.1161/01.CIR.0000138934.28340.ED

*McMurray, J. J. V., Packer, M., Desai, A. S., et al. (2014). Angiotensin–neprilysin inhibition versus enalapril in heart failure. *New England Journal of Medicine, 371*, 993–1004.

Nair, A., Timoh, T., & Fuster, V. (2012). Contemporary medical management of systolic heart failure. *Circulation, 76*, 268–277.

*Packer, M., & Cohn, J. N., on behalf of the Steering Committee and Membership of the Advisory Council to Improve Outcomes Nationwide in Heart Failure. (1999). Consensus recommendations for the management of chronic heart failure. *American Journal of Cardiology, 83*, 1A–38A.

Packer, M., O'Connor, C. M., Ghali, J. K., et al., for the Prospective Randomized Amlodipine Survival Evaluation Study Group. (1996). Effect of amlodipine on morbidity and mortality in severe chronic heart failure. *New England Journal of Medicine, 335*, 1107–1114.

*Pagell, R. L., O'Bryant, C. L., Cheng, D., et al. (2016). Drugs that may cause or exacerbate heart failure, a scientific statement from the American Heart Association. *Circulation, 134*, e32–e69.

*Pasternak, B., Svanström, H., Melbye, M., et al. (2014). Association of treatment with carvedilol vs metoprolol succinate and mortality in patients with heart failure. *JAMA Internal Medicine, 174*(10), 1597–1604. doi: 10.1001/jamainternmed.2014.3258

*Pitt, B., Pfeffer, M., Assmann, S., et al. (2014). Spironolactone for heart failure with preserved ejection fraction. *New England Journal of Medicine, 370*(15), 1383–1392. doi: 10.1056/NEJMoa1313731

Pitt, B., Segal, R., Martinez, F. A., et al. (1997). Randomised trial of losartan versus captopril in patients over 65 with heart failure (Evaluation of Losartan in the Elderly Study, ELITE). *Lancet, 349*, 747–752.

*Pitt, B., Zannad, F., Remme, W. J., et al. (1999). The effect of spironolactone on morbidity and mortality in patients with severe heart failure. *New England Journal of Medicine, 341*(10), 709–717.

Pressler, S. J., Subramanian, U., Kareken, D., et al. (2010). Cognitive deficits and health-related quality of life in chronic heart failure. *Journal of Cardiovascular Nursing, 25*(3), 189–198.

*Savarese, G., Costanzo, P., Cleland, J. G., et al. (2013). A meta-analysis reporting effects of angiotensin-converting enzyme inhibitors and angiotension receptor blockers in patients without heart failure. *Journal American College of Cardiology, 61*(3), 131–142. doi: 10.1016/j.jacc.2012.10.011

*Singh, S. N., Fletcher, R. D., Fischer, S. G., et al. (1995). Amiodarone in patients with congestive heart failure and symptomatic ventricular arrhythmias. *New England Journal of Medicine, 333*, 77–82.

Smith, T. W., Braunwald, E., & Kelly, R. A. (2015). The management of heart failure. In E. Braunwald (Ed.), *Heart disease* (pp. 485–543). Philadelphia, PA: W.B. Saunders.

*Solomon, S. D., McMurray, J. J. V., Anand, I. S., et al. (2019). Angiotensin-neprilysin inhibition in heart failure with preserved ejection fraction. *New England Journal of Medicine, 381*(17), 1609–1620.

*SOLVD Investigators. (1991). Effect of enalapril on survival in patients with reduced left ventricular ejection fractions and HF. *New England Journal of Medicine, 3325*, 303–310.

*Velazquez, E. J., Morrow, D. A., DeVore, A. D., et al. (2019). Angiotensin-neprilysin inhibition in acute decompensated heart failure. *New England Journal of Medicine, 380*(6), 539–548.

*Yancy, C. W., Jessup, M., Bozkurt, B., et al. (2013). 2013 ACCF/AHA guideline for the management of heart failure. *Journal of the American College of Cardiology, 62*(16), e147–e239.

*Yancy, C. W., Jessup, M., Bozkurt, B., et al. (2016). 2016 ACC/AHA/HFSA focused update on new pharmacological therapy for heart failure: An update of the 2013 ACCF/AHA guideline for the management of heart failure. *Journal of the American College of Cardiology, 68*(13), 1476–1488.

*Yancy, C. W., Jessup, M., Bozkurt, B., et al. (2017). 2017 ACC/AHA/HFSA focused update of the 2013 ACCF/AHA guideline for the management of heart failure: A report of the American College of Cardiology/American Heart Association Task Force on Clinical Practice Guidelines and the Heart Failure Society of America. *Circulation, 136*(6), e137–e161.

22 Arrhythmias

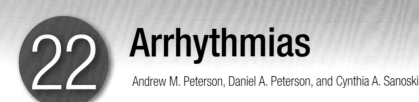

Andrew M. Peterson, Daniel A. Peterson, and Cynthia A. Sanoski

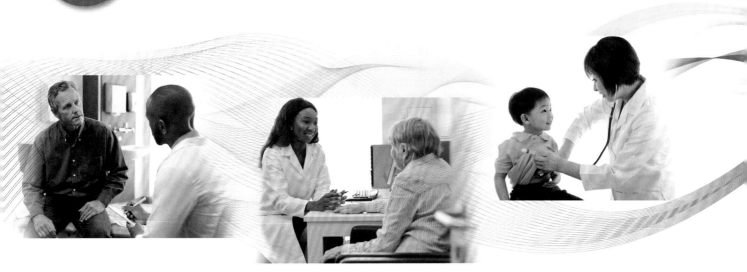

Learning Objectives

1. Describe the mechanisms that cause cardiac arrhythmias.
2. Identify the Vaughan Williams classification of at least three different drugs used in the treatment of arrhythmias.
3. Discuss the basic pharmacological and pharmacokinetic profile of specific antiarrhythmic agents.
4. Select the first-line treatment for common ventricular and supraventricular arrhythmias.
5. Identify common adverse effects of antiarrhythmic agents.

INTRODUCTION

Cardiac arrhythmias are abnormal cardiac rhythms, including tachyarrhythmias (an increase in heart rate) and bradyarrhythmias (a decrease in heart rate). Arrhythmias may be asymptomatic or symptomatic, causing palpitations, weakness, loss of consciousness, heart failure (HF), and sudden death. Searching for a reversible cause of the arrhythmia is the first step in patient care. However, in many cases, antiarrhythmic drugs (AADs) are necessary to permit stabilization until the underlying condition is normalized. Many patients require chronic drug therapy for an arrhythmia due to an underlying disease condition that makes them chronically susceptible to cardiac arrhythmias that are associated with high morbidity and mortality rates.

CAUSES

Arrhythmias may result from structural or electrical/conduction system changes in the heart that may compromise cardiac function and cardiac output. Conditions that give rise to arrhythmias include myocardial ischemia, chronic HF, hypertension, valvular heart disease, hypoxemia, thyroid abnormalities, electrolyte disturbances, drug toxicity, excessive caffeine or ethanol ingestion, anxiety, and exercise. Some of these conditions are reversible, and some cause structural changes that are not reversible.

PATHOPHYSIOLOGY

Basic Electrophysiology

Electrically active myocardial cells (non-pacemaker-type cells) at rest maintain a potential difference between their intracellular fluid and the extracellular fluid. When excited, these cells manifest a characteristic sequence of transmembrane potential changes called the *action potential*. The resting membrane potential is –90 mV with respect to the extracellular fluid. The activity of the sodium–potassium pump and the permeability of the membrane to sodium, potassium, and calcium ions determine the membrane potential of a cardiac cell at any given time. Permeability is defined by the diffusion of ions across the membrane through various ion-selective channels. The phases of the action potential correspond to the excitation state of a myocardial cell (**Box 22.1**).

BOX 22.1   Phases of the Action Potential

- **Phase 0** is when rapid depolarization occurs due to the rapid influx of Na⁺.
- **Phase 1** is a brief initial repolarization period. Inactivation of the inward Na⁺ current and activation of the outward K⁺ current cause this brief but rapid phase of repolarization.
- **Phase 2** is a plateau period during which there is little change in membrane potential. The outward K⁺ current and the influx of Ca²⁺ through calcium channels typify the plateau period. The offsetting effect of these currents creates only a small net change in potential, thus creating a plateau.
- **Phase 3** is a period of repolarization that is characterized primarily by K⁺ efflux.
- **Phase 4** is a gradual depolarization of the cell, with Na⁺ gradually leaking into the intracellular space, balanced by decreasing efflux of K⁺. As the cell is slowly depolarized during this phase, an increase in Na⁺ permeability occurs, which again leads to phase 0.

Arrhythmias can result from disorders of impulse formation and/or impulse conduction. Several factors are believed to be involved in precipitating arrhythmias. There may be a defect in the normal mechanism of spontaneous phase 4 depolarization or an increased automaticity of pacemaker cells. In addition, ectopic pacemakers in normally quiescent tissue are responsible for arrhythmias originating from disorders of impulse formation. Impulse conduction defects occur when the impulse is slowed or blocked because of functional unidirectional block, a change in conduction velocity, or a change in the refractory period. Furthermore, simultaneous abnormalities of impulse formation and conduction may occur.

AADs are used to treat abnormal electrical activity of the heart. The drugs outlined in this chapter are used to treat, suppress, or prevent two major mechanisms of arrhythmias—an abnormality in impulse formation (i.e., increased automaticity) or an abnormality in impulse conduction (i.e., reentry).

Automaticity

Automaticity refers to the ability of the cardiac cells to depolarize spontaneously. Three factors determine automaticity: maximum diastolic depolarization, the rate of depolarization, and the level of the threshold potential. Arrhythmias resulting from abnormal automaticity include sinus tachycardia and junctional tachycardia. The sinoatrial (SA) node has the most rapid rate of depolarization during diastole and reaches threshold first. Cells of the atrioventricular (AV) node and

His–Purkinje system have automaticity but a slower rate of phase 4 depolarization. The primary role of the SA node is as the pacemaker of the heart. The SA node is sensitive to alterations in autonomic nervous system output and in its biochemical surroundings. Catecholamine stimulation leads to a shorter action potential duration and increases the spontaneous rate of depolarization. Vagal stimulus and endogenous purines such as adenosine increase outward potassium currents, thus inhibiting depolarization. Increased adrenergic innervation produces major changes in ionic current activity in the SA node.

Another mechanism for arrhythmias due to abnormal impulse formation is intracellular calcium overload, called *after-depolarization*. If after-depolarizations reach threshold, a new action potential is generated and propagated in adjacent cells. After-depolarizations may occur in response to hypothermia, electrolyte imbalance, catecholamine excess, or stretch. Late after-depolarizations may also be of particular importance in some of the arrhythmias caused by digoxin toxicity.

Reentry

Reentry involves indefinite propagation of the impulse and continued activation of previously refractory tissue. Reentrant foci occur if there are two pathways for impulse conduction: an area of unidirectional block (prolonged refractoriness) in one of these pathways and slow conduction in the other pathway. A refractory period occurs when the cell cannot be activated after having already fired. Excitability determines the strength of a stimulus required to initiate a new action potential at any given point during the action potential cycle.

Types of Arrhythmias

Arrhythmias evolve either above or below the ventricles and can be regular or irregular. *Supraventricular arrhythmias* evolve above the ventricles in the atria, SA node, or AV node. These arrhythmias may present with either tachycardia or bradycardia or with regularity or irregularity. *AV nodal arrhythmias* originate at or within the AV node and are caused by delayed or absent SA node conduction to the AV node. Supraventricular and AV nodal arrhythmias are not usually life threatening; however, they may become troublesome and lead to reduced cardiac output related to decreased ventricular filling.

Ventricular arrhythmias originate in the ventricles or the bundle of His. These types of arrhythmias are usually symptomatic and may cause loss of consciousness or death. Therefore, arrhythmias in this category require immediate intervention. Underlying clinical conditions that usually give rise to these arrhythmias are myocardial ischemia/infarction, dilated and hypertrophic cardiomyopathies, electrolyte disorders, hypoxia, hyperthyroidism, valvular diseases, and drug toxicity. **Box 22.2** lists arrhythmias by category.

BOX 22.2 Categories of Supraventricular, Junctional, and Ventricular Arrhythmias

SUPRAVENTRICULAR ARRHYTHMIAS

AF
AFl
Atrial tachycardia
PSVT (originates above or within the AV node and conducts
    to the His–Purkinje system) (e.g., AV nodal reentrant
    tachycardia, AV reentrant tachycardia)
Premature atrial contractions
Sinus bradycardia
Sinus tachycardia
WPW syndrome

JUNCTIONAL ARRHYTHMIAS

AV dissociation
First-degree heart block
Junctional escape rhythm (heart rate 40–60 beats/min)
Nonparoxysmal AV junctional tachycardia (heart rate >
    60 beats/min)
Premature AV junctional complexes
Second-degree heart block (Mobitz type 1 [Wenckebach],
    Mobitz type 2)
Third-degree (complete) heart block

VENTRICULAR ARRHYTHMIAS

PVCs
TdP (a rapid form of polymorphic VT associated with a long
    QT interval)
VF
Ventricular tachycardia

DIAGNOSTIC CRITERIA

The practitioner must first assess the patient via a thorough and sometimes urgent history and physical examination. There may be no symptoms, or the patient may present with symptoms such as chest pain, shortness of breath, decreased level of consciousness, syncope, confusion, diaphoresis, weakness, and palpitations. The practitioner should ask when the symptoms started, how long they have lasted, their frequency, and how the patient tolerated the symptoms.

It is also important to assess the patient's risk factors for development of arrhythmias, such as previous coronary artery disease (CAD), myocardial infarction (MI), dilated or hypertrophic cardiomyopathy, hypertension, valvular heart disease, alcohol or drug abuse, or prescription drug use (e.g., digoxin, AADs). The practitioner should focus the physical examination on heart rate and blood pressure; presence of extra, irregular, or skipped beats; rate, rhythm, amplitude, and symmetry of peripheral pulses; and response to exercise.

Laboratory and diagnostic studies are also vital in diagnosing arrhythmias. The practitioner should examine the 12-lead electrocardiogram (EKG) for evidence of myocardial ischemia; calculation of the PR interval, QRS interval, and QT interval; presence of premature atrial or ventricular contractions; characteristics of Wolff-Parkinson-White (WPW) syndrome; presence or absence of P waves; and relationship between P waves and QRS complexes. Continuous cardiac monitoring is needed for patients who have episodes of life-threatening arrhythmias so that electrical cardioversion and/or AADs can be administered as immediate interventions.

A complete blood count, basic metabolic profile (to assess electrolyte concentrations), thyroid function tests, and a digoxin level should be performed as necessary to determine any underlying causes of the arrhythmia. In addition, an echocardiogram should be performed to assess left ventricular (LV) function. If myocardial ischemia is suspected as a cause of the arrhythmia, the patient should undergo further evaluation with measurement of cardiac enzymes, performance of cardiac stress testing, and, possibly, cardiac catheterization.

INITIATING DRUG THERAPY

During the past several decades, the treatment approach for both atrial and ventricular arrhythmias has been gradually shifting away from the use of AADs toward the use of various nonpharmacological therapies. Several factors have likely contributed to the decline in AAD use over the years. The negative results of the Cardiac Arrhythmia Suppression Trial (CAST) likely had a significant influence on the downward prescribing patterns of class I AADs. In addition, increasing clinical evidence to support the use of nonpharmacological strategies for the treatment of both supraventricular and ventricular arrhythmias has likely contributed to the decline in the use of AADs as a whole. It is now well established that a rhythm-control regimen does not confer any benefit over a rate-control regimen in patients with persistent atrial fibrillation (AF), and this fact may have also contributed to the decline in AAD use.

Treatable conditions may cause the arrhythmia. Identification of treatable causes before administering an AAD is a priority. Conditions that may cause arrhythmias are electrolyte imbalances (e.g., hypokalemia, hypomagnesemia), drug overdose, drug interactions with other medications or herbal supplements, renal failure, thyroid disorders, metabolic acidosis, hypovolemia, MI, pulmonary embolism, cardiac tamponade, tension pneumothorax, dissecting aortic aneurysm, hypoxemia, and valvular or congenital defects in the heart.

Nonpharmacological therapies, such as radiofrequency catheter ablation and implantable cardioverter–defibrillators (ICDs), are also available to treat various arrhythmias. ICDs are used in the management of ventricular arrhythmias, and their benefits have been demonstrated in several clinical trials (Antiarrhythmics Versus Implantable Defibrillators Investigators, 1997; Bardy et al., 2005; Buxton et al., 1999; Connolly et al., 2000; Kuck et al., 2000; Moss et al., 1996, 2002). Radiofrequency catheter ablation permanently terminates the arrhythmia by ablating the focal area where the arrhythmia occurs. This procedure can be used for AF, atrial flutter (AFl), and symptomatic drug-refractory ventricular tachycardia (VT).

Goals of Antiarrhythmic Drug Therapy

The overall goals of AAD therapy are to relieve the acute episode of irregular rhythm, establish sinus rhythm (SR), and prevent further episodes of the arrhythmia. Typical agents used to treat arrhythmias include AADs (classes I–IV), digoxin, adenosine, and atropine (**Table 22.1**).

Drug Classification

AADs are organized into four classes: I (Ia, Ib, and Ic), II, III, and IV (Vaughan Williams, 1984). Although the Vaughan Williams classification system is the most widely used method for grouping AADs based on their electrophysiologic actions, using this classification system requires some points of exception to be made. This system is somewhat incomplete, and it excludes certain drugs including digoxin, adenosine, and atropine. In addition, the classification is not pure, and there is some overlapping of drugs into more than one category. For instance,

TABLE 22.1

Overview of Selected Antiarrhythmic Agents

Generic (Trade) Name and Dosage	Selected Adverse Effects	Contraindications	Special Considerations
Adenosine (Adenocard) Adult: 6 mg IV push over 1–2 s; repeat with 12 mg IV push if sinus rhythm not obtained within 1–2 min after first dose; may repeat 12-mg dose a second time if no response in 1–2 min	Headache, chest pain, light-headedness, dizziness, nausea, flushing, dyspnea, blurred vision	2nd-/3rd-degree heart block or sick sinus syndrome in the absence of a pacemaker	Monitor EKG during administration. Use cautiously in patients with asthma (bronchoconstriction may occur). Each dose should be immediately followed with a 20-mL saline flush.
Amiodarone (Cordarone, Nexterone, Pacerone) *AF* Adult IV: 150 mg over 10 min, then continuous infusion of 1 mg/min for 6 h, and then 0.5 mg/min; convert to PO when hemodynamically stable and able to take PO medications Adult PO: 400 mg BID–TID for 1 wk, until patient receives ~10 g total and then 200 mg PO daily *Pulseless VT/VF* Adult IV: 300 mg IV push/IO; can give additional 150 mg IV push/IO if persistent VT/VF; if stable rhythm achieved, initiate continuous infusion at 1 mg/min for 6 h and then 0.5 mg/min; convert to PO when hemodynamically stable and able to take PO medications (see PO dose under stable VT) *Stable VT (with a pulse)* Adult IV: 150 mg (diluted in 100 mL of D5W or saline) over 10 min; may repeat dose q10min, if necessary, for breakthrough VT; if stable rhythm achieved, initiate continuous infusion at 1 mg/min for 6 h and then 0.5 mg/min; convert to PO when hemodynamically stable and able to take PO medications Adult PO: 1,200–1,600 mg/d in 2 or 3 divided doses for 1 wk and then 200–400 mg PO daily	IV: hypotension, bradycardia, heart block, phlebitis PO: corneal microdeposits, optic neuritis, nausea, vomiting, anorexia, pulmonary fibrosis, bradycardia, tremor, ataxia, paresthesias, insomnia, constipation, abnormal liver function tests, hypothyroidism, hyperthyroidism, blue-gray discoloration of skin, photosensitivity	2nd-/3rd-degree heart block or sick sinus syndrome in the absence of a pacemaker or bradycardia (in the absence of a pacemaker); cardiogenic shock; hypersensitivity to iodine	Advise patient to apply sunscreen and to minimize areas of exposure to sun. Patients should have chest X-ray performed annually. Liver function and thyroid function tests should be performed every 6 months. Pulmonary function tests and ophthalmologic exam should be performed if patient becomes symptomatic. A chest X-ray, pulmonary function tests, liver function tests, and thyroid function tests should also be performed at baseline. An ophthalmologic exam should be performed at baseline if the patient has significant visual abnormalities. Monitor for drug interactions (CYP3A4 substrate; CYP3A4, 2C9, 2D6, and P-gp inhibitor).
Atropine Adult: 0.5 mg IV q3–5min; not to exceed 3 mg total dose	Palpitations, tachycardia, dry mouth, dizziness	Acute angle-closure glaucoma, obstructive uropathy, tachycardia, obstructive disease of GI tract	Administer IV over 1 min. Monitor EKG during administration.

TABLE 22.1

Overview of Selected Antiarrhythmic Agents (*Continued*)

Generic (Trade) Name and Dosage	Selected Adverse Effects	Contraindications	Special Considerations
Digoxin (Lanoxin) Adult LD (IV or PO): 0.25–0.5 mg over 2 min; may give 0.25 mg q6h to a max of 1.5 mg in 24 h Adult MD: 0.125–0.25 mg IV or PO daily in normal renal function	Anorexia, nausea, vomiting, diarrhea, headache, dizziness, vertigo, visual disturbances (yellow-green halos), confusion, hallucinations, arrhythmias, AV conduction disturbances (heart block, AV junctional rhythm, bradycardia)	2nd-/3rd-degree heart block or sick sinus syndrome in the absence of a pacemaker and VF	Teach patient how to take pulse. Dose adjustment required in renal impairment. Monitor for drug interactions (P-gp substrate).
Diltiazem (Cardizem) Adult IV: 0.25 mg/kg over 2 min; if ventricular rate remains uncontrolled after 15 min, can repeat with 0.35 mg/kg over 2 min; then initiate continuous infusion of 5–15 mg/h Adult PO: Start with 30 mg QID and ↑ to 180–480 mg/d in divided doses (sustained-release can be given once daily)	Dizziness, headache, edema, heart block, bradycardia, HF exacerbation, hypotension	2nd-/3rd-degree heart block or sick sinus syndrome in the absence of a pacemaker, LVSD, acute MI and pulmonary congestion. Severe hypotension (SBP <90 mm Hg)	Teach patient how to take pulse and blood pressure. Monitor for drug interactions (CYP3A4 substrate and inhibitor).
Disopyramide (Norpace) Adult (<50 kg): IR: 100 mg PO q6h; sustained-release: 200 mg PO q12h Adult (>50 kg): IR: 150 mg PO q6h; sustained-release: 300 mg PO q12h; may ↑ up to 800 mg/d	Hypotension, HF exacerbation, nausea, anorexia, dry mouth, urinary retention, blurred vision, TdP	2nd-/3rd-degree heart block or sick sinus syndrome in the absence of a pacemaker, LVSD; congenital long QT syndrome, cardiogenic shock	Dose adjustment required in renal impairment (CrCl ≤ 40 mL/min; sustained-release form not recommended when CrCl ≤ 40 mL/min). Monitor for drug interactions (CYP3A4 substrate).
Dofetilide (Tikosyn) Adult: 125–500 mcg PO BID	Chest pain, headache, dizziness, insomnia, nausea, diarrhea, dyspnea, TdP	CrCl <20 mL/min, QT interval >440 msec, concomitant use of cimetidine, dolutegravir, hydrochlorothiazide, itraconazole, ketoconazole, megestrol, prochlorperazine, QTc-prolonging drugs, trimethoprim/ sulfamethoxazole, or verapamil Congenital or acquired long QT syndrome	Patients must be hospitalized for ≥3 days for therapy initiation. Dose adjustment required in renal impairment (CrCl ≤ 60 mL/min). Dose must also be adjusted based on QT interval. Monitor for drug interactions.
Dronedarone (Multaq) Adult: 400 mg PO BID (with meals)	Nausea, vomiting, diarrhea, HF exacerbation, hepatic impairment, pulmonary toxicity, renal impairment/failure	Permanent AF, NYHA class IV HF, NYHA class II–III HF with recent hospitalization for decompensated HF, 2nd-/3rd-degree heart block or sick sinus syndrome in the absence of a pacemaker, heart rate < 50 beats/min, concurrent use of potent CYP3A4 inhibitors or QTc-prolonging drugs, QT interval ≥ 500 msec, PR interval > 280 msec, severe hepatic impairment, history of amiodarone-induced hepatic or pulmonary toxicity. Pregnancy and nursing mothers	Instruct patient to report adverse reactions or any signs/symptoms of HF immediately. Monitor for drug interactions (CYP3A4 substrate; CYP2D6, CYP3A4, and P-gp inhibitor).

(Continued)

TABLE 22.1

Overview of Selected Antiarrhythmic Agents (*Continued*)

Generic (Trade) Name and Dosage	Selected Adverse Effects	Contraindications	Special Considerations
Esmolol (Brevibloc) Adult: 500 mcg/kg/min IV for 1 min and then maintenance infusion of 50 mcg/kg/min; if inadequate response, rebolus with 500 mcg/kg/min for 1 min and ↑ infusion rate by 50 mcg/kg/min; repeat this process until desired response achieved or maximum infusion rate of 300 mcg/kg/min is reached	Hypotension, heart block, bradycardia, HF exacerbation	2nd-/3rd-degree heart block in the absence of a pacemaker, decompensated HF, sinus bradycardia, cardiogenic shock, pulmonary hypertension. Avoid IV administration of calcium channel blockers in close proximity to esmolol	Use with caution in patients with LVSD.
Flecainide Adult: 50 mg PO q12h up to a maximum of 300 mg/d	Dizziness, headache, light-headedness, syncope, blurred vision or other visual disturbances, dyspnea, HF exacerbation, arrhythmias	2nd-/3rd-degree heart block in the absence of a pacemaker, recent MI, ischemic heart disease, cardiogenic shock, HF, bundle branch block, congenital/acquired long QT prolongation with history of TdP. Concurrent use of ritonavir	Dose adjustment required in renal impairment (CrCl ≤35 mL/min) Monitor for drug interactions (CYP2D6 substrate).
Ibutilide (Corvert) Adult (<60 kg): 0.01 mg/kg IV over 10 min; can repeat with another dose if AF/AFl does not terminate within 10 min after end of initial dose Adult (≥60 kg): 1 mg IV over 10 min; can repeat with another dose if AF/AFl does not terminate within 10 min after end of initial dose	TdP, hypotension, heart block, headache, nausea	Sinus node disease, prolonged QT interval, hypersensitivity to ibutilide	Monitor EKG during administration. Stop infusion if QT interval prolongation or ventricular arrhythmias occur. Correct electrolyte abnormalities before administering.
Lidocaine (Xylocaine) *Pulseless VT/VF* Adult: 1–1.5 mg/kg IV push/IO; may give additional 0.5–0.75 mg/kg IV push/IO q5–10min, if persistent VT/VF (maximum cumulative dose = 3 mg/kg); if stable rhythm achieved, initiate continuous infusion of 1–4 mg/min *Stable VT (with a pulse)* Adult: 1–1.5 mg/kg IV push; may give additional 0.5–0.75 mg/kg IV push q5–10min, if persistent VT (maximum cumulative dose = 3 mg/kg); if stable rhythm achieved, initiate continuous infusion of 1–4 mg/min	Seizures, confusion, stupor, dizziness, bradycardia, respiratory depression, slurred speech, blurred vision, muscle twitching, tinnitus	Hypersensitivity to amide local anesthetics, 2nd-/3rd-degree heart block in the absence of a pacemaker. Wolff-Parkinson-White syndrome	A lower infusion rate (1–2 mg/min) should be used in older adults or patients with HF or hepatic disease. Monitor for drug interactions (CYP1A2 and CYP3A4 substrate)
Metoprolol (Lopressor) Adult IV: 2.5–5 mg over 2 min; can repeat q5min (maximum cumulative dose = 15 mg over 10- to 15-min period) Adult PO: IR: 25 mg BID; sustained-release: 50 mg daily; may ↑ up to 400 mg/d	Bradycardia, HF exacerbation, heart block, bronchospasm, fatigue, ↓ exercise tolerance, dizziness, hypotension	2nd-/3rd-degree heart block in the absence of a pacemaker, decompensated HF, heart rate <45 beats/min	Use IV with caution in patients with LVSD. Teach patient how to take pulse and blood pressure. Instruct patient to not discontinue drug abruptly (may lead to hypertensive crises, angina, or MI). Use metoprolol succinate (sustained-release) when initiating PO therapy in patients with LVSD.

TABLE 22.1

Overview of Selected Antiarrhythmic Agents (*Continued*)

Generic (Trade) Name and Dosage	Selected Adverse Effects	Contraindications	Special Considerations
Mexiletine Adult: 150–200 mg PO q8h; may ↑ up to 400 mg PO q8h	Dizziness, drowsiness, paresthesias, blurred vision, tremor, seizures, confusion, arrhythmias, nausea, vomiting	2nd-/3rd-degree heart block in the absence of a pacemaker, cardiogenic shock	Monitor for drug interactions (CYP1A2 and CYP2D6 substrate).
Procainamide Adult: 10–17 mg/kg IV at a rate of 20–50 mg/min and then continuous infusion of 1–4 mg/min	Bradycardia, heart block, hypotension, HF exacerbation, TdP	Hypersensitivity to procaine, 2nd-/3rd-degree heart block in the absence of a pacemaker. Systemic lupus erythematosus, TdP	Monitor EKG during administration. Stop infusion if QT interval prolongation or ventricular arrhythmias occur. Use with caution, if at all, in renal impairment.
Propafenone (Rythmol) Adult: IR: 150 mg PO q8h (up to a maximum of 300 mg PO q8h); sustained-release: 225 mg PO q12h (up to a maximum of 425 mg PO q12h)	Dizziness, drowsiness, HF exacerbation, blurred vision, arrhythmias, heart block, bradycardia, taste disturbances, bronchospasm	2nd-/3rd-degree heart block in the absence of a pacemaker, bradycardia, cardiogenic shock, HF, bronchospastic disorders	Teach patient how to take pulse and blood pressure. Instruct patient to not discontinue drug abruptly (may lead to hypertensive crises, angina, or MI).
Propranolol Adult IV: 1 mg over 1 min; may repeat q5min up to a total dose of 5 mg In combination with an IV antiarrhytmic, adult PO: IR: 10–40 mg q6h, ER: 60–160 mg q12h; can ↑ to 80–240 mg/d in 2–4 divided doses	Bradycardia, HF exacerbation, heart block, bronchospasm, fatigue, ↓ exercise tolerance, dizziness, hypotension	2nd-/3rd-degree heart block or sick sinus syndrome in the absence of a pacemaker, LVSD, decompensated HR, cardiogenic shock Relatively contraindicated in asthma	Teach patient how to take pulse and blood pressure. Instruct patient to not discontinue drug abruptly (may lead to hypertensive crises, angina, or MI).
Quinidine Adult: Sulfate: 200–400 mg PO q6h, up to a maximum of 600 mg PO q6h Gluconate: 324 mg PO q8–12h, up to a maximum of 648 mg PO q8–12h	TdP, heart block, hypotension, tinnitus, diarrhea, nausea, vomiting, fever, HF exacerbation, thrombocytopenia	Allergy or sensitivity to quinidine or cinchona derivatives, long QT syndrome (may predispose to TdP) Thrombocytopenia, myasthenia gravis, concurrent use of quinolone antibiotics, cisapride, amprenavir or ritonavir	Instruct patient to take drug with food if GI distress occurs. Monitor for drug interactions (CYP3A4 substrate; CYP2D6 inhibitor).
Sotalol (Betapace, Betapace AF) *AF (Betapace AF)* Adult: 80 mg PO BID, up to a maximum of 160 mg PO BID *Ventricular Arrhythmias (Betapace)* Adult: 80 mg PO BID, up to a maximum of 160 mg PO BID	Bradycardia, heart block, HF exacerbation, TdP, bronchospasm	2nd-/3rd-degree heart block in the absence of a pacemaker, bradycardia, HF, asthma, long QT syndrome (may predispose to TdP), cardiogenic shock. Serum potassium <4 mEq/L	Patients must be hospitalized for ≥3 days for therapy initiation. Teach patient how to take pulse and blood pressure. Dose adjustment required in renal impairment (CrCl ≤ 60 mL/min) Instruct patient to not discontinue drug abruptly (may lead to hypertensive crises, angina, or MI).

(Continued)

TABLE 22.1

Overview of Selected Antiarrhythmic Agents (*Continued*)

Generic (Trade) Name and Dosage	Selected Adverse Effects	Contraindications	Special Considerations
Verapamil (Calan) Adult IV: 5–10 mg over 2 min; if ventricular rate remains uncontrolled after 15–30 min, dose may be repeated. If adequate response, then initiate continuous infusion of 5 mg/h to goal HR; may increase to 20 mg/h as needed. Adult PO: 120–180 mg/d in 3–4 divided doses (sustained-release can be given once daily) to a maximum of 480 mg/day	Constipation, bradycardia, heart block, HF exacerbation, hypotension, dizziness, peripheral edema, headache, gingival hyperplasia	2nd-/3rd-degree heart block or sick sinus syndrome in the absence of a pacemaker, LVSD. AF or AFl in an accessory pathway (Wolff-Parkinson-White syndrome, Lown-Ganong-Levine syndrome)	Encourage patient to ↑ fluid and fiber intake to combat constipation. Teach patient how to take pulse and blood pressure. Monitor for drug interactions (CYP3A4 substrate and inhibitor).

AF, atrial fibrillation; AFl, atrial flutter; AV, atrioventricular; CrCl; creatinine clearance; CYP, cytochrome P-450, D5W, 5% dextrose in water; EKG, electrocardiogram; GI, gastrointestinal; HF, heart failure; IO, intraosseous; IR, immediate-release; IV, intravenous; LD, loading dose; LVSD, left ventricular systolic dysfunction; MD, maintenance dose; MI, myocardial infarction; NYHA, New York Heart Association; P-gp, P-glycoprotein; PR; QT; QTc; SBR; TdP, torsades de pointes; VF, ventricular fibrillation; VT, ventricular tachycardia.

amiodarone and dronedarone have electrophysiologic properties of all four Vaughan Williams classes. Furthermore, this system does not take into account the fact that the active metabolites of AADs may have different electrophysiologic effects than their parent drugs. For example, *N*-acetyl procainamide (NAPA), the major active metabolite of procainamide, blocks outward potassium channels and therefore can be considered a class III AAD. Although procainamide blocks outward potassium channels, it also primarily blocks inward sodium currents, thereby making it a class Ia AAD. Therefore, the overall electrophysiologic effect produced by procainamide depends upon the relative concentrations of procainamide and NAPA that are present in the body, which can vary based on several clinical factors. The Vaughan Williams classification scheme (**Box 22.3**) identifies drugs that block sodium channels (classes Ia, Ib, and Ic), those that are beta blockers (class II), those that block potassium channels (class III), and those that are nondihydropyridine calcium channel blockers (CCBs) (class IV). While there have been suggested revisions to this classification scheme (Lei, 2018), it remains in widespread use in the field.

Class I Antiarrhythmic Drugs

This class of drugs, known as the *sodium channel blockers*, may be subdivided into classes Ia, Ib, and Ic according to the rate of sodium channel dissociation. These agents vary in the rate at which they bind and then dissociate from the sodium channel receptor. Class Ib AADs bind to and dissociate from the sodium channel receptor quickly ("fast on–off"), while class Ic AADs slowly bind to and dissociate from this receptor ("slow on–off"). The binding kinetics of the class Ia AADs are intermediate between those of the class Ib and Ic agents. In addition, class I AADs possess rate dependence, whereby sodium channel blockade is greatest at fast heart rates (i.e., tachycardia) and least during slower heart rates (i.e., bradycardia) (see **Table 22.1**).

Class Ia Drugs
Quinidine

Quinidine is a broad-spectrum AAD that may be used to treat supraventricular and ventricular arrhythmias. This drug slows conduction velocity (phase 0), prolongs refractoriness (phase 3), and decreases automaticity (phase 4). Quinidine widens the QRS complex, prolongs the QT interval, and slightly prolongs the PR interval on the EKG. Quinidine has been used in the management of AF, AFl, AV nodal reentrant tachycardia, and VT.

Quinidine has potent anticholinergic properties that affect the SA and AV nodes. Therefore, quinidine can increase the SA nodal discharge rate and AV nodal conduction. Consequently, in patients with AF or AFl, these anticholinergic effects may lead to a more rapid ventricular rate. Therefore, the AV node should be adequately inhibited with the use of an AV nodal blocking drug, such as a beta blocker, nondihydropyridine CCB (e.g., diltiazem or verapamil), or digoxin, prior to administering quinidine in these patients. Quinidine also blocks alpha₁ receptors, which can lead to vasodilation and subsequent dose-related hypotension, especially when administered intravenously.

The most common adverse effects associated with quinidine are gastrointestinal (GI) (nausea, vomiting, and diarrhea). As with other class Ia drugs, quinidine can cause proarrhythmia, specifically torsades de pointes (TdP). Other adverse effects associated with quinidine include thrombocytopenia, hepatitis, cinchonism (tinnitus, blurred vision, headache), worsening of underlying HF, and hemolytic anemia.

Quinidine is a substrate of the cytochrome P-450 (CYP) 3A4 isoenzyme and an inhibitor of the CYP2D6 isoenzyme. Therefore, quinidine can interact with any drug that inhibits or induces CYP3A4 (e.g., inhibitors: ketoconazole, erythromycin, amiodarone, verapamil, diltiazem; inducers: rifampin, phenobarbital, phenytoin) or is a substrate of CYP2D6 (e.g., beta blockers). Quinidine can also significantly increase serum digoxin concentrations.

BOX 22.3 Classification of Antiarrhythmic Drugs

CLASS I—SODIUM CHANNEL BLOCKERS

Ia (intermediate onset/offset)
    Disopyramide
    Procainamide
    Quinidine
Ib (fast onset/offset)
    Lidocaine
    Mexiletine
Ic (slow onset/offset)
    Flecainide
    propafenone[1]

CLASS II—Β-BLOCKERS

Atenolol
Esmolol
Metoprolol
Propranolol

CLASS III—POTASSIUM CHANNEL BLOCKERS

Amiodarone[2]
Dofetilide
Dronedarone[3]
Ibutilide
Sotalol[4]

CLASS IV—CALCIUM CHANNEL BLOCKERS

Diltiazem
Verapamil

---

[1] *Also has β-blocking properties (class II).
[2] Also has sodium channel blocking (class I), β-blocking (class II), and calcium channel blocking (class IV) properties.
[3] Also has sodium channel blocking (class I), β-blocking (class II), and calcium channel blocking (class IV) properties.
[4] *Also has β-blocking properties (class II).

Procainamide

Procainamide has basically the same electrophysiologic effects as those of quinidine, except that procainamide does not have the anticholinergic activity of quinidine. Procainamide slows conduction velocity (phase 0), prolongs refractoriness (phase 3), and decreases automaticity (phase 4). Procainamide widens the QRS complex, prolongs the QT interval, and slightly prolongs the PR interval on the EKG. NAPA, the major metabolite of procainamide, blocks outward potassium currents and thereby has class III electrophysiologic properties. NAPA prolongs the QT interval. Procainamide is a broad-spectrum AAD and has been used to treat supraventricular and ventricular arrhythmias.

Procainamide is only available in the intravenous (IV) formulation; all of its oral formulations have been discontinued. Therefore, adverse effects that would most likely occur with chronic therapy (e.g., systemic lupus erythematosus, agranulocytosis) should no longer be a concern. Most of the adverse effects associated with IV administration of procainamide include bradycardia, AV block, hypotension, worsening of underlying HF, and TdP.

Procainamide and NAPA can accumulate in patients with renal impairment. Therefore, serum concentrations must be monitored regularly to assess for efficacy and toxicity. The therapeutic ranges of procainamide and NAPA are 4 to 10 mcg/mL and 15 to 25 mcg/mL, respectively.

Disopyramide

Disopyramide slows conduction velocity (phase 0), prolongs refractoriness (phase 3), and decreases automaticity (phase 4). These effects are manifested as a prolonged QT interval and a slightly prolonged QRS complex on the EKG. Disopyramide has direct and indirect effects on the heart rate similar to those of quinidine. Disopyramide is a broad-spectrum AAD and has been used to treat supraventricular and ventricular arrhythmias. However, the clinical use of this agent is limited because of its potent anticholinergic and negative inotropic effects. If disopyramide is used to treat AF or AFl, the practitioner should give an AV nodal blocking agent (e.g., beta blocker, diltiazem, verapamil, or digoxin) to minimize its vagolytic effect.

The primary adverse effects associated with disopyramide are precipitation of HF and anticholinergic effects (e.g., dry mouth, urinary retention, constipation, blurred vision). Disopyramide is contraindicated in patients with HF with reduced ejection fraction (HFrEF) (left ventricular ejection fraction [LVEF] of 40% or less) because it can cause significant depression of myocardial contractility. Disopyramide can also cause TdP.

Class Ib Drugs

The class Ib AADs include lidocaine and mexiletine. These agents decrease automaticity and conduction velocity and shorten refractoriness. These AADs primarily exert their electrophysiologic effects on the ventricular myocardium since they have little or no effect on atrial tissue.

Lidocaine

Lidocaine is categorized as a class Ib AAD; however, its electrophysiologic effects are different in that it is selective to ischemic tissue and especially to active, fast sodium channels in the bundle of His, Purkinje fibers, and ventricular myocardium. Thus, lidocaine has little effect on conduction in nonischemic tissue and the atrial myocardium. Lidocaine also has very little effect on the automaticity of the SA node. However, lidocaine does suppress the automaticity of ectopic ventricular pacemakers and Purkinje fibers. In normal tissues, the action potential duration is shortened and conduction velocity shows little change with lidocaine. However, in depolarized fibers or in fibers damaged by ischemia, lidocaine prolongs the action potential and slows conduction.

Lidocaine is primarily effective in treating ventricular arrhythmias, especially those associated with acute MI. Prophylactic administration in patients with acute MI demonstrated a decreased incidence of ventricular fibrillation (VF) but no difference in prehospital treatment outcomes of acute MI and no improvement or even higher mortality rates in hospitalized patients. Selective administration of lidocaine to patients with VF associated with MI or cardiac arrest also demonstrated no improvement in survival rates (Wyse et al., 1988). The use of lidocaine as prophylaxis against VT or VF in patients with MI is not warranted. Its use should be reserved for the treatment of ventricular arrhythmias.

Lidocaine is not effective in the treatment of supraventricular arrhythmias such as AF or AFl. However, lidocaine can be used for the treatment of digoxin-induced arrhythmias (atrial and ventricular) because of its selectivity for depolarized myocardium.

Lidocaine is eliminated primarily by hepatic metabolism with the metabolic rate being proportional to hepatic blood flow. In patients with HFrEF, the volume of distribution in the central compartment is decreased and hepatic blood flow may be reduced if cardiac output is depressed. Hepatic impairment slows lidocaine's clearance rate but does not affect its volume of distribution.

The principal adverse effects associated with lidocaine are central nervous system (CNS) effects (i.e., dizziness, paresthesia, disorientation, tremor, agitation). At higher concentrations, seizures and respiratory arrest may occur with the use of lidocaine. Lidocaine's adverse effects are more frequent in older patients, in patients with HFrEF or hepatic disease, and during prolonged administration (>24 hours). Therefore, these patients should be closely monitored for signs and symptoms of lidocaine toxicity. Lidocaine concentrations should also be closely monitored in these patients. The therapeutic range of lidocaine is 1.5 to 6 mg/L. Lidocaine toxicity is most commonly observed at concentrations greater than 5 mg/L.

Mexiletine

Mexiletine is a structurally related oral analog of and has similar electrophysiologic effects, antiarrhythmic effects, and adverse events to lidocaine. Mexiletine decreases conduction velocity (phase 0) preferentially in ischemic tissue.

Mexiletine is effective in the treatment of VT. Combining mexiletine with a second AAD (class Ia or III) is more effective than mexiletine monotherapy for the treatment of refractory VT. However, its clinical use is limited by a high incidence of GI reactions such as nausea and vomiting. CNS adverse effects such as dizziness, confusion, ataxia, and speech disturbances may lead the practitioner to discontinue treatment with this drug. Mexiletine can also cause proarrhythmia, although the incidence is lower when compared to other AADs.

Class Ic Drugs

Flecainide

Flecainide is a potent blocker of sodium channels during phase 0 of the action potential, thereby slowing conduction velocity in the Purkinje fibers and AV node and diminishing automaticity in the Purkinje fibers. Because of the slowed cardiac conduction, increases in the PR interval and QRS duration may be seen on the EKG.

Flecainide is most commonly used in clinical practice for the treatment of supraventricular arrhythmias such as AF and AFl. Flecainide has very good efficacy in terms of restoring and maintaining SR in patients with AF (Camm et al., 2012; Slavik et al., 2001). Flecainide has been shown to restore SR in 75% to 90% of patients with AF at 8 hours (with single, oral loading doses of 300 mg) as well as maintain SR in up to 77% of patients at 1 year. Although flecainide is approved by the U.S. Food and Drug Administration (FDA) for the treatment of life-threatening sustained VT, it is rarely, if ever, used for this indication, primarily due to its suboptimal efficacy and the potential for proarrhythmic events (Anderson et al., 1983). There may be a resurgence in the use of flecainide for the use of ventricular arrhythmias, as this AAD has shown to be effective in suppressing exercise-induced ventricular arrhythmias in patients with catecholaminergic polymorphic VT that is refractory to beta-blocker therapy (Van der Werf et al., 2011).

The CAST was conducted to determine if suppression of asymptomatic or mildly symptomatic premature ventricular contractions (PVCs) with the class Ic AADs, flecainide, encainide, or moricizine would reduce the incidence of death from arrhythmia in post-MI patients (CAST Investigators, 1989). Despite adequate suppression of ventricular arrhythmias, flecainide significantly increased mortality from arrhythmia or cardiac arrest (presumably due to proarrhythmia) and significantly increased total mortality. Overall, the results of this trial demonstrated that the use of AADs to suppress asymptomatic PVCs in post-MI patients does not improve survival and is most likely detrimental. The use of flecainide should be avoided in patients with any form of structural heart disease (SHD), which includes CAD, HF, or LV hypertrophy.

Adverse effects associated with flecainide include blurred vision, dizziness, headache, tremor, nausea, vomiting, conduction disturbances, and ventricular arrhythmias (sustained VT) that can be quite resistant to cardioversion. Flecainide also has potent negative inotropic effects that may lead to worsening HF.

Propafenone

Propafenone has the same ability to block sodium channels, slow conduction velocity, and diminish automaticity in the AV node and Purkinje fibers as flecainide. However, propafenone also has a mild, nonselective beta-blocking effect. Although propafenone is FDA approved for the treatment of life-threatening ventricular arrhythmias, its use in clinical practice has been limited to the management of supraventricular arrhythmias such as AF. Propafenone has been shown to be effective for restoring and maintaining SR in patients with

AF (Miller et al., 2000; Roy et al., 2000). The use of single, oral loading doses of propafenone (450–600 mg) in patients with recent-onset AF has been associated with conversion rates of 72% to 76% at 8 hours (Slavik et al., 2001). Although propafenone was not evaluated in the CAST and has not been associated with increased mortality in other trials, there still tends to be an overall negative perception of this drug's safety in patients with SHD. Until the safety of propafenone can be demonstrated conclusively in a large, randomized, prospective trial in patients with SHD, its use should be avoided in this population.

Adverse effects associated with propafenone include blurred vision, dizziness, headache, nausea, vomiting, fatigue, bronchospasm, taste disturbances (metallic taste), conduction disturbances (bradycardia, heart block, QRS prolongation), and ventricular arrhythmias (sustained VT) that can be quite resistant to cardioversion. Propafenone also has potent negative inotropic effects that may lead to worsening HF.

Class II Antiarrhythmic Drugs

Beta blockers are useful in suppressing ventricular arrhythmias. They are also used for treating many supraventricular arrhythmias because of their ability to block receptor sites in the conduction system and subsequently slow AV nodal conduction and the SA nodal rate, which in turn slows the ventricular rate. Furthermore, beta blockers are helpful when used in combination with other AADs or in treating the underlying cause of some arrhythmias (ischemia, catecholamine excess) (see **Table 22.1**).

Beta blockers decrease automaticity (decrease the slope of phase 4 depolarization in the sinus node and in the Purkinje fibers) and conduction velocity (phase 0) and prolong refractoriness (phase 3). Changes in the EKG caused by beta blockers are a sinus bradycardia, consisting of a normal or slightly prolonged PR interval and occasional shortening of the QT interval. In addition to being negative chronotropic drugs (decreasing AV nodal conduction), beta blockers are also negative inotropic agents (decreasing cardiac contractility). Both of these properties enable beta blockers to decrease myocardial oxygen consumption, which is useful especially in patients with underlying CAD. Patients with sinus node dysfunction or AV conduction system defects may have significant sinus bradycardia when a beta blocker is initiated.

In general, beta blockers lower the heart rate and blood pressure, decrease myocardial contractility, decrease oxygen consumption in the myocardium, and lower cardiac output. Beta blockers have a diverse range of uses, including paroxysmal supraventricular tachycardia (PSVT), AF, AFl, and arrhythmias caused by catecholamine excess, ischemia, mitral valve prolapse, hypertrophic cardiomyopathy, and MI. Beta blockers also reduce complex ventricular arrhythmias, including VT. The VF threshold is increased with the use of beta blockers in animal models, and beta blockers have been found to decrease VF in patients with acute MI. Beta blockers reduce myocardial ischemia, which may reduce the likelihood of VF.

All beta blockers (without intrinsic sympathomimetic activity) are relatively similar in efficacy for the treatment of supraventricular and ventricular arrhythmias. Selection of a particular beta blocker is usually based on the safety profile of the individual agent.

The adverse effects associated with beta blockers depend on their selectivity for beta$_1$ or beta$_2$ receptors. Bronchospasm may be seen in patients with asthma and chronic obstructive pulmonary disease; this adverse effect is not eliminated by the use of selective beta$_1$ blockers since these agents gradually become nonselective as the dose is increased. HF, hypotension, bradycardia, and depression also are common adverse effects of beta blockers. In addition, patients receiving beta blockers often report fatigue and impotence.

Class III Antiarrhythmic Drugs

Class III AADs include amiodarone, dofetilide, dronedarone, ibutilide, and sotalol. Ibutilide and dofetilide are used to treat AF and AFl. Amiodarone and sotalol can be used to treat both supraventricular and ventricular arrhythmias. Dronedarone is FDA approved to reduce the risk of hospitalization from cardiovascular (CV) causes in patients in SR with a history of paroxysmal or persistent AF.

Patients receiving class III AADs should be monitored closely for EKG changes such as increased ventricular ectopy and changes in PR interval, QRS duration, and QT interval. Practitioners should avoid using class III AADs concomitantly with other drugs that can prolong the QT interval to minimize the risk of TdP (see **Table 22.1**).

Amiodarone

Amiodarone is a unique drug that possesses electrophysiologic characteristics of all four Vaughan Williams classes of AADs. While amiodarone is primarily a potassium channel blocker (blocks the rapid and slow components of the delayed rectifier potassium current), it also blocks sodium channels, has nonselective beta-blocking activity, and has weak calcium channel blocking properties. As a result, amiodarone reduces automaticity (phase 4) and conduction velocity (phase 0) and prolongs refractoriness (phase 3). When administered intravenously, amiodarone's beta-blocking and calcium-channel-blocking activities are more predominant. Amiodarone has minimal to no negative inotropic effects, which makes it one of the few AADs that can be safely used in patients with HFrEF.

Amiodarone is approved by the FDA for the management of life-threatening recurrent ventricular arrhythmias. However, its off-label use for AF has increased over the past decade not only because of its increased efficacy in maintaining SR as compared to other AADs but also because it is one of the few AADs proven to be safe in patients with concomitant SHD. Amiodarone is often given IV for the acute treatment of life-threatening ventricular arrhythmias such as VT or VF. IV amiodarone can also be used to terminate AF acutely. Even though ICDs now play a primary role in the chronic management of ventricular arrhythmias, amiodarone is still used in patients who refuse or are not candidates for these devices. Also, amiodarone (with a beta blocker) can also be used as adjunctive therapy in these patients if frequent ICD discharges occur (Connolly et al., 2006).

Because of amiodarone's poor oral bioavailability, large volume of distribution, and long half-life, its onset of action may not be apparent for several months. To achieve efficacy more quickly, loading doses of oral amiodarone must be initially used to saturate the myocardial stores. Once the patient is appropriately loaded with oral amiodarone, the dose should be reduced to the recommended maintenance dose to minimize the incidence of adverse events.

Because of its extremely large volume of distribution and high lipophilicity, amiodarone has the potential to accumulate and cause adverse effects in numerous organs with chronic use, with the lungs, thyroid, eyes, heart, liver, skin, GI tract, and CNS being most notably affected. Unlike other amiodarone-induced adverse effects, pulmonary toxicity can be life threatening. Pulmonary toxicity can develop in up to 15% of patients receiving amiodarone (Range et al., 2013). Definitive diagnosis of amiodarone-induced pulmonary toxicity is difficult, since many of the subjective and objective findings are nonspecific. Patients may present with cough, dyspnea, or fever. The chest radiograph may reveal diffuse infiltrates, and pulmonary function tests may demonstrate a reduction in the diffusion capacity. If pulmonary toxicity is detected, amiodarone should be immediately discontinued. Corticosteroids may be needed to treat the pulmonary inflammation. To screen for pulmonary toxicity in patients receiving amiodarone, pulmonary function tests and a chest radiograph should be obtained at baseline. Subsequently, a chest radiograph should be obtained on an annual basis, while pulmonary function tests can be repeated if symptoms develop (Goldschlager et al., 2007).

Because it contains approximately 38% iodine by weight, amiodarone may also cause thyroid abnormalities that can manifest as either hypothyroidism or hyperthyroidism (Bogazzi et al., 2012). Hypothyroidism is the more common form of amiodarone-induced thyroid dysfunction. Although patients often report increased lethargy, the diagnosis of amiodarone-induced hypothyroidism is made upon detection of elevated levels of thyroid-stimulating hormone (TSH). Patients developing amiodarone-induced hypothyroidism can usually be treated with thyroid hormone supplementation (i.e., levothyroxine). The diagnosis of amiodarone-induced hyperthyroidism should be suspected if patients present with new or recurrent arrhythmias. Patients developing hyperthyroidism have abnormally low TSH levels and can usually be treated with antithyroid medications. To screen for thyroid dysfunction in patients receiving amiodarone, thyroid function tests should be performed at baseline and then every 6 months throughout therapy (Goldschlager et al., 2007).

Ocular complications induced by amiodarone often manifest as corneal microdeposits, which occur in virtually every patient (Passman et al., 2012). Although these opacities rarely produce visual disturbances, photophobia, halos, and blurred vision have been reported. Because of their relatively benign nature, these opacities do not require routine monitoring or discontinuation of amiodarone when they develop. Chronic amiodarone therapy has also been associated with optic neuritis and optic neuropathy. Since these ocular disturbances are vision-threatening, amiodarone must be discontinued once the diagnosis is confirmed. To screen for these complications, ophthalmologic examinations should be performed at baseline only if patients have significant visual abnormalities and then later only if symptoms develop (Goldschlager et al., 2007).

GI adverse effects are relatively common and occur most frequently when amiodarone-loading doses are administered. Typically, patients report nausea, vomiting, loss of appetite, and abdominal pain. Constipation can also occur during long-term therapy. These GI disturbances can be minimized by dividing the total daily dose into two to three doses and by taking the drug with food. Liver function test abnormalities can also develop. Although elevations in aspartate aminotransferase and alanine aminotransferase levels are relatively common with amiodarone therapy, overt hepatotoxicity rarely occurs (Babatin et al., 2008). Liver enzyme levels usually return to baseline following reduction of the amiodarone dose or discontinuation of the drug. To screen for these hepatic abnormalities, liver function tests should be performed at baseline and then every 6 months throughout therapy (Goldschlager et al., 2007).

Although laboratory tests cannot detect amiodarone-induced CV, neurologic, and dermatologic toxicities, patients should still be clinically evaluated for these adverse effects on a routine basis. Compared with other AADs, amiodarone produces fewer CV adverse effects. The bradycardia and heart block that can develop merely represent an accentuation of amiodarone's pharmacologic and electrophysiologic properties. Additionally, even though amiodarone markedly prolongs the QT interval, TdP is rare. Neurologic toxicities associated with amiodarone occur frequently and may include tremors, ataxia, peripheral neuropathy, fatigue, and insomnia. The most common dermatologic reactions observed during amiodarone therapy are photosensitivity and a blue-gray skin discoloration (Jaworski et al., 2014). Photosensitivity reactions can range from extremely tanned areas to sunburned areas with erythema and edema. Blue-gray skin discoloration, which often appears on the patient's face and hands, may be related to the cumulative dose and duration of therapy. To prevent these dermatologic toxicities, patients receiving amiodarone should use opaque sunscreens such as zinc oxide while outdoors.

Patients receiving amiodarone also need to be monitored for drug interactions. Amiodarone is a substrate of the CYP3A4 isoenzyme, a potent inhibitor of the CYP3A4, 2C9, and 2D6 isoenzymes and an inhibitor of P-glycoprotein. Amiodarone significantly interacts with digoxin and warfarin, which are commonly used in patients with AF. Amiodarone potentiates the anticoagulant effects of warfarin, which results in an increased international normalized ratio (INR) and an increased risk of bleeding (Sanoski &

Bauman, 2002). When amiodarone and warfarin are initiated concurrently or when warfarin is initiated in a patient already receiving amiodarone, warfarin should be started at a dose of 2.5 mg daily. When amiodarone is initiated in a patient already receiving warfarin, the warfarin dose should be empirically reduced by approximately 30% (Sanoski & Bauman, 2002). Amiodarone can also double serum digoxin concentrations. Therefore, the digoxin dose should be empirically reduced by 50% when amiodarone is initiated. Furthermore, to minimize the risk of myopathy or rhabdomyolysis, the doses of simvastatin and lovastatin should not exceed 20 mg/d and 40 mg/d, respectively, when coadministered with amiodarone.

Dronedarone

Like amiodarone, dronedarone is primarily considered a class III AAD, but it exhibits electrophysiological properties of all four Vaughan Williams classes. Although structurally related to amiodarone, dronedarone's structure has been modified through the addition of a methylsulfonyl group and the removal of iodine to potentially limit the risk of toxicity. Dronedarone also has a considerably shorter half-life (24 hours) when compared with amiodarone (>50 days), which allows for steady state to be achieved in 5 to 7 days without the need for loading doses.

The efficacy and safety of dronedarone have been evaluated in several clinical trials. Dronedarone has been shown to be more effective than placebo in maintaining SR in patients with paroxysmal AF or AFl (Singh et al., 2007). In another trial, the use of dronedarone was associated with a significant reduction in the incidence of hospitalization due to CV events or death when compared to placebo in patients with persistent or paroxysmal AF and at least one additional risk factor for death (Hohnloser et al., 2009). A trial that evaluated the efficacy and safety of dronedarone in patients with New York Heart Association (NYHA) class III or IV HF (LVEF of 35% or less) was terminated prematurely after significantly more patients in the dronedarone group died (primarily because of worsening HF) compared with the placebo group (Køber et al., 2008). Based on the results of this particular trial, dronedarone is contraindicated in patients with advanced HF (NYHA class IV or NYHA class II or III with a recent hospitalization for decompensated HF). Dronedarone has also been shown to be significantly less effective than amiodarone in reducing AF recurrences (Le Heuzey et al., 2010). Another trial that enrolled older adult patients with permanent AF and risk factors for major vascular events was terminated prematurely after significantly more patients in the dronedarone group died (primarily from CV causes), were hospitalized for HF, and suffered a stroke when compared with the placebo group (Connolly et al., 2011). Based on the results of this trial, dronedarone is contraindicated in patients with permanent AF (i.e., those who cannot be restored to SR).

Dronedarone is a substrate of the CYP3A isoenzyme, a moderate inhibitor of the CYP3A and CYP2D6 isoenzymes, and an inhibitor of P-glycoprotein. Because of the potential for significantly increasing dronedarone concentrations, concomitant use of potent CYP3A inhibitors (i.e., ketoconazole, itraconazole, voriconazole, cyclosporine, clarithromycin, and ritonavir) or inducers (e.g., rifampin, phenobarbital, phenytoin, carbamazepine, and St. John's wort) should be avoided. No significant interaction has been observed between dronedarone and warfarin. Dronedarone may significantly increase serum digoxin concentrations by about 2.5-fold. Therefore, when concomitantly using dronedarone with digoxin, the digoxin dose should be empirically reduced by 50%. Dronedarone can also significantly increase dabigatran concentrations. The dose of dabigatran should be reduced to 75 mg twice daily in patients with AF who have a creatinine clearance (CrCl) of 30 to 50 mL/min. Concomitant use with dabigatran should be avoided in patients with AF who have a CrCl less than 30 mL/min. To minimize the risk of myopathy or rhabdomyolysis, the doses of simvastatin and lovastatin should not exceed 10 mg/d when administered concomitantly with dronedarone.

The most common adverse effects associated with dronedarone in the clinical trials were GI disturbances, including nausea, vomiting, and diarrhea. However, postmarketing reports have suggested that more significant organ toxicities, including severe hepatic injury, interstitial lung disease (i.e., pneumonitis, pulmonary fibrosis), and acute kidney injury, may also be associated with this AAD. Although a prolonged QT interval can occur with dronedarone, TdP is rare.

Sotalol

Sotalol is a class III AAD that also has nonselective beta-blocking properties. Sotalol blocks the rapid component of the delayed rectifier potassium current, which prolongs atrial and ventricular refractoriness. Sotalol exhibits reverse-use dependence, whereby its action potential–prolonging effects are lessened at higher heart rates and increased at lower heart rates. Sotalol increases the QT interval by prolonging ventricular repolarization and may give rise to TdP. The QT interval prolongation with sotalol is a dose-dependent effect. The QT interval should be closely monitored during treatment. Sotalol should be discontinued if the QT interval exceeds 550 msec. The practitioner should avoid combining sotalol with other drugs that increase the QT interval.

Sotalol is effective for the treatment of supraventricular and ventricular arrhythmias. Although sotalol is not effective for conversion of AF, it is an effective agent for maintaining SR in patients with AF (Roy et al., 2000). Several trials have been conducted to compare the efficacy of sotalol and amiodarone in patients with AF (Roy et al., 2000; Singh et al., 2005). The results of these trials suggest that amiodarone is more effective than sotalol in restoring SR in patients with AF. Amiodarone is also more effective than sotalol in maintaining patients in SR, except in those patients with CAD, where the efficacy of these AADs appears to be similar. In patients with an ICD, sotalol has also been shown to significantly reduce arrhythmia recurrence and discharge from the ICD (Pacifico et al., 1999).

Because sotalol is eliminated primarily by the kidneys, the initial dosing regimen must be based on the patient's CrCl. The practitioner should routinely monitor the patient's renal function throughout therapy to determine if any dosing adjustments are necessary. Sotalol should not be used to treat AF if the patient's CrCl is less than 40 mL/min. The practitioner should also routinely monitor electrolytes, especially if the patient is concomitantly receiving diuretics, since hypokalemia and hypomagnesemia can increase the risk of TdP. Because of concern about TdP when initiating therapy with sotalol, patients must be hospitalized and placed on telemetry for at least 3 days.

Most of the adverse effects associated with sotalol can be attributed to its beta-blocking activity (e.g., bradycardia, fatigue, dyspnea). The beta-blocking effect of sotalol may decrease cardiac contractility; therefore, this drug should be avoided in patients with HFrEF.

Dofetilide

Dofetilide acts as a selective potassium channel blocker, affecting the rapid component of the delayed rectifier potassium current. This results in a prolonged action potential and QT interval. Dofetilide affects the atria more than the ventricles. It also exhibits reverse-use dependence.

Dofetilide is approved for the conversion of AF or AFl to SR and for the maintenance of SR in patients with permanent AF or AFl. In a study comparing the efficacy and safety of dofetilide with those of placebo, patients randomized to dofetilide were more likely to convert to SR with ascending doses (Singh et al., 2000). At 1 year, slightly more than 50% of patients in the group taking 500 mcg of dofetilide remained in SR. Like amiodarone, dofetilide also has been proven to be safe to use in patients with underlying HFrEF (Køber et al., 2000; Torp-Pedersen et al., 1999).

As with other AADs, the main concern with dofetilide is the dose-dependent onset of TdP and other ventricular arrhythmias. Other adverse effects associated with dofetilide include headache and dizziness.

Dofetilide has a number of important drug interactions. The concomitant use of cimetidine, dolutegravir, ketoconazole, hydrochlorothiazide, megestrol, prochlorperazine, trimethoprim–sulfamethoxazole, or verapamil with dofetilide is contraindicated since these drugs can significantly increase plasma concentrations of dofetilide. Additionally, drugs that prolong the QT interval should not be used concomitantly with dofetilide because of the increased risk of a prolonged QT interval and TdP.

Because dofetilide is eliminated primarily by the kidneys, the initial dosage must be based on the patient's CrCl. The dosage of dofetilide should be decreased in patients with renal impairment (CrCl of <60 mL/min). The drug should not be given to patients with a CrCl of less than 20 mL/min or a QT interval greater than 440 msec at baseline. Because of concern about TdP when initiating therapy with dofetilide, patients must be hospitalized and placed on telemetry for at least 3 days.

Ibutilide

Ibutilide is structurally related to L-sotalol, but it has no beta-blocking activity. It prolongs the action potential by increasing the slow inward sodium current and blocking the rapid component of the delayed rectifier potassium current, which prolongs atrial and ventricular refractoriness. Ibutilide is available only in IV form. It is indicated only for the acute termination of AF or AFl.

Ibutilide restores SR in approximately 50% of patients with AF or AFl. However, it is more effective for restoring SR in patients with AFl than in those with AF (Stambler et al., 1996). Ibutilide also appears to be effective for facilitating direct-current cardioversion (DCC) of AF (Oral et al., 1999). The major adverse effect associated with ibutilide is TdP. Patients with HFrEF or electrolyte abnormalities (e.g., hypokalemia or hypomagnesemia) are especially at risk for developing proarrhythmia with ibutilide.

Class IV Antiarrhythmic Drugs

The class IV AADs, verapamil and diltiazem, are nondihydropyridine CCBs used to treat supraventricular arrhythmias, including PSVT, AF, and AFl. By inhibiting the inward movement of calcium through calcium channels located in cell membranes, these drugs slow conduction, prolong refractoriness, and decrease automaticity in the SA and AV nodes. In AF or AFl, these drugs slow conduction through the AV node and thereby slow the ventricular rate. Their cardiac effects are vascular relaxation, a negative inotropic effect, and a negative chronotropic effect. Verapamil has more potent negative inotropic effects than diltiazem.

Because of their potent negative inotropic effects, both verapamil and diltiazem should be avoided in patients with HFrEF because they are likely to precipitate worsening HF symptoms. These drugs also should not be used in patients with an accessory pathway or WPW syndrome because they can shorten the refractory period of the accessory pathway and subsequently increase the ventricular rate, which may lead to VF.

Bradycardia, heart block, headache, flushing, dizziness, and peripheral edema are the most common adverse effects of diltiazem and verapamil. Verapamil can also cause constipation. The practitioner should use caution when using IV verapamil because significant hypotension can occur (Phillips et al., 1997).

The practitioner should be cautious when administering these agents concomitantly with beta blockers, digoxin, or clonidine because of the increased risk of bradycardia and heart block. Since diltiazem and verapamil are substrates and inhibitors of the CYP3A4 isoenzyme, the practitioner should also use caution when concomitantly administering either of these drugs with other agents that are also metabolized by this isoenzyme.

Other Antiarrhythmic Drugs

Several other AADs are commonly used to treat abnormal cardiac impulse formation or conduction. Digoxin, adenosine, and atropine are used in the treatment of various cardiac arrhythmias (see **Table 22.1**).

Digoxin

Digoxin's predominant antiarrhythmic effect is on the AV node of the conduction system. Digoxin affects the autonomic nervous system by stimulating the parasympathetic division, which increases vagal tone. This vagal effect slows conduction through the AV node and prolongs the AV nodal refractory period.

Digoxin is commonly used to slow electrical impulse conduction through the AV node, thus slowing the ventricular rate in supraventricular arrhythmias such as AF or AFl. Digoxin is not effective for converting AF or AFl to SR. Although digoxin is frequently used to control the ventricular rate in patients with HFrEF and concomitant AF or AFl, its use tends to be limited by its relatively slow onset of action and its inability to control the ventricular rate during exercise. Even after an appropriate loading dose is administered, digoxin's peak onset of effect is delayed for up to 6 to 8 hours. Achievement of steady-state concentrations may take up to a week in patients with normal renal function or even longer in patients with renal impairment. The increased sympathetic tone generated during exercise tends to offset the vagal effects of digoxin, which limits its efficacy under these conditions. In patients with HFrEF and concomitant AF or AFl, digoxin can provide effective ventricular rate control without increasing the risk of worsening HF symptoms because of its additional positive inotropic effects.

Digoxin toxicity can be precipitated by declining renal function, electrolyte disturbances, and drug interactions. Because digoxin is primarily excreted unchanged by the kidneys, a decline in the CrCl can predispose a patient to digoxin toxicity. Hypokalemia, hypomagnesemia, and hypercalcemia can also predispose the myocardium to the toxic effects of digoxin. Concomitant drug therapy with agents such as amiodarone, dronedarone, or verapamil can also increase serum digoxin concentrations. Potential signs and symptoms of digoxin toxicity include heart block, ventricular arrhythmias, visual disturbances (e.g., blurred vision, yellow/green halos), dizziness, weakness, nausea, vomiting, diarrhea, and anorexia. Digoxin has a narrow therapeutic index. The therapeutic range for digoxin in patients with AF and normal LV systolic function (LVEF > 40%) is 0.8 to 2 ng/mL. Because of the potential risk of increased mortality with higher serum concentrations, the therapeutic range for digoxin in patients with AF and concomitant HFrEF (LVEF of 40% or less) is 0.5 to 0.9 ng/mL.

Adenosine

Adenosine is an AAD used for converting PSVT to SR. It activates potassium channels and, by increasing the outward potassium current, hyperpolarizes the membrane potential, decreasing spontaneous SA nodal depolarization. Adenosine may also decrease the inward calcium current by blocking adenylate cyclase, which normally increases the inward calcium current. Automaticity (phase 4) and conduction (phase 0) are inhibited in the SA and AV nodes. The most common adverse effects of adenosine include chest discomfort, dyspnea, flushing, and headache. Sinus arrest can also occur. However, because of adenosine's short half-life of 10 seconds, these adverse effects are short lived. Adenosine is administered intravenously because of its short half-life.

Atropine

Atropine is a parasympatholytic drug that enhances both sinus nodal automaticity and AV nodal conduction through direct vagolytic action. Atropine blocks acetylcholine at parasympathetic neuroeffector sites. Atropine is used almost exclusively in the monitored clinical setting for the treatment of symptomatic bradycardia.

Patients who do not experience signs or symptoms of hemodynamic compromise, ischemia, or frequent ventricular ectopy do not require atropine in bradycardic events. Atropine has been reported to be harmful in some patients with AV block at the His–Purkinje level (type 2 AV block and third-degree AV block with a new wide QRS complex). Atropine can be used in these situations, but the practitioner must monitor the patient closely for paradoxical slowing of the heart rate.

Atropine may induce tachycardia, which may result in poor outcomes in patients with myocardial ischemia or an MI. Therefore, atropine should be used cautiously in these patients.

Selecting the Most Appropriate Agent

Determining the cause and type of the arrhythmia is essential to selecting the most appropriate drug therapy. **Figures 22.1** to **22.5**, as well as **Table 22.1**, guide the practitioner in the initial assessment of which drug to use for patients with various types of arrhythmias.

The first main question to ask when selecting drug therapy is whether the slow or fast rate of the arrhythmia makes the patient ill or symptomatic. A symptomatic patient is one with an arrhythmia characterized by low blood pressure, shock, chest pain, shortness of breath, decreased level of consciousness, pulmonary congestion, HF, or acute MI. These patients may require more urgent treatment, perhaps even with nonpharmacological interventions (e.g., DCC, defibrillation) to immediately terminate the arrhythmia. The practitioner should not make clinical decisions based only on the rhythm displayed on the monitor. The practitioner needs to assess the patient's symptoms to determine how urgent the situation is and how quickly treatment needs to be initiated. Treatment of various arrhythmias is discussed in the first-line and second-line therapy sections. **Table 22.2** consolidates the various treatment regimens.

Second, the practitioner must think of treatable conditions that might be causing the arrhythmia. The patient's medical history and laboratory values are important to assess whenever patients present with arrhythmias. Some possible causes of arrhythmias are electrolyte imbalances (i.e., hypokalemia, hypomagnesemia), drug overdose/toxicity, drug

TABLE 22.2

Recommended Order of Treatment for Arrhythmias

Order	Agents	Comments
AF/AFl		
First line	Hemodynamically unstable patient: synchronized DCC Hemodynamically stable patient with rapid ventricular rate: • LVEF > 40%: IV diltiazem, IV verapamil, or IV beta blocker • LVEF ≤ 40%: IV beta blocker or IV digoxin	Premedicate whenever possible when performing DCC. IV amiodarone can be used for ventricular rate control in any patient with AF/AFl who is refractory to or has contraindications to beta blockers, diltiazem, or verapamil; avoid using for ventricular rate control if the AF/AFl has been present >48 h as these patients may be at risk for thromboembolic events induced by conversion to SR.
Second line	Patients with 1st episode of arrhythmia (if likely to convert to and remain in SR): electrical or pharmacological cardioversion can be considered once ventricular rate is acutely controlled. For pharmacological cardioversion, the AAD used depends on the presence of SHD. Decision of whether to proceed acutely with cardioversion depends on the duration of the arrhythmia: • <48 h: May proceed with cardioversion without prolonged period of anticoagulation. • >48 h or unknown duration: Anticoagulate for ≥3 weeks before proceeding with cardioversion. Anticoagulate for ≥4 wk following successful cardioversion. For patients with persistent or recurrent AF, a strategy of ventricular rate control and anticoagulation is a reasonable alternative to rhythm control. Selection of PO drug for ventricular rate control (diltiazem, verapamil, beta blocker, or digoxin) depends on patient's LV function. Anticoagulant therapy should be based on the patient's CHA$_2$DS$_2$-VASc risk score.	A transesophageal echocardiography TEE can be performed in patients with AF >48 h or unknown duration to exclude the presence of thrombi and to facilitate cardioversion. If a thrombus is detected, cardioversion should not be performed and the patient should be anticoagulated indefinitely. If no thrombus is detected, cardioversion can be performed within 24 h without the need for the initial 3-wk period of anticoagulation. These patients will still require anticoagulation after cardioversion for ≥4 wk unless contraindicated. Decisions regarding long-term anticoagulant therapy after this time period should be primarily based on the patient's risk for stroke and not on whether he/she is in SR For AADs to be used for acute pharmacologic cardioversion, see **Figure 22.2**. Goal heart rate is based on patient's LV systolic function: • LVEF > 40% and no or acceptable symptoms of AF: <110 beats/min (at rest) • LVEF ≤ 40%: <80 beats/min (at rest) PO agents for ventricular rate control: • LVEF > 40%: diltiazem, verapamil, or beta blocker • LVEF ≤ 40%: beta blocker (i.e., carvedilol, metoprolol succinate, or bisoprolol) or digoxin
Third line	Chronic AAD therapy can be considered for patients who remain symptomatic despite having adequate ventricular rate control or for those in whom adequate ventricular rate control cannot be achieved. The AAD used depends on patient's LV function and the type of SHD that may be present. For patients with permanent AF, a strategy of ventricular rate control and anticoagulation should be considered. Selection of PO drug for ventricular rate control (diltiazem, verapamil, beta blocker, or digoxin) depends on patient's LV function. Anticoagulant therapy should be based on the patient's CHA$_2$DS$_2$-VASc risk score.	PO AADs for chronic rhythm control: • No SHD: dofetilide, dronedarone, flecainide, propafenone, or sotalol; amiodarone is considered alternative if patient fails or does not tolerate one of the initial AADs. • LVEF ≤ 40%: amiodarone or dofetilide • CAD: dofetilide, dronedarone, or sotalol; amiodarone is considered alternative if patient fails or does not tolerate one of the initial AADs. • Significant LV hypertrophy: amiodarone Avoid flecainide and propafenone in patients with *any* form of SHD.
PSVT (due to AVNRT)		
First line	Vagal maneuvers or IV adenosine	Examples of vagal maneuvers include unilateral carotid sinus massage, Valsalva maneuver, facial immersion in ice water, and coughing. Carotid sinus massage should be avoided in patients with carotid bruits or history of cerebrovascular disease.
Second line	Hemodynamically unstable patient: synchronized DCC Hemodynamically stable patient: IV diltiazem, IV verapamil, or IV beta blocker	Premedicate whenever possible when performing DCC.
Third line	Amiodarone or DCC	

TABLE 22.2

Recommended Order of Treatment for Arrhythmias (*Continued*)

Order	Agents	Comments
Nonsustained VT		
First line	No SHD: • Asymptomatic or minimal symptoms: no drug therapy • Symptomatic: PO beta blocker Post-MI patients: • LVEF > 40%: PO beta blocker regardless of the presence of symptoms • LVEF ≤ 40%: EP testing; if sustained VT/VF, ICD should be placed; if sustained VT/VF noninducible, PO beta blocker or amiodarone may be used.	Correct reversible causes. Post-MI patients with normal LV systolic function should receive a beta blocker even if they have no or minimal symptoms associated with the nonsustained VT to ↓ mortality associated with the MI. If frequent shocks occur in patients with an ICD, PO amiodarone and beta blocker combination therapy or sotalol monotherapy can be used.
Sustained VT		
First line	Hemodynamically unstable patient: synchronized DCC	Premedicate whenever possible when performing DCC. Correct reversible causes.
	Hemodynamically stable patient: IV procainamide, IV amiodarone, or IV sotalol	
Second line	Hemodynamically stable patient: IV lidocaine; synchronized DCC should be considered if AAD therapy fails. Once arrhythmia acutely terminated, patient should be considered for ICD placement. If patient refuses or is not a candidate for an ICD, PO amiodarone can be considered.	If frequent shocks occur in patients with an ICD, PO amiodarone and beta blocker combination therapy or sotalol monotherapy can be used.
Pulseless VT/VF		
First line	Start CPR, establish an airway, and deliver one shock, immediately resume CPR for 2 min and then check rhythm.	Correct reversible causes.
Second line	If patient remains in pulseless VT/VF, deliver one shock and then immediately resume CPR; if pulseless VT/VF persists after at least one shock and CPR, give vasopressor therapy (epinephrine 1 mg IV push/IO q3–5min through pulseless VT/VF episode) (give drug during CPR; do not interrupt CPR to give drug); immediately resume CPR for 2 min and then check pulse.	
Third line	If patient remains in pulseless VT/VF, deliver one shock and then immediately resume CPR; if pulseless VT/VF persists despite defibrillation, CPR, and vasopressor therapy, consider AAD therapy (IV amiodarone; lidocaine may be used as alternative) (give drugs during CPR; do not interrupt CPR to give drugs); immediately resume CPR for 2 min; then check pulse.	
Bradycardia		
First line	Stable: Close observation	Correct reversible causes.
	Signs/symptoms of poor perfusion (e.g., altered mental status, chest pain, hypotension, shock): Immediately administer IV atropine (0.5 mg q3–5min, up to 3 mg total dose). If ineffective, transcutaneous pacing or sympathomimetic continuous infusion (dopamine or epinephrine) should be initiated.	
Second line	If drug therapy and transcutaneous pacing are ineffective, transvenous pacing should be utilized.	

AAD, antiarrhythmic drug; AF, atrial fibrillation; AFl, atrial flutter; AVNRT, atrioventricular nodal reentrant tachycardia; CAD, coronary artery disease; CPR, cardiopulmonary resuscitation; DCC, direct-current cardioversion; EP, electrophysiologic; ICD, implantable cardioverter–defibrillator; IV, intravenous; LV, left ventricular; LVEF, left ventricular ejection fraction; MI, myocardial infarction; PSVT, paroxysmal supraventricular tachycardia; SHD, structural heart disease; SR, sinus rhythm; TEE, transesophageal echocardiogram; VF, ventricular fibrillation; VT, ventricular tachycardia.

interactions, renal failure, hyperthyroidism, metabolic acidosis, hypovolemia, MI, pulmonary embolism, cardiac tamponade, tension pneumothorax, dissecting aortic aneurysm, and hypoxia related to pulmonary disorders, or structural defects in the heart itself. The practitioner may have to correct the cause of the arrhythmia before initiating drug therapy, especially if the patient is asymptomatic. However, time may be a critical factor when treating symptomatic arrhythmias.

Initial vagal maneuvers may serve as both diagnostic and therapeutic purposes for certain arrhythmias. For example, carotid sinus massage may make the flutter waves in AFl more apparent. Appearance of flutter waves allows the practitioner to differentiate AFl from AF, PSVT, or other tachycardias. Examples of vagal maneuvers include unilateral carotid sinus massage, breath holding, facial immersion in ice water, coughing, nasogastric tube placement, gag reflex stimulation by tongue blade or fingers, eyeball massage, squatting, digital sweep of the anus, and bearing down during a bowel movement. Many patients who have recurrent PSVT with disorders such as mitral valve prolapse often learn how to do these maneuvers to terminate the arrhythmia themselves. It is important to note that eyeball massage should never be taught, encouraged, or performed because it may cause retinal detachment. Unilateral carotid sinus massage (firm massage of the carotid sinus that never lasts for more than 5–10 seconds) should be performed only with continuous EKG monitoring and an IV line in place. The procedure should be avoided in older adult patients and should not be performed on patients with carotid bruits because it may occlude already impaired circulation to the brain. Likewise, the practitioner should avoid ice water facial immersion in patients with CAD because of the potential for inducing ischemia.

Atrial Fibrillation/Atrial Flutter

AF and AFl may be stable or unstable. Patients presenting with severe hypotension, syncope, HF, or angina would be considered to be hemodynamically unstable and would require more urgent treatment. When the patient is hemodynamically stable, the practitioner should consider conditions that may be causing the AF or AFl. Such conditions include acute MI, hypoxia, pulmonary embolism, electrolyte imbalance (i.e., hypokalemia, hypomagnesemia), drug toxicity (especially digoxin or sympathomimetic agents), thyrotoxicosis, and alcohol intoxication. Since new-onset AF can be due to acute MI, the practitioner should look for ischemic changes on the 12-lead EKG. If acute ischemic changes appear, admission of the patient to the hospital in a monitored bed may be needed. Obviously, treatment and correction of acute causes of AF or AFl should be a priority.

If untreated, AF and AFl can lead to serious hemodynamic and thromboembolic consequences. A rapid ventricular rate can induce angina in patients with underlying CAD, or worsening signs and symptoms of HF in patients with HFrEF. A persistently rapid ventricular rate may lead to the development of a tachycardia-induced cardiomyopathy. Loss of synchronized atrial contraction can lead to a significant reduction in cardiac output, which can especially affect patients with underlying HF. In addition, loss of coordinated atrial contraction can lead to the pooling of blood and subsequent thrombus formation. Therefore, AF and AFl can lead to serious thromboembolic complications, particularly ischemic stroke. Overall, the treatment goals for AF and AFl are controlling the ventricular rate, preventing thromboembolic events, and, possibly, restoring and maintaining SR. **Figure 22.1** illustrates an algorithm for the management of AF and AFl.

First-Line Therapy

If the patient presenting with AF or AFl is hemodynamically unstable (i.e., severe hypotension, syncope, HF, or angina), immediate DCC is first-line therapy. If the patient is hemodynamically stable and has a rapid ventricular rate, the first priority is to control the ventricular rate. In the acute treatment of AF, the selection of a drug to control the ventricular rate depends on the patient's LV systolic function (January et al., 2019). In patients with normal LV systolic function (LVEF > 40%), IV diltiazem, IV verapamil, or an IV beta blocker is preferred to digoxin because of their relatively quick onset. Beta blockers are especially useful in high adrenergic states (i.e., postoperative patients, hyperthyroidism). The use of digoxin is limited by its relatively slow onset of action and its inability to control heart rate in high adrenergic states (i.e., exercise). In patients with HFrEF (LVEF of 40% or less), an IV beta blocker or IV digoxin is preferred, since these agents are also used to treat HFrEF. Diltiazem or verapamil should be avoided in these patients because their potent negative inotropic effects may precipitate worsening HF symptoms. Beta blockers should be avoided in patients who are exhibiting signs and/or symptoms of decompensated HF. In those patients who are having worsening HF symptoms, IV digoxin or IV amiodarone is recommended as first-line therapy for controlling the ventricular rate. IV amiodarone can also be used for ventricular rate control in any patient with AF who is refractory to or has contraindications to beta blockers, diltiazem, or verapamil. Since amiodarone is a class III AAD, the practitioner should be aware that the patient may convert to SR when using this agent. Patients with AF that has persisted for longer than 48 hours are at risk for thromboembolic events if conversion to SR occurs in the absence of therapeutic anticoagulation. Therefore, in these patients who have not been therapeutically anticoagulated, IV amiodarone should be avoided.

Second-Line Therapy

Once the ventricular rate is acutely controlled, patients should be evaluated for the possibility of restoring SR if AF persists. The results of six landmark clinical trials (Pharmacological Intervention in Atrial Fibrillation, Rate Control versus Electrical Cardioversion for Persistent Atrial Fibrillation, Atrial Fibrillation Follow-Up Investigation of Rhythm Management, Strategies of Treatment of Atrial Fibrillation, How to Treat Chronic Atrial Fibrillation, and Atrial Fibrillation and Congestive Heart Failure) have provided practitioners with

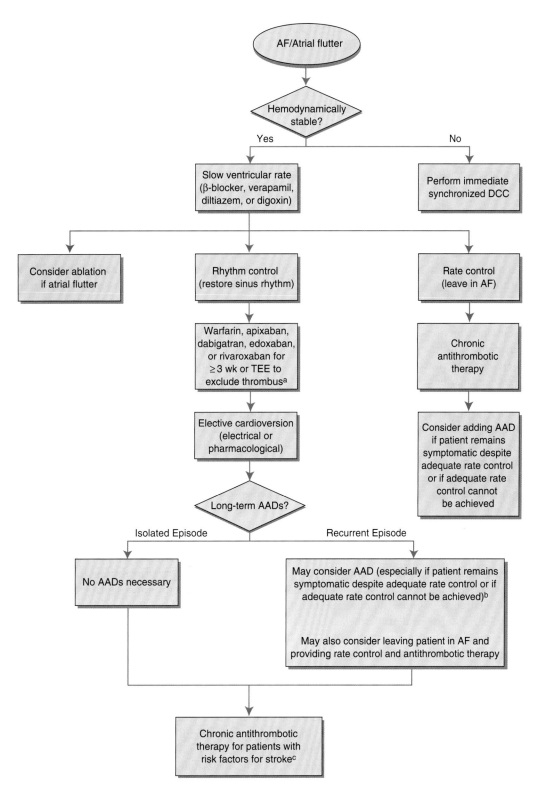

FIGURE 22–1 Treatment algorithm for atrial fibrillation and atrial flutter.

---

[a] If AF < 48 hr, 3 wk of anticoagulation prior to cardioversion is unnecessary in patients at high risk for stroke; initiate unfractionated heparin, a low-molecular weight heparin, apixaban, dabigatran, edoxaban, or rivaroxaban as soon as possible either before or after cardioversion.

[b] Radiofrequency ablation may be considered for patients who fail or do not tolerate >1 AAD.

[c] Chronic antithrombotic therapy should be considered in all patients with AF and risk factors for stroke regardless of whether they remain in sinus rhythm.

AAD, antiarrhythmic drug; AF, atrial fibrillation; DCC, direct-current cardioversion; TEE, transesophageal echocardiogram.

significant insight into the comparative efficacy of rate control (controlling ventricular rate; patient remaining in AF) and rhythm control (restoring and maintaining SR) treatment strategies in patients with AF (Carlsson et al., 2004; Hohnloser et al., 2000; Opolski et al., 2004; Roy et al., 2008; Van Gelder et al., 2002; Wyse et al., 2002). The results of all of these trials essentially demonstrated that there were no significant differences in outcomes between patients who received a rate-control strategy and those who received a rhythm-control strategy. Therefore, based on these findings, a rate-control strategy appears to be a viable alternative to a rhythm-control strategy in patients with persistent or recurrent AF. Consequently, considering the potential toxicities of AADs, it is reasonable to initially consider a rate-control strategy in these patients, including those with concomitant HF. However, a rhythm-control strategy should be considered for those patients who remain symptomatic despite having adequate ventricular rate control or for those in whom adequate ventricular rate control cannot be achieved. The results of the clinical trials mentioned previously do not necessarily apply to patients experiencing their first episode of AF. If these particular patients are likely to convert to and remain in SR, a rhythm-control strategy may be considered.

If the decision is made to restore SR in hemodynamically stable patients with AF, either electrical (i.e., DCC) or pharmacological (i.e., AADs) cardioversion may be used. The decision to use either of these methods is often based on the practitioner's or patient's preference. DCC is associated with higher success rates than pharmacological cardioversion. However, this method requires sedation or anesthesia and may be rarely associated with complications such as sinus arrest or ventricular arrhythmias. Pharmacological cardioversion is associated with adverse effects (e.g., TdP) and drug interactions.

In those patients in whom it is decided to restore SR, it is important to note that the process of cardioverting the patient from AF to SR may place the patient at risk for a thromboembolic event. Restoration to SR may dislodge thrombi in the atria. This risk is present regardless of whether an electrical or pharmacological method is used to restore SR. In patients undergoing DCC or pharmacological cardioversion, it is imperative to determine how long the patient has been in AF because the risk of thrombus formation increases if the AF duration exceeds 48 hours. If AF has been present for more than 48 hours or for an unknown duration, cardioversion should not be performed acutely because of the risk of thromboembolism. These patients should be therapeutically anticoagulated with warfarin (INR target range 2–3) or one of the direct oral anticoagulants (DOAC) for at least 3 weeks (January et al., 2019). After that time, the patient can undergo DCC or pharmacological cardioversion, which should be followed by therapeutic anticoagulation with warfarin (INR target range 2–3) or preferably a DOAC for at least 4 weeks. If the 3 weeks of oral anticoagulant therapy prior to cardioversion is not feasible, the patient may alternatively undergo a transesophageal echocardiogram (TEE) prior to cardioversion to look for any thrombi that may be present in the atria or

ventricles. If no thrombus is observed on TEE, the patient can undergo cardioversion. In these patients, anticoagulant therapy with either IV unfractionated heparin or low molecular weight heparin (subcutaneously at treatment doses) should be initiated at the time the TEE will be performed (You et al., 2012). Cardioversion should then be performed within 24 hours of the TEE. Alternatively, warfarin therapy (INR target range of 2–3) may be used for at least 5 days prior to the TEE and cardioversion. If cardioversion is successful, therapeutic warfarin (INR target range 2–3) or a DOAC should be continued for at least 4 weeks regardless of the patient's baseline risk of stroke (January et al., 2019). Decisions regarding long-term anticoagulant therapy after this 4-week time period should be primarily based on the patient's risk for stroke and not on whether he/she is in SR. If a thrombus is seen on TEE, cardioversion should not be performed, and the patient should be anticoagulated indefinitely. If cardioversion is considered in these patients at a later time, a TEE should again be performed.

When the duration of AF is definitively known to be less than 48 hours, a prolonged period of anticoagulation is not necessary prior to proceeding with electrical or pharmacological cardioversion because the risk of thromboembolism is deemed to be low. In those patients who are at high risk for stroke, IV unfractionated heparin (target activated partial thromboplastin time 60 seconds; acceptable range 50–70 seconds), a low molecular weight heparin (subcutaneously at treatment doses), apixaban, dabigatran, edoxaban, or rivaroxaban should be initiated as soon as possible either before or after cardioversion (January et al., 2019). If cardioversion is successful in these high-risk patients, therapeutic anticoagulation with warfarin (INR target range 2–3) or a DOAC should be continued for at least 4 weeks. While the mentioned previously anticoagulants can also be initiated immediately before or after cardioversion in patients at low risk for stroke, it is also reasonable to not initiate anticoagulant therapy in these patients. Decisions regarding long-term anticoagulant therapy after this 4-week time period should be primarily based on the patient's risk for stroke and not on whether he/she is in SR.

If the practitioner decides to proceed with pharmacological cardioversion as the initial therapy, the selection of drug is primarily based on the presence of SHD (i.e., CAD, HF, LV hypertrophy). Pharmacological cardioversion is most effective when initiated within 7 days of the onset of AF. The AADs with proven efficacy during this time frame include dofetilide, flecainide, ibutilide, propafenone, or amiodarone (oral or IV). The class Ia AADs, disopyramide, procainamide, and quinidine, have limited efficacy or have been incompletely studied for this purpose. Sotalol is not effective for converting AF to SR. Although the use of single, oral loading doses of propafenone or flecainide is effective in restoring SR, these drugs should only be used in patients without underlying SHD. Ibutilide may also be considered in patients without underlying SHD. When utilizing the approach of administering single, oral loading doses of flecainide or propafenone for AF conversion for the first time, patients must be hospitalized to monitor for the development of proarrhythmic adverse effects.

If no adverse arrhythmic events occur during this hospitalization, then patients will be educated to self-administer an oral loading dose of flecainide or propafenone at the onset of AF symptoms (e.g., palpitations) in the future. A patient's ventricular rate should be adequately controlled with AV nodal blocking drugs prior to administering a class Ic (or class Ia) AAD for cardioversion since these AADs can precipitate an increased ventricular response as a result of their vagolytic effects. In patients with SHD, propafenone, flecainide, and ibutilide should be avoided because of the increased risk of proarrhythmia. Instead, amiodarone or dofetilide should be primarily used in this patient population (January et al., 2019).

If the practitioner does not wish to proceed with cardioversion, an initial management strategy of ventricular rate control and anticoagulation is also reasonable. As previously stated, this strategy, whereby the patient is left in AF, has been shown to be an acceptable alternative to rhythm control for the chronic management of AF. The selection of an oral drug for chronic ventricular rate control is primarily based on the patient's LV systolic function. In patients with normal LV systolic function (LVEF > 40%), an oral beta blocker, diltiazem, or verapamil is preferred to digoxin. Digoxin can be added if adequate ventricular rate control cannot be achieved with one of these drugs. In patients with HFrEF (LVEF of 40% or less), an oral beta blocker or digoxin is preferred because these drugs can also concomitantly be used to treat chronic HF. The nondihydropyridine CCBs should be avoided in patients with HFrEF because of their potent negative inotropic effects. In patients with AF and stable HF symptoms (NYHA class II or III), the beta blockers, carvedilol, metoprolol succinate, or bisoprolol should be used as first-line therapy because of their documented survival benefits in patients with HFrEF. Other beta blockers should be avoided in these patients because their effects on survival in HF are unknown. Digoxin should be used as first-line therapy in patients with AF and decompensated HFrEF (NYHA class IV) because beta blocker therapy may exacerbate HF symptoms. Oral amiodarone may also be considered if adequate ventricular rate control cannot be achieved with or the patient has contraindications to beta blockers or nondihydropyridine CCBs (January et al., 2019). In patients with persistent AF who have no or acceptable symptoms and stable LV systolic function (LVEF > 40%), the goal heart rate should be less than 110 beats/min at rest (January et al. 2014; Van Gelder et al., 2010). In patients with LVSD (LVEF of 40% or less), a stricter heart rate goal (<80 beats/min) should be considered to minimize the potential harmful effects of a rapid heart rate response on ventricular function.

Assessing the patient's risk of stroke becomes important for selecting the most appropriate anticoagulant regimen. The most recent guidelines for the treatment of AF have recommended the CHA_2DS_2-VASc scoring system for stroke risk stratification in patients with AF (January et al., 2019). CHA_2DS_2-VASc is an acronym for each of these risk factors—**C**ongestive heart failure, **H**ypertension, **A**ge 75 years or more, **D**iabetes mellitus, **S**troke or transient ischemic attack (TIA), **V**ascular disease, **A**ge 65 to 74 years, **S**ex **c**ategory. With this risk index, patients with AF are given 2 points each if they have a history of a previous stroke, TIA, or thromboembolism or if they are at least 75 years old. Patients are given one point each for being at least 65 to 74 years old, having hypertension, having diabetes, having congestive HF, having vascular disease (e.g., MI, peripheral arterial disease, or aortic plaque), or being female. The points are added up, and the total score is then used to determine the most appropriate anticoagulant therapy for the patient. Patients with a CHA_2DS_2-VASc score of 2 or higher are considered to be at high risk for stroke. In these patients, oral anticoagulant therapy with warfarin (target INR, 2.5; range, 2–3) or a DOAC is preferred to aspirin. Patients with a CHA_2DS_2-VASc score of 1 are considered to be at intermediate risk for stroke. In these patients, oral anticoagulant therapy (warfarin [target INR: 2.5; range: 2–3]), a DOAC, aspirin 75 to 325 mg/d, or no anticoagulant therapy can be selected. Patients with a CHA_2DS_2-VASc score of 0 are considered to be at low risk for stroke. The guidelines state that it is reasonable to not give any anticoagulant therapy to patients who are considered to be at low risk for stroke. Refer to Chapter 50 for a further discussion of anticoagulation in AF.

The need for anticoagulant therapy should be assessed in all patients with AF regardless of whether a rate-control or rhythm-control strategy is initiated. In addition, if patients are considered candidates for anticoagulant therapy, this regimen should be continued if SR is restored because of the potential for patients to have episodes of recurrent AF.

Third-Line Therapy

For those patients who remain symptomatic despite having adequate ventricular rate control or for those patients in whom adequate ventricular rate control cannot be achieved, it is reasonable to consider AAD therapy to maintain SR once they have been converted to SR. The selection of an AAD to maintain SR is primarily based on the presence of SHD (January et al., 2019) (see **Figure 22.2**). In patients without SHD, dofetilide, dronedarone, flecainide, propafenone, or sotalol should be considered initially, since these AADs have the best long-term safety profile. Amiodarone can be used as alternative therapy if the patient fails or does not tolerate one of these initial AADs. In patients with any type of SHD, the class Ic AADs, flecainide and propafenone, should be avoided. In these patients, the selection of AAD therapy is based upon the type of SHD present. In patients with LVSD (LVEF of 40% or less), either oral amiodarone or dofetilide can be used. Both dronedarone and sotalol should be avoided in patients with LVSD because of the risk of increased mortality (dronedarone) or worsening HF (sotalol). In patients with CAD, dofetilide, dronedarone, or sotalol can be used as initial therapy. In these patients, sotalol and dronedarone should only be used if their LV systolic function is normal. Amiodarone can be considered as an alternative therapy in these patients if these AADs are not tolerated. In patients with significant LV hypertrophy, amiodarone is the drug of choice. Patients with symptomatic episodes of recurrent AF who fail or do not tolerate at least one class I or III AAD may also be considered for radiofrequency catheter ablation (January et al., 2019).

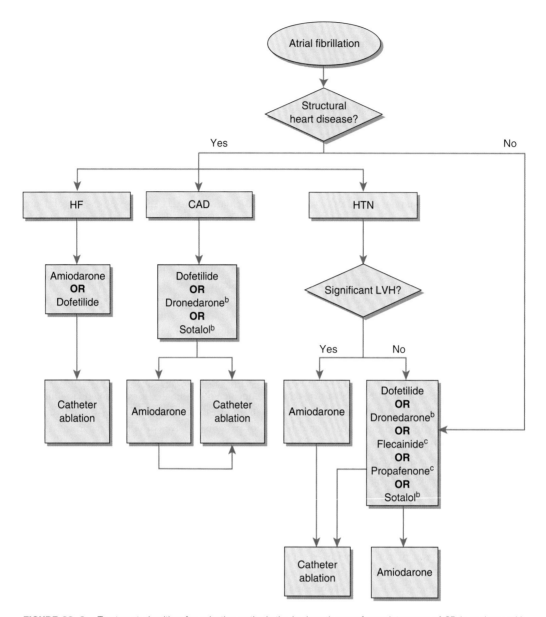

FIGURE 22–2   Treatment algorithm for selecting antiarrhythmic drug therapy for maintenance of SR in patients with recurrent paroxysmal or persistent AF. (Adapted from January, C. T., Wann, L. S., Alpert, J. S., et al. (2014). 2014 AHA/ACC/HRS guideline for the management of patients with atrial fibrillation: A report of the American College of Cardiology/American Heart Association Task Force on Practice Guidelines and the Heart Rhythm Society. *Circulation, 130*, e199–e267.)

[a] Within each of the boxes, the drugs are listed alphabetically, not in order of suggested use. However, the sequence of the boxes does imply the order of suggested use.
[b] Should only be used if patient has normal left ventricular systolic function.
[c] Should only be used if patient has no other form of structural heart disease.

AF, atrial fibrillation; CAD, coronary artery disease; HF, heart failure; HTN, hypertension; LVH, left ventricular hypertrophy.

Paroxysmal Supraventricular Tachycardia (Due to Atrioventricular Nodal Reentrant Tachycardia)

First-Line Therapy

Unless contraindicated, initial management of patients with vagal maneuvers (e.g., unilateral carotid sinus massage, Valsalva maneuver, facial immersion in ice water, and coughing) and/or adenosine may be appropriate. Clinical studies have shown that adenosine is as effective as IV verapamil in initial conversion of PSVT. Adenosine does not produce hypotension to the degree that verapamil does, and it has a shorter half-life. If a total of 30 mg of adenosine does not successfully terminate PSVT, further doses of this agent are unlikely to be effective. Furthermore, consideration may be given to acute treatment with oral beta-blockers, diltiazem, or verapamil in

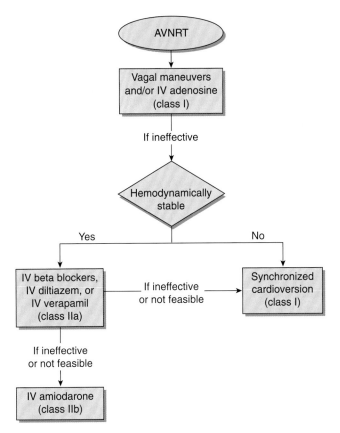

FIGURE 22–3 Treatment algorithm for paroxysmal supraventricular tachycardia (due to atrioventricular nodal reentrant tachycardia). (Adapted from Page, R. L., Joglar, J. A., Caldwell, M. A., et al. (2016). 2015 ACC/AHA/HRS guideline for the management of adult patients with supraventricular tachycardia: Executive Summary: A report of the American College of Cardiology/American Heart Association Task Force on Clinical Practice Guidelines and the Heart Rhythm Society. *Circulation*, *133*(14), e471–e505. https://doi.org/10.1161/CIR.0000000000000310)

AVNRT, atrioventricular nodal reentrant tachycardia; IV, intravenous.

hemodynamically stable patients. **Figure 22.3** illustrates an algorithm for the management of PSVT due to AV nodal reentrant tachycardia.

Second-Line Therapy

If vagal maneuvers or adenosine is unsuccessful or if PSVT recurs, second-line therapy is AADs. Therefore, in patients with persistent PSVT, other AADs will need to be used. In these patients, IV diltiazem, verapamil, or a beta blocker can be used. In hemodynamically unstable PSVT, or if PSVT continues, synchronized DCC to restore SR and correct hemodynamic compromise is warranted.

Third-Line Therapy

Third-line therapy focuses on the management of chronic PSVT. Chronic preventive therapy is usually necessary if the patient has either frequent episodes of PSVT that require therapeutic intervention or infrequent episodes of PSVT that are accompanied by severe symptoms. Radiofrequency catheter ablation is considered first-line therapy for most of these patients because of its effectiveness in preventing recurrence of PSVT and its relatively low complication rate. Drug therapy with oral diltiazem, verapamil, beta blockers, or digoxin can also be considered if the patient is not a candidate for or refuses to undergo radiofrequency catheter ablation.

Nonsustained Ventricular Tachycardia

VT that spontaneously terminates within 30 seconds is known as *nonsustained VT*. Given the poor survival of patients who experience cardiac arrest, it is essential to identify the most effective treatment strategies to prevent the initial episode of sustained VT or sudden cardiac death from occurring.

The presence of nonsustained VT in patients without SHD is not associated with an increased risk of sudden cardiac death. Therefore, drug therapy is not necessary in these patients if they are asymptomatic. However, if these patients do become symptomatic, treatment options include a beta blocker, nondihydropyridine CCB, class Ic AAD, or catheter ablation (depending on the underlying etiology) (Pedersen et al., 2014). Post-MI patients (especially those with LVSD) who develop nonsustained VT are at increased risk for sudden cardiac death. For these patients, the selection of therapy is based on the patient's LV systolic function. In patients who experience nonsustained VT due to prior MI, and have an LVEF greater than 40%, drug therapy is not necessary to treat the arrhythmia if they are asymptomatic. However, these patients should still chronically receive a beta blocker specifically to reduce mortality associated with the MI. Beta blockers are also effective if these patients develop significant symptoms associated with the nonsustained VT. In patients who experience nonsustained VT due to prior MI, and have an LVEF of 40% or less, electrophysiologic testing is often performed when asymptomatic nonsustained VT occurs (Pedersen et al., 2014). If sustained VT or VF is induced, an ICD is then recommended (Epstein et al., 2013). If sustained VT or VF is not induced, a beta blocker or amiodarone can be initiated.

Sustained Ventricular Tachycardia

VT that persists for at least 30 seconds or that requires electrical or pharmacological termination because of hemodynamic instability is known as *sustained VT*. Since sustained VT can degenerate into VF, the treatment goals are to terminate the VT acutely and then prevent recurrence of the arrhythmia.

First-Line Therapy

If the patient is hemodynamically unstable (i.e., severe hypotension, syncope, HF, or angina), immediate synchronized DCC is first-line therapy. If the patient is hemodynamically stable, IV amiodarone, IV procainamide, or IV sotalol can be considered (Neumar et al., 2010). Lidocaine can be used as alternative therapy. Synchronized DCC should be considered if AAD therapy fails.

Second-Line Therapy

Once the acute episode is terminated, measures should be taken to prevent recurrent episodes of VT. Based on the results of several trials, ICDs are clearly indicated as first-line therapy in patients with a history of sustained VT or VF (Epstein et al., 2013). If the patient with an ICD experiences frequent discharges because of recurrent ventricular arrhythmias or new-onset supraventricular arrhythmias (e.g., AF), either amiodarone and a beta blocker or sotalol monotherapy can be used. For the patient who refuses or is not a candidate for an ICD, oral amiodarone should be used as an alternative therapy.

Pulseless Ventricular Tachycardia/Ventricular Fibrillation

The majority of cases of sudden cardiac death can be attributed to VF. Sustained VT usually precedes VF and most commonly occurs in patients with CAD. VF is usually not preceded by any symptoms and always results in a loss of consciousness and eventually death if not treated. Immediate treatment is essential in patients who develop VF or pulseless VT, since survival is reduced by 10% for every minute that the patient remains in the arrhythmia. It is imperative to identify and correct any potential reversible causes for the arrhythmia.

For administration of drug therapy during an episode of pulseless VT/VF, while IV access is preferred, the guidelines recommend the intraosseous (IO) route as an alternative if IV access cannot be established (Neumar et al., 2010). IO access can be used not only for administration of drugs and fluids but also for obtaining blood for laboratory monitoring. If neither IV nor IO access can be established, the endotracheal route can then be used for the administration of only certain agents (i.e., atropine, lidocaine, epinephrine, and vasopressin). **Figure 22.4** illustrates an algorithm for the management of pulseless VT/VF.

First-Line Therapy

In patients with pulseless VT/VF, high-quality cardiopulmonary resuscitation (CPR) should be immediately initiated until a defibrillator or automated external defibrillator (AED) arrives (Kleinman et al., 2015). High-quality CPR is composed of the following components: minimizing interruptions in chest compressions (i.e., providing chest compressions for at least 80% of the time that the patient is in cardiac arrest), delivering 100 to 120 chest compressions per minute, delivering chest compressions at a depth of at least 2 inches (but avoiding a depth of >2.4 inches), minimizing leaning over the patient's chest (leaning can result in a reduction in venous return and cardiac output), and providing a ventilation rate of 10 breaths per minute. Each cycle of CPR involves delivering 30 chest compressions followed by two breaths. If a defibrillator or AED is not readily available, hands-only CPR (compressions only; no ventilations) should be provided if the bystander possesses no CPR training or is trained but lacks confidence in providing effective CPR with rescue breaths. If the bystander possesses CPR training and is confident in their ability to provide

effective CPR with rescue breaths, conventional cycles of CPR (30 chest compressions followed by two breaths) should be delivered until a defibrillator or AED becomes available. Once an advanced airway (e.g., endotracheal tube) is placed, chest compressions should be delivered continuously at a rate of 100 to 120 compressions per minute without pausing for ventilation (should be provided by a separate individual at a rate of one breath every 6 seconds). Once a defibrillator or AED arrives, defibrillation should be administered immediately.

With regard to defibrillation, delivery of only one shock at a time is recommended in patients with pulseless VT/VF to minimize interruptions in chest compressions (Link et al., 2015). For biphasic defibrillators, the dose of the shock is device specific (usually 120–200 J); the maximum dose available can be used for the initial shock if the effective dose range of the defibrillator is unknown. This dose or a higher dose can then be used for any subsequent shocks that may be needed. After delivery of the initial shock in patients with pulseless VT/VF, CPR should be immediately resumed and continued for 2 minutes, after which the patient's pulse and rhythm should be checked. Delaying pulse and rhythm checks until after this period of CPR is administered is intended to minimize interruptions in chest compressions and increase the potential for success with defibrillation. If pulseless VT/VF persists, another shock should be delivered at the appropriate dose, followed by 2 minutes of CPR. This general sequence of resuscitation and defibrillation should be followed as long as the patient remains in pulseless VT/VF.

Second-Line Therapy

If pulseless VT/VF persists after delivery of at least one shock and CPR, vasopressor therapy with epinephrine should be initiated (Link et al., 2015). The recommended dosage of epinephrine for pulseless VT/VF is 1 mg given IV push/IO every 3 to 5 minutes throughout the duration of the pulseless VT/VF episode.

Third-Line Therapy

If pulseless VT/VF persists despite the use of defibrillation, CPR, and vasopressor therapy, AAD therapy can be considered. IV amiodarone or lidocaine is recommended as AAD therapy for the treatment of pulseless VT/VF (Panchal et al., 2018). The recommended dose of lidocaine is 1 to 1.5 mg/kg IV or 300 mg amiodarone IV for the first dose and 0.5 to 0.75 mg/kg IV lidocaine or 150 mg amiodarone IV for the second dose, if needed. The value of using one of these drugs is increased in patients with witnessed arrest. The routine use of IV magnesium sulfate in patients with pulseless VT/VF is not recommended.

If the patient is resuscitated from the pulseless VT/VF episode, measures should be taken to prevent recurrent episodes of cardiac arrest. Based on the results of several trials, ICDs are clearly indicated as first-line therapy in patients with a history of sustained VT or VF (Epstein et al., 2013). If patients with an ICD experience frequent discharges because of recurrent ventricular arrhythmias or new-onset supraventricular arrhythmias (e.g., AF), either amiodarone and a beta blocker or sotalol monotherapy can

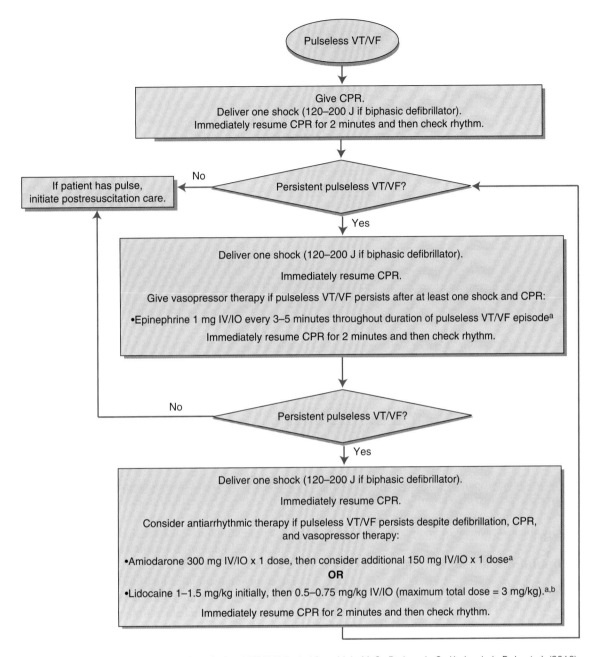

FIGURE 22–4   Treatment algorithm for pulseless VT/VF. (Adapted from Link, M. S., Berkow, L. C., Kudenchuk, P. J., et al. (2010). Part 7: Adult advanced cardiovascular life support: 2015 American Heart Association Guidelines Update for Cardiopulmonary Resuscitation and Emergency Cardiovascular Care. *Circulation, 132*(Suppl. 2), S444–S464.)

[a] If IV or IO access cannot be established, epinephrine and lidocaine may be administered by the endotracheal route. Because of the potential risk of pulmonary toxicity, IV amiodarone should not be administered down an endotracheal tube.

[b] Lidocaine can be used as alternative to IV amiodarone.

CPR, cardiopulmonary resuscitation; IO, intraosseous; IV, intravenous; J, joules; VF, ventricular fibrillation; VT, ventricular tachycardia.

be used. For patients who refuse or are not candidates for an ICD, oral amiodarone should be used as an alternative therapy.

Bradycardia

If patients with bradycardia present with signs and symptoms of adequate perfusion, only close observation is required. If patients with bradycardia develop signs or symptoms of poor perfusion (e.g., altered mental status, chest pain, hypotension, shock), IV atropine (0.5 mg every 3–5 minutes, up to 3 mg total dose) should be immediately administered (Neumar et al., 2010). If atropine is not effective, either transcutaneous pacing or a continuous infusion of a sympathomimetic agent, such as dopamine (2–10 mcg/kg/min) or epinephrine (2–10 mcg/min)

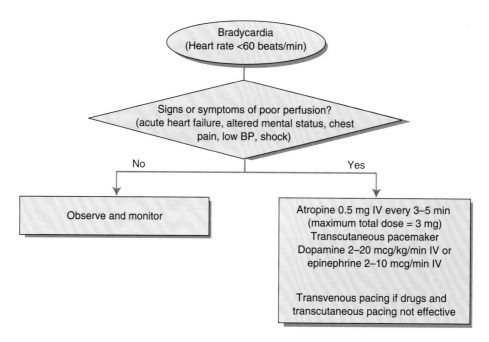

FIGURE 22–5 Treatment algorithm for bradycardia. (Adapted from Page, R. L., Joglar, J. A., Caldwell, M. A., et al. (2016). 2015 ACC/AHA/HRS guideline for the management of adult patients with supraventricular tachycardia: executive summary: A Report of the American College of Cardiology/American Heart Association Task Force on Clinical Practice Guidelines and the Heart Rhythm Society. *Circulation, 133*(14), e471–e505. https://doi.org/10.1161/CIR.0000000000000310)

BP, blood pressure; IV, intravenous.

(i.e., dopamine or epinephrine), should be initiated. If symptomatic bradycardia persists despite any of these measures, transvenous pacing should be utilized. **Figure 22.5** illustrates an algorithm for the management of bradycardia.

Special Population Considerations

Pediatric

The epidemiology of arrhythmias is different between adults and children. Adults have arrhythmias primarily of a cardiac origin, whereas children have arrhythmias primarily of a respiratory origin.

Tachyarrhythmias occasionally compromise infants and young children. PSVT is the most common arrhythmia in young children. It typically occurs during infancy or in children with congenital heart disease. PSVT with ventricular rates exceeding 180 to 220 beats/min can produce signs of shock. If signs of shock appear, synchronized cardioversion or administration of adenosine can be done in an emergency. Common causes of PSVT in young children and infants are congenital heart disease (preoperative) such as Ebstein's anomaly, transposition of the great arteries, or a single ventricle. Postoperative PSVT can also occur after atrial surgery for correction of congenital defects of the heart. Other common causes of PSVT in children are drugs such as sympathomimetics (cold medications, theophylline, beta agonists). WPW syndrome and hyperthyroidism can also cause PSVT. Common causes of AF and AFl in children are

intra-atrial surgery, Ebstein's anomaly, heart disease with dilated atria (aortic valve regurgitation), cardiomyopathy, WPW syndrome, sick sinus syndrome, and myocarditis.

Bradycardia is a common arrhythmia in seriously ill infants or children. It is usually associated with a reduction in cardiac output and is an ominous sign, suggesting that cardiac arrest is imminent. The first-line therapy for this arrhythmia in infants and young children is administration of oxygen, support respiration, epinephrine, and, possibly, atropine.

Pulseless VT and VF are treated much the same way as in adults (de Caen et al., 2015). The recommended dose of epinephrine for a child with pulseless VT/VF is 0.01 mg/kg IV/IO, administered as 0.1 mL/kg of a 1:10,000 concentration every 3 to 5 minutes throughout the duration of the pulseless VT/VF episode. If IV/IO access cannot be established, epinephrine can be administered endotracheally (0.1 mg/kg administered as 0.1 mL/kg of a 1:1,000 concentration).

Geriatric

With aging, body fat increases, lean body tissue decreases, and hepatic and renal system changes set the stage for potential overdosage and toxicity, particularly in the case of AADs. Similarly, declining organ function affects the amount and dosage of the drug prescribed as well as the occurrence of adverse effects. Cardiac disease and chronic conditions such as HF exacerbate the decline in organ function. Together, these factors can increase the risk of an adverse effect from the AADs the practitioner prescribes.

For example, digoxin toxicity is relatively common in older adult patients who are not receiving a reduced dosage to accommodate for the reduced renal function. It is imperative for the practitioner to assess the patient's baseline renal and hepatic function to determine whether certain AADs are safe to use and the most appropriate dosage to use in this patient.

Signs and symptoms of adverse effects of many drugs are confusion, weakness, and lethargy. These signs and symptoms are often attributed to senility or disease. Therefore, it is important for the practitioner to take a thorough drug history and to document accurately the dosages and frequencies prescribed in the patient record. If the practitioner merely attributes confusion to old age, the patient may continue to receive the drug while actually experiencing drug toxicity. Furthermore, the practitioner may add another drug to treat the complications caused by the original AAD, compounding the issue of polypharmacy and excessive medication.

AADs sometimes require accurate and timely dosing. If an older adult patient forgets to take a dose or cannot remember when he or she took the last dose, undermedication or overmedication may occur. This can be dangerous when AADs are prescribed. Many older adults have multiple prescriptions, even for the same medication, and therefore take an overdose of the drug. Consequently, it is essential to review medications with older adult patients and make sure they understand and can follow a safe drug therapy regimen.

MONITORING PATIENT RESPONSE

The goals of AAD therapy are to restore SR and prevent recurrences of the original arrhythmia or development of new arrhythmias. Evaluating the outcomes of AAD therapy requires the practitioner to schedule regular follow-up visits after initial treatment of the arrhythmia. The outcomes to be closely monitored include impulse generation and conduction from the SA node to the AV node, time interval for conduction, heart rate within a normal range that is age specific, and patterns of AV and ventricular conduction.

Data to be monitored to evaluate therapeutic outcomes vary from the simple to complex. The patient may monitor some of them and needs to be taught the signs and symptoms to look for and the expectations from the therapeutic regimen. Patients with arrhythmias may be monitored on a regular or periodic basis with 12-lead EKGs, 24-hour Holter monitors, blood pressure, heart rate, echocardiograms, electrolytes, and serum drug levels (when applicable).

In addition, the patient needs to self-monitor for symptoms such as light-headedness, dizziness, syncopal episodes, palpitations, chest pain, shortness of breath, or weight gain. Other clinical outcomes to be monitored are those that affect quality of life, such as activity tolerance, organ perfusion, cognitive function, fear, anxiety, and depression.

PATIENT EDUCATION

Drug Information

Included in the therapeutic plan for arrhythmias is patient education. Learning outcomes can be evaluated by monitoring compliance with the medication regimen, recurrences of arrhythmia, adverse effects, weight gain, blood pressure, heart rate, and emergency department visits or hospitalizations.

AADs have narrow therapeutic windows. Toxicity is common at normal dosages. Consequently, patient education is essential for providing maximal benefits and avoiding adverse effects and accidental overdosing or underdosing.

The patient, family, and significant others should be taught the basics, such as the name of the drug (both the generic and the trade names), the dose, the frequency and timing of the dose, and the reason the drug is needed. This may avoid duplicate prescribing and administration of AADs. The patient should communicate, either verbally or in writing, the names and dosages of these drugs to all other health care providers and should wear a medical identification device listing all medications. In addition, the patient should inform his or her health care provider when any new prescription, over-the-counter, or complementary or alternative medications are started so that potential drug interactions can be minimized or avoided.

The practitioner should provide written instructions for the medication regimen. Providing instructions in large print and simple language may be helpful to patients who have difficulty with memory, hearing, or vision. Instructions should include what to do when the patient misses a dose of medication, has an adverse response to the medication, or wants to stop taking the drug. If beta blockers are prescribed, the patient should be warned that abrupt discontinuation may result in rebound angina, an increased heart rate, and hypertension. The symptoms associated with these adverse effects should also be identified.

The practitioner can also teach the patient or caregiver how to take blood pressure and pulse readings; how to interpret the readings; and how to recognize and respond to signs and symptoms of hypotension, dizziness, chest pain, shortness of breath, peripheral edema, or palpitations. The patient should take his or her weight each day and call the practitioner if weight gain of over 2 lb occurs. If the patient has difficulty learning these monitoring techniques or cannot perform them, he or she may need to schedule regular follow-up appointments for monitoring. Patients with AF or AFl should know the signs and symptoms of a stroke.

In today's health care environment, the insurance plan's pharmacy provider sometimes makes substitutions with generics or less expensive brands of medications. To prevent harmful drug effects, the patient needs to be aware of this practice and should be cautioned not to change brands of the prescribed AAD or anticoagulant without the approval of the practitioner.

An important teaching point from an ethical and legal perspective is to warn the patient to avoid hazardous activities such as driving, using electrical tools, climbing ladders, or any activity that would put the patient or others in harm's way until the effects of the drug are demonstrated. Patients with an ICD should refrain from driving for at least 6 months after the last arrhythmic event (for devices implanted for secondary prevention) or for at least 7 days following implantation of the ICD (for devices implanted for primary prevention). Documentation of patient teaching on risks, benefits, lifestyle modification, and safety issues with AAD treatment should always be entered in the patient's medical record.

Nutrition

Clear instructions should be given to avoid alcohol, excessive salt intake, and caffeine during treatment for arrhythmias. Many AADs may cause periods of hypotension resulting in dizziness, or the dose of the drug may need to be regulated, especially in the initial weeks.

Complementary and Alternative Medications

The practitioner must emphasize to the patient the importance of reporting the use of any of these agents so that interactions with AAD therapy can be minimized or avoided. While the information regarding potential interactions between AADs and specific complementary and alternative medications is relatively sparse, there are a few notable interactions of which practitioners should be aware. Patients taking AADs should avoid licorice root. Licorice has mineralocorticoid effects, which can promote hypokalemia. In patients taking digoxin, the presence of hypokalemia may predispose the patient to digoxin toxicity. In patients taking other AADs, the presence of hypokalemia may promote the development of atrial or ventricular arrhythmias. In addition, certain licorice preparations have been shown to cause a prolonged QT interval, which may increase the risk for TdP in patients receiving class III AADs. The use of Siberian ginseng or oleander should also be avoided in patients receiving digoxin, as digoxin toxicity may result. The use of St. John's wort may decrease digoxin concentrations; therefore, digoxin concentrations should be closely monitored when concomitant therapy is used. St. John's wort may also decrease plasma concentrations of amiodarone and dronedarone, which may predispose the patient to arrhythmia recurrence. Consequently, the use of St. John's wort in patients receiving amiodarone or dronedarone should be avoided. Patients with a history of atrial or ventricular arrhythmias should also be instructed to avoid the use of any medication containing ephedra (e.g., Ma Huang) because it can promote the development of arrhythmias.

CASE STUDY 1*

H.T. is a 66-year-old man with heart failure with reduced ejection fraction (New York Heart Association class III) who presents to the emergency department with shortness of breath and palpitations. An electrocardiogram reveals atrial fibrillation with a heart rate (HR) of 130 beats/min. He states that these symptoms have been occurring for the past 5 days. H.T. has a medical history of diabetes (A1c, 12.2%) and chronic kidney disease requiring hemodialysis. His current medications include insulin glargine 40 units subcutaneously every evening, insulin lispro 12 units subcutaneously before meals, metoprolol succinate 100 mg orally daily, and lisinopril 5 mg orally daily. His vitals are blood pressure 145/95 mm Hg and HR 130 beats/min.

DIAGNOSIS: ATRIAL FIBRILLATION

1. Which of the following would be the most appropriate treatment to acutely manage this patient's symptoms?
    a. Metoprolol IV
    b. Diltiazem IV
    c. Digoxin IV
    d. Amiodarone IV

2. What additional therapy, if any, should be recommended for this patient to prevent thromboembolic complications?
    a. No anticoagulant therapy is necessary because his CHA_2DS_2-VASc score is 0.
    b. Dabigatran is recommended because his CHA_2DS_2-VASc score is 1.
    c. Apixaban is recommended because his CHA_2DS_2-VASc score is 2.
    d. Warfarin is recommended because his CHA_2DS_2-VASc score is 3.

---

*Answers can be found online.

Bibliography

Starred references are cited in the text.

*Anderson, J. L., Lutz, J. R., & Allison, S. B. (1983). Electrophysiologic and antiarrhythmic effects of oral flecainide in patients with inducible ventricular tachycardia. *Journal of the American College of Cardiology, 2,* 105–114.

*Antiarrhythmics Versus Implantable Defibrillators (AVID) Investigators. (1997). A comparison of antiarrhythmic-drug therapy with implantable defibrillators in patients resuscitated from near-fatal ventricular arrhythmias. *New England Journal of Medicine, 337,* 1576–1583.

*Babatin, M., Lee, S. S., & Pollak, P. T. (2008). Amiodarone hepatotoxicity. *Current Vascular Pharmacology, 6,* 228–236.

*Bardy, G. H., Lee, K. L., Mark, D. B., et al. (2005). Amiodarone or an implantable cardioverter-defibrillator for congestive heart failure. *New England Journal of Medicine, 352,* 225–237.

*Bogazzi, F., Tomisiti, L., Bartalena, L., et al. (2012). Amiodarone and the thyroid: A 2012 update. *Journal of Endocrinological Investigation, 35,* 340–348.

*Buxton, A. E., Lee, K. L., Fisher, J. D., et al. (1999). A randomized study of the prevention of sudden death in patients with coronary artery disease. *New England Journal of Medicine, 341,* 1882–1890.

Cairns, J. A., Connolly, S. J., & Roberts, R. (1997). Randomized trial of outcome after myocardial infarction in patients with frequent or repetitive ventricular premature depolarizations: CAMIAT. *Lancet, 349,* 675–682.

*Camm, A. J., Camm, C. F., & Savelieva, I. (2012). Medical treatment of atrial fibrillation. *Journal of Cardiovascular Medicine, 13,* 97–107.

*Cardiac Arrhythmia Suppression Trial Investigators. (1989). Preliminary report: Effect of encainide and flecainide on mortality in a randomized trial of arrhythmia suppression after myocardial infarction. *New England Journal of Medicine, 321,* 406–412.

*Carlsson, J., Miketic, S., Windeler, J., et al. (2004). Randomized trial of rate-control versus rhythm-control in persistent atrial fibrillation: The Strategies of Treatment of Atrial Fibrillation (STAF) study. *Journal of the American College of Cardiology, 41,* 1690–1696.

*Connolly, S. J., Camm, A. J., Halperin, J. L., et al. (2011). Dronedarone in high-risk atrial fibrillation. *New England Journal of Medicine, 365,* 2268–2276.

*Connolly, S. J., Dorian, P., Roberts, R. S., et al. (2006). Comparison of beta-blockers, amiodarone plus beta-blockers, or sotalol for prevention of shocks from implantable cardioverter defibrillators: The OPTIC study. *Journal of the American Medical Association, 295,* 165–171.

*Connolly, S. J., Gent, M., Roberts, R. S., et al. (2000). Canadian Implantable Defibrillator Study (CIDS): A randomized trial of the implantable cardioverter defibrillator versus amiodarone. *Circulation, 101,* 1297–1302.

Dager, W. E., Sanoski, C. A., Wiggins, B. S., et al. (2006). Pharmacotherapy considerations in advanced cardiac life support. *Pharmacotherapy, 26,* 1703–1729.

*de Caen, A. R., Berg, M. D., Chameides, L., et al. (2015). Part 12: Pediatric advanced life support: 2015 American Heart Association Guidelines Update for Cardiopulmonary Resuscitation and Emergency Cardiovascular Care. *Circulation, 132*(Suppl. 2), S526–S542.

Dorian, P., Cass, D., Schwartz, B., et al. (2002). Amiodarone as compared with lidocaine for shock-resistant ventricular fibrillation. *New England Journal of Medicine, 346,* 884–890.

*Epstein, A. E., DiMarco, J. P., Ellenbogen, K. A., et al. (2013). 2012 ACCF/AHA/HRS focused update incorporated into the ACCF/AHA/HRS 2008 guidelines for device-based therapy of cardiac rhythm abnormalities: A report of the American College of Cardiology/American Heart Association Task Force on Practice Guidelines and the Heart Rhythm Society. *Journal of the American College of Cardiology, 61,* e6–e75.

*Goldschlager, N., Epstein, A. E., Naccarelli, G., et al. (2007). A practical guide for clinicians who treat patients with amiodarone. *Heart Rhythm, 4,* 1250–1259.

*Hohnloser, S. H., Crijns, H. J., van Eickels, M., et al. (2009). Effect of dronedarone on cardiovascular events in atrial fibrillation. *New England Journal of Medicine, 360,* 668–678.

*Hohnloser, S. H., Kuck, K. H., & Lilienthal, J. (2000). Rhythm or rate control in atrial fibrillation—Pharmacological Intervention in Atrial Fibrillation (PIAF): A randomised trial. *Lancet, 356,* 1789–1794.

*January, C. T., Wann, L. S., Alpert, J. S., et al. (2014). 2014 AHA/ACC/HRS guideline for the management of patients with atrial fibrillation: A report of the American College of Cardiology/American Heart Association Task Force on Practice Guidelines and the Heart Rhythm Society. *Circulation, 130,* e199–e267.

*January, C. T., Wann, L. S., Calkins, H., et al (2019). 2019 AHA/ACC/HRS focused update of the 2014 AHA/ACC/HRS guideline for the management of patients with atrial fibrillation: A report of the American College of Cardiology/American Heart Association Task Force on Clinical Practice Guidelines and the Heart Rhythm Society. *Journal of the American College of Cardiology, 74*(1), 104–132. https://doi.org/10.1016/j.jacc.2019.01.011

*Jaworski, K., Walecka, I., Rudnicka, L., et al. (2014). Cutaneous adverse reactions of amiodarone. *Medical Science Monitor, 20,* 2369–2372.

*Kleinman, M. E., Brennan, E. E., Goldberger, Z. D., et al. (2015). Part 5: Adult basic life support and cardiopulmonary resuscitation quality: 2015 American Heart Association Guidelines Update for Cardiopulmonary Resuscitation and Emergency Cardiovascular Care. *Circulation, 132*(Suppl. 2), S414–S435.

*Køber, L., Bloch-Thomsen, P. E., Møller, M., et al. (2000). Danish Investigations of Arrhythmia and Mortality on Dofetilide (DIAMOND) Study Group. Effect of dofetilide in patients with recent myocardial infarction and left-ventricular dysfunction: A randomised trial. *Lancet, 356,* 2052–2058.

*Køber, L., Torp-Pedersen, C., McMurray, J. J., et al. (2008). Increased mortality after dronedarone therapy for severe heart failure. *New England Journal of Medicine, 358,* 2678–2687.

*Kuck, K. H., Cappato, R., Siebels, J., et al. (2000). Randomized comparison of antiarrhythmic drug therapy with implantable defibrillators in patients resuscitated from cardiac arrest: The Cardiac Arrest Study Hamburg (CASH). *Circulation, 102,* 748–754.

Kudenchuck, P. J., Cobb, L. A., Copass, M. K., et al. (1999). Amiodarone for resuscitation after out-of-hospital cardiac arrest due to ventricular fibrillation. *New England Journal of Medicine, 341,* 871–879.

*Le Heuzey, J. Y., De Ferrari, G. M., Radzik, D., et al. (2010). A short-term, randomized, double-blind, parallel-group study to evaluate the efficacy and safety of dronedarone versus amiodarone in patients with persistent atrial fibrillation: The DIONYSOS study. *Journal of Cardiovascular Electrophysiology, 21,* 597–605.

*Lei, M., Wu, L., Terrar, D. A., & Huang, C. L. (2018). Modernized classification of cardiac antiarrhythmic drugs. *Circulation, 138*(17), 1879–1896. doi: 10.1161/CIRCULATIONAHA.118.035455. Erratum in: *Circulation,* 2019 Mar 26, *139*(13), e635. PMID: 30354657.

*Link, M. S., Berkow, L. C., Kudenchuk, P. J., et al. (2015). Part 7: Adult advanced cardiovascular life support: 2015 American Heart Association Guidelines Update for Cardiopulmonary Resuscitation and Emergency Cardiovascular Care. *Circulation, 132*(Suppl. 2), S444–S464.

*Miller, M. R., McNamara, R. L., Segal, J. B., et al. (2000). Efficacy of agents for pharmacological conversion of atrial fibrillation and subsequent maintenance of sinus rhythm: A meta-analysis of clinical trials. *Journal of Family Practice, 49,* 1033–1046.

*Moss, A. J., Hall, W. J., Cannom, D. S., et al. (1996). Improved survival with an implanted defibrillator in patients with coronary disease at high risk for ventricular arrhythmia. *New England Journal of Medicine, 335,* 1933–1940.

*Moss, A. J., Zareba, W., Hall, W. J., et al. (2002). Prophylactic implantation of a defibrillator in patients with myocardial infarction and reduced ejection fraction. *New England Journal of Medicine, 346,* 877–883.

*Neumar, R. W., Otto, C. W., Link, M. S., et al. (2010). Part 8: Adult advanced cardiovascular support: 2010 American Heart Association Guidelines for Cardiopulmonary Resuscitation and Emergency Cardiovascular Care. *Circulation, 122*(Suppl. 3), S729–S767.

*Opolski, G., Torbicki, A., Kosior, D. A., et al. (2004). Rate control vs. rhythm control in patients with nonvalvular persistent atrial fibrillation:

The results of the Polish How to Treat Chronic Atrial Fibrillation (HOT CAFE) Study. *Chest, 126,* 476–486.

*Oral, H., Souza, J. J., Michaud, G. F., et al. (1999). Facilitating transthoracic cardioversion of atrial fibrillation with ibutilide pretreatment. *New England Journal of Medicine, 340,* 1849–1854.

*Pacifico, A., Hohnloser, S. H., Williams, J. H., et al. (1999). Prevention of implantable-defibrillator shocks by treatment with sotalol: Sotalol Implantable Cardioverter-Defibrillator Study Group. *New England Journal of Medicine, 340,* 1855–1862.

*Panchal, A. R., Berg, K. M., Kudenchuk, P. J., et al. (2018). 2018 American Heart Association focused update on advanced cardiovascular life support use of antiarrhythmic drugs during and immediately after cardiac arrest: An update to the American Heart Association guidelines for cardiopulmonary resuscitation and emergency cardiovascular care. *Circulation, 138*(23), e740–e749. https://doi.org/10.1161/CIR.0000000000000613

*Passman, R. S., Bennett, C. L., Purpura, J. M., et al. (2012). Amiodarone-associated optic neuropathy: A critical review. *American Journal of Medicine, 125,* 447–453.

*Pedersen, T. P., Kay, G. N., Kalman, J., et al. (2014). EHRA/HRS/APHRS expert consensus on ventricular arrhythmias. *Heart Rhythm, 11,* e166–e196.

*Phillips, B. G., Gandhi, A. J., Sanoski, C. A., et al. (1997). Comparison of intravenous diltiazem and verapamil for the acute treatment of atrial fibrillation and flutter. *Pharmacotherapy, 17,* 1238–1245.

*Range, F. T., Hilker, E., Breithardt, G., et al. (2013). Amiodarone-induced pulmonary toxicity: A fatal case report and review of the literature. *Cardiovascular Drugs and Therapy, 27,* 247–254.

*Roy, D., Talajic, M., Dorian, P., et al. (2000). Amiodarone to prevent recurrence of atrial fibrillation. *New England Journal of Medicine, 342,* 913–920.

*Roy, D., Talajic, M., Nattel, S., et al. (2008). Rhythm control versus rate control for atrial fibrillation and heart failure. *New England Journal of Medicine, 358,* 2667–2677.

*Sanoski, C. A., & Bauman, J. L. (2002). Clinical observations with the amiodarone/warfarin interaction: Dosing relationships with long-term therapy. *Chest, 121,* 19–23.

*Singh, B. N., Connolly, S. J., Crijns, H. J., et al. (2007). Dronedarone for maintenance of sinus rhythm in atrial fibrillation or flutter. *New England Journal of Medicine, 357,* 987–999.

*Singh, S. N., Singh, B. N., Reda, D. J., et al. (2005). Amiodarone versus sotalol for atrial fibrillation. *New England Journal of Medicine, 352,* 1861–1872.

*Singh, S., Zoble, R. G., Yellen, L., et al. (2000). Efficacy and safety of oral dofetilide in converting to and maintaining sinus rhythm in patients with chronic atrial fibrillation or atrial flutter: The Symptomatic Atrial Fibrillation Investigative Research on Dofetilide (SAFIRE-D) Study. *Circulation, 102,* 2385–2390.

*Slavik, R. S., Tisdale, J. E., & Borzak, S. (2001). Pharmacological conversion of atrial fibrillation: A systematic review of available evidence. *Progress in Cardiovascular Diseases, 44,* 121–152.

*Stambler, B. S., Wood, M. A., Ellenbogen, K. A., et al. (1996). Efficacy and safety of repeated intravenous doses of ibutilide for rapid conversion of atrial flutter or fibrillation. *Circulation, 94,* 1613–1621.

*Torp-Pedersen, C., Moller, M., Bloch-Thomson, P. E., et al. (1999). Dofetilide in patients with congestive heart failure and left ventricular dysfunction. Danish Investigations of Arrhythmia and Mortality on Dofetilide Study Group. *New England Journal of Medicine, 341,* 857–865.

*Van der Werf, C., Kannankeril, P. J., Sacher, F., et al. (2011). Flecainide therapy reduces exercise-induced ventricular arrhythmias in patients with catecholaminergic polymorphic ventricular tachycardia. *Journal of the American College of Cardiology, 57,* 2244–2254.

*Van Gelder, I. C., Groenveld, H. F., Crijns, H. J. G. M., et al. (2010). Lenient versus strict rate control in patients with atrial fibrillation. *New England Journal of Medicine, 362,* 1363–1373.

*Van Gelder, I. C., Hagens, V. E., Bosker, H. A., et al. (2002). The rate control versus electrical cardioversion for persistent atrial fibrillation study group. A comparison of rate control and rhythm control in patients with recurrent persistent atrial fibrillation. *New England Journal of Medicine, 347,* 1834–1840.

*Vaughan Williams, E. M. (1984). A classification of antiarrhythmic actions reassessed after a decade of new drugs. *Journal of Clinical Pharmacology, 24,* 129–147.

*Wyse, D. G., Kellen, J., & Rademaker, A. W. (1988). Prophylactic versus selective lidocaine for early ventricular arrhythmias of myocardial infarction. *Journal of the American College of Cardiology, 12,* 507–513.

*Wyse, D. G., Waldo, A. L., DiMarco, J. P., et al. (2002). A comparison of rate control and rhythm control in patients with atrial fibrillation. *New England Journal of Medicine, 347,* 1825–1833.

*You, J. J., Singer, D. E., Howard, P. A., et al. (2012). Antithrombotic therapy for atrial fibrillation: Antithrombotic therapy and prevention of thrombosis, 9th ed: American College of Chest Physicians Evidence-Based Clinical Practice Guidelines. *Chest, 141,* e531S–e575S.

UNIT
6

Pharmacotherapy for Respiratory Disorders

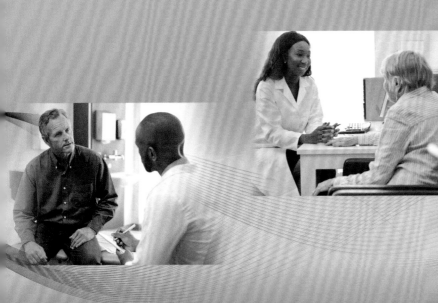

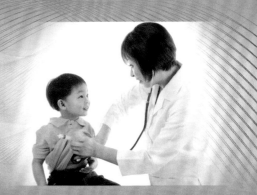

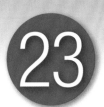

23 Respiratory Infections

Sara Jung, Karleen Melody, Anisha B. Grover, and Andrew J. Grimone

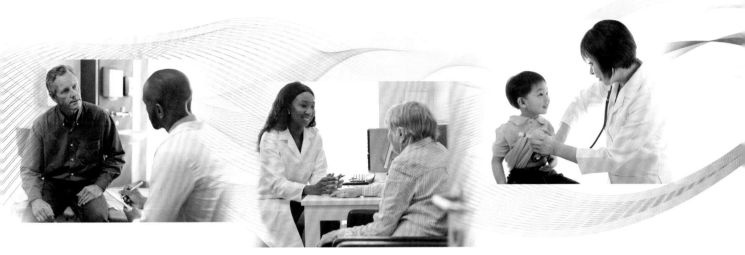

Learning Objectives

1. Differentiate between the common cold and rhinosinusitis.
2. Differentiate between bronchitis and pneumonia.
3. Develop a treatment plan based on symptoms.

INTRODUCTION

Upper respiratory tract infections (URIs), including the common cold and rhinosinusitis, are some of the most common problems seen in primary care. URIs are usually self-limiting, minor illnesses that account for half or more of all acute illnesses. It is difficult to differentiate the common cold from rhinosinusitis or allergic rhinitis. URIs commonly involve rhinitis, which refers to irritation and inflammation of the intranasal mucous membrane and is characterized by nasal congestion, nasal discharge, sneezing, and postnasal drip. Other common URI symptoms include tenderness over the sinuses, fever, headache, malaise, sore throat, myalgias, a full feeling around the eyes and ears, and coughing. Symptoms may present individually or in combination, and it can be difficult to determine whether the cause is viral or bacterial.

URIs can progress to involve acute or chronic complications. In children especially, URIs may progress to otitis media. In a small percentage of cases, the viral or bacterial cause may travel, causing rhinosinusitis and bronchitis. Acute respiratory infections have been projected to kill approximately 3.9 million people annually and represent a leading cause of mortality in children living in developing countries who are less than 5 years of age (Liu et al., 2012). There is also an enormous economic burden associated with URIs.

COMMON COLD

Acute infectious rhinitis, also known as the *common cold*, *nasopharyngitis*, *rhinopharyngitis*, or *acute coryza*, is caused by one of more than 200 viral types and most commonly involves rhinovirus. It is one of the most common infections and is usually minor and self-limiting. Coryza is an acute inflammation of the mucous membranes of the respiratory passages, particularly of the nose, sinuses, and throat, and is characterized by sneezing, rhinorrhea (watery nasal discharge), and coughing.

In 2012, the U.S. Attitudes of Consumers Toward Health, Cough, and Cold survey was developed to collect information regarding participant demographics, basic knowledge of cough and cold symptoms, treatment choices, and treatment preferences (Blaiss et al., 2015). Of the 2,505 survey participants, 84.6% had experienced at least one occurrence of cold in the past year that lasted approximately 1 to 7 days. Cough was the most common cold symptom, affecting 73.1% of participants, and this symptom, along with nasal congestion, was reported as the most bothersome symptom. A subsequent publication examined the data from this study in order to assess the impact of cough and cold on daily activity, productivity, and absenteeism (Dicpinigaitis et al., 2015). Fifty-two percent of participants described the impact on daily life as a "fair amount" to "a lot" for the duration of the illness (Dicpinigaitis et al., 2015). During the time of a cold, participants reported a decrease in productivity by a mean of 26.4%. Almost half of respondents reported absenteeism from work or school lasting 1 to 2 days (Dicpinigaitis et al., 2015). In 2019, the Consumer Healthcare Products Association released a white paper publication estimating annual sales of $4.8 billion on over-the-counter medications in the United States. Another survey published in 2003 estimated that noninfluenza viral respiratory infections result in an annual $40 billion in costs. This includes costs related to cold-related absenteeism, including 70 million missed workdays, 186 million missed school days, and 126 million missed workdays among caregivers of children suffering from colds (Fendrick et al., 2003).

Causes

The pathogen most frequently associated with common colds is human rhinovirus (HRV), a single-stranded ribonucleic acid accounting for one half to two-thirds of common colds (Jacobs et al., 2013). The coronavirus, respiratory syncytial virus (RSV), influenza virus, human parainfluenza virus, human metapneumovirus, and adenovirus can also contribute to cold-like symptoms, but HRVs are the single most pervasive cause of colds and in some cases can increase the susceptibility to bacterial infection within the upper and lower airway epithelial cells (Jacobs et al., 2013).

Predisposition to viral infections can be attributed to many factors, including frequent exposure to viral infectious agents; age, especially in pediatric and older populations; and the inability to resist invading organisms because of allergies, malnutrition, immune deficiencies, physical abnormalities, or other comorbidities. Some experts propose a relationship between the host response to the virus and the production of cold symptoms. Studies show that common colds are more frequent or more severe in those under increased stress, probably as a result of stress weakening the immune system.

Pathophysiology

If there is a breakdown or failure in the protective barriers of the upper respiratory tract (i.e., cough, gag, and sneeze reflexes, lymph nodes, immunoglobulin A antibodies), viral pathogens trigger an acute inflammatory reaction with release of vasoactive mediators and increased parasympathetic stimuli. This produces congestion and rhinorrhea. Viral URIs also trigger inflammatory mediators that increase the sensitivity of afferent sensory nerves in the airway, which may contribute to the cough typically associated with the common cold.

Bradykinin and lysyl-bradykinin contribute to the pathogenesis of HRV infections. An increase in kinin levels is associated with increased permeability of the vasculature. However, histamine levels remain unchanged, indicating the lack of involvement of mast cells and basophils (Jacobs et al., 2013). The involvement of prostaglandins can be elucidated by the demonstrated effectiveness of cyclooxygenase inhibitors in reducing headache, malaise, myalgias, and cough during HRV infection.

Transmission of HRV occurs predominantly by intranasal or conjunctival inoculation and has been attributed to three methods: airborne transmission by small particles (droplets), airborne transmission by large particles, and direct contact. Large particle transmission is not efficient and requires prolonged exposure. Direct contact involves donor nose-to-hand contact, which is then transmitted to a recipient. From there, transmission occurs primarily when the infected hand makes contact with the eyes or nose. Although conjunctival cells are not thought to harbor HRV, it probably can be passed through the tear duct into the nose. HRV can survive indoors for a range of hours to days at room temperature (Jacobs et al., 2013). Rhinoviruses grow in the upper airway and attach and gain entry to host cells by binding to an intracellular adhesion molecule. Infection begins in the adenoidal area and spreads to the ciliated epithelium in the nose. HRVs remain infectious for at least 3 hours after drying on hard surfaces such as telephones or countertops, but they do not last as long on porous surfaces.

Diagnostic Criteria

Available laboratory diagnostic tests include the collection and processing of specimens, detection and serology of antigens, conventional and rapid virus cultures, and many other technologies; however, diagnostic tests are not recommended (Jacobs et al., 2013). In order to evaluate specimens, collection would have to occur as soon as possible after symptom onset, since HRV titers are most elevated during the first 2 days of clinical presentation. The short duration of most colds results in an impractical window of appropriate timing and, therefore, makes the diagnostic process inaccurate.

The most common method of diagnosis involves symptom evaluation. Onset of common cold signs and symptoms occurs 1 to 2 days after viral infection and peaks in approximately 2 to 4 days. A cough may persist following the resolution of other symptoms. Symptoms consist primarily of clear nasal discharge, sneezing, nasal congestion, cough, low-grade fever (below 102°F [38.9°C]), scratchy or sore throat, mild aches, chills, headache, watery eyes, tenderness around the eyes, fullness in the ears, and fatigue. In children, the presentation could also include fever with seizures, anorexia, vomiting, diarrhea, and abdominal pain. Symptoms usually resolve in approximately 1 week, but they may linger for up to 2 weeks.

Initiating Drug Therapy

Improper treatment of the common cold by clinicians is common for several reasons. It is often difficult to determine whether the cause is viral or bacterial. There is no cure for the common cold; therefore, treatment strategies are supportive in nature and consist primarily of symptom relief.

Nonpharmacologic therapies are the first line of treatment, beginning with bed rest. This also helps prevent transmission to others. Adequate fluid intake is encouraged, which can assist with liquefying tenacious secretions, which in turn allows easier expectoration, soothes sore throats, and relieves dry skin and lips. Saline gargles also are effective for soothing sore throats. Saline nasal flushes and irrigation have shown benefit in clearing nasal passages without the risk for rebound congestion; however, evidence remains limited (Fokkens et al., 2012).

Coughing caused by chest congestion can cause a muscular chest pain. Menthol rubs can soothe this ache and open airways for congestion relief. Menthol lozenges also have similar effects. Petrolatum-based ointments can alleviate skin irritation and excoriation around nasolabial areas caused by friction from wiping. Inhalation of steam has not demonstrated benefit in the drainage of mucus or the destruction of the cold virus and is therefore not recommended (Fokkens et al., 2012).

Goals of Drug Therapy

The main goals of treatment for the common cold are relief of symptoms, reduction of the risk for complications, and prevention of spread to others.

Decongestants

Decongestants come in topical or oral preparations and can be somewhat effective for the short-term relief of cold symptoms (Fashner et al., 2012). Topical decongestants, such as oxymetazoline hydrochloride (Afrin) and phenylephrine hydrochloride (Afrin Children's, Little Remedies, Neo-Synephrine), are available in nasal spray and pump mist preparations. Oral decongestants, such as pseudoephedrine (Sudafed) and phenylephrine (Sudafed PE), are also available. Decongestants are typically available OTC. Preparations containing pseudoephedrine can be obtained without a prescription but must be purchased from behind the counter at a pharmacy.

Mechanism of Action

Decongestants are sympathomimetic agents that stimulate alpha- and beta-adrenergic receptors, causing vasoconstriction in the respiratory tract mucosa and thereby improving ventilation. Topical decongestants have little systemic absorption but work locally by slowing ciliary motility and mucociliary clearance. Oral agents have the same mechanism of action and assist in the clearance of nasal mucus and obstruction. Their use may help to prevent rhinosinusitis and eustachian tube blockage in patients susceptible to these conditions.

Dosage

Oxymetazoline hydrochloride 0.05% nasal spray and pump mists can be used in patients who are at least 6 years old at a dosage of 2 to 3 sprays in each nostril not more often than every 10 to 12 hours. Patients should not exceed two doses of oxymetazoline in a 24-hour time period. Phenylephrine nasal sprays are available as 0.125%, 0.25%, 0.5%, and 1% preparations. For specific dosing recommendations, see **Table 23.1**.

TABLE 23.1

Overview of Agents for Upper Respiratory Infections

Generic (Trade) Name and Dosage	Selected Adverse Events	Contraindications	Special Considerations
Decongestants			
Oxymetazoline hydrochloride (Afrin, Mucinex Sinus, Neo-Synephrine, Vicks Sinex) Nasal spray and pump mists (0.05%) ≥6 y: 2–3 sprays per nostril q10–12h	Palpitations, headaches	Hypersensitivity	These drugs may cause rebound congestion. Use only 2–3 d and then switch to oral decongestants.
Phenylephrine hydrochloride (Neo-Synephrine, Sudafed PE, Afrin Children) Nasal spray (0.125%) 2–5 y: 2–3 sprays per nostril q4h Mild nasal spray (0.25%) 6–12 y: 2–3 sprays per nostril q4h Regular nasal spray (0.5%) ≥12 y: 2–3 sprays per nostril q4h Extra strength nasal spray (1%) ≥12 y: 2–3 sprays per nostril q4h Tablet, PO (10 mg) ≥12 y: 10 mg q4h	Palpitations, headaches	Hypersensitivity, urinary retention, severe uncontrolled hypertension, coronary artery disease, MAO inhibitor use within 14 d	These drugs may cause rebound congestion. Use only 2–3 d and then switch to oral decongestants.
Pseudoephedrine (Sudafed) IR tablet, PO (30 mg) ≥12 y: 60 mg q4–6h 6–11 y: 30 mg q4–6h 12-h tablet, PO (120 mg) ≥12 y: 120 mg q12h ER tablet, PO (240 mg) ≥12 y: 240 mg q24h	Palpitations, headaches, increased blood pressure, dizziness, GI upset, tremor, insomnia	Hypersensitivity, narrow-angle glaucoma, severe uncontrolled hypertension, coronary artery disease, MAO inhibitor use within 14 d	Give at least 2 h before bedtime. Do not crush, break, or chew tablets.

(Continued)

TABLE 23.1

Overview of Agents for Upper Respiratory Infections (*Continued*)

Generic (Trade) Name and Dosage	Selected Adverse Events	Contraindications	Special Considerations
Expectorants			

Guaifenesin (Antitussin, Mucinex, Robitussin, Uni-Tussin)
Liquid, PO (100–200 mg/5 mL)
Solution, PO (100 mg/5 mL)
Syrup, PO (100 mg/ 5 mL)
Packet, PO (50 mg, 100 mg)
  6 mo–12 y: 25–50 mg q4h
  2–5 y: 50–100 mg q4h
  6–12 y: 100–200 mg q4h
  ≥12 y: 200–400 mg q4h
IR tablet, PO (200 or 400 mg)
  ≥12 y: 200–400 mg q4h
ER tablet, PO (600 mg)
  ≥12 y: 600–1,200 mg q12h
	Drowsiness, headache, dizziness, GI upset	Hypersensitivity	Not given for prolonged time if cough persists or accompanied by high fever. Oral packet may be swallowed whole or opened and sprinkled on soft food.

Antitussives			

Dextromethorphan (Delsym)
Lozenge, PO (5 mg)
Capsule, PO, 15 mg
Sublingual strip, PO (7.5 mg)
Gel, PO (7.5 mg/5 mL)
Syrup, PO (varying strengths)
IR liquid, PO (varying strengths)
  4–6 y: 2.5–7.5 mg q4–8h
  6–12 y: 5–10 mg q4h
  ≥12 y: 10–20 mg q4h or 30 mg q6–8h
ER liquid, PO (30 mg/5 mL)
  4–6 y: 15 mg q12h
  6–12 y: 15 mg q6–8h
  ≥12 y: 60 mg q12h
	Dizziness, nausea, drowsiness	Hypersensitivity, MAO inhibitor use within 14 d	None.

Benzonatate (Tessalon Perles) Capsule, PO (100 or 200 mg) ≥10 y: 100–200 mg q8h	Constipation, drowsiness, headache, GI upset, confusion	Hypersensitivity	
Antiinflammatories			
Naproxen sodium (Naprosyn, Aleve) Tablet, PO (220 mg) ≥12 y: 220 mg q8–12h	Dizziness, drowsiness, headache, edema, abdominal pain, constipation, nausea, heartburn	Hypersensitivity	Take on full stomach to reduce GI upset.
Anticholinergics			

Ipratropium bromide (Atrovent)
Nasal spray (0.06%)
  ≥12 y: 2 sprays per nostril BID–QID
  5–11 y: 2 sprays per nostril TID
	Headache, epistaxis, pharyngitis, nasal dryness	Hypersensitivity to atropine
		Use caution in patients with narrow-angle glaucoma, BPH, bladder neck obstruction, pregnancy, and lactation.
			Safety and efficacy not established beyond 4 d.

Antihistamines			
Diphenhydramine (Benadryl) Tablet, PO (25 mg) ≥12 y: 25–50 mg q4–6h	Confusion, dizziness, drowsiness, fatigue, paradoxical excitability, nervousness, headache, sedation, blurred vision, dry mouth, hallucinations, tachycardia, urinary retention	Hypersensitivity, patients who are breastfeeding, neonates, premature infants	Caution needed in older patients as it may increase fall risk

TABLE 23.1

Overview of Agents for Upper Respiratory Infections (*Continued*)

Generic (Trade) Name and Dosage	Selected Adverse Events	Contraindications	Special Considerations
Chlorpheniramine (Chlor-Trimeton) IR tablet, PO (4 mg) ≥12 y: 4 mg q4–6h ER tablet, PO (12 mg) ≥12 y: 12 mg q12h	Headache, fatigue, nervousness, dizziness, nausea, dry mouth, GI upset, urinary retention, blurred vision	Hypersensitivity, narrow-angle glaucoma, bladder neck obstruction, symptomatic prostate hypertrophy, during acute asthma attacks, stenosing peptic ulcer, pyloroduodenal obstruction	Caution needed in older patients as it may increase fall risk.
Amoxicillin with clavulanic acid (Augmentin) Adults or children >40 kg: 500 mg q8h Children 3 mo to adolescence who are ≤40 kg: 20 mg/kg/d q8h or 25 mg/kg/d q12h Children <3 mo: 30 mg/kg/d q12h Children with severe ABRS: 40 mg/kg/d q8h or 45 mg/kg/d q12h CrCl 10–30 mL/min: 250–500 mg q12h CrCl < 10 mL/min: 250–500 mg q24h	Common: GI upset, rash, vaginal infections, photosensitivity Rare: Stevens-Johnson syndrome, seizures	Hypersensitivity or allergy to penicillin or cephalosporins Do not use ER formulation in patients with CrCl < 30 mL/min.	"High dose" (2 g q12h) is reserved for patients with risk for antibiotic resistance.*
Doxycycline (Oracea) Adults and children >8 y of age weighing >45 kg: 200 mg daily in 1–2 divided doses	Common: GI upset, rash, vaginal infections, headache Rare: Stevens-Johnson syndrome, hepatotoxicity	Hypersensitivity or allergy to tetracyclines	Not recommended for children ≤8 y of age Take on an empty stomach if tolerated.
Levofloxacin (Levaquin) Adults: 500–750 mg q24h Children: 10–20 mg/kg/d q12–24 h CrCl 20–49 mL/min: 500 mg × 1 followed by 250 mg q24h or 500 mg × 1 followed by 750 mg q48h	Common: GI upset, rash, dyspepsia, headache, chest pain, decreased blood glucose, edema, photosensitivity, vaginal infections Black box warning for tendon inflammation and rupture	Hypersensitivity or allergy to fluoroquinolones	Avoid in patients with myasthenia gravis. Can prolong QTc interval. Avoid concurrent use with other medications that prolong the QTc interval. Avoid taking with corticosteroids due to increased risk of ruptured Achilles tendon. Avoid in patients at risk for aortic aneurysm or dissection.
Moxifloxacin (Avelox) Adults: 400 mg q24h	Same as levofloxacin	Same as levofloxacin	Same as levofloxacin
Clindamycin (Cleocin) Children: 30–40 mg/kg/d divided q8h	Common: GI upset	Hypersensitivity or allergy to lincosamides	Must be taken with third-generation cephalosporins
Cefpodoxime (Vantin) Children >2 mo and <12 y: 5 mg/kg q12h Children ≥12 y: 200 mg q12h	Common: GI upset headache	Caution with penicillin allergy	Interacts with antacids, H_2 antagonists.
Cefixime (Suprax) Children >6 mo and <12 y: 4 mg/kg q12h Children ≥12 y: 400 mg divided q12–24h	Same as cefpodoxime	Same as cefpodoxime	Same as cefpodoxime

*Patients with ABRS from regions with high endemic rates of resistant *S. pneumoniae*, those with severe infection, children in day care, patients of ages < 2 years or > 65 years, immunosuppressed individuals, or those with a recent hospitalization or antibiotic use within the past month.

ABRS, acute bacterial rhinosinusitis; BPH, benign prostatic hyperplasia; CrCl, creatinine clearance; ER, extended-release; GI, gastrointestinal; IR, immediate-release; MAO, monoamine oxidase; QTc, corrected QT interval.

Despite the ability to use the spray every 4 hours, it should generally not be used more than twice to thrice daily. Topical decongestants should not be used for more than 3 days because prolonged use can cause rhinitis medicamentosa (rebound congestion), which is characterized by severe nasal edema, rebound congestion, and increased discharge due to decreased receptor sensitivity. Rebound congestion interferes with ciliary action and dries the nasal mucosa.

Oral pseudoephedrine is available in 30-mg tablets in preparations that vary with regard to duration of action. Adults greater than 12 years of age can take a short-acting preparation at a dose of 60 mg every 4 to 6 hours or a long-acting preparation at a dose of 120 mg every 12 hours. All-day preparations are also available at a dosage of 240 mg and should not be taken more than once in a 24-hour time period. Children who are 4 to 5 years of age can take a 15 mg dose every 4 to 6 hours to a maximum daily dose of 60 mg. Children aged 6 to 12 should take 30 mg every 4 to 6 hours and should not exceed 120 mg within 24 hours. Oral preparations should be given at least 2 hours before bedtime, and extended-release (ER) formulations should not be crushed, broken, or chewed. Oral phenylephrine has not demonstrated consistent benefit and should not be recommended.

Time Frame for Response

Topical decongestants have a rapid onset of action and can begin to work within several minutes. Oral decongestants have a slower onset of action of approximately 30 minutes.

Contraindications

Decongestants are contraindicated in patients with hypersensitivity to any component of the formulation, narrow-angle glaucoma, severe uncontrolled hypertension, and coronary artery disease and in patients who have been treated with a monoamine oxidase (MAO) inhibitor within 14 days. Caution is recommended in patients with hypertension, cardiovascular disease, renal impairment, hyperthyroidism, diabetes, prostatic hypertrophy, and urinary incontinence.

Adverse Events

Adverse drug events (ADEs) include increased blood pressure and heart rate, palpitations, headache, dizziness, gastrointestinal (GI) distress, insomnia, and tremor. These reactions are especially seen at doses above 210 mg. In patients with controlled hypertension, products can be taken for a short course and with frequent monitoring.

Interactions

Decongestants interact with appetite suppressants, MAO inhibitors (hypertensive crisis), and beta-adrenergic agents (hypertension). Decongestants are less effective when taken with drugs that acidify the urine and more effective when taken with drugs that alkalinize the urine.

Expectorants

The most commonly available expectorant is guaifenesin (Antitussin, Mucinex, Robitussin). Some studies have shown this product to have limited advantage over increased fluid intake, and evidence regarding benefit is generally controversial (Fashner et al., 2012). Use of guaifenesin should generally not last beyond one week.

Mechanism of Action

Expectorants, including water, increase the output of respiratory tract fluid by decreasing the adhesiveness and surface tension of the respiratory tract and by facilitating the removal of viscous mucous.

Dosage

Guaifenesin is available in both liquid and tablet oral preparations. Some preparations are available in the form of oral sprinkles, which may be swallowed whole or sprinkled on soft food, such as applesauce. The recommended dose for adults over the age of 12 is 200 to 400 mg every 4 hours to a maximum daily dose of 2.4 grams (g). ER tablets can be taken at a dosage of 600 to 1,200 mg every 12 hours with the same maximum daily dose as the immediate-release (IR) preparations. For children less than 4 years of age, a physician or pharmacist should be consulted prior to treatment with expectorants. If recommended by a health care professional, children aged 6 months to 2 years can be given a dose of 25 to 50 mg every 4 hours to a maximum of 300 mg/d. Children aged 2 to 5 can take a dose of 50 to 100 mg every 4 hours, not to exceed 500 mg/d. Children who are 6 to 12 years of age can be given a dose of 100 to 200 mg every 4 hours to a maximum of 1.2 mg/d.

Time Frame for Response

Expectorants have an onset of action of approximately 1 to 2 hours.

Contraindications

Expectorants are contraindicated in patients with hypersensitivity to any component of the formulation.

Adverse Events

ADEs include drowsiness, headache, dizziness, and GI upset.

Interactions

There are no known drug interactions.

Antitussives

Cough suppressants, such as dextromethorphan (Delsym) and benzonatate (Tessalon Perles), are available in oral preparations, including liquids, gels, capsules, lozenges, and sublingual strips, but studies have shown minimal benefit with the common cold (Fashner et al., 2012). For some patients, these agents may reduce cough frequency and help achieve sleep; however, consistent benefit has not been demonstrated. There is little evidence to favor the use of narcotic antitussives, such as codeine and hydrocodone, over other agents to relieve cough. Many practitioners believe that cough suppressants are ineffective in children.

Mechanism of Action

Antitussives diminish the cough reflex by direct inhibition of the cough center in the medulla.

Dosage

Patients over the age of 12 years can take IR preparations of dextromethorphan at a dose of 10 to 20 mg every 4 hours or 30 mg every 6 to 8 hours. ER products can be taken at a dose of 60 mg twice daily. Adult patients should not exceed a dose of 120 mg within a 24-hour time period. Dextromethorphan is not recommended for children less than 4 years of age. Children who are 4 to 6 years of age may take an IR preparation at a dose of 2.5 to 7.5 mg every 4 to 8 hours or an ER preparation at a dose of 15 mg twice daily to a maximum of 30 mg/d. Children aged 6 to 12 years may take IR preparations at a dose of 5 to 10 mg every 4 hours or 15 mg every 6 to 8 hours. ER preparations can be taken at a dose of 30 mg twice daily. The maximum dose of dextromethorphan for this age range is 60 mg per 24-hour time period.

Benzonatate can be taken by patients greater than 10 years of age at a dose of 100 to 200 mg thrice daily, as needed with total daily doses not to exceed 600 mg.

Time Frame for Response

Onset of action is noted within 15 to 30 minutes.

Contraindications

Antitussives are contraindicated in patients who have hypersensitivity to these agents or have taken an MAO inhibitor within 2 weeks.

Adverse Events

Adverse events include dizziness, nausea, and drowsiness.

Interactions

Drug–drug interactions occur with concomitant use of amiodarone (Cordarone), MAO inhibitors, quinidine, and proserotonergic drugs, such as selective serotonin reuptake inhibitors, serotonin–norepinephrine reuptake inhibitors, or triptans. Caution should also be used with other antidepressants.

Antiinflammatories and Analgesics

Mechanism of Action

Cyclooxygenase inhibitors, such as nonsteroidal antiinflammatory drugs (NSAIDs), inhibit prostaglandin secretions, which can reduce headache, malaise, myalgias, cough, and even sneezing. Naproxen (Naprosyn, Aleve) is available as an oral tablet or suspension and is the NSAID of choice in the American College of Clinical Pharmacy (ACCP) guidelines because it does not impact viral shedding (Jacobs et al., 2013).

Dosage

Naproxen available in an OTC preparation can be taken by patients who are 12 years of age or older at a dose of 220 mg every 8 to 12 hours. Total daily dosage should not exceed 600 mg. NSAIDs should be taken with food to avoid GI upset.

Time Frame for Response

Effects are noted within 1 to 2 hours.

Contraindications

Contraindications include hypersensitivity to any component of the formulation. Caution should be used for patients with active peptic ulcers or GI bleeds, bleeding disorders, asthma, severe hepatic impairment, severe renal impairment involving a creatinine clearance (CrCl) of less than 30 milliliters per minute (mL/min), severe uncontrolled heart failure, hyperkalemia, or those who are in their third trimester or are breastfeeding. Aspirin, a common NSAID, should not be used in children because of the secondary risk of Reye's syndrome. Patients should also refrain from taking acetaminophen (Tylenol) and ibuprofen (Motrin, Advil) because these drugs are believed to shed the virus. NSAIDs are discussed in greater detail in Chapter 7.

Adverse Events

Adverse events include dizziness, drowsiness, headache, edema, abdominal pain, constipation, nausea, and heartburn.

Interactions

Naproxen may increase the therapeutic effect of antiplatelet agents, anticoagulants, lithium, methotrexate, haloperidol, potassium-sparing diuretics, quinolone antibiotics, salicylates, tacrolimus, tenofovir, vitamin K antagonists, and several other drugs. The levels of naproxen may be increased by angiotensin-converting enzyme inhibitors, angiotensin II receptor blockers, tricyclic antidepressants, cyclosporine, ketorolac, omega-3 fatty acids, proserotonergic agents, and several other drugs.

Anticholinergic Agents

Ipratropium bromide (Atrovent) nasal spray is available at concentrations of 0.03% and 0.06% and has been recommended for rhinorrhea associated with the common cold. This agent has not shown consistent benefit for the alleviation of nasal congestion or sneezing (Fokkens et al., 2012).

Mechanism of Action

Local application of anticholinergic agents to the nasal mucosa inhibits vagally mediated reflexes by antagonizing the action of acetylcholine at the cholinergic receptor, thereby inhibiting secretions from the serous and seromucous glands lining the nasal mucosa. The result is a decrease in nasal discharge and rhinorrhea.

Dosage

Adults greater than 12 years of age should use the ipratropium bromide 0.06% nasal spray at a dose of 2 sprays per nostril three to four times daily. Children who are 5 to 11 years of age can use the 0.06% solution at a dose of 2 sprays in each nostril thrice daily. The safety and efficacy of use beyond 4 days for patients with the common cold have not been established.

Time Frame for Response

The onset of action for these products is 30 to 60 minutes.

Contraindications

Ipratropium bromide is contraindicated in patients with hypersensitivity to any component of the formulation, including atropine or its derivatives. Caution should be used in patients with narrow-angle glaucoma, prostatic hyperplasia, or bladder neck obstruction.

Adverse Events

Adverse effects include headache, epistaxis, pharyngitis, and nasal dryness.

Interactions

There are no known drug interactions.

Antihistamines

Antihistamines should not be recommended as monotherapy for the treatment of cough and other cold symptoms as they are ineffective. Antihistamine-induced dryness may even exacerbate symptoms of congestion and cause upper airway obstruction by impairing the flow of mucus. For symptoms of rhinorrhea and a feeling of fullness in the ears, first-generation antihistamines, such as diphenhydramine and chlorpheniramine, may be effective when combined with decongestants. See further commentary below in "Combination Treatments" section. Treatment of cough with second-generation, non-sedating antihistamines, such as loratadine (Claritin) and cetirizine (Zyrtec), is ineffective and is not recommended (Pratter, 2006). Antihistamines are discussed further in Chapter 48.

Mechanism of Action

Antihistamines are theorized to block the release of histamine from mast cells and basophils in the nasal passageways, which is activated by cold virus inoculation. This release of histamine may result in the sneezing symptom that affects patients during the course of a common cold. Antihistamines competitively antagonize histamine at the H_1 receptor, and first-generation antihistamines also competitively antagonize acetylcholine activity at muscarinic receptors.

Dosage

Antihistamines are not recommended for symptoms of the common cold in children less than 12 years of age. Diphenhydramine can be given at a dose of 25 to 50 mg every 4 to 6 hours to a maximum of 300 mg daily. IR preparations of chlorpheniramine can be given at a dose of 4 mg every 4 to 6 hours, and ER preparations can be given at a dose of 12 mg every 12 hours. The total daily dose of chlorpheniramine should not exceed 24 mg.

Time Frame for Response

The onset of action for first-generation antihistamines is typically 30 to 60 minutes.

Contraindications

Diphenhydramine should not be used in patients with hypersensitivity, in patients who are breastfeeding, and in neonates or premature infants. Caution should be used in patients with asthma, cardiovascular disease, increased intraocular pressure, prostatic hyperplasia, bladder neck obstruction, and thyroid dysfunction.

Chlorpheniramine is contraindicated in patients with hypersensitivity, narrow-angle glaucoma, bladder neck obstruction, symptomatic prostate hypertrophy, stenosing peptic ulcer, and pyloroduodenal obstruction and during acute asthma attacks. Use should also be avoided in newborns due to possible association with sudden infant death syndrome.

Neither first-generation antihistamine listed in this section should be used as a sedative to help a child sleep. Additionally, these agents should be used with caution in older patients due to the increased risk for confusion, constipation, and dizziness.

Adverse Events

The ability of first-generation antihistamines to pass the blood–brain barrier and the impact on cholinergic receptors contributes to a higher incidence of anticholinergic and central nervous system ADEs than second-generation products. These can include confusion, dizziness, drowsiness, fatigue, paradoxical excitability, nervousness, headache, sedation, blurred vision, dry mouth, hallucinations, tachycardia, and urinary retention.

Interactions

First-generation antihistamines may potentiate the effects of other sedative drugs or alcohol.

Combination Treatments

A limitless selection of combination products is available for the alleviation of cough and cold symptoms. These products can often be difficult to recommend, as they contain multiple active ingredients, each associated with unique ADEs. If recommending one of these products, it is important to ensure that there is an indication for each active ingredient to avoid overmedicating the patient. Additionally, individual symptoms may last for varying durations; therefore, even if the patient initially presented with symptoms matching each ingredient, they may be overmedicating at some point during the course of their illness if some symptoms persist longer than others. For example, congestion may predominate in the first few days, but a cough may last for up to 2 weeks. Purchasing a product containing only one active ingredient can help with flexibility in targeting specific symptoms for the appropriate amount of time.

For sneezing, rhinorrhea, acute cough, and postnasal drip, a combination of decongestant and first-generation antihistamine may be effective in adult or adolescent patients. Evidence for this combination treatment is generally limited and of poor quality; therefore, clinically significant benefits are difficult to conclude. The benefit of symptomatic relief should be weighed against the risk for adverse effects. This combination has not proven effective in children under the age of 12 (Fokkens et al., 2012).

Several products also combine expectorants and antitussives. This combination is not recommended as the ingredients are associated with opposing mechanisms. As stated previously, expectorants increase respiratory tract fluid output, while antitussives diminish the cough reflex.

Selecting the Most Appropriate Agent

Because symptoms of a cold are manifested individually or in combination, not everyone will present with the same signs and symptoms. Therefore, the therapeutic approach involves treatment of symptoms as specifically as possible (**Figure 23.1**).

First-Line Therapy

Initial therapy consists of symptom relief. For nasal obstruction and rhinorrhea, which are caused by secretions and increased

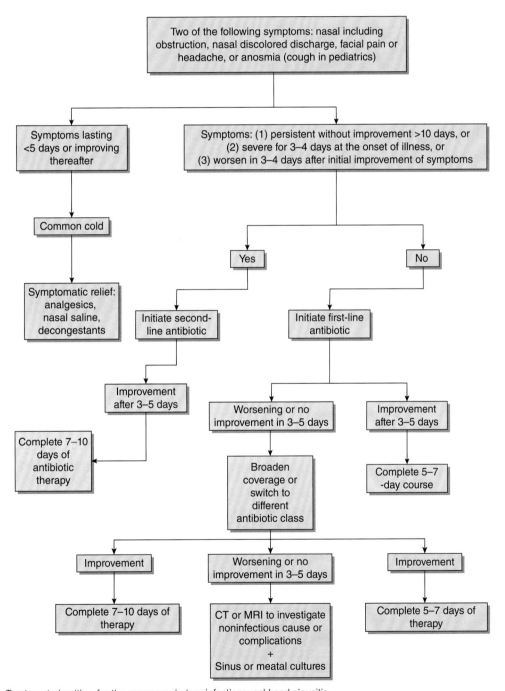

FIGURE 23–1   Treatment algorithm for the upper respiratory infections: cold and sinusitis.

CT, computerized tomography; MRI, magnetic resonance imaging.

vascular permeability with leakage of serum into the nasal mucosa, topical decongestants, such as oxymetazoline hydrochloride (Afrin) or phenylephrine hydrochloride (Neo-Synephrine), are often used for the first 3 days when the patient feels the worst. If other symptoms are diminished but nasal obstruction remains a problem, the use of an oral decongestant, such as pseudoephedrine, or a combination of decongestant and antihistamine, or an antihistamine alone may relieve symptoms and help prevent complications such as sinusitis and eustachian tube blockage. Antiinflammatories, such as naproxen, may be recommended to relieve aches and discomfort.

Second-Line Therapy

Second-line therapy may be instituted if first-line therapy fails to relieve symptoms or if complications, such as secondary infection (ear infections, sinusitis, bronchitis, or pneumonia), develop. The therapy should be specific to the disorder.

Monitoring Patient Response

Patient response is monitored by the decrease of symptoms. If symptoms decrease without onset of complications, then therapy is successful. If the common cold does not improve in 8 to 10 days, a bacterial cause is suspected and antibiotic therapy should be considered. Persistent coughs lasting more than several weeks should be investigated for other infectious or noninfectious causes. Continuation of OTC cough products may mask symptoms of a separate underlying disorder.

RHINOSINUSITIS

Rhinosinusitis is an URI characterized by inflammation of the mucous membranes that line the sinuses and nasal cavity causing nasal blockage, purulent discharge, and facial pain or pressure. Sinusitis and rhinitis are unlikely to occur without inflammation of the nasal cavity membranes, so the term "rhinosinusitis" provides a better description of the inflammatory disease involving the URI (Rosenfield et al., 2015).

Rhinosinusitis is classified by duration of symptoms as either acute rhinosinusitis (ARS), lasting for less than 4 weeks, or chronic rhinosinusitis (CRS), persisting for more than 12 weeks. Rhinosinusitis with symptoms lasting more than 4 weeks and less than 12 weeks is defined as subacute rhinosinusitis (Rosenfield et al., 2015). ARS is typically infectious, whereas CRS is less infectious and more inflammatory mediated (Dykewicz & Hamilas, 2010).

ARS can further be stratified by etiology into acute viral rhinosinusitis (AVRS) or acute bacterial rhinosinusitis (ABRS). ARS is more frequently caused by a viral infection with only 0.5% to 2% of AVRS transitioning to ABRS. However, antibiotics are prescribed in 85% to 98% of ARS cases (Dykewicz & Hamilas, 2010).

ARS has a global prevalence of 6% to 15% and is one of the most common reasons for primary care visits, affecting over 30 million Americans every year (Fokkens et al., 2014; Rosenfield

---

BOX 23.1 Selected Risk Factors for Acute Rhinosinusitis

- Winter season
- Air pollution
- Septal deviation
- Nasal polyps
- Allergic rhinitis
- Tobacco smoke
- Gastroesophageal reflux
- Asthma
- Prior upper respiratory tract infection
- Cystic fibrosis
- Dental infections
- Immunodeficiency
- Intranasal medications or illicit drugs
- Mechanical ventilation
- Nasogastric tubes

---

et al., 2015). ARS is also the fifth most common diagnosis for which an antibiotic is prescribed, even though there is consistent evidence of spontaneous resolutions and recent guidelines recommend restricting antibiotic use (Fokkens et al., 2014; Rosenfield et al., 2015). It is estimated that rhinosinusitis costs the U.S. health care system more than $11 billion on medications, laboratory tests, workplace absenteeism, and outpatient and emergency room visits each year (Rosenfield et al., 2015).

Causes

Most cases of AVRS can be attributed to respiratory viruses including rhinovirus, influenza, and parainfluenza virus. The most common pathogens involved in ABRS include *Streptococcus pneumoniae, Haemophilus influenzae,* and *Moraxella catarrhalis* with the latter being the most common pathogen in pediatric cases (Dykewicz & Hamilas, 2010). Most healthy persons harbor bacteria in their URIs with no problems until the bodily defenses are weakened or drainage from the sinuses is blocked by a cold or other viral infection. Then, bacteria that may have been living harmlessly in the nose can multiply and invade the sinuses, causing a secondary infection. Risk factors for ARS are outlined in **Box 23.1** (Anselmo-Lima & Sakana, 2015).

CRS is believed to be due to a dysfunctional interaction among environmental factors, including allergens, toxins, and microbial agents, and host factors, such as a deficiency of the immune system and anatomical defects. Fungi and bacteria are the most common environmental causes of CRS (Lam et al., 2015). Patients with CRS tend to have a higher immunological response to the *Alternaria* species, which is a fungus commonly found in the sinus mucus. *Staphylococcus aureus* is usually the bacterial pathogen associated with CRS (Dykewicz & Hamilas, 2010). Frequently, patients with CRS will present with other comorbidities including gastroesophageal reflux disease, defects in mucociliary clearance (as in cystic fibrosis), or anatomical abnormalities including nasal septal deviation. Additionally, allergic rhinitis and asthma occur in 60% and 20% of patients with CRS, respectively (Dykewicz & Hamilas, 2010).

Pathophysiology

There are four paired, air-filled cavities that make up the sinuses. Small tubular openings called the *sinus ostia* connect the sinus cavities and facilitate drainage of the sinuses into the nasal cavity using ciliated cells. Proper sinus functioning requires motile cilia, unobstructed ostia, and mucus of a low viscosity that allows transport (Dykewicz & Hamilas, 2010). The nose reacts to the viral invasion by increasing production of mucus and sending white blood cells (WBCs) to the lining of the nasal passage, which causes inflammation. This inflammation results in dysfunctional cilia, obstruction of the ostia, or both. Blocked sinuses provide an ideal environment for bacterial growth, which can lead to a secondary bacterial infection. Air trapped within a blocked sinus, along with pus or other secretions, can increase pressure on the sinus wall. The result is sinus pain, which can sometimes be intense. Similarly, when a swollen membrane prevents air from entering a paranasal sinus cavity, a vacuum can form, causing additional pain.

Diagnostic Criteria

The diagnosis of ARS in adults at primary health care levels is based on the presence of two or more of the following hallmark symptoms: nasal congestion, nasal discharge, facial pain or headache, and anosmia (loss of smell). For pediatric patients, cough replaces decreased sense of smell as one of the four hallmark symptoms. Additionally, a patient may present with painful swallowing, cough, ear pressure, fever, and fatigue (Anselmo-Lima & Sakana, 2015). The clinical presentation of AVRS and ABRS is very similar and therefore difficult to differentiate based on symptoms alone. Therefore, practitioners need to rely on symptom severity, duration, and nature to differentiate between AVRS and ABRS (Fokkens et al., 2014). The European Respiratory Society/European Academy of Allergy and Clinical Immunology rhinosinusitis guidelines characterize ABRS if three of the hallmark symptoms previously mentioned are present (Fokkens et al., 2012). The Infectious Disease Society of America (IDSA) has identified three clinical features to distinguish patients who have ABRS versus AVRS: (1) symptoms persistent greater than 10 days from onset without any clinical improvement, (2) severe symptoms or an elevated temperature (≥102°F) and either facial pain or purulent nasal discharge lasting for 3 to 4 consecutive days at the onset of illness, and (3) worsening symptoms (fever, headache, or increased nasal discharge) following a typical viral URI that lasted 5 to 6 days after an initial improvement of symptoms (Chow et al., 2012). Radiographic imaging in ARS is not recommended (Rosenfield et al., 2015).

Diagnostic tests such as nasal endoscopy or computerized tomography (CT) scan should be used to diagnose CRS.

However, diagnosis in most patients is based on the presence of two or more hallmark symptoms lasting longer than 12 weeks.

Initiating Drug Therapy

Primarily specialists manage CRS; therefore, ARS will be the focus of this section. Before initiating drug therapy, it is critical to determine the etiology of ARS because antibiotic therapy is inappropriate to prescribe for patients with AVRS. For both AVRS and ABRS, it is recommended to provide the patient with symptomatic relief including analgesics, topical intranasal steroids, and/or nasal saline irrigation. For patients meeting diagnosis criteria for ABRS, as previously described, practitioners should offer either watchful waiting or treatment with antibiotics.

While weighing these choices, the practitioner should consider a few points. The first is the ability for the patient to follow up when choosing the watchful waiting option (Rosenfield et al., 2015). Another consideration for deciding whether or not to initiate antibiotics is that systematic reviews have demonstrated that antibiotics did not provide benefits in uncomplicated ARS and only reduced length of disease by less than half a day (Fokkens et al., 2014). This evidence should be weighed against the risk of adverse effects with antibiotics and antibiotic resistance before prescribing antibiotics for ABRS. The need for a specialist referral should also be contemplated when considering drug therapy. Reasons to refer may include mental status changes, visual disturbances, immunosuppressive illness, anatomic defects, recurrent URI, or a history of antibiotic resistance (Chow et al., 2012).

The recommended length of therapy for uncomplicated ABRS in adults is 5 to 7 days, whereas treatment duration in children should be 10 to 14 days (Chow et al., 2012).

Goals of Drug Therapy

The primary treatment goal is to restore sinuses to health. Other goals include decreasing the duration and severity of symptoms, promoting appropriate use of antibiotic treatment, preventing complications and the progression from acute illness to chronic disease, and preventing the transmission of illness to other people.

Antibiotics

Obtaining cultures is only recommended for patients who do not respond to first- or second-line treatment; therefore, management strategies will focus on the empiric treatment of ABRS. Guidelines no longer recommend the regular use of macrolides, third-generation cephalosporins, or trimethoprim–sulfamethoxazole (Bactrim) for empiric treatment due to their high resistance rates with *S. pneumoniae*.

Amoxicillin and Amoxicillin–Clavulanate
Mechanism of Action

Amoxicillin, a beta-lactam antibiotic, inhibits synthesis of the bacterial cell wall by binding to one or more of the penicillin-binding proteins (PBPs), causing the bacteria to lyse. Adding clavulanate to amoxicillin expands its spectrum of activity by inhibiting bacterial beta-lactamases that inactivate amoxicillin.

Dosage

Amoxicillin–clavulanate (Augmentin) is dosed based on the amoxicillin component and is available in 250 mg, 500 mg, or 875 mg IR oral tablets and 1,000 mg ER tablets. Amoxicillin–clavulanate is also available in 125 mg/5 mL, 250 mg/5 mL, 200 mg/5 mL, or 400 mg/5 mL suspension format and 200 mg or 400 mg chewable tablets. For adults or adolescents weighing greater than 40 kg, a dose of 500 mg every 8 hours or 875 mg every 12 hours should be given. Infants less than 3 months old should be given 30 mg/kg/d every 12 hours. Children aged 3 months to adolescents weighing less than 40 kg should be given 20 mg/kg/d every 8 hours or 25 mg/kg/d every 12 hours for mild infections. For severe infections in this pediatric population, a dose of 40 mg/kg/d every 8 hours or 45 mg/kg/d every 12 hours should be prescribed. "High-dose" amoxicillin consists of 2,000 mg every 12 hours and should be reserved for children and adults with ABRS from regions with high endemic rates of resistant *S. pneumoniae*, those with severe infection, children in day care, patients of ages less than 2 or greater than 65, immunosuppressed individuals, and those with a recent hospitalization or antibiotic use within the past month. For patients with a CrCl of 10 to 30 mL/min or less than 10 mL/min, the recommended dose is 250 to 500 mg every 12 hours and 250 to 500 mg every 24 hours, respectively. No dose adjustments are required in hepatic impairment.

Contraindications

Amoxicillin is contraindicated in patients who have a history of an allergic reaction to beta-lactam antibiotics or any component of the formulation (e.g., penicillins, cephalosporins), cholestatic jaundice, or hepatic dysfunction. The ER formulation of amoxicillin–clavulanate has an additional contraindication for use in patients with a CrCl of less than 30 mL/min or those on hemodialysis.

Adverse Events

Diarrhea is the most frequent ADE that patients experience while taking amoxicillin. Other common ADEs include rash or hives, nausea, vomiting, photosensitivity, and vaginal infections.

Interactions

Amoxicillin may increase levels of methotrexate and warfarin and can decrease the effects of mycophenolate and the typhoid vaccine, and therefore, patients should be monitored accordingly. Concurrent use of probenecid and amoxicillin should be avoided as probenecid may increase the levels of amoxicillin. Tetracyclines may reduce the effect of amoxicillin and should also be avoided. Additionally, caution is warranted in patients taking allopurinol because they may have an increased risk of allergic reaction to amoxicillin.

Doxycycline
Mechanism of Action

Doxycycline (Oracea, Vibramycin), a tetracycline antibiotic, binds with the 30S and possibly the 50S ribosomal subunit(s) of the bacteria, which inhibits protein synthesis resulting in bacteriostatic effects.

Dosage

Doxycycline has an off-label use to treat ABRS at a dose of 200 mg daily in one to two divided doses for adults and children older than 8 years of age and weighing greater than 45 kg. It is available in 50 mg, 75 mg, 100 mg, and 150 mg capsules or tablets; 40 mg delayed-release capsules; and 25 mg/5 mL or 50 mg/5 mL suspensions. In children older than 8 years of age weighing less than or equal to 45 kg, the dose is 2 to 5 mg/kg/d in one to two divided doses. Doxycycline is not recommended for children of 8 years and younger. No dose adjustments are necessary in hepatic or renal impairment.

Contraindications

The only contraindication is a hypersensitivity to tetracyclines or any component of the formulation.

Adverse Events

Although GI ADEs such as photosensitivity, nausea, vomiting, diarrhea, and abdominal pain are common ADEs of doxycycline, diarrhea occurs less frequently than with amoxicillin. Other common ADEs include vaginal infections, headache, and rash. Stevens-Johnson syndrome and hepatotoxicity are rare but serious ADEs associated with doxycycline.

Interactions

Antacids, lanthanum, bismuth subsalicylate, sucralfate, bile acid sequestrants, calcium, multivitamins, and quinapril can lower the absorption or concentration of tetracyclines and should be given 2 hours prior or 6 hours after doxycycline. Iron salts may decrease the levels of doxycycline and vice versa, so therapy can be modified to ferrous gluconate, which does not have this interaction. The following medications should be used with caution because of their effect on reducing doxycycline levels: barbiturates, carbamazepine, fosphenytoin, phenytoin, and rifampin. Doxycycline should be avoided in patients on retinoic acid derivatives as well as neuromuscular blocking agents due to enhanced neuromuscular blocking effects and toxicity. Furthermore, chronic alcohol consumption and dairy reduce the serum levels of doxycycline. Patients on warfarin should be monitored closely while on tetracyclines, as they may increase the risk of bleeding.

Levofloxacin and Moxifloxacin
Mechanism of Action

Fluoroquinolone antibiotics such as levofloxacin (Levaquin) and moxifloxacin (Avelox) inhibit topoisomerase IV and deoxyribonucleic acid (DNA) gyrase, which are essential enzymes that maintain the superhelical structure of DNA and are required for DNA replication and transcription, repair, recombination, and transposition.

Dosage

Levofloxacin is available in the following oral preparations: 25 mg/mL suspension and 250 mg, 500 mg, and 750 mg tablets. Recommended dosing of levofloxacin in adults is 500 to 750 mg every 24 hours for 5 to 7 days. Levofloxacin can be used off-label for pediatrics and should be dosed 10 to 20 mg/kg/d every 12 to 24 hours. Patients with a CrCl of 20 to 49 mL/min should be prescribed a 500 mg loading dose followed by 250 mg every 24 hours or 750 mg every 48 hours. Patients with a CrCl of 10 to 19 mL/min or on hemodialysis should be prescribed a 500 mg loading dose followed by 250 mg every 48 hours or a loading dose of 750 mg followed by 500 mg every 48 hours. Hepatic dosing adjustments are not required. Moxifloxacin is recommended for adults at a dose of 400 mg every 24 hours and should not be used in children. It is available in the following oral formulations: 400 mg/250 mL solution or 400 mg tablet.

Contraindications

The only contraindication is a hypersensitivity to quinolones or any component of the formulation.

Adverse Events

The most common ADEs with fluoroquinolones are GI disturbances such as nausea, diarrhea, constipation, abdominal pain, vomiting, and dyspepsia. Less common ADEs are rash, headache, chest pain, decreased blood glucose, edema, photosensitivity, hepatotoxicity, and vaginal infections. A rare but serious ADE of fluoroquinolones involves exacerbations of myasthenia gravis; therefore, this medication should be avoided in patients with this disease. Fluoroquinolones also have a black box warning for tendonitis and tendon rupture, so they should be avoided in patients older than 60 years of age, who are taking concurrent corticosteroids, or those who have had a solid organ transplant. Furthermore, fluoroquinolones may prolong corrected QT (QTc) interval and have been associated with aortic aneurysm ruptures and aortic dissections.

Interactions

Antacids, lanthanum, sucralfate, calcium, sevelamer, didanosine, multivitamins, quinapril, and magnesium, iron, and zinc salts can lower the absorption or concentration of fluoroquinolones and should be given 2 hours prior to or 6 hours after doxycycline. Fluoroquinolones may also prolong the QTc interval; therefore, caution should be used with other medications that can prolong the QTc interval. Fluoroquinolones can also interact with antidiabetic agents resulting in poor blood glucose control. The use of corticosteroids and fluoroquinolones is not recommended due to the increased risk of ruptured Achilles tendon. Patients on warfarin should be monitored closely while on fluoroquinolones as they may increase the risk of bleeding.

Clindamycin
Mechanism of Action

Clindamycin (Cleocin), a lincosamide antibiotic, reversibly binds to 50S ribosomal subunits preventing the formation of a peptide bond, which in turn inhibits bacterial protein synthesis. Clindamycin is predominantly a bacteriostatic agent; however, depending upon drug concentration, infection site, and organism, it can also have bactericidal effects.

Dosage

Since the use of clindamycin is only recommended in pediatric patients after failing initial therapy or in those with an increased risk of antibiotic resistance, only pediatric dosing will be discussed. Clindamycin is available in 75 mg or 150 mg oral capsules and 75 mg/5 mL oral solution and should be dosed at 30 to 40 mg/kg/d divided every 8 hours. Clindamycin is only recommended with concomitant use of cefpodoxime or cefixime for 10 to 14 days (Chow et al., 2012).

Contraindications

The only contraindication is a hypersensitivity to lincosamide antibiotics or any component of the formulation.

Adverse Events

Common ADEs include diarrhea, nausea, vomiting, and abdominal pain.

Interactions

Lincosamide antibiotics may enhance the neuromuscular-blocking effects of neuromuscular-blocking agents and should be avoided.

Cefpodoxime and Cefixime
Mechanism of Action

Cefpodoxime (Vantin) and cefixime (Suprax), third-generation cephalosporin antibiotics, inhibit synthesis of the bacterial cell wall by binding to one or more of the PBPs, causing the bacteria to lyse.

Dosage

Since the use of third-generation cephalosporins is only recommended in pediatric patients after failing initial therapy or in those with an increased risk of antibiotic resistance, only pediatric dosing will be discussed. Recommended dosing of cefpodoxime for children older than 2 months but less than 12 years of age is 5 mg/kg/d, and 200 mg every 12 hours for children 12 years and older. Cefpodoxime is available in 50 mg/5 mL or 100 mg/5 mL oral suspensions or 100 mg or 200 mg oral tablets. Recommended dosing of cefixime for children older than 6 months but less than 12 years of age is 8 mg/kg/d divided every 12 hours, and 400 mg divided every 12 to 24 hours for children 12 years and older. Cefixime is available in 400 mg oral capsules and tablets, 100 mg or 200 mg chewable tablets, as well as in 100 mg/5 mL, 200 mg/5 mL, and 500 mg/5 mL oral suspensions. Both agents must be used in combination with clindamycin for 10 to 14 days (Chow et al., 2012).

Contraindications

The only contraindication is a hypersensitivity to cephalosporins or any component of the formulation.

Adverse Events

Diaper rash and diarrhea are the most common ADEs associated with third-generation cephalosporins. Other common ADEs include nausea, vomiting, abdominal pain, and headache.

Interactions

Cephalosporins may increase the nephrotoxic effect of aminoglycosides and should be monitored with concurrent use. Antacids and histamine-2 receptor antagonists may decrease the absorption of cephalosporins and therefore their dosing should be separated by 2 hours. Additionally, anticoagulant effects of warfarin may be enhanced with cephalosporins, so patients should be monitored carefully.

Symptomatic Therapy

Nonpharmacologic therapies include the following: adequate rest and hydration; elevating the head of the bed while sleeping; use of a humidifier; and avoidance of environmental factors such as allergens, cigarette smoke, and pollution (Peters et al., 2014). Unlike the common cold, topical or oral decongestants or antihistamines should not be used as adjunctive treatment in ABRS (Chow et al., 2012). Intranasal corticosteroids are recommended as adjunctive treatment, particularly in patients with a history of allergic rhinitis (see Chapter 48) (Chow et al., 2012). Even though there is minimal clinical evidence supporting the benefit of nasal lavage in rhinosinusitis to improve ciliary function and reduce inflammation, it is a generally recommended treatment strategy. Surgical intervention is to be avoided in ARS and should be individualized in patients with CRS. A lack of randomized controlled trials has resulted in the absence of a gold standard technique (Anselmo-Lima & Sakana, 2015).

Selecting the Most Appropriate Agent

Due to the increasing levels of antimicrobial resistance worldwide, clinicians must reevaluate their approaches to treating ARS by using evidence-based methods of diagnosis and treatment. As mentioned previously, it is imperative to differentiate AVRS from ABRS. When ABRS pathogen is suspected or diagnosed, antibiotics may not always be the optimal choice; therefore, patients need to be educated regarding the appropriate initial treatment regimens. When prescribing antibiotics, the provider should consider cost, formulation, whether the patient is at risk for resistant bacteria (**Box 23.2**), and if the patient can be compliant with the selected regimen.

First-Line Therapy

Amoxicillin–clavulanate is preferred to amoxicillin for ABRS in adults and children. For penicillin-allergic adults, doxycycline, levofloxacin, or moxifloxacin should be used. Levofloxacin is the antibiotic of choice in children with a penicillin allergy.

Second-Line Therapy

Second-line agents for patients include doxycycline (not recommended for most children), levofloxacin, or moxifloxacin.

BOX 23.2   Risk Factors for Antibiotic Resistance

- Age < 2 years or > 65 years
- Child in day care
- Prior antibiotics in the past month
- Comorbidities
- Immunocompromised

Combination therapy with clindamycin and a third-generation oral cephalosporin such as cefixime or cefpodoxime is an alternative treatment for children with a penicillin allergy.

Monitoring Patient Response

Patients should notice relief within 48 to 72 hours. If there is no relief of symptoms in 3 to 5 days or if symptoms worsen despite treatment, an alternative antibiotic should be selected. It is recommended that patients who fail to respond to first- or second-line treatment should have cultures collected via direct sinus aspiration rather than nasopharyngeal swab. Alternatively, endoscopically guided cultures of the middle meatus could be taken in adults; however, the integrity of this option in pediatric patients has not been established. CT, which is preferred to magnetic resonance imaging, may also be necessary to investigate noninfectious causes (Chow et al., 2012). Once an uncomplicated episode of ARS resolves, there is no further evaluation required (Peters et al., 2014).

Patient Education

The role of the practitioner is to make the patient aware not only of appropriate symptom management but also of prevention. It is essential that patients understand that symptoms of viral and bacterial URIs are similar, that viral URIs and allergies are more prevalent than bacterial URIs, and that antibiotics are not appropriate to treat viral URIs. Education about the importance of completing the full course of antibiotics, should they be prescribed, despite symptoms subsiding in 48 to 72 hours, is also imperative. The patient also needs to know how to recognize and respond to ADEs of antibiotic therapy, especially because allergic reactions are more prevalent with these drugs than other drug classes.

Education needs to begin before cold and flu season so that patients can take steps to prevent disease and to make educated decisions on whether a health care visit is needed or whether the symptoms are likely to be self-limiting. Progress toward the development of vaccines to prevent viral URIs has been difficult due to the abundance of existing viral serotypes (Jacobs et al., 2013). Approved prophylactic antiviral therapies do not currently exist; therefore, prevention consists of behavioral modifications (e.g., appropriate hand hygiene, covering coughs and sneezes, avoiding public spaces).

Drug Information

The ACCP published an evidence-based clinical practice guideline on cough and the common cold (Irwin et al., 2006). The National Institute for Health and Clinical Excellence published a guideline using evidence from randomized placebo-controlled trials in 2008 regarding the prescribing of antibiotics for self-limiting respiratory tract infections (RTI) in adults and children in primary care (Centre for Clinical Practice, 2008). This report describes evidence from randomized placebo-controlled trials that demonstrate the limited efficacy of antibiotics in the treatment of most RTI, including acute otitis media, acute cough/bronchitis, acute sore throat/pharyngitis/tonsillitis, ARS, and the common cold. In 2012, the IDSA published a Clinical Practice Guideline for Acute Bacterial Rhinosinusitis in Children and Adults (Chow et al., 2012). Additionally, in 2012, there was a European Position Paper on Rhinosinusitis and Nasal Polyps (Fokkens et al., 2012). A common theme found in all of these guidelines was to use caution regarding the inappropriate prescribing of antibiotics, which may contribute to drug-related adverse events and an increase in antibiotic-resistant organisms.

Patient-Oriented Information Sources

The American Academy of Family Physicians, American Rhinologic Society, Cleveland Clinic, Mayo Clinic, and Centers for Disease Control and Prevention are organizations that provide patient-oriented information on their Web sites. Another helpful Web site for patient-oriented information resources is www.medicine.net.

Lifestyle Changes

The most important aspect of patient education is to prevent contraction of the virus by practicing good hygiene, such as frequent handwashing, getting adequate sleep and exercise, and avoiding contact with infected people. One study found hand sanitizers containing ethanol to be significantly more effective than handwashing with soap and water (Turner et al., 2010). It is important to consider that handwashing by any method is effective, even without antiseptics. Social distancing can involve avoidance of crowded public spaces or the temporary closing of schools or day cares. Since these strategies can be difficult to execute, utilization of surgical respiratory masks may be a more feasible approach, particularly in health care settings. Another important aspect of patient education is teaching patients to prevent spreading the virus through correct tissue disposal, handwashing, covering the mouth when coughing, and so on.

For persons prone to ARS, it may be uncomfortable to swim in pools treated with chlorine, because it irritates the lining of the nose and sinuses. Divers often get sinus congestion and infection when water is forced into the sinuses from the nasal passages. Air travel may also pose a problem for persons with ARS or CRS. As the air pressure in a plane is reduced, pressure can build up in the sinuses or eustachian tubes. The patient may feel discomfort in the sinus or middle ear during ascent or descent of the airplane.

Alternative Therapies

There is a growing interest in alternative or complementary therapies for treating the common cold. A review of complementary and alternative medicine for the prevention and treatment of the common cold was published in *Canadian Family Physician* in 2011 (Nahas & Balla, 2011). *Echinacea angustifolia*, *Echinacea pallida*, and *Echinacea purpurea* have all been studied, but *E. purpurea* is associated with the most evidence. These products have been investigated for their effects in increasing and enhancing many immune processes, including macrophage activation, cytokine production, phagocytosis, natural killer cell activation, lymphocyte and monocyte production, and antibody response. Among conducted studies, there is a high degree of variability in the species, plant parts, and methods of extraction that have been used. Therefore, despite a moderate level of evidence supporting the use of *E. purpurea* for the treatment of the common cold, it is challenging to recommend specific product formulations or doses. The use of these products for the prevention of cold symptoms has not shown benefit. *Echinacea* products are available in a variety of preparations, including a crude extract at a daily dose of 2,000 to 3,000 mg, a pressed juice at a daily dose of 6 to 9 mL, and a tincture at a daily dose of 0.75 to 1.5 mL. Use should be avoided in patients who are allergic to *Echinacea* or members of the *Asteraceae* or *Compositae* families, including chrysanthemums, daisies, marigolds, and ragweed. Caution should also be used in patients with asthma and seasonal allergies as they may have a higher risk of experiencing allergic reactions. Adverse effects include hives, rash, itching, GI upset, and headache. There are no known drug interactions.

Panax ginseng (Asian ginseng) and *Panax quinquefolius* (North American ginseng) have been studied for the stimulation of macrophages, natural killer cells, and lymphocytes, as well as for increased production of cytokines and antibodies. Data to support the use of ginseng for the prevention or treatment of the common cold are limited and conflicting; therefore, use of these products is not recommended. Side effects include headache, GI upset, anxiety, and insomnia. Drug interactions include phenelzine, involving the induction of mania; warfarin, involving an increase in international normalized ratio; and alcohol, involving increased blood clearance. These products should not be used by pregnant or breastfeeding patients due to the risk of estrogenic effects and teratogenicity.

Vitamin C has been a focus of several studies related to the common cold due to its antioxidant properties, its impact on glutathione regeneration, and its theoretical ability to activate neutrophils and monocytes. Studies have implemented a wide range of doses and have explored the use of this product in both the prevention and treatment of the common cold. An interesting finding involves the potential reduction of colds in study participants who were exposed to subarctic cold or intense physical activity. Patients taking doses of 200 to 2,000 mg daily of vitamin C had half as many colds as those taking placebo, according to a small group of trials studying a total of 642 patients (Nahas & Balla, 2011). Based on the review of many studies, vitamin C can be recommended at a dose of at least 1 g/d for the prevention of colds and may also reduce the duration of symptoms by 1 to 2 days.

Allium sativum, or allicin, is found in garlic and is activated upon chopping or chewing. It is inactivated when cooked. It has been studied for its antiviral properties against HRVs. Evidence supporting the use of this product for the prevention of the common cold is limited, but it can be recommended at a dose of 180 mg of allicin. The use of fresh garlic is not reasonable as each clove contains approximately 5 to 9 mg of allicin. Odor-free formulations are ineffective as these do not contain allicin. The most common ADE is malodorous belching. Evidence does not support the use of this product for treatment.

Probiotics have been investigated for their role in the improvement of mucosal barrier function, GI microflora, and gut-associated lymphoid tissue. They may also interfere with toxin and cell-binding sites. Current literature does not support the use of these products for the prevention or treatment of the common cold.

Several trials have studied zinc due to a proposed mechanism involving the interference with rhinovirus protein cleavage or the disruption of capsid binding to adhesion molecules in the epithelium of the nasal passageways. Results have been variable, but several studies have demonstrated the potential for these products to shorten the duration and severity of cold symptoms. The difficulty exists in selecting the appropriate dose and proper formulation. Lozenges that contain at least 13 mg of elemental zinc can be recommended for use every 2 hours at the immediate onset of cold symptoms. ADEs include bitter taste and nausea. Intranasal zinc should not be used due to its potential association with anosmia. Use of zinc for 6 to 8 weeks may contribute to copper deficiency.

In ARS and CRS, complementary or alternative medicines have also been considerably utilized. As with the common cold, evidence-based recommendations are difficult to suggest due to the scarcity of randomized controlled trials. One study that included 102 patients with ARS examined the use of *Pelargonium sidoides* extract, a common root plant from South Africa. This study concluded that *P. sidoides* may be effective in relieving symptoms; however, some doubt exists because of a poor quality of evidence (Fokkens et al., 2012).

Myrtol, an essential oil derived from pine, lime, and eucalyptus, showed a statistically significant difference in the improvement of sinusitis symptom scores and reduced the need for an antibiotic after treatment with myrtol (Fokkens et al., 2012).

LOWER RESPIRATORY TRACT INFECTIONS

Improving care of patients with lower RTI–usually some form of pneumonia–has been the focus of multiple guidelines and organizations. While URIs are usually self-limiting and viral in nature, the pathogens responsible for causing pneumonia as

well as the host response can be variable, leading to mixed outcomes. Pneumonias remain a common reason for emergency room visits and hospitalizations. Therefore, it is tantamount to be able to recognize pneumonia versus other respiratory syndromes and provide appropriate treatment. This section will focus on the management of bronchitis and community-acquired pneumonia (CAP).

Bronchitis

Bronchitis is a syndrome that manifests in both acute and chronic forms. Acute bronchitis is one of the most common reasons for ambulatory care visits in the United States and accounts for approximately 10 million office visits per year (Harris et al., 2016; Singh et al., 2020; Wenzel et al., 2006).

Causes

Acute bronchitis is defined as a self-limiting inflammation of the bronchi (large airways) that leads to mild symptoms with or without cough. Coughs may or may not be productive but may last up to 6 weeks. Bronchitis may actually be a signal for other RTI such as flu, common cold, or pneumonia. Because symptoms coincide with these other syndromes, it is often difficult to narrow the cause and correctly diagnose. Most cases are viral (e.g., influenza virus, RSV, rhinovirus). Rarely, bronchitis can be caused by atypical bacterial organisms such as *Mycoplasma pneumoniae* and *Chlamydia pneumoniae*.

Patients with chronic bronchitis may have flares exacerbated by other chronic conditions, such as chronic obstructive pulmonary disease, asthma, allergies.

Pathophysiology

Inflammation of the bronchi, which are the large airways branching off the trachea, is triggered by antimicrobial organisms as mentioned earlier as well as noninfectious causes such as allergens and pollution. When exposed to these triggers, lymphocytes and inflammatory mediators will cause mucosal thickening of the bronchi and trachea, epithelial cell desquamation, and denuding of tissue to the basement membrane.

Diagnostic Criteria

Due to similarities in presentation with other RTIs, bronchitis is usually a diagnosis of exclusion. The clinical definition varies across clinical practice guidelines and literature. In general, patients will present with cough as their primary chief complaint. Dyspnea and sputum may or may not be present. Sore throat is usually absent, as well as fever, tachycardia, and tachypnea. Chest radiograph is usually the standard to first rule out pneumonia. Nasopharyngeal or sputum cultures can also be collected. However, availability of Gram staining and rapid diagnostic tests may be limited in certain settings. Furthermore, sample collection is prone to inadequate yield so may not detect any pathogens. Rapid testing may be useful when a suspected organism circulating within the community can be easily treated (e.g., flu test during influenza season).

The clinician should also rule out non-infectious causes of bronchitis. These can include aspiration of foreign bodies, acute decompensated heart failure, and asthma.

Bronchitis is diagnosed as chronic if patients continue to have consistent cough for at least three months for two consecutive years. Acute exacerbation of chronic bronchitis should be approached in the same manner as acute bronchitis.

Initiating Drug Therapy

As diagnosis of bronchitis can oftentimes be vague, treatment strategies should be mostly focused on symptom management and nonpharmacologic supportive care. Furthermore, as bronchitis is usually viral in origin, there is no available targeted treatments outside of influenza. Adequate rest, avoidance of inflammatory triggers (e.g., allergens, pollution, cold air), and lozenges can assist with cough. Using a therapeutic approach or treatment algorithm can further guide decisions, such as the algorithm previously suggested for URIs (**Figure 23.1**). Options for first-line and second-line antimicrobials are further discussed in the text.

Goals of Drug Therapy

The main goals of treatment are mostly targeted to symptom relief. If treating for a specific bacterial or viral organism, treatment will also prevent transmission to others.

Antitussives

Cough suppressants are widely available OTC and utilized for a variety of other cough-inducing syndromes. Commonly used agents are described in Table 24.1 (Chapter 24, Upper Respiratory Infections).

Antimicrobials

Because bronchitis is one of the most common illnesses seen by outpatient physicians, antibiotics are oftentimes prescribed inappropriately, more than any other respiratory tract infection. In general, antimicrobial agents are not recommended. Several clinical practice guidelines recommend against starting antibiotic treatment. Meta-analyses of clinical trials have suggested that there may be a marginal reduction in duration of symptoms, without difference in quality of life or ability to return to daily activities. However, if a specific pathogen is identified, the appropriate antimicrobial drug should be prescribed.

Antivirals

The only available antiviral agent is oseltamivir for the treatment of influenza. Other aforementioned viruses commonly causing bronchitis do not have antiviral agents available.

Mechanism of Action

Oseltamivir (Tamiflu®) acts as a neuraminidase inhibitor. Neuraminidase enzymes are present on the surface of all influenza virus cells and is necessary for viral replication. By inhibiting neuraminidase receptor binding, infected host cells are not able to release progeny virions, thus reducing the viral load and disease progression.

Dosage

Oseltamivir is dosed at 75 mg twice daily for 5 days. Dose adjustments should be made for patients with reduced renal function and end-stage renal disease. Dosage forms include capsule and oral suspension. See **Table 23.2**.

Time Frame for Response

Oseltamivir is most effective when started within 48 hours of symptom onset. Doses are rapidly absorbed from the GI tract and detectable in plasma within 30 minutes. Symptom improvement should be apparent within 24 hours of initiation.

TABLE 23.2			
Overview of Agents for Bronchitis			
Generic (Trade) Name and Dosage	**Selected Adverse Events**	**Contraindications**	**Special Considerations**
Oseltamivir (Tamiflu) 75 mg BID for 5 days	GI upset	Hypersensitivity or allergy to oseltamivir	
Macrolides: Azithromycin (Zithromax) 500 mg one day, then 250 mg daily for 4 days Clarithromycin (Biaxin) 500 mg BID for 7 days Erythromycin, base (Ery-base) 500 mg QID for 14 days	Common: GI upset Rare: hepatotoxicity, Stevens-Johnson syndrome, *C. difficile* colitis	Hypersensitivity or allergy to any macrolides	Strong CYP3A4 inhibitors. Check for drug–drug interactions. Clarithromycin requires renal dose adjustment. May cause QTc prolongation, especially in combination with other QTc-prolonging medications.
Doxycycline (Oracea) 200 mg daily in 1–2 divided doses	Common: GI upset, rash, vaginal infections, headache Rare: Stevens-Johnson syndrome, hepatotoxicity	Hypersensitivity or allergy to tetracyclines	Not recommended for children <8 y of age Take on an empty stomach if tolerated.

GI, gastrointestinal; QTc, corrected QT interval.

Contraindications

Oseltamivir is contraindicated in patients with known serious hypersensitivity to oseltamivir or any of its components.

Adverse Events

Most commonly reported reactions include nausea and vomiting, and diarrhea. Pediatric patients may be at higher risk for confusion and delirium.

Interactions

Oseltamivir has limited food and drug interactions. Patients on probenecid were found to have a 2.5-fold increase in serum concentrations of oseltamivir, but the clinical significance of this effect is unknown.

Macrolides

Macrolide class of antibiotics include azithromycin, clarithromycin, and erythromycin. These antibiotics should be reserved for those who have evidence of atypical bacterial infection– *M. pneumonia*, *C. pneumoniae*, and *Bordetella pertussis*.

Mechanism of Action

Macrolides inhibit bacterial protein synthesis by binding to ribosomal subunit 50S, which inhibits elongation of peptide chains and inhibits ribosomal translation. This results in a bacteriostatic effect, although bactericidal action can be achieved at higher concentrations. All three agents are effective against *Bordetella*, but only azithromycin for *Mycoplasma* and *Chlamydia*.

Dosage

Azithromycin is administered for 5 days at a dose of 500 mg on day one, followed by 250 mg daily on days two through five. Renal dose adjustments are not required.

Clarithromycin is dosed 500 mg twice daily for 7 days. Patients with renal dysfunction with CrCl less than 30 mL/min should reduce dose to 500 mg once daily. CrCl less than 10 mL/min can be dosed 250 to 500 mg once daily. Patients on hemodialysis should use 500 mg once daily.

Erythromycin (base) is dosed 500 mg four times daily for 14 days. Dose adjustments for renal function are not necessary.

Contraindications

Macrolides are contraindicated in patients with history of hypersensitivity to macrolides. Furthermore, use should be avoided if there is history of cholestatic jaundice or hepatic dysfunction with prior azithromycin use.

Adverse Events

GI intolerance (i.e., diarrhea, nausea, abdominal pain) is the most commonly reported effect. Liver function enzymes may become elevated, especially with longer treatment duration, as well as possible QTc prolongation.

Interactions

As macrolides are substrates and inhibitors of CYP3A4, several significant drug interactions exist, namely with human immunodeficiency virus (HIV) protease inhibitors, warfarin, tacrolimus, and cyclosporine. Serum concentrations of these drugs may increase, so patients should be carefully monitored when started on a macrolide.

Doxycycline

Doxycycline is another therapeutic option for treatment of *M. pneumonia* and *C. pneumoniae*. It is previously discussed under "Rhinosinusitis" in the "Antibiotics" section.

Monitoring Patient Response

Patients may not have immediate relief and have persistent cough for weeks to months. If symptoms progress or worsen, clinicians should reevaluate for pneumonia or alternative causes of cough (e.g., heart failure, malignancy).

Patient Education

Antimicrobial stewardship is an important part of patient education. In an effort to decrease health care costs and avoid bacterial resistance, clinicians should emphasize the futility of antimicrobial treatment for bronchitis and avoid prescribing them. Also, education on how to recognize worsening of symptoms can help patients decide whether a follow-up visit or escalation of care is needed.

Community-Acquired Pneumonia

CAPs are a common reason for emergency room visits and hospitalizations. However, CAP can also be managed in an outpatient setting as well. Furthermore, viral illnesses such as influenza can progress to a severe pneumonia, requiring advanced care and supportive measures. For the purposes of this chapter, the diagnosis and management of CAP will be focused on ambulatory care patients, with brief mention of criteria for hospital admission.

Causes

Both bacterial and viral pathogens can cause CAP, either alone or in combination. The most common bacterial pathogens are *S. pneumoniae*, *H. influenzae*, *M. pneumoniae*, *S. aureus*, *M. catarrhalis*, *Legionella* species, and *C. pneumoniae* (Metlay et al., 2019). Common viral etiologies include influenza virus A and B, coronavirus, RSV, parainfluenza virus, and adenovirus. Patients with immunocompromised status due to medications or disease states are at additional risk for other organisms such as *Pneumocystis jerovicii*, Mycoplasma tuberculosis, and fungi (Bartlett, 2019; File, 2020).

Pathophysiology

As the lung is not a sterile site, there are microbes that exist as part of the normal human microbiome. When multiplication of an organism occurs in combination with reduced host defenses, this pathogen can then become virulent and cause an inflammatory cascade. This inflammatory response causes lung tissues to increase permeability, thus allowing for WBCs, neutrophils, lymphocytes, and cytokines to move into the alveolar and pleural spaces. Infection may be limited locally within the alveoli or may go on to cause a systemic response. Systemic inflammation will produce the majority of the patient's clinical signs and symptoms (File, 2020).

Diagnostic Criteria

Diagnosis of CAP requires correlation with clinical symptoms with objective data such as a chest X-ray. Common clinical features include cough with sputum production, fever, chest pain, and dyspnea. Severe CAP is defined by the 2019 IDSA/American Thoracic Society guidelines in **Table 23.3**.

The gold standard for diagnosis of pneumonia is chest radiograph. Although chest X-ray will not differentiate viral versus bacterial pneumonia, the presence of interstitial infiltrates and lobar consolidation should be suspicious for pneumonia. If indicated, a CT scan of the chest may be more accurate as it has a higher sensitivity for detecting CAP.

In general, sputum and blood cultures are not recommended in the outpatient setting. Although it is ideal to provide targeted treatment therapy, the low-yield rates of these tests impede antimicrobial narrowing and do not positively impact overall care. If a patient has prior history of infection with Methicillin-resistant *Staphylococcus aureus* (MRSA) or *Pseudomonas aeruginosa* and was treated with antibiotics in the hospital within the last 90 days, it is reasonable to collect cultures. Furthermore, if there is suspicion for pneumonia secondary to influenza especially during periods of high influenza activity, a rapid influenza molecular assay is recommended. Urine testing for Legionella antigen should be reserved for those with severe CAP or if exposed to a recent outbreak of Legionella.

In recent years, serum procalcitonin assays have emerged as a potential tool to help guide diagnosis of pneumonia and initiation of treatment. If elevated, there is a high likelihood of bacterial infection, whereas lower levels may suggest a viral etiology. However, studies have been inconsistent in proving the sensitivity of the test. Therefore, empiric treatment should be initiated regardless of procalcitonin levels in patients clinically and radiographically suspected of having CAP.

When deciding whether a patient needs escalation of care and admittance to the hospital, there are several prognostic tools that can help clinicians with prognosis. Two of the most well-validated models are the Pneumonia Severity Index and CURB-65 (confusion, urea [blood urea nitrogen level > 20 mg/dL], respiratory rate >30 breaths/min, blood pressure < 90/60, age ≥ 65). Lower scores on both scales suggest that patients are at lower risk for mortality and can receive outpatient care.

Initiating Drug Therapy

Initial treatment strategies should be tailored to the organism most likely to have caused the pneumonia as well as the patient's comorbidities. Bacterial and viral organisms commonly associated with CAP are discussed previously in the "Causes" section for "Community Acquired Pneumonia." Whereas antimicrobial treatment for bronchitis is discouraged, pharmacologic treatment for CAP with antibiotics should first be started and then de-escalated based on the patient's clinical course. Antivirals should be initiated if there is high clinical suspicion. Furthermore, as there can be superimposed bacterial with viral infection, antibiotics will provide antibacterial coverage as most viruses do not have targeted treatment options available.

Nonpharmacologic supportive care includes oral fluids, decongestants, cough suppressants, and expectorants. However, these will only provide symptomatic relief and not a cure for the pneumonia.

Steroids are not recommended.

Goals of Drug Therapy

The primary treatment goal is to decrease the duration of illness, prevent complications and progression of disease severity, and prevent transmission of disease.

Antibiotics

If cultures are obtained and an organism is identified, antimicrobial therapy should be tailored to that microbe. As most patients do not have culture data available at time of diagnosis, it is reasonable to start empiric antibiotics to broadly cover the organisms most likely to cause CAP—*S. pneumoniae*, *H. influenzae*, and atypical organisms. Furthermore, empiric treatment of CAP for outpatients can be divided into those with comorbidities (e.g., chronic renal disease, heart disease, diabetes mellitus, malignancy) or risk factors (e.g., MRSA, *P. aeruginosa*) and those without. Several studies have looked at whether certain treatments are superior to others; however, there has been little evidence of superiority or equivalence of one regimen to another.

Comorbidities include chronic heart, renal, lung, liver disease; diabetes mellitus; alcoholism; malignancy; asplenia.

Beta-Lactams

Beta-lactams have reliable activity against the aforementioned bacterial pathogens and are easily accessible. This group of antibiotics encompasses all the penicillin groups and

---

TABLE 23.3	
Definition for Severe Community-Acquired Pneumonia: Either One Major Criteria or Three Minor Criteria	
Major criteria (At least one)	Septic shock requiring vasopressors Respiratory failure requiring mechanical ventilation
Minor criteria (At least three)	Respiratory rate ≥ 30 breaths/min PaO_2/FiO_2 ratio ≤ 250 Multilobar infiltrates on imaging Confusion/altered mental status Uremia (BUN) ≥ 20 mg/dL White blood cells count < 4000 cells/mcL Platelet count < 10,000 Hypothermia (temperature < 36°C) Hypotension requiring fluid resuscitation

BUN, blood urea nitrogen.

Source: Adapted from Infectious Disease Society of America /American Thoracic Society.

cephalosporins. These agents are referred to as *beta-lactams* due to the presence of a beta-lactam ring within their chemical structure. Examples of recommended agents are amoxicillin, amoxicillin/clavulanate, cefpodoxime, and cefuroxime.

Mechanism of Action.   Beta-lactams inhibit bacterial cell wall synthesis by binding to the PBP, which is essential for cross-linking peptides for the bacterial cell wall. This inhibition of PBP activity eventually leads to bacterial cell lysis and cell death. Bacteria can develop resistance to penicillins by producing an enzyme, beta-lactamase, which hydrolyzes the beta-lactam ring, thus rendering the antibiotic ineffective. Adding a beta-lactamase inhibitor prevents this from occurring and allows for the penicillin to work.

Dosage.   Doses are summarized in **Table 23.4**.

Amoxicillin usual dosing is 1 g once daily. Patients with renal dysfunction with estimated CrCl less than 30 mL/min should be prescribed a reduced dose of 500 mg every 12 hours.

Amoxicillin/clavulanate (Augmentin®) is amoxicillin plus the beta-lactamase inhibitor clavulanate. Recommended dosing is 500 mg/125 mg thrice daily. Patients with CrCl less than 30 mL/min should reduce to twice daily.

Cephalosporins are divided into different "generations" based on their spectrum of activity. Agents that can be empirically used for CAP include cefuroxime (second generation), cefpodoxime (third generation), and cefdinir (third generation). Cefuroxime is dosed 500 mg twice daily. Dose should be reduced to once daily if CrCl is less than 30 mL/min and reduced to every 48 hours if CrCl is less than 10 mL/min.

Cefpodoxime is dosed at 200 mg twice daily. Frequency should be reduced to once daily if CrCl is less than 30 mL/min. Cefdinir can be given 300 mg twice daily with reduction to once daily for CrCl less than 30 mL/min.

All of the drugs mentioned previously are available as oral tablets or capsules, as well as oral suspension.

Time Frame for Response.   Beta-lactams are widely distributed throughout the body, and patients should show clinical improvement within 24 hours.

Contraindications.   All beta-lactams are contraindicated if patients have a history of true immunoglobulin E (IgE)-mediated allergy such as anaphylaxis or angioedema (type 1 hypersensitivity). However, it is generally considered to be safe to give to patients who have a history of non-IgE-mediated reactions, such as rash, depending on the agent and time since reaction. Cross-reactivity risk is low between penicillins and cephalosporins but should still be considered.

Adverse Events.   Beta-lactams are generally well tolerated. Potential adverse effects include diarrhea, nausea and vomiting, seizures, nephritis, and eosinophilia.

Interactions.   Beta-lactams have limited drug–drug interactions. However, patients with renal dysfunction should avoid concomitant nephrotoxic medications.

Macrolides

The two recommended macrolide agents are azithromycin and clarithromycin. Macrolides fulfill a unique immunomodulatory role in addition to their antimicrobial properties. The term "macrolide" refers to the 12-membered lactone ring within its chemical structure.

Mechanism of Action.   Macrolides inhibit bacterial protein synthesis by binding to ribosomal subunit 50S, which inhibits elongation of peptide chains and inhibits ribosomal translation. This results in a bacteriostatic effect, although bactericidal action can be achieved at higher concentrations.

Dosage.   Azithromycin is administered for 5 days at a dose of 500 mg on day one, followed by 250 mg daily on days two through five. Renal dose adjustments are not required.

Clarithromycin is dosed 500 mg twice daily for seven days. Patients with renal dysfunction with CrCl less than 30 mL/min should reduce dose to 500 mg once daily. CrCl less than 10 mL/min can be dosed 250 to 500 mg once daily. Patients on hemodialysis should use 500 mg once daily.

Both drugs are available as oral tablets and suspensions.

Time Frame for Response.   Beta-lactams are widely distributed throughout the body, and patients should show clinical improvement within 24 hours.

Contraindications.   Macrolides are contraindicated in patients with history of hypersensitivity to macrolides. Furthermore, use

TABLE 23.4

Empiric Treatment Strategies

	Suggested Empiric Regimen
No comorbidities or risk for MRSA or Pseudomonas aeruginosa	Amoxicillin 1 g TID *or* Doxycycline 100 mg BID *or* Azithromycin 500 mg for 1 dose, then 250 mg daily for 4 doses *or* Clarithromycin 500 mg BID
With comorbidities*	Combination of amoxicillin/clavulanate or cephalosporin *and* macrolide or doxycycline *or* Respiratory fluoroquinolone monotherapy (see text for drug dosing)

*Comorbidities include chronic heart, renal, lung, liver disease; diabetes mellitus; alcoholism; malignancy; asplenia.

MRSA, Methicillin-resistant *Staphylococcus aureus*.

Source: Adapted from Infectious Disease Society of America/American Thoracic Society.

should be avoided if there is history of cholestatic jaundice or hepatic dysfunction with prior azithromycin use.

Adverse Events. GI intolerance (i.e., diarrhea, nausea, abdominal pain) is the most commonly reported effect. Liver function enzymes may become elevated, especially with longer treatment duration, as well as possible QTc prolongation.

Interactions. As macrolides are substrates and inhibitors of CYP3A4, several significant drug interactions exist, namely with HIV protease inhibitors, warfarin, tacrolimus, and cyclosporine. Serum concentrations of these drugs may increase, so patients should be carefully monitored when started on a macrolide.

Fluoroquinolones

The "respiratory" fluoroquinolones refer to the ones that have anti-streptococcal activity. These are levofloxacin, moxifloxacin, and gemifloxacin. However, gemifloxacin is no longer available in the United States.

Mechanism of Action. Unlike the macrolides, fluoroquinolones exert their antibacterial activity by binding to DNA gyrase and topoisomerase IV. These key enzymes are normally incorporated into the bacterial cell replication process by stabilizing the double-stranded DNA and carrying on replication. Fluoroquinolones will instead inhibit these enzymes and cause DNA strand breakage, eventually leading to cell death.

Dosage. Levofloxacin is dosed 750 mg once daily and moxifloxacin is dosed 400 mg once daily. Levofloxacin does require renal dose adjustment. Patients with a CrCl of 20 to 49 mL/min should be prescribed a 750 mg every 48 hours. Patients with a CrCl of 10 to 19 mL/min or on hemodialysis should be prescribed a 750 mg loading dose followed by either 500 mg every 48 hours or 250 mg every 24 hours. Hepatic dosing adjustments are not required. Levofloxacin is available as both oral tablet and oral suspension. Moxifloxacin is available only as oral tablet.

Time Frame for Response. Fluoroquinolones are well absorbed and widely distributed into tissue. Clinical improvement should be achieved in 48 hours.

Contraindications. Fluoroquinolones are contraindicated in patients with history of hypersensitivity to fluoroquinolones.

Adverse Events. Common ADEs are nausea, diarrhea, and vomiting. There are unfortunately several serious adverse reactions reported as well. These include prolonged QTc interval, aortic dissections, blood glucose dysregulation, hepatotoxicity, photosensitivity, tendon rupture, seizures, and *Clostridium difficile* colitis.

Interactions. In general, drugs that enhance fluoroquinolone adverse effects should be avoided. Some specific examples include amiodarone (enhanced QTc-prolonging effect), warfarin (increased bleeding risk), multivitamins and minerals (decreased absorption of fluoroquinolone).

Antivirals

The only available antiviral agent is oseltamivir for the treatment of influenza.

Mechanism of Action. Oseltamivir (Tamiflu®) acts as a neuraminidase inhibitor. Neuraminidase enzymes are present on the surface of all influenza virus cells and are necessary for viral replication. By inhibiting neuraminidase receptor binding, infected host cells are not able to release progeny virions, thus reducing the viral load and disease progression (Davies, 2010).

Dosage. Oseltamivir is dosed at 75 mg twice daily for 5 days. Dose adjustments should be made for patients with reduced renal function of CrCl of 30 mL/min or lower to 75 mg every other day or 30 mg daily. Use is not recommended in patients with end-stage renal disease. Dosage forms include capsule and oral suspension.

Time Frame for Response. Oseltamivir is most effective when started within 48 hours of symptom onset. Doses are rapidly absorbed from the GI tract and detectable in plasma within 30 minutes. Symptom improvement should be apparent within 24 hours of initiation (Davies, 2010; Fabre & Bartlett, 2019).

Contraindications. Oseltamivir is contraindicated in patients with known serious hypersensitivity to oseltamivir or any of its components.

Adverse Events. Most commonly reported reactions include nausea and vomiting, and diarrhea. Pediatric patients may be at higher risk for confusion and delirium.

Interactions. Oseltamivir has limited food and drug interactions. Patients on probenecid were found to have a 2.5-fold increase in serum concentrations of oseltamivir, but the clinical significance of this effect is unknown.

Monitoring Patient Response

Patients should have symptomatic improvement and achieve clinical stability within 48 to 72 hours of starting therapy. If symptoms persist after 7 days or worsen, alternative antibiotic regimen can be trialed. However, repeated exposure to multiple antibiotics increases risk for developing bacterial resistance. If patients meet criteria for severe CAP, they should be evaluated in the emergency room for inpatient admittance.

Duration of Therapy

In patients who are clinically improving, antibiotics should be continued until the patient is stable or at least for 5 days. Failure to improve after 5 days is correlated with higher mortality and worse clinical outcomes. Therefore, clinicians should promptly assess for possible bacterial resistance or complications (e.g., bacterial and viral superinfection, empyema).

CASE STUDY 1

Jane is a 69-year-old female with past medical history of asthma, hypertension, coronary artery disease, coronary artery bypass graft surgery, and arthritis. She presents to her primary care physician after four days of facial tenderness, rhinorrhea, and "feeling stuff" despite using over-the-counter medications. Her doctor diagnoses her with rhinosinusitis and recommends a course of antibiotics. She has no known allergy history. Which antibiotic therapy is the best option for Jane?

a. None. Continue to use over-the-counter medications.

b. Oral levofloxacin 500 mg daily for 5 days

c. Oral amoxicillin/clavulanate 875 mg every 12 hours for 5 days

d. Go to emergency room for hospital admission.

Bibliography

Starred references are cited in the text.

*Anselmo-Lima, W., & Sakana, E. (2015). Rhinosinusitis: Evidence and experience. *Brazilian Journal of Otorhinolaryngology, 81*, S1–S49.

*Bartlett, G. J. (2019). Diagnostic approach to community-acquired pneumonia in adults. *UpToDate*, www.uptodate.com/contents/diagnostic-approach-to-community-acquired-pneumonia-in-adults

*Blaiss, M. S., Dicpinigaitis, P. V., Eccles, R., et al. (2015). Consumer attitudes on cough and cold: US (ACHOO) survey results. *Current Medical Research and Opinion*, 1–12 (e-publication ahead of print).

Centre for Clinical Practice. (2008). *Respiratory tract infections—Antibiotic prescribing. Prescribing of antibiotics for self-limiting respiratory tract infections in adults and children in primary care.* London, UK: National Institute for Health and Clinical Excellence, NICE Clinical Guideline 69, 1–121.

*Chow, A. W., Benninger, M. S., Brook, I., et al. (2012). ISDA Clinical Practice Guideline for acute bacterial rhinosinusitis in children and adults. *Clinical Infectious Diseases, 54*(8), 1041–1045.

*Davies, B. E. (2010). Pharmacokinetics of oseltamivir: An oral antiviral for the treatment and prophylaxis of influenza in diverse populations. *Journal of Antimicrobial Chemotherapy , 65*, ii5–ii10.

*Dicpinigaitis, P. V., Eccles, R., Blaiss, M. S., et al. (2015). Impact of cough and common cold on productivity, absenteeism, and daily life in the United States: ACHOO Survey. *Current Medical Research and Opinion*, 1–7 (e-publication ahead of print).

*Dykewicz, M., & Hamilas, D. (2010). Rhinitis and sinusitis. *Journal of Allergy and Clinical Immunology, 125*(2), S103–S115.

*Fabre, V., & Bartlett, J. G. (2019). Bronchitis, acute uncomplicated. *Antibiotics Johns Hopkins Guides*, www.hopkinsguides.com/hopkins/index/Johns_Hopkins_ABX_Guide/Antibiotics.

*Fashner, J., Ericson, K., & Werner, S. (2012). Treatment of the common cold in children and adults. *American Family Physician, 86*(2), 153–159.

*Fendrick, A. M., Monto, A. S., Nightengale, B., et al. (2003). The economic burden of non-influenza-related viral respiratory tract infection in the United States. *Archives of Internal Medicine, 163*(4), 487–494.

File, T. M. (2020). Epidemiology, pathogenesis, and microbiology of community-acquired pneumonia in adults. *UpToDate*, www.uptodate.com/contents/epidemiology-pathogenesis-and-microbiology-of-community-acquired-pneumonia-in-adults

*Fokkens, W. J., Hoffmans, R., & Thomas, M. (2014). Avoid prescribing antibiotics in acute rhinosinusitis. *British Medical Journal, 349*, 1–3.

*Fokkens, W. J., Lund, V. J., Mullol, J., et al. (2012). European position paper on rhinosinusitis and nasal polyps 2012. *Rhinology, 23*(3), 1–298.

*Harris, A. M., Hicks, L. A., & Qaseem, A. (2016). Appropriate antibiotic use for acute respiratory tract infection in adults: Advice for high-value care from the American College of Physicians and the Centers for Disease Control and Prevention. *Annals of Internal Medicine, 164*(6), 425. doi: 10.7326/m15-1840

Irwin, R. S., Baumann, M. H., Bolser, D. C., et al. (2006). Diagnosis and management of cough: ACCP evidence-based clinical practice guidelines. *Chest, 129*(Suppl. 1), 1S–23S.

*Jacobs, S. E., Lamson, D. M., St. George, K., et al. (2013). Human rhinoviruses. *Clinical Microbiology Reviews, 26*(1), 135–162.

*Lam, K., Schleimer, R., & Kern, R. (2015). The etiology and pathogenesis of chronic rhinosinusitis: A review of current hypotheses. *Current Allergy and Asthma Reports, 15*(7), 540.

*Liu, L., Johnson, H. L., Cousens, S., et al. (2012). Global, regional, and national causes of child mortality: An updated systematic analysis for 2010 with time trends since 2000. *Lancet, 379*(9832), 2151–2161.

*Metlay, J. P., Waterer, G. W., Long, A. C., et al. (2019). Diagnosis and treatment of adults with community-acquired pneumonia: An official clinical practice guideline of the American Thoracic Society and Infectious Diseases Society of America. *American Journal of Respiratory and Critical Care Medicine, 200*(7). doi: 10.1164/rccm.201908-1581st

*Nahas, R., & Balla, A. (2011). Complementary and alternative medicine for prevention and treatment of the common cold. *Canadian Family Physician, 57*(1), 31–36.

*Peters, A. T., Spector, S., Hsu, J., et al. (2014). Diagnosis and management of rhinosinusitis: A practice parameter update. *Annals of Allergy, Asthma & Immunology, 113*, 347–385.

*Pratter, M. R. (2006). Cough and the common cold: ACCP evidence-based clinical practice guidelines. *Chest, 129*(Suppl. 1), 72S–74S.

*Rosenfield, R. M., Piccirillo, J. F., Chandrasekhar, S. S., et al. (2015). Clinical practice guideline (update): Adult sinusitis executive summary. *Otolaryngology-Head and Neck Surgery, 152*(4), 598–609.

*Singh, A., Avula, A., & Zahn, E. (2020). Acute bronchitis. *StatPearls [Internet]*, U.S. National Library of Medicine. www.ncbi.nlm.nih.gov/books/NBK448067/

Tam, T., Little, P., & Stokes, T. (2008). Antibiotic prescribing for self-limiting respiratory tract infections in primary care: Summary of NICE guidance. *British Medical Journal, 337*, a437.

Torres, A., Ewig, A., Mandell, L., et al. (Eds.). (2006). Cough and acute bronchitis. *Respiratory Infections*, 259–273.

*Turner, R. B., Fuls, J. L., & Rodgers, N. D. (2010). Effectiveness of hand sanitizers with and without organic acids for removal of rhinovirus from hands. *Antimicrobial Agents and Chemotherapy, 54*(3), 1363–1664.

*Wenzel, R. P., & Fowler, A. A. (2006). Acute bronchitis. *New England Journal of Medicine, 355*, 2125–2130.

West, J. V. (2002). Acute upper airway infections. *British Medical Bulletin, 61*, 215–230.

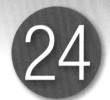

24 Asthma and Chronic Obstructive Pulmonary Disease

Tracy S. Estes and Karen J. Tietze

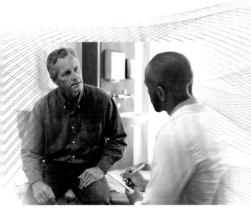
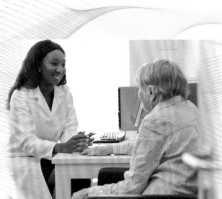
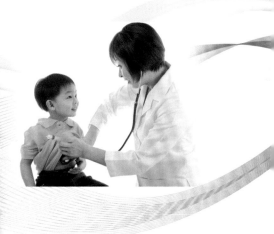

Learning Objectives

1. Define the difference and similarities of asthma and chronic obstructive pulmonary disease.
2. Apply the diagnostic criteria for each condition.
3. Select the most appropriate drug therapy based on clinical criteria for each condition.
4. Rationalize titrating drug therapy for each condition.

INTRODUCTION

Asthma and chronic obstructive pulmonary disease (COPD) are the two most prevalent chronic respiratory diseases in the world (World Health Organization [WHO], 2020). In comparison, asthma is more prevalent in children, while COPD is more prevalent in adults. Both asthma and COPD affect racial and ethnic minority groups more than whites, with asthma reported more in blacks and COPD reported more in American Indians/Alaska Natives and multiracial non-Hispanics (Centers for Diseases Control and Prevention [CDC], 2020a, 2020b). In general, females are more affected than males with both diseases except for pre-pubescent males (CDC, 2020a, 2020b). Interestingly, COPD is more common in patients with a history of asthma (CDC, 2020b).

There are practice guidelines that support evidence-based decisions in the management of asthma and COPD. The Global Initiative for Asthma's (GINA's) Global Strategy for Asthma Management and Prevention 2019 update is the most recent practice guideline in the management of asthma (GINA, 2020). The National Asthma Education and Prevention Program (NAEPP) guidelines for the diagnosis and management of asthma are considered outdated (National Heart, Lung and Blood Institute [NHLBI], 2020). The Global Initiative for Chronic Obstructive Lung Disease (GOLD) Global Strategy for the Diagnosis, Management, and Prevention of Chronic Obstructive Pulmonary Disease (2020 Report) is the most up-to-date practice guideline in the management of COPD (GOLD, 2020). Both guidelines are updated on an annual basis.

CAUSES

The causes of asthma and COPD are quite different. There is no one cause for asthma with a complex interplay of genetic susceptibility with environmental exposures resulting in the disease process (CDC, 2020c). There are three overlapping and interconnected hypotheses that support the theoretical cause of asthma: The Hygiene Hypothesis, the Old Friends Hypothesis, and the Biodiversity Hypothesis. An exaggerated and inappropriate immune response is triggered by the lack of appropriate immune system training (The Hygiene Hypothesis), the lack of beneficial parasitic infection (The Old Friends Hypothesis), and the skewing of bacterial diversity in the human body due to antibiotic use (The Biodiversity Hypothesis) (Brooks et al., 2013; Haahtela, 2019; Rook et al., 2017). In comparison, COPD is thought to be predominantly related to genetic susceptibility and a handful of environmental exposures, mainly tobacco smoke, air pollution, and respiratory infections (CDC, 2020d). Asthma–COPD overlap (ACO) occurs when a person shares characteristic of both asthma and COPD (GINA, 2020).

PATHOPHYSIOLOGY

Personalized and precision medicine is guided by the concepts of endotype, phenotype, theratype, and biomarker (Canonica et al., 2018; Ozdemir et al., 2018). These concepts help to understand the complexity of asthma and COPD pathophysiology. Endotype is the underlying mechanism at the cellular and molecular level, while phenotype is the observable characteristics as a result of the interplay of genetic predisposition and environmental exposures. Theratype is used to designate those patients responding to a specific therapy strategy (Ozdemir et al., 2018). A biomarker is an objective indicator for any pathogenic or biological process to diagnose, determine therapy, and/or monitor therapeutic response (Ozdemir et al., 2018).

Asthma has variable respiratory symptoms (e.g., intermittent cough, wheeze, dyspnea) with airflow limitation caused by an environmental exposure (e.g., allergic, non-allergic) triggering an intermittent inflammatory response (Papi et al., 2018). There are two asthma endotypes: T-helper type 2 (Th2) high or Th2 low (Kuruvilla et al., 2018). Th2 cytokines include interleukin (IL)-4, IL-5, and IL-13, which are higher in eosinophilic inflammation seen in asthma (Kuruvilla et al., 2018). There are four dominant asthma phenotypes: allergic eosinophilic, nonallergic eosinophilic, allergic non-eosinophilic, and nonallergic non-eosinophilic (Humbert et al., 2018; Terl et al., 2017). A biomarker of eosinophilic inflammation is an eosinophil count on a complete blood count. Immunoglobulin E (IgE) is a readily measurable biomarker of atopy (e.g., allergy) in human serum as a total level (e.g., total sIgE) versus specific allergen level (i.e., sIgE cat) (Rath et al., 2018). Atopy is defined as being sensitized to at least one specific allergen.

COPD has persistent respiratory symptoms (dyspnea, chronic cough, sputum, etc.) with airflow limitation caused by noxious particles or gases triggering a chronic inflammatory response (Siafakas et al., 2017). There are four COPD endotypes: Neutrophilic, Th2, alpha-1 antitrypsin deficiency, and systemic inflammation (Russell et al., 2016). Neutrophilic endotype results in an imbalance between tissue repair and destruction, which leads to excessive extracellular matrix digestion (Russell et al., 2016). Th2 endotype occurs when eosinophilic inflammation is present (Agustí et al., 2017). Alpha-1 antitrypsin deficiency endotype results in neutrophil elastase damaging lung tissue due to lack of inhibition (Craig & Henao, 2018). Systemic inflammation endotype results in chronic nonspecific inflammation (e.g., elevated white blood cell count, C-reactive protein, IL-6, fibrinogen) (Woodruff et al., 2015). There are nine phenotypes: Alpha-1 antitrypsin deficiency, frequent exacerbator, upper lobe predominant emphysema, pure emphysema, chronic bronchitis, pulmonary vascular, high systemic inflammation, steroid responsive, and ACO (Russell et al., 2016; Yousuf & Brightling, 2018). There is an ever-evolving body of biomarker evidence for each phenotype of COPD (Moon et al., 2018). The usual features of asthma, COPD, and ACO can be compared in **Table 24.1**.

TABLE 24.1

Usual Features of Asthma, Chronic Obstructive Pulmonary Disease, and Asthma-COPD Overlap

Parameter	Asthma	COPD	ACO
Symptom onset	Childhood onset usually	>40 years of age	Either
Symptom pattern	Variable symptoms with activity limitation. Triggered by exercise, emotions, laughter, dust, or allergen exposure	Chronic symptoms worsening with exercise	Persistent exertional dyspnea but can be variable
Symptomatic spirometry findings	Current or history of reversible obstruction	Persistent obstruction	Partially reversible obstruction
Asymptomatic spirometry findings	Usually normal	Persistent obstruction	Persistent obstruction
Personal or family history	Comorbid allergies; personal history of childhood asthma or family history of asthma	History of noxious particle or gas exposure	Usually a combination of asthma and COPD
Disease trajectory	Spontaneously improves or with therapy, may lead to fixed obstruction	Slow but progressive worsening even with therapy	Symptom improvement with therapy but progressive drug therapy requirements
Chest X-ray	Usually normal	Usually hyperinflation (air trapping)	Usually like COPD
Exacerbations	Exacerbation risk and frequency reduced with therapy	Exacerbation risk and frequency reduced, but comorbidities can contribute to impairment	Exacerbations may be more frequent than COPD but are reduced with therapy. Comorbidities can contribute to impairment

TABLE 24.1

Usual Features of Asthma, Chronic Obstructive Pulmonary Disease, and Asthma-COPD Overlap (*Continued*)

Parameter	Asthma	COPD	ACO
Airway inflammation	Eosinophilic and/or neutrophilic	Neutrophilic with/without eosinophils based on genotype and phenotype. Lymphocyte infiltration of airways with possible systemic inflammation	Eosinophilic and/or neutrophilic

ACO, asthma-COPD overlap; COPD, chronic obstructive pulmonary disease.

DIAGNOSTIC CRITERIA

Asthma's hallmark is the variable and intermittent nature of the symptoms (e.g., wheezing, dyspnea, chest tightness, cough) (GINA, 2020). Symptoms usually do not occur in isolation, vary over time and intensity, worsen overnight or upon waking, and can be triggered by exercise, allergens, extreme temperature, and viral infections. An asthma diagnosis should be made in individuals aged at least 6 years, since children younger than 6 years may show periodic symptoms due to the caliber of their airways, which is not asthmatic in nature. Confirming variable expiratory airflow limitation via spirometry (e.g., forced expiratory volume in 1 second [FEV_1] reduction with FEV_1/forced vital capacity [FVC] reduction) is the first step in the diagnosis of asthma. Spirometry findings coupled with documented expiratory airflow limitation, such as positive bronchodilator reversibility test (e.g., 12% FEV_1 increase, with 200 mL in adults), excessive variability in twice-daily peak expiratory flow over 2 weeks, significant increase in lung function after 4 weeks of antiinflammation drug therapy, positive exercise challenge test, positive bronchial challenge test, or excessive variation in lung function between office visit. The physical examination may be normal in between episodes; however, concomitant atopic conditions may clue the healthcare provider to explore respiratory symptoms (e.g., eczema and allergic rhinoconjunctivitis).

COPD has a constellation of symptoms that hallmark the disease, to include dyspnea, chronic cough or sputum production, and the presence of risk factor(s) (GOLD, 2020). A history of recurrent lower respiratory tract infections increases the index of suspicion for COPD. Risk factors for COPD include genetic predisposition, tobacco smoke exposure, cooking and/or heating smoke, occupational noxious, particulate, or chemical exposures. Family history of COPD and childhood factors such as low birthweight and childhood respiratory infections are important factors to consider when diagnosing COPD. Although symptoms are important, spirometry is required to make a COPD diagnosis (GOLD, 2020). Spirometry must demonstrate persistent obstruction despite bronchodilation (e.g., FEV_1/FVC actual ratio <0.70) to confirm the diagnosis. The physical examination may be normal until significant obstruction is present (e.g., nail clubbing, barrel chest). A diagnosis of COPD should be made when likely differential diagnoses have been excluded. Spirometry findings consistent with asthma, COPD, and ACO must be considered when attempting to understand the underlying pathophysiology (**Table 24.2**).

TABLE 24.2

Spirometry Findings Comparison for Asthma, Chronic Obstructive Pulmonary Disease, and Asthma–COPD Overlap

Spirometry Parameter	Asthma	COPD	ACO
Normal actual FEV_1/FVC ratio pre or post-BD	+	−	−
Post-BD FEV_1/FVC ratio <0.70 actual	+/−	+	+
Post-BD $FEV_1 \geq 80\%$ predicted	+	+	+
Post-BD $FEV_1 < 80\%$ predicted	+/−	+	+
Post-BD $FEV_1 > 12\%$ with 200 mL increase from baseline at initiation of drug therapy	+	+	+
Post-BD $FEV_1 > 12\%$ with 400 mL increase from baseline at initiation of drug therapy	+	−	+

+: Congruent with diagnosis; +/−: Equivocal for diagnosis; −: Not congruent with diagnosis

ACO, asthma–COPD overlap; BD, bronchodilator; COPD, chronic obstructive pulmonary disease; FEV_1, forced expiratory volume in 1 second; FVC, forced vital capacity.

INITIATING DRUG THERAPY

Drugs recommended by GINA and GOLD guidelines to treat asthma and COPD include beta$_2$-adrenergic agonists (short and long acting); muscarinic antagonists (short and long acting); inhaled corticosteroids (ICSs); combination ICS and long-acting beta$_2$-agonists (LABA); combined long-acting inhaled muscarinic antagonists and beta$_2$ agonist; combined ICS, LABA, and long-acting muscarinic antagonist; oral corticosteroids (OCS); leukotriene modifiers; and monoclonal antibodies (**Table 24.3**). Mucolytic agents may help with COPD but are more adjuvant in nature.

TABLE 24.3

Selected Recommended Agents to Treat Asthma and Chronic Obstructive Pulmonary Disease

Generic (Trade) Name and Adult Dosage	Indications	Contraindications	Common Adverse Events	Caution
SABA				
Albuterol (Proventil HFA, Ventolin HFA, ProAir HFA) MDI 90 mcg/inhalation; 1–2 inhalations q4–6h as needed Albuterol (ProAir Respiclick) DPI 90 mcg/inhalation; 1–2 inhalations q4–6h as needed; 2 inhalations 5–30 minutes prior to exercise Albuterol (No trade) nebulizer solution 0.083% (2.5 mg/3 mL), 0.5% (2.5 mL/0.5 mL); 2.5 mg q6–8h as needed; 2.5–10 mg q1–4h with starting 2.5–5 mg every 20 minutes for 3 doses for acute bronchospasm Levalbuterol tartrate (Xopenex HFA) MDI 45 mcg/inhalation; 1–2 inhalations q4–6h as needed Levalbuterol tartrate (Xopenex) nebulizer solution 0.021% (0.63 mg/3 mL); 0.042% (1.25 mg/3 mL); 0.63–1.25 mg q8h as needed	Asthma COPD	Hypersensitivity to drug/class/component Severe hypersensitivity to milk protein for DPI form	Throat irritation, upper respiratory infection symptoms, cough, bad taste, tremor, dizziness, nervousness, nausea/vomiting, headache, palpitations, tachycardia, chest pain, pain, and hyperlactatemia	In persons with MAO inhibitor use within 14 days, TCA use within 14 days, ischemic heart disease, HTN, arrythmias, hypokalemia, diabetes mellitus, seizure disorder, hyperthyroidism, unusually responsive to sympathomimetic amine, renal impairment at higher dosing
SAMA				
Ipratropium bromide (Atrovent HFA) MDI 17 mcg/inhalation; 2 inhalations q6h Ipratropium bromide (no trade) nebulizer solution 0.02% (0.5 mg/2.5 mL); 1 therapy q6–8h for COPD; 1 therapy q20min for 3 doses for moderate to severe asthma exacerbation	Asthma COPD	Hypersensitivity to drug/class/component	Bronchitis, dyspnea, nausea, xerostomia, influenza-like symptoms, sinusitis, dizziness, dyspepsia, urinary tract infection, back pain, and urinary hesitancy/retention	In persons with prostate hypertrophy, bladder neck obstruction, angle-closure glaucoma
Combination of SABA and SAMA				
Ipratropium bromide (Combivent Respimat) SMI 20 mcg/100 mcg/inhalation; 1 inhalation q6h for COPD; 8 inhalations q20min as needed up to 3 hours for moderate to severe asthma exacerbation Ipratropium bromide/albuterol (Duoneb) nebulizer solution 0.017%/0.083% (0.5 mg/2.5 mg/3 mL); 1 therapy q6h for COPD; 1 therapy q20min for 3 doses as needed up to 3 hours for moderate to severe asthma exacerbation	Asthma COPD	Hypersensitivity to drug/class/component	Same as above for each component	Same as above for each component

TABLE 24.3

Selected Recommended Agents to Treat Asthma and Chronic Obstructive Pulmonary Disease (*Continued*)

Generic (Trade) Name and Adult Dosage	Indications	Contraindications	Common Adverse Events	Caution
LMD				
Montelukast (Singulair) tablet 10 mg q24h Zafirlukast (Accolate) tablet 20 mg q12h; 1 hour before or 2 hours after meals Zilueton (Zyflo) tablet 600 mg q6h (Zyflo CR) 1200 mg q12h; give <1 hour after morning and evening meals	Asthma	Hypersensitivity to drug/class/component Active hepatic disease AST or ALT >3x ULN	Headache, upper respiratory infection, fever, influenza-like symptoms, abdominal pain, cough, pharyngo-laryngeal pain, diarrhea, otitis media, otitis, nausea, dyspepsia, rash/urticaria, sinusitis, abdominal pain, elevated liver enzymes, leukopenia, gastroenteritis (in pediatric patients), sleep disorders, anxiety/irritability, restlessness, myalgia, and tremor	Montelukast: In persons with severe asthma, PKU Zafirlukast: In persons with acute asthma, hepatic impairment, caution in tapering systemic steroids Zilueton: In persons history of hepatic disease, alcohol abuse
ICS				
Beclomethason dipropionate (Qvar Redihaler) MDI 40 mcg/inhalation and 80 mcg/inhalation 1–4 inhalations q12h for asthma Budesonide (Pulmicort Flexhaler) DPI 90 mcg/inhalation and 180 mcg/inhalation; 2 inhalations q12h for asthma Budesonide (Pulmicort Respules) nebulizer solution 0.25 mg/2 mL; 0.5 mg/2 mL; 1 mg/2 mL; 1.5–2 mg q6h for COPD exacerbation Ciclesonide (Alvesco) 80 mcg/inhalation and 160 mcg/inhalation; 1–2 inhalations q12h for asthma Fluticasone propionate (Flovent HFA) MDI 44 mcg/inhalation; 110 mcg/inhalation; 220 mcg/inhalation; 2–4 inhalations q12h for asthma Fluticasone propionate (Flovent Diskus) DPI 100 mcg/inhalation and 250 mcg/inhalation; 1–2 inhalations q12h for asthma Fluticasone propionate (ArmonAir Respiclick) DPI 55 mcg/inhalation; 113 mcg/inhalation; 232 mcg/inhalation; 1–2 inhalations q12h for asthma Fluticasone furoate (Arnuity Ellipta) DPI 100 mcg/inhalation; 200 mcg/inhalation; 1 inhalation q24h for asthma	Asthma COPD	Hypersensitivity to drug/class/component Status asthmaticus Acute asthma Acute bronchospasm Avoid abrupt withdrawal Severe hypersensitivity to milk protein for DPI form	Headache, nasopharyngitis, conjunctivitis, upper respiratory infection, influenza, fever, fatigue, rhinitis, nasal congestion, facial edema, sinusitis, bronchitis, pneumonia, pain, abdominal pain, back pain, arthralgia/myalgia, nausea, vomiting, dysphonia, dysmenorrhea, dyspepsia, epistaxis, hematoma, rash/urticaria, pruritus, dry throat, cough, and oral or esophageal candidiasis	In persons with young age, recent long-term systemic corticosteroid therapy, immunocompromised, hepatic impairment, active infection, active or latent TB infection, measles or varicella exposure, osteoporosis, cataracts, glaucoma or at risk, ocular HSV

(Continued)

TABLE 24.3

Selected Recommended Agents to Treat Asthma and Chronic Obstructive Pulmonary Disease (*Continued*)

Generic (Trade) Name and Adult Dosage	Indications	Contraindications	Common Adverse Events	Caution
Mometasone (Asmanex HFA) MDI 100 mcg/inhalation and 200 mcg/inhalation; 2 inhalations q12h for asthma				
Mometasone (Asmanex Twisthaler) 220 mcg/inhalation; 1–2 inhalations q12h for asthma				
LABA				
Arformoterol (Brovana) nebulizer solution 15 mcg/2 mL; 1 therapy q12h for COPD	Asthma COPD	Hypersensitivity to drug/class/component	Similar to SABA, plus back pain, diarrhea, leg cramps, dyspnea, peripheral edema, pulmonary/chest congestion, xerostomia, dizziness	Same as above for SABA, plus QT prolongation or family history of, cardiac disease, recent MI, CHF, prolongation risk, electrolyte abnormalities, labor, and delivery
Formoterol (Performist) nebulizer solution 20 mcg/2 mL; 1 therapy q12h for COPD		Asthma use, if not FDA approved for use; BBW for asthma-related death		
Indacaterol (Arcaptag Neohaler) DPI 75 mcg/inhalation; 1 inhalation q24h for COPD		Acute deteriorating COPD		
Olodaterol (Striverdi Respimat) SMI 2.5 mcg/inhalation; 2 inhalations q24h for COPD		Acute bronchospasm		
Salmeterol (Serevent Diskus) DPI 50 mcg/inhalation; 1 inhalation q12h for asthma and COPD				
LAMA				
Glycopyrrolate (Seebri Neohaler) DPI 15.6 mcg/inhalation; 1 inhalation q12h for COPD	Asthma COPD	Hypersensitivity to drug/class/component	Similar to SAMA, plus upper respiratory infection symptoms, chest pain, abdominal pain, headache, edema, depression, insomnia, constipation, arthralgia/myalgia, vomiting, epistaxis, rash, infection, and candidiasis	Same as above for SAMA, plus renal impairment <60 creatinine clearance, urinary retention risk
Tiopropium bromide (Spiriva Handihaler) DPI 18 mcg/capsule; 2 inhalations from 1 capsule q24h for COPD		Acute deteriorating COPD		
Tiopropium bromide (Spiriva Respimat) SMI 1.25 mcg/inhalation for asthma and 2.5 mcg/inhalation for COPD; 2 inhalations q24h		Acute bronchospasm Severe hypersensitivity to milk protein for DPI form		
Aclininium bromide (Tudorza Pressair) DPI 400 mcg/inhalation; 1 inhalation q12h for COPD				
Umeclidinium bromide (Incruse Ellipta) DPI 62.5 mcg/inhalation; 1 inhalation q24h for COPD				
Combination of LABA and LAMA				
Glycopyrrolate/formoterol fumarate (Bevespi Aerosphere) 9 mcg/4.8 mcg/inhalation; 2 inhalations q12h	COPD	Same as above for LABA and LAMA	Same as above for LABA and LAMA	Same as above for LABA and LAMA, plus torsades de pointes history

TABLE 24.3

Selected Recommended Agents to Treat Asthma and Chronic Obstructive Pulmonary Disease (*Continued*)

Generic (Trade) Name and Adult Dosage	Indications	Contraindications	Common Adverse Events	Caution
Indacaterol/glycopyrrolate (Utibron Neohaler) 27.5 mcg/15.6 mcg/ inhalation; 1 inhalation q12h				
Tiotropium bromide/olodaterol (Stiolto Respimat) SMI 2.5 mcg/2.5 mcg/inhalation; 2 inhalations q24h				
Umeclidinium/vilanterol (Anoro Ellipta) DPI 62.5 mcg/25 mcg/ inhalation; 1 inhalation q24h				
Combination of ICS and LABA				
Budesonide/formoterol (Symbicort HFA) MDI 80 mcg/4.5 mcg/inhalation for asthma and 160 mcg/4.5 mcg/ inhalation for asthma and COPD; 2 inhalations q12h	Asthma COPD	Same as above ICS and LABA	Same as above ICS and LABA	Same as above ICS and LABA
Fluticasone propionate/ salmeterol (Advair Diskus) DPI 100 mcg/50 mcg/inhalation for asthma; 250 mcg/50 mcg/ inhalation for asthma and COPD; 500 mcg/50 mcg/inhalation for asthma; 1 inhalation q12h				
Fluticasone propionate/salmeterol (Advair HFA) MDI 45 mcg/21 mcg/ inhalation; 115 mcg/21 mcg/ inhalation; 230 mcg/21 mcg/ inhalation; 2 inhalations q12h for asthma				
Fluticasone furoate/vilanterol (Breo Ellipta) DPI 100 mcg/25 mcg/ inhalation for COPD and 200 mcg/25 mcg/inhalation for asthma; 1 inhalation q24h				
Mometasone furoate/formoterol fumarate dihydrate (Dulera) MDI 100 mcg/5 mcg/inhalation and 200 mcg/5 mcg/inhalation; 2 inhalations q12h for asthma				
Combination of ICS, LABA, and LAMA				
Fluticasone furoate/umeclidinium/ vilanterol (Trelegy Ellipta) DPI 100 mcg/62.5 mcg/25 mcg/ inhalation for COPD; 1 inhalation q24h	COPD	Same as above ICS, LABA, and LAMA	Same as above ICS, LABA, and LAMA	Same as above ICS, LABA, and LAMA

(*Continued*)

TABLE 24.3

Selected Recommended Agents to Treat Asthma and Chronic Obstructive Pulmonary Disease (*Continued*)

Generic (Trade) Name and Adult Dosage	Indications	Contraindications	Common Adverse Events	Caution
OCS				
Prednisone (No trade) tablet 1 mg, 2.5 mg, 5 mg, 10 mg, 20 mg, 50 mg and solution 5 mg/5 mL, 5 mg/1 mL; 40–60 mg/d divided 1–2 per day for 3–10 days for acute asthma; 7.5 mg–60 mg q24h or q48h for severe persistent asthma; 40 mg q24h for 5–10 days for COPD exacerbation	Asthma COPD	Hypersensitivity to drug/class/component Systemic fungal infection Cerebral malaria Avoid abrupt withdrawal	Length, number of courses, and dosage dependent: Cushingoid appearance, hirsutism, weight gain, erythema, abdominal discomfort, appetite changes, emotional lability, rash/urticaria, nausea/vomiting, sodium and fluid retention, hypokalemia, elevated blood pressure, edema, diaphoresis, muscle atrophy, petechiae/ecchymosis, skin pigmentation abnormality, acne, headache, dizziness/vertigo, insomnia, depression, anxiety, glucose intolerance, menstrual irregularities, and increased intraocular pressure	In persons with young age, immune-compromised, active infection, active or latent TB infection, infection risk, measles or varicella exposure, HTN, pheochromocytoma risk, CHF, recent MI, diabetes mellitus, PUD, ulcerative colitis, diverticulitis, recent intestinal anastomosis, GI perforation risk, seizure disorder, psychiatric disorder, thyroid disorder, osteoporosis or risk of, myasthenia gravis, optic neuritis, ocular HSV, renal impairment, cirrhosis
PDE-4 Inhibitors				
Roflumilast (Daliresp) tablet 250 mcg and 500 mcg; 250 mcg q24h for 1 month then increase to 500 mcg q24h	COPD	Hypersensitivity to drug/class/component Acute bronchospasm Labor and delivery Child-Pugh Class B or C hepatic impairment	Diarrhea, weight loss, nausea, headache, back pain, influenza, insomnia, dizziness, and decreased appetite	In persons with Child-Pugh Class A hepatic impairment, depression or history of, suicidal ideation, smoking habit changes
Methylxanthines*				
Theophylline (Elixophyllin, theo24, Uniphyl) tablet 100 mg, 200 mg, 300 mg, 400 mg, 450 mg, 600 mg; solution 80 mg/15 mL; injection various; 300–600 mg divided q12–24h; start 300–400 mg/d for 3 days then 400–600 mg/d thereafter; maximum 400 mg/d with decrease renal clearance	COPD	Hypersensitivity to drug/class/component	Nausea, vomiting, headache, insomnia, diarrhea, irritability, restlessness, tremor, and transient diuresis	In persons with active PUD, seizure disorder, arrhythmias, CHF, acute pulmonary edema, cor pulmonale, hepatic impairment, hypothyroidism, febrile, sepsis with multi-organ failure, shock, smoking habit changes, neonates or infants, and elderly patients
Mucolytics				
Acetylcysteine (No trade) Solution 10% (100 mg/mL) or 20% (200 mg/mL); 3–5 mL of 20% solution or 6–10 mL of 10% solution nebulized q6–8h; or 200 mg by mouth q8–12h	COPD	Hypersensitivity to drug/class/component	Nausea/vomiting, urticaria, tachycardia, rash, pruritus, flushing, upper respiratory infection symptoms, stomatitis, fever, and drowsiness	In persons with asthma, bronchospasm history, and upper gastrointestinal bleeding risk with oral route

TABLE 24.3

Selected Recommended Agents to Treat Asthma and Chronic Obstructive Pulmonary Disease (*Continued*)

Generic (Trade) Name and Adult Dosage	Indications	Contraindications	Common Adverse Events	Caution
mAB				

Anti-IL-5/5R
Benralizumab (Fasenra) injection
    30 mg; 1 injection q4wk for 3 doses
    then 1 injection q8wk
 	
Mepolizumab (Nucala) injection
    100 mg (auto-injector) and
    100 mg/1 mL (prefilled syringe;
    vial); 1 injection SQ q4wk
 	
Reslizumab (Cinqair) intravenous
    infusion 3 mg/kg/IV q4wk
	Asthma	Anti-IL-5/5R
		Hypersensitivity
		    to drug/class/
		    component
		Acute asthma
		Acute
		    bronchospasm
		Status asthmaticus
			Anti-IL-5/5R
			Benralizumab:
			headache, pharyngitis, fever,
			    hypersensitivity reaction
			    and injection site reaction
			
			Mepolizumab:
			Headache, injection site
			    reaction, back pain,
			    fatigue, influenza, urinary
			    tract infection, abdominal
			    pain, pruritus, eczema,
			    and muscle spasm
			
			Reslizumab:
			Elevated CPK, oropharyngeal
			    pain, and musculoskeletal
			    pain
				Anti-IL-5/5R
				In persons with helminth
				    infection risk,
				    Reslizumab BBW for
				    anaphylaxis, Reslizumab
				    CPK elevation

Anti-IL-4R
Dupilumab (Dupixent) injection
    200 mg–300 mg depending on
    asthma comorbidities; loading
    dose of 400 mg or 600 mg, then
    200 mg–300 mg q2wk
		Anti-IL-4R
		Hypersensitivity
		    to drug/class/
		    component
		Acute asthma
		Acute
		    bronchospasm
		Status asthmaticus
			Anti-IL-4R
			Injection site reaction,
			    conjunctivitis/keratitis,
			    herpes viral infection,
			    arthralgia, eosinophilia,
			    and oropharyngeal pain
				Anti-IL-4R
				In persons with current
				    corticosteroid use,
				    helminth infection risk

Anti-IgE
Omalizumab (Xolair) injection
    75 mg/0.5 mL and 150 mg/1 mL
    (prefilled syringe); 150 mg/1.2 mL
    (vial); 150–375 mg SQ q2–4wk
    based on body weight and IgE levels
		Anti-IgE
		Hypersensitivity
		    to drug/class/
		    component
		Acute
		    bronchospasm
		Status asthmaticus
			Anti-IgE
			Injection site reaction,
			    viral infection, upper
			    respiratory infection
			    symptoms, headache/
			    migraine, arthralgia,
			    nausea, pain, fatigue,
			    dizziness, pruritus,
			    abdominal pain, epistaxis,
			    otitis media, dermatitis,
			    otalgia, myalgia, fractures,
			    peripheral edema,
			    fever, anxiety, alopecia,
			    geohelminth infection, and
			    decreased platelets
				Anti-IgE
				In persons with anaphylaxis
				    history, BBW for
				    anaphylaxis, helminth
				    infection risk

* Not recommended for asthma per GINA guideline. Can be used, but better drug therapy options with less side effects are available.

ALT, alanine aminotransferase; AST, aspartate aminotransferase; BBW, black box warning; CHF, congestive heart failure; COPD, chronic obstructive pulmonary disease; CPK, creatinine phosphokinase; DPI, dry powder inhaler; FDA, food and drug administration; GI, gastrointestinal; HFA, hydrofluoroalkane; HSV, herpes simplex virus; HTN, hypertension; ICS, inhaled corticosteroids; IgE, immunoglobulin E; IL, interleukin; LABA, long-acting beta$_2$-agonists; LAMA, long-acting muscarinic antagonists; LMD, leukotriene modifier drugs; mAB, monoclonal antibodies; MAO, monoamine oxidase; MDI, metered-dose inhaler; MI, myocardial infarction; OCS, oral corticosteroids; PDE-4, phosphodiesterase 4; PKU, phenylketonuria; PUD, peptic ulcer disease; QT, start of the Q wave to the end of the T wave on an eletrocardiogram; SABA, short-acting beta$_2$-agonists; SAMA, short-acting muscarinic antagonists; SMI, soft mist inhaler; SQ, subcutaneous; TB, tuberculosis; TCA, tricyclic antidepressant; ULN, upper limit of normal.

TABLE 24.4

Global Initiative for Asthma Symptom Control for Ages 6 and Above

Asthma Symptom Control			Level of Asthma Symptom Control		
In the last month, have you had:			**Well Controlled**	**Partly Controlled**	**Not Controlled**
Daytime asthma symptom more than twice per week?	Yes	No	None	1–2	3–4
Any night waking due to asthma?	Yes	No			
Reliever needed for asthma symptoms more than twice per week.	Yes	No			
Any activity limitation due to asthma symptoms?	Yes	No			

Asthma drug therapy is initiated according to the age-specific GINA guideline (**Tables 24.4–24.8**) (GINA, 2020). Short-acting beta$_2$-agonists (SABA) or LABA monotherapy is not recommended. All persons with an asthma diagnosis should receive an ICS-containing controller drug, either as needed for mild asthma or daily for more severe asthma to reduce the risk of asthma-related exacerbation, hospitalization, and death. Stepping-up controller drugs are recommended for uncontrolled asthma despite appropriate inhaler technique and good drug adherence. Stepping-down controller drugs are recommended for persons with good asthma control for about 3 months. Risk factors for exacerbation should inform management strategies, to include prescription of daily ICS controller drug, written asthma action plan, more frequent follow-up sessions, addressing modifiable risk factors, and implementing non-pharmacological strategies to help with symptom control and risk reduction. Persons with severe or uncontrolled asthma should be assessed for any contributing factors and should be referred to a specialist for further evaluation.

Before initiating asthma therapy, it is important to document a baseline assessment. The healthcare provider should record all evidence supporting the diagnosis of asthma. Level of symptom control, risk factors for exacerbation, and lung function should be documented. Symptom severity should be measured by a comprehensive disease-specific health status questionnaire, such as the Asthma Control Test (ACT). Factors that influence the healthcare provider's therapy options should be delineated. Choice of initial drug therapy should be individualized based on symptom control, risk factors for exacerbation, patient preference, and practical issues such as insurance formulary restrictions. Initial inhaler training to ensure appropriate technique should be completed and documented. Scheduling an agreed-upon follow-up appointment date is imperative.

COPD drug therapy is initiated according to the GOLD guideline (GOLD, 2020). Smoking cessation is an essential non-pharmacologic therapy to modify disease trajectory. Pharmacologic therapy is tailored to and guided by symptom severity, exacerbation risk, potential side effects, comorbidities, drug formulary and cost, theratype, patient preference, and patient success with drug device use. Severity of airflow limitation is categorized into four classes (**Table 24.9**). Symptom severity should be measured by a comprehensive disease-specific health status questionnaire, such as the Chronic Respiratory Questionnaire, St. George's Respiratory Questionnaire, COPD Assessment Test (CAT), or The COPD Control Questionnaire. Combining spirometry results and severity of airflow limitation with assessment of symptoms or risk of exacerbation helps the healthcare provider to determine the level of pharmacologic therapy to initiate and titrate (**Table 24.10**). See **Box 24.1** for the suggested pharmacologic therapy options.

Supplemental oxygen must be used selectively. When chronic resting hypoxemia occurs, long-term oxygen therapy improves survival rate. Severe chronic hypercapnia with acute respiratory failure hospitalization, decreased mortality, and rehospitalization can be achieved with long-term non-invasive ventilation. Advanced emphysema that is refractory to optimal pharmacologic therapy necessitates surgical or bronchoscopic interventions may be of benefit. End-stage COPD requires palliative care considerations.

Goals of Drug Therapy

Goals of drug therapy for asthma and COPD are similar, yet slightly different. The GINA guidelines for asthma management focus on good symptom control and the minimization of future asthma-related morbidity and mortality, in collaboration with the patient's preferences. A patient–healthcare provider partnership must be established to inform and empower the patient to self-manage their asthma daily. Good communication between the healthcare provider and the patient is essential and will foster patient health literacy. The GOLD guideline goals of COPD management are to reduce symptoms, to reduce exacerbation frequency and severity, and to improve exercise tolerance and overall health status.

Beta$_2$-Adrenergic Agonists (Short and Long Acting)

Mechanism of Action

Beta$_2$-adrenergic agonists stimulate beta$_2$-adrenergic receptors, increasing the production of cyclic 3′5′ adenosine

TABLE 24.5

Global Initiative for Asthma Risk Factor for Poor Asthma Outcomes

Asthma Risk Factors for Poor Asthma Outcomes

Assess risk factors at diagnosis and then periodically thereafter, especially for patients experiencing an asthma exacerbation. Measure FEV_1 with initiation of therapy, after 3–6 months of therapy, and then periodically.

Risk Factors for Exacerbation	Risk Factors for Developing Persistent Airflow Limitation	Risk Factors for Drug Side-effects
Control: • Uncontrolled	History: • Pre-term birth • Low birth weight and greater infant weight gain • Chronic mucus production	Local: • High-dose or potent ICS • Poor inhaler technique
Drugs: • High SABA use • Inadequate ICS or not prescribed • Poor adherence • Incorrect inhaler technique	Drugs: • Lack of ICS therapy	Systemic: • Frequent OCS • Long-term, high-dose, and/or potent ICS • Taking P450 inhibitors
Comorbidities: • Obesity • Chronic rhinosinusitis • GERD • Diagnosed food allergy • Pregnancy	Exposures: • Tobacco smoke • Noxious chemicals • Occupational exposures	
Exposures: • Smoking • Allergen, if sensitized • Air pollution	Testing: • Low initial FEV_1 • Sputum or blood eosinophilia	
Context: • Major psychological problems • Major socioeconomic problems		
Lung function: • Low FEV_1, especially if <60% predicted • High bronchodilator reversibility		
Other testing for Th2 high: • Blood eosinophils • Elevated FeNo, especially for adults taking ICS		
Other: • History of intubation • History of intensive care unit • At least 1 severe exacerbation in last 12 months		

FeNo, fractional exhaled nitric oxide; FEV_1, forced expiratory volume in 1 second; GERD, gastroesophageal reflux disease; ICS, inhaled corticosteroids; OCS, oral corticosteroids; SABA, short-acting beta$_2$-agonists.

TABLE 24.6

Global Initiative for Asthma Severity

Asthma Severity

Mild	Control requires Step 1 or Step 2 therapy
Moderate	Controls requires Step 3 therapy
Severe	Control requires Step 4 or Step 5 therapy

monophosphate (cAMP). Increased cAMP relaxes airway smooth muscle and increases bronchial ciliary activity. Adverse effects of beta$_2$-adrenergic receptor stimulation include increased skeletal muscle activity, central nervous system stimulation, hyperglycemia, and hypokalemia. All beta$_2$-adrenergic agonists have slight cardiovascular stimulatory effects including increased heart rate, increased force of cardiac contractility, and increased cardiac conductivity.

TABLE 24.7

Global Initiative for Asthma Personalized Asthma Management for Ages 12+ Years and Above

	Step 1	Step 2	Step 3	Step 4	Step 5
Controller					
Preferred	As needed low-dose ICS-formoterol*	Daily low-dose ICS, or as needed low-dose ICS-formoterol*	Low-dose ICS-LABA	Medium-dose ICS-LABA	High-dose ICS-LABA Refer for phenotypic assessment ± add on therapy, e.g., tiotropium, anti-IgE, anti-IL-5/5R, anti-IL-4R
Other options	Low-dose ICS taken whenever SABA taken*	LMD or low-dose ICS taken whenever SABA taken*	Medium-dose ICS, or low-dose ICS + LMD‡	High-dose ICS, add on tiotropium, or add on LMD‡	Add low-dose OCS, but consider side effects
Reliever					
Preferred	As needed low-dose ICS-formoterol*		As needed low-dose ICS-formoterol†		
Other options	As needed SABA				

* Off-label.

† Low-dose ICS-formoterol is reliever for patients prescribed budesonide-formoterol maintenance and reliever therapy.

‡ Consider adding house dust mite immunotherapy for sensitized patients with allergic rhinitis and FEV$_1$ >70% predicted.

ICS, inhaled corticosteroids; LABA, long-acting beta$_2$-agonists; LMD, leukotriene modifier drugs; OCS, oral corticosteroids; SABA, short-acting beta$_2$-agonists.

TABLE 24.8

Personalized Asthma Management for Children 6–11 years

	Step 1	Step 2	Step 3	Step 4	Step 5
Controller					
Preferred		Daily low-dose ICS	Low-dose ICS-LABA or medium-dose ICS	Medium-dose ICS-LABA Refer to specialist	Refer for phenotypic assessment ± add on therapy, e.g., anti-IgE
Other options	Low-dose ICS taken whenever SABA taken,* or daily low-dose ICS	LMD or low-dose ICS taken whenever SABA taken*	Low-dose ICS + LMD	High-dose ICS-LABA, or add on tiotropium, or add on LMD	Add on anti-IL-5, or add on low-dose OCS, but consider side effects
Reliever					
Preferred	As needed SABA				

* Off-label.

ICS, inhaled corticosteroids; IgE, immunoglobulin E; IL, interleukin; LABA, long-acting beta$_2$-agonists; LMD, leukotriene modifier drugs; OCS, oral corticosteroids; SABA, short-acting beta$_2$-agonists.

Dosage and Time Frame for Response

The short-acting beta$_2$-adrenergic agonists (e.g., albuterol, levalbuterol) have a quick onset (peak effect 10 minutes) and a short duration of action (3–4 hours). SABA half-life can range from 2.7 hours to 6 hours. The long-acting beta$_2$ adrenergic agonists include formoterol, salmeterol, and vilanterol. LABA half-life can range from 5.5 hours to 11 hours. Formoterol has an onset of action of 3 minutes and a 12-hour duration of action. Salmeterol has an onset of action of about 2 hours and a 12-hour duration of action. Vilanterol has an onset of action of about 15 minutes and a 24-hour duration of action. Arformoterol, the R-enantiomer of formoterol, indacaterol, and olodaterol are approved by the Food and Drug Administration (FDA) for the management of COPD only. Oral (e.g., albuterol syrup and tablets; terbutaline tablets) and parenteral (e.g., terbutaline) dosage forms are available but have limited clinical use due to the quick onset of action, ease of administration, beta$_2$-adrenergic specificity, and minimal systemic exposure

TABLE 24.9

Airflow Limitation Severity Categories for Forced Expiratory Volume in 1 Second/Forced Vital Capacity % Predicted

Category	Severity	FEV$_1$ Predicted (%)
GOLD 1	Mild	≥80
GOLD 2	Moderate	50–<80
GOLD 3	Severe	30–<50
GOLD 4	Very severe	<30

FEV$_1$, forced expiratory volume in 1 second; FVC, forced vital capacity; GOLD, global initiative for chronic obstructive lung disease.

TABLE 24.10

Combined Chronic Obstructive Pulmonary Disease Assessment to Initiate Therapy

Exacerbation History		
≥2 or ≥1 that lead to a hospital admission	C (Few symptoms but high exacerbation risk)	D (More symptoms and high exacerbation risk)
None or 1 that did not lead to a hospital admission	A (Few symptoms with low exacerbation risk)	B (More symptoms but low exacerbation risk)
	CAT < 10	CAT ≥ 10
	Symptom Assessment or Exacerbation Risk	

CAT, COPD assessment test.

with the inhaled route of administration. SABAs are indicated for the relief of acute respiratory symptoms in asthma and COPD. LABAs are indicated for chronic maintenance therapy in COPD but only with an ICS for asthma.

Contraindications

Beta$_2$-adrenergic agonists are contraindicated in persons with a history of hypersensitivity to beta-adrenergic agonists or any component of the formulation. Beta$_2$-adrenergic agonists should be used with caution in patients with known cardiovascular disease, diabetes mellitus, glaucoma, hyperthyroidism, or seizure disorders.

Adverse Events

Serious adverse events associated with SABAs include paradoxical bronchospasm, anaphylaxis, hypersensitivity reaction, angioedema, hypertension, hypotension, angina, cardiac arrest, arrhythmia, hypokalemia, and hyperglycemia. The more common adverse

BOX 24.1 Pharmacologic Options for Chronic Obstructive Pulmonary Disease

- GOLD A:
  - ○ Option 1: As needed SABA or SAMA
  - ○ Option 2: Daily LABA or LAMA
    - One of the above options plus patient education and vaccination, and smoking cessation.
- GOLD B:
  - ○ Option 1: Daily LABA or LAMA
  - ○ Option 2: Daily LABA/LAMA
    - One of the above options plus an as needed SABA or SAMA, patient education and vaccination, smoking cessation, pulmonary rehabilitation, and oxygen.
- GOLD C:
  - ○ Option 1: Daily long acting bronchodilator, LABA or LAMA
  - ○ Option 2: Daily LABA/LAMA
  - ○ Option 3: Daily ICS/LABA
    - One of the above options plus as needed an as needed SABA or SAMA, patient education and vaccination, smoking cessation, pulmonary rehabilitation, theophylline, and oxygen.
- GOLD D:
  - ○ Option 1: Daily LABA/LAMA
  - ○ Option 2: Daily ICS/LABA
    - One of the above options plus as needed SABA or SAMA, patient education and vaccination, smoking cessation, pulmonary rehabilitation, theophylline, oxygen, surgical interventions, and palliative care.
  - ○ Option 3: Daily ICS/LABA/LAMA
    - The above option plus an as needed SABA or SAMA, patient education and vaccination, smoking cessation, pulmonary rehabilitation, theophylline, PDE-4 inhibitor, macrolide antibiotic, oxygen, surgical interventions, and palliative care.

ICS, inhaled corticosteroids; LABA, long-acting beta$_2$-agonists; LAMA, long-acting muscarinic antagonists; PDE-4, phosphodiesterase 4; SABA, short-acting beta$_2$-agonists; SAMA, short-acting muscarinic antagonists.

events include throat irritation, upper respiratory infection symptoms, cough, bad taste, tremor, dizziness, nervousness, nausea/vomiting, headache, palpitations, tachycardia, chest pain, pain, and hyperlactatemia.

Serious adverse events associated with LABAs include paradoxical bronchospasm, asthma exacerbation, asthma related death, laryngospasm, hypersensitivity reaction, anaphylaxis, hypertension, hypotension, angina, cardiac arrest, arrhythmia, hypokalemia, and hyperglycemia. The more common adverse events include headache, throat irritation, nasal congestion, rhinitis, tracheitis/bronchitis, pharyngitis, urticaria, rash, palpitations, tachycardia, tremor, and nervousness.

Adverse effects are more common with high doses of inhaled drug and systemic administration (oral, parenteral). LABA monotherapy is associated with an increased risk of asthma-related death. Previously a black box warning was in place, but surveillance research has established that ICS/LABA combination drugs in asthma patients do not increase asthma-related deaths.

Interactions

Other sympathomimetic drugs (e.g., catecholamines, catecholamine analogs, amphetamines) increase the risk for beta$_2$-adrenergic agonist adverse effects and toxicities. Nonselective and higher doses of beta$_1$-selective adrenergic blocking drugs diminish the bronchodilator effects of the beta$_2$-adrenergic agonists; the risk-to-benefit ratio must be considered before prescribing beta-adrenergic blocking drugs. Concurrent administration of beta-adrenergic agonists and monoamine oxidase inhibitors (MAOIs) or tricyclic antidepressants (TCAs) increases blood pressure and the risk of stroke. MAOIs and TCAs must be discontinued at least 14 days prior to initiating beta$_2$-adrenergic agonists. Thiazide (e.g., hydrochlorothiazide) and loop diuretics (e.g., furosemide) enhance the hypokalemic effect of beta$_2$-adrenergic agonists. The oxazolidinones (e.g., linezolid, tedizolid) enhance the hypertensive effect of beta$_2$-adrenergic agonists. Atomoxetine, a selective norepinephrine reuptake inhibitor indicated for the management of attention-deficit hyperactivity disorder, may increase the tachycardic effect of beta$_2$-adrenergic agonists.

Muscarinic Antagonists (Short and Long Acting)

Mechanism of Action

Muscarinic antagonists, previously referred to as anticholinergic drugs, competitively block acetylcholine at muscarinic receptors, decreasing guanosine cyclic 3',5' monophosphate (cGMP). The decreased cGMP results in a relatively higher proportion of cAMP. Increased cAMP relaxes airway smooth muscle and increases bronchial ciliary activity. Muscarinic antagonists also decrease mucus secretion, dilate the pupil, and prevent acetylcholine-induced release of allergenic mediators from mast cells. Although atropine, the classic muscarinic antagonist, crosses the blood–brain barrier and stimulates the central nervous system, the drugs used to manage asthma and COPD are quaternary amines. Quaternary amines are poorly absorbed after oral administration and unable to cross the blood–brain barrier.

Dosage and Time Frame for Response

The short-acting muscarinic antagonists (SAMA) ipratropium bromide has an onset of action within 15 minutes, a peak effect within 1 to 2 hours, and a duration of action of 2 to 5 hours. SAMA half-life is about 2 hours. The long-acting muscarinic antagonists (LAMAs) aclidinium bromide, glycopyrrolate, revefenacin, tiotropium bromide, and umeclidinium

bromide have a duration of action of 24 hours or more. The LAMA half-life can range from 5 hours to 70 hours.

Contraindications

Muscarinic antagonists are contraindicated in persons with a history of hypersensitivity to muscarinic antagonists or any component of the formulation. Muscarinic antagonists should be used with caution in patients with narrow-angle glaucoma, myasthenia gravis, prostatic hyperplasia, or bladder neck obstruction.

Adverse Events

Serious adverse events associated with SAMAs include hypersensitivity reaction, anaphylaxis, paradoxical bronchospasm, and angle-closure glaucoma. The more common adverse events include bronchitis, dyspnea, nausea, xerostomia, influenza-like symptoms, sinusitis, dizziness, dyspepsia, urinary tract infection, back pain, and urinary hesitancy/retention.

Serious adverse events associated with LAMAs include hypersensitivity reaction, anaphylaxis, paradoxical bronchospasm, and angle-closure glaucoma. The more common adverse events include upper respiratory infection symptoms, xerostomia, chest pain, urinary tract infection, dyspepsia, abdominal pain, headache, edema, depression, insomnia, constipation, arthralgia/myalgia, vomiting, epistaxis, rash, infection, candidiasis, and urinary hesitancy/retention.

Interactions

Concurrent administration of drugs with muscarinic antagonist properties (e.g., first-generation antihistamines) increases the risk of muscarinic antagonist adverse effects.

Leukotriene Modifier Drugs

Mechanism of Action

There are two types of leukotriene modifiers: the 5-lipoxygenase (5-LO) inhibitors and the leukotriene receptor antagonists. Zileuton inhibits 5-LO, preventing the first and second steps in the conversion of arachidonic acid to the bronchoconstrictor and proinflammatory cysteinyl leukotrienes (LTC4, LTD4, and LTE4). Montelukast and zafirlukast bind to cysteinyl leukotriene receptors on eosinophils and other proinflammatory cells, preventing LTC4, LTD4, and LTE4 from binding to the receptors and the subsequent bronchoconstrictor and proinflammatory responses.

Dosage and Time Frame for Response

Leukotriene modifiers, less effective than inhaled glucocorticoids or beta$_2$-adrenergic agonists, are indicated for all asthma patients as a low-intensity maintenance controller therapy. The leukotriene modifier half-life can range from 2.7 hours to 16 hours. The montelukast dose for adolescents older than or aged 15 years and adults is 10 mg daily in the evening; dosages for children of ages 1 year to 15 years depend on the child's age (i.e., 1–5 years: 4 mg; and 6–14 years: 5 mg). The zafirlukast dose for adolescents older than or aged 12 years and adults is 20 mg twice daily; the dose for children of ages 5 to 11 years is 10 mg twice daily. The zileuton dose for adolescents older than or aged 12 years and adults is 600 mg four times daily (immediate-release formulation) or 1,200 mg twice daily (extended-release formulation).

Response to therapy with leukotriene modifiers is gradual, with improved symptoms and lung function observed during the first week of therapy and continued improvement over the following weeks of continued therapy. Intra-class response variability suggests changing agents after a lack of response to one drug.

Contraindications

All leukotriene modifiers are contraindicated in persons with a history of hypersensitivity to the leukotriene modifier or any component of the formulation. The montelukast chewable tablet contains phenylalanine and is contraindicated in persons with phenylketonuria. Zafirlukast and zileuton are contraindicated in persons with hepatic impairment. Zileuton is contraindicated in persons with active liver disease and in persons with transaminase elevations more than or equal to 3 times the upper limit of normal. Baseline liver function tests should be obtained prior to starting zileuton therapy, monthly for 3 months, every 2 to 3 months for 9 months, and then periodically thereafter; zileuton should be discontinued if the serum alanine aminotransferase (ALT) is greater than five times the upper limit of normal.

Adverse Events

Serious adverse events associated with leukotriene modifiers include hypersensitivity reaction, anaphylaxis, severe skin reaction, hepatitis, hepatic failure, hepatotoxicity, hepatic eosinophilic infiltration, pulmonary eosinophilia, eosinophilic granulomatous with polyangiitis (EGPA), angioedema, vasculitis, thrombocytopenia, neuropsychiatric disorders, suicidality, aggressive behavior/behavioral disturbance, hallucinations, and depression. More common adverse events include headache, upper respiratory infection, fever, influenza-like symptoms, abdominal pain, cough, pharyngolaryngeal pain, diarrhea, otitis media, otitis, nausea, dyspepsia, rash/urticaria, sinusitis, abdominal pain, elevated liver enzymes, leukopenia, gastroenteritis (in pediatric patients), sleep disorders, anxiety/irritability, restlessness, myalgia, and tremor.

Interactions

Significant drug interactions are reported for the leukotriene modifiers. Montelukast is CYP2C8, CYP2C9, and CYP4A4 substrate; drugs such as carbamazepine, phenytoin, phenobarbital, and rifampin induce montelukast metabolism, resulting in decreased montelukast drug concentrations and effectiveness. Zafirlukast is a CYP2C9 and CYP2C8 substrate; a weak inhibitor of CYP1A2, CYP2C19, CYP2D6, and CYP3A4; and a moderate inhibitor of CYP2C8/9; drugs such as erythromycin and theophylline decrease zafirlukast drug concentrations and effectiveness. Zileuton is a minor CYP1A2, CYP2C9,

and CYP3A3/4 substrate and a weak inhibitor of CYP1A2. Zileuton decreases theophylline metabolism, doubling the theophylline drug concentration. Zileuton decreases warfarin metabolism, increasing warfarin activity.

Corticosteroids

Mechanism of Action

Corticosteroids reduce airway inflammation by inhibiting or inducing the production of end-effector proteins. An activated intracellular drug–receptor complex binds to glucocorticoid responsive elements in the gene promoter regions of deoxyribonucleic acid, stimulating or inhibiting protein transcription. End-effector proteins alter vascular tone, vascular permeability, and body water distribution; stimulate lipolysis, gluconeogenesis, and glycogen secretion; increase responsiveness of beta-adrenergic receptors; mobilize amino acids from muscles; impair leukocyte migration; and inhibit nuclear factor-kappa, which regulates production of proinflammatory proteins such as cytokines, interleukins, interferons, and chemokines.

Dosage and Time Frame for Response

The dosage and frequency of the ICS depends on many factors for asthma patients. Low-dose ICS provides the most clinical benefit for most patients with asthma. Medium-dose ICS is indicated when asthma remains uncontrolled despite drug adherence and appropriate inhaler technique with or without a LABA. High-dose ICS with or without a LABA should be required in very few patients. Long-term high-dose ICS is associated with increased risk of systemic side effects with little potential benefit. Low-dose OCS (≤7.5 mg/d prednisone equivalent) may be necessary with severe asthma but with substantial side effects. Poor symptom control and/or frequent exacerbations despite adherence to stepping up therapy with appropriate inhaler technique raise clinical concern for chang-ing medication management.

Factors that support initiating ICS therapy in COPD are history of hospitalization for COPD exacerbation, more than or equal to 2 moderate COPD exacerbations per year, blood eosinophils more than 300 cells/mcL, and a history of concomitant asthma. Oral steroids are not recommended in chronic daily COPD therapy due to the lack of benefit with a high rate of systemic complications. A short course of OCS (e.g., prednisone 40 mg daily for 5 days) is indicated for treating acute exacerbations.

The onset of action of ICS and OCS (hours to days) is delayed due to the time it takes for the drug to influence protein expression. The ICS half-life ranges from 2.3 hours to 24 hours. ICS differs in terms of oral bioavailability, pulmonary deposition, on-site activation, receptor binding affinity, lipophilicity, protein binding, and pharmacokinetics. The response to ICS typically begins during the first week of therapy and continues to increase for weeks to months with continued therapy. It takes several hours for lung function to improve in response to systemic (oral or intravenous) corticosteroids. The OCS plasma (measurable) half-life is 2 to 4 hours, but the biologic (effect) is 18 to 36 hours.

Contraindications

Corticosteroids are contraindicated in persons with a history of hypersensitivity to corticosteroids or any component of the formulation.

Adverse Events

Serious adverse events with ICS include hypersensitivity reaction, bronchospasm, eosinophilia, EGPA, and central serous chorioretinopathy. With long-term use, ICS can cause adrenal suppression, angioedema, hypercorticism, immunosuppression, glaucoma, cataracts, osteoporosis, and growth suppression (in pediatric patients). More common adverse events include headache, nasopharyngitis, conjunctivitis, upper respiratory infection, influenza, fever, fatigue, rhinitis, nasal congestion, facial edema, sinusitis, bronchitis, pneumonia, pain, abdominal pain, back pain, arthralgia/myalgia, nausea, vomiting, dysphonia, dysmenorrhea, dyspepsia, epistaxis, hematoma, rash/urticaria, pruritus, dry throat, cough, and oral or esophageal candidiasis.

Serious adverse events with OCS include anaphylaxis, adrenal insufficiency, steroid psychosis, steroid myopathy, Cushing syndrome, infection, diabetes mellitus, pseudotumor cerebri, increased intracranial pressure, seizures, hypokalemic alkalosis, hypertension, congestive heart failure, pancreatitis, gastrointestinal perforation, peptic ulcer disease, exophthalmos, osteonecrosis, and tendon rupture. With long-term use, OCS can cause osteoporosis, glaucoma, cataracts, immunosuppression, Kaposi sarcoma, withdrawal symptoms if abruptly discontinued, and growth suppression (in pediatric patients). More common adverse events include Cushingoid appearance, hirsutism, weight gain, erythema, abdominal discomfort, appetite changes, emotional lability, rash/urticaria, nausea/vomiting, sodium and fluid retention, hypokalemia, elevated blood pressure, edema, diaphoresis, muscle atrophy, petechiae/ecchymosis, skin pigmentation abnormality, acne, headache, dizziness/vertigo, insomnia, depression, anxiety, glucose intolerance, menstrual irregularities, and increased intraocular pressure. With long-term use, OCS can also cause impaired wound healing and skin atrophy.

Interactions

Corticosteroids are metabolized by the hepatic cytochrome P-450 isoenzyme CYP3A4. Corticosteroids induce CYP2C19 and CYP3A4. The healthcare provider should check for potential drug interactions before prescribing corticosteroids and counsel persons to check with the healthcare provider before starting or stopping any nonprescription, prescription, or complementary drug.

Concurrent use of ICS and strong inhibitors of CYP3A4 (e.g., ritonavir, clarithromycin, itraconazole, ketoconazole, telithromycin) increases the risk of OCS adverse effects and is not recommended.

OCSs enhance adverse effects from live vaccines and decrease the response to oral antidiabetic drugs. Antacids decrease the oral bioavailability of OCS, so counsel the patient to wait at least 2 hours between doses of an antacid and OCS.

Phosphodiesterase 4 Inhibitors

Mechanism of Action

Roflumilast inhibits phosphodiesterase 4 (PDE-4), an enzyme commonly found in respiratory inflammatory cells (e.g., neutrophils, monocytes, macrophages, cluster of differentiation 4 (CD4+), cluster of differentiation 8 (CD8+) T lymphocytes) and structural cells (e.g., endothelial cells, epithelial cells, smooth muscle cells, fibroblasts). PDE-4 inhibition increases intracellular cAMP, modifying the inflammatory response in these respiratory cells and structures.

Dosage and Time Frame for Response

Roflumilast reduces moderate to severe exacerbations treated with OCS in patients with chronic bronchitis, severe to very severe COPD with a history of exacerbations. Roflumilast in combination with LABAs in patients not controlled on ICS/LABA combination demonstrates better effects on lung function. The half-life of roflumilast is 30 hours for the active metabolite. There is a titrated dosing regimen with roflumilast, starting at 250 mcg daily for 4 weeks and then increasing to 500 mcg daily thereafter. Titration decreases side effects, and efficacy increases with increased dosing.

Contraindications

Roflumilast is contraindicated in persons with a history of hypersensitivity to roflumilast or any component of the formulation. Roflumilast undergoes hepatic metabolism. Given the risk for serious and potentially life-threatening adverse events, roflumilast is contraindicated in persons with Child-Pugh B or C moderate to severe liver impairment.

Adverse Events

Serious adverse events associated with a PDE-4 inhibitor include suicidality, hypersensitivity reaction, severe diarrhea, atrial fibrillation, pancreatitis, and renal failure. More common adverse events include diarrhea, weight loss, nausea, headache, back pain, influenza, insomnia, dizziness, and decreased appetite.

Interactions

Roflumilast is metabolized by the hepatic cytochrome P-450 isoenzymes CYP3A4 and CYP1A2. CYP3A4 inhibitors and dual CYP3A4 and CYP1A2 inhibitors impair roflumilast hepatic metabolism, increasing the serum concentration of roflumilast and increasing the risk for clinically significant adverse events, and should only be used with caution. The concurrent administration of strong CYP3A4 inducers such as rifampicin, phenobarbital, carbamazepine, and phenytoin is not recommended.

Methylxanthines

Mechanism of Action

Methylxanthine bronchodilators (theophylline, aminophylline) relax bronchial smooth muscle, enhance diaphragmatic contractility, and have a slight antiinflammatory effect; the exact mechanisms of action are not known. Methylxanthines, nonselective PDE inhibitors, increase cAMP by inhibiting PDE 1, 2, 3, 4, and 7. Increased cAMP relaxes airway smooth muscle and increases bronchial ciliary activity. The enhanced diaphragmatic contractility is probably mediated by weak adenosine antagonism. The slight antiinflammatory effect is mediated by other molecular mechanisms.

Dosage and Time Frame for Response

Theophylline and aminophylline, the ethylenediamine salt of theophylline, are dosed to a target serum drug concentration. Aminophylline is about 80% theophylline. Although the therapeutic serum drug concentration range is generally accepted to be 10 to 20 mg/L, persons with COPD may do well with lower serum drug concentrations or experience unacceptable adverse effects with serum drug concentrations within the therapeutic range. The half-life of theophylline is short (approximately 8 hours in nonsmokers); sustained-release dosage formulations (every 12 hours and every 24 hours) are recommended to improve patient adherence. Theophylline is metabolized in the liver; many medical conditions and drugs induce or inhibit theophylline metabolism. It is therefore important to monitor the serum drug concentrations and individualize the dosage based upon patient response, concurrent medical conditions, and drug interactions.

Contraindications

Theophylline and aminophylline are contraindicated in persons with a history of hypersensitivity to theophylline or any component of the formulation. Patients with a history of allergy to aminophylline are most likely allergic to the ethylenediamine component of the drug, not theophylline. Methylxanthines should be used with caution in patients with a history of tachyarrhythmia, peptic ulcer disease, seizure disorders, or hyperthyroidism. Intravenous dosage forms may contain propylene glycol, which can accumulate in persons with renal dysfunction. Large amounts of propylene glycol may cause lactic acidosis, hyperosmolality, seizures, and respiratory depression. Oral dosage forms may contain dyes, alcohol, or sugar.

Adverse Events

Serious adverse events associated with methylxanthines include seizures, arrhythmias, hypotension, shock, and exfoliative dermatitis. Common adverse events include nausea, vomiting, headache, insomnia, diarrhea, irritability, restlessness, tremor, and transient diuresis.

Interactions

Theophylline is primarily metabolized by the hepatic cytochrome P-450 isoenzymes CYP1A2, CYP2E1, and CYP3A3 substrate; theophylline is a minor substrate of CYP2C9 and CYP2D6. Hepatic metabolism can be induced or inhibited by hundreds of drugs and by medical conditions that affect hepatic function. One strict contraindication is coadministration with riociguat, which may lead to increased risk of

severe hypotension. The healthcare provider should check for potential drug interactions before prescribing theophylline and counsel persons with COPD to check with the healthcare provider before starting or stopping any nonprescription, prescription, or complementary drug.

Examples of commonly used drugs that inhibit theophylline metabolism (increase theophylline serum concentration) include ciprofloxacin, cimetidine, erythromycin, and allopurinol. Examples of commonly used drugs that induce theophylline metabolism (decrease theophylline serum concentration) include phenobarbital, diphenylhydantoin, and rifampin. The healthcare provider should check for potential drug interactions before prescribing theophylline and counsel persons with COPD to check with the healthcare provider before starting or stopping any nonprescription, prescription, or complementary drug.

Smoking induces theophylline metabolism, lowering the serum drug concentration. Caffeine and sympathomimetic drugs have similar adverse effects as the methylxanthines; concurrent use increases the risk of adverse effects. Theophylline may antagonize the sedating and anxiolytic effect of benzodiazepines.

Mucolytics

Mechanism of Action

Mucolytics (acetylcysteine) break down the disulfide bonds and thereby decrease mucus viscosity, making it ideal for COPD sputum management.

Dosage and Time Frame for Response

Acetylcysteine has a half-life of 5.6 to 18.1 hours in adults and 11 hours in neonates. Acetylcysteine is metabolized in the liver and is 13% to 38% renally excreted. Coadministration of a bronchodilator is advised. There are no adjustments for renal or hepatic impairment.

Contraindications

Acetylcysteine is contraindicated in persons with a history of hypersensitivity to acetylcysteine or any component of the formulation. Acetylcysteine should be used with caution in patients with a history of asthma, history of bronchospasm, and upper gastrointestinal bleeding risk for the oral route.

Adverse Events

Serious adverse events associated with acetylcysteine include hypersensitivity reaction and bronchospasm. Common adverse events include nausea/vomiting, urticaria, tachycardia, rash, pruritus, flushing, upper respiratory infection symptoms, stomatitis, fever, and drowsiness.

Interactions

Acetylcysteine is extensively metabolized by the liver but minimally through hepatic cytochrome P-450 isoenzymes. There are minimal interactions with other drugs. Caution is advised if prescribing acetylcysteine with auranofin since the combination may decrease level and efficacy of both drugs. Caution is advised if prescribing acetylcysteine with activated charcoal since the combination may decrease acetylcysteine efficacy. The latter caution is more relevant when acetylcysteine is prescribed for acetaminophen overdose.

Monoclonal Antibodies

Mechanism of Action

Anti-Interleukin-5/5R Agents

There are 3 anti-IL-5/5R monoclonal antibodies. Benralizumab, a recombinant humanized monoclonal anti-IL-5 receptor alpha subunit antibody, binds to the IL-5 alpha subunit receptor, thereby leading to eosinophil apoptosis. Mepolizumab and reslizumab, a recombinant humanized monoclonal anti-IL-5 antibody, bind to and interfere with IL-5 cytokine, thereby reducing eosinophil production and survival.

Anti-Interleukin-4R Agent

Dupilumab, a recombinant humanized monoclonal anti-IL-4 receptor alpha subunit antibody, binds to and inhibits with IL-4 and IL-13 cytokines, thereby reducing inflammation and altering immune response.

Anti-Immunoglobulin E Agent

Omalizumab, a recombinant humanized monoclonal anti-IgE antibody, inhibits IgE binding to mast cells and basophils, thereby decreasing mediator release. By binding to IgE, omalizumab decreases free IgE and downregulates IgE receptors.

Dosage and Time Frame for Response

Anti-Interleukin-5/5R Agents

All anti-IL-5/5R agents are indicated for the maintenance therapy in persons with severe asthma with eosinophilic phenotype. Eligibility criteria vary by product and payer, but usually require more than a specified number of severe exacerbations in the last year and blood eosinophils above a specified level (e.g., ≥300/mcL). Patients taking OCS may have a different eosinophil cut point. Benralizumab (≥12 years) dosing is 30 mcg subcutaneous injection every 4 weeks for 3 doses, then every 8 weeks thereafter with a half-life of 15.5 days. Mepolizumab dosing is age dependent. Dosing for patients of ages 6 to 11 years is 40 mg subcutaneous injection every 4 weeks with a half-life of 16 to 22 days. The dosing for patients older than or aged 12 years is 100 mg subcutaneous injection every 4 weeks. In patients with a herpes zoster risk, consider varicella vaccination before starting mepolizumab. Dosing for reslizumab (≥18 years) is 3 mg/kg intravenously every 4 weeks with a half-life of 24 days.

Efficacy is strongly predicted by eosinophil count and exacerbation rate with higher eosinophil counts and number of severe exacerbations demonstrating better outcomes. All anti-IL-5/5R agents demonstrated an approximately 55% reduction in severe asthma exacerbations and improved quality of life, lung function, and symptom control. In patients taking OCS, benralizumab and mepolizumab demonstrated a median OCS dose reduction of approximately 50%. Patients

with adult-onset asthma, comorbid nasal polyps, and maintenance OCS at baseline are more likely to respond. Initial trials of anti-IL-5/5R agents should be at least 4 months.

Anti-Interleukin-4R Agent

Dupilumab (≥12 years) is indicated for moderate to severe asthma with eosinophilic phenotype. Eligibility criteria vary between payers, but usually require more than a specified number of severe exacerbations in the last year and type 2 biomarkers above a specified level (e.g., blood eosinophils ≥300/mcL or fractional exhaled nitric oxide (FeNo) ≥25 ppb), or requirement for maintenance OCS. FeNo is an indirect biomarker of eosinophilic inflammation. Dosing depends on OCS use and other atopic comorbidities. Eosinophilic phenotype alone dosing requires a loading dose of 400 mg to 600 mg subcutaneous injection, then 200 mg to 300 mg every 2 weeks thereafter. Higher dosing should be reserved for more severe asthma. OCS-dependent asthma dosing requires a loading dose of 600 mg subcutaneous injection, then 300 mg every 2 weeks thereafter. Concurrent eosinophilic phenotype with concurrent moderate to severe atopic dermatitis requires a loading dose of 600 mg subcutaneous injection, then 300 mg every 2 weeks thereafter. Initial trials of anti-IL-4R agent should be at least 4 months.

Efficacy is strongly predicted by eosinophil count, with higher eosinophil counts demonstrating better outcomes. Uncontrolled severe asthma with at least one exacerbation in the last year have an approximately 50% reduction in exacerbation rate, improved quality of life, better symptom control, and improved lung function. In patients with OCS-dependent severe asthma without regard to eosinophil count or FeNo, there is 50% reduction in median OCS dose.

Anti-Immunoglobulin E Agent

Omalizumab is indicated for therapy of persons more than or equal to 6 years with moderate to severe allergic asthma with total serum IgE levels from 30 to 700 IU/mL. Eligibility criteria include sensitization to inhaled allergen(s) on skin prick testing or specific IgE, total serum IgE and body weight within local dosing range, and more than a specified number of exacerbations within the last year. The dose and dosing interval are based on the total serum IgE and patient weight. Dosing is usually between 150 mg and 375 mg subcutaneous injection every 2 to 4 weeks with 150 mg maximum per site. The half-life is 26 days.

Efficacy does not depend on the baseline level of IgE. However, if blood eosinophils were more than or equal to 260/mcL or FeNo more than or equal to 20 ppb there is a greater decrease in exacerbations. Patients with childhood-onset asthma or those with allergen-driven symptoms are more likely to respond. Initial trials of anti-IgE agent should be at least 4 months.

Contraindications

Anti-Interleukin-5/5R Agents

All anti-IL-5/5R agent contraindications are hypersensitivity to the specific IL-5/5R agent, class or component, status asthmaticus, acute asthma, and acute bronchospasm.

Anti-Interleukin-4R Agent

Dupilumab contraindications are hypersensitivity to the specific IL-4R agent or component, status asthmaticus, acute asthma, and acute bronchospasm.

Anti-Immunoglobulin E Agent

Omalizumab contraindication is a history of hypersensitivity to the specific anti-IgE agent or component.

Adverse Events

Anti-Interleukin-5/5R Agents

Anti-IL-5/5R agents have slightly different adverse event profiles. Serious adverse events associated with benralizumab include hypersensitivity reaction, anaphylaxis, and helminth infection. The more common adverse events include headache, pharyngitis, fever, hypersensitivity reaction, and injection site reaction. Serious adverse events associated with mepolizumab include hypersensitivity reaction, anaphylaxis, angioedema, herpes zoster, and helminth infection. The more common adverse events include headache, injection site reaction, back pain, fatigue, influenza, urinary tract infection, abdominal pain, pruritus, eczema, and muscle spasm. Serious adverse events associated with reslizumab include anaphylaxis, hypersensitivity reaction, malignancy, and helminth infection. The more common adverse events include elevated creatinine phosphokinase (CPK), oropharyngeal pain, and musculoskeletal pain. Although mepolizumab and benralizumab have been associated with hypersensitivity reaction and anaphylaxis, these agents are FDA approved for home administration without the need for an epinephrine autoinjector. However, reslizumab has a black box warning for anaphylaxis. The risk of anaphylaxis coupled with the need for intravenous access for administration requires reslizumab to be administered in a healthcare setting.

Anti-Interleukin-4R Agent

The more serious adverse events associated with dupilumab include hypersensitivity reaction, anaphylaxis, serum sickness or like reaction, keratitis. Even though dupilumab may be associated with anaphylaxis, there is no black box warning and it is FDA approved for home administration without the need for an epinephrine autoinjector. The more common adverse events include injection site reaction, conjunctivitis/keratitis, herpes viral infection, arthralgia, eosinophilia, and oropharyngeal pain.

Anti-Immunoglobulin E Agent

The more serious adverse events associated with omalizumab include hypersensitivity reaction, anaphylaxis, eosinophilia, EGPA, malignancy risk, cardiovascular event risk, and cerebrovascular event risk. There is an approximately 0.2% risk of anaphylaxis necessitating a black box warning. Anaphylaxis has occurred after the first dose and even after more than 1 year on therapy. Most anaphylactic reactions have occurred in the first 2 hours after the first 3 doses. Most offices administering omalizumab have practices in place requiring patients to stay in the healthcare setting for 2 hours for the first 3 injections and thereafter 30 minutes post injection. An epinephrine autoinjector should be prescribed prior to initiation of omalizumab therapy. More common adverse events include injection site reaction, viral infection, upper respiratory infection symptoms, headache/migraine, arthralgia, nausea, pain, fatigue, dizziness, pruritus, abdominal pain, epistaxis, otitis media, dermatitis, otalgia, myalgia, fractures, peripheral edema, fever, anxiety, alopecia, geohelminth infection, and decreased platelets.

Interactions

Anti-Interleukin-5/5R Agents

All Anti-IL-5/5R agents have no significant drug interactions known or found at this time. However, caution is always advised with multiple drugs.

Anti-Interleukin-4R Agent

Dupilumab is contraindicated in all live vaccine administration. Delay in start or cessation of therapy may need to occur if a live vaccine is required. Non-live vaccinations may require a post-administration titer to confirm adequate antibody response. Combination of dupilumab with immunosuppressive agents (belimumab, cladribine oral, infliximab, or natalizumab, etc.) may increase the risk of serious infection. However, caution is always advised with multiple drugs.

Anti-Immunoglobulin E Agent

Omalizumab has no significant drug interactions known or found at this time. However, caution is always advised with multiple drugs.

Immunizations

GINA and GOLD guidelines recommend all persons with asthma or COPD receive an annual influenza vaccine. Influenza vaccination can reduce exacerbation risk due to lower respiratory tract infection. The GINA guideline does not recommend pneumococcal vaccination in persons with asthma. However, the Center for Disease Control Advisory Committee on Immunization Practices recommends 13-valent pneumococcal conjugate vaccine (PCV-13) and/or 23-valent pneumococcal polysaccharide vaccine (PPSV-23) for asthma patients of ages 2 to 18 years requiring high-dose ICS or OCS therapy (CDC, 2020e). Patients with lung disease (e.g., asthma, COPD) who are older than or aged 19 to 64 years are recommended to get 1 dose of PPSV-23. The GOLD guideline recommends pneumococcal vaccination in immunocompetent patients with PPSV-23 and PCV-13. PPSV-23 has demonstrated a reduction in the incidence of community-acquired pneumonia in patients with COPD aged less than 65 years with an FEV_1 less than 40% predicted and in those with comorbidities. PCV-13 in adults older than or aged 65 years demonstrated a reduction in bacteremia and serious invasive pneumococcal disease.

Oxygen

Supplemental oxygen is not indicated in the routine management of asthma. However, the exchange of oxygen and carbon dioxide worsens as COPD progresses. If peripheral oxygen saturation level via pulse oximetry is less than 92%, an arterial or capillary blood gas should be obtained. Supplemental oxygen may have symptom benefit even if the patient is not hypoxemic. In COPD patients with severe resting chronic hypoxemia, long-term oxygen therapy (>15 hours per day) improves survival. However, supplemental oxygen therapy should not be prescribed for stable COPD with resting or exercise-related desaturation. COPD patients with severe chronic hypercapnia and a history of acute respiratory failure hospitalization, non-invasive positive pressure ventilation may decrease mortality and rehospitalizations. Long-term oxygen therapy should be prescribed when the PaO_2 is at or below 7.3 kPa (55 mmHg) or SaO_2 is at or below 88% on room air confirmed twice in a 3-week period regardless of whether hypercapnia is present or not. Long-term oxygen can also be prescribed when PaO_2 is between 7.3 kPa (55 mmHg) and 8.0 kPa (60 mmHg), or SaO_2 of 88% with pulmonary hypertension, peripheral edema with congestive heart failure, or polycythemia (hematocrit >55%). Re-evaluation at the same oxygen level should take place after 60 to 90 days with arterial blood gas or oxygen saturation.

Antibiotics

Antibiotics are not indicated in the routine management of asthma. However, recent studies have demonstrated that regular use of azithromycin (250 mg per day or 500 mg three times per week) decreased exacerbation risk over 1 year. Azithromycin used in such a manner can increase bacterial resistance and cause corrected QT (QTc) interval prolongation and impaired hearing. Smoking negates any benefit with azithromycin.

Antibiotics for exacerbation therapy can improve recovery time and decrease relapse/therapy failure and hospitalization duration, but are still somewhat controversial. Antibiotics should be reserved for moderate to severe exacerbations when there are clinical signs of bacterial colonization, such as increased sputum purulence, accompanied by increased dyspnea and sputum volume. Antibiotics should be prescribed for 5 to 7 days with the choice of agent depending on local bacterial resistance pattern. Penicillin (e.g., amoxicillin or amoxicillin/clavulanate), macrolide (e.g., azithromycin or clarithromycin), and tetracycline (e.g., doxycycline or tetracycline) agents are good initial empiric therapy options. Fluroquinolones are reserved as secondary options.

Selecting the Most Appropriate Drug

To determine the most appropriate drug therapy, the healthcare provider must process through pertinent patient clinical findings and pertinent guideline recommendations. The first step is to determine if the patient has a chronic airway disease by assessing the clinical history, physical examination, radiological findings if available, and scores on screening questionnaires. Next, the healthcare provider must determine the diagnosis: asthma, COPD, or ACO through an iterative comparison process. There should be a comparison of features and

the number of features that favor one diagnosis over the other. The healthcare provider must consider his or her certainty in the diagnosis considering these features including spirometry results. Once a diagnosis has been made, initiation of drug therapy should be selected.

First-Line Therapy

All patients with asthma, COPD, or ACO should be prescribed a quick reliever drug therapy to treat acute symptoms. This includes SABA and/or SAMA therapy options.

Second-Line Therapy

The type of diagnosis dictates further drug therapy options. For a single asthma diagnosis, the GINA guideline recommendation is for baseline ICS with add-on therapy options as indicated. For a single COPD diagnosis, the GOLD guideline recommendation is for symptomatic therapy with bronchodilators (LABA and/or LAMA) or combination therapy, but not ICS monotherapy. For an ACO diagnosis, the GINA and GOLD guidelines recommend low to moderate dose ICS depending on symptom severity, exacerbation risk, and adverse event risk. Co-administration with LABA and/or LAMA should be initiated. Titration of drug therapy should be determined based on patient response considering exacerbation risk and adverse event risk.

Third-Line Therapy

Referral to a specialist for care should be considered when a patient has persistent symptoms and/or exacerbations despite optimal drug therapy, when there is diagnostic uncertainty and alternative diagnoses must be excluded, when atypical or additional signs or symptoms suggest additional pulmonary diagnoses, chronic airway disease that is not asthma or COPD, difficulty to treat due to comorbidities, and referral arising during the on-going management of asthma, COPD, or ACO for step drug therapy.

Special Considerations
Pediatric

Pediatric considerations when prescribing drugs relate to asthma. Although alpha-1 antitrypsin deficiency causes early onset of COPD, it generally does so in the third decade of life. Not all asthma drugs are FDA approved for pediatric asthma patients. Of those asthma drugs approved for pediatric use, parents and children may have concerns about the effect of ICS on adult height. Growth velocity may be lower in the first 1 to 2 years of ICS therapy; therefore, the minimum effective dose of ICS to achieve asthma control should be prescribed.

Route of drug administration should be considered with pediatric asthma patients. Some respiratory drug delivery devices are limited to older children; younger children may not be able to reliably generate an adequate inspiratory flow rate to disperse the drug (GINA, 2020). Older children (greater than age 8) can effectively use a pressurized metered-dose inhaler.

The combination of a pressurized metered-dose inhaler with a spacer device is appropriate for younger children, including infants. Drug delivery with a nebulizer is effective for all ages. If an ICS is delivered via a facemask or nebulizer, the skin exposed to the ICS should be cleaned shortly after administration to decrease local side effects, such as topical fungal infection or erythema with atrophy.

Assessment of pulmonary status has age limitations. Pulmonary function assessment in younger children may be unreliable. Peak flow meter use and spirometry testing require coordination that younger children may not be able to achieve.

Geriatric

Asthma and COPD may go undiagnosed in the geriatric population due to many factors, including patient poor perception of airflow limitation, symptoms attributed to normal aging process, deconditioning, and sedentary lifestyle. Polypharmacy and multiple comorbidities can complicate the initial diagnosis and continued management. Distinguishing asthma from COPD can be difficult in the geriatric patient, and ACO should be considered in any geriatric asthma patient with history of cigarette smoking or biomass fuel exposure. Patients with ACO have poorer clinical outcomes when compared to patients with asthma or COPD alone. Manual dexterity, motor skills, visual acuity, and inspiratory flow may decline with aging, making it difficult for patients to prepare and self-administer drug with respiratory drug delivery devices.

Women

Women with asthma that are concerned about drug use during and after pregnancy should be advised that poorly controlled asthma with risk of exacerbation is a greater risk to the fetus than reliever and controller asthma drugs (GINA, 2020). The GINA guideline does not recommend stepping-down controller therapy until after delivery. The effect of monoclonal antibodies on the developing fetus is not known. Pregnant asthma patients being therapy with a monoclonal antibody may decide to discontinue until delivery or participate in drug-specific pregnancy registry. The rule of thirds—one-third get better, one-third get worse, and one-third stay the same—provides insight into any therapy adjustments in pregnant women with asthma. Monthly monitoring of asthma control should be assessed via office visit or telephone encounters.

There is no gender-specific recommendation for COPD management.

Ethnic

Culturally specific beliefs regarding cause of disease, acceptance of acute, or chronic drugs, drug color, dosage formulation, and route of administration may influence a person's acceptance and adherence to the prescribed drug and nondrug therapy. Persons with asthma or COPD may seek care from healers and may use natural remedies. It is important to ask about, respect, and integrate these beliefs into the management strategy.

Genomics

At present, there are no gene-specific therapeutic recommendations for managing asthma. Alpha-1 antitrypsin deficiency is a combination of COPD genotype–phenotype and is a rare autosomal inheritance co-dominant disease. Lack of alpha-1 antitrypsin results in ineffective activity of the enzyme responsible for neutralizing neutrophil elastase, which results in inflammatory lung damage. There are an estimated 59,000 patients with COPD with an alpha-1 antitrypsin deficiency in the United States, but only about 10% have been diagnosed. Alpha-1 antitrypsin augmentation therapy has been available since the 1980s and reduces disease progression. Normal alpha-1 antitrypsin alleles are designated MM. A carrier is designated as MZ, while a deficient patient is ZZ. The Z allele is associated with liver disease as well. There is also an S allele, which results in decreased functional expression. An alpha-1 antitrypsin level with reflex can be drawn. If the alpha-1 antitrypsin plasma levels are below 20 mcM/L, the reflex phenotype testing will provide the healthcare provider with variant proteins. An alpha-1 antitrypsin level below 11 mcM/L does not provide adequate protection from inflammatory lung damage. Cigarette smoking is a modifiable risk factor to decrease the impact of alpha-1 antitrypsin deficiency on lung tissue.

MONITORING PATIENT RESPONSE

Maximum benefit with most inhaled controller drugs can take 3 to 4 months for asthma or COPD. The GINA and GOLD guidelines recommend reassessment 1 to 3 months after initiation of therapy and then every 3 to 12 months thereafter depending on the clinical stability and exacerbation risk. Persons experiencing increased symptoms should use their action plan to guide initial therapy and seek additional care. Spirometry is performed at baseline (prior to starting therapy), after 3 to 6 months of therapy, then repeated annually or more frequently if indicated.

PATIENT EDUCATION

Self-Monitoring

A written asthma action plan is an essential component of self-monitoring and self-management. Although an asthma action plan is not recommended for COPD patients, those patients with ACO may benefit from one. Self-management entails monitoring symptoms and peak flow, referencing the written asthma action plan, and following up with his or her healthcare provider for routine care. Self-monitoring and self-management allow the patient to recognize and respond to worsening pulmonary status. Some patients are poor perceivers of pulmonary status and may delay seeking care until severe symptoms are experienced.

Respiratory Drug Delivery Systems

Device-specific patient education regarding the correct use of the specific expiratory drug delivery system is essential. Multiple types of respiratory drug delivery devices are marketed, each with unique drug administration techniques. Respiratory drug delivery systems include metered-dose inhalers, valved holding chambers, non-valved spacers, dry powder inhalers (single-dose inhalers, premetered blisters, and reservoir style),

soft mist inhaler, and small volume nebulizers (jet nebulizers and ultrasonic nebulizers). Each type of device has its own advantages and disadvantages; device selection depends on product availability, patient age, patient ability, cost, and patient preference. General drug delivery device administration techniques are listed in **Table 24.11**; refer to the product package inserts for device-specific drug administration information and device care. Special care should be taken to discuss priming

TABLE 24.11	
Drug Delivery Device Techniques	
Device	**General Technique**
Pressurized metered-dose inhalers	1. Remove dust cap 2. Inspect for debris or possible clogging 3. Clean per package insert instructions if needed 4. Shake vigorously for 5 seconds 5. Hold the device upright with mouthpiece at the bottom 6. Place device in mouth but do not block with the tongue 7. Press down on the canister and breathe in at the same time 8. Complete inhalation and then hold breath for 10 seconds 9. Exhale slowly; repeat dosing based on drug prescribed 10. Replace dust cap
Spacers and valved holding chambers	1. Visually check for debris 2. Prepare metered-dose inhaler 3. Insert metered-dose inhaler in spacer 4. Gently exhale 5. Place spacer/valved holding chamber in mouth holding it level 6. Press the canister once 7. Immediately inspire slowly and deeply (no whistle noise) 8. Remove spacer/ valved holding chamber from the mouth and hold breath for 10 seconds 9. Exhale slowly
Dry powder inhalers	1. Remove cover 2. Prepare dose depending on device activation 3. Exhale softly *away* from device 4. Seal lips around mouthpiece 5. Inhale rapidly and forcefully 6. Remove device from the mouth and hold breath for 10 seconds 7. Exhale softly *away* from device 8. Replace cover
Small volume nebulizers	1. Place the equipment on a stable surface 2. Connect the tubing to the compressor 3. Hold the drug chamber upright; add the premixed drug solution or measure and add drug and saline 4. Place the lid on the drug chamber 5. Connect the tubing to the drug chamber 6. Turn on the air compressor and check for the generation of a fine mist 7. Sit up comfortably straight 8. Seal lips around the mouthpiece; do not block with the tongue 9. Holding the drug chamber upright, breathe in and out normally; take a deeper breath and hold it for a few seconds every minute or so 10. If the fine mist decreases, be sure to periodically shake the chamber to dislodge droplets clinging to the sides 11. Continue until the drug chamber is empty 12. Turn off the compressor 13. Mount the chamber to the nebulizer if being reused shortly or disconnect the drug chamber and tubing and store appropriately 14. Chamber and tubing should be replaced based on manufacturers recommendations

and re-priming of devices since production of a mist may not necessarily contain any drug and just propellant.

Drug Information

The GINA and GOLD guidelines contain pharmacologic class and product-specific drug information. Drug information is available on professional organization (e.g., the American Academy of Allergy, Asthma, and Immunology [AAAAI]), nonprofit organization (e.g., The American Lung Association), and government (e.g., National Institutes of Health) websites. Pharmaceutical company websites often include links to respiratory drug delivery device videos. The package insert for each individual drug provides detailed pharmacologic information pertinent to understand the pharmacokinetic and pharmacodynamic properties. Pharmacy therapeutics and medical pulmonary textbooks provide more in-depth drug information.

Nutrition/Lifestyle Changes

There is no specific diet for asthma or COPD. However, good nutrition is important to maintain overall health. Physical activity is important; persons with asthma and COPD should be encouraged to remain physically active.

Complementary and Alternative Drugs

There are many complementary and alternative medical therapies used for the management of asthma and COPD, including many types of herbal remedies, homeopathic drugs, acupuncture, chiropractic therapy, breathing techniques, relaxation techniques, and yoga. However, the GINA and GOLD guidelines do not recommend any complementary and alternative medical therapies. Healthcare providers should ask persons with asthma or COPD about the use of these therapies, especially herbal and other products, to identify potential disease and drug interactions.

CASE STUDY 1*

S.C. is a 21-year-old college student presenting with intermittent wheezing. She has a history of asthma as a child but had been symptom-free until this year after moving into an old apartment building. She has a remote history of allergy testing supporting sensitization to mold and dust mites. She has symptoms 1 to 2 days/week and may wake-up once per week. She did not have any medication to take for her symptoms but would have used an inhaler each time if she had access. Her symptoms are starting to interfere with her normal activities, especially since they are happening more often and are more severe each time. She has never taken systemic corticosteroids and has never been hospitalized for asthma. On physical exam, you observe soft end–expiratory wheezing at the bases bilaterally. Spirometry today demonstrates a forced expiratory volume in 1 second (FEV_1) = 90% predicted and FEV_1/forced vital capacity (FVC) = 80%. She has no other medical conditions and is

not taking any nonprescription, prescription, or complementary alternative medicines. She has no known environmental or drug allergies.

1. What diagnosis is consistent with S.C.'s spirometry findings and history?
2. What is S.C.'s level of symptom control?
3. What risk factors does S.C. have for poor outcomes?
4. What drug therapy would you prescribe?
5. List specific goals for therapy for S.C.
6. What are the parameters for monitoring success of the therapy?
7. Discuss specific patient education based on the prescribed therapy.
8. List one or two adverse reactions for the selected agent that would cause you to change therapy.
9. What lifestyle changes would you recommend for S.C.?

* Answers can be found online.

Bibliography

Starred references are cited in the text.

*Agustí, A., Celli, B., & Faner, R. (2017). What does endotyping mean for therapy in chronic obstructive pulmonary disease? *The Lancet*, *390*(10098), 980–987. doi: 10.1016/s0140-6736(17)32136-0

Asthma. (2020). In Epocrates 19.11.2 for Android iOS (Version 9) [Mobile application software]. Retrieved from https://online.epocrates.com/diseases/44/Asthma-in-adults

*Brooks, C., Pearce, N., & Douwes, J. (2013). The hygiene hypothesis in allergy and asthma. *Current Opinion in Allergy and Clinical Immunology*, *13*(1), 70–77. doi: 10.1097/aci.0b013e32835ad0d2

*Canonica, G. W., Ferrando, M., Baiardini, I., et al. (2018). Asthma. *Current Opinion in Allergy and Clinical Immunology*, *18*(1), 51–58. doi: 10.1097/aci.0000000000000416

*Centers for Diseases Control and Prevention (CDC). (2020a). Asthma surveillance data. Retrieved from https://www.cdc.gov/asthma/asthmadata.htm

*Centers for Diseases Control and Prevention (CDC). (2020b). Basics about COPD. Retrieved from https://www.cdc.gov/copd/basics-about.html

*Centers for Diseases Control and Prevention (CDC). (2020c). Learn how to control asthma. Retrieved from https://www.cdc.gov/asthma/faqs.htm

*Centers for Diseases Control and Prevention (CDC). (2020d). Basics about COPD. Retrieved from https://www.cdc.gov/copd/basics-about.html

*Centers for Disease Control and Prevention (CDC). (2020e). Immunization schedules. Retrieved from https://www.cdc.gov/vaccines/schedules/hcp/index.html

*Chronic Obstructive Pulmonary Disease (COPD). (2020). In Epocrates 19.11.2 for Android iOS (Version 9) [Mobile application software]. Retrieved from https://online.epocrates.com/diseases/7/COPD

*Craig, T. J., & Henao, M. P. (2018). Advances in managing COPD related to α1-antitrypsin deficiency: An under-recognized genetic disorder. *Allergy*, *73*(11), 2110–2121. doi: 10.1111/all.13558

*Global Initiative for Asthma (GINA). (2020). Global strategy for asthma management and prevention. Retrieved from https://ginasthma.org/wp-content/uploads/2019/06/GINA-2019-main-report-June-2019-wms.pdf

*Global Initiative for Chronic Obstructive Lung Disease (GOLD). (2020). Global strategy for the diagnosis, management, and prevention of chronic obstructive pulmonary disease. Retrieved from https://goldcopd.org/wp-content/uploads/2019/12/GOLD-2020-FINAL-ver1.2-03Dec19_WMV.pdf

*Haahtela, T. (2019). A biodiversity hypothesis. *Allergy*. doi: 10.1111/all.13763

*Humbert, M., Busse, W., & Hanania, N. A. (2018). Controversies and opportunities in severe asthma. *Current Opinion in Pulmonary Medicine*, *24*(1), 83–93. doi: 10.1097/mcp.0000000000000438

*Kuruvilla, M. E., Lee, F. E., & Lee, G. B. (2018). Understanding asthma phenotypes, endotypes, and mechanisms of disease. *Clinical Reviews in Allergy & Immunology*, *56*(2), 219–233. doi: 10.1007/s12016-018-8712-1

*Moon, J.-Y., Filho, F. S. L., Shahangian, K., et al. (2018). Blood and sputum protein biomarkers for chronic obstructive pulmonary disease (COPD). *Expert Review of Proteomics*, *15*(11), 923–935. doi: 10.1080/14789450.2018.1539670

*National Heart, Lung and Blood Institute, National Institutes of Health (NHLBI). (2020). National Asthma Education and Prevention Program (NAEPP). Retrieved from https://www.nhlbi.nih.gov/science/national-asthma-education-and-prevention-program-naepp

*Ozdemir, C., Kucuksezer, U. C., Akdis, M., et al. (2018). The concepts of asthma endotypes and phenotypes to guide current and novel therapy strategies. *Expert Review of Respiratory Medicine*, *12*(9), 733–743. doi: 10.1080/17476348.2018.1505507

*Papi, A., Brightling, C., Pedersen, S. E., et al. (2018). Asthma. *The Lancet*, *391*(10122), 783–800. doi: 10.1016/s0140-6736(17)33311-1

*Rath, N., Raje, N., & Rosenwasser, L. (2018). Immunoglobulin E as a biomarker in asthma. *Immunology and Allergy Clinics of North America*, *38*(4), 587–597. doi: 10.1016/j.iac.2018.06.007

*Rook, G., Bäckhed, F., Levin, B. R., et al. (2017). Evolution, human-microbe interactions, and life history plasticity. *The Lancet*, *390*(10093), 521–530. doi: 10.1016/s0140-6736(17)30566-4

*Russell, D. W., Wells, J. M., & Blalock, J. E. (2016). Disease phenotyping in chronic obstructive pulmonary disease. *Current Opinion in Pulmonary Medicine*, *22*(2), 91–99. doi: 10.1097/mcp.0000000000000238

*Siafakas, N., Corlateanu, A., & Fouka, E. (2017). Phenotyping before starting therapy in COPD? *COPD: Journal of Chronic Obstructive Pulmonary Disease*, *14*(3), 367–374. doi: 10.1080/15412555.2017.1303041

*Terl, M., Sedlák, V., Cap, P., et al. (2017). Asthma management: A new phenotype-based approach using presence of eosinophilia and allergy. *Allergy*, *72*(9), 1279–1287. doi: 10.1111/all.13165

Tripple, J. W., Mccracken, J. L., & Calhoun, W. J. (2017). Biologic therapy in chronic obstructive pulmonary disease. *Immunology and Allergy Clinics of North America*, *37*(2), 345–355. doi: 10.1016/j.iac.2017.01.009

*Woodruff, P. G., Agusti, A., Roche, N., et al. (2015). Current concepts in targeting chronic obstructive pulmonary disease pharmacotherapy: Making progress towards personalised management. *The Lancet*, *385*(9979), 1789–1798. doi: 10.1016/s0140-6736(15)60693-6

*World Health Organization (WHO). (2020). Chronic respiratory diseases. Retrieved from https://www.who.int/health-topics/chronic-respiratory-diseases#tab=tab_2

*Yousuf, A., & Brightling, C. E. (2018). Biologic drugs: A new target therapy in COPD? *COPD: Journal of Chronic Obstructive Pulmonary Disease*, *15*(2), 99–107. doi: 10.1080/15412555.2018.1437897

Pharmacotherapy for Gastrointestinal Disorders

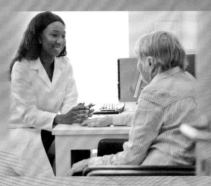

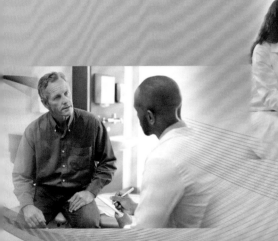

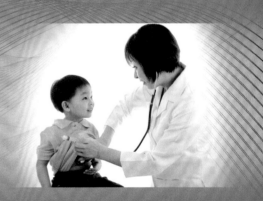

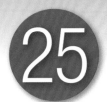

25 Gastric, Functional, and Inflammatory Bowel Disorders

Veronica F. Wilbur

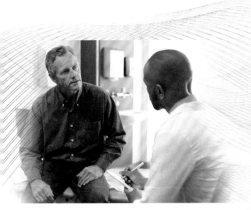
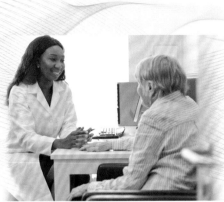
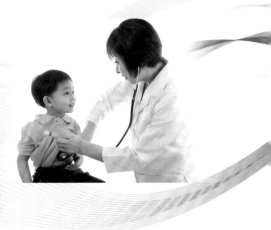

Learning Objectives

After reading this section, the participant will be able to:
1. Describe the pathophysiology and causes of nausea and vomiting.
2. Identify the goals of pharmacologic and nonpharmacologic treatment of nausea and vomiting.
3. Select appropriate drug therapy to treat common causes of nausea and vomiting.
4. Define appropriate symptom monitoring of drug therapy.
5. Distinguish appropriate changes to pharmacologic treatment.

INTRODUCTION

Nausea and vomiting are common complaints in humans. The severity of the event can range from a slight discomfort or queasiness to uncontrollable, forceful vomiting. These symptoms are perceived as uncomfortable, troublesome, and proper and timely treatment is necessary. Patients may refer to this experience by many different names: *upchuck, urp, queasy, throw up*, and *puke*, to name a few. There are many causes of nausea and vomiting, such as motion sickness, pregnancy, and medications. Likewise, many treatment options can be used to manage this complication. People of all ages experience emesis, although the etiology may be related to age-specific factors. Drugs are most frequently used in treating nausea and vomiting, but interventions that emphasize alternative therapies can also decrease emesis. This chapter reviews the pathophysiology and pharmacotherapy of specific types of nausea and vomiting.

CAUSES

There are multiple causes for nausea and vomiting; however, some of the most common is the ingestion or administration of substances or drugs, gastrointestinal (GI) disorders, neurologic processes, and metabolic disorders. The presence of noxious stimuli is frequently a cause of nausea and vomiting. Supratherapeutic digoxin (Lanoxin) and theophylline (Theo-Dur or Slo-Phyllin) are known to produce emesis. Nausea and vomiting occur more frequently with high-dose chemotherapy than with moderate doses of the same drugs. Erythromycin and some penicillin derivatives are acknowledged for inducing uncomfortable GI complications. Emesis can also result from excessive ethanol intake. It is well known that other sensory experiences, such as pungent odors or gruesome sights, can induce nausea and vomiting. **Box 25.1** presents specific etiologies for nausea and vomiting.

Patient-specific factors that increase susceptibility to nausea and vomiting include age, previous nausea and vomiting experiences, and sex. The majority of the research identifying these characteristics was done in patients receiving chemotherapy. Poor control of nausea and vomiting with previous surgeries or chemotherapy predisposes a patient to subsequent episodes of emesis, also referred to as *anticipatory nausea and vomiting*. This form of emesis is often challenging to treat with standard antiemetics drug therapy.

Patients who receive previously received chemotherapy have been noted to experience emesis compared to chemotherapy naive. Additionally, younger female patients appear to have a greater risk of emesis ("Fourth consensus guidelines for the management of postoperative nausea and vomiting: Erratum," 2020). Surprisingly, patients who have higher chronic ethanol intake exceeding 100 g/d (roughly five beers or mixed drinks per day) are associated with better emesis control and decreased

BOX 25.1   Etiologies of Nausea and Vomiting

Therapy-induced causes
  Chemotherapy
  Radiation therapy
  Opiates
  Anticonvulsants
  Ipecac
  Antibiotics
  Digitalis or digoxin toxicity
  Theophylline
  Nonsteroidal anti-inflammatory drugs
  Hormonal therapies
Drug withdrawal
  Opiates
  Benzodiazepines
Metabolic disorders
  Addison disease
  Water intoxication
  Volume depletion
  Diabetic ketoacidosis
  Hypercalcemia
  Renal dysfunction–uremia
GI mechanisms
  Mechanical gastric outlet obstruction
    PUD
    Gastric carcinoma
    Pancreatic disease
  Motility disorders
    Gastroparesis
    Drug-induced gastric stasis
    IBS
    Postgastric surgery
    Idiopathic gastric stasis
  Intra-abdominal emergencies
    Acute pancreatitis
    Acute pyelonephritis
    Acute cholecystitis

Acute cholangitis
Acute viral hepatitis
Intestinal obstruction
Acute gastroenteritis
  Viral gastroenteritis
  Salmonellosis
  Shigellosis
  Staphylococcal gastroenteritis (enterotoxins)
Cardiovascular disease
  Acute myocardial infarction
  Congestive heart failure
  Shock and circulatory collapse
Neurologic processes
  Cerebellar hemorrhage
  Increased intracranial pressure
    Hematoma
    Subdural effusion
    Tumor (benign or malignant)
    Hydrocephalus
    Reye's syndrome
  Headache
    Migraine
    Severe hypertension
  Head trauma
  Vestibular disorders
Psychogenic causes
  Anorexia nervosa
  Anticipatory
Miscellaneous causes
  Pregnancy
  Noxious odors
  Ingestion of an irritant
  Operative procedures
  Septicemia
  Nicotine

vomiting incidence. A history of motion sickness may increase the risks of nausea and vomiting in another situation, such as with chemotherapy or surgery. Children, in general, experience nausea and vomiting more frequently than do adults. Obesity and anxiety have also been associated with heightened emesis incidence ("Fourth consensus guidelines for the management of postoperative nausea and vomiting: Erratum," 2020).

The prevalence of nausea and vomiting may complicate 20% to 70% of surgical procedures ("Fourth consensus guidelines for the management of postoperative nausea and vomiting: Erratum," 2020). Prevalence is also increased using specific inhalation agents, mainly nitrous oxide, and by concomitant use of opiate medications. When propofol is used as an intravenous (IV) anesthetic agent, there is a lower risk of postoperative nausea and vomiting (PONV). PONV is more likely to occur after general than regional anesthesia, and its prevalence increases in parallel with the duration of surgery and anesthesia. Surgical procedures closely associated with PONV include cholecystectomy, gynecological, and the use of laparoscopy. PONV is also more likely in those with a history of PONV or motion sickness.

PATHOPHYSIOLOGY

The pathophysiology of nausea and vomiting is complex (**Figure 25.1**) and involves the modulation of medullary sites and neurotransmitters. Many sensory centers accept

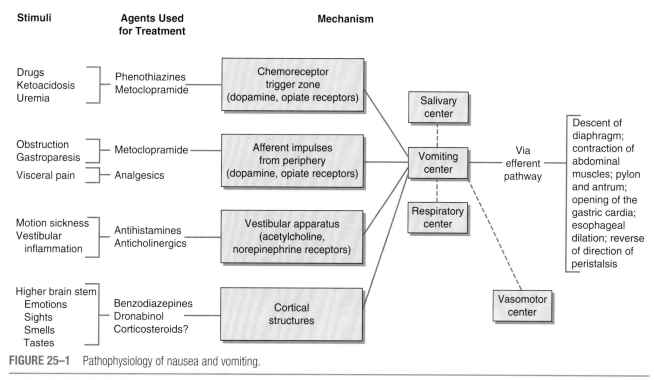

FIGURE 25–1 Pathophysiology of nausea and vomiting.

(Reprinted from Koda-Kimble, M. A., & Young, L. Y. (2012). Nausea and vomiting. In M. A. Koda-Kimble, L. Y. Young, & B. J. Guglielmo (Eds.), *Applied therapeutics: The clinical use of drugs* (10th ed.). Philadelphia, PA: Lippincott Williams & Wilkins, with permission.)

noxious stimuli from the body, including the chemoreceptor trigger zone (CTZ), visceral afferent nerves, cerebral cortex, limbic system, vestibular system, and midbrain intracranial pressure receptors.

Modulation of Nausea and Vomiting

These stimuli are transmitted to the *emetic complex* (EC), a loose group of organized neurons throughout the medulla, which coordinates the sensory inputs and the act of vomiting. The EC is the crucial component in the modulation of nausea and vomiting. Located in the medulla's lateral reticular formation, it receives afferent impulses from the sensory centers. Efferent impulses are sent to the nucleus tractus when the EC is activated, stimulating an intertwined neural network that innervates the salivary, vasomotor, respiratory centers, and cranial nerves VIII and X. The same efferent impulses are also sent to the stomach, abdominal muscles, diaphragm, and associated sphincters to execute the involuntary act of vomiting. Much like the sensory centers that stimulate it, the vomiting center is rich in dopamine, histamine, serotonin, and acetylcholine receptors. It can also be affected by binding to opiate and benzodiazepine receptors. An intact EC is essential for coordination of the vomiting act or the emetic reflex.

Stimulatory Centers

The CTZ is one of the most important chemosensory organs responsible for the detection of noxious stimuli. It is uniquely located in the area postrema on the fourth ventricle floor of the (medulla) brain and is exposed to both blood and cerebrospinal fluid (CSF). Thus, toxins in both the blood and CSF can stimulate a response by the CTZ. These toxins may be drugs (chemotherapy, opiates, and digoxin), poisons, or substances found naturally in the body (excess calcium, hormones). The CTZ is rich in neurotransmitter receptors for dopamine, serotonin, histamine, and acetylcholine. Neurokinin 1 (NK) receptors in the cerebral cortex/thalamus/limbic system also feed in the EC. An antiemetic effect is elicited when these receptors are blocked.

Gastrointestinal Tract

The GI tract and pharynx are sites of origin for the stimulation of nausea and vomiting. Visceral afferent nerves, also referred to as *splanchnic nerves*, from the pharynx and GI tract transmit impulses from local neuroreceptors along the vagus nerve to the vomiting center. The GI tract is rich in local dopamine, histamine, and serotonin receptors. The visceral afferent nerves are also responsible for transmitting stimuli from other peripheral sites such as the heart, lungs, and testes; hence, the vomiting response may occur when a person has been punched in the abdomen or kicked in the groin. Abdominal surgery is another example in which visceral afferent nerves are involved in nausea and vomiting.

Central Nervous System

Motion sickness is primarily a central nervous system (CNS) response mediated by the vestibular system. Acetylcholine and histamine receptors have been found in the vestibular center. Blockade of these receptors provides some degree of protection from emesis. The cerebral cortex, the largest portion of the brain, is responsible for the motor coordination of the body, sensory perception, learning, memory, and many other functions. Afferent impulses from specific sites of the cerebral cortex can result in emesis. The cerebellum is responsible for the regulation of balance, equilibrium, and coordination. Disruption of this portion of the brain can lead to temporary or chronic nausea and vomiting. These structures may also play a role in anticipatory emesis.

Limbic System

The limbic system and the midbrain intracranial pressure receptors can stimulate nausea and vomiting, although their mechanisms are not fully understood. In humans, the limbic system's primary function is associated with the expression of mood, emotions, feelings, and memory recall. Anxiety, fear, and other emotions may play a role at this site in the perception of nausea and vomiting. Head trauma, intracranial bleeding, and mass effect from a benign or malignant tumor can increase brain pressure. This increased intracranial pressure can cause nausea and vomiting. The optimal treatment in these situations is a reduction in intracranial pressure through surgery or corticosteroids.

DIAGNOSTIC CRITERIA

The three identified phases of emesis are nausea, retching, and vomiting. Nausea is the unpleasant physical sensation of impending retching or vomiting. Nausea often occurs without the other two emesis aspects, although all three phases are treated with the same pharmacologic agents. Common symptoms accompanying nausea are flushing, pallor, tachycardia, and hypersalivation. Gastric stasis and decreased pyloric tone, mucosal blood flow, and the duodenum's contractions with reflux into the stomach are physiologic responses to nausea. Retching, the second phase of emesis, is the involuntary synchronized labored movement of abdominal and thoracic muscles before vomiting. Vomiting is the coordinated contractions of the abdominal and thoracic muscles to expel the gastric contents. The lower esophageal sphincter contracts, allowing GI retroperistalsis. The actual expulsion of gastric contents differentiates vomiting from retching.

The acuteness of the symptomatology is based on history and physical examination. Several issues need to be addressed, such as an acute emergency, as found in mechanical obstruction, perforation, or peritonitis. Nonemergent, self-limited causes of vomiting may be caused by viral gastroenteritis or a potentially offending medication. The goal is to determine whether empiric treatment with an antiemetic, a gastric acid–suppressing, or a prokinetic agent would be beneficial or whether the patient should be admitted to the hospital to correct fluid and electrolyte imbalance.

Acute nausea and vomiting differ considerably from chronic nausea and vomiting based on the symptom duration. When the onset of nausea and vomiting is acute, this suggests gastroenteritis, pancreatitis, cholecystitis, or a drug-related side effect. Viral gastroenteritis is associated with diarrhea, headache, and myalgias, and in this instance, symptoms should resolve spontaneously within 5 days or sooner. Insidious onset of nausea without vomiting suggests the etiology could be from gastroparesis, a medication-related side effect, metabolic disorders, pregnancy, or even gastroesophageal reflux disease. When nausea and vomiting are longer than 1 month, this is characterized as chronic.

Timing and description of the vomiting are essential. Vomiting in the morning before breakfast is typically related to pregnancy, uremia, alcohol ingestion, and increased intracranial pressure. Projectile vomiting suggests intracranial disorders, especially those that result in increased intracranial pressure. In this case, vomiting may not be preceded by nausea.

The onset of vomiting caused by gastroparesis or gastric outlet obstruction tends to be delayed, usually by more than 1 hour after meal ingestion. Vomiting may also be suggestive of psychiatric disorders.

Associated symptoms such as abdominal pain, fever, diarrhea, vertigo, or a history of a similar illness among family, friends, or associates are essential data to gather.

The physical examination assesses the vital signs and looks for signs of dehydration. The presence of jaundice, lymphadenopathy, abdominal masses, and occult blood in the stool may reveal features suggestive of thyrotoxicosis or Addison's disease. The abdominal examination should look for distention, visible peristalsis, and abdominal or inguinal hernias. Areas of tenderness are important: tenderness in the mid-epigastrium suggests an ulcer, and in the right upper quadrant, cholecystitis or biliary tract disease. Auscultation may demonstrate increased bowel sounds in obstruction, or absent bowel sounds may indicate an ileus.

INITIATING THERAPY

The treatment of nausea, retching, or vomiting in any patient begins with evaluating and correcting possible causes. Most sources of nausea and vomiting may be reversed or palliated by surgery or medical interventions. Infectious causes should be promptly treated with antibiotics, and metabolic disorders require medical management. Some drug toxicities may be treated with antidotes, such as digoxin toxicity reversed with digoxin immune Fab (Digibind). The following section discusses medications used to treat nausea and vomiting. They should be used with definitive treatments when possible.

Tailoring a patient's daily activities and the use of nonpharmacologic treatments may help manage nausea and vomiting. Changes in a patient's diet may affect the frequency or severity of nausea and vomiting. Examples of dietary changes are avoiding spicy foods and excessive grease or oil and decreased caffeine intake. Professional counseling or group therapy may prove favorable for patients with psychogenic nausea and vomiting. Hypnosis, behavior modification, and imagery are beneficial tools for controlling nausea and vomiting with an anxiety component, such as chemotherapy-related anticipatory emesis. However, the prevention of anticipatory nausea and vomiting is the optimal form of management.

Goals of Drug Therapy

The goals of drug therapy are simple: to alleviate nausea's subjective feeling and the objective act of vomiting and its associated complications (**Box 25.2**). It is important to rely on the patient's subjective response when evaluating the efficacy of specific therapy for nausea. Secondary goals are to minimize drug toxicity and adverse events and contain costs. The prevention of nausea and vomiting is the goal in the setting of chemotherapy and specific surgical procedures. Control or improvement in nausea and vomiting should occur within 5 to 60 minutes of pharmacologic intervention. If this does not ensue, promptly use another method. **Table 25.1** reviews available antiemetic agents, dosages, comparable efficacy, and adverse effects. Pregnancy risk factors are included in each drug class discussion and pregnancy-related nausea and vomiting section.

Phenothiazines

Phenothiazines are a commonly used class of drugs to treat nausea and vomiting. Prochlorperazine (Compazine) and promethazine (Phenergan) are the most frequently used drugs in this class.

Mechanism of Action

Their mechanism of action presumably involves dopamine receptor blockade in the CTZ. Anticholinergic activity in the vomiting and vestibular centers of the brain may also contribute to the mechanism of action.

The phenothiazines may be used as monotherapy for mild-to-moderate nausea and vomiting or in combination with other antiemetics for more symptoms. There is a dose-response quality for this drug class; however, the incidence of adverse effects such as extrapyramidal effects and sedation can also be associated with higher doses. Promethazine has antihistamine antiemetic activities and could also be classified with the antihistamine–anticholinergic class of drugs. The phenothiazines are a viable and practical option for the long-term treatment of nausea and vomiting. Products are available in oral, rectal, and injectable formulations. The drug regime should be tailored to the patient, and oral preparations are available as tablets, sustained-release capsules, and liquids. Rectal suppositories are useful in patients who cannot retain oral medications, and when IV access is not an option. Avoid using suppositories in patients who are thrombocytopenic because of the increased risk of bleeding or hemorrhage.

Contraindications

Caution should be used in patients taking concomitant drugs that cause CNS depression, such as sedatives, hypnotics, and opiates, because additional sedation may result. Phenothiazines may exacerbate the symptoms of Parkinson's disease. The safety of prescribing phenothiazines during pregnancy is controversial; most studies find phenothiazines safe for the mother and fetus if used occasionally in low doses. Care is advised when prescribing these drugs during the third term of pregnancy or when breastfeeding. Phenothiazines may decrease the seizure threshold and should be used cautiously in patients with seizure disorders.

The phenothiazines are relatively inexpensive compared to most other antiemetic drug classes, except for the sustained-release phenothiazine preparations, which tend to be costly.

Adverse Events

The most common adverse event of phenothiazine use is drowsiness or sedation. Also, particularly at high doses, phenothiazines can evoke extrapyramidal symptoms (EPS) by blocking the central dopaminergic receptors involved in motor function. EPS presentation can include dystonic reactions, feelings of motor restlessness, and parkinsonian signs and symptoms. Extreme examples of EPS, parkinsonian type symptoms, are the masklike face, drooling, tremor, cogwheel rigidity, pill-rolling motion, lack of ability to initiate voluntary movement, and gait abnormalities. Dystonic reactions may include spasms of the neck muscles or torticollis, extensor rigidity of back muscles, mandibular tics,

---

BOX 25.2   Complications of Nausea and Vomiting

Metabolic abnormalities
- Dehydration
- Alkalosis
- Hypokalemia
- Hypomagnesemia
- Hyponatremia
- Hypochloremia
- Malnutrition

Structural damage
- Wound dehiscence
- Esophagogastric tears/Mallory-Weiss tears
- Increased bleeding under skin flaps
- Tension on suture lines

Patient dissatisfaction
- Noncompliance
- Poor oral intake; anticipatory nausea and vomiting
- Delayed ambulation after surgery/procedures
- Fatigue
- Depression

Increased use of resources
- Prolongation of hospital stay
- Unexpected hospital admission
- Alteration or additional Therapy

Aspiration pneumonia
Venous hypertension

TABLE 25.1

Overview of Selected Antiemetic Agents

Generic (Trade) Name and Dosage	Selected Adverse Events	Contraindications	Special Considerations
Phenothiazines			
Chlorpromazine (Thorazine) 10–25 mg q4–6h PRN PO, 25–50 mg q4–6h PRN IV, IM, 50–100 mg q6–8h PRN rectal	Sedation or drowsiness EPS symptoms: agitation, insomnia, motor restlessness, spasms of facial muscles, protrusion of tongue, and mandibular tics Anticholinergic effects: dry mouth, urinary retention, and blurred vision	Hypersensitivity Cautious use with other CNS depressants, Parkinson's syndrome, poorly controlled seizure disorder, and severe hepatic dysfunction	Increased incidence of autonomic response with IV administration Higher incidence of EPS symptoms
Fluphenazine (Prolixin) 0.5–5 mg q6–8h PRN PO, IM	Same as those for Chlorpromazine	Same as those for Chlorpromazine	
Perphenazine (Trilafon) 2–6 mg q4–6h PRN PO, 5–10 mg q6h PRN IM	Same as those for Chlorpromazine	Same as those for Chlorpromazine	Higher incidence of EPS symptoms compared with other phenothiazines
Prochlorperazine (Compazine) 5–10 mg q4–6h PRN PO, rectal, IM, IV 10–30 mg BID PO sustained-release capsule	Same as those for Chlorpromazine	Same as those for Chlorpromazine	Sustained-release capsule more expensive Higher incidence of EPS symptoms compared with other phenothiazines
Promethazine (Phenergan) 12.5–25 mg q4–6h PRN PO, rectal, IM, IV	Same as those for Chlorpromazine	Same as those for Chlorpromazine	
Antihistamines and Anticholinergics			
Benzquinamide (Emete-con) 50 mg q3–4h PRN IM 25 mg q3–4h PRN IV	Sedation or drowsiness, confusion Anticholinergic effects: dry mouth, tachycardia, blurred vision, urinary retention, constipation	Hypersensitivity Caution in narrow-angle glaucoma, asthma, prostatic hypertrophy	IV preparation not recommended
Dimenhydrinate (Dramamine) 50–100 mg q4–6h PRN PO, IM, IV	Same as those for Benzquinamide	Same as those for Benzquinamide	Do not exceed 200 mg/d
Diphenhydramine (Benadryl) 25–50 mg q6–8h PRN PO, 10–50 mg q2–4h PRN IM, IV	Same as those for Benzquinamide	Same as those for Benzquinamide	Do not exceed 200 mg/d
Hydroxyzine (Atarax, Vistaril) 25–100 mg q4–6h PRN PO, IM	Same as those for Benzquinamide	Same as those for Benzquinamide	
Meclizine (Antivert, Bonine) 25–50 mg q24h PRN PO	Same as those for Benzquinamide	Same as those for Benzquinamide	
Scopolamine (Transderm Scop) 1.5 mg q3d transdermal patch	Same as those for Benzquinamide	Same as those for Benzquinamide	
Trimethobenzamide (Tigan) 250 mg q6–8h PRN PO 200 mg q6–8h PRN IM, rectal	Same as those for Benzquinamide	Same as those for Benzquinamide	
Benzodiazepines			
Lorazepam (Ativan) 0.5–2 mg q4–8h PRN PO, IM, IV	Drowsiness or fatigue, confusion, constipation	Same as those for Benzquinamide	Dose should be low in frail, older adults, or critically ill patients.
Diazepam (Valium) 2–5 mg BID–QID PRN PO, IM, IV	Same as those for Lorazepam	Same as those for Lorazepam	Same as those for Lorazepam

TABLE 25.1

Overview of Selected Antiemetic Agents (*Continued*)

Generic (Trade) Name and Dosage	Selected Adverse Events	Contraindications	Special Considerations
Serotonin Antagonists			
Dolasetron (Anzemet) 100 mg PO 1 h before chemotherapy 100 mg IV 30 min before chemotherapy 12.5 mg IV 15 min before cessation of anesthesia 100 mg PO 2 h before surgery	Headache, diarrhea, ECG changes	Hypersensitivity Use with caution in patients with severe cardiac dysfunction	Very expensive (IV > PO) Use only when indicated
Granisetron (Kytril) 10 mcg/kg IV 30 min before chemotherapy 1 mg PO BID (q12h)—start before chemotherapy (Sancuso) patch—3.1 mg/24 h (1 patch)	Same as those for Dolasetron	Same as those for Dolasetron	Very expensive (IV > PO) Use only when indicated. IV dose often rounded to 1- or 2-mg doses
Ondansetron (Zofran) 0.15 mg/kg IV 30 min before chemotherapy and at 4 and 8 h Oral—tablet and melt 4 mg, 8 mg	Same as those for Dolasetron	Same as those for Dolasetron	Generic, less expensive than other in the class Approved for NVP
NK1 Antagonist			
Aprepitant (Emend) Oral—40, 80, 125 mg 3 h prior to induction of anesthesia, 1 h prior to chemotherapy	Heartburn, confusion, decreased urination, dizziness Dyspepsia EPS symptoms, fatigue, constipation, erythema, skin allergic reactions	Hypersensitivity to product, contraindication with some chemotherapy agents Possible hypersensitivity to 5-HT_3 component, serotonin syndrome	Interacts with contraceptives Extremely expensive Interactions with dexamethasone, midazolam, oral contraceptives
NK1/Serotonin Antagonist Combo			
Netupitant/palonosetron (Akynzeo) Indicated use with dexamethasone Capsules 300 mg/0.5 mg— approximately 1 h prior to the start of chemotherapy, with or without food. IV: 235 mg fosnetupitant/ 0.25 mg palonosetron as a lyophilized powder in single-dose vial for reconstitution The recommended dosage is one Akynzeo vial diluted and administered as 30-min infusion starting approximately 30 min prior to the start of chemotherapy.	Most common adverse reactions (≥3%) for Akynzeocapsules are headache, asthenia, dyspepsia, fatigue, constipation, and erythema	Pregnancy: May cause fetal harm Hepatic Impairment: Avoid use in patients with severe hepatic impairment Renal impairment: Avoid use in patients with severe renal impairment or end-stage renal disease	Serotonin syndrome has been reported with 5-HT_3 receptor antagonists alone but particularly with concomitant use of serotonergic drugs
Other Antiemetics			
Dexamethasone (Decadron) 8–20 mg IV/PO before chemotherapy; 4–8 mg IV BID (delayed nausea and vomiting)	Hyperactivity, GI irritation, mood swings, depression, hyperglycemia, anxiety	Hypersensitivity Use with caution in patients with diabetes, history of ulcers, young male patients	Give IV over 5–15 min. Administer orally with food. Avoid chronic administration
Methylprednisolone (Solu-Medrol) 125–500 mg IV q6h	Same as those for Dexamethasone	Same as those for Dexamethasone	Same as those for Dexamethasone

(Continued)

TABLE 25.1

Overview of Selected Antiemetic Agents (*Continued*)

Generic (Trade) Name and Dosage	Selected Adverse Events	Contraindications	Special Considerations
Dronabinol (Marinol) 5–15 mg/m^2 PO 1–3 h before chemotherapy and q4h × 6 d 2.5–10 mg PO BID	Sedation, confusion, dysphoria, increased appetite	Use with caution if patient is receiving other CNS depressants	Controlled substance
Antacids 15–30 mL q2–4h PRN	Diarrhea, constipation	Renal dysfunction	May decrease absorption of other drugs
Metoclopramide (Reglan) 20–30 mg PO QID PRN, 1–2 mg/kg IV before chemotherapy and q2–4h (high dose)	EPS symptoms Diarrhea Drowsiness	Avoid use for longer than 12 weeks due to the potential of EPS symptoms.	Side effects are dose dependent. EPS symptoms reversible with diphenhydramine
Doxylamine/pyridoxine (Diclegis) 10 mg each drug	Drowsiness, dizziness, impaired coordination, headache, urinary retention	Use with caution in patients with asthma, increased intraocular pressure, narrow-angle glaucoma, stenosing peptic ulcer, pyloroduodenal obstruction and urinary bladder–neck obstruction	Approved by FDA specifically for NVP Interference with urine drug screen: Diclegis may interfere with urine screening for methadone, opiates, and PCP. Very expensive
Doxylamine/pyridoxine (Bonjesta) 20 mg each drug Start with one pill at bedtime, may increase to twice a day. The maximum recommended dose is 2 tabs daily, one in the morning and one at bedtime	Most common side effect is somnolence.	Use with caution in patients with asthma, increased intraocular pressure, narrow-angle glaucoma, stenosing peptic ulcer, pyloroduodenal obstruction, and urinary bladder–neck obstruction	Approved by FDA specifically for NVP Interference with urine drug screen: Bonjesta may interfere with urine screening for methadone, opiates, and PCP

CNS, central nervous system; ECG, electrocardiographic; EPS, extrapyramidal symptoms; FDA, U.S. Food and Drug Administration; GI, gastrointestinal; IM, intramuscular; IV, intravenous; *NK1*, Neurokinin 1; NVP, nausea and vomiting in pregnancy; PCP, Phencyclidine.

difficulty swallowing or talking, and perioral spasms, often with protrusion of the tongue. Motor restlessness may consist of agitation, jitteriness, tapping of feet, and insomnia. Extrapyramidal reactions can be easily treated with the use of diphenhydramine (Benadryl) 25 mg orally or parenterally three to four times daily or benztropine (Cogentin) 1 to 4 mg orally or parenterally twice a day. Autonomic responses, such as hypotension and tachycardia, have been observed with IV phenothiazine use, particularly chlorpromazine. Hypotension and sedation are less likely to occur with prochlorperazine, thiethylperazine, and perphenazine, but these three agents are associated with a higher frequency of EPS. Dry mouth, urinary retention, blurred vision, and other anticholinergic effects may occur with phenothiazine use. Reversible agranulocytosis is rarely associated (<1%) with phenothiazine therapy. This effect occurs more frequently in women and with chronic phenothiazine use. Cholestatic jaundice and photosensitivity are reactions that can rarely happen within the first few months of regular phenothiazine use. These are more frequently observed when a phenothiazine is used for psychiatric conditions rather than emesis control.

Monitoring parameters include EPS and parkinsonian symptoms. Doses may need to be decreased in severe hepatic dysfunction. Complete blood counts (CBC) should be regularly monitored in chronic phenothiazine use (see **Table 25.1**).

Interactions

These drugs potentiate CNS depression with alcohol and other CNS depressants. They potentiate the action of alpha blockers, and levels of the drug can be increased with propranolol. Anticonvulsant drug doses may have to be adjusted. They may antagonize oral anticoagulants.

Antihistamines–Anticholinergics

There is a wide variety of agents available in the antihistamine–anticholinergic drug class. These agents are most useful for mild nausea, such as motion sickness. Hydroxyzine (Vistaril,

Atarax), meclizine (Bonine, Antivert), dimenhydrinate (Dramamine), and scopolamine (Transderm Scop) are some of the more common agents of this class. Unlike most of the other classes of agents discussed in this chapter, some of the antihistamine–anticholinergic agents are available without a prescription.

Mechanism of Action

The mechanism of action appears to be an interruption of visceral afferent pathways responsible for stimulating nausea and vomiting. These drugs are most frequently administered orally, but some can be given IV, intramuscularly, transdermal, or rectally.

The antihistamines are beneficial for the treatment and prevention of motion sickness. For this indication, it is recommended that a dose be taken at least 30 to 60 minutes before the event (e.g., boating, air flight, car ride) and then repeated at regular intervals several times a day. The scopolamine patch is a beneficial agent for the prevention of motion sickness. A patch should be applied to clean, dry skin 1 to 2 hours before the potentially emetogenic event, and a new patch may be reapplied every 3 days.

Many of the antihistamines and anticholinergics have been used for the treatment of nausea in pregnancy.

Contraindications

Precautions are recommended with asthma, glaucoma, and GI or urinary obstruction. Antihistamines–anticholinergics are not recommended for nursing mothers.

Adverse Events

Adverse effects limit the use of anticholinergics–antihistamines. Patients frequently experience sedation, drowsiness, or confusion. Additional anticholinergic effects are troublesome, including blurred vision, dry mouth, urinary retention, and tachycardia. There is a relationship between the dose and frequency and the extent of the anticholinergic effects. Caution is warranted in patients with narrow-angle glaucoma, prostatic hypertrophy, and asthma because these patients are more prone to the anticholinergic effects of these drugs.

Nondrug therapies may manage anticholinergic effects. Chewing gum or sucking on ice chips or hard candy may refresh a dry mouth. The intake of a high-fiber diet and adequate daily fluid consumption may curb constipation.

Monitoring for anticholinergic effects is of paramount importance. Severe side effects may warrant discontinuation of the drug. Commonly observed overdose symptoms may include dilated pupils, tachycardia, hypertension, CNS depression, flushed skin, or, more seriously, respiratory failure and circulatory collapse. Adverse effects occur more commonly in patients with renal or hepatic dysfunction.

Interactions

These drugs can potentiate CNS depression with alcohol, tranquilizers, and sedative-hypnotics.

Benzodiazepines

Often used for other indications, benzodiazepines offer useful qualities to the treatment of nausea. Not only do these agents treat and prevent emesis, but they can also cause anxiolysis and amnesia. These latter effects are particularly beneficial in anticipatory nausea and vomiting associated with chemotherapy.

Lorazepam (Ativan) is the most frequently used benzodiazepine for nausea and vomiting. Its mechanism of action is not understood; however, it probably acts centrally to inhibit the vomiting center. Lorazepam has only moderate antiemetic properties and is generally used in combination with other agents to control chemotherapy-associated anticipatory and delayed chemotherapy nausea and vomiting.

Dosage

Both oral and parenteral forms of lorazepam are available. Patient-specific variables should be considered when identifying an appropriate dose. Usual oral or IV doses range from 0.5 to 2 mg at least 30 minutes before the start of chemotherapy. As-needed (prn) antiemetic doses range from 0.5 to 3 mg IV or orally every 4 to 6 hours. To prevent excessive sedation, patients who are older adults or frail require low initial doses of lorazepam. Patients with compromised pulmonary or poor cardiac function should receive IV lorazepam with caution and be closely monitored for respiratory and cardiac status.

Contraindications

Lorazepam is not recommended for use in patients with hepatic or renal failure. Several studies have indicated that diazepam (Valium) may also cause fetal toxicity when administered to pregnant women and thus should be avoided in this patient population. These benzodiazepines weigh risk versus benefit due to the potential for teratogenicity. If breastfeeding, monitor infants for risk of infant CNS depression.

Adverse Events

For benzodiazepines, CNS depression occurs most often, with drowsiness, fatigue, memory impairment, impaired coordination, and confusion. Lorazepam has an amnesic effect that, for some patients, is a benefit, whereas others may find it unacceptable. Paradoxical CNS stimulation resulting in restlessness, anxiety, nightmares, and increased muscle spasticity may occur. The drug should be discontinued if paradoxical stimulation occurs. Other adverse effects include constipation, headache, and increased or decreased appetite. Parenteral administration may cause hypotension, bradycardia, or apnea, particularly in the older adults and critically ill (see **Table 25.1**).

Monitoring parameters include cardiovascular and respiratory status for initial doses. Because the liver metabolizes the benzodiazepines, liver function tests should be assessed before dosing. The presence of adverse CNS effects should be evaluated with each clinic or hospital visit.

Interactions

These drugs potentiate CNS depression when used with other drugs that depress the CNS and alcohol.

Serotonin Antagonists

The serotonin antagonists are another class of antiemetics. Ondansetron (Zofran), granisetron (Kytril, Sancuso), palonosetron (Aloxi), and dolasetron (Anzemet) are available in the United States.

Mechanism of Action

These agents work by antagonizing the type 3 serotonin (5-HT$_3$) receptors centrally in the CTZ and peripherally at the vagal and splanchnic afferent fibers from the enterochromaffin cells in the upper GI tract. The serotonin antagonists were initially indicated for the treatment and prevention of chemotherapy-induced nausea and vomiting (CINV). They have changed the way nausea and vomiting are treated and have greatly improved patients' quality of life, receiving highly emetogenic chemotherapy regimens. Radiation-induced nausea and vomiting and PONV are two other areas where the serotonin antagonists have been studied. The unequivocal efficacy and lack of significant adverse effects make these agents ideal for select indications.

The serotonin antagonists are available orally as tablets and liquids and parenterally for IV use. Because these agents are used to prevent nausea and vomiting, oral administration in this situation is encouraged, even with highly emetogenic chemotherapy. There have been few data to support one agent's superior efficacy over another when used at recommended dosages (Barrett et al., 2011). While the serotonin antagonist preparations' cost can be higher than other antiemetics, the recent advent of generic ondansetron (Zofran) has made this class more available to treat nausea and vomiting. However, this class of medication still needs to be used conservatively and appropriately. Many institutions have created antiemetic guidelines to identify serotonin antagonists' approved indications to optimize care and resources. The appropriateness of these agents in specific circumstances is discussed later.

Contraindications

Caution should be used when there is known hypersensitivity to 5-HT$_3$ receptor blockers. Limited study of the 5-HT$_3$ agents in pregnancy reveals little risk of teratogenic defects when used in the first trimester (Andrade, 2020; Parker et al., 2018). The serotonin antagonists should be used with caution in breastfeeding mothers; once again, human data are lacking, but ondansetron is distributed into the milk of lactating rats.

Adverse Events

Mild-to-moderate headaches can occur in patients receiving oral or parenteral serotonin antagonists, followed by diarrhea frequency. A few patients experience severe headaches requiring discontinuation of the drug. Other adverse effects that occur

in less than 10% of patients are abdominal or epigastric pain, increased serum hepatic enzyme levels on liver function tests, hypertension, malaise or fatigue, constipation, pruritus, and fever. Rare cardiovascular effects have been reported, although a definite causal relationship has not been established. All three agents can cause electrocardiographic (ECG) alterations (prolonged PR interval and QT interval and widened QRS complex). Conservatively, in patients with severe cardiac dysfunctions such as arrhythmia and heart block, the serotonin antagonists should be used cautiously.

Important monitoring parameters for serotonin antagonists include baseline and follow-up liver function tests. Dosage reductions may be made for severe hepatic dysfunction. ECG complications can be avoided by assessing electrolytes and correcting hypokalemia and hypomagnesemia (see **Table 25.1**).

Interactions

Caution is used when given with drugs that prolong cardiac conduction interval, diuretics, and a cumulative high-dose anthracycline.

Metoclopramide and Other Antiemetics

Metoclopramide (Reglan) has been used to treat nausea and vomiting caused by several different stimuli. It is a highly useful agent in the treatment of diabetic gastric stasis, postsurgical gastric stasis, and gastroesophageal reflux, which may be associated with some degree of nausea.

Mechanism of Action

For these indications, metoclopramide enhances motility and gastric emptying by increasing the duration and extent of esophageal contractions, the lower esophageal sphincter's resting tone, gastric contractions, and peristalsis of the duodenum and jejunum. Metoclopramide is also used in the prevention and treatment of CINV. Its mechanism of action is dopamine receptor inhibition in the CTZ. The central and peripheral actions of this agent make it efficacious in multiple clinical situations. Metoclopramide can be administered orally, IV, and intramuscularly. A sugar-free syrup exists for patients with diabetes who cannot take the pills. Because metoclopramide is eliminated primarily by the kidneys, when the patient's creatinine clearance is less than 40 mL/min, the dose should be decreased by 50%. Subsequent doses are based on the patient's clinical response. Periodic assessment of renal function is prudent. Patients should be informed of this agent's sedative qualities and that use of other CNS depressants could potentiate this effect.

Adverse Events

The most clinically concerning adverse effects of metoclopramide are the EPS. As with high doses of phenothiazines, facial spasms, rhythmic protrusions of the tongue, involuntary movements of limbs, motor restlessness, agitation, and other dystonic reactions can occur. These effects occur most commonly in children and young adults, in men more than women, and at high doses of metoclopramide. The EPS occurs within 24 to 48 hours of the initial dose and subside within 24 hours of drug discontinuation. High-dose metoclopramide is usually defined as 2 mg/kg per dose. EPS can be prevented or treated with the addition of diphenhydramine 25 to 50 mg IV or orally. IV administration of diphenhydramine is preferred for severe presentations. Other reversal agents are benztropine and diazepam. Secondary to its actions in the intestinal tract, metoclopramide can cause diarrhea. Management of diarrhea includes discontinuation or dosage reduction of metoclopramide, increased fluid resuscitation, and electrolyte replacement. The use of metoclopramide may not be a prudent choice in a patient who already has diarrhea. Metoclopramide may be used during pregnancy and breastfeeding; there is no known risk of fetal harm based on human data.

Interactions

A hypertensive crisis can occur when metoclopramide is used with monoamine oxidase inhibitors. Additive sedation can be seen when used with alcohol or other CNS depressants. These drugs are antagonized by anticholinergics and narcotics. They may diminish gastric and accelerate intestinal absorption of drugs and food.

Corticosteroids

Corticosteroids are usually reserved for CINV and have been shown to create an additive effect in CINV's prevention.

Mechanism of Action

The actual mechanism of action in the relief of nausea and vomiting is unknown, but one postulated theory is prostaglandins' inhibition. In nausea and vomiting secondary to increased intracranial pressure, corticosteroids provide relief by decreasing inflammation. Dexamethasone (Decadron) and methylprednisolone (Solu-Medrol) are the two most common corticosteroids used; however, the addition of prednisone (Deltasone) to lymphoma and leukemia chemotherapy regimens can provide heightened control of emesis. These corticosteroids are almost always used in combination with other agents in the control or prevention of emesis from highly emetogenic regimens.

Corticosteroids are available orally and parenterally. The oral form is beneficial for low doses or prolonged administration but may cause significant GI toxicity. Patients should be encouraged to take oral corticosteroids with food to minimize GI irritation and complications. IV administration is ordinarily used in the prevention of nausea and vomiting, primarily to avoid GI complications. IV preparations should be infused over 5 to 15 minutes to prevent burning, flushing, and itching sensations associated with the phosphate salt dissociation. Of the corticosteroids studied, the utility of dexamethasone has been best defined. In clinical trials, single-agent dexamethasone was superior to prochlorperazine and comparable with high-dose metoclopramide when used for mildly to moderately emetogenic chemotherapy regimens.

The combination of dexamethasone and high-dose metoclopramide was the standard of care for the prevention of cisplatin-induced emesis until the introduction of the serotonin antagonists. IV doses of dexamethasone as a premedication range from 8 to 20 mg.

Corticosteroids should be used with caution in uncontrolled patients with diabetes. Sliding-scale insulin or careful alterations of oral hypoglycemic agent regimens may be used for unacceptably high blood glucose levels.

Adverse Events

Although very useful, the corticosteroids are associated with many toxicities and adverse effects. Mental disturbances range from mood swings, depression, anxiety, and aggression to frank psychosis and personality changes. Men are particularly susceptible to this aggressive behavior. Headache, restlessness, and insomnia are not infrequent, particularly with higher doses of corticosteroids. Patients and family members and loved ones will benefit from knowing that these effects may occur with therapy. However, a recent prospective study by Jakobsen et al. (2020) found that short courses of methylprednisolone, a corticosteroid, did not affect sleep (see Chapter 41 for Sleep Disorders). Variable increases in blood glucose and decreased glucose tolerance also result from glucocorticoid use. Regular evaluation of blood glucose in patients with diabetes is warranted. Glucocorticoids, especially in large or chronic doses, can increase the susceptibility to and mask infection symptoms, such as fever. The long-term consequences of corticosteroid use can be detrimental to the body. Some of the most serious consequences include muscle wasting, adrenocortical insufficiency, fluid and electrolyte disturbances, cataract formation, and atrophy of bone protein matrix resulting in osteoporosis, vertebral compression fractures, aseptic necrosis of femoral or humeral heads, and pathologic fractures. Whenever possible, chronic corticosteroid use should be curtailed.

Interactions

Glucocorticoids may decrease the effects of barbiturates, hydantoins, rifampin, and ephedrine. Potassium levels should be monitored when glucocorticoids are used with potassium-depleting diuretics.

Cannabinoids

Cannabinoids are indicated only for nausea and vomiting associated with chemotherapy. In the 1970s, it was observed that patients on chemotherapy who smoked marijuana experienced a lower incidence of nausea and vomiting. Investigators then determined that tetrahydrocannabinol (THC) has antiemetic properties.

Mechanism of Action

The true mechanism of action of THC is unknown, but it is most likely related to effects on the vomiting center and the opiate receptors in the CNS and cerebral cortex but probably does not involve the CTZ. The agents available in the United States are dronabinol (Marinol) and nabilone (Cesamet).

Cannabinoids can be used to treat and prevent CINV. Because it is necessary to reach therapeutic blood levels of THC before chemotherapy administration to prevent emesis, administration of the cannabinoids should occur at least 6 to 12 hours before chemotherapy. Emesis can be controlled from mildly to moderately emetogenic chemotherapy regimens, and cannabinoids may provide some relief to patients where other agents have failed. When used mildly to moderately emetogenic regimens, THC has been superior to placebo, prochlorperazine, low-dose metoclopramide, and haloperidol. These agents are seldom frontline therapy because of their incidence and severity of adverse effects.

Patients should be cautioned about the deleterious CNS effects and told not to drive or operate machinery. Dosages can be reduced if the patient is experiencing CNS toxicities. Patients should avoid alcohol and other CNS depressants.

Adverse Events

Most of the adverse effects of the cannabinoids are CNS related and include sedation, ataxia, and dysphoria. Dysphoria may be expressed as confusion, hallucinations, anxiety, fear, memory loss, time distortion, and other undesired occurrences. Orthostatic hypotension, blurred vision, and tachycardia have been observed with the use of these drugs. With repeated doses, the patients usually become tolerant to most of the CNS adverse effects, but not to the antiemetic activity. There is a correlation between antiemetic response and a psychological "high." Younger patients and patients who have had previous experiences with recreational cannabinoids appreciate greater antiemetic efficacy from this drug class. The side effects of the cannabinoids occur more frequently than with many of the other agents and are particularly distressing to older adults. One potentially beneficial adverse effect is appetite stimulation, which may prove useful in hematology and oncology patients. Avoid the use of cannabinoids in pregnancy and lactation due to a lack of human data.

Antacids

Over-the-counter (OTC) antacid preparations may provide relief to patients experiencing mild nausea and vomiting. The general mechanism by which these agents exhibit their effects is by coating the stomach and neutralizing gastric acid. Most preparations contain one or several of the following: calcium carbonate, magnesium hydroxide, aluminum hydroxide, or aluminum carbonate. Between 15 and 30 mL orally of an antacid preparation may provide relief. Patients should be encouraged to seek medical attention if they experience continued nausea and vomiting, and the patient may need a medical workup for more serious GI diseases.

Toxicities from OTC antacids are infrequent, but they do exist. The agents containing magnesium may cause diarrhea; conversely, the agents containing aluminum or calcium may cause constipation. These adverse effects are dose dependent. Calcium-containing antacids can cause phosphate depletion. Caution should be used in patients with renal dysfunction because aluminum and magnesium may accumulate. By coating the GI tract, antacids can decrease the absorption of many oral medications such as digoxin, some antibiotics, corticosteroids, and allopurinol (Zyloprim), leading to reduced efficacy of therapy. (For additional information on antacids, see Chapter 26.)

Selecting the Most Appropriate Agent
Nausea and Vomiting Not Chemotherapy Induced

It is necessary for the practitioner to assess the etiology of nausea and vomiting. If an organic cause can be determined, the reason should be corrected to alleviate the symptoms. For example, if nausea and vomiting are side effects of a medication, discontinue the drug. If the cause is diabetic ketoacidosis, insulin is given. **Figure 25.2** shows the treatment algorithm.

First-Line Therapy

An antiemetic is selected based on patient-specific factors. Initially, a phenothiazine is used for mild-to-moderate nausea and vomiting. Promethazine and prochlorperazine are usually sufficient.

Second-Line Therapy

If the earlier mentioned treatment is not effective, an antihistamine or anticholinergic preparation can be used. These are usually not as effective as phenothiazines but may be useful in mild nausea.

Third-Line Therapy

If the first two therapies are not successful, the patient should be reevaluated for a physiological cause that has not been treated and therapy based on patient data.

Table 25.2 lists the recommended order of treatment for nausea and vomiting.

Chemotherapy-Induced Nausea and Vomiting

Nausea and vomiting are two of the toxicities of chemotherapy that patients fear most. Although not usually a life-threatening complication, uncontrolled nausea or vomiting can significantly affect a patient's quality of life and attitude. Fortunately, new agents and combinations of agents make it possible to control emesis.

The severity of chemotherapy-induced emesis depends on numerous factors. Most significant is the intrinsic ability of the chemotherapy regimen to cause nausea and vomiting. Before the U.S. Food and Drug Administration (FDA) approves a drug for use, phase 1 and 2 studies must be performed to prove efficacy and safety and identify adverse effects. The incidence and severity of nausea and vomiting are initially reported when the drug is given as a single agent. Each chemotherapy agent can be identified as having high, moderately high, moderate, relatively low, and low emetogenic potential. Based on this information, antiemetic regimens can

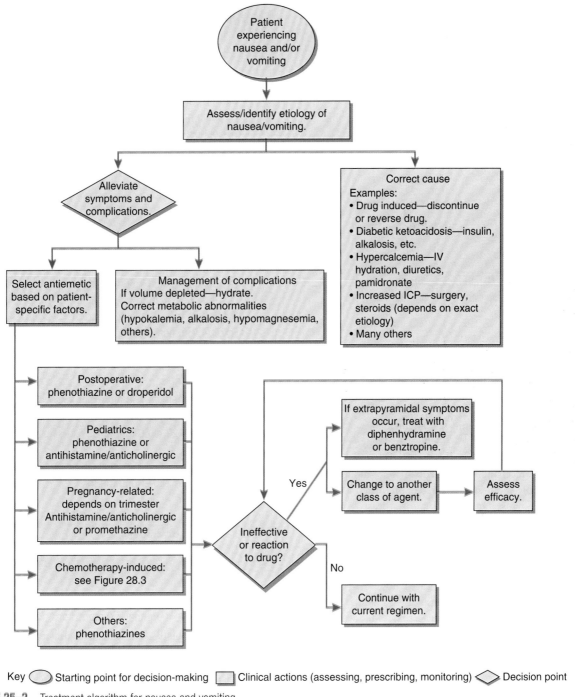

FIGURE 25–2   Treatment algorithm for nausea and vomiting.

be tailored to the chemotherapy regimen to prevent emesis. Mechanisms to identify the emetogenicity of combination chemotherapy regimens are presented in this section. Other factors that may increase the incidence of CINV are previous exposure to chemotherapy, psychosocial factors such as anxiety and depression, low performance status, and younger age (<30 years). A history of alcohol abuse and male sex may correlate with a decreased incidence or severity of nausea and vomiting. The classifications of CINV include acute, delayed, and anticipatory.

Acute Emesis

Acute emesis is vomiting occurring within 24 hours of treatment. The onset of acute emesis is usually within 1 to 2 hours after the start of chemotherapy. It peaks within 4 to 10 hours and resolves within 24 hours, but these factors vary from agent to agent. This most common type of CINV is associated with a higher frequency and severity than the other two classifications. Acute emesis is strongly related to the agent or agents administered and the doses given. (**Box 25.3** identifies the emetogenic potential of specific agents.)

TABLE 25.2
Recommended Order of Treatment for Nausea and Vomiting

Order	Agents	Comments
First line	Phenothiazines	Most frequently used for mild-to-moderate nausea and vomiting Promethazine, prochlorperazine usually effective
Second line	Antihistamine Anticholinergic preparation	Usually not as efficacious as phenothiazines, but may be useful in mild nausea
Third line	Depends on response to other antiemetics	Tailor to patient-specific factors

Note: Consider patient-specific factors when choosing an antiemetic agent.

Highly emetogenic chemotherapy agents are known to induce emesis in greater than 90% of patients receiving that drug without antiemetic premedication. Chemotherapy agents that have moderately high emetogenicity cause emesis in 60% to 90% of patients receiving chemotherapy. Chemotherapy that is moderately emetogenic has an incidence of 30% to 60%, relatively low has a 10% to 30% incidence of emesis, and low emetogenicity is defined as less than 10%.

All patients receiving single agents that are moderately to highly emetogenic should be adequately pretreated to prevent the incidence of nausea and vomiting for at least 24 hours or the expected duration of nausea or vomiting. The current standard of care of antiemetic prophylaxis is the combination of a serotonin antagonist and a corticosteroid, such as granisetron or ondansetron with dexamethasone, at least 30 minutes before chemotherapy administration. Repeated doses may need to be given to prevent and treat emesis for 24 hours, depending on the pharmacokinetics of the agents used. Some practitioners use once-daily administration of serotonin antagonists, claiming that once the receptors are blocked, the duration of receptor binding is the functional component rather than the plasma half-life. Because the purpose of these agents is to prevent nausea and vomiting, and if the patient is not actively experiencing these effects, it is often acceptable to administer antiemetics orally. Combination regimens containing drugs that are moderately to highly emetogenic are given prophylactically in a similar fashion. Although the antiemetic combination is not universally effective, an estimated 70% to 90% of patients experience sufficient control. Examples of challenging clinical situations that may prohibit corticosteroid use include poorly controlled diabetes and uncontrolled hypertension.

Contraindications to serotonin antagonists include hypersensitivity or severe cardiac dysfunction. Alternative prophylactic antiemetics must be chosen for patients who have relative contraindications and are to receive emetogenic chemotherapy.

BOX 25.3
Emetogenic Potential of Chemotherapy Agents

Highly emetogenic (>90%)
  Carmustine more than 250 mg/m^2
  Cisplatin more than 50 mg/m^2
  Cyclophosphamide more than 1,500 mg/m^2
  Dacarbazine
  Lomustine
  Mechlorethamine
  Streptozocin
Moderately high (60%–90%)
  Carboplatin
  Carmustine 250 mg/m^2 or less
  Cisplatin 50 mg/m^2 or less
  Cyclophosphamide 1,500 mg/m^2 or less or 750 mg/m^2 more than
  Cytarabine more than 1,000 mg/m^2
  Doxorubicin more than 60 mg/m^2
  Methotrexate more than 1,000 mg/m^2
  Procarbazine, oral
Moderate (30%–60%)
  Cyclophosphamide 750 mg/m^2 or less
  Cyclophosphamide, oral
  Doxorubicin 20 to 60 mg/m^2
  Idarubicin
  Ifosfamide
  Methotrexate 250–1,000 mg/m^2
  Mitoxantrone
  Topotecan
Moderately low (10%–30%)
  Docetaxel
  Etoposide
  5-fluorouracil
  Gemcitabine
  Methotrexate more than 50 mg/m^2 or <250 mg/m^2
  Mitomycin
  Paclitaxel
Low (<10%)
  Bleomycin
  Busulfan
  Chlorambucil, oral
  Cladribine
  Fludarabine
  Hydroxyurea
  Melphalan, oral
  Thioguanine, oral
  Vinblastine
  Vincristine
  Vinorelbine

High-dose metoclopramide with dexamethasone may be considered an option to a serotonin antagonist with dexamethasone because this was the gold standard for highly emetogenic regimens before the appearance of ondansetron. Once again, the antiemetic regimen should be tailored to the patient and the chemotherapy regimen.

Single-agent or combination chemotherapy regimens that are expected to be moderately low or low in emetogenic potential can be managed less aggressively. These drugs do not warrant the use of a serotonin antagonist. For some chemotherapy regimens and agents, such as the taxanes and fluorouracil, premedication frequently is not necessary; however, patients should be encouraged to use antiemetic medications as needed to control any nausea and vomiting after chemotherapy. Premedication with dexamethasone with or without a phenothiazine or metoclopramide may be used if a patient experiences nausea and vomiting from previous chemotherapy. All these antiemetic drugs may be scheduled for a 24- to 36-hour period to prevent any nausea and vomiting. Patient-specific factors must be considered to identify an appropriate antiemetic regimen.

Regardless of the emetogenicity of a chemotherapy regimen or the use of premedications, antiemetics should be prescribed for as-needed or breakthrough use. The preferred antiemetics are prochlorperazine or metoclopramide, which are effective, inexpensive, and easily administered. These agents provide reliable, safe control of mild nausea. These agents may be used before meals to alleviate anorexia secondary to nausea. Patients should be counseled about these agents' common adverse effects, and each patient should be encouraged to report ineffective control of nausea and vomiting. When adhered to, the basic principles of chemotherapy antiemetic therapy (**Box 25.4**) are tremendously useful.

Delayed Emesis

Delayed nausea and vomiting are defined as emesis that begins or persists more than 24 hours after chemotherapy completion. Some investigators suggest that because there is a "peak" in incidence at 18 hours after cisplatin-based chemotherapy, a revised definition of delayed emesis should include this timetable. The new-found, reliable control of acute emesis from highly to moderately emetogenic chemotherapy regimens has unveiled delayed nausea and vomiting as a more vexing problem. Many chemotherapy agents produce mild delayed nausea and vomiting, but cyclophosphamide, cisplatin, and the anthracyclines are particularly noted for their delayed emesis.

Delayed emesis usually is not as frequent or severe as acute emesis. The mechanism of delayed emesis is believed to be different from that of acute emesis. It is believed that delayed emesis is mediated by neurotransmitters, although serotonin does not play a significant role. Combination antiemetic regimens have proven to be more effective than single-agent therapies. Single-agent serotonin antagonists were found to be equally as effective as metoclopramide or placebo and less effective than dexamethasone, unlike their efficacy in

> ### BOX 25.4 Basic Principles of Chemotherapy Antiemetic Therapy
>
> - Consider emetogenic potential of chemotherapy regimen.
> - Give appropriate antiemetics to prevent nausea and vomiting at least 30 minutes before emetogenic chemotherapy.
> - Schedule antiemetics throughout anticipated period of nausea and vomiting risk.
> - Always prescribe prn antiemetics for breakthrough nausea and vomiting between scheduled doses.
> - Use antiemetic combinations with nonoverlapping mechanisms of action and adverse effects, when possible.
> - Consider patient-specific variables when choosing a regimen (e.g., anxiety, performance status).
> - Reevaluate patients frequently during and between chemotherapy courses for efficacy and toxicity of antiemetic regimen.
> - Consider nonpharmacologic interventions, especially in patients with anticipatory nausea and vomiting.

preventing acute emesis. Regimens identified as most effective for delayed emesis include metoclopramide 0.5 mg/kg orally four times daily for 4 days with dexamethasone 8 mg orally twice a day for 2 days, followed by dexamethasone 4 mg orally twice a day for 2 days.

The use of scheduled phenothiazines (including long-acting phenothiazines) with dexamethasone is another effective option for preventing delayed nausea and vomiting. The addition of a benzodiazepine to the antiemetic regimen may prove useful for the control of emesis in anxious patients or patients with difficulty resting.

Anticipatory Emesis

Anticipatory nausea and vomiting occur in up to 20% to 30% of patients receiving chemotherapy (Molassiotis et al., 2016). It is usually associated with a history of uncontrolled nausea and vomiting with prior chemotherapy and is a conditioned response. Multiple factors can stimulate anticipatory nausea and vomiting, but most aspects remind the patient of the previous unfavorable experience. For example, patients tell stories of becoming nauseated by the sight of their oncologist's office or by a smell that reminds them of receiving chemotherapy. Other triggers may be tastes, sounds, or thoughts of chemotherapy. Anticipatory nausea and vomiting most frequently occur before administering chemotherapy, and it can lead to more inadequate control of nausea and vomiting with subsequent courses. The most effective treatment for delayed nausea and vomiting is prevention. It is crucial to premedicate for highly to moderately emetogenic chemotherapy and to reassess control on a frequent and regular basis. This form of emesis is

TABLE 25.3

Order of Treatment for Chemotherapy-Induced Nausea and Vomiting

Order	Agents	Comments
Acute Prophylaxis for High, Moderately High, and Moderately Emetogenic Regimens		
First line	Serotonin antagonist + dexamethasone	May add other agents as needed
Second line	High-dose metoclopramide + dexamethasone	Prophylaxis for EPS symptoms with metoclopramide
Third line	Depends on response to other antiemetics	Tailor to patient-specific factors
Acute Prophylaxis for Moderately Low and Low Emetogenic Regimens		
First line	No premedication or phenothiazine ± dexamethasone	Depends on chemotherapy regimen
Second line	Metoclopramide ± dexamethasone	Use low-dose metoclopramide
Third line	Depends on response to other antiemetics	Tailor to patient-specific factors
Delayed Nausea and Vomiting		
First line	Metoclopramide + dexamethasone	Continue 3–4 d after chemotherapy
Second line	Long-acting phenothiazine + dexamethasone	Monitor for EPS symptoms
Third line	Depends on response to other antiemetics	Tailor to patient-specific factors

EPS, extrapyramidal symptoms.

frequently refractory to standard antiemetic treatment; however, the benzodiazepines and butyrophenones may provide anxiolysis as well as antiemetogenicity. The addition of one of these agents is strongly encouraged for patients who have had previous unsatisfactory control of nausea and vomiting.

Many practice guidelines are available for the use of antiemetics in CINV. This basis of the guidelines is created by experts and current literature (**Table 25.3** and **Figure 25.3**). To review treatment choices for other types of nausea and vomiting, see **Table 25.2** and **Figure 25.2**.

Special Population Considerations

Pediatric

The treatment of nausea and vomiting in children differs from that in adults. It is crucial in the pediatric population to focus on treating the cause of the problem. The etiology of emesis can vary with age (**Box 25.5**). Because they are smaller, children are predisposed to dehydration and electrolyte abnormalities caused by emesis.

Pediatric patients experience more extrapyramidal or neuromuscular reactions to phenothiazines, mainly when they are administered during an acute viral illness such as chickenpox, measles, or gastroenteritis. Because of its antihistamine quality, promethazine may be a viable phenothiazine option. On a milligram-per-kilogram basis, children experience more extrapyramidal reactions from metoclopramide, even at IV doses as low as 0.5 mg/kg four times daily.

Most antiemetic agents are dosed according to a milligram per kilogram of body weight or the age of the child, and many of the available agents are not recommended for use in patients younger than age 2 or 3. Some agents that are considered safe

and effective in most situations are dimenhydrinate or oral or rectal trimethobenzamide (Tigan; IV not recommended). The phenothiazines are beneficial but should be used cautiously. For pediatric patients receiving chemotherapy, the prevention and treatment of emesis are like that in their adult counterparts, although specific pediatric dosing of the agents applies.

Women

More than 70% of pregnant women experience nausea and vomiting in pregnancy (NVP), especially in the first-trimester gestation; however, they can occur at any time during pregnancy (Fejzo et al., 2017). A few women experience hyperemesis gravidarum, which can present as uncontrollable vomiting with the inability to tolerate oral intake. It is commonly referred to as "morning sickness" but more often 80% of women report it all day.

It has been thought that pregnancy-related emesis is related to the pregnancy hormone human chorionic gonadotropin having CTZ stimulation. A genetic risk factor, GDF15, is being explored as a pathway to the postrema vomiting center; however, further research needs to be completed regarding this theory.

Teratogenicity is the paramount concern when evaluating the safety of an agent in pregnant women. The first trimester of the pregnancy is when drugs or other exogenous substances can most affect embryonic development. Many of the studies performed to study the teratogenic effects of drugs encounter several difficulties. Most fetal malformations occur rarely, and frequently, only a small sample size is obtained and reported. Mothers with underlying diseases, such as seizure disorder, hypertension, diabetes, and cancer, have a higher incidence of

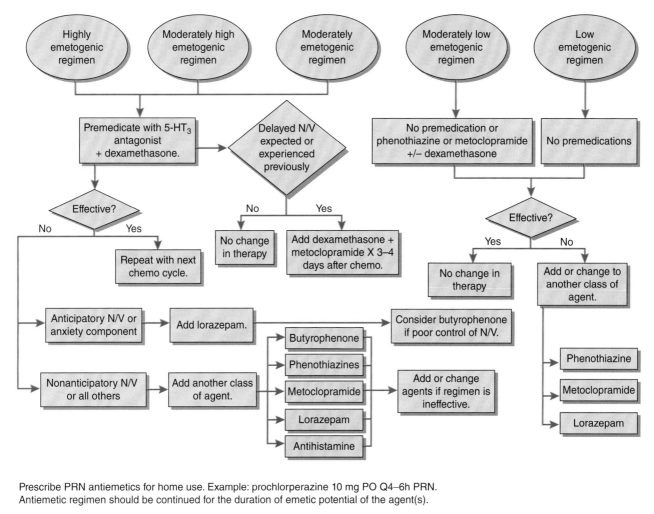

Prescribe PRN antiemetics for home use. Example: prochlorperazine 10 mg PO Q4–6h PRN.
Antiemetic regimen should be continued for the duration of emetic potential of the agent(s).

Key ⬭ Starting point for decision-making ▢ Clinical actions (assessing, prescribing, monitoring) ◇ Decision point

FIGURE 25–3 Treatment algorithm for chemotherapy-induced nausea and vomiting.

infants' malformation. In these patient populations, the role of drugs versus the disease's role in fetal abnormalities is unclear. Recall bias may play a factor in teratogenicity studies as well. Ultimately, the prescriber needs to use current evidence-based information on drugs' safety and risk during pregnancy to make clinical decisions.

Practitioners have several options to treat nausea and vomiting during pregnancy. Approved by the FDA in 2013, the drug most studied in pregnancy is doxylamine/pyridoxine (Dicclegis) and in 2017, Bonjesta. Both are combination pills as the only drugs approved by the FDA to treat nausea and vomiting from pregnancy. It is considered the first line for treatment after attempting conservative measures (American College of Obstetricians and Gynecologists, 2018; DeGeorge & Wiesner, 2017; Ladd, 2017). There are also extensive reassuring studies on ondansetron's fetal safety, but they are contrasted by some studies claiming increased fetal risk.

Other agents that are used for mild-to-moderate NVP include phenothiazines, antihistamine–anticholinergic agents,

metoclopramide, and ondansetron. Antihistamine drugs are generally believed to be safe for the pregnant women and her fetus, although there are incidental findings of malformations in fetuses exposed to antihistamines. Anticholinergic drugs have been proven to cause neonatal meconium ileus. Conversely, some anticholinergic agents such as scopolamine have not been associated with consistent teratogenesis.

Phenothiazines readily cross the placenta, but the bulk of evidence indicates their use is safe in this population. Antacids, such as calcium carbonate, may provide safe and reliable relief from mild nausea. Antihistamines, phenothiazines, metoclopramide, haloperidol, droperidol, and ondansetron have all been used in hyperemesis gravidarum without adverse fetal sequelae. There are also extensive reassuring studies on ondansetron's fetal safety, but they are contrasted by some studies claiming increased fetal risk.

Drug classes that should be avoided in pregnant women are benzodiazepines and cannabinoids. Increased rates of malformations and fetal complications have been associated with the use of these classes of agents; however, the use of other prescribed and illicit drugs by many of these mothers could cloud the picture. Corticosteroids are rarely used for the control of nausea and vomiting in pregnant women. Practitioners must carefully weigh the risks versus benefits of each drug and the presenting situation. The study of prescribing for this patient population is difficult, but an ongoing assessment of safety when prescribing is critical.

MONITORING PATIENT RESPONSE

The best measure of nausea control is how the patient feels. It can be rated as none, mild, moderate, or severe to evaluate nausea more objectively. Another method is to ask the patient to rate nausea on a scale from 0 to 10, with 0 equal to no sickness and 10 equal to severe nausea. These methods may compare nausea from day to day or week to week in the same patient. Episodes per day and volume easily quantify vomiting. If the vomit volume exceeds 200 to 500 mL/d, the patient should be evaluated for electrolyte abnormalities.

PATIENT EDUCATION

It is pivotal to identify the cause of nausea and vomiting and educate the patient about lifestyle actions that help. Many cases of mild nausea and vomiting can be alleviated without additional medications.

Drug Information

Some drugs may be taken with food to avoid GI discomfort, and dietary adjustments may prove to be helpful for some cases of nausea. This knowledge gives patients more control over their well-being. Anxiety and mental illness are components of some occurrences of nausea and vomiting; therefore, counseling and education are the critical components in the treatment of nausea and vomiting of this type. Patients can also be educated about the availability of nonprescription drugs. Realistic goals of nausea control should be set and discussed with the patient.

With antiemetics, usual or severe toxicities should be reviewed with the patient with any other drug therapy. EPS symptoms are frightening and uncomfortable; consequently, patients need to be aware of this potential effect and reversal measures if necessary. Sedation and anticholinergic effects are common with many antiemetics. For most antiemetics, encourage caution when using machinery or driving. The medication's proper administration should be reviewed with the patient; should they take the prescribed medication regularly or only as needed. All of this information ensures that the patient has an optimal benefit from the prescribed medicine.

Nutritional and Lifestyle Changes

Maintenance of proper hydration during all forms of vomiting is important and should be emphasized to patients predisposed to nausea and vomiting (e.g., children, patients following surgery and chemotherapy, patients with GI disorders and infections). Rehydration with clear liquids is preferred over colas, milk, or caffeinated beverages. Patients should be educated on when to seek medical attention because of excessive vomiting or dehydration.

Complementary and Alternative Therapies

Patients suffering from NVP frequently do not receive therapy, in part because of fears of adverse effects of medications on the fetus. Several vitamin-based and herbal treatments are effective and safe. Two randomized trials of vitamin B_6 have shown a benefit in reducing NVP. The recommended daily allowance is 1.3 to 2 mg/d. Women taking prenatal multivitamins are less likely to have severe NVP.

Ginger has been shown to reduce NVP. Ginger appears to work by inhibiting serotonin receptors in the GI tract and CNS. The dose of ginger for the powdered root form in motion sickness is 1 g up to 4 hours before an inciting event; in NVP, 250 mg four times daily; for CINV, 2 to 4 g daily; and for PONV, 1 g 1 hour before anesthesia induction.

Vitamin B_1 (thiamine) deficiency can lead to Wernicke encephalopathy in women with severe NVP. Replacement is needed for all women with vomiting of more than 3 weeks' duration. Prophylaxis with multivitamins and therapy with B_6, with or without doxylamine, are safe and effective therapies for NVP.

FUNCTIONAL BOWEL DISORDERS

Learning Objectives

After reading this section the participant will be able to:
1. Describe the pathophysiology and causes of constipation, diarrhea, and irritable bowel syndrome.
2. Identify the goals of pharmacologic and nonpharmacologic treatment for constipation, diarrhea, and irritable bowel syndrome.
3. Define appropriate symptom monitoring of drug therapy.
4. Distinguish appropriate changes to pharmacologic treatment.

INTRODUCTION

Functional bowel disorders of the lower GI tract can include symptoms of hypogastric cramping, abdominal pain, diarrhea, or constipation. Constipation and diarrhea can be self-limiting or considered symptoms of possibly serious medical problems. Temporary dysfunctions of the bowel can include common GI upsets that can cause short-lived episodes of diarrhea or episodes of constipation. Irritable bowel syndrome (IBS) and chronic idiopathic constipation (CIC) are two of the most common GI complaints globally (Ford et al., 2014; Lacy et al., 2016). Additionally, the increased prescribing of opiates and opioid narcotics has led to an increase in opioid-induced constipation (OIC; Camilleri, 2011; Müller-Lissner et al., 2016). IBS typically presents with vague, crampy hypogastric pain and can be accompanied by constipation, diarrhea, and/or alternating patterns, while CIC presents with issues of stool consistency and problems with defecation but without the presence of abdominal pain. Similar pharmacologic agents are used to treat the symptoms of IBS, CIC, OIC, or diarrhea, whether self-limited or chronic.

CONSTIPATION

Constipation is a common GI symptom that is defined as infrequent or difficult evacuation of stool. Every individual affected by constipation defines it differently, but normal defecation can vary from daily to three times daily or to every 3 days. Constipation can be a consequence of multiple factors, including diet, lifestyle, medications, and many disease states. In a systematic review of the epidemiology of constipation globally, the mean prevalence of constipation in the general population was found to be 14% to 16% (Black & Ford, 2018; Footoran et al., 2018). Constipation affects 2.2 females to 1 male, and the incidence increases with age, especially in those over age 65. Sommers et al. (2015) report a 41.5% increase of emergency room visits and ambulatory care visits for constipation between 2006 and 2011. The incidence of constipation in children is reported between 0.7% and 29% worldwide with prevalence equal between boys and girls (Rajindrajith et al., 2016). Dietary and lifestyle modifications are the preferred therapy for constipation, but many patients use OTC laxatives for relief. Americans spend over $290 million billion for OTC and prescription laxatives and over $7.5 billion annually for treatment (Pomeranz et al., 2013). Most of these laxatives are considered safe and effective, but overuse or abuse may have serious consequences.

Causes

Constipation is a diagnosis based on a thorough history and physical examination. If an identifiable cause is present, constipation is then classified as a secondary symptom. However, constipation may be a symptom of an underlying disease state (**Box 25.6**). The patient's lifestyle (e.g., diet, inactivity) or concomitant medications (**Box 25.7**) may also contribute to constipation. CIC is usually caused by a reduction in the propulsive capacity of the colon (slow transit constipation) or a functional outlet. Another cause of constipation is from the use of opioid drugs and is classified as OIC. Although constipation is often a benign condition, it can be a symptom of a more serious problem. If left untreated in an older patient, constipation may lead to impaction, stercoral ulceration, anal fissures, megacolon, volvulus, and possibly carcinoma of the colon.

BOX 25.6 Disorders Associated with Constipation

Bowel obstruction	Irritable bowel syndrome
Colonic tumors	Megacolon
Depression	Parkinsonism
Diabetes	Spinal injury
Diverticulitis	Stroke
Hypercalcemia	Uremia
Hypothyroidism	

BOX 25.7 Selected Medication Associated with Constipation

Activated charcoal	Diuretics
Antacids (aluminum or calcium containing)	Ferrous salts
	HMG-CoA reductase inhibitors (i.e., statins)
Anticholinergics (sedating)	Narcotic analgesics
Antihistamines	Sodium polystyrene sulfonate
Antipsychotics	Sucralfate
Bile acid sequestrants	Tricyclic antidepressants
Calcium supplements	Verapamil
Clonidine	

Pathophysiology

The absorptive capacity and motility of the colon are major factors of bowel function. Approximately 9 L of fluid enters the small intestine daily from ingestion or intestinal secretions. The small intestine absorbs approximately 80% of this fluid load, which is approximately half of its capacity. The colon absorbs the remainder, except for approximately 0.1 L of water that is passed in the stool. If absorption of the small intestine is reduced, the fluid load adds to the burden of the colon, which can absorb 4 to 5 L of fluid per day. Fluid in excess of this amount results in diarrhea. Likewise, excessive reabsorption of water results in constipation.

The colon can be divided into three distinctive functional areas: (1) the cecum and proximal colon, (2) the transverse colon, and (3) the distal colon and rectum. Each area performs different roles in preparing the chyme for expulsion. The variation in the neurogenic tone of each area affects the capacity of the colon to retain or release the fecal material.

The motility of the bowel is affected by the flow of chyme from the coloileal reflex, and its visceral hypersensitivity can contribute to the sense of urgency and tenesmus of proximal colonic transit. The neurogenic aspects of colon motility are poorly understood and need further study. Some of the stimuli thought to affect colonic activity are awakening from sleep or rest, ingestion of a high-calorie meal, and the sight or smell of food.

With OIC, the opioid receptors in the gut are mediated from the CNS and reduce GI propulsion, thereby altering the autonomic outflow. Additionally, this reduces bowel tone and contractility, ultimately prolonging transit time of the stool. Other characteristics of OIC include increased anal sphincter tone and decreased response to anal distention resulting in difficulty with evacuation.

Diagnostic Criteria

The definition of constipation varies widely between health care providers and patients. Constipation, as previously noted, can be idiopathic or caused by medications, or in rare cases organic. Therefore, a function definition is the infrequent bowel movements accompanied by straining with hard feces that lead to straining and a feeling of incomplete evacuation of the rectum. An important distinction between CIC and IBS is the absence of abdominal pain associated with the bowel pattern.

The diagnosis of constipation stems primarily from the history. A careful history (**Box 25.8**) can help the provider decide which diagnostic tests, if any, may be appropriate. Alarm symptoms include a sudden change in bowel habits after the age of 50 years, blood in stools, anemia, weight loss, and a family history of colon cancer and require further workup.

Initiating Drug Therapy

Lifestyle modifications are preferred over pharmacologic therapy for treating constipation. Diet, exercise, and bowel habit training are usually targeted. However, research is inconclusive as to the value of increasing fluid intake and exercise and is

BOX 25.8	History and Physical Examination for Chronic Constipation

Important history questions:
Onset and duration of symptoms
Patient's definition of constipation
Presence of abdominal cramping relieved by defecation (*if yes, think IBS*)
Presence of blood in the stool

Important aspects of the physical examination:
Evaluation of the perianal area for scars, fistulas, fissures, and external hemorrhoids
Observe the perineum at rest and while the patient is bearing down.
Digital rectal examination—check for fecal impaction, stricture, or rectal masses.

controversial for the increased use of fiber (Emmanuel et al., 2016). The recommendations for dietary fiber originated in 1971 (Burkitt, 1993) and gained widespread acceptance as necessary for a healthy diet and normal bowel movements; however, further study has not substantiated this premise. However, increasing fiber has not proven harmful, and according to the National Health Statistics Report (Clarke et al., 2015), Americans eat 5 to 14 g of fiber daily, far short of the most recent recommendations of 20 to 35 g by the American Dietetic Association (Slavin, 2008). Increased dietary fiber can be recommended for most patients without fear of colon obstruction. Fiber should be both soluble and insoluble in the form of fruits, vegetables, and whole grains, which cannot be digested by the body. Fiber should be slowly increased to 20 to 25 g/d over a 1- to 2-week period to improve compliance with therapy. Dietary fiber is still postulated to increase stool weight and shorten intestinal transit time. Fiber accelerates right colon transit, but there are few treatments for patients where the transit problem is with the left colon. Fiber therapy may not be effective for all patients.

One additional lifestyle modification includes establishing a regular pattern for bathroom visits especially with the older adults. Patients should also be counseled not to ignore the urge to defecate, because this delay increases the time for absorption of fluid from the stool. Biofeedback, a method of retraining the pelvic floor muscles to relax during defecation, may be effective in selected patients.

Measures to treat patients with OIC currently mirror those of acute and chronic constipation; however, there is little research that supports this approach.

Goals of Drug Therapy

An adequate trial of lifestyle modification should be attempted first. If this fails, pharmacologic management with laxatives may be appropriate; however, there is little evidence that laxatives cause dependency and should be withheld from long-term treatment (McRorie et al., 2020; Wald, 2007).

The goal of therapy for constipation is to increase the water content of the feces and increase motility of the intestines to promote comfortable defecation, using the lowest effective dose of a laxative for the least amount of time possible. Only if a patient fails therapy for 3 to 6 months, should the health care provider consider ordering colon transit studies to evaluate the transit time of stool in the intestine (Basson, 2020). Responses to laxatives vary and depend on the patient as well as the preparation. Several classes of laxatives are available for the symptomatic treatment of constipation: bulk-forming agents, saline laxatives, lubricant laxatives, surfactants (emollients), hyperosmotic laxatives, and stimulant laxatives. Proper selection of a laxative should be based on the individual clinical situation (**Table 25.4**).

Bulk-Forming Laxatives

Bulk-forming laxatives work by binding to the fecal contents and pulling water into the stool. This ultimately softens and lubricates the stool, eases its passage, and reduces straining.

Water is reabsorbed from fecal masses that stay in the colon for extended periods, and the result is dry stools. Bulk-forming agents hold water in the stool or swell and increase stool bulk. The bulk stimulates the movement of the intestines and facilitates the passage of intestinal contents. These types of laxatives are not useful when constipation results from the use of opioid medications.

Bulk-forming laxatives generally consist of psyllium seed husk, methylcellulose, polycarbophil, and wheat dextrin, which are made of polysaccharides, cellulose derivatives, or wheat starch such as methylcellulose (Citrucel) or psyllium (Metamucil). Polycarbophil (FiberCon) and wheat dextrin (Benefiber) have significant water-absorptive properties and are used as antidiarrheals. All bulk-forming agents used for constipation should be taken with plenty of fluid (8 ounces) to increase efficacy. Malt soup extract (Maltsupex) made from barley malt reduces fecal pH. This may contribute to its laxative effect. Traditionally, these products have been marketed only as powders, which must be dissolved in water. Now, many fiber products are available in powder, wafer, caplet, and gummy forms. Patients may need to try several before finding one that

TABLE 25.4

Overview of Selected Laxatives and Atypical Agents

Generic (Trade) Name and Dosage	Selected Adverse Events	Contraindications	Special Considerations
Bulk-Forming Laxatives			
Methylcellulose (Citrucel) 2–6 g/d	Flatulence, stomach upset, fullness	GI obstruction	Take with plenty of water. Avoid in patients with GI ulceration
Psyllium (Metamucil) 3.4–10.2 g/d	Same as those for Methylcellulose	Same as those for Methylcellulose	Same as those for Methylcellulose Sugar-free formulation caution with phenylketonuria
Polycarbophil (FiberCon) 1–6 g/d	Same as those for Methylcellulose	Same as those for Methylcellulose	Same as those for Methylcellulose Calcium content may interact with tetracycline or quinolone antibiotics
Malt soup extract (Maltsupex) 12–64 g/d	Same as those for Methylcellulose	Same as those for Methylcellulose	Same as those for Methylcellulose
Wheat dextrin	Same as those for Methylcellulose	Same as those for Methylcellulose	Shelf life of 2 y
(Benefiber) Powder: 1 tbsp daily for age 6 and up Chewables: Age 12—adult: three tabs TID Ages 6–11: 1½ tabs TID		Not a good choice for those with possible celiac disease	Store in a cool environment. Less flatulence production than other bulking agents
Lubricants and Surfactants			
Mineral oil 5–45 mL/d	Rectal seepage, irritation	Do not use with surfactants	Impairs absorption of fat-soluble vitamins Caution in older adults and very young due to potential for development of lipid pneumonia
Docusate sodium (Colace) 50–500 mg/d	Stomach upset	Do not use with mineral oil	Most effective at preventing "straining" in high-risk patients (see text)

(Continued)

TABLE 25.4

Overview of Selected Laxatives and Atypical Agents (*Continued*)

Generic (Trade) Name and Dosage	Selected Adverse Events	Contraindications	Special Considerations
Docusate calcium (Surfak) 50–240 mg	Same as those for Docusate sodium	Same as those for Docusate sodium	Same as those for Docusate sodium
Docusate potassium (Dialose) 100–300 mg	Same as those for Docusate sodium	Same as those for Docusate sodium	Same as those for Docusate sodium
Saline Agents			
Sodium phosphate enema (Fleet) 118 mL/d Only one enema in 24 h	Alterations in fluid/electrolyte balance, diarrhea	Caution in patients with congestive heart failure, hypertension, edema, and renal dysfunction	Care should be taken in the older adults and those with existing electrolyte disturbances
Magnesium citrate 240 mL/d	GI upset, diarrhea	Caution in renal dysfunction	Stagger administration times of tetracycline and quinolone antibiotics
Magnesium hydroxide (Phillips' milk of magnesia) 30–60 mL/d	GI upset, diarrhea	Same as those for Magnesium citrate	Caution in renal dysfunction and the older adults Stagger administration times of tetracycline and quinolone antibiotics
Magnesium sulfate (Epsom salt) 1–2 tsp in ½ glass water	GI upset, diarrhea	Same as those for Magnesium citrate	Caution in renal dysfunction and the older adults Stagger administration times of tetracycline and quinolone antibiotics
Hyperosmotic Agents			
Lactulose (Chronulac, Constilac, Duphalac) 15–60 mL	GI upset, diarrhea, flatulence	Caution in patients with diabetes	Use lactulose with caution in patients with diabetes
Sorbitol 130–150 mL	GI upset, diarrhea, flatulence	Same as those for Lactulose	Caution in patients with diabetes
Stimulants			
Senna (Senokot) Tabs: 2–8/d Supp: 1 QHS Granules: 1–4 tsp/d	Griping, diarrhea, gas, discoloration of urine	GI obstruction	Caution for laxative abuse, cathartic colon
Bisacodyl (Dulcolax) Tabs: 1–3/d Supp: 1 pr daily	Griping, diarrhea, gas	GI obstruction	Do not crush or chew tablets Avoid concomitant administration of antacids and pH-lowering agents
Castor oil 15–60 mL/d	Stomach upset, diarrhea, colic	GI obstruction	Too potent for routine use
Secretagogues—Chloride Channel Activators			
Lubiprostone (Amitiza) 24-mcg capsule BID	Nausea is most common, diarrhea, abdominal pain, abdominal distention, and flatulence.	Known or suspected GI mechanical obstruction	Approved for both genders only for CIC/OIC Capsules must be taken whole and with food and water
Guanylate Cyclase-C Agonist Linaclotide (Linzess) 145 mg capsule daily	Diarrhea, abdominal pain, flatulence, and abdominal distention	Avoid in known or suspected mechanical obstruction.	Dose is different for IBS-C Dose is different for IBS-C Avoid in children <6 years old, but use with caution in 6–17 y
Peripherally Acting Mu-Opioid Receptor Antagonist (PAMORA)			
Naloxegol (Movantik) 12.5–25 mg tab one daily	Abdominal pain, diarrhea, nausea, flatulence, vomiting headache, and hyperhidrosis	Same as those for Guanylate Cyclase-C Agonist Linaclotide	Pregnancy Category C: can cause narcotic withdrawal for fetus Can cause narcotic withdrawal especially with methadone

CIC, chronic idiopathic constipation; GI, gastrointestinal; IBS-C, irritable bowel syndrome-constipation; OIC, opioid-induced constipation.

works for them. Brand names include Metamucil, FiberCon, and Citrucel. Metamucil is the preferred agent because it is the safest and most physiologic. Sugar-free methylcellulose and psyllium products are available for patients with diabetes. Patients with celiac disease or gluten intolerance should avoid using wheat dextrin products.

Contraindications to the use of bulking agents are symptoms of an acute surgical abdomen, intestinal obstruction or perforation, or inability to drink an adequate amount of fluid.

Action for all agents may begin in 12 to 24 hours, but a full effect is not usually seen for up to 3 days.

A half-cup to one bowl daily of wheat bran can provide adequate fiber supplementation, but synthetic forms of fiber are often better absorbed than food. Other foods can also add fiber to the diet and should be reviewed with the patient. The patient should be encouraged to drink adequate amounts of fluid throughout the day; if not contraindicated, up to 2,500 mL is preferred. These agents are more likely to be used as preventive measures. However, given, they can take effect within 12 to 24 hours, and some acute relief of symptoms is possible.

Adverse Events

Overall, these agents are usually well tolerated, but compliance can be a problem because the most common side effect is increased flatulence, and some bloating can occur. With severe constipation, all agents can cause abdominal fullness and cramping. If these agents are used excessively, nausea and vomiting may occur.

Contraindications

Because bulk-forming laxatives have the most physiologic effect and are not systemically absorbed, they are the preferred agents for symptomatic treatment of constipation. However, these agents are not completely benign and should be avoided in patients with strictures of the esophagus, GI ulcerations, or stenosis secondary to the possibility of obstruction from increased bulk of intestinal contents. In addition, some bulk-forming agents may contain as much as 20 g of carbohydrates per dose. Sugar-free bulk-forming agents are available and are recommended for patients with diabetes.

Interactions

The sugar-free preparations may contain aspartame, which is metabolized to phenylalanine and should be used cautiously with patients who must restrict their phenylalanine intake. Wheat gluten is a by-product of extracting the gluten from wheat; however, complete extraction cannot be guaranteed and should be avoided in patients with gluten intolerance. Concomitant administration of calcium-containing bulk laxatives may reduce the effectiveness of quinolone or tetracycline, so patients should separate the administration time of these agents.

Hyperosmotic Laxatives

Lactulose (Cephulac), sorbitol, polyethylene glycol–electrolyte solution (PEG-ES, Colyte), and polyethylene glycol (PEG, MiraLAX) are examples of hyperosmotic laxatives. These agents serve as or are metabolized to solutes in the intestinal tract. The increased concentration of solutes creates osmotic pressure by drawing fluid from a less concentrated gradient to the more concentrated gradient inside the GI tract. This increase in osmotic pressure stimulates intestinal motility and propulsion of fecal contents. The PEG products do not degrade colonic bacteria and therefore produce less bloating. Glycerin (Colace Suppository, Fleet Glycerin Suppository, and Pedia-Lax Suppository) not only helps the stool to evacuate by similar mechanisms, but also provides local rectal stimulation.

In addition to its osmotic effect, glycerin also has a local irritant effect in the suppository form. The irritant action adds to the osmotic action to stimulate bowel movement.

Lactulose is a disaccharide analog that is metabolized by bacteria to acids that increase osmotic pressure and acidify the contents of the colon. The result is increased intestinal motility and secretion.

In addition to its use for the symptomatic treatment of constipation, sorbitol is also used to prevent constipation in combination with activated charcoal for poisoning. Sodium polystyrene sulfonate (Kayexalate), a cation-exchange resin used for treating hyperkalemia, is often combined with sorbitol to reduce the potential for constipation from the resin.

PEG-ES is a nonabsorbable solution that acts as an osmotic agent. It is usually used to evacuate the bowel before a GI examination such as a flexible sigmoidoscopy or colonoscopy. The solution is reconstituted with 1 gallon of tap water and should be chilled before consumption to increase palatability. The patient should begin drinking the solution at 4 PM the day before the procedure. One glass (8 oz) of the reconstituted solution should be consumed every 10 minutes over 3 hours until all 4 L are consumed. The patient should fast for 4 hours before ingesting the solution, and only clear liquids are allowed after ingestion.

Contraindications

Lactulose syrup should be used with caution in patients with diabetes because it contains lactose and galactose. Lactose is also contraindicated in patients with appendicitis, acute surgical abdomen, fecal impaction, or intestinal obstruction. Caution must be used in patients with diabetes because of sugar content.

Other osmotic agents such as magnesium hydroxide (milk of magnesia) or magnesium citrate (Citroma) can be used to promote defecation. Approximately 15% to 30% of the magnesium in these agents may be absorbed systemically; therefore, caution is needed in patients who have renal failure and decreased ability to excrete magnesium.

When taken appropriately, these agents are well tolerated. The most common adverse events are abdominal cramping and nausea. However, the use of these agents may be counterproductive in patients with changes in colonic transit time, IBS, or severe bloating and fullness (Wald, 2007).

In addition, sorbitol as a caloric sweetener has the potential to affect blood glucose levels and should be used with caution in patients with diabetes. PEG-ES is not recommended in patients with gastric obstruction, bowel perforation, or colitis.

Adverse Reactions

Glycerin is among the safest laxative preparations available and is often used in infants and children. Rectal irritation is the most common side effect of glycerin suppositories. The most common side effects associated with lactulose and sorbitol include GI upset and diarrhea. PEG-ES rapidly cleanses the bowel and often causes nausea, abdominal fullness, cramps, and bloating.

Interactions

There are few documented interactions with the osmotic laxatives. However, because antacids may neutralize the acids produced from lactulose and interfere with its mechanism of action, concomitant administration of antacids should be avoided with lactulose. No other medications should be given within 1 hour of consumption of PEG-ES because the medication will likely be flushed from the GI tract.

Saline Laxatives

Like hyperosmotic laxatives, saline laxatives draw water into the intestine through osmosis. This creates an increase in intraluminal pressure and a resultant increase in intestinal motility. Magnesium citrate (citrate of magnesia), magnesium hydroxide (Phillips' milk of magnesia), magnesium sulfate (Epsom salt), sodium phosphate, and sodium biphosphate (Fleet enemas) are examples of saline laxatives (see **Table 25.4**). For treatment of constipation, the dose of sodium phosphate as an enema should not exceed the recommended volume or more than one dose in 24 hours. Magnesium citrate and sodium phosphate and biphosphate are used as bowel evacuants for endoscopic examinations such as flexible sigmoidoscopy or colonoscopy.

Contraindications

Oral sodium phosphate is no longer on the market due to concerns about severe electrolyte imbalances. However, the enema version still exists, but caution in administration should still be exercised. When prescribing sodium phosphate enemas, care should be exercised with individuals who are at higher risk for complications, including young children, individuals over 55 years of age, and those who are dehydrated; have kidney dysfunction or inflammation of the bowel; or are taking medications that can affect the kidneys. In addition, phosphates can accumulate in patients with renal dysfunction, leading to serious complications such as hyperphosphatemia, hypokalemia, hypocalcemia, hypernatremia, metabolic acidosis, and coma.

Magnesium hydroxide and magnesium sulfate are commonly used for the symptomatic treatment of constipation. Because the kidneys eliminate magnesium, magnesium-containing laxatives should be used with caution in the older adults and in patients with decreased renal function. Excessive magnesium levels can result in CNS depression (drowsiness), muscle weakness, decreased blood pressure, and ECG changes.

Adverse Events

Dehydration is a concern with the use of saline laxatives, and these agents must be used with caution in patients who cannot tolerate excessive fluid loss and dehydration.

Interactions

Because milk of magnesia also has antacid properties and can increase the pH of the intestines, it should not be administered at the same time with agents that require an acidic environment to be absorbed. The most common example of this type of interaction is with the antifungals itraconazole (Sporanox) and ketoconazole (Nizoral). Therefore, administration of any antacid should be separated from administration of ketoconazole or itraconazole by at least 2 hours. In addition, the magnesium found in magnesium hydroxide and magnesium sulfate can bind with tetracycline and quinolone antibiotics to form a nonabsorbable complex that may reduce the effectiveness of the antibiotics. Administration of quinolones and tetracyclines should be separated from administration of magnesium-containing compounds.

Stimulant Laxatives

These laxatives vary in effects but act by increasing peristalsis through direct effects on the smooth muscle of the intestines and simultaneously promoting fluid accumulation in the colon and small intestine. Because of the irritating effect of the agents on the musculature, these agents should be avoided in long-term treatment. Stimulant laxatives include bisacodyl (Dulcolax) and senna concentrates (Senokot, Senokot S). Previously, long-term use of stimulant laxatives has been speculated to be addictive and can create permanent injury to the colonic mucosa; however, the research does not support this premise (Kamm et al., 2011).

Contraindications

As with other laxatives, stimulants are contraindicated in patients with appendicitis, acute surgical abdomen, fecal impaction, or intestinal obstruction. Rectal fissures and hemorrhoids can be exacerbated by stimulation of defecation. Action begins 6 to 10 hours after oral administration and 15 minutes to 2 hours after rectal administration.

Adverse Events

These agents are not as well tolerated as the osmotic laxatives or bulking agents because of their side effects, which include nausea, vomiting, and abdominal cramping. These side effects can be more severe with cases of severe constipation. Long-term or excessive use can lead to laxative dependence.

Surfactant Laxatives

This class of laxatives reduces the surface tension of the liquid contents of the bowel. Ultimately, this promotes incorporation of additional liquid into the stool, forming a softer mass, and promotes easier defecation. However, stool softeners have insufficient data to support their efficacy, and fiber products may be superior to improve stool frequency. Examples of this class include docusate sodium (Colace) and docusate calcium (Surfak). For patients who should not strain during defecation, this is the laxative of choice. Emollient laxatives only prevent constipation; they do not treat it. Combining these agents with fiber products helps promote defecation. Administration of emollient laxatives concomitantly with mineral oil is contraindicated because of increased absorption of the mineral oil. Action with these agents usually occurs between 1 and 3 days.

Contraindications

Docusate calcium or docusate potassium may be recommended for patients on sodium-restricted diets (e.g., hypertension, congestive heart failure). The sodium content of Colace (docusate sodium) is quite small (5.2 mg/capsule) and is likely insignificant.

Adverse Events

These agents are extremely well tolerated when used to prevent constipation. The most common side effect is stomach upset; other side effects, such as mild abdominal cramping, diarrhea, and throat irritation, are infrequent. Patients should take surfactants with plenty of water to improve effectiveness.

Interactions

Docusate, as a surfactant emollient laxative, may increase the absorption of mineral oil and potentially increase the risk for liver toxicity; therefore, this combination should be avoided.

Lubricant Laxatives

Mineral oil (liquid paraffin) coats and softens the stool and prevents reabsorption of water from the stool by the colon. Lubricant laxatives are effective at preventing straining in high-risk patients (e.g., rectal surgery, labor and delivery, stroke, hemorrhoids, hernia, myocardial infarction).

Contraindications

Mineral oil may be aspirated and cause lipid pneumonia when administered to young, older adults, or bedridden patients. With the availability of safer laxative preparations, mineral oil should probably be avoided in these populations. If mineral oil is chosen, it should not be administered to patients before bedtime or when they are reclining to prevent aspiration.

Adverse Events

Mineral oil has an unpleasant taste, and because it is not absorbed, large single doses can seep through the anal sphincter and cause irritation. Dividing doses may prevent this.

Interactions

Mineral oil can impair the absorption of fat-soluble vitamins A, D, E, and K. Because warfarin (Coumadin) interferes with the synthesis of vitamin K–dependent clotting factors, a reduction in absorption of vitamin K may increase the effects of the anticoagulant. Although no direct interactions with oral anticoagulants have been reported, prothrombin levels may decrease. The docusates, as surfactant emollient laxatives, may increase the absorption of mineral oil and potentially increase the risk for liver toxicity; therefore, this combination should be avoided.

Secretagogues

Chloride Channel Activators

There is one drug in this class, lubiprostone (Amitiza), that acts on the intestinal lumen and acts to increase intestinal fluid and accelerate colon transit. While the entire mechanism is not understood, it appears to work by enhancing chloride-rich intestinal fluid without altering serum sodium and potassium concentrations. The drug is poorly absorbed systemically and appears to act locally on the intestines, improving stool consistency and motility. Lubiprostone is approved for treatment of adults, men and women with chronic constipation or OIC (see **Table 25.4**).

Contraindications

Lubiprostone is contraindicated in patients with potential mechanical obstruction, severe diarrhea, or hypersensitivity to components of the product. It is contraindicated for children and adolescents <18 years of age.

Adverse Events

Nausea is the most common side effect of lubiprostone. The rate of nausea is dose dependent and was experienced by approximately 29% of patients. Other common GI side effects include diarrhea, abdominal pain, abdominal distention, and flatulence. The most reported neurologic side effect is headache.

Interactions

No drug–drug interactions have been discovered with lubiprostone. In vitro studies showed the cytochrome P-450 isoenzymes are not inhibited by the drug.

Guanylate Cyclase-C Agonist

Linaclotide (Linzess) was the first of this class for the indications of CIC and IBS. In 2017, it was joined by plecanatide (Trulance). The mechanism of action of both is topical rather than system, elevating intracellular cyclic guanosine monophosphate (cGMP), which stimulates secretion of chloride and bicarbonate into the intestinal lumen. Along with the increased fluid, stool transit time is accelerated. Linzess is approved for 18 years and older with CIC.

Contraindications

Linaclotide and plecanatide is contraindicated for children less than 6 years old, and while it may be used off-label, the safety and efficacy between 6 and 17 years old has not been established. The drug should not be used if the patient has known or suspected mechanical obstruction.

Adverse Events

The most common side effect for both drugs is diarrhea, reported by 20% of study participants. Other GI side effects include abdominal pain, flatulence, and abdominal distention. Some (4%) reported headache.

Interactions

Since linaclotide and plecanatide do not interact with the cytochrome P-450 system, no drug–drug interactions have been studied. Administration of recommended clinical doses is encouraged by the prescriber.

Peripherally Acting Mu-opioid Receptor Antagonist

This class acts as antagonist of opioid binding at the mu-opioid receptors. At the prescribed dose, in the GI tract, these agents block the constipating effects of opioids. There are two drugs in this class, naloxegol (Movantik) and naldemedine (Symproic). They are a PEGylated derivative of naloxone and a substrate for the P-glycoprotein transporter. This reduces the passive permeability across the blood–brain barrier and with recommended doses limits potential for interference with centrally mediated opioid analgesia. The indications for naloxegol and naldemedine is OIC.

Contraindications

Naloxegol and naldemedine are contraindicated in patients with known or suspected GI obstruction or potential for GI perforation. Some patients can experience opioid withdrawal especially those who are receiving methadone. Caution is advised during pregnancy when using either naloxegol or naldemedine due to the potential cause withdrawal for the unborn fetus.

Adverse Reactions

The most common reactions are related to the GI system and include abdominal pain, diarrhea, nausea, flatulence, vomiting headache, and hyperhidrosis.

Interactions

Avoid concomitant use of moderate CYP3A4 inhibitors (e.g., diltiazem, erythromycin, verapamil) due to potential increased risk of adverse reactions. Use of strong CYP3A4 inducers (e.g., rifampin, carbamazepine, St. John's wort) is not recommended because they may decrease the efficacy of naloxegol or naldemedine. Avoid concomitant use of either drug with another opioid antagonist due to the increased risk of opioid withdrawal.

Serotonin-4 (5-HT₄) Receptor Agonist

There have been other drugs in this class that were consequently pulled from the market due to effects of cardiac arrhythmias. A new drug in this class, prucalopride (Motegrity), was approved by the FDA in 2018 for the treatment of CIC. Prucalopride, a selective serotonin type 4 (5-HT$_4$) receptor agonist, is a GI prokinetic agent that stimulates colonic peristalsis (high-amplitude propagating contractions), which increases bowel motility. There was no increase of cardiovascular risks with prucalopride (Motegrity).

Contraindications

Prucalopride (Motegrity) is contraindicated in patients with potential mechanical obstruction, severe diarrhea, or hypersensitivity to components of the product. A history of hypersensitivity to prucalopride (Motegrity) includes reactions such as dyspnea, rash, pruritus, urticaria, and facial edema.

Adverse Reactions

The most common adverse reactions include headache at 20%, abdominal pain 16%, nausea 15%, and diarrhea 13%. Monitor patients for suicidal ideation and behavior as well as self-injurious ideation and new onset or worsening of depression. Instruct patients to discontinue prucalopride (Motegrity) immediately and contact their health care provider if they experience any unusual changes in mood or behavior or they experience emerging suicidal thoughts or behaviors.

Interactions

There are no reported drug–drug interactions with prucalopride (Motegrity). Checking for drug–drug interactions is encouraged by the prescriber.

Selecting the Most Appropriate Agent

If lifestyle modification fails to reverse constipation, then selection of an appropriate laxative is necessary. The choice of laxative agent depends on several factors, including the type of constipation (acute, CIC, or OIC), medical history, goal of therapy, concomitant medications, and the potential for side effects, age, and personal preference. **Table 25.4** describes first-, second-, and third-line therapies (**Figure 25.4**).

First-Line Therapy

For all types of constipation, acute, CIC, and OIC, a bulk-forming laxative is recommended, provided no contraindications exist. Bulk-forming laxatives are not systemically absorbed. In addition, their pharmacologic effect is the most physiologic, meaning they have an effect like that of the natural effect of fiber from food on the GI tract. Their side effects are usually mild, and if necessary, they can be administered safely for longer durations than other classes of laxatives such as the stimulants.

When hard or dry stools are the chief complaint or in situations where straining should be avoided (e.g., hernia, cardiovascular disease), a stool softener such as docusate is considered first-line therapy. Stool softeners also are not systemically absorbed, and their side effects are usually minimal.

Glycerin suppositories have a local irritant effect on the rectum and are probably the safest of all preparations. This is preferred as first-line therapy in infants.

Linaclotide (Linzess) and lubiprostone (Amitiza) can be considered as first-line therapy for constipation, especially if it is CIC. Both drugs can increase the incidence of diarrhea, but overall are very well tolerated and have no reported drug–drug interactions. These drugs have been proven to produce rapid and sustained improvement in bowel habits.

For OIC, naldemedine (Symproic) is considered first-line therapy along with bulk-forming laxatives and dietary approaches. Lubiprostone (Amitiza) also has the indication for OIC.

Second-Line Therapy

If a more rapid onset of action is desired, magnesium hydroxide may be chosen. Although it has a faster onset of action, dehydration from excessive use is a concern, particularly in patients unable to tolerate excessive fluid loss. In addition, magnesium-containing preparations should be avoided in patients with renal insufficiency or the older adults.

If the bulk-forming agents and magnesium hydroxide are ineffective or contraindicated, an osmotic laxative such as lactulose or sorbitol may be chosen. However, flatulence

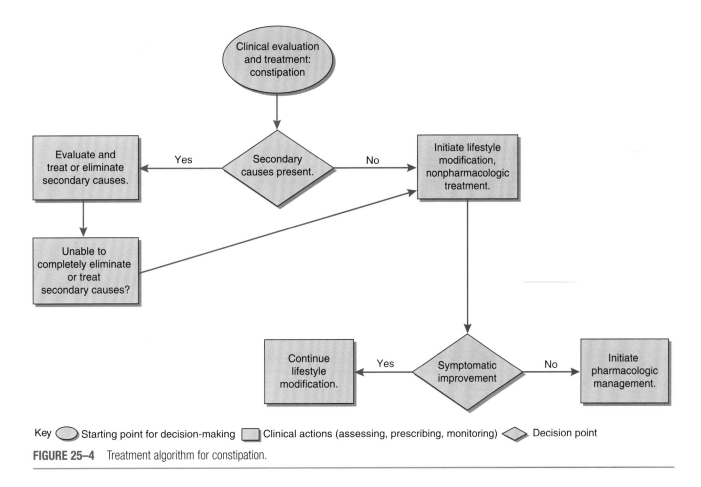

Key ⬭ Starting point for decision-making ▢ Clinical actions (assessing, prescribing, monitoring) ◇ Decision point

FIGURE 25–4 Treatment algorithm for constipation.

and the sweet taste limit compliance. In addition, lactulose and sorbitol should be used with caution in patients with diabetes.

If not used as first-line therapy, consider use of linaclotide (Linzess) and lubiprostone (Amitiza) or Naloxegol (Movantik). Also consider naldemedine (Symproic), however, due to the expense may be difficult to prescribe, or patients may not be able to afford.

Third-Line Therapy

If bulk-forming or osmotic diuretics fail to work, a stimulant laxative may be chosen. Stimulant laxatives are very effective. Mineral oil is effective as a lubricant laxative and may be an option in patients who should avoid straining. However, although mineral oil would seem safe, its ability to impair absorption of necessary vitamins and to cause aspiration pneumonitis limits its use. In addition, seepage is an inconvenient side effect that likely limits compliance. If an agent is necessary to soften the stool to prevent straining, docusate is a safer alternative.

Sodium biphosphate as an enema is another option. These agents have the potential to cause fluid and electrolyte abnormalities and exacerbate concomitant disease states such as hypertension and congestive heart failure. Therefore, these agents should be used only after safer agents have failed. Because sodium biphosphate enemas and magnesium citrate solutions have a rapid onset of action, these agents

are often preferred and are usually reserved for endoscopic procedures.

Castor oil is a potent cathartic that should not be used routinely for treating constipation.

Consider adding prucalopride or any other agent from the novel classes not previously tried (see **Table 25.5**).

Special Populations
Pediatric

Constipation can be distressing for children, particularly young children. Most children do not have an underlying pathophysiologic process. Stress over potty training or painful stools secondary to acute constipation can result in avoidance of defecation by the child. This in turn can result in larger, harder, and more painful stools, which eventually leads to soiling. Constipation and encopresis, a condition where soft stool is involuntarily lost, are often combined. Parents usually pay little attention to their child's bowel frequency unless incontinence occurs. The parents may become angry with the child, leading to further stress. To avoid constipation that may result in soiling, parents should be cognizant of their child's bowel habits.

Constipation may also result in urinary incontinence and urinary tract infections in children, particularly girls. Overflow incontinence may occur when the distended rectum presses on the bladder wall, causing bladder outflow obstruction. Fecal

TABLE 25.5

Recommended Order of Treatment for Constipation

Order	Agents	Comments
First line	Bulk-forming agents (methylcellulose, psyllium, polycarbophil, malt soup extract, wheat dextrin) Docusate derivatives	Avoid in patients with GI obstruction or ulceration Take with plenty of water Most effective at preventing straining at stool in high-risk patients (see text)
	Glycerin Naloxegol (Movantik) Linaclotide or lubiprostone	Used most often in infants and small children Indication for OIC only Consider for first or second line for CIC or OIC
Second line	Milk of magnesia, magnesium sulfate, lactulose, sorbitol Linaclotide or lubiprostone	Caution in renal dysfunction and the older adults Use with caution in patients with diabetes Caution: laxative abuse, cathartic colon Add if not used as first line
Third line	Stimulant laxatives (senna, cascara sagrada, casanthranol, bisacodyl) Mineral oil Sodium biphosphates (only enema available) Magnesium citrate Castor oil	Impairs absorption of fat-soluble vitamins; use with caution in older adults and very young (lipid pneumonia) Use with caution in congestive heart failure, hypertension, edema, and renal dysfunction Used as a bowel evacuant for endoscopic examinations Too potent to be used routinely for constipation

CIC, chronic idiopathic constipation; OIC, opioid-induced constipation.

soiling in the external urethral opening predisposes constipated girls to infection. Treatment of constipation can reduce infection and incontinence.

Initially, manual evacuation of the rectum may be necessary; however, once this is done, it is necessary to use chronic laxative therapy. Treatment with pharmacologic agents in children is controversial, and few well-designed placebo-controlled trials have been conducted on the use of osmotic laxatives, fiber, formula switching, sorbitol-containing juices, rectal stimulation by thermometer, or glycerin suppositories. A Cochrane review of osmotic and stimulant laxatives concluded that PEG preparations may be superior to placebo, lactulose, and milk of magnesia for childhood constipation (Sahn et al., 2016). Liquid paraffin (mineral oil) is also a good alternative. The use of sodium phosphate enemas in children under 2 years of age has been associated with electrolyte disturbances, dehydration, and cardiac arrest.

For infants, malt soup extract or corn syrup (Karo) may be used at a dosage of 5 to 10 mL twice daily. For children older than 6 months, milk of magnesia, lactulose, or sorbitol at a dosage of 1 to 3 mL/kg/d given in one to two doses may be used. Senna syrup at a dosage of 5 to 10 mL/d for children ages 1 to 5 and 10 to 20 mL/d for children ages 5 to 15 is another option.

Geriatric

The choice of a laxative preparation may depend on the patient's attitude or beliefs about normal bowel habits. Normal bowel frequency can range from two or three bowel movements per day to two or three per week. However, many people think that less than one bowel movement per day is abnormal. These patients may seek an OTC laxative to keep them "regular." This concern about regular bowel movements is particularly common in the older adults. The self-reported incidence of constipation increases with advancing age, but the actual bowel movement frequency usually does not decline.

The overuse of laxatives in the older adults can be of particular concern because this population is more intolerant to the fluid and electrolyte abnormalities that accompany laxative abuse. In addition, many of the laxatives should be used with caution in older persons because they are more likely to have the disease states that some laxatives can exacerbate (e.g., heart failure, hypertension). Older patients are also more likely to take medications that may cause constipation, such as antipsychotics, tricyclic antidepressants, calcium supplements, and certain blood pressure medications.

Older patients should be carefully assessed to determine the cause of the constipation, and causative factors should be eliminated. Careful selection and judicious use of laxatives are necessary to avoid complications in this population.

Women

Girls and women with bulimia or anorexia nervosa may abuse laxatives as a means of reducing nutrient absorption to cause weight loss. Bulimia is 10 times more common in women than in men; it affects up to 3% of young women.

For the pregnant woman, the use of laxatives that are not absorbed into the systemic circulation, such as docusate and bulk-forming agents, should be considered as first-line therapy. Docusate sodium has not been found to be associated with fetal malformations and may be safe to use during pregnancy. Lactulose and sorbitol have not been found to be teratogenic in animals and may be safe to administer to pregnant women. Stimulant laxatives should be used only occasionally, if necessary. Cascara sagrada may cause loose stools in breastfed infants. Castor oil should be avoided in pregnant women because of the risk of stimulation of uterine contractions. Mineral oil should be avoided because its use can reduce the absorption of necessary vitamins by the mother, which may result in deficiencies for the neonate.

Monitoring Patient Response

Monitoring the patient's response to laxative therapy usually is accomplished by asking the patient whether they have regained normal bowel patterns after using the laxative. Different patients have different perceptions of what "normal" bowel habits are. Depending on the factors affecting defecation, patients should be informed that the reason for treating with a laxative is not to increase the frequency of defecation but to promote comfortable defecation. Periodic use of laxatives can be safe as there is no substantial evidence of abuse potential.

Patient Education

In most cases, the occasional use of laxatives poses no major problems for the patient. Laxatives are relatively safe when used in moderation. However, the fact that many laxatives are available OTC may give consumers the false impression that constipation is a physiologic condition and there are no other alternatives for treatment. Understanding of constipation has expanded in recent years, and health care providers can provide other options for treatment.

Health care providers should work with patients who have constipation and guide them to the best treatment options. OTC laxatives carry a warning for the consumer not to use them for more than 7 days. For chronic constipation, use of a bulk-forming laxative may be a safer alternative, provided no contraindications exist. However, patients should be counseled that bulk-forming laxatives take time to work (up to 3 days). Because patients are usually looking for an immediate response, they may draw the conclusion that these agents are not effective if a bowel movement has not occurred within the first day.

Patient-Oriented Information Sources

Providing patients with information about constipation can help them understand constipation and their role in treatment. Patient education items are readily available on the Internet through the National Digestive Diseases Information Clearinghouse (NDDIC), which provides information to consumers on a wide variety of GI topics (see **Box 25.16**).

Nutrition/Lifestyle Changes

Patients should be educated on the lifestyle modifications discussed previously to reduce the need for a laxative. An increase in fluid intake improves the efficacy of most laxatives. Patients should also be educated on the potential for side effects of the laxative chosen as well as the appropriate method to administer the laxative.

Complementary and Alternative Medications/Treatments

There is growing evidence that evaluation of the gut microflora can be helpful in the treatment of constipation. The inclusion of prebiotics, probiotics along with synbiotics has shown to be helpful using a traditional Chinese medicine approach can include acupuncture and herbs has been shown to decrease constipation (Xu et al., 2019).

DIARRHEA

True diarrhea is an increase in frequency of loose, watery stools (three or more daily), usually over a period of 24 to 48 hours. It is a relatively common disorder of the GI tract that is experienced occasionally by most people. The organisms that cause diarrhea are easily transferred from person to person through food and water. Globalization and industrialization of the world has increased the ability of these organisms to spread. Experts of infectious diseases estimate that 211 million people experience acute diarrhea every year; an average of 16 million seek medical attention, resulting in 1.2 million hospitalizations and more than 5,000 deaths (Abdoli & Maspi, 2018). Children, the older adults, and those who are immunocompromised are most susceptible to the complications of diarrhea, and serious dehydration can result from the disorder. Proper hydration and symptomatic treatment as well as elimination of causative factors are necessary to prevent these complications. Ultimately, diarrhea can have a profound impact on public health, and proper diagnosis and treatment can prevent an epidemic.

Causes

Diarrhea may be caused by a host of different medications (**Box 25.9**), infective organisms (**Box 25.10**), or disease states or procedures (**Box 25.11**). Prompt attention to causative factors, as well as rehydration, prevents complications.

Medications

Antibiotics may cause diarrhea by direct irritation of the intestinal tract or disruption of the normal intestinal flora. The poor absorption of erythromycin (E-mycin) lends itself to irritation of the GI tract. Clarithromycin (Biaxin) and azithromycin (Zithromax) may cause less diarrhea than erythromycin. The clavulanic acid component of the combination of amoxicillin–clavulanic acid (Augmentin) is also a GI irritant, and diarrhea is a common side effect. Tetracycline and ceftriaxone (Rocephin) cause diarrhea by disrupting the normal balance of the gut flora.

Clostridium difficile, a normal part of the flora of the colon in up to 20% of hospitalized patients, normally does not cause disease unless chemotherapeutic medications or antibiotics trigger its toxins. Only certain antibiotics have been implicated in *C. difficile*–associated diarrhea. Less common causes of *C. difficile* diarrhea are vancomycin (Vancocin), erythromycin,

BOX 25.9 Medications Commonly Causing Diarrhea

Antacids (magnesium containing)
Antibiotics
Antidepressants (SSRIs)
Cholinergic agents
Colchicine
Digoxin
GI stimulants (metoclopramide)
Laxatives
Metformin
Prostaglandins (dinoprostone)
Prostaglandin analog (misoprostol)
Quinidine

BOX 25.10 Infective Organisms Associated with Diarrhea

Aeromonas species
Bacillus cereus
Campylobacter
Chlamydia trachomatis
Clostridium difficile
Cryptosporidium
Escherichia coli
Entamoeba histolytica
Giardia
Mycobacterium avium-intracellulare
Salmonella
Shigella
Staphylococcus aureus
Viral agents
Yersinia

BOX 25.11 Disorders and Procedures Associated with Diarrhea

AIDS
Bowel resection
Colon cancer
Diverticulitis
Enteral feedings
Gastroenteritis
Hyperthyroidism
IBD
IBS
Lactose intolerance
Malabsorption
Pheochromocytoma

BOX 25.12 Treating *Clostridium difficile* Diarrhea

C. difficile diarrhea may occur weeks after stopping antimicrobial therapy. The diarrhea may progress to colitis if left untreated. While awaiting the results of *C. difficile* toxin assay of the stool specimen, empiric therapy with metronidazole (Flagyl) 500 mg orally thrice daily or vancomycin therapy should not be empirically initiated unless there is no clinical improvement within 5 to 7 days.

Because routine use of vancomycin (Vancocin) may contribute to the emergence of vancomycin-resistant *Enterococcus* species, even though oral vancomycin is no longer costly and may be easily prescribed, it should be reserved for cases that fail to respond to oral metronidazole or for patients who are not able to tolerate oral metronidazole. Institute oral doses of vancomycin; start at 125 mg four times daily and increase to 500 mg four times daily for lack of response.

For *C. difficile* diarrhea advancing to colitis, the preferred agent is IV metronidazole 1 g every 24 hours with oral vancomycin at 500 mg four times daily, for 10 days or until colitis has resolved on computed tomography scan. Patients should not be given bowel antispasmodics because this may reduce the elimination of the toxins from the body.

Source: Surawicz, C. M., Brandt, L. J., Binion, D. G., et al. (2013). Guidelines for diagnosis, treatment, and prevention of clostridium difficile infections. *American Journal of Gastroenterology, 108*(4), 478–498. https://doi.org/10.1038/ajg.2013.4

tetracyclines, trimethoprim–sulfamethoxazole (TMP–SMZ), quinolones, and aztreonam (Azactam). The antibiotics most likely to cause *C. difficile* diarrhea are beta-lactam antibiotics (penicillins, cephalosporins, and carbapenems) and clindamycin (Cleocin). **Box 25.12** gives more information.

Infectious Organisms

Patients traveling to a developing region may contract diarrhea from bacterial organisms. *Giardia* should be suspected if the patient travels to mountainous areas, recreational waters, or Russia. Pathogens transmitted by the fecal-to-oral route should be suspected in homosexual men (*Shigella, Salmonella, Campylobacter,* and intestinal protozoa) and in patients exposed to day-care centers (*Shigella, Giardia, Cryptosporidium*).

Travelers' diarrhea (TD) is usually a self-limiting, non–life-threatening illness affecting 20% to 50% of individuals who visit developing countries; however, it can become chronic disease process (Connor, 2013; Steffen, 2017). The cause of TD is ingestion of contaminated food products or water with feces. High-risk areas include Latin America, Africa, Asia, and the Middle East. The typical duration is 2 to 3 days; symptoms include nausea and vomiting, cramps, and bloody stools. The most common pathogen is *Escherichia coli*; *Salmonella*, *Shigella*, and *Campylobacter* are the culprits less frequently.

Dietary restrictions are the main prevention for TD. Travelers should avoid foods and beverages that are not steaming hot, raw vegetables, unpeeled fruit, tap water, and ice.

Pathophysiology

Diarrhea may be classified by duration and category. Acute diarrhea lasts 1 to 14 days and is considered self-limiting. Persistent diarrhea lasts longer than 14 days but less than 30 days, and chronic diarrhea last more than 30 days. Diarrhea may also be categorized as osmotic, secretory, or exudative (inflammatory), or the diarrhea may be related to altered intestinal motility (transit). Some diarrheal illnesses involve more than one of these mechanisms. Diarrhea may also be a defense mechanism against toxins and invading organisms.

Osmotic Diarrhea

Osmotic diarrhea occurs when non-absorbed solutes are retained in the lumen of the intestinal tract. The result is a hyperosmolar state that pulls water and ions into the intestinal lumen. Poorly absorbed salts (magnesium sulfate), lactose (in lactase deficiency), and large amounts of sugar substitutes (sorbitol) found in candy or chewing gum, diet foods, and soft drinks draw fluid into the intestinal tract, resulting in an overload of the colon.

Secretory Diarrhea

In secretory diarrhea, colonic absorption of fluid is secondary to active transport of Na^+ through Na^+–K^+–adenosine triphosphatase activity in the colonic epithelium. The colon absorbs chloride by exchanging it for HCO_3^2 and by uptake of sodium chloride. Any agent that increases concentrations of cyclic adenosine 3, 5-monophosphate in the cells of the colon inhibits sodium chloride uptake and causes secretion of chloride. This results in secretion of fluid in the colon. Prostaglandins E2 and I2 and vasoactive intestinal peptide stimulate adenyl cyclase activity. Cholinergic agents and cholinesterase inhibitors cause secretion of sodium chloride and water. Secretory diarrhea can be classified as pure (e.g., cholera) or a part of a complex disease process (e.g., celiac disease, Crohn's disease [CD]). Other stimuli that can cause secretory diarrhea include bacterial endotoxins, hormones from endocrine neoplasms, dihydroxy bile acids, hydroxylated fatty acids, and inflammatory mediators.

Exudative Diarrhea

Exudative (inflammatory) diarrhea may result from inflammatory diseases of the mucosa. Inflammation occurs due to the compromise of the tight junctions of the epithelial cells in the intestine. These diseases may cause an increase of blood, mucus, pus, and serum proteins that increase fluid and overload the colon, resulting in diarrhea. Enteritis, ulcerative colitis (UC), and carcinoma are examples of inflammatory conditions that may result in exudative diarrhea.

Altered Intestinal Motility

Intestinal contents need to have sufficient time to be in contact with the lining of the intestinal tract for fluid, electrolytes, and nutrients to be absorbed adequately. Any factor that increases or decreases the motility of the intestinal tract may result in decreased absorption of fluid and electrolytes. Resection of the bowels, vagotomy, and certain agents (serotonin, laxatives, prostaglandins, prokinetic agents) can increase intestinal motility. Decreases in motility can result from autonomic injury or smooth muscle injury to the intestine and result in bacterial overgrowth, subsequently leading to diarrhea.

Diagnostic Criteria

A careful travel and social history are important to identify and treat specific causes, such as infection. Use of empiric antibiotic therapy is not recommended due to increasing resistance of many strains of bacteria. However, if a traveler is unable to comply with precautions, it may be prudent to prescribe a fluoroquinolone to hold in reserve. Selective testing of stool will be cost-effective while helping to guide the clinician in the use of specific therapy. According to the most recent guidelines of the Infectious Disease Society of America (Shane et al., 2017), diarrhea can be divided into three categories: community-acquired or TD, nosocomial diarrhea, or persistent diarrhea. Each category can be specifically evaluated, leading to more precise therapy.

The fecal leukocyte, lactoferrin, or Hemoccult blood test is useful in patients with moderate-to-severe cases of acute infectious diarrhea because it supports the use of empiric antibiotic therapy in the febrile patient. However, measuring fecal leukocytes can be unreliable if specimens are transported, refrigerated, or frozen. Fecal lactoferrin, as a measure of polymorphonuclear neutrophils, has an advantage over fecal leukocytes as a highly sensitive and specific testing method for intestinal inflammation. Stool cultures have traditionally been used to identify the pathology of diarrhea, but the positive yields are very poor and incur high costs. Controversy exists regarding when to obtain stool cultures. The absence of vomiting with persistent diarrhea may also indicate the need for stool cultures. Hypotension, tachycardia, orthostasis, bloody stool, and abdominal pain and tenderness were not found to be good predictors of a positive stool culture.

Laboratory evaluation for ova and parasites should be performed in the following:

- A person not previously treated with empiric antiparasitic therapy
- A person with persistent diarrhea for more than 7 days
- A person who recently traveled to mountainous regions, Russia, or Nepal
- A person who was exposed to infants at day-care centers or who was exposed through a community waterborne outbreak
- A person with bloody diarrhea with few or no fecal leukocytes
- Homosexual men or patients with acquired immunodeficiency syndrome (AIDS)

For food- or waterborne pathogens, the incubation period and clinical features can give clues as to the source of infection.

Diarrhea and vomiting 6 hours after exposure to a food item suggests exposure to *Staphylococcus aureus* or *Bacillus cereus*. An incubation period of 8 to 14 hours suggests *Clostridium perfringens*. With an incubation period greater than 14 hours, with vomiting as the predominant feature, viral agents are suspected. In patients with fever greater than 101.3°F (38.5°C) plus leukocyte-, lactoferrin-, or Hemoccult-positive stools, or acute dysentery (grossly bloody stools), the most common pathogens identified by normal stool culture are *Shigella, Salmonella, Campylobacter, Aeromonas,* and *Yersinia.* Additionally, patients with grossly bloody stools should be tested for *E. coli* O157 or hemolytic-uremic syndrome (HUS).

Initiating Drug Therapy

Most cases of diarrhea are self-limiting and can be self-treated. However, patients with profuse, watery diarrhea with dehydration, passage of blood and mucus, and fever exceeding 101.3°F should be evaluated for an inflammation-producing pathogen. These patients may benefit from antimicrobial therapy. In addition, a good history helps to determine the cause of illness. In diarrhea caused by infectious organisms, the pathogen should be identified so that therapy may be initiated to eradicate the organism and to prevent exposure to unnecessary antibiotics.

For TD, prophylactic agents may be given to patients who should not, cannot, or will not comply with dietary restrictions. Chemoprophylaxis of TD is controversial and usually is not recommended for patients unless the patient has an underlying illness (AIDS, prior gastric surgery, other chronic disease process), the purpose of the trip is particularly important (politicians, honeymoon), or the patient cannot or will not comply with dietary restrictions. In such cases, the use of bismuth subsalicylate (BSS; Pepto-Bismol), 2 tablets four times daily, is recommended unless the reason for prophylaxis is a serious underlying illness. In these cases, a quinolone antibiotic or rifaximin should be used.

If prophylactic therapy is not prescribed, at the first symptoms of diarrhea, empiric therapy can be prescribed using a quinolone antibiotic, rifaximin, or azithromycin (**see Table 25.8**). Patients should be properly hydrated, and BSS may be used to treat symptoms. Loperamide (Imodium) is a more effective option than BSS, but loperamide should be used with caution in the presence of fever or bloody stools because the antimotility effects of the drug may prolong disease by reducing the elimination of possible infectious pathogens. If an antidiarrheal medication is necessary, selection should be based on patient-specific variables, including potential side effects, convenience, efficacy, and the patient's symptoms. For patients with moderate or severe TD, empiric antimicrobial therapy with a quinolone antibiotic or rifaximin may be given (see **Table 25.6**). Patients with persistent diarrhea lasting 2 to 4 weeks without systemic symptoms or dysentery may be studied for the cause and treated or given metronidazole (Flagyl) for empiric anti-*Giardia* therapy.

Goals of Drug Therapy

The goals of drug therapy are to reduce the symptoms of diarrhea and to make the patient as comfortable as possible. Causative factors should be identified and eradicated. Fluid and electrolyte replacement is particularly important to avoid serious complications from dehydration. Rehydration is discussed later in this chapter.

Antidiarrheal Agents

Several types of drugs are used for the symptomatic relief of diarrhea; they include antimotility agents, adsorbents and absorbents, and the atypical antisecretory agent BSS. **Table 25.6** provides an overview of these drugs, and **Table 25.7** covers the recommended order of prescription.

Antimotility Agents

The antimotility agent loperamide (Imodium) is an opioid receptor agonist that acts on the mu-opioid receptors of the myenteric plexus of the large intestine, like the action of morphine without action on the CNS. This slows GI motility within the circular and longitudinal muscles of the intestines. Initially, this drug was classified as a controlled substance but in 1982 was declassified. It is not well absorbed and does not provide analgesic or euphoric effects.

Another similar agent is diphenoxylate with atropine (Lomotil). It is also chemically related to the narcotic meperidine. As with loperamide, it acts on decreasing GI motility. However, unlike loperamide, it can cross the blood–brain barrier and cause a euphoric effect. Combining diphenoxylate with atropine causes anticholinergic side effects if too much of the drug is ingested, decreasing the potential for abuse. Due to the potential for abuse, diphenoxylate with atropine is a controlled substance, Schedule V.

Contraindications

The antimotility effects may exacerbate infectious diarrhea by preventing the excretion of the infecting organism, allowing the organism more contact time in the intestines. Caution should be observed in using loperamide in patients with fever, bloody stools, or fecal leukocytes. In nondysenteric forms of diarrhea caused by invasive pathogens, loperamide can be used, provided antimicrobial therapy is administered.

Because loperamide undergoes extensive first-pass metabolism, caution should be used in patients with hepatic dysfunction because excessive side effects (CNS toxicity) may occur in these patients.

Because of the antimotility effects of diphenoxylate, it should be used with caution in patients with infectious diarrhea associated with fever or bloody stools. Diphenoxylate provides euphoric and analgesic effects at high doses but not at therapeutic doses. As previously stated for this reason, diphenoxylate is combined with atropine to discourage abuse. Diphenoxylate should be used with caution in patients with liver impairment because it is extensively metabolized by the liver.

TABLE 25.6

Indications for Empiric and Specific Antimicrobial Therapy in Infectious Diarrhea

Indication for Antimicrobial Therapy	Suggested Antimicrobial Therapy
Fever (oral temperature >101.3°F [38.5°C]) together with one of the following: dysentery (grossly bloody stools) or those with leukocyte-, lactoferrin-, or Hemoccult-positive stools	Quinolone:* NF 400 mg, CF 500 mg (preferred), OF 300 mg BID for 3–5 d
Moderate-to-severe TD	Quinolone:* CF 500 mg, NF 400 mg, OF 300 mg BID for 1–5 d Rifaximin 200 mg TID × 3 d if not complicated by above symptoms
Persistent diarrhea (possible *Giardia* infection)	Metronidazole 250 mg QID for 7 d
Shigellosis	If acquired in the United States, give TMP–SMZ 160/800 mg BID for 3 d; if acquired during international travel, treat as febrile dysentery (above); check to be certain of susceptibility to drug used If not from the United States, give third-generation cephalosporin
Intestinal salmonellosis	If healthy host with mild or moderate symptoms, no therapy; for severe disease or that associated with fever and systemic toxicity or other important underlying conditions, use TMP–SMZ 160 mg/800 mg or quinolone:* NF 400 mg, CF 500 mg, OF mg BID for 5–7 d depending on speed of response
Campylobacteriosis	Erythromycin stearate 500 mg BID for 5 d
Enteropathogenic *Escherichia coli* diarrhea (EPEC)	Treat as febrile dysentery.
Enterotoxigenic *E. coli* diarrhea (ETEC)	Treat as moderate-to-severe TD
Enteroinvasive *E. coli* diarrhea (EIEC)	Treat as shigellosis
Enterohemorrhagic *E. coli* diarrhea (EHEC)	Antimicrobials are usually withheld except in particularly severe cases, in which usefulness of these drugs is uncertain
Aeromonas diarrhea	Treat as febrile dysentery
Noncholera *Vibrio* diarrhea	Treat as febrile dysentery
Yersiniosis	For most cases, treat as febrile dysentery; for severe cases, give ceftriaxone 1 g daily IV for 5 d
Giardiasis	Metronidazole 250 mg QID for 7 d or (if available) tinidazole 2 g in a single dose or quinicine 100 mg TID for 7 d
Intestinal amebiasis	Metronidazole 750 mg TID for 5–10 d plus a drug to treat cysts to prevent relapses: diiodohydroxyquin 650 mg TID for 20 d or paromomycin 500 mg TID for 10 d or diloxanide furoate 500 mg TID for 10 d
Cryptosporidium diarrhea	None; for severe cases, consider paromomycin 500 mg TID for 7 d
Isospora diarrhea	TMP–SMZ 160 mg/800 mg BID for 7 d
Cyclospora diarrhea	TMP–SMZ 160 mg/800 mg BID for 7 d

*Fluoroquinolones include norfloxacin (NF), ciprofloxacin (CF), and ofloxacin (OF).

TMP–SMZ, trimethoprim–sulfamethoxazole.

Reproduced by permission from American Journal of Gastroenterology. (1997). Commercially available oral rehydration solutions. *American Journal of Gastroenterology, 92*, 1962–1975. Copyright © 1997, Rights Managed by Nature Publishing Group.

Adverse Events

Adverse effects of loperamide include abdominal discomfort, constipation, and dry mouth. Although loperamide does not cross the blood–brain barrier, it may still induce drowsiness in some patients. Patients should be warned of the potential for drowsiness before driving or performing activities that require alertness. Although loperamide is usually well tolerated, it is not recommended in children younger than age 4, because shock, enterocolitis, fatal intestinal obstruction, and CNS toxicity have occurred.

Atropine has anticholinergic effects such as dry mouth, dry eyes, urinary retention, constipation, blurred vision, and tachycardia. Diphenoxylate may cause drowsiness or dizziness, and patients should be warned of these effects and should avoid activities that require alertness. The liquid formulation is recommended in children because the dose needs to be carefully tailored to the child based on age and weight. Diphenoxylate with atropine can cause respiratory depression in infants and young children and should be avoided in children younger than age 4.

TABLE 25.7

Overview of Selected Antidiarrheals

Generic (Trade) Name and Dosage	Selected Adverse Events	Contraindications	Special Considerations
Antimotility Agents			
Diphenoxylate/atropine (Lomotil) 2.5–5 mg QID	Dry mouth, dry eyes, urinary retention, blurred vision, drowsiness, dizziness	Caution in patients with liver disease, fever, bloody stool, or fecal leukocytes	Drug Enforcement Administration Class V controlled substance
Loperamide (Imodium) 4–16 mg/d in divided doses	Abdominal discomfort, constipation, drowsiness, dry mouth	Caution in patients with fever, bloody stools, or fecal leukocytes	May induce drowsiness; warn patients about driving or performing activities that require alertness
Selected Antisecretory Agents			
Bismuth subsalicylate (Pepto-Bismol) Start: 2 tabs or 30 mL Range: 2 tabs or 30 mL every 30 min to 1 h up to eight doses	Black stools, darkening of tongue, tinnitus	Caution in patients who are aspirin sensitive or are taking medications that interact with warfarin	Not recommended for children and adolescents due to the presence of salicylate component and potential Reye's syndrome
Polycarbophil (Fiber-Con) 1–6 g/d	Stomach upset, bloating, gas	Caution: potential for drug interactions with tetracycline or quinolones	
Kaolin and bismuth salicylate (Kaopectate) Start: 30–120 mL of liquid or 2 tabs after each bowel movement Range: Up to seven doses a day	Constipation, feeling of fullness, stomach bloating, gas	Do not use with children due to the salicylate component	May adsorb nutrients and medications Separate administration time of adsorbents and other medications
Semisynthetic Antibiotic			
Rifaximin (Xifaxan) TD: 200 mg tabs TID × 3 d	Most common for TD—headache	Known hypersensitivity to rifaximin Bloody diarrhea	Discontinue for diarrhea that worsens or persists >48 h. Consider different antibiotics

TD, travelers' diarrhea.

Interactions

Diphenoxylate may potentiate the action of depressants such as alcohol, barbiturates, or benzodiazepines. In addition, atropine may potentiate the effects of other agents with anticholinergic properties such as tricyclic antidepressants, antipsychotics, and antihistamines. Diphenoxylate has a structure like that of meperidine, and when used concomitantly with monoamine oxidase inhibitors, it can induce a hypertensive crisis.

Atypical Antidiarrheals

Subsalicylate is the active ingredient found in BSS (Pepto-Bismol) and Kaopectate. BSS includes the active ingredients bismuth, which stimulates prostaglandin, mucous, and bicarbonate secretion *in the stomach*, and salicylate, which inhibits prostaglandin and chloride secretion *in the large intestine*. The action of salicylic acid and bismuth on diarrhea is not well understood but is thought to have anti-inflammatory action and antacid and mild antibiotic properties.

Kaopectate is now formulated with the active ingredients of subsalicylic acid and therefore has the same contraindications,

adverse effects, and interactions. Further discussion of Kaopectate as an absorbent is found in the next section.

Contraindications

BSS and Kaopectate are broken down in the intestinal tract to salicylate; therefore, it should be used with caution in patients taking aspirin therapy or those hypersensitive to aspirin. In addition, caution should be used in children and adolescents with the flu or chickenpox because this population is at risk for aspirin-induced Reye's syndrome.

Adverse Effects

Side effects of BSS and Kaopectate with subsalicylate include black stools, darkening of the tongue, and tinnitus, which can be a potential sign of salicylate toxicity.

Interactions

Because BSS and Kaopectate with subsalicylate have a salicylate component, it may interact with other medications that interact with aspirin (e.g., warfarin).

Adsorbents and Absorbents

Mechanism of Action

Kaolinite is a naturally occurring magnesium aluminum silicate and is used in Kaopectate. Previous formulations of Kaopectate included a combination of kaolinite and attapulgite, which was removed from the formulation by the FDA and replaced by subsalicylate (Kim-Jung et al., 2004). Another adsorbent, pectin, has also been removed from the market. The current formulation of Kaopectate adsorbs water along with bacteria and toxins as well as helps to solidify loose stools. As an adsorbent, it is usually given after each bowel movement until diarrhea is relieved or a maximum dose is reached. The dose for adults is 30 mL every 30 to 60 minutes if needed or maximum of eight doses daily. Kaopectate is not approved for children due to the subsalicylate component.

Polycarbophil (FiberCon, Fiberall), an absorbent, absorbs water in the GI tract and is used as an antidiarrheal. Its fiber content also makes it useful as a bulk-forming laxative when taken with plenty of water.

Adverse Events

The most common side effects of the adsorbents are constipation and a feeling of fullness. Absorbents may also produce stomach upset, bloating, and gas. Adsorbents and absorbents are generally considered safe because the medication works locally and is not absorbed systemically. However, adsorbents may not be as effective as antimotility agents at reducing the symptoms of diarrhea.

Interactions

Adsorbents are not selective and may adsorb nutrients and medications. This interaction must be taken into consideration because several doses may be necessary each day. Separating administration times of adsorbents and other medications is advised. Polycarbophil contains calcium and may interact with fluoroquinolone and tetracycline antibiotics.

Semisynthetic antibiotic

Rifaximin

Rifaximin (Xifaxan) is a semisynthetic antibiotic that is only effective against noninvasive strains of *E. coli*. The drug is a derivative of rifampin and acts to block transcription of the bacteria; therefore, it inhibits bacterial protein synthesis and growth. This acts to suppress diarrhea by altering the growth of the bacteria. The recommended dose for TD is 200 mg thrice daily for 3 days and may be administered with or without meals.

Contraindications

Rifaximin is contraindicated in patients with a history of hypersensitivity to rifaximin, rifamycin antimicrobial agents, or any of the components of rifaximin.

Adverse Effects

The most common side effects are peripheral edema, nausea, dizziness, fatigue, and muscle spasms. For TD, the most common side effect was headache. Additional postmarketing side effects include exfoliative dermatitis, rash, angioneurotic edema (swelling of the face and tongue and difficulty swallowing), urticaria, flushing, pruritus, and anaphylaxis.

Interactions

Rifaximin has a low risk of drug interactions because it is poorly absorbed into the bloodstream, and it does not significantly affect the cytochrome P-450 system. Coadministration with cyclosporine in healthy subjects resulted in the increased availability of rifaximin, but overall clinical significance is unknown.

Selecting the Most Appropriate Agent

The choice of antidiarrheal agent should be based on several factors, including the patient's history, potential side effects of the medication, potential for drug interactions, and efficacy of available agents (**Tables 25.6** and **25.8**; **Figure 25.5**).

First-Line Therapy

Although the adsorbents are not absorbed into the systemic circulation and are usually safe and well tolerated, they are not as effective at controlling diarrhea as loperamide. Therefore, loperamide may be considered as first-line therapy secondary to its efficacy. Loperamide is also reasonably well tolerated and has few drug interactions. However, patients should be warned about the potential for loperamide to cause drowsiness (particularly patients who must stay alert).

Because loperamide is an antimotility agent, it should be used with caution in patients with fever or bloody stools to avoid exacerbation of any type of infectious diarrhea. In addition, caution should be used in patients with liver failure.

Appropriate antibiotic therapy should be considered for infectious diarrhea. First line for TD is ciprofloxacin or levofloxacin (see Chapter 6 Principles of Antimicrobial Therapy). Rifaximin can also be considered as a first-line choice.

Second-Line Therapy

For patients who cannot tolerate loperamide or for those with contraindications, an adsorbent or antisecretory agent may be chosen.

Antisecretory agents such as BSS or Kaopectate should be used with caution in patients taking warfarin and should be avoided in children or adolescents with the flu. Antisecretory agents should also be avoided in patients with a documented hypersensitivity to salicylates. Black stools, darkening of the

TABLE 25.8

Recommended Order of Treatment for Diarrhea

Order	Agents	Comments
First line	Loperamide rifaximin (TD)	Easy to use, tablet or liquid Well tolerated, 3-day course
Second line	Adsorbents or antisecretory agent	Selection based on drug–drug interactions or allergies (e.g., aspirin sensitivity and BSS)
Third line	Diphenoxylate	Side-effect profile, especially with atropine added, lowers the utility of this agent

BSS, bismuth subsalicylate; TD, travelers' diarrhea.

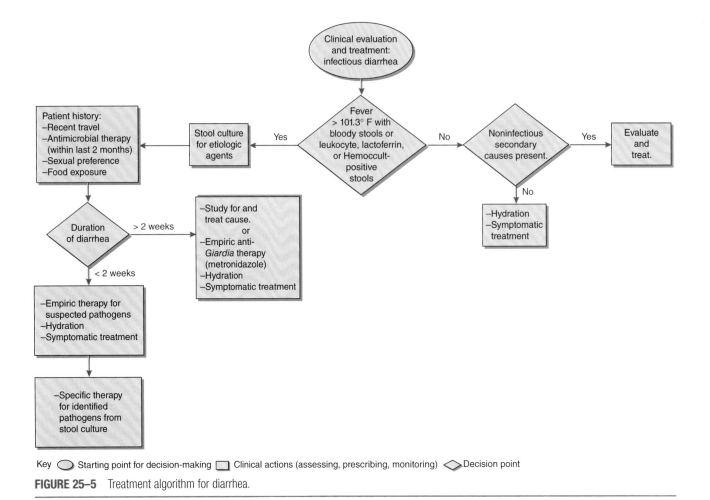

Key ⬭ Starting point for decision-making ▢ Clinical actions (assessing, prescribing, monitoring) ◇ Decision point

FIGURE 25–5   Treatment algorithm for diarrhea.

tongue, and tinnitus are side effects that may be disturbing to the patient. BSS may be useful for prophylaxis against TD and may be preferable over the adsorbents in a patient who also has indigestion or stomach upset that accompanies the diarrhea.

Although adsorbents may inhibit the absorption of nutrients from the diet and can cause some abdominal cramping, they are usually well tolerated.

Second-line antibiotic therapy is rifaximin, if the agent is known to be *E. coli*, and has not responded to ciprofloxacin.

Third-Line Therapy

Although diphenoxylate with atropine is an effective agent for treating diarrhea, the atropine component can cause significant anticholinergic effects that may exacerbate certain conditions and interact with other agents with anticholinergic activity. In addition, diphenoxylate is a Drug Enforcement Administration Schedule V drug, and its potential for abuse limits this agent to third-line therapy. Third-line antibiotic therapy is azithromycin (see Chapter 6).

Special Populations

Pediatric

Recommendations for treatment of diarrhea in children have not changed since 1996 by the American Academy of

Pediatrics, Provisional Committee on Quality Improvement, and Subcommittee on Acute Gastroenteritis. These recommendations apply to children ages 1 month to 5 years who have no previously diagnosed disorders. The focus is on oral rehydration and zinc therapy (Lenters et al., 2013; Nalin & Cash, 2018). Opiate and atropine combination drugs such as diphenoxylate with atropine should be avoided in acute diarrhea in children because of the potential for side effects and the limited scientific evidence for efficacy. Also, loperamide is not recommended based on limited scientific evidence, and BSS or Kaopectate is not appropriate due to the presence of subsalicylate. Adsorbents are also not recommended based on limited evidence. The committee recognized that major toxic effects from adsorbents are in general not a concern, but the potential for poor absorption of nutrients and antibiotics is a potential disadvantage. The final expert conclusion is that oral rehydration is the most important aspect of therapy, and routine use of antidiarrheal agents is not recommended based on lack of evidence or the potential for side effects.

If the health care provider still decides to choose diphenoxylate with atropine, the liquid formulation should be used because specific dosing is required based on the child's weight and age. In addition, diphenoxylate with atropine is contraindicated in children younger than age 2.

Geriatric

As with the pediatric population, rehydration is of paramount importance in the geriatric population. Older patients are likely to have multiple disease states that cause them to be intolerant of dehydration (e.g., congestive heart failure, diabetes, renal insufficiency). In addition, the antidiarrheal preparations may interact with agents that are commonly prescribed in the geriatric population. Diphenoxylate and loperamide may increase the sedative potential of benzodiazepines, antidepressants, anticholinergics, and antipsychotics. Adsorbents can reduce the absorption not only of important nutrients but also of other medications. BSS should be used with caution in older patients taking aspirin and agents that interact with aspirin.

Women

As with constipation, antidiarrheals such as the adsorbents that are not absorbed systemically should be considered as first-line therapy for pregnant women with diarrhea. However, adsorbents can inhibit the absorption of important nutrients. Iron supplementation may be particularly important in pregnant women taking adsorbents for diarrhea. Loperamide has not been shown to be teratogenic in animals but has been inadequately studied in humans; therefore, the routine use of loperamide is not recommended. Diphenoxylate with atropine should be avoided because it has been shown to be teratogenic in animals. In addition, malformations in infants after first trimester exposure have been reported. Both Lomotil and loperamide are excreted in breast milk. Salicylates have been shown to be teratogenic in animals. Therefore, use of BSS in the pregnant woman should be avoided.

Monitoring Patient Response

For most cases of diarrhea, the major concern is dehydration. Fluid and electrolyte depletion can lead to hypotension, tachycardia, and vascular collapse. Vascular collapse may occur quickly in the very old or the very young. Severe dehydration may result in decreased plasma volume and a decrease in perfusion, which may be of clinical significance, particularly in patients with congestive heart failure or chronic renal disease. Bicarbonate loss from excessive diarrhea may result in metabolic acidosis. This may be of particular concern in patients with type 1 diabetes mellitus who may be prone to ketoacidosis.

Patients should be monitored for signs of dehydration, such as orthostatic hypotension and poor skin turgor. The body weight of an infant is mostly water, and therefore, infants may be weighed to determine significant fluid loss and dehydration from severe diarrhea. Monitoring serum electrolytes as well as intake of fluid and output of stools benefits patients who are hospitalized secondary to dehydration.

As stated earlier, the goal of therapy is not only to prevent dehydration but also to make the patient as comfortable as possible. Monitoring the effectiveness of an antidiarrheal preparation requires interviewing the patient to ensure a decrease in stool frequency and improved formation. Frequency and formation of stools vary from patient to patient, and determination of relief is subjective on the patient's part.

Patient Education

To avoid complications, patients should be educated about appropriate rehydration. In most cases, simple replacement of fluid and electrolytes with soda crackers, broths, and soups is all that is necessary in the nondehydrated adult with diarrhea. Oral rehydration therapy (ORT) solutions should also be considered because most sports drinks do not have enough sodium to replace losses from diarrhea (Centers for Disease Control and Prevention, 2020a); however, the palatability of ORT product makes them difficult to administer especially to children. Additionally, food and drink high in sugar content should be avoided because it may increase the osmotic load and worsen the diarrhea. In the older adults or immunocompromised patient, solutions with sodium content in the range of 45 to 75 mEq/L are recommended. Boiled potatoes, noodles, rice, cereals, crackers, bananas, yogurt, soup, and boiled vegetables are recommended during the acute phase of diarrhea. The diet may return to normal as stools become formed.

Infants and children are particularly susceptible to dehydration with diarrhea. Oral replacement therapy is the preferred treatment to replace fluids and electrolytes in children with mild-to-moderate dehydration because it is less expensive than IV therapy and can be administered in many settings, including the home. Oral glucose–ESs available in the United States (**Table 25.9**) are based on physiologic principles and should be recommended over commonly used nonphysiologic solutions such as colas, apple juice, chicken broth, and sports beverages.

Oral replacement solutions (ORSs) have not changed over the years and are recommended for children with mild-to-moderate diarrhea (Centers for Disease Control, 2003). In addition, age-appropriate feeding should be continued, and fluids encouraged. For children with mild-to-moderate dehydration (3%–5% loss of total body weight), 50 to 100 mL/kg of ORS is recommended plus 10 mL/kg for each loose stool to replace continuing fluid losses. Severe dehydration (loss of 10% total body weight) can result in shock and is a medical emergency requiring IV therapy with normal saline or lactated Ringer's solution. In all situations, age-appropriate feeding should begin after dehydration is corrected.

Drug Information

Patients need to be aware of the potential side effects of antidiarrheal medications. Constipation can occur if these agents are taken for too long. Antidiarrheal agents taken in the setting of infectious diseases can prolong or worsen the disease. It is always best to contact a health care provider if diarrhea lasts more than 2 days.

Patient-Oriented Information Sources

Providing patients with information about acute diarrhea and what to expect can help them understand diarrhea and their

TABLE 25.9

Commercially Available Oral Rehydration Solutions

Product	Carbohydrate (g/L)	Na+ (mEq/L)	K+ (mEq/L)	Cl− (mEq/L)	Base (mEq/L)	Calories (kcal)
Infalyte* (Mead Johnson)	30 (rice syrup solids)	50	25	45	34 (citrate)	126
Pedialyte† (Ross Laboratories)	25 (dextrose)	45	20	35	30 (citrate)	100
Rehydralyte (Ross Laboratories)	25 (dextrose)	75‡	20	65	30 (citrate)	100
WHO Solution§ (Ianas Bros. Packing Co.)	20 (glucose)	90‡	20	80	10 (citrate)	80

*Available in hospitals as 6-ounce nursing bottle.

†Available in hospitals as 8-ounce nursing bottle.

‡The American Academy of Pediatrics recommends these solutions with sodium contents of 75–90 mEq/L for replacement of deficit during initial rehydration (*Pediatrics, 75,* 358, 1985).

§Must be mixed with 1 L of boiled or treated water; packets available in stores or pharmacies in all developing countries.

Source: Manufacturer's product information.

Reproduced by permission from American Journal of Gastroenterology. (1997). Commercially available oral rehydration solutions. *American Journal of Gastroenterology, 92,* 1962–1975. Copyright © 1997, Rights Managed by Nature Publishing Group.

role in the treatment. Patient education items are readily available on the Internet through the NDDIC, which provides information to consumers on a wide variety of GI topics. The CDC also has a wide array of patient information about diarrhea (see **Box 25.16**).

Nutrition/Lifestyle Changes

It is not recommended to rest the gut. Oral intake and breast-feeding should continue to replace lost calories during illness. Early feeding will stimulate enterocyte renewal, ultimately promoting a quicker recovery of the gut. Additionally, feeding decreases the potential risk of malnutrition.

Complementary and Alternative Medications

Probiotics have shown some efficacy in the treatment of diarrhea but only shortens the duration for a few days (McFarland & Goh, 2019; Parker et al., 2018). The presumed mechanism of action is to alter the composition of the intestinal microflora and act against enteric pathogens (Guarino et al., 2009). Yogurt is a source of probiotics; however, not all brands have the active ingredients. Acidophilus capsules can be used to treat diarrhea resulting from antibiotic use. It restores the natural flora to the bowel. One to 10 billion viable organisms per day in three or four divided doses are appropriate.

IRRITABLE BOWEL SYNDROME

IBS is a functional bowel disorder that presents with abdominal discomfort and an alteration in bowel pattern. The disorder is an international health problem that can be one of the most perplexing chronic abdominal complaints reported to primary care providers and gastroenterologists. Epidemiologic studies in North America continue to suggest a prevalence of 10% to 15%, with a 4:1 female predominance, while 7% to 10% have IBS worldwide (Brandt et al., 2009; Lovell & Ford, 2012).

Once thought to be associated primarily with psychological problems and stress, research is changing to an emphasis on motility of the gut, autonomic system imbalances, and increased visceral hypersensitivity (Akbara et al., 2009; Quigley, 2018). A syndrome in childhood known as recurrent abdominal pain can be a hallmark of adult IBS. Most patients seeking care are ages 20 to 50, and symptoms can wax and wane over a lifetime.

Causes

For many years, the chief cause of IBS was thought to be primarily psychological. Now, however, research has identified physiologic but not pathologic causes that are accentuated by psychological stress. Symptoms generally are slow in onset, sometimes over weeks or months. Dysregulation occurs between the brain and the gut, leading to typical IBS symptoms. Commonly, the symptoms can be worse during times of physical and emotional stress, including sexual or physical abuse. In addition, some patients can identify foods that exacerbate the condition (e.g., lactose, caffeine, and fatty or spicy foods). Depending on the severity of the illness, pharmacotherapy may not be required, and symptoms may respond solely to lifestyle changes. These lifestyle changes need to become incorporated into the patient's daily routines. Pharmacologic interventions may be required only intermittently to maintain symptom control.

Pathophysiology

In general, the syndrome is believed to have the components of motility and sensory abnormalities. This leads to dysregulation of the bowel as modulated by the CNS. Many neuroimmune and neuroendocrine modulators, such as serotonin (5-HT), substance P, cholecystokinin (CCK), neurotensin, cytokines, and others, contribute to the increase in visceral sensitivity, central mechanisms controlling pain and dysregulation of the brain–gut axis. Local reflex mechanisms can also be responsible for mechanical distention of the gut in response to short-chain fatty acids, affecting the emptying rate of the proximal colon. The prevailing theory is that the emptying rate of the proximal colon may be the key determination of overall colon function. The GI tract is innervated intrinsically and extrinsically by various neurohormonal agents from local or distant sources. Intrinsic factors include the neurons found in the enteric nervous system, which function similarly to the CNS. Bowel motor dysfunction can be associated with inflammation as well as changes in neurotransmitters, such as 5-hydroxytryptamine (5-HT$_3$; serotonin). This neurotransmitter is found in the GI tract, and blocking it pharmacologically can decrease visceral pain, colonic transit, and GI secretions. External factors that can alter colonic activity are eating and drinking, stress, and endogenous hormones. Increased motility and abnormal contractions of the intestinal tract can result in either diarrhea or constipation-predominant IBS, due to either accelerated whole-gut transit times or delays in colonic transit. The IBS patient's sensory perception of colonic activity in response to balloon dilatation is more sensitive than that of patients with normal colonic activity. Sensory perception is also accentuated by external factors that lead to enhanced sensations that differ from those of healthy patients. However, evidence is increasing that IBS is not a psychological illness.

Diagnostic Criteria

The hallmark symptom of IBS is abdominal pain associated with a change in the consistency of stools that is relieved by defecation. Symptoms are usually first noticed in young adulthood and can be persistent or intermittent. Weight loss, rectal bleeding, fever, acute onset, and onset after age 50 are unusual in IBS and should raise suspicion of organic causes, not IBS. Diagnosis can be predominantly based on symptoms and appropriate treatment initiated, with reassessment in 3 to 6 weeks.

In 1978, the original Manning criteria proposed identifying IBS based on the presence of four symptoms: abdominal distention, pain relief with bowel action, more frequent stools with the onset of pain, and looser stools with the onset of pain. These criteria led to the establishment of an international group called the Multinational Working Teams for Diagnosis of Functional GI Disorders that continues work to this day. Previously, the Rome III criteria defined IBS the presenting clinical features may be sporadic, intermittent, or continuous but should be present for at least 3 months. Now the Rome IV criteria no longer classifies by frequency but (**Box 25.13**) defines IBS as recurrent abdominal pain 1 day per week in the last 3 months related to defecation and change in stool frequency and form with the onset at least 6 months prior to diagnosis (Lacey et al., 2016). Classification of the type of stool is also an important aspect of diagnosis. The Bristol Stool Scale provides visual scale that allows patients a way to improve their description and classify stools, therefore, assisting with the plan of care (Riegeler & Esposito, 2001).

The chief complaint most patients report is abdominal discomfort that can be relieved with defecation; however, symptom relief is often short lived. Patients can also report abnormal bowel habits that alternate between diarrhea and constipation or are predominantly diarrhea or constipation; it is much more common to have bowel habits that are predominantly one type. Associated components can be abdominal distention, bloating, and gassiness. Extreme urgency after a meal can be common and can possibly result in an "explosive" bowel movement that relieves the overall discomfort.

Organic symptoms of abdominal pain that do not suggest IBS are those that awaken the patient from sleep, initial onset in the older years, and a change in abdominal pain that is not associated with bowel movements, significant weight loss, rectal bleeding, steatorrhea, and fever. In addition, steadily worsening symptoms should be considered atypical. These symptoms would suggest the need for additional studies.

BOX 25.13 Rome IV Criteria for Irritable Bowel Syndrome

Recurrent abdominal pain at least 1 day per week during the previous 3 months and onset at least 6 months prior. Criteria is associated with two or more of the following:

- Relation to defecation—increased or unchanged
- Associated with change in frequency of stool
- Associated with a change in form or appearance of stool

Source: Palsson, O. S., Whitehead, W. E., van Tilburg, M. A. L., et al. (2016). Development and validation of the Rome IV diagnostic questionnaire for adults. *Gastroenterology, 150*(6), 1481–1491. https://doi.org/10.1053/j.gastro.2016.02.014

However, compared to the general population, IBS patients are not more likely to have organic causes for disease.

A key component of IBS treatment is a thorough history of symptoms, psychosocial stress, medications (because of GI symptoms from many drugs), and dietary habits (to identify nutritional patterns, gaps, and intolerances). Even in the general population, stress can result in GI symptoms. However, in the patient with IBS, these symptoms can become more pronounced. The relationship between psychological distress and GI symptoms has been well researched. Chronic and acute life stresses, including a history of verbal or sexual abuse, especially in childhood, may preclude early symptoms of IBS. These chronic stresses can contribute later in life to IBS symptoms.

Physical examination findings are often normal except for a slight diffuse abdominal tenderness with palpation, especially in the left lower quadrant near the sigmoid colon. Mild abdominal distention may also be present.

In 2009, in an evidence-based position paper on the management of IBS in North America, the American College of Gastroenterology (ACG) Task Force reinforced the recommendation that minimal, if any, testing is necessary. This guidance was again supported by the task force in 2018. The best available data show that only 1% of IBS patients have alarming symptoms signifying serious organic disease. Therefore, for patients without alarming features of IBS, routine diagnostic studies are not necessary. However, patients who are classified as IBS-D (diarrhea) or IBS-M (mixed) should be routinely tested for celiac sprue disease. Other studies such as abdominal ultrasound, flexible sigmoidoscopy, barium enema, or colonoscopy do not lead to any change in the proposed treatment and are therefore not recommended. Additional testing may be indicated for patients with the key symptoms previously identified or if the patient is older than age 50.

Types of Irritable Bowel Syndrome

Once identified according to the Rome IV criteria (see **Box 25.13**), patient definition of further subtypes of constipation (IBS-C), IBS-D, IBS-M, or unspecified (IBS-U) (**Box 25.14**) can further refine the diagnosis and focus for treatment. Symptoms of IBS can vary in frequency. While patients can stay predominately in one category, there is often overlap in symptomatology.

Initiating Drug Therapy

Initial therapy is focused on establishing a therapeutic relationship and mapping out a long-term strategy. This provides the patient with knowledge regarding the disease process and lets the patient know that improvement may be a slow process, taking many months.

Patients with mild symptoms may be responsive to dietary and lifestyle changes (**Box 25.15**). Assessing the diet for potentially offending substances and removing those substances may improve symptoms. Hayes et al. (2014) found in a survey of patients with IBS that cereal products and spicy foods along with vegetables and fatty foods were a predominant cause of symptoms. These substances may be lactose, caffeine, beans,

---

BOX 25.14   Subtyping of Irritable Bowel Syndrome by Predominant Stool Pattern

1. IBS with constipation (IBS-C)—greater than 25% of bowel movements with Bristol Stool Scale Types 1 to 2, 25% with Types 6 to 7.
2. IBS with diarrhea (IBS-D)— greater than 25% of bowel movements with Bristol Stool Scale Types 6 to 7, 25% with Types 1 to 2.
3. IBS mixed (IBS-M)—greater than 25% of bowel movements with Bristol Stool Scale Types 1 to 2, 25% with Types 6 to 7.
4. IBS unclassified (IBS-U)—patients meet diagnostic criteria due to inconsistency to be accurately categorized by any of the earlier mentioned subtypes.

Adapted from Schmulson, M. J., & Drossman, D. A. (2017). What is new in Rome IV. *Journal of Neurogastroenterology and Motility, 23*(2), 151–163. https://doi.org/10.5056/jnm16214

BOX 25.15   Dietary and Lifestyle Changes

Avoid foods that exacerbate the symptoms (e.g., lactose, caffeine, fatty or spicy foods).
Consider dietary restriction of short-chain fermentable carbohydrates (FODMAP).
Incorporate routine exercise into daily activities.
Explore the life stressors that aggravate the symptoms.
Learn ways to deal with stress, such as meditation, counseling, and biofeedback.

---

cabbage, fatty foods, or alcohol (Simren, 2001). Versa and colleagues in 1998 showed a positive correlation between IBS and lactose intolerance, female sex, and abdominal pain in childhood, and these early findings have been supported by additional research (Yang et al., 2014). A 2-week trial of a lactose-free diet is worth pursuing. Aspartame, an artificial sweetener found in many soft drinks and diet foods, may also provoke diarrhea. Trial elimination may also be worthwhile, especially in diarrhea-predominant IBS. Also, consider dietary restriction of short-chain fermentable carbohydrates (fermentable oligosaccharide, disaccharide, monosaccharide, and polyol [FODMAP]) improves IBS symptoms. This type of diet is complex and is best implemented in conjunction with a dietician. However, with most IBS therapies, the placebo effect is often just as successful as the therapy itself.

Maintaining a daily diary of food intake, bowel patterns, and emotional stressors can be helpful in the treatment of IBS. It serves to identify factors that can be addressed and evaluates the effectiveness of treatment. Lifestyle modification requires the patient to understand the stressors in their life and the effect these stressors have on physiologic functions. Identifying ways to reduce stress can be critical to improving IBS symptoms. Biofeedback can be used to decrease gut sensitivity, along with relaxation tapes to decrease stressors. There is some benefit of regular exercise in reducing stress and improving bowel transit. However, as previously discussed in the section on constipation, exercise has little benefit on bowel transit time.

Goals of Drug Therapy

The pharmacologic agents used for IBS are the same as those discussed in the constipation and diarrhea sections of this chapter. The goal of pharmacotherapy for IBS is to alleviate or control the specific symptoms. Generally, clinical trials have been inadequate to establish a definite link between administration of specific drugs and relief of symptoms. In patients with IBS, between 50% and 75% still have symptoms after 10 years (Canavan et al., 2014). In an open-label placebo trial, response rates to a placebo were as high as 53% (Kaptchuk et al., 2010).

Bulk-Forming Laxatives

Previously, administration of dietary fiber in the form of a bulking agent was commonly the first agent prescribed in IBS (**Table 25.10**). However, administration of fiber to patients with IBS has become controversial. While the hypothesis exists that fiber increases colonic transit time and therefore lessens colon wall tension and ultimately abdominal pain, clinical trials on the use of fiber in IBS have had small sample sizes and have been short in duration. Fiber can exacerbate the diarrhea and bloating component of IBS; however, if it is used, the current recommendation by the 2016 ACG Task Force is the use of psyllium, not wheat bran.

Hyperosmotic Laxatives

When the patient requires a laxative, it is preferable to administer one that is osmotic (see **Table 25.10**). These agents can work either as a disaccharide sugar, which produces an osmotic effect in the colon, resulting in colonic distention and promotion of peristalsis, or by an osmotic effect in the small intestine, drawing water into the lumen and softening the stool. Lactulose or sorbitol, disaccharide sugars, can be used for patients with predominant constipation. PEG 3350 (MiraLAX) is a glycolated laxative that can be safely used for a long period without adverse pharmacologic effects.

Contraindications

The same contraindications exist as when using these agents to treat chronic constipation. Lactulose is contraindicated in patients who must restrict their galactose intake and in

TABLE 25.10

Overview of Selected Agents Used to Treat Irritable Bowel Syndrome

Generic (Trade) Name and Dosage	Selected Adverse Events	Contraindications	Special Considerations
Selected Bulk-Forming Laxatives			
Psyllium (Konsyl, Metamucil, Perdiem) Start: 1 tsp in 8 oz liquid BID–TID Range: 1–2 tsp in 8 oz liquid BID–TID	Abdominal fullness, increased flatus	Symptoms of acute surgical abdomen, intestinal obstruction, or perforation Inability to drink adequate amounts of water	Comes in granules, powder, or wafers Takes 12 h to 3 d to work
Calcium polycarbophil (Equalactin, FiberCon, Mitrolan) Start: 500 mg tabs daily) Range: 500–1000 mg QID	Abdominal fullness, increased flatus	Same as those for Psyllium	Takes 12 h to 3 d to work
Methylcellulose (Citrucel) Start: 1 tsp in 8 oz liquid BID–TID Range: 1–2 tsp in 8 oz liquid BID or TID	Nausea, abdominal cramps	Same as those for Psyllium	Takes 12 h to 3 d to work
Hyperosmotic Laxatives			
Lactulose (Duphalac) syrup Start: 15–30 mL PO daily Range: 15–60 mg/d	Flatulence, intestinal cramps, diarrhea, nausea, vomiting, electrolyte imbalances	Galactose-restricted diets, appendicitis, acute surgical abdomen, fecal impaction, or intestinal obstruction Use with caution in patients with diabetes	

(Continued)

TABLE 25.10

Overview of Selected Agents Used to Treat Irritable Bowel Syndrome (*Continued*)

Generic (Trade) Name and Dosage	Selected Adverse Events	Contraindications	Special Considerations
Magnesium citrate (Citroma) oral solution Start: 5 oz QHS Range: 5–10 oz QHS magnesium hydroxide (milk of magnesia/MOM.) Start: 15 mL QHS Range: 15–60 mL QHS	Abdominal cramping, nausea Abdominal cramping, nausea	End-stage renal disease End-stage renal disease	Can cause increased magnesium levels in patients with end-stage renal disease Same as those for Magnesium citrate
Stimulant Laxatives			
Bisacodyl (Dulcolax) Start: 10 mg PO in evening or before breakfast Range: 10–15 mg	Abdominal cramping, nausea, vomiting, burning sensation in rectum with suppositories		Oral: 6–8 h Rectal: 15–60 min
Senna concentrates (Senokot) Start: 2 tabs or 1 level tsp at hs Range: 2–4 tabs or 1–2 tsp QHS	Abdominal cramping, nausea	Signs and symptoms of appendicitis, abdominal pain, nausea, vomiting	Older adults or debilitated, halve the dose
Surfactant Laxatives			
Docusate calcium (Surfak) Start: 240 mg/d Range: 240 mg/d	None	None	May increase the systemic absorption of mineral oil
Docusate sodium (Colace) Start: 50 mg/d Range: 50–200 mg/d	Bitter taste, throat irritation, nausea, rash	Signs and symptoms of appendicitis	Onset: 1–3 d Not to be used for acute relief of constipation
Antidiarrheal Agents			
Diphenoxylate HCl with atropine sulfate (Lomotil) Start: 5 mg QID Range: 5–10 mg QID; maintenance may be 10 mg daily	Sedation, dizziness, dry mouth, paralytic ileus	Pseudomembranous enterocolitis, obstructive jaundice, diarrhea caused by organisms that penetrate intestinal mucosa Under 2 y of age Pregnancy category C	Onset 45–60 min
Loperamide HCl (Imodium) Start: 4 mg after first loose stool then 2 mg after each following stool Range: 4–16 mg/d	Constipation	Acute dysentery	Peak levels 2.5 h after liquid and 5 h after capsule
Selected Antispasmodics (Anticholinergic Agents)			
Belladonna alkaloids (Donnatal) Start: 1 tab or capsule TID or QID Range: 1–2 tabs/capsules TID or QID	Drowsiness, anticholinergic effects, paradoxical excitement	Glaucoma, unstable coronary artery disease, GI or GU obstruction, paralytic ileus, severe ulcerative colitis	Antacids may inhibit absorption. Additive anticholinergic effects with other anticholinergics, antihistamines, narcotics, tricyclic antidepressants
Dicyclomine HCl (Bentyl) Start: 20 mg QID Range: 20–40 mg QID if tolerated	Same as those for Belladonna alkaloids	Same as those for Belladonna alkaloids	Same as those for Belladonna alkaloids
Clidinium (Librax) Start: 1 capsule QID—ac and QHS Range: 1–2 capsules QID—ac and QHS	Drowsiness, anticholinergic effects, paradoxical excitement, ataxia, confusion, jaundice	Glaucoma, GI or GU obstruction	Same as those for Belladonna alkaloids

TABLE 25.10

Overview of Selected Agents Used to Treat Irritable Bowel Syndrome (*Continued*)

Generic (Trade) Name and Dosage	Selected Adverse Events	Contraindications	Special Considerations
Hyoscyamine sulfate (Levsin, Levbid, Levsin SL) *Levsin* Start: 1 tab q4h PRN Range: 1–2 tabs q4h PRN; max 12 tabs/d> *Levbid* Start: 1 tab q12h Range: 1–2 tabs q12h; max 4 tabs/d *Levsin SL* Start: 1 tab swallowed or chewed q4h PRN Range: max 12 tabs/d	Same as those for Clidinium	Same as those for Clidinium	Same as those for Belladonna alkaloids
Secretagogues—Chloride Channel Activators			
Lubiprostone (Amitiza) IBS-C: 8 mcg capsules BID	Nausea, diarrhea, abdominal pain, dyspepsia	Known or suspected mechanical GI obstructions	Pregnancy category C Not approved for children For IBS; only approved for women Must take medication with food and water, swallow whole
Semisynthetic Antibiotic			
Rifaximin (Xifaxan) IBS-D: 500 mg tabs TID × 14 d	Peripheral edema, nausea, dizziness, fatigue, and muscles spasms. Additional post-marketing side effects include exfoliative dermatitis, rash, angioneurotic edema (swelling of face and tongue and difficulty swallowing), urticaria, flushing, pruritus, and anaphylaxis	Known hypersensitivity to rifaximin Bloody diarrhea	If diarrhea continues, consider evaluation for *Clostridium Difficile* May repeat treatment up to two times for recurrent diarrhea at the same dose Can be taken with or without food

GI, gastrointestinal; GU, genitorurinary; IBS, irritable bowel syndrome; IBS-C, IBS-constipation; IBS-D, IBS-diarrhea.

patients with appendicitis, acute surgical abdomen, fecal impaction, or intestinal obstruction. Caution must be used with administration to patients with diabetes because of sugar content.

Other osmotic agents such as magnesium hydroxide (milk of magnesia) or magnesium citrate (Citroma) can be used to promote defecation. Approximately 15% to 30% of the magnesium in these agents may be absorbed systemically; therefore, caution needs to be used in patients who have renal failure and a decreased ability to excrete magnesium.

Adverse Events

When taken appropriately, these agents are well tolerated. The most common adverse events are abdominal cramping or nausea. Extensive, long-term use of these agents can lead to laxative dependence.

Stimulant Laxatives

These laxatives vary in effects but act by increasing peristalsis through a direct effect on the smooth muscle of the intestines and by simultaneously promoting fluid accumulation in the colon and small intestine. The recommendation is to use these agents intermittently due to the irritating effect of the agents on the musculature. Stimulant laxatives include bisacodyl (Dulcolax) and senna concentrates (Senokot, Senokot S). As with other laxatives, stimulants are contraindicated in patients with appendicitis, acute surgical abdomen, fecal impaction, or intestinal obstruction. Rectal fissures and hemorrhoids can be exacerbated by stimulation of defecation. Action begins 6 to 10 hours after oral administration and 15 minutes to 2 hours after rectal administration (see **Table 25.10**).

These agents are not as well tolerated as osmotic laxatives or bulking agents because of their side effects, which include nausea, vomiting, and abdominal cramping. These side effects can be more severe with cases of severe constipation. Several OTC products use the brand name of Dulcolax. One has the main ingredient of bisacodyl, and another is docusate sodium, which is a stool softener. This could be important, especially when the patient has been instructed to use the drug as bowel preparation for a GI study.

Surfactant Laxatives

This class of laxatives reduces the surface tension of the liquid contents of the bowel. Ultimately, this promotes incorporation of additional liquid into the stool, forming a softer mass, and promotes easier defecation. Examples of this class include docusate sodium (Colace, Dulcolax) and docusate calcium (Surfak). This is the laxative of choice for patients who should not strain during defecation. However, emollient laxatives only prevent constipation; they do not treat it. Administration of emollient laxatives concomitantly with mineral oil is contraindicated because of increased absorption of the mineral oil. Action with these agents usually occurs in 1 to 3 days. The practitioner should consider this class for prevention purposes, not for acute treatment (see **Table 25.10**). These agents are extremely well tolerated when used to prevent constipation. Side effects include mild abdominal cramping, diarrhea, and throat irritation, but these are infrequent.

Antidiarrheal Agents

Antidiarrheal agents for patients with IBS with predominant diarrhea can be used on an occasional basis (see **Table 25.10**). Loperamide HCl (Imodium) inhibits peristaltic activity, thereby prolonging transit time, and it can increase anal sphincter tone. Approximately 40% of the drug is absorbed from the GI tract and 75% is metabolized in the hepatic system; excretion is primarily in the feces. As previously discussed, the drug does not cross the blood–brain barrier into the CNS. Because of these properties, it is the preferred agent for treating diarrhea. Conversely, diphenoxylate hydrochloride with atropine (Lomotil) is an opiate similar to meperidine that increases smooth muscle tone in the GI tract, inhibits motility and propulsion, and diminishes gut secretions. It is absorbed orally and extensively metabolized by the liver. It can affect the CNS, and atropine has been added to discourage abuse.

Neither of these antidiarrheal agents should be used in a patient suspected of having diarrhea from pseudomembranous colitis or UC or diarrhea resulting from poisoning or microbial infection. Diphenoxylate hydrochloride is contraindicated in patients who are hypersensitive to atropine or meperidine and

patients with hepatic impairment. The atropine in Lomotil may aggravate glaucoma in patients with this disease. For additional discussion of contraindications and adverse events, see the diarrhea section.

Antispasmodic Agents

Treatment for patients with postprandial abdominal pain may require the use of antispasmodics (see **Table 25.10**). However, the efficacy of these medications remains unproven in controlled studies. The presumed desired action is by direct relaxation of the smooth muscle component of the GI tract. These agents competitively block the effects of acetylcholine at muscarinic cholinergic receptors that mediate the effects of parasympathetic postganglionic impulses. Examples of commonly used anticholinergics are dicyclomine hydrochloride (Bentyl) and hyoscyamine sulfate (Levbid, Levsin SL). Less commonly used are the belladonna alkaloids/phenobarbital (Donnatal) and clidinium/chlordiazepoxide (Librax); while both are still on the market, they can be difficult to find and expensive. These drugs are a combination of older benzodiazepines, antispasmodics, and/or antiepileptics. Dosing of the anticholinergics is variable, and general side effects are associated with the anticholinergic actions.

Contraindications

These agents are contraindicated in patients who have glaucoma, stenosing peptic ulcer, chronic obstructive pulmonary disease, cardiac arrhythmias, impaired liver or kidney function, and myasthenia gravis. Caution should be used in patients with hypertension, hyperthyroidism, and benign prostatic hyperplasia.

Adverse Events

Side effects include dry mouth, altered taste perception, nausea, vomiting, dysphagia, blurred vision, palpitations, and urinary hesitancy and retention. Anticholinergic side effects can be used as a measure of titration to achieve the desired pharmacologic end. It is important to monitor for signs of drug toxicity: CNS signs resembling psychosis, accompanied by peripheral effects that include dilated, nonreactive pupils; blurred vision; hot, dry, flushed skin; dry mucous membranes; dysphagia; decreased or absent bowel sounds; urinary retention; hyperthermia; tachycardia; hypertension; and increased respiration.

Antidepressants

Antidepressants as a class have also been used in the treatment of IBS. It is not clear whether these agents work by improving a concomitant depression or by improving the anxiety and stress often associated with IBS. Initial work was done with use of the tricyclic agents such as imipramine (Tofranil), desipramine (Norpramin), and amitriptyline (Elavil) in patients with severe symptoms. Careful monitoring is important when tricyclic antidepressants are given to patients with IBS in which constipation predominates, because these agents can cause constipation. Newer agents in the selective serotonin reuptake inhibitor (SSRI) class may also prove beneficial. It has been suggested based on current investigations that antidepressants alter perceived pain thresholds, which are often abnormal in patients with IBS. See Chapter 39 for further discussion of these drugs.

Serotonin-3 Receptor Antagonists

This class of drugs is commonly used for nausea but has been found to address the brain–gut–neurotransmitter (5-HT$_3$) connection regarding colonic transit time. The only drug classified specifically for IBS is alosetron. In animal models, serotonin-3 receptor antagonist has been shown to decrease abdominal pain, slow colonic transit time, increase rectal compliance, and improve stool consistency. Indication for use of alosetron is only for women patients who have severe diarrhea and no constipation. The drug was first released in 1999, but later pulled from the market in 2000 due to concerns about ischemic colitis and severe constipation. In 2002, alosetron once again became available with special provisions by the FDA for provider education and distribution. The Weinberg et al. (2014) recommends *conditional* use of alosetron for IBS-D reflecting additional limitations based on FDA requirements.

Secretagogues

Chloride Channel Activators

As previously discussed in the constipation section, lubiprostone (Amitiza) is approved for CIC and OIC for both men and women; however, for treatment of IBS, it is only approved for use in women 18 years and older. Lubiprostone is the only drug in this class. Lubiprostone became approved for IBS in 2008 and is prescribed at a lower strength starting at 0.5 mg twice a day.

Contraindications

Lubiprostone is contraindicated in patients with potential mechanical obstruction or hypersensitivity to components of the product.

Adverse Events

The side-effect profile is like usage in chronic constipation; however, only GI effects are noted. Nausea is the most common side effect of lubiprostone. The rate of nausea is dose dependent and was experienced by approximately 8% of patients. Other common GI side effects include diarrhea, abdominal pain, and abdominal distention.

Interactions

No drug–drug interactions have been discovered with lubiprostone. In vitro studies showed the cytochrome P-450 isoenzymes are not inhibited by the drug.

Guanylate Cyclase-C Agonist

This class has been previously discussed in the constipation section. The mechanism of action for linaclotide (Linzess) is topical rather than systemic, elevating intracellular cGMP, which stimulates secretion of chloride and bicarbonate into the intestinal lumen. Along with the increased fluid, stool transit time is accelerated. Linzess is approved for 18 years and older with IBS. The recommended dosage for IBS is substantially increased to 290 mcg orally once daily, 30 minutes prior to the first meal of the day.

Semisynthetic Antibiotic

Rifaximin

Rifaximin (Xifaxan) is a semisynthetic antibiotic also approved for treatment of IBS-D. It is only effective against noninvasive strains of *E. coli*. The drug is a derivative of rifampin and acts to block transcription of the bacteria; therefore, it inhibits bacterial protein synthesis and growth. Additionally, rifaximin improves IBS-D symptoms of abdominal pain after a 10- to 14-day course of treatment. The recommended dose for IBS-D is 550 mg thrice daily for 14 days; this differs from the TD administration. Rifaximin may be administered with or without meals. Patients with recurrent symptoms can be retreated up to two times with the same regime. If the diarrhea does not improve, providers should consider evaluation for *C. difficile*.

Selecting the Most Appropriate Agent

The emphasis in the care of patients with IBS should be multidimensional. In 2014, the American Gastroenterological Association (AGA) developed pharmacologic guidelines (Weinberg et al., 2014). These recommendations consider the level of available data and analysis of risk/benefits for agents. As patient care evolves toward evidence-based medicine, the AGA notes that few comparative effectiveness studies exist of the various therapeutic alternatives for treatment of IBS. This fact continues to make prescribing for IBS a challenge for clinical care. Therefore, the standard is still the selection of the most appropriate drug therapy based on the presenting symptoms. Each case needs to be evaluated, and treatment should be individualized (**Figure 25.6** and **Table 25.11**).

First-Line Therapy

First-line therapy is selected based on the presenting symptoms. Qualitatively, patients often feel the burden of this disease but believe this is not appreciated by primary care providers and specialists. Pharmacologic agents need to be considered only when an exacerbation of the disease occurs. There is strong evidence that IBS-C should be treated with linaclotide or lubiprostone as a first-line therapy. Consider an osmotic laxative on a long-term basis for those who are averse to the potential incidence of diarrhea with either linaclotide or lubiprostone. Antidiarrheal agents are conditionally recommended in patients with IBS-D. Loperamide is the preferred agent because it causes the least CNS activity and has the added benefit of improving anal sphincter tone.

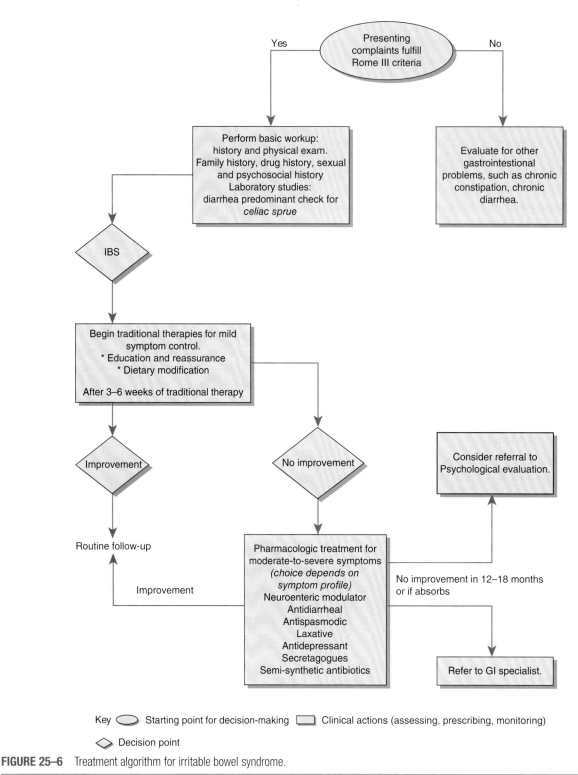

FIGURE 25–6   Treatment algorithm for irritable bowel syndrome.

GI, gastrointestinal; IBS, irritable bowel syndrome.

With the additional problems of pain, gas, and abdominal bloating, a trial of an antispasmodic may relieve symptoms. Dicyclomine is the agent of first choice because of its shorter half-life, which may minimize the anticholinergic side effects of the class. As with any chronic syndrome, use of low-level antidepressants may be helpful for symptom control. Psychological symptoms associated with IBS may be treated by antidepressants. Selection of an antidepressant should be based on the specific symptoms of depression, stress, or anxiety. The SSRIs are the most selected agents because of their safety profile and efficacy.

TABLE 25.11

Recommended Order for Treatment for Irritable Bowel Syndrome

Order	Agents	Comments
First Line		
Predominant constipation (IBS-C)	Osmotic laxative—lactulose syrup, magnesium citrate, magnesium hydroxide	Milk of magnesia is less expensive than citrate
	Consider using psyllium products	Use magnesium products cautiously in patients with renal impairment
		Use lactulose cautiously in patients with diabetes
	Linaclotide or lubiprostone	Consider for first or second line for IBS-C
Predominant diarrhea (IBS-D)	Antidiarrheal—loperamide	May cause constipation
	Hydrochloride (Imodium)	Caution about drowsiness; may have a dry mouth
	Rifaximin	If diarrhea continues after a total of two treatments, consider *C. difficile*
Abdominal bloating/gas	Antispasmodics—dicyclomine hydrochloride (Bentyl)	
Psychological symptoms	Antidepressants—SSRIs	Generally, as a class, these agents may be helpful with chronic syndromes
		Cost may be an issue
Second Line		Generalized CNS effects
Predominant constipation	Continue osmotic laxatives.	
	Add linaclotide or lubiprostone	If not used first line
Predominant diarrhea	Antidiarrheal—diphenoxylate hydrochloride (Lomotil)	Monitor for anticholinergic effects
Abdominal bloating/gas	Antispasmodics—hyoscyamine sulfate (Levsin, Levbid, Levsin SL)	
Psychological symptoms	Antidepressants—tricyclic agents (imipramine, desipramine, amitriptyline) (Tofranil, Norpramin, Elavil)	Onset of action and steady states vary with each drug
Third Line		
Predominant constipation	Laxatives—bisacodyl (Dulcolax), senna concentrates (Senokot), emollient laxatives, docusate sodium (Colace), docusate calcium (Surfak)	Caution with cardiac patients
		Can aggravate abdominal cramping
		Use only as additive to keep stools soft
Abdominal bloating/gas	Antispasmodics—belladonna alkaloids (Donnatal), clidinium (Librax)	More severe generalized anticholinergic effects

CNS, central nervous system; IBS-C, irritable bowel syndrome-constipation; IBS-D, irritable bowel syndrome-diarrhea; SSRIs, selective serotonin reuptake inhibitor

Second-Line Therapy

Unresolved complaints of IBS-D can be treated with diphenoxylate hydrochloride, which has a longer duration of action but can be addictive because of its opioid properties and should be reserved for short-term use. Rifaximin should be tried for those whose diarrhea symptoms do not improve. For postprandial abdominal pain, gas, and abdominal bloating, longer-acting antispasmodics such as hyoscyamine sulfate can be considered. The second-line choice for psychological symptoms is the tricyclic antidepressants; these agents have more side effects than SSRIs.

Third-Line Therapy

The use of stimulant laxatives in cases of IBS-C should be reserved for more resistant cases, but these agents should be used with caution. They should not be used for long periods,

and they can aggravate abdominal cramping. The older anticholinergics such as the belladonna alkaloids and clidinium should be used very sparingly for postprandial abdominal pain, gas, and abdominal bloating because they produce more intense anticholinergic side effects. In addition, both belladonna and clidinium are hard to find and can be expensive. Patients with IBS, no matter which subtype, need to have consistent evaluation and pharmacologic therapies changed as appropriate for their symptoms.

Special Considerations

Pediatric

Children with crampy abdominal pain, constipation, or diarrhea present a challenge to the practitioner. The approach to diagnosis follows the same parameters of adults; however, few if any of the pharmacologic agents are approved for pediatrics. Previously, children were not thought to have IBS but that has changed (Devanarayana & Rajindrajith, 2018; Hyams et al., 2016). Treatment for these symptoms can include some of the same approaches of increasing fiber and use of antidiarrheal agents and the newer antispasmodics. Close follow-up is an important aspect of care.

Geriatric

Initial presentation of IBS in people older than age 50 is rare. Abdominal pain in older patients should be considered a more ominous symptom unless they have been previously diagnosed with IBS or spastic colon, a version of colitis. Older patients may report a long-standing history of bowel trouble with any of these diagnoses.

Women

In Western society, women are more likely to have IBS and to seek care. A history of verbal or sexual abuse may also contribute to IBS. Women have surgery more often when the origins of abdominal pains are unclear.

Monitoring Patient Response

Monitoring the patient's response to therapy should take place within 3 to 6 weeks of the initial evaluation. For all patients, the initial treatment includes working with the patient regarding dietary and lifestyle changes, education about the disease process, and reassurance about lack of organic causes. Patients can easily be managed in the primary care office with close monitoring initially, every 3 to 6 weeks, and then more routine care.

IBS is a disease of exacerbations and remissions, but up to 70% of patients respond to treatment within 12 to 18 months. Those with a shorter duration of symptoms and fewer psychological symptoms have a better prognosis. Referral to a specialist should occur when there is no relief with any therapies or when the patient has atypical symptomatology. Continued symptoms rarely need a reappraisal of the diagnosis, but appropriate testing should be performed.

Patient Education

Patient education needs to cover dietary modifications, psychological stresses, and lifestyle changes. Begin by acknowledging the patient's fears and concerns and show that you take them seriously. According to current evidence-based research, patients can be reassured of the absence of organic disease based on the history and physical examination. The patient should be informed that this is a chronic disease, and that IBS does not lead to cancer, colitis, or an altered life expectancy. Making the necessary dietary changes can be crucial for symptom relief, especially with mild symptoms. A multidisciplinary approach is often the best method of care, using the services of a dietitian and psychological counselor.

Drug Information

A variety of drugs are available to help control symptoms, and most have minimal side effects. However, the drugs need to be used in conjunction with stress relief techniques, identification of influencing factors, and education about the disease to help provide an improved quality of life.

Patient-Oriented Information Sources

Many resources exist for patients with IBS. One of the most comprehensive resources is the ACG, which covers many topics on GI health. The International Foundation of Functional Bowel Disorders also has a comprehensive Web site with resources for both patients and health care providers (**Box 25.16**).

Nutrition/Lifestyle Changes

A major focus of caring for patients with IBS is helping them assess their diet, adjusting as necessary. A trial of removing foods that trigger symptoms such as those containing lactose and gluten from the diet poses no risks to the patient and may have a benefit if it relieves symptoms.

INFLAMMATORY BOWEL DISEASE

Learning Objectives

After reading this section the participant will be able to:
1. Differentiate between ulcerative colitis and Crohn's disease.
2. Select appropriate pharmacologic therapy for treatment of mild, moderate, severe, and fulminant symptoms.
3. Define appropriate symptom monitoring of drug therapy.
4. Distinguish appropriate changes to pharmacologic treatment.

INTRODUCTION

Inflammatory bowel disease (IBD) is a generic term used to describe two main chronic inflammatory conditions of the GI tract: CD and UC. Although these conditions are similar in clinical presentation, CD is a chronic inflammatory disease characterized by transmural lesions located at any point on the GI tract. In contrast, UC is a chronic disease consisting of mucosal inflammation limited to the rectum and colon. IBD affects approximately 1 million Americans. As of 2015, there are 3 million (1.3%) who have the diagnosis of IBD, including either CD or UC (Dahlhamer et al., 2016), which was an increase of 0.9% or over 2 million adults (Nguyen et al., 2016). Both conditions are more common in Whites than in any other race, and those of Jewish descent have a three- to sixfold greater incidence than does the non-Jewish population. IBD shows no gender predilection and is usually first diagnosed in men or women between ages 15 and 35 (Ngo et al., 2014).

Although the mortality rate is low for the disease, it significantly affects the patient's overall mental status, physical health, and quality of life. The most common emotional issues surrounding uncontrolled IBD appear to be anger, frustration, depression, and low self-esteem. These issues usually stem from the patient's inability to participate in routine activities, leading to a decreased quality of life. The disease has a negative impact on social interactions and daily functional status, leading to reduced productivity and attendance at work or school, decreased social engagements, and loss of independence. Health-related issues mirror those related to poor GI absorption, including nutritional deficiencies, electrolyte abnormalities, dehydration, cachexia, and iron deficiency anemia. Fatigue and lack of sleep are also common in patients with IBD. In addition, patients with long-standing CD may also be at risk for adenocarcinoma of the GI tract (Pedersen et al., 2010). All of these may result in frequent hospitalizations, altered lifestyle, and poor general health. Overall, the financial burden of IBD has increased by greater than threefold in the last 5 years with twice the out-of-pocket costs $2213 as previously compared to $979 (Park et al., 2020). IBD had an estimated financial burden of $328 million in indirect health care costs and over $1.8 billion in direct costs (Everhart, 2008).

CAUSES

The etiology of CD and UC is related to the dysregulation of immunologic mechanisms. The condition's inflammatory nature has led researchers to believe that an autoimmune mechanism may predispose patients to IBD. The development of IBD may be attributed to a defect in the GI mucosal barrier that results in enhanced permeability and increased uptake of proinflammatory molecules and infectious agents. Tissue biopsies of the GI mucosal lining from patients with IBD reveal a high proportion of immunologic cytokines, including tumor necrosis factor (TNF), leukotrienes, and interleukin-1 (IL-1). A few bacterial and viral organisms have been associated with disease progression, including *Mycobacterium paratuberculosis*, measles virus, and *Listeria monocytogenes*; however, none has been definitively correlated with IBD.

Much of the recent evidence suggests that IBD is a complex genetic disorder. The high incidence of IBD in the Jewish population supports a genetic component of CD and UC's etiology. A study comparing relatives of patients with IBD with the general population found a tenfold increase in the risk of IBD development in those with familial occurrence. Early work with twins tended to support the notion that CD's disease occurrence was genetically influenced (Halfverson et al., 2007); however, more recent studies continue to support a genotype link, but it is far from straightforward (Gordon et al., 2015). Recently, the NOD2/CARD 15 gene have been associated with CD. Those who carry two copies of the risk alleles have been at higher risk of developing CD than others. The relationship between IBD and other genetic mutations and polymorphisms is currently being investigated. Until there are sufficient data to link a specific genetic mutation to IBD, the identification of genetic polymorphisms remains a research tool and not a clinical diagnostic tool.

Other factors, including psychological well-being and environmental triggers, may contribute to the exacerbation of IBD, although these factors do not have a predictable effect over a large population. Various studies have associated isolated mental instability or stressful events with IBD exacerbations, but a positive correlation between psychiatric illness and IBD is unsupported.

Environmental factors, including geographic location, dietary habits, drug-induced factors, and smoking status, are theorized to affect CD and UC exacerbations. IBD is more prevalent in the northern parts of the United States and England and Scandinavian countries rather than the Mediterranean countries, suggesting that temperature or weather patterns may impact CD or UC. Various dietary habits such as high sucrose consumption have been identified as exacerbating CD or UC. Still, no one food or group of foods seems to have a reliable effect in a large population. Oral contraceptive use and cigarette smoking have variable impacts on CD versus UC; oral contraceptives and nicotine have been found to exacerbate CD, but not UC (Khalili et al., 2013). Previously, the anti-acne product isotretinoin (Accutane) was thought to be associated with the development of IBD. However, Lee et al. (2016) found there is no link between isotretinoin and IBD.

PATHOPHYSIOLOGY

Differentiating CD from UC is difficult because of their similar clinical presentations. Hallmark symptoms of IBD are bloody diarrhea, weight loss, and fever. Generally, CD can be distinguished from UC based only on endoscopic findings. The GI mucosal lining in CD is usually characterized by discontinuous, narrowed, thick, edematous, leathery patches with lesions, ulcerations, fissures, strictures, and granulomas and fibrosis. Fistulas and abscess formation occur most commonly in patients with deep transmural lesions. Granulomas and fistulas usually occur exclusively in patients with CD. UC usually affects the rectum and areas proximal, possibly extending throughout the entire large intestine with continuous, superficial uniform inflammation and ulceration. Other pathologic findings are rare in UC but may occur in patients with chronic, long-standing inflammation (**Table 25.12**).

TABLE 25.12

Common Signs and Symptoms of Crohn's Disease versus Ulcerative Colitis

	Ulcerative Colitis	Crohn's Disease
Signs		
Abdominal mass	0	++
Fistulas	+/−	++
Strictures	+	++
Small bowel involvement	+/−	++
Rectal involvement	++	+/++
Extraintestinal disease		
Arthritis/arthralgia	++	++
Erythema nodosum	+/−	+/−
Abnormal liver function test values	++	++
Iritis/uveitis	+/−	+/−
Ankylosing spondylitis	+	+
Growth retardation	+	+
Toxic megacolon	+	+/−
Recurrence after colectomy	0	+
Malignancy	+	+/−
Symptoms		
Fever	+	++
Diarrhea	++	++
Weight loss	++	++
Rectal bleeding	++	+
Abdominal pain	+	++

Key: +, common; ++, very common; +/−, possible; 0, rare.

Extraintestinal complications, including skin malformations, liver disease, joint deformities, and ocular manifestations, may also occur, although they are more common in CD than UC because of the more aggressive nature of CD, resulting in a higher probability of malabsorption of nutrients (see **Table 25.12**). Because the complications affect a variety of organ systems and result in nonspecific complaints, it is difficult to associate the complaints with CD or UC; however, it is important to be aware of the complications because their presence indicates poorly controlled disease.

DIAGNOSTIC CRITERIA

Because the clinical presentation of patients with CD or UC is nonspecific, definitive diagnosis relies on endoscopic or radiologic studies. Initial diagnosis of IBD must rule out other causes of bloody diarrhea such as infectious causes and other colitis conditions. Visualization techniques must be used to differentiate CD from UC because of their similar clinical presentations. Usually, endoscopic techniques are preferred over radiographs and radioactive isotopes because endoscopy permits direct visualization of the mucosal lining. This increases the specificity as to the extent of lesions, ulcerations, and inflammation and provides the opportunity to obtain mucosal specimens for biopsy and further evaluation. However, the risk of mucosal perforation may limit the use of endoscopic technology in patients with severely active disease.

Sigmoidoscopy or colonoscopy is preferred as a first-line diagnostic procedure; however, for CD, an endogastroduodenoscopy may also be required to visualize the upper GI tract. Radiologic studies with contrast, including either an upper GI series or barium enema, may be preferred in patients with severely active symptoms to decrease the risk of mucosal perforation.

Antibody tests are sometimes helpful in determining the diagnosis of CD or UC. The perinuclear antineutrophil cytoplasmic antibody (pANCA) and/or the anti-*Saccharomyces cerevisiae* antibody (ASCA) tests may be positive in patients with IBD. Still, there is a significant rate of false-negative results since only 60% to 70% of patients with CD, or UC, are antibody positive (Kornbluth & Sachar, 2010). The combination of a positive pANCA and a negative ASCA may indicate the presence of UC, whereas the opposite may indicate CD. However, the combined result still has a significant percentage of false negatives. Therefore, these tests are not used routinely to differentiate UC from CD.

INITIATING DRUG THERAPY

CD and UC share many clinical characteristics with pseudomembranous colitis, irritable bowel disease, peptic ulcer disease (PUD), TD, colon cancer, and hemorrhoids. Evaluation of patients with suspected IBD must include a complete history focusing on the recent use of antibiotics, recent international travel, diet history, use of laxatives or antidiarrheals, frequency and quality of daily bowel movements, history of PUD, and family history of IBD to rule out similar presenting conditions.

Physical examination should include assessing vital signs and weight loss, a thorough abdominal examination, and special attention to extraintestinal complications. Guaiac testing and stool cultures may help rule out PUD or infectious causes. However, there are no reliable surrogate laboratory markers that may indicate CD or UC. Baseline laboratory studies, including electrolytes, liver panel, CBC, and hematology panel, are important in assessing the severity of the condition and patient's well-being.

Initiation of proper drug therapy is based on the severity and extent of the disease. CD may present as a luminal or fistulizing disease. CD confined to the GI lumen can initially present as mild, moderate, or severe disease and is not predictable in its course. The fistulizing disease also has a varied clinical course, whereby certain patients may never experience a fistula, and others may develop one early in the course of the disease. Treatment of fistulizing disease is typically more aggressive than that of luminal disease. It may vary depending on the fistula's location (bowel to the bladder, bowel to the skin, etc.). UC may be confined to the distal colon and rectum or may extend throughout the colon. Due to the disease's location, distal UC treatment options are more significant than for extensive disease.

There are many scales used to assess the severity of UC and can be separated by clinical versus endoscopic scores; however, there is not one gold standard, and none are validated. Each scale highlights specific subjective and objective parameters that should be evaluated when assessing the disease's progression. The Working Definition of Crohn's Disease (Feldman et al., 2007) and Criteria for Severity of Ulcerative Colitis (Feuerstein et al., 2020) are two tools that can be used clinically (**Tables 25.13** and **25.14**). Corticosteroids are used to treat acute exacerbations and should not be used chronically to maintain remission. Immunosuppressive agents are used to maintain

TABLE 25.13
Working Definition of Crohn's Disease

Mild to Moderate
- Ambulatory patients
- Able to tolerate oral alimentation
  - No evidence of the following:
  - Dehydration
  - High fevers
  - Rigors
  - Prostration
  - Abdominal tenderness
  - Painful mass
  - Abdominal obstruction
- 10% weight loss

Moderate to Severe
- Failed treatment for mild-to-moderate disease *or*
- All of the following:
  - High fever
  - >10% weight loss
  - Abdominal pain/tenderness
  - Intermittent nausea or vomiting (without obstructive findings)
  - Significant anemia

Severe to Fulminant
- Persistent symptoms despite outpatient steroid therapy *or*
- All of the following:
  - High fever
  - Persistent vomiting
  - Intestinal obstruction
  - Rebound tenderness
  - Cachexia
  - Abscess

Remission
- Asymptomatic without inflammatory sequelae *or*
- Not dependent on steroids

Adapted from Feldman, P., Wolfson, D., & Barkin, J. (2007). Medical Management of Crohn's Disease. *Clinics in Colon and Rectal Surgery, 20*(4), 269–281. https://doi.org/10.1055/s-2007-991026

TABLE 25.14
Criteria for Severity of Ulcerative Colitis

Mild UC
- <4 stools daily (with or without blood)
- No presence of anemia, fever, or tachycardia
- Normal erythrocyte sedimentation rate (ESR)
- No clinical signs

Moderate UC
- >4 to 6 stools daily (frequent blood)
- Minimal anemia, fever, or tachycardia
- Abdominal tenderness

Severe UC
- >6 bloody stools daily
- Positive fever, tachycardia, anemia, or elevated ESR
- Abdominal tenderness, air in abdomen

Fulminant UC
- >10 stools daily
- Continuous bleeding
- Abdominal tenderness and distention
- Anemia requiring blood transfusion
- Colonic dilation

Adapted from Feuerstein, J. D., Isaacs, K. L., Schneider, Y., Siddique, S. M., Falck-Ytter, Y., Singh, S., Chachu, K., Day, L., Lebwohl, B., Muniraj, T., Patel, A., Peery, A. F., Shah, R., Sultan, S., Singh, H., Singh, S., Spechler, S., Su, G., Thrift, A. P., ... Siddique, S. M. (2020). AGA Clinical Practice Guidelines on the management of moderate to severe ulcerative colitis. *Gastroenterology, 158*(5), 1450–1461. https://doi.org/10.1053/j.gastro.2020.01.006

remission in IBD, whereas IV cyclosporine is used in a limited population to treat severely active, steroid-refractory UC. Antibiotics are reserved for treating and maintaining remission in patients with mild CD. Biologic agents are typically reserved for inducing and maintaining remission in patients with steroid-refractory CD; however, the current recommendation is to use biologics in combination with thiopurines to induce remission in moderately severe CD (**Table 25.15**).

Goals of Drug Therapy

Because no pharmacologic cure is available for CD or UC, treatment goals focus on symptom management and quality-of-life issues. With proper treatment, the patient should be able to

- resume normal daily activities,
- restore general physical and mental well-being,
- attain the appropriate nutritional status,
- maintain remission of the disease,
- decrease the number and frequency of exacerbations,
- decrease side effects related to medications, and
- increase life expectancy.

Ideally, patients should expect to recover from an acute exacerbation within 2 to 4 weeks, have minimal exacerbations throughout the year, and participate in any desired activity.

TABLE 25.15

Overview of Agents Used to Treat Inflammatory Bowel Disease

Generic (Trade) Name and Dosage	Selected Adverse Events	Contraindications	Special Considerations
Aminosalicylates			
Sulfasalazine (Azulfidine, Azulfidine EN) Start: 500 mg BID Range: 1–8 g/d	Stevens–Johnson syndrome, rash, photosensitivity, nausea, vomiting, skin discoloration, agranulocytosis, crystalluria, hepatitis	Sulfa allergy, aspirin allergy, G6PD deficiency	Most efficacious at high doses Drug released in the proximal colon Available in enteric-coated tablets Dosage increases may occur as frequently as every other day
Oral mesalamine (Apriso, Asacol HD, Delzicol, Lialda, Pentasa) Start: depends on product Range: 1–4.8 g/d	Nausea, headache, malaise, abdominal pain, diarrhea	Aspirin allergy, G6PD deficiency	Products released differently in the GI tract May increase dose as frequently as every other day
Rectal mesalamine (Rowasa Enema, Canasa suppository) Suppository Start: 1 g at HS Range: 1 g/d Enema Start: 4 g at HS Range: 1–4 g/d	Malaise, abdominal pain	Aspirin allergy, G6PD deficiency	Only for distal ulcerative colitis, proctitis Suppository is most effective in sigmoid colon, and enema may treat distal and sigmoid colon
Olsalazine (Dipentum) Start: 500 mg BID Range: 1–2 g	Nausea, headache, malaise, abdominal pain, diarrhea	Aspirin allergy, G6PD deficiency	Drug released in proximal colon May increase dose as frequently as every other day Higher incidence of diarrhea
Balsalazide (Colazide) Start: 1.5 g BID Range: 1.5–6.75 g	Headache, abdominal pain, diarrhea	Aspirin allergy, G6PD deficiency	Only approved for treatment of mild-to-moderate ulcerative colitis
Selected Corticosteroids			
Prednisone (Orasone, Deltasone) Start: 40–60 mg daily Range: 10–100 mg	Hyperglycemia, increased appetite, insomnia, anxiety, tremors, hypertension, fluid retention, electrolyte imbalances	Active GI bleeding	Taper patient off steroids within 1–2 mo of initiation to decrease risk of long-term side effects
Oral methylprednisolone (Medrol) Start: 20–50 mg daily Range: 10–100 mg	Same as those for Prednisone	Same as those for Prednisone	Same as those for Prednisone
IV methylprednisolone (Solu-Medrol) Start: 5–10 mg q6h Range: 10–50 mg	Same as those for Prednisone	Same as those for Prednisone	IV treatment used for severe exacerbations Treatment duration should be a maximum of 7–14 d, then switch to oral therapy
Rectal hydrocortisone suppositories (Anusol-HC) Start: 25 mg BID Range: 25–100 mg	Same as those for Prednisone	Used only for distal ulcerative colitis treatment	
Hydrocortisone enema (Cortenema) Start: 100 mg HS Range: 100 mg/d	Enema is more effective than suppositories for distal colitis.		
IV hydrocortisone (Solu-Cortef) Start: 50–100 BID Range: 25–150 BID	Same as those for Hydrocortisone enema	Active GI bleeding	IV treatment used for severe exacerbations Treatment duration should be a maximum of 7–14 d, then switch to oral therapy

TABLE 25.15

Overview of Agents Used to Treat Inflammatory Bowel Disease (*Continued*)

Generic (Trade) Name and Dosage	Selected Adverse Events	Contraindications	Special Considerations
Dexamethasone (Decadron) Start: 5–15 mg daily Range: 2–20 mg/d	Same as those for Hydrocortisone enema	Same as those for Hydrocortisone enema	Has longer onset of action than other agents
Oral budesonide (Entocort EC) Start: 9 mg/d Maintenance: 6 mg/d for 3 mo	Minimal nausea	Same as those for Hydrocortisone enema	Minimal systemic absorption Taper after 8 wk of therapy Effective for mildly to moderately active luminal CD and maintenance
Selected Immunosuppressives			
Azathioprine (Imuran) Start: 50 mg/d Range: 2–2.5 mg/kg	Pancreatitis, fever, arthralgias, nausea, rash, agranulocytosis, diarrhea, malaise, hepatotoxicity	Pregnancy, active liver disease, bone marrow suppression	Decrease dose for patients with severe renal dysfunction
6-mercaptopurine (Purinethol) Start: 50 mg/d Range: 1–2.5 mg/kg	Same as those for Azathioprine	Same as those for Azathioprine	Same as those for Azathioprine
Oral methotrexate (Rheumatrex) Start: 5 mg three times a week Range: 5–7.5 mg three times a week	Hepatic cirrhosis and fibrosis, neutropenia, pneumonitis, skin rash, nausea, diarrhea	Same as those for Azathioprine	Same as those for Azathioprine
IV cyclosporine Start: 4–8 mg/kg/d	Hypertension, nephrotoxicity, superinfection, hypomagnesemia	Renal failure, hepatic failure	Only used for severely acute UC refractory to steroids; total duration of therapy 7–10 d; has many drug interactions
Selected Antibiotics			
Metronidazole (Flagyl) Start: 20 mg/kg/d Range: 10–20 mg/kg/d	Nausea, diarrhea, disulfiram reaction, metallic taste, peripheral paresthesias, dizziness	Liver failure, renal failure, first trimester of pregnancy, uncontrolled seizure disorder	Should not be used with alcohol Most efficacious if used chronically >3 mo
Ciprofloxacin (Cipro) Start: 500 mg BID Range: 500–2,000 mg/d	Dizziness, nausea, diarrhea, photosensitivity	Children <12 y, pregnancy, uncontrolled seizure disorder	May cause arthropathies in patients <12 y Must be administered 2 h before or after divalent and trivalent cations
Tumor Necrosis Factor Inhibitors			
IV infliximab (Remicade) Start: 5 mg/kg Range: 5–10 mg/kg	Infusion reactions (urticaria, dyspnea, hypotension), TB, invasive fungal infections, lymphoma, lupus-like syndrome	Class III/IV heart failure, active TB, hepatitis B or other infections	For severe, refractory UC and luminal and fistulizing CD; administered over 2 h as a single infusion Induction regimen dosed at weeks 0, 2, and 6; maintenance regimen dosed every 8 wk
Adalimumab (Humira) Start: 160 mg SQ Maintenance: 40 week or every other week	Opportunistic infections (TB, fungal, bacterial, viral), lymphoma and other cancers, injection-site reactions (erythema, pain, swelling)	Active TB, hepatitis B, or other infections	For luminal CD; induction regimen 160 mg initially and 80 mg at week 2
Ccrtolizumab pcgol (Cimzia) Start: 400 mg at baseline, week 2, and week 4 Maintenance: 400 mg every 4 wk	Opportunistic infections (TB, fungal, bacterial, viral), lymphoma and other cancers, injection-site reactions (erythema, pain, swelling)	Active TB, hepatitis B, or other infections	For luminal CD

(Continued)

TABLE 25.15

Overview of Agents Used to Treat Inflammatory Bowel Disease (Continued)

Generic (Trade) Name and Dosage	Selected Adverse Events	Contraindications	Special Considerations
Selective Adhesion Molecule Inhibitors			
IV natalizumab (Tysabri) 300 mg IV every 4 wk	Infusion reactions (urticaria, dyspnea, hypotension), opportunistic infections (TB, fungal, bacterial, viral) PML, hepatotoxicity	Active TB, hepatitis B, or other infections, current or history of PML	Taper corticosteroid therapy according to clinical response; discontinue natalizumab if therapeutic benefit is not seen within first 12 wk of therapy
IV vedolizumab (Entyvio) Start: 300 mg IV at baseline, week 2, and week 6 Maintenance: 300 mg IV q8wk	Infusion reactions (urticaria, dyspnea, hypotension), TB, invasive fungal infections, lymphoma, lupus-like syndrome	Active TB, hepatitis B, or other infections	Taper corticosteroid therapy off starting at week 6 of vedolizumab therapy
Other Agents			
Ustekinumab (Stelara) Initial IV infusion based on weight range Up to 55 kg 260 mg ≥55–85 kg 390 mg ≥85 kg 520 mg Then 90 mg subcutaneous dose SQ every 8 wk	Infusion reactions (urticaria, dyspnea, hypotension), TB, invasive fungal infections, lymphoma, lupus-like syndrome, anal abscess, gastroenteritis, ophthalmic herpes zoster, pneumonia, and listeria meningitis	Limited data on use of ustekinumab with pregnancy and lactation from observational studies	Indicated for Crohn's disease and ulcerative colitis

CD, Crohn's disease; G6PD, glucose-6-phosphate dehydrogenase; GI, gastrointestinal; PML, progressive multifocal leukoencephalopathy; TB, tuberculosis; UC, ulcerative colitis.

Aminosalicylates

Aminosalicylates remain the gold standard for the treatment of mild-to-moderate CD and UC. Although the exact mechanism of action is unknown, these drugs decrease inflammation in the GI tract by inhibiting prostaglandin synthesis, which results in a decrease in various immune mediators, including IL-1, cyclooxygenase, and thromboxane synthase. Therapy with these agents may improve symptoms within 1 week of initiating therapy or dosage adjustment. However, patients may need to take these agents long term to prevent exacerbations. Although they are safe for use in most patients, aminosalicylates are contraindicated in patients with aspirin allergy or glucose-6-phosphate dehydrogenase deficiency. Sulfasalazine is also contraindicated in patients who are hypersensitive to sulfa products (see **Table 25.15**). All of these agents must be used at maximum doses for maximum therapeutic benefit, although the incidence of side effects also increases with increased doses.

Sulfasalazine

Sulfasalazine (Azulfidine, Azulfidine EN) is efficacious and cost-effective for CD and UC therapy but has a limited role because of its unfavorable side-effect profile. Sulfasalazine is a combination product that is cleaved in the proximal colon by bacterial azo-reductases to release sulfapyridine and mesalamine. The mesalamine compound is responsible for virtually all of the therapeutic effect, whereas sulfapyridine is responsible for many of the side effects associated with sulfasalazine. Sulfasalazine may be administered up to four times daily; the most effective and maximum daily dosage is 8 g daily.

Mesalamine

Mesalamine (Asacol, Rowasa, Pentasa, Lialda, Apriso, Canasa) is available in various formulations, including oral tablets, oral capsules, enemas, and rectal suppositories. Each formulation is released in multiple GI tract areas, allowing for targeted drug therapy; however, in clinical trials, the capsules and tablets had similar efficacy at equivalent doses. Asacol, one of the oral tablet products, is formulated with an acrylic resin coating that disintegrates at a pH of 7, allowing the active ingredient to be released in the distal ileum and colon. Similarly, Lialda, another oral tablet formulation, has a coating that disintegrates at a pH of 6 to 7, and the core of the tablet forms a matrix that is released across a pH of 6.8 to 7.2. Pentasa, a sustained-release capsule, has ethylcellulose-coated granules that allow for the slow release of the drug beginning in the proximal small intestine and continuing throughout the colon. This formulation has slightly different pharmacokinetics than Apriso, which is also a delayed-release capsule. Apriso capsules are enteric coated; they disintegrate at a pH above 6 and contain granules formulated in a polymer matrix for extended release.

Because each of the oral products has different pharmacokinetics, the dosing interval for the products ranges from one to four times daily (see **Table 25.15**). The rectal suppositories are used primarily for UC-associated proctitis. Use of the enema delivers mesalamine to the distal and sigmoid colon. The enema is typically given at bedtime to allow for the drug's direct contact with the mucosa for at least 8 hours. In patients with distal UC, a combination of oral and rectal mesalamine may be an appropriate therapeutic option. Studies have shown that combination mesalamine therapy is more effective than a single mesalamine formulation.

Olsalazine

Olsalazine (Dipentum) is the third aminosalicylate preparation and consists of two mesalamine molecules joined by an azo-bond. As with sulfasalazine, the azo-bond is cleaved by bacterial azo-reductases in the GI tract, allowing the drug to be released in the proximal colon. It is administered twice daily, with patients taking up to 8 capsules per day for a total dosage of 2 g/d. Although each tablet of olsalazine has twice as much active ingredient as do the mesalamine capsules, the efficacy is minimally enhanced.

Balsalazide

Balsalazide (Colazal) is a combination product consisting of 5-aminosalicylic acid (mesalamine), the therapeutically active portion of the molecule, and 4-aminobenzoyl-alanine, an inert moiety. The product is cleaved by bacterial azo-reductases in the colon to release the active compound. Each capsule contains granules of balsalazide that are insoluble in acid and designed to be delivered to the colon intact. It is administered thrice daily, up to 9 capsules per day, for a total dosage of 6.75 g/d, equaling 2.4 g/d of pure mesalamine. It has been studied only for use in mild-to-moderate UC in both adults and children. Side effects and contraindications are similar to those of mesalamine.

Adverse Events

Mesalamine, olsalazine, and balsalazide are poorly absorbed from the GI tract and thus are considered primarily topical agents, with limited systemic side effects and drug interactions. The major side effects of mesalamine include headache, malaise, abdominal pain, and diarrhea. Olsalazine has a similar side-effect profile but has a higher incidence of diarrhea than mesalamine. Initially, diarrhea may not be easily distinguished from an IBD exacerbation, and therefore close monitoring of improvement of symptoms is essential. If the balsalazide capsules are opened and sprinkled in food, teeth staining may occur. In rare instances, mesalamine, olsalazine, and balsalazide have been associated with renal function impairment; therefore, renal function should be monitored during therapy. Sulfapyridine is absorbed systemically, accounting for many of the side effects and drug interactions incurred by sulfasalazine. Common adverse effects include nausea, vomiting, photosensitivity, oligospermia, and skin discoloration, which may be tolerable for most patients. Severe adverse reactions associated with sulfasalazine include Stevens–Johnson syndrome, agranulocytosis, crystalluria, pancreatitis, and hepatitis, which may necessitate discontinuation of therapy. Sulfasalazine is known to decrease folate levels; therefore, patients taking sulfasalazine should be supplemented with folic acid. Although drug interactions with sulfasalazine are limited, it may significantly reduce the effect of warfarin (Coumadin), and therefore close monitoring of the international normalized ratio is essential.

Corticosteroids

Corticosteroids are used intermittently to treat acute IBD exacerbations only. When the disease fails to respond to aminosalicylate therapy, the use of corticosteroids allows for immunosuppression and prostaglandin inhibition. They can be used in conjunction with aminosalicylates, immunosuppressants, biologic agents, or monotherapy to treat acute exacerbations. Corticosteroids with a relatively quick onset of action and high glucocorticoid activity, such as prednisone (Orasone, Deltasone) and methylprednisolone (Medrol), are desirable in the treatment of CD or UC. Controlled-release oral budesonide (Entocort EC) is a unique corticosteroid due to its long-acting formulation and limited potential for absorption from the GI tract, thus theoretically leading to a localized effect in the GI lumen with minimal systemic side effects. Oral budesonide has been used to treat choice in patients with mild-to-moderate exacerbations of CD in combination with aminosalicylates or as monotherapy.

Dosage

Doses equivalent to oral prednisone 40 to 60 mg/d are initiated in patients with mild or moderate CD or UC exacerbations. A beneficial effect is usually seen with 7 to 10 days of therapy. Patients with mild-to-moderate exacerbations of distal UC can be treated with oral or rectal corticosteroids for approximately 4 to 8 weeks, after which drug dosages are tapered. Hydrocortisone is the only rectal corticosteroid enema formulation available for use in distal UC exacerbations. Many tapering regimens have been studied. The most common is a 5- to 10-mg weekly taper until a daily dose of 20 mg is reached, at which time the amount is tapered by 2.5 mg/wk. In severe exacerbations, patients should receive 3 to 10 days of IV corticosteroid therapy and then switch to oral corticosteroid therapy for the remainder of the treatment period (see **Table 25.15**).

Adverse Events

Short-term corticosteroid use (<3 months) is associated with increased glucose levels, increased appetite, insomnia, anxiety, tremors, and increased fluid retention, leading to increases in blood pressure and electrolyte imbalances. Although discontinuation of therapy due to these side effects is not recommended with short-term corticosteroid treatment, routine monitoring is necessary.

Long-term corticosteroid use is associated with many side effects. These include decreased bone density, osteoporosis, and fat redistribution, leading to the characteristic "buffalo hump"; decreased prostaglandin synthesis; gastric and duodenal ulcers; hypertriglyceridemia; hypokalemia; cataracts; and hirsutism. Therefore, long-term treatment with corticosteroids is not recommended. However, if patients take recurrent steroid therapy for recurrent exacerbations, monitoring these side effects is imperative.

Interactions

Many corticosteroids are substrates of the cytochrome P-450 isoenzyme 3A4, including prednisone, prednisolone, methylprednisolone, and budesonide. Therefore, agents that inhibit or induce this enzyme system, such as ketoconazole, clarithromycin, phenytoin, and pioglitazone, may alter the corticosteroid's efficacy. Budesonide requires an acidic environment (pH < 5.5) to be released, so agents that inhibit acid production or neutralize the acid in the GI tract (i.e., histamine-2 antagonists, proton pump inhibitors, antacids) may limit the effectiveness of budesonide. Corticosteroids may also decrease antidiabetic and antihypertensive agents' effectiveness due to their ability to increase blood glucose levels and blood pressure.

Immunosuppressive Agents

Immunosuppressive agents are used in IBD as adjunctive treatment with aminosalicylates. This combination helps to induce and maintain remission if exacerbations are occurring while the patient is being tapered off corticosteroid therapy. It also helps when frequent exacerbations occur with maximum dosages of aminosalicylates. The exception is IV cyclosporine, which is solely used to treat severe, acute UC refractory exacerbations to corticosteroids.

Azathioprine and 6-Mercaptopurine

Azathioprine (Imuran) and 6-mercaptopurine (Purinethol) are antimetabolites that act as purine antagonists to inhibit the synthesis of protein, ribonucleic acid, and deoxyribonucleic acid (DNA). By doing so, azathioprine and 6-mercaptopurine decrease the production of various inflammatory mediators. Because 6-mercaptopurine is the active metabolite of azathioprine, these agents are similar in efficacy, side-effect profile, and dosing frequency (see **Table 25.15**). Although these agents have a short plasma half-life of approximately 1 to 2 hours, both have active metabolites with long half-lives of 3 to 13 days, resulting in optimal therapeutic effects within 10 to 15 weeks of therapy initiation. 6-mercaptopurine is metabolized by the enzyme thiopurine methyltransferase (TPMT). The activity of this particular enzyme varies in patients based on a genetic polymorphism. Therefore, patients may be at a higher risk for specific side effects if they have low enzyme activity. TPMT testing is available to identify patients who may have low enzyme activity and, in turn, may experience more side effects.

These agents should be initiated during an acute exacerbation once the patient can tolerate oral medications to induce and maintain remission. However, these agents are not sufficient for treating an acute exacerbation because of their slow onset of action. The initial dosage of these agents is 50 mg/d in one dose. The dosage is increased every 2 weeks to target dosage of 1 to 2 mg/kg/d for 6-mercaptopurine and 2 to 2.5 mg/kg/d for azathioprine. Because the renal system clears these agents, a decrease of dosages occurs in patients with creatinine clearance values under 50 mL/min. The dose for azathioprine and 6-mercaptopurine is usually reduced by 50% if the patient's creatinine clearance value falls below 50 mL/min to decrease the risk of accumulation and unwanted effects. Although these agents have the potential to cause significant adverse events, they are generally well tolerated. These agents should not be used in pregnancy or with patients with active liver disease.

Methotrexate

Methotrexate (Rheumatrex) has a therapeutic effect similar to azathioprine and 6-mercaptopurine. This drug inhibits intracellular dihydrofolate reductase, which results in inhibition of purine synthesis and suppression of IL-1 production. The intramuscular and oral preparations of methotrexate are efficacious in the induction and maintenance of CD remission, but similar efficacy has not been shown for UC. Doses of 25 mg/wk injected intramuscularly or 5 mg orally three times a week have effectively induced remission in patients with steroid-dependent CD after 12 to 16 weeks of therapy. At low doses, methotrexate is nearly completely absorbed when administered orally. It is not beneficial to use the intramuscular preparation over the oral formulation with normal GI function.

It is necessary to adjust the methotrexate dosages based on renal function. Patients with creatinine clearance values less than 50 mL/min should receive 50% of the normal dose. Methotrexate should not be prescribed to patients with active liver disease or pregnant women.

Cyclosporine

Cyclosporine (Sandimmune, Neoral) is reserved for the acute treatment of severe, steroid-refractory exacerbations of UC in hospitalized patients. Cyclosporine is a lipophilic, fungus-derived polypeptide that suppresses cell-mediated immunity by predominantly inhibiting IL-2 synthesis and release. The therapeutic effect is correlated with appropriate dosing. IV infusion of cyclosporine has been found effective at dosages of 4 to 8 mg/kg/d for UC. The use of cyclosporine in acute CD exacerbations is reported to have variable results. Because of poor systemic absorption, oral cyclosporine should not be used. Improvement of symptoms with IV therapy usually occurs within 2 to 3 days, and the duration of therapy is usually 7 to 10 days.

Adverse Events

Although azathioprine and 6-mercaptopurine are usually well tolerated, significant side effects may occur. These agents are associated with both allergic- and nonallergic-type side effects. Allergic-type side effects include pancreatitis, fever, rash, arthralgias, malaise, nausea, and diarrhea, which may occur regardless of dose. The main nonallergic-type side effects include bone marrow suppression and hepatotoxicity, which appear to be dose dependent. Pancreatitis may occur at any point in therapy and warrant discontinuation of therapy. The development of pancreatitis precludes the use of either 6-mercaptopurine or azathioprine in the future. Leukopenia and hepatotoxicity usually occur during the initiation phase of therapy and may be managed by decreasing the dose. If a patient experiences side effects with either of these agents, switching the patient to the other agent is not beneficial.

Side effects of methotrexate include hepatic cirrhosis and fibrosis, bone marrow suppression, pneumonitis, folic acid deficiency, and rash. Nausea and diarrhea are also reported, but they occur more frequently with the oral formulation. Bone marrow suppression and liver dysfunction are dose dependent, and doses should be decreased in patients with these disorders. Folic acid should be administered concomitantly to limit folic acid deficiency.

Nephrotoxicity, hypomagnesemia, and hypertension are all associated with cyclosporine. Risk factors for nephrotoxicity are related to high-dose treatment, long-term treatment, and advanced age. Renal function may be restored within 2 weeks of cyclosporine discontinuation. Other side effects of cyclosporine include nausea, vomiting, opportunistic infections, paresthesias, tremor, and seizures. Opportunistic infections occur because of the drug's immunosuppressive effects and may be managed by appropriate antibiotic therapy.

Interactions

Cyclosporine significantly interacts with various agents because of its metabolism through the cytochrome P-450 3A4 isoenzyme system. Enzyme inhibitors, such as erythromycin (Eryc) and ketoconazole (Nizoral), increase blood levels of cyclosporine by inhibiting its metabolism, whereas enzyme inducers, such as phenytoin (Dilantin), carbamazepine (Tegretol), and rifampin (Rifadin), decrease cyclosporine blood levels. Grapefruit juice increases blood levels of cyclosporine, which may increase the incidence of side effects.

Antibiotics

The association between IBD and infectious causes has led to the use of antibiotics. This approach attempts to manipulate the gut microbes. Because the particular organism has not been isolated, it is difficult to determine which antibiotics are most appropriate for treatment. Generally, the selection of an antibiotic includes the action against gram-negative and *Mycobacterium* organisms with a low side-effect profile and poor systemic absorption. Most antibiotic studies focus on CD, specifically, using metronidazole and ciprofloxacin, either individually or together. Other drugs include rifaximin, clarithromycin, and antituberculous regimes. Based on few published controlled trials, mildly to moderately active CD appears to respond only to metronidazole and ciprofloxacin (see **Table 25.15**). The beneficial effects of antibiotic therapy have not been replicated in patients with UC.

Metronidazole showed efficacy in treating perianal CD. Since then, however, a few studies have found beneficial effects of metronidazole in treating mildly to moderately active luminal and fistulizing CD when used in combination with aminosalicylates or alone. The mechanism by which metronidazole alone exerts its beneficial effects in CD is unknown, although it is thought that the immune-modulating effects are more prominent than the antibacterial effects.

The standard dosage for treatment of mildly to moderately active CD is 20 mg/kg/d. Once remission is attained, the dosage is titrated to 10 mg/kg/d for maintenance. The usual therapy duration is up to 12 months, although remission can usually be achieved within 1 to 2 months. There is a report of CD exacerbations when metronidazole is discontinued; however, there are long-term side effects of the drug that have to be considered.

Ciprofloxacin has also been studied for perianal and luminal CD with mixed results. Ciprofloxacin covers gram-negative organisms and *Mycobacterium* species as well as some gram-positive organisms. It is usually well tolerated. Along with inhibiting DNA gyrase, which is its main antibacterial mechanism of action, ciprofloxacin also is reported to have immunosuppressive properties. Dosage of oral ciprofloxacin of 500 mg, twice daily, is as efficacious as 4 g of mesalamine daily in preliminary trials. Remission is attained after approximately 6 weeks of therapy. Ciprofloxacin is contraindicated in children and pregnant women.

Adverse Events

Short-term metronidazole therapy is associated with mild side effects, including dry mouth, metallic taste, nausea, and vomiting. Abdominal distress, including cramping and diarrhea, may also occur, but these effects are difficult to distinguish from IBD symptoms. Long-term use of metronidazole is associated with neurotoxic effects such as peripheral paresthesia, dizziness, pruritus, and vertigo that may warrant therapy discontinuation.

Ciprofloxacin is usually well tolerated. The most common side effects include nausea, diarrhea, dizziness, and rashes secondary to photosensitivity. However, long-term treatment may result in tendinitis and tendon rupture.

Interactions

Metronidazole is associated with severe nausea and vomiting (disulfiram effect) if taken concurrently with alcohol. Ciprofloxacin inhibits theophylline (Slo-Phyllin) metabolism, so theophylline serum levels may need to be monitored with chronic ciprofloxacin use. Any divalent or trivalent cation, such as calcium or iron, may interfere with ciprofloxacin absorption; therefore, at least a 4-hour dosing interval should be maintained between these agents.

Biological Agents

Many biological agents are continuing to be investigated to treat IBD, including TNF-alpha inhibitors, growth factors, lymphocyte inhibitors, and transcription inhibitors. Currently, there are two approved classes for the treatment of severe refractory luminal CD: TNF-alpha inhibitors (infliximab [Remicade], adalimumab [Humira], and certolizumab pegol [Cimzia]) and selective adhesion molecule inhibitors (natalizumab [Tysabri], vedolizumab [Entyvio]).

TNF-α inhibitors

Infliximab (Remicade) is indicated for maintaining remission in CD as well as treating UC and fistulizing CD. The GI mucosal tissues of patients with active CD are found to over-express numerous immunologic cytokines, including TNF. Biological TNF-alpha is a proinflammatory cytokine that stimulates the expression of various immunologic cytokines, such as IL-8 and interferon-gamma. The TNF-alpha inhibitor agents produce their effect by neutralizing soluble forms of TNF-alpha and competitively inhibit its binding to the TNF receptor. In addition, TNF-alpha inhibitors may also induce apoptosis of activated monocytes.

Infliximab is a synthetically derived immunoglobulin (Ig) G monoclonal antibody consisting of 25% murine antibodies and 75% human antibodies (see **Table 25.15**). Infliximab is available only as an IV solution, and it is administered at a dosage of 5 mg/kg over a minimum of 2 hours. A single-infusion dose at baseline, week 2, and week 6 is administered to treat an acute exacerbation; infusions every 8 weeks are used to maintain remission. The infusions may be delivered in an inpatient or a monitored outpatient setting. Repeated doses of the product may increase the risk of immunogenicity and infusion-related reactions due to the product's murine component. Infliximab crosses the placenta and is detected in infants' serum for up to 6 months after in utero exposure and should be held after 30 weeks of gestation in pregnant women. Caution should be used when prescribing to patients with heart failure.

Adalimumab (Humira) is also a TNF-alpha inhibitor; however, it is a fully humanized IgG monoclonal antibody that binds specifically to human TNF. It is approved for maintaining remission of CD in adults and children and for treating and maintaining remission of UC in adults. In general, fully humanized monoclonal antibodies associate with less immunogenicity and infusion-related reactions. Adalimumab is administered as a subcutaneous injection every 2 weeks and can increase to once weekly if necessary (see **Table 25.15**). Adalimumab is effective in patients with CD who may not have responded to infliximab and those who are naive to TNF-alpha inhibitors.

Certolizumab pegol (Cimzia) is also a TNF-alpha inhibitor; however, it is not a fully monoclonal antibody. Certolizumab pegol consists of only the fragment antigen-binding fragment of human-derived IgG, which is attached to PEG. Since certolizumab pegol does not contain certain regions of a full antibody, it cannot cause antibody-dependent cell cytotoxicity or induce apoptosis as with infliximab or adalimumab. The PEG portion of the product allows for a longer duration of action and a longer duration between injections. Certolizumab pegol is administered in two subcutaneous injections initially and at weeks 2 and 4. For those who elicit a clinical response, certolizumab pegol can be used every 4 weeks to maintain remission (see **Table 25.15**). Certolizumab pegol should not be used to treat fistulizing CD, as it is no more effective than placebo. It has not been studied in the treatment of UC or children.

Selective Adhesion Molecule Inhibitors

Selective adhesion molecule inhibitors should be reserved for patients who had an inadequate response or were unable to tolerate conventional CD therapies and TNF-alpha inhibitors. Natalizumab is a humanized monoclonal antibody that is active against the alpha$_4$ integrin subunit, inhibiting leukocyte adhesion and migration into inflamed tissue. Natalizumab (Tysabri) is indicated for CD treatment in adults and is administered intravenously as a 300-mg dose every 4 weeks and should be discontinued if there is no therapeutic benefit achieved within 12 weeks. When initiating natalizumab, patients should be tapered off concomitant corticosteroid use according to clinical response. Antibody formation may occur with natalizumab resulting in infusion reactions, hypersensitivity reactions, and loss of efficacy. Natalizumab is not well studied in pregnant patients and should be enrolled into a pregnancy exposure registry if initiated.

Vedolizumab (Entyvio) is a humanized monoclonal antibody that targets alpha$_4$beta$_7$ integrin, preventing the migration of inflammatory lymphocytes into the gut mucosa. It is indicated for initiating and maintaining remission in adults for both CD and UC. Vedolizumab is administered intravenously as a dose of 300 mg at 0, 2, and 6 weeks, then every 8 weeks after that. In clinical trials, the glucocorticoid doses were left unaltered until week 6 and then tapered according to patient response. If symptoms are not decreased within 14 weeks, discontinuation of therapy is warranted.

Ustekinumab (Stelara) is a human monoclonal antibody active against IL-12 and IL-23. It is approved for use in plaque psoriasis and maintains remission in refractory CD and UC in adults resistant to anti–TNF-alpha therapy. The blocking action of IL-12 and IL-23 activates natural killer cells and CD4 T lymphocytes, which help with chronic inflammatory conditions such as CD. There is a weight-based IV loading dose of 260 mg if weight is 55 kg or less or 390 mg if weight is more than 55 to 85 kg, and 520 mg if weight is more than 85 kg. Administration of a 90-mg subcutaneous dose is performed every 8 weeks. Approximately 3% of CD patients using this drug developed antiustekinumab antibodies (Morita 2020).

Adverse Events

The primary side effects of TNF-alpha inhibitors are injection-site–related reactions, including erythema, itching, and swelling. These agents also have less common but still significant side effects contributing to the development of heart failure, tuberculosis (TB), hepatitis B reactivation, opportunistic infections, lymphoma and other malignancies, hepatotoxicity, vasculitis, and pancytopenia. Patients should be tested for latent TB and treated accordingly prior to treatment with TNF-alpha inhibitors.

TNF-alpha inhibitors are contraindicated in patients with active TB and should be used cautiously in heart failure patients.

Infliximab is also associated with infusion-related reactions, including transient hypersensitivity reactions, flushing, headache, dyspnea, rash, and fever, possibly secondary to the product's murine component. These side effects may be managed by pretreating patients with antihistamines, acetaminophen, and/or corticosteroids. Also, mild-to-moderate infusion reactions may be managed by decreasing the infusion rate.

The primary side effects associated with selective adhesion molecule inhibitors are hypersensitivity and infusion reactions. Patients on natalizumab also have the potential to develop severe hepatotoxicity, and the drug carries a black box warning for increasing the risk of developing progressive multifocal leukoencephalopathy, particularly in patients with a history of John Cunningham virus.

Drug Interactions

Extensive drug interaction studies have not been performed to date, but due to their ability to alter the immunologic response, biologics should not be administered along with live vaccines. Commonly, TNF-alpha inhibitors are administered to patients who are also taking immunosuppressive agents. The administration of other immunosuppressant agents (e.g., azathioprine, methotrexate) with these agents has been shown to be beneficial by decreasing the risk of immunogenicity (development of autoantibodies) and decreasing infusion-related reactions (Lichtenstein et al., 2009a). No significant drug interactions have been reported when TNF-alpha inhibitors are given with conventional IBD therapy.

Selecting the Most Appropriate Agent

There are drug treatment protocols for many diseases and disorders that distinguish between first-line, second-line, and third-line therapies. However, in IBD, the decision to use one therapeutic modality over another is based on the location of the inflammation, the severity and extent of the disease, the patient's tolerance of the therapy, patient compliance, and cost (**Table 25.16**). The American College of Gastroenterology (Rubin et al., 2019) and the American Gastroenterology Association have developed separate guidelines for managing UC (Ford et al., 2018).

Crohn's Disease

Mildly to moderately active luminal CD is typically treated with oral aminosalicylates alone or in combination with antibiotic therapy. However, monotherapy with budesonide has also been used with good results, especially in patients with the ileal or right colonic disease. Oral agents are chosen over rectal

TABLE 25.16

Recommended Treatment Options for Crohn's Disease and Ulcerative Colitis

Severity of Disease	Distal UC	Extensive UC	Luminal CD	Perianal/Fistulizing CD
Mild	Oral/rectal aminosalicylate OR Rectal corticosteroid	Oral aminosalicylate	Oral aminosalicylate WITH/WITHOUT Antibiotic therapy	Surgical drainage AND antibiotic therapy WITH/WITHOUT IV infliximab or SC adalimumab
Moderate	Oral aminosalicylate AND Rectal aminosalicylate Oral/rectal steroid	Oral aminosalicylate AND Oral steroid	Oral aminosalicylate AND Oral steroid (preferably budesonide)	
Severe	IV corticosteroid AND/OR IV cyclosporine	IV corticosteroid AND/OR IV cyclosporine	IV corticosteroid AND/OR biologics	
Fulminant	IV corticosteroids AND/OR IV cyclosporine, IV infliximab, or SC adalimumab*	IV corticosteroid AND/OR IV cyclosporine, IV infliximab, or SC adalimumab*	IV corticosteroid AND/OR biologics	
Remission	Oral/rectal aminosalicylate WITH/WITHOUT Oral immunosuppressive, IV infliximab, or SC adalimumab*	Oral aminosalicylate WITH/WITHOUT Oral immunosuppressive, IV infliximab, or SC adalimumab*	Oral aminosalicylate WITH/WITHOUT Oral immunosuppressive/ biologics	

*Consider selective adhesion molecule inhibitors for inadequate response/failure with TNF-alpha inhibitors.

CD, Crohn's disease; UC, ulcerative colitis.

agents because of CD's random presence along the entire GI tract. Patients may be maintained on aminosalicylates or antibiotic therapy for months to years. Still, the goal is to taper the patient off the medication as soon as possible once remission is attained. Budesonide is indicated for 3 months to maintain remission in CD.

Treatment of moderate-to-severe CD usually consists of combination therapy with aminosalicylates and corticosteroids. Corticosteroid therapy is used acutely on a short-term basis for patients with moderate-to-severe disease to attain remission. Because of their high side-effect profile, chronic use of steroids is avoided to maintain remission. Oral agents may be used for patients with moderate-to-severe disease. The typical therapy duration is 4 to 12 weeks at the full dose, and then doses are tapered by 5 to 10 mg weekly until discontinued. TNF inhibitors may be indicated if patients have had multiple exacerbations that are refractory to steroids or have a fistulizing disease. The 2018 American Gastroenterology Association guideline reaffirmed the recommendation for using TNF-alpha inhibitors in combination with thiopurines over thiopurine monotherapy to induce remission in patients with moderately severe CD (Lichtenstein et al., 2018).

Severe-to-fulminant disease requires definitive drug therapy in addition to substantial supportive care measures due to poor oral absorption and rapid GI transit time. Oral treatment, including aminosalicylates, should not be administered until the patient can tolerate oral alimentation. IV corticosteroids are indicated to decrease inflammation and induce immunosuppression. For patients with moderate-to-severe or severe-to-fulminant disease whose disease is refractory to corticosteroids (either oral or IV), biological agents are an option. Supportive care measures, such as IV fluids, bowel rest, and parenteral nutrition, should also be considered.

Consider ongoing therapy to maintain remission in patients who have frequent exacerbations or who are "steroid dependent." A combination of immunosuppressive agents, such as azathioprine, 6-mercaptopurine, methotrexate, and biologics, may be used with aminosalicylates to maintain remission in patients whose disease is refractory to aminosalicylate monotherapy. The immunosuppressant agents may take effect after 10 to 12 weeks. The therapeutic effect should be seen within 8 weeks of administration of biologics. Patients may be maintained on these agents for months to years, but the goal is to taper the patient off the medication as soon as possible due to the significant side effects. Antibiotics, specifically metronidazole and ciprofloxacin, have proved beneficial in maintaining remission of perianal and fistulizing CD with long-term use (**Figure 25.7**).

Ulcerative Colitis

For UC, guidelines specify various treatment approaches depending on the severity and location of the disease. Distal colitis, identified as lesions below the splenic flexure, may be treated with oral, rectal, or IV agents depending on the disease's severity. Rectal agents should not be used in patients with extensive colitis due to the location of the disease. The decision to use systemic or local preparations for distal colitis largely depends on patient preference; however, topical products allow for less systemic absorption, less frequent dosing, and a quicker onset of effect (**Figure 25.8**). Treatment of mild UC is best achieved with the use of aminosalicylates. The combination of oral and rectal aminosalicylates is more effective than either therapy alone. Corticosteroids may be used concurrently with aminosalicylates for moderate UC exacerbations. Depending on the severity of the exacerbation and the location of the lesions, either rectal or oral preparations may be appropriate. Severe exacerbations may require hospitalization. Discontinuation of oral and topical therapy due to rapid GI transit time and IV corticosteroid therapy initiation are standard. Infliximab may be initiated in an outpatient or inpatient setting in patients with severe exacerbations after an adequate steroid trial.

Surgery may be considered in patients whose disease fails to respond to drug therapy. The management of fulminant exacerbations is very similar to severe exacerbations, but the decision to perform a colectomy is considered a much earlier stage for fulminant exacerbations. Along with definitive therapy, supportive measures including bowel rest, IV fluids, and adequate nutrition should be considered for those with severe and fulminant exacerbations. For those with frequent exacerbations or steroid dependence, immunosuppressive agents such as 6-mercaptopurine and azathioprine should be considered to induce and maintain remission. Typically, immunosuppressive agents are initiated after the patient can tolerate oral medications and are initiated along with aminosalicylate and corticosteroid therapy. The goal is to taper the corticosteroid and continue the aminosalicylate and the immunosuppressive therapy for maintenance of remission.

Methotrexate has not been adequately studied in patients with UC and therefore is not recommended. Antibiotic therapy has not been shown to improve UC symptoms.

Drug Selection

Sulfasalazine was considered the first-line aminosalicylate because of its remarkable efficacy, low cost, and availability in oral liquid and tablet preparations; however, it must be taken four times daily and causes significant adverse drug reactions. For maximum therapeutic benefit, 4 to 8 g/d is necessary, so patients must take up to 16 tablets or 32 teaspoonfuls daily. Also, immediate-release sulfasalazine has activity limited to the colon, making it less effective in conditions affecting the upper GI tract.

Mesalamine has emerged as the aminosalicylate of choice because of its availability. There are many formulations, dosing frequency, and low side-effect profiles, but it is more expensive than sulfasalazine. Depending on the oral formulation and the severity of the disease, patients may need to take 6 to 16 pills daily to attain maximum therapeutic benefit. Standard dosages of oral mesalamine are 2 to 4.8 g/d. Olsalazine and balsalazide are not used as often because of their added cost without any significant clinical benefit.

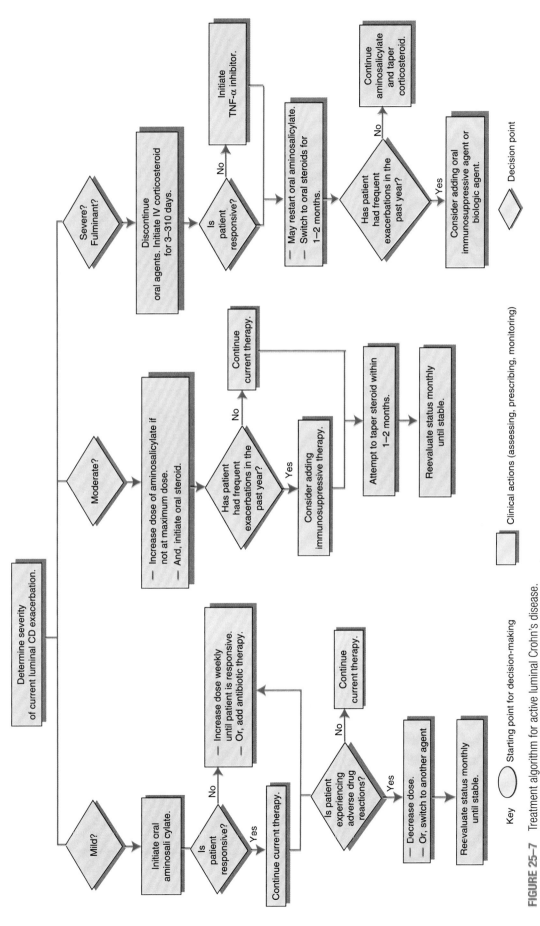

FIGURE 25–7 Treatment algorithm for active luminal Crohn's disease.

CD, Crohn's disease; IV, intravenous; TNF, tumor necrosis factor.

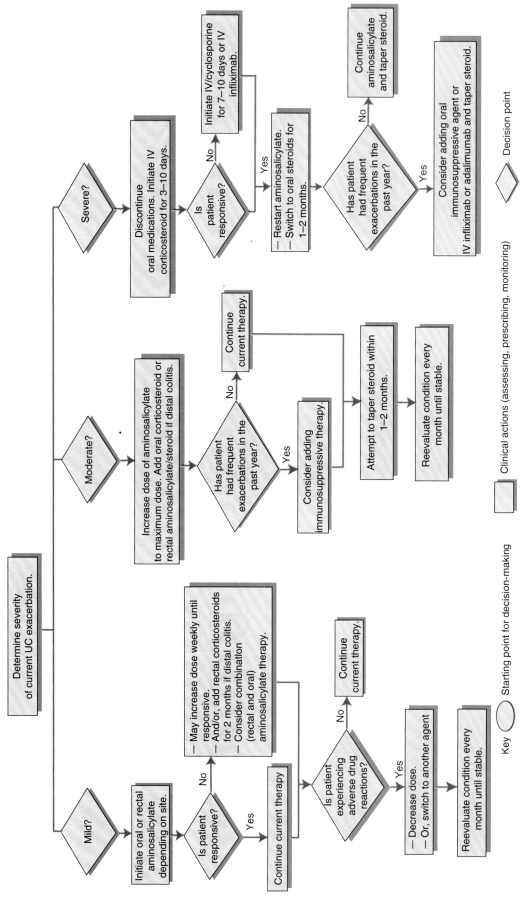

FIGURE 25–8   Treatment algorithm for active ulcerative colitis.

IV, intravenous; UC, ulcerative colitis.

The ideal corticosteroid for treating IBD would have high glucocorticoid activity, a low side-effect profile, and targeted delivery to the diseased site. It would be poorly absorbed from the GI tract, allowing for localized activity. Oral budesonide (Entocort) is explicitly approved for the acute treatment of IBD due to its ideal characteristics. Still, due to its increased cost, other corticosteroids are used frequently to treat an acute exacerbation. The choice of a steroid depends on the route of administration, the onset of action, and glucocorticoid versus mineralocorticoid potency. In general, agents with more glucocorticoid activity are preferred over mineralocorticoid steroids because they have better anti-inflammatory action. Oral agents are used primarily in patients with a localized or generalized disease with mild-to-moderate exacerbations; rectal formulations are reserved for patients with mild-to-moderate distal UC disease exacerbations. An IV treatment may be initiated in patients with severe exacerbations of CD or UC.

The use of immunosuppressive agents varies based on the type of IBD and the severity of the disease. Cyclosporine is reserved for the acute treatment of severe UC exacerbations because of the high cost of therapy and increased incidence of severe side effects. There is a lack of comparative trials of methotrexate and azathioprine or 6-mercaptopurine, making it difficult to identify a first-line agent. However, more data exists to support azathioprine or 6-mercaptopurine than methotrexate for CD and UC. Azathioprine and 6-mercaptopurine are equally efficacious, with similar pharmacokinetics, adverse drug reaction, and cost profiles making no distinction between the two.

The main distinction between methotrexate and the other two agents is its availability as an intramuscular injection and its dosing schedule. The infrequent dosing schedule of oral and intramuscular methotrexate may promote either compliance or noncompliance with the medication, depending on the patient. Combining these agents for the induction and maintenance of remission is not recommended because of overlapping side-effect profiles and lack of improved efficacy data.

If antibiotic therapy is warranted, metronidazole or ciprofloxacin is an acceptable agent, depending on patient-specific factors.

A few differences among the biologics may make one agent more favorable in certain patients than others. In recent years, more biologics have attained the indication for UC. Many agents have FDA approval existing now to treat UC and CD. These include the original drugs, infliximab, and adalimumab, and another addition is Golimumab. Biosimilar agents to infliximab (Infliximab-abda, Infliximab-dyyb, Infliximab-qbtx) and adalimumab (Adalimumab-atto, Adalimumab-adbm) also exist. An option for patients who can self-inject and have luminal CD is either adalimumab or certolizumab pegol. Adalimumab and certolizumab pegol are available as a prefilled syringe for convenience. Both drugs are administered subcutaneously, but adalimumab is one injection every 2 weeks, and certolizumab pegol is two injections every 4 weeks. Infliximab may also be used for luminal CD; however, it must be administered by a health care practitioner in a monitored setting since it is an IV infusion. As fully humanized monoclonal antibodies, adalimumab and certolizumab pegol have increased risk of infusion reactions, hypersensitivity, and the development of autoantibodies. These types of reactions are less likely with infliximab. Adalimumab has also been found effective in patients who have previously not responded to infliximab (Armuzzi et al., 2013; Sandborn et al., 2007). Natalizumab, vedolizumab, and ustekinumab should be considered for patients who failed TNF-alpha therapy and are only available as IV infusions.

Special Population Considerations

Pediatrics

IBD is typically diagnosed early in life, usually during the second or third decade, leading to significant implications of IBD in the pediatric population. Treatment must be aggressive to limit the potential for nutritional deficiencies leading to stunted growth, malnutrition, and anemia. However, many of the medications lead to untoward effects or are not well studied in pediatrics. The use of long-term corticosteroids may lead to growth abnormalities. Ciprofloxacin is contraindicated in children because it can cause arthropathy, resulting in poor bone formation. Infliximab is indicated for inducing or maintaining remission of CD and UC in children older than age 6. Certolizumab pegol has not been studied in children. Adalimumab is indicated for inducing and maintaining remission of CD in children over the age of 6. Adalimumab has been approved for children with CD for ages over 6 years but not for UC. Supplemental therapy, including proper nutrition, iron therapy, and adequate hydration, should also be considered to maintain general health and growth. Treating IBD in children involves aggressively managing the condition and the side effects with the limited options.

Pregnancy

The fertility rate in women with IBD is like the general population, but spontaneous abortions, stillbirths, and developmental defects are more common in pregnant women with active disease. Therefore, IBD should be treated aggressively in pregnant women to limit dehydration, anemia, and nutritional deficiencies that could adversely affect fetal outcomes. However, treatment options are limited for pregnant women due to the risk of teratogenicity or unwanted effects on the fetus. Methotrexate is absolutely contraindicated in pregnancy and lactation due to its potential for spontaneous abortions and teratogenicity. Data are controversial regarding the use of mercaptopurine and azathioprine during pregnancy. If either of these agents is necessary during pregnancy to limit pancytopenia in the fetus, azathioprine dosage of 2 mg/kg/d or less is recommended. Azathioprine and mercaptopurine are contraindicated during nursing due to the potential of fetal immunosuppression. The use of cyclosporine should be reserved for severe refractory cases because it can cause growth retardation. Caution is advised in pregnancy and breastfeeding for all TNF-alpha inhibitors that treat IBD; there is inadequate human data to assess risk. Studies have shown serum levels of

TNF-alpha inhibitors are detectable in the serum of infants for up to 6 months post in utero exposure. Previously, it was recommended to hold therapy after 30 weeks of gestational age (Gisbert, 2010; Zelinkova et al., 2011); however, more recent data shows there is no risk to the pregnant mother or infant (Puchner et al., 2019; Tsao et al., 2018). Selective adhesion molecule inhibitors have not been studied in pregnancy. Ciprofloxacin and metronidazole should also be avoided in pregnancy and lactation because they can cause fetal malformations. Corticosteroids may be used at the lowest doses possible to induce remission for the shortest period to limit adrenal suppression of the fetus. Women taking sulfasalazine should be given higher dosages of folate (2 mg/d) because sulfasalazine interferes with folate absorption. Preconception counseling is imperative to discuss the condition, lifestyle changes, nutritional issues, and treatment options with the patient. Give particular attention to maintaining body weight before conception and preventing exacerbations during pregnancy.

MONITORING PATIENT RESPONSE

Various parameters must be monitored to detect the efficacy and toxicity associated with therapy. Efficacy parameters include signs and symptoms of CD and UC, which are well defined in the Truelove and Witt's Severity Index and Criteria for Severity of Ulcerative Colitis. Nutritional parameters such as weight, albumin, vitamin B_{12} levels, iron levels, and transferrin saturation should also be followed. Mental status and quality-of-life issues such as frequency of social interactions, attendance at work, and completion of daily living activities all may indicate the effectiveness of therapy. Although there are no definitive guidelines for the frequency of monitoring, it is essential to monitor these endpoints when drug therapy is adjusted or when exacerbations occur.

Specific monitoring of drug toxicities is imperative for all pharmacologic agents. As an example, for patients taking sulfasalazine, perform CBC and liver function tests periodically to detect asymptomatic undesired reactions. Also, renal function (i.e., blood urea nitrogen, serum creatinine) should be monitored routinely with aminosalicylates to identify nephrotoxicity.

Corticosteroid treatment is associated with significant drug toxicities, but most occur with long-term use. In general, short-term corticosteroid treatment does not require intense monitoring. However, patients with uncontrolled hypertension or glucose intolerance must have their blood pressure or fasting blood glucose level monitored periodically while taking corticosteroids. For patients taking corticosteroids on a long-term basis, baseline tests including a lipid panel, electrolytes, and fasting blood glucose studies should be performed every 6 to 12 months. A baseline bone density scan may be judicious and repeated yearly if necessary.

Azathioprine and 6-mercaptopurine are both associated with significant side effects, so it is important to acquire a baseline CBC with differential and serum creatinine, amylase, and liver function tests. The CBC should be monitored more frequently during therapy initiation (every 1–2 weeks for the first 3 months) and then less often (every 3–6 months) for therapy duration. Liver function tests are monitored every 3 months for the first year or until a stable dosage has been achieved, then every 4 to 6 months for treatment duration. Creatinine clearance is an essential parameter for guiding the dosing regimen of azathioprine or 6-mercaptopurine, so serum creatinine and creatinine clearance monitor annually if renal function is stable, and more often if fluctuations in dosages or renal function occur. Amylase is not routinely ordered, but it may be checked upon patient complaints due to pancreatitis risk.

During the initial phase of methotrexate therapy, order CBC and liver function test every 2 to 4 weeks. Continuation of methotrexate therapy beyond 16 weeks, monitor CBC and liver function tests every 4 to 8 weeks for therapy duration. Based on dosage adjustments on creatinine clearance, serum creatinine should be monitored first at baseline and every dosage change. If renal function is stable, serum creatinine should be monitored annually at a minimum. Consider once a year liver biopsies if the patient is taking methotrexate, although there is a lack of formal recommendations.

IV cyclosporine is only used in the hospital setting and requires daily monitoring of cyclosporine blood levels (200–400 ng/mL), blood urea nitrogen, serum creatinine, and blood pressure. The metabolism of cyclosporine is through the liver and eliminated through the kidneys. Permanent renal dysfunction is a high associated with the use of cyclosporine; therefore, monitoring creatinine and estimated glomerular filtration rate (eGFR) is essential. The basis of dose adjustment of dosage is renal function and cyclosporine blood levels. Opportunistic infections may occur with high-dose cyclosporine use, monitor temperature, CBC, and signs of infection daily.

Biologics are associated with many side effects; however, most do not occur commonly. Due to the rare incidence of serious side effects, routine laboratory monitoring is not indicated; however, a heightened awareness of adverse events' clinical symptoms is warranted. Regular monitoring by patients and health care professionals for signs of heart failure, vasculitis, TB, infection, hepatotoxicity, and lupus-like syndrome is important. Autoantibodies to the TNF-alpha inhibitors are known to develop and can be monitored via serum levels. Patients who develop autoantibodies may be more likely to develop lupus-like syndrome or have reduced efficacy with the agents (West et al., 2008). Routine administration of biologics and concomitant administration of immunosuppressants limit the development of autoantibodies.

Metronidazole and ciprofloxacin do not require significant drug monitoring, but long-term antibiotic treatment may lead to superinfection, so signs and symptoms of infection should be noted and treated. Patients receiving metronidazole therapy should also be monitored for peripheral paresthesias.

PATIENT EDUCATION

Drug Information

Patients and caregivers need to understand that uncontrolled IBD may affect the quality of life, psychological well-being, and general physical health, so adherence to medication therapy is imperative. Also, due to the increased GI transit time during an exacerbation, patients may not fully absorb oral medications for any of their conditions, leading to poor control of their other conditions during an IBD exacerbation.

Patients should swallow the enteric-coated sulfasalazine or mesalamine tablets and capsules whole so that the dosage form can penetrate the affected area. Sulfasalazine can discolor body fluids (e.g., urine and tears), which may stain clothing and contact lenses. When taking metronidazole, patients must abstain from alcohol to avoid severe nausea and vomiting.

Often, patients request chronic corticosteroid therapy because of its beneficial results. Still, these patients need to be informed of the long-term complications of corticosteroids and advised regarding other medications that may be more appropriate for chronic therapy. Adherence to the medication regimen is imperative even though symptoms resolution will not be apparent for many weeks. The immunosuppressants (azathioprine, 6-mercaptopurine, methotrexate) take 10 to 15 weeks to take effect.

Although the biologics are quite efficacious for IBD, patients must be aware of the significant risks associated with them. If patients are prescribed either adalimumab or certolizumab pegol, they must be instructed on the proper self-administration of subcutaneous injection and sterile technique and safe needle disposal.

Patient-Oriented Information Sources

Along with their health care professionals, there are many other resources available for patients seeking information on IBD. A local support group may be a useful resource for patients having trouble dealing with the illness. Many local hospitals and the Crohn's and Colitis Foundation of America organize support groups for IBD patients. For general medical information regarding IBD, the following Web sites offer helpful patient-specific information:

- AGA: www.gastro.org
- American College of Gastroenterology: www.acg.gi.org
- Crohn's and Colitis Foundation of America: www.ccfa.org
- MedlinePlus: www.nlm.nih.gov/medlineplus/
- National Institute of Diabetes, Digestive, and Kidney Diseases: www.niddk.nih.gov

Preventive Care

Nutritional Status

Nutritional status is a significant issue for patients with active IBD and those with surgical resections. Patients with IBD are at risk for stunted growth, malnutrition, dehydration, weight loss, iron deficiency anemia, macrocytic anemia, osteopenia, and other conditions. Nutrient deficiencies include iron, vitamin B_{12}, zinc, folate, calcium, and vitamin D, resulting from decreased oral intake. There is malabsorption, excessive losses, hypermetabolism due to infection, or drug-induced side effects. To reduce potential nutritional deficiencies from taking corticosteroids, methotrexate, and sulfasalazine, advise the patient to take folate, calcium, and vitamin D. Also, due to

folate deficiencies, patients with IBD are at risk of hyperhomocysteinemia, resulting in an elevated potential for thrombosis. Vitamin B_6 and vitamin B_{12} supplementation are recommended to decrease homocysteine levels. Folate supplementation is essential in women of childbearing age.

Many special dietary agents have been studied in patients with IBD with varying results. Diets high in short-chain fatty acids and fish oils are associated with a small disease severity decrease, potentially due to an anti-inflammatory effect. Fish oils have also been associated with a decreased frequency of exacerbations. An area of new research interest is probiotics such as *Lactobacillus* and *Saccharomyces* in IBD treatment. Altering the GI flora is theorized that probiotic agents assist with controlling IBD exacerbations.

Enteral and parenteral routes of nutrition are used routinely to improve the nutritional status of IBD patients. In general, enteral nutrition is preferred due to the complications of infection, thrombosis, and pancreatitis associated with parenteral nutrition. Besides correcting nutritional deficiencies, enteral nutrition has also been studied as a primary treatment measure combined with aminosalicylates. Parenteral nutrition, however, is advocated in severe exacerbations when bowel rest is necessary for proper healing of the IBD. In general, nutritional supplementation plays a large role in the management of IBD. Depending on the severity of the patient's weight loss and general health status, consider a combination of vitamin and mineral supplementation and either enteral or parenteral nutrition.

Vaccination

Vaccination status in patients with IBD is critical. Since IBD is an autoimmune disease and treatment is focused on immunosuppressant therapy, patients are at higher risk for developing infections. Vaccination records should be reviewed routinely and updated, as necessary. Patients on biologic therapy are at risk for hepatitis B reactivation; therefore, screening patients before treatment may be prudent. Patients taking an immunosuppressant cannot receive live vaccines; however, they are eligible for inactivated vaccines such as influenza, pneumococcal, meningococcal, tetanus, and hepatitis B (Centers for Disease Control, 2020b). Before the initiation of any biologics, consider bringing all immunizations up to date.

Cancer Screening

Patients with IBD are at a higher risk for colorectal cancer (Eaden et al., 2001, Lichtenstein et al., 2018). Due to the increased risk, patients with IBD for a minimum of 8 years should be screened for colorectal cancer with a colonoscopy and biopsy. Although the data are conflicting as to how often patients should be screened, the American College of Gastroenterology recommends either annually or biannually (Lichtenstein et al., 2018; Rubin et al., 2019).

Complementary and Alternative Therapies

Many patients with IBD use alternative therapies; however, there is a lack of controlled studies, and the sample sizes are small (Cheifetz et al., 2017). The use of probiotics, fish oil, marijuana, and mind–body therapy is the most common in IBD. Surgical options are considered in patients at risk for a further decline in physical health and quality of life resulting from frequent exacerbations unresponsive to conventional therapy. These options include proctocolectomy for UC and various ostomy procedures for patients with CD, depending on the disease's location (**Table 25.17**). Proctocolectomy, the removal of the entire colon and rectum, is a curative intervention for UC. However, surgical procedures for CD are not curative because exacerbations may recur in existing areas of the GI tract, and surgery is used only to maintain remission.

For patients who have undergone surgery, the practitioner must pay close attention to general drug therapy issues. Because of the GI tract's resection, these patients have problems similar to short bowel syndrome patients.

TABLE 25.17

Surgical Interventions

Procedure	Area of Resection
Sigmoid colostomy	Distal end of large intestine
Descending colostomy	Descending colon and rectum
Transverse colostomy	Small portion of transverse colon
Proctocolectomy/ileostomy	Entire rectum and large intestine

Rectally administered agents such as suppositories and enemas are ineffective in patients with any lower GI resection. Depending on resection, sustained-release agents and medications targeted to specific GI tract areas are also ineffective in general.

CASE STUDY 1

S.B. is a 57-year-old African American man with newly diagnosed late-stage small cell lung cancer. He has undergone radiation therapy to the brain for his metastases and is to start chemotherapy next week. His past medical history includes hypertension. He has no known drug allergies. A combination chemotherapy regimen has been chosen: cisplatin 100 mg/m^2 for one dose on the first day and etoposide 100 mg/m^2 IV every day for 3 days. He has experienced nausea and vomiting.

DIAGNOSIS: CHEMOTHERAPY-INDUCED NAUSEA AND VOMITING

1. List specific goals for treatment for S.B.
2. What drug therapy would you prescribe? Why?

3. What are the parameters for monitoring success of the therapy?
4. Discuss specific patient education based on the prescribed therapy.
5. List one or two adverse reactions for the selected agent that would cause you to change therapy.
6. What would be the choice for the second-line therapy?
7. What over-the-counter and/or alternative medications would be appropriate for this patient?
8. What dietary and lifestyle changes should be recommended for this patient?
9. Describe one or two drug–drug or drug–food interactions for the selected agent.

Bibliography

Starred references are cited in the text.

Abdalla, M., & Herfarth, H. (2018). Rethinking colorectal cancer screening in IBD, is it time to revisit the guidelines? *Journal of Crohn's and Colitis*, *12*(7), 757–759. https://doi.org/10.1093/ecco-jcc/jjy073

*Abdoli, A., & Maspi, N. (2018). Commentary: Estimates of global, regional, and national morbidity, mortality, and aetiologies of diarrhoeal diseases: A systematic analysis for the global burden of disease study 2015. *Frontiers in Medicine*, *5*, 1211. https://doi.org/10.3389/fmed.2018.00011

*ACOG. (2018). Practice Bulletin No. 189: Nausea and Vomiting of Pregnancy. *Obstetrics & Gynecology*, *131*(1), e15–30.

*Akbara, A., Walters, J. R. F., & Ghosh, S. (2009). Review article: Visceral hypersensitivity in irritable bowel syndrome: Molecular mechanisms and therapeutic agents. *Alimentary Pharmacology & Therapeutics*, *30*(5), 423–435. https://doi.org/10.1111/j.1365-2036.2009.04056.x

Akriche, F., Amlani, B., & Belsey, J. (2020). Polyethylene glycol-based laxatives for chronic constipation. *The Lancet Gastroenterology & Hepatology*, *5*(2), 110. https://doi.org/10.1016/s2468-1253(19)30384-x

Alajbegovic, S., Sanders, J. W., Atherly, D. E., et al. (2012). Effectiveness of rifaximin and fluoroquinolones in preventing travelers' diarrhea (TD):

A systematic review and meta-analysis. *Systematic Reviews*, *1*(1), 39. https://doi.org/10.1186/2046-4053-1-39

Alatab, S., Sepanlou, S. G., Ikuta, K., et al. (2020). The global, regional, and national burden of inflammatory bowel disease in 195 countries and territories, 1990–2017: A systematic analysis for the global burden of disease study 2017. *The Lancet Gastroenterology & Hepatology*, *5*(1), 17–30. https://doi.org/10.1016/s2468-1253(19)30333-4

American Gastroenterology Association. (2001). AGA medical position statement: Nausea and vomiting. *Gastroenterology*, *120*, 261–262. https://doi.org/10.1053/gast.2001.20515

*Andrade, C. (2020). Major congenital malformation risk after first trimester gestational exposure to oral or intravenous ondansetron. *The Journal of Clinical Psychiatry*, *81*(3), e1–e5. https://doi.org/10.4088/jcp.20f13472

*Armuzzi, A., Pugliese, D., Nardone, O. M., et al. (2013). Management of difficult-to-treat patients with ulcerative colitis: Focus on adalimumab. *Drug Design, Development and Therapy*, 289. https://doi.org/10.2147/dddt.s33197

Bai, T., Xia, J., Jiang, Y., et al. (2017). Comparison of the Rome IV and Rome III criteria for IBS diagnosis: A cross-sectional survey. *Journal of Gastroenterology and Hepatology*, *32*(5), 1018–1025. https://doi.org/10.1111/jgh.13642

Baig, M. K., Zhao, R. H., Woodhouse, S. L., et al. (2002). Variability in serotonin and enterochromaffin cells in patients with colonic inertia and idiopathic diarrhoea as compared to normal controls. *Colorectal Disease*, *4*(5), 348–354. https://doi.org/10.1046/j.1463-1318.2002.00404.x

*Barrett, T. W., DiPersio, D. M., Jenkins, C. A., et al. (2011). A randomized, placebo-controlled trial of ondansetron, metoclopramide, and promethazine in adults. *The American Journal of Emergency Medicine*, *29*(3), 247–255. https://doi.org/10.1016/j.ajem.2009.09.028

*Basson, M. D. (2020, March 30). *Constipation: Practice essentials, background, pathophysiology*. Emedicine. https://emedicine.medscape.com/article/184704-overview

Bassotti, G., Usai-Satta, P., & Bellini, M. (2018). Linaclotide for the treatment of chronic constipation. *Expert Opinion on Pharmacotherapy*, *19*(11), 1261–1266. https://doi.org/10.1080/14656566.2018.1494728

Bellido-Blasco, J. B., & Arnedo-Pena, A. (2011). Epidemiology of infectious diarrhea. *Encyclopedia of Environmental Health*, 659–671. https://doi.org/10.1016/b978-0-444-63951-6.00689-6

Berger, M. J., Ettinger, D. S., Aston, J., et al. (2017). NCCN guidelines insights: Antiemesis, version 2.2017. *Journal of the National Comprehensive Cancer Network*, *15*(7), 883–893. https://doi.org/10.6004/jnccn.2017.0117

Bharucha, A. E., Pemberton, J. H., & Locke, G. R. (2013). American Gastroenterological Association technical review on constipation. *Gastroenterology*, *144*(1), 218–238. https://doi.org/10.1053/j.gastro.2012.10.028

Binder, H. J., Brown, I., Ramakrishna, B. S., et al. (2014). Oral rehydration therapy in the second decade of the twenty-first century. *Current Gastroenterology Reports*, *16*(3), 376. https://doi.org/10.1007/s11894-014-0376-2

*Black, C. J., & Ford, A. C. (2018). Chronic idiopathic constipation in adults: Epidemiology, pathophysiology, diagnosis, and clinical management. *Medical Journal of Australia*, *209*(2), 86–91. https://doi.org/10.5694/mja18.00241

Borowitz, S. M., Cox, D. J., Kovatchev, B., et al. (2005). Treatment of childhood constipation by primary care physicians: Efficacy and predictors of outcome. *Pediatrics*, *115*(4), 873–877. https://doi.org/10.1542/peds.2004-0537

Botrel, T., Clark, O., Clark, L., et al. (2011). Efficacy of palonosetron (PAL) compared to other serotonin inhibitors (5-HT$_3$R) in preventing chemotherapy-induced Nausea and vomiting (CINV) in patients receiving moderately or highly emetogenic (MoHE) treatment: Systematic review and meta-analysis. *Support Care Cancer*, *19*, 823–832. https://doi.org/10.1007/s00520-010-0908-8

Bouras, E., & Vazquez-Roque, M. (2015). Epidemiology and management of chronic constipation in elderly patients. *Clinical Interventions in Aging*, 919. https://doi.org/10.2147/cia.s54304

*Brandt, L. J., Schoenfeld, P., Prather, C. M., et al. (2009). An Evidence-Based position statement on the management of irritable bowel Syndrome. *The American Journal of Gastroenterology*, *104*(S1), S1–S35. https://doi.org/10.1038/ajg.2008.122

Bundeff, A. W., & Woodis, C. B. (2014). Selective serotonin reuptake inhibitors for the treatment of irritable bowel syndrome. *Annals of Pharmacotherapy*, *48*(6), 777–784. https://doi.org/10.1177/1060028014528151

*Burkitt, D. P. (1993). Epidemiology of cancer of the colon and rectum. *Diseases of the Colon & Rectum*, *36*(11), 1071–1082. https://doi.org/10.1007/bf02047303

Burri, E., Maillard, M. H., Schoepfer, A. M., et al. (2020). Treatment algorithm for mild and moderate-to-severe ulcerative colitis: An update. *Digestion*, *101*(Suppl. 1), 2–15. https://doi.org/10.1159/000504092

*Camilleri, M. (2011). Opioid-Induced constipation: Challenges and therapeutic opportunities. *American Journal of Gastroenterology*, *106*(5), 835–842. https://doi.org/10.1038/ajg.2011.30

Camilleri, M., Drossman, D. A., Becker, G., et al. (2014). Emerging treatments in neurogastroenterology: A multidisciplinary working group consensus statement on opioid-induced constipation. *Neurogastroenterology & Motility*, *26*(10), 1386–1395. https://doi.org/10.1111/nmo.12417

*Canavan, C., West, J., & Card, T. (2014). The epidemiology of irritable bowel syndrome. *Clinical Epidemiology*, 71. https://doi.org/10.2147/clep.s40245

Cash, B. (2018). Understanding and managing IBS and CIC in the primary care setting. *Gastroenterology & Hepatology*, *14*(5 Suppl 3), 3–15.

Centers for Disease Control. (2019, January 29). *Guidelines for the management of acute diarrhea after a disaster*. Centers for Disease Control and Prevention. https://www.cdc.gov/disasters/disease/diarrheaguidelines.html

*Centers for Disease Control. (2020a, August 111). Inflammatory bowel disease prevalence (IBD) in the United States. https://Www.Cdc.Gov/Ibd/Data-Statistics.Htm.https://www.cdc.gov/ibd/data-statistics.htm

*Centers for Disease Control. (2020b, November 8). ACIP altered immunocompetence guidelines for immunizations | recommendations | CDC. Vaccine Recommendations and Guidelines of the ACIP. https://www.cdc.gov/vaccines/hcp/acip-recs/general-recs/immunocompetence.html#:%7E:text=Inactivated%20Vaccines%3A%20Effectiveness&text=Patients%20vaccinated%20within%20a%2014,immune%20competence%20has%20been%20restored

*Centers for Disease Control and Prevention. (2003). Managing acute gastroenteritis among children: Oral rehydration, maintenance, and nutritional therapy. Atlanta, GA:MMWR.

Chang, J. T. (2020). Pathophysiology of inflammatory bowel diseases. *New England Journal of Medicine*, *383*(27), 2652–2664. https://doi.org/10.1056/nejmra2002697

*Cheifetz, A. S., Gianotti, R., Luber, R., & Gibson, P. R. (2017). Complementary and alternative medicines used by patients With Inflammatory bowel diseases. *Gastroenterology*, *152*(2), 415–429.e15. https://doi.org/10.1053/j.gastro.2016.10.004

Cherniack, E. P. (2013). Use of complementary and alternative medicine to treat constipation in the elderly. *Geriatrics & Gerontology International*, *13*(3), 533–538. https://doi.org/10.1111/ggi.12023

Chey, W. D., Webster, L., Sostek, M., et al. (2014). Naloxegol for opioid-induced constipation in patients with noncancer pain. *New England Journal of Medicine*, *370*(25), 2387–2396. https://doi.org/10.1056/nejmoa1310246

Chey, W. D., & Whelan, K. (2016). Dietary guidelines for irritable bowel syndrome are important for gastroenterologists, dietitians and people with irritable bowel syndrome. *Journal of Human Nutrition and Dietetics*, *29*(5), 547–548. https://doi.org/10.1111/jhn.12413

*Clarke, T., Black, L., Stussman, B., Barnes, P., & Nahin, R. (2015, February). Trends in the use of complementary health approaches among adults: United state, 2002–2012 national health statistics reports (No. 79). National Health Stat Report. https://www.ncbi.nlm.nih.gov/pmc/articles/PMC4573565/

Clave, P. (2011). Treatment of IBS-D with 5-HT3 receptor antagonists vs. spasmolytic agents: Similar therapeutical effects from heterogeneous pharmacological targets. *Neurogastroenterology & Motility*, *23*, 1051–1055. https://doi.org/10.1111/j.136-2982.2011.01808

Cole, J. L. (2020). Steroid-induced sleep disturbance and delirium: A focused review for critically ill patients. *Federal Practitioner*, *37*(6), 260–267.

*Connor, B. A. (2013). Chronic diarrhea in travelers. *Current Infectious Disease Reports*, *15*(3), 203–210. https://doi.org/10.1007/s11908-013-0328-2

D'Inca', R., & Caccaro, R. (2014). Measuring disease activity in Crohn's disease: What is currently available to the clinician. *Clinical and Experimental Gastroenterology*, 151. https://doi.org/10.2147/ceg.s41413

*Dahlhamer, J. M., Zammitti, E. P., Ward, B. W., et al. (2016). Prevalence of inflammatory bowel disease among adults aged ≥18 years—United States, 2015. *Morbidity and Mortality Weekly Report*, *65*(42), 1166–1169. https://doi.org/10.15585/mmwr.mm6542a3

Damas, O. M., & Abreu, M. T. (2020). Are patients with ulcerative colitis still at increased risk of colon cancer? *The Lancet*, *395*(10218), 92–94. https://doi.org/10.1016/s0140-6736(19)33225-8

Dassopoulos, T., Sultan, S., Falck–Ytter, Y. T., et al. (2013). American Gastroenterological Association institute technical review on the use of thiopurines, methotrexate, and Anti–TNF-α biologic drugs for the induction and maintenance of remission in inflammatory Crohn's disease. *Gastroenterology*, *145*(6), 1464–1478.e5. https://doi.org/10.1053/j.gastro.2013.10.046

*DeGeorge, L., & Wiesner, L. (2017). Approach to the patient with nausea and vomiting in pregnancy. In J. Borhart (Ed.), *Emergency Department*

Management of Obstetric Complications. Springer, Cham. https://doi.org/10.1007/978-3-319-54410-6_3

*Devanarayana, N. M., & Rajindrajith, S. (2018). Irritable bowel syndrome in children: Current knowledge, challenges and opportunities. *World Journal of Gastroenterology*, 24(21), 2211–2235. https://doi.org/10.3748/wjg.v24.i21.2211

Dranitsaris, G., Molassiotis, A., Clemons, M., et al. (2017). The development of a prediction tool to identify cancer patients at high risk for chemotherapy-induced nausea and vomiting. *Annals of Oncology*, 28, 1260–1267.

Dulai, P. S., Sandborn, W. J., & Gupta, S. (2016). Colorectal cancer and dysplasia in inflammatory bowel disease: A review of disease epidemiology, pathophysiology, and management. *Cancer Prevention Research*, 9(12), 887–894. https://doi.org/10.1158/1940-6207.capr-16-0124

*Eaden, J. A., Abrams, K. R., & Mayberry, J. F. (2001). The risk of colorectal cancer in ulcerative colitis: A meta-analysis. *Gut*, 48, 526–535.

Einhorn, L. H., Rapoport, B., Navari, R. M., et al. (2017). 2016 updated MASCC/ESMO consensus recommendations: Prevention of nausea and vomiting following multiple-day chemotherapy, high-dose chemotherapy, and breakthrough nausea and vomiting. *Support Care Cancer*, 25, 303–308.

Emmanuel, A., Mattace-Raso, F., Neri, M. C., et al. (2016). Constipation in older people: A consensus statement. *International Journal of Clinical Practice*, 71(1), e12920. https://doi.org/10.1111/ijcp.12920

*Everhart, J. E. (Ed.). (2008). *The burden of digestive diseases in the United States*. US Department of Health and Human Services, Public Health Service, National Institutes of Health, National Institutes of Diabetes and Digestive and Kidney Diseases. Washington, DC: US Government Printing Office; NIH Publication No. 09-6443.

Faegan, B. G., Rutgeerts, P., Sands, B. E., et al. (2013). Vedolizumab as induction and maintenance therapy for ulcerative colitis. *New England Journal of Medicine*, 369, 699–710.

*Fejzo, M. S., Myhre, R., Colodro-Conde, L., MacGibbon, K. W., Sinsheimer, J. S., Reddy, M. P. L., Pajukanta, P., Nyholt, D. R., Wright, M. J., Martin, N. G., Engel, S. M., Medland, S. E., Magnus, P., & Mullin, P. M. (2017). Genetic analysis of hyperemesis gravidarum reveals association with intracellular calcium release channel (RYR2). *Molecular and Cellular Endocrinology*, 439, 308–316. https://doi.org/10.1016/j.mce.2016.09.017

*Feldman, P., Wolfson, D., & Barkin, J. (2007). Medical management of Crohn's disease. *Clinics in Colon and Rectal Surgery*, 20(4), 269–281. https://doi.org/10.1055/s-2007-991026

*Feuerstein, J. D., Isaacs, K. L., Schneider, Y., et al. (2020). AGA clinical practice guidelines on the management of moderate to severe ulcerative colitis. *Gastroenterology*, 158(5), 1450–1461. https://doi.org/10.1053/j.gastro.2020.01.006

*Ford, A. C., Moayyedi, P., Chey, W., et al. (2018). American college of gastroenterology monograph on management of irritable bowel syndrome. *American Journal of Gastroenterology*, 18(1), 1. https://doi.org/10.1038/s41395-018-0084

*Ford, A. C., Moayyedi, P., Lacy, B. E., et al. (2014). American College of Gastroenterology monograph on the management of irritable bowel syndrome and chronic idiopathic constipation. *American Journal of Gastroenterology*, 109, S2–S26. https://doi.org/10.1038/ajg.2014.187

*Forootan, M., Bagheri, N., & Darvishi, M. (2018). Chronic constipation. *Medicine*, 97(20), e10631. https://doi.org/10.1097/md.0000000000010631

Frese, T. (2011). Nausea and vomiting as the reasons for encounter. *Journal of Clinical Medicine Research*, 23–29. https://doi.org/10.4021/jocmr410w

Gade, A. K., Douthit, N. T., & Townsley, E. (2020). Medical management of Crohn's disease. *Cureus*, 1. https://doi.org/10.7759/cureus.8351

Gisbert, J. P. (2010). Safety of immunomodulators and biologics for the treatment of inflammatory bowel disease during pregnancy and breast-feeding. *Inflammatory Bowel Diseases*, 16(5), 881–895. https://doi.org/10.1002/ibd.21154

Gonczi, L., Bessissow, T., & Lakatos, P. L. (2019). Disease monitoring strategies in inflammatory bowel diseases: What do we mean by 'tight control'? *World Journal of Gastroenterology*, 25(41), 6172–6189. https://doi.org/10.3748/wjg.v25.i41.6172

*Gordon, H., Trier Moller, F., Andersen, V., et al. (2015). Heritability in inflammatory bowel disease. *Inflammatory Bowel Diseases*, 1. https://doi.org/10.1097/mib.0000000000000393

Gordon, M., MacDonald, J. K., Parker, C. E., et al. (2016). Osmotic and stimulant laxatives for the management of childhood constipation. *Cochrane Database of Systematic Reviews*, 1. https://doi.org/10.1002/14651858.cd009118.pub3

Grodzinsky, E., Walter, S., Viktorsson, L., et al. (2015). More negative self-esteem and inferior coping strategies among patients diagnosed with IBS compared with patients without IBS - a case–control study in primary care. *BMC Family Practice*, 16(1), 1. https://doi.org/10.1186/s12875-015-0225-x

Guandalini, S. (2020, April 27). Diarrhea: Practice essentials, background, pathophysiology. Retrieved from https://emedicine.medscape.com/article/928598-overview

*Guarino, A., Vecchio, A. L., & Canani, R. B. (2009). Probiotics as prevention and treatment for diarrhea. *Current Opinion in Gastroenterology*, 25(1), 18–23. https://doi.org/10.1097/mog.0b013e32831b4455

*Halfverson, J., Jess, T., Bodine, L., et al. (2007). Longitudinal concordance for clinical characteristics in a Swedish-Danish twin population with inflammatory bowel disease. *Inflammatory Bowel Disease*, 13, 1536–1544.

Hamilton, A. L., Kamm, M. A., De Cruz, P., et al. (2017). Serologic antibodies in relation to outcome in postoperative Crohn's disease. *Journal of Gastroenterology and Hepatology*, 32(6), 1195–1203. https://doi.org/10.1111/jgh.13677

Hardy, J., Skerman, H., Glare, P., et al. (2018). A randomized open-label study of guideline-driven antiemetic therapy versus single agent antiemetic therapy in patients with advanced cancer and nausea not related to anticancer treatment. *BMC Cancer*, 18(1), 1–9. https://doi.org/10.1186/s12885-018-4404-8

Hartman, S., Brown, E., Loomis, E., et al. (2019). Gastroenteritis in children. *American Family Physician*, 99(3), 159–165. https://www.aafp.org/afp/2019/0201/p159.html

Herrick, L. M., Spalding, W. M., Saito, Y. A., et al. (2016). A case-control comparison of direct healthcare-provider medical costs of chronic idiopathic constipation and irritable bowel syndrome with constipation in a community-based cohort. *Journal of Medical Economics*, 20(3), 273–279. https://doi.org/10.1080/13696998.2016.1253584

*Hayes, P., Fraher, M., & Quigley, E. (2014). Irritable bowel syndrome: The role of food in pathogenesis and management. *Gastroenterology & Hepatology*, 10(3), 164.

Hijazi, E. M., Edwan, H., Al-Zoubi, N., et al. (2018). Incidence of nausea and vomiting after Fast-Track anaesthesia for heart surgery. *Brazilian Journal of Cardiovascular Surgery*, 33(4), 371–375. https://doi.org/10.21470/1678-9741-2018-0040

Huguet, J. M., Suárez, P., Ferrer-Barceló, L., et al. (2017). Endoscopic recommendations for colorectal cancer screening and surveillance in patients with inflammatory bowel disease: Review of general recommendations. *World Journal of Gastrointestinal Endoscopy*, 9(6), 255. https://doi.org/10.4253/wjge.v9.i6.255

Huybrechts, K. F., Hernández-Díaz, S., Straub, L., et al. (2018). Association of maternal first-trimester ondansetron use with cardiac malformations and oral clefts in offspring. *JAMA*, 320(23), 2429–2437. https://doi.org/10.1001/jama.2018.18307

*Hyams, J. S., Di Lorenzo, C., Saps, M., Shulman, R. J., Staiano, A., & van Tilburg, M. (2016). Childhood functional gastrointestinal disorders: Child/Adolescent. *Gastroenterology*, 150(6), 1456–1468.e2. https://doi.org/10.1053/j.gastro.2016.02.015

*Jakobsen, G., Engstrøm, M., Hjermstad, M. J., Rosland, J. H., Aass, N., Albert, E., Kaasa, S., Fayers, P., Klepstad, P., & Paulsen, R. (2020). The short-term impact of methylprednisolone on patient-reported sleep in patients with advanced cancer in a randomized, placebo-controlled, double-blind trial. *Supportive Care in Cancer*, 29(4), 2047–2055. https://doi.org/10.1007/s00520-020-05693-6

*Kamm, M. A., Mueller–Lissner, S., Wald, A., et al. (2011). Oral bisacodyl is effective and well-Tolerated in patients with chronic constipation. *Clinical Gastroenterology and Hepatology*, 9(7), 577–583. https://doi.org/10.1016/j.cgh.2011.03.026

*Kaptchuk, T. J., Friedlander, E., Kelley, J. M., Sanchez, M. N., Kokkotou, E., Singer, J. P., Kowalczykowski, M., Miller, F. G., Kirsch, I., & Lembo, A. J. (2010b). Placebos without deception: A randomized controlled trial in irritable bowel syndrome. PLoS ONE, 5(12), e15591. https://doi.org/10.1371/journal.pone.0015591

Keeley, P. W. (2020). Nausea and vomiting in palliative care. Medicine, 48(1), 14–17. https://doi.org/10.1016/j.mpmed.2019.10.009

*Khalili, H., Higuchi, L. M., Ananthakrishnan, A. N., Richter, J. M., Feskanich, D., Fuchs, C. S., & Chan, A. T. (2012). Oral contraceptives, reproductive factors and risk of inflammatory bowel disease. Gut, 62(8), 1153–1159. https://doi.org/10.1136/gutjnl-2012-302362

Khalili, H., Higuchi, L. M., Ananthakrishnan, A. N., et al. (2012). Oral contraceptives, reproductive factors and risk of inflammatory bowel disease. Gut, 62(8), 1153–1159. https://doi.org/10.1136/gutjnl-2012-302362

*Kim-Jong, I. L., Holquist, C, C., & Phillips, J. (2004, April 19). Kaopectate reformulation and upcoming label changes. Retrieved from https://www.fda.gov/media/72651/download

King, C. K., Glass, R., Bresee, J. S., & Duggan, C. (2003, November). Managing acute gastroenteritis among children oral rehydration, maintenance, and nutritional therapy. MMWR (52(RR16);1-16). https://www.cdc.gov/mmwr/preview/mmwrhtml/rr5216a1.htm

*Kornbluth, A., & Sachar, D. B. (2010). Ulcerative colitis practice guidelines in adults: American College of Gastroenterology, practice parameters committee. American Journal of Gastroenterology, 105(3), 501–523. https://doi.org/10.1038/ajg.2009.727

Kumar, L., Barker, C., & Emmanuel, A. (2014). Opioid-Induced constipation: Pathophysiology, clinical consequences, and management. Gastroenterology Research and Practice, 2014, 1–6. https://doi.org/10.1155/2014/141737

Lacy, B. E., Levenick, J. M., & Crowell, M. D. (2012). Linaclotide: A novel therapy for chronic constipation and constipation-predominant irritable bowel syndrome. Advances in Therapy, 8(10), 653–660. https://www.ncbi.nlm.nih.gov/pmc/articles/PMC3969007/

*Lacy, B. E., Mearin, F., Chang, L., et al. (2016). Bowel disorders. Gastroenterology, 150(6), 1393–1407.e5. https://doi.org/10.1053/j.gastro.2016.02.031

Lacy, B. E., Parkman, H. P., & Camilleri, M. (2018). Chronic nausea and vomiting: Evaluation and treatment. American Journal of Gastroenterology, 113(5), 647–659. https://doi.org/10.1038/s41395-018-0039-2

*Ladd, J. (2017). New takes on an old regimen for NVP. Pharmacy Today, 23(4), 36. https://doi.org/10.1016/j.ptdy.2017.03.018

Laskaratos, F.-M., Goodkin, O., Thoua, N. M., et al. (2015). Irritable bowel syndrome. Medicine, 43(5), 266–270. https://doi.org/10.1016/j.mpmed.2015.02.010

Lee, N. M., & Saha, S. (2011). Nausea and vomiting of pregnancy. Gastroenterology Clinics of North America, 40(2), 309–334. http://doi.org/10.1016/j.gtc.2011.03.009

*Lee, S. Y., Jamal, M. M., Nguyen, E. T., et al. (2016). Does exposure to isotretinoin increase the risk for the development of inflammatory bowel disease? A meta-analysis. European Journal of Gastroenterology & Hepatology, 28(2), 210–216. https://doi.org/10.1097/meg.0000000000000496

*Lenters, L. M., Das, J. K., & Bhutta, Z. A. (2013). Systematic review of strategies to increase use of oral rehydration solution at the household level. BMC Public Health, 13(Suppl 3), S28. https://doi.org/10.1186/1471-2458-13-s3-s28

Leonard, J., & Baker, D. E. (2014). Naloxegol. Annals of Pharmacotherapy, 49(3), 360–365. https://doi.org/10.1177/1060028014560191

Levy, E., Lemmens, R., Vandenplas, Y., et al. (2017). Functional constipation in children: Challenges and solutions. Pediatric Health, Medicine and Therapeutics, 8, 19–27. https://doi.org/10.2147/phmt.s110940

Lewis, S. J., & Heaton, K. W. (1997). Stool form scale as a useful guide to intestinal transit time. Scandinavian Journal of Gastroenterology, 32(9), 920–924. https://doi.org/10.3109/00365529709011203

*Lichtenstein, G. R., Diamond, R. H., Wagner, C. L., et al. (2009a). Clinical trial: Benefits and risks of immunomodulators and maintenance infliximab for IBD-subgroup analyses across four randomized trials. Alimentary Pharmacology & Therapeutics, 30(3), 210–226. https://doi.org/10.1111/j.1365-2036.2009.04027.x

*Lichtenstein, G. R., Loftus, E. V., Isaacs, K. L., et al. (2018). ACG clinical guideline: Management of Crohn's disease in adults. American Journal of Gastroenterology, 113(4), 481–517. https://doi.org/10.1038/ajg.2018.27

Loening-Baucke, V., Miele, E., & Staiano, A. (2004). Fiber (glucomannan) is beneficial in the treatment of childhood constipation. Pediatrics, 113(3), e259–e264. https://doi.org/10.1542/peds.113.3.e259

*Lovell, R. M., & Ford, A. C. (2012). Global prevalence of and risk factors for irritable bowel syndrome: A meta-analysis. Clinical Gastroenterology and Hepatology, 10(7), 712–721.e4. https://doi.org/10.1016/j.cgh.2012.02.029

Lynch, W. D., & Hsu, R. (2018, June 20). Ulcerative colitis. StatPearls [Internet], 1. https://www.ncbi.nlm.nih.gov/books/NBK459282/?report=reader#_NBK459282_pubdet_

Mahadevan, U., Long, M. D., Kane, S. V., et al. (2020). Pregnancy and neonatal outcomes after fetal exposure to biologics and thiopurines among women with inflammatory bowel disease. Gastroenterology, 1. https://doi.org/10.1053/j.gastro.2020.11.038

Mahadevan, U., Robinson, C., Bernasko, N., et al. (2019). Inflammatory bowel disease in pregnancy clinical care pathway: A report from the American Gastroenterological Association IBD parenthood project working Group. Gastroenterology, 156(5), 1508–1524. https://doi.org/10.1053/j.gastro.2018.12.022

Martínez-Martínez, M. I., Calabuig-Tolsá, R., & Cauli, O. (2017). The effect of probiotics as a treatment for constipation in elderly people: A systematic review. Archives of Gerontology and Geriatrics, 71, 142–149. https://doi.org/10.1016/j.archger.2017.04.004

Mayhall, E. A., Gray, R., Lopes, V., et al. (2015). Comparison of antiemetics for nausea and vomiting of pregnancy in an emergency department setting. The American Journal of Emergency Medicine, 33(7), 882–886. https://doi.org/10.1016/j.ajem.2015.03.032

*McFarland, L. V., & Goh, S. (2019). Are probiotics and prebiotics effective in the prevention of travellers' diarrhea: A systematic review and meta-analysis. Travel Medicine and Infectious Disease, 27, 11–19. https://doi.org/10.1016/j.tmaid.2018.09.007

*McRorie, J. W., Fahey, G. C., Gibb, R. D., et al. (2020). Laxative effects of wheat bran and psyllium. Journal of the American Association of Nurse Practitioners, 32(1), 15–23. https://doi.org/10.1097/jxx.0000000000000346

MGH Center for Women's Mental Health. (2020, July 23). Ondansetron (Zofran) for Nausea and Vomiting in Pregnancy: Maybe Not for All Women. Retrieved from https://womensmentalhealth.org/posts/ondansetron-pregnancy/

*Molassiotis, A., Lee, P. H., Burke, T. A., et al. (2016). Anticipatory nausea, risk factors, and its impact on Chemotherapy-Induced nausea and vomiting: Results from the Pan European emesis registry study. Journal of Pain and Symptom Management, 51(6), 987–993. https://doi.org/10.1016/j.jpainsymman.2015.12.317

Molodecky, N. A., Soon, I. S., Rabi, D. M., et al. (2012). Increasing incidence and prevalence of the inflammatory bowel diseases with time, based on systematic review. Gastroenterology, 142(1), 46–54.e42. https://doi.org/10.1053/j.gastro.2011.10.001

*Morita, Y., Imai, T., Bamba, S., Takahashi, K., Inatomi, O., Miyazaki, T., Watanabe, K., Nakamura, S., Yoshida, A., Endo, Y., Ohmiya, N., Tsujikawa, T., & Andoh, A. (2020). Clinical relevance of innovative immunoassays for serum ustekinumab and anti-ustekinumab antibody levels in crohn's disease. Journal of Gastroenterology and Hepatology, 35(7), 1163–1170. https://doi.org/10.1111/jgh.14962

Mulder, D. J., Noble, A. J., Justinich, C. J., et al. (2014). A tale of two diseases: The history of inflammatory bowel disease. Journal of Crohn's and Colitis, 8(5), 341–348. https://doi.org/10.1016/j.crohns.2013.09.009

*Müller-Lissner, S., Bassotti, G., Coffin, B., et al. (2016). Opioid-Induced constipation and bowel dysfunction: A clinical guideline. Pain Medicine, 18(10), 1837–1863. https://doi.org/10.1093/pm/pnw255

*Nalin, D. R., & Cash, R. A. (2018). 50 years of oral rehydration therapy: The solution is still simple. The Lancet, 392(10147), 536–538. https://doi.org/10.1016/s0140-6736(18)31488-0

Navari, R. M. (2013). Management of chemotherapy-induced nausea and vomiting. *Drugs*, *73*(3), 249–262. https://doi.org/10.1007/s40265-013-0019-1

*Ngo, S. T., Steyn, F. J., & McCombe, P. A. (2014). Gender differences in autoimmune disease. *Frontiers in Neuroendocrinology*, *35*(3), 347–369. https://doi.org/10.1016/j.yfrne.2014.04.004

Nguyen, G. C., Chong, C. A., & Chong, R. Y. (2014). National estimates of the burden of inflammatory bowel disease among racial and ethnic groups in the United States. *Journal of Crohn's and Colitis*, *8*(4), 288–295. https://doi.org/10.1016/j.crohns.2013.09.001

Nuangchamnong, N., & Niebyl, J. (2014). Doxylamine succinate–pyridoxine hydrochloride (Diclegis) for the management of Nausea and vomiting in pregnancy: An overview. *International Journal of Women's Health*, *6*, 401–409. http://doi.org/10.2147/IJWH.S46653

Ohkusa, T., Koido, S., Nishikawa, Y., et al. (2019). Gut microbiota and chronic constipation: A review and update. *Frontiers in Medicine*, *6*, 1. https://doi.org/10.3389/fmed.2019.00019

Okada, Y., Oba, K., Furukawa, N., et al. (2019). One-day versus three-day dexamethasone in combination with palonosetron for the prevention of chemotherapy-induced nausea and vomiting: A systematic review and individual patient data-based meta-analysis. *The Oncologist*, *24*(12), 1593–1600. https://doi.org/10.1634/theoncologist.2019-0133

Okawa, Y., Fukudo, S., & Sanada, H. (2019). Specific foods can reduce symptoms of irritable bowel syndrome and functional constipation: A review. *BioPsychoSocial Medicine*, *13*(1), 1. https://doi.org/10.1186/s13030-019-0152-5

Olver, I., Ruhlmann, C. H., Jahn, F., et al. (2016). 2016 updated MASCC/ESMO consensus recommendations: Controlling nausea and vomiting with chemotherapy of low or minimal emetic potential. *Supportive Care in Cancer*, *25*(1), 297–301. https://doi.org/10.1007/s00520-016-3391-z

Palsson, O. S., Whitehead, W. E., van Tilburg, M. A. L., et al. (2016). Development and validation of the Rome IV diagnostic questionnaire for adults. *Gastroenterology*, *150*(6), 1481–1491. https://doi.org/10.1053/j.gastro.2016.02.014

Palsson, O. S., Whitehead, W., Törnblom, H., et al. (2020). Prevalence of Rome IV functional bowel disorders among adults in the United States, Canada, and the United Kingdom. *Gastroenterology*, *158*(5), 1262–1273.e3. https://doi.org/10.1053/j.gastro.2019.12.021

*Park, K. T., Ehrlich, O. G., Allen, J. I., et al. (2020). The cost of inflammatory bowel disease: An initiative from the Crohn's & Colitis Foundation. *Inflammatory Bowel Diseases*, *26*(1), 1–10. https://doi.org/10.1093/ibd/izz104

Parker, E. A., Roy, T., D'Adamo, C. R., et al. (2018). Probiotics and gastrointestinal conditions: An overview of evidence from the cochrane collaboration. *Nutrition*, *45*, 125–134.e11. https://doi.org/10.1016/j.nut.2017.06.024

*Parker, S. E., Van Bennekom, C., Anderka, M., et al. (2018). Ondansetron for treatment of nausea and vomiting of pregnancy and the risk of specific birth defects. *Obstetrics & Gynecology*, *132*(2), 385–394. https://doi.org/10.1097/aog.0000000000002679

*Pedersen, N., Duricova, D., Elkjaer, M., et al. (2010). Risk of extra-Intestinal cancer in inflammatory bowel disease: Meta-Analysis of population-based cohort studies. *American Journal of Gastroenterology*, *105*(7), 1480–1487. https://doi.org/10.1038/ajg.2009.760

Pimentel, M., Lembo, A., Chey, W. D., et al. (2011). Rifaximin therapy for patients with irritable bowel syndrome without constipation. *New England Journal of Medicine*, *364*(1), 22–32. https://doi.org/10.1056/nejmoa1004409

*Pomeranz, J. L., Taylor, L. M., & Austin, S. B. (2013). Over-the-counter and out-of-control: Legal strategies to protect youths from abusing products for weight control. *American Journal of Public Health*, *103*(2), 220–225. https://doi.org/10.2105/ajph.2012.300962

Puchner, A., Gröchenig, H. P., Sautner, J., et al. (2019). Immunosuppressives and biologics during pregnancy and lactation. *Wiener Klinische Wochenschrift*, *131*(1–2), 29–44. https://doi.org/10.1007/s00508-019-1448-y

*Quigley, E. (2018). The gut-brain axis and the microbiome: Clues to pathophysiology and opportunities for novel management strategies in irritable bowel syndrome (IBS). *Journal of Clinical Medicine*, *7*, 6. https://doi.org/10.3390/jcm701000

Quigley, E. M. M. (2011). Prucalopride: Safety, efficacy and potential applications. *Therapeutic Advances in Gastroenterology*, *5*(1), 23–30. https://doi.org/10.1177/1756283x11423706

*Rajindrajith, S., Devanarayana, N. M., Crispus Perera, B. J., et al. (2016). Childhood constipation as an emerging public health problem. *World Journal of Gastroenterology*, *22*(30), 6864. https://doi.org/10.3748/wjg.v22.i30.6864

Riddle, M. S., DuPont, H. L., & Connor, B. A. (2016). ACG clinical guideline: Diagnosis, treatment, and prevention of acute diarrheal infections in adults. *American Journal of Gastroenterology*, *111*(5), 602–622. https://doi.org/10.1038/ajg.2016.126

*Riegler, G., & Esposito, I. (2001). Bristol scale stool form. A still valid help in medical practice and clinical research. *Techniques in Coloproctology*, *5*(3), 163–164. https://doi.org/10.1007/s101510100019

*Rubin, D. T., Ananthakrishnan, A. N., Siegel, C. A., et al. (2019). ACG clinical guideline: Ulcerative colitis in adults. *The American Journal of Gastroenterology*, *114*(3), 384–413. https://doi.org/10.14309/ajg.0000000000000152

*Sahn, B., Chen-Lim, M. L., Ciavardone, D., et al. (2016). Safety of a 1-day polyethylene glycol 3350 bowel preparation for colonoscopy in children. *Journal of Pediatric Gastroenterology & Nutrition*, *63*(1), 19–24. https://doi.org/10.1097/mpg.0000000000001072

*Sandborn, W. J., Rutgeerts, P., Enns, R., et al. (2007). Adalimumab induction therapy for Crohn disease previously treated with infliximab. *Annals of Internal Medicine*, *146*(12), 829. https://doi.org/10.7326/0003-4819-146-12-200706190-00159

Sandhu, B. K. (2014). Irritable bowel syndrome in children: Pathogenesis, diagnosis, and evidence-based treatment. *World Journal of Gastroenterology*, *20*(20), 6013. https://doi.org/10.3748/wjg.v20.i20.6013

Saneei Totmaj, A., Emamat, H., Jarrahi, F., et al. (2019). The effect of ginger (Zingiber officinale) on chemotherapy-induced nausea and vomiting in breast cancer patients: A systematic literature review of randomized controlled trials. *Phytotherapy Research*, *33*(8), 1957–1965. https://doi.org/10.1002/ptr.6377

Sanger, G. J., & Andrews, P. L. R. (2018). A history of drug discovery for treatment of nausea and vomiting and the implications for future research. *Frontiers in Pharmacology*, *9*, 1. https://doi.org/10.3389/fphar.2018.00913

Santana, T. A., Trufelli, D. C., de Matos, L. L., et al. (2014). Meta analysis of adjunctive non-NK1 receptor antagonist medications for the control of acute and delayed chemotherapy-induced nausea and vomiting. *Supportive Care in Cancer*, *23*(1), 213–222. https://doi.org/10.1007/s00520-014-2392-z

Sbahi, H., & Cash, B. D. (2015). Chronic constipation: A review of current literature. *Current Gastroenterology Reports*, *17*(12), 1. https://doi.org/10.1007/s11894-015-0471-z

*Schmulson, M. J., & Drossman, D. A. (2017). What is new in Rome IV. *Journal of Neurogastroenterology and Motility*, *23*(2), 151–163. https://doi.org/10.5056/jnm16214

Serban, E. D. (2018). Treat-to-target in Crohn's disease: Will transmural healing become a therapeutic endpoint? *World Journal of Clinical Cases*, *6*(12), 501–513. https://doi.org/10.12998/wjcc.v6.i12.501

Shaikh, S. I., Nagarekha, D., Hegade, G., et al. (2016). Postoperative nausea and vomiting: A simple yet complex problem. *Anesthesia, Essays and Research*, *10*(3), 388–396. https://doi.org/10.4103/0259-1162.179310

*Shane, A. L., Mody, R. K., Crump, J. A., et al. (2017). 2017 Infectious Diseases Society of America clinical practice guidelines for the diagnosis and management of infectious diarrhea. *Clinical Infectious Diseases*, *65*(12), e45–e80. https://doi.org/10.1093/cid/cix669

Sharifzadeh, F., Kashanian, M., Koohpayehzadeh, J., et al. (2017). A comparison between the effects of ginger, pyridoxine (vitamin B6) and placebo for the treatment of the first trimester nausea and vomiting of pregnancy (NVP). *The Journal of Maternal-Fetal & Neonatal Medicine*, *31*(19), 2509–2514. https://doi.org/10.1080/14767058.2017.1344965

Sharma, A., & Rao, S. (2016). Constipation: Pathophysiology and current therapeutic approaches. In M. B. Greenwood-Van (Ed.), *Gastrointestinal pharmacology: Handbook of experimental pharmacology* (Vol. 239, pp. 59–74). Springer International Publishing. https://doi.org/10.1007/164_2016_111

Shawahna, R., & Taha, A. (2017). Which potential harms and benefits of using ginger in the management of nausea and vomiting of pregnancy should be addressed? A consensual study among pregnant women and gynecologists. *BMC Complementary and Alternative Medicine, 17*(1), 1. https://doi.org/10.1186/s12906-017-1717-0

*Simrén, M., Månsson, A., Langkilde, A. M., Svedlund, J., Abrahamsson, H., Bengtsson, U., & Björnsson, E. S. (2001). Food-Related gastrointestinal symptoms in the irritable bowel syndrome. *Digestion, 63*(2), 108–115. https://doi.org/10.1159/000051878

*Slavin, J. L. (2008). Position of the American Dietetic Association: Health implications of dietary fiber. *Journal of the American Dietetic Association, 108*(10), 1716–1731. https://doi.org/10.1016/j.jada.2008.08.007

*Sommers, T., Corban, C., Sengupta, N., et al. (2015). Emergency department burden of constipation in the United States from 2006 to 2011. *American Journal of Gastroenterology, 110*(4), 572–579. https://doi.org/10.1038/ajg.2015.64

Spiegel, B. M. R., Farid, M., Esrailian, E., et al. (2010). Is irritable bowel syndrome a diagnosis of exclusion? A survey of primary care providers, gastroenterologists, and IBS experts. *American Journal of Gastroenterology, 105*(4), 848–858. https://doi.org/10.1038/ajg.2010.47

*Steffen, R. (2017). Epidemiology of travellers' diarrhea. *Journal of Travel Medicine, 24*(suppl_1), S2–S5. https://doi.org/10.1093/jtm/taw072

Sulz, M. C., Burri, E., Michetti, P., et al. (2020). Treatment algorithms for Crohn's disease. *Digestion, 101*(Suppl. 1), 43–57. https://doi.org/10.1159/000506364

Surawicz, C. M., Brandt, L. J., Binion, D. G., et al. (2013). Guidelines for diagnosis, treatment, and prevention of clostridium difficile infections. *American Journal of Gastroenterology, 108*(4), 478–498. https://doi.org/10.1038/ajg.2013.4

Tarbell, S. E., Shaltout, H. A., Wagoner, A. L., et al. (2014). Relationship among nausea, anxiety, and orthostatic symptoms in pediatric patients with chronic unexplained nausea. *Experimental Brain Research, 232*(8), 2645–2650. https://doi.org/10.1007/s00221-014

Theriot, J., Wermuth, H. R., & Ashurst, J. V. (2020). Antiemetic serotonin-5-HT3 receptor blockers. *StatPearls*, 1–11. Retrieved from https://www.ncbi.nlm.nih.gov/books/NBK513318/#article-38853.r4

Tóth, B., Lantos, T., Hegyi, P., et al. (2018). Ginger (Zingiber officinale): An alternative for the prevention of postoperative nausea and vomiting: A meta-analysis. *Phytomedicine, 50*, 8–18. https://doi.org/10.1016/j.phymed.2018.09.007

*Tsao, N. W., Lynd, L. D., Sayre, E. C., et al. (2018). Use of biologics during pregnancy and risk of serious infections in the mother and baby: A Canadian population-based cohort study. *BMJ Open, 9*(2), e023714. https://doi.org/10.1136/bmjopen-2018-023714

Tun, G. S. Z., Cripps, S., & Lobo, A. J. (2018). Crohn's disease: Management in adults, children and young people–concise guidance. *Clinical Medicine, 18*(3), 231–236. https://doi.org/10.7861/clinmedicine.18-3-231

Van den Houte, K., Carbone, F., Pannemans, J., et al. (2018). Prevalence and impact of self-reported irritable bowel symptoms in the general population. *United European Gastroenterology Journal, 7*(2), 307–315. https://doi.org/10.1177/2050640618821804

VanRyckeghem, F. (2016). Corticosteroids, the oldest agent in the prevention of chemotherapy-induced nausea and vomiting: What about the guidelines? *Journal of Translational Internal Medicine, 4*(1), 46–51. https://doi.org/10.1515/jtim-2016-0010

Vesa, T. H., Seppo, L. M., Marteau, P. R., et al. (1998). Role of irritable bowel syndrome in subjective lactose intolerance. *The American Journal of Clinical Nutrition, 67*(4), 710–715. https://doi.org/10.1093/ajcn/67.4.710

*Wald, A. (2007). Appropriate use of laxatives in the management of constipation. *Current Gastroenterology Reports, 9*(5), 410–414. https://doi.org/10.1007/s11894-007-0051-y

*Weinberg, D. S., Smalley, W., Heidelbaugh, J. J., & Sultan, S. (2014). American Gastroenterological Association Institute guideline on the pharmacological management of irritable bowel syndrome. *Gastroenterology, 147*(5), 1146–1148. https://doi.org/10.1053/j.gastro.2014.09.001

*West, R. L., Zelinkova, Z., Wolbink, G. J., Kuipers, E. J., Stokkers, P. C. F., & Van Der Woude, C. J. (2008). Immunogenicity negatively influences the outcome of adalimumab treatment in Crohn's disease. *Alimentary Pharmacology & Therapeutics, 28*(9), 1122–1126. https://doi.org/10.1111/j.1365-2036.2008.03828.x

*Xu, Z., Liu, T., Zhou, Q., et al. (2019). Roles of Chinese medicine and gut microbiota in chronic constipation. *Evidence-Based Complementary and Alternative Medicine, 2019*, 1–11. https://doi.org/10.1155/2019/9372563

*Yang, J., Fox, M., Cong, Y., et al. (2014). Lactose intolerance in irritable bowel syndrome patients with diarrhoea: The roles of anxiety, activation of the innate mucosal immune system and visceral sensitivity. *Alimentary Pharmacology & Therapeutics, 39*(3), 302–311. https://doi.org/10.1111/apt.12582

Yoodee, J., Permsuwan, U., & Nimworapan, M. (2017). Efficacy and safety of olanzapine for the prevention of chemotherapy-induced nausea and vomiting: A systematic review and meta analysis. *Critical Reviews in Oncology/Hematology, 112*, 113–125. https://doi.org/10.1016/j.critrevonc.2017.02.017

Yu, S. W. B., & Rao, S. S. C. (2014). Advances in the management of constipation-predominant irritable bowel syndrome: The role of linaclotide. *Therapeutic Advances in Gastroenterology, 7*(5), 193–205. https://doi.org/10.1177/1756283x14537882

*Zelinkova, Z., de Haar, C., de Ridder, L., et al. (2011). High intra-uterine exposure to infliximab following maternal anti-TNF treatment during pregnancy. *Alimentary Pharmacology & Therapeutics, 33*(9), 1053–1058. https://doi.org/10.1111/j.1365-2036.2011.04617.x

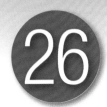

26 Gastroesophageal Reflux Disease and Peptic Ulcer Disease

Alice (Lim) Scaletta

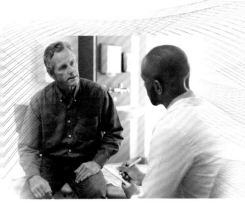
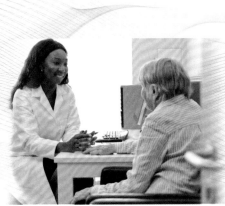
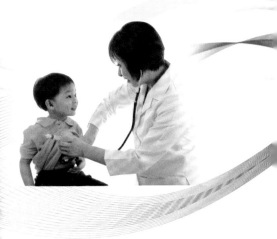

Learning Objectives

1. List the goals of treatment for gastroesophageal reflux disease and peptic ulcer disease.
2. Educate a patient on lifestyle modifications to prevent the worsening of gastroesophageal reflux disease and peptic ulcer disease.
3. Choose appropriate first-line treatment options to manage gastroesophageal reflux disease and peptic ulcer disease, taking into consideration side effects, drug interactions, and patient preference.
4. If patients fail first-line options, identify second-line options to treat gastroesophageal reflux disease and peptic ulcer disease.
5. Recommend appropriate monitoring parameters for safety and efficacy in managing a patient with gastroesophageal reflux disease or peptic ulcer disease.

INTRODUCTION

Gastroesophageal reflux disease (GERD) and peptic ulcer disease (PUD) are two disorders of the gastrointestinal (GI) tract that can cause tissue damage and unpleasant symptoms. They are both commonly encountered in the primary care and gastroenterology settings and can also significantly decrease a patient's health-related quality of life if left unmanaged.

GASTROESOPHAGEAL REFLUX DISEASE

GERD is defined as "troublesome symptoms and/or complications" resulting from the abnormal reflux of gastric contents into the esophagus or beyond, including the oral cavity or lungs. Troublesome symptoms are those that harm the patient's well-being and quality of life.

Depending on how the patient presents, GERD syndromes may be classified into two categories: (1) symptoms present but without erosions seen on the endoscopic exam or (2) those with esophageal tissue injury. Esophageal erosions occur as a result of repeated exposure to refluxed material for prolonged periods.

GERD may occur in all ages, but it most commonly presents in those older than 40 years of age. Patients with mild symptoms do not always seek medical treatment and instead will self-treat with lifestyle changes or over-the-counter remedies. As a result, the true prevalence of the disease is difficult to assess. It is estimated that 18% to 28% of adults in the United States suffer from GERD symptoms weekly (Yamasaki et al., 2018). Prevalence seems to be increasing worldwide, with the highest rates in Western countries and the lowest rates found in East Asia (Nirwin et al., 2020).

CAUSES

Symptoms and/or tissue damage associated with GERD are caused by exposure of the esophagus to gastric contents. This exposure happens because of the relaxation of the lower

523

TABLE 26.1

Risk Factors for Gastroesophageal Reflux Disease

Causes of LES Relaxation

Foods	Drugs
Fatty foods	Anticholinergic agents
Chocolate	Benzodiazepines
Peppermint/spearmint	Caffeine
Garlic	Calcium channel blockers
Onions	(dihydropyridines)
Chili peppers	Dopamine
Alcohol	Estrogen/progesterone
Coffee/caffeinated drinks	Nicotine
Carbonated beverages	Nitrates
	Theophylline
	Tricyclic antidepressants

Causes Direct Irritation of Esophageal Mucosa

Foods	Drugs
Spicy foods	Aspirin
Citrus juices	Bisphosphonates (e.g., alendronate)
Tomato products	Iron
Coffee/caffeinated drinks	NSAIDs
Tobacco chew	Potassium chloride
Alcohol	

LES, lower esophageal sphincter; NSAIDs, nonsteroidal anti-inflammatory drugs.

esophageal sphincter (LES) due to an increase in intra-abdominal pressure (e.g., obesity, pregnancy), delayed gastric emptying, hiatal hernia, or certain medications or foods as listed in **Table 26.1**. Additional risk factors include family history, smoking, alcohol consumption, respiratory diseases, obesity, and reclining or lying down after eating.

PATHOPHYSIOLOGY

Under normal circumstances, the LES serves as a barrier between the esophagus and stomach and, coupled with peristalsis, promotes the forward movement of food. Bicarbonate found in saliva and secreted by the esophageal mucosa buffers acid present in the esophagus. Problems with these standard defense mechanisms contribute to the development of GERD, as illustrated in **Figure 26.1**.

Lower Esophageal Sphincter

The LES is a 3 to 4 cm long smooth muscle located at the distal end of the esophagus. It serves as a high-pressure barrier between the esophagus and stomach and acts to prevent the retrograde passage of gastric contents into the esophagus. The LES relaxes on swallowing, allowing food to enter the stomach. Several mechanisms can disrupt this barrier, such as transient LES relaxation increases in intra-abdominal pressure (e.g., pregnancy, obesity, bending over), delayed gastric emptying, and hiatal hernia. Several foods and medications can also decrease LES tone, as listed in Table 26.1.

Transient LES relaxation is a normal physiological process that allows gas to escape the stomach and facilitate belching. When belching occurs, it is typically accomplished without content escaping from the stomach. In GERD, however, transient LES relaxation occurs more frequently and for more prolonged periods. Over half of the reflux episodes in patients with GERD are due to the relaxation of the LES.

Esophageal Clearance and Protection

The amount of time of exposure of gastric acid to the esophageal mucosa is an essential determinant of GERD risk. Salivation

Pathophysiology of GERD

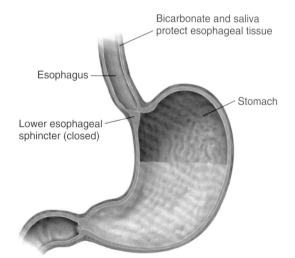

Bicarbonate and saliva protect esophageal tissue

Esophagus

Stomach

Lower esophageal sphincter (closed)

Normal functioning

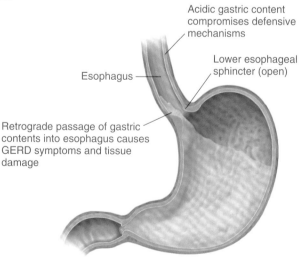

Acidic gastric content compromises defensive mechanisms

Lower esophageal sphincter (open)

Esophagus

Retrograde passage of gastric contents into esophagus causes GERD symptoms and tissue damage

GERD

FIGURE 26–1   Pathophysiology of gastroesophageal reflux disease.

GERD, gastroesophageal reflux disease.

and peristalsis assist the clearance of gastric acid and minimize the duration of contact between the gastric contents and the esophagus. Forty to fifty percent of patients with GERD have abnormal peristalsis. Swallowing saliva, which contains bicarbonate, helps to clear esophageal contents and neutralize acid present. However, some patients have reduced salivary production, especially the older adults or those with Sjögren's syndrome or xerostomia (dry mouth). Additionally, swallowing is hindered during sleep, leading to nocturnal GERD.

The esophageal mucosa contains mucus-secreting glands that act to protect the esophageal wall by secreting bicarbonate. However, repeated exposure to acid can compromise the defense system and result in cellular damage that leads to erosive esophagitis.

Gastric Emptying

Slow emptying of stomach contents can increase intragastric pressure, which consequently contributes to GERD. Factors that are associated with delayed emptying include smoking and high-fat meals. Medications that increase gastric emptying and motility can help.

Refluxate

The refluxate properties, acidity, and volume are important determinants of GERD risk. While the stomach can withstand very low pH levels and enzymatic activity of gastric secretions, the squamous cells lining the esophageal mucosa are more sensitive and readily damaged if exposed to this chemical environment. Gastric acid causes direct damage to the esophageal mucosa. Additionally, pepsin, a gastric enzyme responsible for the breakdown of food proteins, becomes activated in acidic environments, causing further injury to the esophageal lining.

Complications

Complications of GERD occur from repeated exposure to refluxed gastric contents for prolonged periods. These complications are outlined and defined in **Table 26.2**. Barrett's

esophagus is one such complication in which the stratified squamous cells that line the esophagus change and become simple columnar cells, like those that line the intestines. Esophageal adenocarcinoma appears to occur more commonly in older white males with elevated body mass index. Since Barrett's esophagus is a risk factor for esophageal adenocarcinoma, screening for Barrett's esophagus is recommended for this population.

DIAGNOSTIC CRITERIA

Diagnosis is mainly dependent on patient report of symptoms and review of risk factors that are present. Symptoms are commonly classified as typical, atypical, and extraesophageal and are listed in **Table 26.3**. They tend to occur after meals and may be aggravated by reclining or lying down. Since diagnostic testing can be invasive, a diagnosis of GERD can be assumed if patients present with typical symptoms (acid regurgitation and/or heartburn) and if they respond to an empiric trial of acid suppression therapy. Often, patients may present with chest pain, so an evaluation to rule out cardiac causes must be done. Diagnosis of patients who present with atypical symptoms is challenging, since their symptoms may be caused by other conditions, such as PUD and gastroparesis. For these patients, further diagnostic evaluation may be considered before empiric therapy.

Extraesophageal reflux can also be known as silent GERD. In this type of reflux, in addition to the esophagus, other body areas such as the hypopharynx, nasopharynx, oropharynx, larynx, or trachea are affected. Often patients have other associated issues such as chronic cough or laryngitis.

Diagnostic testing with endoscopy should be reserved for patients who do not respond to therapy, those presenting with an extraesophageal syndrome or chest pain to confirm GERD as a cause or to detect complications of GERD. Endoscopy with or without biopsy may be used to assess mucosal injury or other complications like strictures. A biopsy is necessary to detect esophageal adenocarcinoma or Barrett's esophagus. Of note, a normal finding on endoscopy does not rule out GERD.

TABLE 26.2
Complications of Gastroesophageal Reflux Disease

Complication	Definition
Esophagitis	Inflammation of the lining of the esophagus.
Erosive esophagitis	Erosion of the squamous epithelium of the esophagus.
Peptic stricture development	Narrowing or tightening of the esophagus.
Barrett's esophagus	Squamous epithelium of the esophagus is replaced by specialized columnar-type epithelium.
Esophageal adenocarcinoma	Cancer of the esophagus.

TABLE 26.3
Symptoms of Gastroesophageal Reflux Disease

Typical Symptoms	Atypical Symptoms	Extraesophageal Symptoms
Acid regurgitation Heartburn	Epigastric fullness Epigastric pressure Epigastric pain Dyspepsia Nausea Bloating Belching	Chronic cough/ throat clearing Asthma/ bronchospasm Wheezing Hoarseness Sore throat Chronic laryngitis Dental erosions

On the other hand, tissue damage may not be specifically related to GERD. Other tests, such as ambulatory pH monitoring, can help to clarify the diagnosis.

INITIATING DRUG THERAPY

Initial treatment always includes lifestyle modifications like weight loss, avoiding offending foods, elevating the head of the bed, and avoiding meals before bedtime and can alleviate GERD symptoms. However, in many cases, patients will need to supplement lifestyle changes with medication therapy to control their symptoms.

Drug classes used to treat GERD and its symptoms include (1) antacids, (2) histamine-2 receptor antagonists (H_2RA), and (3) proton pump inhibitors (PPI). Generally, a trial of an H_2RA or PPI is given for 2 weeks to confirm the diagnosis of GERD. The dose is increased as needed until symptoms resolve. If the patient responds to therapy, treatment is continued for 4 to 16 weeks. Afterward, the drug is tapered over 1 month to the minimal dose that provides symptom relief if maintenance therapy is warranted. Repeating the initial effective medication is recommended if symptoms reoccur. Diagnostic testing is recommended if the patient does not respond to treatment.

Goals of Drug Therapy

The goals of pharmacologic therapy are to

- relieve symptoms,
- decrease the frequency and duration of reflux,
- heal the esophageal mucosa, and
- prevent complications.

PEPTIC ULCER DISEASE

Peptic ulcer disease (PUD) is characterized by damage to the inner lining of the GI tract caused by exposure to the acidic contents of the stomach. A peptic ulcer often reoccurs, and like GERD, PUD can significantly impair quality of life.

EPIDEMIOLOGY

Causes

There exist three common forms of PUD: *Helicobacter pylori*–positive ulcers, nonsteroidal anti-inflammatory drug (NSAID)–induced ulcers, and stress ulcers. *H. pylori* and NSAID-induced ulcers are chronic conditions that often recur. Stress ulcers usually occur in critically ill patients or just following major trauma or severe illness. Management of stress ulcers is primarily focused on prevention with PPIs or H_2RAs when risk factors are present. Less commonly, peptic ulcers are

TABLE 26.4	
Risk Factors for Nonsteroidal Anti-Inflammatory Drug–Related Peptic Ulcer Disease (American College of Gastroenterology)	
Level of Risk	**Risk Factors**
Low	No risk factors present
Moderate	Presence of 1–2 of the following: • Age greater than 65 years • High-dose NSAID use • History of uncomplicated ulcer • Multiple NSAID use • Concurrent use of aspirin, corticosteroids, or anticoagulants
High	More than 2 of the previously mentioned risk factors History of complicated ulcer

NSAID, nonsteroidal anti-inflammatory drug.

also associated with Zollinger–Ellison syndrome, radiation, chemotherapy, vascular insufficiency, and other chronic diseases. These ulcers develop mostly in the stomach and duodenum, but may occasionally develop in the esophagus, jejunum, ileum, or colon.

The lifetime prevalence is approximately 11% to 14% in men and 8% to 11% in women. An estimated 30% to 40% of the U.S. population is infected with *H. pylori,* with higher rates among non-Hispanic whites (Nagy et al., 2016). Native Americans and Alaskan Natives have the highest incidence of complication from *H. pylori* PUD (Huerta-Franco et al., 2018). The overall prevalence has been decreasing, possibly due to improved therapies and sanitation. *H. pylori* infection typically occurs in the first few years of life and is contracted through the fecal–oral route. Though *H. pylori* infection is common, only 15% of these cases eventually progress to ulcer formation.

PUD occurs in 30% of patients chronically using NSAIDs and aspirin, and 1.5% of these patients experience GI bleeding or perforation. Risk factors for ulcers related to NSAID use are listed in **Table 26.4**.

PATHOPHYSIOLOGY

Normally, the gastric and duodenal environments can maintain a state of homeostasis where food digestion can occur without compromising gastric tissue integrity. Pepsin is the enzyme most involved with protein digestion. Additionally, HCl plays a role in creating the correct pH environment to convert pepsinogen to pepsin. Several defense mechanisms exist to prevent tissue injury from acid and digestive functions of the GI tract. *H. pylori* and NSAIDs can disrupt these processes, leading to the formation of ulcers.

Gastric Acid

HCl and pepsin are responsible for gastric mucosal damage found in PUD. Baseline acid production occurs during fasting states, whereas maximal acid production occurs following meals. Parietal cells in the stomach are stimulated to release acid by histamine, acetylcholine, and gastrin. All of these stimuli are released by the sensation of food, including the sight, smell, and taste. After stimulation, acid is released through the proton pumps located on the parietal cells. In *H. pylori* infection, acid secretion is elevated above normal, while NSAIDs do not affect acid secretion.

Pepsin

In an acidic environment, pepsinogen is converted to active pepsin in the stomach. Pepsin is an enzyme responsible for protein digestion. If pepsin is not deactivated by the protective effect of an adherent layer of bicarbonate-rich mucus lining, the ongoing effect leads to PUD.

Mucosal Protection

The gastric lining contains a mucus layer that works to protect the underlying cells of the gastric wall against gastric acid. Bicarbonate secretion acts as a buffering agent and allows the epithelial lining to maintain a neutral pH despite the acidic levels found in the gastric lumen. Prostaglandins also provide mucosal protection by decreasing gastric acid production and increasing mucus production. Both *H. pylori* and NSAID use can impede these defenses.

Helicobacter pylori

H. pylori is a gram-negative spiral-shaped rod bacterium with flagella that is found on the surface of gastric epithelium. Infection occurs when *H. pylori* penetrates the epithelial cells. The bacterium is able to survive in the acidic environment, mainly due to its ability to hydrolyze urea into carbon dioxide and ammonia through the production of urease. The bacteria cause ulcer formation by increasing acid production, increasing gastrin secretion, and releasing noxious enzymes and toxins. It is also a known carcinogen and, if left untreated, can lead to gastric mucosa–associated lymphoid tissue lymphoma.

Nonsteroidal Anti-Inflammatory Drugs

NSAIDs cause PUD through direct and indirect mechanisms. As weak acids, they are natural irritants against the mucosal wall. NSAIDs also have antiplatelet properties, further compounding the bleeding complications that can occur as a result of PUD.

Nonselective NSAIDs inhibit both cyclooxygenase 1 (COX-1) and cyclooxygenase 2 (COX-2) enzymes. Inhibition of COX-1 in the stomach reduces the production of protective prostaglandin, whereas COX-2 is more associated with the processes that lead to fever and pain. Therefore, selective COX-2 inhibitors are thought to carry less risk for PUD compared to nonselective NSAIDs.

Complications

Complications of PUD include GI bleed (melena or hematemesis), perforation, penetration, or gastric outlet obstruction. Patients who complain of a change in the pain can have a perforation (sharp pain) or an intestinal blockage. Patients who may have a gastric outlet obstruction may experience bloating, anorexia, nausea, vomiting, and weight loss.

DIAGNOSTIC CRITERIA

Though not all patients with PUD present with symptoms, the most common complaints include epigastric pain described as burning, fullness, discomfort, gnawing, cramping, or aching. The severity and frequency of the pain can fluctuate, and some patients report worsening at night. Often, heartburn, belching, and bloating accompany the pain. Symptom presentation is dependent on the location of the ulcer. *H. pylori*–associated ulcers are more commonly found in the duodenum, while stomach ulcers are more often associated with NSAIDs. Symptoms of duodenal ulcers typically occur about 1 to 3 hours following meals and are usually relieved by food intake. In gastric ulcers, nausea, vomiting, and anorexia are common symptoms, and food can precipitate pain generally 10 to 15 minutes after eating.

More severe signs, symptoms, and certain risk factors are described as alarming features. These include prior history or family history of upper GI malignancy, unintentional weight loss, GI bleeding, iron deficiency anemia, dysphagia or odynophagia, early satiety, persistent vomiting, palpable mass, or lymphadenopathy.

Since *H. pylori* produce urease, the enzyme is used as a diagnostic marker to detect *H. pylori*. Endoscopy with biopsy allows access to tissue for rapid urease tests and cultures to detect *H. pylori*. Endoscopy is considered the gold-standard test and is appropriate for the initial evaluation of patients older than 50 years of age who have new-onset dyspepsia or patients of any age who present with alarming features. It should also be considered in those who fail a trial of acid suppression therapy. However, the sensitivity of the rapid urease test may be diminished with the use of medications that reduce urease activity, such as antibiotics or PPIs. Obtaining a culture can provide further guidance, especially if antibiotic-resistant strains are suspected. However, this method is time-consuming and costly.

Less invasive tests are also available and include serologic testing, urea breath testing, and fecal antigen assays. These tests are more appropriate for patients younger than 50 who complain of dyspepsia but without alarming features. Serologic testing can be performed in the office with results returning in 15 minutes. However, it is less sensitive and specific compared to other tests. Moreover, it is not useful in confirming the eradication of the bacteria, since patients can remain seropositive for an extended time following treatment. Given its high specificity and short turnaround time, the urea breath test is the most common noninvasive diagnostic tool for PUD. Since medications can interfere with urease activity, bismuth-containing medications and antibiotics should be held for at least 28 days, and PPIs for 7 to 14 days before testing. Therefore, it is most reliable for confirming eradication 6 to 8 weeks after therapy. Fecal antigen testing is also useful in both diagnosing infection before treatment and to confirm eradication after treatment. Fecal testing is less sensitive to the effects of medications.

INITIATING DRUG THERAPY

Several pharmacologic agents are available for the treatment of PUD, and many overlap with the drugs used in the treatment of GERD. The choice in therapy depends on the etiology, presentation, and presence of complications.

For *H. pylori*–associated ulcers, prescription of the combination of antibiotics and acid suppression therapy is appropriate. Relapses are common and can be prevented only by eradicating *H. pylori*; therefore, the treatment of all patients with *H. pylori*–induced ulcers with antibiotics and PPI is indicated. The empiric use of antisecretory agents for suspected PUD should be used with caution since these can mask the symptoms of severe disease that warrant crucial diagnostic testing and long-term treatment. Thus, it is important to confirm *H. pylori* infection with serologic or urea breath testing before treatment.

Goals of Drug Therapy

The goals of pharmacologic therapy are to

- relieve symptoms,
- reduce acid secretion,
- promote epithelial healing,
- prevent recurrence, and
- prevent complications.

For NSAID-induced PUD, an additional goal is to either identify an alternative for pain management or provide prophylaxis strategies to prevent ulcers if continued treatment with NSAIDs is necessary. Strategies include taking enteric-coated NSAIDs, taking with meals, adding misoprostol, or switching to a selective COX-2 inhibitor.

DRUG CLASSES FOR THE TREATMENT OF GASTROESOPHAGEAL REFLUX DISEASE AND PEPTIC ULCER DISEASE

The drugs used to treat GERD and PUD often overlap. Drug classes and their properties are described in the following sections and in **Table 26.5**.

Antacids

There are numerous antacids available over-the-counter. Common examples include calcium carbonate (e.g., Tums), magnesium salts, and aluminum salts. They may be used for mild, intermittent symptoms (<2 times/week) or break-through therapy for patients taking other acid suppression therapies.

Mechanism of Action

Antacids partially neutralize the HCl in the stomach. By increasing the pH level, the activation of pepsin is also inhibited.

Dosage

Antacid dosage recommendations vary and can be administered on an as-needed basis.

Time Frame for Response

Antacids provide immediate symptom relief in mild GERD and thus are commonly used as self-treatment by patients. However, they have a short duration of action, warranting frequent administration in some patients. When used to treat chronic symptoms or PUD, the sole use of antacids should be avoided since they must be administered many times daily in large doses to achieve symptom relief. Additionally, antacids do not heal ulcers and instead may mask the symptoms of a serious disease and prolong the initiation of other necessary interventions.

Contraindications

There are no contraindications listed for antacids.

Adverse Events

As antacids are minimally absorbed and work locally in the GI tract, the most frequent side effects are chalky taste, cramps, constipation (aluminum-containing products), or diarrhea (magnesium-containing products). Less commonly, calcium carbonate may cause hypercalcemia. Since the kidneys eliminate aluminum and magnesium, antacids containing those elements should be used with caution. Magnesium-containing products can specifically result in hypermagnesium resulting in hypotension, nausea, vomiting, and electrocardiographic changes.

Drug Interactions

Antacids have clinically significant drug interactions by altering the rate and extent of absorption of concomitantly administered drugs, such as iron, sulfonylureas, and tetracycline and quinolone antibiotics. The recommendation is to take antacids 1 to 4 hours after other medications to avoid these interactions.

Histamine-2 Receptor Antagonists

H_2RAs are effective in mild GERD, ulcer healing, and *H. pylori* eradication when combined with other agents and may be used in the prevention of NSAID-related duodenal PUD. Like antacids, these products are available over-the-counter. Because all H_2RAs are equipotent, the choice in therapy depends on the adverse effect profile and drug interactions.

TABLE 26.5

Drugs Used in the Management of Gastroesophageal Reflux Disease and Peptic Ulcer Disease

Generic (Trade) Names	Selected Adverse Effects	Contraindications	Therapeutic Considerations
Antacids			
Calcium-, magnesium-, and aluminum-containing formulations	Rebound hyperacidity, diarrhea with magnesium-containing antacids, constipation with aluminum containing antacids, nausea, stomach pain	None significant	• Monitor for drug interactions • Use magnesium–aluminum combination to avoid diarrhea or constipation • Use caution in renal impairment
Histamine-2 Receptor Antagonists (H₂RAs)			
Cimetidine (Tagamet) Famotidine (Pepcid) Nizatidine (Axid) Ranitidine (Zantac)	Generally well tolerated, may experience headache, dizziness, confusion	Hypersensitivity to H_2RAs	• Take without regard to meals • Monitor for drug interactions • Consider dose reduction in older adults and renal impairment • Reduced efficacy and tolerance may occur with prolonged use
Proton Pump Inhibitors (PPIs)			
Dexlansoprazole (Dexilant) Esomeprazole (Nexium) Lansoprazole (Prevacid) Omeprazole (Prilosec) Omeprazole-sodium bicarbonate (Zegerid) Pantoprazole (Protonix) Rabeprazole (AcipHex)	Diarrhea, constipation, abdominal pain, headache	Hypersensitivity to PPIs	• Take 30–60 minutes before meals (except dexlansoprazole) • Do not crush, chew, or split delayed-release tablets
Antibiotics			
Amoxicillin (Amoxil) Clarithromycin (Biaxin) Metronidazole (Flagyl) Tetracycline	• Amoxicillin: diarrhea, nausea, vomiting • Clarithromycin: diarrhea, abnormal taste, nausea, vomiting • Metronidazole: headache, metallic taste, nausea, peripheral neuropathy • Tetracycline: GI upset, diarrhea, photosensitivity	• Amoxicillin: allergy to penicillin or other beta-lactams • Clarithromycin: allergy to macrolides, QT prolongation, use with astemizole, cisapride, pimozide, simvastatin, or lovastatin • Tetracycline: allergy to tetracycline	• Take without regard to meals, except tetracycline that should be taken on an empty stomach • Avoid clarithromycin in retreatment for those who fail the initial clarithromycin-containing regimen • Avoid alcohol with metronidazole • Avoid dairy, antacids, and iron products within 2 hours of tetracycline administration
Misoprostol			
Misoprostol (Cytotec)	Diarrhea, abdominal pain, cramping, nausea	Hypersensitivity to misoprostol, pregnancy	• Take with food • Reduce dose if diarrhea is intolerable • Avoid in pregnancy
Sucralfate			
Sucralfate (Carafate)	Constipation	Hypersensitivity to sucralfate	• Take on an empty stomach • Monitor for drug interactions
Bismuth Subsalicylate			
Bismuth subsalicylate (Pepto Bismol)	Black stools, darkened tongue, constipation, tinnitus	Hypersensitivity to salicylates	• Avoid in pregnancy and lactation

GI, gastrointestinal.

Mechanism of Action

H_2RAs reversibly inhibit the histamine-2 receptors on gastric parietal cells and thus decrease acid secretion and pepsin activation.

Dosage

Dosing recommendations vary by product and severity of symptoms (see **Table 26.6**). When H_2RAs are used in anti–*H.*
pylori regimens, they are used once or twice daily. Higher doses are required for the prevention of NSAID-related ulcers.

Time Frame for Response

Onset of action is about 1 to 2 hours after administration. Therefore, H_2RAs may be used as needed or on an intermittent basis for mild heartburn. However, if there is a lack of response within 2 weeks, standard twice-daily dosing is

---

TABLE 26.6

Dosing and Administration for Gastroesophageal Reflux Disease Medications

Pharmacologic Agents	Dose	Administration Comments
Mild symptomatic GERD		
Antacids Magnesium-, aluminum-, calcium-containing antacids	Varies depending on product Dosing ranges from hourly to as needed	Use as needed, after meals, or at bedtime to control nocturnal symptoms
Histamine-2 receptor antagonists (over-the-counter) Cimetidine (Tagamet HB) Famotidine (Pepcid AC) Nizatidine (Axid AR) Ranitidine (Zantac 75)	200 mg once daily or BID 10–20 mg once daily or BID 75 mg once daily or BID 75 mg once daily or BID	May be scheduled or used on an as-needed basis
Proton pump inhibitors (over-the-counter) Esomeprazole (Nexium 24H) Lansoprazole (Prevacid 24HR) Omeprazole (Prilosec OTC) Omeprazole/bicarbonate (Zegerid OTC)	20 mg once daily 15 mg once daily 20 mg once daily 20 mg/1,100 mg once daily	Take 30–60 minutes before breakfast or first meal
Persistent mild symptomatic GERD, moderate-to-severe symptomatic GERD		
Histamine-2 receptor antagonists (prescription strength) Cimetidine (Tagamet) Famotidine (Pepcid) Nizatidine (Axid) Ranitidine (Zantac)	400 mg BID 20 mg BID 150 mg BID 150 mg BID	Duration of therapy 6–12 weeks Consider maintenance therapy if symptoms recur
Proton pump inhibitors (prescription strength) Dexlansoprazole (Dexilant) Esomeprazole (Nexium) Lansoprazole (Prevacid) Omeprazole (Prilosec) Omeprazole/bicarbonate (Zegerid) Pantoprazole (Protonix) Rabeprazole (AcipHex)	30 mg once daily 20 mg once daily 15 mg once daily 20 mg once daily 20 mg once daily 20–40 mg once daily 20 mg once daily	Take 30–60 minutes before breakfast or first meal (except dexlansoprazole) Duration of therapy 4–8 weeks Consider maintenance therapy if symptoms recur
Persistent moderate-to-severe symptomatic GERD, healing of erosive GERD, or complications of GERD		
Histamine-2 receptor antagonists Cimetidine (Tagamet) Famotidine (Pepcid) Nizatidine (Axid) Ranitidine (Zantac)	400 mg QID or 800 mg BID 20–40 mg BID 150 mg QID 150 mg QID	Duration of therapy 8–12 weeks Maintenance therapy recommended
Proton pump inhibitors Dexlansoprazole (Dexilant) Esomeprazole (Nexium) Lansoprazole (Prevacid) Omeprazole (Prilosec) Omeprazole/bicarbonate (Zegerid) Pantoprazole (Protonix) Rabeprazole (AcipHex)	60 mg once daily 20–40 mg once daily 30 mg BID 20 mg BID 20 mg/1,100 mg BID 40 mg BID 20 mg BID	Take 30–60 minutes before breakfast or first meal (except dexlansoprazole) Duration of therapy 4–16 weeks Maintenance therapy recommended

GERD, gastroesophageal reflux disease.

reasonable. In standard dosing, symptomatic relief is achieved in 60% of patients, and endoscopic esophageal healing occurs in 50% of patients after 12 weeks. Importantly, prolonged use may lead to reduced efficacy or tachyphylaxis and tolerance to the medication; therefore, intermittent use is preferred.

Contraindications

These agents are contraindicated in hypersensitivity to H_2RAs.

Adverse Effects

H_2RAs are generally well tolerated. Patients may experience headache, drowsiness, fatigue, dizziness, and confusion. The risk of side effects increases in renal impairment, so dosages should be reduced in the older adults and those with an estimated glomerular filtration less than 50 mL/min. Gynecomastia and impotence rarely occurs with cimetidine use and is dose dependent.

Drug Interactions

Many drug interactions exist, and before the initiation of H_2RAs, a thorough review of other medications is essential. Drugs dependent on gastric acid environments for absorption may have decreased effects, such as ketoconazole and protease inhibitors. Cimetidine is a potent inhibitor of cytochrome P450 (CYP450) enzymes and may inhibit the metabolism of warfarin, phenytoin, and other strong substrates in the CYP450 system. Additionally, antacids may decrease the effect of H_2RAs and must be taken 1 to 2 hours after the H_2RA.

Proton Pump Inhibitors

As the most potent acid suppression agents available, PPIs are superior to H_2RAs in moderate-to-severe GERD, prevention of NSAID-induced PUD, and ulcer healing. They are given empirically in the management and diagnosis of GERD and PUD, which are used in anti–*H. pylori* regimens. Several are available in many dosage forms, including intravenous, powder, and orally disintegrating tablets. Currently, omeprazole, omeprazole-sodium bicarbonate, lansoprazole, and esomeprazole are available over-the-counter.

Mechanism of Action

PPIs inhibit gastric proton pumps located on the parietal cells, producing long-lasting suppression of acid secretion.

Dosage

When used empirically to treat GERD, once-daily dosing is recommended. If this is ineffective, the dose may increase to twice-daily dosing. Except for dexlansoprazole, these drugs are most effective when taken in the morning, 30 to 60 minutes before the first meal. Omeprazole-bicarbonate is most effective in controlling nocturnal acid secretion when taken in the evening. The dual delayed-release action of dexlansoprazole allows for its efficacy when taken at any time during the day regardless of food intake. For those with nocturnal symptoms or those taking twice-daily doses, PPIs may be taken in the evening before dinner; however, as-needed dosing is not effective or recommended with PPIs.

Time Frame for Response

A 66% reduction in acid secretion is seen by day 5 of PPI therapy. After 8 weeks of treatment, 83% of patients experience symptom relief, and endoscopic healing of esophageal tissue is seen in 78% of patients.

Contraindications

These agents are contraindicated in hypersensitivity to PPIs.

Adverse Effects

Side effects may include headache, diarrhea, constipation, and abdominal pain. Long-term side effects can occur from PPIs, including hypergastrinemia, fractures, infections (*Clostridium difficile* colitis and bacterial gastroenteritis), vitamin B_{12} deficiency, and hypomagnesemia. Conflicting data exist about the actual risk of chronic PPI use. For patients taking high-dose PPIs or greater than 1 year, the current Food and Drug Administration advisory warnings include the risk of osteoporosis and fractures, hypomagnesemia, and *C. difficile* infections. Generally, the recommendation is to continue PPI therapy in patients with osteoporosis. A careful risk versus benefit needs to be completed for individuals with a higher risk of hip fracture. Patients with low magnesium levels may consider stopping the PPI or adding magnesium supplementation if continuing PPI therapy is necessary. In the short term, PPIs may increase the risk of community-acquired pneumonia; however, this risk appears to disappear after long-term use.

Drug Interactions

Like H_2RAs, PPIs may decrease the efficacy of drugs that depend on an acidic gastric environment for adequate absorption. Additionally, PPIs can be implicated in drug interactions involving the CYP450 system. An example of this is omeprazole and lansoprazole and its possible interaction with clopidogrel. Clopidogrel depends on the CYP2C19 pathway for metabolism; however, these PPIs inhibit CYP2C19. There is a postulated effect that when these PPIs are given concomitantly with clopidogrel that this may result in cardiovascular harm. The clinical significance of this interaction is not well understood, and studies demonstrate mixed results (Demcsák et al., 2018). Decisions regarding concomitant use of these medications should consider both the benefits of acid suppression therapy and the potential risk of cardiovascular complications. Omeprazole likely carries the highest risk for interaction, while pantoprazole has the least risk.

Antibiotics

Antibiotics are used in combination with acid suppression medications to eradicate *H. pylori*–induced PUD. They are ineffective when used as monotherapy due to the high risk of resistance and should therefore be given with other antibiotics and acid suppression therapies. They do not have a role in GERD management.

Amoxicillin

Mechanism of Action

Amoxicillin is an aminopenicillin that kills bacteria by interfering with cell wall synthesis. It is most effective at neutral pH levels and therefore must be administered with an acid suppression agent such as a PPI or H_2RA.

Dosage

It is dosed at 1 g by mouth twice daily.

Time Frame for Response

A 10- to 14-day treatment duration is needed for maximal efficacy.

Contraindications

Amoxicillin must be avoided in those with an allergy to penicillins or other beta-lactams.

Adverse Effects

The most common side effects of amoxicillin are diarrhea, nausea, and vomiting, which may be relieved by taking the medication with food. Patients should be monitored for hypersensitivity reactions.

Drug Interactions

Amoxicillin is not commonly implicated in drug interactions, though it may increase the anticoagulant effects of warfarin therapy.

Clarithromycin

Mechanism of Action

Clarithromycin is a macrolide antibiotic that inhibits bacterial protein synthesis. While highly effective against *H. pylori*, it is susceptible to resistance, so it should be avoided in retreatment if a clarithromycin-containing regimen fails.

Dosage

Clarithromycin is dosed 500 mg by mouth twice daily.

Time Frame for Response

A 10- to 14-day treatment course is needed for maximal efficacy.

Contraindications

Clarithromycin is contraindicated in known allergy to macrolide antibiotics, history of QT prolongation, and concomitant use with astemizole, cisapride, pimozide, simvastatin, or lovastatin.

Adverse Effects

The most common side effects associated with clarithromycin are diarrhea, abnormal taste, nausea, and vomiting, which may be relieved by taking the medication with food.

Drug Interactions

Clarithromycin is a strong CYP3A4 substrate and therefore should be used with caution when used concomitantly with strong CYP3A4 substrates, inducers, and inhibitors.

Metronidazole

Mechanism of Action

Metronidazole kills anaerobic bacteria and protozoa by interfering with deoxyribonucleic acid (DNA) structure, causing inhibition of protein synthesis and subsequent cell death.

Dosage

Depending on the regimen, dosing ranges from 125 to 500 mg taken 2 to 4 times daily.

Time Frame for Response

A 10- to 14-day treatment course is needed for maximal efficacy.

Contraindications

Metronidazole is contraindicated in known allergy to metronidazole.

Adverse Effects

Metronidazole may cause headache, metallic taste, nausea, and peripheral neuropathy.

Drug Interactions

Alcohol consumption with metronidazole should be avoided to prevent disulfiram-like reactions. It may also increase the anticoagulant effect of warfarin.

Tetracycline

Mechanism of Action

Tetracycline inhibits bacterial protein synthesis and is effective against gram-positive and gram-negative bacteria.

Dosage

Tetracycline is dosed at 500 mg 2 to 4 times daily depending on the regimen. It must be given either 2 hours before or 2 hours after food intake to optimize absorption.

Time Frame for Response

A 10- to 14-day treatment course is needed for maximal efficacy.

Contraindications

It is contraindicated in known allergy to tetracycline.

Adverse Effects

Side effects of tetracycline include GI upset, diarrhea, and photosensitivity.

Drug Interactions

Tetracycline is a major substrate and moderate inhibitor of CYP3A4. Antacids, dairy products, and iron may decrease the absorption of tetracycline.

Misoprostol

Misoprostol is used as prophylaxis against NSAID-induced ulcers in patients at high risk for gastric ulcers and its complications.

Mechanism of Action

Misoprostol is a synthetic prostaglandin E_1 analog that inhibits acid secretion and increases mucosal defenses.

Dosage

It is dosed at 200 mcg 4 times daily taken with food.

Time Frame for Response

Time to peak effect is between 6 and 22 minutes.

Contraindications

Misoprostol is contraindicated in hypersensitivity to prostaglandins and pregnancy.

Adverse Effects

GI effects are common and include diarrhea, abdominal pain, flatulence, and nausea. A dose reduction to 100 mcg is warranted if diarrhea persists or is intolerable.

Drug Interactions

Antacids may increase the risk of adverse effects of misoprostol, especially those containing magnesium.

Sucralfate

Sucralfate is approved for the treatment and maintenance of duodenal ulcers and stress ulcer prophylaxis. It is not effective in *H. pylori* eradication.

Mechanism of Action

Sucralfate forms a viscous, adhesive substance that attaches to and protects ulcers against noxious gastric content.

Dosage

Sucralfate is given 1 g by mouth 4 times daily.

Time Frame for Response

Paste formation and symptom improvement occur 1 to 2 hours after administration. Its short half-life necessitates frequent administration.

Contraindications

Sucralfate should not be used in known hypersensitivity to the drug.

Adverse Effects

The most common side effect is constipation. Systemic effects are not common since sucralfate is minimally absorbed from the GI tract. Because it contains aluminum, there is a possibility for aluminum toxicity, particularly in patients with impaired renal function.

Drug Interactions

Because sucralfate coats the GI mucosa, it may decrease the absorption and effect of many medications. Separating sucralfate by 2 hours before or 6 hours after administering other drugs is prudent to avoid interactions.

Bismuth Subsalicylate

Bismuth subsalicylate is highly effective against *H. pylori* when used in combination with antibiotics. It is available both in a chewable tablet and liquid form.

Mechanism of Action

Bismuth subsalicylate has acid secretion suppressing effects. The bismuth component exhibits antimicrobial effects, preventing *H. pylori* adhesion to epithelial cells. The salicylate component may provide anti-inflammatory action as well.

Dosage

Bismuth subsalicylate is administered 525 mg by mouth 4 times daily.

Time Frame for Response

In *H. pylori* eradication regimens, it must be taken for 10 to 14 days to achieve maximal effects.

Contraindications

Bismuth subsalicylate should be avoided with patients sensitive to salicylates.

Adverse Effects

Common side effects include black stools, darkened tongue, and constipation. At higher doses, tinnitus may occur.

Drug Interactions

Due to the salicylate component, which acts similar to aspirin, bismuth subsalicylate may increase bleeding risk when used with anticoagulants or antiplatelets.

SELECTING THE MOST APPROPRIATE AGENT FOR GASTROESOPHAGEAL REFLUX DISEASE

Initial treatment choice depends on the symptom severity, symptom frequency, and the presence of complications.

First-Line Therapy

For patients with mild, typical symptoms, fewer than 3 times a week, lifestyle change should be initiated. Over-the-counter acid suppression therapies with antacids, H_2RAs, or PPIs can be added if lifestyle changes alone do not resolve symptoms. If symptoms are unrelieved after 2 weeks of lifestyle changes alongside acid suppression therapies, the patient should seek medical attention. The goal would be to advance pharmacologic therapy to an empiric acid suppression therapy or diagnostic testing as necessary.

For patients with moderate-to-severe symptomatic GERD or persistent mild GERD symptoms that are troublesome, empiric prescription dosing of acid suppression therapy is first line. There are two general approaches to treatment: step-up versus step-down. The step-up approach begins with lifestyle modifications and the gradual increase of pharmacologic intervention with an H$_2$RA, progressing to PPI therapy or surgery until symptom improvement. The step-down approach begins with PPI therapy, then stepping down to the lowest dose of either a PPI or H$_2$RA that is needed to control symptoms. PPIs are favored in moderate-to-severe GERD since they provide the most rapid relief of symptoms and the most optimal chance of tissue healing. The dosing of these agents is presented in **Table 26.6**. Combination therapy with H$_2$RAs plus PPIs is not more effective and not generally recommended.

Patients with evidence of erosive esophagitis will require high-dose acid suppression therapy for longer durations. Again, PPIs are preferred over H$_2$RAs due to its superiority in tissue healing.

After treatment is complete, patients with moderate-to-severe symptoms or erosive esophagitis are especially susceptible to rebound effects, and often maintenance therapy is necessary for these patients. Additionally, patients who continue to have persistent symptoms after treatment discontinuation should be considered for maintenance therapy. The treatment dose should be titrated down to the lowest most effective strength. The long-standing use of PPIs is limited by the potential for long-term adverse effects, as discussed earlier.

Second-Line Therapy

For patients with incomplete response to acid suppression therapy, adding an H$_2$RA at bedtime may help control overnight symptoms. H$_2$RAs are generally considered second line after PPI therapy for erosive esophagitis and other complications of GERD due to weaker and slower tissue healing. For symptomatic GERD, if maximal doses have been reached with PPI therapy with partial or no response, once-daily PPI dosing may be increased to twice-daily dosing. Switching the PPI to another in the same class may be considered, but limited data support this practice.

Patients who do not respond to twice-daily PPI therapy, who present with atypical symptoms, or who present with alarming symptoms like dysphagia may need endoscopic testing to detect tissue injury and GERD complications.

Third-Line Therapy

Surgery is available as an alternative for refractory symptoms, complications, or those who cannot tolerate long-term acid suppression therapy. Gastric bypass surgery has been shown to improve GERD symptoms in patients with obesity. Fundoplication is the most common anti-reflux procedure that attempts to reposition the LES to optimize intra-abdominal pressure. Ninety percent of patients report a resolution of symptoms following surgery. Rickenbacher et al. (2014), in a meta-analysis, compared the efficacy of anti-reflux surgery versus medical management that showed more favorable effects with surgery in improving quality of life and patient satisfaction. Though fewer patients required maintenance medical management compared to those without surgery, a high proportion of patients still needed maintenance acid suppression

following surgery. Possible adverse effects of the procedure include dysphagia, inability to belch or vomit, flatulence, bloating, and increased abdominal girth. Data on the long-term safety and efficacy of anti-reflux surgery are lacking.

Promotility drugs like metoclopramide have been studied for their use in treating GERD symptoms. Theoretically, they aim to target symptoms that arise due to slow gastric emptying (i.e., gastroparesis). However, results of studies to date have not shown an added benefit to these agents when weighed against their many side effects. Similarly, baclofen, a muscle relaxer, has the potential to improve GERD symptoms (Clarke et al., 2018); but owing to the lack of long-term data and numerous adverse effects, it is not currently recommended. Sucralfate has also been shown to have limited benefit in GERD management.

Special Population Considerations
Pediatric

In infants, regurgitation is known as "spitting up," which occurs daily in 50% of infants younger than 3 months. The cause is likely due to immaturity of the LES, which typically resolves by 12 to 14 months of age. These episodes usually do not cause discomfort or significant clinical consequences for the infant; however, children with chronic gastroesophageal reflux may exhibit poor growth, vomiting, hoarseness, coughing, and chronic sore throat. Management strategies include smaller, more frequent meals and thickening the formula or breast milk with 1 to 2 tablespoons of rice cereal per 2 ounces of liquid. Keeping the infant upright for 30 minutes after feeding and raising the head of the crib may also help. If non-pharmacologic therapies fail, therapy with H$_2$RAs and PPIs may be indicated if the cause of symptoms is confirmed or likely to be GERD. Ranitidine is commonly used, but chronic use may lead to diminished efficacy over time. Overuse of ranitidine has been associated with infections and other adverse effects. PPIs have also been shown to be safe and effective in patients aged 1 to 17, although long-term safety is mostly unknown.

Geriatric

Older patients are at higher risk for GERD due to their decreased ability to produce saliva and decreased gastric motility. Additionally, they are more likely to have comorbidities and medications that can further complicate the presentation of symptoms and treatment availability. Often, older patients do not seek medical care because they feel their symptoms are related to normal aging processes or their symptoms present atypically (dental erosions, chest pain, etc.). Even when they do seek pharmacologic management, drug interactions and adverse effects limit their choice in therapy. Due to declining renal function, exercise caution when recommending aluminum-containing antacids. Older patients are more vulnerable to the central nervous system side effects of H$_2$RAs. PPIs are often prescribed in this patient population due to their efficacy, relative tolerability, and once-daily dosing. However, the long-term impact on bone fractures must be considered when using PPI therapy for a prolonged duration.

Women

Heartburn commonly occurs during pregnancy due to increased intra-abdominal pressure. Over-the-counter antacids may be safely used in moderation. Sodium bicarbonate–containing medications must be avoided due to the risk of metabolic alkalosis and fluid overload.

MONITORING PATIENT RESPONSE

Patients should be evaluated for treatment response within the first few weeks of starting therapy. If symptoms decrease, a full course of treatment should continue. If symptoms do not completely resolve after 6 weeks with an H_2RA or after 4 weeks with a PPI, therapy continues for an additional 6 and 4 weeks, respectively. For erosive GERD, if symptoms do not improve by 8 weeks with an H_2RA or by 4 weeks with a PPI, therapy can extend to 12 weeks with an H_2RA and 16 weeks with a PPI. Patients should be monitored periodically for adverse effects accordingly. For patients who have persistent symptoms, consider endoscopy testing or referral to a gastroenterologist.

After remission is achieved, consider discontinuation of therapy. Most patients, however, will experience recurring symptoms and require retreatment. If recurrence is frequent, initiate maintenance therapy at the lowest effective dose after remission is achieved.

PATIENT EDUCATION

Drug Information

Patients should be educated on possible side effects and instructed to notify their health care providers if they become intolerable. Given the many potential drug–drug interactions, medication profiles must be reviewed, and proper timing of administration of medications should be relayed to the patient.

Nutritional and Lifestyle Changes

Lifestyle changes should be incorporated into any GERD treatment plan. Encouraging weight loss, the elevation of the head of the bed when sleeping, consuming smaller meals, avoiding causative foods, avoiding tight-fitting clothes, smoking cessation, moderation of alcohol, and avoiding recumbency for 3 hours after meals can be helpful. Instead of making all of these changes simultaneously, gradual approaches to lifestyle changes tend to be less overwhelming and more manageable for patients.

Complementary and Alternative Medicine

Peppermint is commonly used for the self-treatment of a variety of GI problems and for its effect on accelerating gastric emptying. However, it is known to decrease esophageal sphincter pressure, so patients should be counseled that it could worsen heartburn. Patients with PUD should avoid peppermint as it may potentiate ulcer formation. Acupuncture was shown to be effective in controlling regurgitation and heartburn in patients with persistent heartburn despite PPI therapy in one study. Electroacupuncture led to a decreased rate of transient LES relaxation in 14 healthy volunteers (Li et al., 2015). Studies with larger sample sizes and longer durations are needed to confirm the benefit of this treatment modality for GERD.

SELECTING THE MOST APPROPRIATE AGENT FOR PEPTIC ULCER DISEASE

Choice in treatment depends on the etiology (*H. pylori* or NSAID induced), resistance patterns, and presence of complications. Because resistance patterns differ geographically, regimens that have been studied and validated in the United States are preferred.

First-Line Therapy

Recommended regimens are listed in **Table 26.7**. Commonly, a PPI-based regimen with two antibiotics is used. Amoxicillin is preferred since it is highly effective against *H. pylori* and resistance rates remain low. However, for patients with a penicillin allergy, metronidazole is a viable substitute for amoxicillin. Eradication rates with first-line regimens are between 70% and 85%, but rates have recently declined due to a rise in clarithromycin resistance. Therefore, clarithromycin-based regimens are not recommended in a place where clarithromycin resistance is greater than 15%. Longer, 14-day durations lead to higher eradication and lower resistance rates.

Another therapy sequence uses a PPI and amoxicillin for 5 days, followed with triple therapy for another 5 days. Evidence exists that this regime is just as effective as standard triple therapy in eradicating *H. pylori*. Though less costly than standard triple therapy, this regimen has not yet been validated in the United States.

In NSAID-induced ulcers, patients should be tested for *H. pylori* and treated with the previously mentioned regimens if positive for infection. The NSAID should be discontinued, and a PPI, H_2RA, or sucralfate should be initiated (doses in **Table 26.8**). The NSAID could also be changed to a lower-dose acetaminophen or a COX-2 inhibitor like celecoxib. If the NSAID must be continued, a PPI or misoprostol should be taken concomitantly with the NSAID to promote healing and for prophylaxis of future ulcers. In cases where patients cannot discontinue the NSAID, H_2RAs are significantly less effective at healing ulcers. PPIs also appear to be more effective than misoprostol when NSAID therapy continues.

Successful eradication alone helps to prevent recurrence of *H. pylori*–induced ulcers; however, in patients who failed eradication therapy, have a history of ulcer-related complications, or have repeated recurrence of ulcers, maintenance therapy with a PPI or H_2RA should be considered.

Second-Line Therapy

For those who fail initial eradication therapy, a PPI-based regimen should be initiated using different antibiotics. Bismuth-based

TABLE 26.7

Treatment for *H. pylori* Eradication

Type	Regimen	Duration	Comments
Triple therapy	1. PPI once daily or BID 2. Amoxicillin 1 g BID 3. Clarithromycin 500 mg BID	7–10 days (up to 14 days)	First line
	Or 1. PPI once daily or BID 2. Metronidazole 500 mg BID 3. Clarithromycin 500 mg BID	10–14 days	Metronidazole can substitute for amoxicillin in penicillin allergy
Sequential therapy	1. PPI once daily or BID for 5 days 2. Amoxicillin 1 g BID for 5 days	10 days (5 days for each regimen)	First line, but has not been validated in the United States
	Followed by 1. PPI once daily or BID for 5 days 2. Clarithromycin 500 mg BID for 5 days 3. Metronidazole 500 mg BID for 5 days		
Quadruple therapy	1. PPI once daily or BID 2. Amoxicillin 1 g BID 3. Clarithromycin 500 mg BID 4. Metronidazole 500 mg BID	10 days	Second line
Bismuth-based quadruple therapy	1. PPI BID 2. Bismuth subsalicylate 525 mg QID 3. Metronidazole 250 mg QID 4. Tetracycline 500 mg QID	10–14 days	Second line or as salvage therapy for persistent infection, or penicillin allergy
Levofloxacin-based triple therapy	1. PPI once daily or BID 2. Amoxicillin 1 g BID 3. Levofloxacin 500 mg daily	10 days	Salvage therapy for persistent infection Has not been validated in the United States

PPI, proton pump inhibitor.

quadruple therapy with bismuth, a PPI, tetracycline, and metronidazole for 10 to 14 days is effective as salvage therapy for treatment failures. It is also preferred if the cost is a significant barrier to treatment or in patients who are allergic to penicillin. Emerging data on levofloxacin-based triple therapy supports its efficacy and tolerability; but since this regimen has not been validated in the United States and resistance rates are increasing, it should be reserved for salvage therapy only.

In areas with high rates of clarithromycin resistance, quadruple therapy with a PPI, amoxicillin, clarithromycin, and metronidazole has high eradication rates despite the regimen containing clarithromycin.

H_2RA-based *H. pylori* eradication regimens are less preferred due to lower eradication rates.

Probiotics have a possible role in *H. pylori* infection when taken alongside eradication regimens. Preliminary data show increased eradication rates and decreased adverse effects, particularly in the case of diarrhea.

Third-Line Therapy

In the case of repeated *H. pylori* eradication treatment failures or persistence of symptoms after 8 to 12 weeks of treatment,

referral to a gastroenterologist for endoscopy and biopsy is warranted to establish the diagnosis and exclude other causes.

Preventative Therapy in Nonsteroidal Anti-Inflammatory Drug–Induced Peptic Ulcer Disease

The risks of GI complications and cardiovascular safety must both be weighed when deciding the appropriate approach to the prevention of PUD, especially when NSAID therapy must be continued. Consequently, the American College of Gastroenterology provides guidance on the choice of therapy when GI and cardiovascular risks are considered (**Table 26.9**). PPIs and misoprostol have both shown efficacy in preventing NSAID-induced ulcers, most of which are gastric ulcers. While PPIs are more commonly used due to its more tolerable side-effect profile compared to misoprostol, large randomized controlled trials of PPI co-therapy are lacking. The trials available to date show promising results in preventing ulcers when taken with NSAIDs and even with COX-2 inhibitors. H_2RAs are not optimal since they are effective in preventing duodenal ulcers, not gastric ulcers. However, if H_2RAs must be used due to cost, high-dose regimens show greater efficacy compared to low doses. Of all NSAIDs, naproxen

TABLE 26.8

Dosing Regimens for Peptic Ulcer Disease Management

Generic (Trade) Name	H. pylori Dose	NSAID-Induced Ulcer Prevention Dose	NSAID-Induced Ulcer Treatment Dose	Usual Range	Dose Adjustments
Proton Pump Inhibitor					
Dexlansoprazole (Dexilant)	30–60 mg daily	30–60 mg daily	30–60 mg daily	30–60 mg/day	Dose adjustment for hepatic impairment
Esomeprazole (Nexium)	40 mg daily or BID	20–40 mg daily	40 mg daily	20–40 mg/day	
Omeprazole (Prilosec) Omeprazole/bicarbonate (Zegerid)	20–40 mg daily or BID	20 mg daily	20–40 mg daily	20–40 mg/day	
Pantoprazole (Protonix)	40 mg daily or BID	20 mg daily	40 mg daily	20–40 mg/day	
Rabeprazole (AcipHex)	20 mg daily or BID	20 mg daily	20 mg daily	20 mg/day	
Histamine-2 Receptor Antagonists					
Cimetidine (Tagamet)	400 mg BID	400 mg daily	300 mg QID or 400 mg BID or 800 mg QHS	800–1,600 mg/day in divided doses	Dose adjustment for renal and hepatic impairment
Famotidine (Pepcid)	40 mg daily	20 mg daily	40 mg daily	20–40 mg/day	Dose adjustment for renal impairment
Nizatidine (Axid)	150 mg BID	150 mg daily	150 mg BID or 300 mg daily	150–300 mg/day	
Ranitidine (Zantac)	150 mg BID	150 mg daily	150 mg BID or 300 mg daily	150–300 mg/day	
Mucosal Protectants					
Sucralfate (Carafate)	N/a	N/a	1 g QID	2–4 g/day	None
Misoprostol (Cytotec)	N/a	200 mcg QID	200 mcg QID	400–800 mcg/day	None

NSAID, nonsteroidal anti-inflammatory drug.

TABLE 26.9

Recommendations for Prevention of Nonsteroidal Anti-Inflammatory Drug–Related Ulcers

Cardiovascular Risk	Gastrointestinal Risk	Recommendation
Low	Low (no risk factors)	NSAID alone
	Moderate (1–2 risk factors)	NSAID plus PPI or misoprostol
	High (>2 risk factors, history of complicated ulcer)	Alternative therapy, or COX-2 inhibitor plus PPI or misoprostol
High	Low (no risk factors)	Naproxen plus PPI or misoprostol
	Moderate (1–2 risk factors)	Naproxen plus PPI or misoprostol
	High (>2 risk factors, history of complicated ulcer)	Avoid NSAID and COX-2 inhibitor, seek alternative therapy

COX-2, cyclooxygenase 2; NSAID, nonsteroidal anti-inflammatory drug; PPI, proton pump inhibitor.

has the least cardiovascular risk associated and is preferred in patients with high risk for cardiovascular events.

Celecoxib is the only COX-2 inhibitor available in the United States and originally was thought to have less GI effects compared to nonselective NSAIDs. However, available evidence shows that it may have the same GI adverse effects compared to other NSAIDs, especially in patients taking concomitant aspirin. Additionally, there is a dose-dependent increase in cardiovascular events, particularly with higher doses and longer durations of treatment.

Special Population Considerations

Pediatric

H. pylori is most often contracted during childhood and has a higher prevalence in areas of lower socioeconomic status and more unsatisfactory sanitation conditions. In children with diagnosed *H. pylori*–associated PUD, pharmacologic eradication is recommended due to high relapse rates if left untreated. If *H. pylori* infection is confirmed in the absence of PUD or if an *H. pylori*–positive child has a first-degree relative with gastric cancer, consider treatment in these children. Triple therapy (PPI plus two antibiotics), sequential treatment, and bismuth-based therapy for 10 to 14 days are viable treatment options in children. Ideally, obtaining susceptibility data will guide therapy. Avoid tetracycline in children younger than 8 years of age due to risk for reduced bone growth and permanent tooth discoloration.

Geriatric

Several factors put the older population at higher risk for PUD and its complications. Because older patients may not present with typical symptoms of *H. pylori* infection, diagnosis and treatment may be delayed. Comorbidities and concomitant medications, especially with NSAIDs, aspirin, bisphosphonates, and anticoagulants, further increase the risk of PUD. Additionally, mucosal defense mechanisms decline with age. Older patients have a higher potential for GI malignancies, and so endoscopy is the preferred method of diagnosis over noninvasive testing. *H. pylori* eradication regimens are similar for the adult population; however, older patients experience more treatment failures due to antibiotic resistance and problems with adherence. They are also more vulnerable to the adverse effects and drug interactions associated with treatment regimens. An individualized treatment plan is critical for each patient including counseling on the importance of adherence to the entire treatment regimen.

Women

Women who are pregnant or planning to become pregnant should avoid misoprostol due to its abortifacient properties. Consider obtaining a negative pregnancy test in women of childbearing age before initiating misoprostol.

MONITORING PATIENT RESPONSE

During treatment, patients should be assessed for the resolution of symptoms, adverse effects, and adherence. Patients can expect resolution of symptoms within 7 days of anti-ulcer therapy and within a few days of discontinuing NSAIDs. If symptoms continue or recur after 14 days of treatment, this signifies treatment failure, and a retreatment plan is necessary. In the case of treatment failures, patients should be assessed for adherence and proper administration of complex regimens.

Most patients with uncomplicated *H. pylori* infection will not need confirmation of eradication. However, consider confirming eradication with a urea breath test 6 to 8 weeks after the end of treatment in patients at risk for complications or who have a frequent recurrence of the disease.

If patients continue NSAID therapy, monitor them closely for complications such as bleeding, obstruction, penetration, or perforation.

PATIENT EDUCATION

Drug Information

Nonadherence to treatment and prevention regimens is a significant cause of treatment failures. These regimens can be complex, can be costly, and can come with intolerable side effects. Additionally, since patients often feel better within several days of treatment initiation, they may feel compelled to discontinue their medications mid-treatment. Counseling patients on the importance of full adherence to recommended therapies is essential in ensuring proper administration and maximal benefit of these therapies. Patients should also be informed of possible side effects to expect and how to manage them appropriately should they occur.

Nutritional and Lifestyle Changes

Encourage patients to avoid causative behaviors such as cigarette smoking and NSAID use if possible. While no foods are known to increase the risk of PUD, some foods may exacerbate the symptoms and discomfort associated with PUD. Advise patients to avoid spicy foods, caffeine, and alcohol to aid in symptom relief. Stress reduction is also encouraged, as psychological stress is sometimes associated with the worsening of symptoms.

Complementary and Alternative Medicine

Few studies exist examining the effect of licorice and its ability to enhance gastric mucosal protective mechanisms. In a recent study, licorice appeared to be just as effective as bismuth when taken with amoxicillin, metronidazole, and omeprazole in the eradication of *H. pylori* (Hajiaghamohammadi et al., 2016). Given the small sample size and lack of data in the United States, more robust studies are needed to confirm its utility in the treatment and prevention of PUD. Adverse effects of licorice include hypertension and hypokalemia.

CASE STUDY 1

Gene is a 42-year-old White man presenting with a 2-month history of intermittent mid-epigastric pain. The pain sometimes wakes him up at night and seems to get better after he eats a meal. He informs you that his doctor told him that he had an infection in his stomach 6 months ago. He never followed up and has been taking over-the-counter *PEPCID* for 2 weeks without relief. He takes no other medications. He is concerned because the pain is continuing. He has no other significant history except he is a 20-pack-year smoker and he drinks 5 cups of coffee a day. He eats late at night and goes to bed about 30 minutes after dinner. He is allergic to penicillin (Learning Objective 3).

1. What drug therapy would you prescribe for Gene? Why?
2. List one or two adverse reactions for the selected agent that would cause you to change therapy.
3. Describe one or two drug–drug or drug–food interaction for the selected agent.

Bibliography

Starred references are cited in the text.

Badillo, R., & Francis, D. (2014). Diagnosis and treatment of gastroesophageal reflux disease. *World Journal of Gastrointestinal Pharmacology and Therapeutics, 5*(3), 105–112.

Bhatt, D. L., Cryer, B. L., Contant, C. F., et al. (2010). Clopidogrel with or without omeprazole in coronary artery disease. *New England Journal of Medicine, 363*(20), 1909–1917.

Bor, S., Kitapcioglu, G., & Kasap, E. (2017). Prevalence of gastroesophageal reflux disease in a country with a high occurrence of *Helicobacter pylori. World Journal of Gastroenterology, 23*(3), 525–532. https://doi.org/10.3748/wjg.v23.i3.525

Bundhun, P. K., Teeluck, A. R., Bhurtu, A., et al. (2017). Is the concomitant use of clopidogrel and proton pump inhibitors still associated with increased adverse cardiovascular outcomes following coronary angioplasty?: A systematic review and meta-analysis of recently published studies (2012–2016). *BMC Cardiovascular Disorders, 17*(1), 3.

Chey, W. D., Leotiadis, G. I., Howden, C. W., & Moss, S. F. (2017). ACG clinical guideline: Treatment of *Helicobacter pylori* infection. *American Journal of Gastroenterology, 112*(2), 212–239.

*Clarke, J. O., Fernandez-Becker, N. Q., Regalia, K. A., & Triadafilopoulos, G. (2018). Baclofen and gastroesophageal reflux disease: Seeing the forest through the trees. *Clinical and Translational Gastroenterology, 9*(3), 137. https://doi.org/10.1038/s41424-018-0010-y

*Demcsák, A., Lantos, T., Bálint, E. R., et al. (2018). PPIs are not responsible for elevating cardiovascular risk in patients on clopidogrel: A systematic review and meta-analysis. *Frontiers in Physiology, 9*, 1–14. https://doi.org/10.3389/fphys.2018.01550

DeMeester, T. R. (2017). Surgical options for the treatment of gastroesophageal reflux disease. *Gastroenterology & Hepatology, 13*(2), 128–129.

El-Serag, H. B., Sweet, S., Winchester, C. C., et al. (2014). Update on the epidemiology of gastroesophageal reflux disease: A systematic review. *Gut, 63*(6), 871–880.

Fashner, J., & Gitu, A. C. (2015). Diagnosis and treatment of peptic ulcer disease and *H. pylori* infection. *American Family Physician, 91*(4), 236–242.

FDA Drug Safety Communication: Possible increased risk of fractures of the hip, wrist, and spine with the use of proton pump inhibitors. Rockville, MD: U.S. Food and Drug Administration. https://www.fda.gov/drugs/postmarket-drug-safety-information-patients-and-providers/fda-drug-safety-communication-possible-increased-risk-fractures-hip-wrist-and-spine-use-proton-pump

FDA Drug Safety Communication: Low magnesium levels can be associated with long-term use of Proton Pump Inhibitor drugs (PPIs). Rockville, MD: U.S. Food and Drug Administration. https://www.fda.gov/drugs/drug-safety-and-availability/fda-drug-safety-communication-low-magnesium-levels-can-be-associated-long-term-use-proton-pump

FDA Drug Safety Communication: Clostridium difficile associated diarrhea can be associated with stomach acid drugs known as proton pump inhibitors (PPIs). Rockville, MD: U.S. Food and Drug Administration. https://www.fda.gov/drugs/drug-safety-and-availability/fda-drug-safety-communication-clostridium-difficile-associated-diarrhea-can-be-associated-stomach

Fox, R. K., & Muniraj, T. (2016). Pharmacologic therapies in gastrointestinal diseases. *Medical Clinics of North America, 100*(4), 827–850.

Gwee, K. A., Goh, V., Lima, G., et al. (2018). Coprescribing proton-pump inhibitors with nonsteroidal anti-inflammatory drugs: Risks versus benefits. *Journal of Pain Research, 11*, 361–374.

Gyawali, C. P., & Fass, R. (2018). Management of gastroesophageal reflux disease. *Gastroenterology, 154*(2), 302–318.

*Hajiaghamohammadi, A. A., Zargar, A., Oveisi, S., et al. (2016). To evaluate of the effect of adding licorice to the standard treatment regimen of *Helicobacter pylori. The Brazilian Journal of Infectious Diseases, 20*(6), 534–538. https://doi.org/10.1016/j.bjid.2016.07.015

He, Y., Chan, E. W., Man, K. K., et al. (2014). Dosage effects of histamine-2 receptor antagonist on the primary prophylaxis of nonsteroidal anti-inflammatory drug (NSAID)-associated peptic ulcers: A retrospective cohort study. *Drug Safety, 37*(9), 711–721.

Heda, R., Toro, F., & Tombazzi, C. R. (2020). Physiology, pepsin. [Updated May 24, 2020]. In: *StatPearls* [Internet]. Treasure Island, FL: StatPearls Publishing.

Hom, C., & Vaezi, M. F. (2013). Extra-esophageal manifestations of gastroesophageal reflux disease: Diagnosis and treatment. *Drugs, 73*, 1281–1295.

Hooi, J. K. Y., Lai, W. Y., Ng, W. K., et al. (2017). Global prevalence of *Helicobacter pylori* infection: Systematic review and meta-analysis. *Gastroenterology, 153*(2), 420–429.

*Huerta-Franco, M. R., Banderas, J. W., & Allsworth, J. E. (2018). Ethnic/racial differences in gastrointestinal symptoms and diagnosis associated with the risk of *Helicobacter pylori* infection in the U.S. *Clinical and Experimental Gastroenterology, 11*, 39–49. https://doi.org/10.2147/CEG.S144967

Kalach, N., Bontems, P., & Cadranel, S. (2015). Advances in the treatment of *Helicobacter pylori* infection in children. *Annals of Gastroenterology, 28*(1), 10–18.

Kim, D., & Velanovich, V. (2014). Surgical treatment of GERD: where have we been and where are we going? *Gastroenterology Clinics of North America, 43*(1), 135–145.

Lanas, A., & Chan, F. K. L. (2017). Peptic ulcer disease. *Lancet, 390*(10094), 613–624.

*Li, H., He, T., Xu, Q., et al. (2015). Acupuncture and regulation of gastrointestinal function. *World Journal of Gastroenterology, 21*(27), 8304–8313.

Malik, T. F., Gnanapandithan, K., & Singh, K. (2020). Peptic ulcer disease. [Updated June 18, 2020]. In: *StatPearls* [Internet]. Treasure Island, FL: StatPearls Publishing.

*Nagy, P., Johansson, S., & Molloy-Bland, M. (2016). Systematic review of time trends in the prevalence of *Helicobacter pylori* infection in China and the USA. *Gut Pathogens, 8*, 8. https://doi.org/10.1186/s13099-016-0091-7

Ness-Jensen, E., Hveem, K., El-Seag, H., et al. (2016). Lifestyle intervention in gastroesophageal reflux disease. *Clinical Gastroenterology and Hepatology, 14*(2), 175–182.

*Nirwin, J. S., Babar, Z., Conway, B. R., & Ghori, M. U. (2020). Global prevalence and risk factors of gastro-oesophageal reflux disease (GoRD): Systematic review with meta-analysis. *Scientific Reports, 10*, 5814. https://doi.org/10.1038/s41598-020-62795-1

Nugent, C. C., Falkson, S. R., & Terrell, J. M. (2020). H2 blockers. [Updated March 25, 2020]. In: *StatPearls* [Internet]. Treasure Island, FL: StatPearls Publishing.

O'Connor, A., Vaira, D., Gisbert, J. P., et al. (2014). Treatment of *Helicobacter pylori* infection 2014. *Helicobacter, 19*(Suppl 1), 38–45.

Patrick, L. (2011). Gastroesophageal reflux disease (GERD): A review of conventional and alternative treatments. *Alternative Medicine Review, 16*(2), 116–133.

Richter, J. E., & Rubenstein, J. H. (2018). Presentation and epidemiology of gastroesophageal reflux disease. *Gastroenterology, 154*(2), 267–276.

*Rickenbacher, N., Kotter, T., Kochen, M. M., et al. (2014). Fundoplication versus management of gastroesophageal reflux disease: A systematic review and meta-analysis. *Surgical Endoscopy, 28*(1), 143–155.

Scally, B., Emberson, J. R., Spata, E., et al. (2018). Effects of gastroprotectant drugs for the prevention and treatment of peptic ulcer disease and its complications: A meta-analysis of randomized trials. *The Lancet Gastroenterology and Hepatology, 3*(4), 231–241.

Scheiman, J. M. (2013). The use of proton pump inhibitors in treating and preventing NSAID-induced mucosal damage. *Arthritis Research & Therapy, 15*(Suppl 3), S5.

Scheiman, J. M. (2016). NSAID-induced gastrointestinal injury: A focused update for clinicians. *Journal of Clinical Gastroenterology, 50*(1), 5–10.

Seo, J. H., Hong, S. J., Kim, J. H., et al. (2016). Long-term recurrence rates of peptic ulcers without *Helicobacter pylori*. *Gut and Liver, 10*(5), 719–725. https://doi.org/10.5009/gnl15262

Shams, R., Oldfield, E. C., Copare, J., et al. (2015). Peppermint oil: Clinical uses in the treatment of gastrointestinal diseases. *JSM Gastroenterology and Hepatology, 3*(1), 1036.

Spechler, S., Hunter, J., Jones, K., et al. (2019). Randomized trial of medical versus surgical treatment for refractory heartburn. *New England Journal of Medicine, 381*, 1513–1523. https://doi.org/10.1056/NEJMoa1811424

*Yamasaki, T., Hemond, C., Eisa, M., et al. (2018). The changing epidemiology of gastroesophageal reflux disease: Are patients getting younger? *Journal of Neurogastroenterology and Motility, 24*(4), 559–569. https://doi.org/10.5056/jnm18140

27 Liver Diseases

Ryan G. D'Angelo and Jennifer Andres

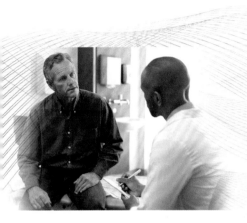
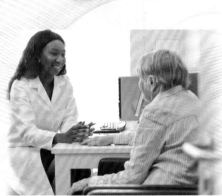
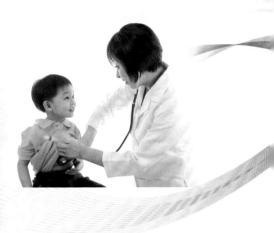

Learning Objectives

1. Recognize diagnostic criteria for common complications of cirrhosis.
2. List appropriate drug therapy choices for each complication of cirrhosis.
3. Compare and contrast diagnostic criteria for hepatitis B and C virus (HCV) infection.
4. Match HCV antiviral agents to their corresponding HCV genotype(s).

INTRODUCTION

Chronic liver disease (CLD) is a worldwide problem and broadly defined as the deterioration of liver functions. Throughout the world, there has been a 13% increase since 2000 in the incidence of liver disease (Moon et al., 2020), and in the United States (2018), there are 1.8 million cases of liver disease and cirrhosis. While the incidence is shifting away from hepatitis B virus (HBV) and C (HCV) toward metabolic syndrome and alcohol abuse, the treatments for CLD are similar (Centers for Disease Control and Prevention, 2020).

CIRRHOSIS

Cirrhosis is most commonly identified in patients aged 45 to 64, predominantly due to HCV. This cohort of the population has been found to be at particularly high risk because of their possible exposure to blood products prior to widely available viral screening. Intravenous drug users and those participating in high-risk sexual activity also have an elevated risk of transmitting HCV and ultimately cirrhosis. In North America, prolonged, excessive alcohol abuse, nonalcoholic fatty liver disease, and nonalcoholic steatohepatitis are additional common causes of cirrhosis. In developing countries, HBV is still a common preventable cause of cirrhosis. CLD and cirrhosis are the ninth leading cause of death in the United States—contributing to 35,000 deaths in the United States each year—and are the eighth leading economic cost among chronic illnesses.

Causes

The liver is an essential organ for many physiologic functions of the human body. It serves to provide metabolic functions, excretion of toxic substances, and synthesis of numerous proteins and macromolecules (**Figure 27.1**). The liver also serves to filter blood arriving from the gastrointestinal tract before reaching the systemic circulation, resulting in what is often referred to as *first-pass metabolism*. The liver is composed of hepatocytes arranged around bile canaliculi, which then allow the drainage of bile into the bile ducts, ultimately traversing to the common bile duct. Additionally, various sinusoids surround clusters of hepatocytes, providing a passage from the portal circulation to the systemic venous circulation. Damage to these various structures can lead to injury of the hepatocytes, and injury to the hepatocytes can lead to functional alteration of these structures.

Acute liver injury describes an episode of abrupt liver dysfunction and should also be further classified as hepatocellular or cholestatic liver injury, which may be identified by the presence of an elevated alkaline phosphatase in addition to aspartate aminotransferase (AST) and alanine aminotransferase (ALT) (**Table 27.1**). Drug-induced liver injury (DILI)

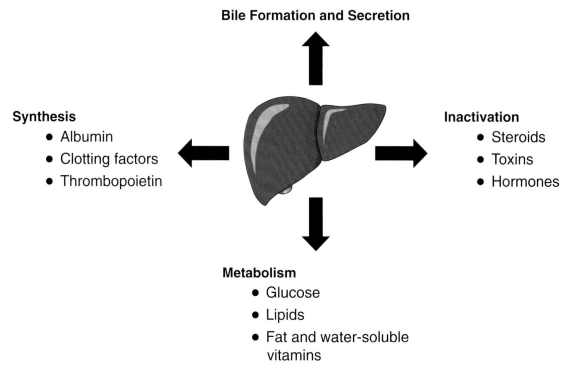

FIGURE 27–1 Functions of the liver.

TABLE 27.1							
Laboratory Findings in Liver Diseases							
Type of Liver Injury	**AST**	**ALT**	**ALP**	**Conjugated Bilirubin**	**Unconjugated Bilirubin**	**Albumin**	**Platelets**
Alcoholic Hepatocellular Injury*	↑↑	↑↑↑↑	N/↑	↑↑	↑↑	N/↓	N/↓
Viral Hepatitis	↑↑↑	↑↑	N/↑	↑↑	↑↑	N	N
Cholestasis	N/↑	N/↑	↑↑↑	↑↑	N/↑	N	N
Cirrhosis	N/↑	N/↑	↑	↑	↑↑	↓↓	↓↓

*AST typically 2x ALT in alcoholic liver injury; N, normal.

ALP, alkaline phosphatase; ALT, alanine aminotransferase; AST, aspartate aminotransferase.

is a frequently encountered medical problem that can lead to acute liver failure. The National Institutes of Health (NIH) maintains a searchable database (http://livertox.nlm.nih.gov) describing the likelihood of drugs for causing DILI, the likely patterns of injury (i.e., hepatocellular vs. cholestatic), and potential management strategies for reversal of acute liver injury.

Cirrhosis is a chronic condition that develops after repeated episodes of injury to the hepatocytes, leading to replacement of healthy liver cells with nonfunctional scar tissue. This leads to progressive liver dysfunction and, overtime, can cause liver failure and hepatocellular carcinoma (HCC).

Pathophysiology

Liver disease is an overarching term often used to describe hepatocyte dysfunction or injury, but unfortunately, the term can be overly vague because it does not incorporate the etiology, chronicity, and/or severity of injury. While acute liver injury and cirrhosis may be related, they are vastly different problems that require different management strategies and patient evaluation.

Cirrhosis is a progressive disease that develops after repeated episodes of liver injury. Over time, normal healthy hepatocytes are replaced with scar tissue, leading to fibrosis within the liver. Not only are hepatocytes replaced with scar tissue but fenestrated endothelia that line the hepatic sinusoids are also decreased as fewer capillary beds are required to supply nutrients and oxygen. These fibrotic changes lead to a cascade of detrimental effects on functions of the liver, which ultimately cause the development of cirrhosis complications: portal hypertension (PH), variceal hemorrhage, ascites, hepatic encephalopathy (HE), spontaneous bacterial peritonitis (SBP), and hepatorenal syndrome (HRS).

The pathophysiology of cirrhosis complications is complex but can be traced back to activation of hepatic stellate cells (**Figure 27.2**). Stellate cell activation causes fibrotic tissue deposition and decreases elasticity within the liver, leading to an increase in vascular resistance within the portal vein, which brings blood from the splanchnic circulation to the liver. As resistance builds within the portal vein, vasodilators such as nitric oxide (NO) are released in an attempt to decrease the

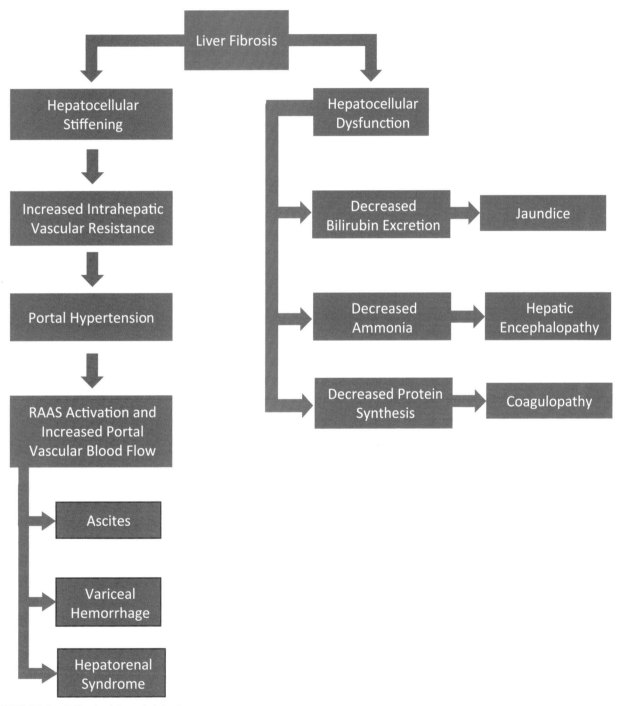

FIGURE 27–2   Pathophysiology of cirrhosis.

blood pressure within the portal vein, but due to the continued fibrotic changes that occur, only limited vasodilation is possible and the portal pressure continues to increase. At some point during the progression of liver fibrosis, this usual local NO production begins, leading to systemic vasodilation without a concomitant portal vein vasodilation, which in turn leads to systemic hypotension. In response, the renin angiotensin aldosterone system (RAAS) activates, triggering aldosterone and angiotensin II release. Angiotensin II has many downstream effects such as arterial vasoconstriction, antidiuretic hormone release, and sodium reabsorption, which are beneficial for improving the systemic vasodilation that has occurred, but ultimately these actions further increase the portal pressure by increasing blood volume delivery to the portal circulation and vasoconstriction of the portal vein. Similarly, aldosterone causes increased sodium and water retention, which then increases the effective circulating volume of blood, increasing volume delivery to the portal circulation, ultimately further increasing the portal pressure.

As fibrosis progresses, hepatic portal venous pressure simultaneously increases. As PH evolves, it causes enlargement of splanchnic vessels in the esophagus and stomach, which are termed *varices*. Ultimately, without reversing the pressure in the varices, there is a risk of rupturing and leading to profuse gastrointestinal hemorrhage. These variceal hemorrhages can be more complicated to control if the patient has more advanced stages of cirrhosis due to the coagulopathies associated with liver dysfunction.

A buildup of fluid in the peritoneum is also a hallmark complication of cirrhosis. A multifactorial mechanism of PH, arterial vasodilation, increased RAAS effects, and low oncotic pressure from reduced albumin synthesis all play a role in the development of ascites. Although the development of ascites in patients with cirrhosis is a common complication, it generally confers a poor prognosis. Nearly 45% of patients who develop ascites will die within 5 years. Identification of ascites should always prompt the clinician to begin considering the potential for liver transplantation (see Chapter 49).

As ascites develop, patients are at an increased risk for SBP, an infection of the peritoneal space. Historically, the mechanism of bacterial inoculation of the peritoneal space in patients with cirrhosis was unclear. Even after nearly 60 years of research, little light has been shed on the exact mechanism for this process. Several theories have suggested a small intestinal bacterial overgrowth and small intestinal dysmotility, leading to increased *Escherichia coli*, *Klebsiella pneumoniae*, and *Streptococcus pneumonia* colonies in the gastrointestinal tract. Increased intestinal permeability likely leads to bacterial translocation from the lumen of the gut to the peritoneal space.

In the late stages of cirrhosis, despite increasing amounts of fluid being retained, it escapes the vasculature and can lead to profound reduction of blood flow to the kidneys. This reduction of blood flow causes HRS, a prerenal acute or subacute kidney injury, which often signifies very late–stage cirrhosis and poor prognosis for patients.

In addition to the vascular and hemodynamic changes associated with cirrhosis, hepatocellular dysfunction leads to additional pathophysiologic alterations, many of which will lead to liver failure. As fibrosis progresses and replaces functioning hepatocytes, metabolic functions of the liver, conjugation and clearance of bilirubin, protein synthesis (predominantly albumin and clotting factors), and production of thrombopoietin all decrease. These changes are associated with the development of neuropsychiatric changes, jaundice, and coagulopathy.

Nearly 45% of patients with cirrhosis are likely to develop HE, the neuropsychiatric complication of cirrhosis. HE, like the other complications of cirrhosis, is multifactorial. Ammonia accumulation plays the most pivotal role in the pathophysiologic manifestation of HE. Ammonia accumulation occurs in patients with cirrhosis as the liver's metabolic capacity declines and ammonia conversion to urea is diminished. As the ammonia concentration increases, it crosses the blood–brain barrier, causing transient damage to astrocytes and neurons. This damage causes a spectrum of neurologic changes, ranging from mild inattention and agitation to coma and death. Interestingly, ammonia levels do not have any direct correlation with the clinical signs or symptoms of HE and thus should not be used as diagnostic tool.

Diagnostic Criteria

Various objective imaging studies may be helpful in confirming a diagnosis of cirrhosis, but often a thorough patient history and evaluation of signs and symptoms is the first step to identifying the likelihood of cirrhosis in a patient. Once a thorough history consistent with cirrhosis is obtained, a full liver panel (AST, ALT, alkaline phosphatase, total bilirubin, and serum albumin), complete blood cell count with platelets, and prothrombin time should be obtained. Additional serologic studies (α1-antitrypsin, antinuclear antibodies [ANA], hepatitis B surface antigen [HBsAg], HCV antibody, alfa fetoprotein, etc.) can be obtained if the patient's history is consistent with other causes, or other common etiologies have been ruled out (**Table 27.1**). Because no radiographic imaging study is considered the standard, often a right, upper quadrant ultrasound is used due to its absence of radiation exposure and relative low cost to identify gross anatomical changes to liver. Typical cirrhotic changes observed from an ultrasound include nodularity, irregularity, and enhanced echogenicity. Computed tomography and magnetic resonance imaging can also identify nodularity and hypertrophic changes within the liver but may lead to unnecessary costs and potential for patient harm; consequently, these tests are infrequently used as the first imaging study to assist in the diagnostic evaluation of cirrhosis. The most invasive diagnostic approach is with a liver biopsy, although it is considered the "gold-standard" diagnostic test. This is generally reserved for situations where the previous steps have been inconclusive despite a high suspicion for cirrhosis. Typically, several tissue samples are obtained to increase the sensitivity and specificity of the results. Additional innovative imaging techniques such as ultrasound elastography are increasing in frequency but are still being formally evaluated to replace previous imaging techniques.

Once the diagnosis of cirrhosis is confirmed, several additional tools may be implemented to evaluate the severity of cirrhosis. Historically, the Child-Turcotte Pugh (CTP) score has been used not only to stage cirrhosis but also as a tool to determine the need for medication dosage adjustment (**Table 27.2**). The Model for End-Stage Liver Disease (MELD) and MELD-Na are tools used to assess the severity of end-stage liver failure, predict 3-month mortality, and prioritize patients for liver transplant (**Table 27.3**). Whereas the CTP scoring tool is limited by some subjectivity of the observer, the MELD and MELD-Na are calculations based on purely objective laboratory measurements of creatinine, bilirubin, international normalized ratio, sodium, and the need for renal replacement therapy within the last week.

Depending on the underlying etiology of cirrhosis, risk factors should be identified and addressed. Alcohol abstinence is pivotal in patients with alcoholic liver disease. Early steatosis may be resolved by simply refraining from alcohol use. In patients with more advance liver injury or cirrhosis, alcohol abstinence can still improve the risk of mortality. Generally, patients with cirrhosis have concomitant nutritional

TABLE 27.2
Child-Turcotte-Pugh Scoring System

Characteristics	Points		
	1	2	3
Encephalopathy	None	Grade 1–2 (or precipitated)	Grade 3–4 (or chronic)
Ascites	None	Mild/moderate (diuretic responsive)	Severe (diuretic refractory)
Bilirubin (mg/dL)	<2	2–3	>3
Albumin (g/dL)	>3.5	2.8–3.5	<2.8
PT or	<4	4–6	>6
INR	<1.7	1.7–2.3	>2.3

CTP score: 5 to 6 points = A; 7 to 9 points = B; >9 points = C

CTP, Child-Turcotte Pugh; INR, international normalized ratio; PT, prothrombin time.

TABLE 27.3
MELD-Na Score Interpretation

Score	90-day Mortality (%)
≤9	1.9
10–19	6.0
20–29	19.6
30–39	52.6
≥40	71.3

deficiencies, which should be addressed when identified. These include folic acid, vitamin B6, vitamin A, thiamine, selenium, zinc, and magnesium.

Portal Hypertension and Varices
Diagnostic Criteria: Liver Fibrosis

PH nearly directly correlates with the progression of liver fibrosis. The primary diagnosis of clinically significant PH is based on a hepatic venous portal gradient (HVPG) of more than 10 mm Hg. A HVPG of more than 12 mm Hg is associated with variceal rupture and hemorrhage and development of ascites. Furthermore, patients with an HVPG of more than 16 mm Hg are associated with a higher risk of mortality. The most reliable method for HVPG measurement is by inserting a balloon catheter and measuring the difference between the wedged hepatic venous pressure, which closely represents the pressure within the portal vein, and the free hepatic vein pressure. This process is similar to what is used to measure the pulmonary capillary wedge pressure in patients with congestive heart failure. Potential complications of measuring the HVPG include transient arrhythmias, pain, and vagal reactions. The HVPG is not only useful in the diagnostic approach for PH but is becoming more frequently used as an additional prognostic marker for CLD and cirrhosis.

Because liver fibrosis and PH develop concurrently, there has been recent interest in using ultrasound elastography to measure the presence of clinically significant PH. As these techniques are still developing and improving, there have been mixed results in their performance to accurately detect the presence PH in all patients with cirrhosis. Finally, any patient with known gastroesophageal varices should be classified as having clinically significant PH since these patients have an HVPG of at least 10 mm Hg.

Gastroesophageal Varices

Identification of patients with varices is a crucial step in the assessment and evaluation of patients with cirrhosis. Most patients diagnosed with cirrhosis should undergo evaluation for gastroesophageal varices via esophagogastroduodenoscopy (EGD). EGD assessment regarding the size of varices and the presence of red wale marks can identify patients with varices that are at a high risk of hemorrhage. When high-risk features (i.e., red wale sign, large varices, coil shaped) are identified, endoscopic variceal ligation can be performed and/or pharmacologic intervention can be implemented to reduce the incidence of bleeding and lengthen the time to first variceal bleed. EGD is not without its own risks and complications; thus, noninvasive tests to determine the likelihood of the presence of high-risk varices have been validated in patients with compensated cirrhosis. The 2017 American Association for the Study of Liver Disease (AASLD) guidelines suggest that patients with a liver stiffness of less than 20 kPa based on transient elastography and a platelet count more than 150,000 cells/mm^3 have less than 5% risk of having high-risk varices and thus can avoid EGD evaluation. Additional non-invasive tests have been proposed based on the varying etiologies of cirrhosis and additional objective measures but are not as well validated.

Initiating Drug Therapy

Because PH is the first consequence of cirrhosis, it is also the first opportunity to initiate pharmacologic therapy. Three nonselective beta blockers (NSBBs), propranolol, nadolol, and carvedilol, are used to cause reduced blood flow through the portal vascular system (**Table 27.4**). A large study identified that the initiation of drug therapy at the stage of mild PH (portal pressure <10 mm Hg) does not impact the development of varices in patients with cirrhosis. Based on this study, guidelines now suggest withholding treatment until gastroesophageal varices are identified (Groszmann, 2005). NSBBs are indicated for either primary prophylaxis of variceal hemorrhage or secondary prophylaxis after having a variceal bleed.

Goals of Drug Therapy

Clinically, the goal of drug therapy for PH is to prevent variceal hemorrhage and reduce mortality. Based on the pathophysiology of cirrhosis, it is thought that reducing the portal pressure may also mitigate or prolong the time to the additional complications of cirrhosis. Objectively, a resting heart rate of 55 to 60 beats per minute should be targeted when using nadolol or propranolol. Based on the studies conducted, when carvedilol is used, rather than target a specific heart rate, a dose of 6.25 mg twice daily should be targeted for maximal efficacy. Additionally, the systolic blood pressure should not decrease below 90 mm Hg for any of the three NSBBs.

Nonselective Beta Blockers

Mechanism of Action

Nadolol, propranolol, and carvedilol are beta-adrenergic receptor agonists. Nadolol and propranolol share a similar affinity for both beta-1 and beta-2 receptors. By blocking the stimulation beta-1 receptors, located primarily on the myocardial tissue, cardiac output can be reduced; thus, the volume of blood delivered to the portal circulation is reduced. Interestingly, the blockade of beta-2 receptors, primarily located in the vasculature, has a counterintuitive mechanism. When beta-2 receptors are antagonized in the vasculature, unopposed alpha-receptor agonism occurs. Specifically, in the splanchnic vasculature, this unopposed alpha-receptor stimulation causes vasoconstriction, thus further reducing the blood flow to the portal vein. Carvedilol, a more potent NSBB, also has additional alpha-1 receptor antagonism. This alpha-1 blockade has a direct effect of the vascular tone of the portal vein and has been shown to be at least as, if not more effective in reducing the portal pressure when compared to nadolol and/or propranolol.

Selecting the Most Appropriate Drug

First-Line Therapy

All three NSBBs (see **Table 27.4**) are indicated for primary prophylaxis of variceal hemorrhage. Due to multiple daily doses required for propranolol and carvedilol, patients may benefit from the once-daily dosing of nadolol. Despite the ease of dosing with nadolol, it is generally more expensive and may lead to additional out-of-pocket costs for patients.

For secondary prophylaxis, nadolol and propranolol are recommended by the AASLD guidelines. Carvedilol is not included, although evidence has suggested that it can be used safely and effectively.

TABLE 27.4

Beta-Blockers for Variceal Hemorrhage Prophylaxis

Drug	Initial Dose	Maximum Dose	Adverse Effects	Contraindications	Drug Interactions
Propranolol	20–40 mg BID	With ascites: 160 mg/d Without ascites: 320 mg/d	CV: bradycardia, hypotension, syncope CNS: fatigue, drowsiness, dizziness Endocrine: hyper/hypoglycemia, hyperkalemia	>1st degree heart block Cardiogenic shock Decompensated cardiac failure Decompensated liver failure	Enhanced effects: amiodarone, dronedarone Reduced efficacy: theophylline
Nadolol	20–40 mg once daily	With ascites: 80 mg/d Without ascites: 160 mg/d			
Carvedilol	3.125 mg BID	With or without ascites: 12.5 mg/d			Enhanced serum concentration: vincristine, topotecan, Reduced efficacy: theophylline

CNS, central nervous system; CV, cardiovascular.

TABLE 27.5
Diuretic Therapy for Ascites

Drug	MOA	Initial Dose	Maximum Dose	Time to Response	Adverse Effects
First Line					
Spironolactone	Aldosterone antagonist	50–100 mg daily (in combination with furosemide)	400 mg daily	2–3 days	CV: hypotension Endocrine: hyperkalemia, gynecomastia Renal: acute kidney injury
Furosemide	Loop diuretic	20–40 mg daily (in combination with spironolactone)	160 mg daily		CV: hypotension Endocrine: hypokalemia Renal: acute kidney injury
Second Line					
Amiloride (in place of spironolactone)	Potassium-sparing diuretic (collecting tubule sodium channel antagonist)	10 mg BID (in combination with furosemide)	30 mg BID	4 days	CV: hypotension Endocrine: hyponatremia, hyperkalemia Genitourinary: impotence

CV, cardiovascular; MOA, mechanism of action.

Nadolol is the only agent of the three that is cleared renally, so close monitoring of renal function is required, and appropriate dosage adjustment should be made based on the creatinine clearance to avoid unnecessary adverse effects.

In patients with known ascites, the maximum daily doses of nadolol and propranolol should be limited due to the risk of causing decompensated liver failure. Some clinicians suggest avoiding beta blockers completely in patients with ascites because some studies have identified increased risk of acute kidney injury and hospital readmissions (**Table 27.5**).

Special Considerations: Geriatrics

Older patients are at a higher risk of bradycardia with NSBBs and should have regular monitoring of their heart rate. It may be prudent to slow the dosage titration to ensure tolerance of increasing doses. Older patients are also particularly susceptible to central nervous system effects (confusion, lethargy, etc.) from propranolol due to its ability to cross the blood–brain barrier.

Monitoring Patient Response

NSBB therapy should be continued indefinitely unless new contraindications develop (see **Table 27.4**). Home blood pressure and heart rate monitoring may help improve the safety of therapy and determine if dose adjustments are required. All providers involved with the care of the patient should ensure

the patient's heart rate is on target at all visits. Patients should also be evaluated for the presence of ascites to ensure doses of NSBBs are appropriate.

Variceal Hemorrhage
Diagnostic Criteria

Unfortunately, for many patients with advanced cirrhosis, acute variceal hemorrhage can be one of the first physical manifestations of cirrhosis. Although variceal hemorrhage is ultimately diagnosed via an EGD, the initial clinical signs and symptoms are similar to that seen in patients with upper gastrointestinal bleed (i.e., decreased hemoglobin and hematocrit, hematochezia, "coffee-ground" emesis, altered mental status, elevated blood urea nitrogen [BUN], hypotension, and tachycardia). After initial episodes of variceal hemorrhage, patients should be monitored at regular intervals by EGD for further development of high-risk varices amenable to nonpharmacologic interventions.

Initiating Drug Therapy

Variceal hemorrhage occurs in approximately 20% of patients with cirrhosis each year and is associated with a mortality rate of upwards of 30%. Increasing size of varices and the presence of red wale marks are associated with augmented risk of bleeding. Without appropriate treatment, variceal hemorrhage can be a recurrent complication of cirrhosis and is one of the most common causes of morbidity and mortality.

Goals of Drug Therapy

The primary goal of drug therapy for variceal hemorrhage is to reduce the risk of mortality at 6 weeks post event. Acutely, the clinician should ensure hemodynamic stability with intravenous fluids, maintain adequate oxygenation with supplemental O_2, maintain hemoglobin between 7 and 9 g/dL with packed red-blood cell transfusion, and control bleeding. In patients with known or suspected ascites, administration of antibiotics is of upmost importance to further reduce the incidence of SBP and mortality. Additional long-term goals include those discussed for varices and PH to prevent future episodes of bleeding.

Selecting the Most Appropriate Drug: First-Line Therapy

Vasoactive agents have been shown to reduce short-term mortality and transfusion requirements in patients presenting with variceal hemorrhage. Several intravenous vasoactive therapies have been studied in patients with variceal hemorrhage, but only octreotide is used frequently in the United States. Vasopressin, in combination with intravenous nitroglycerin, is no longer used due to complications of myocardial and limb ischemia resulting from systemic vasoconstriction.

Octreotide, a synthetic somatostatin analogue, within minutes, causes acute splanchnic vasoconstriction and reduced portal blood flow that leads to a reduction of portal pressure. Octreotide is provided as an initial bolus of 50 mcg, followed by 25 to 50 mcg per hour intravenously. The infusion can be continued for 2 to 5 days and should generally be accompanied by endoscopic evaluation and endoscopic variceal ligation, if possible. Commonly encountered side effects of short-term octreotide use include hyperglycemia and prolonged QTc interval. Patients may be considered for early transjugular intrahepatic portosystemic shunt (TIPS) if endoscopic variceal ligation is unable to control bleeding effectively or if bleeding recurs despite pharmacologic therapy. TIPS forms a shunt between the portal vein and the hepatic vein, thereby significantly reducing portal pressure. TIPS is not frequently performed due to the high incidence of HE and cardiac decompensation that can develop post-procedurally.

Once patients have stopped bleeding, vasoactive therapy should be discontinued and appropriate NSBB therapy should be started for secondary prophylaxis. If TIPS was placed successfully, NSBB can be omitted.

Monitoring Patient Response

During an episode of variceal hemorrhage, patients should have frequent complete blood counts performed, typically every 8 to 12 hours to ensure resolution of acute bleeding and stabilization of hemoglobin. Electrolyte and renal function monitoring should also be performed at least daily while the patient is hospitalized, as many patients presenting with cirrhosis have several deficiencies that can be corrected to prevent additional complications. When patients are admitted to intensive care units, continuous hemodynamic monitoring can allow the clinician to carefully monitor the need for further fluid resuscitation and vasopressors if indicated.

In the setting of acute variceal hemorrhage, octreotide is relatively well tolerated. Short-term use can be associated with mild symptoms such as hyperglycemia and constipation.

ASCITES

Diagnostic Criteria

Ascites, although most frequently associated with cirrhosis, can develop due to additional causes such as heart failure, neoplasm, nephrotic syndrome, and so forth. A thorough physical exam in patients with a distended or protuberant abdomen will assist the clinician in identifying patients with ascites. Approximately 1,500 mL of fluid in the peritoneal space is required to detect the presence of percussed tympanic dullness around the flank. The serum-ascites albumin gradient (SAAG) is a validated approach to categorize the etiology of ascites. An albumin concentration of the ascitic fluid and the serum must be obtained on the same day, and the calculation is simply subtracting the ascitic albumin concentration from the serum. A SAAG value of more than 1.1 g/dL is 97% accurate in classifying ascites due to PH.

Initiating Drug Therapy

Ascites develop due to the hemodynamic changes related to PH and is associated with increasing activity of aldosterone and antidiuretic hormone. No specific criteria have been developed to help guide the clinician in determining the appropriate time to initiate drug therapy; however, once patients develop apparent ascites, treatment should be started.

Goals of Drug Therapy

The primary goal of therapy for ascites is to mobilize and excrete fluid by administration of diuretics while minimizing intravascular volume depletion. Additionally, drug therapy is used to prevent the re-accumulation of fluid. Although the mainstay of treatment is diuretic agents, occasionally, paracentesis is required in patients with large-volume ascites and/or ascites refractory to treatment.

Selecting the Most Appropriate Drug

The aldosterone antagonist spironolactone is considered the gold-standard initial therapy for the treatment of ascites. It is preferred to furosemide monotherapy as it targets the underlying hyperaldosteronism that occurs in patients with ascites and has been shown to be more effective in mobilizing fluid. Due to the frequency of hyperkalemia that occurs with high-dose spironolactone and the longer time to mobilization of fluid, the combination of spironolactone and furosemide is recommended for most patients. The dose of each diuretic can be increased to the maximum dose, but the ratio of spironolactone and furosemide should be maintained at 5:2, respectively, to prevent electrolyte abnormalities. Spironolactone has the propensity to cause tender gynecomastia due to its ability to upregulate estrogen synthesis. In patients who develop gynecomastia, amiloride, another type of diuretic, may be used as an alternative option. Eplerenone, another aldosterone receptor blocker that is used in place of spironolactone in patients with heart failure, has not been studied extensively in patients with cirrhosis and at this time cannot be routinely recommended.

In patients with refractory ascites, serial therapeutic paracenteses every week to two weeks may be required to control ascites' re-accumulation. When paracentesis is performed, it is generally recommended that intravenous albumin be administered when more than 5 L of fluid is removed, which has been shown to reduce mortality by 35%. Albumin is thought to maintain hydrostatic pressure within the vasculature and prevent fluid from shifting from the vasculature into the peritoneal space after paracentesis. When used for this indication, albumin 25% should be used at a dose of 6 to 8 g/L of fluid removed.

Monitoring Patient Response

As with any patient receiving diuretic therapies, blood pressure, orthostatic symptoms, and basic metabolic panel should be monitored at frequent intervals when first starting therapy. Patients should be instructed to weigh themselves daily and notify their provider if they identify a weight change of ±2 kg as this may reflect too aggressive or insufficient volume removal. The dose of most diuretics can be titrated as quickly as every 48 to 72 hours, but appropriate laboratory monitoring should be obtained to ensure serum creatinine, potassium, and sodium levels are maintained appropriately. Specifically, a rise in serum creatinine to a level more than 2.0 mg/dL or 2-fold increase from baseline necessitates temporary diuretic cessation.

Urine electrolyte monitoring can also be useful to help determine if additional titration of diuretics would be useful in patients who do not appear to lose weight appropriately. Current AASLD guidelines recommend that in patients whose spot urine sodium excretion is less than 78 mmol daily, diuretic doses should be escalated. Once euvolemia is achieved, and further changes in diuretic regimens are minimized, frequency of laboratory monitoring can be extended.

SPONTANEOUS BACTERIAL PERITONITIS

Diagnostic Criteria

In patients with known cirrhosis and ascites, the ascitic fluid can become infected, leading to SBP. SBP is diagnosed when an elevated ascitic fluid polymorphonuclear cell count or neutrophil count is 250 cells/mm³ or more without an intra-abdominal source of infection (i.e., perforation). SBP is most commonly caused by enteric gram-negative pathogens (e.g., *E. coli* and *K. pneumonia*) and *S. pneumonia*, and thus

BOX 27.1 Laboratory Analysis of Ascitic Fluid

Routine

- Gross appearance (clear, cloudy, milky, bloody)
- Cell count and differential
  - White blood cell, neutrophils, lymphocytes, eosinophils, red blood cell
- Albumin
- Total protein

Optional

- Gram-stain and culture
- Glucose
- Lactate dehydrogenase
- Amylase

empiric therapy should adequately cover those isolates until sensitivities are available. Even in the absence of culture-positive ascites (culture-negative neutrocytic ascites), prompt antimicrobial therapy should be implemented as these patients have similar presenting signs and symptoms, and more importantly mortality rates are similar. Importantly, ascitic fluid sampling should always be performed prior to administration of empiric antibiotic therapy (as long as such a delay would not cause significant patient harm) as this can increase a positive microbial yield by upwards of nearly 90% (**Box 27.1**).

Initiating Drug Therapy

Once the diagnosis of SBP is made based on ascitic fluid cell counts and patient symptoms, empiric antimicrobial therapy targeting *E. coli*, *K. pneumonia*, and *S. pneumonia* should be started. When patients have survived an episode of SBP, they are also candidates for indefinite secondary antibiotic prophylaxis because upwards of 70% of patients who survive an initial episode of SBP will redevelop the infection within 1 year without prophylaxis. Additionally, certain high-risk populations may warrant primary prophylaxis. These include patients with cirrhosis who present with a gastrointestinal bleed, patients who have ascites and concomitant renal dysfunction (creatinine ≥1.2 mg/dL, blood-urea-nitrogen ≥25 mg/dL, or serum sodium ≤130 mmol/L), or patients with liver failure (CTP score of ≥9 and bilirubin ≥3 mg/dL).

Goals of Drug Therapy

Eradication of active peritoneal infection and improving survival are the primary goals of therapy in SBP. Furthermore, certain patients presenting with SBP are at higher-than-normal risk of mortality as well as kidney injury, which requires additional non-antimicrobial therapies.

Selecting the Most Appropriate Drug—Treatment

First-Line Therapy

In most cases, the third-generation cephalosporins should be used as first-line therapy for the treatment of SBP (**Table 27.6**). These antimicrobials provide excellent coverage of commonly implicated organisms and are well studied in the management of SBP. When used appropriately, cure rates can reach as high as 90%. Although cefotaxime is the primary cephalosporin listed in the guidelines for SBP, many hospitals utilize ceftriaxone as their agent of choice due to its usage for other infections, decreased frequency of administration, and relatively safe side effect profile.

Second-Line Therapy

Fluoroquinolones have also been documented as having excellent empiric coverage in SBP. Unfortunately, due to heightened antimicrobial resistance from their widespread use, these options are not preferred and should be reserved for patients with significant allergies to first-line therapy or in the setting of resistance to first-line therapies. Also, these agents are less-attractive options for routine use due to recent significant safety warnings published related to fluoroquinolones. Increasing rates of acute kidney injury, aortic rupture, severe altered mental status, and significant blood glucose instability have been observed in post-marketing studies. Patients at high risk for these complications include those with base-line renal dysfunction, cardiovascular disease, advanced age, and diabetes mellitus.

Third-Line Therapy

Sulfamethoxazole–trimethoprim may be reserved for patients unable to tolerate first- or second-line therapies. Sulfamethoxazole–trimethoprim is commonly used for urinary tract infections and is one of the most prescribed antibiotics, which has ultimately increased the resistance rates significantly in the past 15 years. Because *E. coli* resistance to sulfamethoxazole–trimethoprim is approximately 20%, this agent is a relatively poor empiric option and should be kept for patients in areas where resistance rates are lower (~ <10%).

TABLE 27.6

Antibiotics for Spontaneous Bacterial Peritonitis

Drug	MOA	Dose	Adverse Effects	Contraindications	Drug Interactions
First Line					
Cefotaxime	Cell-wall synthesis inhibitor (3rd Gen. Cephalosporin)	2 g IV q8h	Renal: Acute interstitial nephritis Misc.: allergic response	Anaphylaxis to beta-lactams	N/A
Ceftriaxone	Cell-wall synthesis inhibitor (3rd Gen. Cephalosporin)	2 g IV once daily (treatment) 1 g IV once daily (prophylaxis)	Hepatic: biliary sludging Misc.: allergic response	Anaphylaxis to beta-lactams	N/A
Second Line					
Levofloxacin	DNA gyrase inhibitor (fluoroquinolone)	750 mg IV/PO once daily	CNS: altered mental status CV: QTc prolongation, aortic rupture Dermatologic: photosensitivity, TEN Endocrine: hyper/hypoglycemia GI: *C. difficile* infection Renal: acute interstitial nephritis	History of tendon rupture; significant cardiovascular disease (non-absolute)	Enhanced QTc prolongation: ondansetron, antiarrhythmics, methadone, varenicline
Third Line (not recommended for empiric therapy)					
Sulfamethoxazole– trimethoprim	Bacterial folic acid synthesis inhibitor	1–2 tablets (double-strength tablet) PO BID	Dermatologic: photosensitivity, TEN Endocrine: hyperkalemia Renal: pseudo-prerenal injury, acute interstitial nephritis	Anaphylaxis to sulfonamide moiety	Enhanced effects: digoxin, dofetilide, methotrexate

CNS, central nervous system; CV, cardiovascular; DNA, deoxyribonucleic acid; GI, gastrointestinal; IV, intravenous; MOA, mechanism of action; TEN, toxic epidermal necrolysis.

Adjunctive Therapy

The study of the addition of albumin to antimicrobial therapy has produced some data to suggest a potential mortality and morbidity benefit among specific SBP patient populations. Patients with a serum creatinine of more than 1 mg/dL, BUN of more than 30 mg/dL, or a total bilirubin of more than 4 mg/dL at the time of diagnosis may benefit from the addition of 1.5 g of albumin per kilogram body weight within 6 hours on day 1 and a second dose of 1 g/kg on day 3. Due to the relatively high cost of albumin for health systems, its use should be restricted to this population as the benefit has not been consistently demonstrated outside of these criteria.

Monitoring Patient Response

Patients should become afebrile and begin to clinically improve within 24 to 48 hours after antibiotic initiation; thus, repeat diagnostic paracentesis is not required unless the patient clinically deteriorates or demonstrates a lack of improvement. If an additional paracentesis is required, additional causes of infection should be evaluated, and surgical intervention may be required. Once patients have become afebrile and hemodynamically stable and the serum white blood cell count is improving, initial intravenous antibiotic therapy can be transitioned to an appropriate oral agent based on culture and sensitivity reports. All the options listed for the treatment of SBP have the propensity to cause renal injury and/or require renal dose adjustment; thus, serum creatinine and urine volume should be closely monitored.

Selecting the Most Appropriate Drug—Prophylaxis

Like the treatment of SBP, primary and secondary prophylaxis should target typical infecting organisms. Current guidelines recommend either norfloxacin (400 mg once daily) or sulfamethoxazole–trimethoprim (800/160 mg once daily) as equally efficacious agents for the prevention of SBP (**Box 27.2**). However, due to the increased adverse effects of fluoroquinolones, the use of sulfamethoxazole–trimethoprim is preferred among most clinicians. Regardless of the agent chosen, daily administration should be used to prevent the development of antimicrobial resistance.

Hepatorenal Syndrome
Diagnostic Criteria

HRS is a complex problem encountered in patients with cirrhosis and ascites, characterized by either an acute or a subacute rise in serum creatinine. Two types of HRS exist. Type 1 HRS is classified as an acute doubling of the serum creatinine or a 50% reduction of the patient's baseline creatinine clearance. Additional features of HRS (**Box 27.3**) are included to ensure other more common causes of acute kidney injury are ruled out; thus, HRS is generally considered a diagnosis of exclusion. Because of the time frame required to make a

---

BOX 27.2 Spontaneous Bacterial Peritonitis Prophylaxis

Indications for Prophylaxis

Active GI bleed in patient with cirrhosis

Duration: 7 days

Ascites and cirrhosis

- Ascitic fluid protein <1.5 g/dL PLUS
  - Creatinine ≥1.2 mg/dL OR
  - BUN ≥25 mg/dL OR
  - Na ≤130 mEq/L

Duration: indefinite

Ascites and liver failure

- CTP score ≥ 9 AND bilirubin ≥ 3

Duration: indefinite

After survival of an episode of SBP

Duration: indefinite

BOX 27.3 Criteria for Diagnosis of Hepatorenal Syndrome

Cirrhosis with ascites
Serum creatine more than 1.5 mg/dL or doubling of baseline serum creatinine within 2 weeks
Absence of shock (mean arterial pressure <65 mm Hg)
Absence of nephrotoxic agents
Absence of proteinuria (<500 mg/d), microscopic hematuria, and abnormal renal ultrasound
Lack of improvement in renal function after 48 hours of diuretic withdrawal and albumin administration

---

diagnosis of HRS and poor prognosis of these patients, there is debate on additional biomarkers or tests that can be used more quickly to confirm the diagnosis: urinary gelatinase-associated lipocalin, urine kidney molecule-1, and kidney biopsy to determine the presence of glomerular tubular reflux, although the latter is associated with bleeding risks due to possible concomitant coagulopathies.

Type 2 HRS is typically a poor prognosis for patients with cirrhosis and is characterized by a subacute or chronic worsening of renal function in a patient with cirrhosis and ascites.

Initiating Drug Therapy

Treatment of HRS is often delayed because of the lack of formal diagnostic criteria but should be implemented as soon as possible as short-term mortality is significant. Because HRS is most frequently triggered by infection, a careful infectious workup and prompt antimicrobial therapy should be implemented. The clinician should carefully review the patient's medication list to ensure nephrotoxic agents are discontinued to prevent further renal injury.

Goals of Drug Therapy

The primary focus of treatment is to successfully bridge the patient to liver transplant. During the bridge period, renal function can be maintained through either pharmacologic therapy or renal replacement therapies. If a reversible cause of acute liver dysfunction is identified, treatment should also be initiated to reverse the cause.

Selecting the Most Appropriate Drug

First-Line Therapy

Due to the lack of formalized diagnostic criteria, randomized control trials are lacking, but a combination of albumin, octreotide, and midodrine (**Table 27.7**) has been shown to be effective in increasing mean arterial blood pressure, which may improve renal blood flow and may also improve short-term mortality. This medication regimen is suitable as it can be used in patients admitted in general medical floors as well as intensive care units. There may be a dose-related benefit with midodrine; thus, it is commonly titrated up to a target dose of 15 mg thrice daily. These agents are generally administered for 15 to 20 days and then discontinued.

Second-Line Therapy

For patients admitted to an intensive care unit, limited studies have shown a beneficial impact on renal function with the use of intravenous norepinephrine and albumin. As with any patient receiving vasopressor therapy, careful cardiac monitoring with electrocardiogram and continuous blood pressure monitoring should be employed to minimize adverse effects. Norepinephrine can be titrated to achieve an increase in the mean arterial pressure of 10 mm Hg. In most situations, this regimen should be trialed only after failure of first-line therapy due to the potential of arrhythmias that can occur from beta-adrenergic stimulation.

Monitoring Patient Response

Regardless of the treatment regimen utilized in the management of HRS, close evaluation of the serum creatinine and urine output will assist the clinician in determining the efficacy of therapy. If severe electrolyte derangements (i.e., sodium, potassium), uremia, or overt volume overload develop, renal replacement therapy should be considered to stabilize the patient. Although some improvement may occur within days of initiating treatment, a full return to baseline renal function is not likely, particularly in those with type 2 HRS. Patients should continue to be evaluated for liver transplant throughout the treatment course, and patients who require dialysis for more than 8 weeks prior to transplant are recommended both liver and kidney transplants.

HEPATIC ENCEPHALOPATHY

Diagnostic Criteria

As discussed briefly in prior sections, HE is a wide-ranging constellation of neurologic signs and symptoms displayed in patients with cirrhosis. In its most mild forms, patients may

TABLE 27.7			
Drug Therapy for Hepatorenal Syndrome			
Drug	**MOA**	**Dose**	**Adverse Effects**
First Line			
Albumin	Enhancement of intravascular osmotic pressure	1 g/kg on day 1, then 20–40 g/d thereafter	Miscellaneous: infusion-related reactions; Anaphylaxis; fever
Octreotide	Somatostatin analogue	100–200 mcg subcutaneously TID	CV: bradycardia, hypertension CNS: headache Endocrine: hyperglycemia GI: diarrhea, cramping
Midodrine	Alpha-1 agonist	5–15 mg TID	CV: hypertension CNS: paresthesia
Second Line			
Norepinephrine (used with albumin)	Noradrenergic agonist	0.5–3 mg/h continuous IV infusion	CV: arrhythmia, bradycardia Respiratory: dyspnea Miscellaneous: extravasation necrosis

CNS, central nervous system; CV, cardiovascular; GI, gastrointestinal; IV, intravenous; MOA, mechanism of action.

display inattention, agitation, and general confusion. As HE progresses, dyskinesia, parkinsonian tremors, and loss of deep tendon reflexes may become apparent. Assessing for asterixis, a flapping tremor, in a patient with cirrhosis may help in the clinical diagnosis of HE, but it is important to understand that this can be a nonspecific test as asterixis can be present from several other causes such as electrolyte derangements and drug intoxication. Overt HE is truly a clinical diagnosis made by careful clinical examination and correlation with the patient's history. Serum ammonia levels do not correlate with the presence and/or severity of HE and should not be used as an objective data point in the diagnostic evaluation of HE. Appropriate classification according to the etiology or underlying disease, severity of manifestations, time course, and presence of precipitation factors is pivotal to determine whether treatment is appropriate and additional precipitating risks can be minimized.

Initiating Drug Therapy

Initiation of drug therapy is the last step in the management of overt HE. For those with grade 4 overt HE or those with an altered level of consciousness, the initial treatment should target protection of the airway and maintenance of breathing. Once encephalopathy is identified, reversible toxic-metabolic causes should be tested for and corrected. As alternative causes are ruled out, the clinician should not only initiate treatment but also continue exploring for precipitating causes. The most common causes precipitating overt HE include treatment noncompliance, dehydration, infection, electrolyte abnormalities, and constipation. Both medicinal and recreational drugs, specifically opioids, benzodiazepines, and cocaine, are also frequently identified as drugs that lead to overt hepatic encephalopathy (OHE).

Goals of Drug Therapy

Although serum ammonia levels are not used for the initial diagnosis of OHE, a decrease in their level may correlate with drug therapy efficacy. Ultimately, treatment should provide a return to baseline mental status. Some of the specific drug therapies used have explicit target doses or parameters that have been shown to be beneficial in clinical studies. Often the clinician will be required to use both these objective and subjective parameters to individualize therapy for the patient.

Selecting the Most Appropriate Drug

First-Line Therapy

First-line therapy includes lactulose administered orally or rectally to facilitate two to three soft bowel movements each day for chronic therapy (Table 27.8). In the acute stage of treatment, augmented dosing should be used to facilitate rapid stool output. Oral treatment should be initiated prior to discontinuation of a rectal regimen to ensure oral onset of action is achieved. Lactulose is cost-effective and is considered the standard of care for OHE.

TABLE 27.8				
Drug Therapy for Overt Hepatic Encephalopathy				
Drug	**MOA**	**Dose**	**Time to Response**	**Adverse Effects**
Lactulose (Oral)	Acidification of GI tract, resulting in inhibiting diffusion of NH_3 into the blood	20–30 g PO q1–2h until bowel movement occurs, then 20–30 g TID–QID	Hours	GI: abdominal cramping, diarrhea Endocrine: hypokalemia, metabolic acidosis
Lactulose (Rectal retention enema)		200 g via balloon catheter, retained for 30–60 minutes, q4–6h		
Second Line				
Rifaximin (as add-on to lactulose for refractory OHE)	Bacterial RNA synthesis inhibitor resulting in reduced bacterial generation of NH_3	550 mg BID	Variable	GI: nausea, irritable bowel syndrome (diarrhea) Hematologic: anemia Hepatic: elevated ALT Respiratory: nasopharyngitis
Third Line				
Polyethylene glycol 3350	Osmotic laxative inducing large-volume catharsis	280 g in 4 L of water administered over 4 hours	Hours	GI: dyspepsia Endocrine: electrolyte derangements

ALT, alanine aminotransferase; GI, gastrointestinal; MOA, mechanism of action; OHE, overt hepatic encephalopathy; RNA, ribonucleic acid.

Second-Line Therapy

For patient's refractory to lactulose therapy, rifaximin, which is an antibiotic, can be added as an adjunctive agent. Rifaximin works by inhibiting the growth of organisms in the bowel that produce ammonia. Although some studies suggest a possible benefit when used alone, cost is often prohibitive for patients. Rifaximin can be used during episodes of recurrent OHE as well as for prevention of episodes.

Third-Line Therapy

Polyethylene glycol solution, a common stool-softening agent, has recently been studied as monotherapy and add-on therapy for the acute treatment of OHE. Because of its cathartic properties, it is thought to allow enhanced removal of ammonia through the gastrointestinal tract. The dose is significantly larger than that that used for daily catharsis, and many of these patients require administration via nasogastric enteral access. Smaller, more frequent doses have not been well studied and are not indicated for preventative treatment. Further study of this economically friendly and relatively benign drug is currently ongoing (U.S. National Library of Medicine, n.d.).

Other antimicrobial agents such as metronidazole and neomycin have been used historically and have shown benefit, but significant adverse effects such as neurotoxicity, and nephrotoxicity and ototoxicity, respectively, deter their use in current practice.

Branched-chain amino acids (BCAA), a dietary supplement, can be added to parenteral nutrition and has shown more rapid improvement in neuropsychiatric symptoms, although no standard dose exists. Patients with severe protein malnutrition may benefit from BCAA supplementation, but the short- and long-term benefit remains to be seen.

Monitoring Patient Response

For acute episodes of OHE, close monitoring is required to ensure that drug therapy targets are achieved and progression into more severe grades of OHE does not occur. Daily ammonia levels may be used to determine response to drug therapy but is not routinely used. Clinical evaluation of mental status through the Glasgow Coma Scale is the most reliable assessment of patient response to therapy and can be used at the bedside without additional resources.

Patient Education

Drug Information

Patients can obtain information about cirrhosis from the National Institute of Diabetes and Digestive and Kidney Diseases at https://www.niddk.nih.gov/health-information/liver-disease/cirrhosis and through the U.S. Department of Veterans Affairs at https://www.hepatitis.va.gov/pdf/cirrhosis_handbook.pdf. The handbook provided by the Veterans Affairs provides guidance on when to seek care, as well as a guide of care, so patients can be active contributors to their health.

Nutrition/Lifestyle Changes

Of all the dietary recommendations for patients with cirrhosis, the single most important instruction should be to abstain from any alcohol use. Avoidance of alcohol can slow the progression of cirrhosis and minimize episodes of decompensation. Other dietary recommendations revolve around prevention and management of specific complications of cirrhosis. Like patients with heart failure, patients with cirrhosis and ascites should be instructed to limit sodium intake to 2,000 mg/day or lower. Fluid restriction should not be routinely employed unless the serum sodium is less than 125 mmol/L while patients are taking diuretics for ascites. Patients should be counseled to avoid potassium-rich foods to minimize the risk of developing hyperkalemia, particularly if spironolactone monotherapy is utilized.

Patients with ascites should abstain from the use of prescription and over-the-counter, nonsteroidal, antiinflammatory agents as these products can not only contribute to increasing risk of acute kidney injury but also lead to accumulation of fluid through its effects on the renal vasculature.

Current guidelines recommend optimization of nutrition to minimize recurrent HE, as nearly 75% of these patients have some degree of protein-calorie malnutrition because of the significant catabolic state of patients with cirrhosis. Although seemingly counterintuitive, it is pivotal for patients with or at risk of HE to ensure adequate protein intake to prevent further muscle breakdown, which is a frequent contributor to HE. Milk or vegetable-based protein is currently recommended over meat-based proteins. Current nutritional targets include protein of 1.2 to 1.5 mg/kg/day and a total of 35 to 40 kcal/kg of ideal body weight (divided between fats and carbohydrates). Patients will likely need small meals divided across the waking hours and can be augmented with supplemental nutritional drinks to achieve these targets.

Complementary and Alternative Medications

Although the use of complementary and alternative medications for the management of cirrhosis have increased in the recent years, many of these therapies carry a significant risk of hepatotoxicity and are not proven to be effective. Commonly used agents such as valerian, vitamin A, nonsteroidal antiinflammatory drugs, and acetaminophen, even in appropriate doses, are associated with higher risk of hospitalization and/or liver injury.

VIRAL HEPATITIS

Causes

HBV and HCV are blood-borne pathogens and are spread via transmission of infected blood and body fluids. Risk factors for HBV and HCV are similar and include exposure to blood or blood-contaminated body fluids, injection drug use, unprotected sexual intercourse with an infected person, men who have sex with men, household contacts or sexual partners of known persons with chronic HBV or HCV infection, hemodialysis, infants born to infected mothers. Additional risk factors for HCV acquisition include clotting factor concentrate receipt prior to 1987 and blood transfusion or organ transplant receipt prior to 1992. Screening for HCV was not implemented until this time.

Pathophysiology

Hepatitis viruses replicate preferentially in the hepatocytes of the liver. In general, acute and chronic hepatitis can be differentiated based on the duration of inflammation in the liver. Acute hepatitis lasts less than 6 months, and chronic hepatitis lasts longer than 6 months. HBV and HCV are not cytopathic to the hepatocytes; rather, they induce an immune response, which causes hepatic inflammation and damage, leading to fibrosis, and cirrhosis.

HBV and HCV infection can be acute or chronic. Acute HBV infection is defined as the presence of HBsAg less than 6 months, while chronic HBV infection is defined as the presence of HBsAg more than 6 months. Acute HCV infection can be defined by a positive HCV ribonucleic acid (RNA) for up to 6 months following the initial infection. Chronic HCV infection is defined as a persistently positive RNA for more than 6 months (lower limit of detection is generally <15 IU/mL). HCV is more likely to become a chronic infection than HBV with up to 85% of patients who acquire acute HCV developing chronic infection. The likelihood of HBV chronicity depends on the age at acquisition. The highest risk is in infants who acquire HBV perinatally. If HBV is acquired during childhood, it is likely to become a chronic infection (~30%). If HBV is acquired during adulthood, it is also less likely to become a chronic infection (~5%).

Hepatitis B Virus

Blood circulation allows the HBV virion to reach the liver. There, it attaches to the hepatocyte for transport into the nucleus. The HBV deoxyribonucleic acid (DNA) is converted into covalently closed circular (ccc) DNA, which integrates with the host DNA and is a template for RNA to be transcribed. This cccDNA is the reason why HBV persists in hepatocytes. Drugs used to treat HBV infection target transcription; by competitively inhibiting HBV polymerase, the viral DNA strand is prematurely terminated. Once RNA is transcribed, it can be transported to the cytoplasm where it can be exported out of the cell to infect other cells. Several proteins and enzymes are required for viral replication. These proteins can also aid in diagnosis.

Hepatitis C Virus

HCV reaches the liver via lymphatic and blood circulation. Once it enters the hepatocyte, structural and non-structural proteins are responsible for replication, including NS5A protease, NS5B polymerase, and NS3/4A protein, which are used as drug targets. HCV does not possess a proof-reading polymerase; thus, viral mutations are frequent. Once replication is complete, the virus is exported from the hepatocyte and into the circulation to infect other cells.

Diagnostic Criteria

Patients with acute HBV or HCV may be asymptomatic or may exhibit nonspecific symptoms including right upper quadrant pain, fatigue, myalgia/arthralgia, fever, nausea, jaundice, pruritis, and dark urine. When HBV or HCV becomes chronic, hepatic symptoms and extrahepatic manifestations may occur. As liver disease progresses, symptoms of cirrhosis may become present.

Hepatitis B Virus

To evaluate the presence of HBV, various proteins made by the HBV and antibodies can be found (**Tables 27.9** and **27.10**).

For patients with chronic HBV infection, further evaluation is required to determine the likelihood of liver disease progression. This will often determine the need for antiviral therapy to prevent cirrhosis (**Table 27.11**).

Hepatitis C Virus

To evaluate the presence of HCV infection, serologic markers and a viral load can be assessed (**Table 27.12**):

- Antibody to HCV (anti-HCV)—It develops in patients who have been exposed to the HCV virus regardless of chronicity and becomes detectable in approximately 6 weeks. Patients are screened for HCV infection using anti-HCV. It does not confer immunity and will remain present, even if the patient is not chronically infected with HCV.
- HCV RNA—It is detectable during acute and chronic infections.

Initiating Drug Therapy

Hepatitis B Virus

Treatment for HBV infection is not given to all patients. AASLD and The European Association for the Study of the Liver have clinical guidelines that recommend times to consider the initiation of treatment. Certain laboratory characteristics must be evaluated prior to initiating therapy to assist in treatment decisions (**Table 27.13**).

Hepatitis C Virus

Treatment for HCV infection should be initiated in all patients, regardless of duration of infection. Treatment should not be initiated in patients who have a limited life expectancy (generally less than 6–12 months) from a complication unrelated to HCV.

TABLE 27.9

Hepatitis B Serologic Markers and Interpretation

Serologic Marker	Abbreviation(s)	Description
Hepatitis B surface antigen	HBsAg	Detectable at the onset of clinical symptoms; when present for >6 months indicates a chronic infection
Antibody to HBsAg	Anti-HBsAg, Anti-HBs	Development of an antibody to HBsAg denotes immunity to HBV; detectable in patients who have been vaccinated against HBV
Hepatitis B e-antigen	HBeAg	Present in an acute infection; generally, a marker of viral replication and infectivity; however, some HBV infections never express HBeAg.
Antibody to HBeAg	Anti-HBeAg/Anti-HBe	Develops once an HBeAg-positive infection is resolved. Also termed *seroconversion*
Hepatitis B core antigen	HBcAg	A nucleocapsid protein that promotes immune-mediated cell death
Antibodies to HBcAb	HBcAb/anti-HBc	Detectable once exposed to HBV infection; does not determine if infection is active
Hepatitis B virus DNA	HBV DNA	Detectable during acute and chronic infections

DNA, deoxyribonucleic acid.

TABLE 27.10

Interpretation of Hepatitis B Serologic Results

HBsAg	Anti-HBs	HBeAg	HbeAb	Anti-HBc	HBV DNA	Interpretation
+	−	+/−	+/−	+	+	Acute infection
+	−	+/−	+/−	+	+	Chronic infection
−	+	−	−	−	−	Immune due to vaccination
−	+	−	−	+	−	Immune due to natural infection
−	−	−	−	−	−	Susceptible to infection

Note: + indicates presence of a serologic marker; − indicates a serologic marker is not present.

Once a patient is determined to have chronic HBV infection, further differentiation can be made to determine chronic infection from chronic hepatitis. Terminology for classifying these types of infection has changed in recent years.

Anti-HBc, hepatitis B core antibody; Anti-HBs, hepatitis B surface antibody; DNA, deoxyribonucleic acid; HbeAb, hepatitis B e-antigen antibody; HBeAg, hepatitis B e-antigen; HBsAg, hepatitis B surface antigen; HBV, hepatitis B virus.

TABLE 27.11

Classification of Chronic Hepatitis B Infection

	ALT	HBV DNA	HBeAg	HBsAg	Active Liver Disease	Disease Progression
Chronic infection	WNL	Increased (>1 million IU/mL)	Present	High	None/minimal	Low
Chronic hepatitis	Increased	Increased (>20,000 IU/mL)	Present	High-intermediate	Present	Moderate-high
Chronic Infection	WNL	<2,000 IU/mL	Not present	Low	None	Low
Chronic hepatitis	Increased	Increased (>2,000 IU/mL)	Not present	Low-intermediate	Present	Moderate-high

ALT, alanine aminotransferase; DNA, deoxyribonucleic acid; HBeAg, hepatitis B e-antigen; HBsAg, hepatitis B surface antigen; HBV, hepatitis B virus; WNL, within normal limits.

TABLE 27.12

Interpretation of Hepatitis C Serologic Results

		HCV RNA	
		Detectable	Undetectable
HCV antibody	Positive	Acute/chronic infection (depending on duration of detectable HCV RNA)	Resolved HCV infection
	Negative	Acute infection/chronic infection in immunocompromised host	No infection

Note: HCV antibody does not confer immunity and is not protective against future HCV infections.

HCV, hepatitis C virus; RNA, ribonucleic acid.

TABLE 27.13

Current Recommendations for Treatment Initiation

HBeAg (+)			HBeAg (−)		
HBV DNA, IU/mL	ALT, U/L	Histologic Disease Presence	HBV DNA, IU/mL	ALT, U/L	Histologic Disease Presence
Any	>2 × ULN	N/A	Any	>2 × ULN	N/A
>20,000	Any	Any	>2,000	Any	Any
Any	Any	Cirrhosis	Any	Any	Cirrhosis

ALT, alanine aminotransferase; DNA, deoxyribonucleic acid; HBeAg, hepatitis B e-antigen; HBV, hepatitis B virus.

Goals of Drug Therapy

Hepatitis B Virus

Goals of therapy for HBV include suppression of viral replication to the point of undetectable HBV DNA, loss of HBsAg, prevention of cirrhosis and related complications of end stage liver disease, prevention of HCC, and minimization and mitigation of drug therapy adverse effects and toxicity. In patients with hepatitis B e-antigen (HBeAg) disease, attaining seroconversion loss of HBeAg and development of anti-HBe should also be achieved.

Hepatitis C Virus

Similar goals of preventing liver-related morbidity and mortality exist in the treatment of patients with HCV. Additionally, achieving sustained virologic response (SVR) at 12 weeks (SVR12), defined as an undetectable level of HCV RNA (<15 IU/mL) 12 weeks after completing treatment, is the primary marker of successful HCV treatment.

Selecting the Most Appropriate Drug—Hepatitis B Virus

Several antiviral agents have been approved for the treatment of HBV infection (**Table 27.14**).

First-Line Therapy

Peginterferon, entecavir (ETV), or Tenofovir disoproxil fumarate (TDF) and tenofovir alamfenamide (TAF) are preferred first-line options. The pegylated form of interferon is preferred to non-pegylated formulations due to improved patient tolerance and less frequent administration. ETV, TAF, and TDF may be preferred in patients unwilling to receive injections and should be preferentially used in patients with or at risk of bone and renal complications (i.e., osteoporosis, osteomalacia, chronic kidney disease). If tenofovir is chosen, TAF should be avoided if the creatinine clearance is less than 15 mL/min or hemodialysis is required.

Second-Line Therapy

Alternative drug therapy options for the treatment of HBV include lamivudine (3TC) and adefovir (ADV). These agents are not preferred to first-line options because of their lower barrier to resistance. 3TC does have the potential to be useful in some patients with HBV-human immunodeficiency virus (HIV) coinfection.

Time Frame for Response

Interferon products are administered for a finite period, usually 48 weeks. Response will be assessed at this time. Patients who respond to interferon therapy are unlikely to relapse. Oral products are administered until patients achieve seroconversion in those with HBeAg present at baseline. Generally, therapy would be stopped 6 months after achieving seroconversion, provided HBV DNA remains undetectable. If HBeAg is not present at baseline, then treatment should be continued indefinitely as HBsAg loss is uncommon. Relapse is common after therapy is discontinued. Patients with cirrhosis should be treated indefinitely, regardless of HBeAg status.

TABLE 27.14

Drug Therapy for Hepatitis B Virus

Generic	Class	MOA	Dose	Adverse Events
Interferon alfa-2b Peginterferon alfa-2a	Immuno-modulator	Induces immune system to exert antiviral activity	5 million IU sq daily 10 million IU sq 3×/week 180 mcg sq once weekly	Systemic effects (flu-like syndrome, fever/chills, myalgias/arthralgias, fatigue) Mood disturbances (depression, irritability, insomnia) Hematologic (myelosuppression—neutropenia, anemia, thrombocytopenia) Endocrine (hypo/hyperthyroidism) Dermatologic (alopecia, injection site reactions) Gastrointestinal (anorexia, nausea, weight loss, LFT increases)
3TC	Reverse transcriptase inhibitor	Nucleoside analog	100 mg PO daily 300 mg PO daily for HIV-infected	Headache Fatigue Nausea/vomiting/diarrhea Insomnia Myalgias/CK elevation/rhabdomyolysis LFT increases Pancreatitis
ADV	DNA polymerase inhibitor	Acyclic nucleoside analog	10 mg PO daily	Headache Weakness Abdominal pain Hematuria Rash Nephrotoxicity
ETV	DNA polymerase inhibitor	Guanosine nucleoside analog	0.5 mg PO daily treatment - naïve 1 mg PO daily 3TC resistance Dose adjust when CrCl < 50 mL/min	Peripheral edema Pyrexia Ascites LFT increases Hematuria Nephrotoxicity/SCr increases
LdT	Reverse transcriptase inhibitor/DNA polymerase inhibitor	Nucleoside analog	600 mg PO daily	Upper respiratory tract infection/nasopharyngitis Headache Fatigue Myopathy/CK elevation Lactic acidosis
TDF	Reverse transcriptase inhibitor	Nucleotide analog	300 mg PO daily Dose "adjust" when CrCl <50 mL/min.	Headache Depression Nausea/vomiting/diarrhea Loss of bone density (osteopenia) Nephrotoxicity (Fanconi syndrome) LFT and CPK increases
TAF	Reverse transcriptase inhibitor	Nucleotide analog	25 mg PO daily Dose "adjust" when CrCl <10 mL/min (give after dialysis)	Less likely to cause adverse effects than TDF formulation Headache Abdominal pain Nausea Fatigue Cough Loss of bone density (osteopenia) LFT increases

3TC, lamivudine; ADV, adefovir; CK, creatinine kinase; CPK, creatinine phosphokinase; DNA, deoxyribonucleic acid; ETV, entecavir; HIV, human immunodeficiency virus; LdT, Telbivudine; LFT, liver function tests; MOA, mechanism of action; TAF, tenofovir alamfenamide; TDF, tenofovir disoproxil fumarate.

Contraindications

Interferon products should be avoided in patients with autoimmune disorders, uncontrolled psychiatric disorders, decompensated hepatic disease, cardiac disease, hematologic abnormalities, and uncontrolled seizures. Oral nucleotide reverse transcriptase inhibitors (NRTIs) for HBV, except for telbivudine, can cause HIV resistance in patients with untreated HIV infection due to their activity against HIV.

Interactions

Interferon products have many significant interactions with drugs, leading to enhanced side effect profiles and thus increasing the likelihood of toxicities. Oral NRTIs for HBV are eliminated by the kidneys. Drugs that are eliminated by active tubular secretion may increase concentrations of the oral NRTI and/or the coadministered drug. Drugs that decrease renal function may increase concentrations of the oral NRTI.

Selecting the Most Appropriate Drug—Hepatitis C Virus

The direct acting antivirals (DAAs) have revolutionized HCV care since their introduction to the market in 2011. There are three classes of DAAs including the NS3/4A protease inhibitors (glecaprevir [GLE], grazoprevir, and voxilaprevir), the NS5A inhibitors (elbasvir, ledipasvir [LDV], pibrentasvir [PIB], and velpatasvir), and the NS5B polymerase inhibitors (sofosbuvir [SOF]) (**Table 27.15**). Ribavirin, an antiviral agent, may be added to some DAA regimens to increase SVR rates. DAAs are administered as multidrug regimens.

All patients with HCV infection should be screened for HBV infection prior to DAA initiation. Risk factors for acquisition are similar. When a patient with HBV and HCV coinfection who was previously HBsAg negative and hepatitis B core antibody (anti-HBc) positive is started on DAA treatment, an abrupt increase in HBV DNA level or detection of HBsAg can occur. This can be followed by fulminant hepatitis. Patients with current or prior HBV infection should be monitored for clinical and laboratory signs (HBsAg, HBV DNA, liver function tests [LFTs], bilirubin) of hepatitis flare or HBV reactivation during DAA treatment and post-treatment follow-up.

Guidelines exist to help guide the care of patients with HBV and HCV. The American Association of Liver Disease has published guidelines to assist with care of HBV. First-line therapy for HBV includes pegylated interferon and the oral nucleos(t)ide inhibitors, ETV, TAF, and TDF. These agents are preferred due to a low risk of resistance. Factors to consider when selecting an agent include patient factors (age, renal impairment, comorbidities such as osteoporosis, drug–drug interaction, and cost). Interferon-based products, because of their toxicity, should be used in patients who have minimal disease and do not have contraindications.

TABLE 27.15

Currently Available Direct Acting Antiviral Products

Drug	MOA	Dosage	Genotype Coverage	Interactions
Sofosbuvir (SOF)	NS5B polymerase inhibitor	400 mg	1 to 6	Coadministration with amiodarone can cause symptomatic and severe bradycardia. Use not recommended.
Sofosbuvir/Ledipasvir (LDV/SOF; LED/SOF)	NS5B polymerase inhibitor/NS5A inhibitor	400 mg/90 mg	1, 4, 5, 6	Acid-suppressing agents decrease concentrations of ledipasvir. Substrate of P-gp
Elbasvir/Grazoprevir (ELB/GRZ)	NS5A inhibitor/NS3/4A protease inhibitor	50 mg/100 mg	1, 4	Substrate of CYP3A, OATP1/B1/3
Sofosbuvir/Velpatasvir (SOF/VEL)	NS5B polymerase inhibitor/NS5A inhibitor	400 mg/100 mg	1 to 6	Acid- suppressing agents decrease concentrations of velpatasvir. Substrate of P-gp, CYP2B6, CYP2C8, CYP3A4
Sofosbuvir/ Velpatasvir/ Voxilaprevir (SOF/VEL/VOX)	NS5B polymerase inhibitor/NS5A inhibitor/NS3/4A protease inhibitor	400 mg/100 mg/100 mg	1 to 6	Acid-suppressing agents decrease concentrations of velpatasvir. Substrate of P-gp, CYP2B6, CYP2C8, CYP3A4, CYP1A2
Glecaprevir/ Pibrentasvir (GLE/ PIB; G/P)	NS3/4A protease inhibitor/NS5A inhibitor	100 mg/40 mg (total daily dose 300 mg/120 mg)	1 to 6	Substrate of P-gp, OATP1B1/3 Inhibitor of P-gp, BCRP, OATP1B1/3 Weak inhibitor of CYP3A, CYP1A2, UGT1A1

BCRP, breast cancer resistance protein; MOA, mechanism of action; OATP1B1, organic anion transporter family member 1B1.

The American Association of Liver Disease and Infectious Disease Society of America has collaborated on guidelines for HCV care, which are freely available at www.hcvguidelines.org. The guidelines are organized by genotype and other patient characteristics such as presence or absence of cirrhosis and treatment history. First-line treatment is a combination therapy of at least two DAAs. Factors that should be considered when selecting a regimen include viral factors (HCV genotype and subtype, baseline HCV RNA, resistance), treatment factors (ribavirin eligibility, treatment history), hepatic disease (Meta-analysis of Histological Data in Viral Hepatitis fibrosis stage, cirrhosis status), coinfection and comorbidities (HIV, drug–drug interactions), financial considerations (insurance approval, preferred formulary agent, cost to the patient), and social/behavioral considerations (alcohol and drug use, ongoing risk of infection, and patient adherence).

Overall, DAAs are well tolerated. Frequently occurring adverse effects with the DAA drug class include headache, fatigue, and nausea. Nausea occurs more frequently in patients on DAAs containing a protease inhibitor. Patients should be educated about eating habits along with administration of DAAs containing protease enzymes to decrease the likelihood of nausea. DAAs containing a protease inhibitor also have a risk of hepatic decompensation and should be avoided in patients with decompensated cirrhosis.

Special Considerations

Pediatric

Hepatitis B Virus

Clinicians should consider treatment with antiviral therapy in HBeAg-positive children (ages 2–18 years) with both elevated ALT and measurable HBV DNA levels, with the goal of achieving sustained HBeAg seroconversion.

If treating children, interferon-alpha-2b is approved for children of 1 year of age and older and should be continued for 24 weeks. 3TC and ETV are approved for children of 2 years of age and older and should be continued until seroconversion occurs. TDF is approved for children of 12 years of age and older and should be continued until seroconversion occurs. TAF has not been studied in children to date.

Hepatitis C Virus

If DAA treatment is available for a child's age group and infecting genotype, all children over the age of 3 years should be treated, independent of disease severity.

GLE/PIB is FDA approved for pediatric patients with any genotype more than 12 years of age and more than 45 kg. SOF/LDV can be used in patients as young as 3 years of age with dose adjustments, provided they have genotype 1, 4, 5, or 6 infection.

Geriatric

Geriatric patients may have renal impairment or may be on medications that interact. Ensure that medications are dosed appropriately for degree of renal impairment.

The baby boomers, or those born between 1945 and 1965, have a high rate of HCV. All patients in this birth cohort should be tested for HCV.

Women

Hepatitis B Virus

HBV treatment during pregnancy is not routinely recommended. HBV can be treated during pregnancy if HBV DNA is more than 200,000 IU/mL. First-line treatment during pregnancy is TDF. Other choices include telbivudine or 3TC. Antiviral treatment can be discontinued 3 months post-partum with continued ALT monitoring.

Following birth to a HBsAg-positive mother, the infant should be provided the first dose of hepatitis B vaccine and a hepatitis B immunoglobulin to prevent perinatal infection.

Breastfeeding can be performed without risk of HBV transmission since infants are vaccinated and given immunoglobulin. Limited data exist on the safety of tenofovir and 3TC in lactation.

Hepatitis C Virus

HCV treatment is not currently recommended during pregnancy. Women of child-bearing age should be treated prior to pregnancy to prevent transmission.

Ribavirin is teratogenic. If using a DAA regimen that includes ribavirin, women and the female partners of treated males will need to wait at least 6 months after therapy completion to conceive to prevent birth defects.

Following birth to a mother who is HCV positive, the infant should be tested for an HCV antibody after 18 months of age. If positive, HCV RNA should be evaluated after the age of 3 to determine chronicity of infection. Breastfeeding can be performed without risk of HCV transmission except when the mother has cracked, damaged, or bleeding nipples. No data exist about the safety of DAAs in lactation.

Genomics: Hepatitis C Virus

Resistance-associated variants or substitutions (RAV and RAS) are common in patients with HCV infection since it lacks a proofreading polymerase. Some RAV and RAS may decrease efficacy of DAA treatment. Concern for resistance will vary depending on the infecting genotype and the DAA class being used (**Table 27.16**).

RAV and RAS are common in patients with HCV infection since it lacks a proofreading polymerase. Some RAV and RAS may decrease efficacy of DAA treatment.

- **NS5A Inhibitors**—The presence of NS5A RAS (specifically Y93H) can cause a reduction in efficacy of some DAA combinations in genotype 1a or genotype 3 infection. These RAS tend to persist over many years.
- **NS3/4A Protease Inhibitors**—The presence of NS3/4A RAS can cause a reduction of efficacy in some DAA combinations in genotype 1a infection. RAS disappear within several months of medication discontinuation.
- **NS5B Polymerase Inhibitors**—No clinically occurring RAS that decrease response to DAAs have been discovered. RAS disappear within several months of medication discontinuation.

Prior to utilizing certain DAA combinations in patients with genotype 1a or 3 infections, RAV and RAS should be checked depending on drug therapy choice (**Table 27.17**). If a patient does

TABLE 27.16

Direct Acting Antiviral Class and Risk of Resistance

DAA Class	Resistance Concern
NS5A Inhibitors	The presence of NS5A RAS (specifically Y93H) can cause a reduction in efficacy of some DAA combinations in genotype 1a or genotype 3 infection. These RAS tend to persist over many years.
NS3/4A Protease Inhibitors	The presence of NS3/4A RAS can cause a reduction of efficacy in some DAA combinations in genotype 1a infection. RAS disappear within several months of medication discontinuation.
NS5B Polymerase Inhibitors	No clinically occurring RAS that decrease response to DAAs have been discovered. RAS disappear within several months of medication discontinuation.

DAA, direct acting antivirals; RAS, resistance-associated substitutions.

not have genotype 1a or 3 infection or is not using one of the listed regimens, evaluating RAV or RAS is not clinically necessary.

Monitoring Patient Response

Hepatitis B Virus

Monitoring of patients on HBV treatment will depend on therapy selection. Patients on interferon products will have more frequent monitoring performed for adverse effects than those on oral therapy. In patients who initiate HBV treatment, LFTs should be monitored every 3 to 4 months for 1 year and then can be checked every 6 months. Serologic markers such as HBV DNA and HBeAg can be evaluated on a similar time frame. Patients who have undetectable HBV DNA can be evaluated for anti-HBe (in patients who are HBeAg positive) and HBsAg. If HBsAg is negative, hepatitis B surface antibody (anti-HBs) can be tested. Clinical monitoring for decompensation and HCC should be performed at regular intervals.

Hepatitis C Virus

On-treatment monitoring depends on the DAA regimen that is used. DAA regimens are generally well tolerated, but adverse effect monitoring should be performed as clinically indicated. Current practice guidelines recommend evaluating HCV RNA 4 weeks into treatment. At this time, HCV RNA should be undetectable. If HCV RNA is still detected, an additional HCV RNA should be drawn 6 weeks into treatment, though the utility of continuing treatment is unknown. Patients who have initiated DAA therapy should have HCV RNA checked 12 weeks after completing drug treatment. The absence of HCV RNA at 12 weeks determines "cure" and is termed *SVR*. If a patient has underlying hepatic impairment, they will need to have future hepatic follow-up to assess for hepatic function and evaluate for HCC.

Patient Education

Drug Information

The Centers for Disease Control and Prevention and NIH have several up-to-date disease and drug information resources freely available to patients at https://www.cdc.gov/hepatitis/resources/patientedmaterials.htm,https://www.niddk.nih.gov/health-information/liver-disease/viral-hepatitis/what-is-viral-hepatitis.

TABLE 27.17

Evaluation of Resistance-Associated Variants and Substitutions in Direct Acting Antiviral Regimens

Genotype 1a		
	Grazoprevir/elbasvir	Evaluate for NS5A RAS in all treatment-naïve or -experienced patients. If RAS are present, treatment will need to be extended to 16 weeks and ribavirin will need to be added or an alternate regimen should be considered.
	Ledipasvir/sofosbuvir—	Evaluate for NS5A RAS in treatment-experienced patients. If RAS are present (>100 fold resistance), an alternate regimen should be considered.
	Simeprevir	Evaluate for Q80K, which can cause a decreased response to simeprevir in patients with genotype 1a. Note that the use of simeprevir is not recommended and the agent is no longer available in the United States.
Genotype 3		
	Sofosbuvir/velpatasvir	Evaluate for NS5A RAS (Y93H) in treatment-naïve patients with cirrhosis and all treatment-experienced patients. If present, addition of ribavirin or use of sofosbuvir/velpatasvir/voxilaprevir should be considered.
	Daclatasvir + sofosbuvir	Evaluate for NS5A RAS (Y93H) in treatment-experienced patients without cirrhosis and treatment-naïve patients with cirrhosis. If present, addition of ribavirin or use of an alternate agent should be considered. Note that the use of daclatasvir is not recommended and the agent is no longer available in the United States.

RAS, resistance-associated substitutions.

Nutrition/Lifestyle Changes

Patients should be encouraged to avoid hepatotoxic medications including alcohol. No amount of alcohol has been shown to be safe in a patient with HBV or HCV.

Patients who have HBV/HCV should be educated on prevention of transmission, including not sharing products that have blood on it, which could include syringes and needles (for illicit drug use, health care–associated transmission, tattoos, etc.) toothbrushes, shaving equipment, fingernail clippers, among others. Patients should also be educated on the risk of sexual transmission, which, although low with HCV, is increased in patients with HIV, in those with sexually transmitted infections/diseases, and in those with multiple partners.

Obesity and the metabolic syndrome can hasten fibrosis progression, so appropriate dietary and exercise modifications should be encouraged.

Complementary and Alternative Medications

Several complementary and alternative medicines, including milk thistle (silymarin) and licorice root (glycyrrhizin), have been used as hepatoprotectants and/or antivirals for hepatitis. No proven benefit exists with any complementary and alternative medicine. All have potential side effects, drug interactions, and/or risk. The Hepatitis C Antiviral Long-Term Treatment Against Cirrhosis trial of 1,145 people infected with HCV found that 23% of responders were using herbal supplements for HCV despite limited to no evidence of clinical benefit (Halegoua-DeMarzio, 2014).

CASE STUDY 1

Otis Jakobsen is a 68-year-old man with a past medical history significant for hypertension and type 2 diabetes mellitus, for which he takes lisinopril 30 mg daily and metformin 1,000 mg twice daily, respectively. He is known to have several hospital admissions for alcohol intoxication and withdrawal. He presents to the emergency department today with complaints of abdominal distention and dull abdominal tenderness. His wife reports that he has not been sleeping well, and during the day, he is agitated and can become disoriented, which is new for him.

An abdominal ultrasound is ordered, which reveals nodular appearance of the liver and approximately 1.5 L of peritoneal fluid. Labs return with the following significant values: while blood cell (WBC) 12 cells/mm^3, blood urea nitrogen 42 mEq/L, creatinine 1.0 mg/dL (baseline ~0.8 mg/dL), bilirubin 4.9 mg/dL, albumin 2.9 g/dL, and international normalized ratio 1.2.

His ascitic fluid is also run for cytology, and the results are as follows:

Gross appearance: cloudy
WBC: 635 cells/mm^3
Lymphocytes: 20%
Neutrophils: 40%
Red blood cell: 20 cells/mm^3
Albumin: 1.0 g/dL

1. What is the patient's current ascitic fluid polymorphonuclear (PMN) count? If antibiotic therapy is indicated for spontaneous bacterial peritonitis (SBP), which agent would be appropriate to start empirically?
2. Based on the available information, what other major complications of cirrhosis are present, and what intervention(s) would be appropriate at this time?
3. Assuming the patient recovers from this admission, what drug therapy should be initiated to manage his complications of cirrhosis?

Bibliography

Starred references are cited in the text.

AASLD-IDSA HCV Guidance Panel. (2018). Hepatitis C guidance 2018 update: AASLD-IDSA recommendations for testing, managing, and treating hepatitis C virus infection. *Clinical Infectious Diseases, 67*(10), 1477–1492.

Bass, L. M. (2018). Variceal bleeding and morbidity- considerations for primary prophylaxis. *Journal of Pediatric Gastroenterology and Nutrition, 67*(3), 312–313.

Bernardi, M., Angeli, P., Claria, J., et al. (2020). Albumin in decompensated cirrhosis: New concepts and perspectives. *Gut, 69*(6), 1127–1138.

Bourlière, M., Gordon, S. C., Flamm, S. L., et al. (2017). Sofosbuvir, velpatasvir, and voxilaprevir for previously treated HCV infection. *New England Journal of Medicine, 376*(22), 2134–2146.

*Centers for Disease Control and Prevention. (2020, October 30). *FastStats*. Chronic Liver Disease or Cirrhosis. https://www.cdc.gov/nchs/fastats/liver-disease.htm.

Chancharoenthana, W., & Leelahavanichkul, A. (2019). Acute kidney injury spectrum in patients with chronic liver disease: Where do we stand? *World Journal of Gastroenterology, 25*(28), 3684–3703.

Charlton, M., Everson, G. T., Flamm, S. L., et al. (2015). Ledipasvir and sofosbuvir plus ribavirin for treatment of HCV infection in patients with advanced liver disease. *Gastroenterology, 149*(3), 649–659.

Feld, J. J., Jacobson, I. M., Hézode, C., et al. (2015). Sofosbuvir and velpatasvir for HCV genotype 1, 2, 4, 5, and 6 infection. *New England Journal of Medicine, 373*(27), 2599–2607.

Garbuzenko, D. V., & Arefyev, N. O. (2019). Current approaches to the management of patients with cirrhotic ascites. *World Journal of Gastroenterology, 25*(28), 3738–3752.

Garcia-Tsao, G., Abraldes, J. G., Berzigotti A., et al. (2017). Portal hypertensive bleeding in cirrhosis: Risk stratification, diagnosis, and management: 2016 practice guidance by the American Association for the Study of Liver Diseases. *Hepatology, 65*(1), 310–335.

*Groszmann, R. J., Garcia-Tsao, G., Bosch, J., et al. (2005). Beta-blockers to prevent gastroesophageal varices in patients with cirrhosis. *NEJM, 353*(21), 2254–2261.

*Halegoua-DeMarzio, D. L., & Finkel, J. M. (2014). Complementary and alternative medication in hepatitis C infection. *World Journal of Hepatology, 6*(1), 9–16.

Li, T., Ke, W., Sun, P., et al. (2016). Carvedilol for portal hypertension in cirrhosis: Systematic review with meta-analysis. *BMJ Open, 6*(5), e010902.

Long, B., & Koyfman, A. (2018). The emergency medicine evaluation and management of the patient with cirrhosis. *The American Journal of Emergency Medicine, 36*(4), 689–698.

*Moon, A. M., Singal, A. G., & Tapper, E. B. (2020). Contemporary epidemiology of chronic liver disease and cirrhosis. *Clinical Gastroenterology and Hepatology, 18*(12), 2650–2666. doi: 10.1016/j.cgh.2019.07.060

Moreau, R., Elkrief, L., Bureau, C., et al. (2018). Effects of long-term norfloxacin therapy in patients with advanced cirrhosis. *Gastroenterology, 155*(6), 1816–1827.e9.

Sauerbruch, T., Mengel, M., Dollinger, M., et al. (2015). Prevention of rebleeding from esophageal varices in patients with cirrhosis receiving small-diameter stents versus hemodynamically controlled medical therapy. *Gastroenterology, 149*(3), 660–668.e1.

Shehata, H. H., Elfert, A. A., Abdin, A. A., et al. (2018). Randomized controlled trial of polyethylene glycol versus lactulose for the treatment of overt hepatic encephalopathy. *European Journal of Gastroenterology & Hepatology, 30*(12), 1476–1481.

Terrault, N. A., Lok, A. S. F., McMahon, B. J., et al. (2018). Update on prevention, diagnosis, and treatment of chronic hepatitis B: AASLD 2018 Hepatitis B Guidance. *Hepatology, 67*(4), 1560–1599.

*U. S. National Library of Medicine. (2020). Clinical trials. Retrieved from www.clinicaltrials.gov. on June 3, 2020.

Zeuzem, S., Ghalib, S., Reddy, K. R., et al. (2015). Grazoprevir–elbasvir combination therapy for treatment-naive cirrhotic and noncirrhotic patients with chronic hepatitis C virus genotype 1, 4, or 6 infection: A randomized trial. *Annals of Internal Medicine, 163*(1), 1–13.

Pharmacotherapy for Genitourinary Tract Disorders

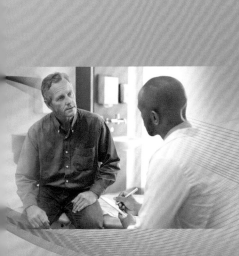

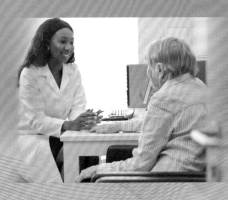

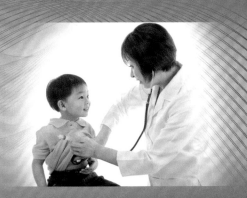

28 Urinary Tract Infection

Veronica F. Wilbur

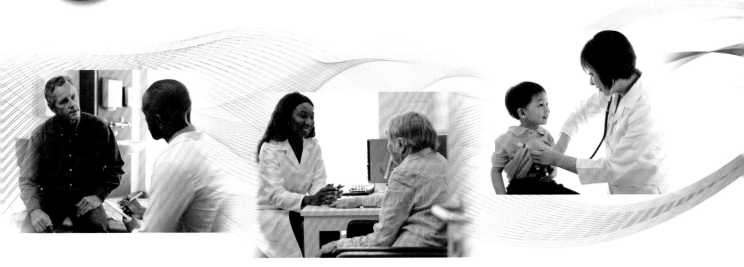

Learning Objectives

1. Identify common bacterial agents that cause urinary tract infections in children, men, and women.
2. Select an appropriate antibiotic based on the current evidence-based guidelines.
3. Distinguish appropriate changes to pharmacologic therapy for acute cystitis, pyelonephritis, and complicated urinary tract infection.

INTRODUCTION

Urinary tract infection (UTI) is a broad term used to describe inflammation of the urethra, bladder, and kidney. Bacteria, yeast, or chemical irritants can cause inflammation in the urinary tract. UTIs are a common problem encountered in health care. It is estimated that each year there are at least 150 million cases of symptomatic UTIs worldwide (Foxman, 2014). UTIs occur across the life span. UTI is more prevalent in women who are greater than 65 years old compared to the overall population (Chu & Lowder, 2018). As many as 10% of women experience at least one episode of acute uncomplicated urinary infection in a year, 50% to 60% have at least one episode during their lifetime. The peak incidence of infection occurs in young, sexually active women ages 18 to 24. In later years, UTI incidence in men and women older than 60 years is approximately equal. Recurrent episodes of UTI are experienced by as many as 10% of women during their lifetime (Medina & Castillo-Pino, 2019).

PATHOPHYSIOLOGY

In general, the urinary tract is resistant to invading bacteria and rapidly eliminates organisms that reach the bladder. As previously stated, UTI is a broad term that describes the inflammation of the urinary system. However, when an infection develops, it can be classified as either cystitis (of the bladder) or pyelonephritis (of the kidneys). Of the two infections, cystitis is the most common type of UTI that targets the bladder.

The infection mechanism is most commonly the ascension of pathogens into the urinary tract from the urethra into the bladder. These microorganisms generally come from bacteria that colonize the gut and feces, but the vagina is also an important source of infecting organisms. Once the bacteria are in the bladder, they multiply and travel up the urethra into the bladder. From the bladder, the microorganisms can ascend into the renal pelvis and parenchyma, especially if there is vesicoureteral reflux. The severity of the UTI depends on the bacterial virulence and the host defenses. Virulence involves bacterial adherence to the bladder wall and the production of toxins, and the formation of biofilm. The primary defenses of the host depend mainly on the native immunity and inflammatory factors.

Anatomically, men are at less risk for UTIs due to the longer urethra to the bladder. This length increases the distance between the rectum and the urethral meatus. The drier environment around the urethra and the antibacterial activity of prostatic fluid also decrease UTI risk in men. Later in life, men who are greater than 50 years old have an increased potential for UTIs mostly due to the enlarging prostate (see Chapter 29).

Clinical Spectrum of Urinary Tract Infection

UTIs' clinical spectrum ranges from asymptomatic bacteriuria to symptomatic and recurrent UTIs, to sepsis associated with UTI requiring hospitalization. Recent evidence helps differentiate asymptomatic bacteriuria from symptomatic UTI. Asymptomatic bacteriuria is transient in older women, often resolves without any treatment, and is not associated with morbidity or mortality. The diagnosis of symptomatic UTI is made when a patient has clinical features and laboratory evidence of a urinary infection. Absent other causes, patients presenting with any two of the following meet the clinical diagnostic criteria for symptomatic UTI: fever, worsened urinary urgency or frequency, acute dysuria, suprapubic tenderness, or costovertebral angle pain or tenderness. A positive urine culture (≥ 105 CFU/mL) with no more than two uropathogens and pyuria confirms UTI diagnosis. Risk factors for recurrent symptomatic UTI include diabetes, functional disability, recent sexual intercourse, prior history of urogynecology surgery, urinary retention, and urinary incontinence. Testing for UTI is easily performed in the clinic using dipstick tests.

> **BOX 28.1**
> ## Underlying Conditions that Predispose Individuals to Urinary Tract Infections
>
> - Female sex
> - Pregnancy
> - Diabetes
> - Chronic degenerative neurologic conditions
> - Paralysis
> - Recurrent UTI
> - Ineffective bladder emptying
> - Estrogen deficiency
> - Constipation
> - Delayed postcoital micturition
> - History of recurrent childhood UTI
> - Sickle cell disease
> - Polycystic kidney disease
> - Structural defects of the urinary system
> - Renal transplant

CAUSES

Women contract UTIs more often than men because of their anatomy of a short urethra and the proximity to the rectum. Sexual intercourse is also a contributing factor. With intercourse, periurethral and urethral bacteria may ascend into the bladder. UTI risk factors in men include homosexuality, intercourse with an infected partner, and an uncircumcised penis.

Normal urine is sterile. Infection occurs when microorganisms, usual bacteria from the digestive tract, cling to the opening of the urethra, and multiply. *Escherichia coli* is the causative pathogen in 85% to 90% of community-acquired UTIs. *Staphylococcus saprophyticus* accounts for approximately 5% to 15% of UTIs in young women. The microbial spectrum of complicated UTIs is broader and includes *Pseudomonas, Enterococcus, Staphylococcus, Serratia, Providencia*, and fungi.

Bacterial growth is decreased by dilute urine and a low urine pH. Glucose in urine is an enhanced medium for the development of *E. coli*. The urine from pregnant women has a more suitable pH for the growth of *E. coli*. Diaphragm and spermicide use (nonoxynol 9), estrogen deficiency, and constipation also are risk factors for UTIs. Inefficient bladder emptying causes UTIs because of stagnating urine. Underlying conditions that predispose to UTI are listed in **Box 28.1**.

In the average male urethra, the distance between the end of the urethra and the bladder is too long to allow ascending bacteria to the bladder. Therefore, bacteriuria in men should always be considered abnormal, and men's UTI is still classified as complicated infections.

DIAGNOSTIC CRITERIA

In women of childbearing age, the most frequent cystitis presentation is the classic triad of urinary urgency, frequency, and dysuria, with symptoms of abrupt onset. There may also be pressure or fullness in the suprapubic area and back pain. Pyelonephritis presents with flank pain, nausea and vomiting, and temperature greater than 100.4°F (38°C) with or without cystitis symptoms.

Differentiation must be made between complicated and uncomplicated UTI before progressing with diagnostic evaluation. An uncomplicated UTI is defined as occurring in a premenopausal, sexually active, nonpregnant woman who has not recently had a UTI. A complicated UTI occurs in a man, a postmenopausal or pregnant woman, or a patient with urinary structural defects, neurologic lesions, or a catheter. A UTI also is considered complicated if symptoms have persisted for more than seven days. In sexually active men with symptoms of cystitis, urethritis must be considered and ruled out. Pyelonephritis presents with recurrent fevers, chills, flank pain, and a positive urine culture.

The diagnosis of UTI is made after a careful history, physical examination, and limited laboratory studies. Because UTI is the most common infection for which adults receive antibiotics, the evaluation and management must be cost-effective. Cultures do not need to be performed if the criteria for an uncomplicated UTI are met because antimicrobial susceptibility profiles are predictable, and culture results do not return until the symptoms have been resolved. However, knowing local antibiotic grams help guide appropriate treatment selection for UTIs.

The leukocyte dipstick test is 75% to 95% sensitive in detecting pyuria. Microscopic examination of spun or unspun urine that does not show leukocytes should suggest a diagnosis other than UTI. Hematuria occurs in approximately half of all acute UTIs. Pretreatment and posttreatment cultures should be performed for male patients. Pretreatment cultures are ordered in suspected pyelonephritis; posttreatment cultures are performed only if symptoms recur within 2 weeks or if the symptoms do not resolve with treatment initially.

INITIATING DRUG THERAPY

Without treatment, 25% to 42% of uncomplicated acute cystitis cases in women resolve spontaneously. However, the standard therapy for all UTIs is antibiotic treatment.

Urine culture with 10^5/mL organisms or greater is a diagnostic indicator of UTI with or without symptoms. A patient who has symptoms and a culture with 10^2/mL organisms or greater is treated. All symptomatic UTIs should be treated. The purpose of early treatment of cystitis is to reduce the risk of progression to pyelonephritis, although the incidence is small. Treatment does not affect the duration of symptoms, which is 3 to 4 days. In patients with pyelonephritis, early treatment is important to reduce the duration of symptoms, eliminate microorganisms from the renal parenchyma, and reduce the risk of dissemination to the blood.

For some patients with cystitis, a urinary analgesic may be useful to relieve discomfort caused by severe dysuria. A 2-day course is usually sufficient to allow time for symptomatic response to antimicrobial therapy and minimize inflammation. Dysuria is usually diminished within a few hours after the start of antimicrobial therapy.

Although most UTIs resolve spontaneously even if not treated, they are treated for symptom relief. The treatment for UTI is antibiotics. The choice of antibiotic and the length of treatment depend on whether the infection is uncomplicated or complicated and on the sex and age of the patient.

A short course of treatment increases compliance and decreases the cost and side effects. For women infected with susceptible *E. coli*, cure rates of 90% to 95% are achieved with 1 to 3 days of therapy. There is no benefit to treatment exceeding 3 days in uncomplicated UTIs in women unless nitrofurantoin is used; this drug's length of treatment is 5 to 7 days.

Evidence exists regarding increasing resistance to fluoroquinolones in treating UTIs and has fallen from favor as first-line therapy for these types of infections (Khoshnood et al., 2017). Resistance to trimethoprim–sulfamethoxazole (TMP–SMZ) is up to 20% in some areas of the United States, but resistance to nitrofurantoin continues to remain low.

Goals of Therapy

The goals of therapy for UTIs are to destroy the offending organism, relieve symptoms, and prevent complications.

Antibiotics are discussed in detail in Chapter 6. Those used to treat UTIs are listed in **Table 28.1**.

Urinary Analgesics

This class of drugs is used for the symptomatic relief of pain, urgency, burning, frequency, and discomfort associated with trauma to the lower urinary tract mucosa. They are used in infection, trauma, surgery, endoscopic procedures, and catheterization. They should not be used for more than 2 days and are not used for treatment of a UTI per se, but for symptom relief.

The azo dye in this class is excreted in the urine and exerts a rapid topical analgesic effect on the mucosa of the urinary tract. The urinary analgesics are used with caution in pregnancy and lactation and are contraindicated in renal insufficiency. For additional information, see **Table 28.1**.

Selecting the Most Appropriate Agent

Antibiotics are selected by identifying the uropathogen, knowing local resistance rates, and considering adverse effect profiles. The treatment recommendations arise from the last guidelines for treatment of uncomplicated UTI. Nitrofurantoin monohydrate/macrocrystals (100 mg twice daily for 5 days) is the recognized first-line agent due to minimal resistance and adverse drug reactions. Despite heavy use, very little resistance to nitrofurantoin has developed.

Another option is a 3-day course of TMP–SMZ or TMP alone for first-line treatment. There are concerns, however, about rare but serious skin reactions to the sulfa component and about growing resistance (about 10% in Canada). This drug should be avoided in patients treated within 6 months because they are more likely to have resistant organisms.

Another choice for first-line therapy is Fosfomycin (Monurol). This is a powder dissolved in water. The advantage of this drug is the one-time dosing.

While used in the past, fluoroquinolones have more recently been introduced to treat UTIs, and they are very effective in a 3-day course. Their cost and the potential for developing resistance, however, suggest that they should remain a second-line choice for treatment. Cephalosporins, ampicillin, and amoxicillin should not be used unless the cultured organism is sensitive to these agents.

Cystitis and pyelonephritis are treated with the same antibiotic, but the treatment course for pyelonephritis is longer. The most desirable antibiotic is one that is low in cost with an infrequent dosing schedule, lack of resistance in local pathogens, long duration in the urinary tract, and the potential to decrease the number of *E. coli* in the vaginal and fecal reservoirs. The antibiotic selected should spare the protective, natural bacterial flora of the vagina and gastrointestinal tract, and there should be a low side-effect profile. Nonpregnant women with uncomplicated cystitis may be treated with a 3-day course of antibiotics (except with nitrofurantoin, which is 5–7 days). Postmenopausal women should be treated for 7 days (**Figure 28.1**; **Tables 28.2** and **28.3**). Men also require a 7-day treatment because of the increased chance of a complicated infection and prostatic infection.

TABLE 28.1

Overview of Selected Agents for Urinary Tract Infection

Generic (Trade) Name and Dosage	Selected Adverse Events	Contraindications	Special Considerations
Antibiotics			
Trimethoprim–sulfamethoxazole (Bactrim, Bactrim D.S.) *Dosing is based on TMP component Children: 8–12 mg/kg/d TMP PO divided q6–12h for 7–14 days; Max: 320 mg/d TMP Adults: 160 mg TMP PO/IV q12h for 3 days for uncomplicated cystitis—longer if complicated	Nausea, vomiting, anorexia, diarrhea Rash, urticaria, hypersensitive reaction, photosensitivity	Megaloblastic anemia Folate deficiency G6PD deficiency Caution with hepatic and renal dysfunction. Sulfa allergy	G6PD-deficient patients can have hemolysis. **Pregnancy** Sulfamethoxazole consider an alternative in 1st trimester, otherwise caution advised in 3rd trimester. Trimethoprim consider an alternative during pregnancy; possible risk of spontaneous abortion based on limited human data; possible risk of congenital neural tube and cardiovascular defects based on conflicting human data and drug's mechanism of action. **Lactation Sulfamethoxazole:** Avoid use while breastfeeding infant with G6PD deficiency, otherwise caution advised while breastfeeding. **Trimethoprim:** may use while breastfeeding
Trimethoprim (Trimpex) 100 mg q12h for 3 days	Same as mentioned earlier	Same as mentioned earlier except for sulfa allergy	Can give to patients who have sulfa allergy May cause falsely elevated creatinine independent of eGFR which is reversible Increase fluid intake.
Nitrofurantoin (Macrobid, Macrodantin) Macrobid—100 mg q12h for 7 days Macrodantin—100 mg QID for 7 days	Nausea, vomiting, anorexia, diarrhea, abdominal pain Possible hemolytic, megaloblastic, or aplastic anemia if used long term	Anuria Oliguria Caution if renal or hepatic impairment. Chronic pulmonary conditions can occur with treatment more than 6 months.	**Pregnancy** Contraindicated at 38–42 weeks gestation, consider alternative in 1st trimester, otherwise may use during pregnancy **Lactation** Breastfeeding for infant <1 month with hyperbilirubinemia or G6PD deficiency Take with food to increase absorption. Avoid use with live vaccines.
Fosfomycin tromethamine (Monurol) 3 gram powder packet for 1 day	Diarrhea, nausea, vaginitis Rhinitis, headache, dizziness	Caution if recent antibiotic-associated colitis.	Pregnancy and Lactation—may use risk of fetal/infant harm not expected Mixed in 4 ounces or 120 milliliters of cold water and stir to dissolve. Do not use warm or hot water. Drink all the mixture right away.
Ciprofloxacin (Cipro) 250 mg q12h for 3 days for uncomplicated cystitis and 7 days for complicated cystitis and 500 mg for 10–14 days for uncomplicated pyelonephritis	Nausea, diarrhea, altered taste, dizziness, drowsiness, headache, insomnia, agitation, confusion Serious: pseudomembranous colitis, Stevens–Johnson syndrome, aggravation of myasthenia gravis Avoid use for UTI unless no other options	Black box warning for the class: Disabling, potentially irreversible serious reactions Fluoroquinolones associated with tendinitis/tendon rupture, peripheral neuropathy, and CNS effects that may occur together; affects all ages but especially older patients >60 years. Risk of prolongation of the QT_c.	Raises serum level of theophylline Avoid taking with aluminum- or magnesium-containing antacids. Food slows absorption. Drug interacts with antacids, theophylline, warfarin, probenecid, digoxin, glucocorticoids. **Pregnancy** Weigh risk/benefit during pregnancy; no known risk of teratogenicity based on human and animal data **Lactation** Consider avoiding breastfeeding for 3–4 hours after dose if anthrax use, otherwise consider avoiding breastfeeding during tx and for 2 days after D/C.

TABLE 28.1

Overview of Selected Agents for Urinary Tract Infection (*Continued*)

Generic (Trade) Name and Dosage	Selected Adverse Events	Contraindications	Special Considerations
Ofloxacin (Brand is discontinued.) 200 mg q12h for 3 days for uncomplicated cystitis and 7 days for complicated cystitis and 200–300 mg for 10–14 days for uncomplicated pyelonephritis	Nausea, diarrhea, headache, insomnia, photosensitivity	Black box warning—see earlier mentioned.	**Pregnancy** and **Lactation** as mentioned earlier Food slows absorption. Avoid taking with aluminum- or magnesium-containing antacids or sucralfate, iron, and multivitamins with zinc because these can decrease absorption. Increase fluid intake significantly.
Levofloxacin (Levaquin) 250 mg daily for 3 days for uncomplicated cystitis and 7 days for complicated cystitis and 10–14 days for uncomplicated pyelonephritis	Nausea, diarrhea, photosensitivity	Black box warning—see earlier mentioned.	Same as mentioned earlier
Urinary Analgesics			
Methenamine Hippurate (Hiprex, Urex) 1 g BID Methanamine mandelate (only generic) 1 g QID	Rash, anticholinergic effects, xerostomia, flushing, difficulty in urinating, acute urinary retention with benign prostatic hyperplasia, tachycardia, dizziness, blurry vision, urine, or fecal discoloration	Glaucoma Not recommended in patients <6 years Pregnancy (category C) Breastfeeding Bowel obstruction Urinary obstruction Cardiospasm	May cause blue-green discoloration of urine or feces Is not antibacterial but can be preventative for recurrent UTI Pregnancy and Lactation—may use risk of fetal/infant harm not expected
Phenazopyridine (Pyridium) 200 mg TID	Headache, rash, GI upset, hemolytic anemia	Renal insufficiency Pyelonephritis in pregnancy	Discolors urine and clothes (red-orange) Is not antibacterial Take after meals. May use in pregnancy unless pyelonephritis Lactation—avoid use.
Flavoxate (Urispas) 100–200 mg TID–QID	Nausea and vomiting, anticholinergic side effects, vertigo, headache, drowsiness, urticaria, confusion, tachycardia	GI obstruction Obstructive uropathies Glaucoma	Reduce dose on improvement. Caution advised in both pregnancy and lactation.

CNS, central nervous system; eGFR, estimated glomerular filtration rate; GI, gastrointestinal; G6PD, glucose-6-phosphate dehydrogenase; TMP, trimethoprim; UTI, urinary tract infection.

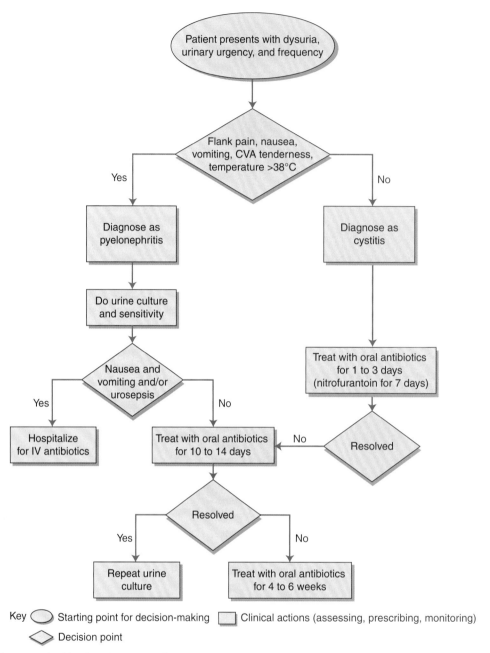

FIGURE 28–1 Treatment algorithm for urinary tract infection.

CVA, costovertebral angle; IV, intravenous.

First-Line Therapy

There are multiple agents for the first-line choice for acute cystitis. Choice should always be based on patient allergies, cost, and local resistance patterns. According to the most recent guidelines, nitrofurantoin is the first-line choice for treatment (Gupta et al., 2011). The drug is favored due to its action on multiple aspects of biochemical processes and is bactericidal at therapeutic doses. The broad-based nature of the action helps to explain the lack of antibiotic resistance.

The next best choice for cystitis is TMP–SMZ (Bactrim). This drug combination has little impact on normal vaginal flora but decreases the number of *E. coli* in vaginal and fecal reservoirs, decreasing the chance of reinfection. TMP appears to be similar in efficacy but with fewer side effects; it can also be used in patients with sulfa allergies. The sulfa ingredient may be more important for complicated cystitis and pyelonephritis.

Fosfomycin (Monaural) is also used in first-line therapy. It is dissolved in water. This is a one-time drug. The disadvantage is that the price is high. There is no generic substitute.

Patients with cystitis can also be given urinary tract analgesics. This group includes methenamine (Urised), phenazopyridine (Pyridium, Uristat), or flavoxate (Urispas).

TABLE 28.2

Recommended Order of Treatment for Uncomplicated Cystitis

Order	Agent	Comments
First line	3-day oral therapy of	Drink at least 8 glasses of fluids.
	• TMP–SMZ	Initiate 7-day therapy in postmenopausal women and in men.
	Or 7-day therapy of nitrofurantoin (preferred)	May use urinary analgesics in combination with antibiotics
		Higher incidence of treatment failure with nitrofurantoin for 3 days, so 7-day use is recommended
	Or fosfomycin tromethamine (Monurol)	Mixed in 4 ounces or 120 milliliters of cold water and stir to dissolve
		Do not use warm or hot water. Drink all the mixture right away.
Second line	7-day oral therapy of • TMP–SMZ May also use 7-day oral therapy of • ciprofloxacin • levofloxacin • ofloxacin • norfloxacin	Consider the risk versus benefits of this drug class
Third line	Culture and sensitivity/ testing, then treat based on results.	

TMP–SMZ, trimethoprim–sulfamethoxazole.

TABLE 28.3

Recommended Order of Treatment for Uncomplicated Pyelonephritis

Order	Agents	Comments
First line	Oral for varies for the agent between 5–7 days: • ciprofloxacin • levofloxacin • norfloxacin • ofloxacin • cefixime • cefpodoxime proxetil	Urine culture and sensitivity testing should be performed before treatment.
Second line	• TMP–SMZ for 14 days • Amoxicillin-clavulanate (Augmentin) for 14 days • Cefaclor for 7 days	Oral beta-lactams are not as effective for treating pyelonephritis; however, if they are used, administer with a single dose of ceftriaxone (Rocephin) 1 g IM
Third line	Hospitalization for IV therapy	For severe illness or possible urosepsis

IM, intramuscular; IV, intravenous; TMP–SMZ, trimethoprim–sulfamethoxazole.

Uncomplicated pyelonephritis is usually treated in the outpatient setting because of the available oral antibiotics. The patient with pyelonephritis is admitted to the hospital only if they cannot take oral fluids or oral antibiotics, have a high fever or marked debility, or have a social situation incompatible with outpatient treatment. First-line therapy for pyelonephritis is an antibiotic, as mentioned previously, for 10 to 14 days. Fluoroquinolones are usually given first if culture results are not available because of their broad spectrum of activity. No follow-up is required if the symptoms resolve.

Second-Line Therapy

Fluoroquinolones are options for empiric therapy of recurrent cystitis. If symptoms of cystitis do not resolve after 3 days of therapy, a 7-day course of antibiotics is recommended. Fluoroquinolones are not recommended as first-line agents for uncomplicated cystitis because of the increased cost and concerns over development of quinolone resistance along with potential cardiac side effects of this class. They should be reserved for treatment of UTIs in men and postmenopausal women and for patients with complicated UTIs and pyelonephritis.

In pyelonephritis, a culture is obtained after treatment. If the urine is not free of bacteria after initial therapy, 4 to 6 more weeks of therapy is prescribed.

Third-Line Therapy

The recurrence rate for UTIs is approximately 20%. At this point, a urine culture is done and treatment is based on the culture results. If the patient has fewer than two UTIs a year, treatment can be based on the previous culture results. Women who have three or more recurrences annually may be offered the option of self-treatment of recurrences. Postcoital use of antibiotic prophylaxis is effective for women who have recurrences related to intercourse. Continuous antibiotic prophylaxis in a single bedtime dose is also accepted practice for women who have frequent recurrences. Antibiotics that have been shown to reduce the number of recurrences to 0.3 or fewer per year are TMP–SMZ 40 mg/200 mg, TMP 100 mg, and nitrofurantoin macrocrystals 50 to 100 mg.

Special Population Considerations
Geriatric

In older patients, UTIs are commonly asymptomatic but should be strongly considered as a diagnostic possibility for individuals who have changes in mentation. Postmenopausal women are more prone to UTIs because there is uropathogen-dominant vaginal flora with the loss of estrogen. Lactobacilli diminish and pH increases. Older patients are at increased risk for UTIs. Vaginal estrogen therapy effectively reduces symptomatic UTI episodes in the older population.

Approximately 10% to 20% of the population older than age 65 has bacteriuria related to factors such as fecal incontinence, incomplete bladder emptying, malnutrition, and increased urine pH. Any UTI in a man is considered complicated. *E. coli* and *Enterobacter* species are the usual organisms. In older men, *Proteus, Klebsiella, Serratia, Pseudomonas,* and *Enterococcus* species are also responsible for UTIs. UTIs in men are most often seen in conjunction with prostatic hyperplasia with partial obstruction or persistent prostatitis.

Nitrofurantoin is not recommended in the older adults because it requires a creatinine clearance of 40 mL/min. Treatment is for 7 to 10 days in women and 10 to 14 days in men with uncomplicated UTIs.

Pregnancy

Asymptomatic bacteriuria occurs in approximately 7% of pregnant women. Of these, pyelonephritis develops in 30% if the bacteriuria is not treated. Untreated UTIs can contribute to prematurity or stillbirth. Amoxicillin is effective in approximately two thirds of UTIs in pregnant women and is safe for the fetus. Also safe are cephalexin and nitrofurantoin (only during the first and second trimesters). Sulfonamides are safe except in the last trimester. In pregnancy, the urine is cultured 1 week after treatment and every 4 to 6 weeks during the pregnancy.

Physiologic changes in pregnancy increase the risk for pyelonephritis. The ureters become obstructed because of blockage from the enlarged uterus. In addition, increased progesterone relaxes the smooth muscles of the ureter and bladder. Bacteriuria in pregnancy has been associated with a 20% to 30% incidence of pyelonephritis and premature delivery, intrauterine growth retardation, increased risk for death in the perinatal period, and congenital anomalies.

In 5% to 10% of women with UTI, there are no symptoms. Pregnant women should be screened for UTIs, and they must be treated regardless of whether they are symptomatic.

Children

UTIs in children may indicate a genitourinary anomaly. Accurate diagnosis usually requires invasive collection of urine, especially in very young children. It is important to start treatment quickly, especially in young children, because there is an increased risk of renal scarring in children under age 5 from UTIs. UTIs recur in 32% to 40% of children.

UTI should be suspected in febrile infants without an obvious source. Urine specimens collected with a bag are considered insufficient to make a diagnosis. Transurethral and suprapubic catheterization are accepted methods of urine collection in children. All children younger than 3 years diagnosed with a first UTI should have a renal ultrasound scan and a voiding cystourethrogram (VCUG). Boys older than 3 years

can either have ultrasonography with VCUG or a renal cortical scan with follow-up VCUG as indicated based on the results. Girls between the ages of 3 and 7 years should have either ultrasonography with VCUG or a renal scan if febrile or observation without imaging if afebrile. Girls older than 7 years can be observed without imaging.

First-line antimicrobial agents include the β-lactams amoxicillin–clavulanate (25–45 mg/kg/d, divided every 12 hours), cephalexin (25–50 mg/kg/d, divided every 6–12 hours), and cefpodoxime (10 mg/kg/d, divided every 12 hours) as well as TMP–SMX (8–10 mg/kg/d, divided every 12 hours). Two-day to 4-day courses have been shown to be as effective as 7 to 14 days.

MONITORING PATIENT RESPONSE

Prescribers need to evaluate for cystitis that does not resolve or that recurs within a week after treatment, which requires culture and sensitivity testing and treatment with a fluoroquinolone for 7 days. UTIs recur within a year in approximately half of all women, although there is a very low incidence of pyelonephritis that develops as a result.

If pyelonephritis recurs within 2 weeks after treatment, a urine culture and sensitivity test and renal ultrasound or computed tomography scan should be performed to determine whether there is a urologic abnormality. If the organism is the same as the first, a 4- to 6-week course of antibiotics is recommended.

Patients who have three or more UTIs a year should be given prophylaxis, either continuous or postcoital. Continuous prophylaxis usually consists of TMP–SMZ 40 to 200 mg daily or three times a week. Postcoital therapy is indicated in women who identify intercourse as the cause of infection; the selected therapy is taken after intercourse. The use of estrogen replacement therapy in postmenopausal women decreases the number of recurrent UTIs. In cases of true relapse, the culture is repeated and therapy is prescribed for 2 to 4 weeks.

In pyelonephritis, a culture is repeated 1 to 2 weeks after completion of therapy. If there is a recurrence, therapy is recommended for 6 to 12 months.

PATIENT EDUCATION

Drug Information

Patients can get information about UTIs at http://www.nlm.nih.gov/medlineplus/urinarytractinfections.html, http://kidney.niddk.nih.gov/KUDiseases/topics/uti.aspx, and http://www.healthline.com/health/urinary-tract-infection-adults.

Lifestyle Changes

The most important advice is for sexually active women to urinate shortly after sexual intercourse. In doing so, they wash out the increased number of bacteria in the distal urethra. Another useful suggestion is for patients with recurrent UTIs to practice double or triple voiding and changing positions while urinating to rid the bladder of residual urine.

Other behavioral factors to consider are the direction of toilet paper use after bowel movements, the type of menstrual protection used, and the method of contraception. The use of spermicides changes the vaginal flora, increasing the colonization of *E. coli* and the frequency of UTIs. Women with recurrent UTIs should use a method of birth control that does not involve spermicides.

Other preventive measures include avoiding bubble baths and "feminine hygiene" products. Urinating every 2 hours, taking the time to empty the bladder, also helps prevent UTIs. Foods that irritate the bladder should be avoided, including tea, coffee, alcohol, cola, chocolate, and spicy foods.

Patients with frequently recurring cystitis can benefit from early self-treatment if they are well informed and compliant. If treatment is started very shortly after the onset of symptoms, a 3-day course or even a single dose of antimicrobial provides rapid relief of symptoms.

Complementary and Alternative Medicine

Cranberry juice concentrate or cranberry concentrate capsules have been recognized as alternatives to antibiotics or UTIs prevention. Cranberry is believed to have anti-adherence properties in the urinary tract and acidifies the urine. In the past, there has been conflicting evidence that cranberry makes any difference; however, a more recent study shows there is a benefit from both cranberry juice and pills (Jensen et al., 2017; Leblanc et al., 2020). Taking a 300–400 mg capsule two times a day with a glass of water is beneficial. Additionally, 8 to 16 ounces of preparations with at least 30% of cranberry juice can be taken. Vitamin C, 500 mg every 4 hours for the UTI duration, has been suggested, with 1,000 to 1,500 mg/d for the prevention of UTIs.

Probiotics may decrease UTIs by restoring normal vaginal flora. Lactobacillus is thought to prevent colonization with *E. coli*.

CASE STUDY 1

J.S., a 65-year-old woman with diabetes, seeks treatment for dysuria, frequent urination, flank pain, and costovertebral angle tenderness. She has a temperature of 102°F, and under the microscope, her spun urine contains a large number of leukocytes.

DIAGNOSIS: CYSTITIS WITH POSSIBLE PYELONEPHRITIS

1. List specific goals for treatment for J.S.
2. What drug therapy would you prescribe? Why?
3. What are the parameters for monitoring the success of the therapy?

4. Discuss specific patient education based on the prescribed therapy.
5. List one or two adverse reactions for the selected agent that would cause you to change therapy.
6. What would be the choice for second-line therapy?
7. What over-the-counter and/or alternative medications would be appropriate for J.S.?
8. What lifestyle changes would you recommend to J.S.?
9. Describe one or two drug-drug or drug-food interactions for the selected agent.

Bibliography

Starred references are cited in the text.

Anger, J., Lee, U., Ackerman, A. L., et al. (2019). Recurrent uncomplicated urinary tract infections in women: AUA/CUA/SUFU guideline. *Journal of Urology, 202*(2), 282–289. https://doi.org/10.1097/ju.0000000000000296

Beerepoot, M. A., ter Riet, G., Nys, S., et al. (2011). Cranberries vs antibiotics to prevent urinary tract infections: A randomized double-blind noninferiority trial in premenopausal women. *Archives of Internal Medicine, 171*(14), 1270–1278.

*Chu, C. M., & Lowder, J. L. (2018). Diagnosis and treatment of urinary tract infections across age groups. *American Journal of Obstetrics and Gynecology, 219*(1), 40–51. https://doi.org/10.1016/j.ajog.2017.12.231

Chwa, A., Kavanagh, K., Linnebur, S. A., et al. (2019). Evaluation of methenamine for urinary tract infection prevention in older adults: A review of the evidence. *Therapeutic Advances in Drug Safety, 10,* 2042098619876749. https://doi.org/10.1177/2042098619876749

Clark, C., Kennedy, W., & Shortliffe, L. (2010). Urinary tract infections in children: When to worry. *Urologic Clinics of North America, 37*(2), 229–241.

Daley, M. F., Arnold Rehring, S. M., Glenn, K. A., et al. (2020). Improving antibiotic prescribing for pediatric urinary tract infections in outpatient settings. *Pediatrics, 145*(4), e20192503. https://doi.org/10.1542/peds.2019-2503

Doern, C. D., & Richardson, S. E. (2016). Diagnosis of urinary tract infections in children. *Journal of Clinical Microbiology, 54*(9), 2233–2242. https://doi.org/10.1128/jcm.00189-16

Flores-Mireles, A., Walk, J., Caparon, M., et al. (2015). Urinary tract infections: Epidemiology, mechanisms of infection and treatment options. *Nature Reviews Microbiology, 13,* 269–284. https://doi.org/10.1038/nrmicro.3432

*Foxman, B. (2014). Urinary tract infection syndromes: Occurrence, recurrence, bacteriology, risk factors, and disease burden. *Infectious Disease Clinics of North America, 28,* 1–13. http://dx.doi.org/10.1016/j.idc.2013.09.003

*Guptal, K., Hooton, T. M., Naber, K. G., et al. (2011). International clinical practice guidelines for the treatment of acute uncomplicated cystitis and pyelonephritis in women: A 2010 update by Infectious Diseases Society of America and the European Society for Microbiology and Infectious Diseases. *Clinical Infectious Diseases*, *52*(5), e103–e120.

Horton, J. (2015). Chapter 36: Urinary Tract Agents: Nitrofurantoin, Fosfomycin, and Methenamine. In *Mandell, Douglas, and Bennett's Principles and Practice of Infectious Diseases* (Vol. 1, pp. 447–451.e1). Elsevier. https://doi.org/10.1016/B978-1-4557-4801-3.00036-9

*Jensen, H. D., Struve, C., Christensen, S. B., et al. (2017). Cranberry juice and combinations of its organic acids are effective against experimental Urinary tract infection. *Frontiers in Microbiology*, *8*, 1. https://doi.org/10.3389/fmicb.2017.00542

*Khoshnood, S., Heidary, M., Mirnejad, R., Bahramian, A., Sedighi, M., & Mirzaei, H. (2017). Drug-resistant gram-negative uropathogens: A review. *Biomedicine & Pharmacotherapy*, *94*, 982–994. https://doi.org/10.1016/j.biopha.2017.08.006

Korbel, L., Howell, M., & Spencer, J. D. (2017). The clinical diagnosis and management of urinary tract infections in children and adolescents. *Paediatrics and International Child Health*, *37*(4), 273–279. https://doi.org/10.1080/20469047.2017.1382046

Lashkar, M. O., & Nahata, M. C. (2018). Antimicrobial pharmacotherapy management of urinary tract infections in pediatric patients. *Journal of Pharmacy Technology*, *34*(2), 62–81. https://doi.org/10.1177/8755122518755402

*Leblanc, V., Babar, A., Moore, L., et al. (2020). Standardized high versus low dose cranberry proanthocyanidin extracts for prevention of urinary Tract infection confirmed by pyuria in women: A Randomized clinical trial. *Current Developments in Nutrition*, *4*(Supplement_2), 423. https://doi.org/10.1093/cdn/nzaa045_056

Loubet, P., Ranfaing, J., Dinh, A., et al. (2020). Alternative therapeutic options to antibiotics for the treatment of urinary tract infections. *Frontiers in Microbiology*, *11*, 1. https://doi.org/10.3389/fmicb.2020.01509

*Medina, M., & Castillo-Pino, E. (2019). An introduction to the epidemiology and burden of urinary tract infections. *Therapeutic Advances in Urology*, *11*, 3. https://doi.org/10.1177/1756287219832172

Mody, L., & Juthani-Mehta, M. (2014). Urinary tract infections in older women: A clinical review. *The Journal of the American Medical Association*, *311*(8), 844–854.

Nguyen, H. M., & Graber, C. J. (2020). A critical review of cephalexin and cefadroxil for the treatment of acute uncomplicated lower urinary tract infection in the era of "Bad bugs, few drugs." *International Journal of Antimicrobial Agents*, *56*(4), 106085. https://doi.org/10.1016/j.ijantimicag.2020.106085

Nicolle, L. E., Gupta, K., Bradley, S. F., et al. (2019). Clinical practice guideline for the management of asymptomatic bacteriuria: 2019 update by the Infectious Diseases Society of America. *Clinical Infectious Diseases*, *68*, 83. https://doi.org/10.1093/cid/ciy1121

Paul, R. (2018). State of the globe: Rising antimicrobial resistance of pathogens in urinary tract infection. *Journal of Global Infectious Diseases*, *10*(3), 117–118. https://doi.org/10.4103/jgid.jgid_104_17

Pujades-Rodriguez, M., West, R. M., Wilcox, M. H., et al. (2019). Lower urinary tract infections: Management, outcomes and risk factors for antibiotic re-prescription in primary care. *EClinicalMedicine*, *14*, 23–31. https://doi.org/10.1016/j.eclinm.2019.07.012

Stapleton, A. E. (2016). Urine culture in uncomplicated UTI: Interpretation and significance. *Current Infectious Disease Reports*, *18*(5), 15. https://doi.org/10.1007/s11908-016-0522-0

Stapleton, A. E., Wagenlehner, F. M. E., Mulgirigama, A., et al. (2020). Escherichia coli resistance to fluoroquinolones in Community-Acquired uncomplicated urinary tract infection in women: A systematic review. *Antimicrobial Agents and Chemotherapy*, *64*(10), 1. https://doi.org/10.1128/aac.00862-20

Ulchaker, J. C., & Martinson, M. (2017). Cost-effectiveness analysis of six therapies for the treatment of lower urinary tract symptoms due to benign prostatic hyperplasia. *ClinicoEconomics and Outcomes Research*, *10*, 29–43. https://doi.org/10.2147/ceor.s148195

Walsh, C., & Collyns, T. (2017). The pathophysiology of urinary tract infections. *Surgery (Oxford)*, *35*(6), 293–298. https://doi.org/10.1016/j.mpsur.2017.03.007

Wang, A., Nizran, P., Malone, M. A., et al. (2013). Urinary tract infections. *Primary Care; Clinics in Office Practice*, *40*(3), 687–706.

Zhang, Y., Wu, J.-G., Zhou, H.-J., et al. (2020). Efficacy of nonsteroidal anti-inflammatory drugs for treatment of uncomplicated lower urinary tract infections in women: A meta-analysis. *Infectious Microbes and Diseases*, *2*(2), 77–82. https://doi.org/10.1097/im9.0000000000000020

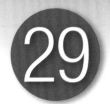

29 Prostatic Disorders and Erectile Dysfunction

Veronica F. Wilbur

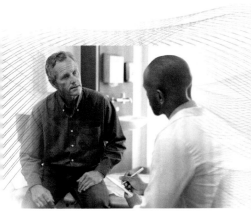
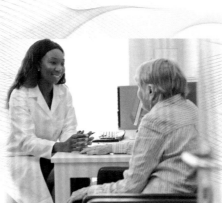
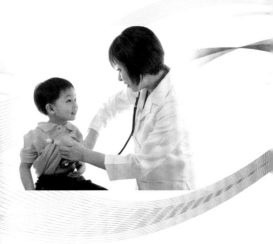

Learning Objectives

1. Differentiate between benign prostatic hypertrophy (BPH), prostatitis, and prostate cancer.
2. Identify the goals of pharmacologic and nonpharmacologic treatment of BPH and prostatitis and erectile dysfunction (ED).
3. Base selection of pharmacologic agents on patient symptoms in the treatment of BPH prostatitis and ED.
4. Define appropriate symptom monitoring of drug therapy.
5. Distinguish appropriate changes to pharmacologic treatment.

INTRODUCTION

Disorders of the prostate generally appear as men age and can be divided into benign prostatic hypertrophy, prostatitis, and prostate cancer. Generally, the prostate enlarges as part of the normal aging process. Often, it is not until age 40 that a man begins to show some form of prostatic disorder, with an increasing incidence for each decade of life and by the 9th decade over 80% of men have prostate enlargement that affects the urinary tract (Lim, 2017). In contrast, prostate cancer usually is found after age 50. As many as 14 million men have BPH in the United States (Egan, 2016). Prostate cancer is the second most common type of cancer affecting men and the fifth leading cause of death in the world (Rawla, 2019). In the United States, black men have the highest incidence of prostate cancer, 163.8 per 100,000 while White males have 96.7 per 100,000. Asian and Hispanic men are at lower risk than White men.

In addition to race, other risk factors for prostate cancer are age and family history. The disease rarely occurs before age 45, but the incidence rises exponentially thereafter; nearly 70% of cases are diagnosed in men age 65 and older. There are 106.5 per 100,000 cases of newly diagnosed prostate cancer per year (U.S. Department of Health and Human Services, Centers for Disease Control and Prevention and National Cancer Institute, 2020). Prostate disorders are diagnosed through clinical manifestations and screening procedures used to detect or rule out prostate cancer. Lack of knowledge about prostate cancer and lack of available screening procedures are the major deterrents to accurate and timely diagnosis of prostate cancer.

Treatment of prostatic disorders itself may result in some untoward side effects, which must then also be managed. Often, the man postpones seeking medical intervention and blames aging for many of the manifestations, thus delaying treatment. Some difficulties in seeking treatment can relate to the man's culture; sexuality—specifically, masculinity—can be perceived as synonymous with virility. For this reason, a man may choose not to discuss (even with a health care worker) clinical manifestations.

Prostatic disorders and lower urinary tract symptom (LUTS) occur because of inflammation or infection (prostatitis), BPH, and prostate cancer; prostatitis can involve the bladder neck, thus becoming prostatocystitis. A bacterial infection is often the cause of prostatitis, although some nonbacterial forms of prostatitis do exist. Inflammation can be chronic or acute.

Adenocarcinoma is the most common type of prostate cancer. Metastasis can follow slowly or quickly, and often, the symptoms of metastasis are what lead the man to seek medical intervention.

Presenting manifestations of prostatic disorders are usually specific to the urinary tract and include difficulty in onset of urine flow with or without a low flow of urine, frequency or urgency in voiding, incontinence, distention of the bladder, and hematuria. Management of prostatic disorders is specific to the disorder (cancerous vs. noncancerous), with some overlap in treatment.

PROSTATITIS

Causes

Prostatitis is a common condition that involves inflammation of the prostate and surrounding area. The condition of prostatitis is categorized by the National Institutes of Health system that was established through and international process (Weidner & Anderson, 2008) (see **Table 29.1**).

Most patients with prostatitis are found to have either nonbacterial prostatitis or prostatodynia, which can be acute or chronic. With acute bacterial prostatitis, the chief organisms involved are *Escherichia coli* and *Pseudomonas* species, although strains of staphylococci or streptococci also are seen. Chronic bacterial prostatitis is associated with *Pseudomonas, E. coli, Proteus mirabilis, Klebsiella pneumoniae,* and *Enterococcus* species, particularly *Enterococcus faecalis.* Nonbacterial prostatitis is essentially an inflammatory disorder.

Pathophysiology

Acute Prostatitis

Acute prostatitis (AP) is attributable to bacteria ascending from the urethra. The most likely cause of AP is reflux of urine from the urethra into the intraprostatic ducts. In acute bacterial prostatitis, as with any type of bacterial invasion, the prostate becomes overwhelmed by the bacteria, leading to inflammatory response activation. Usually, acute bacterial prostatitis is seen as an infection ascending up the urinary tract, and younger men, age 30 to 50, can be affected with this illness. It is also thought that bacteria may chronically colonize in the prostate gland and can remain, promoting low-grade glandular infection. In young men, the most common cause is after anal or vaginal intercourse. Atypical pathogens can be attributed to sexually transmitted infections such as *Neisseria gonorrhoeae, Chlamydia trachomatis,* or *Mycoplasma genitalium.* The most common causes of AP in the older adults are prolonged catheterization and biopsy.

Chronic Prostatitis and Pelvic Pain Syndrome

Chronic prostatitis (CP) is the manifestation of recurrent bacterial infections with or without complete resolution. Symptoms tend to be milder than acute but persistently problematic. As with AP, inflammatory process is causing the painful sensations. In CP, the presence of inflammation produces high amounts pro-inflammatory cytokines and reactive oxygen species (Paulis, 2018).

Diagnostic Criteria

Symptom manifestation revolves around urinary tract signs. There is pain in the lower abdomen, difficulty in bladder emptying with or without a small stream during urination, nocturia, and fever to 104°F (40°C). Along with the febrile state, as with other infections, general arthralgia and malaise can occur.

On examination and interview, the man often admits to painful ejaculation and pain in the rectal or perineal areas. All the symptoms are due to the edema associated with acute inflammation of the prostate. Because of the risk of generalized septicemia, pharmacotherapeutics are urgently warranted.

Culture isolation of prostatic urine is the most accurate method of diagnosis. Prostatic urine is defined as the third and fourth (urine) secretion specimens of four serial urine sample because prostatic fluid is at a significantly higher concentration in these last two of four serial voids. The four urine samples are obtained sequentially, beginning with the initial void, followed by a midstream urine specimen, prostatic massage secretion, and finally the urine voided after the prostatic massage. Standard laboratory culture techniques are applied to establish the causative organism.

Nonbacterial prostatitis is confirmed by negative prostatic urine cultures with a positive elevated white blood cell count and the presence of inflammatory cells in prostatic secretions. This condition and another nonbacterial type of prostatitis known as *prostatodynia* have the same symptoms as does bacterial prostatitis. Treatment of the nonbacterial forms usually consists of symptom management without the use of antibiotics.

TABLE 29.1	
4 Categories of Prostatitis per the National Institutes of Health Classification of Prostatitis Syndromes	
Category	**Definition**
I. Acute bacterial prostatitis	Acute infection of the prostate
II. Chronic bacterial prostatitis	Recurrent urinary tract infection and/or chronic infection of the prostate
III. Chronic pelvic pain syndrome	Chronic pelvic syndrome ≥3 months in the absence of bacteria localized to the prostate
IIIA. Inflammatory	Significant WBC in semen, or expressed prostatic secretions or midstream bladder specimen
IIIB. Noninflammatory	Insignificant WBC in semen, or expressed prostatic secretions or midstream bladder specimen
IV. Asymptomatic prostatitis	WBC count and/or bacteria in the expressed prostatic secretions, voided bladder, semen, or histologic specimens

WBC, white blood cell.

Initiating Drug Therapy

Antibiotics are the required pharmacotherapy (see Chapter 8). Given that causative organisms are usually gram negative and, less commonly, gram positive, appropriate antibiotics are needed. The overall course of antibiotic therapy is of longer duration than that used to treat other systemic infections. Usually, antibiotics are given for 4 to 6 weeks, but up to 12 weeks of therapy may be necessary due to poor penetration of prostate tissue. Because chronic bacterial prostatitis is a bacterial infection, an appropriate antibiotic with good tissue penetration in the prostate should be selected. Fluoroquinolones have demonstrated the best tissue concentration and are recommended as first-line agents. Although trimethoprim–sulfamethoxazole (TMP–SMZ) may be considered, the tissue penetration may not be as effective, and in many areas of the United States, there is evidence of increasing uropathogenic resistance.

Second-line drugs include doxycycline, azithromycin, and clarithromycin. A 4- to 6-week course of therapy is usually recommended; however, a 6- to 12-week course is often needed to eradicate the causative organism and to prevent recurrence, especially if symptoms persist after completion of the initial therapy. No guidelines exist for treating gram-positive bacterial infections, but ciprofloxacin and levofloxacin have adequate gram-positive coverage as well as excellent gram-negative coverage, and both medications penetrate the prostate tissue well.

Adjunctive therapies that may be beneficial include the use of sitz baths, analgesics, stool softeners, and antipyretics, along with rest. Prostatic massage, voiding in a warm bath (to relax pelvic muscles), and discontinuation of alcohol and caffeinated beverages can also help to relieve symptoms. If possible, withdrawal from antidepressants, anticholinergics, or sedatives may also help bladder function.

Goals of Drug Therapy

The goal of pharmacotherapy for prostatitis is to eradicate the causative organism and restore the prostate to health. Prostatitis often becomes chronic and, therefore, repeated trials with antibiotics or prolonged dosage schedules may be warranted.

Anti-infectives

Table 29.2 depicts dosage information, adverse events, contraindications, and special considerations for the anti-infective management of bacterial prostatitis.

Trimethoprim–Sulfamethoxazole. This drug is a bacteriostatic combination product and is more powerful than its two components given separately. Also, when given as the combined form, resistance on the part of the causative organism arises less frequently. This agent ultimately adversely affects the production of proteins and nucleic acids of bacteria at the target (prostate) site. TMP–SMZ further inhibits growth of bacteria because of its antimetabolite property toward *para*-aminobenzoic acid. Drug–drug interactions can present when the patient is also taking phenytoin (Dilantin), oral hypoglycemics, or warfarin (Coumadin). Close monitoring of the seizure threshold, serum glucose level, or partial thromboplastin time is important in the patient on TMP–SMZ, who is also taking these other agents.

TABLE 29.2			
Overview of Selected Antibiotics Used to Treat Acute Bacterial Prostatitis			
Generic (Trade) Name and Dosage	**Selected Adverse Events**	**Contraindications**	**Special Considerations**
Trimethoprim–sulfamethoxazole (Septra, Bactrim) 160 mg of TMP with 800 mg SMZ PO q12h	GI distress, rash	Allergy to sulfa and sulfa products	May prolong the INR for patients on oral anticoagulants
Fluoroquinolones Ciprofloxacin (Cipro) 500 mg BID Norfloxacin (Noroxin) 400 mg BID Levofloxacin (Levaquin) 250 mg daily	Headache, diarrhea, nausea, drowsiness, altered taste, insomnia, agitation, confusion Serious: pseudomembranous colitis, Stevens–Johnson syndrome	Allergy to macrolides Pregnancy and lactation Use with caution in patients with severe hepatic or renal disease.	May interfere with theophylline metabolism
Doxycycline (Vibramycin) 200 mg PO as first dose, thereafter 100–200 mg PO q12h	GI distress, potential acute hepatotoxicity, potential for nephrotoxicity	Hypersensitivity to any of the tetracyclines Pregnancy and lactation	Decreased effectiveness with food and dairy products, so do not take with food unless side effects are significant Can lead to diabetes insipidus because of antagonistic effect with antidiuretic hormone

GI, gastrointestinal; INR, international normalized ratio; SMZ, sulfamethoxazole; TMP, trimethoprim.

Fluoroquinolones.   Fluoroquinolones are also effective for bacterial prostatitis. Effective against gram-negative anaerobes and some gram-positive bacteria, these agents decrease the growth and replication of bacteria by inhibiting bacterial deoxyribonucleic acid during synthesis. These agents may be the first choice for someone sensitive or allergic to TMP–SMZ.

The absorption of fluoroquinolones is reduced by milk, antacids (aluminum or magnesium based), iron or zinc salts, and sucralfate. For the patient who is also taking any of these medications, the dose should be taken either 2 hours after or 4 hours before the other medication.

Fluoroquinolones also affect the use of theophylline and warfarin. Elevated levels can occur, and thus, a lower dosage of theophylline or warfarin may be necessary.

Doxycycline.   A long-acting tetracycline, doxycycline (Vibramycin), acts by inhibiting protein synthesis: binding of peptidyl transfer ribonucleic acid (tRNA) is blocked at ribosomal messenger ribonucleic acid (mRNA).

Many of the metal ions—aluminum, calcium, iron, magnesium, and zinc—can interfere by creating chelates with doxycycline. Thus, if these metals are given (and they often are as components of antacids), at least 2 hours should separate their use from the ingestion of doxycycline.

Azithromycin and Clarithromycin.   These are macrolide antibiotics. Macrolides inhibits RNA-dependent protein synthesis by reversibly binding to the 50S ribosomal subunits of susceptible microorganisms. They induce dissociation of tRNA from the ribosome during the elongation phase. Thus, RNA-dependent protein synthesis is suppressed, and bacterial growth is inhibited. Macrolides are mainly bacteriostatic but can be bacteriocidal depending on bacterial sensitivity and antibiotic concentration.

Selecting the Most Appropriate Agent

Oral antibiotics are the treatment agents of choice.

First-Line Therapy

The primary choice for first-line antibiotic therapy is a fluoroquinolone (**Table 29.3**). Therapy lasts for 4 to 6 weeks. See **Figure 29.1** for more information. TMP–SMZ may also be

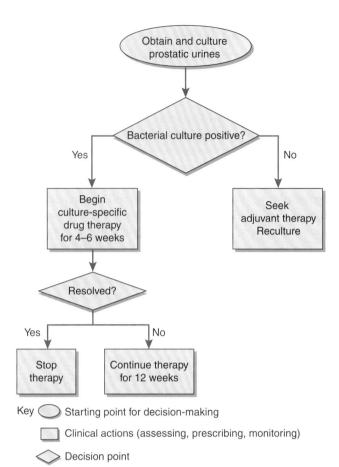

FIGURE 29–1   Treatment algorithm for Prostatitis.

considered if treatment is in an area where there is not a high incidence of resistance.

Second-Line Therapy

Doxycycline, azithromycin, and clarithromycin are second-line agents. If the infection is not resolved with 4 to 6 weeks of drug treatment, therapy can be continued for up to 12 weeks.

Special Population Considerations

In older men who are taking fluoroquinolones, creatinine clearance must be monitored.

Monitoring Patient Response

As a group, anti-infective agents should begin to elicit results after the first week of therapy. Subjective response from the patient indicating alleviation of symptoms is helpful in monitoring the effectiveness of these medications. Some patients may not notice symptom resolution until after 2 weeks; they should be told this and encouraged to continue taking the medication. Ultimately, 12 weeks of therapy may be required. Follow-up cultures may be obtained at the practitioner's discretion. Further diagnostic criteria may also be recommended for ongoing symptom manifestation.

TABLE 29.3		
Recommended Order of Treatment for Prostatitis		
Order	**Agents**	**Comments**
First line	Fluoroquinolones or TMP–SMZ	Ineffective against enterococci Treat for 4–6 weeks.
Second line	Doxycycline or azithromycin or clarithromycin	

TMP–SMZ, trimethoprim–sulfamethoxazole.

Patient Education

The patient should understand potential side effects, interactions, and appropriate use of the medications. Literature can provide patients with a guide for such potential concerns as well as dosing information. With a prepared and knowledgeable patient, these medications are effective against prostatitis. Cost also can be a factor of concern to the patient. The practitioner should be aware of any financial constraints the patient may have because compliance with medication is important for effective treatment of bacterial prostatitis.

BENIGN PROSTATIC HYPERPLASIA

BPH is the most common prostate problem in men older than age 50; the disease rarely causes symptoms before age 40. As life expectancy rises, so does the occurrence of BPH—an estimated 6.3 million men have BPH. In the United States alone, the disease accounts for 6.4 million doctor visits and more than 400,000 hospitalizations annually. Approximately 90% of men age 80 and older have histologic evidence of BPH, and more than 80% have BPH-related symptoms. Approximately 25% of men older than age 55 and 50% of men older than age 75 experience decreased urinary flow.

Causes

The cause of BPH is not well understood. It has been observed that BPH does not develop in men whose testes were removed before puberty. For this reason, some researchers believe that factors related to aging and the testes may spur the development of BPH. Men produce both testosterone and small amounts of estrogen. As men age, the amount of active testosterone in the blood decreases, leaving a higher proportion of estrogen. Studies performed on animals have suggested that BPH may occur because the higher amount of estrogen within the gland increases the activity of substances that promote cell growth. Another theory focuses on dihydrotestosterone (DHT), a substance derived from testosterone in the prostate, which may help control its growth. Some research has indicated that even with a drop in the blood's testosterone level, older men continue to produce and accumulate high levels of DHT in the prostate. This accumulation of DHT may encourage the growth of cells. Researchers have also noted that men who do not produce DHT do not develop BPH.

Pathophysiology

The dynamic component of BPH and LUTS is based on autonomic input to the smooth muscles in the lower urinary tract, including the bladder, prostate, and urethra. These areas have a large concentration of alpha$_1$-adrenergic receptors that, when stimulated by various stressors, cause increasing smooth muscle tone. This increased smooth muscle tone leads to increased urethral resistance and contributes to the bladder outlet obstructive symptoms of BPH. This physiology leads to the

basis for a main class of drugs to treat BPH, the use of alpha$_1$-adrenergic blockers.

An underlying pathophysiologic process of BPH is the formation of large, nonmalignant lesions at the periurethral region of the prostate gland. Prostatic hyperplasia is an overgrowth of normal cells in the stromal and epithelial tissues of the prostate gland. The hyperplasia originates in the transition zone of the prostate, which surrounds the prostatic urethra between the bladder and the anus. The etiology of the hyperplastic process is unknown, but it has been speculated that it is hormone related because it occurs only in older men. The male aging process involves a decrease in testosterone production with a concomitant increase in estrogen; estrogen may be a sensitizer for the escalating hyperplasia. Bladder control involves reflex activity of the peripheral autonomic nervous system (ANS). The reflex for normal micturition is housed in the brain stem and supported by descending and ascending pathways from the spinal cord. Both the external sphincter and the detrusor muscle are needed for bladder control. Reflex micturition is innervated at the S2 to S4 and T1 to L1 levels in the spinal cord. The cortical center of the brain appears to be important for inhibition or control of the micturition center to modulate contractile, filling, and expulsion activity.

Parasympathetic and sympathetic innervation is crucial to the role of the ANS in voiding. Parasympathetic interplay allows for the detrusor muscle to maintain tone and to contract, whereas sympathetic interplay allows for the bladder to expand and maintain a large filling capacity. The dynamic component of BPH and LUTS is based on autonomic input to the smooth muscles in the lower urinary tract, including the bladder, prostate, and urethra. These areas have a large concentration of alpha$_1$-adrenergic receptors that, when stimulated by various stressors, cause increasing smooth muscle tone. This increased smooth muscle tone leads to increased urethral resistance and contributes to the bladder outlet obstructive symptoms of BPH. This physiology leads to the basis for a main class of drugs to treat BPH, the alpha$_1$-adrenergic blockers.

BPH disease manifests as urinary tract symptoms. Obstructed urine outflow, the predominant pattern, includes diminished force of the urine stream, an urgent need for nocturnal voiding, residual urine with or without overflow incontinence, and even a feeling of pressure in the abdomen. These manifestations result from either partial or complete compression of the urethra by the hyperplastic prostate. Bladder wall hypertrophy occurs, and herniation into the bladder can occur. Ultimately, if treatment is not initiated, a postrenal cause of acute renal failure can develop because of back pressure on the renal system (i.e., the ureters) and the onset of hydronephrosis.

Diagnostic Criteria

Diagnosis of BPH usually begins with the patient seeking medical intervention because of the annoying symptoms. Along with a complete social history and physical examination, a digital rectal examination (DRE) can be performed to palpate the

TABLE 29.4

American Urological Association Symptom Index Scale

Questions to Be Answered	AUA Symptom Score (Circle 1 Number on Each Line)					
	Not at All	Less than 1 Time in 5	Less than Half the Time	About Half the Time	More than Half the Time	Almost Always
1. Over the past month, how often have you had a sensation of not emptying your bladder completely after you finished urinating?	0	1	2	3	4	5
2. Over the past month, how often have you had to urinate again <2 hours after you finished urinating?	0	1	2	3	4	5
3. Over the past month, how often have you found that you stopped and started again several times when you urinated?	0	1	2	3	4	5
4. Over the past month, how often have you found it difficult to postpone urination?	0	1	2	3	4	5
5. Over the past month, how often have you had a weak urinary stream?	0	1	2	3	4	5
6. Over the past month, how often have you had to push or strain to begin urination?	0	1	2	3	4	5
7. Over the past month, how many times did you most typically get up to urinate from the time you went to bed at night until the time you got up in the morning?	0 (None)	1 (1 time)	2 (2 times)	3 (3 times)	4 (4 times)	5 (5 times or more)

AUA, American Urological Association.

prostate but it recently has become optional. The degree of prostate enlargement has not been found to correlate with the severity of symptoms; rather, the location of the enlargement is what leads to symptom manifestation.

BPH severity is assessed using validated, self-administered symptom questionnaires such as the American Urological Association Symptom Index (AUASI) (Barry et al., 2017) (**Table 29.4**) or International Prostate Symptom Score. Mild or non-bothersome symptoms do not require treatment. Bothersome symptoms are managed with lifestyle modifications, medications, and surgery.

In the AUASI, symptoms are scored as mild (0–7 points), moderate (8–19 points), or severe (20–35 points). The American Urological Association (AUA) recommends that this scale be used on initial assessment and then for following the course of illness by periodic ongoing assessment of the patient. Such follow-up management enables the practitioner to initiate more acute or intensive therapy when the score increases. Patients with severe BPH symptoms should not be managed by this scale.

Postvoid catheterization is performed to ascertain the degree of urine retention; any amount of residual urine beyond 100 mL is considered significant. Uroflowmetry provides information about the force of the urine stream. Urodynamics can also be assessed using noninvasive pneumatic technology.

Other diagnostic tools include x-ray films, digital ultrasound, computed tomography (CT) scans, magnetic resonance imaging (MRI), and radionuclide scans. Biopsies can be added to the diagnostic workup for further clinical assessment of any hardened prostatic areas found by DRE. Laboratory monitoring of creatinine and blood urea nitrogen should be incorporated to determine whether renal involvement exists and, if so, to what degree. Prostate-specific antigen (PSA) levels can be elevated in patients with BPH.

Many symptoms of BPH stem from obstruction of the urethra and gradual loss of bladder function, which results in incomplete emptying of the bladder. The symptoms of BPH vary, but the most common ones involve changes or problems with urination, including a hesitant, interrupted, or weak stream; urgency, dribbling, or urinary retention; more frequent urination, especially at night; painful urination; and incontinence.

It is extremely important to evaluate men at risk for these symptoms. In 8 out of 10 cases, these symptoms suggest BPH, but they also can signal more serious conditions, such as prostate cancer.

Initiating Drug Therapy

There are three major classes of drugs used to treat BPH. One group is alpha-adrenergic antagonists or alpha-blockers (doxazosin, terazosin, tamsulosin, alfuzosin, and silodosin). Tamsulosin, silodosin, and alfuzosin are selective alpha$_1$-adrenoreceptor antagonists, selective for alpha$_{1A}$-adrenergic receptor. While causing smooth muscle relaxation in the lower urinary tract, it minimizes blood pressure–related adverse effects. These relax the smooth muscle fibers of the bladder neck and prostate, thereby reducing the dynamic components of prostatic obstruction.

Another group is 5-alpha-reductase inhibitors (finasteride and dutasteride). Five-alpha-reductase inhibitors decrease levels of intracellular DHT (the major growth-stimulatory hormone in prostate cells) without reducing testosterone levels. This leads to prostatic size reduction of 20% to 30%. Symptom relief occurs within 2 weeks of initiating alpha-blockers, compared with several months with finasteride.

The third category is phosphodiesterase type 5 (PDE5) inhibitor. The only drug in this class approved for this use is tadalafil (Cialis). PDE5 inhibitors have been found to regulate smooth muscle tone in human prostate. These are useful in patients who do not respond to alpha-blockers, especially in men with concomitant erectile dysfunction (ED).

Management of BPH can include medical, surgical, and a combination of medical and surgical intervention. Choosing the right treatment should be guided by patients' symptoms, comorbidities, and potential side effects of available drugs. Silodosin is a valid option for older adults and for people taking antihypertensive drugs. BPH patients affected by ED can target both conditions with continuous tadalafil therapy.

Pharmacotherapy is prescribed with both medical and surgical approaches to care. The progression of BPH is unique to the individual; the man often will "watch and wait" before proceeding further into active therapy because the process of hyperplasia can be slow. This is acceptable as long as the AUA score is 19 or less.

The Medical Therapy of Prostatic Symptoms (MTOPS) trial tested whether finasteride (Proscar), doxazosin (Cardura), or a combination of the drugs could prevent progression of BPH and the need for surgery or other invasive treatments (Marberger, 2006; Slawin, 2003). Physicians at 17 MTOPS medical centers treated 3,047 men with BPH for an average of 4.5 years. Participants were randomly assigned to receive doxazosin, finasteride, combination therapy, or a placebo. Vital signs, urinary symptoms, urinary flow, adverse effects, and medication use were assessed every 3 months. DRE, serum PSA level, and urinalysis were performed yearly. Prostate size was measured by ultrasound at the beginning and end of the study. Progression of disease was defined by one of the following: a four-point rise in the AUA score, urinary retention, recurrent urinary tract infection, or urinary incontinence.

Finasteride, a 5-alpha-reductase inhibitor, and doxazosin, an alpha$_1$-receptor blocker, together reduced the overall risk of BPH progression by 66% compared with a placebo. The combined drugs also provided the greatest symptom relief and improvement in urinary flow rate. Doxazosin alone reduced the overall risk of progression by 39% and finasteride alone by 34% relative to a placebo. The risk of urinary retention was reduced by 81% with combination therapy and 68% with finasteride alone. Doxazosin alone did not reduce the risk of urinary retention. The risk of incontinence was reduced by 65% with combination therapy. Only five men developed urinary tract or blood infections. No patients developed impaired kidney function related to BPH.

Twenty-seven percent of men taking doxazosin, 24% of men taking finasteride, and 18% of men taking combination therapy stopped treatment early, primarily because of adverse effects. The most common adverse effects included sexual dysfunction in men treated with finasteride and dizziness and fatigue in men treated with doxazosin.

Goals of Therapy

The goals of therapy include reduced bladder outlet obstruction, improved quality of life, fewer symptoms, and decreased residual urine volume.

The mainstay of medical management is pharmacotherapy. Pharmacotherapy is used for both controlling hyperplasia and managing annoying side effects, either as primary therapy or as an adjunct to surgical intervention. Management of hyperplasia is based on the premise that there are hormonal changes related to aging and that alpha-adrenergic receptors are present in prostate tissue, specifically smooth muscle. Pharmacotherapeutic interventions consist of hormonal manipulation and blocking effects achieved by alpha-adrenergic blockers. For dosage, adverse events, contraindications, and special considerations of drugs used for BPH, see **Table 29.5**.

5-Alpha-Reductase Inhibitors

Finasteride (Proscar) and dutasteride (Avodart), androgen hormone inhibitors, are used for managing the symptoms of BPH. They aid in the inhibition of androgen transformation from their steroid precursors. On average, most men achieve 20% to 40% reduction in prostate size after at least 6 months of use. In general, these agents are most effective in men with prostate glands more than 30 g (or cm^3). Both drugs lower PSA levels by about 50% after 6 months of use. This is critical to consider when screening for prostate cancer. If the PSA level does not fall by one half and the patient has been compliant with medication, the patient should be referred to a urologist for a workup.

Mechanism of Action

5-alpha-reductase inhibitors act by specifically blocking 5-alpha-reductase, the enzyme that activates testosterone in the prostate. It impairs prostate growth by inhibiting the conversion of testosterone to DHT and causes changes in the epithelial cells of the transition zone. By preventing testosterone activation, 5-alpha-reductase inhibitors lessen or prevent urinary system symptoms. They also decrease prostatic volume and prevent the progression of the disease in men with a significantly enlarged prostate. There is a slow reduction of 80% to 90% in the serum DHT level. As a result, prostatic volume decreases by about 20% over 3 to 6 months of treatment. Dutasteride blocks both types 1 and 2 5-alpha-reductase.

Studies have been done to determine the efficacy of finasteride and placebo. The larger Proscar Safety Plus Efficacy

TABLE 29.5

Overview of Selected Agents Used to Treat Benign Prostatic Hyperplasia

Generic (Trade) Name and Dosage	Selected Adverse Events	Contraindications	Special Considerations
Alpha-Adrenergic Blockers			
Terazosin (Hytrin) 1–20 mg PO daily	Orthostatic hypotension, somnolence, dizziness	Hypersensitivity to terbutaline Tachyarrhythmias, hypertension, pregnancy, lactation Use with caution in patients with cardiac insufficiency.	Take at bedtime to avoid hypotension.
Doxazosin (Cardura) 4–8 mg PO daily	Dizziness, headache, fatigue, malaise	Lactation Use with caution in patients with CHF, renal failure, hepatic impairment.	May have secondary benefit to client with cardiac disease Avoid combination with alcohol, nitrates, or other antihypertensive drugs.
Tamsulosin HCl (Flomax) 0.4 mg/d PO daily; increase to 0.8 mg/d PO daily Silodosin (Rapaflo) 8 mg PO daily	Orthostasis, headache, problems with ejaculation Orthostatic hypotension, priapism, headache, URI symptoms	Allergy to tamsulosin Prostatic cancer, pregnancy, lactation Hepatic impairment Severe renal impairment	Ejaculatory problems more common in higher dosage (0.8 mg/d) Interaction with cimetidine decreases clearance of tamsulosin. Contraindicated with clarithromycin
5-alpha-Reductase Inhibitor			
Finasteride (Proscar) 5 mg daily Dutasteride (Avodart) 0.5 mg daily Dutasteride/tamsulosin (Jalyn) 1 capsule (0.5/0.4) daily	Impotence, decreased libido, smaller ejaculate Orthostatic hypotension, priapism, increased risk for prostate cancer	Not to be handled by pregnant women Caution if sensitivity to sulfonamides	Inform patient that effective outcome of therapy may take up to 6 months. Avoid handling if pregnant or potentially pregnant.

CHF, congestive heart failure; HCl, hydrochloride; URI, upper respiratory infection.

Canadian Two-Year Study (PROSPECT) found that treatment with finasteride led to significant improvements in urinary symptoms and flow rates (Nickel et al., 1996). However, in the PROSPECT study, the improvements with finasteride were significantly less than those with any alpha-blocker or surgery.

5-alpha-reductase inhibitors decrease PSA levels by 40% to 50%. In a patient taking finasteride who has PSA screening, PSA levels should be doubled and then compared in the usual fashion to age-related norms.

Dosage

The dosage for finasteride is 5 mg/d; that for dutasteride is 0.5 mg/d. These dosages are recommended for use as long-term therapy; studies have shown benefit beyond the usual 2-year period, with beneficial effects in the third year.

Adverse Events

Adverse events include decreased libido, impotence, ejaculatory failure, and gynecomastia. Finasteride can also falsify the PSA level after 6 months of therapy.

Alpha-Adrenergic Blockers

Alpha-adrenergic blockers include terazosin (Hytrin), doxazosin (Cardura), prazosin (Minipress), tamsulosin (Flomax), and silodosin (Rapaflo). It is recommended to use alpha-blockers in men with smaller prostate glands (≤30–35 g

or cm^3), in younger men, and in patients in whom rapid effect is needed. Side effects of this class include headache, dizziness, asthenia, drowsiness, and retrograde ejaculation. Silodosin is an alpha$_1$-adrenoreceptor antagonist that is selective for alpha$_{1A}$-adrenergic receptor. While causing smooth muscle relaxation in the lower urinary tract, it minimizes blood pressure–related adverse effects.

Mechanism of Action

As a pharmacologic classification, alpha-adrenergic blockers are functional antihypertensives with potential effects on glomerular filtration rate, renal perfusion, and heart rate. They are strongly linked with fluid retention. These agents relax the smooth muscle of the prostate and bladder neck without interfering with bladder contractility, thereby decreasing bladder resistance to urinary outflow. In general, weeks to months may pass before benefits from these medications are noted. However, benefits may last for up to 2 years, in some cases longer.

Adverse Events

Side effects can be a major concern, especially considering the potential for hypotension, specifically orthostatic hypotension, and fluid retention. However, cardiac output can improve, thus preventing heart failure. Of the four agents, prazosin has more potential for causing orthostatic hypotension than the others.

Side effects such as dizziness, postural hypotension, fatigue, and asthenia affect 7% to 9% of patients treated with nonselective alpha-blockers. Side effects can be minimized by bedtime administration and slow titration of the dosage.

Tamsulosin (Flomax) is a highly selective alpha$_{1A}$-adrenergic antagonist that was developed to avoid the side effects of nonselective agents. Some patients who do not respond to nonselective alpha-blockers may respond to tamsulosin and, because of the selectivity, may have fewer side effects.

Dutasteride/tamsulosin (Jalyn) is a combination of 5-alpha-reductase inhibitor and alpha$_1$-adrenergic antagonist for the treatment of symptomatic BPH. The complementary mechanisms affect hormonal and smooth muscle pathways, inhibiting enlargement of the prostate and producing muscular relaxation resulting in a decrease of symptoms. Although monotherapy with dutasteride or tamsulosin is beneficial for many men, the combination drug is slightly better than either component alone at decreasing symptom scores. In carefully diagnosed, selected, and monitored patients who do not respond to monotherapy, Jalyn may produce clinical benefit.

Phosphodiesterase-5 Inhibitors (See Erectile Dysfunction)

The use of tadalafil (Cialis) at a dose of 5 mg daily has been approved for BPH.

Selecting the Most Appropriate Agent

The most appropriate agent is the one that achieves symptom control and produces the fewest adverse effects (**Table 29.6** and **Figure 29.2**).

First-Line Therapy

If symptoms are mild (AUA score <7), no medical treatment is recommended. The man should limit his fluid intake after dinner, avoid decongestants, massage the prostate after intercourse, and void frequently.

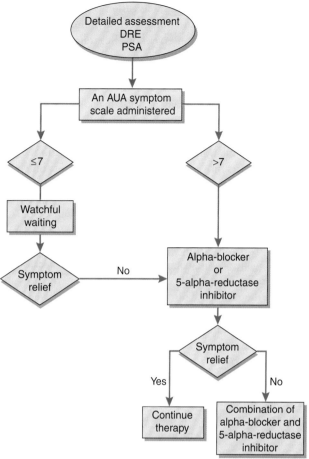

Key ◯ Starting point for decision-making

▢ Clinical actions (assessing, prescribing, monitoring)

◇ Decision point

FIGURE 29–2   Treatment algorithm for benign prostatic hyperplasia.

AUA, American Urological Association; DRE, digital rectal examination; PSA, prostate-specific antigen.

Second-Line Therapy

Pharmacotherapy is initiated when the AUA score is more than 7. An alpha-adrenergic blocker is effective first-line pharmacotherapy. The addition of a 5-alpha-reductase inhibitor is effective in men with moderate-to-severe symptoms and a documented enlarged prostate when an alpha-adrenergic blocker is not effective. Choosing the right treatment should be guided by patients' symptoms and comorbidities and potential side effects of available drugs. Silodosin is a valid option for older adults and for people taking antihypertensive drugs. BPH patients affected by ED can target both conditions with continuous tadalafil therapy.

Third-Line Therapy

Combination therapy with a 5-alpha-reductase inhibitor and alpha blocker may show greater improvement.

Fourth-Line Therapy

Referral to urology for possible surgery is recommended if other therapy fails.

TABLE 29.6		
Recommended Order of Treatment for Benign Prostatic Hyperplasia		
Order	**Agents**	**Comments**
First line	If AUA score is 7 or less, watchful waiting	
Second line	Alpha-adrenergic blocker or 5-alpha-reductase inhibitor or PDE5 inhibitor	Alpha-adrenergic blocker can be prescribed for patients with hypertension; 5-alpha-reductase inhibitor is recommended if prostate enlargement exceeds 40 g.
Third line	Combination of alpha-blocker and 5-alpha-reductase inhibitor or PDE5 inhibitor	

AUA, American Urological Association; PDE5, phosphodiesterase-5.

The prevailing surgical intervention is prostatic resection or prostatectomy. Transurethral resection of the prostate is the most common surgical intervention. Regardless of the surgical technique used (i.e., retrograde, perineal, or suprapubic approach), removal of the prostate is not without potential complications. The primary side effect, which can be permanent, is impotence from nerve damage. Incontinence is rare and usually only temporary; retrograde ejaculation can occur. Prostatectomy using laser technique is also an option, as is balloon dilation or urethral stent implantation. Laser surgery requires only an overnight stay; stent insertion is recommended for the man with cardiac or pulmonary morbidities, although it does not address the underlying problem of BPH itself.

Transurethral microwave thermotherapy is performed on an outpatient basis. Although anesthesia is not required, use of a local or general antianxiety agent may be helpful because the procedure is performed by catheter insertion into the prostate, through the urethra. This procedure uses heat derived from microwave energy (~45°C) to remove or destroy excess cells of the prostate while cool water is circulated to preserve surrounding tissue.

Monitoring Patient Response

As noted previously, the AUA symptom score can be used to monitor men with mild or even moderate BPH. A three- or four-point improvement in the AUASI score is clinically significant. Abatement of symptoms is used to evaluate the success of pharmacotherapy. If side effects become evident with a chosen agent, a different agent can be tried. The patient's blood pressure should be monitored frequently during the first 2 weeks of treatment to observe for an untoward hypotensive response. In addition, the practitioner should not pass off subjective complaints related to sexual health, because it could lead to medication noncompliance.

Patient Education

Drug Information

With terazosin use, an improvement in urine flow may begin within 1 to 2 weeks; thus, the patient must be informed that urine flow improvement will not occur overnight. The man should rise slowly from a sitting or standing position and quickly sit down or recline if abrupt vertigo occurs.

Lifestyle Changes

Patients with BPH can obtain symptomatic relief with regular, relaxed, and frequent voiding; decreasing fluid intake several hours before bedtime; and avoiding diuretics and alcohol. Other medications to avoid include anticholinergics, antihistamines, and antidepressants.

Alternative Therapies for BPH

Many men are using herbal and nutritional therapies to support prostate health although there is no scientific proof

TABLE 29.7	
Alternative Therapies for Benign Prostatic Hyperplasia	
Agent	**Dosage**
Saw palmetto	Doses vary based on manufacturer.
Pygeum	50–100 mg PO BID
Zinc	150 mg PO daily for 2 months, 50–100 mg daily thereafter

that these are effective. Men are encouraged to lose weight if overweight; to eat a low-fat, high-fiber diet; and to drink a minimum of two quarts of water daily. Supplements to maintain prostate health include saw palmetto, pygeum, and zinc (**Table 29.7**). Because these are not found in standard pharmacologic compendiums, dosages for saw palmetto and pygeum should follow the manufacturer's recommendations.

Saw palmetto, a herb derived from the dark berries of a palm tree native to the Southern United States, is reported to have been in use since the 1700s. Purportedly, it is useful for the management of prostate inflammation by a threefold mechanism. First, it inhibits testosterone conversion to DHT, resulting in the prevention of prostate enlargement. Second, it stops DHT binding to receptor sites; third, it has a general inhibitory effect on both estrogen and androgen receptors. There is no evidence of deleterious effects on PSA levels with the use of saw palmetto. Saw palmetto is available in capsule, liquid, or softgel form and as a tea; the tea is not believed to be effective for BPH. Saw palmetto often is used in combination with pygeum (http://www.sawpalmetto.com).

Pygeum is the ground and powdered bark of the pygeum tree, an evergreen of Southern Africa. It is prepared as a tea for easing complaints related to the genitourinary system. Widely used in Europe for symptom relief in BPH and thus postponement of surgery or the use of stronger medications, the efficacy of pygeum is being researched at the University of Southern California. Dosage recommenations are 50 to 100 mg twice daily; gastrointestinal irritation is a rare side effect.

Zinc also plays a role in BPH, improving general prostate health by preventing or even decreasing prostate enlargement. Research has supported that doses of zinc sulfate lead to the inhibition of 5-alpha-reductase, the enzyme for conversion of testosterone to DHT. The recommended dosage for zinc sulfate is 150 mg/d for 2 months followed by a maintenance dose of 50 to 100 mg/d.

PROSTATE CANCER

In the decade from 1980 to 1990, the incidence of prostate cancer increased by 50%, although this is perceived as a positive development, indicating enhanced screenings rather than a truly increased incidence of disease. In the United States, prostate cancer is the third leading cause of cancer deaths in men (Siegel et al., 2017). Between 2008 and 2017, the U.S. Preventive Services Taskforce (USPST) downgraded to a D recommendation for prostate cancer, which led to a decline in testing. It is projected that if this trend continues, distant-stage disease will return to pre-PSA screening levels by 2025. The focus now is a mutual decision between the provider and patient about the need for screening (Catalona, 2018).

Causes

The disease seems to be closely aligned with the aging process; the exact cause is not well understood, although a genetic predisposition has been found. Thus, sons of men who have had prostate cancer are at higher risk for developing prostate cancer themselves. No link between prostate cancer and BPH has been uncovered. From an environmental and occupational perspective, association with cadmium in the workplace is correlated with the later onset of prostate cancer.

Essentially, 95% of prostate cancers are adenocarcinomas, with most occurring at the prostate's periphery. How aggressive the neoplasm becomes seems to be more highly correlated with the degree of anaplasia, or lack of differentiation, of the cancer cells as opposed to tumor size. Progression of the cancer begins with local extension, but metastasis to distant sites occurs through blood and lymphatic vessels. Given the anatomic location of the prostate, it is easily understood how progression to the pelvis and rectum, lumbar and thoracic spine and ribs, and femur can ensue.

Pathophysiology

In many cases, symptoms present only with advanced disease. As with BPH, bladder-associated problems occur first—slow urine stream, inadequate emptying of bladder, painful urination, frequency, and nocturia. However, with prostate cancer, unlike BPH, there is no remission from these symptoms. Difficulty in defecation, and even obstruction of the large bowel, can also occur depending on how the tumor is spreading, but again this is usually seen with advanced disease.

Diagnostic Criteria

While early detection of prostate cancer is crucial, routine screening is controversial depending on age, and according to the USPSTF, AUA, and needs to be a shared decision for men between 55 and 69 years of age (Eggener et al., 2015). That being said, prostate cancer remains a significant problem specifically for African American men who tend to be diagnosed at a more advanced stage, and their rate of survival is poorer than among Whites (Carter et al., 2010; Lehto et al., 2010). Thus, public education targeting African American men is of paramount importance.

Three screening methods are commonly used. The first is the DRE; the second is the serum level of PSA. When either result is abnormal, an ultrasound study is performed transrectally. The man should be cautioned to avoid ejaculation for 48 hours before obtaining a PSA because false-positive results may be obtained. The diagnostic yield rises dramatically when ultrasound is incorporated with DRE and PSA. It is recommended that all men older than age 45 undergo an annual DRE and all men older than age 50 have a conversation about annual testing of their PSA level in addition to the DRE. Normal PSA values should be less than 2.7 in men younger than age 40 and 4.0 or less in men older than age 40.

However, for confirmation of cancer, and with suspect findings, further diagnostic investigation is warranted. This includes a biopsy to confirm the diagnosis and identify the cancer's histologic type, after which MRI and CT scans are necessary to determine the extent of metastasis.

Treatment options include surgery, chemotherapy, and radiation, either alone or in combination. Regardless of the treatment modality, loss of physiologic function can occur. This loss of function varies from temporary loss of urinary control to permanent incontinence. In addition to loss of urinary control, fecal incontinence can also result. Sexual dysfunction frequently occurs and involves the ability to attain an erection or have emission or ejaculation. Return to normal physiologic function often occurs over time, but some permanent dysfunction can result.

Initiating Drug Therapy

Pharmacologic intervention can also help the patient return to normal physiologic function after other treatments, such as partial or radical prostatectomy, which are options based on the cancer's histologic type and the extent of metastasis. Often, surgery is performed after a period of radiation or chemotherapy. A main postoperative concern is that bladder dysfunction will persist; this manifests as incomplete emptying, incontinence, decreased force of stream, and urinary scarring.

Bilateral orchiectomy has also been used for advanced disease to decrease the risk of complications and spread of prostate cancer, but it is not considered curative in the setting of metastasis or advanced disease. Bilateral orchiectomy is radical surgery used to extend the man's life; it provides relief from symptoms. There is minimal morbidity and mortality associated with the surgery, but it may have a negative impact on the man's self-esteem and sense of identity. Postsurgical pharmacologic management is crucial to promoting the man's self-esteem and correcting, as much as possible, the altered physiologic function.

ERECTILE DYSFUNCTION

ED is the most common sexual problem in men. It is defined as the repeated inability to achieve or maintain an erection that is firm enough for sexual intercourse. ED can be a total inability to achieve erection, an inconsistent ability to do so, or a tendency to sustain only brief erections. Approximately

30 million men in the United States over age 20 are affected by ED. The estimation is 1 in 10 men will have ED in their lifetime. The incidence of ED ranges from approximately 22% at age 40 to 49% by age 70. Although less common in younger men, erectile dysfunction still affects 5% to 10% of men below the age of 40 (Mulhall et al., 2016). The presence of comorbid diseases, diabetes and hypertension, also increases the incidence of ED. An organic cause can be found in about 80% of men with ED. The other 20% have psychogenic causes.

The cost and coverage of ED treatment varies widely amongst insurance carriers. Even if the condition is considered medically necessary, equity in care does not exist (Burnett et al., 2020). Lifestyle choices associated with ED include being sedentary, obese, smoking, and abuse of either illicit substances (e.g., cocaine) or alcohol. Lower education levels are also associated with higher prevalence of ED.

Causes

An erection requires a precise sequence of events, and ED can occur when any of the events are disrupted. The sequence includes nerve impulses in the brain, the spinal column, and the area around the penis and response in muscles, fibrous tissues, veins, and arteries in and near the corpora cavernosa. As men age, libido decreases, probably because of a decline in testosterone levels. Cardiovascular diseases encompass vascular damage associated with diabetes, hypertension, coronary heart disease, and dyslipidemia. Any history of psychological or psychiatric problems including depression, anxiety, sexual abuse, or stress predisposes to developing ED. Damage to nerves, arteries, smooth muscles, and fibrous tissues (often as a result of disease) is the most common cause of ED. Chronic diseases such as diabetes, kidney disease, chronic alcoholism, multiple sclerosis, atherosclerosis, vascular disease, and neurologic disease account for about 70% of ED cases. Between 35% and 50% of men with diabetes experience ED. Psychological issues can also lead to ED, and it is often a combination of physical and psychological issues. See **Box 29.1** for a list of risk factors for ED.

Surgery (especially radical prostate surgery for cancer) can injure nerves and arteries near the penis, thus causing ED. Injury to the penis, spinal cord, prostate, bladder, and pelvis can lead to ED by harming nerves, smooth muscles, arteries, and fibrous tissues of the corpora cavernosa.

Many common drugs such as antihypertensives, antihistamines, antidepressants, tranquilizers, appetite suppressants, and cimetidine can have ED as an adverse event. Psychological factors such as stress, anxiety, guilt, depression, low self-esteem, and fear of sexual failure cause 10% to 20% of ED cases. Other possible causes of ED include smoking, which affects blood flow in veins and arteries, and hormonal abnormalities, such as low testosterone levels.

Pathophysiology

Sexual performance in men has four stages: libido (desire), erection (arousal or engorgement), ejaculation, and detumescence.

> **BOX 29.1   Risk Factors for Erectile Dysfunction**
>
> Advancing age
> Cardiovascular disease
> Cigarette smoking
> Diabetes mellitus
> History of pelvic irradiation or surgery, including radical prostatectomy
> Hormonal disorders (e.g., hypogonadism, hypothyroidism, hyperprolactinemia)
> Hypercholesterolemia
> Hypertension
> Illicit drug use (e.g., cocaine, methamphetamine)
> Medications (e.g., antihistamines, benzodiazepines, selective serotonin reuptake inhibitors)
> Neurologic conditions (e.g., Alzheimer's disease, multiple sclerosis, Parkinson's disease, paraplegia, quadriplegia, stroke)
> Obesity
> Peyronie's disease
> Psychological conditions (e.g., anxiety, depression, guilt, history of sexual abuse, marital or relationship problems, stress)
> Sedentary lifestyle
> Venous leakage

Problems in any stage can result in male sexual dysfunction. The basic mechanical or primary focus of ED is on stage 2. Erection is a complex neuroendocrine psychophysiological event that can occur even during sleep, indicating that sexual stimulation is not required.

Nitric oxide (NO) is essential for erection. The release of NO in the cells of the corpus cavernosa following parasympathetic stimulation leads to the conversion of guanylate cyclase to cyclic guanosine monophosphate (cGMP). This causes smooth muscle relaxation that permits the influx of blood causing engorgement of the penis. This mechanism also slows the outflow of venous blood from the penis thus enhancing penile engorgement. Other contributors to vasodilation during erection include vasoactive intestinal peptide and prostaglandins E1 and E2 (PGE1 and PGE2).

The penis is innervated by both autonomic and somatic nerves. Sympathetic and parasympathetic fibers in the cavernous nerves regulate blood flow into the corpus cavernosum during erection and detumescence. Erection, at the level of the penis, begins with transmission of impulses from parasympathetic nerves and nonadrenergic, noncholinergic nerves. This neural stimulus leads to the release of NO from the nonadrenergic, noncholinergic nerves and possibly the endothelial cells. NO increases intracellular levels of cGMP in the cavernosal smooth muscle, which acts to relax cavernosal tissue, perhaps by activating protein kinase G and stimulating phosphorylation of the proteins that regulate corporal smooth muscle tone. The actions of the parasympathetic nervous system, NO, and cGMP permit rapid blood flow into the penis and the development of an erection. As pressure within the corporal body increases, small emissary veins traversing the tunica albuginea are occluded, trapping blood in the corpus cavernosum. The erection is maintained until ejaculation, which usually leads to detumescence.

PDEs are hydrolytic enzymes that play a critical role in regulating physiologic processes by terminating signal transduction through their hydrolytic action on cyclic nucleotides. They play a key role in the physiology of erection.

Significant changes in penile structure occur with aging. Collagen and elastic fibers in the tunica albuginea are key structures that permit increases in the girth and length of the penis during tumescence, and ultrastructural analysis of penile biopsies has shown that the concentration of elastic fibers decreases with age. This decrease results in a reduction in elasticity, which could contribute to ED in older men. Additionally, there is a decrease of up to 35% in the smooth muscle content of the penis in men older than age 60. Decreases in the ratio between corpus cavernosum smooth muscle and connective tissue have been associated with increased likelihood of diffuse venous leak that may contribute to ED. It has also been noted that the concentration of type III collagen decreases and that of type I collagen increases in the aging penis. It has been suggested that this change makes the corpus cavernosum less compliant, reduces filling of vascular spaces, and contributes to veno-occlusive dysfunction. It has also been hypothesized that changes in the collagen content of the penis may result in chronic ischemia that leads to loss of smooth muscle cells. Any condition, disease, medication, or injury or surgery that affects the ability to initiate erections or to fill the lacunar space or store blood may cause ED.

ED involves multiple organic and psychogenic factors, which often coexist. Psychogenic factors are the most common causes of intermittent ED in younger men, but these are usually secondary to or may coexist with organic factors in older men. Other factors contributing to ED include vasculogenic, neurogenic, endocrinologic, structural (traumatic), and pharmacologic causes and lifestyle factors, such as obesity, a sedentary lifestyle, and alcohol and tobacco use. Many of the conditions that contribute to ED are chronic and systemic, involving multiple avenues of damage. These conditions include cardiovascular disease, hypertension, diabetes mellitus, and depression. Many of the diseases linked to ED involve endothelial dysfunction.

There are many drugs that can affect erectile function. These include

- alcohol,
- analgesics,
- anticholinergics,
- anticonvulsants,
- antidepressants,
- antihistamines,
- antihypertensives,
- anti-Parkinson agents,
- corticosteroids,
- diuretics,
- nicotine, and
- tranquilizers.

Diagnostic Criteria

A thorough history is paramount to diagnosing ED. Every male patient should be asked about medical conditions, medications, and sexual function. Initial diagnostic workup should usually be limited to a fasting serum glucose level and lipid panel, thyroid-stimulating hormone test, and morning total testosterone level.

Initiating Drug Therapy

ED can be very traumatic to men. There are now drugs that can assist with achieving and maintaining an erection that is firm enough for sexual intercourse. Testosterone levels should be determined, and a complete cardiac history and evaluation should be done to determine whether there are contraindications to these medications. Approximately one third of men with ED do not respond to therapy with PDE5 inhibitors.

Goals of Drug Therapy

The goals of drug therapy for ED are to enable the patient to achieve sexual satisfaction and to achieve and maintain an erection.

Phosphodiesterase-5 Inhibitors

PDE5 inhibitors promote penile erection by inhibiting the breakdown of one of the messengers involved in the erectile response. PDE5 is the main cGMP-catalyzing enzyme in human trabecular smooth muscle. It is also expressed in vascular smooth muscle, lung, platelets, and a wide variety of other tissues but is not present in cardiac muscle cells. Human corpus cavernosum also contains PDE types 2, 3, and 4 enzymes. PDE5 inhibitors are contingent on the presence of cGMP in the smooth muscle cell. In the presence of sexual stimulation, PDE5 inhibitors reinforce the normal cellular signals that increase cyclic nucleotide concentrations by blocking cyclic nucleotide hydrolysis, thereby facilitating the initiation and maintenance of an erection.

Dosage

The recommended dosage of sildenafil is 50 mg 30 to 60 minutes before intercourse, but doses range from 25 to 100 mg. The maximum is one dose a day. Food can delay absorption, especially if taken close to a fatty meal.

The recommended dose of tadalafil is 10 mg, but doses range from 5 to 20 mg. Tadalafil can be taken without restriction on food or alcohol intake.

The recommended dose of vardenafil is 10 mg, but doses range from 2.5 to 20 mg. It is taken 60 minutes before intercourse. Food can delay absorption.

Avanafil (Stendra) is a new novel second-generation PDE5 inhibitor with a much shorter half-life. The recommended dose is 100 mg, but doses range from 50 to 200 mg. It is taken 15 minutes prior to intercourse. Dosing is not restricted by food intake, but alcohol intake should be limited.

Time Frame for Response

Sildenafil (Viagra) and vardenafil (Levitra) are rapidly absorbed, reaching maximum plasma concentrations within 30 to 120 minutes (median 60 minutes) of oral dosing in the fasted state; a high-fat meal has been found to reduce the rate of absorption. The elimination half-life is approximately 4 hours, and no more than one dose should be taken per 24-hour period.

Tadalafil (Cialis) has an onset of action of 30 minutes and allows intercourse for at least 30 hours. This is significant because it may eliminate the need for planning sexual activity.

Avanafil (Stendra) has an onset of action of 30 to 45 minutes. Absorption occurs quickly following oral administration elimination half-life of 5 hours. As with sildenafil and vardenafil, no more than one dose should be taken in 24 hours.

Contraindications

PDE5 inhibitors can potentiate the vasodilatory properties of nitrates, so their administration in patients who use nitrates in any form is contraindicated. In an emergency, nitrates can be used 24 hours after administration of sildenafil and vardenafil and 48 hours after tadalafil.

PDE5 inhibitors are contraindicated in patients with unstable angina, hypotension with a systolic blood pressure below 90 mm Hg, uncontrolled hypertension of more than 170/110 mm Hg, history of recent stroke, life-threatening arrhythmia, myocardial infarction (MI) within 6 months, and severe cardiac failure. They are also contraindicated in patients with severe hepatic impairment or end-stage renal disease requiring dialysis.

Sildenafil has a relative contraindication with the concomitant use of alpha-blockers and should not be taken within 4 hours of an alpha-blocker and at a dose no greater than 25 mg. Tadalafil should not be taken with an alpha-blocker other than tamsulosin, 0.4 mg once daily. Vardenafil is contraindicated with any alpha-blocker. Avanafil should be administered cautiously with an alpha-blocker, preferably at the 50 mg dose.

Adverse Events

Most adverse events are vasodilatory, including headache, flushing, and nasal congestion. Dyspepsia has also been reported. With sildenafil, abnormal color vision has been reported.

Interactions

Potent CYP4503A4 inhibitors can cause increased levels of PDE5 inhibitors. They may also be affected by amlodipine, beta blockers, cimetidine, diuretics, and erythromycin.

Selecting the Most Appropriate Agent

It is important to include the significant other in counseling about ED. A complete cardiac history must be taken. If there is any question as to the stability of the cardiac status, further testing must be done. Testosterone, serum glucose (or alternatively glycosylated hemoglobin), and serum lipid levels must be determined in all cases of ED. Depending on patient history and physical examination findings, more extensive laboratory tests may be necessary. If testosterone levels are abnormal, testosterone replacement is needed. See **Table 29.8** for selected agents.

TABLE 29.8

Overview of Selected Agents Used to Treat Erectile Dysfunction

Generic (Trade) Name and Dosage	Selected Adverse Events	Contraindications	Special Considerations
Tadalafil (Cialis) 5–20 mg/d	Headache, flushing, GI disturbance, nasal congestion, rash, priapism	Nitrates and alpha-blockers except tamsulosin 0.4 mg once daily	Food and alcohol make no difference in absorption; may remain in system for 36 hours.
Vardenafil (Levitra, Staxyn) 5–20 mg/d	As mentioned earlier	Nitrates and alpha-blockers	High-fat meal delays absorption.
Sildenafil (Viagra) 25–100 mg/d	As mentioned earlier and color disturbances	Nitrates and within 4 hours of an alpha-blocker and at a dose no >25 mg	As mentioned earlier
Avanafil (Stendra) 50–200 mg/d	As mentioned earlier	Nitrates and alpha-blockers	Food makes no difference in absorption. Caution with alcohol.

GI, gastrointestinal.

The patient with the following factors is considered at low risk for a cardiac event with the use of PDE5 inhibitors: fewer than three risk factors for coronary artery disease; controlled hypertension; mild, stable angina; uncomplicated MI more than 8 weeks previously; mild valvular disease; and New York Heart Association class 1 heart failure (see **Box 29.2** and **Figure 29.3**).

First-Line Therapy

First-line therapy for ED is aimed at lifestyle changes and modifying pharmacotherapy that may contribute to ED. A PDE5 inhibitor is also prescribed (**Table 29.9**).

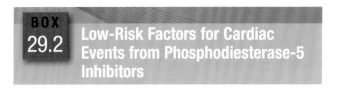

BOX 29.2   Low-Risk Factors for Cardiac Events from Phosphodiesterase-5 Inhibitors

Fewer than three risk factors for coronary artery disease
Controlled hypertension
Stable angina
Uncomplicated MI more than 8 weeks previously
Mild valvular disease
New York Heart Association class 1 heart failure (see Chapter 22)

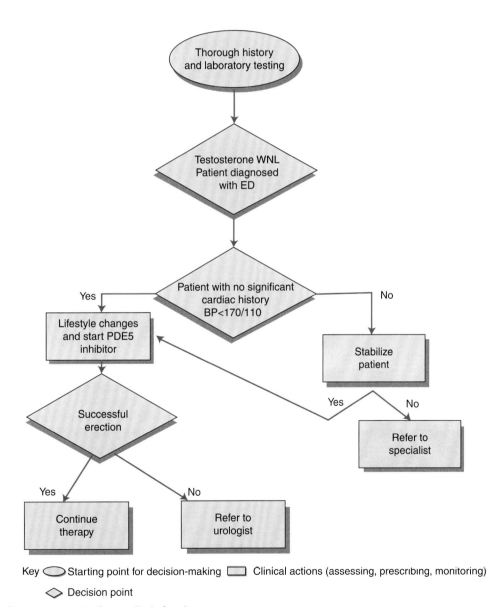

FIGURE 29–3   Treatment algorithm for erectile dysfunction.

BP, blood pressure; ED, erectile dysfunction; PDE5, phosphodiesterase-5; WNL, within normal limits.

TABLE 29.9

Recommended Order of Treatment for Erectile Dysfunction

Order	Agent	Comment
First line	PDE5 inhibitors	Contraindicated if on nitrates, unstable hypertension, unstable cardiac condition
Second line	Referral to urologist	Procedures available include penile intracavernosal injection therapy, medical intraurethral system for erections, vacuum erection device, penile prostheses.

PDE5, phosphodiesterase-5.

Second-Line Therapy

If PDE5 inhibitors are not successful in treating ED, the patient should be referred to an urologist. Alternative therapies include penile intracavernosal injection therapy, a medical intraurethral system for erections, a vacuum erection device, and penile prostheses.

Monitoring Patient Response

The patient should be followed in 6 months to determine the effectiveness of therapy and to reevaluate his cardiac status. If the patient does not meet the criteria for low risk, the PDE5 inhibitors are discontinued.

Patient Education

Drug Information

With sildenafil and vardenafil, a high-fat meal has been found to reduce the rate of absorption. Food and alcohol have no effect on the absorption of tadalafil.

Sildenafil has a relative contraindication with the concomitant use of alpha-blockers and should not be taken within 4 hours of an alpha-blocker and at a dose no greater than 25 mg. Tadalafil should not be taken with an alpha-blocker other than tamsulosin 0.4 mg once daily. Vardenafil is contraindicated with any alpha-blocker.

Complementary and Alternative Medicine

Yohimbine, an agent derived from the bark of the African yohimbe tree, has been found to be beneficial in some cases of ED. It is reported to act by both peripheral and central mechanisms, acting peripherally as a presynaptic stimulant at parasympathetic nonnoradrenergic, noncholinergic transmitter nerves and presynaptically as an adrenergic depressant at sympathetic $alpha_1$-adrenoceptors, both mechanisms augmenting penile blood flow. It also appears to have central nervous system activity, with blockade of the erection-suppressing $alpha_2$-adrenoceptors; several studies have reported a more favorable response with yohimbine compared with placebo in ED of psychogenic origin. Ginkgo biloba, ginseng, human chorionic gonadotropin, and l-arginine are some of the popular supplements advertised for ED. Patient should be asked about use of these therapies, and those patients who choose to continue use should be monitored for adverse effects and potential drug–drug interactions.

CASE STUDY 1

M.P., age 45, works as an accountant in a busy firm. He is of African American descent. He and his wife have been married for 25 years and have 2 children, age 21 and 18. His father is alive and well at age 68 but was diagnosed with benign prostatic hypertrophy (BPH) 5 years ago. M.P. considers himself to be in good health and has no allergies; he is approximately 15% overweight. His wife insisted that he seek medical intervention because of urinary symptomatology: He has difficulty starting his stream of urine, burning on urination, nocturia, and lower back and pelvic discomfort. The result of a prostate-specific antigen (PSA) test, his first in over 2 years, is 3.1.

DIAGNOSIS: BPH

1. List specific goals for treatment for M.P.
2. What drug therapy would you prescribe? Why?

3. What are the parameters for monitoring the success of the therapy?
4. Discuss specific patient education based on the prescribed therapy.
5. List one or two adverse reactions for the selected agent that would cause you to change therapy.
6. What would be the choice for second-line therapy?
7. What over-the-counter and/or alternative medications would be appropriate for this patient?
8. What dietary and lifestyle changes should be recommended for this patient?
9. Describe one or two drug–drug or drug–food interactions for the selected agent. Use caution if on another antihypertensive because alpha-blockers may intensify the effect.

Bibliography

Starred references are cited in the text.

Ahuja, S. (2014). Chronic bacterial Prostatitis. Retrieved from http://emedicine.medscape.com/article/458391-overview#a8

Barry, M. (2009). Screening for prostate cancer: The controversy that refuses to die. *New England Journal of Medicine, 360,* 1351–1354.

*Barry, M. J., Fowler, F. J., O'leary, M. P., Bruskewitz, R. C., Holtgrewe, H. L., Mebust, W. K., & Cockett, A. T. K. (2017). The American Urological Association Symptom Index for benign prostatic hyperplasia. *Journal of Urology, 197*(2S), S189–S197. doi: 10.1016/j.juro.2016.10.071

Bullock, B. A., & Henze, R. L. (2000). *Focus on pathophysiology.* Philadelphia, PA: Lippincott Williams & Wilkins.

*Burnett, A. L., Edwards, N. C., Barrett, T. M., Nitschelm, K. D., & Bhattacharyya, S. K. (2020). Addressing Health-Care system inequities in the management of erectile dysfunction: A call to action. *American Journal of Men's Health, 14*(5), 155798832096507. https://doi.org/10.1177/1557988320965078

*Carter, V., Tippett, F., Anderson, D., et al. (2010). Increasing prostate cancer screening among African American men. *Journal of Health Care for the Poor and Underserved, 21*(3), S91–S106. doi: 10.1353/hpu.0.0366

*Catalona, W. J. (2018). Prostate cancer screening. *The Medical Clinics of North America, 102*(2), 199–214. doi: 10.1016/j.mcna.2017.11.001

Church, D. (n.d.). Prostatitis – Infectious disease and antimicrobial agents. http://www.antimicrobe.org/e53.asp#top

Davis, N. G., & Silberman, M. (2020, January). *Bacterial acute prostatitis. [Updated May 28, 2020].* In: *StatPearls* [Internet]. Treasure Island, FL: StatPearls Publishing.

Deters, L. (2015). Benign prostatic hypertrophy. Retrieved from http://emedicine.medscape.com/article/437359-overview

Djavan, B., Eckersberger, E., Finkelstein, J., et al. (2010). Benign prostatic hyperplasia: Current clinical practice. *Primary Care: Clinics in Office Practice, 37*(3), 583–597.

Eardley, I., Donatucci, C., Corbin, J., et al. (2010). Pharmacotherapy for erectile dysfunction. *Journal Sex Medicine, 7,* 524–540. doi: 10.1111/j.1743-6109.2009.01627.x

*Egan, K. B. (2016). The epidemiology of benign prostatic hyperplasia associated with lower urinary tract symptoms. *Urologic Clinics of North America, 43*(3), 289–297. doi: 10.1016/j.ucl.2016.04.001

*Eggener, S., Cifu, A., & Nabhan, C. (2015). JAMA clinical guidelines synopsis: Prostate cancer screening. *Journal American Medical Association, 314*(8), 825–826.

Gacci, M., Andersson, K.-E., Chapple, C., Maggi, M., Mirone, V., Oelke, M., Porst, H., Roehrborn, C., Stief, C., & Giuliano, F. (2016). Latest evidence on the use of phosphodiesterase type 5 inhibitors for the treatment of lower urinary tract symptoms secondary to benign prostatic hyperplasia. *European Urology, 70*(1), 124–133. doi: 10.1016/j.eururo.2015.12.048

Gammoch, J. (2010). Lower urinary tract symptoms. *Clinics in Geriatric Medicine, 26*(2), 249–260.

Grant, P., Jackson, G., Baig, I., et al. (2013). Erectile dysfunction in general medicine. *Clinical Medicine, 13*(2), 136–140. doi: 10.7861/clinmedicine.13-2-136

Gupta, B. P., Murad, M., Clifton, M. M., et al. (2011). The effect of lifestyle modification and cardiovascular risk factor reduction on erectile dysfunction: A systematic review and meta-analysis. *Archives of Internal Medicine, 171*(20), 1797–1803. doi: 10.1001/archinternmed.2011.440

Heidelbaugh, J. (2010). Management of erectile dysfunction. *American Family Physician, 81*(3), 305–312.

Howlader, N., Noone, A. M., Krapcho, M., et al. (2014). SEER Cancer Statistics Review, 1975–2011, National Cancer Institute. Bethesda, MD. http://seer.cancer.gov/csr/1975_2011/, based on November 2013 SEER data submission, posted to the SEER web site, April 2014.

Jiwrajka, M., Yaxley, W., Ranasinghe, S., Perera, M., Roberts, M. J., & Yaxley, J. (2018). Drugs for benign prostatic hypertrophy. *Australian Prescriber, 41*(5), 150–153. doi: 10.18773/austprescr.2018.045

Katz, E., Tan, R., Rittenberg, D., et al. (2014). Avanafil for erectile dysfunction in elderly and younger adults: Differential pharmacology and clinical

utility. *Therapeutics and Clinical Risk Management, 10,* 701–711. doi: 10.2147/TCRM.S57610

Lee, S., Chan, E., & Lai, Y. K. (2017a). The global burden of lower urinary tract symptoms suggestive of benign prostatic hyperplasia: A systematic review and meta-analysis. *Scientific Reports, 7*(1), 7984. doi: 10.1038/s41598-017-06628-8

Lee, C. L., & Kuo, H. C. (2017b). Pathophysiology of benign prostate enlargement and lower urinary tract symptoms: Current concepts. *Ci ji yi xue za zhi = Tzu-chi Medical Journal, 29*(2), 79–83. doi: 10.4103/tcmj.tcmj_20_17

*Lehto, R., Song, L., Stein, K., & Coleman-Burns, P. (2010). Prostate cancer screening in African American men. *Western Journal of Nursing Research, 32*(6), 779–793. doi: 10.1177/0193945910361332

*Lim, K. B. (2017). Epidemiology of clinical benign prostatic hyperplasia. *Asian Journal of Urology, 4*(3), 148–151. doi: 10.1016/j.ajur.2017.06.004

*Marberger, M. (2006). The MTOPS study: New findings, new insights, and clinical implications for the management of BPH. *European Urology Supplements, 5,* 628–633. doi: 10.1016/j.eursup.2006.05.002.

*Mulhall, J. P., Luo, X., Zou, K. H., Stecher, V., & Galaznik, A. (2016). Relationship between age and erectile dysfunction diagnosis or treatment using real-world observational data in the USA. *International Journal of Clinical Practice, 70*(12), 1012–1018. doi: 10.1111/ijcp.12908

McNicholas, T., & Kirby, R. (2012). Benign prostatic hyperplasia and male lower urinary tract symptoms. *American Family Physician, 86*(4), 359–360.

McVary, K. T., Roehrbom, C. G., Avins, A. L., et al. (2010). American Urological Association guideline: Management of benign prostatic hyperplasia (BPH). Retrieved from http://www.auanet.org/common/pdf/education/clinical-guidance/Benign-Prostatic-Hyperplasia.pdf

Mobley, D., Feibus, A., & Baum, N. (2015). Benign prostatic hypertrophy and urinary symptoms: Evaluation and treatment. *Postgraduate Medicine, 127*(3), 301–307.

*Nickel, J. C., Fradet, Y., Boake, R., et al. (1996). Efficacy and safety of finasteride therapy for benign prostatic hyperplasia: Results of a 2-year randomized controlled trial (the PROSPECT study). *Canadian Medical Journal, 155*(9), 1251–1259.

Nunes, K. P., Labazi, H., & Webb, R. C. (2012). New insights into hypertension-associated erectile dysfunction. *Current Opinion in Nephrology and Hypertension, 21*(2), 163–170. doi: 10.1097/MNH.0b013e32835021bd

Olesovsky, C., & Kapoor, A. (2016). Evidence for the efficacy and safety of tadalafil and finasteride in combination for the treatment of lower urinary tract symptoms and erectile dysfunction in men with benign prostatic hyperplasia. *Therapeutic Advances in Urology, 8*(4), 257–271. doi: 10.1177/1756287216650132

*Paulis, G. (2018). Inflammatory mechanisms and oxidative stress in Prostatitis: The possible role of antioxidant therapy. *Research and Reports in Urology, 10,* 75–87. doi: 10.2147/RRU.S170400

Pearson, R., & Williams, P. M. (2014). Common questions about the diagnosis and management of benign prostatic hyperplasia. *American Family Physician, 90*(11), 769–774B.

Pirola, G. M., Verdacchi, T., Rosadi, S., Annino, F., & De Angelis, M. (2019). Chronic Prostatitis: Current treatment options. *Research and Reports in Urology, 11,* 165–174. doi: 10.2147/RRU.S194679

*Rawla, P. (2019). Epidemiology of prostate cancer. *World Journal of Oncology, 10*(2), 63–89. doi: 10.14740/wjon1191

Rensing, A. J., Kuxhausen, A., Vetter, J., & Strope, S. A. (2017). Differences in the treatment of benign prostatic hyperplasia: Comparing the primary care physician and the urologist. *Urology Practice, 4*(3), 193–199. doi: 10.1016/j.urpr.2016.07.002

Russo, A., LaCroce, G., Capogrosso, P., et al. (2014). Latest pharmacotherapy options for benign prostatic hyperplasia. *Expert Opinion on Pharmacotherapy, 15*(16), 2319–2328.

Shamloul, R., & Ghanem, H. (2013). Erectile dysfunction. *The Lancet, 381*(9861), 153–165. doi: 10.1016/s0140-6736(12)60520-0

Sharp, V., Takas, E., & Powell, C. (2010). Prostatitis: Diagnosis and treatment. *American Family Physician, 82*(4), 397–406.

*Siegel, R. L., Miller, K. D., & Jemal, A. (2017). Cancer statistics, 2017. *CA: A Cancer Journal for Clinicians, 67*(1), 7–30. doi: 10.3322/caac.21387

*Slawin, K. M. (2003). The medical therapy of prostatic symptoms study: What will we learn? *Reviews in Urology, 5*(Suppl. 4), S42–S47.

Unnikrishnan, R., Almassi, N., & Fareed, K. (2017). Benign prostatic hyperplasia: Evaluation and medical management in primary care. *Cleveland Clinic Journal of Medicine, 84*(1), 53–64. doi: 10.3949/ccjm.84a.16008

U.S. Cancer Statistics Working Group. (2015). United States Cancer Statistics: 1999–2012 incidence and mortality web-based report. Atlanta, GA: Department of Health and Human Services, Centers for Disease Control and Prevention, and National Cancer Institute.

*U.S. Department of Health and Human Services, Centers for Disease Control and Prevention and National Cancer Institute. (2020, June 30). *U.S. Cancer Statistics Working Group. U.S. cancer statistics data visualization tool based on 2019 submission data (1999–2017):* United States Cancer Statistics: Data Visualizations.https://www.cdc.gov/cancer/dataviz

Wang, X. H., Wang, X., Shi, M. J., Li, S., Liu, T., & Zhang, X. H. (2015). Systematic review and meta-analysis on phosphodiesterase 5 inhibitors and α-adrenoceptor antagonists used alone or combined for treatment of LUTS due to BPH. *Asian Journal of Andrology, 17*(6), 1022–1032. doi: 10.4103/1008-682X.154990

*Weidner, W., & Anderson, R. (2008). Evaluation of acute and chronic bacterial Prostatitis and diagnostic management of chronic prostatitis/chronic pelvic pain syndrome with special reference to infection/inflammation. *International Journal of Antimicrobial Agents, 31S*(2008), S91–S95.

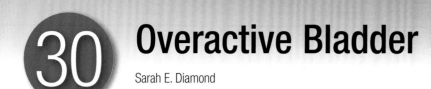

30 Overactive Bladder

Sarah E. Diamond

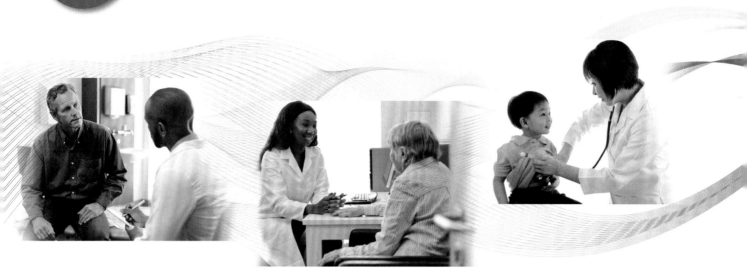

Learning Objectives

1. Describe the epidemiology and pathophysiology of overactive bladder (OAB).
2. Summarize the approach to treating OAB.
3. Compare pharmacotherapeutic agents used to manage OAB.
4. Recommend appropriate pharmacotherapy for the treatment of OAB based on patient-specific characteristics.

INTRODUCTION

Overactive bladder (OAB) is a highly prevalent yet underreported condition that transcends the boundaries of race, gender, and socioeconomic class. OAB is loosely defined by the International Continence Society (ICS) as a constellation of symptoms that include primarily urinary urgency usually accompanied by frequency (voiding eight or more times per 24 hours) and nocturia (awakening two or more times at night to void), with or without urge urinary incontinence (UUI). It is a symptom syndrome and not a discrete diagnosis. Data from the National Overactive Bladder Evaluation study suggest that OAB affects between 16% and 17% of adults in the United States (Stewart et al., 2003). However, given the substantial underreporting and the inherent challenges in identifying sufferers of OAB, the actual prevalence is likely markedly higher. Women and men tend to be affected by OAB proportionately; however, women are more likely than men to present with the symptom of incontinence as part of their clinical picture.

The incidence of OAB increases linearly with age and is predicated on a number of factors that are impacted by aging. However, OAB with or without incontinence is not considered a normal part of aging; OAB symptomatology and any instance of urgency are always considered pathologic.

OAB syndrome has extensive ramifications with respect to morbidity, mortality, and economic impact. A preponderance of literature supports the assertion that OAB is associated with increased rates of depression, decreased self-esteem, social isolation, general fragility, and falls and fracture. Upon development of OAB symptoms, patients tend to engage in avoidance behaviors in order to escape the social stigma and embarrassment associated with urinary incontinence (UI) or urinary urgency. Eventually, this translates into substantial lifestyle changes and the potential for social isolation. Total annual direct and indirect costs attributable to OAB are estimated to be $19.5 billion in the United States (Faiena et al., 2015). A leading cause of morbidity in the older population and the most commonly cited reason for assisted living and long-term care facility admission, OAB needs to be assessed in the primary care setting preemptively.

The terms *OAB*, *detrusor overactivity* (DO), and *UI* are frequently used interchangeably erroneously. UI is a possible symptom as part of the symptomatology construct that constitutes OAB; it does not necessarily need to be present in patients diagnosed with OAB. While urgency is the cardinal symptom of OAB and must be present in order to yield a diagnosis of OAB, only about 25% to 35% of patients experience *incontinence* as well. DO implies an involuntary and inappropriate contraction of the bladder; however, it is considered a surrogate marker of OAB that may or may not correlate with urgency. DO is further delineated into idiopathic (absence of an identifiable cause) or neurogenic (an underlying neurological condition, deficit, or injury is the causative factor). There is considerable overlap between nonpharmacologic and pharmacologic treatments for OAB, UI, and DO; therefore, UI subtypes will be discussed. The accepted nomenclature for UI differentiates between the underlying pathophysiology and the nature of the urine loss. UUI implies a strong and sudden urge to urinate that cannot be deferred and results in involuntary loss of urine. Stress urinary incontinence (SUI) occurs when an internal or external force impacts the bladder or the musculature that supports it. Common examples of such pressures include coughing, sneezing, heavy lifting, or prolapsed pelvic organs. Mixed UI is a combination of both SUI and UUI. The historical term *overflow incontinence*, which suggested some level of obstruction or voiding difficulty, has been replaced with bladder outlet obstruction (BOO) and is no longer part of the classification schema.

CAUSES

The exact cause of the OAB symptom constellation is multifactorial and not completely elucidated. There are numerous underlying anatomic, physiologic, and comorbidity-related

factors that precipitate or exacerbate OAB. The majority of cases are considered idiopathic, with the remainder being attributed to myogenic or neurogenic causation.

PATHOPHYSIOLOGY

The bladder and the corresponding micturition cycle are controlled by a complex, coordinated interplay among the central nervous system (CNS), peripheral nervous system, and the anatomic components of the lower urinary tract (LUT). The LUT is composed of the bladder, urethra, bladder outlet, internal and external urethral sphincters, and the musculature of the pelvic floor (**Figure 30.1**). The discord between the continuous production of urine (1–2 L/d) and the episodic nature of voiding necessitates the storage of urine. The bladder (detrusor muscle) is a highly compliant, viscoelastic hollow organ that expands to accommodate the storage of urine while maintaining a constant pressure throughout this filling phase. As the bladder fills, it maintains a pressure that is lower than that of the urethra, thereby facilitating the development of a pressure gradient that prevents urine from being expelled. The normal urge to void is under voluntary control, and therefore only when the bladder reaches a critical volume, or about 75%

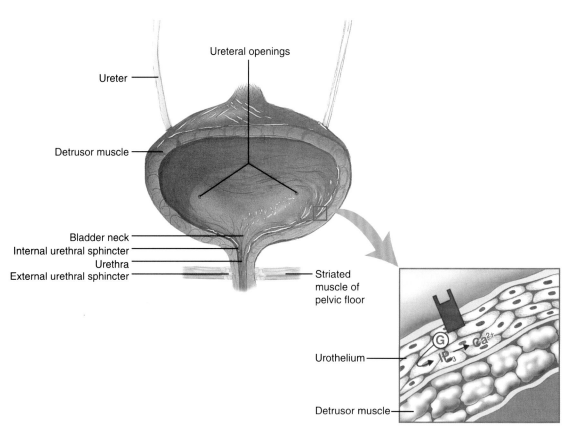

FIGURE 30–1 M_3 receptors are coupled to G proteins, which activate phospholipase, generating inositol triphosphate. Inositol triphosphate causes the release of stored Ca^{2+}, which stimulates bladder contraction.

IP$_3$, inositol triphosphate.

TABLE 30.1

Bladder and Urethral Innervation

Nerve	Anatomic Location	Nervous System	Spinal Cord Origin	Physiologic Function
Pudendal	External sphincter	Somatic	S2, S3, S4	Maintains tone in pelvic floor Excitatory innervation to external urethral sphincter
Pelvic	Urethra	Parasympathetic	S2, S3, S4	Relaxes sphincter
Hypogastric	Urethra	Sympathetic	T1–L2	Stimulates sphincter closure
Pelvic	Bladder neck	Parasympathetic	S2, S3, S4	Relaxes sphincter
Hypogastric	Bladder neck	Sympathetic	T1–L2	Stimulates sphincter closure
Pelvic	Bladder	Parasympathetic	S2, S3, S4	Contraction of detrusor during micturition
Hypogastric	Bladder	Sympathetic	T1–L2	Relaxes detrusor during filling phase

of total capacity, will an individual feel the desire to void. This urge, which is different from pathologic urgency and is under different neural control, can be deferred until an appropriate time. Upon conscious and deliberate urination, the urethral resistance decreases, and phasic contractions in the bladder result in increased bladder pressure and the subsequent voiding of urine.

The LUT is innervated by efferent and afferent neuronal complexes involving sympathetic, parasympathetic, and somatic nerves. The *sympathetic* nervous system primarily stimulates urethral sphincter closure and detrusor relaxation during filling, while the *parasympathetic* system influences contraction of the detrusor and relaxation of the urethral sphincters during the emptying phase. Somatic innervation maintains the tone of the striated pelvic floor muscles and the external urethral sphincter (**Table 30.1**). The bladder is continuously bombarding the CNS with afferent signals during the filling phase via A-delta fibers and C fibers. These normal impulses indicate when the bladder is filling and also when it is nearing capacity. The impulses are transmitted to higher brain centers such as the cortex, pons, and brain stem, which also exert some level of control over micturition. The sensations generated by this neurotransmission will result in variable degrees of the normal urge to urinate. The A-delta fibers generally respond to the mechanical stretch of the bladder during the filling phase. However, during pathologic conditions, it is thought that the unmyelinated C sensory fibers may precipitate abnormal OAB sensations. The C sensory fibers are dappled with vanilloid receptors (which can be stimulated by capsaicin), purinergic receptors or $P2X_2$ and $P2X_3$ (which can be stimulated by adenosine triphosphate), and neurokinin receptors (which can be stimulated by neurokinin A and substance P) (see **Figure 30.2**).

Acetylcholine-mediated activation of muscarinic receptors is the predominant physiologic mediator of detrusor contraction. Muscarinic receptor subtypes M_1, M_2, and M_3 are found in the urinary bladder; however, it is the M_3 subtype that is primarily responsible for bladder contraction. These receptors, particularly the M_3 subtype, have become drug targets for purposes of treating OAB.

Any aberration of any individual component or combination of components involved in the micturition reflex can result in OAB or UI, as can separate comorbid conditions or physiologic states. Transient and reversible conditions or behaviors may contribute to symptoms consistent with OAB, namely, increases in fluid intake or increases in caffeine or alcohol consumption. Benign prostatic hyperplasia (BPH) or obstruction can manifest in incontinence. Sacral nerve damage can lead to urinary retention. Irrespective of the etiology of OAB, the common themes include increased bladder pressure at low volumes during filling, altered response to stimuli, amplified myogenic activity and contraction, and changes in the smooth muscle anatomy.

Owing to the poor electrical coupling between smooth muscle bundles in the bladder, the highly innervated bladder is able to ignore some of the errant impulses that would otherwise cause unwanted contraction. Patchy denervation and morphologic changes in the electrical coupling may result in bladder hypertrophy and incomplete emptying. Abnormal micturition can be stimulated by damage to the afferent neurons in the dorsal root ganglia as well, which can then confer an abbreviated delay in the micturition reflex. Ischemic conditions such as diabetic neuropathy, peripheral vascular disease, and urethral stricture may also result in compromised blood flow and ultimately neuronal death with subsequent detrusor hyperactivity. Inevitable physiologic changes that occur during the aging process may also contribute to impaired cortical inhibition of bladder contraction. Stroke, Alzheimer's disease, and multiple sclerosis have been implicated in contributing to the disease process as well. Nonneurogenic conditions may also yield OAB symptoms; polyuria may be produced by uncontrolled diabetes, and nocturia may be precipitated by sleep apnea (**Box 30.1**).

Once OAB symptoms have emerged, a self-propelling cycle of factors can further exacerbate the condition. Urgency, a central feature of OAB, increases the frequency of micturition and therefore reduces the volume of each micturition,

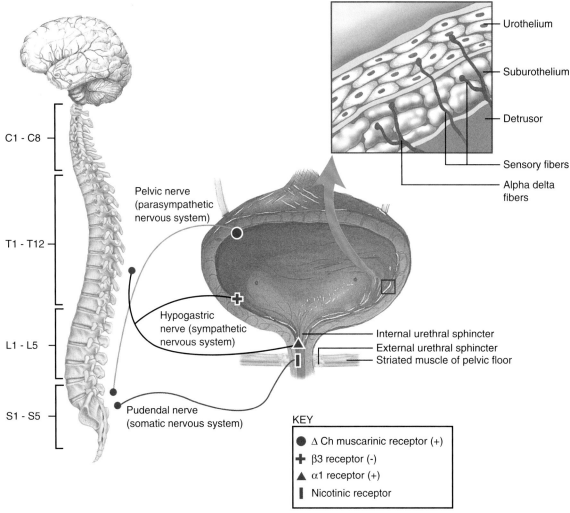

FIGURE 30–2 The bladder is innervated by the sympathetic, parasympathetic, and somatic nervous systems. The pudendal nerve maintains external sphincter and pelvic muscle tone. The pelvic nerve stimulates bladder contraction. The hypogastric nerve stimulates internal sphincter closure and detrusor relaxation.

provided that fluid intake remains constant. This sometimes leads to incomplete bladder emptying and subsequent residual volume that promotes the urgency and increased frequency of urination. Similarly, DO can result from neurogenic or myogenic causes. The contractions tend to be weak, which results in incomplete bladder emptying, a reduced bladder capacity, and therefore increased urinary frequency.

DIAGNOSTIC CRITERIA AND EVALUATION

OAB is a markedly underreported condition, owing mostly to the embarrassment and stigma with which it is associated. It tends to elude the typical clinical assessments and patient interviews that constitute the primary care visit and is generally diagnosed only when it is reported by the patient. The only

diagnostic criteria that have been firmly established are the presence of urgency with or without nocturia and frequency. These criteria are inherently subjective; however, there have been attempts to impose objective measurements and ratings in order to determine whether a symptom is pathologic.

Current recommendations suggest that pointed questioning should be integrated into the patient interview during routine primary care visits in order to capture urinary symptoms that may otherwise be overlooked. If patient complaints or interview-generated information is suggestive of OAB, the practitioner should perform a genitourinary exam and urinalysis as well as a more in-depth medical history that is germane to urinary health. One of the major goals of this interview would be the establishment of potential causative factors acutely or chronically (acute infection, changes in fluid intake, menstrual history, obstetric history, prostate pathology). The urinalysis is intended to assist in ruling out hematuria or an infection.

BOX 30.1 Factors That May Precipitate or Worsen Overactive Bladder

NEUROLOGIC CONDITIONS

Stroke
Spinal cord injury
Diabetic neuropathy
Alzheimer's disease
Multiple sclerosis

SYSTEMIC OR METABOLIC CONDITIONS

Sleep disorders (apnea)
Venous insufficiency/heart failure
Diabetes mellitus

BEHAVIORAL CONSIDERATIONS

Excessive fluid or caffeine consumption
Constipation
Impaired mobility

PSYCHOLOGICAL CONDITIONS

Depression

MEDICATIONS

Diuretics
Narcotic pain relievers
Calcium channel blockers
Alpha-adrenergic antagonists
Anticholinergics
Alpha-adrenergic agonists

MISCELLANEOUS

Prostate enlargement
Estrogen deficiency

URINARY TRACT PATHOLOGY

Urinary tract infection
Urinary obstruction

Since abnormalities or pathology in the LUT can precipitate OAB symptoms, it is imperative to evaluate the bladder, urethra, and pelvic floor muscles as well. In patients at risk for urinary retention (diabetics, spinal cord injury patients, patients with BPH), more invasive testing may be required. A residual urine volume of more than 100 mL suggests urinary retention, and these patients may need to be evaluated by cystoscopy to rule out malignancy. OAB is a constellation of symptoms, all of which could be reasonably attributed to other conditions. Therefore, OAB is often diagnosed after the exclusion of other pathology. Primarily, infections, cancers (bladder, prostate), structural abnormalities (urethral, prostate), and urinary retention should be ruled out during the evaluation process.

A neurologic exam, with emphasis on the sacral neuronal pathways, is recommended because OAB may be caused by neurogenic LUT dysfunction. In addition to assessments of gait, abduction/dorsiflexion of toes, and sensory innervation to the LUT, a rectal exam will provide some information relevant to voluntary sphincter control. In males specifically, a measurement of prostate-specific antigen (PSA) and administration of the American Urological Association's (AUA) subjective symptoms assessment (AUA-7) should occur (**Box 30.2**).

One of the tools with the highest level of clinical evidence is the *bladder diary* or *voiding diary*, a patient-generated daily log that includes fluid intake and urinary output with corresponding times. Typically, entries are made by the patient over

BOX 30.2 Diagnostic Differential

Bladder cancer, bladder calculus, interstitial cystitis
Endometriosis
Prostate cancer
Urethral calculus
Bacterial cystitis, prostatitis, urethritis
Urinary retention, polyuria, psychogenic urinary frequency

either a 3- or 7-day period. It yields information regarding urinary habits, estimation of bladder capacity, volume voided with each micturition, diurnal and nocturnal frequency, urgency, and incontinence. A number of clinical trials have used this tool to assess outcomes and have found that bladder diaries are an accurate measure of OAB symptoms, including urgency. Another parameter that is thus far not validated is "warning time," the length of time between an initial perception of the urge to void and the time at which it can no longer be deferred.

The use of urodynamic testing (UDT), the comprehensive evaluation of bladder and urethral performance during micturition, has been met with some controversy. UDT consists of

TABLE 30.2

Urodynamic Testing

Component	Description	Clinical Utility
Uroflowmetry	Measurement of the volume over urine voided, speed at which voiding occurs, and duration of void	Obstruction is likely if speed is <10 mL/s.
PVR	After voiding, determination of PVR made via ultrasound or through catheterization	<25 mL is considered normal and >100 mL is abnormal.
Multichannel filling cystometry	Evaluation of bladder capacity, bladder compliance, and at what volume the urge to void occurs; accomplished by filling the bladder with normal saline and measuring detrusor pressure	Bladder pressure during filling should be <10 cm H_2O; dysfunction is diagnosed if the pressure rises at an unacceptable rate.
Leak point pressure	Evaluation of the first urine leakage and the abdominal pressure at which it occurs; the patient is instructed to perform Valsalva maneuver (e.g., coughing); patient is observed for urine leakage.	Low readings (<40 cm H_2O) are associated with sphincter weakness.
Pressure flow study	Assessment of the interaction among the bladder, bladder outlet, pelvic floor, and urethra during voiding; patient is instructed to void with all catheters in place (catheters include urethral catheterization and possibly vaginal or rectal catheterization).	Useful for diagnosing bladder outlet obstructions
Electromyography	Assessment of the coordination between the perineal muscles and the bladder	Useful in diagnosing neurogenic etiology of OAB

OAB, overactive bladder; PVR, postvoid residual.

a collection of urodynamic assessments that range from simple direct observations to complex, sophisticated, invasive evaluations. In order to best assess a LUT dysfunction or OAB, the symptoms need to be reproducible in a clinical setting. **Table 30.2** provides a list of the possible components of UDT. UDT is not required for a diagnosis of OAB; however, it may be indicated if there is suspicion of a BOO, neurogenic voiding dysfunction, or an uncertain diagnosis.

INITIATING DRUG THERAPY

Once a diagnosis of OAB has been established, the subsequent steps include an assessment of the degree of impairment or annoyance resulting from OAB, initiation of empiric or disease-specific therapy if required, treatment of comorbid conditions, and referral to a specialist if warranted. If it is determined that the patient is significantly bothered by OAB and/or has begun to engage in avoidance behaviors that are compromising quality of life, therapy should be initiated. The 2019 AUA guidelines recommend utilizing behavioral therapies as the first-line intervention, a series of behaviors that are intended to change patient behavior or the environment (Lightner et al., 2019). The most common behavioral interventions are bladder training, pelvic floor muscle exercises, and weight loss. The nondrug therapies usually are ultimately combined with pharmacologic therapy (**Table 30.3**).

The *anticholinergic* or antimuscarinic drugs (oxybutynin, tolterodine, trospium, darifenacin, solifenacin, fesoterodine) have the greatest level of evidence with respect to their safety and efficacy in treating OAB and are recommended as

first-line pharmacologic therapy by the 2019 AUA guidelines along with beta$_3$-adenoceptor agonists. Their clinical use is sometimes limited, however, by their inherent anticholinergic adverse effects, most commonly dry mouth, blurred vision, constipation, cognitive dysfunction, and urinary retention. This is particularly challenging because the population with the highest prevalence of OAB is the older adult population, an age cohort that is also more predisposed to cognitive dysfunction, urinary retention, and visual disturbances.

If tolerability issues preclude the use of anticholinergic drugs, tricyclic antidepressants (TCAs; imipramine), desmopressin, topical estrogens for females, and alpha-adrenergic antagonists for males are appropriate alternatives. There is emerging evidence about the role of selective serotonin reuptake inhibitors (SSRIs) and serotonin norepinephrine reuptake inhibitors (SNRIs) in treating OAB syndrome. Vanilloids and afferent nerve inhibitors such as capsaicin or resiniferatoxin are in the investigation phases to assess their utility in managing OAB.

The combination of pharmacologic and nonpharmacologic treatment tends to yield superior outcomes and clinical success. *Bladder training* encompasses pelvic floor exercises, scheduled voiding, urge suppression skills, and extensive patient education (Willis-Gray et al., 2016). Benefit may still be derived from prompted scheduled voiding in patients who are cognitively impaired. In refractory cases of OAB, biofeedback devices that deliver electrical stimulation via vaginal or rectal probes augment the pelvic floor exercises. In severe or refractory patients, surgical interventions, such as neural ablation, slings, and neuromodulating device implantation, may be attempted. This will be further discussed.

TABLE 30.3

Overactive Bladder Medication Overview

Medication	Usual Dose	Uroselectivity	Clinical Considerations
Anticholinergics/Antimuscarinics			
Oxybutynin (Ditropan)	5–15 mg PO TID	No	Dry mouth occurs in up to 66% of patients. Indicated for neurogenic and nonneurogenic detrusor overactivity
Oxybutynin ER (Ditropan XL)	5–15 mg PO once daily	No	Dry mouth occurs in up to 66% of patients. Indicated for neurogenic and nonneurogenic detrusor overactivity
Oxybutynin (Oxytrol transdermal patch)	3.9 mg/patch twice weekly (q3–4d)	No	Dry mouth occurs half as frequently as compared to the oral formulation.
Tolterodine (Detrol)	2 mg PO BID	Yes	Incidence of dry mouth is 20%–25%.
Tolterodine ER (Detrol LA)	4 mg PO once daily	Yes	Dry mouth occurs in <20% of patients.
Trospium (Sanctura)	20 mg PO BID	Yes	Take before meals or on an empty stomach. No CYP P-450 metabolism
Trospium extended-release (Trospium XR)	60 mg PO once daily	Yes	Take before meals or on an empty stomach. No CYP P-450 metabolism
Solifenacin (VESIcare)	5–10 mg PO once daily	Yes	
Darifenacin hydrobromide (Enablex)	7.5–15 mg once daily (may titrate up to 15 mg after 2 wk if tolerated)	Yes	Possibly less impact on cognitive function than other antimuscarinics
Fesoterodine (Toviaz)	4–8 mg PO daily	No	Less CYP2D6 interaction potential
Beta-3-Adrenoreceptor Agonists			
Mirabegron (Myrbetriq)	25–50 mg PO once daily	Yes	Less incidence of anticholinergic and cognitive adverse effects
OnabotulinumtoxinA		Yes	Efficacy maintained for several months; possible risk of urinary retention and voiding dysfunction
100 U injections (interval undetermined but generally q6–9mo) OnabotulinumtoxinA (Botox)			
SNRIs			
Duloxetine (Cymbalta)	40–80 mg PO once daily	No	Avoid concomitant administration with other serotonergic drugs.
Alpha-Adrenergic Antagonists			
Alfuzosin (Uroxatral)	2.5 mg PO TID	No	
Doxazosin (Cardura)	1–16 mg PO once daily	No	Dizziness occurs in up to 20% of patients.
Prazosin (Minipress)	1–10 mg PO BID	No	
Tamsulosin (Flomax)	0.4–0.8 mg PO once daily	No	
Terazosin (Hytrin)	1–10 mg PO HS	No	
Silodosin (Rapaflo)	8 mg PO once daily	No	Retrograde ejaculation occurs in up to 28% of patients.
Miscellaneous			
Estrogen	Vaginal tablet: 1 tablet vaginally daily for 2 weeks and then 1 tablet twice weekly Vaginal cream: 0.5 g applied nightly for 2 weeks and then twice weekly Vaginal ring: 2 mg intravaginally; following insertion, ring should remain in place for 90 d.	No	Risk of worsening estrogen-responsive malignancies Potential for CHD risk
Desmopressin	20–40 mg spray intranasally at bedtime 0.1–0.4 mcg PO 2 h prior to bedtime	No	Risk of worsening estrogen-responsive malignancies Potential for CHD risk

CHD, coronary heart disease; CYP, cytochrome P-450; ER, extended release; SNRIs, serotonin norepinephrine reuptake inhibitors.

BOX 30.3 Behavioral Modifications

Reduce fluid consumption
Reduce alcohol consumption
Reduce caffeine consumption
Start bladder training
Perform pelvic floor exercises

Compensatory behaviors such as limiting fluid intake or reducing the frequency of diuretics are not recommended, although patients frequently engage in these behaviors. Self-imposed fluid restriction may precipitate dehydration and subsequent increased fall risks, cognitive impairment, worsened renal function, and changes in drug metabolism. Altering diuretic administration could negatively impact the treatment of other conditions or result in fluid overload. The use of absorbent pads or undergarments may help to mitigate the social stigma aspect of OAB, especially in patients who experience incontinence. Rushing to find a restroom when urgency occurs also predisposes patients to falls and fractures (**Box 30.3**).

Goals of Drug Therapy

The intended outcome of pharmacologic therapy is primarily resolution of symptoms (urgency, frequency, nocturia), cessation of incontinence episodes (if present), and a full return to previous level of social functioning. In the event of a comorbid mood disorder (depression, anxiety) that emerged as a consequence of OAB, goals of therapy would include resolution of this disorder as well. Patients suffering from OAB are at an increased risk for urinary tract infections, and those with associated incontinence are at risk for perineal skin infections. These corresponding issues may resolve spontaneously upon treatment of the OAB and/or incontinence; however, additional drug therapy may be required (**Table 30.4**).

Anticholinergic/Antimuscarinic Drugs

As a class, antimuscarinic drugs are the mainstay of pharmacologic therapy for OAB and UI. Anticholinergic drugs are considered first-line therapy and typically will be used even after clinical failure or intolerance to an initial anticholinergic medication. The class is divided into tertiary and quaternary amines, differing with respect to lipophilicity, molecular size, and charge. High lipophilicity, small molecular size, and low charge confer upon the tertiary amines (oxybutynin, tolterodine, solifenacin, darifenacin, fesoterodine) easy transfer into

TABLE 30.4
Medication Pharmacokinetics and Clinical Considerations

Drug	Metabolism	Interactions	Contraindications	Clinical Considerations
Antimuscarinics				
Oxybutynin	Minor substrate of CYP3A4	CYP3A4 inhibitors or inducers Pramlintide may enhance the anticholinergic effects of anticholinergics.	Narrow-angle glaucoma, urinary retention	Xerostomia (29%–71%; dose related) Constipation (7%–15%)
Tolterodine	Major substrate of CYP2D6 and 3A4 Minor substrate of CYP2C9 and 2C19	Strong CYP2D6 or 3A4 inhibitors or inducers Systemic azole antifungals may decrease metabolism of tolterodine. Tolterodine may enhance the anticoagulant effect of warfarin.	Urinary retention, narrow-angle glaucoma	Prolonged QTc interval at supratherapeutic doses CYP2D6 poor metabolizers more likely to exhibit QTc prolongation Dosage adjustment for renal impairment Dry mouth (35%; ER capsules, 23%)
Trospium	Not fully elucidated; thought to be metabolized by esterase hydrolysis and conjugation	Pramlintide may enhance the anticholinergic effect of anticholinergics.	Bladder flow obstruction, narrow-angle glaucoma	Dosage adjustment of IR trospium in renal impairment Avoid use of ER trospium in patients with renal impairment.
Solifenacin	Major CYP3A4 substrate	Major inhibitors or inducers of CYP3A4 Grapefruit juice may increase the serum-level effects of solifenacin.	Bladder flow obstruction, narrow-angle glaucoma	Dosage adjustment for severe renal impairment (CrCl < 30 mL/min)

TABLE 30.4

Medication Pharmacokinetics and Clinical Considerations (*Continued*)

Drug	Metabolism	Interactions	Contraindications	Clinical Considerations
Darifenacin	Major substrate of CYP3A4 and minor substrate of 2D6 Moderate inhibitor of 2D6 and minor inhibitor of 3A4	CYP3A4 or 2D6 inhibitors or inducers	Uncontrolled narrow-angle glaucoma; urinary retention, paralytic ileus, GI or GU obstruction Concomitant administration of thioridazine	Xerostomia (19%–35%), constipation (15%–21%)
Fesoterodine	Parent compound metabolized to active metabolite (5-HMT) by nonspecific esterases 5-HMT metabolized by CYP2D6 and CYP3A4	CYP3A4 or 2D6 inhibitors or inducers	Bladder flow obstruction, narrow-angle glaucoma	Dosage adjustment for severe renal impairment (CrCl < 30 mL/min)
Beta-3-Adrenoreceptor Agonists				
Mirabegron	Substrate of CYP2D6 and CYP3A4 Moderate inhibitor of CYP2D6 Minor inhibitor of CYP3A4	Drugs metabolized by CYP2D6 May increase levels of digoxin	Hypersensitivity to mirabegron	Dosage adjustment for severe renal impairment (CrCl < 30 mL/min)
OnabotulinumtoxinA				
OnabotulinumtoxinA (Botox). No metabolism. Neuromuscular blocking agents and aminoglycoside antibiotics can potentiate the neuromuscular effect of onabotulinumtoxinA.			Hypersensitivity to onabotulinumtoxinA	Black box warning for distant spread (can result in muscle weakness, life-threatening breathing issues)
SNRIs				
Duloxetine	Major substrate of CYP1A2 and 2D6 Moderate inhibitor of 2D6	CYP1A2 or 2D6 inhibitors or inducers MAO inhibitors or thioridazine	Concomitant use or within 2 wk of MAO inhibitors; uncontrolled narrow-angle glaucoma	Ulcerogenic potential increased with NSAIDs (increased risk of bleeding) Serotonin syndrome or neuroleptic malignant syndrome risk Not recommended when CrCl <30 mL/min
Alpha-Adrenergic Antagonists				
Alfuzosin	Major substrate of CYP3A4	Strong CYP3A4 inhibitors	Strong CYP3A4 inhibitors (itraconazole, ketoconazole, ritonavir)	Avoid concomitant use with other alpha-1-antagonists. Potential to cause dizziness
Doxazosin	Major substrate of CYP3A4	Strong CYP3A4 inhibitors	Strong CYP3A4 inhibitors (itraconazole)	Dizziness may occur in up to 28% of patients.
Prazosin	Major substrate of CYP3A4	Strong CYP3A4 inhibitors	Strong CYP3A4 inhibitors (itraconazole)	Dizziness
Tamsulosin	Major substrate of CYP3A4	Strong CYP3A4 inhibitors	Strong CYP3A4 inhibitors (itraconazole)	Dizziness
Terazosin	Major substrate of CYP3A4	Strong CYP3A4 inhibitors	Strong CYP3A4 inhibitors (itraconazole)	Dizziness
Silodosin	Major substrate of CYP3A4	Strong CYP3A4 inhibitors	Strong CYP3A4 inhibitors (itraconazole)	Retrograde ejaculation

CrCl, creatinine clearance; CYP, cytochrome P-450; ER, extended release; GI, gastrointestinal; GU, genitourinary; IR, immediate-release; NSAIDs, nonsteroidal antiinflammatory drugs; MAO, monoamine oxidase; 5-HMT, 5-hydroxymethyl tolterodine; QTc, corrected Q-T interval.

TABLE 30.5

Molecular Properties of Antimuscarinic Drugs

Drug	Molecular Classification	Corresponding Molecular Characteristics	Clinical Characteristics
Oxybutynin Tolterodine Solifenacin Darifenacin Fesoterodine	Tertiary amine	High lipophilicity Small molecular size Low charge	Extensive transfer into CNS Increased risk of cognitive adverse effects
Trospium	Quaternary amine	Low lipophilicity Large molecular size High charge	Limited transfer into CNS Reduced risk of cognitive adverse effects

CNS, central nervous system.

the CNS via the blood–brain barrier. The quaternary amine trospium tends to not be as well absorbed and has limited ability to cross the blood–brain barrier (**Table 30.5**).

Mechanism of Action

The mechanism of action of each of the medications is relatively similar, with the exception of oxybutynin. Generally, anticholinergics mediate a pharmacologic action by antagonizing the parasympathetic muscarinic receptors in the bladder with relative selectivity for the M_3 and M_1 subtypes. Antagonism of the M_3 muscarinic receptors manifests as a reduction in spontaneous myocyte activity, a decrease in frequency, and a reduction in contraction intensity. They effectively increase bladder capacity, decrease the intensity and frequency of bladder contractions, and delay the initial urge to void. Oxybutynin is both an antimuscarinic and an antispasmodic (secondary to direct muscle relaxation) as well as a local anesthetic.

Oxybutynin boasts a lengthy and robust history of efficacy with respect to OAB and UI. A tertiary amine, oxybutynin is highly lipophilic and easily crosses the blood–brain barrier, thereby conferring higher rates of CNS and anticholinergic adverse effects. The potential for cytochrome P-450 (CYP) enzyme interactions is relatively high as well. Secondary to these adverse effects and interaction potential, oxybutynin may not be well tolerated in all patient populations. Oxybutynin undergoes extensive first-pass metabolism to its active metabolite, *N*-desmethyl oxybutynin, which is purported to produce most of the pharmacologic activity and adverse effects. Up to 80% of patients will report at least one significant muscarinic-mediated adverse effect during therapy, up to 20% of whom will subsequently discontinue therapy. Xerostomia, experienced by up to 70% of patients, is dose related but is also the most common reason cited for discontinuing oxybutynin therapy. Despite these inherent limitations, the use of oxybutynin remains prevalent among all available formulations. The extended-release (ER; Ditropan XL) formulation of oxybutynin has been clinically shown to be equally efficacious but is associated with less adverse effects than the conventional formulation. The transdermal oxybutynin patch (Oxytrol) causes roughly 75% less dry mouth as compared to ER tolterodine and is now available without a prescription.

The transdermal system releases drug constantly over 96 hours at which time the patch is replaced.

Tolterodine (Detrol) is a competitive antagonist of muscarinic receptors that causes increased residual urine volume and decreased detrusor pressure. It is associated with clinically meaningful reductions in micturition frequency as well as incontinence episodes. In comparison to oxybutynin, tolterodine use yields less dosage changes, adverse effects, and treatment-related therapy discontinuations. Tolterodine ER (Detrol LA) has shown superior efficacy compared to the immediate-release (IR) formulation (Leron et al., 2018). ER oxybutynin, however, is significantly more efficacious than ER tolterodine in reducing micturition frequency.

Trospium (Sanctura) is a nonselective muscarinic receptor antagonist that improves urinary frequency, episodes of incontinence, urgency, and volume voided. A quaternary ammonium compound, trospium crosses the blood–brain barrier only to a limited extent, which confers a reduced likelihood of cognitive sequelae. Trospium may possess a therapeutic advantage in patients with comorbidities that require drug therapy, given its negligible hepatic metabolism and low risk of drug interactions.

Solifenacin (VESIcare) is a bladder-selective M_3 receptor antagonist that has been shown to be statistically significantly more efficacious than ER tolterodine with respect to urge incontinence, overall incontinence, and urgency. In another pivotal study, solifenacin was shown to reduce episodes of urgency and increase warning time. It is postulated that solifenacin may provide a greater level of efficacy as compared to other drugs within the class. However, despite its bladder selectivity, solifenacin is associated with increased dose-dependent adverse events (Leron et al., 2018).

Darifenacin (Enablex), a tertiary amine, is a highly selective M_3 receptor antagonist that is effective in reducing frequency of micturition, increasing bladder capacity, reducing frequency and severity of urgency, and reducing the number of episodes of incontinence. A comparative advantage associated with darifenacin is its lack of cognitive impairment, as evidenced in multiple randomized controlled trials.

Fesoterodine (Toviaz), a prodrug, is converted to its active metabolite 5-hydroxymethyl tolterodine (5-HMT), which exerts a pharmacologic effect as a competitive antagonist at the muscarinic receptors. Tolterodine (Detrol) is metabolized to 5-HMT via a CYP2D6-mediated oxidation, and both tolterodine and 5-HMT are responsible for the pharmacologic effect of Detrol. Fesoterodine, however, does not require CYP2D6 activation and therefore may have less potential for pharmacokinetic variability and CYP2D6-specific drug interactions.

The AUA recommends initiating an ER anticholinergic as first-line therapy but does not recommend a specific product.

Time Frame for Response

Expected therapeutic response is variable among members of this class. Generally, a meaningful response would be realized within about 2 weeks. However, evidence suggests that patients taking tolterodine ER experienced reduced micturition, urgency episodes, and incontinence by day 5 of therapy. Trospium may exert a clinical effect as early as day 1 with regard to incontinence, day 3 for urgency, and day 5 for micturition frequency.

Contraindications

Anticholinergic medications are capable of precipitating or worsening urinary retention as well as worsening narrow-angle glaucoma. Both of these conditions, if present in the patient prior to therapy, represent contraindications to the use of antimuscarinics. Antagonism of muscarinic receptors and subsequent downregulation of acetylcholine activity can result in paralysis of smooth muscle in the bladder or gastrointestinal tract. Additionally, mydriasis can occur with increased intraocular pressure; therefore, anticholinergics should be avoided in patients with narrow-angle glaucoma. Tolterodine, trospium, solifenacin, and fesoterodine require a dosage reduction in the case of severe renal impairment (creatinine clearance [CrCl] less than 30 mL/min). However, the ER formulation of trospium should be avoided in patients with severe renal impairment (**Table 30.6**).

Adverse Events

The expected adverse event profile includes traditional anticholinergic effects such as xerostomia, constipation, and urinary retention. Antimuscarinic drugs exert an action mainly during the storage phase of the micturition cycle when there is an absence of parasympathetic activity in the detrusor. During the emptying phase of micturition, there is a massive release of acetylcholine, which effectively blunts the drug's action. If this did not occur, the presence of the active drug would undoubtedly decrease the ability of the bladder to contract to promote urinary retention. Prescribing these drugs within the confines of acceptable dosing typically does not precipitate urinary retention; however, overdose or pharmacokinetic interactions may do so.

Interactions

Most antimuscarinic drugs are metabolized by one or more CYP P-450 isoenzymes, the most common of which are CYP3A4 and CYP2D6. Heterozygous or CYP2D6 homozygous patients are considered "extensive metabolizers," which implies an innate ability to appropriately metabolize drugs via this isoenzyme. However, patients who are poor metabolizers with respect to CYP2D6 may be at an increased risk for drug-related toxicity secondary to their inability to fully metabolize CYP2D6-metabolized drugs. Trospium is metabolized exclusively by nonspecific esterases independent of the hepatic CYP P-450 system. Notable drug interactions within the anticholinergic class tend to involve pharmacokinetic interactions at the enzyme level and typically manifest as increases or decreases in drug metabolism. Solifenacin and tolterodine are capable of causing prolonged corrected Q-T interval (QTc), particularly in supratherapeutic dosing. Concomitant administration of other QTc-prolonging medications can potentiate a pharmacodynamic interaction that may result in arrhythmia.

Beta-Adrenoreceptor Agonists

Mirabegron (Myrbetriq) is a selective beta-3-adrenoreceptor agonist that increases bladder capacity and decreases the frequency of micturition without impacting micturition pressure or residual volume. Detrusor relaxation is achieved in part by activation of beta-3-adrenoreceptors by norepinephrine, which subsequently results in activation of adenylyl cyclase, and formation of cyclic adenosine monophosphate, which produces smooth muscle relaxation. Bladder relaxation is crucial during the storage phase of micturition as it allows for compliance and low intravesical pressure during filling. Mirabegron, through its interaction with the beta-3-adrenoreceptor, promotes relaxation during filling and therefore increases bladder capacity, which then influences frequency of micturition. This is the first novel compound for the treatment of OAB, which has been able to produce a therapeutic effect without engaging the muscarinic receptors and producing anticholinergic adverse effects, a limiting factor associated with the mainstay of therapy, the antimuscarinic drugs.

Mirabegron, in daily doses of 25 to 200 mg, was evaluated in several 12-week randomized, placebo-controlled phase III studies, which support its efficacy, safety, and tolerability. Treatment with mirabegron resulted in decreased incontinence episodes, decreases in the number of micturitions, decreases in urgency episodes, and increases in mean volume voided per urination. Therapeutic effects were observed as early as week 4 and persisted throughout the duration of the studies. Meaningful and statistically significant improvements in these micturition parameters and in quality-of-life measures were observed in patients who were treatment naive and in patients who had failed or were intolerant to the antimuscarinics. Several studies that utilized tolterodine ER 4 mg as an active control reported similar efficacy and tolerability among the mirabegron and tolterodine groups, although no direct statistical comparisons occurred. Rates of xerostomia were significantly higher in patients treated with tolterodine, however. Evaluation of the available literature suggests that mirabegron is similar in efficacy to the antimuscarinics but with a lower incidence of adverse effects.

TABLE 30.6

Antimuscarinic Medication Dosing Considerations

	Oxybutynin	Tolterodine	Trospium	Solifenacin	Darifenacin	Fesoterodine
Usual dose	IR: 5–15 mg PO TID ER: 5–15 mg PO once daily Patch: 3.9 mg/patch twice weekly (q3–4d)	IR: 2 mg PO BID ER: 4 mg PO once daily	IR: 20 mg PO BID ER: 60 mg once daily ≥75: 20 mg PO once daily	5–10 mg PO once daily Dosage adjustment with concomitant CYP3A4 inhibitors: maximum dose 5 mg/d	7.5–15 mg once daily Dosage adjustment with concomitant potent CYP3A4 inhibitors (e.g., azole antifungals, erythromycin, protease inhibitors): 7.5 mg/d	4–8 mg PO daily
Renal insufficiency		**CrCl 10–30 mL/min IR: 1 mg BID ER: 2 mg daily	CrCl ≤30 mL/min IR: 20 mg once daily HS ER: use not recommended	CrCl <30 mL/min Maximum dose 5 mg/d		Severe renal impairment (CrCl <30 mL/min): 4 mg
Hepatic insufficiency		IR: 1 mg BID ER: 2 mg daily		Moderate (Child-Pugh class B): maximum dose 5 mg/d Severe (Child-Pugh class C): use not recommended	Moderate impairment (Child-Pugh class B): daily dosage should not exceed 7.5 mg/d. Severe impairment (Child-Pugh class C): use not recommended	Severe hepatic impairment (Child-Pugh class C): use not recommended
CYP interactions	CYP3A4 inhibitors or inducers	Strong CYP2D6 or 3A4 inhibitors or inducers Azole antifungals		Major inhibitors or inducers of CYP3A4	CYP2D6 and 3A4 inhibitors	Strong CYP3A4 inhibitors

**Use with caution.

CrCl, creatinine clearance; CYP, cytochrome P-450; ER, extended release; IR, immediate-release.

Dosage

Mirabegron is available as a 25- or 50-mg ER 24-hour tablet, which is formulated as an oral-controlled absorption system. Generally, 25 mg daily is sufficient to control symptoms of urgency, frequent urination, and UI. An increase to 50 mg daily can be considered dependent upon observed efficacy and tolerability in the individual patient. Maximum daily doses of 25 mg are recommended for patients with severe renal impairment or moderate hepatic impairment. It is not recommended in patients with end-stage renal disease or severe hepatic impairment. Mirabegron is approximately 70% bound to albumin and alpha-1-acid glycoprotein and is extensively metabolized through multiple pathways including dealkylation, glucuronidation, oxidation, and hydrolysis, as well as enzymatically metabolized through CYP3A4 and CYP2D6. Metabolism of mirabegron produces 10 pharmacologically inactive metabolites. The 50-hour elimination half-life allows for once-daily dosing.

Time Frame for Response

A therapeutic effect is usually realized within the first 8 weeks of therapy, at which point a decision regarding the need to a dosage increase can be considered. Meaningful improvements in parameters of micturition were observed in studies as early as week 4, however.

Contraindications

Mirabegron does not have specifically labeled contraindications; however, dose-related QT prolongation has been observed in clinical studies. Prolongation of the QT interval was observed in female patients on the 200-mg dose of mirabegron, a dose that is supratherapeutic and is not available in the market. Doses of 50 to 100 mg daily did not elicit any electrocardiogram abnormalities in any evaluation. However, patients with QT prolongation or at risk of QT prolongation (taking concurrent medications that prolong QT) should avoid mirabegron.

Adverse Events

Long-term safety and tolerability studies suggest that the rate of treatment-emergent adverse effects is similar between mirabegron and placebo and tends to be mild to moderate in intensity. As compared to tolterodine, mirabegron causes less xerostomia, constipation, urinary retention, and blurred vision. It also does not induce neurological adverse effects such as cognitive impairment, which tends to be associated with the antimuscarinics. Meaningful increases in blood pressure were observed during clinical studies, although hypertension is not considered a contraindication. Monitoring blood pressure is recommended, however.

Interactions

There are no clinically meaningful drug interactions related to the hepatic metabolism with the exception of drugs metabolized by CYP2D6, as mirabegron is a moderate inhibitor of this isoenzyme.

Given mirabegron's efficacy in treatment-experienced and treatment-naive patients as well as its low potential for drug interactions, mild adverse effect profile, and absence of cognitive impairment-related sequelae, mirabegron may become a first-line option. Mirabegron can be considered an appropriate intervention in patients at risk of cognitive impairment and older patients. Treatment discontinuation is a frequent and unfortunate reality with regard to the antimuscarinic drugs, the current treatment of choice. There is no evidence thus far related to treatment adherence with mirabegron, though one of its advantages is its low incidence of adverse effects.

OnabotulinumtoxinA: Botox

Botulinum toxin serotype A, a purified version of *Clostridium botulinum*, is a neurotoxin, which has demonstrated utility in OAB and DO. Two noninterchangeable products are currently approved and marketed for both neurogenic bladder and urge incontinence: Botox (onabotulinumtoxinA) and Dysport (abobotulinumtoxinA). The preponderance of evaluation and evidence focuses on the Botox product. Generally, the use of injectable botulinum toxin is reserved for patients who have failed more than one of the recommended initial drug therapies (anticholinergics or mirabegron) and are considered refractory. The 2019 AUA guidelines have officially incorporated botulinum toxin into its therapeutic recommendations and consider it a third-line option.

Mechanism of Action

Botulinum toxin, when injected into the detrusor muscle, inhibits calcium-dependent release of acetylcholine, adenosine triphosphate, and substance P and reduces the expression of capsaicin receptors on motor neurons. The resulting desensitization of the motor neurons ultimately causes inhibition of the afferent and efferent pathways that influence DO. In addition to the motor effects, botulinum toxin also modulates the sensory aspect of DO by reducing the expression of vanilloid and muscarinic (M_1, M_2, and M_3) receptors in the suburothelium. The resulting flaccid paralysis in the detrusor reduces bladder pressure, increases bladder capacity, reduces incontinence episodes, and reduces perceived urgency. The effect is permanent and persists until the motor endplate units regenerate after 3 to 24 months, necessitating additional treatment.

Randomized controlled studies have demonstrated onabotulinumtoxinA's sustained efficacy over 6 months in reducing incontinence episodes and improving nocturia, voiding frequency, urgency episodes, and quality-of-life indicators. Clinical success was achieved in upwards of 70% of patients. Voiding dysfunction and urinary tract infections were the most commonly reported adverse effects.

Optimal dosing and dosing interval have yet to be established; however, there appears to be a balance between efficacy and tolerability at doses of 100 U per injection. Higher doses demonstrated similar efficacy and much appreciably higher rates of adverse effects, namely, urinary retention. The duration of therapeutic effect is dependent upon the regrowth of the motor end units on the affected neurons and, therefore, is highly variable. Most patients require retreatment after 6 to 9 months.

Contraindications, Adverse Events, and Interactions

Adverse effects tend to be restricted to urinary tract infections and urinary retention secondary to the localized placement of the botulinum toxin. Urinary tract infection has been observed in 18% to 49% of patients and urinary retention in 6% to 17% of patients. A condition of treatment, as recommended by the product labeling and the AUA guidelines, is willingness and ability of the patient to self-catheterize. Education on technique should be provided prior to initiating therapy. Systemic adverse effects do not occur unless there is unintended spread of the botulinum toxin beyond the site of injection. A black box warning includes statements related to the blurred vision, dysarthria, muscle weakness, ptosis, dysphagia, and life-threatening breathing difficulties that could indicate unintentional spread of the toxin from its injection site.

Contraindications include sensitivity to the product or patients with existing urinary retention. Botulinum toxins are not metabolized, and therefore, interactions are limited to other drugs that may potentiate the neuromuscular-blocking effects such as anticholinergics, neuromuscular-blocking drugs, and aminoglycoside antibiotics.

Serotonin Norepinephrine Reuptake Inhibitors

Venlafaxine (Effexor) and duloxetine (Cymbalta), both SNRIs, have been evaluated as nontraditional therapies for OAB.

Mechanism of Action

Serotonin facilitates urine storage, augmenting parasympathetic innervation and inhibiting sympathetic innervation to the bladder. During the filling phase, glutamate is released and acts upon Onuf nucleus. Onuf nucleus is a discrete confluence of neurons in the anterior horn of the sacral region of the spinal cord, which is involved in the micturition reflex, continence, and muscular contraction during orgasm. The action of glutamate in Onuf nucleus activates the pudendal nerve and subsequent release of acetylcholine, which elicits contraction of the external urethral sphincter. The dense population of the nucleus with serotonin and norepinephrine receptors implies a facilitator role for these monoamines with regard to the micturition reflex and urine storage. Duloxetine enhances urethral sphincter activity and is associated with dose-dependent decreases in episodes of incontinence and improvements in quality of life. It is believed that duloxetine exerts this effect by increasing the availability of serotonin and norepinephrine in the synaptic clefts of Onuf nucleus. Nausea occurs in about 25% of patients but tends to subside by day 7 of treatment. Numerous studies support the use of SNRIs alone or in combination with pelvic floor muscle exercises.

Contraindications, Adverse Events, and Interactions

Duloxetine may not be used concurrently with monoamine oxidase (MAO) inhibitors or within 2 weeks of discontinuing an MAO inhibitor. Duloxetine is metabolized in the liver by CYP3A4 and CYP2D6 and therefore is subject to pharmacokinetic interactions with strong inhibitors of these isoenzymes. It is not to be coadministered with thioridazine because there is a significant CYP2D6-mediated interaction that may result in increased concentrations and toxicity in both drugs. Concomitant administration of duloxetine with other medications that have serotonergic or noradrenergic actions may increase the risk of serotonin syndrome or neuroleptic malignant syndrome.

Alpha-Adrenergic Antagonists

The alpha-adrenergic antagonists have proven efficacy and tolerability with respect to treating BPH in males. However, some studies suggest that tamsulosin may reduce bladder pressure, increase the flow rate, and provide symptomatic improvement in patients with OAB and a confirmed obstruction. The extent to which OAB symptoms are relieved is appreciably less than the resolution of symptoms of obstruction. Use in women is controversial because alpha-adrenergic antagonists may precipitate stress incontinence in female patients.

Mechanism of Action

Alpha-adrenergic antagonists, or alpha-blockers, competitively inhibit postsynaptic alpha-1-adrenergic receptors in prostate and bladder tissue. The antagonism reduces the sympathetic-mediated urethral stricture that is associated with BPH or BOO symptoms.

Adverse Events

Postural hypotension is one of the most clinically relevant adverse effects that may occur. All of the drugs in this class have the potential to induce this effect; however, doxazosin precipitates postural hypotension in upwards of 30% of patients. It is of special concern since the majority of patients who would likely be taking an alpha-1-antagonist are older adults and are predisposed to postural hypotension and subsequent falls.

Interactions

The alpha-1-antagonists are metabolized by CYP3A4, and concomitant administration with strong CYP3A4 inhibitors should be avoided. Also, secondary to the potential to cause hypotension, more than one alpha-blocker should not be used concurrently.

Estrogens

Despite the dearth of anecdotal evidence supporting the use of estrogens for symptomatic improvement of OAB and incontinence in females, randomized controlled trials have yielded contradictory results at best. Unopposed systemic estrogen therapy or combination estrogen/progesterone therapy is associated with an increase in SUI and UUI episodes, as was evidenced by several large multinational studies. Topical estrogen therapy in the form of vaginal estradiol tablets (Vagifem) or the estrogen-releasing vaginal ring (Estring) has, however, demonstrated some symptomatic improvement. The vaginal tablet improved urgency, frequency, urge incontinence, and stress incontinence. The vaginal ring improved urge incontinence, stress incontinence, and nocturia. The therapeutic effect is attributed to increasing the maximum urethral pressure, although some clinicians hypothesize that it is due to reversal of urogenital atrophy and not direct bladder or urethral activity.

Mechanism of Action

Topical estradiol exerts a local action that improves tone and elasticity of female urogenital anatomy by increasing secretion of the cervical mucosa, thickening vaginal mucosa, and proliferation of the endometrium. Both the vaginal tablet and the vaginal ring are indicated for urinary urgency and dysuria.

Contraindications

Patients with undiagnosed vaginal bleeding, a history of breast carcinoma or estrogen-dependent tumors, and thromboembolic disorders (deep vein thrombosis, pulmonary embolism, stroke, myocardial infarction) and patients who are pregnant should not use estrogens.

Adverse Events

Administration of topical estrogens for OAB and incontinence symptoms is not without risk. Well-designed, large-scale, randomized, controlled trials have clearly demonstrated the cardiovascular sequelae that can result from utilizing hormone replacement therapy (HRT) for primary prevention of cardiovascular disease. Since the advent of the Women's Health Initiative study, the use of HRT has dramatically declined. However, in selected individuals, HRT is still used for the treatment of menopause-related symptoms, which include urogenital complaints (vaginal atrophy, dysuria, incontinence).

Risks of administration include the potential for thromboembolic complications, aggravation of existing estrogen-responsive malignancies or development of estrogen-responsive cancers, changes in libido, mood dysregulation, irritability, or syncope.

Antidiuretic Drugs

Mechanism of Action

Desmopressin (1-desamino-8-D-arginine vasopressin; DDAVP), a synthetic vasopressin analogue, had been indicated for nocturnal enuresis in adults and children. It possesses profound antidiuretic properties without any appreciable pressor activity; DDAVP can diurese without impacting blood pressure in a clinically significant way. Exploiting the hypothesis that a relative absence of nocturnal vasopressin and subsequently increased nocturnal urine production underlies the predisposition to suffer from enuresis, DDAVP reduces urine volume and osmolality. In addition to the established indication for enuresis in children, DDAVP has been shown to be efficacious in treating adult patients with nocturia of polyuric origin.

Contraindications and Adverse Events

Patients with hyponatremia or a history of hyponatremia or moderate to severe renal impairment (CrCl < 50 mL/min) should avoid DDAVP. Adverse effects are mild and rare. However, there is a risk of water retention with or without hyponatremia. Sodium monitoring is recommended in older patients prior to treatment and several days into therapy.

Interactions

There are no significant drug interactions associated with DDAVP. Several medications (lithium, TCAs, SSRIs, nonsteroidal antiinflammatory drugs, carbamazepine) may enhance the toxic effects of DDAVP, but none of the risks are particularly likely.

New and Emerging Therapies

Vanilloid receptors on afferent neurons that innervate the bladder and urethra may be acted upon by capsaicin or resiniferatoxin. Capsaicin-mediated activation of the afferent neurons results in an initial excitation phase immediately followed by a protracted blockade that effectively desensitizes the neurons to normal stimuli. A capsaicin analogue, resiniferatoxin, can also impact the afferent neurons and the A-delta fibers. This transient physiologic "damage" to sensory nerves results in more prolonged retention of urine and improvement in OAB and DO of neurogenic and idiopathic origin.

Botulinum toxin A blocks the release of acetylcholine from the presynaptic neuron, which, in turn, decreases muscle contractility and increases muscle atrophy locally.

Selecting the Most Appropriate Agent

First-Line Therapy

The AUA 2019 guidelines for the management of OAB recommend initiating behavioral therapy in all patients prior to commencing drug therapy. In the absence of contraindications, anticholinergic medications are considered first-line pharmacologic therapy for OAB and symptoms of incontinence. Nonpharmacologic interventions, such as bladder training, typically are recommended prior to initiating drug therapy. Oftentimes, if the behavioral modifications do not suitably resolve the symptoms of OAB, a medication will be added to the nondrug intervention.

Antimuscarinics as a class have an established reputation with regard to efficacy and safety. They effectively reduce bladder pressure, increase bladder capacity and compliance, increase the volume threshold for desire to urinate, and reduce inappropriate bladder contractions. Tolerability issues involving anticholinergic adverse effects (dry mouth, constipation) may limit clinical utility in some patient populations but largely do not significantly impact therapy. There is no unequivocal evidence that recommends the use of one member of this class over another; however, there have been smaller studies that suggest some differential benefits. In terms of efficacy, the larger body of literature supports relative equivalence among antimuscarinics. ER formulations have demonstrated improved efficacy compared to their IR counterparts. When considering the anticholinergic side effect potential, oxybutynin is undeniably responsible for the most xerostomia and constipation. Trospium and darifenacin promote fewer cognitive sequelae than oxybutynin, tolterodine, or solifenacin. Trospium is not metabolized by the CYP P-450 system and therefore is associated with far fewer drug interactions than the rest of this class, which is metabolized primarily by CYP. New evidence suggests that fesoterodine may be more effective than tolterodine in terms of efficacy and improvement in quality of life. Tolterodine is currently the market leader in the majority of countries. The AUA recommends initiating an ER formulation of any of the anticholinergic drugs. If therapeutic failure occurs or tolerability issues arise, it is recommended that another member of the class be initiated before attempting another drug class.

Mirabegron is now also considered an appropriate first-line pharmacologic intervention, according to the guidelines. Mirabegron is a novel entity, which acts upon beta-3-adrenoreceptors in the detrusor muscle to promote relaxation during the filling phase, thereby reducing urgency, increasing the bladder capacity, and decreasing the number of micturitions. Clinical studies have consistently demonstrated efficacy that is similar to that of the anticholinergics and also improved tolerability comparatively, with a remarkably decreased risk of anticholinergic adverse effects and cognitive impairment. The once-daily dosing, coupled with the efficacy and tolerability advantages, low incidence of drug–drug interactions, and absence of anticholinergic effects, confers upon mirabegron a possible therapeutic advantage.

Second- and Third-Line Therapies

Failure or intolerance to the initial anticholinergic medication generally warrants the trial of a second anticholinergic medication. Since there are some appreciable differences among anticholinergics in terms of side effect profiles and tolerability, a switch to another anticholinergic typically precedes a switch to a different class. The transdermal oxybutynin patch is available without a prescription and may also be considered if oral therapy is not well tolerated but is not recommended as the initial pharmacologic intervention.

Botulinum A toxin is indicated for neurogenic and nonneurogenic DO as well as neurogenic spasm of the urethra due to spinal cord injury or secondary to DO. Injections of 100 U directly into the detrusor muscle promote an effect for 6 to 9 months secondary to the resulting flaccid paralysis of the bladder. Retreatment after dissipation of therapeutic effect is recommended, and the interval at which this occurs has not been established. There is a low risk of drug–drug interactions but a relatively significant risk of serious adverse effects such as urinary retention requiring catheterization. Botulinum toxin is recommended after failure of at least two first-line pharmacologic options.

Duloxetine has demonstrated some success in OAB, but to a greater extent with stress incontinence. Incontinence (generally urge incontinence) is part of the OAB symptom constellation and is alleviated by duloxetine treatment. A similar scenario exists for the use of estrogens for OAB. Estrogens are primarily used for SUI and other urogenital symptoms but have demonstrated utility in OAB. Neither the SNRIs nor estrogen is recommended in the guidelines.

Surgical intervention is arguably the last option in terms of management of OAB; it is generally attempted after failure of all reasonable pharmacologic options. This is mostly due to the inherent risks in abdominal or pelvic operation, namely impacts on renal function, on sexual function, and on any abdominal or pelvic pathology. In addition, surgical intervention is generally most effective in cases of isolated stress incontinence where there is underlying bladder or urethral pathology. In females, surgery usually involves repositioning the urethra so that it is more amenable to pressure changes or providing artificial support or resistance to the urethra by way of a sling. In males, surgery involves implantation of a manually controlled artificial silicone urethral sphincter.

Refractory Overactive Bladder

Depending upon the underlying etiology of OAB, some patients may not be successfully treated with first- or even second-line options. If multiple antimuscarinic drugs fail, as well as appropriate second- and third-line options, more invasive interventions might become necessary. Implantable neurostimulator devices or sacral neuromodulator placement is moderately

successful but costly alternatives. Electrical stimulation of the peripheral nervous system has been shown to positively impact urinary urgency and urge incontinence. Both anal and vaginal transcutaneous stimulations play a role in the treatment of OAB. Direct electrical stimulation of the third and sometimes fourth sacral nerves via a surgically implanted modulator delivers continuous stimulation directly to a nerve with which it is in close contact. Augmentation cystoplasty surgery involves the anastomosis of a segment of bowel to the bisected bladder. This procedure increases bladder capacity and decreases bladder pressure. Serious risks include kidney or bladder infections, new recurrent urinary tract infections, or metabolic abnormalities. Surgical augmentation cystoplasty, neobladder construction, and urinary diversion techniques involve more risk and tend to be reserved for severe, refractory cases.

Another therapeutic consideration is the somewhat controversial dual antimuscarinic drug therapy. This has been studied in both adults and children and has been found to be safe and effective. A meta-analysis evaluated the combination of solifenacin with mirabegron. Combination therapy yielded improved efficacy rates with similar rates of side effects of solifenacin (Kelleher et al., 2018).

In male patients with OAB in the setting of BOO secondary to BPH, the combination of alpha-adrenergic blockers and 5-alpha-reductase inhibitors (finasteride, dutasteride) may offer some clinical utility (see Chapter 33 for further discussion of BPH).

Special Considerations
Pediatric

Isolated incontinence tends to manifest in young children as nocturia or enuresis. This is generally due to underlying deficits in learned neural control, delayed development of the nervous system, or potentially a more complex issue involving multiple systems. OAB symptoms of urgency or frequency in children commonly occur as a result of fecal impaction or underlying structural abnormalities. Children can present with voiding dysfunction, urgency, frequency, or incontinence. Oxybutynin IR and ER formulations are the only pharmacologic options approved by the U.S. Food and Drug Administration for OAB in children, although tolterodine IR and ER and trospium have been evaluated in clinical trials. All of the medications yielded successful outcomes in terms of reductions in diurnal incontinence, urgency episodes, micturition, and increases in bladder capacity. The adverse effects are similar to those experienced by adults and consisted mainly of dry mouth. Cognitive effects are not significant with respect to memory, cognition, speed of processing, or attention. DDAVP nasal spray has been the cornerstone of therapy for children with enuresis and has demonstrated clinical efficacy, safety, and tolerability.

Geriatric

As was previously mentioned, there is an inherent challenge with regard to OAB in older patients. Numerous nonurinary factors such as anatomic, physiologic, age-related, or iatrogenic elements predispose older patients to the development of OAB or the worsening of existing OAB. The incidence of OAB is highest in the older population, and yet the preferred pharmacologic modality for treating this syndrome tends to impact cognition to an extent that may limit utility in this population. Despite these clinical considerations, antimuscarinic therapy is still considered first line. If the adverse effects are intolerable or if the antimuscarinic agent aggravates an existing condition, an alternate medication should be given. If pharmacologic options are exhausted or are not feasible, surgical interventions can be considered in surgical candidates, or the syndrome can be managed less aggressively. Less aggressive options include scheduled voiding, bladder training, and the use of absorbent pads or undergarments.

Women

True OAB syndrome affects men and women relatively equally; however, the symptom of incontinence tends to present more frequently in women. Furthermore, within postmenopausal symptomatology, vaginal atrophy and other urogenital changes may underlie urgency, frequency, and urge or stress incontinence that frequently accompanies menopause. SUI affects the majority of women with incontinence episodes (Aoki et al., 2017). SUI may be predicated on intrinsic urethral sphincter deficiency or urethral hypermobility secondary to the loss of vaginal support structures. Antimuscarinic medications are first line; however, in appropriately selected patients, topical estrogens may offer some therapeutic benefit. Duloxetine has been extensively studied in women with stress incontinence secondary to urethral dysfunction or vaginal atrophy. There is an established correlation between SUI and female sexual dysfunction.

MONITORING PATIENT RESPONSE

Despite the seemingly impressive efficacy of anticholinergic drug therapy, there is roughly a 50% placebo response rate, which complicates the assessment of patient response. As the majority of OAB symptomatology is subjective in nature, patient-generated feedback is the most valuable assessment tool with which to measure success. The domains related to the pathology itself that should be assessed include symptoms, symptom severity, and quality of life. If drug therapy has been initiated, drug-specific parameters such as treatment-emergent side effects or drug interactions need to be assessed as well.

There are numerous validated symptom inventories and quality-of-life assessment tools that have been employed in clinical trials as well as in practice to monitor patient response to treatment. The ICS highly recommends that symptom assessment and quality-of-life inventories be used throughout the treatment process in order to assess and guide therapy. The OAB-q assesses both the symptoms and quality-of-life impact in men and women. The reduced version of this scale includes 8 bladder symptom items and 25 health-related quality-of-life (HRQOL) items, which include symptom bother, coping skills, concerns and worries, sleep, social interaction, and HRQOL total. In females, the Urogenital Distress Inventory-6 (UDI-6),

the Incontinence Severity Index (ISI), and the Bristol Female Lower Urinary Tract Symptoms (BFLUTS) questionnaire are used to assess the symptom of UI specifically. In males, the ICS_{male} and Danish Prostatic Symptom Score (DAN-PSS) will assess the symptom of UI. The UDI-6 assesses 19 LUT symptoms as well as the degree of anxiety or bother that is experienced as a result of the incontinence episodes. This scale may have predictive value with respect to urodynamic studies, especially in stress incontinence, BOO, and DO. The ISI is a simple index that generates a numerical product based on frequency and volume of urine loss. The product is associated with the level of severity of the incontinence. BFLUTS evaluates incontinence symptoms and LUT symptoms as well as the degree of bother associated with each. Both the ICS_{male} and DAN-PSS assess LUT symptoms and the extent to which the patient is bothered. Unfortunately, there is no consensus regarding at which point or how frequently these assessment tools should be administered to yield optimal information about treatment response.

Ongoing assessment of potential treatment-related adverse effects is highly recommended. This can be accomplished by clinician-led patient interviews or patient-generated complaints. The drugs most frequently used to treat OAB have the potential to cause bothersome or sometimes serious adverse effects. Since the patient population most often affected by OAB is usually also affected by polypharmacy, multiple medical conditions, predisposition to falls, and predisposition to anticholinergic adverse effects, diligent monitoring of iatrogenic effects is paramount. A review of medical claims revealed that after one year, only 5% to 9% of patients continued on antimuscarinic therapy, which underscores the importance of anticipating and then mitigating adverse effects and other barriers to successful treatment (Kim & Lee, 2016).

PATIENT EDUCATION AND PATIENT-ORIENTED INFORMATION SOURCES

Although OAB tends to affect older patients more frequently than younger patients and may be partially caused or worsened by seemingly normal processes associated with aging, OAB is *not* considered a normal part of aging. Patients need to be made aware of this, and their symptoms need to be validated. One of the challenges in diagnosing OAB is the reluctance of patients to complain of the symptoms or the patient's misconception about the symptoms being a normal part of aging. Once a patient is diagnosed with OAB, it is exceptionally important to emphasize that the symptoms need not be tolerated and that ongoing assessment of symptoms and symptom bother is essential to successful treatment.

Once a treatment modality has been mutually agreed upon by the patient and the care provider, the risks and benefits need to be clearly explained to the patient. More often than not, the treatment will consist of a medication and lifestyle changes or bladder training. The medications used to treat OAB (usually anticholinergics) will likely cause at least some minor anticholinergic adverse effects such as dry mouth or constipation. Severe xerostomia can be treated with adequate hydration as well as saliva substitutes. Constipation can be avoided by maintaining adequate hydration or remedied by using a stool softener (docusate) or a stimulant laxative (senna, bisacodyl). Patients should be warned about potentially severe anticholinergic effects such as urinary retention and advised to seek medical attention if symptoms consistent with urinary retention present. Antimuscarinic drugs may potentially augment anticholinergic effects of other anticholinergic medications. Therefore, in the case of multiple physicians, patients should be advised to make their care providers aware of any and all medications prescribed by all members of the health care team.

Aside from the OAB and medication information that may be provided by the patient's care provider, there are numerous reputable sources for patient-oriented information. The American Urogynecology Society maintains a patient-friendly Web site that explains pelvic floor disorders, incontinence, and OAB. It also provides a list of frequently asked questions, tools for patients, bladder diary support, medications and other treatment options, and a search engine for locating a care provider. The National Association for Continence is another reputable Web site that offers useful information regarding underlying causes of OAB, treatment options, frequently asked questions, and a public bathroom finder. The bathroom finder tool is a Google Maps™–powered application that allows the user to input a city or zip code and will then generate a graphical representation of the location of public restrooms.

Nutrition/Lifestyle Changes

Generally before the initiation of drug therapy, patients will be encouraged to adopt some clinician-guided lifestyle changes to minimize the impact of diet or behavior on OAB. It is *not* recommended that patients attempt to remedy OAB on their own by modifying behavior as was previously discussed. Uninformed and unmonitored changes (such as cessation of diuretic use) may detrimentally impact other aspects of the patient's care or may instigate a nascent problem. All of the nutritional or lifestyle changes should be recommended by the care provider and should be monitored; none of these changes should be initiated by the patient.

Compounds that irritate the bladder may exacerbate or precipitate OAB. Tomatoes, artificial sweeteners, grapes,

carbonated beverages, strawberries, apple juice, vinegar, weight-loss supplements, and spicy foods all may contribute to OAB pathology. Alcohol and caffeine not only act as bladder irritants but also inhibit antidiuretic hormone release, which, in turn, will increase the production of urine and contribute to urgency and frequency. Moderation of the consumption of these foods, beverages, or products will likely reduce some of the added pressures that may be contributing to OAB symptoms.

Maintenance of a healthy body weight will also aid in the mitigation of OAB symptoms as excess weight puts increased pressure on the bladder. Pelvic floor exercises and bladder training are also shown to be effective in treating OAB as monotherapy or in combination with medications.

Complementary and Alternative Medications

Numerous natural compounds and botanicals have been evaluated for purposes of treating OAB; however, there is a paucity of evidence to support their use. OAB or urinary dysfunction that is associated with BPH may be further remedied by adjunctive treatment with saw palmetto extract. Saw palmetto or American dwarf plant (*Serenoa repens*) is thought to inhibit 5-alpha-reductase as its primary pharmacologic action. 5-alpha-reductase is responsible for the conversion of testosterone to dihydrotestosterone (DHT). DHT is among the androgens that contribute to prostate growth, and, in BPH, DHT contributes to pathologic prostate growth. Inhibition of 5-alpha-reductase opposes the pathologic enlargement of the prostate and subsequently eases the pressure on the urethra at the bladder neck. This effectively reduces or removes the BOO and improves LUT symptoms in males. Saw palmetto extract would not be an appropriate therapeutic option in patients who do not have an underlying BPH-mediated BOO.

To date, three active comparator trials have evaluated the efficacy and safety of saw palmetto extract as compared to 5-alpha-reductase inhibitors or alpha-1-receptor antagonists. Saw palmetto and finasteride both improved the score on the International Prostate Symptom Score (IPSS), improved quality of life, and increased peak urinary flow rate. Unlike finasteride, saw palmetto did not impact prostate volume or PSA. The trial comparing saw palmetto to tamsulosin did not find a difference between the two groups in terms of IPSS reduction, maximal flow rate, and irritative or obstructive symptoms (Suzuki et al., 2009).

CASE STUDY 1

C.J. is a 55-year-old postmenopausal woman presenting with a 2-year history of incontinence. She reports that she often cannot get to the bathroom in time when she feels the urge to urinate. She also experiences incontinence most frequently when she laughs or sneezes. This has caused significant embarrassment and has decreased her social interactions. She drinks four cups of coffee daily. Current prescription medications include hydrochlorothiazide for

hypertension. C.J. denies the use of any nonprescription medications or supplements.

DIAGNOSIS: STRESS INCONTINENCE

1. List specific goals for treatment for C.J.
2. What drug therapy would you prescribe? Why?

3. What are the parameters for monitoring the success of the therapy?

4. Discuss specific patient education based on the prescribed therapy.

5. List one or two adverse reactions for the selected agent that would cause you to change therapy.

6. What would be the choice for second-line therapy?

7. What over-the-counter and/or alternative medications would be appropriate for this patient?

8. What dietary and lifestyle changes should be recommended for this patient?

9. Describe one or two drug–drug or drug–food interactions for the selected agent.

Bibliography

Starred references are cited in the text.

*Aoki, Y., Brown, H., Brubaker, L., et al. (2017). Urinary incontinence in women. *Nature Reviews Disease Primers, 3,* 17042. doi: 10.1038/nrdp.2017.42

Corcos, J., Przydacz, M., Campeau, L., et al. (2017). CUA guideline on adult overactive bladder. *Canadian Urological Association Journal, 11*(5), E142–E173.

Drake, M., Nitti, V., Ginsberg, D., et al. (2017). Comparative assessment of the efficacy of onabotulinumtoxinA and oral therapies (anticholinergics and mirabegron) for overactive bladder: A systematic review and network meta-analysis. *BJU International, 120*(5), 611–622.

Eapen, R. & Radomski, S. (2016). Review of the epidemiology of overactive bladder. *Research and Reports in Urology, 8,* 71–76.

*Faiena, I., Patel, N., Parihar, J., et al. (2015). Conservative management of urinary incontinence in women. *Reviews in Urology, 17*(3), 129–139.

*Kelleher C., Hakimi Z., Zur, R., et al. (2018). Efficacy and tolerability of mirabegron compared with antimuscarinic therapy or combination therapies for overactive bladder: A systematic review and network meta-analysis. *European Urology, 74*(3), 324–333.

*Kim, T., & Lee, K. (2016). Persistence and compliance with medication management in the treatment of overactive bladder. *Investigative and Clinical Urology, 57*(2), 84–93.

Kosilov, K., Loparev, S., Ivanovskaya, M., et al. (2016). Influence of different doses of trospium and solifenacin on manageability of OAB symptoms with different severity in elderly men and women. *Journal of Clinical Urology, 9*(3), 180–188.

*Leron, E., Weintraub, A., Mastrolia, S., et al. (2018). Overactive bladder syndrome: Evaluation and management. *Current Urology, 11*(3), 117–125.

*Lightner, D., Gomelsky, A., Souter, L., et al. (2019). Diagnosis and treatment of overactive bladder (non-neurogenic) in adults: AUA/SUFU guideline. *The Journal of Urology, 202*(3), 558–563.

Maund, E., Guski, L., & Gotzsche, P. (2017). Considering benefits and harms of duloxetine for treatment of stress urinary incontinence: A meta-analysis

of clinical study reports. *Canadian Medical Association Journal, 189*(5), E194–E203.

Peyronnet, B., Mironska, E., & Chapple, C. (2019). A comprehensive review of overactive bladder pathophysiology: On the way to tailored treatment. *European Urology, 75*(6), 988–1000.

Powell, L., Szabo, S., Walker, D., et al. (2018). The economic burden of overactive bladder in the United States: A systematic literature review. *Neurotology and Urodynamics, 37*(4), 1241–1249.

Rossanese, M., Novara, G., Challacombe, B., et al. (2015). Critical analysis of phase II and III randomised control trials (RCTs) evaluating efficacy and tolerability of a beta$_3$-adrenoceptor agonist (mirabegron) for overactive bladder (OAB). *BJU International, 115*(1), 32–40.

*Stewart, W., Van Rooyen, J., Cundiff, G., et al. (2003). Prevalence and burden of overactive bladder in the United States. *World Journal of Urology, 20*(6), 327–336.

*Suzuki, M., Ito, Y., Fujino, T., et al. (2009). Pharmacological effects of saw palmetto extract in the lower urinary tract. *Acta Pharmacologica Sinica, 30*(3), 227–281.

Vij, M., & Drake, M. (2015). Clinical use of the β$_3$ adrenoceptor against mirabegron in patients with overactive bladder syndrome. *Therapeutic Advances in Urology, 7*(5), 241–248.

Wang, C., Liao, C., & Kuo, H. (2015). Clinical guidelines for male lower urinary tract symptoms associated with non-neurogenic bladder. *Urological Science, 26*(1), 7–16.

*Willis-Gray, M., Dieter, A., Geller, E., et al. (2016). Evaluation and management of overactive bladder: Strategies for optimizing care. *Research and Reports in Urology 8,* 113–122.

Yehoshua, A., Chancellor, M., Vasavada, S., et al. (2016). Health resource utilization and cost for patients with incontinent overactive bladder treated with anticholinergics. *Journal of Managed Care & Specialty Pharmacy, 22*(4), 406–413.

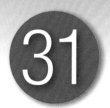

31 Sexually Transmitted Infections

Caragh E. Clayton and Virginia P. Arcangelo

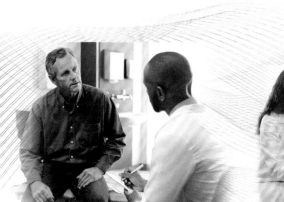
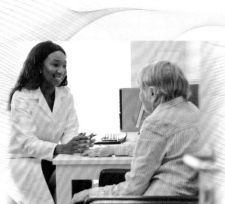
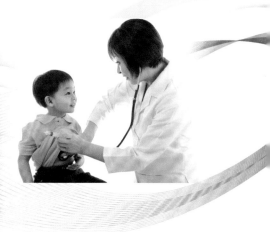

Learning Objectives

1. Be able to recognize common signs and symptoms associated with sexually transmitted infections.
2. Be able to interpret laboratory and diagnostic tests.
3. Be able to prescribe the most appropriate drug therapy regimen and monitoring plan based on patient and current guidelines.
4. Be able to educate patients on drug-specific information, safe-sex practices, notification of sexual partners, and when to seek reevaluation for persistent symptoms.

INTRODUCTION

Sexually transmitted infections (STIs) are among the most common illnesses in the world. They have far-reaching health, social, and economic consequences. Our knowledge about the global prevalence and incidence of these infections is limited by the quality and quantity of data available from throughout the world. STIs remain a major public health concern in the United States. The economic burden is impressive: Centers for Disease Control and Prevention's (CDC) new estimates show that there are about 20 million new infections in the United States each year, with a total of more than 110 million among men and women. STIs cost the American healthcare system nearly $16 billion in direct medical costs alone (Barrow et al., 2020).

It is estimated that half of all new STIs in the country occur among young men and women. Those at the highest risk for contracting STIs are those between 15 and 24 years and gay and bisexual men. Gay and bisexual men have the highest rate of syphilis infections. While most STIs will not cause harm, some have the potential to cause serious health problems, especially if not diagnosed and treated early.

In 2015, the CDC updated the guidelines for treating STIs (**Table 31.1**). Available from the CDC, these guidelines are one of the most widely used documents published by that organization. The guidelines emphasize the development of management strategies that are adaptable to the managed care environment. Because these guidelines are considered the gold standard for treating STIs, most of the information in this chapter is based on them. The goals of therapy for all STIs are to eradicate the causative organism and prevent complications.

The accurate and timely reporting of STIs is integrally important for assessing morbidity trends, targeting limited resources, and assisting local health authorities in partner notification and treatment. STIs, human immunodeficiency virus (HIV), and acquired immunodeficiency syndrome (AIDS) cases should be reported in accordance with state and local statutory requirements. Syphilis, gonorrhea, chlamydia, chancroid, HIV infection, and AIDS are reportable diseases in every state. The requirements for reporting other STIs differ by state, and clinicians should be familiar with state and local reporting requirements. Reporting can be provider or laboratory based.

Intrauterine or perinatally transmitted STIs can have severely debilitating effects on pregnant women, their partners, and their fetuses. All pregnant women and their sex partners should be asked about STIs, counseled about the possibility of perinatal infections, and ensured access to treatment, if needed.

All pregnant women in the United States should be tested for HIV infection as early in pregnancy as possible. Testing should be conducted after the woman is notified that she will be tested for HIV as part of the routine panel of prenatal tests, unless she declines the test.

TABLE 31.1

Pharmacotherapy for Sexually Transmitted Infections

Infection	Treatment	Comments
Chlamydial infection	Azithromycin 1 g PO once *or* doxycycline 100 mg PO BID for 7 days *Alternative:* Erythromycin base 500 mg PO QID for 7 days *or* erythromycin ethylsuccinate 800 mg PO QID for 7 days *or* ofloxacin 300 mg BID for 7 d *or* levofloxacin 500 mg PO for 7 days	Use amoxicillin, erythromycin, *or* azithromycin in pregnancy.
Genital herpes	*Initial episode treatment* for 7–10 days Acyclovir 400 mg PO TID *or* acyclovir 200 mg PO 5 times daily *or* valacyclovir 1 g PO BID *Recurrent treatment:* Acyclovir 400 mg PO TID for 5 days *or* acyclovir 800 mg BID for 5 days *or* acyclovir 800 mg TID for 2 days *or* famciclovir 125 mg PO BID for 5 days *or* famciclovir 100 mg BID for 1 day Valacyclovir 500 mg PO BID for 3 days *or* valacyclovir 1 g once daily for 5 days *Suppressive treatment:* Acyclovir 400 mg BID *or* famciclovir 250 mg BID *or* valacyclovir 500 mg or 1,000 mg daily	Treatment can be extended if healing is not complete after 10 days.
Gonorrhea	Ceftriaxone 250 mg IM once PLUS Azithromycin 1 g PO once *or* doxycycline 100 mg PO BID for 7 days *Alternative:* Cefixime 400 mg once	
Human papillomavirus	*Patient applied:* Podofilox 0.5% solution or gel for 3 days and then 4 days of no therapy Imiquimod 5% cream three times a week up to 16 weeks	Solution applied with cotton swab and gel with finger to visible warts. This is done for 3 days and then 4 days with no therapy and may be repeated four times.
	Provider applied: Podophyllin resin 10%–25% in compound of tincture of benzoin weekly as needed	Area should be washed with mild soap and water 6–10 hours after application. Allow to air-dry. Wash off 1–4 hours after application.
	Trichloroacetic acid or bichloracetic acid 80%–90% weekly as needed	Apply only on warts and let dry; white "frosting" appears; powder with talc or sodium bicarbonate to remove unreacted acid.
Pelvic inflammatory disease	Ceftriaxone 250 mg IM once *or* cefoxitin 2 g IM *and* probenecid 1 g PO once *and* doxycycline 100 mg PO BID for 14 days PLUS Doxycycline 100 mg PO BID for 14 days WITH OR WITHOUT Metronidazole 500 mg PO BID for 14 days	
Syphilis	*Early primary, secondary, or latent syphilis <1 year* Adult: benzathine penicillin G 2.4 million U, IM single dose Child: 50,000 U/kg, IM, single dose up to 2.4 mil unit *Latent disease >1 year or unknown duration* Adult: benzathine penicillin G 2.4 million U, IM, for 3 doses at 1-week intervals Child: 500,000 U/kg, IM, for 3 doses at 1-week intervals *Allergic to penicillin and not pregnant:* doxycycline 100 mg PO BID for 14 days *or* tetracycline 500 mg PO BID for 14 days *Allergic to penicillin and pregnant:* desensitization followed by treatment with penicillin	

IM, intramuscular.

CHLAMYDIAL INFECTION

Chlamydial infection is the most prevalent STI in the United States, with 1.8 million cases reported to the CDC in 2018. The detection and treatment of this disease are important because the complications can be serious.

CAUSES

Chlamydial infection is caused by *Chlamydia trachomatis*, which shares properties of both bacteria and viruses. The organism is transmitted sexually or perinatally. Repeated infections are common.

In infants, perinatal exposure to the mother's cervix causes the infection. The prevalence is greater than 5% regardless of race, ethnicity, or socioeconomic status. In preadolescent children, sexual abuse must be considered as a causative factor for chlamydial infection; infection of the nasopharynx, urogenital tract, and rectum may persist for greater than 1 year. Because criminal investigation is always a possibility, cultures should be confirmed by microscopic fluoroscopy, which can detect conjugated monoclonal antibodies specific for *C. trachomatis*.

Chlamydial infections occur most frequently in women younger than age 25. All adolescents and young women should be screened for chlamydia yearly, as should any woman who has new or multiple sex partners.

PATHOPHYSIOLOGY

Chlamydial organisms are like viruses in that they are obligate, intracellular parasites. They resemble bacteria by containing both deoxyribonucleic acid (DNA) and ribonucleic acid, by dividing by binary fission, and by having cell walls that resemble those of gram-negative bacteria. Species of chlamydial organisms include *Chlamydia psittaci* and *C. trachomatis*, the latter of which has a number of serotypes. These species cause numerous diseases, including lymphogranuloma venereum, blinding trachoma, conjunctivitis, nongonococcal urethritis, cervicitis, salpingitis, proctitis, epididymitis, and newborn pneumonia.

DIAGNOSTIC CRITERIA

Chlamydia is sometimes referred to as a "silent" infection, as many patients are asymptomatic. In symptomatic women, the clinical presentation includes vaginal discharge, mucopurulent cervicitis with edema and friability, urethral syndrome or urethritis, pelvic inflammatory disease (PID), ectopic pregnancy, infertility, and endometritis. Less than 10% of men report symptoms that may include a thin, clear discharge and dysuria. Chlamydial organisms are the major causes of nongonococcal urethritis and epididymitis in young men.

Since the infection is often asymptomatic, it is recommended that all women less than 25 years and older women with new sexual partners be screened. The nucleic acid amplification test (NAAT) is the gold standard. NAATs can also be done using various body fluid such as clean catch urine sample or vaginal swab.

In infants aged 1 to 3 months, chlamydial infection presents in the mucous membranes of the eye, oropharynx, urogenital tract, and rectum and as subacute, afebrile pneumonia; in neonates, it presents as an asymptomatic infection of the oropharynx, genital tract, and rectum. However, chlamydial infection most commonly presents as conjunctivitis 5 to 12 days after birth and is the most frequent identifiable infectious cause of ophthalmia neonatorum. Therefore, for all infants with conjunctivitis who are no older than 30 days, a chlamydial etiology should be considered.

Diagnostic tests for chlamydial ophthalmia neonatorum include tissue cultures and nonculture tests. Ocular exudate should also be tested for *Neisseria gonorrhoeae*.

Chlamydial infection is diagnosed by examination, culture, and antigen detection methods, including direct fluorescent monoclonal antibody staining, enzyme-linked immunosorbent assay, DNA probe assay, and polymerase chain reaction.

INITIATING DRUG THERAPY

Treatment for all STIs consists of antimicrobial therapy followed by preventive education.

Goals of Drug Therapy

Patients are treated to eradicate the organism and prevent transmission to sex partners or to a newborn during birth. Because chlamydial infections often are accompanied by gonococcal infections, patients may be treated for both infections.

Antibiotic Therapy

Antibiotic treatments are prescribed to cure infection and usually relieve symptoms (CDC, 2015). Azithromycin (Zithromax), erythromycin (E-Mycin), macrolide antibiotics; doxycycline (Vibramycin), a tetracycline antibiotic; and ofloxacin (Floxin), a fluoroquinolone, are drugs of choice for chlamydial infections.

If therapeutic compliance is in question, azithromycin should be used for treatment because it is prepared as a single-dose drug. Doxycycline, however, has been used more extensively and is less expensive. An alternative regimen can be erythromycin, but it is less efficacious and has gastrointestinal (GI) side effects. Other alternatives include fluoroquinolones such as ofloxacin and levofloxacin (**Table 31.2**).

In infants, erythromycin base treatment has an efficacy of 80%. A second course of therapy may be required, and follow-up of the infant is recommended.

TABLE 31.2

Overview of Drugs Used to Treat Chlamydial Infections*

Generic (Trade) Name and Dosage	Selected Adverse Events	Contraindications	Special Considerations
Azithromycin (Zithromax) Adult: 1 g PO single dose Pregnancy: 1 g PO in a single dose Child (≥45 kg, <8 y): 1 g PO in a single dose Child (≥8 y): 1 g PO in a single dose (or doxycycline as below)	GI upset, abdominal pain, pseudomembranous colitis, angioedema, cholestatic jaundice	Hypersensitivity to azithromycin, erythromycin, or any macrolide antibiotic Use with caution for impaired hepatic function.	Do not take with aluminum- or magnesium-containing antacids.
Doxycycline (Vibramycin) Adult: 100 mg BID for 7 days Child (≥8 y): 100 mg PO BID for 7 days	Superinfection, photosensitivity, GI upset, enterocolitis, rash, blood dyscrasias, hepatotoxicity	Pregnancy, lactation, hypersensitivity to any of the tetracyclines	Use of drug during tooth development may discolor teeth in pediatric patients. Advise patient to avoid excessive sunlight or ultraviolet light. Caution patient that drug absorption is reduced when taken with food or bismuth subsalicylate.
Amoxicillin (Augmentin) Pregnancy: 500 mg TID for 7 days	Hypersensitivity reactions, pseudomembranous colitis, GI upset, rash, urticaria, vaginitis	History of Augmentin-associated cholestatic jaundice, hepatic dysfunction, or allergic reactions to any penicillin	Monitor blood, renal, and hepatic function in long-term use.
Ofloxacin (Floxin) 300 mg BID for 7 days	Rash, hives, rapid heartbeat, difficulty swallowing or breathing, photosensitivity, angioedema, dizziness, light-headedness	Pregnancy, hypersensitivity to ofloxacin or quinolones Use with caution for hepatic or renal insufficiency.	Do not take with food. Drink fluids liberally.
Levofloxacin (Levaquin) 500 mg daily for 7 days	Same as above	Same as above	Same as above
Erythromycin base (E-Mycin) Adult: 500 mg QID for 7 days Pregnancy: 500 mg QID for 7 days or 250 mg QID for 14 days Children: 50 mg/kg/d PO divided into 4 doses daily for 10–14 days	GI upset, pseudomembranous colitis, hepatic dysfunction, cardiac dysrhythmias, CNS disturbances, urticaria, skin eruptions, hearing loss, superinfection and local irritation	Known hypersensitivity to erythromycin Prescribe with caution for patients with impaired hepatic function and children who weigh <45 kg.	Effectiveness of treatment is ~80%; a second course of therapy may be required. Use for prophylaxis of ophthalmia neonatorum and infant pneumonia.
Erythromycin ethylsuccinate (EES) Adult: 800 mg QID for 7 days Pregnancy: 800 mg QID for 7 days or 400 mg QID for 14 days	Same as above	Same as above	Same as above

Note: *In adults, pregnant women, children, ophthalmia neonatorum, and infant pneumonia.

CNS, central nervous system; GI, gastrointestinal.

Mechanism of Action

Azithromycin and erythromycin bind to bacterial ribosomes to block protein synthesis. The drugs are also bactericidal, depending on their concentration. (For more information on antibiotic actions, see Chapter 6.) Doxycycline is thought to act in a similar way, whereas ofloxacin kills bacteria by blocking DNA gyrase and inhibiting DNA synthesis.

Dosages

A single 1-g dose of azithromycin or 100 mg of doxycycline twice daily for 7 days is the usual initial therapy.

Contraindications

Sensitivity to erythromycin or other macrolides is the main contraindication to therapy.

The safety and efficacy of azithromycin in pregnant and lactating women are not known. Doxycycline and ofloxacin are contraindicated in pregnant women.

Adverse Events

In some patients, GI side effects (nausea, vomiting, diarrhea, abdominal discomfort) cause them to discontinue therapy.

Selecting the Most Appropriate Agent

The most appropriate therapy is the one that best matches the needs of the patient in different situations or stages of life. **Figure 31.1** and **Tables 31.1** and **31.2** summarize treatment options.

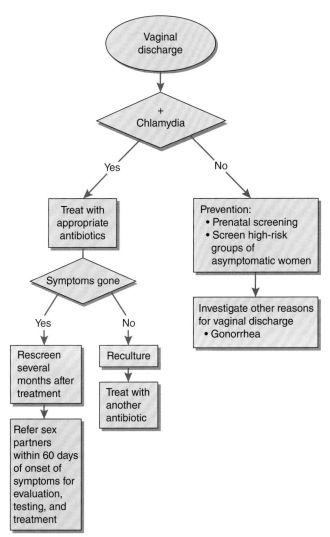

Key ⬭ Starting point for decision making

▢ Clinical actions (assessing, prescribing, monitoring)

◇ Decision point

FIGURE 31–1   Treatment algorithm for chlamydial infection.

Special Population Considerations

Pediatric

To prevent chlamydial infection among neonates, prenatal screening is recommended. In general, patients appropriate for screening include pregnant women younger than age 25 with new or multiple sex partners.

C. trachomatis infection of neonates results from perinatal exposure to the mother's infected cervix. The prevalence of *C. trachomatis* infection among pregnant women does not vary by race/ethnicity or socioeconomic status. Neonatal ocular prophylaxis with silver nitrate solution or antibiotic ointments does not prevent perinatal transmission of *C. trachomatis* from mother to infant. However, ocular prophylaxis with those agents does prevent gonococcal ophthalmia and therefore should be continued.

Initial *C. trachomatis* perinatal infection involves mucous membranes of the eye, oropharynx, urogenital tract, and rectum. *C. trachomatis* infection in neonates is most often recognized by conjunctivitis that develops 5 to 12 days after birth. Chlamydia is the most frequent identifiable infectious cause of ophthalmia neonatorum. *C. trachomatis* is also a common cause of subacute, afebrile pneumonia with onset from ages 1 to 3 months. Asymptomatic infections can also occur in the oropharynx, genital tract, and rectum of neonates.

A chlamydial etiology should be considered for all infants aged 30 days or less who have conjunctivitis. Sexual abuse should be considered for infants and children who test positive for chlamydial infections.

Pregnancy

The recommended regimen for pregnancy is a single dose of azithromycin 1 g or amoxicillin 500 mg orally thrice daily for 7 days.

Alternative regimens are erythromycin base 250 mg orally four times daily for 14 days, erythromycin ethylsuccinate 800 mg orally four times daily for 7 days or 400 mg orally four times daily for 14 days, or azithromycin 1 g orally as a single dose. Erythromycin estolate is contraindicated during pregnancy because of drug-related hepatotoxicity. Doxycycline is contraindicated in the second and third trimesters. All pregnant women who have chlamydia should be retested within 3 to 4 weeks after finishing treatment, and again at 3 months, which is contrary to the discussion in monitoring patient responses. If infection persists, it can severely affect the mother and neonate.

MONITORING PATIENT RESPONSE

Because therapy with azithromycin or doxycycline is highly efficacious, patients do not need to be retested after treatment is completed unless they are pregnant (see section titled Pregnancy). If alternative agents, such as erythromycin, are used for treatment, repeat testing for cure is no longer recommended unless therapeutic adherence is in question, symptoms persist, or reinfection is suspected (CDC, 2015).

Screening for *C. trachomatis* should be performed in high-risk groups when the practitioner performs a pelvic examination. High-risk groups include sexually active adolescents and women aged 15 to 24, particularly those who have new or multiple sex partners; those attending family planning clinics, prenatal clinics, or abortion facilities; or those in juvenile detention centers. Screening for high-risk men should be considered when they seek healthcare.

PATIENT EDUCATION

The patient's sex partner must be treated; current guidelines (CDC, 2015) recommend presumptive treatment for all partners. Patients should abstain from sexual intercourse for 7 days after single-dose therapy or until the 7-day regimen is completed. Abstinence should also continue until the patient's sex partner has been treated to prevent reinfection. Sex partners should be treated if they have had sexual contact with the patient during the 60 days preceding onset of the symptoms in the patient or the diagnosis of chlamydial infection. The most recent sex partner should be treated even if the time of the last sexual contact was greater than 60 days before onset or diagnosis.

GONORRHEA

N. gonorrhoeae is the second most commonly reported STI in the United States after chlamydia (CDC, 2019). Like chlamydia, gonorrhea is a major cause of PID, tubal scarring, infertility, ectopic pregnancy, and chronic pelvic pain in the United States. Most men seek treatment before serious complications develop, but not soon enough to prevent transmission to others. In women, symptoms may not develop until complications such as PID occur. Screening of men and women at high risk for STIs is an important component of gonorrhea control (CDC, 2015). Patients infected with *N. gonorrhoeae* frequently are coinfected with *C. trachomatis*; this finding has led to the recommendation that patients treated for gonococcal infection also be treated routinely with a regimen that is effective against uncomplicated genital *C. trachomatis* infection. Because the majority of *gonococci* in the United States are susceptible to doxycycline and azithromycin, routine cotreatment might also hinder the development of antimicrobial-resistant *N. gonorrhoeae*.

CAUSES

Gonorrhea is caused by *N. gonorrhoeae*, a gram-negative diplococcal bacterium. It is transmitted by sexual contact, and the rate of male-to-female transmission is higher than that of female-to-male or male-to-male transmission. Women with gonorrhea have a high prevalence of other STIs including chlamydial infection, trichomoniasis, bacterial vaginosis, and herpes genitalis.

Uncomplicated anogenital gonorrhea in women can involve the endocervix, urethra, Skene glands, Bartholin glands, and anus. The endocervix is the most common site of infection. Pharyngeal infection can also occur and is usually asymptomatic.

PATHOPHYSIOLOGY

Several strains of gonorrhea have been identified. Gonococcal sensitivity and resistance to antibiotics are clinically significant. Certain strains of the organism are resistant to sulfonamides. Penicillinase-producing *N. gonorrhoeae* and chromosomal-resistant *N. gonorrhoeae* are resistant to penicillin, and tetracycline-resistant *N. gonorrhoeae* is resistant to tetracycline.

DIAGNOSTIC CRITERIA

In the United States, 583,405 new *N. gonorrhoeae* cases were reported to the CDC in 2018, over a 60% increase since 2014. Most infections among men produce symptoms that cause them to seek curative treatment soon enough to prevent serious sequelae, but this may not be soon enough to prevent transmission to others. Among women, many infections do not produce recognizable symptoms until complications such as PID have occurred. Up to 30% of women with gonorrheal infection have symptoms. Signs and symptoms include purulent or mucopurulent cervical discharge, dysuria, anal bleeding, menorrhagia, and pelvic discomfort. Men with gonococcal urethritis present with penile burning, purulent discharge, and itching.

Gonorrhea is diagnosed by examination and culture for *N. gonorrhoeae*. Culture can be obtained from endocervical (women) or urethral (men) swabs or urine (from both men and women). NAAT is the gold standard for diagnosis. A culture is useful only if susceptibilities are needed as cultures have a longer turnaround time.

INITIATING DRUG THERAPY

Preventive education is always offered. Sex partners should be referred for evaluation and treatment of *N. gonorrhoeae* and *C. trachomatis* infection if their last contact with the patient was within 60 days before onset of the symptoms or diagnosis of infection. The patient's most recent sex partner should be treated even if the patient's last sexual intercourse was more than 60 days before onset of the symptoms or diagnosis. Patients and their sex partners should refrain from unprotected sexual intercourse for 7 days after initiation of therapy, resolution of symptoms, and until sex partners have been successfully treated. All patients diagnosed with gonorrhea should be tested for syphilis.

Patients treated for gonococcal infection are also treated for chlamydial infection because patients with gonorrhea are commonly coinfected with *C. trachomatis*. Patients with treatment failure should undergo culture and susceptibility testing, and the local health department should be notified (CDC, 2015).

Goals of Drug Therapy

The goal of drug therapy is to eradicate disease and prevent complications and spread of infection to others.

Antibiotics

The CDC describes recommended regimens for uncomplicated gonococcal infections of the cervix, urethra, and rectum (**Table 31.3**).

Ceftriaxone

A single injection of 250 mg of ceftriaxone provides sustained, high antibacterial levels in the blood. Extensive clinical experience shows that the drug is safe and effective for treating uncomplicated gonorrhea at all sites with a cure rate of 99.1% in clinical trials for uncomplicated urogenital and anorectal infections.

Cefixime

Cefixime (Suprax) covers an antimicrobial spectrum similar to that of ceftriaxone (Rocephin). Due to increasing minimum inhibitory concentrations for oral cephalosporins to *N. gonorrhoeae*, cefixime is no longer recommended as a first-line treatment option. Cefixime can be given as an alternative therapy to ceftriaxone if the latter is not available. Cefixime given as a single 400-mg oral dose in combination with azithromycin will require a test of cure 1 week after treatment.

Azithromycin

Due to the development of antimicrobial resistance of *N. gonorrheae*, treatment with dual antibiotics with different mechanisms of action is required. Azithromycin (Zithromax) is given as one-time dose of 1 g in addition to IM ceftriaxone.

TABLE 31.3

Overview of Selected Drugs Used to Treat Uncomplicated Gonococcal Infections in Adults and Children*

Generic (Trade) Name and Dosage	Selected Adverse Events	Contraindications	Special Considerations
Ceftriaxone (Rocephin) Adult: 250 mg IM in a single dose	Pseudomembranous colitis, rash, GI upset, hematologic abnormalities	Known allergy to cephalosporins Prescribe with caution for penicillin-sensitive patients.	Use for uncomplicated gonococcal infection of the pharynx.
Child: Ophthalmia neonatorum: 25–50 mg/kg IV or IM in a single dose, not to exceed 125 mg Child: 125 mg IM in a single dose or 50 mg/kg (maximum dose 1 g) IM or IV in a single dose daily for 7 days or 50 mg/kg (maximum dose 2 g) IM or IV in a single dose daily for 10–14 days Child (<45 kg with bacteremia or arthritis): 50 mg/kg, max 1 g IM or IV in a single daily dose for 7 days Child (>45 kg with bacteremia or arthritis): 50 mg/kg, max 2 g, IM or IV in a single daily dose for 10–14 days		Prescribe with caution for hyperbilirubinemic infants, especially premature infants.	Prescribe prophylactically for infants whose mothers have gonococcal infection.
Cefixime (Suprax) 400 mg PO in single dose	Pseudomembranous colitis, GI upset, skin rash, headache, dizziness	Known allergy to cephalosporins Prescribe with caution for penicillin-sensitive patients and patients with renal impairment or GI disease. Prescribe with caution for patients on dialysis.	Only use if IM ceftriaxone not available. Requires a test of cure 1 week after treatment.
Azithromycin (Zithromax) 1 g PO in a single dose	GI upset, abdominal pain, pseudomembranous colitis, angioedema, cholestatic jaundice	Hypersensitivity to azithromycin, erythromycin, or any macrolide antibiotic Prescribe with caution for patients with impaired hepatic function.	Take 1 hour before or 2 hours after meals for greatest absorption. Avoid taking with aluminum- or magnesium-containing antacids. Comes in powder form

(Continued)

TABLE 31.3

Overview of Selected Drugs Used to Treat Uncomplicated Gonococcal Infections in Adults and Children (Continued)

Generic (Trade) Name and Dosage	Selected Adverse Events	Contraindications	Special Considerations
Doxycycline (Vibramycin) 100 mg PO BID for 7 days	Superinfection, photosensitivity, GI upset, enterocolitis, rash, blood dyscrasias, hepatotoxicity	Pregnancy, lactation, hypersensitivity to any of the tetracyclines	Monitor blood, renal, and hepatic function in long-term use. Because of photosensitivity, patients should avoid sunlight or UV light. Use of drug during tooth development may discolor teeth. Absorption is reduced when drug is taken with food or bismuth subsalicylate (Pepto-Bismol). Prescribe for uncomplicated gonococcal infection of the pharynx.
Gemifloxacin (Factive) 320 mg given as a single oral dose Alternative agent for patients with cephalosporins allergies	GI upset, diarrhea, photosensitivity, QTc prolongation, peripheral neuropathy, CNS effects, superinfection, tendon rupture	Pregnancy, lactation, hypersensitivity to gemifloxacin or other quinolones	May need to be renally adjusted
Gentamicin (Garamycin) 240 mg IM in a single or 5 mg/kg <45 kg Alternative agent for patients with cephalosporins allergies	Renal toxicity, ototoxicity, neurotoxicity	Hypersensitivity to gentamicin or other aminoglycosides	No need to monitor gentamicin levels since a single dose is given.

Note: *Infections of the cervix, urethra, and rectum; uncomplicated gonococcal infection of the pharynx; ophthalmia neonatorum; and gonococcal infection in children.

CNS, central nervous system; GI, gastrointestinal; IM, intramuscular; IV, intravenous; QTc, Corrected QT interval; UV, ultraviolet.

Azithromycin is preferred to doxycycline due to efficacy and ease of a single-dose regimen.

The CDC also recognizes other antimicrobials for use against *N. gonorrhoeae* in cases of cephalosporin or Immunoglobulin E (IgE) meditated penicillin allergy. Azithromycin 2 g PO is given in combination with either 240 mg IM gentamicin or 320 mg PO gemifloxacin and is an effective treatment regimen for uncomplicated gonococcal infection. If there is an azithromycin allergy, doxycycline can be considered; however, some isolates are resistant to this class of antibiotic.

The regimen recommended by the CDC for uncomplicated gonococcal infections of the pharynx is summarized in **Table 31.1** and **Figure 31.2**. These infections are more difficult to treat than urogenital and anorectal infections. Few drugs can reliably cure these infections more than 90% of the time. Treatment for gonorrhea and chlamydial infection is suggested even though chlamydial coinfection of the pharynx is unusual.

Selecting the Most Appropriate Agent

Therapy for uncomplicated gonococcal infections includes a two-drug regimen as follows:

- Single-dose ceftriaxone 250 mg IM
- PLUS
- Single-dose azithromycin 1 g or
- Doxycycline 100 mg orally twice daily for 7 days

The choice is based on the practitioner's assessment of the patient's reliability, allergies, and preferences. If there is a question regarding the patient's reliability, ceftriaxone IM may be the treatment of choice because it is administered in the office.

Special Population Considerations

Pediatric

Gonococcal infection may be transmitted to infants exposed to infected cervical exudate at birth. The infection presents

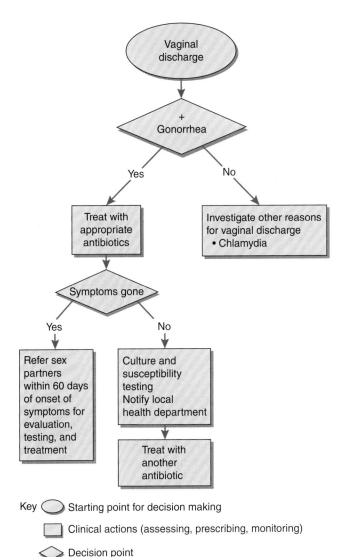

Key ⬭ Starting point for decision making

　　　▭ Clinical actions (assessing, prescribing, monitoring)

　　　◇ Decision point

FIGURE 31–2   Treatment algorithm for gonorrheal infection.

diplococci are identified in conjunctival exudate, and testing for chlamydial organisms should be done in all cases of neonatal conjunctivitis. Presumptive treatment can be given for newborns who are at increased risk for gonococcal ophthalmia or who have conjunctivitis but no *gonococci* in a gram-stained smear of conjunctival exudate. Infants with gonococcal ophthalmia should be hospitalized and monitored for signs of disseminated infection. Many physicians prefer to continue therapy until cultures are negative for gonococcal organisms at 48 to 72 hours.

To prevent ophthalmia neonatorum, erythromycin is used as a prophylactic agent and installed in the eyes within 24 hours of delivery; this is required by law in most states, regardless of whether delivery was vaginal or cesarean (**Table 31.4**).

In preadolescent children, sexual abuse is the most frequent cause of gonococcal infection. Vaginitis is the most common manifestation, followed by anorectal and pharyngeal infections, which are commonly asymptomatic. Standard culture procedures should be used to diagnose the infection, and nonculture gonococcal tests should not be used alone.

Follow-up cultures are not needed if ceftriaxone is used. Only parenteral cephalosporins are recommended for use in children. Quinolones are not approved for use in children because of concerns regarding toxicity. A follow-up culture is needed to ensure that treatment was effective if spectinomycin is used. All children with gonococcal infections should be evaluated for syphilis and chlamydial coinfection.

MONITORING PATIENT RESPONSE

Patients who have had uncomplicated gonorrhea and who were treated with any of the recommended regimens do not need to return for test of cure. If symptoms persist after treatment, the patient is evaluated by culture for *N. gonorrhoeae*, and isolated *gonococci* should be tested for antimicrobial susceptibility. If infection is identified, its source is usually reinfection rather than treatment failure.

PATIENT EDUCATION

Patient education concentrates on prevention. All patients should be encouraged to adopt meticulous hygiene and practice safe sex, to insist that partners seek treatment, and to schedule and keep follow-up healthcare appointments.

as an acute illness 2 to 5 days after birth. The prevalence in infants depends on the prevalence of infection in pregnant women, whether pregnant women are screened for gonorrhea, and whether newborns receive prophylactic treatment. Manifestations of the infection in newborns include ophthalmia neonatorum, which may result in perforation of the ocular globe and blindness, sepsis with arthritis, and meningitis, rhinitis, vaginitis, urethritis, and inflammation at fetal monitoring sites. Cultures should be taken when typical gram-negative

TABLE 31.4			
Prophylaxis for Ophthalmia Neonatorum			
Topical Agent	**Adverse Events**	**Contraindications**	**Special Considerations**
Erythromycin (Ilotycin) 0.5% ophthalmic ointment in a single application	Sensitivity reactions	Hypersensitivity to erythromycin	Instill into both eyes as soon as possible after birth. Use single tubes for administration.

SYPHILIS

In the 1990s, syphilis reemerged in endemic forms in the United States with a significant increase in the incidence of primary, secondary, and congenital syphilis. The increase has been attributed to greater use of illicit drugs, most notably crack cocaine, and high-risk sexual behavior related to drug use. Approximately 35,000 new cases of primary and secondary syphilis occur annually in the United States (CDC, 2018). Gay and bisexual men are at greatest risk.

CAUSES

Syphilis is a chronic, infectious disease caused by the spirochete *Treponema pallidum*. Infection may be active, and characterized by symptoms, or inactive (latent). The latent stage has no clinical symptoms. During the latent stage, infections can be detected by serologic testing. Early latent syphilis is defined as latent syphilis acquired within the preceding year. Any other cases of latent syphilis are either late latent syphilis or syphilis of unknown duration (CDC, 2015).

PATHOPHYSIOLOGY

T. pallidum is considered a bacterium because of its cell wall and response to antibiotic therapy. *T. pallidum* is not readily grown in vitro and cannot be seen by light microscopy.

DIAGNOSTIC CRITERIA

Patients who contract syphilis may seek treatment for signs or symptoms of primary infection, which include an ulcer or chancre at the infection site. The chancre erupts approximately 3 weeks after exposure. Signs and symptoms of secondary syphilis are low-grade fever, malaise, sore throat, hoarseness, headache, anorexia, rash, mucocutaneous lesions, alopecia, and adenopathy. Signs and symptoms of tertiary infection include cardiac, neurologic, ophthalmic, auditory, or gummatous lesions. Definitive methods for diagnosing early syphilis include dark-field examination and direct fluorescent antibody study of the chancre's exudate or tissue. The serologic tests used to confirm the syphilis diagnosis are nontreponemal and treponemal. The nontreponemal tests are the Venereal Disease Research Laboratory (VDRL) test and the rapid plasma regain test. The treponemal tests include the fluorescent treponemal antibody absorption test and the microhemagglutination assay for antibody to *T. pallidum*. The two serologic tests are necessary because false-positive nontreponemal test results occur on occasion secondary to certain medical conditions. Treponemal test antibody titers do not correlate accurately with disease activity and should not be used to assess treatment response.

A single test cannot be used to diagnose all cases of neurosyphilis. The diagnosis is made using a combination of tests including combinations of reactive serologic test results, abnormalities of cerebrospinal fluid (CSF) cell count or protein, or reactive VDRL-CSF with or without clinical manifestations (CDC, 2015).

INITIATING DRUG THERAPY

Although sexual transmission occurs only when mucocutaneous syphilitic lesions, including the rash, are present, people exposed in any stage should be evaluated clinically and serologically. Treatment should be given to those who were exposed within 90 days preceding the diagnosis of primary, secondary, or early latent syphilis in a sex partner, because the partner might be infected even if he or she is seronegative. Treatment should also be given to those who were exposed more than 90 days before the diagnosis of primary, secondary, or early latent syphilis in a sex partner if serologic test results are unavailable and follow-up tests and treatments are uncertain. Patients who have syphilis of unknown duration and who have high nontreponemal serologic test titers are considered to have early syphilis. Sex partners should be notified and treated. Long-term partners of patients with late syphilis should have a clinical and serologic evaluation and should be treated based on the findings.

For all stages of syphilis, penicillin is the preferred treatment. The stage and clinical manifestations of the disease determine the preparation used as well as the dosage and duration of treatment. However, no adequate trials have been performed to determine the optimal penicillin regimen. The only therapy with documented efficacy for syphilis during pregnancy or neurosyphilis is parenteral penicillin G benzathine. Penicillin G has been used for the past five decades to achieve a local cure and to prevent late sequelae.

Goals of Drug Therapy

The goal of treatment for primary and secondary syphilis is cure. The goal of treatment for latent syphilis is to prevent occurrence or progression of late complications. There is limited evidence supporting specific regimens for penicillin even though clinical experience has shown the effectiveness of penicillin in achieving these goals.

Antibiotics

Penicillin

Adults with primary or secondary syphilis should be treated with penicillin G benzathine (Bicillin). Other choices for unusual situations include doxycycline, tetracycline (Achromycin), ceftriaxone, and erythromycin (**Table 31.5**).

Mechanism of Action

Penicillins are bactericidal. They disrupt synthesis of the bacterial cell wall and bind to enzyme proteins, interfering with the biosynthesis of mucopeptides and preventing the structural components of the cell wall from leaking out. As such,

TABLE 31.5

Overview of Selected Drugs Used to Treat Syphilis

Generic (Trade) Name and Dosage	Selected Adverse Events	Contraindications	Special Considerations
Nonallergic Adults			
Penicillin G benzathine (Bicillin) *Primary, secondary, and early latent infection:* 2.4 million U IM single dose *Late latent infection, infection of unknown duration, or tertiary infection:* 2.4 million U q7d × 3 weeks (if dosing late by >2 days restart from first dose)	Hypersensitivity, urticaria, laryngeal edema, fever, eosinophilia, serum sickness–like reactions, anaphylaxis, hemolytic anemia, leukopenia, thrombocytopenia, neuropathy, nephropathy	Hypersensitivity to any penicillin or procaine	Use with caution for patients with allergies or asthma. Do not inject into or near an artery or nerve.
Nonallergic Children			
Penicillin G benzathine (Bicillin) *Primary, secondary, and early latent infection:* 50,000 U/kg IM up to adult dose of 2.4 million U in a single dose *Late latent infection, infection of unknown duration:* 50,000 U/kg IM up to adult dose of 2.4 million U administered as 3 doses at q7d × 3 weeks (total 150,000 U/kg up to adult dose of 7.2 million U)	Same as above	Same as above	Same as above
Nonpregnant, Penicillin-Allergic Patients			
Doxycycline (Vibramycin) 100 mg PO BID for 14 days *Latent syphilis:* 100 mg PO BID for 28 days (if infection is <1 year, give for 2 weeks)	Superinfection, photosensitivity, GI upset, enterocolitis, rash, blood dyscrasias, hepatotoxicity	Pregnancy, lactation Hypersensitivity to any of the tetracyclines	Monitor blood, renal, and hepatic function in long-term use. Avoid sunlight or UV light. Use of drug during tooth development may cause dental discoloration. Absorption is reduced when taken with food or bismuth subsalicylate.
Tetracycline (Achromycin) 500 mg PO QID for 14 days *Latent syphilis:* 500 mg PO QID for 28 days (if infection is <1 year, give for 2 weeks)	Photosensitivity, GI upset, glossitis, dysphasia, enterocolitis, pancreatitis, anogenital lesions, elevated hepatic enzymes, hepatic toxicity, rash, hypersensitivity, dizziness, tinnitus, visual disturbances	Hypersensitivity to any tetracyclines	Use of drug during tooth development may cause dental discoloration. Use of tetracycline may render oral contraceptives less effective.
Ceftriaxone (Rocephin) 1–2 g IV/IM q24h for 10–14 days	Pseudomembranous colitis, rash, GI upset, hepatologic abnormalities	Known allergy to cephalosporins	Prescribe with caution for penicillin-sensitive patients. Limited data for use

GI, gastrointestinal; IM, intramuscular; IV, intravenous; UV, ultraviolet.

the bacteria cannot lay protein cross-links in the cell wall. In addition, autolytic enzymes, which promote lysis of bacteria, are activated.

Contraindications

Penicillin is contraindicated in patients with hypersensitivity reaction. There is a small percentage of a possible cross-reactivity allergic reaction with penicillin and those that have a reported allergy to other classes of beta-lactam antibiotics (e.g., cephalosporins).

Adverse Events

Hypersensitivity, urticaria, laryngeal edema, fever, eosinophilia, anaphylaxis, hemolytic anemia, leukopenia, thrombocytopenia, neuropathy, and nephropathy are some of the adverse effects of the penicillins.

Interactions

Penicillin decreases the effect of oral contraceptives. Hyperkalemia can result from concurrent use of potassium-sparing diuretics, angiotensin-converting enzyme inhibitors, and potassium supplements with parenteral penicillin G.

Doxycycline, Tetracycline, and Others

Nonpregnant patients with latent syphilis who are allergic to penicillin should be treated with doxycycline or tetracycline. Both drugs should be given for 2 weeks if the infection is of less than 1 year's duration; otherwise, they should be given for 4 weeks. Patients who are not pregnant but who are allergic to penicillin and who have primary or secondary syphilis should be treated with doxycycline or tetracycline. For patients who cannot tolerate these, ceftriaxone is recommended. Although erythromycin is less effective than other regimens, it can be used for nonpregnant, compliant patients. Patients whose compliance is questionable or pregnant patients who are allergic to penicillin should be desensitized and treated with penicillin. For more information, see Chapter 6.

Jarisch-Herxheimer Reaction

Some patients may experience Jarisch-Herxheimer reaction (fever, headache, myalgias) within the first 24 hours of treatment for syphilis due to the release of exotoxins from the killed spirochetes. Premedication with a nonsteroidal antiinflammatory drug such as ibuprofen or naproxen may be helpful.

Selecting the Most Appropriate Agent

Penicillin G therapy is the most efficacious treatment for patients who have syphilis. If a patient reports a penicillin allergy with an unknown reaction, a penicillin skin test may be considered to confirm allergy. If a patient has a true penicillin allergy and resources are available, the patient may undergo penicillin desensitization first before trying an alternative regimen; this would require the patient be admitted inpatient for observation for possible anaphylactic reaction. There are no proven alternative drugs for pregnant women who have syphilis and who are allergic to penicillin. These women should be desensitized and then treated with penicillin (**Figure 31.3**).

Special Population Considerations

Pediatric

Children with syphilis should have a CSF examination for asymptomatic neurosyphilis. To assess for congenital or acquired syphilis, birth and maternal records should be reviewed. Children who have primary or secondary syphilis should have an evaluation, consultation with child protection services, and treatment with a pediatric regimen.

Women

Pregnant women should be screened and treated for syphilis to protect the fetus and the newborn from exposure to syphilis. Screening is performed at the time pregnancy is confirmed. If the patient is in a high-risk group, testing should also occur at 28 weeks and at delivery. Pregnant patients who are allergic to penicillin should be desensitized and treated with penicillin.

At-Risk Populations

All patients with syphilis should be tested for HIV infection. In areas where the prevalence of HIV is high, patients with primary syphilis should be retested for HIV after 3 months if the first HIV result was negative.

MONITORING PATIENT RESPONSE

Patients should have a clinical and serologic examination at 6 and 12 months or more frequently if follow-up results are uncertain. Those who fail to respond to treatment or who were reinfected, those who have signs that persist or recur, or those who have a sustained fourfold increase in nontreponemal test titer values within 6 months after treatment for primary or secondary syphilis should be retreated after evaluation for HIV infection. Treatment with three weekly injections of penicillin G benzathine is recommended if additional follow-up results are uncertain, unless CSF examination identifies neurosyphilis.

Patients with latent syphilis should be evaluated for tertiary disease. All patients with latent syphilis should have quantitative nontreponemal serologic tests repeated at 6, 12, and 24 months.

Patients should be evaluated for neurosyphilis and treated if titer values increase fourfold, an initially high titer fails to decrease at least fourfold within 12 to 24 months, or signs and symptoms related to syphilis develop. Patients with symptoms of neurologic or ophthalmic disease should be evaluated for neurosyphilis and syphilitic eye disease and treated appropriately according to the results (**Table 31.6**).

PATIENT EDUCATION

Teaching patients about preventive strategies is important in deterring the transmission of disease. All patients with a diagnosis of syphilis should be advised to undergo HIV testing as well.

GENITAL HERPES SIMPLEX VIRUS INFECTION

In the United States, genital herpes simplex virus (HSV) is the most prevalent genital ulcer disease with approximately 50 million persons infected. It is associated with a higher risk of HIV infection. More than 500,000 new cases occur each year. Most infected people remain undiagnosed. They have mild

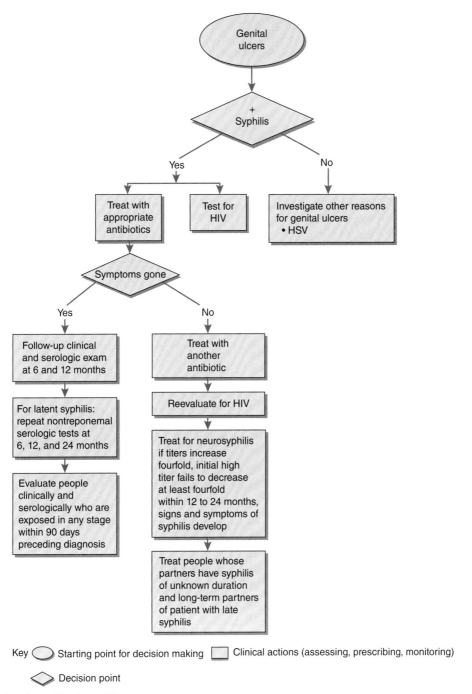

FIGURE 31–3 Treatment algorithm for syphilis.

HIV, human immunodeficiency virus; HSV, herpes simplex virus.

or unrecognized infections that shed the virus in the genital tract intermittently. Although some first episodes of genital herpes may be characterized by severe disease requiring hospitalization, many people are unaware they have the infection or are asymptomatic when transmission occurs. The disease can be controlled, not cured. It recurs periodically. Viral infections, for which curative therapy is not available, have been stable or increasing in prevalence. With 500,000 new cases each year, HSV is one of the most common viral STIs.

CAUSES

Genital herpes simplex is caused by HSV, which has two serotypes: HSV-1 (genital) and HSV-2 (anorectal). The infection is transmitted by contact with an infected person by kissing or sexual intercourse, or during vaginal birth. Recurrent outbreaks may be triggered by injury to the infected area, an illness that alters immune status, emotional stress, or menses.

TABLE 31.6

Overview of Drugs Used to Treat Neurosyphilis

Generic (Trade) Name and Dosage	Selected Adverse Events	Contraindications	Special Considerations
Aqueous crystalline penicillin G 18–24 million U/d, give as 3–4 million U IV q4h for 10–14 days	Similar to penicillins	Hypersensitivity to penicillin	This penicillin preparation is the drug of first choice in treating neurosyphilis; second-line therapy is procaine penicillin.
Procaine penicillin (Bicillin with probenecid, Benemid) 2.4 million U IM/d, plus probenecid 500 mg PO QID, both for 10–14 days	Similar to other penicillins *Probenecid:* Headache, dizziness, GI upset, hypersensitivity reactions, acute gouty arthritis, nephrotic syndrome, uric acid stones	Hypersensitivity to penicillin or probenecid Children <2 years: blood dyscrasias, uric acid kidney stones	If compliance can be ensured, avoid IV, intravascular, or intra-arterial administration. *Probenecid:* Use caution in prescribing for patients with peptic ulcer.

GI, gastrointestinal; IV, intravenous.

PATHOPHYSIOLOGY

Recurrent genital herpes is usually caused by HSV-1, while anorectal is HSV-2. After the virus enters the body through a susceptible mucosal surface, it resides and remains dormant in the cells of the nervous system until activated later. Exacerbations of varying frequency may or may not occur. In general, recurrent outbreaks are less severe than the initial episode.

DIAGNOSTIC CRITERIA

A diagnostic evaluation for herpes includes a health history and physical examination. In addition to serologic testing for HSV, patients should have a serologic test for syphilis. HIV testing should be considered as well. Specific tests for genital herpes include culture or antigen test for HSV. In addition, a POCkit HSV-2 test can be performed.

The patient seeking treatment may report any one of three genital HSV syndromes. The first is primary infection, which is the first infection with genital HSV characterized by no preexisting antibodies to either HSV-1 or HSV-2. Symptoms include genital pain, vesicles, fever, malaise, regional adenopathy, and, in women, lesions on the cervix. The second syndrome is nonprimary first-episode infection, which is the first clinically evident infection in women who have had a previous infection with heterologous strains. The symptoms include fewer lesions, few constitutional symptoms, and a shorter, milder course. The third syndrome is recurrent infection, which usually has no constitutional symptoms but has a shorter duration of viral shedding and a shorter healing time.

INITIATING DRUG THERAPY

The only effective therapy for genital herpes is drug therapy. Patient education is an important measure for preventing spread of the disease.

Goals of Drug Therapy

Treatment goals for first clinical episodes, recurrent episodes, and daily suppressive therapy aim to control the symptoms of the herpes episodes. The drugs *do not eradicate* the latent virus, and once discontinued, they do not affect the risk, frequency, or severity of recurrences. Treatment trials show acyclovir (Zovirax), valacyclovir (Valtrex), and famciclovir (Famvir) to be beneficial for treating genital herpes. The use of topical acyclovir is discouraged because it is substantially less effective than the systemic drug. The recommended acyclovir dosing regimens have been approved by the U.S. Food and Drug Administration and reflect substantial clinical experience and expert opinion for initial and recurrent episodes (**Table 31.7**).

Antivirals: Acyclovir, Famciclovir, and Valacyclovir

The three first-line systemic agents used to control genital herpes infections are acyclovir, famciclovir, and valacyclovir. These drugs inhibit viral DNA replication and are highly effective.

Acyclovir, which has low bioavailability, works only in the cells infected by HSV. Famciclovir, a prodrug of penciclovir, is well absorbed. It is converted to penciclovir by first-pass metabolism. Valacyclovir, a prodrug of acyclovir, is converted rapidly by first-pass metabolism to acyclovir. It has a 50% bioavailability; it also deactivates viral DNA polymerase.

Because antiviral medications are excreted by the renal system, caution should be used in patients with renal disease. They should also be prescribed cautiously for pregnant patients and are contraindicated in breast-feeding patients. These antivirals interact with probenecid, which increases the effect of the antiviral agent, and with zidovudine (Retrovir), which may cause drowsiness. For a detailed discussion of the roles that acyclovir, famciclovir, and valacyclovir play in controlling HSV-1 and HSV-2, see Chapter 13.

TABLE 31.7

Overview of Selected Drugs to Treat Genital Herpes

Generic (Trade) Name and Dosage	Selected Adverse Events	Contraindications	Special Considerations
Acyclovir (Zovirax) *First clinical episode:* 400 mg TID for 7–10 days or 200 g five times daily for 7–10 days *Recurrence:* 400 mg TID for 5 days or 200 mg five times daily for 5 days or 800 mg BID for 5 days *Daily suppressive therapy:* 400 mg BID *Severe disease:* 5–10 mg/kg IV q8h for 5–7 days or until clinical resolution occurs	GI upset (nausea, vomiting), headache, CNS disturbances, rash, malaise, vertigo, arthralgia, fatigue, viral resistance	Hypersensitivity to acyclovir Use with caution for renal impairment, pregnancy, breast-feeding mothers.	Do not exceed maximum dose.
Famciclovir (Famvir) *First clinical episode:* 250 mg TID for 7–10 days *Recurrence:* 125 mg BID for 5 days *Daily suppressive therapy:* 250 mg BID	Headache, fatigue, GI upset With chronic use: pruritus, rash, laboratory test abnormalities, paresthesias	Hypersensitivity to famciclovir Pregnancy, lactation Use with caution in patients with renal dysfunction.	Easy to administer for prolonged treatment May be affected by drugs metabolized by aldehyde oxidase
Valacyclovir (Valtrex) *First clinical episode:* 1 g PO BID for 7–10 days *Recurrent episodic infection:* 500 mg PO BID for 5 days *Daily suppressive therapy:* 500 mg PO daily (<9 episodes a year) or 1,000 mg PO daily	GI upset, headache, dizziness, abdominal pain	Hypersensitivity to valacyclovir Do not use in children. Use with caution for renal impairment, pregnancy, lactation.	Valacyclovir 500 mg daily is less effective than other valacyclovir regimens in patients with ≥10 episodes yearly. Be alert for renal or CNS toxicity in patients taking other nephrotoxic drugs.

CNS, central nervous system; GI, gastrointestinal.

Selecting the Most Appropriate Agent

Therapy progresses from selecting treatment for the first clinical episode of infection to prescribing an antiviral agent for suppressive therapy (**Figure 31.4**).

First-Line Therapy

Treatment for the first clinical episode of genital herpes includes antiviral therapy and counseling about the natural history of the virus, sexual and perinatal transmission, and methods to reduce transmission. Antiviral therapy for the initial outbreak includes the following:

- Acyclovir 400 mg thrice daily for 7 to 10 days or
- Acyclovir 200 mg five times daily for 7 to 10 days or
- Famciclovir 250 mg thrice daily for 7 to 10 days or
- Valacyclovir 1 g twice daily for 7 to 10 days

The choice is based on the cost of medication, patient preference, or scheduling issues.

Second-Line Therapy: Recurrent Episodes

Most patients with genital herpes infection have recurrent episodes of genital lesions. Episodic or suppressive antiviral therapy may shorten the duration of lesions or prevent recurrences. Episodic therapy is beneficial for recurrent disease if the treatment is started during the prodromal phase or within 1 day after onset of the lesions. When given episodic treatment, the patient should also be given additional antiviral therapy so the treatment can be initiated at the first sign of prodrome or genital lesions. Recurrent episodes are treated with the following:

- Acyclovir 400 mg thrice daily for 5 days or
- Acyclovir 800 mg twice daily for 5 days or
- Acyclovir 800 mg thrice daily for 2 days or
- Famciclovir 125 mg twice daily for 5 days or
- Famciclovir 1,000 mg twice daily for 1 day or
- Valacyclovir 500 mg twice daily for 3 days or
- Valacyclovir 1 g once daily for 5 days

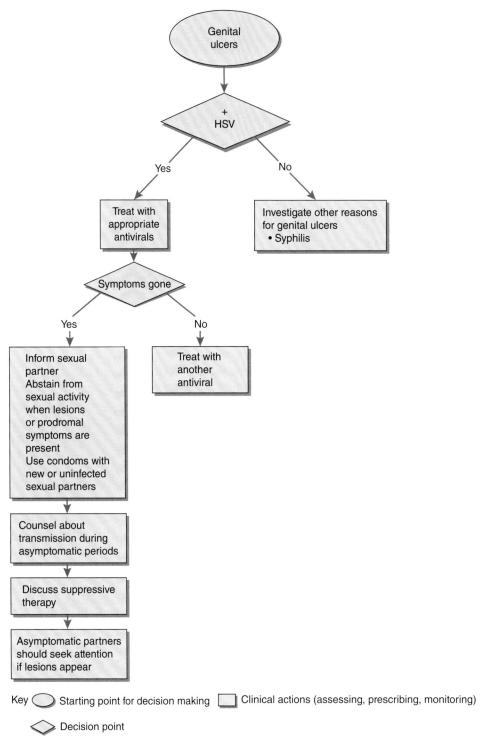

FIGURE 31–4   Treatment algorithm for genital herpes.

HSV, herpes simplex virus.

Third-Line Therapy: Suppressive Therapy

Third-line therapy is also known as suppressive therapy for HSV. The frequency of recurrent symptoms, or outbreaks, can be reduced by 75% or more with daily suppressive therapy, although suppressive therapy does not eliminate subclinical viral shedding. This therapy is used for patients with more than six episodes a year. Acyclovir has documented safety and efficacy for use for as long as 6 years, and valacyclovir and famciclovir for 1 year. Discontinuation of therapy should be discussed with the patient after 1 year of continuous suppressive therapy to determine the rate of recurrence and the patient's psychological adjustment. In many patients, the frequency of recurrence decreases over time.

Asymptomatic viral shedding is reduced but not eliminated with suppressive treatment with acyclovir. Therapy is not discontinued in patients who are HIV positive.

Suppressive therapy is as follows:

- Acyclovir 400 mg twice daily, or
- Famciclovir 250 mg twice daily, or
- Valacyclovir 500 or 1,000 mg once daily

Valacyclovir 500 mg once daily may be less effective than other regimens for prolonged suppression.

Severe or Complicated Disease

For patients with severe disease or complications requiring hospitalization, intravenous (IV) therapy is indicated. The recommended regimen is acyclovir 5 to 10 mg/kg body weight IV every 8 hours for 5 to 7 days or until clinical resolution is attained.

Special Population Considerations

Pediatric

The risk of HSV infection in the neonate is not completely eliminated with cesarean delivery. Infants exposed to HSV during birth should be followed up carefully. The CDC recommends that before clinical signs develop the infant have surveillance cultures of mucosal surfaces to detect HSV infection. Infants born to women who acquired genital herpes near term should receive acyclovir therapy. Infants with neonatal herpes should be treated with acyclovir 30 to 60 mg/kg/d for 10 to 21 days.

Women

During pregnancy, the first clinical episode of genital herpes may be treated with oral acyclovir. IV administration of acyclovir is indicated for life-threatening maternal HSV infection. Acyclovir is not recommended for routine administration in pregnant women who have a history of recurrent genital herpes. The safety of systemic acyclovir and valacyclovir in pregnant women is unknown.

Women who acquire genital herpes close to the time of delivery (30%–50%) are at high risk for transmitting the disease to the neonate. Those who have recurrent herpes at term or those who acquire genital HSV during the first half of pregnancy (3%) are at low risk for transmitting the disease to the neonate.

Sex partners who are symptomatic should have an evaluation and treatment similar to patients who have genital lesions. Most people who have genital HSV infection have no history of genital lesions. Therefore, asymptomatic sex partners of patients with newly diagnosed genital herpes should be interviewed regarding histories of typical and atypical genital lesions and encouraged to perform examinations and seek medical attention immediately if lesions appear.

MONITORING PATIENT RESPONSE

Response to therapy is monitored by symptom relief and resolution of lesions.

PATIENT EDUCATION

Patients should inform their sex partners that they have genital herpes and should abstain from sexual activity when lesions or prodromal symptoms are present. The practitioner can also discuss use of condoms with sex partners. Patients should also be counseled about transmission of HSV during asymptomatic periods. A diagnosis of genital herpes can be devastating to the individuals involved, so counseling should include helping patients cope with their infection and prevention of transmission.

Effective episodic treatment of recurrent herpes requires initiation of therapy within 1 day of lesion onset or during the prodrome that precedes some outbreaks. The patient should be provided with a supply of drug or a prescription for the medication with instructions to initiate treatment immediately when symptoms begin.

The risk of neonatal infection should be discussed with both sexes, and women who are pregnant should advise their healthcare providers about the infection. Patients should also be advised that episodic antiviral therapy may shorten the duration of lesions during recurrent episodes and that recurrent outbreaks can be ameliorated or prevented with suppressive antiviral therapy. Prevention of neonatal herpes should be emphasized during late pregnancy and counseling provided regarding unprotected genital and oral sexual contact at this time.

Patients who have genital herpes should be educated about the natural history of the disease, with emphasis on the potential for recurrent episodes, asymptomatic viral shedding, and the attendant risks of sexual transmission. All persons with genital HSV infection should be encouraged to inform their current sex partners that they have genital herpes and to inform future partners before initiating a sexual relationship. Persons with genital herpes should be informed that sexual transmission of HSV can occur during asymptomatic periods. Asymptomatic viral shedding is more frequent in genital HSV-2 infection than in genital HSV-1 infection and is most frequent in the first 12 months of acquiring HSV-2.

PELVIC INFLAMMATORY DISEASE

It is estimated that PID affects 1 million women each year. Approximately 250,000 of these women are hospitalized and more than 150,000 major surgical procedures are performed. The disease is associated with significant long-term consequences including tubal factor infertility, ectopic pregnancy, and chronic pelvic pain. Risk factors for PID include previous episodes of PID; presence of *N. gonorrhoeae*, *C. trachomatis*, or bacterial vaginosis in the lower genital tract; multiple sex partners; use of an intrauterine contraceptive device; adolescence; sexual intercourse during the last menstrual period; douching;

and cigarette smoking. Oral contraceptives are thought to afford some protection against PID.

CAUSES

The most common etiologic agents for PID are *N. gonorrhoeae* and *C. trachomatis*. Other microorganisms that are part of the vaginal flora can also cause PID, as well as *Mycobacterium hominis* and *Ureaplasma urealyticum*.

PATHOPHYSIOLOGY

PID consists of several inflammatory disorders of the upper female genital tract that include any combination of endometritis, salpingitis, tubo-ovarian abscess, and pelvic peritonitis. It is an ascending infection that spreads from the lower genital tract to the endometrium, to the fallopian tubes, and to the peritoneal cavity.

DIAGNOSTIC CRITERIA

In all settings, no single historical, physical, or laboratory finding is sensitive and specific enough to make the diagnosis of acute PID. Many cases of PID are not recognized because they are asymptomatic or because the patient or healthcare provider fails to recognize mild or nonspecific symptoms.

The following diagnostic criteria are from the CDC (2015) guidelines. Empiric treatment of PID should be given to sexually active young women and others who are at risk for STIs if all of the following minimum criteria are present with no other causes for the illness: lower abdominal tenderness, adnexal tenderness, and cervical motion tenderness. Additional criteria may be used to enhance the specificity of the minimum criteria including oral temperature exceeding 101°F (38.3°C), abnormal cervical or vaginal discharge, elevated erythrocyte sedimentation rate, elevated C-reactive protein, and laboratory documentation of cervical infection with *N. gonorrhoeae* or *C. trachomatis*. In selected cases, the following definitive criteria for diagnosing PID are warranted: histopathologic evidence of endometritis on endometrial biopsy; transvaginal sonography or other imaging techniques showing thickening, fluid-filled tubes with or without free pelvic fluid or tubo-ovarian complex; and laparoscopic abnormalities consistent with PID.

INITIATING DRUG THERAPY

Treatment for PID is prescribed when the patient's signs and symptoms meet the diagnostic criteria. Treatment includes empiric, broad-spectrum coverage of likely pathogens including *N. gonorrhoeae*, *C. trachomatis*, anaerobes, gram-negative facultative bacteria, and streptococci. The CDC (2015) recommends patients be hospitalized when surgical emergencies cannot be excluded and when the patient is pregnant; does not respond clinically to oral antimicrobials; cannot tolerate an outpatient oral regimen; has severe illness, nausea and vomiting, or high fever; has a tubo-ovarian abscess; or is immunodeficient. There are no efficacy data that compare parenteral with oral regimens, and clinical experience should guide the decision to switch from parenteral to oral therapy, which may occur within 24 hours of clinical improvement.

Goals of Drug Therapy

In addition to ameliorating infection or preventing the progression of disease, the goal of drug therapy is to preserve the patient's reproductive health or at least minimize the effects of infection. Treatment should begin as promptly as possible because prevention of long-term sequelae has a direct correlation with immediate antibiotic coverage. Factors to consider in selecting treatment include drug availability and cost, patient acceptance, and antimicrobial susceptibility.

Antimicrobials and Appropriate Treatment Choices

For the most part, antimicrobial regimens for PID are those used for patients with chlamydial and gonorrheal infections. Refer to the sections on chlamydial infection and gonorrhea in this chapter and also see **Table 31.8** for an overview of drug therapy in PID and **Figure 31.5** for a synopsis of the treatment. For women with PID of mild or moderate severity, parenteral therapy and oral therapy appear to have similar clinical efficacy. Patients with severe PID who are treated with parental therapy may be transitioned to an oral regimen within 24 to 48 hours with symptom improvement.

Mild to moderate PID (oral/outpatient regimens):

- Cefoxitin 2 g IM single dose + probenecid 1 g PO single dose + doxycycline 100 mg PO q12h × 14 d ± metronidazole 500 mg PO q12h ×14 d, or
- Ceftriaxone 250 mg IM single dose + probenecid 1 g PO single dose + doxycycline 100 mg PO q12h × 14 d ± metronidazole 500 mg PO q12h ×14 d, or
- Third-generation oral cephalosporin (e.g., cefdinir or cefpodoxime) + probenecid 1 g PO single dose + doxycycline 100 mg PO q12h × 14 d ± metronidazole 500 mg PO q12h ×14 d.

Severe PID (parental/inpatient regimens):

- Cefotetan 2 g IV q12h or cefoxitin 2 g IV q6h + doxycycline 100 mg q12h IV/PO, or
- Clindamycin 900 mg IV q8h + gentamicin IV/IM 2 mg/kg loading dose, then 1.5 mg/kg IV q8h or 3 to 5 mg/kg IV once daily dosing.

Special Population Considerations

Pregnant women with suspected PID should be hospitalized and treated with parenteral antibiotics so that the mother and fetus can be closely monitored.

TABLE 31.8

Overview of Selected Drugs to Treat Pelvic Inflammatory Disease

Generic (Trade) Name and Dosage	Selected Adverse Events	Contraindications	Special Considerations
Cefoxitin (Mefoxin) 2 g IV q6h	Pseudomembranous colitis, thrombophlebitis, rash, pruritus, eosinophilia, fever, dyspnea, hypotension, GI upset	Hypersensitivity to cefoxitin or cephalosporins	Prescribe with caution to penicillin-sensitive patients and those with GI disease. Monitor blood, renal, and hepatic function in long-term use.
Cefotetan (Cefotan) 2 g IV q12h	Same as above	Hypersensitivity to cefotetan or cephalosporin	Same as above
Doxycycline (Vibramycin) 100 mg q12h IV or PO for 14 days	Superinfection, photosensitivity, GI upset, enterocolitis, rash, blood dyscrasias, hepatotoxicity	Pregnancy, lactation, hypersensitivity or doxycycline or tetracyclines	Avoid sunlight or UV light. Use of drug during tooth development may cause dental discoloration. Absorption is reduced when taken with food or bismuth subsalicylate.
Probenecid 1 g PO single dose	GI upset, flushing, headache, dizziness	Avoid use in G6PD deficiency and blood dyscrasias, hypersensitivity to probenecid, children <2 years of age, aspirin therapy, uric acid kidney stone	Take with food to minimize GI upset. Advise patient to drink plenty of fluids.
Clindamycin (Cleocin) 900 mg IV q6h or 450 mg PO QID for 14 days			Clindamycin is used with tubo-ovarian abscess rather than doxycycline.
Gentamicin (Garamycin) IV/IM 2 mg/kg loading dose, then 1.5 mg/kg IV q8h or 3–5 mg/kg IV once daily dosing	Renal toxicity, ototoxicity, neurotoxicity	Hypersensitivity to gentamicin or other aminoglycosides.	Requires monitoring of renal function
Metronidazole (Flagyl) 500 mg PO BID for 14 days	CNS stimulation, phototoxicity, GI upset, insomnia, headache, dizziness, tendinitis or tendon rupture, local reactions	Hypersensitivity to metronidazole Pregnancy, lactation	Take on empty stomach with full glass of water and maintain adequate hydration throughout therapy. Avoid alcohol, excessive sunlight or UV light. Monitor blood, renal, and hepatic function in long-term use. Use with caution for CNS disorders that increase risk of seizure and for renal or hepatic impairment.
Ceftriaxone (Rocephin) 250 mg IM once	Pseudomembranous colitis, rash, GI upset, hematologic abnormalities	Known allergy to cephalosporins	Prescribe with caution to penicillin-sensitive patients.

CNS, central nervous system; G6PD, glucose-6-phosphate dehydrogenase; GI, gastrointestinal; IM, intramuscular; IV, intravenous; UV, ultraviolet.

MONITORING PATIENT RESPONSE

Patients treated with oral or parenteral therapy should demonstrate substantial clinical improvement within 3 days after therapy has been initiated. Those who do not improve in this period usually require additional diagnostic tests or surgical intervention. The patient should be seen after 1 week of antibiotic therapy to check for residual pelvic abnormalities. Outpatient oral or parenteral therapy also requires a follow-up examination performed within 72 hours, using the criteria for clinical improvement.

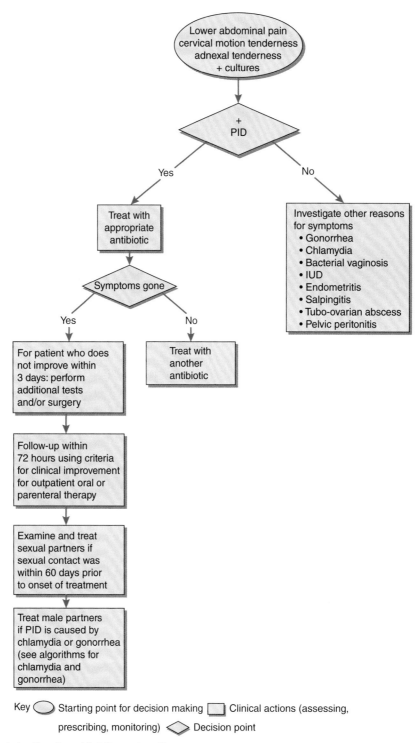

FIGURE 31–5   Treatment algorithm for pelvic inflammatory disease.

IUD, intrauterine devices; PID, pelvic inflammatory disease.

PATIENT EDUCATION

If *N. gonorrhoeae* or *C. trachomatis* is present, the practitioner needs to explain to patients with PID that their sex partners should be examined and treated if they have had sexual contact with the patient during the 60 days before the onset of the patient's symptoms. Male partners of women with PID caused by *C. trachomatis* or *N. gonorrhoeae* are often asymptomatic and should be treated empirically with regimens that are effective against both infections.

HUMAN PAPILLOMAVIRUS INFECTION

The detection of human papillomavirus (HPV) infection has increased in frequency in the genital tracts of men and women. Genital warts, known as *condylomata acuminata*, have been detected with widely increasing frequency as well. About 14 million new cases of HPV are diagnosed each year, and the prevalence of this disease is estimated to be 79 million cases (CDC, 2018).

CAUSES

There are over 100 identified types of HPV, in which 40 are genital. The sexual transmission of HPV is well documented, with the highest prevalence in young, sexually active adolescents and adults. Risk factors include the presence of other STIs, an increased number of sex partners, and use of oral contraceptives without other protection.

PATHOPHYSIOLOGY

Most HPVs cause no symptoms, are subclinical, or remain unrecognized. Warts that are visible in the genital tract are usually caused by HPV type 6 or type 11, which also causes warts (that cannot be seen externally) on the uterine cervix and in the vagina, urethra, and anus. These viruses, which can produce symptoms, have also been associated with conjunctival, nasal, oral, and laryngeal warts. They are rarely associated with invasive squamous cell carcinoma of the external genitalia. Genital warts can be painful, friable, or pruritic, depending on their size and anatomic location.

Cervical dysplasia has been strongly associated with other HPV types in the anogenital region, including types 16, 18, 31, 33, and 35. These are found occasionally in visible genital warts and have been associated with external genital squamous intraepithelial neoplasia and vaginal, anal, and cervical intraepithelial dysplasia and squamous cell carcinoma. Visible genital warts can be infected simultaneously with multiple HPV types. The body's immune system clears most HPV naturally within 2 years (about 90%), though some infections persist.

DIAGNOSTIC CRITERIA

Genital warts are diagnosed definitively by biopsy, which is needed only if the diagnosis is uncertain; if the lesions do not respond to standard therapy; if the disease worsens during therapy; if the patient is immunocompromised; or if the warts are pigmented, indurated, fixed, and ulcerated. The literature does not support HPV nucleic acid tests for use in the routine diagnosis or management of visible genital warts. For women who have exophytic cervical warts, high-grade squamous intraepithelial lesions must be ruled out before initiating treatment for genital warts (CDC, 2015).

INITIATING DRUG THERAPY

There is no evidence that current treatments eradicate or affect the natural history of HPV infection or the development of cervical cancer. Removal of warts may or may not decrease infectivity. Warts that are not treated may resolve on their own, remain unchanged, or increase in number and size. Treatment is guided by patient preference, cost of treatment and available resources, experience of the healthcare practitioner, wart size and number, anatomic location of wart, wart morphology, convenience, and adverse effects. No single treatment is ideal for all patients, nor is one superior to another.

Visible genital warts may be self-treated by the patient if they are accessible or by the healthcare practitioner. Nonpharmacologic therapies include surgery or laser therapy. Carbon dioxide laser is used for extensive warts or intraurethral warts and for patients who do not respond to other treatments. Pharmacotherapy may include podophyllin resin (Podofin), imiquimod (Aldara), trichloroacetic acid (TCA), bichloracetic acid (BCA), or intralesional interferon (Intron A).

Goals of Drug Therapy

The primary goal in treating visible genital warts is the removal of symptomatic warts and prevention of HPV transmission. Removal can induce wart-free periods in most patients. Often, genital warts are asymptomatic. Pharmacologic therapy may include podofilox (Condylox), imiquimod, TCA, and BCA (**Table 31.9**).

Podofilox and Podophyllin Resin

Visible genital warts can be self-treated by the patient with podofilox. The patient must be able to identify and reach the warts to be treated. Podofilox in 0.5% solution or gel is safe, inexpensive, easy to use, and efficacious on mucosal surfaces.

A stronger preparation for application only by the healthcare provider is podophyllin resin, which may be administered at a 10% to 25% concentration in a compound with tincture of benzoin. The CDC does not recommend use of podophyllin by the patient because of rare but potential toxicity involving systemic absorption, bone marrow suppression, or serious GI upset. The preparation is applied weekly as needed. Again, to guard against potential toxicities, the CDC recommends washing the preparation from the application site 1 to 4 hours after application. The most common adverse effect, which indicates the preparation is working, is local irritation. The preparation has not been established as safe for use during pregnancy.

Imiquimod

Like podofilox, imiquimod may be self-administered by the patient. This antimitotic preparation enhances the immune response to HPV. Imiquimod can be topically applied thrice weekly for 3 to 4 months. As with podophyllin, the imiquimod site should be washed with mild soap and water 6 to 10 hours after application. Warts should disappear in 8 to 10 weeks.

TABLE 31.9

Overview of Selected Drugs and Procedures Used to Treat Genital Warts

Generic (Trade) Name and Dosage	Selected Adverse Events	Contraindications	Special Considerations
Patient Applied			
Podofilox solution or gel (Condylox) 0.5% BID for 3 days followed by 4 days of no therapy; repeat cycle as needed for a total of 4 cycles.	Mild or moderate pain or local irritation	The safety of podofilox during pregnancy has not been established.	Apply solution with cotton swab or apply gel with finger. Total wart area should not exceed 10 cm², and total volume of podofilox should not exceed 0.5 mL/d.
Imiquimod cream (Aldara) 5% cream applied three times a week for up to 16 weeks	Mild to moderate local inflammatory reactions	The safety of imiquimod during pregnancy has not been established.	Apply with finger at bedtime. Wash area with mild soap and water 6–10 hours after application of cream. May clear area of warts in 8–10 weeks or sooner.
Practitioner Applied			
Cryotherapy	Pain, necrosis, blistering	Use of cryoprobe in the vagina is not recommended because of risk of vaginal perforation and fistula formation.	Repeat applications every 1–2 weeks. Use local anesthetic. Indicated for urethral meatus warts, anal warts, oral warts
Podophyllin or resin in compound tincture of benzoin 10%–25% (Podofin)	Local irritation	The safety of podophyllin during pregnancy has not been established. Use with caution vaginally because of potential systemic absorption.	Apply small amount on each wart and allow site to air-dry. Limit to ≤0.5 mL of podophyllin or ≤10 cm² of warts per therapy session.
			Wash off preparation 4 hours after application to reduce local irritation.
			Repeat application weekly if necessary.
			With vaginal warts, allow to dry before removing speculum and treat with ≤2 cm² per session.
			For warts on the urethral meatus, treatment area must be dry before preparation comes in contact with normal mucosa.
Trichloroacetic acid or bichloracetic acid 80%–90%	Can spread rapidly and damage adjacent tissue; pain		Apply only small amount on warts and allow site to dry. White "frosting" will develop. Use talc with baking soda to remove unreacted acid if an excess amount is applied. Repeat treatment weekly as needed. Indicated for vaginal warts

During imiquimod therapy, sexual contact should be avoided to prevent viral transmission. Adverse effects include a local inflammatory reaction. The safety of use during pregnancy has not been established.

Trichloroacetic Acid and Bichloracetic Acid

TCA and BCA are applied by the healthcare provider. These are strong 80% to 90% acids that flow onto the wart site quickly, and the fluid can spread equally quickly. Application requires particular care and skill. The acid is applied only to the warts and left to air-dry. A white "frosting" appears at the site. The practitioner can use talc or sodium bicarbonate powders to neutralize acid that falls on healthy tissue. TCA and BCA can be used effectively on keratinized areas and are safe for use during pregnancy. They are associated with low systemic toxicity.

Intralesional Interferon

Interferon is ineffective when used systemically. However, the use of intralesional interferon appears to be effective, and recurrence rates after therapy are comparable to those with other treatment modalities. Intralesional therapy appears to be effective because of interferon's antiviral or immunostimulating effects.

Selecting the Most Appropriate Agent

Treatment of genital warts should be guided by the preference of the patient, the available resources, and the experience of the healthcare provider. No definitive evidence suggests that any one of the available treatments is superior to the others, and no single treatment is ideal for all patients or all warts. Most patients have 10 or fewer genital warts. These warts respond to most treatment modalities. Factors that may influence selection of treatment include wart size, wart number, and anatomic site of wart, wart morphology, patient preference, and cost of treatment, convenience, adverse effects, and provider experience.

Many patients require a course of therapy rather than a single treatment. In general, warts located on moist surfaces or in intertriginous areas respond better to topical treatment than do warts on drier surfaces. **Figure 31.6** outlines the most appropriate patient- or practitioner-applied drug therapies in the most appropriate order.

Special Population Considerations
Pediatric

Laryngeal papillomatoses in infants and children are caused by HPV-6 and HPV-11. The prevention value of cesarean section is unknown, and the route of transmission is not completely understood.

Women

Many experts recommend removing warts during pregnancy because they can proliferate and become friable.

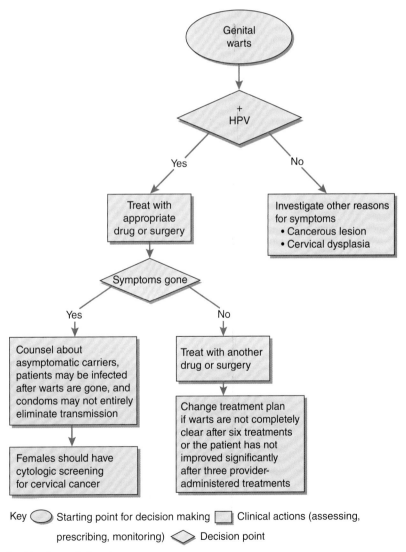

FIGURE 31–6   Treatment algorithm for genital warts.

HPV, human papillomavirus.

MONITORING PATIENT RESPONSE

If the warts are not completely clear after six treatments or the patient has not improved significantly after three practitioner-administered treatments, the treatment plan should be changed. Evaluation of the risk–benefit ratio of treatment should occur throughout the course of therapy to avoid overtreatment. Women with genital warts should have cytologic screening for cervical cancer.

Once warts are eradicated, follow-up evaluations are not mandatory. Patients should monitor for recurrences, especially in the first 3 months. Patients who have concerns regarding recurrences can have a follow-up evaluation 3 months after treatment. Earlier follow-up visits may help to verify a wart-free state and monitor or treat complications and can be used for patient education and counseling.

PATIENT EDUCATION

Most sexually active men and women will get HPV at some point in their lives. This means that everyone is at risk for the potential outcomes of HPV and many may benefit from the prevention that the HPV vaccine provides. HPV vaccines are routinely recommended for 11- or 12-year-old boys and girls and protect against some of the most common types of HPV that can lead to disease and cancer, including most cervical cancers. The HPV vaccination should be recommended to anyone aged 9 to 26, regardless of gender. The HPV vaccination can be considered for adults 27 to 45 years of age who were not previously vaccinated, after a shared clinical decision between the patient and clinician. HPV vaccines are most effective if they are provided before an individual ever has sex.

The practitioner needs to provide precise instruction and guidance for applying topical antimitotic preparations, such as by showing how to apply podofilox solution with a cotton swab and the gel with a finger on visible warts. Patients should also be informed that HPV organisms persist despite resolution of lesions. Sex partners do not need to be examined because reinfection is most likely minimal and treatment to reduce transmission is not realistic in the absence of curative therapy. However, partners should be counseled about having a partner with genital warts and should be informed that the patient may remain infectious even when the warts are gone. The use of condoms may not eliminate the risk of transmission.

Patients should be warned that ablative therapies may cause scarring in the form of persistent hypopigmentation or hyperpigmentation. Depressed or hypertrophic scars rarely occur. Disabling chronic pain syndromes can also occur but are rare.

CASE STUDY 1

John is a 25-year-old male with no significant past medical history. He presents to an emergency care walk-in with complaints of several days of mild dysuria, genital itching, and penile discharge. John's physical exam is unremarkable; there is no rash or genital ulcers. John expresses concerns: "I may have got what my ex had." Upon further questioning, John tells you that his now ex-girlfriend was treated several weeks ago for an STI a few days after she had gone for her yearly gynecological exam (Learning Objectives 1–4).

1. What sexually transmitted infection (STI) does John appear to have?
2. If you have decided to test John for his current STI, what diagnostic test would you choose?
3. You decide to treat John empirically for both gonorrhea and chlamydia. What is the most appropriate antimicrobial regimen you would prescribe?
4. John asks you when he can have sexual intercourse again. What education would you provide to John?

Bibliography

Starred references are cited in the text.

*Barrow, R. Y., Ahmed, F., Bolan, G. A., et al. (2020). Recommendations for providing quality sexually transmitted diseases clinical services. *MMWR Recommendations and Reports, 68*(No. RR-5), 1–20. Retrieved from https://www.cdc.gov/mmwr/volumes/68/rr/rr6805a1.htm

*Centers for Disease Control and Prevention (CDC). (2015). Sexually transmitted treatment guidelines, 2015. *Morbidity and Mortality Weekly Report, 64*(RR3), 1–137.

*Centers for Disease Control and Prevention (CDC). (2019). Sexually transmitted disease surveillance, 2018. Atlanta, GA: Department of Health and Human Services. Retrieved from https://www.cdc.gov/std/stats18/default.htm

Gibson, E. J., Bell, D. L., & Powerful, S. A. (2014). Common sexually transmitted infections in adolescents. *Primary Care; Clinics in Office Practice, 41*(3), 631–650.

LeFevre, M. L. (2014). Behavioral counselling interventions to prevent sexually transmitted infection: U.S. Preventive Services Task Force recommendations. *Annals of Internal Medicine, 161*(12), 894–901.

Meites, E., Szilagyi, P. G., Chesson, H. W., et al. (2019). Human Papillomavirus Vaccination for adults: Updated recommendations of the advisory committee on immunization practices. *Morbidity and Mortality Weekly Report, 68*, 698–702.

O'Connor, E. A., Lin, J. S., Burda, B. U., et al. (2014). Behavioral sexual risk-reduction counseling in primary care to prevent sexually transmitted infections: A systematic review for the U.S. Preventive Services Task Force. *Annals of Internal Medicine, 161*(12), 874–883.

Rompalo, A. (2011). Preventing sexually transmitted infections: Back to basics. *Journal of Clinical Investigation, 121*(12), 4580–4583.

Pharmacology for Musculoskeletal Disorders

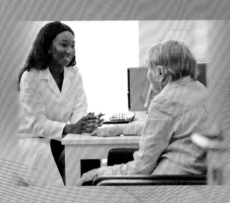

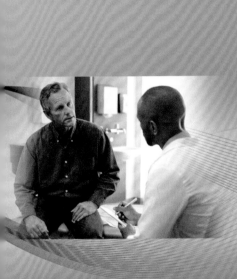

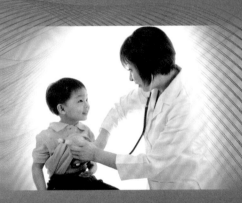

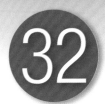

32 Osteoarthritis and Gout

Rachael DiMeo, Daniel Purzycki, and Sarah F. Uroza

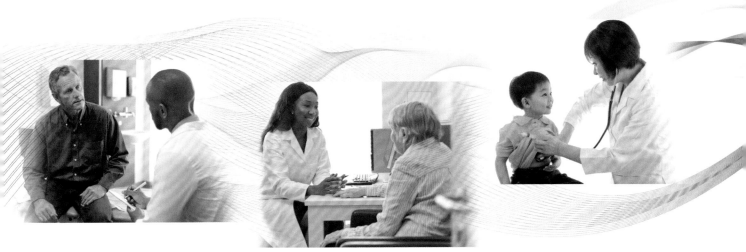

Learning Objectives

1. Describe the different pharmacologic options for the treatment of osteoarthritis.
2. Recommend appropriate therapy for osteoarthritis based on a patient's affected joint(s) and comorbidities.
3. Recommend initial treatment options for gout.
4. Educate patients on proper lifestyle modifications to reduce acute gout attacks.

OSTEOARTHRITIS

Introduction

Osteoarthritis (OA), formerly known as *degenerative joint disease*, is the most common joint problem in the United States. The Centers for Disease Control and Prevention estimates that 54.4 million U.S. adults suffer from arthritis, of which 27 million adults of age 25 years and older have clinical OA. Although prevalent, OA is often undiagnosed because clinical signs and symptoms are typically attributed to the normal aging process. In population-based studies in which asymptomatic patients were screened, the incidence of radiographic-defined OA was consistently higher than the incidence of symptomatic OA in the hands, knees, and hips.

OA is a progressive disease that can result in chronic pain, restricted range of motion, and muscle weakness, especially if a weight-bearing joint is affected. The joints commonly affected by OA include the knees, hips, cervical and lumbar spine, distal interphalangeal (DIP) joints, and the carpometacarpal joint at the base of the thumb.

Causes

There are two forms of OA. *Primary*, or idiopathic, OA arises from physiologic changes that occur with normal aging. *Secondary* OA usually results from traumatic injuries or inherited conditions and may present as hemochromatosis, chondrodystrophy, or inflammatory OA.

There are several modifiable and nonmodifiable risk factors that contribute to the development of OA. Of all the risk factors, obesity is the greatest in the development of OA of the knees and hips, especially in women. This is due to mechanical stress on weight-bearing joints. There may also be a metabolic effect of excess fat on articular cartilage that may account for some of the significance of obesity as a systemic risk factor. Other modifiable risk factors include prior joint injury and occupations that require excessive mechanical stress or heavy lifting. For patients with a past knee injury, the lifetime risk of knee OA is 57% compared to 45% in patients with no previous injury.

The nonmodifiable risk factors include gender, age, race, and genetics. Women have a higher overall risk for developing OA, but men tend to have disease onset at an earlier age. Increasing age is a risk factor until age 75, at which point the risk equilibrates. OA of the DIP and carpometacarpal joints is more common in white women; OA of the knees occurs more frequently in African American women. Genetics may determine approximately one fourth of knee OA cases and one half of hip and hand OA cases.

Pathophysiology

OA must be differentiated from other forms of arthritis because the physiologic changes specific to the condition dictate disease management. Although most forms of arthritis, including

641

OA, result in degeneration of articular cartilage, the subsequent formation of new bone is a change specific to OA.

The physiologic changes associated with OA begin with deterioration of the articular cartilage, which reduces joint friction during movement by diffusing mechanical stress to the underlying bone. Normal articular cartilage is smooth and is supported by subchondral bone. The subchondral bone serves as a flexible base to absorb mechanical force.

Articular cartilage consists of chondrocytes, connective tissue cells that are embedded in an extracellular matrix. The matrix is made up of collagen, water, and proteoglycans (macromolecules). The proteoglycans provide elasticity and flexibility to the matrix, which allows the articular cartilage to resist direct pressure. In OA, there is a reduction in proteoglycans in the extracellular matrix, leading to a decrease in resiliency to mechanical stress. In time, the articular cartilage becomes friable. The underlying subchondral bone responds to this change through a process termed *remodeling*. Remodeling involves the production of new bone that is thicker than the original bone. If remodeling occurs at the joint margins, an osteophyte (bone spur) may develop. The adjacent cortical bone becomes fortified with new bone, resulting in an irregular narrowing of the joint space. Sclerosing and cyst formation may ensue.

In addition to cartilaginous changes, concomitant changes in the synovial fluid must be considered. Synovial fluid, the main lubricant of joints, is produced and excreted from the cartilage. Destruction of the proteoglycans in OA renders the mechanism of synovial release ineffective, thereby further impairing the smooth mechanical operation of the joint. **Figure 32.1** demonstrates the mechanism of cartilage destruction.

Diagnostic Criteria

Joints commonly affected by OA include the hip, knee, hand, and cervical and lumbosacral spine. The American College of Rheumatology (ACR) published criteria for the diagnosis of OA of the knee (1986), hip (1991), and hand (1990) (**Box 32.1**). Often, a thorough history and physical examination provide enough data to diagnose OA. The most common symptom is joint pain; the patient in an early stage of OA usually describes the pain as insidious, intermittent, and mild. As the disease progresses, the patient may describe the pain as more constant and more disabling. Most patients report remittance of pain with rest and exacerbation of pain with joint movement.

BOX 32.1   Diagnostic Criteria for Osteoarthritis

- Hand: Pain, aching, or stiffness and three of the following:
  Hard tissue enlargement of more than two joints
  Hard tissue enlargement of more than two DIP joints
  Less than three swollen metacarpophalangeal joints
  Deformity of more than one selected joint
- Hip: Pain and two of the following
  Erythrocyte sedimentation rate (ESR) less than 20 mm/h
  Radiographic femoral or acetabular osteophytes
  Radiographic joint space narrowing
- Knee
  Clinical diagnosis: Knee pain and three of the following
      More than 50 years old
      Stiffness less than 30 minutes
      Crepitus
      Bony tenderness
      Bony enlargement
      No palpable warmth
  Clinical and radiographic diagnosis: Knee pain + osteophytes and one of the following:
      More than 50 years old
      Stiffness less than 30 minutes
      Crepitus
  Clinical and laboratory diagnosis: Knee pain and five of the following:
      Age more than 50 years old
      Stiffness less than 30 minutes
      Crepitus
      Bony tenderness
      Bony enlargement
      No palpable warmth
      ESR less than 40 mm/h
      RF less than 1:40
      Synovial fluid signs of OA (clear, viscous, or WBC count <2,000/mm^3)

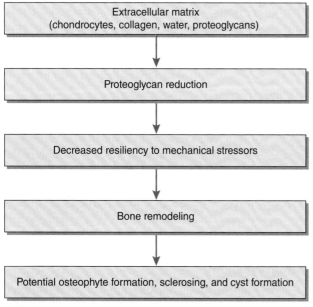

FIGURE 32–1   Destruction of cartilage in osteoarthritis.

Although the symptoms of OA are localized, associated pain may be referred. For example, it is common for OA of the hip to be referred to the medial knee. Another symptom associated with OA is crepitus, a painless "crackling" in the joint. Crepitus most commonly affects the knee, but it may be heard in other joints affected by OA as well. As OA progresses to later stages of articular damage, deformity of the joint may be observed. The deformity usually appears as an enlargement of the joint, which may result from either increased bone production or synovitis. Other deformities resulting from OA of the knee include varus (bow-legged knees) and valgus (knock-kneed legs).

OA of the cervical spine may present with pain that radiates to the supraclavicular or upper trapezius areas. Depending on the level of nerve involvement, symptoms may progress to include pain in the distal upper extremities. OA of the lumbar spine may produce symptoms of neurogenic claudication.

On physical examination, decreased range of motion is the most common finding. This finding may be absent in the early stages of the disease but gradually progresses as the condition worsens. In later stages of the disease, joint contractures may occur, resulting in varus and valgus deformities. Patients with severe OA of the hip may present with gait disturbances.

Because OA is a progressive disease, complications such as joint effusion and enlargement may occur. Occasionally, radicular problems may occur secondary to changes in the cervical vertebrae.

Joint enlargement due to the formation of osteophytes may be observed. Osteophyte formation in the DIP joint is called *Heberden nodes*; in the proximal interphalangeal joint, it is referred to as *Bouchard nodes*.

Radiologic findings in OA may be used to confirm the suspected diagnosis. Narrow joint spaces with osteophyte formation are common findings.

Initiating Drug Therapy

Before initiating drug therapy, the practitioner should recommend appropriate physical activity or physical therapy. The goals in managing OA are to reduce pain, improve motion, and maintain functional ability. The 2019 ACR/Arthritis Foundation guidelines for the management of OA of the hand, hip, and knee recommend a multimodal approach including behavioral, physical, pharmacotherapy, and lifestyle interventions including weight loss (**Box 32.2**) (Kolasinski et al., 2020).

The goals of pharmacotherapy for OA are to maintain function, prevent further joint damage, and diminish associated pain. The degree of joint involvement and the severity of the symptoms and concomitant comorbidities usually dictate proper interventions for individual patients.

Topical Agents
Topical Nonsteroidal Antiinflammatory Drugs
Topical therapy is preferred to systemic therapy by the European League Against Rheumatism (EULAR) and the Osteoarthritis Research Society International (OARSI; Fernandes et al., 2013).

BOX 32.2 Recommended Nonpharmacologic Therapies for Osteoarthritis

- Strongly recommended by the ACR for hand, knee, and hip OA
  - Exercise (more effective when supervised)
  - Self-efficacy and self-management programs
- Strongly recommended for knee and hip
  - Weight loss
  - Tai Chi
  - Cane
- Certain orthotic devices are strongly recommended for both hand and knee
- Conditionally recommended for hand, knee, and hip
  - Heat/cooling
  - Cognitive behavioral therapy
  - Acupuncture
  - Kinesiotaping (hand and knee)
  - Balance training (knee and hip)

Topical nonsteroidal antiinflammatory drugs (NSAIDs) are strongly recommended by the ACR for knee OA and conditionally for hand OA. Due to concerns with absorption in hip OA, topical therapy is typically not recommended. Systemic therapy may be more effective depending on the number and location of joints affected. Topical therapy is an attractive option due to the relatively benign side effect profiles.

Diclofenac is currently the only commercially available topical NSAID. It is available as a 1.5% solution (Klofensaid II) and as a 2% solution (Pennsaid) for the relief of OA pain of the knee and as a 1% topical gel (Voltaren) for the relief of OA pain in joints amenable to topical therapy.

Mechanism of Action. The mechanism of action for topical diclofenac is the same as for oral NSAIDs. The benefit is that minimal diclofenac is absorbed when applied topically, which then decreases the risk of adverse events. Data have shown that only 6% to 10% of the topical gel and 2% to 3% of the solution is absorbed.

Dosage. The dosage of topical diclofenac is dependent on the formulation and location. For the gel, if used on the lower extremities, 4 g should be applied four times a day; if used on the upper extremities, 2 g should be applied four times a day. The entire total daily dose should not exceed 32 g/d. For the 1% topical solution, 40 drops should be applied to the affected knee(s) four times a day. The solution should be applied in 10-drop increments to limit spillage. It can be first applied to the hand and then rubbed on the knee. The 2% solution should be applied as two pump actuations to the affected knee twice daily. Regardless of formulation, it is imperative that the entire affected area be covered to achieve maximal effect.

Contraindications. Topical diclofenac carries the same warnings and contraindications as oral NSAIDs, although the risk is less. Also, topical diclofenac is contraindicated on non-intact or damaged skin.

Adverse Events. The most common adverse events are application site reactions and include pruritus, rash, dry skin, pain, and exfoliation.

Interactions. Topical diclofenac should be used cautiously with medications that interact with oral NSAIDs since some of the topical medication is absorbed.

Capsaicin

Mechanism of Action. For the relief of arthritic pain, capsaicin exerts its effect through the depletion of substance P. Initially, capsaicin releases substance P from the peripheral sensory neurons. However, with repeated use, substance P becomes depleted, and capsaicin prevents reaccumulation of substance P. Substance P is a chemomediator responsible for pain transmission from the periphery to the central nervous system (CNS). Therefore, by depleting peripheral neurons of substance P, the pain impulse will not be transmitted centrally.

Dosage. Capsaicin is available as an over-the-counter (OTC) product in a patch, cream, gel, liquid, or lotion. The directions for the patch are to apply it to the affected area three to four times a day for 7 days. The patch can remain on the area for up to 8 hours. The cream, gel, liquid, and lotion forms should be applied at least thrice daily for maximal efficacy.

Time Frame for Response. The maximal effect is seen after 2 to 4 weeks of continual use.

Contraindications. There are no absolute contraindications for topical capsaicin. Patients should be advised to not apply capsaicin to broken or irritated skin. Use for hand OA is not recommended due to the risk of eye contamination.

Adverse Events. The most common adverse event is burning and irritation at the application site. The burning typically subsides within days of continual use. Due to the initial release of substance P, patients may experience some pain with initial use and should be advised to expect this.

Nonsteroidal Antiinflammatory Drugs

Second-line therapy for OA includes oral NSAIDs. NSAIDs are further classified according to their chemical structure (**Table 32.1**). Although these classes have subtle differences, they all exhibit cyclooxygenase (COX) inhibition.

Mechanism of Action

There are two mechanisms by which NSAIDs exert their antiinflammatory action. One is by inhibiting the conversion of arachidonic acid to prostaglandin, prostacyclin, and thromboxanes—all of which are mediators of pain and inflammation.

The other is by interfering with protein kinase activation (especially when taken at higher doses).

COX is the enzyme that converts arachidonic acid to prostaglandin G_2. The COX enzyme is present in two forms: COX-1 and COX-2. Most NSAIDs nonselectively inhibit both COX-1 and COX-2, except for celecoxib, which is more selective for COX-2. COX-1 enzymes are found in the gastrointestinal (GI) tract and kidney and produce protective prostaglandins, which is why most research focuses on preserving the activity of COX-1. COX-2 is produced at nonspecific sites of inflammation as well as in the kidneys. Inhibition of COX-2 produces antiinflammatory and analgesic effects without affecting the GI tract. COX-2 produces protective prostaglandins in the kidney that are responsible for maintaining adequate blood perfusion via vasodilation of the afferent arteriole. Therefore, inhibition of either COX-1 or COX-2 can result in decreased renal perfusion and impaired kidney function.

Dosage

Dosing of NSAIDs is variable. The drugs are classified into short-, intermediate-, and long-acting categories. NSAIDs require five half-lives to reach peak therapeutic levels and five half-lives to be fully excreted. Categories with a longer half-life require longer periods to reach therapeutic levels.

Some common agents used to treat OA are diclofenac, ibuprofen, and the COX-2 inhibitor celecoxib. Due to concerns for adverse reactions, NSAIDs should be used at the lowest effective dose for the shortest duration of time. **Table 32.1** gives information about other agents and dosing considerations.

Time Frame for Response

Patients' responses to NSAIDs are quite variable. Patients who do not respond to one NSAID may respond to another, even one in the same class. This response variability is also seen in the side effect profile of NSAIDs. The practitioner should be familiar with several of the NSAIDs from each class and should try to individualize therapy based on symptom management and side effects.

Contraindications

NSAIDs are contraindicated in patients allergic to aspirin, in patients with alcohol dependence, or in pregnant patients. Furthermore, since celecoxib contains a sulfa moiety, it is contraindicated in patients with a sulfa allergy. Caution should be used when prescribing NSAIDs to patients with renal or hepatic impairment or older patients. Due to the increase in cardiovascular adverse events, all NSAIDs carry a black box warning emphasizing that they are contraindicated for perioperative pain treatment in patients undergoing coronary artery bypass graft surgery and should be avoided in patients with cardiovascular disease or risk factors.

Adverse Events

NSAIDs have gained a reputation as innocuous agents because of their OTC availability and widespread use. However,

TABLE 32.1

Overview of Selected Nonsteroidal Antiinflammatory Agents Used to Treat Osteoarthritis and Rheumatoid Arthritis

Generic (Trade) Name	Dosage	Contraindications	Special Considerations	Short, Intermediate, or Long Acting
Acetic Acid NSAIDs				
Etodolac (Lodine)	IR: 400–500 mg PO BID, 300 mg PO BID–TID ER: 400–1,000 mg/d PO	Pregnancy and lactation; use cautiously with allergies, renal, hepatic, CV, and GI conditions.		Intermediate
Indomethacin (Indocin)	IR: 50–200 mg/d PO in 2–3 divided doses Maximum daily dose 200 mg/d Rectal: 25 mg PR: 2–3 times/d ER: 75 mg PO 1–2/d maximum dose 150 mg/d	Same as etodolac, and also GI bleeding with history of proctitis or rectal bleeding	Decreased diuretic effect with loop diuretics; potential decreased antihypertensive effect with beta blockers; increased CNS adverse effects due to lipophilicity	Short
Nabumetone (Relafen)	Initial dose 1,000 mg PO daily may increase to 2,000 mg/d in 1–2 divided doses. Dose >2,000 mg not studied	Pregnancy and lactation; use cautiously with allergies, hepatic, CV, and GI conditions; significant renal impairment		Long
Sulindac (Clinoril)	150 mg PO BID. Maximum dose 400 mg/d	Pregnancy and lactation; use cautiously in patients with asthma, chronic urticaria, CV dysfunction, hypertension, GI bleeding, peptic ulcer, impaired hepatic or renal function	May take with meals if GI upset occurs.	Intermediate
Tolmetin (Tolectin)	Initial 400 mg PO TID Adjust dose per patient response after 1–2 weeks Maintenance dose 600–1,800 mg/d in 3 divided doses Maximum dose 1,800 mg/d	Pregnancy, lactation; use cautiously with allergies, renal, hepatic, CV, and GI conditions.	May affect results (false positive) of proteinuria tests using acid precipitation tests; patient should have ophthalmic examination periodically during long-term therapy.	Intermediate
Enolic Acid NSAIDs				
Piroxicam (Feldene)	10–20 mg PO once daily	Pregnancy and lactation; use cautiously with allergies, renal, hepatic, CV, and GI conditions	Because therapeutic response progresses over several weeks, evaluate response after 2 wk. NSAID with the longest half-life	Long
Fenamic Acid NSAID				
Meclofenamate (Meclomen)*	200–400 mg/d PO in 3–4 divided doses Maximum dose 400 mg/d Maximum clinical benefit may not be seen for 2–3 wk	Same as piroxicam and in patients undergoing CABG surgery	Patients should have ophthalmic examination periodically during long-term therapy.	Short
Phenylacetic Acid NSAIDs				
Diclofenac sodium (Voltaren)	IR: 50 mg PO BID–TID DR: 50 mg PO BID–TID or 75 mg BID ER: 100 mg PO once daily	Significant renal impairment, pregnancy, lactation; use cautiously with impaired hearing; allergies; hepatic, CV, and GI conditions	NSAID with the shortest half-life Maximum recommended dose due to risk for vascular events is 100 mg/d	Short
Diclofenac potassium (Cataflam)				

(Continued)

TABLE 32.1 Overview of Selected Nonsteroidal Antiinflammatory Agents Used to Treat Osteoarthritis and Rheumatoid Arthritis (Continued)

Generic (Trade) Name	Dosage	Contraindications	Special Considerations	Short, Intermediate, or Long Acting
Propionic Acid NSAIDs				
Fenoprofen (Nalfon/Fenortho)	400–600 mg PO TID–QID. Adjust dose based on patient response. Maximum dose 3,200 mg/d	Same as diclofenac	Patients should have ophthalmic examination periodically during long-term therapy.	Short
Ibuprofen (Motrin/Advil)	400–800 mg PO TID–QID Maximum 3,200 mg daily	Same as diclofenac	Therapeutic response may occur over several weeks.	Short
Naproxen (Naprosyn)	IR: 500–1,500 mg/d PO in 2 divided doses ER: 750–1,000 mg PO daily May increase to 1,500 mg/d for a limited course (<6 months).	Same as diclofenac	May take with meals if GI upset occurs.	Intermediate
Salicylic Acid NSAIDs				
Diflunisal (Dolobid)	500–1,500 mg/d PO in 2 divided doses Maximum 1,500 mg/d	Pregnancy and lactation; use cautiously with allergies, renal, hepatic, CV, and GI conditions		Intermediate
Aspirin (Bayer, others)	Arthritis associated w/ rheumatic disease: IR: 4–8 g/d PO in 4–5 divided doses. Continue up to 8 wk. Analgesic: IR: 325–1,000 mg/d q4–6h as needed Maximum dose 4 g/d	Allergy to salicylates, other NSAIDs, tartrazine, hemophilia, and other bleeding disorders, pregnancy (possibly teratogenic), and more; do not use in children after illness because of association with Reye syndrome. High doses (4–8 g/d) may be limited by adverse effects	Increased risk of bleeding when taken concomitantly with anticoagulants and other NSAIDs Consult package insert for extensive list of interacting drugs and effects.	Short
COX-2 Selective NSAIDs				
Celecoxib (Celebrex)	200 mg PO once daily or 100 mg BID	Allergy to the drug or to sulfonamides, NSAIDs, or aspirin; significant renal impairment; pregnancy, lactation	Elimination of the drug occurs primarily through hepatic metabolism; therefore, patients with symptoms suggesting liver dysfunction should be carefully monitored. Consider dose reduction of 50% in CYP2C9 poor metabolizers.	Intermediate

*Brand name only available in Canada.

CABG, coronary artery bypass graft; CNS, central nervous system; CV, cardiovascular; GI, gastrointestinal; NSAIDs, nonsteroidal antiinflammatory drugs.

NSAIDs are associated with risk, and patient education should include potential adverse events.

Visual changes, weight gain, headache, dizziness, nervousness, photosensitivity, weakness, tinnitus, easy bruising or bleeding, and fluid retention are adverse events that have been associated with use of NSAIDs. Cautious use and frequent monitoring, particularly of older patients, are important for safe NSAID use. The most common adverse events of NSAIDs occur in the GI and renal systems.

Adverse GI events range from minor GI irritation to ulcers, GI bleeding, perforation, and gastric outlet obstruction. NSAIDs carry a black box warning of increased risk of serious GI adverse events including bleeding, ulceration, and perforation of the stomach or intestines. Concomitant use of misoprostol (Cytotec) has been shown to decrease the incidence of ulcer disease and GI complications. Misoprostol, a prostaglandin analog, is given at 100 to 200 mcg orally four times daily. Its use should be limited to patients at high risk for GI complications (age > 65, comorbid medical conditions, history of peptic ulcer disease or upper GI bleeding, oral glucocorticosteroids, or anticoagulants).

Studies of the treatment of GI effects as a result of NSAIDs have compared the efficacy of proton pump inhibitors and histamine-2 (H_2) receptor antagonists. Yeomans et al. (1998) determined that omeprazole (Prilosec), a proton pump inhibitor, healed existing ulcers and prevented further ulcer development more effectively than did ranitidine (Zantac), an H_2 receptor antagonist. Similarly, Hawkey et al. (1998) found omeprazole and misoprostol equally successful at treating ulcers and other GI symptoms associated with NSAID use. However, omeprazole was better tolerated and was associated with an improved relapse rate. Some studies suggest that alterations in intestinal microbiota may be related to NSAID-induced enteropathy. Long-term use of acid suppression may exacerbate NSAID-induced small bowel injury. Long-term use of both NSAIDs and acid suppressive therapy should be evaluated based on the risks and benefits to the patient.

Another option for patients experiencing GI adverse events with nonselective NSAIDs is celecoxib. In a study conducted by Chan et al. (2010), patients randomized to celecoxib had a lower incidence of upper or lower GI events compared with patients treated with diclofenac plus omeprazole. Celecoxib is also preferred to nonselective NSAIDs in patients with GI comorbidities such as a history of gastric ulcer disease.

Patients with renal disease, congestive heart failure (CHF), cirrhosis, and volume depletion may experience renal aberrations, particularly related to renal blood flow. These adverse events underscore the need for frequent monitoring of patients on long-term NSAID therapy.

All NSAIDs carry a black box warning regarding an increase in serious cardiovascular thrombotic events, including myocardial infarction and stroke. This increased risk led to the market removal of two COX-2 selective agents, rofecoxib and valdecoxib. In multiple analyses, naproxen appears to have little to no increased cardiovascular risk, whereas diclofenac consistently demonstrates an increased risk.

Interactions

NSAIDs have the potential to increase bleeding, so they need to be used cautiously with anticoagulants. Also, due to the risk of hypertension (HTN), NSAIDs may counteract the effect of antihypertensives. If possible, patients with HTN should not be on NSAIDs. The combination of NSAIDs and angiotensin-converting enzyme (ACE) inhibitors or angiotensin receptor blockers may result in decreased renal function and should be avoided. For patients who take aspirin daily, ibuprofen must be taken 30 minutes to 2 hours after or 8 hours before the aspirin in order for the aspirin to be cardioprotective. If taken concurrently with lithium, NSAIDs may increase the drug concentrations of lithium, and caution is advised.

Nonacetylated Salicylates

Nonacetylated salicylates (**Box 32.3**) are especially beneficial in patients who are sensitive to the GI irritation caused by long-term aspirin use. Diflunisal (Dolobid), the most commonly used nonacetylated salicylate, is an effective COX-1 inhibitor with antiinflammatory and analgesic properties, but its antipyretic activities are weak. In terms of symptom relief, the nonacetylated salicylates are probably as effective as aspirin in treating inflammatory disorders.

Acetaminophen

Acetaminophen (Tylenol) is conditionally recommended by the 2019 ACR guidelines and considered an option by the EULAR recommendations due to its possible efficacy and relatively safe side effect profile and affordability. Acetaminophen is not recommended in the 2019 OARSI guidelines due to questionable efficacy and risk for hepatotoxicity (Bannuru et al., 2019). It is however an option in patients with limited pharmacologic options due to intolerance or contraindications to the use of NSAIDs. Acetaminophen is best used for short-term infrequent use.

Mechanism of Action

Acetaminophen exerts its action within the CNS. It is thought to inhibit central COX, which results in decreased prostaglandin synthesis. Through this prostaglandin inhibition, acetaminophen exerts analgesic and antipyretic effects but does not have antiinflammatory effects.

BOX 32.3 Nonacetylated Salicylates

- Diflunisal
- Sodium salicylate
- Choline salicylate
- Magnesium salicylate
- Choline magnesium trisalicylate
- Salsalate

Dosage

The recommended dose is 325 to 650 mg orally every 4 to 6 hours or 1,000 mg every 6 to 8 hours around the clock. The recommended dose of up to 4 g/d is safe for patients with normal liver function. Higher doses have been associated with hepatotoxicity. Patients with a history of liver disease or who are chronic alcohol drinkers should not take more than 1,800 to 2,000 mg/d. All patients should be counseled regarding the need to avoid other products that contain acetaminophen.

Time Frame for Response

If taken as scheduled, patients can experience pain relief within 1 week of initiation.

Contraindications

The only absolute contraindication to acetaminophen use is hypersensitivity to acetaminophen. Acetaminophen should be used cautiously in patients with hepatic disease or who drink more than three alcoholic drinks daily and in patients taking other products containing acetaminophen.

Adverse Events

Acetaminophen is typically well tolerated with the most common adverse events being dizziness and rash. For patients who take more than the recommended daily dose, acetaminophen can induce hepatic failure as a result of the accumulation of a hepatotoxic metabolite. Also, patients need to be educated about the risk of accidental overdose with combination products that also contain acetaminophen. Renal toxicity has also been observed with chronic overdosages.

Interactions

With chronic doses of greater than 1.3 g daily, acetaminophen can increase the international normalized ratio (INR) of a patient on warfarin. If a patient is on chronic acetaminophen and warfarin, the INR should be monitored more frequently upon initiation and discontinuation of acetaminophen. The risk of hepatotoxicity with acetaminophen may also increase with concomitant use of isoniazid.

Analgesics

When the pain associated with OA progresses and is no longer responsive to acetaminophen or NSAIDs, analgesics are an option. Analgesics can also be used in patients who cannot tolerate acetaminophen or NSAIDs or in whom they are contraindicated. Analgesics only decrease pain and have no effect on inflammation. These drugs should be prescribed in the lowest effective dose for a limited time because of potential dependence and withdrawal symptoms. Opioids are strongly not recommended by the OARSI due to the risk of chemical dependency.

Tramadol

Mechanism of Action. Tramadol exerts multiple effects to induce pain relief. It is a mu-opioid receptor agonist similar to other opioids such as morphine. By binding to the mu-opioid receptor, ascending pain pathways are inhibited, resulting in decreased pain sensation. In addition, tramadol also inhibits the reuptake of serotonin and norepinephrine. These neurotransmitters are also involved in the ascending pain pathway.

Dosage. Tramadol is available as an immediate-release tablet (Ultram), extended-release tablet (Ultram ER), and in combination with acetaminophen (Ultracet). For the immediate-release tablet, patients can take 25 to 100 mg every 4 to 6 hours as needed for pain with a maximum daily dose of 400 mg. For patients taking the extended-release tablet, the starting dose is 100 mg daily with an increase by 100 mg increments every 5 days to the maximum of 300 mg/d. All forms of tramadol need to be dose-adjusted for renal and hepatic dysfunction.

Time Frame for Response. Patients may feel a decrease in pain as soon as 1 hour after taking an immediate-release tramadol dose with a maximum effect at 2 hours. The extended-release tablet takes about 12 hours for the maximum effect to be seen.

Contraindications. Patients with an opioid dependency should not take tramadol since it has opioid effects. Also, patients with acute intoxication with alcohol, hypnotics, central-acting analgesics, opioids, or psychotropic drugs should not be given tramadol. Tramadol has the ability to lower the seizure threshold. Therefore, tramadol should not be used in patients with a history of seizures and needs to be used cautiously with other medications that may lower the seizure threshold. Tramadol, like all opioids, carries several black box warnings including life-threatening respiratory depression; risk for concomitant CNS depression; and risk for addiction, abuse, and misuse.

Adverse Events. Unlike NSAIDs, tramadol does not produce serious GI adverse events nor does it aggravate existing HTN, CHF, or renal disease. The most common side effects of tramadol include nausea, dizziness, drowsiness, and sweating. Due to the opioid receptor agonism, tramadol has the potential to exert similar adverse events as other opioids, such as constipation, dependency, euphoria, and respiratory depression.

Interactions. Tramadol is metabolized by CYP2D6, and any medication that inhibits or induces this enzyme will interact with tramadol. Also, because it inhibits serotonin reuptake, tramadol has the potential to induce serotonin syndrome when used in combination with other serotonergic agents, such as selective serotonin reuptake inhibitors, tricyclic antidepressants, monoamine oxidase inhibitors, or linezolid.

Duloxetine

Mechanism of Action. Duloxetine is a serotonin and norepinephrine reuptake inhibitor. By enhancing serotonin and norepinephrine, duloxetine works in the CNS to reduce pain transmission. Duloxetine is a relatively balanced serotonin and norepinephrine reuptake inhibitor.

Dosage. The dosing approved by the Food and Drug Administration (FDA) for chronic musculoskeletal pain is 30 mg orally daily for 7 days and then increased to 60 mg orally daily, which is the listed maximum dose for this indication. However, the trials that resulted in duloxetine's approval for this indication increased the dose to 120 mg orally daily in patients not having an adequate response to the 60-mg dose.

Time Frame for Response. The benefit of duloxetine was seen as early as 4 weeks in the clinical trials. Time points sooner than this were not assessed, so it is not known if its effect starts sooner.

Contraindications. Due to the risk for serotonin syndrome, duloxetine should not be started while a patient is on a monoamine oxidase inhibitor (MAOI) or within 14 days of stopping an MAOI. Also, starting duloxetine while a patient is receiving linezolid and intravenous methylene blue may increase the risk of serotonin syndrome and is contraindicated.

Adverse Effects. Some of the precautions and warnings associated with duloxetine risk include hepatotoxicity, orthostatic hypotension, serotonin syndrome, abnormal bleeding, and activation of mania. These are considered the rarest but have serious adverse effects. More common adverse effects seen in the clinical trials include nausea, constipation, somnolence, and hyperhidrosis. Duloxetine carries a black box warning with all antidepressants for increased risk of suicidal thinking and behavior in children, adolescents, and young adults with major depressive disorder.

Interactions. Duloxetine is metabolized through CYP1A2 and CYP2D6; therefore, medications that inhibit these enzymes may cause increased duloxetine concentrations. Due to the serotonergic effects of duloxetine, there is a risk for serotonin syndrome if other serotonergic agents are used concomitantly. Heavy alcohol use should be discouraged due to an increased risk of hepatotoxicity.

Intra-Articular Therapy

If symptoms of OA are restricted to one or two joints that have not responded to first- or second-line treatment, intra-articular corticosteroids may be helpful. Aseptic technique and a local anesthetic are required. The dose of drug injected depends on the size of the joint. It is imperative to use careful technique that avoids the surrounding soft tissues to avoid tissue atrophy. Patients may develop localized pain as an adverse effect that may be treated with an NSAID or another appropriate analgesic. Intra-articular injection of corticosteroids usually produces symptom relief within a few days, and the relief may last a few weeks to several months.

Recent data have suggested specific formulations of corticosteroids, or certain frequencies of corticosteroid administration may lead to cartilage loss. The data provided by the 2019 ACR guideline available at the time of publication were insufficient to recommend long-acting formulations over short-acting formulations. Intra-articular corticosteroids are more commonly recommended for knee OA especially in patients with GI or cardiovascular comorbidities who may have contraindications to systemic therapy.

The 2019 ACR guideline generally recommends against the use of intra-articular hyaluronic acid largely due to limited evidence of benefit and the potential for harm. However, hyaluronic acid may be considered in patients who do not find satisfactory relief or after alternatives have been exhausted.

Selecting the Most Appropriate Agent

In selecting therapies for OA, the prescriber should consider patient variables such as age, childbearing status, progression of arthritis, and underlying illnesses. The most recent guidelines suggest a multimodal patient-centered approach is needed including both pharmacologic and nonpharmacologic therapies.

Table 32.2 compares pharmacotherapy recommendations from several prominent guidelines-producing bodies including the ACR, EULAR, and OARSI. The ACR released the 2019 guidelines for the management of OA of the hand, hip, and knee. The EULAR published a 2018 update on the management of hand OA and a 2013 guideline for the nonpharmacologic management of knee and hip OA, while the OARSI published guidelines on the nonsurgical management of knee, hip, and polyarticular OA in 2019.

Nonpharmacologic therapies are often recommended over pharmacologic ones due to lower risk of side effects. The type and level of evidence of these nonpharmacologic therapies vary but include, as some examples, weight loss, cognitive behavioral therapy with exercise, aquatic exercise, tai chi, acupuncture, balance training, and various orthotic devices.

If pharmacologic therapy is appropriate, topical treatments are generally considered first line for hand and knee OA. For all forms of OA, oral NSAIDs are preferred to opioids and acetaminophen due to better proven efficacy and more favorable side effect profile. The choice of NSAID and the addition of an acid-suppressive therapy should be based on a patient's history and comorbid illnesses. COX-2 selective agents may be preferred in patients with GI comorbidities.

First-Line Therapy

Historically, acetaminophen was considered first line; however, there is conflicting data regarding the analgesic effect of acetaminophen compared to NSAIDs for OA pain. Many trials indicate that NSAIDs are superior, especially in patients with more severe disease. The EULAR continues to recommend acetaminophen as first-line therapy for hip and knee OA (last updated in 2005 and 2003 respectively). Due to questionable efficacy and risk for hepatotoxicity, more recent guidelines recommend topical therapies as first line, followed by oral NSAIDs as first or second line depending on the affected joint.

Second-Line Therapy

Oral nonselective NSAIDs are generally considered second line after topical therapy depending on the patient's comorbidities.

TABLE 32.2

Pharmacotherapy Guideline Recommendations for the Treatment of Osteoarthritis*

	ACR: 2019 Guidelines	EULAR	OARSI: 2019 Guidelines
Hand	**Strongly recommended** Oral NSAIDs **Conditionally recommended** Topical NSAIDs IACS Acetaminophen Tramadol Duloxetine Chondroitin	**2018 guideline update** **Initial treatment options:** Topical NSAIDs Topical capsaicin Oral NSAIDs **Additional recommendations** Chondroitin sulfate IACS (interphalangeal joints only)	
Hip	**Strongly recommended** Oral NSAIDs IACS (with imaging guidance) **Conditionally recommended** Acetaminophen Tramadol Duloxetine	**1st line:** APAP **2nd line:** NSAIDs ± astroprotection **3rd line:** opioid APAP IA steroids for flares unresponsive to analgesia and NSAIDs	**Without comorbidities** **Strong recommendations** Nonselective NSAIDS Conditional recommendations Nonselective NSAIDS + PPI COX-2 inhibitors **With comorbidities** **Strong recommendations** COX-2 inhibitors (for GI comorbidities) Conditional recommendations Nonselective NSAID + PPI
Knee	**Strongly recommended** Oral NSAIDs Topical NSAIDs IACS **Conditionally recommended** Acetaminophen Tramadol Duloxetine Topical capsaicin	**1st line:** APAP, topical NSAIDs, capsaicin **2nd line:** NSAIDs gastroprotection **3rd line:** opioid APAP IA steroids for flares with effusions	**Without comorbidities** **Strong recommendations** Topical NSAIDs **Conditional recommendations** Nonselective NSAIDS PPI COX-2 inhibitors IACS **Low consensus** IAHA **With comorbidities** **Strong recommendations** Topical NSAIDs **Conditional recommendations** COX-2 inhibitors (GI comorbidities) IACS/IAHA (GI, CV comorbidities or frailty) Widespread pain/depression Conditional recommendations Nonselective NSAIDS PPI COX-2 inhibitors **Low consensus recommendation** Duloxetine IACS/IAHA Topical NSAIDs

*All guidelines recommend exercise-based programs as well as weight management.

ACR, American College of Rheumatology; APAP, acetaminophen; COX, cyclooxygenase; CV, cardiovascular; EULAR, European League Against Rheumatism; GI, gastrointestinal; IA, intra-articular; IACS, intra-articular corticosteroid; IAHA, intra-articular hyaluronic acid; NSAIDs, nonsteroidal antiinflammatory drugs; OARSI, Osteoarthritis Research Society International; PPI, proton pump inhibitor.

For patients without risk factors for GI disturbance, ibuprofen or a similar nonselective NSAID should be considered for second-line therapy as monotherapy. Since there is no evidence that one NSAID is more effective than another, the choice of the specific NSAID should be based on the cost and convenience of therapy. For patients at increased risk for GI disorders, such as peptic ulcer disease, a COX-2 inhibitor may be a better second-line choice. Alternatively, the use of a nonselective NSAID coupled with a proton pump inhibitor may be sufficient to provide analgesia along with gastric protection.

Third-Line Therapy

Third-line therapies vary by affected joint but include acetaminophen, intra-articular corticosteroids, duloxetine, chondroitin, tramadol, and perhaps intra-articular hyaluronic acid. In general, opioid analgesics are not recommended due to the risk of dependence and abuse.

Special Populations

Geriatric

For older patients, topical therapies are preferred when appropriate. Additionally, the practitioner may prescribe an NSAID with a shorter half-life in a smaller dosage than for a younger adult. Patients over age 65 should be considered at risk for GI hemorrhage and treated with either a COX-2 inhibitor or a combination of a nonselective NSAID and a gastric protective agent, such as misoprostol or a proton pump inhibitor.

Women

Many of the NSAIDs are pregnancy category C agents during the first 30 weeks of gestation. After gestational week 30, most NSAIDs are categorized as class D agents, indicating that there is evidence of harm to the fetus and should only be used in life-threatening illnesses.

Monitoring Patient Response

In addition to routine questions about the efficacy of the drug (e.g., pain relief), baseline and ongoing monitoring for specific drug therapy should be done. If a patient is taking acetaminophen, baseline liver function tests should be checked and monitored periodically. Monitoring for NSAID therapy includes a complete blood count, urinalysis, and serum creatinine. These studies should be repeated at 1 to 3 months and then every 3 to 6 months thereafter for the duration of therapy. In patients at risk for GI hemorrhage, the clinician should consider evaluating the patient for stool occult blood, anemia, and other signs of bleeding.

Patient Education

Drug Information

For patients taking acetaminophen, patients need to be cognizant of other products that may contain acetaminophen and ensure they are not exceeding the daily limit. Additionally, for patients taking scheduled acetaminophen, alcohol intake should be minimized or avoided.

Patients taking NSAIDs need to be aware of their potentially harsh effects on the GI system, ranging from mild GI discomfort to gastric bleeding. The practitioner may emphasize strategies for dealing with some of these adverse events, including taking NSAIDs with food or milk or at meals. Patients should be reminded that NSAIDs are recommended to be used at the lowest effective dose for the shortest amount of time.

Patients receiving a corticosteroid injection for joint pain need to be informed that a single joint should not be injected more frequently than every 6 months. Patients should be cautioned to limit the activity of the injected joint for several days after the injection. Otherwise, the reduced pain perception of the joint may allow the patient to cause further joint damage, enhancing the progression of OA.

Patient-Oriented Information Sources

The National Institute of Arthritis and Musculoskeletal and Skin Diseases is a government-sponsored group that provides information on OA and its treatment (http://www.niams.nih.gov/hi/topics/arthritis/oahandout.htm). This information is also available in Spanish. The Arthritis Foundation (http://www.arthritis.org/about-arthritis/types/osteoarthritis/) provides information on the web and in print.

Nutrition/Lifestyle Changes

The practitioner should provide the patient with information about the continued use of physical therapy, exercise, and weight loss. All of the guidelines stress the importance of nonpharmacologic recommendations in the treatment of OA (**Figure 32.2**).

Complementary and Alternative Medications

Glucosamine, a form of an amino acid, is a naturally occurring substance in the body. It is believed to be involved in the development and repair of cartilage. Exogenous replacement of this substance is thought to help build on existing cartilage. Evidence-based reviews of this agent suggest that moderate improvements in pain relief and function can be achieved

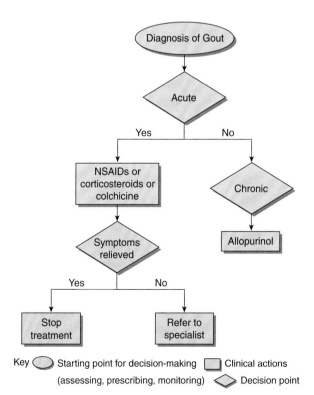

FIGURE 32–2   Treatment algorithm for osteoarthritis.

NSAIDs, nonsteroidal antiinflammatory drugs.

when administered at 1,500 mg/d. This effect is thought to be similar in magnitude to that of low-dose NSAIDs or acetaminophen.

Chondroitin, a large protein-like molecule that can impart elasticity to collagen, has shown similar, but slightly less, efficacy compared to glucosamine. The dosage of chondroitin used in most of the studies was 800 to 1,200 mg/d. The ACR recommends strongly against the use of chondroitin for knee and hip OA but conditionally recommends its use in hand OA due to a single trial suggesting efficacy.

The most common adverse effects associated with these products are GI discomfort, including diarrhea, heartburn, nausea, and vomiting. A concern exists that glucosamine may negatively affect blood glucose; however, this has not been proven in trials. Also, because of its uncertainty, glucosamine is not recommended in patients with poorly controlled diabetes. Since they are considered food supplements, there is little U.S. FDA regulation, and the preparations may vary in potency and effectiveness.

Trials that have examined the use of glucosamine and chondroitin for the treatment of OA have failed to consistently show a benefit of the combination versus placebo. In a subgroup analysis of the GAIT trial conducted by Clegg et al. (2006), for patients with moderate to severe symptoms, the use of combination of glucosamine and chondroitin resulted in decreased pain scales. However, this was a subgroup analysis that has not yet been verified with a subsequent trial. The ACR is strongly against the use of glucosamine for the treatment of OA of the hip, knee, and hand due to a lack of proven efficacy.

GOUT

Introduction

Historically, gout has been called the "disease of kings." For years, it was believed that gout was caused by an overindulgence in food and alcohol that only the rich could afford. While dietary factors can play a role, they are not the only risk factor leading to the development of gout.

Gout is the most common form of inflammatory arthritis in the United States. The incidence of gout in America has increased over the last 20 years and is now estimated to affect 8.3 million Americans (4%). This increase is thought to be due to the improved diagnosis but also the increasing number of patients with obesity, HTN, thiazide diuretic use, and alcohol intake.

Gout is an inflammatory condition that results from monosodium urate crystals precipitating in the synovial fluid between joints due to hyperuricemia. The monosodium urate crystals form due to hyperuricemia either from overproduction or underexcretion of uric acid. The most common joint affected is the metatarsophalangeal joint. Other common affected joints include the midtarsal joints, ankles, knees, fingers, wrists, and elbows.

Causes

The overproduction or underexcretion of uric acid in the body leads to hyperuricemia. Hyperuricemia is defined as serum urate concentrations greater than 6.8 mg/dL. At levels greater than 6.8 mg/dL, serum uric acid concentrations exceed the natural saturation point, which leads to the development of monosodium urate crystals. These crystals precipitate in patients' joints causing pain, arthritis, and inflammation.

The underexcretion of uric acid through insufficient renal clearance is the most common cause of hyperuricemia. Patients with diseases that can affect the kidneys (i.e., diabetes, chronic kidney disease [CKD], etc.) or those taking drugs that can alter uric acid excretion such as thiazide diuretics and aspirin can also have insufficient renal clearance of uric acid leading to hyperuricemia.

Genetic and dietary factors play a role in the overproduction of uric acid. Typically, dietary factors alone will not cause a significant enough increase in serum urate levels to cause hyperuricemia. Foods and beverages associated with increasing urate levels can cause an acute elevation in patients who are already experiencing hyperuricemia due to genetic overproduction or renal underexcretion leading to a gout attack. A further discussion of dietary modifications that can be made to decrease gout attacks can be found in the Nutrition/Lifestyle Changes (p. 22) section of this chapter.

There are many other factors that can play a role in the development of gout. Female sex hormones increase the excretion of uric acid in premenopausal women. This may explain why gout is seen more in male patients than in female patients. As female patients go through menopause and sex hormones change, this can decrease their excretion of uric acid leading to postmenopausal women developing gout. Gout is also associated with advancing age in men, obesity, and comorbidities such as HTN, CHF, and organ transplantation. A full list of risk factors for the development of gout can be found in **Box 32.4**.

Pathophysiology

When hyperuricemia leads to the development of monosodium urate crystals being released into joint spaces, these crystals are phagocytized by macrophages. This phagocytosis causes the activation and release of IL-1-beta. IL-1-beta binds to synovial endothelium and causes the release of proinflammatory cytokines. Neutrophils are recruited to the synovium, which causes further release of IL-1-beta and other proinflammatory cytokines that perpetuates the gouty arthritis inflammatory process.

In some cases, the monosodium urate crystals alone may not be sufficient to trigger the activation and release of IL-1-beta from macrophages. In these cases, they require additional stimulation from free fatty acids or lipopolysaccharides to release IL-1-beta. When patients consume alcohol or a large meal, this can increase the free fatty acid concentration in the body and trigger the release of IL-1-beta.

> ### BOX 32.4 Risk Factors for the Development of Gout
>
> - Males
> - Advancing age
> - Menopausal women
> - Obesity
> - Dietary factors
>   - Organ meat
>   - Seafood
>   - Sweetened beverages
>   - Fructose
>   - Ethanol
> - Drugs
>   - Thiazide diuretics
>   - Loop diuretics
>   - Cyclosporine
>   - Aspirin (<1 g/d)
> - Insulin resistance
> - Renal insufficiency
> - HTN
> - CHF
> - Organ transplantation

> ### BOX 32.5 American College of Rheumatology Diagnostic Criteria for Gout
>
> More than one acute arthritis attack
> Maximum joint inflammation develops within 1 day
> Monoarticular arthritis attack
> Joint redness
> Pain or swelling of first metatarsophalangeal joint
> Unilateral first metatarsophalangeal joint attack
> Unilateral tarsal joint attack
> Suspected tophus
> Hyperuricemia
> Radiography of asymmetric swelling within a joint
> Radiography of subcortical cysts without erosions
> Monosodium urate crystals in joint fluid during attack
> Negative culture for organisms within joint fluid during an
>   attack

Chronic gout and acute inflammation from gouty flares can lead to chronic pain, joint damage, and potential disability. As the disease progresses, joints may look deformed due to the development of tophi. Tophi are nodules created by monosodium urate crystals in a matrix of lipids, proteins, and mucopolysaccharides, and they may form in joint spaces. Tophi are most commonly found in the metatarsophalangeal joint, but they can also be found in other common joints affected by gout and throughout the body. Tophi can protrude through the skin and resemble a chalky substance. These urate crystals can also be found in other areas of the body, such as soft tissue, vertebrae, or skin. When they are located outside of the common joints, these crystals can mimic other disease states.

Diagnostic Criteria

Diagnosis of gout usually occurs clinically when a patient is experiencing rapid monoarticular arthritis, typically in the first metatarsophalangeal joint. This arthritis is accompanied by swelling and redness of the joint. The ACR diagnostic criteria that were developed in 1977 are still the most widely used form of diagnosis for patients with gout. Patients experiencing six or more of the clinical, laboratory, or radiologic criteria found in **Box 32.5** are considered to have gout.

Confirmation of a gout diagnosis can be made by aspirating monosodium urate crystals from the synovial fluid of the inflamed joint, but this is a painful and often unnecessary procedure if the patient is already displaying characteristic symptoms. Radiography can also be done using ultrasounds,

magnetic resonance imaging, or computed tomography, but often it takes over 10 years of untreated chronic gout before crystals can be seen using one of these methods.

Initiating Drug Therapy

The treatment of gout can be divided into treatment of chronic gout and treatment of acute gout attacks. The goals of drug therapy in chronic gout are to decrease the serum urate level to less than 6 mg/dL and to decrease the occurrence of acute gout attacks. The goal of less than 5 mg/dL may be preferred in patients with multiple risk factors or with a history of frequent acute gout attacks. Decreasing the serum urate level will help to reach the clinical goal of less pain and inflammation in the joints. For an acute gout attack, the goals are to relieve pain, terminate the attack, and maintain joint function.

The sections that follow are divided based on chronic gout treatment and acute gout attack treatment.

Chronic Gout

Urate-lowering therapies (ULT) are the primary pharmacologic treatment for chronic gout. Often, gout flares can occur when initiating ULT due to the redistribution of uric acid. To prevent these gout flares, patients should take NSAIDs or colchicine for the first 6 months of therapy. After 6 months, the number of gout flares should decrease due to the initiation of ULT. At this time, NSAIDs and colchicine can be discontinued until it is required for gouty flares.

Xanthine Oxidase Inhibitors

According to the 2012 ACR guidelines, the first-line therapy for the management of chronic gout is xanthine oxidase inhibitors (XOIs). There are currently two XOIs available today: allopurinol and febuxostat. Allopurinol has been used as first-line therapy among clinicians for decades. However, allopurinol therapy is associated with a rare, and sometimes life-threatening, hypersensitivity reaction and must be dose-adjusted in patients with decreased kidney function. When febuxostat became FDA-approved for chronic gout treatment in 2009, many expert clinicians viewed it as an attractive, alternative agent to allopurinol without the risk of hypersensitivity reaction or the need for a renal dose adjustment. However, a postmarketing study on the safety of febuxostat published in 2018 revealed febuxostat therapy was associated with an increased risk of cardiovascular death. Subsequently, the FDA updated the labeling for febuxostat to include this risk in a black box warning and significantly limited its approved use. According to the FDA, febuxostat should only be considered in patients who have had an inadequate response to a maximally titrated dose of allopurinol, patients who are intolerant to allopurinol, or patients for whom treatment with allopurinol is otherwise not appropriate.

Mechanism of Action. XOIs decrease uric acid levels by selectively inhibiting xanthine oxidase. Xanthine oxidase is the enzyme responsible for the conversion of hypoxanthine to xanthine to uric acid. Hypoxanthine and xanthine are then excreted in the urine with little risk of precipitation. By inhibiting the conversion to uric acid, uric acid levels are decreased, thereby reducing the risk of crystallization and a gout attack.

Dosage. Allopurinol is initially dosed 100 mg orally once daily and should be gradually titrated by 100 mg/d in 2- to 5-week increments until uric acid is less than 6 mg/dL. The usual dosage is 300 mg daily either once daily or taken in divided doses up to four times daily. The maximum dose is 800 mg/d. Patients with stage 4 or worse CKD should start at 50 mg/d and titrate up to a therapeutic dosage.

Febuxostat is dosed 40 mg orally once daily and may be increased to the FDA-approved maximum dose of 80 mg once daily in patients who do not achieve a serum uric acid level less than 6 mg/dL after 2 weeks. According to the 2012 ACR guidelines, febuxostat may be considered to be increased up to 120 mg daily in refractory cases. Febuxostat is metabolized through the liver and can be used in patients with mild to moderate kidney impairment without dose reduction.

Time Frame for Response. Serum urate levels can begin to decrease as early as 2 weeks following initiation of chronic gout therapy. Serum uric acid levels should be drawn every 2 to 5 weeks during dose titration until desired level is reached, which may take up to 6 months. Once goal serum uric acid levels are achieved, the patient should have levels drawn every 6 months throughout treatment.

Contraindications. Pegloticase should not be administered with allopurinol or febuxostat. Using both agents could increase the risk of infusion site reactions or anaphylaxis

with the pegloticase. Allopurinol should not be used with didanosine as it may increase the serum concentrations of didanosine leading to toxicity. Allopurinol and febuxostat can inhibit the metabolism of azathioprine and mercaptopurine leading to toxic doses and should not be used concurrently.

Adverse Events. Common adverse reactions that can occur with the use of XOIs include rash, arthralgias, and GI complications, which can be reduced by taking the medication with food.

Allopurinol is generally well tolerated. However, allopurinol therapy is associated with a rare and sometimes life-threatening risk of hypersensitivity reaction. Allopurinol hypersensitivity syndrome consists of a severe rash, which can include features of Stevens-Johnson syndrome or toxic epidermal necrolysis, fever, impaired liver and kidney function, leukocytosis, and eosinophilia. The risk of allopurinol hypersensitivity syndrome is highest in patients who have recently been on allopurinol in the previous 6 to 8 weeks, patients with decreased renal function, patients treated concomitantly with diuretics, and patients of certain ethnicities with a genetic predisposition. Genetic testing for the HLA-B*5801 allele is recommended prior to initiating allopurinol by the 2012 ACR guidelines in patients of the following descent: Koreans with stage 3 or worse CKD, Han Chinese and Thai peoples. Patients who report HLA-B*5801 positive should be prescribed an alternative therapy to allopurinol. Patients should be counseled to report a rash immediately to their health care provider. Allopurinol has also been associated with liver function abnormalities. Liver function tests should be performed at baseline and repeated if clinically indicated.

Febuxostat therapy has been associated with an increased risk of cardiovascular death in a postmarketing safety study, and its use should generally be reserved for patients not adequately controlled on maximally dosed allopurinol or patients not safe for allopurinol therapy. Febuxostat also has been associated with an increased risk of hepatic failure in postmarketing reports, and liver function tests should be performed at baseline and repeated if clinically indicated. Also, of note, postmarketing reports have described serious skin and hypersensitivity reactions in patients taking febuxostat. Many patients with a hypersensitivity reaction to febuxostat also reported a similar reaction to allopurinol.

Interactions. The use of ACE inhibitors, thiazide, and loop diuretics along with allopurinol may increase the levels of allopurinol and increase the risk of allopurinol hypersensitivity syndrome. Drug–drug interactions should also be evaluated before initiating allopurinol with patients taking concomitant antineoplastic agents. Multiple antineoplastic agents are affected by allopurinol, and the effects can range from non-effective antineoplastic treatment to toxicity. Allopurinol may also decrease the metabolism of warfarin subsequently leading to an increased INR and increased risk of bleeding. Patients maintained on warfarin who are newly started on allopurinol should have the INR monitored closely. As previously mentioned, both allopurinol and febuxostat inhibit the metabolism of mercaptopurine and azathioprine. Concurrent use should be avoided if possible. Febuxostat is contraindicated with these agents. However, allopurinol may be used, but the azathioprine or mercaptopurine dose needs to be reduced to one third to one fourth of the typical dose, and patients should be monitored closely for toxicity.

Uricosuric Agents

If at least one XOI is contraindicated or not tolerated well, practitioners should use probenecid for the treatment of chronic gout. The 2012 update to the ACR guidelines also recommends the addition of probenecid to a XOI if serum uric acid levels are not at goal with a XOI alone.

Mechanism of Action.   Probenecid increases the excretion of serum uric acid by inhibiting transporter proteins responsible for the reabsorption of uric acid in the kidneys.

Dosage.   The initial dose of probenecid is 250 mg twice daily for 1 week, and the dose is then increased to 500 mg twice daily if needed. The dose can be increased in 500-mg increments every 4 weeks to a maximum of 2 g/d. Once serum uric acid levels are within normal limits and no gout attacks have occurred for 6 months, the dose can be reduced by 500 mg every 6 months. Probenecid should not be recommended in patients with CrCl less than 50 mL/min due to a paucity of safety and efficacy data.

Time Frame for Response.   As with the XOIs, serum uric acid levels with uricosuric agents will begin to decrease within 2 weeks but may take up to 6 months to see full effect.

Contraindications.   Probenecid should not be given during an acute gout attack as it could exacerbate the symptoms when initiated. It also should not be given to patients who have been diagnosed with blood dyscrasias, those with uric acid kidney stones, children less than 2 years old, or anyone who has a past medical history of a reaction with probenecid. Patients should also not use ketorolac while taking probenecid, because it may increase the concentration of ketorolac leading to toxic symptoms such as nausea, gastric ulcers, headache, and edema.

Adverse Events.   There are a variety of adverse effects associated with probenecid. Serious reactions that can occur include hemolytic anemia and aplastic anemia in patients with G6PD deficiency, hepatic necrosis, and anaphylaxis. Other less serious but common reactions include headache, dizziness, anorexia, nausea vomiting, gingival soreness, urinary frequency, renal colic, nephrotic syndrome, dermatitis, pruritus, flushing fever, and gout exacerbations.

Interactions.   Avoid the use of probenecid with antibiotics including penicillin derivatives, cephalosporins, and fluoroquinolones as probenecid may increase the concentrations of the antibiotics increasing the risk of adverse effects and toxicities associated with these drugs. The use of methotrexate with probenecid may result in methotrexate toxicity including leukopenia, thrombocytopenia, anemia, and nephrotoxicity. Using citalopram with probenecid may increase citalopram concentrations, increasing the risk of QT prolongation, and its use with lorazepam can also increase lorazepam concentrations leading to toxicity. The use of probenecid with aspirin and other salicylates may diminish the uricosuric effect of probenecid. As with XOIs, probenecid should not be used with pegloticase due to an increased risk of anaphylaxis and infusion reactions of the pegloticase.

Pegloticase

Pegloticase is used as last-line therapy for patients with chronic gout that has not successfully been treated with either XOIs or probenecid. It must be administered intravenously in a health care facility every 2 weeks and costs more than $5,000 per dose.

Mechanism of Action.   Pegloticase is a pegylated recombinant form of uricase. Uricase is an enzyme typically absent in humans but is found in high levels in primates. Uricase converts uric acid to allantoin, which is an inactive, water-soluble metabolite of uric acid allowing uric acid to be easily excreted by the kidneys.

Dosage.   The recommended dose for pegloticase is 8 mg IV over at least 2 hours every 2 weeks. Before beginning pegloticase infusions, patients should discontinue the use of any oral antihyperuricemic agents and should not begin taking oral medications for chronic gout throughout the course of therapy.

Gouty flares can occur from initiating a new therapy and can be prevented by using NSAIDs or colchicine. It is recommended to begin this prophylaxis at least 1 week prior to initiating pegloticase and to continue for 6 months.

Patients should also be pretreated with antihistamines and corticosteroids prior to the infusion. This will help patients with any infusion reactions and potential anaphylaxis.

Time Frame for Response.   The reduction of uric acid concentrations can be seen as soon as 1 day after the infusion. For patients who are responders to pegloticase, the reduction can be maintained for at least 6 months.

Contraindications.   Pegloticase is contraindicated in patients with glucose-6-phosphate dehydrogenase deficiency.

Adverse Events.   As with all of the chronic gout medications, pegloticase can cause potential gout flares within the first few months of treatment. Prophylaxis for these gout flares is recommended for the first 6 months of treatment with colchicine or an NSAID.

Injection site reactions such as bruising, urticaria, erythema, and pruritus are also common. Administering antihistamines and corticosteroids with each infusion can decrease these injection site reactions in most patients.

Some patients also experience GI-related symptoms such as nausea, vomiting, and constipation with pegloticase.

Antipegloticase antibodies form in 92% of patients and Antipegloticase antibodies antibodies in 42%. These antibodies may result in a loss of response to pegloticase as early as 4 months into treatment.

Pegloticase does hold a black box warning for hypersensitivity and anaphylaxis reactions. Anaphylaxis has been reported during and after administration. Due to these reactions, patients should receive pegloticase infusions in a health care facility while being closely monitored during and for a period of time after administration. Most reactions occur within 2 hours of administration, but some patients have had delayed hypersensitivity reactions. The risk of these infusion reactions increases in patients whose uric acid level is greater than 6 mg/dL. Health care practitioners should monitor serum uric acid levels prior to infusion and discontinuing treatment if patients' concentrations are greater than 6 mg/dL on two consecutive measurements.

Interactions. Patients taking pegloticase should discontinue all other chronic gout medications. Allopurinol, febuxostat, and probenecid may increase the levels of pegloticase and increase the risk of infusion reactions and anaphylaxis.

Selecting the Most Appropriate Drug

In 2012, the ACR developed guidelines for the management of gout and the treatment of hyperuricemia (Khanna, 2012a). In addition to outlining the treatment options, they defined which patients should be initiated on chronic ULT. The criteria for initiating long-term ULT include patients with a diagnosis of gouty arthritis and one of the four following criteria: tophi or tophus, two or more gouty attacks yearly, CKD stage 2 or worse, or past urolithiasis. For those meeting criteria for chronic ULT, the options include XOIs, probenecid, and pegloticase.

First-Line Therapy

Allopurinol should be used as first-line therapy for chronic management of gout. Although the 2012 update to the ACR guidelines made no preference of one XOI over another, FDA warnings released subsequent to this guideline update have determined febuxostat should only be considered in patients who have had an inadequate response to a maximally titrated dose of allopurinol, patients who are intolerant to allopurinol, or patients for whom treatment with allopurinol is otherwise not appropriate. A 2020 update to the ACR guidelines is not available at the time of this writing.

XOIs can effectively lower serum uric acid in patients who are underexcretors or overproducers. The XOIs are considered first-line agents due to their efficacy and relative safety.

As previously mentioned, regardless of the agent selected, patients need to be initiated on acute gout prophylaxis when chronic ULT is started. This acute gout prophylaxis could include NSAIDs or colchicine and should be continued for 6 months.

Second-Line Therapy

If a patient is on a XOI at maximal appropriate dose and the goal serum urate concentration is not achieved, probenecid may be added to the XOI.

If at least one XOI is contraindicated or not tolerated well, probenecid monotherapy may be used as a second-line agent if no other contraindications are present.

Third-Line Therapy

For patients unable to achieve their uric acid goal and who continue to have disease activity, pegloticase can be initiated after discontinuation of other ULT.

Acute Gout

Patients with chronic gout will commonly experience gout attacks. Making dietary modifications and discontinuing the usage of medications that can induce gout attacks and weight loss and controlling other diseases states will help decrease the frequency of attacks, but they will occur in gout patients. When an acute gout attack occurs, patients can rest the joint and apply ice as needed to help with pain. They can also use short courses of NSAIDs, corticosteroids, or colchicine to reduce pain.

Nonsteroidal Antiinflammatory Drugs

NSAIDs can help decrease inflammation and pain during acute gout attacks. Naproxen, indomethacin, and sulindac are the three NSAIDs indicated for the treatment of acute gout. NSAIDs should be initiated at onset of the gout attack and continued for 24 hours after the resolution of symptoms. The usual course of treatment is 3 to 7 days. See the discussion of NSAIDs in the OA section of this chapter for more information about NSAIDs. See **Table 32.3** for appropriate dosing for acute gout attacks.

TABLE 32.3 Nonsteroidal Antiinflammatory Drug Dosing for Acute Gout	
Drug	**Dose**
Naproxen	750 mg initially followed by 250 mg q8h until attack subsides
Indomethacin	50 mg TID until pain is tolerable and then reduce dose
Sulindac	200 mg BID

Systemic Corticosteroids

Systemic corticosteroids can be given to patients to help decrease inflammation during an acute gout attack. Most patients will tolerate a short duration of oral corticosteroids; those who do not may benefit from an intramuscular dose. If a patient's gout attack is focused in 1 to 2 large joints, the clinician may choose to provide an intra-articular dose alone or in addition to oral corticosteroids.

Mechanism of Action. Corticosteroids decrease inflammation by suppressing the migration of polymorphonuclear leukocytes. Leukocytes cause a further release of IL-1-beta and other proinflammatory cytokines that lead to the inflammation associated with gouty arthritis.

Dosage. For oral doses, patients can take prednisone or methylprednisolone. Patients taking prednisone should use 0.5 mg/kg for 5 to 10 days or 0.5 mg/kg for 2 to 5 days and then taper 7 to 10 days. Clinicians can also choose to use a methylprednisolone dose pack. This dose pack contains (21) 4-mg tablets. These are tapered from six tablets on day 1, five tablets on day 2, and so forth until the patient is only taking one tablet on day 6.

For patients unable to take oral corticosteroids, an intramuscular dose of methylprednisolone 0.5 to 2 mg/kg for one dose can be given. This dose can be repeated as clinically indicated.

For patients experiencing pain in 1 to 2 large joints, an intra-articular dose of triamcinolone acetonide can be given. The dose is dependent on the size of the joint being treated. Large joints such as knees can be given 40 mg of triamcinolone, medium joints such as wrist ankles and elbows can be given 30-mg injections, and smaller joints can be given 10-mg injections.

Time Frame for Response. Patients should start to feel pain relief in 1 to 2 days. It may take up to a week for complete resolution.

Contraindications. Oral corticosteroids should be used with caution in patients with suppressed immune systems, diabetes, uncontrolled HTN, cardiovascular disease, and psychiatric disorders. If patients are requiring a corticosteroid and have one of these conditions, they may be a candidate for an intra-articular dose as these will have less of a systemic effect.

Adverse Events. Adverse effects of corticosteroids are extensive. By limiting the duration of treatment, many of the more chronic adverse effects will be avoided. However, even using corticosteroids for 5 to 10 days may result in acute adverse effects. These acute adverse effects include hyperglycemia, HTN, fluid retention, CNS stimulation, and dyspepsia. Patients at risk for these conditions need to be monitored closely while on corticosteroids.

Interactions. Interactions associated with corticosteroids are more severe when associated with long-term treatment. With the short-term use of corticosteroids being used to treat gout, there are few interactions. Interaction monitoring should be tailored to the patient's specific disease states. Diabetic patients should monitor their blood sugar more closely as corticosteroids may cause an increase in blood sugar levels. Patients with HTN, CHF, and fluid retention should also monitor their blood pressure and symptoms as corticosteroids can cause edema leading to worsening HTN and CHF. Corticosteroids also cause immunosuppression, so use caution in patients where immunosuppression needs to be avoided.

Colchicine

Colchicine has been used for the treatment of gout, Mediterranean fever, and multiple cardiovascular diseases for centuries. Although colchicine has had widespread use for many years, it was only approved by the FDA in 2009 under the unapproved drugs initiative. With this approval, there were changes to the dosing regimen and a new focus on safety related to comorbidities and drug–drug interactions.

Mechanism of Action. Colchicine inhibits the activation, degranulation, and migration of neutrophils to the area of a gout attack. This then decreases the inflammation and pain associated with a gout attack.

Dosage. For acute gout attacks, patients should be given their first dose within 24 hours of symptom onset. Colchicine is not strongly recommended if symptoms began more than 36 hours prior to presentation. Patients without organ dysfunction or concomitant interaction medications should take colchicine 1.2 mg orally for one dose at the first sign of gout flare followed by 0.6 mg 1 hour later.

Patients on strong CYP3A4 inhibitors who are to be treated with colchicine for acute gout attacks should receive a reduced dose of colchicine at 0.6 mg orally for 1 dose followed by 0.3 mg orally 1 hour later. Patients on moderate CYP3A4 inhibitors should receive colchicine 1.2 mg orally for one dose. Patients on P-glycoprotein (P-gp) inhibitors should receive a significantly reduced dose of colchicine 0.6 mg orally for one dose. Patients on these medications may have a dose repeated no earlier than every 3 days. Also, of note, patients with end-stage renal disease should receive colchicine 0.6 mg orally for one dose.

Most patients without organ dysfunction or concomitant interacting medications may take prophylactic colchicine at a dose of 0.6 mg daily or twice daily starting 12 hours later and continue until the attack resolves. Patients with severe renal failure (CrCl < 30 mL/min) should have the dose reduced to 0.3 mg daily. Patients with either renal or hepatic impairment should be monitored closely for adverse effects and should not repeat a treatment course more frequently than once every 2 weeks.

Prophylactic doses of colchicine to prevent gout attack during initiation of chronic gout treatment are 0.6 mg once or twice daily for up to 6 months after achieving target serum urate levels. If a patient is receiving prophylactic dosing and

TABLE 32.4

Prophylactic Colchicine Dosing Dependent on Interactions

Usual Treatment	Strong 3A4 Inhibitor	Moderate 3A4 Inhibitor	P-gp Inhibitor	CrCl < 30 mL/min
0.6 mg BID	0.3 mg daily	0.3 mg BID or 0.6 mg daily	0.3 mg daily	0.3 mg daily
0.6 mg daily	0.3 mg QOD	0.3 mg daily	0.3 mg QOD	

experiences a gout attack, they can begin the acute gout dose. They should wait 12 hours from their last dose of acute gout treatment before resuming the prophylactic dosing.

If patients are taking P-gp or CYP3A4 inhibitors, prophylactic dosing needs to be altered to prevent colchicine toxicities. See **Table 32.4** for dosage adjustments with P-gp or CYP3A4 inhibitors (**Figure 32.3**).

Patients with renal or hepatic impairment should not be given colchicine with concomitant P-gp or strong CYP3A4 inhibitors. Life-threatening and fatal colchicine toxicities have been reported in these patients.

Time Frame for Response.   Colchicine begins to provide its pain relief within 18 to 24 hours. It can take up to 48 hours to have its full antiinflammatory effect.

Contraindications.   Patients who have renal or hepatic impairment or those taking P-gp inhibitors or strong CYP3A4 inhibitors should be monitored closely and may be best served with lower doses of colchicine. Patients with a history of either renal or hepatic impairment who are also taking a P-gp inhibitor or strong CYP3A4 inhibitor are contraindicated for colchicine therapy as this may lead to fatal colchicine toxicity.

Adverse Events.   The most common adverse effect of colchicine is diarrhea. Some patients also experience pharyngolaryngeal pain, fatigue, and headache when being treated for gout flares. Other more uncommon but serious adverse effects of colchicine include blood dyscrasias and neuromuscular toxicity including rhabdomyolysis.

Interactions.   Colchicine is a substrate of the efflux transporter P-gp, and it is mainly metabolized by CYP3A4. Because of these pharmacokinetic properties, colchicine has many drug interactions with P-gp and CYP3A4 inhibitors. If P-gp or CYP3A4 inhibitors are coadministered with colchicine, it can increase serum concentrations of colchicine. Fatal colchicine toxicities attributed to drug–drug interactions have been described in literature. In addition to its antiinflammatory effects, colchicine inhibits cell mitosis. Significant inhibition of cell mitosis can lead to organ system dysfunction and failure. Cardiac effects are most commonly seen in patients who have taken increased concentrations of

colchicine. Since many drugs are P-gp and CYP3A4 inhibitors, it is imperative to evaluate each medication for drug–drug interactions and understand the strength of enzymatic inhibition for each medication. These factors will help a clinician decide if a patient should be monitored closely while taking the drugs concomitantly, if the colchicine dose should be reduced, or if colchicine therapy should be avoided entirely. **Figure 32.3** lists some common drug interactions with colchicine and the degree to which each drug inhibits P-gp or CYP3A4, although this list is not all-inclusive. **Table 32.4** lists the dose adjustments for prophylactic colchicine based on the clinician's assessment of the drug interaction and renal function.

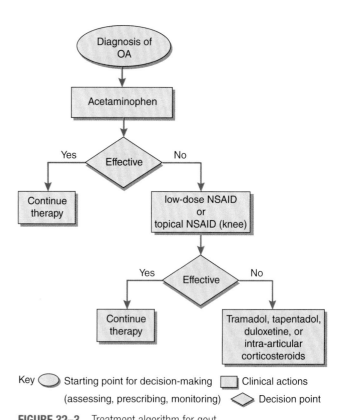

FIGURE 32–3   Treatment algorithm for gout.

NSAIDs, nonsteroidal antiinflammatory drugs; OA, osteoarthritis.

Selecting the Most Appropriate Drug

The ACR created guidelines for the treatment of acute gout attacks in 2012 (Khanna, 2012b). Prior to determining appropriate therapy, the patient's attack needs to be classified as mild, moderate, or severe. This is determined based on the patient's reported pain score with mild being less than or equal to 4, moderate being 5 to 6, and severe being greater than or equal to 7. Also, the location needs to be considered. The ACR breaks down the extent of the attack into one or few small joints, one or two large joints (ankle, knee, wrist, elbow, hip, or shoulder), or polyarticular (four or more joints). Based on the location and severity of pain, the appropriate treatments can be determined.

First-Line Therapy

For patients with mild to moderate pain in small joints or one to two large joints, initial therapy includes NSAIDs, systemic corticosteroids, or colchicine. If the pain started more than 36 hours prior, then colchicine is no longer a preferred agent. For patients with diabetes, heart failure, HTN, or other conditions predisposing them to adverse effects of corticosteroids, steroids would not be the preferred agent. Patients may also want to supplement pharmacologic treatment with topical ice applied to the affected joint(s) as needed.

For patients with severe pain or polyarticular attacks, combination therapy is recommended as initial therapy. **Box 32.6** lists common combinations recommended for acute gout treatment.

Second-Line Therapy

If monotherapy is not effective, the patient can switch to another first-line therapy or switch to combination therapy (**Box 32.6**). NSAIDs and corticosteroids are not recommended as a combination due to the overlap in toxicities and should be avoided in the treatment of gout.

Special Considerations

Ethnic/Genomics

As mentioned in the discussion of allopurinol, Korean, Han Chinese, and Thai patients have a higher probability of having an allopurinol hypersensitivity reaction due to the

---

HLA-B*5801 genetic allele. All Han Chinese and Thai patients and Korean patients with stage 3 or worse CKD should be genetically tested for the HLA-B*5801 allele before beginning allopurinol therapy. If the patients test positive, they should be given alternative therapy to allopurinol.

Monitoring Patient Response

Patients should have their serum urate levels monitored during the titration of XOIs or probenecid every 2 to 5 weeks. Once the target serum urate level has been achieved (<6 mg/dL or <5 mg/dL), the patients should be monitored every 6 months.

It is very common for patients with gout to also have HTN and renal insufficiency, so it is important that they also undergo appropriate assessments for their renal and cardiovascular systems. Baseline lab tests should include complete blood cell count, urinalysis, serum creatinine, blood urea nitrogen, and serum uric acid measurements.

Nephrolithiasis occurs in approximately 10% to 25% of patients with primary gout. The solubility of uric acid crystals increases when the urine pH becomes more alkaline. Acidic urine saturated with uric acid crystals may result in spontaneous stone formation. Patients should be warned about this complication and should be treated appropriately if stones occur.

Patient Education

To prevent acute gout attacks, patients can follow some nutritional and lifestyle modifications listed in the following. During an acute attack, patients should be counseled to elevate, ice, and rest the affected joint(s).

Drug Information
Patient-Oriented Information Sources
The ACR Web site has a section targeted to patients with gout (https://www.rheumatology.org/practice/clinical/patients/diseases_and_conditions/gout.as). There is a page regarding gout that includes basic facts and lists of other resources for patients.

Nutrition/Lifestyle Changes
Dietary modifications can help to decrease the risk and frequency of acute gout attacks. Decreasing purine-rich foods, sweetened beverages, and alcohol will help decrease the serum urate levels. **Box 32.7** has a full list of foods to decrease or avoid the consumption of in patients with gout. Patients should also increase their consumption of water, vegetables, and nonfat dairy as they have been shown to lower the risk of gout. Improving overall health status through weight loss and smoking cessation and closely monitoring and treating comorbidities, such as coronary artery disease, obesity, diabetes, hyperlipidemia, and HTN, can also help decrease the risk of gout and prevent gouty flares.

> **BOX 32.6 Combination Therapy for Acute Gouty Arthritis**
>
> Colchicine + NSAID
> Oral corticosteroid + colchicine
> Intra-articular steroid + (NSAID or colchicine or oral corticosteroid)

BOX 32.7 Foods and Beverages That Can Increase Serum Urate Levels

Red meat (specifically organ meat):
    Kidney
    Liver
    Sweetbreads
Seafood:
    Sardines
    Shellfish
High-fructose corn syrup:
    Sodas or sports drinks
    Foods containing high levels
Alcohol:
    Especially beer
    Also wine and spirits

Complementary and Alternative Medicine

Studies have shown that vitamin C inhibits uric acid synthesis and lowers serum uric acid levels. In a 2011 meta-analysis by Juraschek et al. (2011) of 13 trials, researchers studied the effect of oral vitamin C supplementation on serum uric acid levels. This trial showed that a mean dose of 500 mg/d of vitamin C reduced serum urate levels to 0.32 mg/dL. This dose is well over the recommended dietary allowance for vitamin C (90 mg/d men; 75 mg/d women) but is still under the maximum tolerable intake of 2 g/d. Vitamin C along with dietary modifications may be an option for some patients who do not tolerate pharmacologic therapy or wish to have an additional benefit with their pharmacologic therapy.

CASE STUDY 1

G.P., a 66-year-old, right-handed white man, seeks treatment for swelling and decreased range of motion in the right knee. He tells you that he has retired at age 65, after 40 years of assembly-line work. He reports that his physical activity has decreased and his weight has increased 20 lb since retiring. His hobbies include woodworking and playing cards and playing with his two grandchildren. He denies tobacco use and alcohol use.

Although he describes several years of joint pain that gradually worsened, his activities were not limited until approximately 6 months ago, when he noted an insidious onset of swelling in the right knee. Over the years, he has sporadically taken acetaminophen, aspirin, and ibuprofen to control the pain. He reports that none of the drugs provided better relief than the others. His medical history is remarkable for hypertension and three episodes of gout.

1. List specific goals of treatment for G.P.
2. What treatment recommendations would you make—both pharmacologic and nonpharmacologic?
3. What are the parameters for monitoring success of the therapy?
4. Discuss specific patient education based on the prescribed therapy.
5. What would be the choice for second-line therapy?
6. What side effects should be considered with your choice of second-line therapy?
7. What counseling points would you discuss with the patient regarding your choice of second-line therapy?

Bibliography

Starred references are cited in text.

Altman, R., Alarcon, G., Appelrouth, D., et al. (1991). The American College of Rheumatology criteria for the classification and reporting of osteoarthritis of the hip. *Arthritis and Rheumatism, 34,* 505–514.

Altman, R., Asch, E., Bloch, D., et al. (1986). The American College of Rheumatology criteria for the classification and reporting of osteoarthritis of the knee. *Arthritis and Rheumatism, 29,* 1039–1049.

Altman, R. D., & Barthel, H. R. (2011). Topical therapies for osteoarthritis. *Drugs, 71*(10), 1259–1279.

American College of Rheumatology. (1977). Criteria for the classification of acute arthritis of primary gout. Retrieved from https://www.rheumatology.org/ACR/practice/clinical/classification/gout.asp on May 15, 2015.

*Bannuru, R. R., Osani, M. C., Vaysbrot, E. E., et al. (2019). OARSI guidelines for the non-surgical management of knee, hip and polyarticular osteoarthritis. *Osteoarthritis and Cartilage, 27,* 1578–1589.

Bannuru, R. R., Schmid, C. H., Kent, D. M., et al. (2015). Comparative effectiveness of pharmacologic interventions for knee osteoarthritis: A systematic review and network meta-analysis. *Annals of Internal Medicine, 162,* 46–54.

Barbour, K. E., Helmick, C. G., Boring, M., & Brady, T. J. (2017). Vital signs: Prevalence of doctor-diagnosed arthritis and arthritis-attributable activity limitation—United States, 2013–2015. *MMWR Morbidity and Mortality Weekly Report, 66,* 246–253. doi: 10.15585/mmwr.mm6609e1External

*Chan, F. K., Lanas, A., Scheiman, J., et al. (2010). Celecoxib versus omeprazole and diclofenac in patients with osteoarthritis and rheumatoid arthritis (CONDOR): A randomized trial. *Lancet, 376,* 173–179.

Chappell, A. S., Desaiah, D., Liu-Seifert, H., et al. (2010). A double-blind, randomized, placebo-controlled study of the efficacy and safety of duloxetine for the treatment of chronic pain due to osteoarthritis of the knee. *Pain Practice, 11*(1), 33–41.

*Clegg, D. O., Reda, D. J., Harris, C. L., et al. (2006). Glucosamine, chondroitin sulphate, and the two in combination for painful knee osteoarthritis. *New England Journal of Medicine, 354*(8), 795–808.

Cymbalta [package insert]. (2014). Indianapolis, IN: Eli Lilly and Company.

Danelich, I. M., Wright, S. S., Lose, J. M., et al. (2015). Safety of nonsteroidal anti-inflammatory drugs in patients with cardiovascular disease. *Pharmacotherapy, 35*(5), 520–535. doi: 10.1002/phar.1584

Doherty, M., Hawkey, C., Goulder, M., et al. (2011). A randomised controlled trial of ibuprofen, paracetamol or a combination tablet of ibuprofen/paracetamol in community-derived people with knee pain. *Annals of the Rheumatic Diseases, 70*, 1534–1541.

Felson, D. T. (2015). Osteoarthritis. In D. Kasper, A. Fauci, S. Hauser, et al., (Eds.), *Harrison's principles of internal medicine* (19th ed.). Retrieved from http://accesspharmacy.mhmedical.com/content.aspx?bookid=1130&Sectionid=79751047 on May 7, 2015.

Finkelstein, Y., Aks, S. E., Juurlik, D. N., et al. (2010). Colchicine poisoning: The dark side of the ancient drug. *Clinical Toxicology, 48*(5), 407–414.

Gonzalez, E. B. (2012). An update on the pathology and clinical management of gouty arthritis. *Clinical Rheumatology, 31*, 13–21.

Grosser, T., Smyth, E., & FitzGerald, G. A. (2011). Anti-inflammatory, antipyretic, and analgesic agents; pharmacotherapy of gout. In L. L. Brunton, B. A. Chabner, & B. C. Knollmann (Eds.), *Goodman & Gilman's the pharmacological basis of therapeutics* (12th ed., Chapter 34). Retrieved May 18, 2015. New York, NY: McGraw-Hill.

Guo, C. G., & Leung, W. K. (2019). Prevention of NSAID-related lower GI injury. *Gut Liver, 14*(2), 179–189 Published online.

Hainer, B. L., Matheson, E., & Wilkes, R. T. (2014). Diagnosis, treatment, and prevention of gout. *American Family Physician, 90*(12), 831–836.

*Hawkey, C. J., Karrasch, J. A., Szczepanski, L., et al. (1998). Omeprazole compared with misoprostol for ulcers associated with nonsteroidal antiinflammatory drugs. *New England Journal of Medicine, 338*, 727–734.

Helmick, C. G., Felson, D. T., Lawrence, R. C., et al. (2008). Estimates of the prevalence of arthritis and other rheumatic conditions in the United States: Part 1. *Arthritis and Rheumatism, 58*(1), 15–25.

Hochberg, M. C., Altman, R. D., April, K. T., et al. (2012). American College of Rheumatology 2012 recommendations for the use of nonpharmacologic and pharmacologic therapies in osteoarthritis of the hand, hip and knee. *Arthritis Care and Research, 64*(4), 465–474.

Hochberg, M. C., Martel-Pelletier, J., Monfort, J., et al. (2015). Combined chondroitin sulphate and glucosamine for painful knee osteoarthritis: A multicentre, randomised, double-blind, non-inferiority trial versus celecoxib. *Annals of the Rheumatic Diseases, 75*(1), 37–44. doi: 10.1136/annrheumdis-2014-206792

Jordan, K. M., Arden, N. K., Doherty, M., et al. (2003). EULAR recommendations 2003: An evidence based approach to the management of knee osteoarthritis: Report of a Task Force of the Standing Committee for International Clinical Studies Including Therapeutic Trials (ESCISIT). *Annals of the Rheumatic Diseases, 62*, 1145–1155.

*Juraschek, S. P., Miller, E. R., & Gelber, A. C. (2011). Effect of oral vitamin C supplementation on serum uric acid: A meta-analysis of randomized controlled trials. *Arthritis Care and Research, 63*(9), 1295–1306.

*Khanna, D., Fitzgerald, J. D., Khanna, P. P., et al. (2012a). American College of Rheumatology guidelines for management of gout. Part 1: Systematic nonpharmacologic and pharmacologic therapeutic approaches to hyperuricemia. *Arthritis Care and Research, 64*(10), 1431–1446.

*Khanna, D., Khanna, P. P., Fitzgerald, J. D., et al. (2012b). American College of Rheumatology guidelines for management of gout. Part 2: Therapy and anti-inflammatory prophylaxis of acute gouty arthritis. *Arthritis Care and Research, 64*(10), 1447–1461.

Kim, S. C., Newcomb, C., Margolis, D., et al. (2013). Severe cutaneous reactions requiring hospitalization in allopurinol initiators: A population-based cohort study. *Arthritis Care and Research, 65*(4), 578–584.

*Kolasinski, S. L., Neogi, T., Hochberg, M. C., et al. (2020). 2019 American college of rheumatology/arthritis foundation guidelines for the management of osteoarthritis of the hand, hip, and knee. *Arthritis Care & Research, 72*(2), 149–162.

Loeser, R. F., Goldring, S. R., Scanzelloo, C. R., et al. (2012). Osteoarthritis: A disease of the joint as an organ. *Arthritis and Rheumatism, 64*(6), 1697–1707.

McAlindon, T. E., Bannuru, R. R., Sullivan, M. C., et al. (2014). OARSI guidelines for the non-surgical management of knee osteoarthritis. *Osteoarthritis and Cartilage, 22*(3), 363–388.

Murphy, L., & Helmick, C. G. (2012). The impact of osteoarthritis in the United States: A population-health perspective. *American Journal of Nursing, 112*(3), S13–S17.

Myers, J., Wielage, R. C., & Han, B. (2014). The efficacy of duloxetine, non-steroidal anti-inflammatory drugs, and opioid in osteoarthritis: A systematic literature review and meta-analysis. *BMC Musculoskeletal Disorders, 15*, 76.

National Center for Chronic Disease Prevention and Health Promotion. (2010). *Arthritis: Meeting the challenge.* Retrieved from www.cdc.gov/arthritis

Neogi, T. (2011). Gout. *New England Journal of Medicine, 364*, 443–452.

Silverstein, F. E., Faich, G., Goldstein, J. L., et al. (2000). Gastrointestinal toxicity with celecoxib vs nonsteroidal anti-inflammatory drugs for osteoarthritis and rheumatoid arthritis: The CLASS study: A randomized controlled trial. *Journal of the American Medical Association, 284*(10), 1247–1255.

Singh, J. A., Reddy, S. F., & Kundukulam, J. (2011). Risk factors for gout and prevention: A systematic review of the literature. *Current Opinion in Rheumatology, 23*(2), 192–202.

Slobodnick, A., Shah, B., Pillinger, M. H., et al. (2015). Colchicine: Old and new. *The American Journal of Medicine, 128*, 461–470.

Sundy, J. S., Baraf, H. S., Yood, R. A., et al. (2011). Efficacy and tolerability of pegloticase for the treatment of chronic gout in patients refractory to conventional treatment: Two randomized controlled trials. *Journal of the American Medical Association, 306*(7), 711–720.

Towheed, T., Maxwell, L., Judd, M., et al. (2009). Acetaminophen for osteoarthritis (review). *Cochrane Database of Systematic Reviews, 1*, CD004257.

U.S. Food and Drug Administration. (2012). Full Prescribing Information for colchicine. Retrieved from http://www.accessdata.fda.gov/drugsatfda_docs/label/2014/022352s017lbl.pdf on May 15, 2015.

Wallace, S. L., Robinson, H., Masi, A. T., et al. (1977). Preliminary criteria for the classification of the acute arthritis of primary gout. *Arthritis and Rheumatism, 20*(3), 895–900.

*Yeomans, N. D., Tulassay, Z., Laszlo, J., et al. (1998). A comparison of omeprazole with ranitidine for ulcers associated with nonsteroidal anti-inflammatory drugs. *New England Journal of Medicine, 338*, 719–726.

Zhang, W., Doherty, M., Arden, N., et al. (2005). EULAR evidence based recommendations for the management of hip osteoarthritis: Report of a Task Force of the Standing Committee for International Clinical Studies Including Therapeutic Trials (ESCISIT). *Annals of the Rheumatic Diseases, 64*, 669–681.

Zhang, W., Doherty, M., Leeb, B. F., et al. (2007). EULAR evidence based recommendations for the management of hand osteoarthritis: Report of a Task Force of the Standing Committee for International Clinical Studies Including Therapeutic Trials (ESCISIT). *Annals of the Rheumatic Diseases, 66*, 377–388.

Zhang, W., Moskowitz, R. W., Nuki, G., et al. (2008). OARSI recommendations for the management of hip and knee osteoarthritis, Part II: OARSI evidence-based, expert consensus guidelines. *Osteoarthritis and Cartilage, 16*, 137–162.

Zhu, Y., Pandya, B. J., & Choi, H. K. (2011). Prevalence of gout and hyperuricemia in the US general population. *Arthritis and Rheumatism, 61*(10), 3136–3141.

33 Osteoporosis

Jola Salavaci and Virginia P. Arcangelo

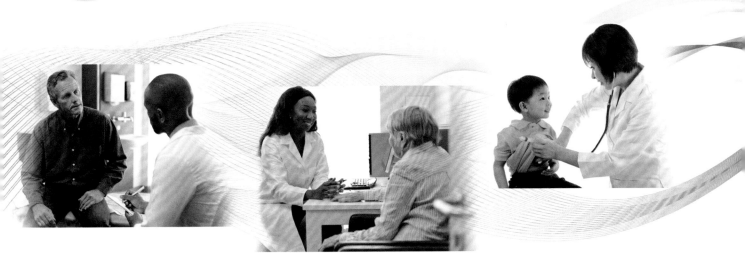

Learning Objectives

1. Identify the risk factors associated with osteoporosis.
2. Discuss lifestyle modifications and alternative treatment options.
3. Demonstrate an understanding of available drug therapy and choose optimal therapy that is patient specific.

INTRODUCTION

Osteoporosis is a progressive systemic disease characterized by a decrease in bone mass and microarchitectural deterioration of bone tissue, resulting in bone fragility and increased susceptibility to fractures. Bone loss occurs at the rate of about 10% every 10 years after the age of 30. Each decade after 40 years is associated with a fivefold increase in the incidence of osteoporosis. Osteoporosis, or low bone mass (osteopenia), is estimated to occur in approximately 54 million Americans aged 50 years and older, 80% of whom are women (National Osteoporosis Foundation, 2021). Women are more likely than men to develop osteoporosis because of thinner, lighter bones, changes associated with menopause, and greater longevity than men.

One in four men will have an osteoporotic-associated fracture. Men develop osteoporosis because of the inability to convert testosterone into estrogen through enzyme deficiency leading to decreased bone mass. They also may develop it because of medication side effects.

Bone fracture is the major cause of mortality and morbidity in patients with osteoporosis. The most common fractures are vertebral compression fractures and fractures of the distal radius and proximal femur.

CAUSES

The three types of osteoporosis are postmenopausal, senile, and secondary (**Box 33.1**). Many risk factors are associated with osteoporosis (**Box 33.2**).

Skeletal growth and the majority of bone mass are achieved during the first two decades of life, with bone density peaking around age 30. Between age 30 and menopause, bone mass remains relatively stable. At menopause, women have a period of 5 or more years during which there is an accelerated rate of bone loss. Some women lose up to 5% of their bone mass per year during this time.

PATHOPHYSIOLOGY

Two types of bone are discerned at the macroscopic level: cortical bone and trabecular bone. Cortical bone has a dense structure, whereas trabecular bone has a sponge-like appearance. Long bones have a thick outer layer of cortical bone and a thin inner layer of trabecular bone, whereas short bones consist of mostly trabecular bone with a thin layer of cortical bone.

Bone is in a constant state of remodeling (reforming). Osteoblasts are responsible for bone formation and osteoclasts for bone resorption. A balance is normally achieved between osteoblast and osteoclast activity. When bone resorption occurs at a faster rate than bone remodeling, osteoporosis is the result because the bones then become brittle and prone to fracture. Bone loss is greater in trabecular bone than in cortical bone.

The skeleton undergoes continuous remodeling throughout life. Bone remodeling involves the removal of mineralized bone by osteoclasts followed by the formation of bone matrix

BOX 33.1   Types of Osteoporosis

TYPE I: POSTMENOPAUSAL OSTEOPOROSIS

- Occurs in postmenopausal women between ages 51 and 75.
- Decreased estrogen causes an accelerated rate of bone loss, especially trabecular bone loss.
- The most common fractures are of the vertebrae and distal femur. There is also tooth loss.

TYPE II: SENILE OSTEOPOROSIS

- Occurs in men and women older than age 70.
- There is a proportional loss of cortical and trabecular bone.
- The most common fractures are hip, pelvic, and vertebral.

TYPE III: SECONDARY OSTEOPOROSIS

- Occurs in men and women at any age.
- Secondary to other conditions such as drug therapy and other diseases.

BOX 33.2   Risk Factors for Osteoporosis

PATIENT CHARACTERISTICS

- Female gender
- Advanced age
- Asian or white race
- Family history
- Low body weight

MEDICAL CONDITIONS/DISEASES

- Anorexia nervosa
- Diabetes
- GI diseases (e.g., inflammatory bowel disease [IBD], celiac disease, gastric bypass, and other malabsorption syndromes)
- Hyperthyroidism
- Hypogonadism (in males)
- Menopause (either natural or surgical) without hormone replacement
- Rheumatoid arthritis and other autoimmune diseases
- Others (e.g., HIV/AIDS, Parkinson's disease, epilepsy)

LIFESTYLE FACTORS

- Smoking
- Physical inactivity or sedentary lifestyle
- Low calcium and/or vitamin D intake
- Excess alcohol intake (>3 drinks/day)

MEDICATIONS

- Anticonvulsants (e.g., carbamazepine, phenytoin, phenobarbital)
- Aromatase inhibitors
- Thyroid hormones
- Depot medroxyprogesterone (Depo-Provera)
- Lithium
- GnRH (gonadotropin-releasing hormone) agonists
- PPIs
- Steroids (≥5 mg daily of prednisone or equivalent for >3 months)
- Others (e.g., heparin, loop diuretics, selective serotonin reuptake inhibitors [SSRIs], thiazolidinediones [TZDs])

through the osteoblasts that become mineralized. There are three phases of remodeling: resorption, during which osteoclasts digest old bone; reversal, when mononuclear cells appear on the bone surface; and formation, when osteoblasts lay down new bone until the resorbed bone is completely replaced. Bone remodeling serves to maintain skeletal integrity and repairs microdamages in bone matrix, preventing the accumulation of old bone. Additionally, it serves to maintain plasma calcium homeostasis. Bone remodeling takes place at the systemic and the local levels. The major systemic regulators include parathyroid hormone (PTH), calcitriol, and other hormones such as growth hormone, glucocorticoids, thyroid hormones, and sex hormones. Factors such as insulin-like growth factors, prostaglandins, tumor growth factor-beta, bone morphogenetic proteins (BMPs), sclerostin, and cytokines are involved as well. At the local level, there are cytokines and growth factors that affect bone cell functions. Through the RANK/receptor activator of NF-kappa B ligand (RANKL)/osteoprotegerin (OPG) system, the processes of bone resorption and formation are closely interwoven, allowing bone formation to follow each cycle of bone resorption to maintain skeletal integrity.

An imbalance in bone remodeling causes osteoporosis. This can be due to numerous factors targeting both osteoblasts and osteoclasts that result in greater resorption than formation. One cause is the decreased estrogen levels during menopause, causing an upregulation of RANKL. OPG secretion is suppressed, which then leads to a greater osteoclastogenesis and accelerated bone resorption. Since bone formation is coupled to resorption, the entire remodeling unit is activated. Bone resorption is a rapid process, taking about 2 weeks for the osteoclasts to attach and resorb matrix. Formation is much more deliberate, meaning that with the release of soluble cytokines, an imbalance in remodeling immediately occurs, and this favors bone resorption. The loss is faster than remodeling causing bone loss. Estrogen administration can prevent bone loss by enhancing OPG production as well as by suppressing RANKL expression.

BMPs are a family of proteins found on the surface of osteoblast precursor cells and are potent inducers of bone formation. Low-density lipoprotein (LDL)–related protein 5 (LRP5) is another cell surface receptor that is of interest for bone formation. Sclerostin, which is expressed by osteocytes, binds to LRP5 receptors on osteoblasts and inhibits the wingless-related integration site (Wnt) signaling, leading to a decrease in bone formation. Therefore, inhibition of sclerostin leads to increased bone formation and strength.

Maximal mineral content of cortical bone occurs between the second and fourth decades of life, followed by a slow decline. In general, women have less bone mass than men, so even a small loss is more significant in women. Cortical bone loss in women is approximately 3% per decade until menopause, when the rate of bone loss accelerates to 9% per decade. Women lose approximately 15% of trabecular bone during the first 5 to 7 years after menopause. The rate returns to normal approximately 20 years after menopause. Generalized bone loss in men occurs at a rate of approximately 4% per decade throughout life.

DIAGNOSTIC CRITERIA

Medical history and a drug history are essential in the diagnosis. Bone mineral density (BMD) is related to bone mass at maturity and subsequent bone loss. Dual-energy x-ray absorptiometry (DEXA) scan measures BMD of the spine and hip and calculates a T-score or a Z-score. The T-score compares a person's measured BMD to the average peak BMD of a healthy, young white adult of the same sex. The Z-scores are calculated the same way, but they compare the patient's measured BMD to the mean BMD of an age-, sex-, and ethnicity-matched population.

T-scores are used to diagnose osteoporosis and are expressed in negative numbers, a score at or above –1 (closer to zero) correlates with stronger and denser bones, which are less likely prone to fractures.

A normal T-score is ≥ –1, whereas osteopenia (low bone mass) is diagnosed with a T-score of –1 to –2.4. Osteoporosis is diagnosed with a T-score of ≤ –2.5, meaning that if a patient's T-score is < –2.5, the patient's BMD is at least 2.5 standard deviations below an average BMD of healthy, young, white adults. Initial screening is recommended for the following populations:

- All women ≥65 years and men ≥70 years should have BMD measured, preferably with a DEXA scan.
- Women <65 years and men aged 50 to 69 years should have BMD checked if there is a history of having a fragility fracture (e.g., fall from standing height or less that results in fracture) after the age of 50 years.
- Anyone with risk for disease or drug-induced bone loss.
- Parental history of hip fracture or other clinical risk factors (see **Box 33.2**).

The guidelines use fracture risk calculations derived from a computerized algorithm developed by the World Health Organization (WHO) called FRAX (Fracture Risk Assessment Tool), which is a free online tool (available at www.nof.org or www.shef.ac.uk/FRAX). It assesses the likelihood a patient will experience an osteoporotic fracture in the next 10 years. FRAX has been well validated, and the U.S. version has adapted versions available for Caucasian, black, Hispanic, and Asian patients. This tool is intended for postmenopausal women and men >50 years of age. Clinical risk factors included in the tool are age, gender, weight, height, fracture history, parental hip fracture history, femoral neck BMD, smoking status, steroid use, alcohol intake, disorders strongly associated with osteoporosis (e.g., type 1 diabetes, chronic liver disease, premature menopause), and diagnosis of rheumatoid arthritis.

TREATMENT AND PREVENTION OF OSTEOPOROSIS

Lifestyle Measures

Fall prevention measures should be taken for patients who are at increased fall risk, such as those with a history of recent falls, those taking medication that causes sedation or orthostasis, those with neurologic disorders or conditions that cause physical instability or poor coordination, those with poor or impaired vision or hearing, and those with poor health/frailty and urinary/fecal urgency. Home safety assessment should ensure floors are safe (e.g., removal of rugs/cords), lighting is appropriate, storage is at appropriate heights, bathrooms have safety bars and nonskid floors, stairs have handrails and are well lit with nonskid carpeting. If a disability is present, canes or walkers are strongly recommended. All patients with low bone density should be encouraged to perform muscle strengthening (e.g., weight training, yoga, Pilates, and boot camp programs) and weight-bearing exercises (e.g., walking, jogging, Tai Chi, stair climbing, dancing, and tennis)to enhance bone mass, stop smoking and avoid secondhand smoke, reduce alcohol intake, and adopt fall prevention strategies at home.

Vitamin D and Calcium Intake

Prevention of osteoporosis should begin early in life with adequate intake of calcium and vitamin D. Adequate calcium intake is critically important in children (who can build bone stores), during pregnancy (when fetus depletes mother's stores), and during menopause (when bone loss is rapid). Children ages 9 to 18 years should consume 1,300 mg of calcium daily. Adults ages 19 to 49 years need 1,000 mg of calcium per day, whereas women ≥50 years and men ≥70 years require 1,200 mg each day. Dietary calcium intake is preferred with supplements used if needed. Excess intake over the recommended amounts, however, may contribute to kidney stones, cardiovascular disease, and stroke, although evidence remains controversial in this area.

Vitamin D Deficiency

Vitamin D is required for calcium absorption, and low levels can contribute to various health conditions. Vitamin D deficiency in children causes rickets, and in adults it causes osteomalacia (softening of the bones with low levels of collagen and calcium). The National Osteoporosis Foundation (NOF) recommends 800 to 1,000 mg international units (IU) of vitamin D daily for adults >50 years of age. Other organizations recommend 600 IU for adults up to 70 years old and 800 IU for those ≥71 years. However, these recommendations are controversial, and many endocrinologists may recommend even higher intakes of vitamin D with a safe upper limit of 4,000 IU daily for adults, as recommended by the Institute of Medicine. A serum vitamin D level [25(OH)D] should be measured and vitamin D deficiency diagnosed for those with 25(OH)D levels <30 ng/mL. Cholecalciferol (vitamin D_3) or ergocalciferol (vitamin D_2) 50,000 IU weekly or 5,000 to 7,000 IU daily for 8 to 12 weeks is recommended in adults with deficiency to replenish stores; maintenance therapy with 1,500 to 2,000 IU daily is recommended to maintain 25(OH)D levels above 30 ng/mL.

Calcium Supplementation

Sufficient calcium intake is necessary for the prevention of osteoporosis. Dietary calcium is generally not sufficient and to reach recommended levels, most women need an additional 600 to 900 mg daily. Doses above 500 to 600 mg of calcium should be divided and taken multiple times a day, as calcium absorption is saturable. Patients should not take calcium with meals that are high in fiber or with bulk-forming laxatives because such materials decrease absorption. Calcium carbonate (e.g., TUMS®) has 40% elemental calcium and must be taken with meals; its absorption is acid dependent. Calcium citrate (e.g., Calcitrate) has a lower amount of elemental calcium (21%) but better absorption as it is not acid dependent and can be taken with or without food. Calcium products are available in many formulations: capsules, tablets, chewables, liquids, granules, and powder; a common side effect is constipation. If simple measures such as increased fluids and fiber intake do not relieve constipation, another form of calcium should be tried. Calcium supplement intake should be increased gradually over several weeks.

INITIATING DRUG TREATMENT

NOF recommends that health care providers consider U.S. Food and Drug Administration (FDA)–approved medical therapies in patients with the following conditions:

1. A hip or vertebral (clinical or morphometric) fracture
2. Low bone mass (T-score from –1.0 to –2.5 at the femoral neck, total hip, or spine) and a 10-year probability of hip fracture of ≥3% or more or a 10-year probability of any major osteoporosis-related fracture of ≥20%
3. T-score ≤ –2.5 at the femoral neck, total hip, or spine by DEXA scan

There are various FDA-approved medications for treatment and/or prevention of osteoporosis, and they fall under two categories: antiresorptives and anabolics. Resorption-inhibiting agents or antiresorptives include bisphosphonates (alendronate ± D, ibandronate, risedronate, and zoledronic acid), a receptor activator of nuclear factor kappa-B (RANK) ligand inhibitor (denosumab), calcitonin, estrogen-based therapies, and estrogen agonist/antagonist (raloxifene). These work by slowing down the breakdown of the remodeling cycle. When these agents are taken, the rate of bone resorption decreases within weeks and the rate of bone formation increases within months. Remodeling spaces fill in, and an increase of BMD of 5% to 10% occurs with treatment. This process takes 2 to 3 years. Anabolic agents include the PTH analog (teriparatide), a PTH-related protein analog (abaloparatide), and a sclerostin inhibitor (romosozumab-aqqg). Anabolics work by helping to stimulate the formation of the remodeling process, which leads to more bone formed, making stronger bones, which are less prone to fractures/break.

Selecting the Most Appropriate Agent

Adequate supplementation of calcium and vitamin D should always augment any of the prescribed medications. Results of the DEXA scan guide the provider's decision in selecting therapy for osteoporosis. If the T-score is ≥ –1, the patient is said to have no osteoporosis or osteopenia and considered low risk, but calcium and vitamin D intake as well as weight-bearing and muscle-strengthening exercises are encouraged. A T-score from –1 to –2.5 indicates osteopenia and is considered moderate risk. Treatment with calcium and vitamin D should begin and initiation of preventive resorption-inhibiting therapy (e.g., bisphosphonates) should be considered. Pharmacologic treatment is recommended for high risk patients: those with a T-score ≤ –2.5, those who have had a prior hip or vertebral fracture, those with a 10-year hip fracture risk of ≥3% or a 10-year major osteoporostic risk of ≥20%. High-risk patients can be initiated on bisphosphonates, denosumab, teriparatide, or abaloparatide along with adequate calcium and vitamin D supplementation. If these patients experience any intolerance or the initial therapy is a no longer appropriate, alternative therapy such as SERMs, calcitonin, and sclerostin inhibitor should be considered. The risk of fracture almost doubles for each BMD decrease of 1 SD; therefore, close monitoring of BMD is recommended. The DEXA scan should be repeated in 2 years or sooner if medically indicated. Patients' compliance with prescribed medication should be checked at least annually and modifications in therapy should be made if any adverse effects or intolerance occurs. Therapy chosen should be individualized based on the patient's characteristics, and risk versus benefit assessment should be done if any preexisting conditions or contraindications are present (**Figure 33.1**).

Goals of Drug Therapy

The goals of drug therapy are minimizing bone loss, delaying the progression of osteoporosis, and preventing fractures and fracture-related morbidity and mortality. Once osteoporosis is diagnosed and drug therapy is started, patients should

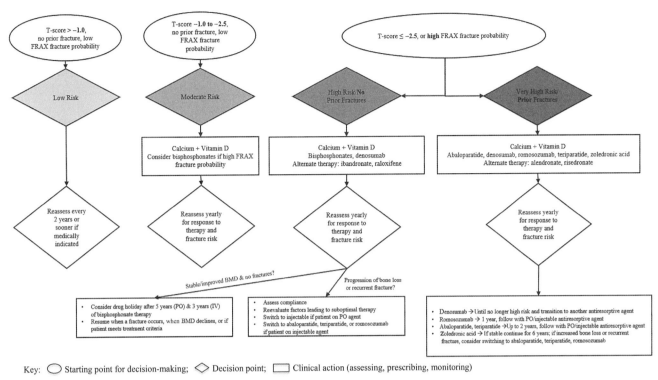

FIGURE 33-1   Risk assessment and treatment algorithm.

be reevaluated and have BMD levels checked every 2 years or sooner if medically indicated. No pharmacologic treatment should be considered indefinite. **Tables 33.1** and **33.2** provide an overview of the drugs used.

Bisphosphonates

Alendronate ± D (Fosamax ± D, Binosto), risedronate (Actonel, Atelvia), ibandronate (Boniva), and zoledronic acid (Reclast) are bisphosphonates used for preventing and treating osteoporosis.

Mechanism of Action

These drugs inhibit bone resorption and increase bone density. They are deposited in the bone at sites of mineralization and in resorption lacunae. The bone resorption and fracture rates decline, whereas bone density increases. In studies of alendronate, an increase in bone mass was shown in the spine and hip, with a 48% decrease over 3 years in the rate of vertebral compression fractures. Bone turnover increases to previous levels after 6 to 9 months when the patient takes alendronate for 6 months and then stops. If the patient takes alendronate for 6 years, no decrease in bone mass is noted for 2 years after therapy stops. These drugs have been used successfully for prevention and treatment of decreased bone mass as a result of long-term use of glucocorticoids.

In large, randomized, controlled trials, alendronate showed consistent increases in BMD irrespective of the severity of the underlying bone density levels, and it reduced the incidence of both vertebral and nonvertebral fractures (Cummings et al., 1998; Liberman et al., 1995). Among women

with osteoporosis, the incidence of symptomatic vertebral fractures was decreased by 44% over 4 years and clinical fractures were reduced by 36% (Cummings et al., 1998). Risedronate similarly reduced the incidence of vertebral fractures by 41% over 3 years (Harris et al., 1999) and reduced hip fractures by 40% in older women who had low BMD but not in women who had risk factors alone (McClung et al., 2001).

Dosage

The dosage for alendronate is 5 mg/d for prevention or 35 mg once a week for postmenopausal women. It has been approved for treatment in postmenopausal women and men at 10 mg/d or 70 mg once a week +/- vitamin D (2,800 IU or 5.600 IU). It has also been approved at 5 mg/d for men/women taking glucocorticoids and 10 mg/d for postmenopausal women not on hormone therapy. The dosage for ibandronate is 150 mg once a month or 3 mg/3 mL solution for intravenous (IV) use every 3 months. Zoledronic acid is an IV medication given once a year. The dose is 5 mg/100 mL. The dosage for treatment with risedronate is 5 mg/d (or 35 mg once a week) or 75 mg on 2 consecutive days each month (or 150 mg monthly); it has been approved at 5 mg/d or 35 mg once a week for prevention. It has also been approved at 5 mg/d for men/women taking glucocorticoids.

Dose Administration and Patient Education

Intestinal absorption of the alendronate and ibandronate is poor, so patients should take it on awakening with 8 oz of water and 30 minutes before consuming any food or other drink. If taken weekly or monthly, it should be taken on the same day each week or month. These medications must be taken while sitting

TABLE 33.1

Overview of Selected Agents Used to Prevent or Treat Osteoporosis

Generic (Trade) Name and Dosage		Selected Adverse Events	Contraindications	Special Considerations
Bisphosphonates				
Alendronate ± D (Fosamax ± D) effervescent tablets (Binosto)		GI disturbance, hypocalcemia, hypophosphatemia, esophagitis, diarrhea, abdominal and musculoskeletal pain	Esophageal abnormalities, inability to be upright for 30 min, hypocalcemia, CrCl < 35 mL/min	Swallow whole. Take with 8 oz of water 30 min before eating or drinking (do not lie down until after eating) Calcium supplements and aluminum- or magnesium-containing antacids may interfere with absorption, so it should be given at different times.
Prevention	PO: 5 mg/d or 35 mg/wk			
Treatment	PO: 10 mg/d or 70 mg/wk ± vit D3 2,800 or 5,600 IU/wk			
Glucocorticoid-induced osteoporosis:	PO: 5 mg/d or 10 mg/d (women not on hormonal therapy)			
Risedronate (Actonel, Atelvia)			Esophageal abnormalities, inability to be upright for 30 min, hypocalcemia, CrCl < 30 mL/min	Risedronate is more tolerable for patients with GI problems than alendronate. If taken monthly, take the same day each month. IV medications are given over at least 15 min.
Prevention	PO: 5 mg/d, 35 mg/wk			
Treatment	PO: 5 mg/d, 35 mg/wk, 75 mg 2 d/mo, 150 mg/mo			
Glucocorticoid-induced osteoporosis:	PO: 5 mg/d			
Ibandronate (Boniva)			Esophageal abnormalities, inability to be upright for 60 min, hypocalcemia	
Prevention	PO: 150 mg/mo			
Treatment	PO: 150 mg/mo IV: 3 mg/3 mL q3mo			
Zoledronic acid (Reclast)				
Prevention	IV: 5 mg/100 mL q2yrs		Hypocalcemia, CrCl < 35 mL/min or acute renal impairment	
Treatment	IV: 5 mg/100 mL every year			
Glucocorticoid-induced osteoporosis:	IV: 5 mg/100 mL every year			
Calcitonin (Miacalcin)				
Treatment	IN: 200 units/d SC/IM: 100 units/d (women > 5 yr post menopause)	Rhinitis, GI upset, arthralgia, facial flushing (with injection)	Allergy to calcitonin-salmon	Perform periodic nasal examination to check for ulceration. Switch nostrils each day. Injection recommended at bedtime because of possible facial flushing and nausea.

TABLE 33.1

Overview of Selected Agents Used to Prevent or Treat Osteoporosis (Continued)

Generic (Trade) Name and Dosage		Selected Adverse Events	Contraindications	Special Considerations
Selective Estrogen Receptor Modulators				
Raloxifene (Evista)		Hot flashes, leg cramps, deep vein thrombosis, arthralgias	Lactation or pregnancy, thromboembolic events (active or past history)	Separate raloxifene and levothyroxine by several hours as it can inhibit levothyroxine absorption.
Prevention	PO: 60 mg/d			Discontinue raloxifene 72 hours before prolonged immobilization.
Treatment	PO: 60 mg/d			
Conjugated estrogens/bazedoxifene (Duavee)		Nausea, diarrhea, abdominal pain, dyspepsia, muscle spasms	Conjugated estrogens/bazedoxifene is also contraindicated in women with endometrial/breast cancer, patients with dementia, and patients taking other estrogens	
Prevention	PO: (0.45/20 mg)/d (women with uterus)			
PTH and PTH-Related Protein Analog				
Teriparatide (Forteo)		Increased calcium levels and risk of digoxin toxicity with teriparatide	Paget's disease, children, previous bone radiation therapy, history of skeletal malignancy, metabolic bone disease, hypercalcemia, hyperparathyroidism	Rotate injection sites (thigh or abdomen area).
Treatment	SC: 20 mcg/d			Sit or lie down for first doses.
Glucocorticoid-induced osteoporosis	SC: 20 mcg/d	Dizziness, nausea, leg cramps, arthralgia, hyperuricemia		Treatment for > 18–24 months is not recommended for both agents.
Abaloparatide (Tymlos)				
Treatment	SC: 80 mcg/d			
Sclerostin Inhibitor				
Romosozumab-aqqg (Evenity)		Arthralgia, headache, injection site reactions, muscle spasms, peripheral edema	Hypocalcemia	Must be administered by health care professional.
Treatment	SC: 210 mg q/mo for 12 mo			Rotate injection sites (abdomen, thigh, upper arm).
				Treatment for >12 months is not recommended.
RANK Ligand Inhibitor				
Denosumab (Prolia)		Musculoskeletal pain, skin infection, arthralgia, myalgia, abdominal pain	Pregnancy, hypocalcemia	Must be administered by a health care professional.
Treatment	SC: 60 mg q6mo			
Glucocorticoid-induced osteoporosis	SC: 60 mg q6mo			

GI, gastrointestinal PTH, parathyroid hormone.

TABLE 33.2

Overview of Selected Agents Based on Indication and Gender

	Prevention	Treatment	Glucocorticoid-Induced Osteoporosis
Postmenopausal Women	Alendronate PO 5 mg/d Alendronate PO 35 mg/wk Risedronate PO 5 mg/d Risedronate PO 35 mg/wk Ibandronate PO 150 mg/mo Zoledronic Acid IV 5 mg/100 mL q2yr Raloxifene PO 60 mg/d Conjugated Estrogens/bazedoxifene PO (0.45/20 mg)/d (women with uterus)	Alendronate PO 10 mg/d Alendronate PO 70 mg/wk Alendronate PO 70 mg + vit D 2,800 or 5,600 IU/wk Risedronate PO 5 mg/d Risedronate PO 35 mg/wk Risedronate PO 75 mg 2 d/mo Risedronate PO 150 mg/mo Ibandronate PO 150 mg/mo Ibandronate IV 3 mg/3 mL q3mo Zoledronic Acid IV 5 mg/100 mL q/yr Calcitonin IN 200 units/d or calcitonin SC/IM 100 units/d (women > 5 yr post menopause) Raloxifene PO 60 mg/d Teriparatide SC 20 mcg/d Abaloparatide SC 80 mcg/d Romosozumab-aqqg SC 210 mg q/mo for 12 mo Denosumab SC 60 mg q6mo	Alendronate PO 5 mg/d Alendronate PO 10 mg/d (women not on estrogen) Risedronate PO 5 mg/d Zoledronic acid IV 5 mg/100 mL q/yr Teriparatide SC 20 mcg/d Denosumab SC 60 mg q6mo
Men		Alendronate 10 mg/d Alendronate 70 mg/wk Alendronate 70 mg + vit D 2,800 IU/wk Alendronate 70 mg + vit D 5,600 IU/wk Risedronate 35 mg/wk Zoledronic acid 5 mg/100 mL IV q/yr Teriparatide SC 20 mcg/d Denosumab SC 60 mg q6mo	Alendronate PO 5 mg/d Risedronate PO 5 mg/d Zoledronic acid IV 5 mg q/yr Teriparatide SC 20 mcg/d Denosumab SC 60 mg q6mo

up or standing and staying upright for at least 30 minutes after (60 minutes with monthly ibandronate [Boniva]).

Alendronate effervescent tablets (Binosto) must be dissolved in 4 oz of room temperature water; the patient needs to wait 5 minutes for the medication to dissolve and then stir for 10 seconds before taking on an empty stomach.

Risedronate (Atelvia), delayed-release alendronate, must be taken after breakfast with 4 oz of water; the patient should remain upright for 30 minutes. As it requires acidic gut for absorption, the patient should avoid histamine 2 receptor antagonists (H2RAs) and proton-pump inhibitors (PPIs) completely.

Separate supplements or antacids, which contain calcium, iron, or magnesium, from oral bisphosphonates by at least 2 hours

The prefilled syringe of ibandronate is given IV over 15 to 30 seconds.

Zoledronic acid 5 mg/100 mL is infused IV over at least 15 minutes, and patients should be well hydrated and may be pretreated with acetaminophen to reduce the risk of acute phase reaction.

Warnings and Contraindications

Bisphosphonates affect the renal function and are contraindicated in patients with CrCl < 35 mL/min for alendronate and zoledronic acid (CrCl < 30 mL/min for risedronate) or patients with evidence of acute renal impairment.

Osteonecrosis of the jaw (ONJ) has been reported with long-term use of bisphosphonates, and risk appears to increase when patients are treated for more than 5 years.

Atypical femur fractures with long-term (>5 years) bisphosphonate use have been reported.

Esophagitis, esophageal ulcers, erosions, stricture, or perforation may happen with improper administration of oral bisphosphonates, and injectable bisphosphonates are preferred if esophagitis is present.

Bisphosphonates are contraindicated in patients with abnormalities of the esophagus, with difficulty swallowing or at high risk of aspiration, with an inability to stand or sit upright for at least 30 minutes (60 minutes for ibandronate), and with hypocalcemia.

Adverse Events

Adverse events include gastrointestinal (GI) disturbance, hypocalcemia and hypophosphatemia, esophagitis, diarrhea, and abdominal and musculoskeletal pain.

Calcitonin

Salmon calcitonin (Miacalcin, Fortical) is another drug used in treating osteoporosis.

Mechanism of Action

Calcitonin works by directly inhibiting osteoclast bone resorption. It is available in injectable form and as a nasal spray. It is FDA approved for treatment of osteoporosis in postmenopausal women (at least 5 years post menopause) when alternative treatment is not suitable. The intranasal (IN) spray has not been shown to be effective in increasing BMD in the early postmenopausal periods. In one study of postmenopausal women who used calcitonin daily, new vertebral fractures were decreased by 33% compared with placebo, though only a small increase was noted in BMD (Chesnut et al., 2000). Continuous therapy needs to be reevaluated periodically due to an association between calcitonin use and malignancy.

Dosage

The IN dosage of calcitonin is 1 spray (200 units) in one nostril daily. The injectable dosage is 100 U subcutaneously (SC) or intramuscularly (IM) each day.

Dose Administration and Patient Education

Keep unused bottles in the refrigerator; opened bottles may be kept at room temperature for 30 days.

Prime the new bottle by releasing at least 5 sprays and alternate nostrils each day with IN calcitonin. The nasal mucosa should be inspected every 6 months for ulceration. Patients should perform injections at bedtime because facial flushing and nausea may occur.

Warnings

Hypocalcemia, increased risk of malignancy with long-term use, or hypersensitivity reactions may occur.

Adverse Events

With both inhalation and injection, myalgia, nausea, dizziness, and back pain may occur. Rhinitis, epistaxis, and allergic reactions have been reported with the use of IN calcitonin. Injection can cause local irritation, flushing, and injection site reactions.

Selective Estrogen Receptor Modulator

Raloxifene (Evista) is a selective estrogen receptor modulator (SERM) or estrogen agonist/antagonist that is indicated for treating and preventing osteoporosis and reducing risk of breast cancer in postmenopausal women with osteoporosis. Raloxifene has been shown to reduce the risk of vertebral fractures but does not appear to have an effect on hip fractures.

Conjugated estrogens/bazedoxifene (Duavee) is indicated for prevention in postmenopausal women with a uterus and has shown increase in lumbar spine and total hip BMD in postmenopausal woman 1 to 5 years post menopause.

Mechanism of Action

SERMs mimic the effects of estrogen on bones without replicating the stimulating effects of estrogen on the breasts and uterus. They decrease bone resorption and bone turnover. Conjugated estrogens are combined with bazedoxifene (an equine/horse estrogen agonist/antagonist), which reduces the risk of endometrial hyperplasia from estrogens.

Dosage

The dose of raloxifene (Evista) is 60 mg/d for treatment and prevention in postmenopausal women. Conjugated estrogens/bazedoxifene (Duavee)'s dose is 1 tablet (0.45/20 mg) daily for prevention in postmenopausal women with a uterus.

Dose Administration and Patient Education

Take raloxifene and conjugated estrogens/bazedoxifene without regard to food.

Separate raloxifene from levothyroxine by several hours as raloxifene can inhibit levothyroxine absorption.

The patient must discontinue raloxifene 72 hours before prolonged immobilization, such as surgery requiring bed rest.

Warnings and Contraindications

Raloxifene and conjugated estrogens/bazedoxifene are contraindicated in women who are lactating or who may become pregnant. They are also contraindicated in women who have a history of thromboembolic events, as a black box warning exists for increased risk of deep vein thrombosis (DVT, pulmonary embolism [PE]) events and death due to stroke similar to that of estrogens.

Conjugated estrogens/bazedoxifene is also contraindicated in women with endometrial and breast cancer (from use of unopposed estrogen in women with a uterus), patients with dementia (not recommended for patients >75 years of age), and those using additional estrogens.

Adverse Events

Adverse events of raloxifene include hot flashes, peripheral edema, flu-like symptoms, leg cramps, DVT, and arthralgias.

Adverse effects of conjugated estrogens/bazedoxifene include nausea, diarrhea, abdominal pain, dyspepsia, and muscle spasms.

Parathyroid Hormone and Parathyroid Hormone-Related Protein Analog

PTH (1-34) analog teriparatide (Forteo) and PTH-related protein analog abaloparatide (Tymlos) are indicated for treatment in postmenopausal women and men (teriparatide only) at high risk of fractures or those who have failed to respond to or who are intolerant of other therapies. Teriparatide is also indicated in glucocorticoid-induced osteoporosis.

Mechanism of Action

PTH is the primary regulator of calcium and phosphate metabolism and regulates bone metabolism, renal tubular reabsorption of calcium and phosphates, and intestinal calcium absorption. It stimulates new bone formation in trabecular and cortical bone surface by preferential stimulation of osteoblastic activity over osteoclastic activity. This causes an increase in skeletal mass and an increase in markers of bone formation and resorption and bone strength.

A study showed that women using teriparatide had an increased density of the spine of 10% to 14% and of the hip of 5%. In 18 months, vertebral fractures were reduced by 60% to 70% and nonvertebral fractures by 55% (Dempster et al., 2001). It has been shown that teriparatide can prevent back pain in women with osteoporosis for up to 18 months beyond the end of treatment.

Dosage

Teriparatide is administered SC at a dosage of 20 mcg daily, whereas abaloparatide is administered at 80 mcg SC daily.

Dose Administration and Patient Education

Inject into thigh or abdomen area; injection sites must be rotated. Sit or lie down for first doses.

Bone loss can be rapid with discontinuation of treatment; alternative agents should be used (usually a bisphosphonate) to maintain BMD levels.

Keep refrigerated and protect from light and discard pen after up to 30 days from starting.

Warnings and Contraindications

Teriparatide and abaloparatide are contraindicated in the following populations: patients with Paget's disease, children, and patients with previous bone radiation therapy, a history of skeletal malignancy (increased risk of osteosarcoma in rat studies), metabolic bone disease, hypercalcemia (which is usually transient), and hyperparathyroidism. They should be used cautiously in patients with a history of kidney stones. Treatment for >18 months is not recommended for both agents.

Adverse Events

Common adverse events include dizziness, nausea, leg cramps, arthralgia, and hyperuricemia. Teriparatide may increase calcium levels and increase the risk of digoxin toxicity.

Sclerostin Inhibitor

Romosozumab-aqqg (Evenity) is indicated in treatment of postmenopausal women at high risk of fractures or those who have failed to respond to or who are intolerant of other therapies.

Mechanism of Action

IgG2, a monoclonal antibody, binds to sclerostin a regulatory factor in bone metabolism. When sclerostin inhibition occurs, there is an increase in bone formation and a decrease in bone resorption. Romosozumab-aqqg has shown to stimulate new bone formation by stimulating osteoblasts' activity, resulting in increased bone mass and strength.

Dosage

The dosage is 210 mg SC every month for 12 months.

Dose Administration and Patient Education

Romosozumab-aqqg must be administered by a health care professional (2 prefilled syringes for a total dose of 210 mg) into the abdomen, thigh, or upper arm; the injection site should be rotated.

It should be kept refrigerated and not be shaken; it should be used within 30 days from removal from refrigerator.

Warnings and Contraindications

It may increase risk of myocardial infarction (MI), stroke, and cardiovascular (CV) death; do not initiate in patients who have had a stroke or MI within a year. It is contraindicated in women who are lactating or who may become pregnant. Hypocalcemia (must be corrected prior to initiation) and systemic hypersensitivity (e.g., angioedema, rash, urticaria) may occur. Atypical femur fractures and ONJ have been reported. Treatment for >12 months is not recommended.

Adverse Events

Common adverse effects include arthralgia, headache, injection site reactions, muscle spasms, and peripheral edema.

RANK Ligand Inhibitor

Denosumab (Prolia) is a RANK ligand inhibitor.

Mechanism of Action

In postmenopausal osteoporosis, decreased estrogen leads to increased RANK ligand, an essential mediator of osteoclast activity. Denosumab is a monoclonal antibody that binds to the RANK ligand and blocks its interaction with RANK to prevent osteoclast formation (which increases bone loss and fracture risk), thus preventing bone resorption. It has been shown to reduce incidence of vertebral, nonvertebral, and hip fractures. Denosumab is indicated in treatment of postmenopausal women and men. It is also indicated in treatment of glucocorticoid-induced osteoporosis in men and women at high risk of fracture, treatment of bone loss in men receiving androgen deprivation therapy for prostate cancer, and treatment in women receiving aromatase inhibitor therapy for breast cancer.

Dosage

The dosage is 60 mg SC every 6 months.

Dose Administration and Patient Education

It must be administered by a health care professional.

Bone loss can be rapid with discontinuation of treatment; alternative agents should be used (usually a bisphosphonate) to maintain BMD levels.

Keep refrigerated and protect from light; use within 14 days of removal from the refrigerator.

Warnings and Contraindications

Denosumab is contraindicated in pregnancy and hypocalcemia. Caution is necessary in patients with CrCl < 30 mL/min and those predisposed to hypocalcemia. Increased risks of skin infections and dermatologic reactions (skin rash) have been reported with denosumab use, as well as atypical femur fractures and ONJ when used to treat patients with cancer at higher doses.

Adverse Events

Denosumab can cause musculoskeletal pain, fatigue, hypophosphatemia, dyspnea, nausea, diarrhea, and headache.

MONITORING PATIENT RESPONSE

It is important to assess the patient's compliance to the prescribed medications and to encourage continuous compliance with fall prevention, lifestyle modifications, and adequate calcium and vitamin D intake in order to help reduce risk of fractures. Follow-up is recommended 1 to 2 months after the start of therapy and then every 3 to 6 months if the patient has osteoporosis. Patients should be assessed at least annually on the need for continued pharmacologic treatments for the treatment of osteoporosis. The DEXA scan should be repeated every 2 years. Measurement of the density of the proximal femur is most helpful in predicting fractures, and measurement of the density of the lumbar spine is most effective in measuring the response to therapy. Within 2 years, resorption-inhibiting drugs increase the BMD of the lumbar spine by 5% to 10% in women with postmenopausal osteoporosis, causing the incidence of fractures to decrease by 50% (Cummings et al., 1998; Melton et al., 1993).

Even if the medication is stopped, its positive effects can persist. That's because after taking a bisphosphonate for a period of time, the medicine remains in your bone. Because of this lingering effect, experts believe that it is reasonable for people who are doing well during treatment—those who have not broken any bones and are maintaining bone density—to consider taking a holiday from bisphosphonate after taking it for 5 years.

INFORMATION ACCESS FOR PATIENTS

Information about osteoporosis can be obtained from the NOF Web site (http://www.nof.org) or the National Institutes of Health Osteoporosis and Related Bone Disease National Resource Center (http://www.osteo.org).

CASE STUDY 1

J.D., a 72-year-old woman of Asian descent, has just transferred to your practice. She is 5 ft 2 in. tall and weighs 102 lb. She is diabetic and has a sedentary lifestyle (she was a secretary and retired 2 years ago) and has not had any previous fractures. She drinks 4 glasses of wine a day. Her mother died at age 62 from complications of a hip fracture. J.D. tells you that she takes aspirin, atorvastatin, and Lantus. You prescribe a dual-energy x-ray absorptiometry scan, and the T-score is –2.6.

DIAGNOSIS: OSTEOPOROSIS

1. List some of the risk factors for J.D.
2. What drug therapy would you prescribe? Why?
3. Discuss specific patient education based on the prescribed therapy.
4. What are some lifestyle modifications that you can recommend for J.D.?

Bibliography

Starred references are cited in the text.

Bolland, M. J., Grey, A., & Reid, I. R. (2013). Calcium supplements and cardiovascular risk: 5 years on. *Therapeutic Advances in Drug Safety, 4*(5), 199–210.

Camacho, P. M., Petak, S. M., Binkley, N., et al. (2020). American Association of Clinical Endocrinologists/American College of Endocrinology clinical practice guidelines for the diagnosis and treatment of postmenopausal osteoporosis-2020 update Executive Summary. *Endocrine Practice, 26*(5), 564–570.

*Chesnut, C. H., III, Silverman, S., Andriano, K., et al. (2000). A randomized trial of nasal spray salmon calcitonin in postmenopausal women with established osteoporosis: The Prevent Recurrence of Osteoporotic Fractures Study. PROOF Study Group. *American Journal of Medicine, 109*, 267–276.

Cosman, F., de Beur, S. J., LeBoff, M. S., et al. (2014). Clinician's guide to prevention and treatment of osteoporosis. *Osteoporosis International, 25*, 2359–2381.

*Cummings, S. R., Black, D. M., Thompson, D. E., et al. (1998). Effect of alendronate on risk of fracture in women with low bone density but without vertebral fractures: Results from the Fracture Intervention Trial. *Journal of American Medical Association, 280*, 2077–2082.

*Dempster, D. W., Cosman, F., & Kurland, E. S. (2001). Effects of daily treatment with parathyroid hormone on bone microarchitecture and turnover in patients with osteoporosis: A paired biopsy study. *Journal of Bone and Mineral Research, 16*, 1846–1853.

Eastell, R., Rosen, C. J., Black, D. M., et al. (2019). Pharmacological management of osteoporosis in postmenopausal women: An endocrine society clinical practice guideline. *Journal of Clinical Endocrinology and Metabolism, 104*(5), 1595–1622.

Föger-Samwald, U., Dovjak, P., Azizi-Semrad, U., Kerschan-Schindl, K., & Pietschmann, P. (2020). Osteoporosis: Pathophysiology and therapeutic options. *EXCLI Journal, 19*, 1017–1037.

*Harris, S. T., Watts, N. B., Genant, H. K., et al. (1999). Effects of risedronate treatment on vertebral and nonvertebral fractures in women with postmenopausal osteoporosis: A randomized controlled trial. Vertebral Efficacy with Risedronate Therapy (VERT) Study Group. *Journal of American Medical Association, 282*, 1344–1352.

*Liberman, U. A., Weiss, S. R., Broll, J., et al. (1995). Effect of oral alendronate on bone mineral density and the incidence of fractures in postmenopausal osteoporosis. The Alendronate Phase III Osteoporosis Treatment Study Group. *New England Journal of Medicine, 333*, 1437–1443.

*McClung, M. R., Geusens, P., Miller, P. D., et al. (2001). Effect of risedronate on the risk of hip fracture in elderly women. *New England Journal of Medicine, 344*, 333–340.

*Melton, L. J., Atkinson, E. J., O'Fallon, W. M., et al. (1993). Long-term fracture prediction by bone mineral assesses at different skeletal sites. *Journal of Bone and Mineral Research, 8*, 1227–1233.

*National Osteoporosis Foundation. (2021, April 12). Learn what osteoporosis is and what it's caused by. Retrieved from www.nof.org/patients/what-is-osteoporosis/

Nelson, H. D. (2014). Osteoporosis. In H. Sloane, et al., (Eds.), *Ham's primary care geriatrics* (pp. 445–455). Philadelphia, PA: W.B. Saunders.

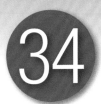

34 Rheumatoid Arthritis

Lauren K. McCluggage and Kelsey C. Haines

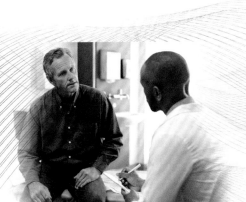
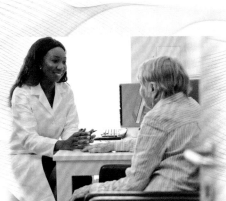
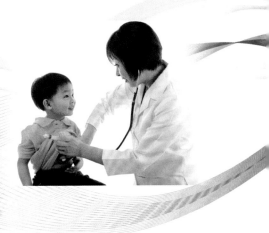

Learning Objectives

1. Discuss the causes and pathophysiology of rheumatoid arthritis.
2. Identify criteria for diagnosis of rheumatoid arthritis.
3. Describe the goals and overall treatment algorithms for patients with rheumatoid arthritis.
4. Describe the characteristics of medications used to treat rheumatoid arthritis.
5. Explain how rheumatoid arthritis treatment should be modified in special populations.

INTRODUCTION

Rheumatoid arthritis (RA) is a chronic autoimmune inflammatory disease characterized by symmetric polyarthritis and joint changes including erythema, effusion, and tenderness. The course of RA is characterized by remissions and exacerbations. RA can affect several organs, but it usually involves synovial tissue changes in the freely movable joints (diarthroses). RA most commonly affects small joints, including the wrists, second through fifth metatarsophalangeal joints, proximal interphalangeal joints, and metacarpophalangeal joints. RA may also affect large joints, including the elbows, shoulders, neck, hips, knees, and ankles.

In 2014, approximately 1.3 million adults in the United States had RA, with the prevalence in women more than twice that of men (Hunter et al., 2017). RA can be diagnosed at any age, including infancy, but most cases occur in the fifth or sixth decade of life. Previous data have shown that patients with RA have a higher rate of disability and mortality compared to patients of similar age without RA. However, with the increased use of disease-modifying antirheumatic drugs (DMARDs), especially early in the disease process, many patients are able to achieve remission or low disease activity.

CAUSES

The cause of RA continues to be the subject of research. Theories of causation include genetic factors, infectious agents, environmental factors, and an antigen–antibody response. It is unlikely that a single factor is responsible for all cases of RA.

PATHOPHYSIOLOGY

The major physiologic changes associated with RA include synovial membrane proliferation followed by erosion of the subarticular cartilage and subchondral bone. Although the precise etiology of RA is unknown, mounting evidence points to a series of immunologic events. It is unclear whether an infectious, viral, or genetic agent prompts these events.

Specific major histocompatibility complex class II alleles and human leukocyte antigen are seen more frequently in patients with RA. These molecules are responsible for processing and presenting antigenic material to CD4$^+$ T cells. The exact antigen that initiates the following cascade is unknown but could be an exogenous or endogenous protein. T-cell activation stimulates monocytes, macrophages, and synovial fibroblasts to produce proinflammatory cytokines, including tumor necrosis factor (TNF) alpha, interleukin (IL)-1, and IL-6. During this process, matrix metalloproteinases are also released, causing major destruction in the joint cartilage. The activated T cells stimulate B cells, which then produce immunoglobulins, including rheumatoid factor (RF) and anticitrullinated protein antibody (ACPA). The activation of the macrophages, monocytes, and synovial fibroblasts along with the release of cytokines stimulates angiogenesis in the synovial membrane. TNF-alpha is a key inflammatory mediator because it induces further production of proinflammatory-cytokines and stimulates expression of adhesion molecules on endothelial cells. The expression of adhesion molecules promotes recruitment of leukocytes and more inflammatory cells. The result is a self-perpetuating inflammatory cycle.

Early Phase

In the early phase of RA, the synovium becomes more vascularized, and proliferation and hypertrophy begin. This results in the synovial tissue becoming edematous and exhibiting frond-like villi. As leukocytes proliferate, the synovial fluid becomes less viscous.

Progression

As RA progresses to the chronic form, continued hyperplasia and hypertrophy of the synovial lining occur. The thickness of the synovial lining increases up to fivefold from the normal one or two cell layers. The proliferation of the synovium persists, with lymphocytic tissue and plasma cells forming around blood vessels. This proliferative tissue extends into the joint space, joint capsule, ligaments, and tendons.

Severe, Chronic Rheumatoid Arthritis

In severe RA, pannus forms as a result of the release of lysosomal enzymes. Pannus is granulation tissue composed of lymphocytes, plasma cells, fibroblasts, and macrophages. Growing much like a tumor, pannus can invade the cartilage, activate chondrocytes, and release enzymes that can degrade cartilage and bone. This destructive process begins at the synovium and extends to the unprotected area at the junction of the cartilage and subchondral bone. These inflammatory cells can erode surrounding tissue, tendons, and cartilage. When pannus invades the joint margins, decreased range of motion and ankylosis may ensue. Pannus is a specific feature of RA, differentiating it from other forms of arthritis.

DIAGNOSTIC CRITERIA

In 2010, the American College of Rheumatology (ACR) and the European League Against Rheumatism (EULAR) collaborated on defining classification criteria for RA (**Table 34.1**). The goal of the criteria is to identify patients early who have a high probability of persistent RA and in whom early treatment would be beneficial. The emphasis of the classification criteria is on new patients with synovitis not explained by other conditions. Components of these criteria include joint involvement,

serologic testing, acute phase reactants, and duration of symptoms. Patients that score 6 or higher are classified as having RA, but a lower score does not exclude diagnosis.

The serology test can be either RF or ACPA, and the acute phase reactant test can be either erythrocyte sedimentation rate (ESR) or C-reactive protein (CRP). For serology tests, results are divided into three categories: negative, low positive (above normal but less than three times the upper limit of normal [ULN]), or high positive (greater than three times the ULN). The acute phase reactants are either normal or abnormal. None of these tests alone are sufficient to diagnose RA, but each is a component of diagnosis.

Other classic symptoms experienced by patients with RA include morning stiffness in involved joints persisting for at least 1 hour and subsiding with activity, symmetric joint involvement, and painful, swollen joints. Although RA characteristically affects joint structures, it is a systemic disease with potential extra-articular manifestations. Throughout the disease, the patient also may have generalized symptoms such as weakness, fatigue, mild fever, anorexia, and weight loss. End-organ involvement may occur in patients with high RF titers.

The most common extra-articular manifestation of RA is joint nodules. These occur in 15% to 20% of patients with RA and are most commonly seen in patients with erosive disease. These subcutaneous nodules may develop in any area of the body exposed to pressure. Some of these areas are the olecranon bursa, knuckles, ischial spines, Achilles tendon, extensor surfaces of the forearm, and the bridge of the nose (in patients who wear glasses). These nodules may also form internally on the heart, lungs, and intestinal tract. The nodules are firm and rubbery, occur in clusters, and may be either freely mobile or attached to underlying connective tissue. The treatment of the nodules is confined to the treatment of the underlying disease. These nodules may occur in other connective tissue diseases (e.g., systemic lupus erythematosus), so alone they are not criteria for diagnosing RA.

An ocular manifestation of RA is sicca syndrome; patients have a sensation of grittiness in the eyes, accumulation of dried mucus, and decreased tear production. Scleritis and episcleritis are occasional sequelae of sicca syndrome. Additional extra-articular manifestations of RA include vasculitis, pulmonary fibrosis, and pericarditis.

INITIATING DRUG THERAPY

Physical and occupational therapies are considered mainstays of nonpharmacologic therapy in patients with RA. These therapies help protect the joints and maintain strength, function, and mobility. Reduction of joint stress is an additional goal of therapy. Patients should engage in activity to their fullest possible extent with adequate rest after activity, but they should avoid vigorous exercise and heavy labor during acute exacerbations of the disease. Hydrotherapy and hot and cold packs may be used to relax muscle spasms and facilitate joint movement. Warm showers and paraffin treatments may help relieve morning stiffness.

TABLE 34.1

2010 American College of Rheumatology/European League Against Rheumatism Classification Criteria for Rheumatoid Arthritis

	Score
Target population (Who should be tested?):	
1. Patients who have at least one joint with definite clinical synovitis (swelling)*	
2. Patients with synovitis not better explained by another disease[†]	
Classification criteria for RA (score-based algorithm: add score of categories A–D; a score ≥6/10 is needed for classification of a patient as having definite RA)[‡]	
A. Joint involvement[§]	
1 large joint[‖]	0
2–10 large joints	1
1–3 small joints[#]	2
4–10 small joints	3
>10 joints with at least 1 small joint**	5
B. Serology (at least one test is needed for classification)[††]	
Negative RF and negative ACPA	0
Low-positive RF or low-positive ACPA	2
High-positive RF or high-positive ACPA	3
C. Acute phase reactants (at least 1 test results is needed for classification)[‡‡]	
Normal CRP and ESR	0
Abnormal CRP or abnormal ESR	1
D. Duration of symptoms[§§]	
<6 wk	0
≥6 wk	1

*The criteria are aimed at classification of newly presenting patients. In addition, patients with erosive disease typical of RA with a history compatible with prior fulfillment of the 2010 criteria should be classified as having RA. Patients with long-standing disease, including those whose disease is inactive (with or without treatment) and who, based on retrospectively available data, have previously fulfilled the 2010 criteria, should be classified as having RA.

[†]Differential diagnosis varies among patients with different presentations but may include conditions such as systemic lupus erythematosus, psoriatic arthritis, and gout. If it is unclear about the relevant differential diagnoses to consider, an expert rheumatologist should be consulted.

[‡]Although patients with a score <6/10 are not classifiable as having RA, their status can be reassessed and the criteria might be fulfilled cumulatively over time.

[§]Joint involvement refers to any swollen or tender joint on examination, which may be confirmed by imaging evidence of synovitis. Distal interphalangeal joints, first carpometacarpal joints, and first metatarsophalangeal joints are excluded from assessment. Categories of joint distribution are classified according to the location and number of involved joints, with placement into the highest category possible based on the pattern of joint involvement.

[‖]Large joints refer to shoulders, elbows, hips, knees, and ankles.

[#]Small joints refer to metacarpophalangeal joints, proximal interphalangeal joints, second through fifth metatarsophalangeal joints, thumb interphalangeal joints, and wrists.

**In this category, at least one of the involved joints must be a small joint; the other joints can include any combination of large and additional small joints, as well as other joints not specifically listed elsewhere (e.g., temporomandibular, acromioclavicular, sternoclavicular, etc.).

[††]Negative refers to IU values that are less than or equal to the ULN for the laboratory and assay; low positive refers to IU values that are higher than the ULN but less than or equal to three times the ULN for the laboratory and assay; high positive refers to IU values that are greater than three times the ULN for the laboratory and assay. When RF is only available as positive or negative, a positive result should be scored as low positive for RF.

[‡‡]Normal/abnormal is determined by local laboratory standards.

[§§]Duration of symptoms refers to patient self-report of the duration of signs and symptoms of synovitis (e.g., pain, swelling, tenderness) of joints that are clinically involved at the time of assessment, regardless of treatment status.

ACPA, anticitrullinated protein antibody; CRP, C-reactive protein; ESR, erythrocyte sedimentation rate; RA, rheumatoid arthritis; RF, rheumatoid factor.

Source: Redrawn with permission from Aletaha, D., Neogi, T., Silman, A. J., et al. (2010). 2010 rheumatoid arthritis classification criteria. *Arthritis and Rheumatism, 62*(9), 2569–2581.

In 2012, the ACR updated their guidelines for the treatment of RA, and in 2019, the EULAR provided updated recommendations for the management of RA with synthetic and biological DMARDs (bDMARDs). Both organizations indicated the importance of starting patients on DMARDs as early in the disease process as possible. Evidence has shown that the earlier in the disease process that DMARDs are started, the greater the chance of reducing disability and disease progression. Ideally, patients should be started on DMARD therapy within 3 months of diagnosis. The use of nonsteroidal anti-inflammatory drugs (NSAIDs) can still be considered for symptom control, but these do not have disease-modifying characteristics.

Goals of Drug Therapy

The goals of drug therapy for RA include reducing pain, stiffness, and swelling; preserving mobility and joint function; and preventing further joint damage. Due to advancements in the treatment of RA, the ACR and EULAR now recommend treating to a goal of remission. If remission is not possible, it is recommended to aim for low disease activity. In 2011, the ACR and EULAR developed a definition for remission, which includes a swollen joint count, tender joint count, CRP level and patient global assessment of 1 or less each, or a simplified Disease Activity Score of 3.3 or less. Low disease activity can be assessed in a variety of ways via the Patient Activity Scale (0.28–3.7), Clinical Disease Activity Index (>2.8–10.0), Disease Activity Score in 28 joints (2.6–3.2), or the simplified Disease Activity Index (>3.3–11).

Nonsteroidal Anti-Inflammatory Drugs

NSAIDs are typically used to help relieve immediate pain and improve symptoms during the diagnostic process. These agents are continued through the initiation of a DMARD to maintain reduced symptoms. This approach allows NSAIDs to exert their anti-inflammatory action while the DMARD takes effect. See the discussion of NSAIDs in Chapter 32 Osteoarthritis and Gout (**Table 32.1**).

Corticosteroids

Low-dose corticosteroids (≤prednisone 10 mg or equivalent) are beneficial in patients who are beginning DMARD therapy. Because the therapeutic effect of DMARDs may not be seen until several weeks to months after initiating therapy, corticosteroids may be used to provide almost immediate symptom relief and bridge patients until DMARDs take effect. Higher doses of corticosteroids can also be beneficial in acute flares to regain control of inflammation and pain. In either circumstance, corticosteroids should be tapered off as soon as possible.

Injectable corticosteroids can be used if symptoms are restricted to one or two joints that have not responded to first-line treatment. They may also be of limited benefit for acute flare-ups of RA.

The most common adverse events of corticosteroid therapy include restlessness, insomnia, weight gain, and cutaneous atrophy. Less common adverse events include myopathy, hypothalamic–pituitary–adrenal axis dysfunction, glaucoma, and osteoporosis. Osteoporosis may be avoided by taking a calcium supplement (1,500 mg/d) along with vitamin D (800 mg/d).

Disease-Modifying Antirheumatic Drugs

As stated previously, the early use of DMARDs is advocated because of the high degree of inflammation that is present early in the disease (**Table 34.2**). Radiographic evidence of joint damage usually is present in the first year of the disease, and functional deterioration due to this damage may be irreversible. Therefore, early initiation of DMARD therapy may be the best course of action to take in meeting the long-range goals of treatment. DMARD therapy should be initiated within 3 months after onset of symptoms, if not immediately after diagnosis. There are several DMARDs to select from; the

TABLE 34.2

Overview of Selected Disease-Modifying Antirheumatic Drugs

Generic (Trade) Name and Dosage	Selected Adverse Events	Contraindications	Special Considerations
Preferred csDMARDs			
Methotrexate (Rheumatrex) 7.5 mg/wk in single dose, up to 25 mg/wk	GI effects, leukopenia, oral ulcers, thrombocytopenia, pulmonary toxicity, hepatotoxicity	Pregnancy and 1 mo before conception; caution in alcohol drinkers and liver disease	May take 3–8 wk to achieve clinical benefit; can induce spontaneous abortion and birth defects; monitoring includes CBC, serum creatinine, and liver function tests.
Sulfasalazine (Azulfidine) 1,000 mg/d in divided doses; may increase up to maximum 3 g/d	GI effects, heartburn, dizziness, headache, rash, neutropenia, thrombocytopenia	Contraindicated in intestinal or urinary obstruction as well as sulfa or salicylate allergy	May take 1–4 mo to achieve clinical effect; causes reversible sterility in men; recommend that men cease therapy 90 d before starting a family; monitoring includes liver enzyme evaluation; CBC is necessary early in therapy but required less with prolonged use.

TABLE 34.2

Overview of Selected Disease-Modifying Antirheumatic Drugs (*Continued*)

Generic (Trade) Name and Dosage	Selected Adverse Events	Contraindications	Special Considerations
Hydroxychloroquine (Plaquenil) 400–600 mg/d in divided doses	GI effects, rash, CNS effects, ocular effects	Contraindicated in patients with preexisting retinal field changes	Six months may be needed for clinical effect. Can trigger exacerbation of psoriasis; prolonged therapy may cause retinal damage. Monitoring should include periodic CBC and eye examinations.
Leflunomide (Arava) 100 mg PO daily for 3 d; 20 mg daily thereafter	Diarrhea, hair loss, weight loss, rash, infection	Pregnancy	If 20 mg daily is not tolerated, then 10 mg daily may be used. Long half-life; cholestyramine will enhance elimination if agent is to be discontinued.
Nonpreferred csDMARDs (removed from RA guidelines)			
D-Penicillamine (Depen, Cuprimine) 125 mg/d as single dose; may increase at monthly intervals to maximum daily dose of 1.5 g	GI effects, rash, itching, renal effects, autoimmune reactions, cytopenia	Not recommended in pregnancy or lactation—causes damage to fetal connective tissue	From 4 to 6 mo may be needed to establish clinical effect of therapy. Monitoring should include CBC with differential and platelets and urinalysis q2–6 wk.
Anakinra (Kineret) 100 mg SQ daily	Redness, swelling, bruising, or pain at the site of injection, headache, upset stomach, diarrhea, infection, rash	Sensitivity to *Escherichia coli*–derived proteins; preexisting infection	Routine monitoring of WBCs is recommended; concomitant immunosuppressants can increase risk of serious infection.
Azathioprine (Imuran) 50–100 mg in single daily dose; can increase after 6–8 wk; 3.5 mg/kg is maximum daily dose	GI effects, bone marrow suppression, infection, hepatotoxicity, alopecia	Renal disease; avoid during pregnancy and lactation	From 6 to 8 and up to 12 wk may be needed to establish clinical effect. Monitoring should include CBC with differential and platelets weekly for the first month, then biweekly for the second and third months, then monthly.
Cyclophosphamide (Cytoxan, Neosar) 1 mg/kg/d increased to 2 mg/kg/d after 6 wk	Alopecia, hemorrhagic cystitis, sterility, GI effects, increased susceptibility to infection, thrombocytopenia	Contraindicated for RA during pregnancy and lactation	In renal impairment, decrease dose. Four months may be needed to establish clinical effect. Monitoring includes CBC with differential, platelets, urinalysis for blood repeatedly, ESR, BUN, serum creatinine.
Cyclosporine A (Sandimmune, Neoral) 5 mg/kg/d divided into 2 doses	Hypertension, tremor, nephrotoxicity, hepatotoxicity, increased susceptibility to infection, hyperkalemia	Contraindicated for RA during pregnancy and lactation	Approximately 8 wk may be needed to establish clinical effect. Decrease dose by 50% if hypertension or nephrotoxicity results. Monitoring includes CBC with differential, BUN, serum creatinine, serum bilirubin, liver enzymes repeatedly.
Gold compounds *Injectable*: aurothioglucose (Solganal); gold sodium thiomalate (Myochrysine) 10 mg/wk IM, up to a total dose of 1 g; maintenance dose ~50 mg/mo *Oral*: auranofin (Ridaura) 3 mg BID	GI effects, rash, itching, stomatitis, vasomotor reactions, bone marrow suppression, nephritis, pneumonitis, exfoliative dermatitis, proteinuria	Uncontrolled diabetes; liver and renal disease, systemic lupus erythematosus, blood dyscrasias; lack of long-term studies in pregnant women, so not recommended during pregnancy or lactation	May take 6–8 wk for injectable form and 3–6 mo for oral form of drug to establish effectiveness. Monitoring includes routine CBC with differential, platelet count; urinalysis to measure protein; renal and liver function tests.

TABLE 34.2

Overview of Selected Disease-Modifying Antirheumatic Drugs (*Continued*)

Generic (Trade) Name and Dosage	Selected Adverse Events	Contraindications	Special Considerations
tsDMARD			
Tofacitinib (Xeljanz) 5 mg PO BID; baricitinib (Olumiant) 2 mg PO daily; upadacitinib (Rinvoq) 15 mg PO daily	Bone marrow suppression (lymphopenia, neutropenia, anemia), GI perforations, infections	Coadministration with strong CYP3A4 inducers, lymphocytes <500 cells/mm^3, ANC <1,000 cells/mm^3, Hgb< 8 g/dL	Not to be used in combination with bDMARDs. Dose adjustments for coadministration with CYP3A4 inhibitors and CYP2C19 inhibitors
Biologic DMARDs			
Etanercept (Enbrel) 25 mg SQ twice weekly or 50 mg SQ weekly	Upper respiratory tract infections, pain at the injection site, headache	Concurrent infections or hypersensitivity to medication	Use caution in patients predisposed to infection. Concomitant immunosuppressants can increase risk of serious infection.
Infliximab (Remicade) 3 mg/kg IV infusion at baseline, 2 wk, 6 wk, then q8wk thereafter	Urticaria, infusion reactions, dyspnea, hypotension	Same as mentioned earlier	Same as mentioned earlier
Adalimumab (Humira) 40 mg SQ every other week; 40 mg weekly as monotherapy	Redness, swelling, bruising, or pain at the site of injection, headache, upset stomach, diarrhea, infection, rash	Same as mentioned earlier	Same as mentioned earlier
Golimumab (Simponi) 50 mg SQ monthly in combination with methotrexate	Injection site reactions, infection, dizziness, antibody formation	Same as mentioned earlier	Same as mentioned earlier
Certolizumab pegol (Cimzia) 400 mg SQ at weeks 0, 2, and 4 then 200 mg every other week	Injection site reactions, headache, nausea, infection	Same as mentioned earlier	Same as mentioned earlier
Abatacept (Orencia) 500–1,000 mg (based on weight) IV at weeks 0, 2, and 4, and then q4 wk; 125 mg SQ weekly	COPD exacerbations, headache, hypertension, infusion reactions, infections, anaphylaxis	Hypersensitivity to abatacept; use caution in patients with history of infections or COPD.	Concomitant immunosuppressants increase risk of infection.
Tocilizumab (Actemra) 4–8 mg/kg IV q4wk; 162 mg SQ every other week—weekly (weight based); sarilumab (Kevzara) 200 mg SQ q2 wk	Increased LDL and transaminase, decreased WBC, infusion-related reactions	Untreated latent TB or hepatitis; ANC <2,000 cells/mm^3, low platelets, LFTs > 1.5x ULN	Monitoring includes CBC, lipid panel, and LFTs. It may take up to 3 months for symptomatic improvement.
Rituximab (Rituxan) 1,000 mg IV on days 1 and 15	Infusion reactions (may be severe)	Avoid in patients with hepatitis B or severe, active infection.	Give methylprednisolone prior to infusion.

ANC, absolute neutrophil count; BUN, blood urea nitrogen; CBC, complete blood count; CNS, central nervous system; COPD, chronic obstructive pulmonary disease; csDMARDs, conventional synthetic DMARDs; ESR, erythrocyte sedimentation rate; GI, gastrointestinal; IM, intramuscularly; IV, intravenous; LDL, low-density lipoprotein; LFTs, liver function tests; RA, rheumatoid arthritis; TB, tuberculosis; tsDMARD, targeted synthetic DMARDs; ULN, upper limit of normal; WBCs, white blood cell.

ones described here are the DMARDs currently recommended by the ACR and EULAR. Due to lack of data or high adverse events profile, cyclophosphamide, D-penicillamine, cyclosporine, azathioprine, gold compounds, and anakinra are not currently recommended for patients with RA.

Due to the development of new DMARDs, a modified nomenclature for the DMARDs has been developed. DMARDs are first divided into synthetic and biologic DMARDs. The synthetic DMARDs are then further divided in conventional synthetic DMARDs (csDMARDs) (methotrexate, leflunomide, sulfasalazine, hydroxychloroquine) and targeted synthetic DMARDs (tsDMARDs) (tofacitinib, baricitinib, and upadacitinib). Biologic DMARDs are also further divided into biologic originator DMARD (boDMARD) and biosimilar DMARD (bsDMARD).

Methotrexate

The most commonly prescribed DMARD is methotrexate. Unless contraindicated, methotrexate should be part of a patient's initial treatment plan.

Mechanism of Action

Methotrexate, a folic acid antagonist, is thought to affect leukocyte suppression, decreasing the inflammation that results from immunologic by-products. When treatment stops, exacerbation of symptoms may occur as early as 2 weeks after cessation.

Dosage

Methotrexate is available for oral, subcutaneous, and intramuscular use for the treatment of RA. It may also be given intravenously or intrathecally when used for oncologic indications. For most patients, a starting dose of 7.5 mg orally once per week is recommended. If a significant decrease in symptoms is not noted, the dose should be increased every few weeks to a maximal dose of 25 to 30 mg weekly. The patient needs to be on the maximal dose for at least 8 weeks before someone can be considered a methotrexate failure. Most patients respond to 12.5 to 15 mg per week. Injectable methotrexate may be used if there is an inadequate response to oral therapy or if the weekly dose needs to exceed 25 mg.

Time Frame for Response

Approximately 70% to 75% of patients respond favorably to methotrexate therapy, but it may take 3 to 8 weeks before improvement is noted. More than 50% of patients stay on the treatment for more than 5 years. However, if patients have difficulty tolerating side effects, methotrexate should be discontinued or the dosage should be lowered.

Contraindications

Methotrexate is contraindicated in pregnant and breastfeeding patients and those with leukopenia (white blood cell [WBC] count <3,000 cells/mm^3) and other blood dyscrasias. It is also not recommended in immunodeficiency syndromes, renal impairment (creatinine clearance <30 mL/min), and liver disease. Methotrexate has many black box warnings, including the risk of hepatotoxicity, renal impairment, pneumonitis, bone marrow suppression, diarrhea, ulcerative stomatitis, dermatologic reactions, and opportunistic infections. The ACR also lists acute serious bacterial infections, latent or active tuberculosis (TB), active fungal infections, active herpes zoster viral infection, platelets less than 50,000 cells/mm^3, treated lymphoproliferative disease within 5 years, and acute or chronic hepatitis B or C as contraindications to methotrexate therapy.

Adverse Events

The most commonly reported adverse events of methotrexate are nausea and abdominal pain. These effects may be minimized by switching to parenteral therapy. Oral ulcers, leukopenia, anemia, and thrombocytopenia are also common. However, these adverse reactions may be minimized by administering 1 to 5 mg of folic acid daily. Although methotrexate may inhibit folic acid metabolism, it does not seem to affect the efficacy of the therapy.

The most serious adverse event of therapy is liver toxicity, which occurs more frequently in patients with diabetes, obesity, alcohol use, and existing liver disease. Pneumonitis is another potentially serious side effect of therapy. A baseline chest x-ray may be obtained, and patients should be instructed to report the new onset of a dry cough, dyspnea, or fever. Methotrexate should be immediately discontinued if the patient has pulmonary problems because irreversible pulmonary damage may occur.

Baseline laboratory values should be obtained before initiation of therapy and should include a complete blood count (CBC), liver function tests, blood urea nitrogen (BUN), and serum creatinine. Screening for hepatitis B and C should also be done for high risk patients. During therapy, monitoring should occur every 2 to 4 weeks initially, followed by every 8 to 12 weeks for patients on methotrexate for 3 to 6 months, and every 12 weeks in patients on therapy for over 6 months. A transient yet marked increase in liver enzymes may be seen, with stabilization occurring with continued treatment or dose reduction. If liver enzymes persist at concentrations of two to three times the ULN, then methotrexate should be discontinued and a liver biopsy obtained.

Methotrexate has a black box warning that classifies the use of this agent as unsuitable due to the risk of fetal death or severe abnormalities and has implications for both males and females. Therefore, women who wish to conceive should stop taking methotrexate at least one ovulatory cycle before attempting to become pregnant. Men must discontinue methotrexate at least 3 months before trying to conceive. Men and women of childbearing age who are not sterilized should use a reliable form of contraception.

Interactions

Concurrent use with NSAIDs may increase the risk of bone marrow suppression and gastrointestinal (GI) toxicity. The combination should be avoided when taking moderate-to-high doses of methotrexate seen in oncologic indications and used cautiously with lower doses seen in the treatment of RA. Medications such as penicillins, tetracyclines, probenecid, and sulfonamides that compete with methotrexate for renal tubular secretion will enhance the effects of methotrexate and should be used cautiously. Methotrexate may increase the concentrations of mercaptopurine and theophylline. Concomitant use of cholestyramine decreases the absorption of methotrexate.

Sulfasalazine

Like methotrexate, sulfasalazine (Azulfidine) is an effective DMARD that relieves symptoms relatively quickly. It should be considered as initial treatment in patients with a contraindication or intolerance to methotrexate.

Mechanism of Action

Sulfasalazine's mechanism of action is not clearly understood but is thought to be due to its conversion to sulfapyridine and 5-acetylsalicylic acid in the gut. The sulfapyridine component is thought to be responsible for the disease-modifying activity. Research has shown the anti-inflammatory features of this conversion, as well as its ability to decrease inflammatory cytokine production.

Dosage

Sulfasalazine is available as 500-mg tablets. Dosing is started at 1,000 mg/d in two divided doses. The daily divided dose is gradually increased to 2,000 mg over 2 weeks. After 12 weeks of 2,000 mg daily, if the response is still not adequate, then the dose can be increased to 3,000 mg daily. Enteric-coated tablets are recommended for the treatment of RA to reduce the risk of GI-related adverse events.

Time Frame for Response

Patients may start to notice an effect as early as 1 month, but the full effect may take up to 4 months.

Contraindications

Due to its sulfa component, sulfasalazine is contraindicated in patients with a sulfonamide or salicylate allergy. Patients with a GI or genitourinary tract obstruction or those with porphyria should not use this medication. The ACR guidelines recommend avoiding use in patients with a platelet count of less than 50,000 cells/mm^3 or liver enzymes greater than two times the ULN, as well as in patients with hepatitis B or C infection resulting in Child-Pugh class B or C hepatic function.

Adverse Events

The most common adverse events to sulfasalazine are dose dependent and include nausea and diarrhea. Other reported adverse events include dizziness, intestinal or urinary obstruction, oral ulcers, thrombocytopenia, skin rash, and headache. Any of these common adverse events may become intolerable and cause discontinuation of the drug. Reversible sterility has been reported in men; therapy should be discontinued 3 months before attempting to father a child.

Agranulocytosis, the gravest adverse event to sulfasalazine, has been reported in fewer than 2% of patients, but it dictates immediate discontinuation. Before initiating sulfasalazine therapy, the practitioner should obtain baseline laboratory test values, including a CBC and liver enzymes. These values should be monitored every 2 to 4 weeks for the first 3 months after initiation of therapy and then every 8 to 12 weeks during months 3 to 6. If laboratory values remain stable for the first 6 months of therapy, a CBC should be checked every 3 months.

Interactions

The risk of bone marrow suppression will be enhanced if used with other suppressive agents such as azathioprine, methotrexate, or mercaptopurine, and additional monitoring is warranted. Sulfasalazine may increase the effects of oral anticoagulants; therefore, patients should be monitored closely if on concurrent therapy. Sulfasalazine may decrease the concentration of cyclosporine.

Antimalarials

The antimalarial agent's hydroxychloroquine (Plaquenil) and chloroquine are attractive because of their tolerable adverse event profile, with these medications being discontinued in fewer than 9% of patients. However, because they cannot limit the progression of RA, they are currently used as an adjunct to methotrexate therapy or as single-agent therapy in early, mild RA without bone erosion. Hydroxychloroquine is the preferred agent in this class.

Mechanism of Action

Antimalarials inhibit antigen processing by elevating cellular pH, which changes antigen degeneration. Thus, the presentation of the antigen to T cells is impaired.

Dosage

Hydroxychloroquine is available as tablets that are rapidly and completely absorbed. Dosing is calculated by patient weight, but the typical dosage for hydroxychloroquine is 200 to 400 mg daily as a single daily dose or two divided doses.

Time Frame for Response

Therapeutic effects are usually noted within 2 to 6 months of treatment.

Contraindications

Patients with preexisting retinal field changes should not use antimalarials due to the ocular effects of long-term therapy.

Adverse Events

The most common adverse events associated with antimalarials are nausea, diarrhea, and abdominal discomfort. Less common adverse events include photosensitivity and skin pigmentation changes. A maculopapular, pruritic rash encompassing the entire body may occur and cause extreme discomfort. Although neuromyopathy has been reported rarely, deep tendon reflexes should be monitored regularly for diminished activity.

After absorption, these drugs concentrate in the retina, kidneys, bone marrow, and liver. The concentration of antimalarials in specific organs dictates baseline and ongoing monitoring during therapy. Specifically, patients need a baseline eye examination with a follow-up exam 5 years later and then annually thereafter because of potential retinal accumulation of the drug.

Interactions

Antimalarial agents can decrease the metabolism of most beta-blockers with the exception of atenolol, nadolol, and sotalol. As a result, patients should be monitored for increased effects of these medications (lower blood pressure, lower heart rate) when started on hydroxychloroquine. Also, cyclosporine and digoxin concentrations may be increased, requiring more frequent monitoring.

Leflunomide

Leflunomide (Arava) exerts anti-inflammatory and antiproliferative actions, retarding erosions and joint space narrowing.

Mechanism of Action

Leflunomide is a prodrug that undergoes rapid conversion to its active metabolite. The drug is a competitive inhibitor of dihydrofolate reductase. This inhibition decreases the production of pyrimidines (amino acid building blocks), decreasing T-cell and B-cell proliferation. This action is similar to methotrexate, making this agent a reasonable alternative for patients who cannot tolerate or who have an inadequate response to methotrexate. Since leflunomide inhibits pyrimidine synthesis and methotrexate inhibits purine synthesis, these agents may be used in combination.

Dosage

Since the half-life of the active metabolite is 15 to 18 days, therapy with leflunomide is usually initiated with a 100-mg daily loading dose for 3 days, and then the agent is continued at 20 mg/d if tolerated. If the patient cannot tolerate 20 mg/d, the dose can be lowered to 10 mg/d. The loading dose can be omitted in patients at increased risk for hepatic or hematologic toxicity.

Time Frame for Response

Benefit from leflunomide can be seen as early as 4 weeks but may take up to 3 months.

Contraindications

Like other DMARDs, leflunomide is contraindicated in pregnancy. Since the half-life is so long, a typical washout period for women who wish to conceive is about 2 years. However, agents interrupting the enterohepatic recirculation (e.g., activated charcoal or cholestyramine) can be used to reduce the half-life of the metabolite to about 1 day. The dosing of cholestyramine, as recommended by the manufacturer, is 8 g thrice daily for 11 days. To ensure appropriate clearance, plasma concentrations should be less than 0.02 mg/L measured twice at least 14 days apart.

Due to hepatotoxicity, patients with a history of alcoholism or with preexisting liver disease should not take leflunomide.

Adverse Events

About 5% of patients receiving leflunomide mono therapy have elevated liver enzymes. While this number appears low, there are reports of more than 10 patients dying while on leflunomide therapy; the deaths are thought to be related to the hepatotoxicity of the agent.

More common adverse events include GI symptoms, alopecia, and hypertension. Leflunomide also has been associated with bone marrow suppression, including anemia, thrombocytopenia, and agranulocytosis.

A CBC and liver function tests should be monitored every 2 to 4 weeks in the first 3 months of therapy, followed by every 8 to 12 weeks during months 3 to 6. Once a patient has been on leflunomide for more than 6 months, monitoring may be done every 12 weeks.

Interactions

Leflunomide is a weak inhibitor of the CYP2C9 enzyme and therefore may increase the levels of agents metabolized through this pathway, including warfarin. Rifampin may increase the concentration of leflunomide's active metabolite. The use of bile acid sequestrants decreases the enterohepatic recycling of leflunomide, decreasing its effectiveness.

Janus Kinase Inhibitors

Tofacitinib was the first tsDMARD available and targets Janus kinase (JAK) activity. Other JAK inhibitors include baricitinib and upadacitinib.

Mechanism of Action

These medications interfere with JAK1, JAK2, JAK3, and Tyk2. They are competitive, reversible inhibitors. The JAK inhibitors prevent the phosphorylation and activation of signal transducers and activators of transcription. This results in decreased signal transduction for cytokines and decreases propagation of the inflammatory response via decreased leukocyte maturation and activation and cytokine production.

Dosage

The typical dose of tofacitinib is 5 mg orally twice daily. However, if used in combination with a strong CYP3A4 inhibitor (e.g., ketoconazole) or concomitant moderate CYP3A4 inhibitor with a potent CYP2C19 inhibitor (e.g., fluconazole), the recommended dose is 5 mg orally daily. Also, for patients with moderate-to-severe renal or hepatic impairment, the dose is 5 mg orally daily. The dose of baricitinib is 2 mg orally once daily. If the patient has moderate renal impairment or is also on a strong organic anion transporter 3 (OAT3) inhibitor such as probenecid, the dose should be 1 mg once daily. For upadacitinib, the dose is 15 mg orally once daily.

Contraindications

There are no absolute contraindications to JAK inhibitor therapy; however, there are many warnings associated with its use. Due to the risk of bone marrow suppression, tofacitinib should not be initiated if a patient has a lymphocyte count less than 500 cells/mm^3, absolute neutrophil count of less than 1,000 cells/mm^3, or hemoglobin less than 8 g/dL. A CBC should be monitored at baseline, 4 to 8 weeks after initiation and then every 3 months thereafter. These agents may cause hepatotoxicity and patients should be monitored for this. Similar to other DMARDs, JAK inhibitors may increase the risk of infection including TB, fungal infections, and opportunistic infections. Patients should be screened for latent TB prior to initiating therapy.

Adverse Events

Common adverse effects include headache, diarrhea, hypertension, and upper respiratory infections. Tofacitinib may increase lipid parameters such as total cholesterol, low-density lipoprotein (LDL), and high-density lipoprotein (HDL), and a lipid panel should be checked 4 to 8 weeks after initiating therapy as well as periodically thereafter.

Interactions

Tofacitinib and upadacitinib are not recommended to be used with strong CYP3A4 inducers such as rifampin. Baricitinib is not recommended for use in patients taking strong OAT3 inhibitors such as probenecid. Due to the risk of infection, these medications should not be used with any biologic DMARDs. Live vaccines should not be administered while a patient is receiving a JAK inhibitor.

Biologic Disease-Modifying Antirheumatic Drugs

Biologic agents are developed from living sources, such as humans, animals, or microorganisms. The introduction of various biologics effective against RA has changed the management of RA. These agents target multiple components involved in the pathogenesis of RA, such as TNF-alpha, T-cell activation, IL-1, and IL-6. Prior to initiating bDMARDs, patients should be screened for latent TB and hepatitis B due to the increased risk of reactivation.

Tumor Necrosis Factor Inhibitors

Etanercept (Enbrel), infliximab (Remicade), adalimumab (Humira), golimumab (Simponi), and certolizumab pegol (Cimzia) are TNF-alpha inhibitors used in RA treatment.

Mechanism of Action

These agents act by binding the circulating TNF-alpha and render it inactive. This then reduces the chemotactic effect of TNF-alpha by reducing IL-6 and CRP, resulting in reduced infiltration of inflammatory cells into joints. Also, when these agents bind to surface TNF-alpha, cell lysis occurs.

Dosage

All five of these agents are injectable. Etanercept is self-administered subcutaneously at 25 mg twice weekly or 50 mg weekly as combination therapy or monotherapy. Infliximab is an intravenous infusion with a recommended dose of 3 mg/kg at 0, 2, and 6 weeks and then every 8 weeks thereafter. Doses of infliximab have ranged from 3 to 10 mg/kg every 4 to 8 weeks. Infliximab is indicated in conjunction with methotrexate because infliximab antibodies develop when administered as monotherapy. Adalimumab is given at 40 mg every other week as a subcutaneous injection. Adalimumab may be administered concomitantly with methotrexate, glucocorticoids, or NSAIDs. It may also be used as monotherapy; however, the dose may need to be increased to 40 mg weekly. Certolizumab pegol is administered as a subcutaneous injection at a dose of 400 mg at 0, 2, and 4 weeks and then 200 mg every other week thereafter. An alternative maintenance dosing regimen is 400 mg every 4 weeks. Golimumab is only indicated for use in combination with methotrexate, and the recommended dose is 50 mg subcutaneously once a month.

Time Frame for Response

All of the TNF-alpha inhibitors produce a rapid response, within days to weeks.

Contraindications

Patients should be assessed at baseline for infections or risk factors for infections. There have been reports of TB developing in patients taking infliximab; the theory is that the immunomodulation allows latent TB to flare. This usually occurs within the first 2 to 5 months of therapy. Therefore, all patients must be evaluated for latent TB with a tuberculin skin test or interferon gamma release assay prior to beginning therapy. Other serious infections, including fungal, bacterial, viral, and other opportunistic infections, have also occurred with these agents, and careful consideration of the patient's history is important when prescribing them. This class of medications is not recommended for patients with untreated hepatitis B or treated hepatitis B with Child-Pugh score of B or higher. In addition, patients with New York Heart Association class III or IV heart failure should not be initiated on TNF inhibitors.

Adverse Events

Adverse events include injection-site reactions (certolizumab pegol, golimumab, etanercept, adalimumab) or infusion reactions (infliximab). Caution must be used when administering these agents to patients predisposed to infection. Sepsis and fatal infections have occurred in patients receiving TNF-alpha inhibitors. If a patient develops an infection while taking a TNF-alpha inhibitor, the agent should be discontinued until the infection resolves. Other serious but more rare adverse events include demyelinating central nervous system diseases, autoimmune disorders such as lupus-like syndrome, and lymphomas. The risk of lymphoma is increased in children and adolescents, and it is not elucidated if the increased risk is due to the medication or the disease. Due to this risk, these agents are not recommended for the treatment of RA in patients with a treated solid malignancy within the last 5 years or treated lymphoproliferative malignancy.

Interactions

TNF-alpha inhibitors should not be used in combination with other biologic DMARDs due to the increased risk of infection. As a result of immunosuppressive effects, patients should not receive live vaccinations while being treated with a TNF-alpha inhibitor. Also, the response to other vaccines may be diminished while on therapy.

Abatacept

Abatacept (Orencia) is indicated for the treatment of moderate-to-severe RA as monotherapy or in combination with csDMARDs.

Mechanism of Action

Abatacept is a costimulation modulator that binds to CD80 and CD86 on antigen-presenting cells. This binding blocks the CD28 interaction between the antigen-presenting cell and

T cells necessary for T-cell activation. Therefore, abatacept decreases the activation of T cells.

Dosage

Abatacept is given as an IV infusion over 30 minutes and is dosed based on weight (<60 kg, 500 mg; 60–100 kg, 750 mg; >100 kg, 1,000 mg). It is dosed at weeks 0, 2, and 4 and then every 4 weeks thereafter. It is also available as a subcutaneous injection which can be initiated with or without receiving an IV dose. If a patient receives an IV loading dose (based on weight), the subcutaneous dose is 125 mg within 24 hours of the IV dose followed by 125 mg weekly thereafter. If the patient does not receive an IV loading dose, the dose is 125 mg subcutaneously weekly. If a patient had been receiving the IV formulation and wishes to convert to the subcutaneous formulation, the recommendation is to start the 125 mg by subcutaneous weekly at the time of their next scheduled IV dose.

Time Frame for Response

The onset of action for abatacept ranges from 1 to 3 months.

Contraindications

The only absolute contraindication associated with abatacept is hypersensitivity to it or any component of the formulation. Abatacept should be used cautiously in patients with a history of infection or chronic obstructive pulmonary disease (COPD). Patients need to be screened for hepatitis and latent TB prior to initiation due to the risk of reactivation.

Adverse Events

Patients with COPD experienced a higher rate of exacerbations, cough, pneumonia, and dyspnea. Common adverse events include headache, hypertension, and infusion-related reactions. Similarly to other immunomodulators, abatacept is associated with a higher risk of infections. Although rare, abatacept can cause anaphylaxis.

Interactions

Patients should not receive a live vaccine while on abatacept or for up to 3 months after discontinuing the drug. Abatacept should not be used in combination with other bDMARDs due to the increased risk of immunosuppression.

Interleukin-6 Receptor Antagonists

Tocilizumab (Actemra) was the first IL-6 receptor inhibitor on the market. Since then, sarilumab (Kevzara) has also been released.

Mechanism of Action

Tocilizumab and sarilumab are anti-IL-6 receptor monoclonal antibodies. By inhibiting IL-6 activity, B-cell and T-cell activation is decreased as well as acute phase reactant production and osteoclast activation.

Dosage

Tocilizumab is available as an IV infusion or a subcutaneous injection. For the IV infusion, tocilizumab is initiated at a dose of 4 mg/kg every 4 weeks with an option to increase to 8 mg/kg if needed based on clinical response. For the subcutaneous formulation, the dose for a patient weighing less than 100 kg is 162 mg every other week with the option to increase to weekly dosing if needed. For patients weighing 100 kg or more, the recommended starting dose is tocilizumab 162 mg subcutaneously every week. For a patient wishing to transition from IV to subcutaneous, they would initiate the subcutaneous dose at the time of their next scheduled IV dose. For sarilumab, the dose is 200 mg subcutaneously once every 2 weeks.

Time Frame for Response

It may take up to 3 months for symptomatic improvement with IL-6 receptor antagonists.

Contraindications

These medications should not be initiated if patients have an absolute neutrophil count less than 2,000 cells/mm^3, platelets less than 100,000/mm^3 for tocilizumab or less than 150,000/mm^3 for sarilumab, or alanine transaminase (ALT) or aspartate aminotransferase (AST) greater than 1.5 times the ULN. Similar to the other biologic agents, patients should be screened for TB and hepatitis prior to initiation.

Adverse Events

Overall, these agents are well tolerated. There have been laboratory abnormalities associated with tocilizumab and sarilumab that include increased low-density lipoprotein cholesterol, elevated transaminases, and decreased WBCs. Infusion reactions and injection site reactions can also be seen.

Based on laboratory abnormalities, a CBC and liver function tests need to be monitored at baseline and then every 4 to 8 weeks while on therapy. A lipid panel should be checked at baseline, 4 to 8 weeks into therapy, and then every 6 months while being treated with tocilizumab or sarilumab.

Interactions

Avoid using tocilizumab with leflunomide due to concern for increased hematologic toxicity. Patients should not receive live vaccines while on therapy and for at least 3 months after discontinuing treatment. Also, patients may not be able to respond appropriately to inactivated vaccines administered while on therapy. Due to the risk of infection, tocilizumab should not be used with any TNF-alpha inhibitors, anakinra, abatacept, or other immunosuppressants.

Rituximab

Rituximab (Rituxan) is a monoclonal antibody sometimes used in combination with methotrexate to help improve response.

Mechanism of Action

Rituximab is an antibody directed against the CD20 antibody on B lymphocytes. By binding to CD20, rituximab activates complements that lead to B-cell cytotoxicity. In RA, B-cells are thought to play a role in disease severity and progression.

Dosage

The recommended dose is 1,000 mg as an IV infusion on days 1 and 15 in combination with methotrexate. After that, subsequent courses may be given every 16 to 24 weeks. Patients should also receive methylprednisolone 100 mg IV prior to the start of the infusion.

Contraindications

Although rituximab has no major contraindications, it should be avoided in patients with hepatitis B, or severe, active infection (including TB).

Adverse Events

The most common side effects of rituximab are infusion reactions. Patients must receive vital sign monitoring upon arrival, after the start of the medication, every 15 minutes for an hour, every 30 minutes thereafter, upon discontinuing the infusion, and before the patient departs. Additionally, patients must be monitored for signs and symptoms such as flushing, chills, rigors, hives, difficulty breathing, and chest pain. Depending on the severity, patients may require intervention.

Interactions

Rituximab should not be used in combination with bDMARDs. Patients should not receive live vaccines while on therapy or before starting treatment. Also, patients may not be able to respond appropriately to inactivated vaccines administered while on therapy.

Selecting the Most Appropriate Agent

In 2008, the ACR published recommendations regarding the use of nonbiologic and biologic DMARDs for the treatment of RA, and this guideline was updated in 2012. Due to emerging evidence and a number of new therapies, new guidelines were released in 2015. It is important to note that anakinra, gold, azathioprine, cyclosporine, and minocycline were not included due to infrequent use and lack of relevant new data. Decisions regarding appropriate therapy are based on disease duration and disease activity. Disease duration is divided into early (<6 months) or established (>6 months). Disease activity is divided into low, moderate, or high based on several questionnaire instruments. Treatment algorithms are displayed in **Figures 34.1** and **34.2**.

In 2019, the EULAR published recommendations regarding the management of RA with synthetic and biologic DMARDs (**Table 34.3**). These guidelines break treatment into three phases based on response to therapy. Unlike the ACR guidelines, the EULAR guidelines differentiate treatment for patients with or without poor prognostic factors.

In selecting a DMARD or combining DMARDs, the clinician needs to consider the toxicities of the medications, including the interactions with other prescribed drugs. Some patients may have difficulty adhering to monitoring requirements for some of the more toxic drugs. Other patients may not be able to adhere to a strict dosing schedule. In addition, the time required to achieve benefit can be protracted with certain DMARDs, which may be unacceptable to the patient. Finally, the cost of the various therapies varies widely.

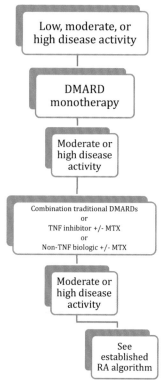

FIGURE 34–1 2015 American College of Rheumatology recommendations for the treatment of DMARD-naïve early RA. DMARD, disease-modifying antirheumatic drug (includes hydroxychloroquine [HCQ], leflunomide [LEF], methotrexate [MTX], and sulfasalazine); TNF, tumor necrosis factor. Consider using short-term glucocorticoids for flares, and may also consider adding low-dose glucocorticoids in patients with moderate or high disease activity when starting DMARDs and in patients with DMARD or biologic failure. (Adapted from Singh, J. A., Saag, K. G., Bridges, Jr. S. L., et al. (2016). 2015 American College of Rheumatology Guideline for the treatment of rheumatoid arthritis. *Arthritis Care & Research, 68*(1), 1–25.)

TABLE 34.3		
European League Against Rheumatism Treatment Recommendations		
Phase I	Initial treatment	Methotrexate monotherapy. If contraindication to methotrexate: leflunomide or sulfasalazine.
Phase II	Failure of phase I	With poor prognostic factors: bDMARD or JAK inhibitor. Without poor prognostic factors: change to or add a second csDMARD.
	Failure of second csDMARD regimen	bDMARD or JAK inhibitor.
Phase III	Failure of first bDMARD	Change the bDMARD or JAK inhibitor.
	Failure of ≥2 bDMARD	Replace bDMARD or JAK inhibitor.

bDMARD, biological DMARDs; csDMARD, conventional synthetic DMARDs; JAK, Janus Kinase.

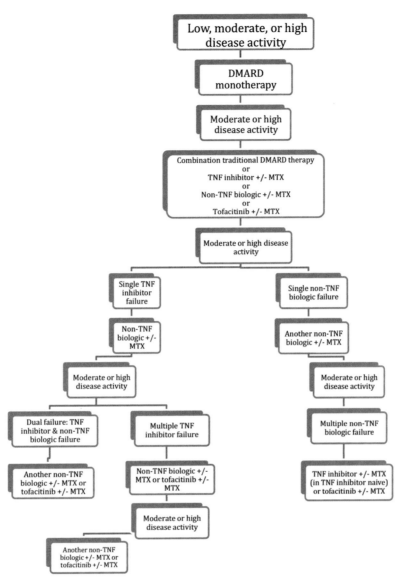

FIGURE 34–2   2015 American College of Rheumatology recommendations for the treatment of DMARD-naïve established RA. DMARD, disease-modifying antirheumatic drug (includes hydroxychloroquine [HCQ], leflunomide [LEF], methotrexate [MTX], and sulfasalazine); TNF, tumor necrosis factor. Consider using short-term glucocorticoids for flares, and may also consider adding low-dose glucocorticoids in patients with moderate or high disease activity when starting DMARDs and in patients with DMARD or biologic failure. When patients are in remission, consider tapering RA treatments, but do not discontinue all RA treatments. (Adapted from Singh, J. A., Saag, K. G., Bridges, Jr. S. L., et al. (2016). 2015 American College of Rheumatology Guideline for the treatment of rheumatoid arthritis. *Arthritis Care & Research, 68*(1), 1–25.)

Symptomatic Treatment

NSAIDs and/or corticosteroids are recommended for acute symptoms associated with RA. These agents are particularly helpful while a patient is undergoing diagnostic assessment. NSAIDs do not have disease-modifying abilities, and steroids often have intolerable adverse effects; therefore, once a definite diagnosis is made, DMARD therapy should be started. NSAIDs and steroids can be continued until the DMARD takes effect.

First-Line Therapy

For patients with early disease, the recommended first-line treatment from the ACR (**Figure 34.1**) is monotherapy csDMARD for patients with low, moderate, or high disease activity. If

patients still experience moderate or high disease activity despite DMARD monotherapy, it is recommended to use combination DMARDs or a TNF-alpha inhibitor or a non-TNF biologic. These agents can be used with or without methotrexate.

The EULAR guidelines state that methotrexate should be a part of the initial treatment strategy for patients with active disease. If patients have a contraindication to methotrexate, leflunomide or sulfasalazine can be substituted.

Second-Line Therapy

Based on the ACR recommendations, options for those with established disease or those not responding to primary treatment vary depending on previous treatments and disease activity.

Figure 34.2 outlines the specific recommendations based on these criteria. If disease activity remains moderate or high despite initial treatment, it is recommended to use combination DMARDs or a TNF-alpha inhibitor or a non-TNF biologic or tofacitinib. These treatment options can be used with or without methotrexate.

For those not responding to first-line treatment appropriately, the EULAR outlines second-line treatment based on the presence of poor prognostic factors. For those patients without poor prognostic factors, changing csDMARD strategy is preferred, and for those with poor prognostic factors, adding a bDMARD or JAK-inhibitor is preferred.

Third-Line Therapy

As seen in **Figure 34.2**, The ACR recommends subsequent treatment choices based on the medications that patients have failed previously as well as disease activity. Another option recommended by the EULAR guidelines is changing the bDMARD or JAK-inhibitor.

Special Populations
Geriatric

Caution should be used when starting older patients on NSAIDs due to the increased risk of GI hemorrhage. Further, many older patients have decreased renal function, and NSAIDs may contribute to a decline in this function. Several DMARDs and some immunomodulators are renally excreted, and doses should be adjusted in the older adults due to decreased renal function.

Women

Women with RA who plan on having children need to discuss treatment options with their physician and understand the risks of conception. Certain medications, including methotrexate, leflunomide, abatacept, and rituximab, cannot be used during pregnancy because of known teratogenicity. DMARDs with the most data to support their use during pregnancy are antimalarials, sulfasalazine, azathioprine, and cyclosporine. These medications can be used as monotherapy or in combination with corticosteroids or NSAIDs. If corticosteroids are used during pregnancy, the dose should not exceed 15 mg/d because higher doses increase the risk of intrauterine infection and premature delivery. NSAIDs should be avoided after 30 weeks of gestation because of the increased risk of premature closure of the ductus arteriosus in the fetus. TNF-alpha inhibitors have shown no teratogenic effects in animals and limited or no data in humans. There have been case reports of congenital malformations in children exposed to TNF-alpha inhibitors as a fetus. Therefore, TNF-alpha inhibitors need to be used cautiously in pregnant women.

MONITORING PATIENT RESPONSE

Because the drugs used for treating arthritis have many adverse events and because most are used for long-term treatment, monitoring should include baseline studies against which later results can be compared. CBC with differential, urinalysis, creatinine, serum bilirubin, liver enzymes, ESR, BUN, platelet studies, and eye examinations are among the tests performed periodically during therapy.

Patients should follow the treat-to-target approach, which requires more intensive follow-up and monitoring. Patients started on DMARD therapy should be assessed at least every 3 months and as soon as 1 month to have disease activity assessed. If goals are not met at 3 months, therapy should be adapted until the goal or remission or low disease activity is met. Once the goal is met, patients can be reassessed every 3 to 6 months to ensure their goals are sustained.

PATIENT EDUCATION

Patient education depends on the type of agent selected. The patient should know that routine blood work is important to detect adverse events before they become serious and life-threatening. Patients taking DMARDs and immunomodulators should report illness immediately, as the risk of serious infections is increased in these patients. Patients need to understand that there is a delay between initiating therapy and experiencing the full clinical effects and that therapy must be continued in order to be effective.

Patient-Oriented Information Sources

Support groups, education of family members, and assistive devices can help with activities of daily living. The ACR has patient information available on their website regarding a variety of topics such as medications, research, advocacy, and exercise (https://www.rheumatology.org/I-Am-A/Patient-Caregiver/Patient-and-Caregiver-Resources). In addition, the Arthritis Foundation has information directed at patients regarding different aspects of living with arthritis (www.arthritis.org). The National Institutes of Health, in conjunction with the American Society of Health-System Pharmacists and the United States Pharmacopeia, has a drug information website with information about thousands of medications (http://www.nlm.nih.gov/medlineplus/druginformation.html).

Nutrition/Lifestyle Changes

Weight loss programs and healthy habits such as adequate rest are keys to the success of a treatment program. Patients should consider occupational therapy as needed to help with household chores. Additionally, they should avoid repetitive joint motion and vibrations from electrical appliances or tools to reduce exacerbations. Splinting the affected joint helps relieve pain and prevent deformity, but splints should be removed at least once daily and for any exercise activities. Patients should also be instructed on strategies to avoid physical and emotional stress, which may precipitate an exacerbation.

Complementary and Alternative Medications

Folk remedies have been used for RA for many years. Although most of these remedies cause no harm, there is little scientific evidence supporting their efficacy. Some of the more commonly used approaches include shark cartilage, chondroitin, herbs, vitamins, acupuncture, magnet therapy, climate therapy, and several diets. Clinicians should be aware of the therapies being considered or used by the patient; joint treatment goals should be established and monitored. Just as in traditional medicine, patients using complementary approaches either alone or as adjunctive therapy require ongoing monitoring for safety and efficacy of the selected approach.

CASE STUDY 1

J.W., a 46-year-old African American woman, presents to your office with the chief complaint of bilateral stiffness of the shoulders, hands, and wrists in the morning. She reports she is otherwise healthy, takes no medications, and is employed as a systems analyst for a large bank. She recalls having some minor flulike symptoms approximately 3 weeks before her visit. The stiffness makes it difficult for her to work for any extended period. She has also started wearing a wig because she cannot raise her arms in the morning to fix her hair. She has lost 10 pounds over the past 8 months but has not consciously dieted. She finds it increasingly difficult to drive, particularly when making turns and driving in reverse.

Pertinent laboratory results:

Erythrocyte sedimentation rate 89 mm/hr (0–29 mm/hr), anti–citrullinated protein antibody 65 EU/mL (<20 EU/mL), SCr 1.0 mg/dL

DIAGNOSIS: RHEUMATOID ARTHRITIS WITH MODERATE DISEASE ACTIVITY (LEARNING OBJECTIVES 3 AND 4)

1. List specific goals of treatment for J.W.
2. Which drug therapy would you prescribe, and why?
3. What are the parameters for monitoring success of the therapy?
4. Discuss specific patient education based on the prescribed therapy.
5. List one or two adverse reactions for the selected agent that would cause you to change therapy?

Bibliography

Starred references are cited in the text.

Aletaha, D., Neogi, T., Silman, A. J., et al. (2010). 2010 rheumatoid arthritis classification criteria. *Arthritis and Rheumatism, 62*(9), 2569–2581.

American College of Rheumatology Ad Hoc Committee on Clinical Guidelines. (1996). Guidelines for monitoring drug therapy in rheumatoid arthritis. *Arthritis and Rheumatism, 39*, 723–731.

Anderson, J. J., Wells, G., Verhoeven, A. C., et al. (2000). Factors predicting response to treatment in rheumatoid arthritis: The importance of disease duration. *Arthritis and Rheumatism, 43*(1), 22–29.

Feist, E., & Burmester, G. R. (2013). Small molecules targeting JAKs: A new approach in the treatment of rheumatoid arthritis. *Rheumatology, 52*, 1352–1357.

Felson, D. T., Smolen, J. S., Wells, G., et al. (2011). American College of Rheumatology/European League Against Rheumatism provisional definition of remission in rheumatoid arthritis for clinical trials. *Arthritis and Rheumatism, 63*(3), 573–586.

Gruber, S., Lezcano, B., & Hylland, S. (2020). Rheumatoid arthritis. In J. T. Dipiro, et al. (Eds.), *Pharmacotherapy: A pathophysiologic approach* (11th ed.). New York, NY: McGraw-Hill.

*Hunter, T. M., Boytsov, N. N., Zhang, X., et al. (2017). Prevalence of rheumatoid arthritis in the United States adult population in healthcare claims databases, 2004–2014. *Rheumatology International, 37*, 1551–1557.

Kavanaugh, A., & Wells, A. F. (2014). Benefits and risks of low-dose glucocorticoid treatment in the patient with rheumatoid arthritis. *Rheumatology, 53*, 1742–1751.

Kroot, E. J., van Leeuwen, M. A., van Rijswijk, M. H., et al. (2000). No increased mortality in patients with rheumatoid arthritis: Up to 10 years of follow up from disease onset. *Annals of the Rheumatic Disease, 59*, 954–958.

McInnes, I. B., & Schett, G. (2011). The pathogenesis of rheumatoid arthritis. *The New England Journal of Medicine, 365*, 2205–2219.

Nell, V. P., Machold, K. P., Eberl, G., et al. (2004). Benefit of very early referral and very early therapy with disease-modifying anti-rheumatic drugs in patients with very early rheumatoid arthritis. *Rheumatology, 43*(7), 906–914.

Ostensen, M. (2009). Management of early aggressive rheumatoid arthritis during pregnancy and lactation. *Expert Opinion on Pharmacotherapy, 10*(9), 1469–1479.

Ruderman, E. M. (2012). Overview of safety of non-biologic and biologic DMARDs. *Rheumatology, 51*, vi37–vi43.

Saag, K. G., Teng, G. G., Patkar, N. M., et al. (2008). American College of Rheumatology 2008 recommendations for the use of nonbiologic and biologic disease-modifying antirheumatic drugs in rheumatoid arthritis. *Arthritis and Rheumatism, 59*(6), 762–784.

Singh, J. A., Furst, D. E., Bharat, A., et al. (2012). 2012 Update of the 2008 American College of Rheumatology Recommendations for the use of disease-modifying antirheumatic drugs and biologic agents in the treatment of rheumatoid arthritis. *Arthritis Care & Research, 64*(5), 625–639.

Singh, J. A., Saag, K. G., Bridges, Jr. S. L., et al. (2016). 2015 American College of Rheumatology Guideline for the treatment of rheumatoid arthritis. *Arthritis Care & Research, 68*(1), 1–25.

Smolen, J. S., Aletaha, D., Bijlsma, J. W., et al. (2010). Treating rheumatoid arthritis to target: Recommendations of an international task force. *Annals of the Rheumatic Diseases, 69*(4), 631–637.

Smolen, J. S., Breedveld, F. C., Burmester, G. R., et al. (2016). Treating rheumatoid arthritis to target: 2014 update of the recommendations of an international task force. *Annals of the Rheumatic Diseases, 75*, 3–15.

Smolen, J. S., Landewe, R. B. M., Bijlsma, J. W., et al. (2020). EULAR recommendations for the management of rheumatoid arthritis with synthetic and biological disease-modifying antirheumatic drugs: 2019 update. *Annals of Rheumatic Diseases, 79*, 685–699.

Smolen, J. S., van der Heijide, D., Machold, K. P., et al. (2014). Proposal for a new nomenclature of disease-modifying antirheumatic drugs. *Annals of the Rheumatic Diseases, 73*(1), 3–5.

Soeken, K. K., Miller, S. A., & Ernst, E. (2003). Herbal medicines for the treatment of rheumatoid arthritis. *Rheumatology, 42*(5), 652–659.

Upchurch, K. S., & Kay, J. (2012). Evolution of treatment of rheumatoid arthritis. *Rheumatology, 51*, vi28–vi36.

Wolters Kluwer Clinical Drug Information, Inc. (Lexi-Drugs). Wolters Kluwer Clinical Drug Information, Inc.; March 7, 2020.

Pharmacotherapy for Neurological Disorders

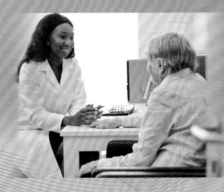

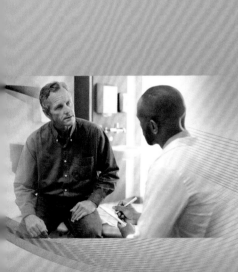

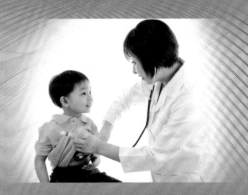

35 Headaches

Kelleen N. Flaherty

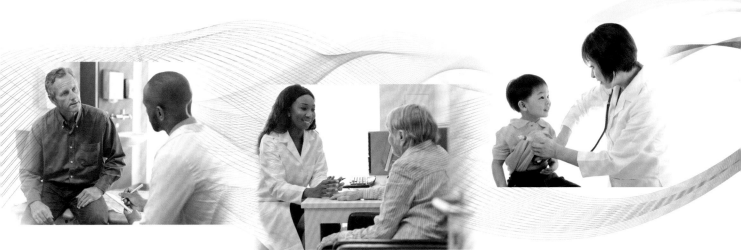

Learning Objectives

1. Describe the pathophysiologic and distinguishing characteristics of the primary headaches.
2. Differentiate between the types of headaches based on patient presentation and appropriate diagnostic testing.
3. Select appropriate pharmacotherapy based on indication, symptoms, duration of headache, previous treatment failure, contraindications, and patient expectations.

INTRODUCTION

Headache is one of the most common complaints presenting in primary care. The pain of a headache can range from mild to severe, can be acute or chronic, and may last hours to days. Severe headache and migraine are estimated to afflict one in seven individuals in the United States based on multiple population-wide studies and have a significant impact on quality of life and health care resource utilization (Burch et al., 2015, 2018). While there are three main categories of headaches according to the most recent *International Classification of Headache Disorders* (ICHD-3) (Headache Classification Subcommittee of the International Headache Society [IHS], 2018), the most commonly encountered headaches seen in primary care are the primary and secondary headaches (**Box 35.1**). A primary headache is one with no identifiable, underlying organic disease process; a secondary headache

is one for which a specific etiology has been identified. The practitioner must first rule out a secondary headache (or more serious cause of headache pain) and then accurately diagnose the type of primary headache. In some instances, both primary and secondary headaches can occur simultaneously. Primary headaches include tension-type headache (TTH), migraine, and cluster headache (CH). This chapter will focus on diagnosing and treating TTH and migraine, the most common forms of primary headache presenting in clinical practice.

Tension headaches have a dull quality, with pain that radiates bilaterally from the forehead to the occiput in a band-like fashion. The pain often radiates down the neck and sometimes even into the trapezius muscle. The pain is mild to moderate and can last from 30 minutes to several days in severe cases. Tension headaches are not typically present upon awakening but begin later in the day and progress with time. The pain of these headaches is rarely debilitating, but it can affect a person's ability to function, especially if prolonged or chronic. There are no associated symptoms of nausea, vomiting, photophobia, or phonophobia.

Migraine is a neurologic syndrome causing not only throbbing head pain but also often nausea, appetite change, photophobia, and phonophobia. The pain generally ranges from moderate to severe and can be disabling. The Global Burden of Disease Study in 2017 ranked headache (primarily migraine) as the second most prevalent and seventh highest specific cause of disability in the world (Institute for Health Metrics and Evaluation, 2018). According to epidemiologic studies, migraine occurs in one in seven individuals in the United States and is two to three times more common in females than in males. The National Health Interview Survey

Primary and Secondary Headaches, International Classification of Headache Disorders, Third Edition

Primary Headaches

Migraine

Tension-type headache (TTH)

Trigeminal autonomic cephalalgias (includes CH, paroxysmal hemicranias, short-lasting unilateral neuralgiform headache attacks, hemicranias continua)

Other primary headache disorders (primary cough headache, primary exercise headache, primary headache associated with sexual activity, primary thunderclap headache, cold-stimulus headache, external pressure headache, primary stabbing headache, nummular headache, hypnic headache, and new daily-persistent headache)

Secondary Headaches

Headache attributed to trauma or injury to the head and/ or neck

Headache attributed to cranial and/or cervical vascular disorder

Headache attributed to nonvascular intracranial disorder

Headache attributed to a substance or its withdrawal

Headache attributed to infection

Headache attributed to disorder of homeostasis

Headache or facial pain attributed to disorder of cranium, neck, eyes, ears, nose, sinuses, teeth, mouth, or other facial or cervical structure

Headache attributed to psychiatric disorder

Painful lesions of the cranial nerves and other facial pains

Other headache disorders

Source: Modified from Headache Classification Committee of the International Headache Society (IHS). (2018). The International Classification of Headache Disorders, 3rd ed. *Cephalalgia, 38*(1), 1–211.

(2018) estimated a national prevalence of 15.9%, 21% in females and 10.7% in males, with migraine occurring disproportionately higher in at-risk groups such as the unemployed, the uninsured, or those in lower socioeconomic strata (Burch et al., 2018; National Health Interview Survey, 2018). Large population-based studies have shown a 3:1 incidence of migraine or higher in women versus men (Ford et al., 2017). The age of onset is from 15 to 35, but peak prevalence is from ages 35 to 45. A family history of migraine has shown to be diagnostic in 60% of cases and is considered to be a significant risk factor. Significant comorbidity has also been demonstrated in population studies, including psychiatric disorders, respiratory disorders, cardiovascular disorders, digestive disorders, endocrine disorders, and other central nervous system (CNS) disorders (D'Amico et al., 2018; Ford et al.,

2017; Lipton et al., 2019b). Combined direct and indirect costs for migraine have been estimated to be $36 billion in the United States for 2016 (Bonafede et al., 2018). In a large study (N = 150,971 after inclusion/exclusion criteria applied) assessing direct and indirect health care resource utilization and costs among patients with migraine in the United States, it was found that individuals with migraine spent $8,924 per year in direct and indirect costs compared to migraine-free matched controls (Bonafede et al., 2018). Patients with migraine had twice as many pharmacy claims as those without migraine (26.5 vs. 13.2) and had, unfortunately, twice as much opioid use—45.5% versus 21.9% (Bonafede et al., 2018). Decreased productivity and absenteeism contribute significantly to the indirect cost burden of migraine, accounting for one quarter of total costs. Migraine is often misinterpreted by its sufferers and therefore underreported, is frequently underdiagnosed, and is consequently undertreated.

CHs represent one of the most severe, excruciating types of headaches (Brandt et al., 2020). The pain is disabling, burning, or boring and is centered around one eye and is described by patients as being more severe than childbirth or passing a kidney stone. They are unilateral, accompanied by ipsilateral symptoms such as ptosis or flushing, last from 15 minutes to 3 hours, can occur several times a day or every other day, and predominantly occur at night (Brandt et al., 2020). Two forms exist: chronic CH (cCH), which generally occurs without remission, and episodic CH (eCH), which can remit for years at a time (Brandt et al., 2020). Patients suspected of having CHs should be promptly referred to a neurologist to exclude potentially serious differential diagnoses (Lee et al., 2018). CH is far less common than migraine or tension headaches, occurring in less than 1% of the population. It is approximately three times more common in males than in females, and eCH is approximately six times more common than cCH (Brandt et al., 2020). Significant disability and comorbidity including cognitive impairment, anxiety, depression, agoraphobia, and even suicidal tendencies may be associated with CH (Torkamani et al., 2015). While the pathophysiology of CH is incompletely understood, hypothalamic dysfunction is believed to be involved, with hypothalamic activation serving as an "attack generator" (Brandt et al., 2020).

CAUSES OF TENSION HEADACHES

Tension headaches are highly prevalent in the population, with a worldwide lifetime prevalence of 46% to 78% demonstrated in a variety of population studies, and TTH causes greater disability and absenteeism than migraine (Scripter, 2018). Headaches are classified as frequent episodic, infrequent episodic, or chronic (ICHD-3, 2018). Chronic TTH is a serious, disabling disease, contributing to a significantly decreased quality of life (ICHD-3, 2018). Prevalence is approximately twice as high in females as it is in males (ICHD-3, 2018). The high prevalence of TTH results in a more significant and costly socioeconomic burden than that of migraine (ICHD-3, 2018).

Chronic TTH has a global prevalence of 0.5% to 4.8%. While stress has been shown to be the most common precipitant of TTH, other precipitants have been identified (ICHD-3, 2018; Yu & Han, 2015). Sleep dysregulation has been shown to have a bidirectional relationship with TTH, with lack of sleep being a precipitant of TTH and TTH being a precipitant of insomnia. Other sleep disturbances associated with TTH include poor sleep quality, excessive daytime sleepiness, and insufficient sleep. Many studies have shown that disrupted sleep is present more often than not in TTH and that clinical presentation of TTH is worse in individuals with disrupted sleep (Cho et al., 2019). Environmental triggers are more common in TTH than in migraine and may include sunlight, fatigue, anxiety, temperature (cold and warm), activity, traveling, and reading. Pericranial muscle tenderness and disorders of the neck and spine may also contribute (Rizzoli & Mullally, 2018). Unlike migraine, food does not appear to be a trigger. Cigarette smoking has also been correlated with an increased number of days of headache per week.

Although more common in migraine patients, one cause of recurrent tension headaches is the overuse of over-the-counter (OTC) and prescription analgesic medications, leading to medication overuse headache (MOH) (ICHD-3, 2018). The headache recurs as each dose of medication wears off, causing the patient to take another analgesic and thus continue the cycle of pain. Treating more than two headaches with an OTC analgesic for either migraine or TTH per week can lead to development of chronic daily headache. Other modifiable risk factors include obesity, caffeine overuse, alcohol consumption, and temporomandibular issues. Nonmodifiable risk factors include female gender, genetics, socioeconomic status, head or neck injury, age, and life events (Cho & Chu, 2015; Yu & Han, 2015).

PATHOPHYSIOLOGY OF TENSION HEADACHES

While TTH was originally assumed to be psychogenic in nature, evidence now suggests that these headaches have neurobiologic etiologies (ICHD-3, 2018) and may be a consequence of both centrally (chronic) and peripherally (episodic) processed pain. Central pain processing may result in increased tenderness and lower pain thresholds in pericranial and myofascial muscles. There may also be genetic, comorbid (e.g., chronic pain, depression, etc.), vitamin D deficiency, and vascular components to TTH (Rizzoli & Mullally, 2018).

DIAGNOSTIC CRITERIA

The first step in determining the type of headache a patient has is to take a detailed headache history. The history should include the patient's age; the time of day when the attack(s) occur(s); the duration and frequency of attacks; precipitating or relieving factors; the quality, location, and intensity of the pain; use of OTC analgesics; and associated symptoms. The social history and family history are also important. The results of physical and neurologic examinations should be unremarkable in a patient with primary headache, other than revealing possible tenderness of pericranial muscles. Diagnosis is mostly of exclusion: all possible secondary headaches, migraine headache, and CHs are ruled out. Tension headaches may be diagnosed as primary, secondary, or both. The ICHD characterizes TTH by "frequent episodes of headache, typically bilateral, pressing or tightening in quality and of mild to moderate intensity, lasting minutes to days. The pain does not worsen with routine physical activity and is not associated with nausea, but photophobia or phonophobia may be present" (ICHD-3, 2018).

Diagnostic alarms in the evaluation of a headache patient that require further testing include headache onset after age 50, sudden-onset headache, accelerating headache pattern, headache with fever and stiff neck, headache accompanying signs of a systemic illness, posttraumatic headache, and abnormal results on the neurologic examination (Clinch, 2015). In the absence of red flags (e.g., suspicion of hemorrhage, etc.), neuroimaging (e.g., electroencephalograpy, computed tomography scan, or magnetic resonance imaging) is not recommended (Clinch, 2015). The ICHD-3 diagnostic criteria for frequent episodic tension headache can be seen in **Box 35.2**.

BOX 35.2

Diagnostic Criteria for Frequent Episodic Tension Headache, *International Classification of Headache Disorders,* **Third Edition**

A. At least 10 episodes of headache occurring on 1 to 14 days per month on average for greater than 3 months (≥12 and <180 days per year) and fulfilling criteria B–D
B. Lasting from 30 minutes to 7 days
C. At least two of the following four characteristics:
   1. Bilateral location
   2. Pressing or tightening (nonpulsating) quality
   3. Mild or moderate intensity
   4. Not aggravated by routine physical activity such as walking or climbing stairs
D. Both of the following:
   1. No nausea or vomiting
   2. No more than one of photophobia or phonophobia
E. Not better accounted for by another ICHD-3 diagnosis

Source: Headache Classification Committee of the International Headache Society (IHS). (2018). The International Classification of Headache Disorders, 3rd ed. *Cephalalgia, 38*(1), 1–211.

INITIATING DRUG THERAPY FOR TENSION HEADACHES

Before initiating drug therapy, it is critical to determine the type and frequency of OTC medication use. Patients with tension headaches and headaches in general frequently self-medicate and may be presenting with MOH. Again, treating more than two headaches per week for more than a few consecutive weeks can lead to development of a chronic daily headache pattern. Caffeine and butalbital products are notorious contributors to MOH. The initial treatment of MOH consists of withholding all OTC analgesics for 1 to 2 weeks.

It is also important to help identify headache triggers and to encourage a healthy lifestyle. Often, simple changes, such as eating and sleeping in a consistent pattern, decreasing alcohol and tobacco use, and using good posture, can decrease headache severity and frequency.

Adjuncts to pharmacotherapy include relaxation therapy, biofeedback, self-hypnosis, cognitive behavioral therapy, exercise, and manual therapy (massage)—physical therapy is the most common nonpharmacologic approach to managing headache (Jensen, 2018).

Headache sufferers (TTH and migraine) use a substantial amount of complementary and alternative/integrative medicine (CAM) for the self-management of headache. The alternative approaches include acupuncture, chiropractic, massage, yoga, homeopathy, and use of dietary supplements such as herbal compounds and vitamins. In one large literature review, some 30% to 70% of CAM users report the therapy to be effective. Most practitioners use CAM as adjunctive therapy to pharmacotherapy, rather than prior to or after treatment with medications. While there have been some studies on the efficacy of CAM, they are methodologically weak. Furthermore, many patients are using CAM therapies concomitantly with conventional treatment and may not report its use to the health care practitioner. Health care practitioners should be vigilant and inquire about CAM use to anticipate and avoid any potential adverse reactions (Adams et al., 2012).

Goals of Drug Therapy for Tension Headaches

The primary goals of drug therapy should be to reduce the severity and frequency of headaches, thus improving the patient's quality of life and ability to function. The goals for patients with episodic tension headaches are to select appropriate analgesic agents that will have the fewest side effects. Prophylactic therapy should be considered in addition to abortive analgesic agents for patients with more than two significant headaches per week. In a patient with MOH, it is appropriate to start a prophylactic agent and abruptly stop abortive analgesic medications simultaneously (other than barbiturate drugs, which must be tapered). It is important to educate patients about MOH and to limit the use of analgesics to 2 days per week. Again, regular and frequent treatment with analgesics may cause development of chronic headache.

It is important that patients do not overuse analgesics as this is likely to interfere with the efficacy of preventive treatment (ICHD-3, 2018).

Acetaminophen and Aspirin

Acetaminophen functions as both an analgesic and an antipyretic but has no effect on inflammation. It is used for the management of mild to moderate and sometimes severe pain and is well tolerated by pediatric, adult, and older individuals (Ishitsuka et al., 2020; Prescriber's Digital Reference [PDR], 2020). Acetaminophen at a dose of 1,000 mg can be very effective in treating mild to moderate tension headaches; although given the hepatotoxic qualities of the drug, the recommended single dose was lowered to 650 mg in 2009 (making 1,000-mg tablets available by prescription only) and the maximum daily limit was lowered to 3,250 mg. Acetaminophen is available as both an OTC and a prescription agent, in several different oral formulations and suppositories and injectable formulations (Ishitsuka et al., 2020). Injectable acetaminophen carries a boxed warning for potential liver failure, transplant, and death (PDR, 2020). The advantages of acetaminophen are that it is well tolerated and has far fewer hematologic, gastrointestinal (GI), and renal effects and fewer drug–drug interactions and side effects as compared with the nonsteroidal antiinflammatory drugs (NSAIDs) (PDR, 2020). Acetaminophen should be avoided in patients with heavy alcohol consumption, alcoholic liver disease, or chronic liver disease, as the drug is metabolized through the liver. Consumption of three or more alcoholic drinks a day in conjunction with acetaminophen use can have hepatotoxic effects. Chronic use of acetaminophen or use of acetaminophen at high doses can cause liver damage, particularly in older persons; the leading cause of acute liver failure in the United States is acetaminophen overdose (and the leading drug overdose seen in emergency departments is with acetaminophen). Acetaminophen overdose is often accidental; patients need to be cautioned not to exceed 4,000 mg/d and to take care not to take other acetaminophen-containing medications in the same day. Prolonged use of acetaminophen and aspirin or NSAIDs should be avoided. Given its superior GI profile, acetaminophen is preferred first line over aspirin, although trials show essentially equivocal efficacy between aspirin and acetaminophen.

Aspirin is also an antipyretic/analgesic indicated for the alleviation of mild to moderate tension headaches. It is available in oral and rectal formulations (PDR, 2020). It inhibits prostaglandin synthesis via nonspecific and irreversible deactivation of both cyclooxygenase 1 (COX-1) and cyclooxygenase 2 (COX-2), reducing the inflammatory response and platelet aggregation. Contraindications to aspirin use include a history of bleeding disorders, asthma, and hypersensitivity to salicylates or NSAIDs. Patients should avoid combining aspirin with other NSAIDs because decreased serum concentrations of NSAIDs result when these drugs are used together. The most common adverse effects associated with aspirin are GI in nature, such as nausea, vomiting, or heartburn. Aspirin has also been recommended as first-line treatment for TTH and migraine, regardless of headache severity.

Aspirin and acetaminophen are the first-line mainstays for the management of TTH. They are also frequently used in combination with other agents such as caffeine, codeine, sedatives, or tranquilizers, although these are not necessarily indicated for TTH and come with the risk of developing dependency or MOH (Jensen, 2018).

Nonsteroidal Antiinflammatory Drugs

NSAIDs work well for moderate tension headaches. They work by selectively inhibiting COX-2, responsible for prostaglandin synthesis, thereby reducing inflammation. These drugs take effect in 30 to 60 minutes, like aspirin and acetaminophen. Commonly used NSAIDs for the management of TTH include ibuprofen, naproxen, ketoprofen, and diclofenac (Jensen, 2018). Many studies have shown that these NSAIDs perform quite well against placebo and tend to be more effective in managing TTH pain than either aspirin or acetaminophen (Jensen, 2018).

Common side effects of NSAIDs are abdominal cramps, nausea, indigestion, and even headache. Occasionally, these drugs cause peptic ulcers and GI hemorrhage. Many NSAIDs contain boxed warnings about cardiovascular effects, GI effects, and/or use in patients with renal impairment. COX-2-specific inhibitors are not indicated specifically for headache.

Any given NSAID should be tried in a patient twice before deciding whether it is successful or not. It is not uncommon for a patient to respond poorly to one NSAID and extremely well to another. Route of administration may also be a consideration to improve NSAID response with certain NSAIDs available in oral, topical, and/or injected formulations (PDR, 2020).

Other Abortive Agents

For patients whose headaches do not respond to the agents mentioned previously, certain combination agents can be considered. Some patients have a good response to OTC agents containing acetaminophen, aspirin, and caffeine (such as Excedrin Extra Strength). However, these agents have a high rate of analgesic MOH when used regularly and should not be used more than 1 to 2 days per week.

Prescription combinations that can be used include butalbital/acetaminophen/caffeine (Fioricet and others) and butalbital/aspirin/caffeine (Fiorinal and others). Butalbital is a barbiturate, which is sedating and potentially habit forming; these medications should not be used in patients with a history of substance abuse. Fiorinal and Fioricet very commonly cause MOH and should not be used for more than 3 days per month. If a patient is taking many butalbital-containing pills per day, they must be slowly tapered to avoid withdrawal symptoms. Patients taking these medications should be closely monitored.

Combination acetaminophen/narcotic products such as Vicodin and Percocet are not recommended. Opioid- or butalbital-containing medications should not be prescribed as first-line treatment for recurrent headache disorders. **Table 35.1** gives an overview of selected drugs used to abort TTH.

Prophylaxis of Tension Headaches

If a patient has more than two tension headaches per week, prophylaxis should be considered. Antidepressant medications are commonly used for headache prophylaxis. Abundant evidence exists for the efficacy of amitriptyline with individuals experiencing relief even at low doses. Its antinociceptive effects are independent from its antidepressant effects (Jensen, 2018; Yu & Han, 2015). There are data supporting the use

TABLE 35.1			
Overview of Selected Drugs to Abort Tension-Type Headaches			
Generic (Brand) Name and Dosage	**Selected Adverse Events**	**Contraindications**	**Special Considerations**
Acetaminophen (Tylenol) 325–650 mg q4–6h limit dose to 3,250 mg/d	Severe hepatotoxicity on acute overdose, potential liver damage with chronic daily dosing, nephrotoxicity, agranulocytosis, rash (including potentially fatal Stevens-Johnson syndrome)	Chronic alcohol use, alcoholic liver disease, impaired liver or renal function, G6PD deficiency	Avoid using with alcohol
Aspirin 325–650 mg q4–6h, not to exceed 4,000 mg/d	GI upset (stomach pain, nausea, heartburn, vomiting); GI bleeding and angioedema (uncommon)	Platelet or bleeding disorders, renal dysfunction, erosive gastritis, peptic ulcer disease, asthma, rhinitis, nasal polyps, severe hepatic or renal failure, or sensitivity to salicylates	Avoid using with NSAIDs, alcohol, during pregnancy, and in children <16 y with viral infections; discontinue 1–2 wk prior to surgery.

(Continued)

TABLE 35.1

Overview of Selected Drugs to Abort Tension-Type Headaches (*Continued*)

Generic (Brand) Name and Dosage	Selected Adverse Events	Contraindications	Special Considerations
NSAIDs			
Ibuprofen (Advil)			
200–400 mg q4–6h, not to exceed 1,200 mg/d; under clinical supervision not to exceed ≤2,400 mg/d *Note*: Use lower doses in patients with renal or hepatic disease.	3%–9%: dizziness, rash, epigastric pain, heartburn, nausea, tinnitus	*Boxed Warning: NSAIDs are associated with an increased risk of adverse cardiovascular thrombotic events, including MI, stroke, and new onset or worsening of preexisting HTN. Use is contraindicated for treatment of perioperative pain in the setting of CABG surgery.* Recent GI bleed, third trimester of pregnancy, renal disease	Use with caution if history of CHF, HTN, GI bleeding; monitor for anemia with long-term use; older persons are at increased risk for AEs even at low doses; withhold for at least 4–6 half-lives prior to dental or surgical procedures; may increase risk of GI irritation, inflammation, ulceration, bleeding, and perforation
Naproxen (Aleve)			
Initial: 500 mg, then 250 mg q6–8h not to exceed 1,250 mg/d *Note*: Enteric-coated formulations not recommended for acute migraine	3%–9%: edema, dizziness, drowsiness, headache, pruritus, skin eruption, ecchymosis, fluid retention, abdominal pain, constipation, nausea, heartburn, hemolysis, tinnitus, dyspnea	Same as ibuprofen, including *boxed warning*	Same as ibuprofen
Ketoprofen			
25–50 mg q6–8h	>10%: dyspepsia, abnormal LFTs; 3%–9%: headache, abdominal pain, constipation, diarrhea, flatulence, nausea, renal dysfunction	Same as ibuprofen, including *boxed warning*	Same as ibuprofen
Barbiturates			
Butalbital 50 mg, caffeine 40 mg, acetaminophen 325 mg (Fioricet) 1–2 tabs q4h, not to exceed 6 tabs/d *Note*: Do not use butalbital for the management of acute migraine.	Drowsiness, light-headedness, dizziness, sedation, shortness of breath, nausea, vomiting, abdominal pain, intoxicated feeling	Hepatic or renal dysfunction, peptic ulcer disease, history of substance abuse, porphyria, pregnancy, concomitant use with alcohol or other CNS depressants	Contains acetaminophen; use with caution when taking other acetaminophen-containing drugs; do not exceed a total daily dose of 3,250-mg acetaminophen; may be habit forming or subject to abuse; avoid prolonged use or using with other sedating medications; not recommended for use in older persons
Butalbital 50 mg/caffeine 40 mg/aspirin 325 mg (Fiorinal) 1–2 tabs q4h, not to exceed 6 tabs/d *Note*: Do not use butalbital for management of acute migraine.	Same as butalbital	Hemorrhagic diathesis (e.g., hemophilia, hypoprothrombinemia, von Willebrand disease, thrombocytopenias, thrombasthenia and other ill-defined hereditary platelet dysfunctions, severe vitamin K deficiency, and severe liver damage); nasal polyps, angioedema, and bronchospastic reactivity to aspirin or other NSAIDs; peptic ulcer or other serious GI lesions; porphyria	Use with caution in the debilitated; severe impairment of renal or hepatic function, coagulation disorders, head injuries, elevated intracranial pressure, acute abdominal conditions, hypothyroidism, urethral stricture, Addison's disease, or prostatic hypertrophy; not recommended for use in older persons

AEs, adverse events; CABG, coronary artery bypass graft; CHF, congestive heart failure; CNS, central nervous system; GI, gastrointestinal; HTN, hypertension; LFT, liver function tests; MI, myocardial infarction; NSAIDs, nonsteroidal antiinflammatory drugs.

of venlafaxine and mirtazapine, but data supporting the use of other antidepressants for headache prophylaxis (including migraine) are lacking. Both mirtazapine and venlafaxine have both noradrenergic and seratonergic actions, which may be what contributes to their efficacy (Jensen, 2018). Smaller noncontrolled trials or case studies have shown efficacy with other tricyclic antidepressants (TCAs), such as imipramine, doxepin, and protriptyline. While there have been trials conducted on the efficacy of fluoxetine as headache prophylaxis, neither it nor the other selective serotonin reuptake inhibitors (SSRIs) have been shown to be effective as headache prophylaxis despite having a more favorable side effect profile compared with TCAs (Jensen, 2018). Other antidepressants, such as monoamine oxidase inhibitors (MAOIs) and serotonin antagonists, have been studied, but safety issues and side effect profiles make them an inappropriate choice for headache prophylaxis. Antidepressants for which little support exists for the management of headache should only be considered if the headache being treated is comorbid with depression. Alleviation or palliation of one comorbidity, however, will not necessarily resolve the other. Prophylactic medications should be started at low dosages and increased slowly. It can take 4 to 8 weeks before the full effect of these medications is seen. Finding the appropriate prophylactic agent for a patient is a process of trial and error, as medications work differently in different patients. Efficacy of preventive agents may only be modest, so it is important to consider the risk versus benefit of medication use. Discontinuation (typically as a taper) should be attempted every 6 to 12 months (Jensen, 2018).

Amitriptyline, a TCA, is the medication most commonly used to prevent tension headaches and considered to be a first-line, gold-standard drug. It can be used in doses much lower than those used for treating depression, ranging from 10 to 75 mg. Common side effects include sedation, constipation, blurred vision, and dry mouth. Amitriptyline should be used with caution in patients with a history of coronary artery disease (CAD), urinary retention, glaucoma, and seizures. Usually, only low doses of amitriptyline are needed, making discontinuation because of side effects uncommon. Higher doses of amitriptyline are typically used in headache patients with concomitant depression. Given its anticholinergic properties, amitriptyline is an inappropriate choice for use in older patients.

Second-line drugs that have been determined to be effective include venlafaxine (Effexor, a serotonin/norepinephrine reuptake inhibitor [SNRI]) and mirtazapine (Remeron, a tetracyclic antidepressant) at 150 and 30 mg, respectively (Jensen, 2018).

These drugs may also concurrently treat depression and anxiety. Common side effects of venlafaxine include nausea, somnolence, and insomnia, which often diminish after a few weeks. Patients may also experience sexual dysfunction, increased sweating, or nervousness, which may or may not diminish with time. Venlafaxine can also interact with many medications and should be tapered upon discontinuation,

as withdrawal symptoms may occur with abrupt discontinuation. An additional caution when considering the use of any antidepressant is that of suicidal ideation, particularly in adolescents. For this reason, all antidepressants carry boxed warnings.

Recently, data have emerged on the use of local anesthetics injected into pericranial myofascial trigger points. Lidocaine and bupivacaine are the most commonly used, with the most commonly injected muscles being the trapezius, sternocleidomastoid, and temporalis. While there are not many data on this approach, some studies have shown substantial efficacy in headache prophylaxis. Contraindications include pregnancy, infection, open skull defect or any condition in which injection landmarks become difficult to identify (e.g., obesity). Adverse events (AEs) are typically mild (associated with injection in general), and severe AEs are rare (but have been reported, e.g., pneumothorax) (Robbins et al., 2014). **Table 35.2** lists prophylactic agents for TTH.

First-Line Therapy for Tension Headaches

Aspirin and acetaminophen are appropriate first-line agents. They should be used no more than 2 days per week, as with any other analgesic agent, to avoid MOH. Acetaminophen should be used at a maximum single dose of 650 mg and a maximum daily dose of 3,250 mg. If used judiciously, these agents have few adverse effects and are very well tolerated. They work best for mild to moderate headaches. Again, the "Choosing Wisely" guideline of the American Headache Society (AHS) specifically counsels against the use of opioid- or butalbital-containing analgesics as first-line therapy (Loder et al., 2013).

Second-Line Therapy for Tension Headaches

NSAIDs are the next option for treatment of TTH. If one agent fails for two consecutive headaches, another agent in this class should be tried. NSAIDs seem to work well for more stubborn TTHs. If they provide incomplete relief, an antiemetic agent may be added to augment their effect.

Caffeine-containing analgesics available OTC such as Excedrin Extra Strength can also be an effective treatment. These medications should be used infrequently to obviate MOH and may be alternated with NSAIDs for different headaches.

Third-Line Therapy for Tension Headaches

If the agents mentioned earlier fail, then butalbital-containing compounds (Fioricet or Fiorinal) may be used in patients without specific risk factors for these medications. These agents may also be reserved as backup if the agents mentioned previously fail to relieve a more severe TTH. Again, butalbital-containing agents should never be used more than 3 days per month as they easily trigger MOH. As mentioned earlier, any patient requiring treatment for two or more headaches per week or who has particularly severe TTH should be considered for a prophylactic agent.

TABLE 35.2

Overview of Selected Drugs Used to Prevent Tension-Type Headaches

Generic (Brand) Name and Dosage	Selected Adverse Events	Contraindications	Special Considerations
Amitriptyline (Elavil)			
Initial: 10–25 mg QHS, usual dose 150 mg QHS; reported dosing ranges 10–400 mg/d (higher doses in patients with concomitant depression)	Degree of anticholinergic effects (urinary retention, dry mouth, constipation) are higher in amitriptyline than in other TCAs; drowsiness/ sedation (sometimes significant), orthostasis, conduction abnormalities	*Boxed Warning: Antidepressants increase the risk of suicidal thinking and behavior in children, adolescents, and young adults (ages 18–24) with major depressive disorder and other psychiatric disorders.* Not FDA approved for children aged <12	Most widely used; use with caution in patients with history of CVD (stroke, MI, tachycardia, or conduction abnormalities); use with caution in patients with BPH, glaucoma, urinary retention, xerostomia, visual problems, constipation, or history of bowel obstruction; use with caution in patients with diabetes, seizures, hyperthyroidism or thyroid supplementation), or hepatic or renal dysfunction; effects may be intensified by use of other CNS drugs or alcohol; use with caution in older persons.
Venlafaxine XR (Effexor XR)			
150 mg/d; taper discontinuation to obviate discontinuation syndrome.	>10%: nausea, somnolence, insomnia (often diminish after a few weeks); sexual dysfunction, increased sweating, nervousness (may or may not diminish with time)	*Boxed Warning: Antidepressants increase the risk of suicidal thinking and behavior in children, adolescents, and young adults (18–24 y of age) with major depressive disorder (MDD) and other psychiatric disorders.* Not FDA approved for use in children; monitor for serotonin syndrome, tachycardia, hypertension, and bleeding.	Often used because it usually has fewer side effects than amitriptyline; use with caution in older persons.
Mirtazapine (Remeron)			
15–30 mg/d; taper discontinuation to obviate discontinuation syndrome.	>10%: somnolence, increased cholesterol, xerostomia, increased appetite, constipation, weight gain	*Boxed Warning: Antidepressants increase the risk of suicidal thinking and behavior in children, adolescents, and young adults (18–24 y of age) with major depressive disorder (MDD) and other psychiatric disorders.* Not FDA approved for use in children; monitor for serotonin syndrome.	Use with caution in seizure disorders or in patients predisposed to seizure (e.g., brain damage, alcoholism, concomitant use with drugs that lower seizure threshold), hepatic or renal dysfunction, and in older persons; may actually help with nausea

BPH, benign prostatic hyperplasia; CNS, central nervous system; CVD, cardiovascular disease; FDA, U.S. Food and Drug Administration; MDD, major depressive disorder; MI, myocardial infarction; TCA, tricyclic antidepressants; XR, extended-release.

CAUSES OF MIGRAINE HEADACHE

The ICHD-3 characterizes migraine headaches as a "recurrent headache disorder manifesting in attacks lasting 4 to 72 hours. Typical characteristics of the headache are unilateral location, pulsating quality, moderate or severe intensity, aggravation by routine physical activity and association with nausea and/or photophobia and phonophobia" (ICHD-3, 2013). A large (N = 6,045) study assessing the most bothersome symptoms in migraine showed that the most bothersome symptom was photophobia (49.1%), followed by nausea in 28.1% and phonophobia in 22.8% of participants (Munjal et al., 2020). Why some patients experience migraines while others do not

is unknown, but it is clear that there is a genetic component to migraines and that migraines tend to cluster in families (Cho & Chu, 2015). Migraines are qualified as episodic (≤14 days per month) or chronic (≥15 days per month) (ICHD, 2018). There are many possible migraine triggers, and each patient's triggers are unique. Triggers range from certain foods to too much or too little sleep to medications to hormonal factors and others. In some patients, no obvious triggers are found. Estrogen is thought to play a role in the development of migraines, which explains the predominance of migraines in females. About 25% of migraine attacks occur within 4 days of menses when estrogen has fallen to a low level. The best way to pinpoint triggers is to have the patient keep a diary of

BOX 35.3 Factors That May Trigger Migraine Headaches

PSYCHOLOGICAL FACTORS

Anxiety
Depression
Stress (and relaxation after stress or the "letdown" hypothesis)
Intense emotion
Crisis; postcrisis letdown

MEDICATIONS

Vasodilators (e.g., blood pressure medications, medications for erectile dysfunction)
Hormones (contraceptives, hormone replacement therapy)
Caffeine
Vitamins

DIETARY FACTORS

Alcohol
Aspartame
Caffeine
Chocolate
Monosodium glutamate
Tyramine-containing foods (e.g., red wine)
"Certain foods" (patient-specific reports)

ENVIRONMENTAL/MECHANICAL FACTORS

Head movements
Bright, flashing lights, glare, or sunlight (photophobia)
High altitude
Loud noises (phonophobia)
Strong odors, perfume
Tobacco smoke (smoking or passive smoking) (nicotine)
Weather changes (hot or cold)

LIFESTYLE FACTORS

Dieting, skipping meals or fasting (hunger)
Obesity
Strenuous exercise/physical effort
Sleep problems: too much or too little sleep, insomnia, bruxism, snoring, daytime sleepiness
Fatigue
Smoking
Excessive alcohol consumption

HORMONAL FACTORS

Ovulation
Menopause
Menses
Pregnancy

Sources: Cho, S. J., & Chu, M. K. (2015). Risk factors of chronic daily headache or chronic migraine. *Current Pain and Headache Reports, 19*(1), 465; Lipton, R. B., Pavlovic, J. M., Haut, S. R., et al. (2014). Methodological issues in studying trigger factors and premonitory features of migraine. *Headache, 54*(10), 1661–1669; Pavlovic, J. M., Buse, D. C., Sollars, C. M., et al. (2014). Trigger factors and premonitory features of migraine attacks: Summary of studies. *Headache, 54*(10), 1670–1679.

what he or she ate and did in the 12 hours before getting the headache to see if any patterns emerge. A large literature review covering 15 studies evaluating triggers (in males and females, with either spontaneous reporting of triggers or selection from a list) identified a large variety of triggers experienced by individuals, reporting them anywhere from 8% of the time to 90% of the time. Some triggers are nonmodifiable (e.g., menstruation, gender, age, etc.), while others are modifiable (e.g., sleep deprivation) (Cho & Chu, 2015; Lipton et al., 2014; Pavlovic et al., 2014). **Box 35.3** lists migraine triggers.

PATHOPHYSIOLOGY OF MIGRAINE HEADACHES

The pathophysiology of migraine is thought to involve a "complex interplay between three distinct systems: the nervous system (the trigeminal nerve), the immune system (satellite glial cells), and the vascular system (intracranial dural arteries)" (p. 66601) (Ashina et al., 2019; Dubowchik et al., 2020; Edvinsson et al., 2019; Goadsby et al., 2019). Studies have shown an interaction of a large number of factors that result in the phenomenon, including genetics, afferent pain processing, anatomy and physiology of the trigeminal system, modulatory influence on trigeminal pain transmission, and various pain-processing phenomena (Goadsby, 2012). While previously believed to be vasculogenic in nature ("a good story ruined by the facts," as Goadsby says), neurogenic mechanisms are now recognized as the underlying cause of migraine pathophysiology, including atypical pain processing, central sensitization, hyperexcitability in the cortex, and inflammation (Schwedt, 2014). Recurring migraine may serve to sensitize the trigeminal system, lowering pain thresholds and possibly contributing to chronic migraine (CM). A network of primarily unmyelinated nerve fibers largely arising from the ophthalmic branch of the trigeminal nerve surrounds large cranial blood vessels, blood sinuses, the pia, and the dura in close proximity. The trigeminovascular system is an initiator and promoter of tissue inflammation and, when activated, releases neuropeptides such as substance P and calcitonin gene–related peptide (CGRP) that cause vasodilation and inflammation (which has significant implications for antimigraine therapy) (Ashina et al., 2019). Stimulation of these vessels and sinuses has been shown to be quite painful. Noradrenergic (from the locus ceruleus) and, more significantly, serotonergic neurons (from the dorsal raphe) regulate this activity; the periaqueductal gray region also contributes to pain modulation. Once triggered, impulses travel out through cranial nerve V and ultimately result in dilated meningeal blood vessels and release of neuroinflammatory and nociceptive compounds (Goadsby, 2012; Schwedt, 2014).

Some 80% of people with migraine report premonitory symptoms (e.g., nausea, bloating, fatigue, stiff neck, etc.) prior to the development of aura. Approximately 30% of migraines are accompanied by a prodromal aura, a focal neurologic phenomenon associated variously with visual, sensory, or motor symptoms, but typically affecting the visual field in a spreading fashion, traveling at approximately 3 mm/min from central to peripheral vision. Aura is not typically associated with pain (Charles, 2013; Goadsby, 2012).

In summary, migraine is a heritable disorder of episodic sensory sensitivity, associated with acute, throbbing pain and enhanced sensitivity to light, motion, sound, and odors. Migraine can be accompanied by nausea and unsteadiness. In different people with migraine, migraines can occur more or less frequently and vary in duration.

DIAGNOSTIC CRITERIA FOR MIGRAINE HEADACHE

The first step in making a precise diagnosis of migraine is to obtain a thorough headache history. Evaluation of the history should include age at onset; time of day when attacks occur; duration of attacks; precipitating or relieving factors; nature, intensity, and location of headache pain; and any associated symptoms. The patient should also be questioned about any aura symptoms, such as visual symptoms (flashing lights, loss of peripheral vision, diplopia, etc.) or other sensory symptoms (vertigo, tinnitus, paresthesias, or hemiparesis). Having patients keep a migraine diary helps identify triggers and premonitory symptoms. Because a family history is evident in many patients, asking if anyone in the family experiences migraines aids in the diagnosis. Note that some patients may fulfill criteria for both migraine with aura and migraine without aura (ICHD-3, 2018). Specific diagnostic criteria for migraine with aura (classic migraine) and without aura (common migraine) are given in **Box 35.4**.

Patients most frequently experience migraines in the early morning, but a migraine attack can come at any time of the day. Migraines are more often unilateral than bilateral with the pain occurring around the eye or the temple. Migraine pain generally peaks 2 to 12 hours into the attack. Common

---

BOX 35.4   Diagnostic Criteria for Migraine, International Classification of Headache Disorders, Third Edition

MIGRAINE WITHOUT AURA

A. At least five attacks fulfilling criteria B–D
B. Headache attacks lasting 4 to 72 hours (untreated or unsuccessfully treated)
C. Headache has at least two of the following four characteristics:
   1. Unilateral location
   2. Pulsating quality
   3. Moderate or severe pain intensity
   4. Aggravation by or causing avoidance of routine physical activity (e.g., walking or climbing stairs)
D. During headache, at least one of the following:
   1. Nausea and/or vomiting
   2. Photophobia and phonophobia
E. Not better accounted for by another ICHD-3 diagnosis

MIGRAINE WITH AURA

A. At least two attacks fulfilling criteria B and C
B. One or more of the following fully reversible aura symptoms:
   1. Visual
   2. Sensory
   3. Speech and/or language
   4. Motor
   5. Brain stem
   6. Retinal
C. At least three of the following six characteristics:
   1. At least one aura symptom spreads gradually over 5 minutes or more.
   2. Two or more symptoms occur in succession.
   3. Each individual aura symptom lasts 5 to 60 minutes.
   4. At least one aura symptom is unilateral.
   5. At least one aura symptom is positive.
   6. The aura is accompanied, or followed within 60 minutes, by headache.
D. Not better accounted for by another ICHD-3 diagnosis

Source: Modified from Headache Classification Committee of the International Headache Society (IHS). (2018). The International Classification of Headache Disorders, 3rd edition. *Cephalalgia, 38*(1), 1–211.

---

symptoms accompanying migraine include nausea, anxiety, depression, irritability, fatigue, light and noise sensitivity, diarrhea or constipation, and hunger or anorexia. Patients may describe the pain of migraine as pounding, pulsating, or throbbing. A migraine sufferer often seeks refuge in a dark, quiet place.

INITIATING DRUG THERAPY FOR MIGRAINE HEADACHES

Practitioners must consider many factors when designing a treatment regimen for patients with migraine, such as the severity of the pain, duration of attack, concomitant disease states, current medication use, and any triggers. Migraine treatment needs to be highly individualized. **Table 35.3** gives an overview of selected drugs used for abortive treatment of migraine headaches.

The most effective treatment for migraines involves both nonpharmacologic and pharmacologic approaches. Nonpharmacologic approaches include various psychological techniques that aid in managing the migraine attack. Relaxation, stress management, and biofeedback are some techniques used to reduce migraine severity and frequency. Progressive muscle relaxation and the use of autogenic phrases are examples of relaxation techniques (see section on tension headaches).

Goals of Drug Therapy

The main goal of pharmacologic therapy is to prevent or relieve the migraine attacks with minimal or no side effects. Short-term goals include decreasing the severity, frequency, and number of migraine days of the headache and relieving nausea, if present. Long-term goals established by the U.S. Headache Consortium include reducing attack frequency and severity, reducing disability, improving quality of life, preventing headache, avoiding headache medication escalation, and educating and enabling patients to manage their disease (Silberstein et al., 2012). Efficacy endpoints in the management of migraine (i.e., in clinical trials) are generally recognized as being pain free (no pain) or headache relief (improvement) response at 2 hours post dose, reduction in 24-hour recurrence rate, and favorable AE profile.

Nonsteroidal Antiinflammatory Drugs

NSAIDs and aspirin are qualified by the AHS as having established efficacy (AHS, 2019). These medications, like all migraine medications, work best when taken early in the attack. The most common side effects are GI. The same doses as used for tension headaches are appropriate for migraines (American Academy of Neurology [AAN] guidelines have not changed since 2000) (Marmura et al., 2015). Aspirin may be used in initial dosages of up to 900 mg. Aspirin alone is effective in up to 40% of migraine patients. As AAN guidelines have not been updated since 2000, a starting dose of 1,000 mg acetaminophen is still reported as an effective intervention for acute migraine, although recommended doses of acetaminophen in general have been reduced. As with tension headaches, a given NSAID should be used on more than one occasion before deciding whether it is efficacious.

Caffeine-Containing Compounds

OTC caffeine-containing compounds (such as Excedrin Extra Strength or Excedrin Migraine) are also effective for milder migraines, but they can easily cause MOH and should be used

no more than 3 days per month or for more than 48 hours at a time. These preparations also contain acetaminophen (250 mg per tablet), so caution is required if acetaminophen or many of the other OTC or prescription acetaminophen-containing preparations are being used, especially concomitantly.

5-HT$_{1b/d}$ Receptor Agonists (Triptans)

Triptans are migraine-specific drugs that work as 5-HT$_1$ serotonin receptor agonists. These receptors are located on intracranial blood vessels, presynaptically on CNS sensory neurons, and trigeminal terminals. Peripherally, triptans binding to the 5-HT$_{1b}$ receptors cause cerebral vasoconstriction and can treat both the pain and nausea of migraine. Binding to 5-HT$_{1d}$ is associated with blockage of the vasoactive peptides that trigger neurogenic inflammation. Triptans also have central effects, interfering with afferent nociceptive signaling (Ong & De Felice, 2018).

Triptans are indicated for acute treatment of migraine with or without aura, and they are used for moderate to severe migraines or for milder migraines that do not respond to NSAIDs, aspirin, or the combination drugs mentioned previously. Triptans vary in their time to onset of action, peak concentration, half-lives, AE profiles, formulation, and route of administration, which helps guide the selection of a triptan for a particular patient. Given the highly individualized nature of migraine, different medications may be more effective than others in any given patient. If a triptan fails on two separate occasions, another triptan should be tried. Triptans work best when given early during a migraine, but unlike many other agents, they may be effective even when given late in the course of a migraine (Ong & De Felice, 2018).

Triptans should not be used more than 9 days per month and should not be used within 24 hours of any other vasoconstricting drug such as ergotamine. Use of these medications is considered to be a better choice than use of the ergot derivatives, as potency is similar but AEs are significantly fewer in number (Khoury & Couch, 2010). In a meta-analysis of 133 randomized controlled trials of triptans, standard dose triptans provided 42% to 76% 2-hour pain relief and 18% to 50% pain freedom (Cameron et al., 2015). Triptans should be avoided in patients with basilar, hemiplegic, or retinal migraines; they must also be avoided in patients with CAD, cerebrovascular disease, or severe peripheral vascular disease (PVD). Concomitant use of ergotamines and dihydroergotamine (DHE) is also contraindicated, and while serotonin syndrome is rare, the possibility for it exists with concomitant use of triptans and SSRIs or SNRIs. No more than one triptan at a time should be used within 24 hours.

The seven triptan drugs are sumatriptan, zolmitriptan, naratriptan, rizatriptan, almotriptan, eletriptan, and frovatriptan. A combination sumatriptan/naproxen formulation is also available. Sumatriptan and zolmitriptan are available as a nasal spray, and sumatriptan is also available in subcutaneous and nasal powder formulations. These are useful for patients with severe nausea, who cannot tolerate an oral medication.

TABLE 35.3

Overview of Selected Drugs for Acute/Abortive Migraine Treatment

Generic (Trade) Name and Dosage	Selected Adverse Events	Contraindications	Special Considerations
Aspirin 325–900 mg q4–6h, not to exceed 4,000 mg/d	GI upset (stomach pain, nausea, heartburn, vomiting); GI bleeding and angioedema (uncommon)	Platelet or bleeding disorders, renal dysfunction, erosive gastritis, peptic ulcer disease, asthma, rhinitis, nasal polyps, severe hepatic or renal failure, or sensitivity to salicylates	Avoid using with NSAIDs, alcohol, during pregnancy, and in children <16 y with viral infections; discontinue 1–2 wk prior to surgery.
NSAIDs			
See **Table 35.1**.	See **Table 35.1**.	See **Table 35.1** (including *boxed warning*).	See **Table 35.1**.
OTC caffeine-containing compounds (Excedrin Extra Strength or Excedrin Migraine; acetaminophen 250 mg/aspirin 250 mg/caffeine 65 mg) 1–2 tabs q24h; do not use for longer than 48 h.	Insomnia, agitation	Uncontrolled HTN	Avoid use with other vasoconstrictive agents; use sparingly to obviate MOH.
Triptans			
Sumatriptan (Imitrex and Alsuma) 25, 50, 100 mg PO at headache onset, may repeat dose up to 100 mg in 2 h	PO: 3%–>10%: Malaise/fatigue, jaw pain/lightness/pressure, paresthesia, pressure/lightness/heaviness, warm/cold sensation	Pregnancy, uncontrolled HTN, ischemic heart disease, stroke, TIA, PVD, severe hepatic impairment, basilar or hemiplegic migraine; use within 24 h of use of ergot derivatives, or within 2 weeks of (or concomitant) use of MAOIs; do not use as prophylactic treatment for migraine; not for IV use Contraindications are ischemic CAD or coronary artery vasospasm, including Prinzmetal's angina or Wolff-Parkinson-White syndrome or arrhythmias associated with other cardiac accessory conduction pathway disorders History of stroke, TIA, or hemiplegic or basilar migraine; PVD; ischemic bowel disease; or uncontrolled hypertension Recent (i.e., within 24 h) use of ergotamine-containing or ergot-type medication, or another 5-HT$_1$ agonist; or concurrent or recent (within 2 weeks) use of an MAO inhibitor; known hypersensitivity to sumatriptan (angioedema and anaphylaxis seen) or severe hepatic impairment	Use with caution in history of CAD, HTN, seizure disorder (or low seizure threshold), or hepatic impairment; use caution with concomitant use of other serotonergic drugs (SSRIs, SNRIs, other triptans) or proserotonergic drugs (e.g., tryptophan); use at lowest possible doses ONZETRA may cause myocardial ischemia/infarction, Prinzmetal's angina; arrhythmias; sensations of chest/throat/neck/jaw pain, tightness, pressure, or heaviness; cerebral hemorrhage, subarachnoid hemorrhage, and stroke; other vasospasm reactions; MOH; serotonin syndrome; increased BP, anaphylaxis, and seizures (use with caution in epilepsy or lowered seizure threshold)
Imitrex, Zembrace, 6 mg subcutaneous, may repeat dose in 2 h	SC: >10%: dizziness, warm/hot sensation, pain at injection site, paresthesia; 3%–10%: chest pain/lightness/ heaviness/pressure, burning, feeling of heaviness, flushing, pressure sensation, feeling of tightness, drowsiness, neck, throat, and jaw pain/lightness/pressure, mouth/tongue discomfort, weakness, numbness, throat discomfort		
Imitrex, Tosymra; 5, 10, or 20 mg intranasal spray; may repeat dose in 2 h (to 30 mg maximum per day)	IN powder: >2%: abnormal taste, nasal discomfort, rhinorrhea, and rhinitis		
Onzetra Xsail; 22 mg intranasal powder; may repeat dose in 2 h	IN: >10%: bad taste, nausea, vomiting; 5%–10%: nasal discomfort/disorder		

TABLE 35.3

Overview of Selected Drugs for Acute/Abortive Migraine Treatment *(Continued)*

Generic (Trade) Name and Dosage	Selected Adverse Events	Contraindications	Special Considerations
Zolmitriptan (Zomig) Tablet: 2.5 mg at onset, not to exceed 10 mg q24h ODT: 2.5 mg at onset, not to exceed 10 mg q24h Nasal spray: 1 spray (2.5 mg) at onset, not to exceed 10 mg q24h	PO: 3%–10%: chest pain, dizziness, somnolence, pain, nausea, xerostomia, dyspepsia, paresthesia, weakness, warm/cold sensation, neck/throat/jaw pain, diaphoresis	Pregnancy, ischemic heart disease or vasospastic CAD, uncontrolled HTN, symptomatic Wolff-Parkinson-White syndrome or other arrhythmias associated with accessory cardiac conduction pathway disorders; do not use within 24 h of (or concomitant with) use of another 5-HT$_1$ agonist, or use within 2 weeks of (or concomitant with) use of MAOIs; do not use with with ergot derivatives; do not use for management of basilar or hemiplegic migraine; additional contraindications for IN use: stroke, TIA, PVD	High-risk factors for heart disease (HTN, high cholesterol, obesity, diabetes, smoking, strong family history of heart disease, postmenopausal women, and males >40 y old)
Naratriptan (Amerge) 1 mg or 2.5 mg q4h to maximum of 5 mg/d (used off-label for menstrual migraine prophylaxis, 1 mg BID for 5 days, starting 2 days before menses onset)	1%–10%: dizziness, drowsiness, malaise/fatigue, nausea, vomiting, paresthesia, pain/pressure in throat or neck	Pregnancy, uncontrolled HTN, ischemic heart disease, PVD, severe hepatic or renal impairment; do not use within 24 h of (or concomitant) use of ergot derivatives; do not use for treatment of basilar or hemiplegic migraine.	Use with caution in patients with risk factors for CAD, smoking, cerebral/subarachnoid hemorrhage, stroke, peripheral vascular ischemia, and history of HTN; not recommended for use in older persons; use lowest possible dose.
Rizatriptan (Maxalt oral tablet and Maxalt-MLT, ODT) Tablet: 5 mg and 10 mg q2h to maximum of 30 mg/d (patients taking concomitant propranolol: maximum of 15 mg/d) ODT: 5 and 10 mg q2h to maximum of 30 mg (patients taking concomitant propranolol: maximum of 15 mg/d) *Note:* Patients with cardiac risks should be administered first dose in the physician's office under observation.	>10%: dizziness, drowsiness, fatigue (dose dependent); 1%–10%: paresthesia, chest or neck/throat/jaw pain (tightness/pressure and/or heaviness), xerostomia, nausea	Documented ischemic heart disease or Prinzmetal angina or uncontrolled HTN; do not use within 24 h of (or concomitant) use of another 5-HT$_1$ agonist, or use within 2 weeks of (or concomitant) use of MAOIs, or concomitant use with ergot derivatives; do not use for treatment of basilar or hemiplegic migraine.	Reconsider migraine diagnosis if patient does not respond to first dose; patients with symptoms of angina post dose should be evaluated for CAD or Prinzmetal angina before receiving a second dose; do not administer to patients with risk factors for CAD (e.g., HTN, hypercholesterolemia, smoking, obesity, diabetes, strong family history of CAD, menopause, males >40 y) without adequate cardiac workup; use with caution in older persons or in patients with hepatic or renal impairment (including dialysis); evaluate cardiovascular status periodically; avoid concomitant use of other serotonergic drugs (SSRIs/SNRIs, other triptans) and serotonin precursors (e.g., tryptophan).

(Continued)

TABLE 35.3

Overview of Selected Drugs for Acute/Abortive Migraine Treatment *(Continued)*

Generic (Trade) Name and Dosage	Selected Adverse Events	Contraindications	Special Considerations
Almotriptan (Axert) 6.25 and 12.5 mg q2h to maximum of 25 mg/d *Note:* Patients taking potent CYP3A4 inhibitors should only take 6.25 mg as a starting dose to a maximum of 12.5 mg/d	3%–10%: somnolence, dizziness, nausea	Pregnancy, known or suspected ischemic heart disease, stroke TIA, PVD, uncontrolled HTN; do not use within 24 h of (or concomitant) use of another 5-HT$_1$ agonist or concomitant use with ergot derivatives, MAOIs, or sibutramine; do not use for treatment of basilar or hemiplegic migraine.	Do not use for migraine prophylaxis or cluster headache; if patient doesn't respond to first dose, reconsider migraine diagnosis; use with caution in patients with sulfonamide allergy; do not administer to patients with risk factors for CAD (e.g., HTN, hypercholesterolemia, smoking, obesity, diabetes, strong family history of CAD, menopause, males >40 y) without adequate cardiac workup; evaluate cardiovascular status periodically; use with caution in patients with hepatic or renal impairment, avoid concomitant use of other serotonergic drugs (SSRIs/SNRIs, other triptans).
Eletriptan (Relpax) 20 and 40 mg q2h to maximum of 80 mg/d	3%–10%: chest pain/tightness, dizziness, somnolence, headache, nausea, xerostomia, weakness, paresthesia	Pregnancy, ischemic heart disease or signs or symptoms of ischemic heart disease, stroke, TIA, PVD, or uncontrolled HTN; do not use in severe hepatic impairment or with concomitant use within 24 h of an ergot derivative or another 5-HT$_1$ agonist, or within 72 h of potent CYP3A4 inhibitors or sibutramine; do not use for treatment of basilar or hemiplegic migraine or for migraine prophylaxis.	Do not administer to patients with risk factors for CAD without adequate cardiac workup; evaluate cardiovascular status periodically; use with caution in patients with mild to moderate hepatic impairment; avoid concomitant use of other serotonergic drugs (SSRIs/SNRIs, other triptans) or serotonin precursors (e.g., tryptophan).
Frovatriptan (Frova) 2.5 mg q2h to maximum of 7.5 mg/d	3%–10%: flushing, dizziness, fatigue, headache, hot or cold sensation, xerostomia, paresthesia, skeletal pain	Ischemic heart disease or signs and symptoms of ischemic heart disease, stroke, TIA, PVD, or uncontrolled HTN; do not use with concomitant use within 24 h of an ergot derivative or another 5-HT$_1$ agonist; do not use for treatment of hemiplegic or basilar migraine.	Not intended for migraine prophylaxis or cluster headache; rule out underlying neurologic disease in patients with atypical headache or migraine (with no prior history of migraine), or inadequate clinical response to first dose; do not administer to patients with risk factors for CAD without adequate cardiac workup; evaluate cardiovascular status periodically; slow onset, longest half-life of the triptans
Triptan plus NSAID			
Sumatriptan plus naproxen (Treximet) 85 mg sumatriptan and 500 mg naproxen, maximum 2 tab/24h	See individual **Selected Adverse Events** for sumatriptan and naproxen given previously.	See individual **Contraindications** for sumatriptan and naproxen given previously. Contraindicated in hepatic impairment	See individual **Special Considerations** for sumatriptan and naproxen given previously. Not recommended in patients with a CrCl <30 mL/min

TABLE 35.3

Overview of Selected Drugs for Acute/Abortive Migraine Treatment (*Continued*)

Generic (Trade) Name and Dosage	Selected Adverse Events	Contraindications	Special Considerations
Ditans			
Lasmiditan (Reyvow) 50 mg, 100 mg, or 200 mg PRN; maximum of 1 dose/24 h	AEs reported at ≥2% in clinical trials include dizziness, fatigue, paresthesia, sedation, nausea/vomiting, and muscle weakness	None	May cause significant driving impairment; may cause CNS depression (dizziness, sedation); may cause serotonin syndrome (e.g., agitation, hallucinations, coma, tachycardia, labile blood pressure, hyperthermia, hyperreflexia, incoordination, nausea, vomiting, diarrhea); may cause MOH
Gepants (Oral CGRP Inhibitors)			
Ubrogepant (Ubrelvy) 50 mg and 100 mg PRN; a second dose may be administered at least 2 h after initial dose; maximum 200 mg/24 h Severe hepatic or renal impairment: 50 mg; a second dose 2 h after the initial dose	AEs >2% most commonly reported in clinical trials were nausea and somnolence	Concomitant use with strong CYP3A4 inhibitors	Avoid concomitant administration of strong and moderate CYP3A inducers
Rimegepant (Nurtec) ODT: 75 mg; maximum dose/24 h, 75 mg	AE reported in ≥1% in clinical trials was nausea.		Severe hypersensitivity reactions (dyspnea and rash) Drug interactions: strong CYP3A4 inhibitors (avoid concomitant administration); moderate CYP3A4 inhibitors (avoid another dose within 48h); strong and moderate CYP3A inducers (avoid concomitant administration); inhibitors of P-gp or BCRP (avoid concomitant administration)
Ergot Derivatives			
Ergotamine tartrate (Ergomar) 6 mg/24 hours or per attack SL; not to exceed 10 mg/wk	Serious vasoconstrictive distress (ischemia, cyanosis, absence of pulse, cold extremities, gangrene, precordial distress and pain, ECG changes and muscle pains), transient tachycardia or bradycardia and hypertension, nausea, vomiting, paresthesias, numbness, weakness, vertigo, localized edema, itching, rare fibrosis (retroperitoneal, pleuropulmonary, and heart valve)	*Boxed warning: Serious and/or life-threatening peripheral ischemia has been associated with the coadministration of ergotamine tartrate with potent CYP3A4 inhibitors, including protease inhibitors and macrolide antibiotics. Because CYP3A4 inhibition elevates the serum levels of ergotamine tartrate, the risk for vasospasm leading to cerebral ischemia and/or ischemia of the extremities is increased. Hence, concomitant use of these medications is contraindicated.* Pregnancy category X; do not use in patients with PVD, coronary heart disease, or HTN, impaired hepatic or renal function, or sepsis.	Withdrawal and MOH may occur with prolonged use.

(Continued)

TABLE 35.3

Overview of Selected Drugs for Acute/Abortive Migraine Treatment (*Continued*)

Generic (Trade) Name and Dosage	Selected Adverse Events	Contraindications	Special Considerations
Dihydroergotamine (Migranal) IM/SC: 1 mg first sign of headache, repeat hourly to a maximum dose of 3 mg total, to a maximum dose of 6 mg/wk IV: 1 mg first sign of headache, repeat hourly to a maximum dose of 2 mg total, to a maximum of 6 mg/wk Intranasal: 1 spray (0.5 mg) each nostril, repeat q15min if necessary, to a maximum of 4 sprays to a maximum of 6 sprays/d and a maximum of 8 sprays/wk	3%–10%: dizziness, somnolence, nausea, taste disturbance, vomiting, application-site reaction, pharyngitis Nasal spray >10%: rhinitis	See *boxed warning* of ergotamine. Pregnancy category X; do not use in patients with ischemic heart disease (angina pectoris, history of MI, or documented silent ischemia) or in patients with clinical symptoms or findings consistent with coronary artery vasospasm, including Prinzmetal variant angina; do not use in uncontrolled HTN; do not use with concomitant use of 5-HT$_1$ agonists, or other ergotamine-containing or ergot-type medications or methysergide within 24 h; do not use for treatment of hemiplegic or basilar migraine, PAD, sepsis, following vascular surgery, or in severely impaired hepatic or renal function.	Use only when a clear diagnosis of migraine headache has been established; not for prolonged use; use with caution in older persons.
Caffeine/Ergotamine (Cafergot) PO: 1 mg ergotamine/100 mg caffeine; 1–2 tabs at onset; may repeat after 1 h to maximum of 6 tabs/d Rectal: 2 mg ergotamine/100 mg caffeine; 1 supp PR; may repeat after 1 h to maximum 2 supp/d	Nausea, vomiting, irritability, palpitations, paresthesias, MOH, dizziness, tingling of the extremities, rare MI	*Boxed warning: Serious and/or life-threatening peripheral ischemia has been associated with coadministration of Cafergot with potent CYP3A4 inhibitors (e.g., protease inhibitors, macrolide antibiotics). Because CYP3A4 inhibition elevates serum levels of Cafergot, the risk of vasospasm leading to cerebral ischemia and/or ischemia of the extremities is increased. Concomitant use of these medications is contraindicated.* Pregnancy category X; do not use in HTN, PVD, and CAD; do not use with impaired hepatic or renal function or in sepsis.	Use with caution with concomitant use of less potent CYP3A4 inhibitors; avoid excessive or prolonged use; not indicated for migraine prophylaxis; monitor use in mild to moderate hepatic impairment; MOH may be associated with prolonged and uninterrupted use.

Barbiturates (see **Table 35.1**)

Opioids

Butorphanol Nasal spray (1 mg) 1 spray in 1 nostril, may repeat in 1 h; can repeat initial dosing sequence q3–4h PRN Adjust for renal and hepatic impairment: 1 mg at onset, 1 mg 60–90 min later, then at intervals of no <6 h	>10%: somnolence, dizziness, nausea and/or vomiting, nasal congestion, insomnia	History of substance abuse	Use with caution in impaired renal, hepatic, or pulmonary function; use with caution in older persons; use sparingly—not recommended as a first-line drug.

TABLE 35.3

Overview of Selected Drugs for Acute/Abortive Migraine Treatment (Continued)

Generic (Trade) Name and Dosage	Selected Adverse Events	Contraindications	Special Considerations
Acetaminophen with codeine (Tylenol with codeine) 1–2 tabs q4h to a maximum of 12 tabs/d Tylenol with codeine 3: 30-mg codeine, 300-mg acetaminophen Tylenol with codeine 4: 60-mg codeine, 300-mg acetaminophen	Severe hepatotoxicity on acute overdose, potential liver damage with chronic daily dosing, nephrotoxicity, agranulocytosis, rash, drowsiness, constipation	Chronic alcohol use, alcoholic liver disease, or impaired liver or renal function; G6PD deficiency; history of substance abuse; do not use for pregnancy for prolonged use or high doses at term.	May be used sparingly in pregnancy; do not exceed 3,250-mg acetaminophen/d (including concomitant use with other acetaminophen-containing products); decrease dose in patients with renal impairment; use with caution in patients with respiratory disorders, CNS depression/ coma, head trauma, morbid obesity, prostatic hyperplasia, urinary stricture, thyroid dysfunction, or severe renal or liver insufficiency; may cause CNS depression or hypotension; use with caution in patients with hypovolemia or cardiovascular disease; abrupt discontinuation after prolonged use may result in withdrawal.
Steroids			
Dexamethasone Single dose of 4 or 4 mg BID × 2 d then 4 mg daily × 3 d with tapered discontinuation	Nausea, GI upset, insomnia, mood swings, rare and serious steroid psychosis, peptic ulcer disease, CHF	Pregnancy; systemic fungal infections or acute head injury; avoid concomitant use with aldesleukin, BCG, dronedarone, everolimus, natalizumab, nilotinib, nisoldipine, pazopanib, ranolazine, romidepsin, tolvaptan, and live vaccines.	Use as rescue medication only; use with caution in thyroid disease, hepatic and renal impairment, CVD, DM, glaucoma, cataracts, myasthenia gravis, GI diseases, and in patients at risk for osteoporosis or seizures; use with caution in older persons at the lowest possible dose for a short duration.

AEs, adverse events; BCG, Bacillus Calmette-Guerin vaccine; BCRP, breast cancer resistance protein; BP, blood pressure; CAD, coronary artery disease; CGRP, calcitonin gene–related peptide; CNS, central nervous system; DM, dextromethorphan; ECG, electrocardiogram; GI, gastrointestinal; HTN, hypertension; IM, intramuscular; IV, intravenous; MAOIs, monoamine oxidase inhibitors; MOH, medication overuse headache; NSAID, nonsteroidal antiinflammatory drug; ODT, orally disintegrating tablets; OTC, over-the-counter; PAD, peripheral arterial disease; PVD, peripheral vascular disease; SC, subcutaneous; SL, sublingual; SNRIs, serotonin/norepinephrine reuptake inhibitor; SSRIs, serotonin reuptake inhibitors; TIA, transient ischemic attack.

Zolmitriptan and rizatriptan are also available as orally disintegrating tablets (ODT). The injectable form of sumatriptan has the fastest onset of action of any of the triptans but has a short half-life, often giving limited headache relief. Sumatriptan is also associated with more AEs than the other triptans. Frovatriptan has the longest half-life (but one of the slowest onsets) of the triptans, at 25 hours, making it useful for patients with long-lasting migraines (frovatriptan also binds to 5-HT$_{1f}$ in addition to 5-HT$_{1b}$ and 5-HT$_{1d}$). Use of the triptans in the early, mild stages of migraine (but not during aura) results in greater relief (up to 70% pain free in clinical trials) than use of the drugs during moderate or severe migraine (up to 30% pain free in clinical trials), but the patient needs to be able to recognize onset of migraine and distinguish it from TTH. Use of a triptan for more than 9 days per month may result in MOH, during which time, preventive therapy will be ineffective (Ong & De Felice, 2018).

Sumatriptan

Sumatriptan (Imitrex) was the first triptan on the market (approved by U.S. Food and Drug Administration [FDA] in 1992 and now available as a generic) and still offers the fastest relief of all the triptans presently available. In its subcutaneous form, it offers the highest therapeutic gain of all the triptans in clinical trials (Cameron et al., 2015; Ong & De Felice, 2018). It is safe and well tolerated (available OTC in the United Kingdom) (Antonaci et al., 2010; Johnston & Rapoport, 2010). Sumatriptan is available in tablets (25, 50, and 100 mg), a powder nasal spray (20 mg), a nasal powder (11 mg), and a subcutaneous injection (4 and 6 mg). A transdermal formulation was removed from the market in 2016 (see **Table 35.3**).

Injectable sumatriptan offers the quickest onset of action (10 minutes), whereas onset of effect of the tablet takes longer (30–90 minutes). Sumatriptan is the only triptan with a subcutaneous formulation, making it the fastest-onset triptan available, but it also has the shortest half-life of the triptans (2 hours), limiting the longer-term relief associated with some of the other triptans with longer half-lives. Injectable sumatriptan is associated with more AEs than oral sumatriptan (Ong & De Felice, 2018). If the headache recurs, the patient can take a second dose of medication, but only after a certain time and without exceeding the maximum dose of 200 mg/d. Patients with migraine with aura cannot take sumatriptan until the headache actually begins because the drug has no effect on relieving aura symptoms. Patients with nausea and vomiting tend to find the nasal formulations easier to take (Ong & De Felice, 2018). Pain relief may be dose dependent, but with increased doses come increased AEs. AEs vary by mode of delivery, but most occurred in less than 10% of trial subjects. Concomitant use of sumatriptan with MAOIs is contraindicated.

Zolmitriptan

Zolmitriptan (Zomig) (FDA approved in 1997 and now available as a generic) is available in tablet, nasal spray, and orally disintegrating formulations and can be used for migraine with or without aura and as prophylaxis for menstrual migraine (Ong & De Felice, 2018). The recommended initial dose of zolmitriptan is 2.5 to 5 mg; a maximum high dose of 10 mg is possible. The onset of effect is attained within 45 minutes, resulting in a rapid therapeutic response. Its half-life is 2.5 to 3 hours, longer than that of sumatriptan, and it is extremely potent at serotonin receptors. Zolmitriptan has been shown in clinical trials to be similar in efficacy to sumatriptan (5 vs. 100 mg, respectively), and at a dose of 2.5 mg, it is similar in efficacy to sumatriptan 50 mg, almotriptan 12.5 mg, eletriptan 40 mg, and rizatriptan 10 mg. Therapeutic gain is slightly higher in nasal and orally disintegrating formulations. Efficacy may be dose dependent with a concomitant increase in AEs. Dosage should be adjusted down to 1.25 mg in patients with moderate to severe hepatic impairment. Contraindications and adverse effects are similar to the other triptans, and zolmitriptan carries a specific contraindication in patients with Wolf-Parkinson-White syndrome (Ong & De Felice, 2018). MAOIs should also not be used with zolmitriptan, nor should CYP1A2 inhibitors such as cimetidine, fluvoxamine, and ciprofloxacin (see **Table 35.3**).

Naratriptan

Naratriptan (Amerge) (FDA approved in 1998 and now available as a generic) is marketed as an alternative agent for patients who are taking repeated doses of other migraine therapies, specifically those who have recurrent headache or chest tightness when using oral sumatriptan. Naratriptan is available only in 1 and 2.5 mg tablet formulations (see **Table 35.3**) and reaches peak serum concentrations in 2 to 3 hours. While onset is slow (1–2 hours), duration of action is longest of all the triptans; because of its long half-life of 5 to 6.3 hours, headache recurrences are not common. An initial dose of 1 to 2.5 mg should be used; if headache does not resolve, a second dose can be administered within 4 hours, not to exceed a total dose of 5 mg (Ong & De Felice, 2018). The safety of treating more than four migraines per month with naratriptan has not been established. Therapeutic gain at 4 hours (as compared with 2 hours) tends to be higher in this triptan. In the original clinical trial, headache relief was experienced by 68% of patients 4 hours post dose and was maintained for 8 to 24 hours. Given its availability only in low dosages, its side effect profile in clinical trials was comparable to placebo, making this triptan a good option for patients experiencing intolerable side effects with other triptans (Ong & De Felice, 2018).

Rizatriptan

Rizatriptan (Maxalt) (FDA approved in 1998 and now available as a generic) is available in a tablet (5 and 10 mg) and as an ODT (Maxalt-MLT; 5 and 10 mg), offering an alternative way to treat a migraine. Onset of action is rapid (half an hour to 2 hours), particularly with the ODT. Rizatriptan 10 mg produces faster relief than do sumatriptan 50 mg and naratriptan 2.5 mg and is similar in efficacy to almotriptan 12.5 mg, eletriptan 40 mg, and zolmitriptan 2.5 mg. Effects of rizatriptan can be observed within 30 minutes and last from 14 to 16 hours (half-life of 2–3 hours). In the original clinical trial, 62% of patients taking the 5-mg dose and 71% of patients taking the 10-mg dose experienced pain relief 2 hours post dose. Complete relief was achieved in 33% of patients taking a 5-mg dose and 42% of patients taking the 10-mg dose. The drug is well tolerated even at 10 tablets per month. A second dose can be taken within 2 hours of the first dose if the headache is not resolving; 30 mg should not be exceeded per 24 hours. Rizatriptan should not be used concomitantly with MAOIs, and if used concomitantly with propranolol, only a 5 mg dose of rizatriptan should be used, to a maximum dosage of 15 mg per 24 hours (Ong & De Felice, 2018) (see **Table 35.3**).

Almotriptan

Almotriptan (Axert) (FDA approved in 2001; now available only as a generic) is a rapidly absorbed triptan with a moderately long half-life (3–4 hours) but comparatively slow onset (1–3 hours). Its efficacy is similar to that of the other triptans, but its potential for drug–drug interactions is reduced, given that it is metabolized by three separate metabolic pathways. It is a well-tolerated drug with few AEs and is a good choice for triptan-naive patients or as an alternate drug for patients who need to be switched over from other triptans due to intolerable side effects (Ong & De Felice, 2018). Use of almotriptan is contraindicated in patients with renal impairment with concomitant use of a potent CYP3A4 inhibitor. Dose of almotriptan should be adjusted down to 6.25 mg in a single dose, to a maximum dose of 12.5 mg in any patient taking a potent CYP3A4 inhibitor (e.g., ketoconazole, itraconazole, clarithromycin, etc.) (see **Table 35.3**).

Eletriptan

Eletriptan (Relpax) (FDA approved in 2002 and available as a generic) is available in 20 and 40 mg tablets. The recommended initial dose is 40 mg at the onset of migraine. If relief is not obtained in 2 hours, the dose may be repeated to a maximum of 80 mg/d. Onset of action is rapid (less than an hour), and elimination half-life is moderately long (4 hours)—shorter only than naratriptan and frovatriptan. While essentially comparable in efficacy to the other triptans, eletriptan at a dose of 40 mg is the only triptan shown to have greater efficacy than sumatriptan at 100 mg. Both efficacy and AEs are dose dependent, although trials have reported AEs to be transient and mild to moderate in nature. Contraindications and adverse effects are similar to those of the other triptans, but eletriptan is metabolized exclusively by CYP3A4 and therefore should not be used within 72 hours of use of potent CYP3A4 inhibitors (e.g., conivaptan, systemic fusidic acid, itraconazole, systemic ketoconazole, posaconazole, and voriconazole) (Ong & De Felice, 2018) (see **Table 35.3**).

Frovatriptan

Frovatriptan (Frova) (FDA approved in 2001 and now available as a generic) has a half-life of 26 hours—by far the longest of all the triptans. Hence, its therapeutic gain is better assessed

at 4 hours rather than 2; the 40-hour headache response rate for frovatriptan is 66%. Frovatriptan is unique among the triptans as it is the only one that binds to 5-HT_{1f} in addition to 5-HT_{1b} and 5-HT_{1d}. Like naratriptan, its onset is somewhat slower (1–2 hours, although this is not the case in all patients taking the medication in early migraine), but its effects are more sustained. Frovatriptan is also metabolized both by the kidney and hepatic CYP1A2, reducing the likelihood for drug–drug interactions. It has also been shown to be particularly effective in menstrual-related migraine, not only for acute relief but also as a 2-day "miniprophylaxis" (Allais et al., 2015). It is available as a 2.5-mg tablet, which is the recommended dose. If a first dose provides some relief but the headache recurs, another dose may be taken no sooner than 2 hours after the preceding dose, to a maximum of 7.5 mg/d. Contraindications and adverse effects are similar to the other triptans (Ong & De Felice, 2018) (see **Table 35.3**).

Sumatriptan and Naproxen

Sumatriptan and naproxen (Treximet) (FDA approved in 2008 and now available as a generic) is an oral tablet combination medication containing 85 mg sumatriptan and 500 mg naproxen used for treating migraine with or without aura. It is more efficacious than monotherapy with sumatriptan or naproxen alone (as is combined use of individual sumatriptan and naproxen tablets). Sustained pain relief at 24 hours was also significantly better than monotherapy with either sumatriptan or naproxen in clinical trials. It follows the sumatriptan dosing recommendations (one tablet at migraine onset; if relief is not obtained, a second dose may be taken at least 2 hours later with a maximum of two tablets in 24 hours), and its AEs, contraindications, and warnings are the same as those for each of its individual components (including the boxed warning for the naproxen component) (Khoury & Couch, 2010). Use of sumatriptan/naproxen is not recommended in patients with a creatinine clearance of less than 30 mL/min, and its use is contraindicated in hepatic impairment (PDR, 2020) (see **Table 35.3**).

5-HT_{1f} Receptor Agonists (Ditans)

Ditans represent a new class of migraine agents, comprised of a single agent approved in late 2019. While related to the triptans, the ditans are associated with fewer vasoconstrictive effects, given their preferential affinity for the 5-HT_{1f} receptor. The triptans have some weak affinity for 5-HT_{1f} but primarily exert their effects via agonism of $5\text{-HT}_{1b/d}$, which are more predominantly located on vascular structures. Ditans, therefore, offer a new option for people with migraine who have not responded to the triptans or who have underlying cardiovascular comorbidities (Oswald & Schuster, 2018).

Lasmiditan

Lasmiditan (Reyvow) was the first serotonergic migraine agent preferential for 5-HT_{1f}. It was approved in October of 2019 and is the only member of its new class and is indicated for the acute treatment of migraine with or without aura (lasmiditan PI, 2020). The percentage of patients treated within 4 hours of migraine onset achieving pain freedom and freedom from most bothersome symptoms (self-identified as photophobia, phonophobia, or nausea) 2 hours after treatment was significantly greater in the lasmiditan group as compared to the placebo group (lasmiditan PI, 2020). Lasmiditan is an orally dosed tablet, taken at a dose of 50, 100, or 200 mg, not to exceed a single dose per day. The most common AEs reported in trials were dizziness, fatigue, paresthesia, and sedation. Given these concerns, lasmiditan has some warnings and precautions, primarily regarding driving impairment. Patients should be advised not to drive or operate machinery until at least 8 hours after taking each dose. Ensure that patients are capable of following this advice, taking into account the fact that they may not be able to assess their own driving competence and the degree of impairment caused by the drug. Given its CNS depressant effects, lasmiditan should be used with caution if used concomitantly with alcohol or other CNS depressants. Some patients experienced reactions consistent with serotonin syndrome; if this occurs, lasmiditan should be discontinued (lasmiditan PI, 2020) (see **Table 35.3**).

Calcitonin Gene–Related Peptide Receptor Antagonists

CGRP is a widely distributed proinflammatory neuropeptide, modulating nociception in migraine by binding to fibers in the trigeminovascular system. Consequently, pain is both centrally and peripherally mediated, contributing to vasodilation, plasma extravasation, neurogenic inflammation, mast cell degranulation, and regulation of gene expression (Ceriani et al., 2019). The CGRP receptor antagonists (RAs) are thought to be mediating the vasodilatory component of neurogenic inflammation in migraine (Lew & Punnapuzha, 2020). There are two novel groups of CGRP RAs: the gepants (used in acute treatment) and the monoclonal antimigraine agents (used in migraine prophylaxis).

Gepants

The gepants are a novel class of CGRP RA antimigraine agents. They have no active vasoconstrictor effects, therefore making them attractive options for patients who are not candidates for triptan therapy due to cardiovascular risk factors (Ceriani et al., 2019; Goadsby et al., 2019). They are orally administered small molecules with efficacy at least equivalent to the triptans and ditans, but with improved tolerability (Negro & Martelletti, 2019). Presently, there are two approved gepants (a third, atogepant, is in late-stage clinical trials; NCT03700320, 2020).

Ubrogepant

Ubrogepant (Ubrelvy) (FDA approved in December 2019) is a potent small-molecule tablet indicated for the treatment of acute migraine with or without aura in adults. Tablets are available in 50 or 100 mg. No more than 200 mg should be taken in 24 hours. Pharmacologic availability is 11 minutes after

dosing, peak plasma concentration is 1.5 hours after dosing, and elimination half-life is 5 to 7 hours. Its only contraindication is concomitant use with strong CYP3A4 inhibitors (which can decrease serum ubrogepant concentration). AEs are minor, most commonly nausea and somnolence (ubrogepant PI, 2019). In clinical trials, ubrogepant demonstrated superiority over placebo on both of its primary endpoints, headache pain freedom and absence of the most bothersome migraine-associated symptom at 2 hours post dose for the 50 and 100 mg doses (Lipton et al., 2019a). Pain freedom at 2 hours was reported by 21.8% of trial participants in the ubrogepant 50 mg group, 20.7% in the ubrogepant 25 mg group, and 14.3% in the placebo group, and absence of the most bothersome associated symptom at 2 hours was reported by 38.9% in the ubrogepant 50 mg group, 34.1% in the ubrogepant 25 mg group, and 27.4% in the placebo group (Lipton et al., 2019a). A post-hoc analysis of patient-reported outcomes, including functional disability, satisfaction, and patient global impression of change, also demonstrated significant improvement with ubrogepant as compared to placebo (Dodick et al., 2020) (see **Table 35.3**).

Rimegepant

Rimegepant (Nurtec ODT) (FDA approved in February 2020) is an ODT available in a single strength of 75 mg for the acute treatment of migraine with or without aura in adults. No more than 75 mg should be taken in a 24-hour period. While there are no contraindications, concomitant administration with CYP3A4 inhibitors should be avoided. The most common adverse reaction is nausea, occurring in few patients (rimegepant PI, 2020). In clinical trials, a single 75-mg dose of rimegepant demonstrated superiority over placebo with regard to freedom from pain (21% in the rimegepant group vs. 11% in the placebo group) and freedom from the most bothersome symptom (35% vs. 27%) at 2 hours post dose (Croop et al., 2019). Rimegepant is not approved for migraine prevention, although it is presently in late-stage clinical trials assessing it for that indication (NCT03732638, 2020) (see **Table 35.3**).

Ergot Derivatives

The first migraine-specific drugs to be developed were the ergot derivatives (ergotamine tartrate and DHE with a variety of trade names). They are generally recognized as safe and effective but have fallen out of favor because of unpredictable patient responses and greater AEs as compared with the safer triptans. Ergot derivatives have partial agonist, antagonist, or both types of activity for serotonergic, dopaminergic, and alpha-adrenergic receptors, resulting in constriction of peripheral and cranial vessels. Ergot derivatives are typically used to treat infrequent, long-standing migraines in patients who have had multiple relapses when using triptans, but care should be taken to prescribe the medication infrequently, at recommended doses, and in careful consideration of contraindications (e.g., they are contraindicate in pregnancy and are absolutely contraindicated in patients with cardiovascular or cerebrovascular and in patients taking concomitant medications metabolized by the CYP3A4 pathway, such as protease inhibitors, azole antifungals, and certain macrolide antibiotics). While generally found to be less efficacious than oral sumatriptan in clinical trials, rectal ergotamine was found to have superior efficacy than rectal sumatriptan (73% vs. 63%, respectively; rectal sumatriptan is not available as an approved medication). Ergotamine/caffeine combinations are also available in oral, sublingual, and rectal formulations, although evidence of efficacy for these preparations is inconsistent or conflicting (Ong & De Felice, 2018).

Ergotamine tartrate (Ergomar; Ergostat has been discontinued) is available in 2-mg sublingual tablets. Ergotamine is not an optimal choice, given its side effect profile (nausea may be sufficient enough for discontinuation). It is associated with more side effects than DHE, and use of the medication more than 10 times per month may cause MOH. DHE (Migranal) is available intramuscularly (1 mg), intravenously (1 mg), subcutaneously (1 mg), and as a nasal spray (0.5 mg). There are no oral formulations. This drug is mainly used to treat severe, refractory migraines, recurring migraines, MOH, or status migrainosus (debilitating migraine attacks lasting longer than 72 hours) and is usually managed by specialists. Cafergot, a combination of caffeine and ergotamine, is available in oral (1 mg ergotamine, 100 mg caffeine) and suppository (2 mg/100 mg) formulations. The lowest effective dose of these medications should be used (PDR, 2020). Cafergot can also increase the incidence of migraines and should be used infrequently. Use of these agents is contraindicated in severe renal impairment and carries a boxed warning for serious and/or life-threatening peripheral ischemia with coadministration of ergotamine tartrate and potent CYP 3A4 inhibitors including protease inhibitors and macrolide antibiotics, since CYP 3A4 inhibition elevates the serum levels of ergotamine tartrate, increasing the risk for vasospasm leading to cerebral ischemia and/or ischemia of the extremities (Ergotamine Tartrate and Caffeine PI, 2002). (PDR, 2020) (see **Table 35.3**).

Barbiturates

Butalbital-containing compounds such as Fiorinal (butalbital 50 mg/aspirin 325 mg/caffeine 40 mg; tablets and capsules) and Fioricet (butalbital 50 mg/acetaminophen 325 mg/caffeine 40 mg; tablets, capsules, or liquid) are C-III controlled substances and should be used sparingly and only if the migraine-specific agents have repeatedly failed. There are no data to support the efficacy of these medications, and if overused (as infrequently as five times per month), these agents can lead to addiction, MOH, development of chronic daily headache, and withdrawal symptoms. These drugs have been removed from the market in the European Union, Asia, and Latin America due to their associated risks and their lack of efficacy (Ong & De Felice, 2018). Fioricet should particularly be used with caution given its acetaminophen content if it is used concomitantly with other acetaminophen-containing drugs. The "Choosing Wisely" Task Force of the AHS identified

overuse of butalbital-containing and opioid medications for the treatment of migraine as a problem (Loder et al., 2013). See **Table 35.3** for side effects and contraindications.

Opioids

Opioids have been used as rescue medications for severe migraines that do not respond to the medications given earlier. They are also used in patients who have infrequent migraines and have contraindications to other agents. They are used sparingly for moderate to severe migraines during pregnancy. However, they are in general not recommended for the treatment of migraine and, if used as rescue medications, should be used only a few times per year. Overuse can lead to MOH, status migrainosus, or development of chronic daily headache (Ong & De Felice, 2018). These are C-IV medications, and the potential for dependence or abuse should also be taken into account when considering them for use. Examples of these medications include butorphanol (generic nasal spray, 1 mg/spray), tramadol (generic tablet, 100 mg daily; can be titrated to a maximum of 300 mg daily), and acetaminophen plus codeine (Tylenol plus codeine; acetaminophen 300 mg/codeine 30 mg or 40 mg) for mild to moderate pain. The acetaminophen content per dose is 300 mg, which needs to be considered when used concomitantly with other acetaminophen-containing drugs so that a maximum daily dose of 3,250 mg is not exceeded. As with the butalbital-containing drugs, use of opioid medications for migraine was the second most identified problem by the "Choosing Wisely" Task Force. Use of opioids is rare (seen most frequently in emergency departments) and has even been described as contributing to disease progression, increased use of health care resources, and comorbidity (Loder et al., 2013; Minen et al., 2014; Ong & De Felice, 2018). Opioids are not a good choice for managing migraine pain. See **Table 35.3** for side effects and contraindications.

Steroids

If a patient has a severe, persistent migraine or status migrainosus that seems refractory to any abortive medications, a brief course of steroids (typically dexamethasone 6 mg for 5 days or IV 4 mg–16 mg) may be used as a rescue medication until the patient is headache free for 24 hours. There are few good data supporting the efficacy of steroid use (AHS level of evidence category C: "possibly effective"), but they have been used with good results and may serve as effective outpatient management of acute migraine (AHS, 2019; Marmura et al., 2015). See **Table 35.3** for side effects and contraindications.

Antiemetic Agents

The antiemetic agents prochlorperazine, metoclopramide, and droperidol as well as the antipsychotic chlorpromazine are effective adjunctive therapies for patients experiencing an acute migraine with or without nausea and vomiting. These agents are dopamine antagonists and may be acting on dopamine hypersensitivity associated with migraine (Ong & De Felice, 2018). Prochlorperazine comes in a suppository form, which is useful for patients unable to tolerate oral medications. Droperidol carries a boxed warning for QT prolongation and torsade de pointes. These medications augment the effects of abortive agents (possibly through contributing to increase absorption of migraine medications) and may be taken before or together with these medications (Ong & De Felice, 2018).

PREVENTIVE TREATMENT FOR MIGRAINES

Preventive migraine medications are used to prevent the occurrence of migraine by reducing the frequency and severity of migraine attacks. Epidemiologic studies have shown that some 38% of people with migraine require some form of preventive therapy, yet only 3% to 13% are receiving prophylactic treatment (AHS, 2019; Marmura et al., 2015). A therapeutic trial of a given agent should last for 2 to 3 months before the efficacy of the agent is assessed. The main classes of agents used for migraine prophylaxis are anticonvulsants, beta blockers, triptans, angiotensin-converting enzyme inhibitors, angiotensin II receptor blockers, calcium channel blockers, antidepressants (TCAs and SSRIs/SNRIs), and antihistamines, although strength of evidence for efficacy has been determined for individual medications and not for entire medication classes. The 2018 AHS consensus statement advocates use of evidence-based preventive therapies. Oral medications with established efficacy include divalproex sodium, sodium valproate, topiramate, metoprolol, propranolol, and timolol (AHS, 2019). Medications determined to be "probably effective" include amitriptyline, venlafaxine, atenolol, and nadolol (AHS, 2019). "Possibly effective" preventive therapies include lisinopril, clonidine, guanfacine, carbamazepine, propranolol, nebivolol, timolol, pindolol, cyproheptadine, and candesartan. Five injectable medications have been approved for migraine prevention: the neurotoxin onabotulinumtoxinA (for CM) and four monoclonal antibodies (for both episodic and CM), erenumab, fremanezumab, galcanezumab, and eptinezumab (AHS, 2019). **Table 35.4** gives an overview of selected drugs used to prevent migraines.

According to the AHS's 2019 updated position statement, the goal of preventive therapy is to reduce attack frequency, severity, duration, and disability; improve responsiveness to and avoid escalation in use of acute treatment; improve function and reduce disability; reduce reliance on poorly tolerated, ineffective, or unwanted acute treatments; reduce overall cost associated with migraine treatment; enable patients to manage their own disease to enhance a sense of personal control to improve health-related quality of life (HRQoL); and reduce headache-related distress and psychological symptoms (AHS, 2019). Preventive therapy for migraine is indicated for and should be offered to patients who have attacks that continue to interfere with their daily routines and functioning despite treatment; patients who have frequent attacks (≥4 MHDs); patients who have contraindications for or failure or overuse of acute treatments (defined by AHS as 10 or more days per month for ergot derivatives, triptans, opioids, combination analgesics, and a combination of drugs from different classes that are not individually overused, or 15 or more days per month for nonopioid analgesics, acetaminophen, and NSAIDs); patients who are experiencing AEs with acute therapies; and patients who prefer preventive therapy. Preventive therapy is mostly driven by level of patient impairment and frequency of attacks (AHS, 2019).

Oral medications should be started at low doses and titrated slowly until the desired effects occur. Dosages may need to be lowered if side effects occur. A full therapeutic trial takes at least 2 months. It may take months until an effective agent is found. It is important to help the patient develop realistic expectations (e.g., 50% reduction in headaches as compared to 100% reduction, etc.) and to emphasize the importance of adherence to therapy (AHS, 2019).

Anticonvulsants

Valproic acid (Depakene) and divalproex sodium (Depakote) can reduce the frequency, severity, and duration of migraines. Use of these drugs is contraindicated in patients with liver disease. Side effects such as tremor, weight gain, nausea, and hair loss may limit their use as agents for prophylaxis. Numerous drug interactions can result when valproic acid or divalproex sodium is administered with other anticonvulsants. Increased effects or toxicity of valproic acid is seen with the administration of CNS depressants and aspirin. Valproic acid is contraindicated in pregnancy because it is toxic to the fetus.

Topiramate (Topamax) has been shown to be effective in migraine prophylaxis and is particularly effective for patients who have chronic daily headache or who have failed to respond to many other prophylactic treatments. Topiramate was also shown in trials to be at least as or more effective as other migraine prophylactic therapies such as propranolol, valproate, and amitriptyline. A retrospective claims analysis of oral migraine prevention medications revealed that topiramate was the most commonly prescribed oral migraine prevention medication and the preventive agent for which there was the greatest amount of patient adherence (Hepp et al., 2015). Topiramate has many potential side effects that limit its use, such as concentration and memory impairment, significant somnolence, mood disturbance, and tremor. It should be used with caution in patients with renal or hepatic impairment.

Beta Blockers

Beta blockers are often considered first-line agents for prophylactic treatment of migraine with many studies showing a 50% reduction or more in occurrence of migraine. Propranolol (Inderal), metoprolol (Lopressor), and timolol are classified as having "established efficacy," based on AAN criteria, while atenolol (Tenormin) and nadolol (Corgard) are classified as "probably effective" (AHS, 2019). They have all been used for

TABLE 35.4

Overview of Selected Drugs Used for Migraine Headache Prophylaxis

Generic (Brand) Name and Dosage	Selected Adverse Events	Contraindications	Special Considerations
Anticonvulsants			
Valproic acid (Depakene, Stavzor) Depakene 250 mg soft gel capsule Stavzor delayed release 125, 250, and 500 mg soft gel capsules initial dose: 250 mg BID to a maximum of 1,000 mg/d	≥5%: headache, asthenia, fever, nausea, vomiting, abdominal pain, diarrhea, anorexia, dyspepsia, constipation, somnolence, tremor, dizziness, diplopia, amblyopia/blurred vision, ataxia, nystagmus, emotional lability, abnormal thinking, amnesia, flu syndrome, infection, bronchitis, rhinitis	*Boxed warning: May cause teratogenic effects such as neural tube defects (e.g., spina bifida). Hepatic failure resulting in fatalities has occurred in patients; children < age 2 are at considerable risk. Cases of life-threatening pancreatitis, occurring at the start of therapy or following years of use, have been reported in adults and children.* Hepatic disease or significant hepatic dysfunction or with urea cycle disorders	Monitor for hypothermia and thrombocytopenia; monitor psychiatric patients for suicidal ideation; use with caution with concomitant use of carbapenem, topiramate, aspirin, or lamotrigine; drug interactions are also known for felbamate, rifampin, amitriptyline/nortriptyline, carbamazepine, clonazepam, diazepam, ethosuximide, phenobarbital, phenytoin, tolbutamide, warfarin, and zidovudine; use with caution in older persons.
Divalproex (Depakote) Initial: 250 mg BID, up to 1,000 mg/d	>10%: nausea, somnolence, dizziness, vomiting; >5%–10%: asthenia, abdominal pain, dyspepsia, rash	See *boxed warning* of valproic acid	Same as valproic acid
Topiramate (Topamax) Initial: 25 mg QHS for first week, increased weekly by increments of 25 mg; recommended therapeutic dose 100 mg/d in two divided doses *Note*: Taper gradually.	>5%: paresthesia, anorexia, weight decrease, fatigue, dizziness, somnolence, nervousness, psychomotor slowing, difficulty with memory, difficulty with concentration/attention, confusion; renal calculi, rare acute-angle glaucoma; >5% in migraine trials: paresthesia, taste perversion	None	Decreases effectiveness of oral contraceptives; monitor for acute myopia, oligohidrosis and hyperthermia, suicidal behavior and ideation, metabolic acidosis, cognitive/neuropsychiatric dysfunction, and hyperammonemia; use caution with concomitant administration of valproic acid, oral contraceptives, metformin, lithium, and other carbonic anhydrase inhibitors
Beta Blockers			
Propranolol (Inderal) (long acting) Start 80 mg daily; goal 160–240 mg daily; increase dose gradually and taper discontinuation, discontinue after 6 weeks if no satisfactory response. *Note*: Adjust dose in hepatic impairment	Common: drowsiness or fatigue, cold hands and feet, weakness or dizziness, dry mouth, eyes, and skin	*Boxed warning: Beta blocker therapy should not be withdrawn abruptly (particularly in patients with CAD), but gradually tapered to avoid acute tachycardia, hypertension, and/or ischemia.* Pregnancy, uncompensated CHF, cardiogenic shock, severe sinus bradycardia or second- or third-degree heart block or with severe asthma or COPD	Useful if there is history of coexisting HTN or CAD; use with caution in patients with PVD or with concomitant beta blocker use; use with caution in patients with T2D, myasthenia gravis, psychiatric disease, and renal or hepatic dysfunction.

(Continued)

TABLE 35.4

Overview of Selected Drugs Used for Migraine Headache Prophylaxis (*Continued*)

Generic (Brand) Name and Dosage	Selected Adverse Events	Contraindications	Special Considerations
Timolol (Betamol) Initial: 10 mg BID to a maximum of 30 mg/d	Anaphylaxis (serious); >3%: fatigue/tiredness, bradycardia; AEs in CAD population more numerous; asthenia or fatigue, heart rate <40 beats/min, cardiac failure—nonfatal, hypotension, claudication, cold hands and feet, nausea or digestive disorders, dizziness	See *boxed warning* of propranolol. Bronchial asthma or history of bronchial asthma, or severe COPD; sinus bradycardia, second- and third-degree AV block, overt cardiac failure, or cardiogenic shock	Use with caution in impaired hepatic or renal function, marked renal failure, muscle weakness, or cerebrovascular insufficiency; use with caution with concomitant use of catecholamine-depleting drugs, NSAIDs, calcium antagonists, digoxin and either diltiazem or verapamil, quinidine, and clonidine
Tricyclic Antidepressants			
Amitriptyline (see **Table 35.1**)			
Calcium Channel Blockers			
Verapamil 40–80 mg TID	>1%: headache, URI, fatigue, nausea, constipation, dizziness, edema	Severe left ventricular dysfunction, hypotension or cardiogenic shock, sick sinus syndrome, second- or third-degree AV block, atrial flutter or atrial fibrillation and an accessory bypass tract (e.g., Wolff-Parkinson-White, Lown-Ganong-Levine syndromes)	Useful if there is coexisting HTN; monitor LFTs periodically, use with caution in patients with impaired renal or hepatic function and in patients with decreased neuromuscular transmission; use caution with concomitant administration of erythromycin, ritonavir, alcohol, aspirin, grapefruit juice, beta blockers, digitalis, other antihypertensive agents, disopyramide, flecainide, quinidine, lithium, carbamazepine, and rifampin, phenobarbital, cyclosporine, theophylline, inhalation anesthetics, neuromuscular-blocking agents, telithromycin, or clonidine.
OnabotulinumtoxinA			
OnabotulinumtoxinA (Botox) Five cycles over a period of 12 weeks (155–195 U/cycle); does not require dose titration Adults only	AEs >5% in clinical trials were neck pain and headache (other AEs reported in trials for other indications)	*Boxed warning: Distant spread of toxin effect. May spread from the area of injection to produce symptoms consistent with botulinum toxin effects. These symptoms have been reported hours to weeks after injection. Swallowing and breathing difficulties can be life threatening and there have been reports of death. The risk of symptoms is probably greatest in those patients who have an underlying condition that would predispose them to these symptoms.*	Spread of toxin effects; swallowing and breathing difficulties can lead to death. Seek immediate medical attention if respiratory, speech, or swallowing difficulties occur (see *boxed warning*); potency units are not interchangeable with other preparations of botulinum toxin products; potential serious adverse reactions after injections for unapproved uses; concomitant neuromuscular disorder may exacerbate clinical effects of treatment; use with caution in patients with compromised respiratory function.

TABLE 35.4

Overview of Selected Drugs Used for Migraine Headache Prophylaxis (*Continued*)

Generic (Brand) Name and Dosage	Selected Adverse Events	Contraindications	Special Considerations
Injectable (mAb) CGRP inhibitors			
Erenumab-aooe (Aimovig) SC; 70 and 140 mg/mL. Both available in autoinjector pens and prefilled syringes Recommended dosage is 70 mg once monthly. Administer in the abdomen, thigh, or upper arm subcutaneously.	AEs in clinical trials ≥3% were injection-site reactions and constipation	None apart from hypersensitivity to drug or its excipients	Needle shield within the white or orange cap of the prefilled autoinjector and the gray needle cap of the prefilled syringe contain dry natural rubber (a derivative of latex), which may cause allergic reactions in individuals sensitive to latex; hypersensitivity reactions (may occur within hours to >1 week after administration): if serious hypersensitivity reaction occurs, discontinue administration and initiate appropriate therapy; constipation with serious complications may occur; new onset or worsening of preexisting HTN may occur.
Fremanezumab-vfrm (Ajovy) SC; 225 mg/ 1.5 mL monthly, or 675 mg every 3 months (675 mg dose administered as three consecutive injections of 225 mg/1.5 mL each) Available in autoinjector or as a prefilled syringe Administer in the abdomen, thigh, or upper arm	AEs in clinical trials ≥5% were injection-site reactions	None apart from hypersensitivity to drug or its excipients	If hypersensitivity occurs, consider discontinuing and institute appropriate therapy.
Galcanezumab-gnlm (Emgality) SC; 120 mg/mL: 240 mg loading dose (administered as two consecutive injections of 120 mg each), followed by monthly doses of 120 mg Available in autoinjector or as a prefilled syringe Administer in the abdomen, thigh, back of the upper arm, or buttocks subcutaneously. (*Note*: also approved for cluster headache with different dosing)	AEs in clinical trials ≥2% were injection-site reactions.	None apart from hypersensitivity to drug or its excipients	If a serious hypersensitivity reaction occurs, discontinue administration and initiate appropriate therapy; hypersensitivity reactions can occur days after administration and may be prolonged.
Eptinezumab-jjmr (Vyepti) IV (note that this is IV, not SC); must dilute before use; dilute in 100 mL of 0.9% sodium chloride injection Recommended dose 100 mg/ IV infusion over approximately 30 minutes every 3 months; some patients may benefit from 300-mg dose.	AEs in clinical trials ≥2% were nasopharyngitis and hypersensitivity.	None apart from hypersensitivity to drug or its excipients	Hypersensitivity reactions have included angioedema, urticaria, facial flushing, and rash; if hypersensitivity reaction occurs, consider discontinuing and initiating appropriate therapy.

AEs, adverse events; AV, atrioventricular; CAD, coronary artery disease; CGRP, calcitonin gene–related peptide; CHF, congestive heart failure; COPD, chronic obstructive pulmonary disease; HTN, hypertension; IV, intravenous; LFTs, liver function tests; NSAIDs, nonsteroidal antiinflammatory drugs; PVD, peripheral vascular disease; SC, subcutaneous; T2D, type 2 diabetes; URI, upper respiratory infection.

migraine with similar efficacy. Nebivolol (Bystolic) and pindolol are classified as "possibly effective." Only propranolol and timolol have been approved by FDA for migraine prophylaxis. Beta blockers are contraindicated in patients with uncompensated congestive heart failure, bradycardia, second- or third-degree atrioventricular block, and asthma. Side effects include fatigue, vivid dreams, depression, impotence, bradycardia, and hypotension. Many pathways of the cytochrome P450 enzyme system metabolize beta blockers. Beta blockers have numerous drug interactions, so careful consideration of polypharmacy is necessary prior to prescribing them.

Tricyclic Antidepressants

TCAs can also be used as first-line agents for migraine prophylaxis. Only amitriptyline (Elavil) and venlafaxine (Effexor) are characterized by AAN/AHS as "possibly effective" (AHS, 2019). Patients usually need only low doses for prophylaxis, lower than those generally used to treat depression. Patients should avoid use if they are currently taking an MAOI, have glaucoma, or are pregnant. Anticholinergic side effects commonly occur and include sedation, constipation, blurred vision, hypotension, and slowed conduction in the atrioventricular node. These agents also have many potential drug interactions; prescribers should consult a reference before administering them.

Calcium Channel Blockers

Verapamil (Calan) is the calcium channel blocker most commonly used in migraine prophylaxis; however, it provides only a slight benefit in reducing the frequency of attacks (AAN category U; not recommended) (Loder et al., 2012). It is often considered a second- or third-line agent for use when other agents are ineffective or contraindicated. The mechanism of action is believed to be the inhibition of serotonin release, which may not be achieved until after 8 weeks of therapy. Its use is contraindicated in patients with bradycardia, heart block, ventricular tachycardia, or atrial fibrillation. Side effects include constipation, fluid retention, bradycardia, and hypotension. Numerous drug interactions are associated with calcium channel blockers; prescribers must consult a reference before administering.

OnabotulinumtoxinA (Intramuscular Injectable)

OnabotulinumtoxinA (Botox) (FDA approved for CM in October 2010) is a neurotoxin approved for a variety of indications (including spasticity and overactive bladder) that function by inhibiting release of acetylcholine and effecting neuromuscular blockade. In clinical trials, onabotulinumtoxinA injected in up to five cycles over a period of 12 weeks (155–195 U/cycle) resulted in statistically significant and clinically meaningful improvements in headache symptoms, acute headache pain medication usage, headache impact, overall functioning and HRQoL in adults with CM, as well as significantly reduced headache-related disability and medication overuse (Dodick, et al., 2010; Frampton & Silberstein, 2018).

Two-thirds of trial participants had acute medication overuse, and another one-third had failed to respond to three or more prior oral preventive therapies (Frampton & Silberstein, 2018). Longer-term studies (up to nine treatment cycles over a period of 2 years) have substantiated medication effectiveness (Frampton & Silberstein, 2018). OnabotulinumtoxinA is characterized by AHS as having established efficacy and represents a good preventive option for patients who have CM and who have failed (or are intolerant to or have contraindications for) prior oral preventive therapies (Frampton & Silberstein, 2018). As an injectable agent, onabotulinumtoxinA does not require titration in dose. In trials, AEs were mild to moderate in nature with neck pain and muscular weakness occurring in over 5% of trial participants. The most commonly reported additional AEs included ptosis, musculoskeletal pain, injection-site pain, headache, myalgia, and musculoskeletal stiffness (Dodick et al., 2010). OnabotulinumtoxinA has a boxed warning for distant spread of toxin effect. It may spread from the area of injection to produce symptoms consistent with botulinum toxin effects. These symptoms have been reported hours to weeks after injection. Swallowing and breathing difficulties can be life threatening, and there have been reports of death (onabotulinumtoxinA PI, 2019).

Injectable Biologic Calcitonin Gene–Related Peptide Inhibitors

Three new preventive agents for migraine received FDA approval in 2018, and a fourth received approval in 2020, providing people with chronic migraine with a variety of new options. These are biologic agents: monoclonal antibodies requiring injection or infusion (the 4-letter drug name suffix is an FDA pharmacovigilance mandate). These were originally approved for migraine (i.e., were not previously approved for other indications). Like the oral gepants, these target the CGRP receptor or ligand. These medications offer benefit in that the doses do not need to be titrated up slowly over time, onset of therapeutic benefit is rapid, and tolerability is good (AHS, 2019).

Erenumab-aooe

Erenumab-aooe (Aimovig) (FDA approved in September 2018) is a humanized monoclonal antibody (mAb) CGRP RA approved for preventive therapy for episodic and CM (erenumab PI, 2019; Zhu et al., 2019). Erenumab is dosed at 70 mg/mL or 140 mg/mL and comes in a prefilled autoinjector or prefilled syringe for monthly subcutaneous injection. The prefilled syringe needs to be refrigerated and brought to room temperature 30 minutes prior to injection. Recommended dose is 70 mg/mL; some patients may benefit more from the higher dose. Erenumab should be injected into the abdomen, thigh, or upper arm. The most common AE reported in clinical trials were injection-site reactions and constipation (the latter being more common in the higher dose). Constipation with serious complications (including surgery, in some cases) was reported in postmarketing surveillance, earning erenumab a warning on its package insert (erenumab PI, 2019). In clinical trials, both doses of erenumab were associated with a significant reduction in the 50% responder rate, reduced migraine-specific medication days, and reduced migraine-specific medication days from baseline (Zhu et al., 2019).

Fremanezumab-vfrm

Fremanezumab-vfrm (Ajovy) (FDA approved in September 2018) is a humanized mAb that functions by binding to CGRP, interfering with its binding to the CGRP receptor. Fremanezumab is also available in a prefilled autoinjector pen at a dose of 225 mg/mL, which can be administered once a month or 675 mg/mL once every three months (quarterly) as three consecutive doses of 225 mg/mL into the thigh, abdomen, or upper arm (fremanezumab PI, 2020). Fremanezumab is approved to treat both episodic and CM. Both monthly and quarterly dosing options were shown in clinical trials to significantly reduce migraine frequency, requirement for acute headache medication use, and headache-related disability (Hoy, 2018).

Galcanezumab-gnlm

Galcanezumab-gnlm (Emgality) (FDA approved in September 2018; approved in June 2019 for CH) is a mAb CGRP antagonist that binds to the ligand, preventing binding to the receptor, and is indicated for the preventive treatment of both episodic and CMs, as well as for the treatment of episodic CH (galcanezumab PI, 2018). It is also provided in a prefilled pen for subcutaneous delivery (120 mg/mL) and in prefilled syringes (120 mg/mL). For episodic migraine, the clinical trial showed a significantly reduced number of migraine headache days as compared to placebo (4.7 days vs. 2.8 days, $P < .001$) (Stauffer et al., 2018). For CM, the clinical trial showed a significantly reduced number of migraine headache days as compared to placebo (4.8 days vs. 2.7 days, $P < .001$) (Detke et al., 2018). The only AE was injection-site reactions, and the only warning/precaution was for hypersensitivity reactions (including dyspnea, urticaria, with cases of anaphylaxis and angioedema reported in the postmarketing setting; hypersensitivity reactions can occur days after administration and may be prolonged) (galcanezumab PI, 2018).

Eptinezumab-jjmr

Eptinezumab-jjmr (Vyepti) (FDA approved in February 2020) is a mAb CGRP antagonist that binds to the CGRP ligand, interfering with binding to its receptor, and is indicated for migraine prevention (eptinezumab PI, 2020). Unlike the other preventative CGRP agents, eptinezumab is an IV drug, infused over 30 minutes, every 3 months. In a clinical trial, treatment with eptinezumab showed a statistically significant dose-dependent reduction in migraine headache days as compared to placebo (100 mg, 7.7 days; 300 mg, 8.2 days; vs. placebo, 5.6 days, all $p < .0001$) (Lipton et al., 2020). Treatment-emergent adverse events (TEAEs) were also dose dependent, occurring at 43.5% (100 mg) and 52.0% (300 mg) versus 46.7% (placebo). Nasopharyngitis was the

only TEAE reported for greater than 2% of eptinezumab-treated patients and only at the 300-mg dose. Warnings and precautions pertain to hypersensitivity reactions as with the others, including angioedema, urticaria, facial flushing, or rash (eptinezumab PI, 2020).

CLUSTER HEADACHES

The goals of therapy for CH include acute management, preventive management, and transitional management during titration to effective levels of preventive medications (Brandt et al., 2020). There is clinical evidence for the efficacy of several medications for the acute treatment of CH. Subcutaneous sumatriptan 6 mg to 12 mg, zolmitriptan nasal spray 5 mg to 10 mg, and 100% inhaled oxygen 10 L/min to 15 L/min are recommended for the management of acute attacks and have Level A ("established efficacy") from the AHS treatment guidelines for CH (Robbins et al., 2016). Drugs with AHS Level B recommendations ("probably effective") include intranasal sumatriptan (20 mg) and oral zolmitriptan (5 to 10 mg). Subcutaneous octreotide, a somatostatin receptor agonist, has also been shown to be efficacious at 100 mcg, as has intranasal lidocaine 4% (Brandt et al., 2020; Robbins et al., 2016). Both of these medications carry AHS Level C recommendations (Robbins et al., 2016). For individuals with repeated CH, preventive medications should be considered. There are data supporting the use of a variety of medications, including verapamil and lithium, the most commonly used preventive medications (Level C recommendations). Other Level C recommended agents include warfarin (INR 1.5–1.9) and melatonin (10 mg). Suboccipital steroid injections are effective CH prophylaxis and the only intervention presently with a Level A AHS recommendation (Robbins et al., 2016). Several other agents have been used, but only with limited, inconclusive, or negative research support (Robbins et al., 2016). Galcanezumab, as previously mentioned, is a new mAb CGRP antagonist approved by FDA in 2019 for preventive therapy for CH (approved in 2018 for migraine) with strong clinical trial support for efficacy. Ergotamines, long used for the management of CH, are not recommended. Preventive therapies may take some time and may possibly require upward titration to become effective, during which time transitional agents may be needed (Brandt et al., 2020). Intravenous DHE is FDA approved for the management of CH and has been shown to be up to 100% effective when used for a minimum of three consecutive days. Intravenous DHE is particularly effective as a transitional agent. Prednisolone has also shown some efficacy, but its use should be limited to the short term given the risk for serious AEs. Nonpharmacologic neuromodulatory approaches to treating CH have also been shown to be effective, including sphenopalatine ganglion stimulation, occipital nerve stimulation, and noninvasive vagal nerve stimulation. A noninvasive vagal nerve stimulator has been approved by FDA both for management of acute attacks and as preventive treatment for eCH (Brandt et al., 2020; Leone et al., 2017; Robbins et al., 2016).

SPECIAL POPULATION CONSIDERATIONS

Pediatric

The most common headache type seen in children is migraine. Migraines may present differently in children than in adults. Prevalence is higher in boys prior to puberty, but higher in girls thereafter. Epidemiologic studies have shown that prevalence increases with age, hitting a peak in adolescence. Average age of onset is 7 in boys and 11 in girls, and the incidence of migraine with aura peaks before migraine without aura (Straube & Andreou, 2019). Recurrent headache in adolescents is associated with being overweight, caffeine and alcohol use, lack of physical activity, poor sleep habits, tobacco exposure, and depression (Oskoui et al., 2019a, 2019b). The pain is throbbing and pulsating but tends to be bifrontal or bitemporal. Children may have severe nausea and vomiting along with the pain. The headache usually persists for 1 to 3 hours but may last for longer than a day. A particular challenge with pediatric patients is distinguishing migraine from a host of other possible disorders (e.g., other headache, epilepsy, or vascular or metabolic disorders), further complicated by interpreting the complaint from the child or his or her parents. Another complication is that in clinical trials of young children, often "migraine" was not a specific category, rather than "headache" or "primary headache" (Straube & Andreou, 2019). Cheese, chocolate, and citrus fruits are common triggers of migraine in children. Nonpharmacologic approaches to migraine management, such as developing good sleeping habits and routines, are important. Biofeedback and relaxation therapy are the most commonly used behavioral approaches and have shown some efficacy in reducing frequency and severity of headaches. Clinical trial data for the pharmacologic management of pediatric migraine are limited, and most trials do not show significant improvement in migraine symptoms or reduction in migraine days as compared with placebo (Straube & Andreou, 2019). Placebo response rates, however, are high (Oskoui et al., 2019a, 2019b). Pediatric migraines are usually best managed by simple analgesics such as acetaminophen and ibuprofen with an antiemetic added, if necessary. Patients and their caregivers, however, need to be cautioned not to use the medication too frequently; use of OTC analgesics more than five times per week can lead to MOH or development of chronic daily headache. Triptans are not indicated for use in children, although safety and efficacy of the nasal formulations of sumatriptan and zolmitriptan and oral formulations of rizatriptan and almotriptan have been demonstrated in clinical trials in patients aged 12 to 17. Topiramate is presently the only FDA-approved medication for children over the age of 12, but other agents have some limited efficacy. Amitriptyline is a popular drug of choice for prevention of pediatric migraine (Kacperski, 2015). Involving the family in counseling is critical, as topiramate is associated with significant fetal harm so should be used in pediatric patients of childbearing age with caution, and amitriptyline—as do other antidepressants—comes with a warning for suicidal thinking (Oskoui et al., 2019b). Prophylactic medications may require tapering up or down, and, while most of these agents are well tolerated, patients should be monitored for adverse effects. Many of the pediatric formulations are available as suspensions (Kacperski, 2015). Weight loss (in children who are overweight or obese) and cognitive behavioral therapy have also shown benefit in reducing pediatric migraine frequency (Oskoui et al., 2019a, 2019b).

Tension headaches do occur in children. Recurrent tension headaches should prompt a search for underlying stressors at home or at school. A vision examination should also be performed. Tension headaches are usually best managed by simple analgesics, taking care not to overuse the medication.

Geriatric

New-onset migraines are rare in the older population, although prevalence of headache in older adults remains high (Berk et al., 2018). Symptoms tend to change in older adults with less frequent nausea, vomiting, and a pulsating headache and pain more likely in the neck (Straube & Andreou, 2019). Changes in renal and hepatic function often occur with advancing age, so if an older patient is experiencing migraines, adjustment of drug dosages is recommended.

A new headache pattern in an older patient should make the practitioner suspicious of organic disease or a medication side effect. While triptans are recommended in general, it is important to note that evidence of efficacy is limited, given that most clinical trials are conducted in individuals younger than age 65. Supposedly, therapeutic benefit from the triptans has been reported to increase with age, but given that the triptans are associated with vasoconstriction, they are contraindicated in individuals who have had stroke, or who have CAD, or PVD (Berk et al., 2018). Many of the medications used to treat migraine are contraindicated for use in older populations (naratriptan is not recommended for use in older persons, and rizatriptan should be used with caution) or need to be used at a lower dose. Comorbidities, underlying physiologic changes associated with aging, and polypharmacy need to be considered carefully prior to choosing pharmacologic management (Berk et al., 2018).

Women

As noted earlier, migraines occur more frequently in women than in men (approximately three times as much): likely an estrogen-related phenomenon. Migraine without aura and menstrual-related migraine are the most common types of migraine in women (Todd et al., 2018). Pregnancy is a primary concern if drug therapy is to be initiated, even though migraines can diminish during the second and third trimesters. Practitioners should consider drug therapy for pregnant women using the risk-versus-benefit approach. The agents selected should be those that are safe to use during pregnancy. Triptans and ergot derivatives are *strongly contraindicated* in pregnancy. Acetaminophen is the safest analgesic to use during pregnancy, but it is usually minimally effective. For more severe migraines, ibuprofen may be used in the first and second trimesters only. Tylenol with codeine may be used sparingly throughout the pregnancy. Valproic acid is contraindicated in pregnancy for migraine prophylaxis.

Menstrual migraines are a common problem that may be particularly responsive to triptans. Frovatriptan, in particular, has been used with success as "miniprophylaxis" for menstrual-related migraine (Allais et al., 2015; Johnston & Rapoport, 2010). Women may also be particularly vulnerable to migraine during perimenopause and menopause when estrogen levels dramatically decline. Oral contraceptive pills are considered safe options in women younger than 45 years with no cardiovascular risk factors and may, in fact, improve migraine symptoms. Unfortunately, migraine symptoms may also worsen (Todd et al., 2018). If a woman wishes to stay on hormone replacement therapy despite migraines, she can be given a reduced dose and can be switched to pure estradiol or synthetic ethinyl estradiol. Using continuous dosing instead of interrupted dosing may also reduce migraine frequency.

MONITORING PATIENT RESPONSE

Careful monitoring of therapy is important. The practitioner should document the frequency, intensity, and duration of migraines before starting any new therapy and should evaluate the patient periodically after implementing any drug or lifestyle change to assess its effectiveness. Prescribers should monitor how frequently patients are taking abortive therapies to ensure they are not using them excessively to obviate MOH and other potential complications. Patients should return to the office after a few attempts with a therapy to assess its effectiveness, and practitioners should switch to another agent if the therapy is unsuccessful. Practitioners also need to evaluate prophylactic therapies for patient compliance and effectiveness. They should note side effects to therapy and treatment failures in a chart to avoid repeating ineffective therapies. Patients should also be queried directly about the use of dietary supplements as they may not volunteer the information (i.e., not considering it to be a "drug").

PATIENT EDUCATION

Drug Information

Practitioners need to educate patients about their headaches and what they should realistically expect from treatment (AHS, 2019). The prescriber should attempt to identify headache triggers (i.e., diet, medication, or environmental factors) by encouraging patients to keep diaries and to pay close attention when migraines start and should encourage the patient to avoid or minimize these triggers.

Practitioners must also educate patients about their drug therapy. They should tell patients how frequently they can take an abortive therapy, what the maximum daily dose is, and what side effects to expect from the medication. If the patient will be using a nasal spray or injectable medication, the prescriber should demonstrate proper administration technique. Also, prescribers need to encourage patients to take their prophylactic therapies as scheduled, emphasizing that taking prophylactic therapies on an as-needed basis will not improve the condition. If switching to a new therapy, the prescriber should remind the patient to stop using the old therapy and not to use the two therapies simultaneously (unless this is intended). For patients starting preventive therapy with the newer drugs (ditan or CGRP antagonists), thorough education is required, particularly if a novel delivery mechanism (e.g., autoinjector pen) is used. Patients must be strongly cautioned about drug–drug interactions, the dangers of concomitant use with some medications, and the use of any medications or dietary supplements they may not report. Acetaminophen overdose is common; patients must ensure that they are not taking a combined dose of acetaminophen from two or more medications that exceed a maximum daily dose of 3,250 mg.

Nutrition

Foods that can trigger headaches include aspartame, caffeine, chocolate, monosodium glutamate, and red wine and other alcohol. The patient should be aware of any foods that trigger his or her headaches (a migraine diary is helpful for this) and should avoid them. Some medications should be taken with food, and taking some (oral) medications on a full stomach may slow down absorption of the drug.

Complementary and Alternative/Integrative Medicine

There is mostly low to moderate evidence in support of the efficacy of some complementary and alternative practices to manage migraine, including acupuncture, massage, yoga, biofeedback, some nutritional supplements and botanicals, diet alteration, and hydrotherapy (Millstine et al., 2017). It is important that people with migraine inform their physicians of any dietary supplement that they may be taking, as there may be interactions with prescribed or OTC medications. Several herbal agents have been used and studied in migraine. A large recent meta-analysis found studies assessing feverfew, butterbur, curcumin, menthol/peppermint oil, coriander, citron, Damask rose, chamomile, and lavender (Lopresti et al., 2020). Most studies had low-quality results, including for feverfew, a popular herbal approach (Lopresti et al., 2020). There were limited data on positive efficacy for butterbur. For prophylactic supplements, there were some positive preliminary findings for curcumin, citron, and coriander, and for acute use, there were some positive data for menthol and chamomile. However, authors found a high risk of bias in many of the studies (Lopresti et al., 2020). Other agents that have been identified to manage migraine include riboflavin, coenzyme Q10, magnesium, and omega-3 polyunsaturated fatty acids (Millstine et al., 2017).

CASE STUDY 1

Cristina H., age 30, is on a follow-up visit to your office. She has been a patient of yours for 2 years. She smokes half a pack of cigarettes a day but is otherwise in good health, although she reports a high level of stress and over-work in her job and reports being "kind of worn out." She was diagnosed 10 years earlier with migraine without aura that was not responding well to over-the-counter (OTC) analgesics, including OTC analgesics with caffeine. Given that her headaches were "near-crippling," particularly right when they started, she was prescribed sumatriptan subcutaneous 6 mg. She reports that it "worked for a while," but she was frequently using it twice a day and was starting to use OTC analgesics more frequently as well. She said that when she was on birth control pills, she hardly had any migraines, but she had stopped taking them as she and her spouse were trying to have a baby. She reports a minimum of 10 headaches per month varying in intensity from moderate to severe. The headaches are causing her to miss work and interfere with her time with her young daughter, and she is also afraid she will lose her job (Learning Objectives 2 and 3).

1. What options and recommendations would you discuss with Cristina at this point?
2. What kind of therapy would you select at this point in time for Cristina?
   a.

Bibliography

Starred references are cited in text.

*Adams, J., Barbery, G., & Lui, C. W. (2012). Complementary and alternative medicine use for headache and migraine: A critical review of the literature. *Headache, 53*(3), 459–473.

*Allais, G., Bussone, G., Tullo, V., et al. (2015). Frovatriptan 2.5 mg plus dexketoprofen (25 mg or 37.5 mg) in menstrually related migraine. Subanalysis from a double-blind, randomized trial. *Cephalalgia, 35*(1), 45–50.

*American Headache Society. (2019). The American Headache Society position statement on integrating new migraine treatments into clinical practice. *Headache, 59*(1), 1–18.

*Antonaci, F., Dumitrache, C., De Cillis, I., et al. (2010). A review of current European treatment guidelines for migraine. *Journal of Headache and Pain, 11*(1), 13–19.

*Ashina, M., Hansen, J. M., Do, T. P., et al. (2019). Migraine and the trigemino-vascular system-40 years and counting. *Lancet Neurology, 18*(8), 795–804.

*Berk, T., Ashina, S., Martin, V., et al. (2018). Diagnosis and treatment of primary headache disorders in older adults. *Journal of the American Geriatric Society, 66*(12), 2408–2416.

*Bonafede, M., Sapra, S., Shah, N., et al. (2018). Direct and indirect healthcare resource utilization and costs among migraine patients in the United States. *Headache, 58*(5), 700–714.

*Brandt, R. B., Doesborg, P. G. G., Haan, J., et al. (2020). Pharmacotherapy for cluster headache. *CNS Drugs, 34*(2), 171–184.

*Burch, R. C., Loder, S., Loder, E., et al. (2015). The prevalence and burden of migraine and severe headache in the United States: Updated statistics from government health surveillance studies. *Headache, 55*(1), 21–34.

*Burch, R., Rizzoli, P., & Loder, E. (2018). The prevalence and impact of migraine and severe headache in the United States: Figures and trends from government health studies. *Headache, 58*(4), 496–505.

*Cameron, C., Kelly, S., Hsieh, S. C., et al. (2015). Triptans in the acute treatment of migraine: A systematic review and network meta-analysis. *Headache, 55*(Suppl 4), 221–235.

*Ceriani, C. E. J., Wilhour, D. A., & Silberstein, S. D. (2019). Novel medications for the treatment of migraine. *Headache, 59*(9), 1597–1608.

*Charles, A. (2013). The evolution of a migraine attack—A review of recent evidence. *Headache, 53*(2), 413–419.

*Cho, S. J., & Chu, M. K. (2015). Risk factors of chronic daily headache or chronic migraine. *Current Pain and Headache Reports, 19*(1), 465.

*Cho, S. J., Song, T. J., & Chu, M. K. (2019). Sleep and tension-type headache. *Current Neurology and Neuroscience Reports, 19*(7), 44.

*Clinch, C. R. (2015). Chapter 29: Evaluation & management of headache. In J. E. South-Paul, S. C. Matheny, & E. L. Lewis (Eds.), *CURRENT diagnosis & treatment: Family medicine*, 4th ed. (293–297). New York, NY: McGraw-Hill.

*Croop, R., Goadsby, P. J., Stock, D. A., et al. (2019). Efficacy, safety, and tolerability of rimegepant orally disintegrating tablet for the acute treatment of migraine: A randomised, phase 3, double-blind, placebo-controlled trial. *Lancet, 394*(10200), 737–745.

*D'Amico, D., Sansone, E., Grazzi, L., et al. (2018). Multimorbidity in patients with chronic migraine and medication overuse headache. *Acta Neurologica Scandinavica, 138*(6), 515–522.

*Detke, H. C., Goadsby, P. J., Wang, S., et al. (2018). Galcanezumab in chronic migraine: The randomized, double-blind, placebo-controlled REGAIN study. *Neurology, 91*(24), e2211–e2221.

*Dodick, D. W., Lipton, R. B., Ailani, J., et al. (2020). Ubrogepant, an acute treatment for migraine, improved patient-reported functional disability and satisfaction in 2 single-attack phase 3 randomized trials, ACHIEVE I and II. *Headache, 60*(4):686–700.

*Dodick, D. W., Turkel, C. C., DeGryse, R. E., et al. (2010). OnabotulinumtoxinA for treatment of chronic migraine: Pooled results from the double-blind, randomized, placebo-controlled phases of the PREEMPT clinical program. *Headache, 50*(6), 921–936.

*Dubowchik, G. M., Conway, C. M., & Xin, A. W. (2020). Blocking the CGRP pathway for acute and preventive treatment of migraine: The evolution of success. *Journal of Medicinal Chemistry, 63*, 6600–6623. doi: 10.1021/acs.jmedchem.9b01810

*Edvinsson, L., Haanes, K. A., & Warfvinge, K. (2019). Does inflammation have a role in migraine? *Nature Reviews Neurology, 15*(8), 483–490.

*Eptinezumab-jjmr (Vyepti) [prescribing information]. Lundbeck Seattle BioPharmaceuticals, Inc.: Rev. February, 2020. Retrieved from https://www.lundbeck.com/upload/us/files/pdf/Products/Vyepti_PI_US_EN.pdf on May 10, 2020.

*Erenumab-aooe (Aimovig) [prescribing information]. Amgen Inc.: Rev. October 2018. Retrieved from https://www.pi.amgen.com/-/media/amgen/repositorysites/pi-amgen-com/aimovig/aimovig_pi_hcp_english.ashx on April 12, 2020.

*Ergotamine Tartrate and Caffeine (Cafergot) [prescribing information]. (2002). Novartis Pharmaceuticals Corporation: Rev. June 2002. Retrieved from https://www.accessdata.fda.gov/drugsatfda_docs/label/2002/9000s22s23lbl.pdf on January 31, 2021.

*Ford, J. H., Jackson, J., & Milligan, G. (2017). A real-world analysis of migraine: A cross-sectional study of disease burden and treatment patterns. *Headache, 57*(10), 1532–1544.

*Frampton, J. E., & Silberstein, S. (2018). OnabotulinumtoxinA: A review in the prevention of chronic migraine. *Drugs, 78*(5), 589–600.

*Fremanezumab-vfrm (Ajovy) [prescribing information]. (2020). Teva Pharmaceuticals USA Inc.: Rev. January 2020. Retrieved from https://www.ajovyhcp.com/globalassets/ajovy/ajovy-pi.pdf on April 12, 2020.

*Galcanezumab-glnm (Emgality) [prescribing information]. (2018). Eli Lilly and Company: Rev. September 2018. Retrieved from http://uspl.lilly.com/emgality/emgality.html#pi on May 10, 2020.

*Goadsby, P. J. (2012). Pathophysiology of migraine. *Annals of Indian Academy of Neurology, 15*(Suppl. 1), S15–S22.

Goadsby, P. J., Holland, P. R., Martins-Oliveira, M., et al. (2019). Pathophysiology of migraine: A disorder of sensory processing. *Physiological reviews, 97*(2), 553–622.

Harvey, P., Shah, P., & Shipley, S. (2020). An overview of new biologics for migraine prophylaxis. *US Pharmacist, 45*(1), 21–24.

*Headache Classification Committee of the International Headache Society (IHS). (2018). *The international classification of headache disorders*, 3rd edition. *Cephalalgia, 38*(1), 1–211.

*Hepp, Z., Dodick, D. W., Varon, S. F., et al. (2015). Adherence to oral migraine-preventive medications among patients with chronic migraine. *Cephalalgia, 35*(6), 478–488.

*Hoy, S. M. (2018). Fremanezumab: First global approval. *Drugs, 78*(17), 1829–1834.

*Institute for Health Metrics and Evaluation (IHME). (2018). *Findings from the Global Burden of Disease Study 2017*. Seattle, WA: IHME.

*Ishitsuka, Y., Kondo, Y., & Kadowaki, D. (2020). Toxicological property of acetaminophen: The dark side of a safe antipyretic/analgesic drug? *Biological and Pharmaceutical Bulletin, 43*(2), 195–206.

*Jensen, R. H. (2018). Tension-type headache—the normal and most prevalent headache. *Headache, 58*(2), 339–345.

*Johnston, M. M., & Rapoport, A. M. (2010). Triptans for the management of migraine. *Drugs, 70*(12), 1505–1518.

*Kacperski, J. (2015). Prophylaxis of migraine in children and adolescents. *Paediatric Drugs, 17*(3), 217–226.

*Khoury, C. K., & Couch, J. R. (2010). Sumatriptan–naproxen fixed combination for acute treatment of migraine: A critical appraisal. *Journal of Drug Design, Development and Therapy, 18*(4), 9–17.

*Lasmiditan (Reyvow) [prescribing information]. (2020). Eli Lilly and Company: Rev. January 2020. Retrieved from http://pi.lilly.com/us/reyvow-uspi.pdf March 10, 2020.

Lee, V., Ang, L. L., Soon, D., et al. (2018). The adult patient with headache. *Singapore Medical Journal, 59*(8), 399–406.

*Leone, M., Proietti Cecchini, A., Messina, G., et al. (2017). Long-term occipital nerve stimulation for drug-resistant chronic cluster headache. *Cephalalgia, 37*(8), 756–763.

*Lew, C., & Punnapuzha, S. (2020) Migraine medications. *StatPearls* [Internet]. Treasure Island, FL: StatPearls Publishing.

*Lipton, R. B., Dodick, D. W., Ailani, J., et al. (2019a). Effect of ubrogepant vs. placebo on pain and the most bothersome associated symptom in the acute treatment of migraine: The ACHIEVE II randomized clinical trial. *Journal of the American Medical Association, 322*(19), 1887–1898.

*Lipton, R. B., Fanning, K. M., Buse, D. C., et al. (2019b). Migraine progression in subgroups of migraine based on comorbidities: Results of the CaMEO Study. *Neurology, 93*(24), e2224–e2236.

*Lipton, R. B., Goadsby, P. J., Smith, J., et al. (2020). Efficacy and safety of eptinezumab in patients with chronic migraine: PROMISE-2. *Neurology, 94*(13), e1365–e1377.

*Lipton, R. B., Pavlovic, J. M., Haut, S. R., et al. (2014). Methodological issues in studying trigger factors and premonitory features of migraine. *Headache, 54*(10), 1661–1669.

Loder, E., & Rizzoli, P. (2018). Pharmacologic prevention of migraine: A narrative review of the state of the art in 2018. *Headache, 58*(Suppl 3), 218–229.

*Loder, E., Weizenbaum, E., Frishberg, B., et al. (2013). Choosing wisely in headache medicine: The American Headache Society's list of five things physicians and patients should question. *Headache, 53*(10), 1651–1659.

*Lopresti, A. L., Smith, S. J., & Drummond, P. D. (2020). Herbal treatments for migraine: A systematic review of randomised-controlled studies. *Phytotherapy Research, 34*(10), doi: 10.1002/ptr.6701

*Marmura, M. J., Silberstein, S. D., & Schwedt, T. J. (2015). The acute treatment of migraine in adults: The American Headache Society evidence assessment of migraine pharmacotherapies. *Headache, 55*(1), 3–20.

*Millstine, D., Chen, C. Y., & Bauer, B. (2017). Complementary and integrative medicine in the management of headache. *British Medical Journal, 357*, j1805.

*Minen, M. T., Tanev, K., & Friedman, B. W. (2014). Evaluation and treatment of migraine in the emergency department: A review. *Headache, 54*(7), 1131–1145.

*Munjal, S., Singh, P., Reed, M. L., et al. (2020). Most bothersome symptom in persons with migraine: Results from the Migraine in America Symptoms and Treatment (MAST) Study. *Headache, 60*(2), 416–429.

*National Health Interview Survey. (2018). Table A-5a. Age-adjusted percentages (with standard errors) of migraines and pain in neck, lower back, face, or jaw among adults aged 18 and over, by selected characteristics: United States. Centers for Disease Control and Prevention: National Health Interview Survey. Retrieved from https://ftp.cdc.gov/pub/Health_Statistics/NCHS/NHIS/SHS/2018_SHS_Table_A-5.pdf on February 23, 2019.

*NCT03700320. (2020). To evaluate the safety and tolerability of treatment with atogepant 60 mg daily for the prevention of migraine in participants with episodic migraine. ClinicalTrials.gov. Retrieved from https://clinicaltrials.gov/ct2/show/NCT03700320?term=atogepant&draw=2&rank=2 on March 26, 2020.

*NCT03732638. (2020). Efficacy and safety trial of rimegepant for migraine prevention in adults. ClinicalTrials.gov. Retrieved from https://clinicaltrials.gov/ct2/show/NCT03732638 on March 26, 2020.

*Negro, A., & Martelletti, P. (2019). Gepants for the treatment of migraine. *Expert Opinion on Investigational Drugs, 28*(6), 555–567.

*OnabotulinumtoxinA (Botox) [prescribing information]. (2019). Allergan, Inc.: Rev October 2019. Retrieved from https://media.allergan.com/actavis/actavis/media/allergan-pdf-documents/product-prescribing/20190620-BOTOX-100-and-200-Units-v3-0USPI1145-v2-0MG1145.pdf on March 10, 2020.

*Ong, J. J., & De Felice, M. (2018). Migraine treatment: Current acute medications and their potential mechanisms of action. *Neurotherapeutics, 15*(2), 274–290.

*Oskoui, M., Pringsheim, T., Holler-Managan, Y., et al. (2019a). Practice guideline update summary: Acute treatment of migraine in children and adolescents: Report of the guideline development, dissemination, and implementation subcommittee of the American Academy of Neurology and the American Headache Society. *Headache, 59*(8), 1158–1173.

*Oskoui, M., Pringsheim, T., Billinghurst, L., et al. (2019b). Practice guideline update summary: Pharmacologic treatment for pediatric migraine prevention: Report of the guideline development, dissemination, and implementation subcommittee of the American Academy of Neurology and the American Headache Society. *Neurology, 93*(11), 500–509.

*Oswald, J. C., & Schuster, N. M. (2018). Lasmiditan for the treatment of acute migraine: A review and potential role in clinical practice. *Journal of Pain Research, 11*, 2221–2227.

*Pavlovic, J. M., Buse, D. C., Sollars, C. M., et al. (2014). Trigger factors and premonitory features of migraine attacks: Summary of studies. *Headache, 54*(10), 1670–1679.

*Prescriber's Digital Reference. (2020). Retrieved from https://www.pdr.net/ on March 10, 2020.

*Rimegepant (Nurtec ODT) [prescribing information]. (2020). Biohaven Pharmaceuticals: Rev. March 2020. Retrieved from https://www.nurtec.com/pi on January 31, 2021.

*Rizzoli, P., & Mullally, W. J. (2018). Headache. *American Journal of Medicine, 131*(1), 17–24.

*Robbins, M. S., Kuruvilla, D., Blumenfeld, A., et al. (2014). Trigger point injections for headache disorders: Expert consensus methodology and narrative review. *Headache, 54*(9), 1441–1459.

*Robbins, M. S., Starling, A. J., Pringsheim, T. M., et al. (2016). Treatment of cluster headache: The American Headache Society evidence-based guidelines. *Headache, 56*(7), 1093–1106.

*Schwedt, T. J. (2014). Chronic migraine. *British Medical Journal, 348,* g1416.

*Scripter, C. (2018). Headache: Tension-type headache. *FP Essentials, 473,* 17–20.

*Silberstein, S. D., Holland, S., Freitag, F., et al. (2012). Evidence-based guideline update: Pharmacologic treatment for episodic migraine prevention in adults. *Neurology, 78*(17), 1337–1345.

Spierings, E. L., Brandes, J. L., Kudrow, D. B., et al. (2018). Randomized, double-blind, placebo-controlled, parallel-group, multi-center study of the safety and efficacy of ADAM zolmitriptan for the acute treatment of migraine. *Cephalalgia, 38,* 215–224.

*Stauffer, V. L., Dodick, D. W., Zhang, Q., et al. (2018). Evaluation of galcanezumab for the prevention of episodic migraine: The EVOLVE-1 randomized clinical trial. *JAMA Neurology, 75*(9), 1080–1088.

*Straube, A., & Andreou, A. (2019). Primary headaches during lifespan. *Journal of Headache Pain, 20*(1), 35.

Tepper, S. J. (2018a). History and review of anti-calcitonin gene-related peptide (CGRP) therapies: From translational research to treatment. *Headache, 58*(Suppl 3), 238–275.

Tepper, S. J. (2018b). Anti-calcitonin gene-related peptide (CGRP) therapies: Update on a previous review after the American Headache Society 60th Scientific Meeting, San Francisco, June 2018. *Headache, 58*(Suppl 3), 276–290.

*Todd, C., Lagman-Bartolome, A. M., & Lay, C. (2018). Women and migraine: The role of hormones. *Current Neurology and Neuroscience Reports, 18*(7), 42.

*Torkamani, M., Ernst, L., & Cheung, L. S., (2015). The neuropsychology of cluster headache: Cognition, mood, disability, and quality of life of patients with chronic and episodic cluster headache. *Headache, 55*(2), 287–300.

*Ubrogepant (Ubrelvy) [prescribing information]. (2019). Allergan USA Inc.: Rev. December 2019. Retrieved from https://media.allergan.com/products/Ubrelvy_pi.pdf on March 27, 2020.

*Yu, S., & Han, X. (2015). Update of chronic tension-type headache. *Current Pain and Headache Reports, 19*(1), 469.

*Zhu, C., Guan, J., Xiao, H., et al. (2019). Erenumab safety and efficacy in migraine: A systematic review and meta-analysis of randomized clinical trials. *Medicine* (Baltimore), *98*(52), e18483.

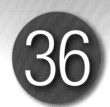

36 Seizure Disorders

Jesse Chen and Quinn A. Czosnowski

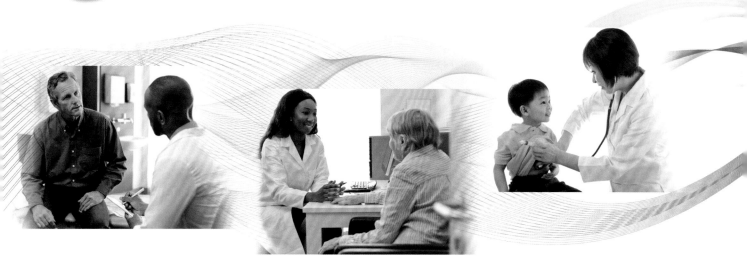

Learning Objectives

1. Describe the different types of seizures based on the new seizure classification system of the International League Against Epilepsy.
2. Describe the pharmacotherapeutic properties, along with risk versus benefits, of antiepileptic medications.
3. Review the treatment algorithm for managing seizures and status epilepticus.

INTRODUCTION

Epilepsy is a common neurologic condition affecting an estimated 2.9 million people in the United States and is the nation's fourth most common neurologic disorder. Every year, approximately 150,000 new cases are diagnosed, with the highest rate occurring in children and older adults. Epilepsy is a complex neurologic disorder best defined as recurrent seizure activity. A single seizure does not constitute epilepsy unless a brain abnormality is identified, which may result in future seizure episodes. It is a multifaceted disease with various physical manifestations, prognoses, outcomes, and responses to treatment. Frequent seizures can lead to neuronal damage, which may lead to changes in memory and other cognitive functions. Therefore, it is important for the practitioner to be aware of the various etiologies and to screen patients appropriately with accurate and reliable diagnostic testing. With appropriate diagnosis and treatment, more than 90% of people with epilepsy lead normal, healthy, and productive lives.

CAUSES

Seizures can occur at any age, with etiology varying by age. The most common cause of epilepsy is idiopathic, accounting for about 65% of all cases. Other causes of epilepsy include vascular abnormalities (11%), congenital malformations (8%), and trauma (5%). Seizures from degeneration, infection, and neoplasm are considerably less prevalent. In newborns and infants, perinatal injuries, metabolic defects, congenital malformations, and infection are more likely causes of epilepsy, but still less frequent than the idiopathic diagnoses.

Some cases of epilepsy are hereditary or congenital (present at birth), and some are acquired (e.g., serious head injury, a central nervous system [CNS] infection, stroke, or dementia). However, not all people with these disorders develop epilepsy. This suggests that there is a certain threshold that plays a role in the development of epilepsy and may be based on individual biochemistry. Why a person may have a seizure at one time rather than another relates to cause. This further suggests that there may be immediate triggers that can provoke an attack in a predisposed person (e.g., sudden seizure activity in people who are playing video games, working with a calculator, or listening to a particular piece of music). These sensory triggers are uncommon and are often referred to as *reflex epilepsy*.

Predisposing factors that may cause epilepsy more often are sleep deprivation, hyperventilation, fever from underlying illness, hormonal changes occurring during menses, and drug or alcohol ingestion. All of these may lower the seizure threshold and provoke seizures in people who are predisposed.

Several acute metabolic, infectious, medication-related, and other disorders (e.g., alcohol or drug withdrawal, viral meningitis, or hypoglycemia from an overdose of insulin) are associated with seizures. However, upon recovery from these disorders, a person is not necessarily predisposed to future seizures. These are known as *secondary* or *acute* seizures rather than epilepsy.

PATHOPHYSIOLOGY

To understand the pathophysiologic process of an epileptic seizure, it is necessary to understand normal neuronal conduction. Normal cellular transmission between nerve cells is dependent on a normal distribution of positively or negatively charged ions between the inside and the outside of the cell. In normal human physiology, there is a resting membrane potential (70 mcV) that leaves the inside of the cell negatively charged with respect to the outside of the cell. A stimulus is needed to produce a cellular discharge, and once stimulated, an action potential is generated. After the generation of the action potential, there is a brief period during which the nerve cell membrane is hyperpolarized, which makes it more difficult for a second action potential to be generated until the normal resting membrane ionic gradient is restored.

Communication between neurons occurs through highly specialized structures called *synapses*. There are hundreds of synapses on each neuron. In these synapses, neurotransmitters are released from vesicles in the neurons, where they are stored and then diffuse across the synaptic region to contact specific receptors. Once stimulated, the receptors can open or close a specific ion channel. There are two types of ion channels—excitatory and inhibitory. The channels consist of a number of different protein substances. The main inhibitory neurotransmitter in the CNS is gamma-aminobutyric acid (GABA). There are several excitatory neurotransmitters as well, including glutamate and aspartate. These chemicals can activate several different receptors that, depending on their action, can excite or inhibit a group of nerve cells.

To produce an actual seizure, a large group of nerve cells (neurons) must fire abnormally and together. It is thought that this firing occurs within certain highly organized areas of the brain that tend to support seizure activity. This is known as an *epileptic focus*. When epileptic discharges (focus) occur, normal inhibitory circuits (GABA-ergic) begin to fire, which tends to limit the size of the focus. The implication is that a seizure may result from impairment of the inhibitory brain nerve cells or conditions in which there is abnormal excitation. The epileptic focus that is produced may lead to a focal seizure only in the involved area of the brain, or the discharge may travel through other pathways to become more generalized and involve the entire brain. Clinical manifestations of a seizure can be classified by type of seizure, but the manifestations depend on the balance among abnormal, excitatory, and inhibitory neuronal firing; the location of the epileptic focus; and the patterns and degree of spread of the epileptic focus.

Classification of Seizures

The International League Against Epilepsy (ILAE) recently updated to a new basic classification system, which categorizes seizures based on where seizures begin in the brain, level of awareness during a seizure, and other features of a seizure. While there are many other features or symptoms that can occur during a seizure, the new system simply separates them into groups based on movement. ILAE now categorizes seizures into three major groups: focal onset, generalized onset, and unknown onset. The terminology used by the ILAE, however, is not always the same as that used by many clinicians. For instance, many practitioners call the ILAE "absence" seizure a *petit mal*, and the designation "tonic–clonic" is often referred to as a *grand mal* seizure. A focal onset impaired awareness seizure (previously called complex partial seizure) is often referred to as a *psychomotor* or *temporal lobe* seizure.

Furthermore, classifying epileptic seizures by seizure type is difficult because seizures often appear within a cluster of other signs and symptoms. To help classify seizure type, physicians may look for precipitating factors, age of onset, severity, chronicity, diurnal or circadian cycling, anatomic location of seizure focus, and physical manifestations to help define the patient's treatment and prognosis.

Focal Onset Seizures (Partial Seizures)

Focal onset seizures begin in a localized area of the brain, although there may be generalization to involve both hemispheres. Focal onset aware seizures (simple partial seizures) typically result in no alteration of consciousness, and the first clinical and electro-encephalogram (EEG) change indicates an initial activation of nerve cells in a limited part of one cerebral hemisphere.

The patient's symptoms are determined by the anatomic location of the seizure focus. There may be motor, sensory, autonomic, psychic, or other non-motor symptoms. These may evolve into focal onset impaired awareness seizures (complex partial seizures) or focal-to-bilateral seizures (secondary generalized tonic–clonic seizures). An EEG recorded during this time may show some low-voltage, fast activity; rhythmic spikes; and slow-wave activity.

Focal onset impaired awareness seizures are associated with impaired consciousness and with some form of automatic behavior (automatisms). This type of seizure can evolve from a focal onset aware seizure and can generate into a focal-to-bilateral seizure. The EEG may show a unilateral or bilateral, low-voltage, fast activity with rhythmic spikes and slow waves. Focal onset impaired awareness seizures may be preceded by an aura.

Generalized (Motor or Non-Motor) Seizures

Generalized seizures involve both hemispheres of the brain from the onset, and they result in early loss of consciousness. Generalized seizures can be further classified into generalized non-motor seizures, which may involve only loss of consciousness (similar to absence seizures), or generalized motor seizures (tonic–clonic, clonic, or myoclonic seizures).

Absence seizures (petit mal) usually have a sudden onset, are brief (often lasting <10 seconds), and interrupt ongoing activities. The patient exhibits a blank stare and is usually unresponsive when spoken to, although at times the patient may be able to relate what was said to him or her during the initial phase of the seizure. There may be some mild clonic or tonic jerking, but it is not prolonged. There is abrupt onset and discontinuation. There is no postictal confusion, which may be characteristic of other seizure types, and there are no other associated symptoms. The EEG shows a very rhythmic, 3 cycles/s spike-wave discharge during the event. There is often confusion as to the diagnosis of absence seizures versus complex partial seizures. Absence seizures are usually restricted to childhood and are provoked by hyperventilation.

A subtype of absence seizure is the atypical *absence seizure*, in which the alteration of consciousness may not be complete. A child experiencing this type of seizure may continue with some activities. There may be an associated loss of muscle tone of the face and neck muscles, and there may be mild clonic twitching of the eyelids and mouth. The onset and discontinuation of this type of seizure is gradual.

Tonic–clonic seizures (grand mal) are associated with abrupt loss of consciousness. There may be some vague, ill-defined warning signs but no true aura. The patient experiences a sudden, sharp, bilaterally symmetric contraction of muscles and may cry, fall, or do both. The patient's head may be extended and appear cyanotic. There may be associated tongue biting and incontinence. Depressed consciousness that can be prolonged (several hours) characterizes the postictal period, during which the patient exhibits bilaterally symmetric clonic jerking of the extremities, increased salivation and frothing at the mouth, and deep respiration and relaxation of muscles. After the postictal period, the patient usually reports waking with muscle stiffness and headache. The EEG typically shows generalized high-voltage, spike-wave activity.

Clonic seizures consist of rapidly repetitive bilateral jerking of the extremities and facial muscles with loss of consciousness. The postictal phase is usually short.

Atonic seizures (drop attacks or astatic seizures) are characterized by a sudden loss of muscle tone, which may be only fragmentary. This type of seizure may be brief and not associated with loss of consciousness. It can occur in a repetitive, rhythmic, and successive manner and may be seen in patients with more diffuse neurologic insult and psychomotor retardation. Atonic seizures are frequently associated with Lennox–Gastaut syndrome, a pediatric epilepsy associated with multiple seizure types, mental retardation, and abnormal EEG findings.

Myoclonic seizures are sudden, brief, shock-like muscular contractions. They may be generalized or they may be confined to the face and trunk muscles, to one or more of the extremities, or to individual muscle groups. Myoclonic seizures can occur regularly in a repetitive manner, or they can be sporadic. These seizures may accompany other neurologic conditions, such as metabolic or toxic states, as well as epilepsy.

Tonic seizures consist of brief, generalized tonic contractions with associated head extension, possible stiffening of the back, and stiffening of all four extremities. These seizures can be associated with autonomic symptoms, a rapid heart rate, and cessation of breathing followed by cyanosis. This type of seizure is also seen in Lennox-Gastaut syndrome and may be precipitated during slow-wave sleep.

Unknown Onset Seizures

Unknown onset seizures occur when the beginning of a seizure is not known or witnessed by anyone, for example, when seizures occur in a person living alone or at night. Even when the onset of a seizure is unknown, the new classification offers a system to describe whether the features are motor or nonmotor. Unknown onset seizures may be diagnosed as focal or generalized seizures later on when more information about the seizure is available.

Status Epilepticus

Status epilepticus (SE) is a life-threatening emergency that requires immediate identification and treatment. The standard definition is seizure activity persisting for more than 30 minutes or two or more sequential seizures without recovery between them. Clinical practice and recent guidelines define SE as continuous clinical and/or electrographic seizure activity persisting for more than 5 minutes or recurrent seizure activity without recovery between seizures. Thirty-day mortality of convulsive SE is estimated to be 19% to 27% and as high as 65% in nonconvulsive status. Significant morbidity is also associated with SE with the poorest functional outcomes in patients with refractory seizures. Precipitating factors include drug noncompliance and sudden withdrawal from antiepileptic drugs (AEDs), CNS infection, withdrawal from alcohol or sedative drugs, metabolic disturbances, sleep deprivation, stroke, trauma, or encephalitis.

DIAGNOSTIC CRITERIA

The accurate diagnosis of a seizure helps the health care provider decide whether to initiate or withhold drug treatment and which medications to prescribe. A well-conducted history and physical and neurologic examinations may allow a diagnosis of epilepsy to be made without further diagnostic or laboratory testing. The initial assessment should include associated factors (e.g., age, medical history, precipitating events), symptoms during the seizure (e.g., aura, behavior, motor symptoms, loss of consciousness), and symptoms following a seizure (e.g., postictal state). Unfortunately, many of the manifestations of epilepsy are subtle, making diagnosis and classification difficult. In fact, no single test, clinical finding, or symptom is reliable by itself to discriminate between epilepsy and nonepileptic events.

One of the most useful and standard tests for assisting in the diagnosis of epilepsy is the EEG. The EEG is a brainwave tracing showing voltage fluctuations versus time that is recorded from scalp electrodes placed in specific locations on the head (i.e., montages). An EEG is recommended as part of the neurodiagnostic evaluation of children and adults presenting with an apparent unprovoked first seizure.

Neurologic imaging studies also help in the diagnosis of epilepsy. Computed tomography (CT) scanning of the brain is used to detect masses or lesions, bleeding, or stroke-like conditions. Magnetic resonance imaging (MRI), although helpful in diagnosing lesions, bleeding, and stroke-like states, also helps find more subtle brain abnormalities, including medial temporal sclerosis. Current guidelines recommend the use of CT or MRI as part of the initial neurodiagnostic evaluation of adults presenting with an apparent unprovoked first seizure. MRI is the preferred imaging study for use in children. Other less frequently used tests include cerebral arteriography and positron emission tomography (PET). Cerebral arteriography may detect vascular malformation, aneurysms, and significant vascular disease. PET helps particularly in diagnosing partial epilepsy. PET scans measure regional cerebral blood flow and metabolism both during and between seizures. However, PET scanning is expensive, and some insurance carriers do not approve the test for reimbursement.

INITIATING DRUG THERAPY

The selection of the ideal AED depends on several factors, including seizure type, classification, and frequency. Other factors include sex of the patient, age, comorbidities, potential side effects, and willingness to adhere to treatment. Treatment with AEDs starts after the diagnosis is confirmed and the patient has experienced two or more seizures. If a patient has one or more risk factors for recurrent seizures (EEG abnormalities, structural lesions, partial seizures, or a family history), then pharmacotherapy can be initiated.

Many epilepsy specialists advocate monotherapy as the first principle of management. If monotherapy fails, replacement by a second AED is recommended. Monotherapy has several advantages, including increased compliance. The most frequent cause of failure to control seizure activity is the patient's lack of adherence to drug therapy. Management of toxicity is easier with monotherapy because adverse events often can be correlated with serum drug levels. Some epilepsy specialists report that up to 75% of their patients have had complete seizure control on monotherapy.

Usually, when monotherapy with several drugs has failed, polytherapy may be tried. In contrast to monotherapy, polytherapy may increase the risk of chronic toxicity in the patient. Whenever two or more drugs are used simultaneously, decisions regarding therapy become more complex, and there is an increased risk of adverse events and drug interactions.

The particular drug selected depends on the seizure type and toxicity. **Table 36.1** and **Figure 36.1** outline the recommended treatment order and algorithm of treatment.

Surgical Treatment of Epilepsy

The surgical treatment of epilepsy has become an important therapeutic modality. Candidates for surgery may include patients who have failed multiple medical therapies, with refractory SE, or experience intolerable drug side effects. Various surgical procedures can be performed, including anterior temporal lobectomy, amygdalohippocampectomy, extratemporal focus removal, lesionectomy, corpus callosotomy, and hemispherectomy. Outcomes are generally good with approximately 70% of patients seizure free after a temporal lobectomy.

Goals of Drug Therapy

The drug treatment of patients with epilepsy is designed to reduce the number of seizures while limiting adverse effects of the medication. A realistic goal for most patients is to completely control seizures, ideally achieved with monotherapy. In addition to controlling seizures, another goal should be improving the patient's quality of life by allowing a return to normal activities of daily living without restriction (except driving; see Patient Education).

Hydantoins: Phenytoin and Fosphenytoin
Indications/Uses

One of the oldest and most effective AEDs is phenytoin (Dilantin). fosphenytoin (Cerebyx), a prodrug, was approved

---

TABLE 36.1
Recommended Order of Treatment for Epileptic Seizures

	Focal Onset (both aware and impaired awareness) Seizures	Generalized Tonic–Clonic Seizures	Absence Seizures	Atypical Absence, Myoclonic, and Atonic Seizures
First-line therapy	Carbamazepine, phenytoin, fosphenytoin, valproic acid, lamotrigine, lacosamide, topiramate, oxcarbazepine	Carbamazepine, lacosamide phenytoin, valproic acid, fosphenytoin	Ethosuximide, valproic acid, lamotrigine	Valproic acid
Second-line therapy (alternative therapy)	Eslicarbazepine, felbamate, gabapentin, levetiracetam, perampanel, phenobarbital, pregabalin, primidone, tiagabine, vigabatrin	Felbamate, gabapentin, lamotrigine, levetiracetam, phenobarbital, primidone, ethotoin, mephobarbital, mephenytoin, vigabatrin	Clonazepam, paramethadione, trimethadione, methsuximide, phensuximide	Clonazepam, levetiracetam

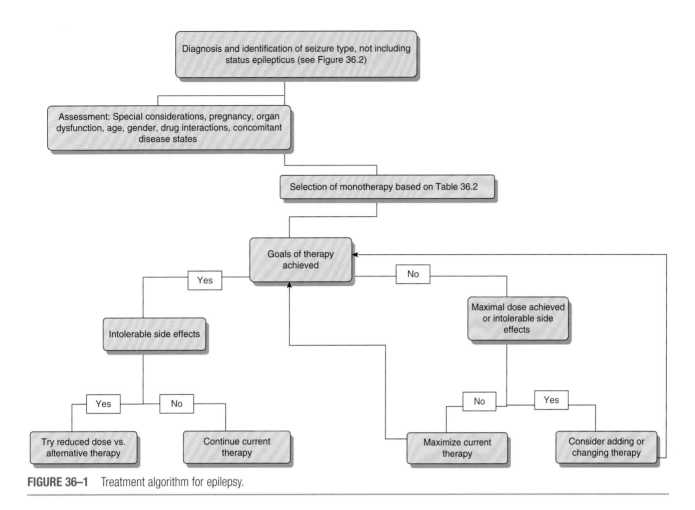

FIGURE 36–1 Treatment algorithm for epilepsy.

40 years later and is used for the same indications as its parent compound, phenytoin. Hydantoins are effective in treating a wide range of seizure types, including generalized tonic–clonic as well as focal seizure activity. In either case, they can be used as first-line agents for monotherapy. Phenytoin is one of the most commonly used anticonvulsants for generalized tonic–clonic (grand mal) seizure activity and for focal onset seizures. It can also be used to prevent early posttraumatic seizures occurring within 7 days after a traumatic brain injury. Phenytoin is not effective against generalized myoclonic or absence seizures and can even exacerbate these types of seizures.

Mechanism of Action

Phenytoin blocks posttetanic potentiation by stabilizing neuronal membranes. It decreases seizure activity by increasing the efflux or decreasing the influx of sodium ions across cell membranes in the motor cortex during generation of nerve impulses. It also regulates neuronal excitability by inhibiting calcium conduction through altering calcium uptake in presynaptic terminals and preventing cyclic nucleotide accumulation and cerebellar stimulation. Phenytoin is the active moiety of fosphenytoin, after administration fosphenytoin is converted to phenytoin by plasma esterases.

Dosage

Phenytoin is available in multiple dosage forms, including chewable tablets, extended-release capsules, suspension, and intravenous (IV). Regardless of dosage form, a loading dose of phenytoin is typically given to achieve a therapeutic level as quickly as possible. The loading dose is 15 to 20 mg/kg/d in both adults and children. The maximum infusion rate for IV administration of phenytoin is 50 mg/min to avoid cardiac arrest or 25 mg/min in patients with preexisting cardiac disease. If given orally, it is usually divided into three doses given every 2 to 4 hours to increase tolerability with a max of 400 mg per dose secondary to absorption. Following a loading dose, the normal maintenance dose is 4 to 6 mg/kg/d in adults and 5 to 12 mg/kg/d in children based on age. Absorption is also impaired when administered in patients on continuous enteral nutrition; therefore, it is recommended to hold enteral nutrition feeds 1 to 2 hours before and after each phenytoin dose given per feeding tube.

The dose, concentration in solutions, and infusion rates for fosphenytoin are expressed as phenytoin sodium equivalents. Fosphenytoin should always be prescribed in phenytoin sodium equivalents: 75 mg of fosphenytoin sodium = 50 mg of phenytoin sodium (see **Table 36.2**). Fosphenytoin is given as a loading dose of 15 to 20 phenytoin equivalents/kg followed

TABLE 36.2

Overview of Antiepileptic Drugs

Generic (Trade) Name	Significant Metabolic/ Transporter Interactions	Selected Adverse Events	Contraindications	Special Considerations
Phenytoin (Dilantin) Loading dose: 15–20 mg/kg IV. If PO, give in divided doses q2–4h to decrease GI adverse events SE: 20 mg/kg IV loading dose Maintenance dose: 300 mg/d or 4–7 mg/kg/d in three divided doses or daily–BID using an extended release form of the drug	Strong inducer: CYP3A4 Major substrate: CYP2C19, CYP2C9	Nystagmus, ataxia, cognitive impairment, lethargy, gingival hyperplasia, increase in body hair, coarsening of facial features, acne, folate deficiency, skin rash	Heart block; sinus bradycardia Pregnancy Category D	Avoid IM and SQ administration due to pain, erratic absorption, and risk of local tissue damage An in-line 0.22–5 mcg filter is recommended for IVPB solutions Therapeutic ranges: Neonates: 8–15 mcg/mL total phenytoin, 1–2 mg/mL free phenytoin Children and adults: Total concentration: 10–20 mcg/mL Free: 1–2.5 mcg/mL
Fosphenytoin (Cerebyx) See dosing recommendation of phenytoin, order in PE	See phenytoin	See phenytoin	See phenytoin	See phenytoin
Carbamazepine (Tegretol) Immediate-release formulation: Infants and children <6 y: 10–20 mg/kg/day in 2–3 divided doses; maximum 35 mg/kg/day 6–12 y: 100 mg BID; usual dose is 400–800 mg/d in 3–4 divided doses; maximum 1 g/d 12 y–adult: usual dose 800–1,200 mg/d in 3–4 divided doses	Inducer: CYP1A2, CYP2B6, CYPC19, CYP3A4 (strong) Major substrate: CYP3A4 (causes autoinduction starting between days 3 and 5 of therapy and maximal effects within 4 wk)	Hematologic abnormalities, drowsiness, fatigue, ataxia, SIADH, rash (SJS), GI upset, confusion, nystagmus, and tinnitus	Hypersensitivity to tricyclic antidepressants, bone marrow suppression, recent use of an MAO inhibitor (≤14 d) Pregnancy Category D	Oral suspension should not be administered simultaneously with other liquid medicinal agents or diluents To avoid GI upset, take with food or water and divide doses The appearance of a rash does not automatically rule out using carbamazepine Therapeutic ranges: 4–12 mcg/mL; 4–8 mg/mL if used in combination with other AEDs; toxic >15 mcg/mL
Oxcarbazepine (Trileptal) Initial dose: 300 mg BID; increased by 600 mg/d at weekly intervals Children 4–16 y: 8–10 mg/kg in 2 divided doses/d, not to exceed 600 mg/d	Weak inducer: CYP3A$	Dizziness, diplopia, ataxia, headache, weakness, rash, hyponatremia	Pregnancy Category C	Commonly leads to hyponatremia; older adults at higher risk Conversion from immediate release to extended release may require higher doses

TABLE 36.2

Overview of Antiepileptic Drugs *(Continued)*

Generic (Trade) Name	Significant Metabolic/ Transporter Interactions	Selected Adverse Events	Contraindications	Special Considerations
Eslicarbazepine (Aptiom) Initial dose: 400 mg daily; increased to 800 mg/d after 1 wk Maintenance dose 800 mg to 1,600 mg Dose adjustment for CrCl <50 mL/min	Moderate inducer of CYP3A4 Weak inhibitor of CYP2C19 Substrate of UGT2B4	Dizziness, somnolence, diplopia, fatigue, nausea, ataxia, cognitive dysfunction, vomiting, abnormal vision, abdominal pain, tremor, dyspepsia, abnormal gait, and hyponatremia (decrease >10 mEq/L)	History or presence of second- or third-degree AV block (Canadian labeling; not in U.S. labeling) Oxcarbazepine use Pregnancy Category C	Dosage may need to be increased when used with enzyme-inducing AED (phenobarbital, phenytoin, primidone)
Valproic acid (Depakote, Depakene) Children and adults: 30–60 mg/kg/d in 2–3 divided doses SE: 20–40 mg/kg loading dose Dose adjustment: Reduce dose in hepatic impairment and avoid in severe impairment	Weak inducer: CYP2A6 Weak inhibitor: CYP2A6 Minor substrate: CYP: 2A6, 2B6, 2C19, 2C9, 2E1	Lethargy, GI upset, weight gain, alopecia, hepatitis	Hepatic dysfunction; hepatic failure resulting in death has occurred, and children <2 y are at considerable risk Pregnancy Category X for migraine prophylaxis and Category D for other indications	Therapeutic range: total concentration 50–100 mcg/mL; toxic >200 mcg/mL Free: 5–15 mcg/mL Seizure control may improve at levels >100 mcg/mL Toxicity may occur at levels of 100–150 mcg/mL Take with food or milk; do not administer with carbonated drinks Oral formulations: IR (3–4 doses per day); DR (2–3 doses per day); ER (once daily)
Ethosuximide (Zarontin) Children 3–6 y: 20 mg/kg/d in 2 divided doses Children >6 y and adults: 20–40 mg/kg/d in 2 divided doses	Major substrate: CYP3A4	Nausea, GI upset, hiccups, headache	Pregnancy Category C	Seldom-used drug for absence seizures in children Therapeutic range: 40–100 mcg/mL; levels up to 150 mcg/mL reported without toxicity
Phenobarbital Infants and children <5 y: 3–5 mg/kg/d in 1–2 divided doses Children 5–12 y: 2–3 mg/kg/d in 1–2 divided doses Children >12 y–adults: 1–3 mg/kg/d in 2–3 divided doses or 50–100 mg BID–TID SE: 20 mg/kg loading dose; may give additional 5–10 mg/kg after 10 min	Weak inducer: CYP1A2, CYP2A6, CYP2B6, CYP2C9 Strong inducer: CYP3A4 and P-glycoprotein Major substrate: CYP2C19	Ataxia, cognitive impairment, hyperactivity, rash, problems with sleep, megaloblastic anemia (responds to folic acid)	Use caution in patients with hypovolemic shock, congestive heart failure, hepatic impairment, respiratory dysfunction or depression, previous addiction to the sedative/hypnotic group, chronic or acute pain, renal dysfunction, and the older adults (Because of its long half-life and addiction potential, phenobarbital is not recommended as a sedative in older adults.) Pregnancy Category D	Avoid rapid IV administration (>50 mg/min) Do not add IV form to acidic solutions Tolerance, or psychological and physical dependence, may occur with prolonged use Abrupt withdrawal in patients with epilepsy may precipitate status epilepticus Therapeutic ranges: Infants and children: 15–30 mcg/mL Adults: 10–40 mg/mL Toxic range: >40 mcg/mL

(Continued)

TABLE 36.2

Overview of Antiepileptic Drugs (Continued)

Generic (Trade) Name	Significant Metabolic/ Transporter Interactions	Selected Adverse Events	Contraindications	Special Considerations
Primidone (Mysoline) Children <8 y: Maintenance dose: 125–250 mg TID Children >8 y–adults: Start at 100–125 mg QHS for 3 d; then, increase to 100–125 mg BID for 3 d; then, increase to 100–125 mg TID for 3 d; then 750 mg to 1,500 mg/day in 3–4 doses	Weak inducer: CYP1A2, CYP2A6, CYP2B6, CYP2C9 Strong inducer: CYP3A4 and P-glycoprotein	Same as phenobarbital	Porphyria Use caution in renal or hepatic impairment or pulmonary insufficiency Pregnancy Category D	Folic acid as a supplement to avoid folic acid deficiency and megaloblastic anemia: Adults: 5–12 mcg/mL Children <5 y: 7–10 mcg/mL Toxic level: >15 mcg/mL Be consistent with protein intake during primidone therapy (Low-protein diets increase the duration of action.) Avoid foods high in vitamin C because of displacement of drug from binding sites
Pregabalin Initial dose: 150 mg/day in 2–3 divided doses, maximum dose of 600 mg/d	None Known	Peripheral edema, dizziness, drowsiness, weight gain, xerostomia, blurred vision	Hypersensitivity to pregabalin	FDA is warning that serious and fatal respiratory depression may occur in patients using gabapentinoids (pregabalin) Risk is increased in older adults and use with opioids or other CNS depressants
Gabapentin (Neurontin) Children ≥12 y and adults: 900–1,800 mg/d in 3 divided doses Dose adjustment: renal failure (CrCl < 60 mL/min)	None known	Ataxia, fatigue, dizziness, somnolence, weight gain, GI upset	Pregnancy Category C	Dosage adjustments for patients with renal impairment (depends on maintenance dose): CrCl >60 mL/min: 1,200 mg/d CrCl 30–60 mL/min: 600 mg/d CrCl 15–30 mL/min: 300 mg/d CrCl <15 mL/min: 125 mg/d

TABLE 36.2

Overview of Antiepileptic Drugs (*Continued*)

Generic (Trade) Name	Significant Metabolic/Transporter Interactions	Selected Adverse Events	Contraindications	Special Considerations
Tiagabine (Gabitril) Children 12–18 y: 4 mg daily for 1 wk; may increase to 8 mg daily in 2 divided doses for 1 wk; then may increase by 4–8 mg weekly to response or up to 32 mg in 2–4 divided doses/d Adults: 4 mg daily for 1 wk; may increase by 4–8 mg/wk to response or up to 56 mg in 2–4 divided doses/d	Major substrate: CYP3A4	Dizziness, somnolence, asthenia, confusion, GI upset, anorexia, fatigue, impaired concentration, speech or language problems, confusion	Hypersensitivity to tiagabine Pregnancy Category C	Dose recommendations are for patients also receiving enzyme-inducing AED regimens Patients not receiving enzyme-inducing AED regimens should be started on lower doses with slower titration Do not use loading doses, rapid or large dose titration in any patient Should be taken with food
Lamotrigine (Lamictal) Children 2–12 y with concomitant AEDs without valproic acid therapy: 4.5–7.5 mg/kg/d; max 300 mg/d in 2 divided doses Adults: 100–400 mg/d in 1–2 doses/d Dose adjustment is necessary for patients taking with valproic acid or interacting AEDs	Inhibits OCT2	Dizziness, headache, rash, ataxia, tremor, GI upset, diplopia, SJS (rare)	Use with caution with lactation, hepatic, or cardiac dysfunction, and in children Pregnancy Category C	Take without regard to meals; drug may cause GI upset Immediately report development of a rash Gradually decrease dosage (taper) over at least 2 weeks when discontinuing drug therapy If doses held for >5 half-lives, consider restarting using initial titration recommendations
Perampanel (Fycompa) Initial dose: 2 mg/d HS; increase by 2 mg q7d Maximum dose 12 mg/d If on enzyme-inducing AEDs: Initial dose 4 mg/d HS Dose reduction in mild-to-moderate hepatic impairment Avoid if CrCl <30 mL/min	Major substrate: CYP3A4	Perampanel carries a black box warning due to its potential to cause serious life-threatening neuropsychiatric events (aggression, anger, homicidal thoughts, and hostility) Common side effects include dizziness, somnolence, headache, fatigue, gait/balance disturbances, and falls	Pregnancy Category C	Watch for neuropsychiatric symptoms with initiation and titration
Levetiracetam (Keppra) 500 mg BID; max 3,000 mg SE: loading dose of 1,000–3,000 mg	None known	Somnolence, asthenia, fatigue, dizziness, ataxia, anorexia, cognitive difficulties, tremor, dizziness, ataxia, headache, fatigue, GI upset, renal calculi	Hypersensitivity to levetiracetam or any component of the formulation Pregnancy Category C	Limited drug interactions Concentrations only helpful to assess compliance to therapeutic regimen; no therapeutic range Maintain adequate fluid intake

(Continued)

TABLE 36.2

Overview of Antiepileptic Drugs (Continued)

Generic (Trade) Name	Significant Metabolic/Transporter Interactions	Selected Adverse Events	Contraindications	Special Considerations
Lacosamide (Vimpat) Initial dose monotherapy: 100 mg BID, increased by 100 mg/d at weekly intervals Initial dose adjunctive therapy: 50 mg BID; increased by 100 mg/d at weekly intervals Maximum dose of 300 mg/d in patient with CrCl <30 mL/min or mild/moderate hepatic impairment	Substrate: CYP3A4, CYP2C9, CYP2C19	Dizziness, fatigue, somnolence, blurred vision, diplopia, nausea, and tremor Increases in PR interval, second- and third-degree AV block, syncope, atrial fibrillation, and atrial flutter may occur, especially in patients with a history of cardiovascular disease	History of/current second- or third-degree AV block (Canadian labeling; not in U.S. labeling) Pregnancy Category C	Use caution in patients with cardiac history Consider ECG monitoring at baseline and when at steady state in patients with significant cardiac history
Topiramate (Topamax) Adults: initial: 50 mg/d; titrate by 50 mg/d at 1-wk intervals to a target dose of 200 mg BID Dose adjustment: CrCl <70 mL/min: administer 50% of dose and titrate more slowly	None known	Cognitive difficulties, tremor, dizziness, ataxia, headache, fatigue, GI upset, renal calculi	Hypersensitivity to topiramate or any of its components Pregnancy Category D	Maintain adequate fluid intake It is not recommended to crush, break, or chew immediate-release tablets due to bitter taste
Zonisamide (Zonegran) Initial dose: 100 mg daily, titrated by 100 mg q2wk for a maintenance dose of 400–600 mg/d Not recommended in GFR <50 mL/min	Major substrate: CYP3A4	Fatigue, dizziness, ataxia, and anorexia Psychiatric symptoms, psychomotor slowing, fatigue, and somnolence more common with doses >300 mg/d	Hypersensitivity to zonisamide or any component of the formulation	In chronic therapy, withdraw gradually to avoid potential of increased seizure frequency and withdrawal symptoms
Felbamate Initial dose: 1,200 mg/d in 3–4 divided doses. Titrate q2wk to 2,400 mg/d, maximum 3,600 mg/d	Major substrate: CYP3A4	Drowsiness, headache, dizziness, vomiting, upper respiratory infection, chest pain	Hypersensitivity to felbamate, history of any blood dyscrasia or hepatic dysfunction	U.S. black box warning for increase of incidence of aplastic anemia and acute liver failure associate with felbamate When starting felbamate therapy, decrease dose of concomitant carbamazepine, phenobarbital, phenytoin, or valproic acid by 20%

TABLE 36.2

Overview of Antiepileptic Drugs (Continued)

Generic (Trade) Name	Significant Metabolic/ Transporter Interactions	Selected Adverse Events	Contraindications	Special Considerations
Vigabatrin Initial dose: 500 mg BID, increase by 500 mg weekly, maintenance dose 1.5 g BD	None known	Drowsiness, irritability, weight gain, vomiting, tremor, visual field loss	Hypersensitivity to vigabatrin, pregnancy, breastfeeding (only in the Canadian labeling; not in U.S. labeling)	U.S. black-box warning for permanent vision loss associated with vigabatrin use Consider discontinuing if vision loss is reported
Rufinamide (Banzel) Adults: initial dose 400–800 mg/d divided in two doses Titrated by 400–800 mg/d QOD until max dose of 3,200 mg/d If on concurrent valproate, start at <400 mg/d Children: 10 mg/kg/d in two divided doses; titrate by 10 mg/kg/d QOD until 45 mg/kg/d or 3,200 mg reached Consider supplemental doses following hemodialysis	Weaker inducer: CYP3A$	QT shortening, somnolence, fatigue, coordination abnormalities, dizziness, gait disturbances, ataxia, nausea, vomiting, and rash Less common: multiorgan hypersensitivity reactions, DRESS, SJS, and leukopenia	Familial short QT syndrome, history or presence of short QT due to risk of sudden cardiac death Hypersensitivity to triazole derivatives Pregnancy Category C	Must be taken with food
Cannabidiol Initial dose: 2.5 mg/kg BID; may increase after 1 wk to 5 mg/kg BID, max 10 mg/kg BID	Minor substrate: CYP2C19, CYP3A4 Moderate inhibitor: CYP2C19	Drowsiness, lethargy, sedation, sleep disorder, weight loss, diarrhea, increased hepatic enzyme levels	Hypersensitivity to cannabidiol	Assess ALT, AST, and total bilirubin prior to starting treatment, dose changes, or changes with other hepatotoxic medications
Brivaracetam (Briviact) Initial dose for patients >16 y of age: 50 mg BID, maximum 200 mg/d	Major substrate: CYP2C19	Drowsiness, abnormal gait, lethargy, fatigue, equilibrium disturbance, nystagmus, vomiting, psychiatric disturbance	Hypersensitivity to brivaracetam	If taking with rifampin, recommendation is to double the brivaracetam dose Food may delay but does not affect the extend of absorption

AEDs, antiepileptic drugs; ALT, alanine transaminase; AST, aspartate aminotransferase; AV, atrioventricular; CNS, central nervous system; DR; DRESS, drug reaction with eosinophilia and systemic syndromes; ECG, electrocardiogram; ER, extended release; FDA, U.S. Food and Drug Administration; GFR, glomerular filtration rate; GI, gastrointestinal; IM, intramuscular; IV, intravenous; IVPB, intravenous piggyback; MAO, monoamine oxidase; OCT, organic cation transporter; PE, phenytoin equivalents; SIADH, syndrome of inappropriate diuretic hormone secretion; SJS, Stevens-Johnson syndrome; SQ, subcutaneous.

by a maintenance dose of 4 to 6 phenytoin equivalents/kg/d. Advantages include the ability to give it as an intramuscular injection in those without IV access and at a maximum infusion rate of 150 phenytoin equivalents/min.

Phenytoin is unique because it is metabolized in a nonlinear manner, exhibiting Michaelis-Menten enzyme kinetics. The enzymes that metabolize phenytoin are saturable, meaning that as the amount of drug approaches this saturation point, small incremental increases in a dose can result in disproportionately high serum levels. Further, as the concentrations reach closer to the saturation point, the half-life of phenytoin increases. This must be considered when adjusting phenytoin doses.

The therapeutic serum concentration of phenytoin is 10 to 20 mcg/mL in a person with a normal albumin level, while the therapeutic level of free, unbound phenytoin is 1 to 2.5 mcg/mL. In clinical scenarios in which protein binding is impaired, such as hypoalbuminemia or when concurrent medication therapy competes for protein-binding sites, the free fraction and pharmacologically active component are increased. Equations have been developed to help prescribers estimate free fraction in states of hypoalbuminemia, renal failure, and critical illness.

Contraindications

There are no absolute contraindications for phenytoin other than allergy (**Table 36.2**). It carries a black box warning for severe cardiovascular events (hypotension and arrhythmias) with rapid IV administration.

Adverse Events

Phenytoin exhibits adverse effects specific to dosage form and serum concentration in addition to other adverse effects. Common adverse events across dosage forms and concentrations include hypertrichosis, gingival hyperplasia, hirsutism, coarsening of facial features, vitamin D deficiency, peripheral neuropathy, and osteopenia. Concentration-related adverse effects include rash, ataxia, altered coordination, nystagmus, confusion, hepatitis, and mild sensory polyneuropathy. Serious but less common adverse events include blood dyscrasias (anemia, neutropenia, leukopenia, thrombocytopenia), hepatitis, Stevens-Johnson syndrome (SJS), drug reaction with eosinophilia and systemic syndromes (DRESS), and systemic lupus erythematosus (SLE). The IV forms of phenytoin and fosphenytoin carry boxed warnings for cardiovascular events with rapid infusion including hypotension, bradycardia, cardiac arrhythmias, cardiovascular collapse (especially with rapid IV use), venous irritation, thrombophlebitis, and possibly death. The IV formulations of phenytoin are also associated with local tissue necrosis following extravasation. Concentration-specific adverse effects of phenytoin are listed in **Table 36.3**.

Interactions

Phenytoin is a cytochrome P450 CYP2C9 and CYP2C19 enzyme substrate and a CYP1A2, CYP2C9, CYP2D6, and

TABLE 36.3

Relationship between Total Serum Concentration of Phenytoin and Adverse Events

Serum Concentration (mcg/mL)	Adverse Events
>20	Far lateral nystagmus
>30	45° lateral gaze nystagmus and ataxia
>40	Decreased mentation and lethargy
>100	Lethal

CYP3A3/CYP3A4 enzyme inducer. In addition to enzyme interactions, because of the high protein binding exhibited by phenytoin, it may be displaced by other highly protein-bound drugs, such as valproic acid and salicylic acid. Drug interactions occur frequently with phenytoin and can have a significant impact on therapeutic outcomes. **Box 36.1** contains a list of non-AEDs that interact with phenytoin, and **Table 36.2** lists AEDs that may interact with phenytoin.

Carbamazepine

Indications/Uses

Carbamazepine is indicated for the treatment of focal onset seizures and generalized tonic–clonic seizures. It is a first-line drug choice for monotherapy in focal onset seizures.

Mechanism of Action

Carbamazepine's mechanism of action is not completely understood. It is believed to alter synaptic transmission by limiting the influx of sodium ions across cell membrane channels. Other potential mechanisms of action include depressing activity in the nucleus ventralis of the thalamus or decreasing summation of temporal stimulation.

BOX 36.1   Nonantiepileptic Drugs That Interact with Phenytoin

NON-AEDs AFFECTING PHENYTOIN LEVELS

Decreases Phenytoin Levels
    Alcohol (long-term use)
    Antacids, folic acid, rifampin, tube feedings
Increases Free Phenytoin Levels
    Aspirin, diazoxide, tolbutamide
Increases Total Phenytoin Levels
    Alcohol (shortly after intake), amiodarone, chloramphenicol, chlordiazepoxide, chlorpheniramine, cimetidine, disulfiram, fluconazole, fluoxetine, imipramine, isoniazid, metronidazole, omeprazole, propoxyphene, sulfonamides, ticlopidine, trazodone

Dosage

Carbamazepine is available as an immediate-release tablet, extended-release tablet, extended-release capsule, and oral suspension. The usual starting dosage of carbamazepine is 200 mg twice daily as tablets or 100 mg four times daily as a suspension. Doses should be increased weekly by increments of no more than 200 mg. The usual maintenance dose is 800 to 1,200 mg divided into 2 to 4 doses, depending on the dosage form chosen. The therapeutic plasma concentration is 4 to 12 mg/L. Carbamazepine undergoes autoinduction, which begins 3 to 5 days into therapy, and is complete after 21 to 28 days of therapy. This results in a variable drug half-life and time to steady. Patients' serum concentrations will often vary significantly from week 1 of therapy to week 4 of therapy despite remaining on the same dosage of carbamazepine. As a result, frequent monitoring may be required following initiation or changes in dosing. Practitioners should be wary of decreasing a dose for a slightly elevated level during the first month of therapy due to a high likelihood that the serum concentration will decrease as a result of autoinduction. However, if a serum level is low during the first month of therapy, it is highly likely that the patient's level will drop further and a dosage increase is warranted.

Contraindications

Contraindications to carbamazepine include hypersensitivity to carbamazepine or tricyclic antidepressants, bone marrow suppression, recent use of a monoamine oxidase (MAO) inhibitor (≤14 days), and concurrent use of nefazodone, delavirdine, or other nonnucleoside reverse transcriptase inhibitors that are substrate of CYP3A4.

Carbamazepine has black box warnings due to the risk of serious dermatologic reactions in patients with the human leukocyte antigen (HLA)-B*1502 allele. Asian patients should be screened for the variant HLA-B*1502 allele prior to initiating therapy because this variant is associated with a significantly increased risk of SJS and toxic epidermal necrosis. It also has a black box warning for aplastic anemia and agranulocytosis. Baseline complete blood count should be checked with periodic monitoring. Those patients demonstrating decreased white blood count or platelets should be monitored more closely for the development of significant bone marrow suppression.

Adverse Events

Common adverse events associated with carbamazepine include pruritus, rash, constipation, nausea, vomiting, ataxia, dizziness, somnolence, blurred vision, urinary retention, xerostomia, and hyponatremia. Serious but less common adverse events include blood dyscrasias, syndrome of inappropriate diuretic hormone secretion (SIADH), cardiac conduction abnormalities, SJS, and DRESS (see **Table 36.2**). Carbamazepine is not effective in the treatment of myoclonic seizures and may in fact exacerbate seizures in these patients. Concentration-related adverse effects include dizziness, ataxia, drowsiness, nausea, vomiting, tremors, agitation, nystagmus, urinary retention, arrhythmias, coma, seizures, respiratory depression, and cardiac conduction disturbances.

> **BOX 36.2** **Nonantiepileptic Drugs That Interact with Carbamazepine**
>
> ### NON-AEDs AFFECTED BY CARBAMAZEPINE
>
> *Decreased Levels due to Carbamazepine*
> Benzodiazepines, corticosteroids, cyclosporine, doxycycline, folic acid, haloperidol, oral contraceptives, theophylline, warfarin
>
> ### NON-AEDs AFFECTING CARBAMAZEPINE LEVELS
>
> *Increases Carbamazepine Level*
> Cimetidine, danazol, diltiazem, erythromycin, fluoxetine, imipramine, isoniazid, propoxyphene, verapamil, nicotinamide
>
> *Decreases Carbamazepine Level*
> Alcohol (long-term use), folic acid

Interactions

Carbamazepine is a significant inducer of numerous CYP450 enzymes, including CYP1A2, CYP2B6, CYP2C9, CYP2C19, and CYP3A4. Caution should be used when administering other medications metabolized via these pathways. It is also a major substrate of CYP3A4. Since it induces CYP3A4 and is metabolized by CYP3A4, it can induce its own metabolism resulting in decreased serum concentrations over time. This effect is complete after approximately 3 to 4 weeks of therapy. **Table 36.2** and **Box 36.2** list drug interactions among carbamazepine, AEDs, and other drugs.

Oxcarbazepine

Indications/Uses

Oxcarbazepine (Trileptal) is indicated for monotherapy or as adjunctive therapy in treating focal onset seizures in adults or in children ages 4 or older and as adjunctive therapy for focal onset seizures in children ages 2 and above.

Mechanism of Action

Oxcarbazepine's pharmacologic effect is exerted through oxcarbazepine and the 10-monohydroxy metabolite (MHD) of oxcarbazepine. The exact mechanism by which oxcarbazepine and MHD work is unknown. However, studies indicate that the drug blocks sodium channels, resulting in stabilization of hyperexcited neural membranes and inhibition of repetitive neuronal firing. These actions are thought to decrease the propagation of synaptic impulses and prevent the spread of seizures. Increased potassium conductance and modulation of high-voltage activated calcium channels may contribute to the anticonvulsant effect.

Dosage

The typical starting dosage for the immediate-release product is 300 mg twice daily (extended release is 600 mg once daily), increasing by 600 mg/d at weekly intervals. The target maintenance dosage is 600 to 2,400 mg/d. There are no therapeutic levels established for this agent.

Contraindications

Oxcarbazepine is contraindicated in patients with a hypersensitivity to the drug or any of its components. Oxcarbazepine should be avoided in patients who have had a hypersensitivity reaction to carbamazepine because there is a cross-reactivity of about 30%.

Adverse Events

Common adverse events include dizziness, somnolence, diplopia, fatigue, nausea, ataxia, vomiting, abnormal vision, abdominal pain, tremor, dyspepsia, and abnormal gait (see **Table 36.2**). Clinically significant hyponatremia (<125 mmol/L) has been reported. Older adults are at an increased risk. Oxcarbazepine has been linked to fatal dermatologic reactions, including SJS, and patients with toxic epidermal necrolysis (TEN) should be monitored for signs and symptoms. Other rare adverse effects include blood dyscrasia (agranulocytosis, leukopenia, and pancytopenia), bone disorders, hepatic dysfunction, and hypothyroidism.

Interactions

Oxcarbazepine is a weak inducer CYP3A4. This leads to potential interactions with numerous AEDs, including valproic acid, lamotrigine, carbamazepine, phenytoin, and phenobarbital. Strong inducers of CYP enzymes (carbamazepine, phenytoin, and phenobarbital) have been shown to decrease plasma levels of the metabolite MHD (29%–40%). Oxcarbazepine also interacts with non-AEDs metabolized by CYP3A4, including dihydropyridine calcium antagonists and oral contraceptives, leading to decreased plasma concentrations. Avoid concomitant use of oxcarbazepine with any of the following: dolutegravir, doravirine, elvitegravir, eslicarbazepine, ledipasvir, rilpivirine, selegiline, simeprevir, sofosbuvir, and tenofovir alafenamide.

Eslicarbazepine

Indications/Uses

Eslicarbazepine is a newer agent approved for both monotherapy and adjunctive therapy for focal onset seizures in adults and children 4 years or older.

Mechanism of Action

Eslicarbazepine acetate is primarily converted to the major active metabolite eslicarbazepine along with minor active metabolites of R-licarbazepine and oxcarbazepine. The exact mechanism for eslicarbazepine is unknown but it is thought to block voltage-gated sodium channels resulting in stabilization of hyperexcited neural membranes and inhibition of repetitive neuronal firing.

Dosage

The recommended initial starting dose is 400 mg once daily, which can be increased after 1 week in increments of 400 to 600 mg to the recommended maintenance dose of 800 to 1,600 mg once daily. Patients with CrCl < 50 mL/min should receive an initial dose of 200 mg once daily, and titration should occur no more frequently than every 2 weeks by no more than 200 mg with a max dose of 600 mg once daily. There are no published data for use in hemodialysis or severe hepatic impairment.

Contraindications

Contraindications to eslicarbazepine include a history of hypersensitivity to oxcarbazepine or carbamazepine or the presence or history of second- or third-degree atrioventricular (AV) block.

Adverse Events

Common adverse events include dizziness, somnolence, diplopia, fatigue, nausea, ataxia, cognitive dysfunction, vomiting, abnormal vision, abdominal pain, tremor, dyspepsia, abnormal gait, and hyponatremia (decrease >10 mmol/L). Severe but less common adverse effects including SJS/TEN, DRESS, severe hyponatremia (<125 mmol/L), dose-dependent decreases in serum T3 and T4, and increased liver transaminases and bilirubin have been reported.

Interactions

Eslicarbazepine is a substrate of UGT2B4 as well as a weak inhibitor of 2C19 and a moderate inducer of CYP3A4. Eslicarbazepine may increase the concentrations of a number of medications that are substrates of CYP2C19; of particular importance is phenytoin. Due to its ability to induce CYP3A4, concomitant use with CYP3A4 substrates should be avoided if possible due to a decrease in their serum concentrations. Eslicarbazepine concentrations may be increased by carbamazepine and decreased by carbamazepine, phenytoin, phenobarbital, and primidone.

Valproic Acid and Derivatives: Divalproex

Indications/Uses

Valproic acid and its derivatives (divalproex) are approved as monotherapy and adjunctive therapy in focal onset and generalized onset seizures and as adjunctive therapy in patients with multiple seizure types, including absence seizures. It is considered first-line therapy for generalized tonic–clonic, focal onset aware, focal onset impaired awareness, and absence seizures. It has also been used in the treatment of partial myoclonic seizures, atonic seizures, infantile spasms, and SE.

Mechanism of Action

The exact mechanism is not completely understood but is believed to work by affecting GABA. It has been postulated to affect GABA in numerous ways, including increasing GABA availability, enhancing the action of GABA, and mimicking its action at postsynaptic sites.

Dosage

There are three specific forms of valproic acid available in the United States. While the dosage forms and dosing intervals vary, the total daily starting dose is the same (see **Table 36.2**). The recommended initial dose is 15 mg/kg/d increasing at 1-week intervals by 5 to 10 mg/kg/d. The dose is titrated to a desired therapeutic effect or toxicity, whichever occurs first. Doses above 60 mg/kg/d are not recommended. The therapeutic range is 50 to 100 mg/L with some patients requiring levels higher than 100 mg/L to achieve seizure control.

Contraindications

Valproic acid is contraindicated in patients with hypersensitivity to valproic acid, divalproex, derivatives, or any component of the formulation, significant hepatic disease, and in those with urea cycle disorders.

It carries several black box warnings including the potential for hepatic failure leading to death in all patients as well as an increased risk of hepatotoxicity in patients with known mitochondrial disorders due to mutations in mitochondrial deoxyribonucleic acid polymerase gamma (POLG). There is a warning for major congenital malformations, in particular spina bifida. It should not be given to women of childbearing age or during pregnancy unless other medications have failed to control their seizures. The last black box warning is for severe life-threatening pancreatitis that can occur at any time during therapy.

Adverse Events

Common adverse events include fatigue, tremor, gastrointestinal (GI) upset, alopecia, behavioral changes, and weight gain. Severe adverse effects include thrombocytopenia, pancreatitis, hyperammonemia/encephalopathy, and hepatotoxicity, which may occur at various times in therapy. Severe hepatotoxicity has been reported, especially in children age 2 and younger who are also taking other anticonvulsants. Patients taking valproic acid should be monitored for symptoms of hepatotoxicity, including malaise, weakness, facial edema, anorexia, jaundice, and vomiting. Other adverse events include a change in the menstrual cycle, ataxia, drowsiness, impaired judgment, headache, erythema multiforme, prolonged bleeding time, transient increased liver enzymes, tremor, nystagmus, SIADH, and fever. Levels above 100 mg/L are associated with increased adverse effects.

Valproic acid is teratogenic and produces neural tube defects (e.g., spina bifida) in 1% to 2% of pregnancies. It is a Pregnancy Category X drug for migraine prophylaxis and a category D drug for all other indications and should be avoided if possible during pregnancy.

Interactions

Minor interactions may occur with drugs that affect the CYP2C19, CYP2C9, CYP2A6, and CYP3A4 enzyme systems. Valproic acid may increase free phenytoin levels through displacement from protein-binding sites. Carbamazepine, lamotrigine, and possibly clonazepam reduce serum concentrations of valproic acid, while aspirin may increase valproic acid levels. Increased effects and possibly toxicity have been associated with the concomitant use of diazepam, CNS depressants, and alcohol.

Concurrent administration with carbapenems (e.g., meropenem) will cause a rapid decline in valproate plasma concentrations, producing an average drop of 66% within 24 hours.

Ethosuximide

Indications/Uses

Ethosuximide (Zarontin) is one of the drugs of choice for absence seizures. It should always be used in combination with another agent. It also is used for managing akinetic epilepsy and myoclonic seizures.

Mechanism of Action

The exact mechanism of ethosuximide is not completely understood, but it suppresses the paroxysmal spike-and-wave pattern in absence seizures and depresses nerve transmission in the motor cortex.

Dosage

The usual adult dosage is 500 mg daily adjusted by 250 mg every 4 to 7 days. The average daily maintenance dose is 20 to 30 mg/kg/d. The initial dose for children ages 3 to 6 is 250 mg daily with the same titration schedule and usual maintenance dose as adults. Doses greater than 1.5 g/d are not recommended and, if necessary, should be used only under the strict supervision of a physician. Serum concentrations should be monitored periodically with a therapeutic range of 40 to 100 mg/L (see **Table 36.2**).

Contraindications

Allergy is the only absolute contraindication to taking ethosuximide.

Adverse Events

Common adverse events are GI upset and fatigue. Ethosuximide has been associated with blood dyscrasias, CNS depression, SLE, and cutaneous reactions.

Interactions

Ethosuximide is a major substrate of CYP3A4 and, therefore, serum concentrations are affected by inducers and inhibitors of CYP3A4.

Barbiturates

Barbiturates have a relatively broad spectrum of antiepileptic activity and can be used as alternative monotherapy in generalized tonic–clonic seizures as well as in focal onset seizures with or without secondary generalization. Barbiturates are usually sedating and have long-term cognitive, memory, and behavioral effects, and drug dependence may develop. Therefore, it is usually best to try exhausting other alternatives before initiating barbiturate therapy.

Phenobarbital

Indications/Uses

Phenobarbital is the most commonly used barbiturate-based anticonvulsant. In addition to the indications listed previously, phenobarbital is used for myoclonic epilepsies, SE, and neonatal and febrile seizures in children.

Mechanism of Action

Phenobarbital works by binding to the barbiturate-binding site at the GABA receptor complex, leading to enhanced GABA activity. It interferes with the transmission of impulses from the thalamus to the cerebral cortex, resulting in an imbalance in central inhibitory and facilitatory mechanisms.

Dosage

In SE, phenobarbital is commonly given as a 15 to 20 mg/kg loading dose to more rapidly achieve therapeutic levels. The loading dose should be given no faster than 1 mg/kg/min with a maximum infusion of 30 mg/min for infants and children and 60 mg/min for adults. The recommended adult maintenance dose is 2 to 3 mg/kg/d or 60 to 200 mg/d. The recommended maintenance dose in children is highly variable based on age and ranges from 1 to 5 mg/kg/d. Serum concentrations should be monitored periodically with the usual therapeutic range being 10 to 40 mg/L.

Contraindications

The drug should be administered cautiously to patients with severe liver disease because of increased side effects. It is also contraindicated in patients with porphyria and respiratory disease with dyspnea or obstruction and those with a history of sedative or hypnotic addiction.

Adverse Events

The principal adverse events—drowsiness and fatigue—make phenobarbital difficult to use (see **Table 36.2**). It also may cause ataxia and blurred vision, nausea, vomiting, constipation, and, over a long period, cognitive impairment and behavioral disturbances. Other major adverse events include cardiac arrhythmias, bradycardia, dizziness, light-headedness, CNS excitation or depression, and gangrene with inadvertent intra-arterial injection. To a lesser extent, hypotension, hallucinations, hypothermia, SJS, rash, agranulocytosis, megaloblastic anemia, thrombocytopenia, laryngospasm, respiratory depression, and apnea (especially with rapid IV use) also may occur.

If an overdosage or toxicity occurs, the expected signs and symptoms include unsteady gait, slurred speech, confusion, jaundice, hypothermia, hypotension, respiratory depression, and coma. Patients may require an IV vasopressor to treat hypotension. Repeated doses of activated charcoal significantly reduce the half-life of phenobarbital; the usual dose is 0.1 to 1 g/kg every 4 to 6 hours for 3 to 4 days unless the patient has no bowel movement, causing the charcoal to remain in the GI tract. Urinary alkalinization with IV sodium bicarbonate helps promote elimination. Patients in stage 4 coma due to high serum barbiturate levels may require charcoal hemoperfusion.

Interactions

Phenobarbital is a weak inducer of CYP1A2, CYP2B6, CYP2A6, CYP2C8, and CYP2C9 and a strong inducer of CYP3A4 and P-glycoprotein. It is also a major substrate of CYP2C19. As a result, it interacts with a number of other AEDs. Other drug interactions include increased toxicity of propoxyphene (Darvon), benzodiazepines, CNS depressants, and methylphenidate (**Box 36.3**).

Primidone

Indications/Uses

Primidone (Mysoline) is structurally related to the barbiturates. It is metabolized to phenobarbital and to phenylethylmalonamide (PEMA). PEMA may enhance the activity of phenobarbital. Primidone is used in the management of generalized tonic–clonic (grand mal), and focal onset seizures.

Mechanism of Action

Its mechanism of action is similar to phenobarbital and is thought to decrease neuronal excitability and raise the seizure threshold.

Dosage

The adult dose of primidone is 125 mg/d increased by increments of 125 mg every 3 days. The usual dose is 750 to

---

BOX 36.3 **Nonantiepileptic Drugs That Interact with Phenobarbital**

NON-AEDs AFFECTED BY PHENOBARBITAL

Decreases Phenobarbital Level
Beta-blockers, chloramphenicol, chlorpromazine, cimetidine, corticosteroids, cyclosporine, desipramine, doxycycline, folic acid, griseofulvin, haloperidol, meperidine, methadone, nortriptyline, oral contraceptives, quinidine, theophylline, warfarin

NON-AEDs AFFECTING PHENOBARBITAL LEVELS

Increases Phenobarbital Levels
Chloramphenicol, propoxyphene, quinine
Decreases Phenobarbital Levels
Chlorpromazine, folic acid, prochlorperazine

INCREASED TOXICITY

Benzodiazepines, CNS depressants, methylphenidate

1,500 mg/d in 3 or 4 divided doses with a maximum recommended dose of 2,000 mg/d. The usual serum level for primidone is 5 to 12 mg/L; however, serum phenobarbital levels are typically used for monitoring purposes (see **Table 36.2**).

Contraindications

See the contraindications for phenobarbital.

Adverse Events

Primidone has an adverse event profile similar to phenobarbital. Dose-related adverse events include fatigue, cognitive impairment, and ataxia. Other adverse events include nausea, vomiting, hematologic abnormalities, and an SLE-like syndrome. A skin rash may develop, and over time, further cognitive impairment and behavioral changes may develop. Patients who have GI upset while taking primidone may take the medication with food.

Interactions

Drug interactions with primidone are similar to those with phenobarbital.

Pregabalin

Indications/Uses

Pregabalin (Lyrica) is approved as adjunctive therapy for focal onset seizures in adult patients.

Mechanism of Action

Pregabalin binds to the voltage-gated calcium channels in the brain, inhibiting excitatory neurotransmitter release.

Dosage

Pregabalin is typically started at a dose of 150 mg daily in two or three divided doses and should be titrated based on efficacy and side effects to a maximum dose of 600 mg/d. It requires dosage adjustment in patients with impaired renal function to avoid accumulation and increased adverse effects.

Contraindications

Hypersensitivity to pregabalin or any component of the formulation is a contraindication. Caution should be used in patients with a history of angioedema, heart failure, hypertension, or diabetes due to the risks of weight gain and edema.

Adverse Events

Peripheral edema and weight gain are common adverse effects. Other common adverse events include dizziness, somnolence, ataxia, and blurred vision. Serious, life-threatening, and fatal respiratory depression may occur in patients, especially with concomitant use of opioids or other CNS depressants. The older adults are at a higher risk.

Interactions

Pregabalin may enhance the sedative effects of other CNS depressants and may enhance the fluid-retaining effects of thiazolidinediones.

Lamotrigine

Indications/Uses

Lamotrigine (Lamictal) is approved for focal onset seizures (monotherapy or adjunctive therapy), primary generalized tonic–clonic seizures (adjunctive therapy only), and Lennox-Gastaut syndrome (adjunctive therapy only). Lamotrigine is commonly used off-label for other seizure types.

Mechanism of Action

Although its mechanism of action is not completely clear, lamotrigine stabilizes neuronal membranes by inhibiting the release of glutamate (an excitatory amino acid) and inhibiting voltage-sensitive sodium channels.

Dosage

The starting dosage for lamotrigine is 25 mg daily, with a slow titration every 2 weeks to a maintenance dose of 300 to 400 mg/d. In patients taking valproic acid, the starting dosage is 25 mg every other day. Slower titration can be used to help lower the risk for rash.

Contraindications

Lamotrigine is contraindicated in patients with a hypersensitivity to lamotrigine or any of its components.

Adverse Events

Overall, lamotrigine is well tolerated and does not appear to have any long-term cognitive side effects. The principal adverse events include nausea, fatigue, dizziness, diplopia, and ataxia (see **Table 36.2**). In approximately 5% to 10% of patients (most often in children), a rash may develop. If a rash develops, the drug should be discontinued immediately per U.S. Black Box warning. SJS and TEN have been reported with the majority of cases occurring in the first 8 weeks of therapy. The risk may be increased by coadministration with valproic acid, higher than recommended starting doses, and rapid dose increases. However, isolated cases have been reported with prolonged therapy or without these risk factors. Other adverse events include angioedema, nystagmus, and hematuria.

Interactions

The combined use of lamotrigine and carbamazepine may result in increased serum concentrations of carbamazepine and carbamazepine 10/11 epoxide. Valproic acid inhibits lamotrigine metabolism, whereas carbamazepine and phenytoin induce its metabolism. These enzyme interactions may result in significant changes in the half-life of lamotrigine. When used with valproic acid, the half-life is extended to 48 hours (from 24 hours when used alone), and with carbamazepine or phenytoin, it is reduced to 12 hours. Phenobarbital and primidone tend to decrease lamotrigine levels by approximately 40%. Although acetaminophen (Tylenol) may decrease lamotrigine levels, caution must be used when giving lamotrigine concomitantly with a folate inhibitor because it is an inhibitor of dihydrofolate reductase.

Levetiracetam

Indications/Uses

Levetiracetam (Keppra) has shown efficacy in the adjunctive treatment of adults with focal onset, myoclonic, or primary generalized tonic–clonic seizures. The immediate-release tablet and oral solution formulation are also U.S. Food and Drug Administration (FDA) approved in monotherapy for focal onset seizures and generalized onset seizures.

Mechanism of Action

The mechanism of action of levetiracetam is not known, but it is theorized to inhibit voltage-dependent N-type calcium channels, facilitate GABA-ergic inhibitory transmission, reduce delayed potassium currents, and bind to synaptic proteins that modulate neurotransmitter release.

Dosage

Levetiracetam is started at a dosage of 500 mg twice daily with immediate-release formulations (1,000 mg daily with extended release) and titrated up to 3,000 mg/d. Dosages of greater than 3,000 mg/d have been used in clinical trials with good tolerability but without evidence of additional benefit. When switching to oral therapy, dose and frequency remain the same.

Contraindications

Levetiracetam is contraindicated in patients with a hypersensitivity to levetiracetam or any of its components.

Adverse Events

The primary adverse events associated with levetiracetam therapy include somnolence, asthenia, headache, and infection. Most of these occur within the first 4 weeks of therapy, with no dose–toxicity relationship seen. Another common adverse event is changes in behavior, including aggression, neurosis, and psychosis, which may require a dose reduction. Serious but rare adverse events include anemia, neutropenia, eosinophilia, and SJS/TEN.

Interactions

Since levetiracetam does not undergo significant metabolism, there are no clinically relevant enzymatic drug interactions with this agent.

Lacosamide

Indications/Uses

Lacosamide is approved for monotherapy and adjunctive therapy of focal onset seizures.

Mechanism of Action

Lacosamide stabilizes neuronal membranes and enhances the slow inactivation of sodium channels leading to inhibition of repetitive neuronal firing.

Dosage

The initial dose of lacosamide when used as monotherapy is 100 mg twice daily and as adjunctive therapy is 50 mg twice daily. The dose may be increased at weekly intervals by 50 mg twice daily to a maintenance dose of 200 to 400 mg/d. An initial loading dose of 200 to 400 mg has been used in some patient with SE. When switching to oral therapy, dose and frequency remain the same. In patients with creatinine clearance of less than 30 mL/min or mild-to-moderate hepatic impairment, the dose should not exceed 300 mg/d. Lacosamide should be avoided in patients with severe liver disease.

Contraindications

There are no contraindications to lacosamide according to the manufacturer.

Adverse Events

Common adverse events seen with lacosamide include dizziness, fatigue, somnolence, blurred vision, diplopia, nausea, and tremor. Less commonly, increases in PR interval, second- and third-degree AV block, syncope, atrial fibrillation, and atrial flutter may occur, especially in patients with a history of cardiovascular disease.

Interactions

Phenytoin, carbamazepine, and phenobarbital may decrease the serum concentration of lacosamide.

Tiagabine

Indications/Uses

Tiagabine (Gabitril) is used as adjunctive therapy in adults and children older than age 12 with focal onset seizures.

Mechanism of Action

Its mechanism of action is not known; however, in vitro experiments show that it enhances GABA activity by binding to the GABA uptake carrier, inhibiting the uptake of GABA into presynaptic carriers.

Dosage

The starting dosage of tiagabine is 4 mg once daily and is titrated 4 to 8 mg weekly to response or up to 56 mg daily in 2 to 4 divided doses. The maintenance dose typically ranges from 32 to 56 mg/d.

Contraindications

Avoid using tiagabine in patients with hypersensitivity to any components of the formulation. Caution should be used in patients with hepatic impairment.

Adverse Events

Adverse events of tiagabine include infection, dizziness, headache, somnolence, CNS depression, memory disturbance, ataxia, confusion, tremors, weakness, and myalgia (see **Table 36.2**). Rarely, severe dermatologic reactions such as SJS may occur.

Interactions

Tiagabine is a CYP2D6 and CYP3A3/4 enzyme substrate and is cleared more rapidly when given with other hepatic enzyme–inducing AEDs (i.e., carbamazepine, phenytoin, primidone, and phenobarbital).

Perampanel

Indications/Uses

Perampanel (Fycompa) is approved for monotherapy or adjunctive therapy for focal onset seizures in patients greater than 4 years of age and adjunctive therapy for primary generalized tonic–clonic seizures in patients greater than 12 years of age.

Mechanism of Action

The exact mechanism of perampanel's antiseizure activity wis unknown, but it is a noncompetitive antagonist of the α-amino-3-hydroxy-5-methyl-4-isoxazolepropionic acid glutamate receptor on postsynaptic neurons.

Dosage

The recommended initial starting dose in patients not on enzyme-inducing AEDs is 2 mg once daily at bedtime, which can be increased in 2-mg increments every 7 days to a maximum recommended dose of 8 to 12 mg daily. Patients on enzyme-inducing AEDs (phenytoin, carbamazepine, oxcarbazepine) should start on an initial dose of 4 mg with the same titration of 2 mg weekly with a maximum dose of 8 to 12 mg daily. Older patients should have their dose titrated no more frequently than every 2 weeks.

Use is not recommended in patients with a CrCl less than 30 mL/min or on hemodialysis. Patients with mild-to-moderate hepatic impairment should be started on no more than 2 mg once daily and titrated no more frequently than every 2 weeks. The maximum dose is 6 mg once daily in Child-Pugh Class A impairment and 4 mg once daily in Class B impairment. Use should be avoided in Class C impairment due to lack of data.

Contraindications

Avoid use in patients with hypersensitivity to perampanel or any component of the formulation. Perampanel carries a black box warning due to its potential to cause serious life-threatening neuropsychiatric events (aggression, anger, homicidal thoughts, and hostility).

Adverse Events

Common side effects include dizziness, somnolence, headache, fatigue, gait/balance disturbances, weight gain, and falls. Neuropsychiatric events (aggression, anger, homicidal thoughts, hostility) are more common with initiation of therapy and following dosage titrations. Therapy should be adjusted or discontinued if this develops.

Interactions

Perampanel is a minor substrate of CYP1A2 and 2B6 and a major substrate of CYP3A4. In addition, it is a weak inducer of 3A4. Strong inducers of CYP3A4 should be avoided due to their potential to decrease perampanel concentrations. The use of other AEDs, which are enzyme inducers (carbamazepine, oxcarbazepine, phenytoin, etc.), may decrease perampanel concentrations and starting doses should be increased as a result. Concomitant use of CNS depressants may increase the risk of sedation.

Topiramate

Indications/Uses

Topiramate (Topamax) is used as monotherapy or adjunctive therapy for focal onset seizures and primary generalized tonic–clonic seizures. It is also used as adjunctive therapy for seizures associated with Lennox-Gastaut syndrome.

Mechanism of Action

It is thought to decrease seizure frequency by blocking voltage-dependent sodium channels in neurons, by enhancing GABA activity, and by blocking glutamate activity.

Dosage

The dosage starts at 25 to 50 mg/d and is increased to 200 to 400 mg/d in weekly increases of 25 to 50 mg/d up to 200 mg/d and, thereafter, may increase in 100 mg increments. In patients with a creatinine clearance of below 70 mL/min, the dosage should be lowered by 50%.

Contraindications

Extended release: Recent alcohol use 6 hours prior to and after administration.

Immediate release: There are none listed by the manufacturer's labeling.

Caution must be used in patients with hepatic or renal impairment, during pregnancy, and in breastfeeding mothers.

Adverse Events

Prominent adverse events are fatigue, dizziness, ataxia, somnolence, psychomotor slowing, nervousness, memory difficulties, speech problems, nausea, paresthesias, tremor, nystagmus, and upper respiratory infections (see **Table 36.2**). These may occur more frequently in patients taking more than 600 mg/d of topiramate or when titration occurs too rapidly (3–4 weeks to maintenance dose). Other adverse events include chest pain, edema, confusion, depression, difficulty concentrating, hot flashes, dyspepsia, abdominal pain, anorexia, xerostomia, gingivitis, myalgia, back pain, leg pain, rigors, nephrolithiasis, and epistaxis.

Therapy should never be withdrawn abruptly. Proper hydration is essential to decrease the risk of kidney stones.

Interactions

Topiramate is a CYP2C19 enzyme substrate inhibitor; thus, concurrent administration with phenytoin can decrease topiramate concentrations by as much as 48%, administration with carbamazepine reduces them by 40%, and administration with valproic acid reduces them by 14%. Digoxin (Lanoxin) and norethindrone (Aygestin) blood levels are decreased when given with topiramate, and concomitant administration with other CNS depressants increases topiramate's sedative effects. If used with carbonic anhydrase inhibitors, the risk of nephrolithiasis increases.

Zonisamide

Indications/Uses

Zonisamide is a broad-spectrum, sulfonamide-derivative AED approved as adjunctive therapy in focal onset seizures in adults.

Mechanism of Action

Zonisamide stabilizes neuronal membranes through blockage of sodium channels and select calcium channels.

Dosage

The initial dosage of zonisamide is 100 mg once daily, giving it a distinct compliance advantage over other agents requiring more frequent dosing. The titration to the daily maintenance dose of 400 to 600 mg is slow, at a rate of 100 mg daily every 2 weeks. There are no guidelines for dose adjustment in patients with renal or hepatic impairment, though it is not recommended for use in patients with glomerular filtration rate of less than 50 mL/min.

Contraindications

Use should be avoided in patients with a history of hypersensitivity to sulfonamide agents or any components of the zonisamide formulation.

FDA-approved product labeling states that zonisamide is contraindicated with other sulfonamide-containing drug classes; however, the scientific basis has been challenged as potential for cross-reactivity between antibiotic sulfonamides and nonantibiotic sulfonamides is extremely low.

Adverse Events

Potentially fatal reactions such as SJS, TEN, and agranulocytosis have been reported. Other important adverse events include fatigue, dizziness, ataxia, and anorexia. In children, there have been reports of high fever secondary to hyperhidrosis; zonisamide is not approved for use in children.

Interactions

Zonisamide is a major substrate of CYP3A4. Concentrations may be decreased when using inducers, such as phenytoin, phenobarbital, and rifampin. Serum levels may be increased when used concomitantly with protease inhibitors, azole antifungals, and macrolide antibiotics.

Felbamate

Indications/Uses

Felbamate can be used as either monotherapy or adjunctive therapy in the treatment of focal seizures. It is also used as adjunctive therapy in the treatment of focal onset and generalized onset seizures associated with Lennox-Gastaut syndrome in children. Due to an increased risk of life-threatening adverse effects, the American Academy of Neurology has published a practice advisory directing use.

Mechanism of Action

The mechanism of action is unknown but is believed to have weak inhibitory effects on GABA and benzodiazepine receptor binding.

Dosage

The initial dose of felbamate is 1,200 mg/d in divided doses three or four times a day for both monotherapy and adjunctive therapy. For monotherapy, the dose may be titrated in 600-mg increments every 2 weeks to 2,400 mg/d based on response and to 3,600 mg/d if clinically indicated. For adjunctive therapy, the dose may be titrated in 1,200-mg increments every week up to 3,600 mg/d. Prior to prescribing felbamate, an "informed consent" form needs to be signed by the patient and physician.

Contraindications

Avoid use in patients with hypersensitivity to felbamate or any component of the formulation or with a known sensitivity to other carbamates. It has black box warnings for an approximately 100-fold increased risk of aplastic anemia in addition to an increased risk of acute hepatic failure. As a result, its use should be avoided in patients with a history of blood dyscrasias or hepatic dysfunction.

Adverse Events

Common adverse effects of felbamate include somnolence, headache, dizziness, ataxia, skin rash, nausea, vomiting, anorexia, and miosis. Rarely, felbamate has been associated with cases of hepatic failure and therefore should not be used in patients with a history of liver disease. An increased risk of developing aplastic anemia is present as well, and routine hematologic monitoring should be performed to detect evidence of bone marrow suppression.

Interactions

Felbamate is a major substrate for CYP3A4 and may be affected by concomitant use of drugs such as phenytoin. In addition, felbamate may increase concentrations of valproic acid and phenobarbital and may decrease the effectiveness of oral contraceptives. It is recommended to decrease the dose of concomitant carbamazepine, phenobarbital, phenytoin, or valproic acid by 20% when starting felbamate therapy.

Vigabatrin

Indications/Uses

Vigabatrin (Sabril) is an AED approved for the treatment of infantile spasms and refractory focal onset impaired awareness (complex partial) seizures in patients 10 years old or above not controlled with usual treatments. It is only available in the United States through a restricted distribution program called Vigabatrin Risk Evaluation and Mitigation Strategy (REMS) program. Only prescribers and pharmacies registered with the program are able to prescribe and distribute the drug.

Mechanism of Action

Vigabatrin irreversibly inhibits GABA transaminase, increasing the levels of GABA in the brain.

Dosage

The adult dose of vigabatrin is 500 mg as an oral tablet twice daily. The dose should be titrated by increments of 500 mg weekly based on the patient's response and adverse effects. The recommended maintenance dose is 1,500 mg twice daily. Upon discontinuation, the drug should be tapered by 1,000 mg weekly. The dose for the treatment of refractory focal onset impaired awareness seizures in children 10 years and above is dependent on weight and/or age. The dose for the treatment of infantile spasms is 50 mg/kg/d divided twice daily titrated by increments of 25 to 50 mg/kg/d every 3 days. The maximum dose for infants is 150 mg/d. Dose adjustments are necessary in renal impairment.

Contraindications

Hypersensitivity to vigabatrin or any component of the formulation contraindicates its use. Vigabatrin has a black box warning for its ability to cause permanent bilateral concentric visual field constriction.

Adverse Events

Common adverse effects of vigabatrin include somnolence, headache, dizziness, irritability, insomnia, weight gain, and diarrhea. Vigabatrin can cause permanent vision loss in patients receiving the drug. Patients who do not show substantial benefit within a short time after initiation (2–4 weeks for infantile spasms, <3 months for adults) should have the drug discontinued to avoid this adverse effect. Vision loss increases with larger doses and cumulative exposure and can affect more than 30% of patients. Vision should be assessed at baseline, at 4 weeks, and every 3 months thereafter.

Interactions

Vigabatrin may increase the sedative effects of other drugs and alcohol.

Rufinamide

Indications/Uses

Rufinamide (Banzel) is indicated for adjunctive treatment of seizures associated with Lennox Gastaut syndrome in patients 1 year of age or older.

Mechanism of Action

Rufinamide is a triazole derivative whose precise mechanism is unknown. In vitro data suggest it prolongs the inactive state of sodium channels and limits repetitive firing of sodium-dependent action potentials.

Dosage

The starting dose in patients less than 17 years old is 10 mg/kg/d divided into twice-daily doses. The dose should be increased by 10 mg/kg/d every other day until a maximum of 45 mg/kg/d or 3,200 mg, whichever is lower, is reached. Patients on concomitant valproate should start on doses less than 10 mg/kg/d in divided doses.

The starting dose in patients 17 years or older is 400 to 800 mg daily divided into twice daily doses. The dose should be increased by 400 to 800 mg every other day to a maximum dose of 3,200 mg/d. Patients on concomitant valproate should start at 400 mg daily in divided doses.

The extent of absorption is decreased with increasing doses. It should be taken with food as food significantly increases absorption. While no dosage adjustments are provided by the manufacturer, approximately 30% of a dose is removed by a 4-hour run of hemodialysis. A supplemental dose may need to be considered based on clinical response.

Contraindications

Patients with familial short QT syndrome and presence or history of short QT syndrome should not take rufinamide due to a potential for increased risk of sudden cardiac death. Its use is contraindicated in patients with hypersentivity to triazole derivatives or any component of the formulation.

Adverse Events

Common adverse events in clinical trials included QT shortening, somnolence, fatigue, coordination abnormalities, dizziness, gait disturbances, ataxia, nausea, vomiting, SE, and rash. Less common but clinically important adverse events include multiorgan hypersensitivity reactions, DRESS, SJS, and leukopenia.

Interactions

Rufinamide undergoes extensive hydrolysis via carboxylesterases with no appreciable CYP-mediated metabolism. It is a weak inhibitor of CYP2E1 and a weak inducer of CYP3A4. Despite no appreciable CYP-mediated metabolism, carbamazepine, phenytoin, phenobarbital, and primidone may decrease levels of rufinamide. Rufinamide may decrease levels of carbamazepine and estrogen or progestin-based contraceptives. Rufinamide concentrations are significantly increased with concomitant administration of valproic acid. If given together, initiate at lower doses and consider slower dosage titration. Levels of phenytoin and phenobarbital may be increased with coadministration. Food significantly increases the extent of absorption, and patients should be instructed to take it with a meal.

Benzodiazepines

The benzodiazepine antianxiety agents are discussed in depth in Chapter 41.

Clobazam

Indications/Uses

Clobazam (Onfi) is indicated for adjunctive treatment of seizures associated with Lennox-Gastaut syndrome in patients 2 years of age or older.

Mechanism of Action

Clobazam is thought to act as an agonist at the $GABA_A$ receptor to enhance GABA action, thereby depressing nerve transmission in the motor cortex area.

Dosage

Initial clobazam doses are determined by patient weight. Patients weighing 30 kg or less should start on 5 mg daily, while patients weighing more than 30 kg should start on 10 mg/d. Doses greater than 5 mg daily should be given in divided doses twice daily. Dose increases should occur no more frequently than every 7 days and by no more than 100% of the previous dose. Maximum doses per package labeling are 20 mg/d for patients weighing 30 kg or less and 40 mg/d for patients weighing more than 30 kg. Dose decreases should occur slowly and no more frequently than weekly to avoid withdrawal symptoms. Poor metabolizers of CYP2C19 should be started at the lowest recommended doses and titrate slowly to half of the recommended maximum dose.

Contraindications

Contraindications include hypersensitivity to clonazepam, any of its components, or other benzodiazepines.

Adverse Events

Constipation, somnolence, sedation, pyrexia, lethargy, and drooling occurred at least 10% more frequently than placebo in clinical trials. Physical and psychological dependence are possible with all benzodiazepines.

Interactions

Clobazam is primarily metabolized by not only CYP3A4 but also 2C19 and 2B6 to its active metabolite N-desmethyl, which is metabolized by 2C19. Strong 2C19 inducers (e.g., theophylline) may decrease clobazam activity, while strong (e.g., fluconazole) to moderate (e.g., omeprazole) 2C19 inhibitors may increase clobazam activity. Alcohol may increase clobazam concentrations by as much as 50%.

Clobazam is a weak inducer of CYP3A4 and may reduce the effectiveness of some hormonal contraceptives. Nonhormonal forms of contraception should be considered when using clobazam. In addition, clobazam inhibits CYP2D6 in vivo, and drugs metabolized by this pathway may require dosage adjustment. Concomitant use of CNS depressants may increase the risk of sedation.

Clonazepam

Indications/Uses

Clonazepam (Klonopin) is effective as an adjunctive drug in some patients with myoclonic, atonic, and generalized tonic–clonic seizures. It also is used for prophylaxis of absence, Lennox-Gastaut, akinetic, and myoclonic seizures.

Mechanism of Action

Clonazepam is thought to act at the GABA receptor to enhance GABA action, thereby depressing nerve transmission in the motor cortex area.

Dosage

Clonazepam is given in three divided doses with an initial daily starting dose of up to 1.5 mg in adults. The dose may be increased by 0.5 to 1 mg every third day until seizures are controlled or adverse effects are evident (maximum, 20 mg/d). The initial daily dose is 0.01 to 0.03 mg/kg/d in divided doses in infants and children less than 10 years old or weight less than 30 kg. The dose may be increased by no more than 0.25 to 0.5 mg every third day until a daily maintenance dose of 0.1 to 0.2 mg/kg/d. Tolerance to this drug is common.

Contraindications

Contraindications include hypersensitivity to clonazepam, any of its components, or other benzodiazepines; severe liver disease; and acute narrow-angle glaucoma. Caution must be used in patients with chronic respiratory disease or impaired renal function and in patients who are mentally challenged (may have more frequent drug-induced behavioral symptoms).

Adverse Events

Fatigue, sedation, and behavioral changes (e.g., aggressiveness and confusion) are the principal adverse reactions. Tachycardia, chest pain, headache, constipation, nausea, and decreased salivation are other adverse reactions.

Interactions

Medications that induce CYP3A4 enzyme substrates, such as phenytoin and barbiturates, may increase clonazepam clearance. Concomitant use of CNS depressants may increase the risk of sedation.

Lorazepam

Indications/Uses

Lorazepam (Ativan) is used intravenously to treat SE and has an unlabeled use for focal onset impaired awareness seizures.

Mechanism of Action

The drug is believed to depress all levels of the CNS, including the limbic system and reticular formation, probably through the increased action of GABA.

Dosage

In the treatment of SE, lorazepam may be given as a 4-mg slow IV bolus (maximum rate of 2 mg/min). Doses may be repeated every 3 to 5 minutes until seizures stop.

Contraindications

Lorazepam is contraindicated in patients with a hypersensitivity to lorazepam or to any of its components. It is also contraindicated in patients with hypersensitivity to polyethylene glycol, propylene glycol, or benzyl alcohol. There is also a risk of cross-sensitivity with other benzodiazepines. It should not be used in comatose patients; patients with preexisting CNS depression, narrow-angle glaucoma, severe, uncontrolled pain, and severe hypertension; and pregnant women. Caution must be used in patients with renal or hepatic impairment, organic brain syndrome, myasthenia gravis, or Parkinson's disease.

Adverse Events

Common adverse reactions include tachycardia, chest pain, drowsiness, confusion, ataxia, amnesia, slurred speech, paradoxical excitement, headache, and depression. Light-headedness, rash, decreased libido, xerostomia, bradycardia, cardiovascular collapse, syncope, constipation, nausea, vomiting, decreased salivation, phlebitis, and blurred vision also may occur. Menstrual irregularities, increased salivation, blood dyscrasias, and physical and psychological dependence occur with prolonged use.

Interactions

Lorazepam has a decreased effect with oral contraceptives (combination products), cigarette smoking, and levodopa. Its effects are increased with morphine or other narcotic analgesics. An increased risk of toxicity occurs with the concomitant use of alcohol, CNS depressants, MAO inhibitors, loxapine (Loxitane), and tricyclic antidepressants. There is a U.S. black box warning regarding concomitant use of benzodiazepines and opioids warning of profound sedation, respiratory depression, coma, and potentially death. Reserve use of both for when alternative treatments are inadequate.

Diazepam

Indications/Uses

Diazepam is used to treat SE and as an adjunct in convulsive disorders.

Mechanism of Action

Its mechanism of action is the same as that of lorazepam.

Dosage

Diazepam may be given intravenously 5 to 10 mg as a single dose with a maximum infusion rate of 5 mg/min repeated every 3 to 5 minutes if seizures continue (maximum dose of 30 mg). It may also be given as a rectal gel out of hospital as a 10-mg, one-time dose and may be repeated once if necessary.

Contraindications

Diazepam should not be used by patients with severe or acute liver disease. Contraindications include hypersensitivity to diazepam or to any of its components. Other contraindications are similar to those for lorazepam. Caution should be used in patients taking other CNS depressants, patients with low albumin levels or hepatic dysfunction, and older patients and infants. Because of its long-acting metabolite and the risk for falls in the older population, diazepam is not considered a drug of choice.

Adverse Events

Adverse drug effects resemble those of lorazepam.

Interactions

Diazepam is a CYP1A2 and CYP2C9 enzyme substrate. It is also a major enzyme substrate for CYP3A4 and CYP2C19. Enzyme inducers may increase the metabolism of diazepam, resulting in decreased efficacy. Increased toxicity, sedation, and respiratory depression may result when diazepam is given with CNS depressants (e.g., alcohol, barbiturates, and opioids). Cimetidine (Tagamet) may decrease the metabolism of diazepam. Valproic acid may displace diazepam from binding sites, which may result in an increase in sedative effects. Selective serotonin reuptake inhibitors (e.g., fluoxetine [Prozac], sertraline [Zoloft], paroxetine [Paxil]) greatly increase diazepam levels by altering its clearance.

Cannabidiol

Indications/Uses

Cannabinoids used to be one of the most discussed alternative medication therapies for treatment of refractory seizures. Cannabidiol recently gained approval for the treatment of Lennox-Gastaut syndrome seizures in patients 2 years or older.

Mechanism of Action

The exact mechanism is not well understood. However, it does not appear to bind to the cannabinoid 1 and 2 receptors in the brain and lack the psychotropic side effects as other cannabinoids.

Dosages

Cannabidiol (Epidiolex) is available as an oral solution. The recommended initial dosage is 5 mg/kg/day given twice daily. After one week, the dosage can be increased to a maintenance dosage of 10 mg/kg/day given twice daily. The maximum recommended maintenance dose is 20 mg/kg/day given twice daily. Dosage adjustments are recommended for patients with moderate or severe hepatic impairment.

Contraindications

Cannabidiol is contraindicated in patients with hypersensitivity to cannabidiol or any of its ingredients.

Adverse Events

Some of the most common adverse events include somnolence, decreased appetite, diarrhea, liver enzyme elevations, fatigue, malaise, rash, insomnia, sleep disorder, and infections.

Interactions

If given with moderate or strong inhibitors of CYP3A4 or CYP2C19, consider dose reduction of cannabidiol. If given with strong inducers of CYP3A4 or CYP2C19, consider dose increase of cannabidiol. Due to the risk of transaminase elevations, concomitant use of valproic acid and its derivatives with cannabidiol should be monitored closely and doses adjusted if necessary.

Brivaracetam

Indication

Brivaracetam (Briviact) tablets or oral solution is indicated for the treatment of focal onset seizures (monotherapy or adjunctive therapy) in patients 4 years and older. The injection formulation is only indicated for patients 16 years and older.

Mechanism of Action

The exact mechanism by which brivaracetam exerts its antiseizure activity is unknown. Brivaracetam does have a selective and high affinity for synaptic vesicle protein 2A (SV2A) in the brain, which has been shown to minimize epileptic effect.

Dosages

In patients 16 years and old, the recommended initial dosage for monotherapy or adjunctive therapy is 50 mg twice daily (100 mg/d). The dose may actually be titrated down to 25 mg twice daily or up to 100 mg twice daily depending on individual patient tolerability and therapeutic response. In patients between the ages of 4 to 16 years old, the recommended dosage is based on body weight and given twice daily. The dosage for IV formulation is the same as the oral regimen. Dose adjustment is recommended for all stages of hepatic dysfunction. If brivaracetam needs to be stopped for any reason, brivaracetam should be gradually withdrawn.

Contraindications

Brivaracetam is contraindicated in patients with hypersensitivity to brivaracetam or any of the inactive ingredients in brivaracetam.

Adverse Events

Most common adverse reactions seen are somnolence, sedation, dizziness, fatigue, and nausea/vomiting. Patients should be monitored for suicidal behavior and ideation, aggressive behavior, depression, anxiety, or psychotic symptoms while on this medication.

Interactions

Brivaracetam is the major substrate of CYP2C19. It is recommended to increase the dose of brivaracetam while on concomitant rifampin. Carbamazepine may decrease the concentration of brivaracetam. At the same time, brivaracetam may increase concentration of the active metabolite of carbamazepine. Dose reduction of carbamazepine is recommended if tolerability issues arise with concomitant use. Phenytoin may also decrease the concentration of brivaracetam and phenytoin concentrations may also increase while on brivaracetam, so phenytoin levels should be monitored.

Selecting the Most Appropriate Agent

There are several excellent AEDs from which to choose for various seizure types. The goal of monotherapy is to promote patient compliance, minimize side effects and toxicity, and reduce cost. In general, first-line monotherapy drugs are tried before using second-line monotherapy drugs, and first-line drugs may be first combined before trying the various second-line, adjunctive agents. Whether the second-line, adjunctive agents will be effective in monotherapy is still to be determined. The choice of an AED is determined by ease of use (i.e., dosing regimen), pharmacokinetics, interactions, need for monitoring, and toxicity (which could be dose related, idiosyncratic, chronic, or teratogenic). Ultimately, the optimal treatment for a given patient can be established by a process of trial and error and by knowledge of prior AEDs used.

First-Line Therapy

Selecting the appropriate therapy for each patient is difficult, but there is a science to choosing the best treatment:

- Select the appropriate drug and dose for the type and severity of the seizure being treated.
- Consider the patient's characteristics. For example, does the patient have hepatic or renal insufficiency, liver disease, hypoalbuminemia, burns, pregnancy, or malnutrition? What concomitant medications does the patient take? How old is the patient? Does the patient comply with the medication regimen? What adverse events are associated with the medication?
- Determine the patient's socioeconomic status.

If the initial AED fails, the practitioner should taper this drug's dosage while starting another first-line AED, if available. A list of commonly used first-line drugs for different seizure types can be found in **Table 36.1**.

Second-Line Therapy

Before switching to a second-line agent, the practitioner must optimize treatment with the selected first-line drug (unless the patient experiences intolerable adverse effects) and exhaust all possible first-line drug therapy choices. The practitioner at this point may, based on the patient's past medical history, initiate combination therapy with two or more first-line drugs or a first-line drug and a second-line drug. **Table 36.1** contains a list of second-line drugs.

Third-Line Therapy

If all medications fail and the patient experiences intractable seizures, surgery may be a third-line treatment option. Before recommending surgery, the practitioner should make sure drug treatment errors such as inappropriate drug selection, drug interactions, or inappropriate dosage are not contributing.

Special Population Considerations

Status Epilepticus

Guidelines recommend achieving definitive control of SE within 60 minutes of onset. All patients with an epileptic cause

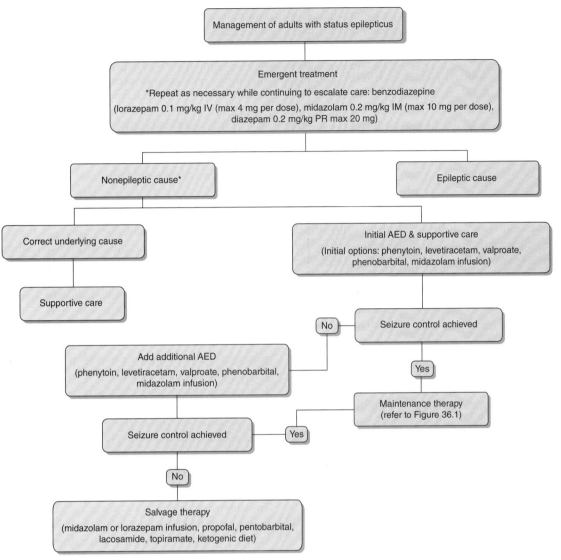

FIGURE 36–2   Treatment algorithm for status epilepticus.

AED, antiepileptic drug; IM, intramuscular; IV, intravenous; PR, per rectal.
*While repeating benzodiazepines consider additional supportive therapies or AEDs.

will need emergent, abortive therapy, as well as an antiepileptic medication to maintain or achieve seizure control. The goal of treatment is to stop clinical and electrographic seizure as quickly as possible using a combination of benzodiazepines and AEDs (see **Figure 36.2**). Concurrently, acute supportive care measures including airway management, IV access, hemodynamic support, and identification of the underlying cause must be provided in the stabilization phase (0–5 minutes of seizure activity).

In the initial therapy phase (5–20 minutes of seizure activity), benzodiazepines are the first-line treatment option to emergently abort seizure activity. IV administration is preferred; however, if unable to obtain IV access, IM, per rectal (PR), or intranasal options can be utilized. First-line therapy, lorazepam 0.1 mg/kg IV up to 4 mg per dose, doses can be repeated as needed based

on clinical response. All benzodiazepines can cause respiratory depression; therefore, careful monitoring is required especially with escalating or repeated doses. Midazolam is the preferred IM agent; 0.2 mg/kg up to a maximum of 10 mg can be given to adults. Diazepam PR is often administered in prehospital setting and is often used in pediatric population; adults can receive 0.2 mg/kg (maximum of 10 mg/dose) up to a maximum of 20 mg. An EEG is necessary to ensure treatment has adequately controlled both convulsive and electrographic seizure activity. If epileptic cause is identified, initial AED therapy should be urgently instituted. Treatment options for the second therapy phase (20–40 minutes of seizure activity) include phenytoin or fosphenytoin, levetiracetam, valproic acid, or phenobarbital. Refer to **Table 36.2** for additional information regarding loading and maintenance doses in SE.

Refractory SE is defined as either persisting clinical or electrographic seizures after the administration of a benzodiazepine and appropriate antiepileptic medication. Treatment options for refractory patients in the third therapy phase (40–60 minutes of seizure activity) include midazolam, propofol, pentobarbital, valproic acid, levetiracetam, phenytoin or fosphenytoin, and/or phenobarbital. Treatment of refractory SE is a challenge and there is not a defined treatment algorithm for therapy escalation, for treatment duration, or to drive therapeutic selection.

Pediatric

The most common seizure syndrome in childhood is Lennox-Gastaut syndrome. This usually is associated with mental retardation. Characteristically, multiple seizure types can occur, including atypical absence, atonic (drop attacks), secondarily generalized tonic–clonic, and myoclonic and tonic seizures. EEGs show considerable slow-wave and spike-wave activity. Although patients respond to valproic acid, benzodiazepines, and lamotrigine, there is a poor prognosis for seizure control.

Simple febrile seizures are another important category of seizures that affect children between ages 6 months and 5 years. Febrile seizures occur in 4% of all children and are preceded by high fevers, underlying the importance of controlling high fevers in children. The seizure is generalized and usually lasts under 15 minutes. Approximately 33% of children experience a recurrence, although almost never within the first 24 hours. These patients usually have no preceding neurologic abnormality or family history of epilepsy. Long-term anticonvulsant therapy is not indicated for this seizure type.

Geriatric

Understanding the basic pharmacologic principles involved in the administration of AEDs is the key to the optimal use of these drugs in older patients. Drug clearance and metabolism are significant issues in this population. Many older patients have decreased renal and liver function, which may have a profound effect on drug metabolism and excretion. Consequently, AED dosages may need to be adjusted.

AEDs are bound to different degrees by plasma proteins, particularly albumin. If a patient has a low albumin level (as older adults tend to have), higher free-drug concentrations are present in the blood and may lead to an increased risk of adverse events.

In patients with liver disease, which is common in the geriatric population, the rates of hepatic biotransformation of drugs and of hepatic blood flow are decreased. Therefore, protein binding of AEDs may also be affected by low protein and displacement by bilirubin or other substances. This has the net effect of increasing the serum concentration of free drug. In renal disease, there may be a decrease in the clearance of drugs eliminated entirely by the kidney. Renal failure also may complicate elimination of drugs principally cleared by the liver. Studies have shown that in the patients with uremia who are taking phenytoin, hepatic biotransformation processes continue or accelerate during the renal failure, but renal excretion of metabolites is decreased. Therefore, uremic patients tend to have lower total serum phenytoin concentrations but higher serum concentrations of the oxidized principal metabolite (hydroxyphenyl-phenylhydantoin).

Women

For women taking anticonvulsant therapy, a major point for discussion is the risk during pregnancy. Several anticonvulsants are listed as Pregnancy Category C or D (i.e., phenytoin, fosphenytoin, phenobarbital, primidone, valproic acid, ethosuximide, topiramate, and tiagabine), indicating a greater risk for fetal abnormalities. Pregnancy risk categories for each drug are listed in **Table 36.2**. The practitioner must work closely with women who wish to become, or are, pregnant to assess the risks involved and to choose the most effective drug that's safest for the fetus. In order to minimize the risk of congenital malformations, valproic acid and polytherapy should be avoided during the first trimester of pregnancy. Conversely, topiramate, oxcarbazepine, and lamotrigine may decrease serum concentrations of progestins and lead to oral contraceptive failure.

Pharmacogenetics

A patient's response to a given AED is dependent on both environmental and genetic factors. Pharmacogenetic variations exist that may impact therapeutic response, enzyme activity, transporter activity, or even drug-related toxicity. It is an area of increasing focus for many disease states including epilepsy. While pharmacogenetics may have a number of potential impacts on AED therapy, most available data focus on HLA alleles and risk for serious immune-mediated drug reactions. The presence of the HLA-B*1502 allele in patients of Chinese, Thai, Malaysian, and Indian populations has shown a strong association with carbamazepine-induced SJS/TEN. The FDA specifically recommends that HLA testing be completed prior to initiating carbamazepine in patients of Asian ancestry due to this risk of SJS/TEN. HLA variants and risk of serious immune-mediated reactions have been investigated with other AEDs including oxcarbazepine, lamotrigine, valproic acid, zonisamide, phenytoin, and phenobarbital with variable results. While pharmacogenetic testing is not routine, it is an ever-expanding field and may become a routine part of AED selection. The NIH-funded Web site pharmGKB.org provides useful resources on pharmacogenetics and drug dosing considerations with specific recommendations for carbamazepine and phenytoin.

MONITORING PATIENT RESPONSE

For patients taking an AED, the health care practitioner should monitor

- the frequency and severity of seizures,
- adverse drug events, and
- plasma drug levels, if applicable.

Therapy is considered to be a failure if the AED dosage achieves and maintains optimal blood concentrations and seizures are still uncontrolled and/or adverse effects become intolerable. Some patients have good clinical responses at serum drug concentrations below the therapeutic range, while others can exhibit toxicity within the therapeutic range. Some require serum concentrations above normal therapeutic values for seizure control, and these patients may tolerate very high levels without signs of toxicity.

Drugs should be added or subtracted as needed. Whenever a new AED is started or a dosage change is made, it takes five elimination half-lives before the new steady-state serum concentration is achieved. It is at this point the full therapeutic impact of the new medication or dosage change can be assessed. Therefore, too much haste in changing an AED or discarding it as ineffective may have significant therapeutic implications.

When AEDs are administered in combination, it is important to note the types of drug interactions that may occur. Even when monotherapy is used, some AEDs alter their own biotransformation when they are administered chronically (e.g., carbamazepine, valproic acid). The existence of these interactions complicates the design of the therapeutic regimen when more than one AED is used, underscoring the desirability of using monotherapy whenever possible.

PATIENT EDUCATION

More than 90% of patients with epilepsy lead normal lives. The patient should avoid sleep deprivation and excessive alcohol use, both of which can lower the seizure threshold and make recurrent seizure activity likely. The patient should avoid jobs that involve working at heights or near heavy machinery, flames, burners, or molten material, so there are some restrictions on careers (e.g., firefighter, commercial driver, or airline pilot). Patients should never swim alone. Most sports are permitted, but those with an increased risk of a sudden loss of consciousness, such as skydiving, hang gliding, mountain climbing, and scuba diving, could be deadly and should probably be avoided.

Drug Information

The American Academy of Neurology's practice guideline center (https://www.aan.com/Guidelines/) provides information about epilepsy and medications for practitioners. Other sources of information on AEDs include the American Epilepsy Society (https://www.aesnet.org/clinical_resources) and the National Institute of Neurological Disorders and Stroke (http://www.ninds.nih.gov/).

Patient-Oriented Information Sources

Patients often have questions about epilepsy prognosis and treatment, first aid, educational needs, pregnancy, and driving and insurance. The American Epilepsy Foundation or the many epilepsy societies around the country can help answer those questions. These organizations provide both professional and lay support assistance, including counseling and psychotherapy, access to social workers, and financial assistance.

Nutrition/Lifestyle Changes

The ketogenic diet has been advocated as a means of treatment for patients with epilepsy. This diet, high in fat and low in carbohydrates, is usually used in children refractory to AEDs. However, there does not appear to be reliable evidence supporting the use of the ketogenic diet in people with epilepsy.

Driving is, of course, one of the most serious restrictions. Laws concerning driving vary from state to state, but in general, driving is not advised for 6 months after the last seizure. Some exceptions are strictly nocturnal seizures or those related to the discontinuation of an anticonvulsant on a physician's advice. Individual state laws regarding the driving restriction need to be reviewed by the practitioner.

First aid for seizure activity consists primarily of protecting the patient's head and body from injury. It usually is not advisable to try to open the patient's mouth or to put objects in the patient's mouth. This can result in injury to the patient's mouth and airway as well as to the bystander. However, removing dentures, excessive secretions, and foreign materials from the mouth after a tonic–clonic seizure phase is completed may be helpful. Turning the patient into a semiprone position in the postictal period helps to prevent aspiration.

Complementary/Alternative Medicine

Self-reported use of complementary and alternative medicine (CAM) in patients with epilepsy has been described to be as high as 70%. CAM therapies utilized for epilepsy are wide ranging and include but are not limited to acupuncture, classical music, oxygen, herbal supplements, homeopathic regimens, meditation, aromatherapy, chiropractic manipulation, cranial–sacral therapy, and marijuana. Data showing benefit to these therapies are limited but patient-reported satisfaction is often high.

CASE STUDY 1

M.S., age 29, accompanied by her boyfriend, visits your office. Her boyfriend states, "She hasn't been herself the last month. She has headaches and is completely confused and tired for no reason." M.S. denies using illicit drugs and any recent traumatic injuries. She thinks her problem started approximately a month ago when she was at the gym lifting weights. Her friends told her that she became confused and began tugging at her clothes. Then she fell down and was unconscious for a few minutes. When she awoke, she felt extremely tired and did not know what was going on. Her boyfriend recalls that she had been hit in the head with a softball during a game the day before they went to the gym.

Past medical history discloses insulin use since early childhood (currently 10 units neutral protamine hagedorn in the morning and 8 units regular insulin before meals). She is interested in becoming pregnant in the next 12 to 24 months. The patient says she has no allergies and does not drink or use recreational drugs or tobacco.

On physical examination, it is found that B.C. is 5 ft 6 in. and 140 lb. Her temperature is 37.2°C, pulse rate 77, blood pressure 110/70, and glucose level 90. Skin appears normal. Head and neck are normal; chest is clear for anterior and posterior sounds; cardiovascular, regular rate and rhythm, and (2) rubs, murmurs, and gallops; and laboratory values are within normal limits. Electroencephalogram (EEG) findings include sharp-wave discharges.

At a follow-up visit 2 months later, M.S. and her boyfriend report that things have gotten worse. The boyfriend states that as M.S. was eating dinner one night, she had a seizure. She was completely stiff for a short time, and then her arms and legs began moving. He believes that she was unconscious for a few minutes. M.C. says she could not remember what had happened when she woke up (Learning Objective 2).

DIAGNOSIS: GENERAL ONSET TONIC–CLONIC SEIZURE

1. Which of the following should be true regarding your initial antiepileptic drug (AED) regimen?
   a. Initial combination therapy is warranted due to increased success rates.
   b. Drugs that are taken two to three times daily are preferred due to a lower risk of seizure if a dose is missed.
   c. Levetiracetam is the preferred agent for all seizure types and patients.
   d. The risks of pregnancy must be discussed prior to starting any AED.

2. Which of the following is the most appropriate initial antiepileptic regimen for this patient?
   a. Levetiracetam 500 mg orally daily
   b. Phenytoin 100 mg orally thrice daily
   c. Pregabalin 50 mg orally thrice daily
   d. Valproic acid 250 mg once daily

3. The patient fails to respond and has significant side effects to her initial therapy. Her initial therapy is to be discontinued. Which of the following would be the *most* appropriate replacement?
   a. Valproic acid 500 mg twice daily
   b. Lamotrigine 100 mg twice daily
   c. Lacosamide 100 mg twice daily
   d. Rufinamide 200 mg twice daily

4. After several different AEDs, the patient ends up on carbamazepine and phenytoin. A serum concentration on week 2 of therapy was 6 mcg/mL. The patient presents after 8 weeks of therapy with increased seizures and she is found to have a serum concentration of 2 mcg/mL. Which of the following is a likely cause?
   a. Autoinduction of CYP3A4.
   b. Patient has the HLA-B*1502 subtype.
   c. The oral contraceptive that she recently started.
   d. Coadministration with alcohol.

Bibliography

Birbeck, G. L., French, J. A., Perucca, E., et al. (2012). Evidence based guideline: Antiepileptic drug selection for people with HIV/AIDS. *Neurology, 78*(2), 139–145.

De Silva, M., McArdle, B., McGowan, M., et al. (1996). Randomized comparative monotherapy trial of phenobarbitone, phenytoin, carbamazepine or sodium valproate for newly diagnosed childhood epilepsy. *Lancet, 347,* 709–713.

French, J., Kanner, A. M., Ashman E., et al. (2018a). Practice guideline update summary: Efficacy and tolerability of the new antiepileptic drugs I: Treatment of new-onset epilepsy. Report of the guideline development, dissemination, and Implementation Subcommittee of the American Academy of Neurology and the American Epilepsy Society. *Neurology, 91*(2), 74–81.

French, J., Kanner, A. M., Ashman E., et al. (2018b). Practice guideline update summary: Efficacy and tolerability of the new antiepileptic drugs II: Treatment-resistant epilepsy. Report of the guideline development, dissemination, and Implementation Subcommittee of the American Academy of Neurology and the American Epilepsy Society. *Neurology, 91*(2), 82–90.

French, J., Smith, M., Faught, E., et al. (1999). Practice advisory: The use of felbamate in the treatment of patients with intractable epilepsy. *Neurology, 52,* 1540–1545.

Glauser, T., Ben-Menachem, E., Bourgeois, B., et al. (2013). Updated ILAE evidence review of antiepileptic drug efficacy and effectiveness as initial monotherapy for epileptic seizures and syndromes. *Epilepsia, 54,* 551–563.

Glauser, T., Shinnar, S., Gloss, D., et al. (2016). Evidence-based guideline: Treatment of convulsive status epilepticus in children and adults: Report of the Guideline Committee of the American Epilepsy Society. *Epilepsy Currents, 16*(1), 48–61.

Kane, S. P., Bress, A. P., & Tesoro, E. P. (2013). Characterization of unbound phenytoin concentrations in neurointensive care unit patients using a revised winter-tozer equation. *Annals of Pharmacotherapy, 47*, 628–636.

Krumholz, A., Wiebe, S., Gronseth, G., et al. (2015). Evidence-based guideline: Management of an unprovoked first seizure in adults. Report of the Quality Standards Subcommittee of the American Academy of Neurology and the American Epilepsy Society. *Neurology, 84*(16), 1705–1713.

LaRoche, S. M., & Helmers, S. L. (2004a). The new antiepileptic drugs: Clinical applications. *Journal of American Medical Association, 291*(5), 615–620.

LaRoche, S. M., & Helmers, S. L. (2004b). The new antiepileptic drugs: Scientific review. *Journal of American Medical Association, 291*(5), 605–614.

Lowenstein, D. H., & Allredge, B. K. (1998). Current concepts: Status epilepticus. *New England Journal of Medicine, 338*(14), 970–976.

Manci, E. E., & Gidal, B. E. (2009). The effect of carbapenem antibiotics on plasma concentrations of valproic acid. *Annals of Pharmacotherapy, 43*(12), 2082–2087.

Parker, D., Sanders, E. J., Burghardt, K. J., et al. (2016). Pharmacogenetics of antiepileptic drugs: A brief review. *Mental Health Clinician, 6*(1), 28–34.

Riviello, J. J., Ashwal, S., Hirtz, D., et al. (2006). Practice parameter: Diagnostic assessment of the child with status epilepticus (an evidence based review): Report of the Quality Standards Subcommittee of the American Academy of Neurology and the Practice Committee of the Child Neurology Society. *Neurology, 67*, 1542–1550.

Silvestro, S., Mammana, S., Cavalli, E., et al. (2019). Use of cannabidiol in the treatment of epilepsy: Efficacy and security in clinical trials. *Molecules, 24*(8), 1459.

Tomson, T., Battino, D., Bromley, R., et al. (2019). Management of epilepsy in pregnancy: A report from the International League Against Epilepsy Task Force on Women and Pregnancy. *Epileptic Disorders, 21*, 497–517.

von Winckelmann, S. L., Spriet, I., & Willems, L. (2008). Therapeutic drug monitoring of phenytoin in critically ill patients. *Pharmacotherapy, 28*, 1391–1400.

Vossler, D. G., Weingarten, M., & Gidal, B. E. (2018). Summary of antiepileptic drugs available in the United States of America. *Epilepsy Currents, 18*(4), 1–26.

37 Alzheimer's Disease

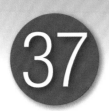

Emily R. Hajjar, Brooke Salzman, and Michael Weisberger

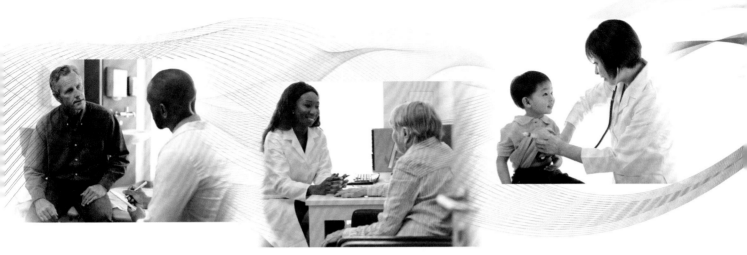

Learning Objectives

1. Describe the pathophysiology of Alzheimer's disease.
2. Identify an appropriate treatment plan for an Alzheimer's patient.
3. Monitor the response to treatment.

INTRODUCTION

Alzheimer's disease (AD), also known as neurocognitive disorder, is the most common cause of dementia accounting for approximately 60% to 80% of all cases of dementia. AD is characterized by a slow, progressive decline in cognitive functions including memory and thinking. Patients initially complain of short-term (recent) memory loss, forgetfulness, and a decreased ability to learn and retain new information.

Estimates suggest that approximately 5.8 million people in the United States and 30 to 40 million people worldwide have AD (Alzheimer's Association, 2019). The number is expected to grow to 13.2 to 16 million in the United States by 2050 as the population continues to age (Quefurth & LaFerla, 2010). A majority of individuals with AD are residing in the community, which represents a huge emotional and financial burden on the patient, friends, and family members, as well as on society as a whole. The cost of care is estimated at approximately $290 billion each year in the United States. This number does not include the cost of unpaid care given by family members or loved ones.

Early onset AD occurs in patients younger than 65 years of age and is much less common, comprising approximately 1% or less cases of AD. Late-onset AD accounts for the majority of cases and occurs in patients age 65 or older. Symptoms of AD can be divided between cognitive symptoms and noncognitive symptoms, and treatment is based on the particular domain of the symptoms. Cognitive symptoms, such as loss of short-term memory, usually present first in mild AD, whereas the noncognitive behavioral symptoms are seen in more moderate-to-severe AD (see algorithm "Diagnosis of Alzheimer's disease"). Currently, AD is incurable although pharmacologic agents have been used to temporarily improve symptoms associated with AD. The average life span for patients with AD is reduced by as much as 70% with a mean duration of approximately 4 to 8 years from the time of diagnosis (Kua et al., 2014; Tom et al., 2015). However, some individuals live as long as 20 years after diagnosis. In the United States, AD is the sixth leading cause of death among all adults and the fifth leading cause for those 65 and older. Women are at a slightly higher risk for developing AD than men. Prevalence increases with age, with AD affecting approximately 40% to 50% of those older than age 85. AD is a fatal illness; however, it is difficult to determine the number of deaths caused by AD because of the way deaths are reported and the underreporting of AD as the cause of death. Severe stages of dementia frequently lead to loss of functions, such as walking and swallowing. As a result, individuals with advanced disease suffer complications of immobility and malnutrition, which in turn increase the risk of acute conditions, such as pneumonia or sepsis, which can be the immediate cause of death. Therefore, death reports may reflect reported immediate causes of death while the underlying cause of death is AD (Alzheimer's Association, 2019). Still, a portion of individuals with AD will die from causes unrelated to AD such as cardiovascular disease (Kua et al., 2014).

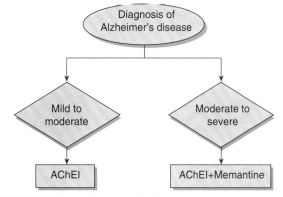

ALGORITHM 37–1   Treatment algorithm.

AChEI, acetylcholinesterase inhibitors.

BOX 37.1   Risk Factors for Alzheimer's Disease

Risk Factors

Advanced age
ApoE-e4 gene
Family history (e.g., genetic abnormalities)
Mild cognitive impairment
Cardiovascular disease
Low education
Traumatic brain injury
Lack of social and cognitive engagement

Source: Data from http://www.alz.org/facts/downloads/facts_figures_2019.pdf

CAUSES

Genetic causes of AD involving mutations of three specific genes, amyloid precursor protein (APP), presenilin-1, and presenilin-2, are more likely to present with early onset AD. Trisomy 21 is a unique risk factor for AD, with 50% of people with Down syndrome having AD in their 60s (Alzheimer's Association, 2019). Apolipoprotein E (ApoE), a protein involved in cholesterol transport, is linked to the development of AD. The E4 allele (homozygote E4/E4) is thought to increase the risk of AD, whereas the E2 allele may be protective. Carrying the E4 from of the ApoE gene and having a family history of AD increase risk for developing late-onset AD but does not guarantee that an individual will develop AD. Advanced age is the most significant risk factor for AD, and other risk factors are listed in **Box 37.1**.

PATHOPHYSIOLOGY

Pathologic changes in AD include formation of neurofibrillary tangles and plaques, cortical atrophy, and neuronal (cholinergic, glutamatergic) destruction and loss. In AD patients, acetylcholine levels are decreased and an excessive stimulation of glutamate causes neuronal toxicity. These changes affect several areas of the brain, including the hippocampus, amygdala, cerebral cortex, and ultimately the motor cortex. As a result of these changes, short- and long-term memory, learning, language, behavior, and eventually motor skills are impaired.

Neurofibrillary Tangles

Neurofibrillary tangles and neuritic or β-amyloid plaques are the hallmark pathologic lesions in AD. Tau protein, the principal component of neurofibrillary tangles, becomes hyperphosphorylated in AD. The abnormal phosphorylation of tau protein leads to the formation of paired helical filaments and finally neurofibrillary tangles. As a result, microtubule assembly is inhibited and critical organelles may collapse, causing abnormal intracellular transport and neuronal cell death.

Plaques

Plaques are brain lesions that contain a core of β-amyloid protein (BAP) and a shell of damaged neurites. APP is the parent protein of BAP. Proteases normally cleave APP through the BAP region, which prevents intact BAP from entering the extracellular fluid. When abnormal proteolysis occurs, leaving BAP intact, increased extracellular BAP becomes involved in plaque formation and neuronal degeneration. Plaques are also composed of neurofibrillary tangles, ApoE, and glial cells, which may be involved in the pathologic process of AD and are areas of interest to researchers. Neurofibrillary tangles and plaque density correlate with increased severity of AD.

Neuronal Destruction

The neuronal cell damage and death seen in AD results in impaired neurotransmitter function. The cholinergic and glutamatergic systems are significantly involved. Destruction of cholinergic neurons leads to decreased levels of acetylcholine, a neurotransmitter that aids in learning and memory. The symptomatic presentation of AD (memory loss and cognitive impairment) appears to be associated with acetylcholine deficiency. The cholinergic system has been the subject of a vast amount of research and pharmacologic development (e.g., acetylcholinesterase inhibitors). Overstimulation of the glutamatergic system in the synapse via the N-methyl-D-aspartate (NMDA) receptor causes neuronal toxicity leading to neuronal death. This disruption is thought to impair learning and memory.

The autoimmune system or inflammatory mediators may be linked to late-onset AD. Glial cells, complement cascade components, and cytokines are present in plaque areas. These cells and inflammatory mediators may contribute to neuronal cell damage and loss. Their role in AD is under investigation, as is the use of intravenous immunoglobulins for the treatment of AD.

Diagnostic Criteria

The clinical diagnosis of AD can be made using the criteria from the *Diagnostic and Statistical Manual of Mental Disorders*, Fifth

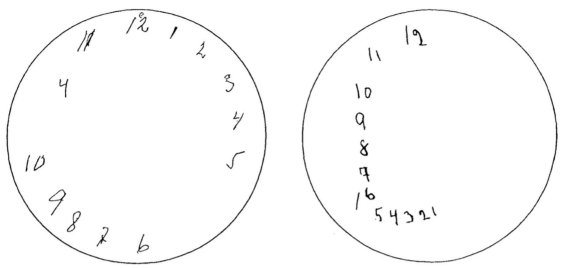

FIGURE 37–1 Clock-drawing task completed by various older subjects. (Reproduced with permission from Agrell, B., & Dehlin, O. (1998). The clock-drawing test. *Age and Ageing, 27*, 399–403).

Edition, known as the *DSM-5*. The diagnosis can be *confirmed* only by autopsy. Diagnostic criteria include concern for loss of memory by the patient, caregiver, or provider, insidious onset, performance below normal on standardized cognition assessments, deficits in one or more cognitive domains that impair a person's ability to function in daily life, and the absence of other diseases that may account for the symptoms of AD.

Patients and their caregivers should be closely involved in the diagnostic process. A complete history and physical examination that includes a neurologic examination and mental status evaluation is essential. The Mini-Cog (including the clock-drawing task in **Figure 37.1**), Sweet 16, and Verbal Fluency tests may be used to screen for cognitive impairment. The Mini–Mental State Examination (MMSE) and the Montreal Cognitive Assessment (MOCA) are longer assessment tools designed to detect impaired cognition.

INITIATING DRUG THERAPY

A careful assessment of baseline diagnostic findings is essential before initiating drug therapy. The patient, family, and caregiver should be informed of the severity of cognitive and functional impairment. Baseline scores on cognitive testing and functional status can help guide decisions related to drug therapy. Reversible causes of dementia must also be considered and eliminated because several medications and medical conditions may cause or aggravate dementia (**Box 37.2**).

Before starting drug therapy for the cognitive symptoms of AD, the patient or family should demonstrate a clear understanding of the efficacy and expected outcomes of treatment, as well as the potential adverse events, costs, and incurability of the disease. The choice not to initiate drug therapy is also a reasonable option as many patients only experience modest benefits from drug therapy and incur side effects and expenses from the medications.

BOX 37.2 Potentially Reversible Causes of Dementia

Medications

Anticholinergics (e.g., benztropine, diphenhydramine)
Antipsychotics (e.g., olanzapine, thioridazine)
Benzodiazepines (e.g., diazepam, lorazepam)
Histamine (H$_2$) blockers (e.g., cimetidine)

Metabolic Disorders

Dehydration
Hyperthyroidism and hypothyroidism
Hyponatremia
Hypercalcemia

Intracranial Infection or Disease

Meningitis
Neurosyphilis
Normalpressure hydrocephalus
Subdural hematoma
Tumor
Toxoplasmosis

Miscellaneous

Toxins (e.g., lead, mercury, alcohol)
Vitamin B$_{12}$ deficiency
Depression
Psychoses

Source: Data from Wiser, T. H. (1994). Alzheimer's disease. *US Pharmacist, 63* and AGS 2019 Beers Criteria.

Pharmacologic management of the noncognitive symptoms is tailored to the individual symptom. These medications may be initiated when the patient demonstrates an impairment in their instrumental activities of daily living or basic activities of daily living (ADLs). The use of both noncognitive and cognitive therapies may be necessary as the disease progresses.

Nonpharmacologic psychotherapies, such as behavior-oriented, emotion-oriented, cognition-oriented, and stimulation-oriented approaches, can be useful for some patients with AD. Other nonpharmacologic interventions include using calendars, timers and clocks, and written notes or instructions. The caregiver should attempt to maintain a predictable routine with the patient. Drastic changes in the environment, as well as confrontation and arguments, should be avoided. Recognition of precipitants of agitation, psychosis, and anxiety can assist the caregiver and health care provider to best develop a patient-specific treatment plan.

The patient's ability to drive should be evaluated, and as AD progresses, the patient should be advised to stop driving because dementia may increase the risk of accidents. The patient's use of a stove and other heavy machinery should be evaluated due to risk. Families should be educated that falling and wandering may become concerns. They should also be informed about the possibility of physical violence and caregiver stress associated with more severe disease. Capable patients may want to discuss with their families advance directives, living wills, desires for nursing home placement, and powers of attorney.

Patient and family education are the most important nonpharmacologic interventions for AD. Depending on the stage of impairment, the patient requires some or full assistance with ADLs, such as dressing, toileting, and, particularly, driving. Support for patients and families is vitally important at any stage of AD (**Box 37.3**), and anyone involved with a patient with AD should be educated on the availability of support groups to deal with the wide variety of issues associated with AD. Other resources for the caregiver include the use of respite care centers and day care centers.

BOX 37.3   Alzheimer's Disease Support Groups and Resources

Alzheimer's Association

Web site: http://www.alz.org

Alzheimer's Disease Education and Referral (ADEAR) Center

Web site: http://www.nia.nih.gov/alzheimers

Eldercare Locator Service (ELS)

Web site: http://www.eldercare.gov

Goals of Drug Therapy

The optimal goal of drug therapy is to maintain and maximize the patient's functional ability, quality of life, and independence for as long as possible while minimizing adverse events and cost (APA, 2017). A multidisciplinary approach to therapy, which includes the patient and family, a prescriber, a psychiatric, neurologic or geriatrician specialist, a nurse, a social worker, and a pharmacist, is the ideal. Drug therapy choices for the cognitive symptoms primarily include the cholinesterase inhibitors (CIs) and memantine.

SELECTED AGENTS FOR COGNITIVE SYMPTOMS

Cholinesterase Inhibitors

CIs, also known as the *acetylcholinesterase inhibitors,* play a key role in the pharmacologic treatment of AD. This drug class includes donepezil (Aricept), rivastigmine (Exelon), and galantamine (Razadyne, Razadyne ER). These agents are used to slow the progression of the cognitive, functional, and behavioral domains of AD.

If no effect is seen within 3 to 6 months of treatment or the patient is experiencing an adverse effect, another agent from this class may be tried. The effects of these medications are to slow the progression of AD, not to cure the disease. There is no definitive recommendation as to when these agents should be started and how long treatment with these agents should be continued. However, once a patient progresses to moderate or severe AD, these agents are no longer solely recommended or may be discontinued due to lack of benefit. Additional pharmacologic therapy may be necessary once the disease progresses into the moderate-to-severe stages to help with behavioral symptoms. Thoughtful discussions with caregivers or families may guide the decision to discontinue therapy.

CIs inhibit one or both types of the cholinesterase enzymes, butyrylcholinesterase or acetylcholinesterase. Butyrylcholinesterase is primarily found in the periphery, and inhibition of this enzyme leads to many of the adverse effects of the cholinesterase agents. Acetylcholinesterase is found more centrally and thus is the primary focus of inhibition for the use in AD.

Rivastigmine is a CI with its potential advantage of being pseudo-irreversible. It inhibits the enzyme for about 10 hours, making this an intermediate-acting agent. It is notable that oral formulation of rivastigmine is the only CI that is approved to treat both mild-to-moderate AD and mild-to-moderate dementia associated with Parkinson's disease. The rivastigmine patch has a labeled indication that includes mild, moderate, and severe AD. Galantamine is indicated to treat mild-to-moderate AD. Besides inhibiting the cholinesterase enzyme, it also allosterically modulates the nicotinic receptor. Donepezil is labeled to treat mild, moderate, and severe AD.

The CIs have been shown to slow the progression of AD. These medications have also had positive effects on the noncognitive or behavioral symptoms of AD. They have been shown to reduce apathy, psychosis, anxiety, depression, and agitation. Although these medications appear to improve the cognitive function of patients with AD, there is no evidence that they alter the course of the disease.

Dosage

The CIs may modestly improve cognitive function or delay decline in cognitive function. The observed delay in cognitive decline correlates with approximately a 6-month decline in patients treated with placebos. Donepezil therapy is initiated at a dose of 5 mg daily. The dosage may be increased after 4 to 6 weeks to a maximum dose of 10 mg/d if tolerated. Donepezil 10 mg/d is slightly more effective than the 5-mg dose; therefore, increasing to 10 mg/d is appropriate for patients who do not respond within 6 weeks of treatment with the 5-mg dose. A 23-mg dose may be tried in moderate-to-severe patients that have been stable on 10 mg daily for at least 3 months. Donepezil is available as a tablet as well as an orally disintegrating tablet for patients who have trouble swallowing. Rivastigmine doses should be started at 1.5 mg twice daily and should increase to 3 mg twice daily after 2 weeks of treatment for the capsule and oral solution formulations. Further dose increases should be based on clinical response and can be attempted on a biweekly basis. The maximum dose is 6 mg twice daily for the capsule and oral solution formulations. If the patch formulation of rivastigmine is started, the dose should be 4.6 mg/24 h and can be titrated to 9.5 mg/24 h after 4 weeks and then to 13.3 mg/24 h after another 4-week period, if tolerated. Galantamine is available as an immediate-release tablet and oral solution as well as in extended-release capsules. The immediate-release forms of galantamine are started at a dose of 4 mg twice daily and titrated up every 4 weeks as tolerated to a maximum dose of 24 mg/d (12 mg twice daily). The extended-release formulation of galantamine is started at 8 mg daily and can be titrated up to a dose of 24 mg/d in 4-week intervals.

Time Frame for Response

While CIs may slow the progression of AD, the effects may not be immediately noticeable. Patients and families may report improvement—or lack of continued decline—within 3 to 6 weeks of beginning treatment. Response may also be seen in repeated cognitive assessment measures done in 3- to 6-month intervals.

Contraindications

Contraindications to using a CI include hypersensitivities to any of the compounds. Precautions to using the CIs include anorexia, neuroleptic malignant syndrome, bradycardia, peptic ulcer disease, conduction abnormalities, asthma or chronic obstructive pulmonary disease, urinary tract obstruction, and

seizure disorders. Patients weighing less than 55 kg may also experience more profound gastrointestinal (GI) side effects such as nausea and vomiting.

Adverse Events

The major adverse effects of the CIs are cholinergic, most commonly nausea, vomiting, and diarrhea (5%–47%). Oral formulations of rivastigmine have been associated with the highest incidence of these GI disturbances (19%–47%); the patch is associated with much lower rates (6%–20%). These effects are dose dependent and can be minimized by slowly titrating to higher doses (**Table 37.1**).

Bradycardia can occur with the use of the CIs, and they should be used with caution in patients with sick sinus syndrome or baseline bradycardia. Hyperacidity can also occur with CIs, and they should be used with caution in patients with a history of peptic ulcer disease, especially in those who currently take nonsteroidal anti-inflammatory drugs. CIs should also be used cautiously in patients with a history of current seizure disorder. Although these effects are not common, they are of concern and should be closely monitored in patients who are at risk. Donepezil is also associated with insomnia or nightmares. If these conditions occur, the dosing of donepezil before bed should be changed to a morning administration. Despite the GI effects associated with a rapid increase in dose, these agents appear to be well tolerated.

Interactions

Drug interactions with CIs include synergy with other cholinergic agents (e.g., succinylcholine). Concomitant use of any anticholinergic agents (e.g., diphenhydramine) may negate the effects of the CI and should be avoided for optimal medication benefit. Donepezil and galantamine are metabolized by the P450 enzyme system. Donepezil and galantamine are substrates for 2D6 and 3A4. A potential advantage of rivastigmine is that it is metabolized by hydrolysis and thus is not susceptible to the drug interactions associated with the P450 enzyme system. Inhibitors of these isoenzymes would cause an increased drug concentration of the CI and thus more susceptible to cholinergic adverse effects.

Memantine (Namenda)

Memantine is an NMDA receptor antagonist. This drug was approved for the treatment of moderate-to-severe AD. Memantine blocks the activation of the NMDA receptor during an abundance of glutamate. Thus, this blocks overstimulation of the NMDA receptor, and neuronal degeneration is inhibited. It does not interfere with the pathologic activation of the NMDA receptor during learning and memory formation.

Clinical trials have shown that memantine used alone in patients with moderate-to-severe AD has produced a modest reduction in clinical deterioration. The immediate release form of memantine should be started at 5 mg once daily and titrated every week, if tolerated, to a maximum dose of

TABLE 37.1

Overview of Cholinesterase Inhibitors and Memantine

Generic (Trade) Name and Dosage	Selected Adverse Events	Contraindications	Special Considerations
Donepezil (Aricept) Start: 5 mg daily Range: 5–23 mg/d Start 5 mg daily × 4 wk then 10 mg daily. If stable for 3 mo, may increase to 23 mg/d.	*GI:* nausea, vomiting *CV:* bradycardia, syncope	Hypersensitivity to agent or piperidine derivatives	If nightmares occur, dose in the morning.
Rivastigmine (Exelon) Oral: Start 1.5 mg BID for 2 wk, then increase by 1.5 mg BID; max. 6 mg BID. Range: 3–6 mg BID Patch: Start one patch (4.6 mg/24 h) daily × 4 wk, then increase to one patch (9.5 mg/24 h) daily × 4 wk, then increase to one patch (13.3 mg/24 h).	Nausea, vomiting, anorexia, dyspepsia, fatigue, headache malaise	Hypersensitivity to agent or carbamate derivatives	Initial response seen within 12 wk of therapy Patches are removed and replaced every 24 h.
Galantamine (Razadyne, Razadyne ER) IR: Start 4 mg PO BID × 4 wk. Range: 4–12 mg PO BID ER: Start 8 mg daily × 4 wk. Range: 8–24 mg	Nausea, vomiting, diarrhea, anorexia, abdominal pain, dyspepsia, dizziness, sleep disturbances	Hypersensitivity to agent Severe hepatic, renal impairment	Moderate hepatic, renal impairment should not exceed a dose of 16 mg/d.
Memantine (Namenda, Namenda XR) IR: Start 5 mg PO daily, increase by 5 mg daily every week to a target of 20 mg PO daily. XR: Start 7 mg PO daily; increase dose 7 mg each week to a maximum dose of 28 mg PO daily. Memantine/donepezil (Namzaric)	Dizziness, confusion, headache, anxiety, hypertension. diarrhea	Hypersensitivity to agent	XR capsules may be opened up and sprinkled on applesauce.

CV, cardiovascular; ER, extended-release; GI, gastrointestinal; INR, international normalized ratio; IR, immediate release; XR, extended release.

10 mg twice daily. The extended-release product is started at a dose of 7 mg daily and increased by 7 mg each week to a maximum dose of 28 mg daily. Memantine is available in a combination tablet with donepezil. Patients should be stabilized on 10 mg on donepezil before starting the combination tablet and the titration follows the extended-release product at weekly increments. Food has no effect on the onset or absorption of memantine. In general, memantine was well tolerated compared to a placebo. Memantine is minimally metabolized by the P450 enzyme system and thus not susceptible to P450 enzyme interactions. It is largely excreted renally via tubular secretion and necessitates a lower maximum dose once the patient's creatine clearance falls below 30 mL/min.

With a different mechanism of action and indication for moderate-to-severe AD, memantine has a unique role for treatment of AD. In the past, once a CI failed, no other viable option for therapy was available. Now, the addition of memantine to a CI may be an option, but patients and families should be educated that the effect is similar to that of the CIs.

SELECTED AGENTS FOR NONCOGNITIVE SYMPTOMS

Antipsychotic Agents

The noncognitive symptoms of AD include agitation, psychosis, anxiety, depression, and sleep disorders. Approximately one-half of patients with dementia experience agitation. Many patients with AD also experience psychotic symptoms, such as delusions, hallucinations, and paranoia. Agitation and psychosis, which may be particularly frightening for families and caregivers, should be treated if the patient is causing harm to self or others.

The choice of an antipsychotic agent is based on adverse events. Choosing an agent with a low degree of anticholinergic activity seems warranted in patients with AD. Atypical antipsychotics are associated with less extrapyramidal symptoms than the typical agents; thus, these agents are preferred.

Although atypical antipsychotics are used, none of the agents are approved to treat the noncognitive symptoms of dementia, and they all contain a black box warning alerting patients and caregivers to the fact that they are associated with an increased risk of death in patients with dementia-related psychosis. Risperidone (Risperdal) and olanzapine (Zyprexa) have also been associated with an increased risk of stroke in patients using these agents for behavioral disturbances associated with dementia. It is important for the practitioner to weigh the risks versus benefits of using these agents. Regardless of the agent chosen, the lowest effective dose should be used. The practitioner should reassess the need for these medications periodically (every 3–6 months).

Benzodiazepines

Benzodiazepines have been prescribed to treat behavioral problems related to dementia and are often reserved for treating symptoms of anxiety or for episodic agitation. These agents can be used as needed in situations where anxiety or agitation are occurring or prior to an event where anxiety may occur.

If a benzodiazepine is prescribed, shorter-acting agents like lorazepam (Ativan) or alprazolam (Xanax) are preferred. Older patients often experience extended effects from benzodiazepines, so shorter-acting agents are preferred to prevent long periods of sedation. All benzodiazepines should be started at the lowest dose and used sparingly.

Adverse effects of benzodiazepines include falls, sedation, delirium, and loss of inhibition. Routine use is not recommended because of limited efficacy, adverse effects, and potential for worsening AD symptoms. The use of benzodiazepines for anxiety associated with dementia should be reevaluated periodically.

Data on using various other agents (trazodone [Desyrel], valproate [Depakene], carbamazepine [Tegretol], buspirone [BuSpar], and beta blockers) for treating anxiety associated with AD are limited. These agents may have a role in treating agitation in patients who do not tolerate or respond to antipsychotic agents or benzodiazepines.

Antidepressants

Because there is a high incidence of depression associated with dementia, pharmacologic treatment is often necessary. Patients may not meet explicit criteria for a depressive syndrome, but it is recommended that these patients still be offered treatment. Treatment may improve cognition, mood, apathy, function, behavior, appetite, sleep, and overall quality of life. Because there is no evidence that one class of antidepressants is superior to another in treating depression,

the prescriber may base the choice of an agent on the individual patient, cost, side-effect profile, and potential drug interactions.

In many clinical practices, selective serotonin reuptake inhibitors (SSRIs), such as sertraline or escitalopram, have become preferred agents for clinically significant depression in the older adults with AD. SSRIs in general have fewer side effects (particularly anticholinergic) than tricyclic antidepressants (TCA) or monoamine oxidase inhibitors and are better tolerated.

SELECTING THE MOST APPROPRIATE AGENT FOR COGNITIVE SYMPTOMS

First-Line Therapy

Once the decision has been made to initiate drug therapy, CIs may be tried for those with mild AD. Donepezil is often considered the first choice because fewer adverse events are associated with its use and the once-daily dosing schedule is easier to follow. However, any CI may be tried as a first-line option. Patients with moderate-to-severe AD may be offered memantine in conjunction with a CI (**Table 37.2**), but like with single-agent therapy, only a modest benefit is expected.

Monitoring Patient Response

Primary care appointments involving both patients with AD and families every 3 to 6 months may be used to monitor cognitive and behavioral symptoms and to assess the patient's response to pharmacotherapy. If clinical improvement does not occur with a CI after 3 to 6 months of treatment, the practitioner may consider switching to another CI. The MMSE or MOCA are useful objective measures of cognitive response to therapy, but input from family and caregivers must also be recognized. Discontinuing the medication may be considered at any time during therapy if there is a perceived lack of efficacy or presence of intolerable side effects. If a marked decline in cognitive

TABLE 37.2

Recommended Order of Treatment of the Cognitive Symptoms Associated with Alzheimer's Disease

Order	Agents	Comments
First line	CIs	Once-daily CIs will be most likely first-line agents for mild-to-moderate AD.
	Memantine	Memantine is reserved for patients with moderate-to-severe AD; may be used in conjunction with a CI.
Second line	CIs	A trial of second CI may be warranted.

AD, Alzheimer's disease; CIs, cholinesterase inhibitors.

function is noted within the first 3 to 6 weeks after discontinuing drug therapy, the practitioner may consider restarting the acetylcholinesterase inhibitor. When patients progress to severe impairment, addition of memantine may be an option.

Ability to perform ADLs, such as bathing, dressing, toileting, and feeding, and instrumental ADLs, such as transferring, housekeeping, shopping, and paying bills, should be assessed to help determine the functional status of the patient and response to treatment. Assessment of the noncognitive symptoms of AD could be a sign of disease progression.

In patients receiving antipsychotic medications, response is usually seen within the first day of therapy. If patients continue to have delusions, hallucinations, or agitation, doses can be gradually increased at 4- to 7-day interval. In contrast, response to antidepressant medications is seen within 4 to 6 weeks. Evidence of suicidal ideation should be taken seriously and immediately addressed by the practitioner.

Treatment with any of these agents may be continued until the risk of pharmacotherapy outweighs the benefit to the patient or family. Clear communication with the patient, family, and caregivers cannot be overemphasized because evaluation of pharmacotherapeutic efficacy and decisions to stop or continue treatment depend on this input.

Patient Education

Regardless of the agents chosen for AD treatment, patients, families, and caregivers must have realistic goals of drug therapy. Their goals should include increasing length of time of self-sufficiency, delaying the need for nursing home placement, and reducing the burden on the caregiver. It is important that the family and patients understand the available agents are expected to minimally slow the disease progression. They need to understand that no currently available agents are curative and only modest improvements can be expected.

Donepezil may be taken with or without food, and patients taking donepezil should be instructed that if insomnia or nightmares occur, the drug may be given in the morning. Rivastigmine is taken with food to have a slow dose titration to minimize the GI side effects. Galantamine can be taken without regard to food and should be slowly titrated to minimize adverse effects. Memantine appears to be well tolerated. Because vitamin E may predispose certain patients (e.g., those with vitamin K deficiency) to bleeding, patients and families should be informed to report unusual bruising, blood in urine or stool, bleeding gums, and the like immediately to their health care provider.

Patient-Oriented Information Sources

The various support resources available for patients and families of patients with AD are shown in **Box 37.3**.

COMPLEMENTARY AND ALTERNATIVE MEDICATIONS

Vitamin E

Vitamin E, an antioxidant, may be useful in AD treatment. Due to its antioxidant effects, vitamin E can stabilize free radicals and the damage they produce. Patients with moderate AD started on vitamin E may expect approximately a 7-month delay in reaching a poor functional outcome or end point (i.e., death, institutionalization, loss of the ability to perform basic ADLs, or severe dementia; Sano et al., 1997). This difference is seen within 2 years of initiating treatment. Indefinite treatment with vitamin E is a reasonable approach.

Vitamin E may be effective because of its antioxidant effects. A starting dose of 1,000 international units given orally twice daily appears to be appropriate because this was the regimen used in the trial supporting its efficacy (Sano et al., 1997). Vitamin E, because of its benign side-effect profile, minimal cost, and lack of significant drug interactions, has become a good choice for treating AD.

Minimal adverse effects are associated with vitamin E. Because vitamin E may worsen coagulation problems (causing bleeding) in patients with vitamin K deficiency or taking warfarin (Coumadin), it is suggested that these patients receive lower doses (200–800 international units/day). An increase in syncope and falls was also noted for vitamin E (and selegiline) in the study by Sano and colleagues (1997). Patients should be monitored for an increase in such events if they are receiving either of these agents.

Herbal Agents

Ginkgo biloba extract, thought to have antioxidant properties, has been studied in patients with mild-to-severe AD or multi-infarct dementia. Modest improvement of cognition was recorded in the results of the AD assessment scale. Caregivers also recognized improvement in function (Le Bars et al., 1997).

Treatment was well tolerated, with some GI side effects reported. Additional well-designed studies should be conducted before routine use is recommended. Because this product is not regulated by the Food and Drug Administration as a medication, its safety remains unknown, and ginkgo biloba products may vary in extract concentrations and contents. Patients who choose to take this product should be cautioned that it may interact with warfarin or aspirin, increasing their risk of bleeding.

CASE STUDY 1

M.W. is a 70-year-old White woman with a medical history of hypertension, osteoarthritis, atrial fibrillation, and total hysterectomy, who lives by herself in a two-storeyrow home. She visits the primary care clinic with her daughter, who is concerned because M.W. has "bounced" a few checks and can no longer pay her bills without assistance. M.W. admits that she has been forgetful and appears anxious as she describes an incident in which she went shopping and could not remember where she parked her car. Her daughter states that her mother's memory has progressively worsened over the past year. M.W.'s medications include fosinopril 20 mg orally daily, metoprolol succinate ER 50 mg orally daily, warfarin 5 mg orally daily, vitamin D 1,000 IU daily daily, and acetaminophen 325 mg 2 tablets (650 mg) orally thrice daily. A careful evaluation and workup was ordered.

DIAGNOSIS: MILD ALZHEIMER'S DISEASE WITH AN MINI–MENTAL STATE EXAMINATION SCORE OF 22

1. List specific goals of treatment for M.W.
2. What drug therapy would you prescribe for M.W.? Why?
3. What are the parameters for monitoring success of therapy?
4. Discuss specific patient education based on the prescribed therapy.
5. List one or two adverse reactions for the selected agent that would cause you to change therapy.
6. What would be the choice for second-line therapy?
7. Would there be any over-the-counter and/or alternative agents appropriate for MW?
8. What lifestyle changes would you recommend to M.W.?
9. Describe one or two drug–drug or drug–food interactions for the selected agent.

Bibliography

Starred references are cited in the text.

*Agrell, B., & Dehlin, O. (1998). The clock-drawing test. *Age and Ageing*, *27*, 399–403.

*Alzheimer's Association. (2019). Alzheimer's disease fact and figures. *2019*, Chicago, IL: The Alzheimer's Association.

American Psychiatric Association. (2007). American Psychiatric Association practice guideline for the treatment of patients with Alzheimer's disease and other dementias. Second edition. *American Journal of Psychiatry*, *164*(Suppl. 12), 5–56.

American Psychiatric Association. (2013). *Diagnostic and statistical manual of mental disorders* (5th ed.). Washington, DC: American Psychiatric Association.

*American Psychiatric Association. (2017). American Psychiatric Association practice guideline for the treatment of patients with Alzheimer's disease and other dementias. *Focus* (Am Psychiatr Publ), *15*(1): 110–128. Published online January 11, 2017. doi: 10.1176/appi.focus.15106

Birks, J. (2006). Cholinesterase inhibitors for Alzheimer's disease. *Cochrane Database of Systematic Reviews*, (*1*), CD005593.

De-Paula, V. J., Radanovic, M., Diniz, B. S., et al. (2012). Alzheimer's disease. *Subcellular Biochemistry*, *65*, 329–352.

*Kua, E. H., Ho, E., Tan, H. H., et al. (2014). The natural history of dementia. *Pscyhogeriatrics*, *14*, 196–201.

Kurz, A., & Grimmer, T. (2014). Efficacy of memantine hydrochloride one-daily in Alzheimer's disease. *Expert Opinion in Pharmacotherapy*, *15*, 1955–1960.

*Le Bars, P. L., Katz, M. M., Berman, N., et al. (1997). A placebo-controlled, double-blind, randomized trial of an extract of ginkgo biloba for dementia. *Journal of the American Medical Association*, *278*, 1327–1332.

Lendon, C. L., Ashall, F., & Goate, A. M. (1997). Exploring the etiology of Alzheimer's disease using molecular genetics. *Journal of the American Medical Association*, *277*, 825–831.

McShane, R., Areosa Sastre, A., & Minakaran, N. (2006). Memantine for dementia. *Cochrane Database of Systematic Reviews*, (*2*), CD003154.

Nyth, A. L., & Gottfries, C. G. (1990). The clinical efficacy of citalopram in treatment of emotional disturbances in dementia disorders: A Nordic multicenter study. *British Journal of Psychiatry*, *157*, 894–901.

*Quefurth, H. W., & LaFerla, F. M. (2010). Alzheimer's disease. *New England Journal of Medicine*, *362*, 329–344.

*Sano, M., Ernesto, C., Thomas, R. G., et al. (1997). A controlled trial of selegiline, alpha-tocopherol, or both as treatment for Alzheimer's disease. *New England Journal of Medicine*, *336*, 1216–1222.

Shah, S., & Reichman, W. E. (2006). Treatment of Alzheimer's disease across the spectrum of clinical activity. *Clinical Interventions in Aging*, *1*, 131–142.

Talbot, C., Lendon, C., Craddock, N., et al. (1994). Protection against Alzheimer's disease with ApoE2. *Lancet*, *343*, 1432–1433.

*Tom, S. E., Hubbard, R. A., Crane, P. K., et al. (2015). Characterization of dementia and Alzheimer's disease in an older population: Updated incidence and life expectancy with and without dementia. *American Journal of Public Health*, *105*(2), 408–413.

*Wiser, T. H. (1994). Alzheimer's cognitive disturbances: A case study. *US Pharmacist*, *19*, 52–78.

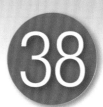

38 Parkinson's Disease

David Dinh, Karleen Melody, and Anisha B. Grover

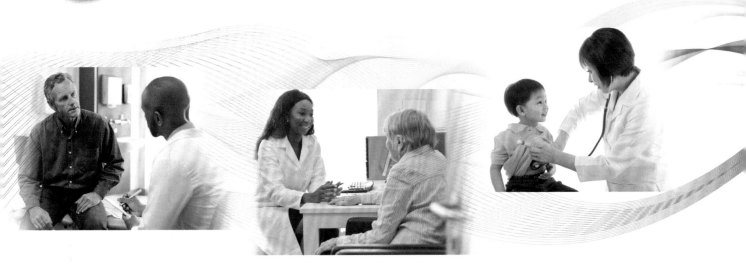

INTRODUCTION

Parkinson's disease (PD) is a neurodegenerative disorder characterized by a set of hallmark motor and nonmotor symptoms and was originally described in the "Essay on the Shaking Palsy," written by James Parkinson (1817). The mean age of onset is 65 years, with the typical age of diagnosis ranging between 55 and 65 years and peaking between 85 and 89 years (Armstrong & Okun, 2020). The incidence is reportedly higher in males, with a male-to-female ratio of 1.4:1. The estimated prevalence among the total population is 0.3%, and the prevalence increases with age, affecting 1% of patients over the age of 60 years. Approximately 1 million people live with PD in the United States (Marras et al., 2018).

CAUSES

The underlying etiologies of PD are not well understood but likely include factors related to aging, genetic expression, and the environment.

As a preliminary step, drug-induced parkinsonism (DIP) must be considered and ruled out prior to the initiation of treatment for PD. The prevalence and incidence are difficult to determine, as it can be challenging to differentiate DIP from PD. Existing research has demonstrated that DIP may be the second most common etiology of parkinsonism (Shin & Chung, 2012). DIP is associated with agents that deplete or antagonize dopamine, such as first-generation "typical" antipsychotics or neuroleptic drugs. This drug class includes chlorpromazine, promazine, haloperidol, perphenazine, fluphenazine, and pimozide. Up to 80% of patients taking a drug from this class present with more than one kind of extrapyramidal side effect (EPS). Second-generation or "atypical" antipsychotic drugs, such as risperidone, olanzapine, and aripiprazole, were thought to carry a decreased risk than first-generation antipsychotic drugs; however, studies have shown otherwise. Of the available second-generation antipsychotics, only clozapine and quetiapine are associated with lower rates of DIP among older patients. Other offending agents include metoclopramide, valproic acid, methyldopa, and prochlorperazine. Amiodarone and lithium may cause tremor, which can appear similar to Parkinson-like symptoms (Shin & Chung, 2012). Management of these cases involves discontinuation of the responsible medication, as the associated parkinsonism is typically reversible. Up to 10% of patients with DIP may experience persistent symptoms, even after discontinuation of the offending drug, but this is usually explained as an unmasking of symptoms rather than as a direct cause of the drug therapy. The reversibility can occur within hours or days but can take up to 2 years. These agents can also worsen symptoms in existing idiopathic PD and should be avoided when possible in diagnosed patients (Shin & Chung, 2012).

The natural aging process is likely associated with some of the neuron degeneration seen in PD. Other contributors include oxidative stress, which may be associated with increased monoamine oxidase-B (MAO-B) metabolism or decreased glutathione clearance of free radicals, mitochondrial dysfunction, inflammation, and signal-mediated apoptosis.

Approximately 15% of patients with PD have a first-degree relative with the disease. The inheritance of Mendelian genes has been linked to 10% or less of PD cases but may be associated with both familial and sporadic PD. At least 23 loci and 19 disease-causing genes for parkinsonism have been identified (Deng et al., 2018).

Although PD is typically considered sporadic or familial, there is a broad body of epidemiologic research related to PD, which associates risk factors that may contribute to developing PD.

Factors for increased risk for developing PD include high diary consumption, chronic pesticide exposure, and traumatic brain injury. Protective factors against PD include caffeine intake, tobacco use, increased physical activity, nonsteroidal antiinflammatory drugs, and statin usage (Ascherio & Schwarzchild, 2016; Marras et al., 2019).

PATHOPHYSIOLOGY

PD is associated with several cardinal pathologic findings within the substantia nigra pars compacta (SNpc), including the depigmentation, or degeneration, of dopaminergic neurons, autophagy dysfunction, and the formation of Lewy bodies in the residual neurons.

The extrapyramidal motor system regulates the movement of muscles. Dopamine is a neurotransmitter associated with movement control and is produced and stored in cells within the midbrain structure called the SNpc. At the point of diagnosis, patients have typically already lost at least half of the dopaminergic neurons in the SNpc. This leads to the depletion of dopamine in the corpus striatum, resulting in a breakdown of communication to the motor regulators within the brain. Additional neuronal dysfunction typically manifests in the basal ganglia, neurocortex, and spinal cord.

Autophagy describes an intracellular process in which cytoplasmic proteins and organelles are gathered in vacuoles that are transported into lysosomes, where they can be degraded and recycled. This process facilitates the elimination of damaged proteins and organelles and is one of the main routes of elimination of alpha-synuclein, a component of Lewy bodies. Dysfunction in this process may also be linked with the neurodegeneration of dopaminergic neurons, contributing to the pathogenesis of PD (Moors et al., 2017).

Lewy bodies, named for Frederick Lewy, are round, eosinophilic aggregates located within neuronal nuclei. These structures are made primarily of alpha-synuclein and ubiquitin and consist of a dense core, surrounded by fibrillary elements. Lewy bodies are found in a small percentage of normal older adult brains and are also found in patients with Down syndrome, Alzheimer's disease, dementia, and other neurodegenerative conditions. In PD, Lewy bodies can be found within the SNpc, cerebral cortex, basal ganglia, cardiac plexus, and gastrointestinal (GI) system. The distribution and anatomical location of these protein inclusions vary among individuals with PD and are closely linked to the presentation and extent of clinical features (Halliday et al., 2012). The early stages of PD involve Lewy body formation in the medulla oblongata, locus coeruleus, raphe nuclei, and even the olfactory bulb. This is directly associated with depression, anxiety, difficulty sleeping, and sensory impairment that may manifest initially. PD progression is marked by Lewy body presence in the SNpc, correlating with hallmark motor symptoms. In advanced cases, Lewy bodies form in the cortex, resulting in cognitive changes. Lewy body accumulation in the lateral collateral pathway within the sacral spinal dorsal horn may contribute to urinary urgency and frequency and constipation associated with PD (VanderHorst et al., 2015). Nonmotor symptoms may also result from the loss of a wide range of neurotransmitters, including dopamine, norepinephrine, serotonin, and acetylcholine, which can decrease as various regions of the brain degenerate.

DIAGNOSTIC CRITERIA

The clinical history of the patient, including risk factors, medical history, medication history, and review of systems, provides the most useful information for the diagnostic process, despite technological advances in imaging and nuclear techniques. In evaluating the patient, it is important to first exclude DIP.

Patients and caregivers provide valuable information when establishing a diagnosis, including the onset of tremor, stiffness or rigidity in arms or legs, speed of movement, and description of changes in facial expressions, posture, and gait. Hallmark or cardinal motor symptoms include a slowing of movement termed *bradykinesia*, resting or postural tremor, cogwheel rigidity, and difficulty maintaining balance, also known as postural instability. A neurological exam includes the assessment of facial expressiveness, posture, tone, balance, tremor, and speed of extremity movements (Postuma et al., 2015). Patients should also be evaluated for any associated nonmotor symptoms or conditions, including depression, anxiety, psychosis, fatigue, sleep disturbances, urinary complaints, increased salivation, orthostatic hypotension, cognitive changes, and GI problems, such as constipation.

The Movement Disorder Society Clinical Diagnostic Criteria for Parkinson's Disease (MDS-PD Criteria) can be utilized for the diagnosis PD. The first essential criterion is parkinsonism, defined by bradykinesia in combination with rest tremor, rigidity, or both. Once parkinsonism is diagnosed, the absence or presence of 26 criteria places the diagnosis of clinically established PD or clinically probable PD (Postuma et al., 2015). The MDS-PD criteria should be used in combination with the MDS-sponsored revision of the Unified Parkinson's Disease Rating Scale (MDS-UPDRS) to monitor the degree of disability and impairment (Goetz et al., 2008). This tool can be used at the time of diagnosis to establish a baseline score, so that patient progress can be measured over time. This 65-item tool has demonstrated validity and reliability and is accompanied by a detailed set of instructions to standardize the use of the tool internationally. It contains four parts: (1) nonmotor experiences of daily living, (2) motor experiences of daily living, (3) motor examination, and (4) motor complications. The patient or caregiver completes a total of 20 questions from parts I and II. Both rater and patient involvement are required for the remaining portions. The total rater time requirement to administer the tool is 30 minutes.

Functional magnetic resonance imaging (MRI) or nuclear imaging techniques may be useful in ruling out other conditions, such as essential tremor, vascular parkinsonism, multiple systems atrophy, and progressive supranuclear palsy. These tools can also help form an earlier and more precise diagnosis, preventing a delay in therapy and helping to continually improve the individualization of disease management strategies for patients with PD. Dopamine transporter (DAT) imaging, sometimes used in combination with contrast agents, can be used to assess the degree of DAT loss in patients with PD, which correlates with disease staging, severity, and duration (Badoud et al. 2016). Although patients diagnosed with PD can look similar at baseline, the clinical subtypes can be differentiated by the variances in dopaminergic degeneration. DAT imaging can be used to diagnose presynaptic parkinsonism because even in early PD, DAT uptake in the striatum is significantly decreased. Utilizing DAT imaging can help to differentiate PD from DIP, which involves drug-induced changes in postsynaptic dopaminergic receptors (Yomtoob et al., 2018). It can also guide the formation of patient-specific treatment strategies. Additional studies have explored whole-brain functional connectivity.

INITIATING DRUG THERAPY

Traditionally, treatment of patients with newly diagnosed PD would be deferred until the patient has developed functional disability interfering with activities of daily living (National Institute for Health and Care Excellence [NICE], 2017). This is largely driven by the lack of available disease-modifying or neuroprotective agents; however, in recent years, there is emerging evidence that points to several advantages of initiating pharmacotherapy early on in PD. Early intervention may delay or diminish both motor and nonmotor symptoms, as well as delay the initiation of levodopa (**Figure 38.1**). By the time motor symptoms present, dopamine has been depleted by 60% to 80%, further strengthening the recommendation to initiate treatment earlier rather than waiting for functional disability (Stocchi et al., 2015).

Patients with untreated or inadequately treated PD will experience significant symptomatic deterioration contributing to a reduced quality of life. Even though motor symptoms are more identifiable in PD, nonmotor symptoms have been shown to have a more negative impact on quality of life

because they represent the majority of PD symptoms and tend to emerge early in PD often before motor symptoms appear. A patient presenting with significant nonmotor symptoms may warrant early treatment intervention to improve quality of life (Grimes et al., 2019).

There are several factors that need to be considered in determining when to initiate treatment as well as which treatment option to use. These factors include age, cognitive function, psychiatric issues, comorbidities, lifestyle, symptom severity, and employment, with the latter two factors being the strongest predictors of need for dopaminergic therapy. The patient's symptom severity and levels of impairment and disability should be assessed upon diagnosis and throughout treatment using a validated scale such as the MDS-UPDRS, to objectively evaluate the motor features of PD (Ossig & Reichmann, 2015).

Goals of Drug Therapy

The ultimate goal of drug therapy for PD is to maintain quality of life by alleviating motor and nonmotor symptoms. Other desired outcomes include maintaining patient independence, preserving the ability to perform activities of daily living, and minimizing adverse drug events and treatment complications (Grimes et al., 2019). As with any disease state, it is important to provide cost-effective therapy; involve and educate the patient, family, and caregivers when creating a patient-centered treatment plan; and connect the patient with reliable and accurate resources.

Selected Agents for Motor Symptoms

Mild-Potency Drugs

Anticholinergics

Indications/Use. The use of anticholinergics in PD is controversial. There is some evidence that they are useful in some patients with PD, particularly for symptoms of drooling and tremor. However, other randomized controlled studies conclude that the benefits on tremor are inconclusive (Connolly & Lang, 2014). They are indicated for PD symptoms as well as drug-induced EPS.

Mechanism of Action. Anticholinergics antagonize acetylcholine receptors to decrease the release of acetylcholine, which regulates muscle movement. The resulting decrease in activity of acetylcholine muscarinic receptors can also decrease salivation, providing an explanation for its potential role for the management of drooling.

Dosage. Two anticholinergics used in PD are trihexyphenidyl and benztropine. Trihexyphenidyl, available in an oral tablet and an elixir, is initiated at 1 mg and is titrated in 2-mg increments every 3 to 5 days. A typical maintenance dose is 6 to 10 mg daily in 3 to 4 divided doses to a maximum dose of 15 mg/d. Benztropine, available in an oral tablet, injection, and solution formulation, should be started at 1 mg daily, which

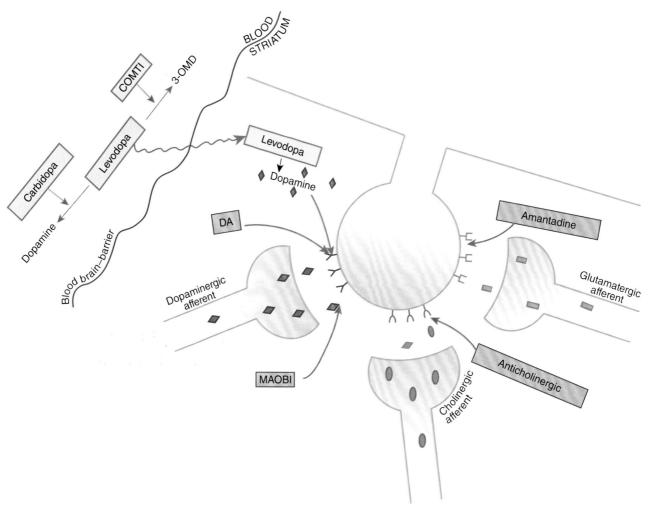

FIGURE 38–1 Sites of action of drugs used in the management of Parkinson's disease. Parkinson's disease is characterized by a deficiency in dopamine, and many drugs work to increase the activity of this neurotransmitter. In the periphery, COMTIs block the degradation of levodopa to 3-*O*-methyldopa, and carbidopa prevents the conversion of levodopa into dopamine, increasing the amount of levodopa that can cross the blood–brain barrier. Once levodopa has entered the striatum, it undergoes central conversion to dopamine. Other drugs that act primarily in the striatum include DAs, which bind to and activate dopamine receptors, and monoamine oxidase type B inhibitors, which inhibit the breakdown of dopamine. In addition to dopamine, other neurotransmitters serve as drug targets in Parkinson's disease. Anticholinergic drugs bind to and block acetylcholine receptors. Amantadine binds to and blocks *N*-methyl-ᴅ-aspartate glutamate receptors and increases the release of dopamine in other ways.

3-OMD, 3-*O*-methyldopa; COMTI, catechol-*O*-methyltransferase inhibitors; DA, dopamine agonists; MAOBI, monoamine oxidase type B inhibitors.

can be divided into 2 to 4 divided doses. Benztropine can be gradually increased every 5 to 6 days by increments of 0.5 mg to a maximum of 6 mg daily. Abrupt discontinuation of either agent can exacerbate adverse effects, so it is recommended to taper the dose. For an overview of selected agents for motor symptoms, see **Table 38.1**.

Time Frame for Response. Anticholinergics have an onset of approximately 1 hour.

Contraindications. Both agents are contraindicated in narrow-angle glaucoma. Benztropine is also contraindicated in children less than 3 years of age.

Adverse Drug Events. Anticholinergics commonly cause impaired memory, confusion, hallucinations, nausea, blurred vision, dry mouth, urinary retention, and constipation, which often limit their use in PD.

Interactions. Potassium chloride should be avoided with anticholinergics because concurrent use increases the risk of ulcers. The risk of GI adverse effects may also be increased in patients on anticholinergics when glucagon is administered. Due to additive side effects, other anticholinergics such as ipratropium, tiotropium, and umeclidinium should be avoided in patients on benztropine or trihexyphenidyl.

TABLE 38.1

Overview of Drugs Used in the Management of Parkinson's Disease

Generic (Trade) Name and Initial Dosage	Dose Adjustments	Selected Adverse Events	Contraindications	Special considerations
Trihexyphenidyl (Artane) 1 mg once daily; titrate by 2 mg q3–5d; maximum 15 mg/d	None.	Impaired memory, confusion, hallucinations, nausea, blurred vision, dry mouth, urinary retention, constipation	Narrow-angle glaucoma	Avoid with potassium chloride, glucagon, and other anticholinergics
Benztropine (Cogentin) 1 mg once daily; titrated by 0.5 mg; maximum 6 mg/d	None.	Same as trihexyphenidyl	Narrow-angle glaucoma; use in <3 y of age	Same as trihexyphenidyl
Amantadine IR (Symmetrel) 100 mg BID; maximum 400 mg/d	Serious concomitant illness or high doses of other PD drugs: start 100 mg once daily. CrCl 30–50 mL/min: 200 mg × 1 and 100 mg daily thereafter. CrCl 15–29 mL/min: 200 mg × 1 and 100 mg every other day thereafter. CrCl <15 mL/min or HD: 200 mg q7d.	Hallucinations, confusion, ankle edema, livedo reticularis, blurred vision, dry mouth, constipation, insomnia	None	Caution with use with memantine or drugs that prolong the QT interval
Amantadine ER Capsule (Gocovri) 137 mg once daily; maximum 274 mg/d	CrCl 30–59 mL/min: 68.5 mg once daily; after 1 week increase to 137 mg once daily if needed. CrCl 15–29 mL/min: 68.5 mg once daily. CrCl <15 mL/min or HD: Contraindicated.	Same as amantadine IR	ESRD or HD	Same as amantadine IR
Amantadine ER tablet (Osmolex ER) 129 mg once daily; maximum 322 mg/d	CrCl 30–59 mL/min: 129 mg QOD; may be increased to q3wk to a maximum of 322 mg QOD. CrCl 15–29 mL/min: 129 mg q96h; may be increased to q4wk to a maximum of 322 mg q96h. CrCl <15 mL/min or HD: Contraindicated.	Same as amantadine IR	ESRD or HD	Same as amantadine IR
Selegiline (Eldepryl) 5 mg BID	None.	Headache, nausea, dizziness, hallucinations, dyskinesia, insomnia	Meperidine, methadone, propoxyphene, tramadol, St. John's wort, cyclobenzaprine, dextromethorphan, other MAO-B inhibitors, carbamazepine, SSRIs, SNRIs, clomipramine, imipramine	Caution with use with other serotonergic agents, alcohol, and tyramine-containing foods

(Continued)

TABLE 38.1

Overview of Drugs Used in the Management of Parkinson's Disease (*Continued*)

Generic (Trade) Name and Initial Dosage	Dose Adjustments	Selected Adverse Events	Contraindications	Special considerations
Rasagiline (Azilect) 1 mg once daily; maximum 1 mg/d	If used with levodopa, initial dose should be decreased to 0.5 once daily.	Headache, nausea, dizziness, hallucinations, dyskinesia, orthostatic hypotension, dyspepsia, depression, flu-like symptoms, and arthralgia	Meperidine, methadone, propoxyphene, tramadol, St. John's wort, cyclobenzaprine, dextromethorphan, and other MAO-B inhibitors	Same as selegiline
Safinamide (Xadago) 50 mg daily; maximum 100 mg/d	Moderate hepatic impairment (Child-Pugh class B): Maximum dose: 50 mg once daily. Severe hepatic impairment (Child-Pugh class C): Use is contraindicated (not studied).	Dyskinesia, hypertension, orthostatic hypotension, nausea	Severe hepatic impairment (Child-Pugh class C), meperidine, methadone, propoxyphene, tramadol, St. John's wort, cyclobenzaprine, dextromethorphan, and other MAO-B inhibitors	Same as selegiline
Pramipexole IR (Mirapex) 0.125 mg TID; titrated q5–7d	CrCl 30–50 mL/min: start 0.125 BID. CrCl 15–29 mL/min: start 0.125 once daily.	Fatigue, nausea, constipation, orthostatic hypotension, hallucinations, lower extremity edema, ICD, sleep attacks	None	
Pramipexole ER (Mirapex ER) 0.375 mg once daily; titrated by 0.75 mg q5–7d; maximum 4.5 mg	CrCl 30–50 mL/min: start 0.375 mg QOD	Same as pramipexole IR	None	Dose should be tapered before discontinuing
Ropinirole IR (Requip) 0.25 mg TID; titrated weekly; maximum 24 mg/d	HD: 0.25 mg TID; maximum 18 mg/d	Same as pramipexole IR	None	Avoid use with CYP1A2 inhibitors and inducers
Ropinirole ER (Requip XL) 2 mg once daily; titrated weekly by 2 mg; maximum 24 mg/d	HD: 2 mg once daily; maximum 18 mg/d	Same as pramipexole IR	None	Dose should be tapered before discontinuing. Avoid use with CYP1A2 inhibitors and inducers.
Rotigotine (Neupro) 2 mg/24 h; titrated by 2 mg/24 h weekly; maximum 6 mg/24 h	None.	Same as pramipexole IR	None	Dose should be tapered before discontinuing.
Apomorphine (Apokyn) 2- or 4-mg test dose; titrated by 1 mg every few days; maximum 6 mg/dose	Renal impairment: start 1-mg test dose.	Same as pramipexole IR	None	4-mg test dose administered 2 h after 2-mg test dose if tolerated but does not respond.

TABLE 38.1

Overview of Drugs Used in the Management of Parkinson's Disease (Continued)

Generic (Trade) Name and Initial Dosage	Dose Adjustments	Selected Adverse Events	Contraindications	Special considerations
Carbidopa/levodopa IR (Sinemet) or ODT (Parcopa) Preferred: 25/100 mg TID; alternative: 10/100 mg TID–QID; titrated by 1 tablet daily or QOD; maximum 8 tablets/d or 200 mg/d carbidopa or 2,000 mg/d levodopa	None.	Nausea, vomiting, constipation, dizziness, headache, peripheral edema, insomnia, orthostatic hypotension, dyskinesias	Narrow-angle glaucoma	Protein consumption and constipation may reduce the absorption of levodopa, so patients should avoid meals high in protein, take levodopa 1 h before or 2 h after meals, and maintain an appropriate bowel regimen.
Carbidopa/levodopa CR (Sinemet CR) 50/200 mg BID; titrated by 1 tablet q3d; maximum 8 tablets/d	Levodopa doses >700 mg should be divided into at least 3 daily doses.	Same as carbidopa/levodopa IR	Narrow-angle glaucoma	Same as carbidopa/levodopa IR.
Carbidopa/levodopa ER (Rytary) 23.75/95 mg TID for 3 d, then 36.25/145 mg TID starting day 4; titrated as tolerated to maximum 612.5/2,450 mg/d	None.	Same as carbidopa/levodopa IR	Narrow-angle glaucoma	Same as carbidopa/levodopa IR.
Carbidopa/levodopa 4.63/20 mg/mL (16 hour enteral infusion) suspension (DUOPA); refer to manufacturer's labeling for morning, continuous, and titration dosing	None.	Same as carbidopa/levodopa IR	Narrow-angle glaucoma	Same as carbidopa/levodopa IR.
Entacapone (Comtan) 200 mg with each dose of levodopa; maximum 8 doses/d	None.	Dyskinesia, hypotension, nausea, diarrhea, dark-colored urine, somnolence, sleep disorders, hallucinations, headache, confusion	None	Only used adjunct to carbidopa/levodopa therapy. May be necessary to reduce dose of levodopa when adding COMTI.
Carbidopa, levodopa, and entacapone (Stalevo) Carbidopa/levodopa ratio of 1:4 plus entacapone 200 mg	See individual components.	See individual components	See individual components	See individual components.
Tolcapone (Tasmar) 100 mg TID	None.	Same as entacapone Black box warning for hepatotoxicity	History of liver disease, nontraumatic rhabdomyolysis or hyperpyrexia and confusion potentially related to medication	Same as entacapone Bioavailability is decreased by 10%–20% when taken with food.

COMTI, catechol-O-methyltransferase inhibitor; CR, controlled-release; CrCl, creatinine clearance; ER, extended-release; ESRD, end-stage renal disease; HD, hemodialysis; ICD, impulse control disorder; IR, immediate-release; MAO-B, monoamine oxidase-B; PD, Parkinson's disease; SNRIs, serotonin–norepinephrine reuptake inhibitors; SSRIs, selective serotonin reuptake inhibitors.

Amantadine

Indications/Uses. Amantadine is indicated for the treatment of mild PD and most frequently used in a patient experiencing dyskinesia. Evidence supporting the use of amantadine in PD is conflicting. Expert opinion supports its use as monotherapy and adjunctive therapy; however, a 2009 Cochrane review concludes that there is insufficient evidence for its use (Connolly & Lang, 2014).

Mechanism of Action. The precise mechanism of amantadine in PD is unknown, although it is hypothesized that its inhibition on N-methyl-D-aspartate receptors potentiates dopaminergic responses to reduce PD symptoms.

Dosage. Amantadine is available as an oral capsule and tablet in immediate and extended-release (ER) formulations and as a solution. The immediate-release (IR) formulation is typically started at a dose of 100 mg twice daily. It can be titrated to a maximum of 400 mg daily in divided doses with careful monitoring. In the presence of a serious concomitant illness, or for patients who are receiving high doses of other PD drugs, an initial dose of 100 mg daily is recommended, which can be titrated to 100 mg twice daily after 1 to 2 weeks. The dose of amantadine needs to be adjusted in patients with renal dysfunction. For patients with a creatinine clearance (CrCl) of 30 to 50 mL/min, a loading dose of 200 mg should be started, followed by 100 mg/d as a maintenance dose. For patients with a CrCl between 15 and 29 mL/min, a 200-mg loading dose should be given, followed by 100 mg every other day. Patients with a CrCl less than 15 mL/min or on hemodialysis (HD) should be given 200 mg every 7 days.

Time Frame for Response. The onset of amantadine is within 48 hours of administration.

Contraindications. The ER formulations are contraindicated in end-stage renal disease or HD.

Adverse Drug Events. Adverse effects of amantadine include hallucinations, confusion, ankle edema, livedo reticularis, a blotchy, and purple-colored skin condition with a net-like pattern, in addition to anticholinergic effects like blurred vision, dry mouth, and constipation. Amantadine may also affect sleep–wake cycles, causing insomnia or reduction in daytime sleepiness.

Interactions. Caution should be used when amantadine is used concurrently with memantine because of an increased risk of QT prolongation and psychosis. Other drugs that prolong the QT interval should also be used with caution in combination with amantadine.

Monoamine Oxidase-B Inhibitors

Indications/Uses. MAO-B inhibitors are used for mild PD. When used as monotherapy in early PD, MAO-B inhibitors provide a modest improvement in motor symptoms, which may be seen as early as 1 week after initiation. In more advanced PD, MAO-B inhibitors are used as adjunctive therapy. MAO-B inhibitors also delay the need for levodopa by a few months, but they do not prevent or delay clinical progression of PD (Goetz & Pal, 2014). The MAO-B inhibitors available for the treatment of PD are selegiline, rasagiline, and safinamide.

Mechanism of Action. MAO-B plays a major role in the metabolism of dopamine. By inhibiting this metabolism, concentrations of dopamine are increased, allowing more dopamine to reach the brain and ultimately reducing motor symptoms of PD. Selegiline also inhibits the uptake of catecholamines and the release of catecholamine by amphetamine metabolites.

Dosage. Selegiline is available in multiple formulations, including an oral capsule, an oral tablet, a patch, and an orally disintegrating tablet (ODT), whereas rasagiline and safinamide are only available as oral tablets. Of note, the patch is only indicated for depression, and the ODT has insufficient efficacy for symptom improvement in PD, so these dosage forms will not be discussed further. Selegiline therapy is initiated at a dose of 5 mg twice daily with breakfast and lunch. The recommended dose of rasagiline as monotherapy or adjunctive therapy (except with levodopa) is 1 mg once daily, which is the maximum daily dose. If rasagiline is used adjunctively with levodopa, the initial dose is 0.5 mg once daily, which could be increased to 1 mg once daily based on response and tolerability. Safinamide is initiated at 50 mg once daily and can be increased to 100 mg once daily after 2 weeks. If discontinuing therapy, safinamide should be decreased to 50 mg for 1 week prior to stopping. The half-life of safinamide is approximately 20 to 26 hours (compared to 3 hours and 10 hours for rasagiline and selegiline, respectively), which may make it advantageous in patients undergoing prolonged procedures (Bette et al., 2018).

Time Frame for Response. MAO-B inhibitors have an onset of approximately 1 week, with moderate improvement in motor symptoms seen within 1 week after initiation.

Contraindications. MOA-B inhibitors are contraindicated with meperidine, methadone, propoxyphene, tramadol, St. John's wort, cyclobenzaprine, dextromethorphan, and other MAO-B inhibitors. Additional contraindications with selegiline only include concomitant therapy with carbamazepine, selective serotonin reuptake inhibitors (SSRIs), serotonin–norepinephrine reuptake inhibitors, clomipramine, and imipramine.

Adverse Drug Events. Adverse effects seen with MOA-B inhibitors include headache, nausea, dizziness, hallucinations, or dyskinesia. Selegiline can also cause insomnia because it is metabolized to amphetamines, which is not true of rasagiline. Rasagiline may additionally cause orthostatic hypotension, dyspepsia, depression, flu-like symptoms, and arthralgia. Safinamide is relatively well tolerated with fewer side effects compared to its counterparts.

MAO-B inhibitors have additional adverse-event concerns that warrant caution with their use. The risk of developing melanoma is increased in patients with PD, although no clear association with dopaminergic drugs has been established. New or worsening mental status or behavioral changes, including impulse control disorders (ICDs), have also been noted with MAO-B inhibitor use. Somnolence, which may impair physical or mental abilities, has been reported with MAO-B inhibitor use particularly in older patients, patients with current sleep disorders, and patients taking concomitant sedating medications. MAO-B inhibitors may also potentiate the dopaminergic side effects of levodopa and may cause or worsen dyskinesia. Rasagiline labeling also contains a warning that it can exacerbate or precipitate hypertension. Proper screenings for the concerns listed previously should be conducted regularly.

Interactions. The impact of cytochrome P450 (CYP) isoforms on the metabolism of MAO-B inhibitors is important to consider. Selegiline is metabolized primarily by CYP2B6 and to a lesser extent by CYP3A4. Selegiline does not inhibit enzymes in the CYP450 system; however, CYP3A4 inducers, such as phenytoin and carbamazepine, could reduce selegiline concentrations. Rasagiline is metabolized by CYP1A2; therefore, CYP1A2 inhibitors, such as ciprofloxacin and cimetidine, reduce rasagiline concentrations. Rasagiline does not inhibit or induce enzymes in the P450 system. Safinamide is predominantly metabolized to inactive metabolites by non-microsomal enzymes, while CYP3A4 plays only a minor role in its overall metabolism. Caution should be used when MAO-B inhibitors are used concomitantly with alpha/beta agonists, stimulants, and buprenorphine. Additionally, potentially fatal serotonin syndrome has occurred when serotonergic agents are used concomitantly with MAO-B inhibitors. Alcohol- and tyramine-containing foods should also be avoided due to their increased risk of serotonin syndrome.

Moderate-Potency Drugs
Dopamine Agonists
Indications/Uses. Compared to levodopa, dopamine agonists (DAs) are less effective but cause dyskinesia or motor fluctuations less frequently (Reich & Savitt, 2019). They are classified as either ergot or nonergot derivatives. The nonergot-derived agents have superior safety profiles and are therefore the preferred choice, so they will be the focus of this section. Pramipexole, ropinirole, and rotigotine are the DAs available to treat moderate symptoms of PD. Apomorphine is an injectable DA that is only approved to treat acute intermittent hypomobility in patients with advanced PD. When used adjunctively to levodopa, a DA has improved efficacy compared to monotherapy and can reduce "wearing-off" phenomena but has an increased risk of dyskinesia (Connolly & Lang, 2014).

Mechanism of Action. The exact mechanism of action of DAs is unknown; however, it is believed that stimulation of dopamine D2-type receptors results in improved dopaminergic transmission in the motor area of the basal ganglia.

Dosage. Pramipexole and ropinirole are available in IR and ER oral tablet formulations. Pramipexole IR tablet is initiated at 0.125 mg thrice daily and titrated every 5 to 7 days. The typical maintenance dose is 0.5 to 1.5 mg thrice daily. The ER formulation of pramipexole is started at 0.375 mg daily and titrated by 0.75 mg daily every 5 to 7 days to a maximum dose of 4.5 mg once daily. Patients with renal impairment require a dose reduction. Pramipexole IR should be initiated at 0.125 mg twice daily and 0.125 mg once daily for patients with a CrCl of 30 to 50 mL/min and CrCl of 15 to 29 mL/min, respectively. Pramipexole IR should not be used in patients with a CrCl less than 15 mL/min or in those requiring HD. For patients with a CrCl of 30 to 50 mL/min, pramipexole ER should be initiated at 0.375 mg every other day, which can be titrated to 0.375 mg daily after at least 1 week of therapy. Pramipexole ER can further be titrated by 0.375 mg every 7 days to a maximum dose of 2.25 mg daily. Patients with a CrCl less than 30 mL/min or on HD should not take pramipexole ER. To discontinue pramipexole, it is recommended to decrease the dose by 0.75 mg/d until the daily dose is 0.75 mg once daily and then to reduce dose by 0.375 mg once daily thereafter until discontinued.

The starting dose of ropinirole IR tablet is 0.25 mg thrice daily. For the first month of therapy, the daily dosage should increase by 0.75 mg (divided into 3 doses) on a weekly basis. After week 4, the daily dosage may be increased by 1.5 mg/d on a weekly basis up to a dose of 9 mg/d and then by 3 mg/d on a weekly basis up to a total dose of 24 mg/d. When discontinuing ropinirole, it must be tapered over 7 days by reducing the administration to twice daily for 4 days and then once daily for the remaining 3 days. The starting dose of the ER tablet is 2 mg once daily for 1 to 2 weeks, which is then titrated by 2 mg/d on a weekly basis to a maximum of 24 mg daily. Neither formulation has been studied in patients with a CrCl less than 30 mL/min, and use of these agents should be avoided in this population. For patients requiring HD, the initial dose of ropinirole IR should be 0.25 mg thrice daily and ropinirole ER should be 2 mg once daily. The maximum daily dose in patients requiring HD for both formulations is 18 mg daily.

Rotigotine is available as a transdermal patch and should be initiated at 2 mg/24 hours. The dose may be increased by 2 mg/24 hours on a weekly basis to a maximum dose of 6 mg/24 hours. If discontinuation of rotigotine is warranted, the dose should be reduced by 2 mg/24 hours every other day. Rotigotine does not require any dose adjustments for hepatic and renal insufficiency.

Since apomorphine is used for acute hypomobility, this medication is administered thrice daily as needed. When initiating apomorphine, a test dose of 2 mg subcutaneously is administered under medical supervision. If the patient tolerates the dose but does not respond, a second test dose of 4 mg should be administered 2 hours later. If the 4-mg dose is tolerated and the patient responds, a maintenance dose of 3 mg should be administered thereafter. If the patient tolerates and responds to either the 2-mg or the 4-mg test dose, the maintenance dose can be titrated in 1-mg increments every few days to a maximum of 6 mg. For patients with mild to moderate renal impairment, the initial test dose and starting dose should be reduced to 1 mg as needed.

Time Frame for Response. Pramipexole and ropinirole have an onset of action within 1 hour of administration. Rogigotine has a slower onset action of 4 to 18 hours with a full treatment benefit seen within 1 week. Apomorphine has a rapid onset of action of 10 to 20 minutes.

Contraindications. There are no contraindications for pramipexole, ropinorole, or rotigotine. Apomorphine is contraindicated with concomitant use of 5-HT3 antagonists.

Adverse Drug Events. Adverse effects are similar among all DAs and include fatigue, nausea, constipation, orthostatic hypotension, hallucinations, and lower extremity edema. Severe side effects may include ICD, or sleep attacks. ICD may improve upon reduction or discontinuation of the DA, but switching to a different agent is not recommended as all DAs have a similar risk of ICD. Since sleep attacks can occur at any time, including while driving, eating, and talking, patients should be counseled about driving safety. Because of these significant adverse drug events, DAs are typically avoided in older patients.

Interactions. Pramipexole and rotigotine do not have any major drug interactions, but caution should be used with antipsychotics as the efficacy of both agents can be diminished. Ropinirole is a major substrate of CYP1A2, so its use should be avoided with any CYP1A2 inducers, such as carbamazepine and rifampin, or inhibitors, such as ciprofloxacin and cimetidine.

High-Potency Drugs

Levodopa

Indications/Uses. Nearly all patients with PD require treatment with levodopa, as it is the most effective treatment for symptomatic relief of PD. Levodopa also has the fastest onset of action compared to other PD medications. After several years of levodopa treatment, patients can begin to experience a "wearing-off" phenomenon, which involves the return of motor and nonmotor symptoms prior to the next dose of levodopa. As PD progresses, patients may find a shortening in the length of time with a good response to the medication, also known as "on time," and a lengthening of time with a poor response, also known as "off time." As PD progresses, patients have a diminished capacity to produce dopamine and store converted levodopa for release when needed, resulting in a reappearance of symptoms. Although "wearing off" can occur with many

different drugs, it is most commonly associated with levodopa. At high doses and with continued use, patients' inability to store excess dopamine can manifest in the form of motor fluctuations and dyskinesia, so it is typically reserved for severe motor symptoms of PD.

Mechanism of Action. Dopamine itself is not used to treat PD because it cannot cross the blood–brain barrier. Levodopa, a dopamine precursor, can cross the blood–brain barrier, where it is then converted via decarboxylation to dopamine. The converted dopamine is then stored in the presynaptic neurons until stimulated for release, when it binds to dopamine receptors. Levodopa is administered in combination with carbidopa, which limits the peripheral breakdown of levodopa. This allows roughly a fourfold increase in circulating levodopa to cross the blood–brain barrier and reduces the undesirable adverse effects of nausea and vomiting caused by dopamine in the periphery.

Dosage. Carbidopa/levodopa is available in many formulations, including an IR tablet, an ODT, a controlled-release (CR) tablet, a suspension, and an ER tablet and capsule and as an enteral suspension infusion. The CR formulation has a more variable absorption profile, resulting in a slower and less predictable onset of action than the IR formulation. The half-life of levodopa is only 60 to 90 minutes, so the daily dosage is divided into 3 to 6 doses.

The preferred initial dosing of the IR or ODT formulations is carbidopa 25 mg/levodopa 100 mg thrice daily, although carbidopa 10 mg/levodopa 100 mg three to four times daily may also be initiated. This can be titrated upward by 1 tablet daily or every other day as necessary to a maximum of 8 tablets of any strength or 200 mg of carbidopa and 2,000 mg of levodopa.

Patients initiating the CR formulation should start at a dose of carbidopa 50 mg/levodopa 200 mg twice daily at intervals not less than 6 hours apart. If doses of levodopa are greater than 700 mg daily, it should be divided into three or more daily doses. Intervals between doses should be 4 to 8 hours while awake, with the smaller doses given toward the end of the day, if the divided doses are not equal. This can be titrated upward by 1 tablet every 3 days to a maximum of 8 tablets daily.

For levodopa-naive patients, ER capsule dosage should be initiated at carbidopa 23.75 mg/levodopa 95 mg thrice daily for 3 days and then increased to carbidopa 36.25 mg/levodopa 145 mg thrice daily on the 4th day. Since ER tablets are not interchangeable with other carbidopa/levodopa products, patients switching from other formulations to the ER formulation are dosed based on their previous total daily dose (TDD) of levodopa. If the TDD was between 400 and 549 mg, initiate 3 capsules of carbidopa 23.75 mg/levodopa 95 mg thrice daily; if the TDD was between 550 and 749 mg, initiate 4 capsules of carbidopa 23.75 mg/levodopa 95 mg thrice daily; if the TDD was between 750 and 949 mg, initiate 3 capsules of carbidopa 36.25 mg/levodopa 145 mg thrice daily; if the TDD was between 950 and 1,249 mg, initiate

4 capsules of carbidopa 36.25 mg/levodopa 145 mg thrice daily; if the TDD is 1,250 mg or more, initiate 4 capsules of carbidopa 48.75 mg/levodopa 195 mg thrice daily. Titration of the ER formulations as tolerated can continue to a maximum daily dose of carbidopa 612.5 mg/levodopa 2,450 mg.

The enteral suspension is infused via a percutaneous endoscopic gastrostomy with jejunal tube directly into the jejunum. Prior to initiation of therapy, patients must be converted from all forms of levodopa to oral IR carbidopa/levodopa tablets (1:4 ratio) to determine the TDD, expressed in the levodopa component. Refer to the manufacturer's labeling for full conversion instructions. Each cassette provides a maximum dose of 2,000 mg of the levodopa component over 16 hours. Patients should receive their routine nighttime dosage of oral IR carbidopa/levodopa after discontinuation of the daily infusion.

Time Frame to Response. The onset of levodopa is approximately 1 hour.

Contraindications. Carbidopa/levodopa is contraindicated in patients with narrow-angle glaucoma.

Adverse Drug Events. The most common side effects of carbidopa/levodopa include nausea, vomiting, constipation, dizziness, headache, peripheral edema, insomnia, and orthostatic hypotension. Carbidopa/levodopa can also cause motor fluctuations and dyskinesia, which are more commonly seen when initiated in younger patients.

Interactions. Carbidopa/levodopa does not have any major drug interactions, but caution should be used with antipsychotics as the efficacy of both agents can be diminished. Additionally, levodopa may enhance the effect of MAO-B inhibitors. In some cases, protein consumption may reduce the absorption of levodopa from the intestine, so patients should avoid meals high in protein. Patients may also try taking levodopa 1 hour before or 2 hours after meals. It is important for patients to increase fluid and fiber intake, as constipation may reduce levodopa absorption as well.

Catechol-O-Methyltransferase Inhibitors
Indications/Uses. Catechol-O-methyltransferase inhibitors (COMTIs) are used in combination with levodopa to decrease PD-associated disability by improving "wearing-off" phenomena; however, they can increase the risk of dyskinesia.

Mechanism of Action. Catechol-O-methyltransferase breaks down levodopa in the periphery. By inhibiting this action, levodopa plasma levels are increased and the half-life is prolonged.

Dosage. Two oral COMTIs, entacapone and tolcapone, are available for adjunctive therapy to carbidopa/levodopa in the treatment of patients with PD who experience "wearing-off" symptoms. Tolcapone was withdrawn from the market in Canada; however, it is still available in the United States for patients who have tried and failed entacapone. The initial dose of

entacapone is 200 mg, administered with each dose of levodopa, to a maximum of 8 doses daily. Tolcapone should be initiated at 100 mg thrice daily and does not have to be taken at the same times as levodopa. If no benefit is seen after 3 weeks, tolcapone should be discontinued. COMTIs can exacerbate the adverse effects of levodopa, so it may be necessary to reduce the dose of levodopa when adding a COMTI to the patient's regimen.

Time Frame to Response. The onset of COMTIs is approximately 1 hour.

Contraindications. There are no contraindications for use with entacapone. Tolcapone is contraindicated in patients with a history of liver disease, nontraumatic rhabdomyolysis, or hyperpyrexia and confusion potentially related to medication.

Adverse Drug Events. Common adverse effects of COMTIs include dyskinesia, hypotension, nausea, diarrhea, dark-colored urine, and central nervous system (CNS) disturbances such as somnolence, sleep disorders, hallucinations, headache, and confusion. These adverse effects are more prevalent with tolcapone. Additionally, tolcapone has a black box warning for hepatotoxicity and requires written consent for its use as well as liver function tests every 2 to 4 weeks for the first 6 months of therapy and periodically thereafter.

Interactions. Because COMTIs commonly cause CNS disturbances, they should be used with caution with other CNS depressants. The bioavailability of tolcapone is decreased by 10% to 20% when taken with food. Therefore, it should be administered at least 1 hour before or 2 hours after meals.

Selecting the Most Appropriate Drug
There are no pharmacologic agents that provide disease-modifying or neuroprotective effects; therefore, therapy selection is based on symptoms causing the greatest disability, age, comorbidities, and side effect profile (Goetz & Pal, 2014). Patients requiring therapy for mild motor symptoms should be started first on a MAO-B inhibitor before trying a DA or levodopa due to the increased risk of major adverse drug events with the latter agents. Patients who are experiencing moderate to severe impairment will usually be initiated on a DA or levodopa. Although levodopa is more efficacious than a DA and is associated with less hallucinations, somnolence, and ICDs, DAs have a decreased risk of dyskinesia. DAs are typically chosen over levodopa in younger patients, because the onset of PD at a younger age is a risk factor for developing dyskinesia (Connolly & Lang, 2014). Careful consideration must be given to the patient's age, level of disability, treatment goals, and potential for late complications of dyskinesia and hallucinations before starting levodopa (Goetz & Pal, 2014).

The stepwise treatment approach for PD is dependent on the symptom that is causing the greatest disability. An algorithm that outlines treatment options deemed first-, second-, and third-line therapies for treating PD is shown in **Figure 38.2**.

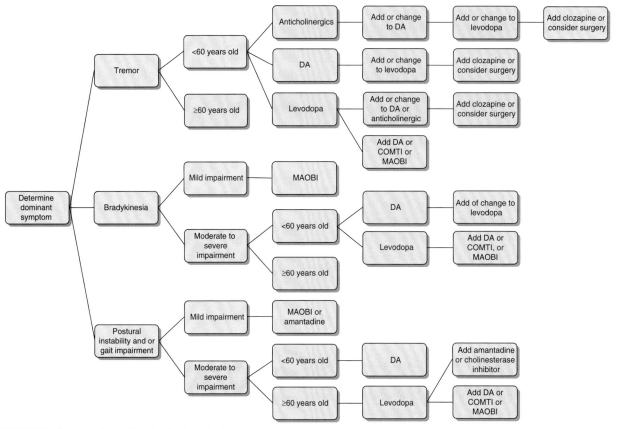

FIGURE 38–2   Treatment algorithm for Parkinson's disease.

COMTI, catechol-*O*-methyltransferase inhibitors; DA, dopamine agonists; MAOBI, monoamine oxidase type B inhibitors.

If symptoms are uncontrolled on an adequate trial of therapy and if there were other treatment options listed in the previous step, all of those alternative agents should be tried before moving to the next step in the algorithm. For a patient with a suboptimal benefit, defined as an improvement in symptoms yet still experiencing bothersome or disabling symptoms, the current medication dose should be increased until maximized before moving to the next step in the algorithm. If the patient is not experiencing any improvement with the medication, the agent should be discontinued and an agent listed in the next step should be initiated (Connolly & Lang, 2014).

Considerations with Mild- and Moderate-Potency Agents

Because of the cognitive side effects associated with anticholinergics and the conflicting evidence related to efficacy, the use of these agents is generally avoided. In younger patients presenting with tremor and fatigue, amantadine should be chosen over MAO-B inhibitors. However, MAO-B inhibitors are favored over amantadine in older patients and those with renal dysfunction. Selegiline may be preferred over rasagiline if cost or a positive urine test for amphetamine is a concern (Goetz & Pal, 2014).

Considerations with Moderate-Potency Agents

Cost and convenience typically direct the selection of a therapeutic option because there is no strong evidence of any agent being more effective than another in this class. Since most adverse drug effects are class effects, switching to another agent within the same class is unlikely to alleviate the problem. If adherence is an issue, selecting an ER formulation is recommended. The transdermal DA can reduce the risk of food or drug interactions within the GI system (Goetz & Pal, 2014).

Considerations with High-Potency Agents

The IR formulation is most effective particularly in early PD, since the other formulations have a more variable absorption rate, resulting in a less predictable improvement in symptoms. Patients having difficulty with nighttime mobility may benefit from the CR formulation because the peak concentration is lower, causing less insomnia (Goetz & Pal, 2014).

Other Considerations

Mild- and even moderate-potency agents may not be the most appropriate choice for employed patients, regardless of symptom severity, since they can take several weeks to see the full effect, whereas levodopa has a rapid onset of action (Goetz & Pal, 2014).

For patients who experience the "wearing-off" phenomena, a few recommended management strategies include increasing the dose of the dopaminergic agent, adding on another dopaminergic medication, increasing the number of daily administrations, or adding a MAO-B or COMTI. Studies have compared the effectiveness of adding a MAO-B or COMTI, which have concluded that both therapeutic options similarly reduce "wearing-off" time (e.g., Connolly & Lang, 2014).

Special Considerations

Geriatric

A DA used as monotherapy can cause confusion and psychosis in older patients and should be avoided, especially in patients with dementia. Geriatric patients, specifically those with cognitive dysfunction, are at the greatest risk for developing psychiatric adverse drug events and may benefit more from levodopa than a DA. Adverse effects of anticholinergics contribute to poor tolerability of this class of medications, and it is therefore not recommended in older patients (Connolly & Lang, 2014).

Advanced Therapies for Motor Symptoms

Deep brain stimulation and MRI-guided focused ultrasound may be beneficial in patients who are responsive to medications but experience "off" periods or dyskinesia or patients who do not respond well to pharmacotherapy. Both therapies require specialty center assessments to determine patient eligibility. Deep brain stimulation requires surgery to place unilateral or bilateral leads in the subthalmic nucleus or the globus pallidus interna, and patients must attend programming visits to optimize stimulation parameters and medications. MRI-guided ultrasound is useful for tremor-predominant PD, which uses highly focused ultrasound beams to burn the thalamus under MRI to target and monitor the lesion (Armstrong & Okun, 2020).

Genomics

As mentioned previously, there is a genetic link in the development of PD. Researchers have identified more than 23 genetic risk factors contributing to PD, including five "PARK" genes (Deng et al., 2018). Because of this discovery, it is hypothesized that pharmacogenomics is going to play a huge role in emerging therapies for PD. One particular area of clinical development is using viral vectors to silence overexpressing genes that contribute to PD (Axelsen & Woldbye, 2018).

Treatment of Selected Nonmotor Symptoms

Psychological Symptoms

Psychological symptoms include depression, psychosis, and dementia, which occur in about 25%, 55%, and 80% of patients, respectively (Connolly & Lang, 2014). Evidence in the literature for treating depression in PD is conflicting. Pramipexole and venlafaxine have been shown to be efficacious, while tricyclic antidepressants and dopaminergic drugs have been labeled as likely efficacious. There is unsatisfactory evidence to support the use of other agents, including SSRIs, MAO-B inhibitors, omega-3 fatty acids, atomoxetine, and nefazodone. Clozapine and quetiapine have the most evidence to support their use in psychosis. Quetiapine is typically preferred, due to the agranulocytosis and frequent blood-monitoring requirements associated with clozapine. Olanzapine, risperidone, and aripiprazole should not be used in PD because they do not reduce the incidence of hallucinations and actually increase the risk of motor deterioration. Donepezil, rivastigmine, and ziprasidone were also shown to be effective in reducing hallucinations. Patients with PD often develop cognitive impairment due to cholinergic dysfunction. Rivastigmine and donepezil have been shown to have some degree of cognitive improvement with PD related dementia; however, larger studies are needed to confirm their effect (Szeto & Lewis, 2016).

Sleep Problems

Insomnia, involving difficulty with initiation, duration, and/or maintenance of sleep, is the most common sleep disorder that affects patients with PD. Only the short-term treatment of insomnia in PD has been assessed with agents, including carbidopa/levodopa, rotigotine, eszopiclone, melatonin, and modafinil. Of these agents, rotigotine has been deemed possibly useful. Similarly, only short-term studies have evaluated the treatment of fatigue in PD with modafinil and methylphenidate, which have inconclusive efficacy (Seppi et al., 2019).

Autonomic or Other Problems

A patient with PD should be regularly evaluated for orthostatic hypotension, as it can be a significant issue in PD. Hypotension is not only a nonmotor symptom; it is also an adverse effect of some PD drugs. This can complicate the treatment of hypertension in a patient with PD, so it is essential to monitor supine blood pressure in these patients. Fludrocortisone, midodrine, and indomethacin have been shown to be mildly effective at treating hypotension in patients with PD, with droxidopa being efficacious for short-term use. Drooling can be an embarrassing nonmotor symptom that may affect patients with PD. Sublingual atropine drops, glycopyrrolate, and botulinum toxin injections can aid in reducing drooling symptoms. Constipation is a significant problem in patients with PD. Not only can it be very uncomfortable for the patient, but over time, it can also lead to more serious complications, such as bowel obstruction, if left untreated (Connolly & Lang, 2014). To alleviate symptoms of constipation, stimulant laxatives and stool softeners can be utilized.

MONITORING PATIENT RESPONSE

The monitoring of patient response is multifactorial, considering the broad range of associated symptoms. The previously mentioned scales, such as MDS-UPDRS, can be used to assess disability and impairment, including motor and nonmotor symptoms, complications, and impact on daily living (Goetz et al., 2008). Monitoring plans should engage patients and caregivers, and symptom journals might help provide therapy-guiding information. It is important to establish appropriate therapy expectations early on, so that patients and caregivers understand the progressive nature of PD and which symptoms may be more likely to respond to drug therapy. Patient responses to varying medication doses, presence of dyskinesia, "on" and "off" times, dizziness, nausea, visual hallucinations, "wearing-off" effects, falls, sleep disturbances, abnormal behaviors, and mood or memory changes should be recorded and discussed. Practitioners should ensure that the patient and caregivers understand the prescribed medication regimen, and administration instructions and treatment adherence should be gauged. Practitioners should evaluate and remedy adherence barriers, such as cost, adverse effects, regimen convenience, or understanding of regimen. Additionally, all health care professionals should monitor for drugs that can exacerbate parkinsonism or cognitive ability.

PATIENT EDUCATION

For a patient with PD, navigating a complex daily routine of medications and symptom management can be challenging. Patient needs and priorities will continue to change throughout disease progression, and it is important that patients have access to accurate, reliable information that is conveyed in understandable terms.

Drug Information

The MDS released evidence-based medicine review updates for motor and nonmotor symptoms of PD (Fox et al., 2018; Seppi et al., 2019). A recent review of pharmacological treatment of PD written by Connolly et al. was published in the *Journal of the American Medical Association* in 2014 (Connolly & Lang, 2014). This publication contains several figures, tables, and algorithms that clarify the complex approaches to the medication management of PD. The American Academy of Neurology (AAN, 2015) lists current guidelines and tools for both health care professionals and patients.

Patient-Oriented Information Sources

Organizations that provide patient-oriented information sources include the American Academy of Neurology, Parkinson's Disease Foundation, and Michael J. Fox Foundation for Parkinson's Research. The National Parkinson Foundation offers several publications, including manuals and checklists. This Web site also offers a smartphone application and allows patients to search for local chapters by indicating their state or zip code. The American Parkinson Disease Association also offers many patient-oriented publications, including books, educational supplements, and brochures. The U.S. Department of Transportation has a posting on their Web site entitled "Driving When You Have Parkinson's Disease."

Nutrition/Lifestyle Changes

Nutrition and lifestyle considerations will vary based on patient-specific factors and should complement drug therapy. In more advanced stages of PD, patients may have speech or swallowing difficulties. Dysarthria is a motor speech disorder comprised of an assortment of speech characteristics. Speech therapy may show benefit with some symptoms of dysarthria, specifically with reduced vocal volume, imprecise articulation, and monotony of both pitch and loudness. Other elements of dysarthria, including hoarseness, may not improve. Speech therapy can also focus on drooling and swallowing issues,

which can include slowed chewing, choking on liquids, and inability to eat food of various consistencies. The Lee Silverman Voice Treatment can have positive effects on voice quality, respiration, articulation, and even swallowing (McDonnell et al., 2018). For patients with swallowing issues, a speech therapist can provide individualized dietary recommendations and recommend appropriate management strategies.

Patients may also have to manage bowel irregularities, which may develop with disease progression or as a result of medication side effects. For constipation, patients can make dietary adjustments to help alleviate this symptom. Increased fluid intake and consumption of high-fiber foods, such as fruits, vegetables, whole grains, beans, and prunes, can be helpful in maintaining bowel regularity. If dietary measures are insufficient in managing constipation, patients can use pharmacological agents, as mentioned previously.

Additional medication side effects that may require management include nausea and loss of appetite. These side effects may diminish over time, but patients can take some medications with a small snack to alleviate discomfort, initially. Other nutrition-related medication considerations involve treatment with levodopa. As mentioned previously, high-protein meals can decrease the effectiveness of levodopa. Patients should not aim to eliminate dietary protein but can instead limit protein portions to 3 to 4 ounces per meal, which is approximately the size of a bar of soap or a deck of cards. Additionally, patients should separate the administration of levodopa from meals, as described previously, and could shift protein consumption to the evening. Iron supplements may also decrease levodopa absorption, so patients should separate these by at least 2 hours. Long-term effects of altered diets should be carefully considered, along with the possible inconveniences.

Patients taking MAO-B inhibitors such as rasagiline, selegiline, and safinamide should avoid or limit tyramine-rich foods, as this can increase the risk of serotonin syndrome. These include aged cheeses, soybean products, red wine, tap beer, and cured, fermented, or air-dried meats or fish. Patients should work with nutritionists or dieticians when making significant dietary adjustments.

It is important for patients with PD to maintain bone density, as these individuals may be at a higher risk for developing osteoporosis and may also have an increased fall risk due to motor symptoms, which can result in fractures. Adults over 50 years of age should incorporate calcium-rich products, such as low-fat milk or yogurt or hard cheeses. Patients should also consume vitamin D in the form of fortified dairy or juice products, egg yolks, breakfast cereal, or fatty fish, such as salmon, trout, mackerel, tuna, and eel. A 3-ounce salmon fillet contains approximately 450 IU of vitamin D. Sun exposure can increase vitamin D, although this should be balanced with the risk for skin cancer. Weight-bearing exercise can also contribute to the maintenance of bone health.

In addition to fortifying bones, high-intensity resistance exercises can improve muscle force production and mobility. A variety of exercise regimens have been studied, including progressive resistance exercise, which has a proposed impact on the mechanisms impacting bradykinesia and muscle weakness.

Physical therapy is also beneficial in improving mobility and strengthening muscles for patients with PD. Benefits of physiotherapy have been described in six core areas: (1) gait; (2) transfers, such as rising from a chair or rolling over in bed; (3) balance; (4) body posture; (5) reaching and grasping; and (6) physical inactivity (Fox et al., 2018).

There appears to be insufficient evidence to support or refute the use of acupuncture; biofeedback; manual therapy, including chiropractic and osteopathic manipulation; or Alexander technique, which involves the development of awareness of posture in order to make improvements. However, this may result from a general lack of conducted studies (Dong et al., 2016). These therapies are unlikely to induce harm, and patients may find them helpful in the establishment of a holistic PD management plan. Examples of other complementary therapies include tai chi to improve balance, qigong to help patients focus on breathing patterns, meditation and massage to help with relaxation, and acupuncture to help with sleep disturbances. The extent of benefit may vary among patients, but patients should be encouraged to work with their health care team to individualize and optimize their PD management strategies.

Complementary and Alternative Medications

Several nonstandard pharmacologic and nonpharmacologic therapies have been explored in patients with PD. The seeds of the *Mucuna pruriens* plant contain levodopa.

Although several small trials demonstrated effectiveness, the American Academy of Neurology concluded that there is currently insufficient evidence to support or refute the use of *M. pruriens* (AAN, 2015). *Vicia faba*, also known as fava beans, has also been shown to contain a minimal amount of levodopa and have been suggested for short-term benefit in PD, but evidence is lacking for the benefit of this product in PD.

In the early stages of PD, creatine has been explored as an option to strengthen muscles and slow the progression of PD; however, its benefit has not been demonstrated with this product. Neuroprotective effects of vitamin E at doses of 2,000 IU and coenzyme Q10 at doses ranging from 300 to 2,400 mg/d have been studied, but effectiveness has not been demonstrated for either supplement.

For patients experiencing orthostatic hypotension, increasing salt and fluid consumption, along with elevating the head of the bed, and wearing compression stockings can be beneficial. Rapid consumption of two 8-ounce glasses of cold water can also result in a prompt response.

A successful PD treatment approach, management strategy, and monitoring plan should ideally incorporate a complete team of interprofessional experts. This team may include primary care and specialist physicians, pharmacists, nurse practitioners, nurses, physician assistants, psychologists, occupational therapists, physical therapists, speech language pathologists, nutritionists, dieticians, social workers, chaplains, and others.

CASE STUDY 1

T.K. is a 62-year-old woman with a past medical history of bipolar disorder, hypertension, and diabetes, for which she takes lithium, valproic acid, lisinopril, and metformin. She states that she was diagnosed a week ago with dyslipidemia but is currently trying to control it with a strict diet. She presents to the clinic with feeling much weaker and has noticed increased arm tremors while she is resting after performing household duties for the past few months. Upon examination, it is found that she is able to walk with a normal gait, which she describes as "slow" for her, and has a slight tremor in her arms at rest, which persists with movement. She states her friend was recently diagnosed with Parkinson's disease (PD) and thinks she may have it as well.

1. What is the *most* appropriate first step in evaluating T.K. for PD?
   a. Diagnose her for PD as she meets criteria for diagnosis
   b. Perform a Movement Disorder Society–sponsored revision of the Unified Parkinson's Disease Rating Scale to establish a baseline score of disability and impairment.
   c. Rule out other causes of possible tremor and weakness.
   d. Perform a dopamine transporter imaging test.

2. What is the *most* appropriate recommendation for T.K.?
   a. Initiate selegiline 5 mg twice daily and reassess in 2 weeks.
   b. Perform genetic testing for disease-causing genes for PD.
   c. Perform laboratory testing for routine labs and therapeutic drug levels.
   d. Encourage increased nutritional intake and reassess in 2 weeks.

T.K. returns to the clinic 2 weeks later. Her laboratory results reveal elevated low-density lipoprotein and triglycerides, as well as elevated lithium and valproic acid levels. Her psychiatrist has since decreased the dosages of her lithium and valproic acid. She is still concerned about PD and asks if there is anything she can do to prevent it from developing.

3. What is the *most* appropriate initial therapy for T.K.?
   a. Initiate atorvastatin 10 mg daily.
   b. Encourage weight-bearing exercises to increase strength.
   c. Increase calcium and vitamin D dietary intake.
   d. All of the above.

Bibliography

Starred references are cited in the text.

Abbvie Inc. (2019). DUOPA (carbidopa and levodopa) enteral suspension: Highlights of prescribing information. North Chicago, IL: Author.

Ahmed, H., Abushouk, A. I., Gabi, M., et al. (2017). Parkinson's disease and pesticides: A meta-analysis of disease connection and genetic alterations. *Biomedicine & Pharmacotherapy, 90,* 638–649.

*American Academy of Neurology. (2015). Practice guidelines: Movement disorders. Retrieved from https://www.aan.com on January 20, 2020.

American Parkinson's Disease Association. (2020). Download publications. Retrieved from http://www.apdaparkinson.org/resources-support/download-publications on January 20, 2020.

*Armstrong, M. J., & Okun, M. S. (2020). Diagnosis and treatment of Parkinson disease: A review. *Journal of the American Medical Association, 323*(6), 548–560.

*Ascherio, A., & Schwarzschild, M. A. (2016). The epidemiology of Parkinson's disease: Risk factors and prevention. *Lancet, 15,* 1257–1272.

*Axelsen, T. M., & Woldbye, D. P. (2018). Gene therapy for Parkinson's disease, an update. *Journal of Parkinson's Disease, 8,* 195–215.

*Badoud, S., Nicastro, N., Garibotto, V., et al. (2016). Distinct spatiotemporal patterns for disease duration and stage in Parkinson's disease. *European Journal of Nuclear Medicine and Molecular Imaging, 43,* 509–516.

Berardelli, A., Wenning, G. K., Antonini, A., et al. (2013). EFNS/MDS-ES/ENS [corrected] recommendations for the diagnosis of Parkinson's disease. *European Journal of Neurology, 20*(1), 16–34.

*Bette, S., Shpiner, D. S., Singer, C., et al. (2018). Safinamide in the management of patients with Parkinson's disease not stabilized on levodopa: A review of the current clinical evidence. *Therapeutics and Clinical Risk Management, 14,* 1737–1745.

Chen, Y., Yang, W., Long, J., et al. (2015). Discriminative analysis of Parkinson's disease based on whole-brain functional connectivity. *PLoS One, 10*(4), e0124153.

*Connolly, B. S., & Lang, A. E. (2014). Pharmacological treatment of Parkinson disease: A review. *Journal of the American Medical Association, 311*(16), 1670–1683.

*Deng, H., Wang, P., & Jankovic, J. (2018). The genetics of Parkinson disease. *Ageing Research Reviews, 42,* 72–85.

Dibble, L. E., Foreman, K. B., Addison, O., et al. (2015). Exercise and medication effects on persons with Parkinson disease across the domains of disability: A randomized clinical trial. *Journal of Neurologic Physical Therapy, 39,* 85–92.

*Dong, J., Cui, Y., & Le, W. (2016). Current pharmaceutical treatments and alternative therapies of Parkinson's disease. *Current Neuropharmacology, 14,* 339–355.

Drug Information Handbook (2019–2020, 28th ed.). Hudson, OH: Lexicomp, Inc.

*Fox, S. H., Katzenschlager, R., Lim, S. Y., et al. (2018). International Parkinson and movement disorder society evidence-based medicine review: Update on treatments for the motor symptoms of Parkinson's disease. *Movement Disorders, 33*(8), 1248–1266.

*Goetz, C. G., & Pal, G. (2014). Initial management of Parkinson's disease. *British Medical Journal, 349,* g6258.

*Goetz, C. G., Tilley, B. C., Shaftman, S. R., et al. (2008). Movement Disorder Society-sponsored revision of the Unified Parkinson's Disease Rating Scale (MDS-UPDRS): Scale presentation and clinimetric testing results. *Movement Disorders, 23*(15), 2129–2170.

*Grimes, D., Fitzpatrick, M., Gordon, J., et al. (2019). Canadian guideline for Parkinson disease. *Canadian Medical Association Journal, 191*(36), E989–E1004.

*Halliday, G., McCann, H., & Shepherd, C. (2012). Evaluation of the Braak hypothesis: How far can it explain the pathogenesis of Parkinson's disease? *Expert Review of Neurotherapeutics, 12*(6), 673–686.

*Marras, C., Beck, J. C., Bower, J. H., et al. (2018). Prevalence of Parkinson's disease across North America. *NPJ Parkinson's Disease, 4*(21), 1–21.

*Marras, C., Canning, C. G., & Goldman, S. M. (2019). Environment, lifestyle, and Parkinson's disease: Implications for prevention in the next decade. *Movement Disorders, 34*(6), 801–811.

*McDonnell, M. N., Rischbieth, B., Schammer, T. T., et al. (2018). Lee Silverman Voice Treatment (LSVT)-BIG to improve motor function in people with Parkinson's disease: A systematic review and meta-analysis. *Clinical Rehabilitation, 32*(5), 607–618.

Michael J. Fox Foundation. (2020a). Diet & nutrition. Retrieved from https://www.michaeljfox.org/news/diet-nutrition on January 20, 2020.

Michael J. Fox Foundation. (2020b). Parkinson's books and resources. Retrieved from https://www.michaeljfox.org/books-resources on January 20, 2020.

*Moors, T. E., Hoozemans, J. J., Ingrassia, A., et al. (2017). Therapeutic potential of autophagy- enhancing agents in Parkinson's disease. *Molecular Neurodegeneration, 12*(11), 1–18.

Movement Disorder Society-sponsored revision of the Unified Parkinson's Disease Rating Scale (MDS-UPDRS). (2008). Retrieved from https://www.movementdisorders.org/MDS-Files1/PDFs/Rating-Scales/MDS-UPDRS_English_FINAL_Updated_August2019.pdf on January 20, 2020.

*National Institute for Health and Care Excellence. (2017). Parkinson's disease in adults (NICE Guideline 71). Retrieved from www.nice.org.uk/guidance/ng71. Accessed January 20, 2020.

National Parkinson Foundation. (2020). Managing Parkinson's. Retrieved from https://www.parkinson.org/Living-with-Parkinsons/Managing-Parkinsons on January 20, 2020.

*Ossig, C., & Reichmann, H. (2015). Treatment strategies in early and advanced Parkinson disease. *Neurology Clinics, 33,* 19–37.

*Parkinson, J. (1817). *An essay on the shaking palsy.* London, UK: Sherwood, Neely, and Jones. The Journal of Neuropsychiatry and Clinical Neurosciences. Retrieved from https://neuro.psychiatryonline.org/doi/full/10.1176/jnp.14.2.223 on January 20, 2020.

*Postuma, R. B., Berg, D., Stern M., et al. (2015). MDS clinical diagnostic criteria for Parkinson's disease. *Movement Disorders, 30*(12), 1591–1599.

*Reich, S. G., & Savitt, J. M. (2019). Parkinson's disease. *Medical Clinics of North America, 103,* 337–350.

*Seppi, K., Chaudhuri, K. R., Coelho, M., et al. (2019). Update on treatments for nonmotor symptoms of Parkinson's disease: An evidence-based medicine review. *Movement Disorders, 34*(2), 180–198.

*Shin, H. W., & Chung, J. S. (2012). Drug-induced parkinsonism. *Journal of Clinical Neurology, 8*(1), 15–21.

*Stocchi, F., Vacca, L., & Radicati, F G. (2015). How to optimize the treatment of early stage Parkinson's disease. *Translational Neurodegeneration, 4*(4), 1–7.

Subramanian, I. (2017). Complementary and alternative medicine and exercise in nonmotor symptoms of Parkinson's disease. *International Review of Neurobiology, 134,* 1163–1188.

*Szeto, J. Y., & Lewis, S. J. (2016). Current treatment options for Alzheimer's disease and Parkinson's disease dementia. *Current Neuropharmacology, 14,* 326–338.

U.S. Department of Health and Human Services, National Institute of Neurologic Disorders and Stroke. (2019). NINDS Parkinson's disease information page. Retrieved from https://www.ninds.nih.gov/disorders/all-disorders/parkinsons-disease-information-page on January 20, 2020.

U.S. Department of Transportation. (2015). Driving when you have Parkinson's disease. Retrieved from https://www.nhtsa.gov/sites/nhtsa.dot.gov/files/10900f-drivewell-handout-parkinsons.pdf on January 20, 2020.

*VanderHorst, V. G., Samardzic, T., Saper, C. B., et al. (2015). α-Synuclein pathology accumulates in sacral spinal visceral sensory pathways. *Annals of Neurology, 78*(1), 142–149. doi: 10.1002/ana.24430

Verschuur, C. V., Suwijn, S. R., Boel, K. A., et al. (2019). Randomized delayed-start trial of levodopa in Parkinson's disease. *New England Journal of Medicine, 380*(4), 315–324.

*Yomtoob, J., Koloms, K., & Bega, D. (2018). DAT-SPECT imaging in cases of drug-induced parkinsonism in a specialty movement disorders practice. *Parkinsonism and Related Disorders, 53,* 37–41.

Pharmacotherapy for Mental Health Disorders

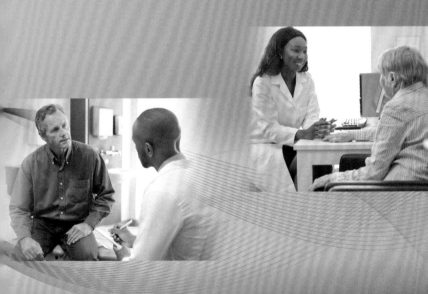

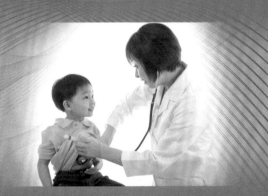

39 Major Depressive Disorder and Bipolar Disorders

Priya M. Shah

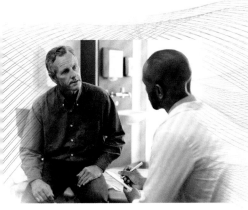
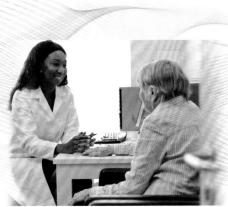
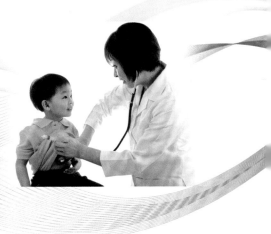

Learning Objectives

1. Select appropriate nonpharmacologic and/or pharmacologic therapy for a patient with major depressive disorder.
2. List adverse drug events, contraindications, and significant counseling points for common antidepressants.
3. Identify lifestyle modifications that can be implemented by a patient with major depressive disorder.
4. List adverse drug events, contraindications, and significant counseling points for common agents used in the management of bipolar disorder.

INTRODUCTION

Major depressive disorder (MDD) is a mood disorder characterized by alterations in cognition, behavior, and physical functioning. It is a constellation of symptoms that interfere with normal function and may render an individual unable to perform psychologically, emotionally, and cognitively at previously attainable levels. The cardinal symptoms associated with a depressive episode are depressed mood, sadness, hopelessness, sleep disturbance, change in appetite and weight, loss of interest, guilt, difficulty concentrating, and suicidal ideation. Further delineated by its recurrence and chronicity, depression results in functional impairment in multiple life domains and is a leading predictor of worsened morbidity and mortality. The clinical course is further complicated by the strong correlation of depression to psychiatric and physical comorbidity.

It is estimated that MDD affects 151 million individuals worldwide. Findings from a national survey published in 2018 demonstrated that among 36,309 U.S. adults, there was a 20.6% lifetime prevalence of MDD (Hasin et al., 2018).

In the United States, mental health and substance abuse disorders exceed $190 billion in yearly spending (Dieleman et al., 2016). Initial onset of depression may occur at any time throughout life; however, the peak onset is considered to be during the fourth decade of life. Earlier onset of presentation is inversely associated with successful treatment outcome; younger patients with depression tend to have a more severe and complicated clinical course with less likelihood of remission and an increased likelihood of recurrence. Today, although 80% to 90% of those affected can be treated effectively, only one third seek treatment.

CAUSES

A single causative factor for the development of depression has not been elucidated. Rather, the development of depression is thought to be a multifactorial, complicated interplay among numerous physiologic, social, genetic, environmental, and biochemical factors. First-degree relatives of an individual with MDD have a 2.8 times greater relative risk of developing MDD than the general population. More than 50% of patients who have experienced one episode of major depression will experience a second, and over 80% of patients who experience a second episode will experience a third.

PATHOPHYSIOLOGY

Most current research focuses on neurochemical aspects of depression and has spurred several theories relating to the generation and maintenance of specific neurotransmitters in the central nervous system (CNS). The basis for these neurochemical theories is the hypothesis that abnormal neurotransmitter release or decreased postsynaptic receptor sensitivity is affected before and during a major depressive episode. At least four theories relate to this hypothesis (**Box 39.1**). Three of the four theories focus on a functional or absolute deficiency in the neurotransmitters serotonin, norepinephrine, or both. A functional deficiency suggests that neurotransmitters are produced but the postsynaptic receptors cannot fully transmit the neural impulse. This is in contrast to an absolute deficiency in which no neurotransmitters are produced or the postsynaptic receptors cannot transmit the signal at all.

Similar to the theories associated with the monoamine catecholamines norepinephrine and serotonin, new evidence suggests that dopamine may play a significant role in the pathogenesis and symptomatology of MDD. Genetic polymorphisms in the genes associated with dopamine transmission may contribute to an increased susceptibility to depression. Deficits in dopamine release or transmission have been linked to dysphoria, one of the most prominent features of MDD. The permissive hypothesis, a more contemporary theory, suggests that reduced serotonin activity sets the stage for a mood disorder, such as depression or mania, depending on the underlying norepinephrine level. A low serotonin level coupled with a low norepinephrine level suggests that depression results from an increased beta-adrenergic receptor sensitivity. This alteration in postsynaptic receptor sensitivity results in an imbalance between the effects of norepinephrine and serotonin and may

create a functional deficiency in serotonin. Secondary to the interplay among the catecholamines within the monoaminergic network, any impact on one of the monoamines will likely impact the others. This is applicable to the predisposition and development of MDD as well as the therapeutics of MDD.

DIAGNOSTIC CRITERIA

Mildly depressed patients meet the minimum criteria for diagnosis, whereas moderately depressed patients display a greater degree of dysfunction. Severely depressed patients experience symptoms well in excess of the diagnostic criteria. Their symptoms often greatly interfere with social and occupational functioning. A 2013 update of the American Psychiatric Association's publication *The Diagnostic and Statistical Manual of Mental Disorders, Fifth Edition* (*DSM-5*), has established criteria for the diagnosis of depression, which are listed in **Box 39.2**. A patient must exhibit at least five of these signs or symptoms in the

---

BOX 39.1 Pathophysiologic Hypotheses of Depression

SEROTONIN HYPOTHESIS

A functional or an absolute deficiency in the neurotransmitter serotonin

CATECHOLAMINE HYPOTHESIS

A functional or an absolute deficiency in the neurotransmitters norepinephrine, serotonin, or dopamine

PERMISSIVE HYPOTHESIS

Diminished serotonin gives "permission" for a superimposed norepinephrine deficiency to manifest as depression

BETA-ADRENERGIC RECEPTOR HYPOTHESIS

Depression results from increased beta-adrenergic receptor sensitivity

---

BOX 39.2 Diagnostic and Statistical Manual of Mental Disorders, Fifth Edition: Criteria for Diagnosing Major Depressive Episode

A. Five (or more) of the following symptoms have been present during the same 2-week period and represent a change from previous functioning. At least one of the symptoms must be #1 or #2.
   1. Depressed mood most of the day. In children or adolescents, the mood can be irritable instead of depressed.
   2. Diminished interest or pleasure in all or almost all of usual activities.
   3. Significant weight loss or weight gain or decrease or increase in appetite.
   4. Insomnia or hypersomnia.
   5. Psychomotor agitation or retardation as observed by others.
   6. Fatigue or loss of energy.
   7. Feelings of worthlessness or excessive or inappropriate guilt.
   8. Diminished ability to think or concentrate, indecisiveness.
   9. Recurrent thoughts of death, suicidal ideation, suicide attempt, or a specific plan for suicide.
B. The symptoms cause clinically significant distress or impairment in social, occupational, or other important areas of functioning.
C. The symptoms are not due to the direct physiologic effects of a substance or a medical condition.

same 2-week period along with symptoms of depressed mood or anhedonia, the inability to gain pleasure from normally pleasurable experiences (American Psychiatric Association, 2013).

In addition to the *DSM-5* diagnostic criteria, numerous rating scales are employed in clinical practice to assess the severity of depression as well as response to treatment. The 17-item Hamilton Depression Scale (HAM-D) and the Beck Depression Inventory (BDI) are clinician-rated scales that are frequently used for this purpose.

Subtypes of MDD delineate the etiology and severity of the illness or episode. These subtypes include mild, moderate, and severe depression. The descriptors (known as *specifiers*) refer to the severity of dysfunction and delineate comorbid or distinguishing features, such as melancholy, catatonia, and psychosis.

TYPES OF DEPRESSION

The *DSM-5* slightly modified the categorization of depressive disorders in its most recent version. MDD and dysthymia are now both included under the singular category of persistent depressive disorder. Dysthymia is a chronic but less severe form of depression that is characterized by 2 years of depressive symptoms and functional impairment. It shared the same common core set of features with MDD and potentially did separate clinically from MDD, which led to its absorption into a larger category and its cessation as an independent diagnosis. The diagnostic criteria for MDD did not change. However, two new specifiers (terms or qualifiers that further narrow the MDD presentation and allow for more tailored treatment based on symptomatology) have been added: "with mixed features," which refers to MDD with the coexistence of at least three manic symptoms not meeting criteria for bipolar disorder, and "with anxious distress," which suggests the presence of an anxious component. Bereavement has been removed as an MDD specifier in the *DSM-5*. The remainder of the depression categories and subtypes remain unchanged. The focus of this chapter will be MDD, as this is the most common presentation; however, the other types are reviewed in the following.

Postpartum Depression

The onset is usually within 6 weeks after childbirth, and symptoms last from 3 to 14 months. Prevalence of postpartum depression ranges from 5.2% to 74% in developed countries (Norhayati et al., 2015). Women with a history of postpartum depression have a 50% risk of recurrence, and 30% of women with a history of depression not related to childbirth have postpartum depression.

Seasonal Affective Disorder

Seasonal affective disorder (SAD) is a pattern of depressive or manic episodes that occurs with the onset of winter. As the days become shorter and the weather colder, there is an increase in depressive symptoms. SAD causes individuals to eat more, sleep more, experience chronic fatigue, and gain weight. In pronounced cases, significant social withdrawal may occur.

Major Depression with Melancholic Features

Melancholic depression is a severe form of depression characterized by a profoundly depressed mood, nonreactivity, and neurovegetative symptoms. This type of depression is markedly more difficult to treat; however, it tends to be highly responsive to drug therapy.

Major Depression with Psychotic Features

Patients suffering from psychotic depression, in addition to the typical depressive symptoms, will also experience mood-congruent delusions and hallucinations.

UTILIZING NONPHARMACOLOGIC THERAPY

Nonpharmacologic therapy for depression includes several psychotherapeutic techniques such as cognitive-behavioral therapy (CBT) and interpersonal therapy (IPT). Psychotherapy is traditionally reserved for patients with concurrent psychosocial stressors. The most common and effective type of psychotherapy, CBT helps to identify and modify dysfunctional thoughts that contribute to depression. It can be administered in individual or group settings and is usually short term.

IPT is a specific intervention studying social issues that can trigger depression. It is similar in structure to CBT. Another type of nonpharmacologic therapy is problem-solving therapy (PST), which focuses on identifying one's personal problems, formulating multiple solutions, choosing a solution to implement, and then reviewing its effectiveness. Meta-analyses that have compared the efficacy of CBT, IPT, and PST show no significant differences among these treatments.

Although psychotherapy alone may be effective, patients meeting the criteria for major depression should be evaluated for medication therapy. Moderately depressed patients often need a combination of medication and psychotherapy. Severely depressed patients may be refractory to psychotherapy, and their risk for suicide should be assessed.

Electroconvulsive therapy (ECT) is another nonpharmacologic treatment modality that consists of delivering brief electrical stimulation pulses to the patient's brain while the patient is maintained under anesthesia. This therapy is often utilized as adjunctive therapy for a variety of psychological illnesses when patients have failed to adequately respond to pharmacologic and psychotherapy. It is also highly effective in patients with severe but uncomplicated MDD, producing significant improvement in up to 80% of patients. Despite reports of favorable outcomes, ECT continues to be one of the most controversial treatment modalities due to the concern about memory loss and confusion that can potentially result from treatment. ECT must be administered in a health care setting under the supervision of trained professionals. Although ECT treatments may be very effective in some patients, ongoing treatment in conjunction with either pharmacologic therapy or repeated sessions is usually required to maintain remission.

INITIATING DRUG THERAPY

The most current guideline for the management of MDD is the American Psychiatric Association's practice guideline for the treatment of patients with MDD, third edition, published in 2010. When prescribing drug therapy, practitioners consider many indicators, among them the severity of symptoms (e.g., mild, moderate, or severe), type of depression (major, acute episode, postpartum, seasonal, dysthymia), duration of therapy, the patient's age, sex, comorbid conditions, and concomitant medications. In addition, if the patient has experienced depressive episodes in the past, the choice of drug may depend on what drug or drug class the patient responded to previously. An abundance of evidence supports the relative efficacy equivalence among antidepressant drug classes. Therefore, selection of the initial drug is generally not based on efficacy but rather on the side-effect profile, patient preference, and target symptoms.

Initial staging of depression severity and ongoing assessment of response to treatment is generally accomplished by utilizing patient- or clinician-rated scales. The 17-item clinician-rated HAM-D is traditionally considered the inventory of choice for monitoring response to therapy. Other tools used in assessing the severity or source of depression include a typical health and medication history. Also useful is a physical examination with documentation of the patient's height, weight, and pertinent laboratory test findings, such as a complete blood count with differential, electrolytes, and kidney and liver function. Caution must be exercised in diagnosing MDD since certain medications and illnesses can induce depression. These conditions must be ruled out prior to making the diagnosis (**Box 39.3**).

Goals of Drug Therapy

Although historically, nearly unattainable secondary to poor tolerability of available drugs, the ultimate goal of therapy for depression is *remission* and resolution of residual symptoms. A *response* to therapy, defined as a 50% reduction in the HAM-D score from baseline, was previously accepted as an appropriate therapeutic outcome. However, with the advent of newer and more tolerable drug therapies, the paradigm has shifted such that full remission is considered the only acceptable goal of therapy. Remission represents a complete resolution of depressive symptoms and a full return to previous level of functioning. Patients who have remitted will no longer fulfill the *DSM-5* diagnostic criteria for depression and will score 7 or below on the HAM-D (consistent with normal).

Residual symptoms refer to symptomatology suggestive of depression that persists after a response to treatment. Even upon a successful course of treatment and clinical remission, some patients may continue to experience cognitive depressive symptoms, such as forgetfulness or apathy, or physical symptoms like fatigue. Patients who do not remit or who continue to have residual symptoms are at a greater risk

---

BOX 39.3   Selected Conditions and Medications Associated with Depression

Endocrine disorders

Addison's disease
Cushing syndrome
Hypothyroidism

Gastrointestinal disease

Irritable bowel syndrome
Inflammatory bowel disease
Cirrhosis

Infections

AIDS
Influenza
Meningitis

Cardiovascular diseases

Congestive heart failure
Myocardial infarction

Neurologic disorders

Alzheimer's disease
Multiple sclerosis
Parkinson's disease
Stroke
Chronic headache

Cancer
Alcoholism
Drug use

Alcohol
Antihypertensives
    Reserpine
    Methyldopa
    Diuretics
    Propranolol
    Clonidine
Oral contraceptives
Steroids

Rheumatologic

Systemic lupus erythematosus
Chronic fatigue syndrome
Fibromyalgia
Rheumatoid arthritis

---

for relapse or recurrence, have a shorter duration between depressive episodes, and have a worsened overall mortality. Optimal drug therapy not only resolves the acute symptoms of depression but also reduces the risk of relapse (American Psychiatric Association, 2010).

MONITORING PATIENT RESPONSE

Drug therapy for depression consists of three phases: acute, continuation, and maintenance. Usually, the patient needs additional contact with the practitioner or other health care provider (psychologist, social worker) during all phases of drug therapy. Assessments of efficacy, side effects, and adherence to the drug regimen should be made weekly, if possible.

Acute Treatment Phase

The goal of drug therapy in the acute treatment phase is to treat the patient until full remission and a return to the premorbid level of function. The duration of this phase is 6 to 8 weeks and potentially up to 12 weeks with apparent improvements occurring within the first 1 to 2 weeks. Though some clinicians attribute early response to a placebo effect, there is a preponderance of evidence that supports a true therapeutic effect within the first 14 days. In fact, newer research suggests that improvement by week 2 of therapy is a highly sensitive predictor of eventual response and remission.

Patients should have frequent contact with their practitioner throughout therapy, but especially in the first few weeks. Lack of efficacy early on may negatively impact patient adherence and motivation. Early improvements tend to include sleep satisfaction, appetite normalization, and recovery of cognitive function. Eventually, patients will experience an elevation in mood and resolution of anhedonia. Full assessment of the effects of the antidepressant should occur at the 4- to 6-week interval after drug therapy begins. At this point, the practitioner evaluates improvements in the target signs and symptoms, assesses adverse drug effects, and determines whether dosage increases or decreases are necessary. To assist the evaluation, several depression rating scales, such as the HAM-D, the Zung Self-Rating Scale for Depression, and the BDI, may again be used as an objective measure of the change, or lack thereof, in a depressive state.

Continuation Phase

The continuation phase represents the time after a treatment response is seen in the acute phase and usually lasts 9 months to 1 year. The practitioner should continue antidepressant therapy for 4 to 6 months after symptom resolution. Failure to continue medication beyond symptom resolution confers an increased risk of relapse. When therapy is eventually discontinued, the medication is typically tapered over a few weeks to avoid physical or psychological effects that occur with abrupt discontinuation of the medication (discontinuation syndrome). During this time, the patient should be monitored closely for reemergence of symptoms.

Maintenance Phase

For some patients, long-term or even indefinite therapy is indicated. Maintenance therapy should be considered in all patients with three or more prior episodes or any patient with two episodes within the past 5 years, a comorbid substance abuse or anxiety disorder, a family history of recurrent depression, or onset of depression earlier than age 20 or later than age 40. This phase of therapy uses the same effective antidepressant used during the acute and continuation phases for a minimum of 3 and up to 5 years or longer. The risk for recurrence increases with every subsequent episode of depression (Bulloch et al., 2014). Patients who have had two or more episodes of depression are candidates for indefinite antidepressant therapy.

Modification of Drug Therapy

Despite the availability of pharmacologic therapies for depression and the relative equivalence in efficacy among the classes, approximately 50% of patients will not respond to the first trial of a first-line antidepressant (American Psychiatric Association, 2010). Overall response rates to antidepressants in general are 50% to 75%. As evidenced by the pivotal STAR*D trial, subsequent trials of alternate medications after the initial failure yield success rates of 20% with a gradual decrease in rates of response and remission with each trial. Only about one third of patients will remit after the first trial, and almost 30% of patients will not remit even after a series of sequential therapies (Papakostas, 2009; Rush et al., 2003).

Initiation of an appropriate drug at an optimal dose, giving the drug an adequate trial (6 to 12 weeks), and educating the patient about the time frame for response and the importance of adherence are critically essential therapeutic concepts. If the patient is started on an appropriate drug for an adequate period, has been compliant with therapy, and does not respond or remit in a reasonable amount of time, drug therapy may need to be adjusted.

There are four common strategies used to modify drug therapy in the depressed patient: dosage increase/optimization, switching to a different drug within the same class or switching to a drug in a different class, augmenting the current drug, or combining medications. Increasing the dose of a drug is typically recommended if the patient has had a response or a partial response during the first few weeks. If an inadequate response or lack of response occurs within the first few weeks of therapy, a switch to a different drug may be warranted. Within-class and between-class switches are viable options depending upon the patient presentation. Lack of response to one drug within a class does not necessarily confer lack of response to all drugs within a class; therefore, switching within a class may be appropriate. Augmentation of the initial drug preserves any benefit experienced by the patient during the trial and also targets side effects or residual symptoms. The combination of two or more drugs with differing mechanisms of action has also been shown to be efficacious.

Antidepressant Drugs

Several drug classes are available for treating depression: selective serotonin reuptake inhibitors (SSRIs), serotonin norepinephrine reuptake inhibitors (SNRIs), tricyclic antidepressants (TCAs), monoamine oxidase (MAO) inhibitors, and atypical agents. They all exert a pharmacologic effect by impacting one or more of the primary neurotransmitters theorized to contribute to depression. In theory, each of the antidepressants increases the relative amount of neurotransmitter available in the synapse, either by inhibiting its metabolic degradation or by decreasing the rate at which it is recycled (by the process called *reuptake*) back into the presynaptic neuron (**Figure 39.1**). For example, SSRIs inhibit the reuptake of select isoforms of serotonin, thereby increasing the functional availability of serotonin in the synaptic cleft. SNRIs increase the relative concentrations of both serotonin and norepinephrine, with more serotonergic or noradrenergic activity depending upon the dose. TCAs are thought to work by inhibiting the reuptake of norepinephrine and serotonin from the synaptic cleft, thereby increasing the amount available to stimulate the postsynaptic neuron. Conversely, MAO inhibitors limit the metabolism of monoamines such as dopamine, serotonin, and norepinephrine. This nonselective inhibition also increases the relative amounts of each of these catecholamines available to stimulate the postsynaptic neurons. However, this nonselectivity may contribute to side effects.

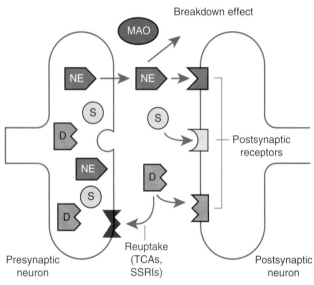

FIGURE 39–1 Schematic representation of the mechanism of action of antidepressant agents. Neurotransmitters (norepinephrine, serotonin, dopamine) are released from the presynaptic neuron into the synaptic space. They interact with the postsynaptic receptors and continue the neuronal transmission. After release from the postsynaptic neuron, these agents can be broken down by the enzyme monoamine oxidase and the components recycled into the presynaptic neuron, or they can be taken up again through the reuptake mechanism. Antidepressant agents can (1) block the monoamine oxidase enzymes and monoamine oxidase inhibitors; (2) inhibit the reuptake of the neurotransmitter; or (3) agonize or antagonize an associated receptor. In effect, each mechanism increases the available concentration of the neurotransmitter.

D, dopamine; MAO, monoamine oxidase; NE, norepinephrine; S, serotonin; SSRI, selective serotonin reuptake inhibitors; TCAs, tricyclic antidepressants.

Table 39.1 presents the antidepressants and the neurotransmitters primarily affected. Because all of these agents appear to have relatively equal efficacy, the practitioner should select the most appropriate initial therapy based on side-effect profiles, predicted patient compliance, and cost of therapy. The following discussion and accompanying tables and charts will help the practitioner in selecting the optimal initial agent for treating depression.

Selective Serotonin Reuptake Inhibitors

The development of SSRIs changed the landscape of depression pharmacotherapy. Just as effective as TCAs and older antidepressants, SSRIs boast improved tolerability and reduced lethality in overdose. The leading cause of death in the depressed patient population is suicide, and therefore utilizing a drug class with minimal risk of successful overdose is paramount. The tolerability profile, relative safety in overdose, and the need for fewer titrations have resulted in SSRIs effectively replacing TCAs as the drug class of choice for treating depression. SSRIs work primarily by binding to the serotonin transporter and inhibiting the reuptake of this neurotransmitter into the presynaptic neurons. Relative efficacy is comparable within the class. **Table 39.2** identifies starting dosages and expected dosage ranges of SSRIs.

Time Frame for Response

The effects of these drugs become apparent within 4 to 6 weeks of treatment. The length of therapy for the first episodes of depression is 4 to 6 months after recovery. Continued treatment beyond the point of recovery drastically reduces the relapse potential over 1 to 3 years. Measures of efficacy include improved scores in the initial rating scales, self-reported improvement in the target symptoms originally described by the patient, and improved affect observed by the practitioner.

Adverse Events

SSRIs are usually administered in the morning because of the potential to induce anxiety and insomnia. Serotonin and serotonin receptors have diverse and variable effects on sleep architecture. SSRI-induced insomnia is thought to be largely related to the suppression of rapid eye movement sleep, which results in an overall decrease in sleep quality and total sleep time. Insomnia that presents as part of the clinical picture of depression itself or that is treatment emergent may be treated with a sedative–hypnotic drug such as a benzodiazepine or a nonbenzodiazepine GABA-A receptor agonist (zolpidem, etc.). Some patients do, however, experience sedation with an SSRI, and these patients may be advised to take their medication at bedtime.

SSRIs have virtually no potential for inducing orthostatic hypotension or cardiac conduction abnormalities, which makes them ideal for older patients or those with a history of arrhythmias. They do have epileptogenic potential, so caution must be used in patients with a history of seizures. Weight gain is another common adverse effect that occurs with various frequencies depending upon the medication. Gastrointestinal (GI)

TABLE 39.1

Classification of Antidepressant Agents and Neurotransmitters Affected

Generic Name	Brand Name	Primary Neurotransmitters Affected		
		NE	5-HT	D
Tricyclic Antidepressants				
Amitriptyline	Elavil	+ + + +	+ + + +	0
Desipramine	Norpramin	+	+ + +	0
Doxepin	Sinequan	+	+ + +	0
Imipramine	Tofranil	+ + +	+ +	0/+
Nortriptyline	Pamelor	+ +	+ + +	0
Protriptyline	Vivactil	+	+ + + +	0
Trimipramine	Surmontil	+ +	+ +	0
Selective Serotonin Reuptake Inhibitors				
Citalopram	Celexa	0	+ + + +	0
Fluoxetine	Prozac	0	+ + + +	0
Fluvoxamine	Luvox	0	+ + + +	
Paroxetine	Paxil	0	+ + + +	0
Sertraline	Zoloft	0	+ + + +	0
Escitalopram	Lexapro	0	+ + + +	0
Serotonin Norepinephrine Inhibitors				
Venlafaxine	Effexor	+ + + +	+ + +	+
Desvenlafaxine	Pristiq	+ + + +	+ + +	+
Duloxetine	Cymbalta	+ + + +	+ + +	+
Levomilnacipran	Fetzima	+ + + +	+ + + +	0
Monoamine Oxidase Inhibitors				
Phenelzine	Nardil	++	++	++
Atypicals				
Amoxapine	Asendin	+ + +	+ + +	0
Bupropion	Wellbutrin	+	0/+	+
Maprotiline	Ludiomil	+ + + +	0	0
Mirtazapine	Remeron	+	+ + + +	0
Nefazodone	Serzone	0/+	+ + +	0
Trazodone	Desyrel	0	+ +	0
Novel Drugs				
Vilazodone	Viibryd	0	+ + + +	0
Vortioxetine	Trintellix	0	+ + + +	0

NE, norepinephrine; 5-HT, 5-hydroxytryptamine (serotonin); D, dopamine; + + + +, highly potent effect; +, minimally potent effect; 0, no effect.

upset occurs transiently during the onset of therapy in approximately one third of patients

Among the most commonly reported SSRI-associated adverse effects is pervasive sexual dysfunction, which may impact any or all of the phases of sexual response and function. This is potentially due to the increased serotoninergic activity at the 5-HT2c receptor. Sexual dysfunction is often a reason cited by patients for prematurely stopping their antidepressants. All SSRIs have the potential to induce sexual dysfunction. The incidence varies from about 24% to 73%, depending on the individual drug. Paroxetine is comparatively associated with the highest rate of sexual side effects, and fluvoxamine may be the least likely in the class to cause sexual dysfunction. The manifestations include reduced

TABLE 39.2

Overview of Antidepressant Agents

Generic (Trade) Name and Dosage	Selected Adverse Events	Contraindications	Special Considerations
Tricyclic Antidepressants			

Amitriptyline (Elavil)
  Start: 25 mg TID
  Range: 50–300 mg
	Sedation, dry mouth	History of cardiovascular disease	Therapeutic plasma concentration range: 60–200 ng/mL

Amoxapine (Asendin)
  Start: 50 mg TID
  Range: 100–600 mg
	Anticholinergic, sedation	History of epilepsy or cardiac dysfunction	Therapeutic plasma concentration range: 180–600 ng/mL

Clomipramine (Anafranil)
  Start: 25 mg QHS
  Range: 150–200 mg
	Sedation, orthostatic hypotension	History of cardiovascular disease	Blood levels not used clinically

Desipramine (Norpramin)
  Start: 25 mg TID
  Range: 50–300 mg
	Sedation, dry mouth	Same as clomipramine	Therapeutic plasma concentration range: 125–250 ng/mL

Doxepin (Sinequan)
  Start: 25 mg TID
  Range: 75–300 mg
	Sedation, orthostatic hypotension	Same as clomipramine	Therapeutic plasma concentration range: 110–250 ng/mL

Imipramine (Tofranil)
  Start: 25 mg TID
  Range: 50–300 mg
	Sedation, orthostatic hypotension	Risk of falling, history of cardiovascular disease	Therapeutic plasma concentration: 180 ng/mL

Maprotiline (Ludiomil)
  Start: 25 mg TID
  Range: 50–300 mg
	Anticholinergic effects, sedation, seizures	History of epilepsy or cardiac dysfunction	Therapeutic plasma concentration range: 200–400 ng/mL

Nortriptyline (Pamelor)
  Start: 25 mg TID
  Range: 50–200 mg
	Sedation	History of cardiovascular disease	Therapeutic plasma concentration range: 50–150 ng/mL

Protriptyline (Vivactil)
  Start: 5 mg TID
  Range: 15–60 mg
	Sedation, orthostatic hypotension	Same as nortriptyline	Therapeutic plasma concentration range: 100–200 ng/mL

Trimipramine (Surmontil)
  Start: 25 mg TID
  Range: 15–90 mg
	Sedation, cardiac conduction disturbances	Same as nortriptyline	

Selective Serotonin Reuptake Inhibitors			

Citalopram (Celexa)
  Start: 20 mg daily
  Range: 20–40 mg daily
	Nausea, dry mouth, increased sweating, somnolence, insomnia	MAO inhibitor therapy	In trials, ~6% of men experienced difficulty with ejaculation, and 3% reported impotence

Fluoxetine (Prozac)
  Start: 10–20 mg each morning
  Range: 10–80 mg
	Insomnia	Same as citalopram	Take in morning to avoid insomnia

Fluvoxamine (Luvox)
  Start: 75 mg BID
  Range: 100–300 mg
	Increases in blood pressure	Same as citalopram	Monitor blood pressure

Paroxetine (Paxil)
  Start: 20 mg daily
  Range: 10–50 mg
	Mild sedation, delayed ejaculation	Same as citalopram	May be useful in patients displaying insomnia as depressive symptom

Sertraline (Zoloft)
  Start: 50 mg daily
  Range: 50–200 mg
	Insomnia	Same as citalopram	Take in morning to avoid insomnia; may be agitating

Escitalopram (Lexapro)
  Start: 10 mg daily
  Range: 10–20 mg daily
	Nausea, diarrhea, increased sweating, somnolence, insomnia, fatigue	Same as citalopram	Extensively metabolized in the liver; the dose for hepatic impairment is 10 mg daily

TABLE 39.2

Overview of Antidepressant Agents (*Continued*)

Generic (Trade) Name and Dosage	Selected Adverse Events	Contraindications	Special Considerations
Serotonin Norepinephrine Reuptake Inhibitors			
Venlafaxine (Effexor) Start: 25 mg TID or 37.5 mg BID Range: 75–375 mg	Increases in blood pressure, sexual dysfunction	Do not use within 14 d of MAO inhibitor therapy; caution in narrow-angle glaucoma	Monitor blood pressure closely
Desvenlafaxine (Pristiq) Start: 50 mg Range: 50–100 mg (no additional benefit above 50 mg)	Same as venlafaxine	Same as venlafaxine	May cause significant dose-related increases in total cholesterol, LDL, and triglycerides; nausea occurs in up to 30% of patients
Duloxetine (Cymbalta) Start: 40–60 mg Range: 60–120 mg (no additional benefit above 60 mg)	Same as venlafaxine	Same as venlafaxine	May worsen psychosis in some patients or precipitate a shift to mania or hypomania in patients with bipolar disorder; nausea occurs in up to 30% of patients
Levomilnacipran (Fetzima) Start: 20 mg daily (increase by 20–40 mg intervals every 2 days per schedule) Range: 40–120 mg	Orthostatic hypotension (dose related), nausea, erectile dysfunction (dose related)	Same as venlafaxine	Specific dosing titration over several days
Atypicals			
Trazodone (Desyrel) Start: 50 mg TID Range: 50–600 mg	Orthostatic hypotension, priapism	Contraindicated in recovery phase of myocardial infarction	
Bupropion (Wellbutrin, Wellbutrin SR, Wellbutrin XL) Start: 100 mg BID (IR); 150 mg daily (SR) Range: 300–450 mg	Headache, insomnia, xerostomia	Do not use within 14 d of MAO inhibitors; do not use during an abrupt cessation of sedatives or ethanol	Lowers seizure threshold at dose >450 mg; avoid concomitant alcohol ingestion
Novel Drugs			
Vilazodone (Viibryd) Start: 10 mg daily (increase to 20 mg after 7 days and to 40 mg after more days) Usual dosing: 40 mg daily	Diarrhea, nausea, dizziness	Do not use within 14 d of MAO inhibitors; do not use during an abrupt cessation of sedatives or ethanol	Significantly less risk of sexual dysfunction compared to other antidepressants with similar mechanisms
Vortioxetine (Trintellix) Start: 10 mg daily (increase to 20 mg daily as tolerated) Range: 10–20 mg daily (5 mg available for patients intolerant of usual doses)	Sexual dysfunction, nausea	Do not use within 14 d of MAO inhibitors; do not use during an abrupt cessation of sedatives or ethanol	Metabolized primarily by CYP2D6-specific dosing adjustments recommended when concomitantly prescribed with strong inducers or inhibitors of CYP2D6
Esketamine (Spravato) Start: 56 mg (2 sprays) twice a week for the first four weeks of therapy Range: Decrease the number of weekly administrations (56–84 mg, 2–3 sprays) once weekly then keep as once weekly or further reduce to 56–84 mg (2–3 sprays) q2wk	Hypertension, cognitive impairment, impaired ability to drive and operate machinery	Do not prescribe in patients with a history of abusing prescription or illicit drugs; avoid in pregnancy	REMS program; Add-on treatment in conjunction with an oral antidepressant for refractory depression; can cause fetal toxicity, counsel patients on using effective birth control when using this drug

CYP, cytochrome P-450; LDL, low-density lipoprotein; MAO, monoamine oxidase; REMS, risk evaluation and mitigation strategy.

libido, arousal difficulties, and delayed or absent orgasm in both men and women. Risk of this side effect must be communicated to the patient prior to starting therapy. Treatment of this dysfunction is available but lowering the dose without compromising efficacy may be the first strategy. If the symptoms persist, one pharmacologic strategy to consider is the addition of bupropion, which has been successfully used to mitigate the sexual dysfunction and provide an additive and different antidepressant mechanism of action. In addition, sildenafil (Viagra), tadalafil (Cialis), or vardenafil (Levitra) may benefit some male patients who suffer from erectile dysfunction. Patients often become tolerant to the sedation and the GI adverse effects, but rarely do patients become tolerant to the sexual dysfunction, and therefore it tends to persist throughout the course of therapy.

The SSRIs are associated with a discontinuation syndrome, particularly upon abrupt discontinuation, but sometimes even after an appropriate taper. The constellation of symptoms include not only a worsening and return of depressive symptoms but also a flu-like presentation, insomnia, irritability, GI effects, and anxiety.

Recently, the question of increased suicidality has been raised with respect to SSRIs and antidepressants in general. SSRIs specifically are associated with an increase in attempted and completed suicide in patients younger than age 25. They have no effect on suicidality in patients ages 25 to 64, and they reduce suicidal behaviors in patients over age 65.

Interactions

The selection of a specific SSRI for an individual patient is determined by the drug interaction profile. SSRIs inhibit various components of the cytochrome P-450 (CYP450) system, thus causing elevations in other medications that are metabolized by this system. Before prescribing an SSRI, the practitioner should conduct a medication history and identify the potential for altering the pharmacokinetics or pharmacodynamics of medications that the patient will be taking concomitantly (**Table 39.3** offers a guide to the major drug–drug interactions with common SSRIs.).

Of special note, SSRIs are contraindicated with MAO inhibitors because the combination can lead to a sudden increase in systemic serotonin. The MAO inhibitor–mediated inhibition of the serotonin metabolism (thereby increasing its circulating availability) coupled with the action of the SSRI itself can result in serotonin excess. The manifestation of excessive serotonin, which is potentially life threatening, is termed *serotonin syndrome*. Signs and symptoms include heat stroke, vascular collapse, fever, and tachycardia.

Serotonin Norepinephrine Reuptake Inhibitors

The pharmacologic effect of SNRIs is primarily mediated through the potent inhibition of neuronal uptake of serotonin and norepinephrine and the weak inhibition of dopamine reuptake. SNRIs have no significant activity for muscarinic cholinergic, H_1-histaminergic, or alpha$_2$-adrenergic receptors and do not possess MAO inhibitor activity. Since the inception of SNRIs, there has been clinical debate regarding whether or not this newer class is superior to SSRIs because of its dual inhibition of serotonin and norepinephrine. It is postulated that this confers a broader antidepressant effect. Venlafaxine (Effexor), the first drug developed in this class, has been extensively studied in terms of its comparative efficacy to SSRIs. Numerous studies suggest that there may in fact be a slight but significant advantage in using venlafaxine over SSRIs with respect to remission rates. Literature also supports the use of SNRIs in more severe depression and in treatment-resistant depression (Bauer et al., 2009). There are currently four SNRIs available in the United States: venlafaxine, desvenlafaxine (Pristiq), duloxetine (Cymbalta), and the newly approved levomilnacipran (Fetzima). Desvenlafaxine, the R-isomer of venlafaxine, differs from its parent compound with respect to its simpler dosing regimen, greater bioavailability, and improved ability to inhibit norepinephrine reuptake. Duloxetine has a once-daily dosing schedule, reduced risk of treatment-emergent hypertension, and fewer discontinuation symptoms. An enantiomer of milnacipran, levomilnacipran is a potent and selective inhibitor of serotonin and norepinephrine reuptake, with preferential inhibition of norepinephrine over serotonin. Its efficacy, as evidenced in multiple clinical trials, is similar and possibly slightly less impressive than that of other members of this class. However, it has demonstrated weight neutrality and good tolerability (see **Table 39.2**).

Time Frame for Response

Similar to SSRIs, SNRIs require approximately 4 to 6 weeks (and potentially up to 12 weeks) to exert a full pharmacologic effect. Some cognitive and physical symptoms of depression may begin to remit within the first week of therapy, but the full effect is slightly more protracted. As with any of the antidepressants, SNRIs should be taken through the continuation and maintenance phases to reduce the risk of relapse.

Adverse Events

SNRIs have the potential to produce more adverse effects as compared to SSRIs secondary to the noradrenergic activity; there are higher rates of dry mouth, constipation, nausea, and insomnia. Treatment-emergent hypertension has occurred in patients taking venlafaxine, although the majority of cases occur in patients who are predisposed to developing hypertension. Increases in blood pressure of approximately 10 mm Hg have also been reported in patients who are hypertensive prior to starting venlafaxine therapy. Two dose-related side effects occur with venlafaxine: nausea and hypertension. Starting therapy with lower doses and gradually increasing the dose as tolerated minimizes the nausea. The prevalence of sexual dysfunction in patients taking venlafaxine, desvenlafaxine, or duloxetine approximates that of SSRIs.

Abrupt discontinuation of SNRI therapy is not recommended, especially venlafaxine. This can produce a discontinuation syndrome similar to that of SSRIs. Duloxetine has not been shown to elicit these types of symptoms to the extent that the other two members of this class have.

TABLE 39.3

Selected Antidepressant Drug Interactions Involving the Cytochrome P-450 System

Agent–Drug Interaction Potential	Isozyme Inhibited	Drugs Affected
Addition of this agent...	*Will inhibit this isoenzyme...*	*Resulting in increased levels of these drugs:*
Fluoxetine—moderate	3A4	Type 1A antiarrhythmics
Mirtazapine—low		Clozapine
Nefazodone—high		Benzodiazepines (alprazolam, triazolam, clonazepam)
Paroxetine—low		Calcium channel blockers
Sertraline—low		Cannabinoids
Venlafaxine—low		Carbamazepine
		Cyclosporine
		Estrogens
		Fentanyl
		HIV-1 protease inhibitors
		HMG-CoA reductase inhibitors
		Macrolide antibiotics
		Ondansetron
		Tricyclic antidepressants (amitriptyline, clomipramine, imipramine)
		R-warfarin
		Zolpidem
Fluoxetine—high	2D6	Narcotic analgesics
Mirtazapine—low		Chlorpromazine
Paroxetine—high		Fluphenazine
Sertraline—low		Haloperidol
Venlafaxine—low		Perphenazine
		Risperidone
		Beta-blockers (labetalol, metoprolol, pindolol, propranolol, timolol)
		Benztropine
		Cyclobenzaprine
		Dextromethorphan
		Donepezil
		Glimepiride
		Trazodone
		Tricyclic antidepressants
Fluoxetine—low	1A2	Clozapine
Fluvoxamine—high		Haloperidol
Mirtazapine—low		Thioridazine
Nefazodone—low		Olanzapine
Paroxetine—low		Chlorpromazine
Sertraline—low		Trifluoperazine
Venlafaxine—low		Caffeine
		Diazepam
		Metoclopramide
		Ondansetron
		Propranolol
		Tacrine
		Theophylline
		Tricyclic antidepressants (amitriptyline, clomipramine, imipramine)
		Verapamil
		Warfarin
		Zolpidem

HIV, human immunodeficiency virus; HMG-CoA, beta-hydroxy-beta-methylglutaryl coenzyme A.

Interactions

SNRIs are metabolized by the CYP450 system, namely, the CYP1A2, CYP3A4, and CYP2D6 isoenzymes. Coadministration of SNRIs with other drugs that are substrates of or that otherwise impact those isoenzymes may result in drug interactions. Concomitant administration of MAO inhibitors with SNRIs is contraindicated because this may result in serotonin syndrome.

Tricyclic Antidepressants

Prior to the emergence of SSRIs, TCAs were the mainstay of therapy for MDD. There are no proven significant differences in terms of efficacy between TCAs and SSRIs; however, the improved tolerability of the SSRIs has served as the impetus for a shift away from the TCAs. TCAs are potent inhibitors of the reuptake of norepinephrine and serotonin, with differences in the extent to which each member of this class impacts each neurotransmitter. Clomipramine (Anafranil) is a potent serotonin reuptake blocker, and its metabolite is a potent norepinephrine reuptake blocker (see **Table 39.2**). Amitriptyline (Elavil), for example, significantly increases the amount of norepinephrine and serotonin available to the postsynaptic neuron. In contrast, nortriptyline (Pamelor) has a relatively low effect on both norepinephrine and serotonin. These drugs, therefore, attempt to restore the balance of neurotransmitters and work in accord with several of the aforementioned theories.

TCAs are also active at acetylcholine and histamine receptors, which contribute to their adverse-effect profile. This complex pharmacology, coupled with the anticholinergic side effects, relegates TCAs to second- or third-line therapy for MDD.

Adverse Events

The selection of a TCA for treating depression is based on the adverse-effect profile (**Table 39.4**) in addition to response to previous treatments, if applicable. In varying degrees, all TCAs can cause sedation, which is an important consideration, especially if the depression is characterized by insomnia. Administering a TCA at bedtime may help alleviate this symptom.

In addition, the hypotensive effect of each agent varies and should be considered when selecting a particular agent. For example, nortriptyline and desipramine (Norpramin) have less potential for inducing orthostatic hypotension, making them advantageous in older patients. Anticholinergic adverse effects are common among this class as is weight gain. Moreover, the epileptogenic potential and life-threatening cardiac conduction abnormalities associated with the TCAs must be considered. TCAs may contribute to atrioventricular block, QT prolongation, and ventricular tachycardia. Preexisting epilepsy and cardiac conduction abnormalities are often considered contraindications to the use of TCAs. TCAs are traditionally lethal in overdose secondary to their proarrhythmic properties.

Therapeutic Ranges

Because the pharmacokinetic properties of the individual agents may vary according to the patient and few TCAs have established therapeutic ranges, routine monitoring of drug levels is not common. However, establishing the drug level at which a patient has improved is reasonable. In this way, the practitioner has documentation of an effective drug concentration for that patient. Later, if needed, changes in drug therapy may be determined based on this baseline information. Otherwise, drug levels should be evaluated only if the practitioner suspects that the patient is not adhering to therapy or if drug toxicity becomes a concern.

Interactions

Drug interactions with TCAs tend to be pharmacodynamic, although some pharmacokinetic interactions do occur. Pharmacokinetically, TCA drug levels may increase in combination with certain SSRIs (see **Table 39.3**) and other CYP450 enzyme inhibitors, such as cimetidine (Tagamet), human immunodeficiency virus protease inhibitors, and some antipsychotic agents. There are additive CNS effects with TCAs and anticholinergic drugs, such as diphenhydramine (Benadryl). In addition, TCA–MAO inhibitor interactions may significantly increase the level of circulating catecholamines and lead to a potentially fatal hypertensive crisis.

Monoamine Oxidase Inhibitors

MAO inhibitors were the first effective medications that were developed for the treatment of depression. They work by nonspecifically and irreversibly inhibiting type A and type B MAO, leading to a decreased degradation of norepinephrine, serotonin, and dopamine in the synapse. However, the adverse-effect profile and potential for life-threatening hypertensive crises have limited their use and relegated them a last-line treatment in clinical practice. Only skilled practitioners with extensive clinical expertise should prescribe MAO inhibitors. See **Table 39.2** for starting dosages and dosage ranges.

Adverse Events

Adverse reactions to MAO inhibitors are more common than in any other class of antidepressant. Orthostatic hypotension occurring with high-dose therapy is probably the most common adverse effect. Attempts to prevent this reaction by applying support stockings, prescribing stimulants such as methylphenidate, or adding the mineralocorticoid have met with reasonable success. However, caution must be used and the patient must be monitored carefully, especially when receiving the corticoid or the stimulant drug concomitantly. Hypertensive crisis can occur when MAO inhibitors are taken with medications that stimulate excessive release of the neurotransmitters dopamine, epinephrine, and norepinephrine. In addition, patients taking MAO inhibitors must be on a strict diet that eliminates tyramine-containing foods.

TABLE 39.4

Major Adverse-Event Profile of Antidepressant Agents

Drug		Major Adverse Events				
	Anticholinergic	Cardiac Conduction	Seizures	Orthostatic Hypotension	Sedation	Sexual Dysfunction
Selective Serotonin Reuptake Inhibitors						
Citalopram (Celexa)	0	0	+	0	0	+ +
Fluoxetine (Prozac)	0	0	+ +	0	0	+ + +
Fluvoxamine (Luvox)	0	0	+ +	0	0	+ + + +
Paroxetine (Paxil)	+	0	+ +	0	+	+ + + +
Sertraline (Zoloft)	0	0	+ +	0	0	+ + +
Escitalopram (Lexapro)	0	0	+ +	0	0	+ +
Serotonin Norepinephrine Inhibitors						
Venlafaxine (Effexor)*	+	+	+ +	0	0	+ + + +
Desvenlafaxine (Pristiq)*	+	+	+	0	0	+ +
Duloxetine (Cymbalta)*	+	0	0	0	0	+ +
Levomilnacipran (Fetzima)*	+	+	0	+ +	0	+ + +
Tricyclic Antidepressants						
Amitriptyline (Elavil)	+ + + +	+ + +	+ + +	+ + +	+ + + +	+
Desipramine (Norpramin)	+ +	+ +	+ +	+ +	+ +	+
Doxepin (Sinequan)	+ + +	+ +	+ + +	+ +	+ + +	0
Imipramine (Tofranil)	+ + +	+ + +	+ + +	+ + + +	+ + +	+
Nortriptyline (Pamelor)	+ +	+ +	+ +	+	+ +	+
Protriptyline (Vivactil)	+ +	+ + +	+ +	+ +	+	+
Trimipramine (Surmontil)	+ + + +	+ + +	+ + +	+ + +	+ + + +	+
Monoamine Oxidase Inhibitors						
Phenelzine (Nardil)	+ +	+	+ +	+ +	+ +	0
Tranylcypromine (Parnate)	+ +	+	+ +	+ +	+ +	0
Atypical Antidepressants						
Amoxapine (Asendin)	+ + +	+ +	+ + +	+ +	+ + +	0
Bupropion (Wellbutrin, Wellbutrin SR, Wellbutrin XL)	+	+	+ + + +	0	+ + + +	0
Maprotiline (Ludiomil)	+ + +	+ +	+ + + +	+ + +	+ + + +	0
Mirtazapine (Remeron)	+ +	+	+	+ + + +	+	0
Nefazodone (Serzone)	0	+	+ +	+ + +	+ +	0
Trazodone (Desyrel)	0	+	+ +	+ + + +	+ +	0
Novel Drugs						
Vilazodone (Viibryd)*	+	0	0	0	+	+
Vortioxetine (Trintellix)*	+ + +	0	0	0	0	+ + + +
Esketamine (Spravato)	0	+	0	0	+ + + +	0

*High rate of nausea and diarrhea.

+ + + +, highly potent effect; +, minimal effect; 0, no effect.

- Aged cheese (cheddar, blue, Gouda, Swiss)
- Yeast products
- Aged meats, processed meats, non-fresh meat
- Beef liver or chicken liver
- Sauerkraut
- Licorice
- Tap beer

Box 39.4 identifies certain foods that have an extremely high tyramine content and, if ingested by patients taking MAO inhibitors, may cause a hypertensive crisis.

Concomitant use of TCAs and MAO inhibitors can lead to a hyperpyretic crisis resulting in seizures and death. Similarly, using SSRIs or SNRIs and MAO inhibitors together can lead to a serotonergic syndrome. Carefully monitored, these agents can be used together safely, but they should be prescribed and monitored only by experienced clinicians.

Atypical Antidepressants

The class of drugs labeled *atypical* represents compounds used to treat depression that elude the traditional classification schema. The mechanisms of action are not consistent within the atypical group but all impact one or more monoamines. These agents are generally considered alternatives to SSRIs, SNRIs, or TCAs; however, the utilization of bupropion has rivaled that of the SSRIs and SNRIs. See **Table 39.2** for starting dosages and dosage ranges.

Bupropion

Bupropion (Wellbutrin) is a structurally distinct compound from the aminoketone class. It is a relatively weak inhibitor of neuronal uptake of norepinephrine and dopamine, and its metabolite also inhibits the reuptake of norepinephrine. It does not inhibit the reuptake of MAO, and unlike all of the other available drugs, it does not impact the serotonergic system. Bupropion is among the preferred pharmacologic agents, possibly second only to SSRIs and SNRIs. Owing to its virtual absence of sexual adverse effects, bupropion is frequently used in patients who cannot tolerate the sexual adverse effects of SSRIs and SNRIs or may be used adjunctively with these drugs to diminish sexual dysfunction. Rates of somnolence, fatigue, and weight gain are markedly reduced compared to SSRIs, TCAs, and SNRIs (Papakostas, 2009). Bupropion has been implicated in lowering the seizure threshold, especially when combined with alcohol. This tends to occur when dosing exceeds 450 mg daily or more than 150 mg per dose, although the reported risk is less than 1%.

Trazodone

Trazodone (Desyrel) is a weak serotonin receptor antagonist that also blocks serotonin reuptake to a lesser degree. Trazodone is highly sedating at therapeutic doses secondary to its antihistamine properties. Patients whose target symptoms or residual symptoms include insomnia may benefit from the use of trazodone as adjunctive therapy. Trazodone monotherapy is not recommended secondary to modest efficacy. Antidepressant effects will be realized within a few weeks; however, the intended sedative effects occur several hours after the first dose. Also an anxiolytic drug, trazodone has a place in therapy for anxiety disorders as well as depression with comorbid anxiety. Important adverse effects include orthostatic hypotension, nausea, blurred vision, and priapism.

Nefazodone

Nefazodone (Serzone), structurally related to trazodone, acts similarly to trazodone but also inhibits the reuptake of norepinephrine and produces fewer side effects. Because it lacks significant anticholinergic and antihistamine effects, reports of blurred vision, urinary retention, and weight gain are relatively infrequent. Nefazodone interferes with the CYP3A4 system, and caution should be used in patients taking drugs metabolized by this enzyme system. In addition, nefazodone increases the levels of agents such as alprazolam (Xanax) and triazolam (Halcion); practitioners should avoid prescribing these agents concomitantly (see **Table 39.3**). Prior to initiating nefazodone, the washout period after discontinuing an SSRI should generally be 4 to 5 days for paroxetine (Paxil) and sertraline (Zoloft) and several weeks for fluoxetine (Prozac). Nefazodone carries a black box warning for hepatotoxicity, which led to the removal of the brand-name product Serzone from the market. Generic nefazodone remains available but has fallen out of favor in practice secondary to its risk of liver damage because safer and more efficacious antidepressants are available.

Mirtazapine

Mirtazapine (Remeron) is a selective alpha$_2$-adrenergic receptor antagonist affecting both the norepinephrine and serotonergic systems. The role of mirtazapine in treating depression is similar to that of the TCAs. It has significant histamine-1 receptor blocking activity, thus causing sedation. In addition, because of its appetite stimulation, it may be a good choice for low-weight older or ill patients. This agent may be useful in combination therapy because there have been no reports of drug interactions. However, there have been rare cases of reversible agranulocytosis.

Novel Drugs
Vilazodone

Vilazodone (Viibryd) is a novel compound and a potent SSRI and partial 5-HT1A receptor agonist. Approved in the United States for the treatment of depression at doses of 10 to 40 mg once daily, vilazodone's antidepressant effects are attributed to its modulation of serotonergic activity at pre- and postsynaptic serotonin transporters. Vilazodone is classified as a SSRI/5-HT1A receptor partial agonist and not a pure SSRI.

Traditional antidepressants (SSRIs, SNRIs, TCAs) increase the amount of available serotonin by inhibiting its reuptake or otherwise modulating its transmission. In doing so, they also stimulate the 5-HT1A autoreceptors, which acutely decreases the amount of available serotonin, as stimulation of an autoreceptor would facilitate the reuptake of serotonin back into the presynaptic neuron. Only after several weeks do the autoreceptors become desensitized and begin to function normally again, thereby normalizing serotonergic transmission. Traditional antidepressants' effects at the 5-HT1A autoreceptor may underlie the delay in therapeutic effect (of several weeks). Vilazodone, in contrast, is a *partial* agonist at the 5-HT1A autoreceptor and does not seem to induce this effect, resulting in an onset of effect that is significantly earlier than traditional antidepressants.

Time Frame for Response. In multiple randomized, double-blinded, placebo-controlled studies, vilazodone-treated patients experienced a response as early as week 1. This may represent a therapeutic advantage over traditional antidepressants, which generally produce a therapeutic effect after 4 to 6 weeks of treatment. To date, all clinical trials involving vilazodone have been placebo controlled and have not included an active comparator, thereby limiting a comparison to existing therapy with respect to efficacy.

Adverse Events. Vilazodone has demonstrated good tolerability and safety in all of the published clinical trials. The most commonly reported adverse effects have consistently been nausea and diarrhea, both occurring in approximately 25% of patients enrolled in trials. These GI disturbances emerged early in treatment and tended to dissipate within a few days. Vilazodone does not appear to produce treatment-related effects on sexual function, and, based on score reductions over the course of the pivotal studies, it may have resulted in a slight improvement of sexual functioning. The partial agonism at the 5-HT1A receptor is thought to be the pharmacologic reason for the low risk of sexual dysfunction. Sexual dysfunction is frequently part of the clinical picture in depressed patients, independently of treatment-emergent sexual dysfunction. The majority of pharmacotherapeutic treatment options have the potential to induce some level of sexual dysfunction in patients in whom it exists already and in patients who did not previously experience sexual dysfunction. As previously discussed, the rates of sexual dysfunction associated with the SSRIs are greater than 70%. This is an important consideration when selecting drug therapy, as worsening of existing sexual dysfunction or development of new-onset sexual dysfunction can directly influence medication compliance and therapeutic outcomes.

Another important consideration in the selection of drug therapy for MDD is impact on weight. Many existing drug therapies cause weight gain, sometimes significant, which may influence treatment adherence. Thus far, vilazodone is considered weight neutral, resulting in approximately a 1.7-kg (3.74-lb) increase in weight after 1 year of treatment.

Interactions. Vilazodone is a major substrate of CYP3A4, and it weakly inhibits CYP2C8 and weakly induces CYP2C19. The clinically relevant drug–drug interactions are limited to strong CYP3A4 inhibitors, which have the ability to increase serum concentrations of vilazodone. In particular, ketoconazole, a prototypical strong CYP3A4 inhibitor, increases the C_{max} and AUC of vilazodone by 50%, necessitating a dose reduction to 20 mg of vilazodone daily. A 20-mg maximum daily dose of vilazodone is recommended when vilazodone is administered concurrently with a strong CYP3A4 inhibitor. Because of extensive hepatic metabolism and lack of renal elimination, mild to moderate renal impairment does not impact vilazodone concentrations. Vilazodone has not been studied in patients with severe renal dysfunction. Mild to moderate hepatic impairment does not result in a clinically meaningful impact on vilazodone concentrations.

Vortioxetine

Vortioxetine (Trintellix) is a multimodal antidepressant, which acts as an inhibitor of serotonin reuptake by antagonizing the 5-HT3, 5-HT7, and 5-HT1D receptors; agonizing the 5-HT1A receptor; partially agonizing the 5-HT1B receptor; and inhibiting the 5-HT transporter. Vortioxetine's activity at multiple receptors results in modulation of the serotonergic, noradrenergic, dopaminergic, and histaminic systems, which results in antidepressant effects. Similar to vilazodone, vortioxetine's action at the 5-HT1A receptor is thought to cause an earlier onset of action as compared to traditional antidepressants. Results from several randomized controlled trials are inconsistent with regard to efficacy and tolerability. Response to 2.5 to 20 mg daily was demonstrated in most of the studies, but not all. Remission rates tended to not differ from placebo.

Time Frame for Response. Onset of therapeutic effect, as evidenced by available clinical studies, is variable. Some evidence suggests that an onset of effect occurs as early as week 1 of treatment. Other studies failed to see a difference until week 4 or 6; and some studies did not observe a difference at all through study end. To date, there are no published trials that directly compare vortioxetine to another antidepressant.

Adverse Events. The most commonly reported adverse effects include dizziness, diarrhea, vomiting, and xerostomia. Sexual dysfunction in men and women occurs at a rate of 34% to 50%.

Interactions. Vortioxetine is a major substrate of CYP3A4 and does not inhibit or induce any of the CYP isoenzymes. Bupropion and buspirone, however, should not be used concurrently with vortioxetine due to their ability to enhance the serotonergic effects of vortioxetine.

Esketamine

Esketamine (Spravato) is one of the newest U.S. Food and Drug Administration (FDA)—approved medications for add-on therapy for treatment refractory major depression. Esketamine, the S-enantiomer of ketamine, is based off a drug that has been used for hundreds of years as an anesthetic. It is an NMDA receptor antagonist that is marketed in the form of a nasal spray. The exact mechanism of action is unknown. Esketamine is approved to be taken in conjunction with an oral antidepressant for adult patients only. There is a black box warning for risk of sedation and dissociation as observed with ketamine with its use, potential for abuse and misuse, and increased risk of suicidal thoughts. The drug is a Schedule 3 controlled substance in the United States and requires the use of a Risk Evaluation and Mitigation Strategy (REMS) drug program to obtain for use.

Time Frame for Response. The induction phase for esketamine consists of instructing the patient to administer 56 mg of the drug twice a week for the first four weeks of therapy. The patient decreases the number of weekly administrations during the maintenance phase: 56 to 84 mg (2–3 sprays) once weekly, then continue regimen as once weekly dosing or further reduce to 56–84 mg every two weeks. The goal of therapy is to individualize frequency of therapy to your patient to allow for the least frequent dosing that maintains a positive response.

Unlike many of the other classes of antidepressants, esketamine does not take several weeks to observe the full activity of the drug. Maximum drug concentrations occur 20 to 40 minutes after the last nasal spray of a treatment session. Patients must be monitored in a health care setting for at least two hours at the conclusion of a treatment session due to the risks of sedation and dissociation.

Adverse Events. Warnings include increases in blood pressure, cognitive impairment and impaired ability to drive and operate machinery due to the risks of sedation and dissociation, and embryo-fetal toxicity. Patients of childbearing potential should be counseled on the risk of fetal harm while using esketamine. The most common adverse events observed in clinical studies in patients treated with esketamine in combination with an oral antidepressant include dissociation, sedation, nausea, vertigo, hypertension, and feeling drunk.

Interactions. Concomitant use with CNS depressants such as opioids, benzodiazepines, and alcohol may increase the risk of sedation. Instruct patients to take caution when driving or operating machinery. Use with psychostimulants such as amphetamine, methylphenidate, modafinil, and MAOIs can increase the risk of hypertension. Closely monitor blood pressure especially patients with baseline hypertension.

Esketamine is a substrate of CYP2B6 and CYP3A4 enzymes and, to a lesser extent, CYP2C19 and CYP2C9.

Selecting the Most Appropriate Drug

Selection of an initial pharmacotherapeutic treatment option involves numerous factors, the most important of which include the patient's target symptoms, comorbid medical or psychiatric conditions, concomitant medications, previous response to an antidepressant, and potential adverse effect and drug interaction profile. A patient's past experience with antidepressants should impact the decision regarding the choice of initial drug because past response tends to predict future response. Another consideration is the patient's perception about the efficacy and side effects she, he, or a family member has experienced. A negative perception of a drug may suggest potential for lack of adherence to drug therapy or an erosion of confidence in the therapy.

Scores of meta-analyses have evaluated the relative efficacy among antidepressants and assert that SSRIs consistently demonstrate relative efficacy as compared to SNRIs, TCAs, bupropion, trazodone, mirtazapine, and nefazodone. Patient-specific considerations will dictate the choice of drug as opposed to efficacy.

First-Line Therapy

Multiple large-scale trials have demonstrated that efficacy within drug classes and among drug classes is relatively equal, save for a few exceptions. Safety, tolerability, and lethality in overdose are the considerations that tend to drive drug selection, not efficacy. SSRIs and SNRIs are considered first-line therapy for depression and are generally used initially in patients without contraindications. In the absence of specific target symptoms, any of the available SSRIs or SNRIs are acceptable first choices. Recent studies purport the superiority of escitalopram over other members of its class, although this claim has not been substantiated with large randomized, controlled trials. If insomnia is problematic in the patient, paroxetine (Paxil) may be the best choice within the SSRI class. If the patient is taking drugs metabolized by CYP3A4, then avoiding fluoxetine (Prozac) is recommended. If the spectrum of depression-related symptoms includes sexual dysfunction, SSRIs and SNRIs should be avoided. If weight gain needs to be avoided, then bupropion is arguably a more appropriate option versus SSRIs (particularly paroxetine, which has the greatest potential to induce weight gain) or mirtazapine. See **Figure 39.2** and **Table 39.5** for an overview of treatment of a patient with depression. Furthermore, combining psychotherapy with pharmacotherapy, especially in patients with psychosocial stressors, leads to better short-term outcomes compared to single option treatment.

Second-Line Therapy

When a patient fails an adequate trial of a first-line antidepressant and therapy needs to be modified, options include dose optimization, augmentation, and switching. If some clinical benefit, but not a true response or remission, is derived from the initial medication and it is well tolerated, an *increase in dose* is appropriate.

If the dose is optimized and some benefit (a response, but not remission) is realized, then *augmentation* with another agent that is not an antidepressant may be appropriate. Lithium, thyroid hormone, and stimulant medications have

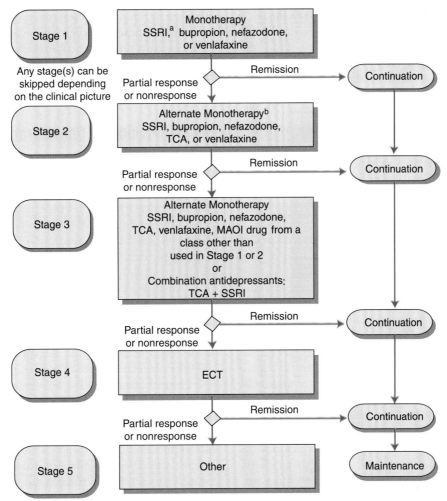

FIGURE 39–2   Amalgam of the Texas Medication Algorithm Project Recommendations (2008) and Recommendations from the American Psychiatric Association (2010). Texas Medication Algorithm Project: Major depressive disorder. (Adapted from Suehs, B. T., Argo T. R., Bendele, S. D., et al. [2008]. *Texas medication algorithm project procedural manual: Major depressive disorder algorithms.* Austin, TX: Texas Department of State Health Services. [The Texas Medication Algorithm Project algorithms are in the public domain, and this figure may be reproduced without permission, but with the appropriate citation.] American Psychiatric Association [APA]. [2011]. *Practice guideline for the treatment of patients with major depressive disorder* [3rd ed., p. 152]. Arlington, VA: American Psychiatric Association [APA].)

ECT, electroconvulsive therapy; MAOI, monoamine oxidase inhibitor; SSRI, selective serotonin reuptake inhibitor; TCA, tricyclic antidepressant.
[a]SSRIs preferred.
[b]Consider TCA or venlafaxine if not tried.

TABLE 39.5

Recommended Order of Treatment in Antidepressant Therapy

Order	Agents	Comments
First line	SSRIs	Fluoxetine and sertraline may be good for patients with somnolence.
		Paroxetine may be good for patients with insomnia.
		Selection of agent should be based on patient's past experiences with medications and drug interactions.
		Cost may be a consideration.
Second line	TCA (desipramine or nortriptyline) or atypical antidepressant	These agents have the better side-effect profile of the class and should be considered as agents of choice for the TCA class.
Third line	Atypical antidepressant or TCA	Depending on past response to other agents and side-effect profile.

SSRI, selective serotonin reuptake inhibitors; TCA, tricyclic antidepressants.

been used traditionally to augment the response to the initial antidepressant. Not common in practice any longer, this recommendation remains in the treatment guidelines.

If a patient fails an SSRI or an SNRI (does not realize any benefit or cannot tolerate the drug), then *switching* to another member of the same class could serve as the second choice, as each member of the class is chemically distinct from the others. Switching to a medication in a different class can also be an option. Atypical antidepressants (bupropion, mirtazapine, etc.) are generally chosen prior to attempting TCAs given the safety and tolerability concerns associated with the TCAs.

Combination therapy implies adding a second drug with a different mechanism of action to the initial therapy. Drugs that are commonly used adjunctively to the initial medication include trazodone, bupropion (though this is often used as initial therapy), mirtazapine, buspirone, and the atypical antipsychotics (AAPs). Generally, the second drug is tailored to address residual symptoms that did not improve on initial therapy; residual symptoms like insomnia or anxious symptoms. There is clinical controversy surrounding the use of AAPs to treat depressed patients that do not have a psychotic component. Even though aripiprazole (Abilify) now carries an FDA indication for the adjunctive treatment of depression, many practitioners are reluctant to use them, given their extensive adverse-effect profile. Quetiapine and risperidone are sometimes used off-label as an adjunctive medication. The AAPs have activity at serotonergic, noradrenergic, dopaminergic, and histaminergic receptors, all of which contribute to their therapeutic effects as well as their adverse effects. AAPs as a class are associated with serious and often irreversible metabolic sequelae including significant weight gain, insulin resistance, new-onset diabetes, and dyslipidemia. QT prolongation has also been observed. Given the serious nature of these adverse effects, and the extent to which they occur, the use of AAPs as an augmentation strategy is frequently met with resistance, particularly by psychiatrists.

The definitive selection should include an assessment of the patient's underlying cardiac, neurologic, and comorbid conditions. For example, venlafaxine should be avoided in patients with uncontrolled hypertension because of its potential to increase blood pressure. Similarly, for an older man with a history of benign prostatic hyperplasia, TCAs and atypical agents with significant anticholinergic activity should be avoided because this action aggravates the condition.

Current treatment guidelines have not been updated since the approval of vilazodone, vortioxetine, and levomilnacipran; therefore, there is no official guidance on their place in therapy. Given the available efficacy and safety data and the absence of direct comparison to existing therapy, these newer medications will probably be integrated into the second-line tier.

Third-Line Therapy

If the first- and second-line agents fail and augmentation strategies are unsuccessful, the clinician can attempt a medication from one of the remaining classes (TCAs, MAOIs). Again, patient-specific indicators help the clinician decide on the next treatment regimen. For the most part, inexperienced general practitioners should not prescribe MAO inhibitors. The side effects and the potential for dangerous drug and food interactions suggest that only clinicians well versed in managing this kind of therapy prescribe these agents.

Special Population Considerations
Children and Adolescents

The risk for underdiagnosis and undertreatment is extremely prevalent in this patient population. Children of parents who have been diagnosed with serious depression are at risk for developing anxiety and MDD in childhood. Early childhood depression may manifest as acting out, changes in eating or sleeping patterns, or social withdrawal. These patients can seldom communicate a feeling of sadness because of the early language development level. From ages 5 to 8, low self-esteem, underachievement at school, and aggressive or antisocial behaviors (including stealing and lying) may indicate depression. Depressed adolescents experience symptoms similar to depressed adults such as sleep disturbances, irritability, difficulty concentrating, and loss of energy.

Currently, fluoxetine (Prozac) is the only SSRI approved by the FDA for the treatment of depression in children age 8 and up. Escitalopram (Lexapro) is labeled for use in children age 12 and older. Caution has been recommended in using other agents, such as paroxetine (Paxil) or venlafaxine (Effexor), with depressed children and adolescents given lack of data showing efficacy and overall higher adverse-effect burden. Compared to adults, adolescents are more likely to become agitated or to develop a mania while they are taking an SSRI. The FDA has issued a black box warning due to increased risk of suicide in children and adolescents taking SSRIs. Non-SSRIs could be considered as a third-line agent in adolescents with treatment refractory depression.

Geriatrics

Late-onset depression commonly occurs in older patients, with nursing home residents nearly three times more likely to be depressed than the general population. These patients may also have an underlying neurologic or vascular disorder. Determining the root of the depression is essential to resolution. Older patients tend to endorse more vegetative symptoms and cognitive disturbances than they do subjective dysphoria, which differs from the presentation in a younger patient. Recognition and appropriate treatment of depression in this population are essential as the occurrence of depression worsens morbidity and mortality and worsens outcomes of somatic diseases.

Effort should be made to minimize pharmacologic burden on older patients and to proactively address possible drug interactions and adverse effects when selecting pharmacotherapy. "Start low and go slow." Geriatric patients often have significant changes in physiologic function, including reduced renal and hepatic function, decreased muscle mass, decreased serum albumin, and dietary alterations. These changes may affect the absorption, distribution, metabolism, and excretion of a variety of drugs, particularly antidepressants. Older patients are also more sensitive to anticholinergic effects and orthostatic hypotension, adverse effects that are associated with several of the antidepressant drug classes. Most practitioners agree that antidepressant therapy should be prescribed at one third to one half the usual starting adult dosage.

Women

As noted earlier, younger women are more likely to experience depression than older women or men in general. Women of childbearing age are at the greatest risk; however, some women are especially sensitive to hormonal fluctuations and therefore may experience new-onset depression associated with menopause. The decision to initiate antidepressant medication in a pregnant woman is a difficult one, and the risk of fetal exposure to the drug must be balanced against the risk of continued depression.

Pregnancy-related and postpartum depression is especially prevalent in women with a history of depression and a previous episode of postpartum depression, although the independent prevalence is 10% to 15%. The risk is increased with concomitant marital problems, lack of social support, and medical issues with newborn children. The decision about which drug to use depends on the factors previously discussed as well as on the issue of breast-feeding and the risk of transmission of drugs through breast milk. The potential for antidepressant-associated fetal harm varies by drug and varies by trimester.

Ethnic

There are genetic variations in the metabolism of drugs in patients with varying ethnicity. The CYP2D6 enzyme system, responsible for the metabolism of many psychotherapeutic agents, is influenced by age, gender, and ethnicity. Up to 10% of whites and nearly 19% of African Americans are considered "poor metabolizers" of drugs via CYP2D6. Similarly, 33% of African Americans and 37% of Asians are poor metabolizers of drugs metabolized by CYP2C19. The result of this poor metabolism can include quicker responses to drugs, greater-than-expected action of the agent, or even more pronounced side effects. As more data accrue on the effects of genetics on depression and CYP450 metabolism, the effects of race and ethnicity on treating depression and selecting antidepressants will play a more prominent role.

Emergencies

Suicide is the most feared consequence of inadequately treated (or unrecognized) depression. Up to two thirds of depressed patients have suicidal ideation, and 10% to 15% commit suicide (**Box 39.5**). The practitioner should be ever vigilant for suicidal ideation and the potential for suicide. This is another reason for frequent contact between the practitioner and the patient. If the patient discloses thoughts of suicide, the practitioner and patient need to develop a plan for psychiatric referral or hospitalization. Contracting with the patient, such as by developing a written agreement to continue treatment without doing self-harm, may also be an effective means for minimizing the risk of suicide. All plans and actions should be documented in the patient's medical record.

| BOX 39.5 | **Warning Signs of Suicidal Ideation** |

- Pacing, agitated behavior, frequent mood changes, and chronic episodes of sleeplessness
- Actions or threats of assault, physical harm, or violence
- Delusions or hallucinations
- Threats or talk of death (e.g., "I don't care anymore" or "You won't have to worry about me much longer")
- Putting affairs in order, such as giving possessions away or writing a new will
- Unusually risky behavior (e.g., unsafe driving, abuse of alcohol, or other drugs)

Monitoring Patient Response

Treatment should have been administered at an appropriate dose or frequently as well as for a sufficient duration when interpreting a patient's response to an agent. If treatment does not show symptomatic improvement after a month of use, it needs to be modified, either by increasing the dose, adding another agent, or switching agents if the initial agent is intolerable or not effective at a higher dose. The adverse-effect profile should be taken into consideration as well as the patient's compliance to the regimen. You can maximize initial treatment by incorporating several different treatment modalities for maximum benefit, that is, an antidepressant + CBT.

PATIENT EDUCATION

Patients and caregivers should be instructed on the full range of issues surrounding depression and antidepressant therapy. Patients should be assured that depression is a biologic illness that occurs in a variety of people, and they should not feel ashamed of the disease. Moreover, the caregivers or significant others should also be counseled on the role they play in aiding in the patient's recovery. The more informed patients and significant others are of the illness, the more likely they will adhere to recommendations.

Expectations for a quick recovery can be detrimental to the healing process. Patients and caregivers should be informed that the antidepressant medication takes several (4 to 6) weeks to begin working and the patient might be required to continue taking the medication.

Teaching patients to recognize early signs and symptoms of behavior that may indicate a recurrence is crucial. Patients and family members should be instructed to contact the clinician if symptoms resume. A support group may also be a good resource for family and patients as a strategy for managing the illness.

Antidepressants and Suicide

Depression is the leading cause of suicide, and up to 80% of depressed patients experience suicidal impulses. Since 1990, whether antidepressant drugs are linked to suicide has been an acrimonious debate. Some argue that depressed adolescents who are suicidal and treated with antidepressants may regain initiative and energy before improvement in cognition and mood, thereby becoming mobilized to attempt suicide. Others argue that the medication prescribed to treat depression is responsible for causing adolescents to attempt suicide. In 2003, British drug regulators warned that SSRIs, with the exception of fluoxetine, were unsuitable in minors experiencing depression. As a result, the FDA began public hearings in February 2004 to discuss this controversy. Currently, fluoxetine (Prozac) is the only FDA-approved antidepressant in patients as young as age 8. However, other antidepressants, such as sertraline (Zoloft), venlafaxine (Effexor), and paroxetine (Paxil), have been widely prescribed for adolescent depression. Current data suggest that the increase in suicidality impacts patients younger than age 25 to a greater extent than patients older than age 25. Therefore, a practitioner needs to be diligent in assessing the patient's risk of suicide.

Patient Information

The National Foundation for Depressive Illness, Inc. (http://www.depression.org), was established in 1983 to educate the public and health care professionals about depression. This Web site contains useful information on the signs and symptoms of depression and provides public awareness on depression through a national "800" number.

The National Institute of Mental Health's Web site (http://www.nimh.nih.gov/publicat/depressionmenus.cfm), also available in Spanish, is an excellent resource for depression. It describes the different types of depression along with the causes and treatments. This Web site also offers valuable information on how family and friends may contribute and assist in therapy.

The National Mental Health Association (http://www.nmha.org) is a nonprofit organization that provides beneficial information to the public and practitioners on mental illness. This Web site contains news releases along with an online bookstore. A calendar notes coming events relating to mental health. This Web site provides access to comprehensive mental health care and increases public awareness of mental health issues.

The Depression and Bipolar Support Alliance (DBSA) (http://www.dbsalliance.org) is a nonprofit organization that provides a wide range of information and support on depression and bipolar disorders. Their mission, as stated on the Web site, is to improve the lives of those affected by depression and bipolar disorder. The DBSA is a patient-directed national organization focusing on the most prevalent mental illnesses, with a network of approximately 1,000 support groups. This Web site is updated regularly to provide up-to-date, scientifically based information. The DBSA is guided by a scientific advisory board comprising researchers and clinicians in the field of mood disorders.

Complementary and Alternative Medications

The use of herbal products in the United States has dramatically increased in the past few decades, resulting in consumer sales of $250 million in 2007. Subsequent research with respect to drug–drug interactions and safety concerns made available to consumers caused a significant decrease in sales over the next decade. Depression is the most common diagnosis associated with complementary and alternative medication use. Despite the decline in popularity of St. John's wort, herbal sales continue to steadily rise. The FDA does not classify herbal products as drugs, and as such they are not regulated under the same scrutiny as other medications.

St. John's wort (*Hypericum perforatum*) has been used for centuries for a variety of illnesses, but it is currently used almost exclusively as an herbal antidepressant. Most clinical trials have studied 300 to 1,800 mg/d of standardized extract (usually standardized to 0.3% hypericin content) divided in three daily doses. The clinical effect is usually seen within 2 to 3 weeks of initiating therapy. The mechanism of action is unknown, although it is theorized that it inhibits MAO and the synaptosomal uptake of serotonin, dopamine, and noradrenaline.

St. John's wort appears to be well tolerated, with the most frequent side effects reported as nausea, fatigue, restlessness, rash, and photosensitivity. There have been reported cases of increase in heart rate, but no significant effect was seen on the PR interval. Efficacy has not been well established, with some evidence to support its use and a wealth of studies in which it did not separate from placebo.

St. John's wort may activate hepatic CYP450, so it has the potential to interact with medication that is metabolized by the CYP450 system. Therefore, it has been reported that St. John's wort decreases serum levels of theophylline, cyclosporine, warfarin, oral contraceptives, and indinavir. St. John's wort should not be taken in combination with any other antidepressant because of the risk of serotonin syndrome, especially in older patients. Symptoms include changes in mental status, tremor, GI disturbances, myalgia, restlessness, and headache.

S-adenosylmethionine is a naturally occurring methyl donor in the synthesis of dopamine and serotonin. Though not regulated by the FDA and not recommended in any of the treatment guidelines, there is some data that supports the use of this compound in MDD. Omega-3 fatty acids have also been evaluated as an adjunctive therapy for MDD. Cardiovascular benefits of omega-3 fatty acids have been established and, given their relative safety and tolerability, could be added to conventional therapy. However, their efficacy in MDD has not been affirmed. Folate, however, has been associated with a positive response to antidepressant therapy. When used adjunctively to antidepressants, folate is recommended in patients who have not fully responded to their initial drug therapy. This is considered a low-risk intervention, given its general health benefits and lack of safety concerns.

BIPOLAR DISORDER

Introduction

Bipolar disorder affects about 1.8% of the population in the United States (*DSM-5*, 2013). As classified by the *DSM-5*, bipolar disorders are a group of psychiatric disorders that are characterized by a significant fluctuation in a person's energy, mood, and ability to function. The word "bipolar" is utilized to describe this illness as it is known by variation in an individual's mood from extreme highs to extreme lows.

Individuals with bipolar disorders experience periods of mania and depression and relatively fluctuate between these two periods. Mania consists of periods of euphoria, overactivity, and excitement, while depression consists of feelings of sadness, hopelessness, and underactivity. The degree of time a person can spend in each state and addition of other factors such as the presence of psychotic episodes can help distinguish the specific subset of bipolar disorder.

Causes

Similar to major depression, there is not a single, specific causative factor that leads to the development of bipolar disorder. Bipolar disorder stems from multiple genetic, physiologic, social, environmental, and biochemical factors that can affect susceptible individuals. Nonetheless, certain factors, such as the family prevalence of bipolar disorder, do affect the rate at which an individual is likely to develop bipolar disorder in their lifetime. A first-degree relative of a person with bipolar disorder has a tenfold greater relative risk of developing bipolar disorder compared to the general population.

Pathophysiology

Most current research focuses on neurochemical aspects of depression and has spurred several theories relating to the generation and maintenance of specific neurotransmitters in the CNS. The basis for these neurochemical theories is the hypothesis that abnormal neurotransmitter release or decreased postsynaptic receptor sensitivity is affected before and during a major depressive episode. At least four theories relate to this hypothesis (**Box 39.1**). Three of the four theories focus on a functional or absolute deficiency in the neurotransmitters serotonin, norepinephrine, or both. A functional deficiency suggests that neurotransmitters are produced but the postsynaptic receptors cannot fully transmit the neural impulse. This is in contrast to an absolute deficiency in which no neurotransmitters are produced or the postsynaptic receptors cannot transmit the signal at all.

Similar to the theories associated with the monoamine catecholamines, norepinephrine and serotonin, new evidence suggests that dopamine may play a significant role in the pathogenesis and symptomatology of MDD. Genetic polymorphisms in the genes associated with dopamine transmission may contribute to an increased susceptibility to depression. Deficits in dopamine release or transmission have been linked to dysphoria, one of the most prominent features of MDD. The permissive hypothesis, a more contemporary theory, suggests that reduced serotonin activity sets the stage for a mood disorder, such as depression or mania, depending on the underlying norepinephrine level. A low serotonin level coupled with a low norepinephrine level suggests that depression results from an increased beta-adrenergic receptor sensitivity. This alteration in postsynaptic receptor sensitivity

results in an imbalance between the effects of norepinephrine and serotonin and may create a functional deficiency in serotonin. Secondary to the interplay among the catecholamines within the monoaminergic network, any impact on one of the monoamines will likely impact the others. This is applicable to the predisposition and development of MDD as well as the therapeutics of MDD.

Diagnostic Criteria

According to the *Diagnostic and Statistical Manual of Mental Disorders, Fifth Edition* (*DSM-5*), bipolar disorders are categorized as bipolar I, bipolar II, and cyclothymic disorders. For a full definition of the various psychiatric disorders, please search and review the *DSM-5* manual online.

Bipolar I disorder consists of a manic-depressive disorder in which neither a major depressive episode nor psychosis is a requirement. It is distinguished from other bipolar disorders by the presence of mania in addition to depressive episodes. On the contrary, bipolar II disorder, which is more common among individuals diagnosed with bipolar disorder, does consist of a lifetime experience of at least one major depressive episode and a hypomanic episode. Although bipolar II disorder does not typically consist of manic episodes, it tends to be characteristic of more severe impairment in social functioning and the ability to work. This is likely due to the greater time these individuals spend in the depressive period of their illness.

Cyclothymic disorder is the subset of bipolar disorder that is diagnosed when an adult experiences depressive and hypomanic episodes for at least 2 years but does not fulfill the criteria for mania or major depression. The onset of bipolar disorders tends to be during adolescence and early adulthood; however, they have been diagnosed in children.

Mania is defined as a period of abnormally and persistently elevated or irritable mood that accompanies a persistently elevated increase in activity or energy throughout the day that lasts for at least 1 week. A manic episode must be severe enough to cause significant impairment in social or occupational functioning and hospitalization or is present with psychotic features and cannot be due to a medical- or substance-related cause.

Hypomania is a type of disorder that it is not severe enough to cause significant social and occupational impairment or hospitalization, although others are still able to identify the change in mood.

For a full definition of major depressive episode, please search and review the *DSM-5* online. In addition, there are a few scales that can help diagnose bipolar disorder, such as the Bipolar Spectrum Diagnostic Scale, which consists of statements pertaining to bipolar disorders that individuals check off if it applies to them as well as narratives that the individual chooses between as it describes their experience. These scales can especially be helpful in diagnosing individuals that may be on the lower end of the bipolar disorder spectrum.

This chapter focuses on the diagnosis and pharmacotherapy for adult patients with bipolar disorder.

Pharmacotherapy

Pharmacotherapy for bipolar disorder comprises several classes of drugs, including mood stabilizers, anticonvulsants, antipsychotics, and antidepressants to treat the various aspects of bipolar disorder. Usually a combination of at least two agents from different classes is used. The choice of specific agents is an individualized choice based on tolerability, adverse effects, and other comorbidities.

The efficacy of pharmacologic agents tends to be similar over classes; however, atypical antipsychotics and newer anticonvulsants tend to be common choices due to their better adverse effect profile and tolerability. On the contrary, some clinicians will utilize older agents, such as lithium, which have decades of data for the treatment of bipolar disorder. Many relapse prevention randomized controlled trials show strong support for lithium as the initial choice of maintenance treatment, followed by use of valproate, lamotrigine, and atypical antipsychotics, such as olanzapine and quetiapine. **Table 39.6** highlights common drugs used for bipolar disorder.

TABLE 39.6			
Overview of Common Bipolar Disorder Agents			
Generic (Trade) Name and Dosage	**Selected Adverse Events**	**Contraindications**	**Special Considerations**
Mood Stabilizer			
Lithium (Lithobid) Start: 200–300 mg TID Range: 600–1800 mg	CNS depression, hypercalcemia, hypothyroidism, renal dysfunction	Severe cardiovascular or renal disease, dehydration, or concurrent use with diuretics	Therapeutic plasma concentration range: acute mania: 0.8–1.2 mEq/L Maintenance: 0.6–1.0 mEq/L **Toxicity is closely related to serum levels** Taper over 1–2 weeks dose if planning to switch to alternate agent.
Anticonvulsants			
Carbamazepine (Tegretol) Start: 100–400 mg daily in divided doses Range: 600–1800 mg	**Severe dermatologic reactions including Stevens–Johnson syndrome and toxic epidermal necrolysis, significant hematologic abnormalities including aplastic anemia and agranulocytosis,** hepatotoxicity, CNS depression, hyponatremia	Bone marrow suppression	**Check for HLA-B*1502 allele in genetically high-risk patients of Asian ethnicity prior to initiating therapy.** Risk of teratogenicity in pregnant patients
Lamotrigine (Lamictal) *Without interacting medications* Start: weeks 1 and 2: 25 mg daily; weeks 3 and 4: 50 mg daily; week 5: 100 mg daily; week 6: 200 mg daily; further increases up to 400 mg daily *With valproate (inhibitor)* Start: weeks 1 and 2: 25 mg QOD; weeks 3 and 4: 25 mg daily; week 5: 50 mg daily; week 6: 100 mg daily *With carbamazepine, phenytoin, not valproate (inducer)* Start: weeks 1 and 2: 50 mg daily; weeks 3 and 4: 100 mg daily; week 5: 200 mg daily; week 6: 300 mg daily Range: 25–400 mg	**Severe dermatologic reactions including Stevens–Johnson syndrome and toxic epidermal necrolysis,** hematologic abnormalities, CNS depression	N/A	Titrated to clinical response rather than serum concentration Careful titration of medications is required when adjusting lamotrigine or lamotrigine inducer/inhibitor doses. Taper over at least 2 weeks is required when discontinuing.

TABLE 39.6

Overview of Common Bipolar Disorder Agents (*Continued*)

Generic (Trade) Name and Dosage	Selected Adverse Events	Contraindications	Special Considerations
Valproate (Depakote) Start: 500–750 mg daily in divided doses Range: 1500–2500 mg	**Severe hepatotoxicity potentially leading to hepatic failure** and **pancreatitis**, hematologic abnormalities, CNS depression, brain atrophy, elevated ammonia levels in the blood/encephalopathy	Severe hepatic impairment or hepatic disease, **certain mitochondrial disorders**	**Risk of teratogenicity in pregnant patients** Therapeutic plasma concentration range (total valproic acid level): mania: 50–125 mcg/mL; up to 90 mcg/mL has been suggested in the older adults.
Typical Antipsychotics			
Haloperidol (Haldol) Start: 2–15 mg daily Range: 2–30 mg	Cardiac conduction abnormalities (use caution in patients with altered cardiac conduction including QTc prolongation), anticholinergic effects, CNS depression, extrapyramidal symptoms	Parkinson's disease, dementia with lewy bodies, severe CNS depression	**Increased risk of death in older patients with dementia-related psychosis**
Chlorpromazine (Thorazine) Start: 30–400 mg daily in divided doses Range: 30–800 mg	Same as above	Severe CNS depression	Same as above
Atypical Antipsychotics			
Aripiprazole (Abilify, Abilify Maintena is an intramuscular long-acting injectable.) *Oral Formulation:* Start: 10–15 mg BID Range: 10–30 mg *Abilify Maintena:* 400 mg monthly	Cardiac conduction abnormalities (use caution in patients with altered cardiac conduction including QTc prolongation), CNS depression, extrapyramidal symptoms, dyslipidemia, hyperglycemia, hematologic abnormalities	N/A	**Increased risk of death in older patients with dementia-related psychosis** **Increased risk of suicidality in children, adolescents, and young adults** Assess tolerability of oral aripiprazole before initiating therapy with injectable. Overlap oral aripiprazole or alternative antipsychotic for 14 days when starting the injectable.
Olanzapine (Zyprexa) Start: 5–10 mg BID Range: 5–50 mg	Same as above	N/A	**Increased risk of death in older patients with dementia-related psychosis** **Increased risk of suicidality in children, adolescents, and young adults** Zyprexa Relprevv (long-acting injectable) must be administered in a registered health care facility (**via REMS**) due to significant sedation and delirium being observed following administration.
Paliperidone (Invega) Start: 3–6 mg daily Range: 3–12 mg	Same as above	N/A	**Increased risk of death in older patients with dementia-related psychosis** Use caution in patients with renal impairment and seizures.
Quetiapine (Seroquel) Start: 100–200 mg daily Range: 100–1200 mg	QTc prolongation, CNS depression, extrapyramidal symptoms, dyslipidemia, hyperglycemia, hematologic abnormalities	N/A	**Increased risk of death in older patients with dementia-related psychosis** **Increased risk of suicidality in children, adolescents, and young adults**

(*Continued*)

TABLE 39.6

Overview of Common Bipolar Disorder Agents (*Continued*)

Generic (Trade) Name and Dosage	Selected Adverse Events	Contraindications	Special Considerations
Risperidone (Risperdal) Start: 1–3 mg daily Range: 1–8 mg	Cardiac conduction abnormalities (use caution in patients with altered cardiac conduction including QTc prolongation), CNS depression, extrapyramidal symptoms, dyslipidemia, hyperglycemia, hematologic abnormalities, anticholinergic effects	N/A	**Increased risk of death in older patients with dementia-related psychosis**
Ziprasidone (Geodon) Start: 40 mg BID Range: 80–160 mg	Hematologic abnormalities, CNS depression, severe dermatologic reactions including Stevens–Johnson syndrome and drug reaction with eosinophilia and systemic symptoms, dyslipidemia, extrapyramidal symptoms, hyperglycemia, QTc prolongation	History of or current QTc prolongation, congenital long QT syndrome, concurrent use of other QTc-prolonging agents, recent myocardial infarction, uncompensated heart failure	**Increased risk of death in older patients with dementia-related psychosis** Administer with a meal containing at least 500 calories. Measure baseline weight, body mass index, lipid levels, EKG, vital signs and repeat all as clinically indicated or at least within 3 months of treatment initiation.

* Bolded terms refer to U.S. Black Box Warnings.

CNS, central nervous system.

CASE STUDY 1

L.B. is a 55-year-old white female who presents to her family physician's office for a yearly routine physical. Her husband passed away 5 months ago after a 2-year battle with lung cancer. She has three children, two of whom are still in college. Her daughter accompanies her to the doctor's office and says she is concerned about her mother's recent behavior. She explains that her mother has been "sleeping all the time" and has lost 25 lb in the past 2 months without being on a diet. When the doctor examines L.B., she explains that she has become increasingly fatigued and complains of a lack of energy. She no longer has any desire to participate in her lifelong hobbies of painting and photography because of frequent feelings of sadness. L.B.'s medical history is significant for hypothyroidism, hypercholesterolemia, and recently diagnosed hypertension. Her medications are levothyroxine 0.075 mg daily, simvastatin 20 mg daily, hydrochlorothiazide 25 mg daily, lisinopril 10 mg daily, multivitamins 1 tab daily,

and aspirin 81 mg daily. In the office today, L.B.'s blood pressure is 138/88 mm Hg.

1. List specific goals for treatment for L.B.
2. What drug therapy would you prescribe? Why?
3. What are the parameters for monitoring success of the therapy?
4. Discuss specific patient education based on the prescribed therapy.
5. List one or two adverse reactions for the selected agent that would cause you to change therapy.
6. What would be the choice for second-line therapy?
7. What over-the-counter and/or alternative medications would be appropriate for L.B.?
8. What lifestyle changes would you recommend to L.B.?
9. Describe one or two drug–drug or drug–food interaction for the selected agent.

Bibliography

Starred references are cited in the text.

2019 American Geriatrics Society Beers Criteria Update Expert Panel. (2019). American Geriatrics Society 2019 updated AGS Beers criteria for potentially inappropriate medication use in older adults. *Journal of American Geriatrics Society, 67*(4), 674–694.

*American Psychiatric Association (APA). (2010). *Practice guideline for the treatment of patients with major depressive disorder* (3rd ed.). Arlington, VA: American Psychiatric Publishing (APA).

*American Psychiatric Association (APA). (2011). *Practice guideline for the treatment of patients with major depressive disorder* (3rd ed., p. 152). Arlington, VA: American Psychiatric Association.

*American Psychiatric Association (APA). (2013). *Diagnostic and statistical manual of mental disorders* (5th ed.). Arlington, VA: American Psychiatric Publishing.

*Bauer, M., Tharmanathan, P., Volz, H., et al. (2009). The effect of venlafaxine compared with other antidepressants and placebo in the treatment of major depression: A meta-analysis. *European Archives of Psychiatry and Clinical Neuroscience, 259*(3), 172–185.

Ben-Sheetrit, J., Aizenberg, D., Csoka, A. B., et al. (2015). Post-SSRI sexual dysfunction: Clinical characterization and preliminary assessment of contributory factors and dose-response relationship. *Journal of Clinical Psychopharmacology, 35*(3), 273–278.

*Bulloch, A., Williams, J., Lavorato, D., et al. (2014). Recurrence of major depressive episodes is strongly dependent on the number of previous episodes. *Depression and Anxiety, 31*(1), 72–76.

Butterweck, V. (2003). Mechanism of action of St. John's Wort in depression. *CNS Drugs, 17*(8), 539–562.

*Dieleman, J. L., Baral, R., & Birger, M. (2016). U.S. spending on personal health care and public health. *Journal of the American Medical Association, 316*(24), 2627–2646.

Fava, G. A., Gatti, A., Belaise, C., et al. (2015). Withdrawal symptoms after selective serotonin reuptake inhibitor discontinuation: A systematic review. *Psychotherapy and Psychosomatics, 84*(2), 72–81.

Geddes, J. R., Calabrese, J. R., & Goodwin, G. M. (2009). Lamotrigine for treatment of bipolar depression: Independent meta-analysis and meta-regression of individual patient data from five randomised trials. *The British Journal of Psychiatry, 194*(1), 4–9.

Gitlin, M. (2016). Lithium side effects and toxicity: Prevalence and management strategies. *International Journal of Bipolar Disorders, 4*(27), 1–10.

Goodwin, G. M., Haddad, P. M., Ferrier, I. N., et al. (2016). Evidence-based guidelines for treating bipolar disorder: Revised third edition recommendations from the British Association for Psychopharmacology. *Journal of Psychopharmacology, 30*(6), 495–553.

Halverson, J., Beevers, C., & Kamholz, B. (2016). Clinical practice review for major depressive disorder. Anxiety and Depression Association of America. https://adaa.org/resources-professionals/practice-guidelines-mdd

Hamilton, M. (1967). Development of a rating scale for primary depressive illness. *British Journal of Social and Clinical Psychology, 6*, 278–296.

Harris, P. A. (2004). The impact of age, gender, race and ethnicity on the diagnosis and treatment of depression. *Journal of Managed Care Pharmacy, 10*(2 Suppl.), S2–S7.

*Hasin, D. S., Sarvet, A. L., Meyers, J. L., et al. (2018). Epidemiology of adult DSM-5 major depressive disorder and its specifiers in the United States. *Journal of the American Medical Association Psychiatry, 75*(4), 336–346.

Janssen. (2019). *Spravato: Highlights of prescribing information.* Titusville, NJ: Author.

Jauhar, S., & Morrison, P. (2019). Esketamine for treatment resistant depression. *British Medical Journal, 366*, 155–172.

Koenig, A., & Thase, M. (2009). First-line pharmacotherapies for depression—What is the best choice? *Polskie Archiwum Medycyny Wewnętrznej, 119*(7–8), 478–486.

Matthews, J. D., & Fava, M. (2000). Risk of suicidality in depression with serotonergic antidepressants. *Annals of Clinical Psychiatry, 12*(1), 43–50.

Munoz-Lopez, F., Shen, W. W., D'Ocon, P., et al. (2018). A history of the pharmacological treatment of bipolar disorder. *International Journal of Molecular Sciences, 19*(7), 2143–2180.

Nassir Ghaemi, S., Miller, C. J., Berv, D. A., et al. (2005). Sensitivity and specificity of a new bipolar spectrum diagnostic scale. *Journal of Affective Disorders, 84*, 273–277.

National Institute for Health and Care Excellence (NICE). (2019). *Depression in children and young people: Identification and management.* London: National Institute for Health and Care Excellence.

*Norhayati, M. N., Nik Hazlina, N. H., Asrenee, A. R., et al. (2015). Magnitude and risk factors for postpartum symptoms: A literature review. *Journal of Affective Disorders, 175C*, 34–52.

Oltedal, L., Kessler, U., Ersland, L., et al. (2015). Effects of ECT in treatment of depression: Study protocol for a prospective neuroradiological study of acute and longitudinal effects on brain structure and function. *BioMed Central Psychiatry, 15*, 94.

*Papakostas, G. (2009). Managing partial response or nonresponse: Switching, augmentation, and combination strategies for major depressive disorder. *Journal of Clinical Psychiatry, 70*(Suppl. 6), 16–25.

Rickels, K., Athanasiou, M., Robinson, D. S., et al. (2009). Evidence for efficacy and tolerability of vilazodone in the treatment of major depressive disorder: A randomized, double-blind, placebo-controlled trial. *The Journal of Clinical Psychiatry, 70*(3), 326–333.

Robinson, D. S., Kajdasz, D. K., Gallipoli, S., et al. (2011). A 1-year, open-label study assessing the safety and tolerability of vilazodone in patients with major depressive disorder. *Journal of Clinical Psychopharmacology, 31*(5), 643–646.

*Rush, A. J., Trivedi, M., & Fava, M. (2003). Depression, IV: STAR*D treatment trial for depression. *American Journal of Psychiatry, 160*(2), 237.

Tadić, A., Helmreich, I., Mergl, R., et al. (2010). Early improvement is a predictor of treatment outcome in patients with mild major, minor or subsyndromal depression. *Journal of Affective Disorders, 120*(1–3), 86–93.

Trivedi, M. (2009). Tools and strategies for ongoing assessment of depression: A measurement-based approach to remission. *Journal of Clinical Psychiatry, 70*(Suppl. 6), 26–31.

Trivedi, M., Rush, A., Wisniewski, S., et al. (2006). Evaluation of outcomes with citalopram for depression using measurement-based care in STAR*D: Implications for clinical practice. *American Journal of Psychiatry, 163*(1), 28–40.

von Wolff, A., Hölzel, L. P., Westphal, A., et al. (2013). Selective serotonin reuptake inhibitors and tricyclic antidepressants in the acute treatment of chronic depression and dysthymia: A systematic review and meta-analysis. *Journal of Affective Disorders, 144*(1–2), 7–15.

Willner, P., Scheel-Krüger, J., & Belzung, C. (2013). The neurobiology of depression and antidepressant action. *Neuroscience and Biobehavioral Reviews, 37*(10 Pt 1), 2331–2371.

Zajecka, J. (2003). Treating depression to remission. *Journal of Clinical Psychiatry, 64*(Suppl. 15), 7–12.

40 Anxiety Disorders

Sarah Jung and Laura A. Mandos

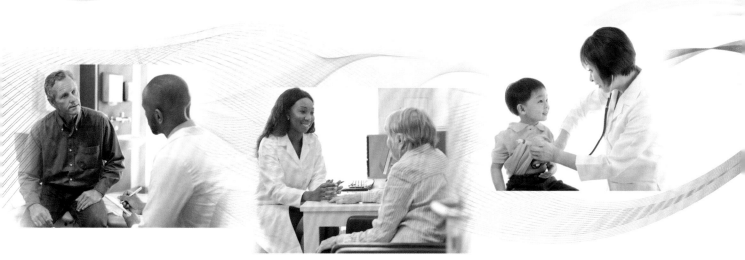

Learning Objectives

1. Distinguish various types and diagnostic criteria of anxiety disorders.
2. Identify therapeutic goals and treatment methods, both pharmacologic and nonpharmacologic.
3. Understand preferred treatment regimens and monitoring parameters.

INTRODUCTION

Though related and with some inherent overlap, the anxiety disorders are a compendium of similar but clinically distinct disorders that share clinical features of excessive fear, worry, anxiety, and associated behavioral manifestations. Patients with anxiety disorders generally endorse psychic and somatic symptoms at varying degrees, which may include tension, apprehension, fear, restlessness, and worry along with physical symptoms such as increased heart rate, pupillary dilation, trembling, and increased perspiration.

One of the complications in identifying the presence of an anxiety disorder is that the core symptoms are mainly normal experiences in the human condition; but what delineates "normal" feelings of anxiety, worry, or fear is the extent to which they occur (severity and frequency) and the extent to which they impact functionality.

With 10 different types, the anxiety disorders represent the largest group of psychiatric disorders (**Table 40.1**). The focus of this chapter will be primarily generalized anxiety disorder (GAD), with an additional review of panic disorder (PD) and social anxiety disorder (SAD, also known as social phobia). There were several meaningful changes in the classification of anxiety disorders in the newest iteration of the *Diagnostic and Statistical Manual (DSM)*, with the publication of the *DSM-5* in 2013. Obsessive–compulsive disorder is no longer considered part of the anxiety disorder spectrum and will not be covered in this chapter. The agoraphobia specifier has been removed from PD and now is considered an independent diagnosis under the anxiety disorder umbrella.

More than 30 million Americans have a lifetime history of anxiety, and anxiety disorders cost an estimated $42 billion per year in the United States, counting direct and indirect costs. Epidemiologic studies report that 2% to 6% of adults and twice as many women as men have GAD. Approximately 1% of all patients have PD with resulting significant impairment, and 4% to 5% have agoraphobia. Approximately 12% of patients seen in anxiety disorder clinics present with GAD. Between 35% and 50% of individuals with major depression meet criteria for GAD. Coexisting anxious distress (formerly referred to as comorbid GAD in depressed patients), now considered a specifier for major depressive disorder (MDD), in depressed patients may worsen the outcome by increasing the suicide rate, worsening overall symptoms, conferring a poorer response to treatment, increasing the number of unexplained symptoms, and increasing functional disability.

The neurobiological and conceptual models that form the basis for anxiety disorders are grounded in the belief that pathologic anxiety is a result of abnormal fear processing, intolerance of uncertainty, anxiety about worry itself, or emotional

TABLE 40.1

Summary of Anxiety Disorders

Anxiety Disorder	Definition
Panic disorder	Recurrent unexpected panic attacks (discrete periods, in which there is a sudden onset of intense apprehension, fearfulness, or terror, often associated with feelings of impending doom, shortness of breath, palpitations, chest pain or discomfort, choking or smothering sensations, and fear of "going crazy" or losing control).
Agoraphobia	Anxiety about, or avoidance of, places or situations from which escape might be difficult (or embarrassing) or in which help may not be available in the event of having a panic attack or panic-like symptoms.
Separation anxiety	Recurrent, excessive distress when anticipating or experiencing separation from home or from an attachment focus (person, object, etc.) or worry about losing attachment figures.
Selective mutism	Failure to speak in specific social situations in which there is an expectation to do so.
Specific phobia	Clinically significant anxiety provoked by exposure to a specific feared object or situation, often leading to avoidance.
Social anxiety disorder (social phobia)	Clinically significant anxiety provoked by exposure to certain types of social or performance situations, often leading to avoidance behavior.
Generalized anxiety disorder	Characterized by at least 6 months of persistent and excessive anxiety and worry.
Anxiety disorder due to a general medical condition	Characterized by prominent symptoms of anxiety that are judged to be a direct physiological consequence of a general medical condition.
Substance-/medication-induced anxiety disorder	Characterized by prominent symptoms of anxiety that are judged to be a direct physiological consequence of a drug abuse, a medication, or toxin exposure.
Anxiety disorder not otherwise specified	Used for coding disorders with prominent anxiety or phobic avoidance that do not meet the criteria for any of the specific anxiety disorders defined in this list (or anxiety symptoms about which there is inadequate or contradictory information).

Adapted from American Psychiatric Association. (2013). *Diagnostic and statistical manual of mental health disorders: DSM-5* (5th ed.). Washington, DC: American Psychiatric Publishing.

hyperarousal. Humans have naturally evolved to be able to apply past experiences and responses to new experiences. For a simple example, if an individual had a traumatic experience with a small animal at some point in his or her life and escaped that fearful situation by running away, that individual may repeat that behavior when faced with a small animal in the future. While evolutionarily helpful in some respects, this response may be maladaptive in that the responses may not only be exaggerated and inappropriate but also may extend beyond a specific experience, hence generalization.

Anxiety disorders most commonly begin in early adulthood. They tend to be chronic, with interspersed periods of remissions and relapses of varying degrees, and they frequently continue into old age. Late onset of an anxiety disorder is rare, although the prevalence of GAD increases with increasing age. In the elderly, anxiety disorders as a whole are the most common psychiatric disorders. It is unknown whether they are a continuation of an illness with an onset from a younger age or whether they appear for the first time in old age.

GAD is a highly prevalent, chronic, debilitating, relapsing, and often underdiagnosed anxiety disorder. Characterized by excessive and pathological worry that is difficult to control, a diagnosis of GAD also incorporates physical, psychological,

and cognitive symptoms as well as a potentially profound functional impairment. The core symptom of excessive worry must be present for a minimum of 6 months and must occur in conjunction with at least three of six physiological arousal symptoms: restlessness, fatigue, muscle tension, irritability, concentration deficit, and sleep disturbance. As the most commonly occurring anxiety disorder with a lifetime prevalence of 4% to 7%, GAD is characterized by a waxing and waning episodic clinical course with periods of remission and relapse. Many patients with GAD report feeling as though they have "felt anxious" for their entire lives. The median onset, however, is 30 years; though age of onset is spread over a broad age range, this represents the latest age of onset of all the anxiety disorders (American Psychiatric Association [APA], 2013).

The pathologic worry is typically based on dangers with an overestimated likelihood of realistically occurring (e.g., a loved one being kidnapped), which then rapidly devolves into generalized worry that involves multiple life domains. For some patients, this worry leads to avoidant behavior where activities or places with perceived danger are avoided. Left untreated, the patient's sphere of comfort may continue to constrict until daily activities become limited and normal function is impaired.

CAUSES

Physiologic Factors

The majority of patients with GAD initially seek attention from a primary health care provider with vague somatic complaints, such as pain, headaches, or gastrointestinal (GI) disturbances. Patients also may casually endorse a nonspecific complaint of insomnia, irritability, sexual dysfunction, or trouble concentrating or remembering.

Although the etiology of anxiety disorders is largely unknown, a wide range of medical illnesses, such as cardiovascular disease, respiratory disease, hyperthyroidism, hypothyroidism, hyperadrenocorticism, pheochromocytoma, Cushing disease, hypoglycemia, vitamin B_{12} deficiency, and neurologic conditions, may cause symptoms of anxiety. In addition, amphetamines, cannabis, caffeine, cocaine, bronchodilators, corticosteroids, sympathomimetics, and thyroid hormone may cause substance-induced anxiety.

Genetic Factors

A family history is seen frequently in people with anxiety disorders. Twin studies suggest that heredity accounts for 30% of the cases of various anxiety disorders; environmental factors seem to be responsible for the remaining cases. More than 50% of people with PD have relatives with the disorder. A twin study reported that anxiety disorder with panic attacks occurs five times more frequently in monozygotic twins than in heterozygotic twins.

PATHOPHYSIOLOGY

Anxiety is a phenomenon that all people experience. One type of anxiety, fear, is a normal fight-or-flight response to an observable threat. In contrast, pathologic anxiety is a fight-or-flight response to an internal or external threat that is real or imagined and causes the person to experience an unpleasant emotional state. During this response, the person's autonomic nervous system, which consists of the sympathetic and parasympathetic nervous systems, prepares the person to deal with a threat (**Box 40.1**).

Neurobiologic Factors

The modulation of normal and pathologic anxiety states is associated with multiple regions of the brain and dysregulation in several neurotransmitter systems (norepinephrine [NE], serotonin [5-HT], gamma-aminobutyric acid [GABA], corticotrophin-releasing factor, alpha$_2$ adrenergic receptors, and cholecystokinin). Furthermore, treatment with medications that modulate these systems have produced short-term and sustained anxiolytic responses, further substantiating the implication of noradrenergic, serotonergic, and GABA system involvement.

NE, 5-HT, and GABA are the major neurotransmitters studied in relation to the pharmacologic treatment of anxiety. People with anxiety disorders, especially PD, are found to have

> ### BOX 40.1 Physiologic Reactions to the Fight-or-Flight Response
>
> The fight-or-flight response causes the following:
>
> 1. Epinephrine, NE, and cortisol are released into the blood.
> 2. The liver releases stored sugar into the blood to meet energy needs.
> 3. Digestion slows, allowing blood to be shifted to the brain and the muscles.
> 4. Breathing becomes rapid to allow for greater oxygen supply to the muscles.
> 5. The heart rate and blood pressure increase.
> 6. Perspiration increases to cool the body.
> 7. Muscles tense in preparation for action.
> 8. The pupils dilate.
> 9. All senses become more acute.
> 10. Blood flow to the extremities becomes constricted to protect the body from bleeding from injury.
>
> This response is appropriate for extremely threatening situations, but the response would cause considerable damage to the body if people responded to all stressful situations in this manner.

malfunctioning noradrenergic systems with a low threshold for arousal. This, coupled with an unpredictable increase in activity, causes the anxiety symptoms.

GABA and its associated receptors function as central nervous system (CNS) inhibitors. Although psychopharmacologic interventions support this role, the exact pharmacology of GABA receptors is still being examined.

DIAGNOSTIC CRITERIA

Anxiety disorders most commonly begin in early adulthood, tend to be chronic with waxing and waning periods of remission and relapse, and frequently continue into old age. In children, anxiety may develop, particularly in relation to school, and late onset of an anxiety disorder is rare but can occur. In the elderly, anxiety disorders are the most common psychiatric disorders seen.

Prior to diagnosis of an anxiety disorder, a medical evaluation should be conducted to rule out medical disease, neurologic problems, current medications that may be anxiogenic, vitamin B_{12} deficiency, and drug or alcohol misuse. The history should focus on anxiety disorders in family members, environmental factors, family dynamics, cognitive functioning, work or school situations, or exposure to chemical substances.

If the anxiety is not reasonably related to a physical or exogenous chemical (drug, alcohol, etc.) consideration, the practitioner should apply the American Psychiatric Association's

BOX
40.2   American Psychiatric Association
DSM-5 Criteria for Diagnosing
Generalized Anxiety Disorder

A. Excessive anxiety and worry (apprehensive expectation), occurring more days than not for at least 6 months, about a number of events or activities (such as work or school performance).
B. The person finds it difficult to control the worry.
C. The anxiety and worry are associated with three (or more) of the following six symptoms (with at least some symptoms present for more days than not for the past 6 months).
   Note: Only one item is required in children.
   1. Restlessness or feeling keyed up or on edge
   2. Being easily fatigued
   3. Difficulty concentrating or mind going blank
   4. Irritability
   5. Muscle tension
   6. Sleep disturbance (difficulty falling or staying asleep, or restless, unsatisfying sleep)
D. The anxiety, worry, or physical symptoms cause clinically significant distress or impairment in social, occupational, or other important areas of functioning.
E. The disturbance is not attributable to the physiological effects of a substance (e.g., a drug of abuse and a medication) or another medical condition (e.g., hyperthyroidism).
F. The disturbance is not better explained by another mental disorder (e.g., anxiety or worry about having panic attacks in PD, negative evaluation in SAD social phobia, contamination or other obsessions in obsessive–compulsive disorder, separation from attachment figures in separation anxiety disorder, reminders of traumatic events in posttraumatic stress disorder, gaining weight in anorexia nervosa, physical complaints in somatic symptom disorder, perceived appearance flaws in body dysmorphic disorder, having a serious illness in illness anxiety disorder, or the content of delusional beliefs in schizophrenia or delusional disorder).

(APA) *Diagnostic and Statistical Manual of Mental Disorders, 5th Edition* (DSM-5, 2013) diagnostic criteria. See **Boxes 40.2**, **40.3**, and **40.4** for the diagnostic criteria for GAD, PD, and SAD, respectively.

Comorbidity with major depression, bipolar disease, and other psychotic disorders is common in patients with anxiety. These patients may self-medicate with alcohol or other substances to relieve their symptoms.

BOX
40.3   American Psychiatric Association
DSM-5 Criteria for Diagnosing
Panic Disorder

A. Recurrent unexpected panic attacks. A panic attack is an abrupt surge of intense fear or intense discomfort that reaches a peak within minutes and during which time four (or more) of the following symptoms occur:
   Note: The abrupt surge can occur from a calm state or an anxious state.
   1. Palpitations, pounding heart, or accelerated heart rate
   2. Sweating
   3. Trembling or shaking
   4. Sensations of shortness of breath or smothering
   5. Feelings of choking
   6. Chest pain or discomfort
   7. Nausea or abdominal distress
   8. Feeling dizzy, unsteady, lightheaded, or faint
   9. Chills or heat sensations
   10. Paresthesias (numbness or tingling sensations)
   11. Derealization (feelings of unreality) or depersonalization (being detached from oneself)
   12. Fear of losing control or "going crazy"
   13. Fear of dying
   Note: Culture-specific symptoms (e.g., tinnitus, neck soreness, headache, uncontrollable screaming or crying) may be seen. Such symptoms should not count as one of the four required symptoms.
B. At least one of the attacks has been followed by 1 month (or more) of one or both of the following:
   1. Persistent concern or worry about additional panic attacks or their consequences (e.g., losing control, having a heart attack, "going crazy")
   2. A significant maladaptive change in behavior related to the attacks (e.g., behaviors designed to avoid having panic attacks, such as avoidance of exercise or unfamiliar situations)
C. The disturbance is not attributable to the physiological effects of a substance (e.g., a drug of abuse, a medication) or another medical condition (e.g., hyperthyroidism, cardiopulmonary disorders).
D. The disturbance is not better explained by another mental disorder (e.g., the panic attacks do not occur only in response to feared social situations, as in SAD; in response to circumscribed phobic objects or situations, as in specific phobia; in response to obsessions, as in obsessive–compulsive disorder; in response to reminders of traumatic events, as in posttraumatic stress disorder; or in response to separation from attachment figures, as in separation anxiety disorder).

> **BOX 40.4** **American Psychiatric Association *DSM-5* Criteria for Diagnosing Social Anxiety Disorder**
>
> A. Marked fear or anxiety about one or more social situations in which the individual is exposed to possible scrutiny by others. Examples include social interactions (e.g., having a conversation, meeting unfamiliar people), being observed (e.g., eating or drinking), and performing in front of others (e.g., giving a speech).
>
> B. The individual fears that he or she will act in a way or show anxiety symptoms that will be negatively evaluated (e.g., will be humiliating or embarrassing; will lead to rejection or offend others).
>
> C. The social situation(s) almost always provoke fear or anxiety. **Note**: In children, the fear or anxiety may be expressed by crying, tantrums, freezing, clinging, shrinking, or failure to speak in social situations.
>
> D. The social situation(s) are actively avoided or endured with intense fear or anxiety.
>
> E. The fear or anxiety is out of proportion to the actual threat posed by the social situation and the sociocultural context.
>
> F. The fear, anxiety, or avoidance is persistent, typically lasting 6 or more months.
>
> G. The fear, anxiety, or avoidance causes clinically significant distress or impairment in social, occupational, or other important areas of functioning.
>
> H. The fear, anxiety, or avoidance is not attributable to the physiological effects of a substance (e.g., a drug of abuse, a medication) or another medical condition.
>
> I. The fear, anxiety, or avoidance is not better explained by the symptoms of another mental disorder such as PD, body dysmorphic disorder, or autism spectrum disorder.
>
> J. If another medical condition (e.g., Parkinson's disease, obesity, disfigurement from burns or injury) is present, the fear, anxiety, or avoidance is clearly unrelated or is excessive.
>
> Specify if: **Performance only**: If the fear is restricted to speaking or performing in public.
>

INITIATING DRUG THERAPY

A multitude of special challenges exists with respect to the diagnosis and successful treatment of GAD. As previously discussed, many patients present with physical complaints and no recognition whatsoever of an emotional or psychiatric component. Patients may lack an understanding of mental illness, may deny symptoms or its existence when given the diagnosis of a mental illness, or may be so ashamed of the stigma associated with mental illness that they are prevented from being open to discussing treatment options. Careful, tactful interventions on the part of the clinician will set the stage for a healthy patient–provider relationship, which will increase the likelihood of successful outcomes. This may be achieved by creating an environment in which the patient is comfortable discussing personal and potentially uncomfortable topics. Empathetic listening, open-mindedness, and acknowledgment that psychiatric disease is a legitimate medical disorder and not a personality flaw are critical. Also, aside from misconceptions about mental illness itself, many patients are reluctant to accept drug therapy as a treatment option. Although there is certainly a place in the treatment spectrum for psychotherapy, drug therapy often is a necessary component in achieving true remission of symptoms.

Successful treatment of anxiety disorders also implies a longer-term commitment from the patient and the clinician, as GAD and the other anxiety disorders are chronic illnesses. Thorough explanation at the beginning of therapy is crucial. The patient education from the outset should include not only explanations of the illness itself but also what the patient should expect during treatment in terms of duration of therapy, when to follow-up, expected length of time before pharmacotherapy will be optimized, and how to respond to potential adverse drug effects. Nonpharmacologic therapy includes psychoeducation, supportive counseling, behavioral therapy, cognitive therapy, stress management techniques, meditation, and exercise. Today, in many cases, these therapies can be helpful and useful in conjunction with drug therapy.

Behavioral therapists treat anxiety as a learned behavior, arguing that anxiety is an internal conditioned response to a perceived threat or stimulus in the environment. They propose that people with anxiety learn to avoid the stimulus in order to reduce anxiety; therefore, behavior modification is the vehicle for changing behavior. Systematic desensitization is used to control external stimuli and internal sensations as well as anticipation of fear of a panic attack.

Cognitive therapists treat anxiety as a faulty thought pattern that evokes the physiologic symptoms of anxiety, feelings of loss of control, and fear of dying. Cognitive–behavioral therapy (CBT) and drug therapy complement each other and tend to produce a greater therapeutic response. CBT is considered the most effective psychotherapy for GAD, according to the literature. CBT for GAD involves self-monitoring of worry, cognitive restructuring, relaxation training, and rehearsal of coping skills. However, CBT requires special training and may not be readily available to all patients.

Goals of Drug Therapy

The long-term goal of therapy for GAD is remission: a complete resolution of anxious symptoms and a return to premorbid functionality and quality of life. In GAD specifically, *response* to treatment is realized by 50% to 60% of patients, yet *remission* is achieved by approximately one-third to one half of patients who respond. Failure to remit fully confers a greater risk of relapse, a reality experienced by 45% of patients with generalized anxiety. Acutely, the goal is to reduce the severity and duration of the anxious symptoms and improve overall functioning. Once target symptoms are improved or resolved, the focus shifts to chronic or maintenance therapy, the goal of which is to completely resolve symptoms and return the patient to a premorbid level of social and occupational functionality (remission). Coupled with the goal of remission is also relapse prevention.

The ideal anxiolytic medication should promote calmness without resulting in daytime sedation and drowsiness and without producing physical or psychological dependence. Pharmacologic options used in the treatment of anxiety disorders can be classified into the following categories: antidepressants, benzodiazepines (BZDs), azapirones, novel antianxiety agents, and atypical antipsychotics (AAPs).

For most anxiety disorders, a single drug, generally an antidepressant, is initiated at a low dose and is titrated upward according to clinical response and tolerability. Four to eight weeks is the generally accepted time at which a preliminary assessment of response can be gauged. Patients who endorse some level of appreciable symptom resolution and are tolerant of the medication are considered to have achieved a durable remission. This is considered predictive of an eventual sustained remission, which persists for several months beyond this acute treatment phase.

Absence of response at the initial 4- to 8-week follow-up visit or intolerance of adverse effects may prompt either a reevaluation of diagnosis or an adjustment in medication therapy. Reasonable interventions include increasing the dose of medication (if the initial drug was tolerated but the clinical effect was not of the magnitude desired), switching to a different drug within the same pharmacologic class (if there was some level of improvement but questionable tolerability), switching to a drug outside of the pharmacologic class (if there was lack of response and/or poor tolerability), or augmenting the initial drug (if the dose of the initial drug was already optimized but the full therapeutic effect has not been achieved).

Upon resolution of the presenting anxious symptoms, it is recommended that treatment be continued beyond initial symptom resolution for 12 months, particularly in GAD, in order to minimize the risk of relapse. In some anxiety disorders, treatment may continue indefinitely depending on the level of severity. The follow-up intervals also may differ based upon individual patient presentation.

Antidepressants

Antidepressants are generally considered first-line pharmacotherapeutic options for the chronic management of patients with anxiety disorders (see **Table 40.2**).

TABLE 40.2		
Antidepressants Used in Treating Anxiety Disorders		
Generic (Trade) Name	**Initial Dose (mg)**	**Usual Dose (mg)**
Tricyclic Antidepressants		
Imipramine (Tofranil)	10–50	150–300
Selective Serotonin Reuptake Inhibitors		
Citalopram (Celexa)	10	10–40
Escitalopram (Lexapro)	10	10–20
Fluoxetine (Prozac)	10	20–60
Fluvoxamine IR	50	100–300
Fluvoxamine ER	100	100–300
Paroxetine (Paxil)	10	10–50
Paroxetine CR (Paxil CR)	12.5	12.5–75
Sertraline (Zoloft)	25	50–200
Vortioxetine (Trintellix)*	10	5–20
Serotonin–Norepinephrine Reuptake Inhibitors		
Venlafaxine (Effexor, Effexor XR)	37.5–75	75–225
Duloxetine (Cymbalta)	60	60–120
Monoamine Oxidase Inhibitors		
Phenelzine (Nardil)	15	45–90

*Not indicated for use in treating anxiety disorder.

CR, controlled-release; ER or XR, extended-release; IR, immediate-release.

Selective Serotonin Reuptake Inhibitors

Considered one of the two first-line pharmacotherapeutic options for the management of GAD in the United States, the selective serotonin reuptake inhibitors (SSRIs) are thought to improve anxiety symptoms by inhibiting the reuptake of 5-HT in the synaptic cleft. While the 2- to 4-week delay until onset of therapeutic effect may be discouraging and may impact patient compliance, significant reductions in "anxious mood" have been documented as early as week 1 in **paroxetine** (Paxil) trials. Remission rates in paroxetine responders at 32 weeks are as high as 73% with only 11% relapsing, a statistic that demonstrates much improvement over the spontaneous remission rate of 20% to 25%. In patients with moderate to severe GAD, **sertraline (Zoloft)** 50 to 100 mg/d has demonstrated superiority to placebo. Clinical response criteria were met by 55% of patients in the sertraline group as compared to 32% in the placebo group by week 12. **Escitalopram** (Lexapro) has been evaluated for the long-term treatment of GAD and prevention of relapse. A randomized, double-blind, placebo-controlled study reported significantly superior results for escitalopram at every time point starting at week 1. **Fluoxetine** (Prozac) and **citalopram** (Celexa) have both shown improvements in anxiety symptoms, especially in patients with comorbid depression, in both adult and pediatric populations. Furthermore, **vilazodone** (Viibryd) and **vortioxetine** (Trintellix) are two new SSRIs that are indicated for the treatment of MDD. Newer evidence for both medications suggests efficacy in decreasing anxiety symptoms in these patients. However, U.S. Food and Drug Administration (FDA)–labeled indication is limited to only MDD at this time.

Adverse Events

Class adverse effects include weight gain, insomnia, GI sequelae, and agitation. Sexual dysfunction, often a presenting symptom in anxious patients, may be exacerbated or caused by SSRIs in up to 40% or 50% of patients. Clinical experience shows that this adverse effect is likely underreported. Another unfortunate pharmacologic phenomenon of the SSRI class is its ability to cause agitation and jitteriness in the acute phase of treatment.

Paroxetine (Paxil) may cause more weight gain and sexual inhibition than the other drugs. Approximately 15% of patients discontinue treatment because of side effects. Caution should be used when SSRIs are given in combination with tricyclic antidepressants (TCAs) because SSRIs can inhibit one or more liver microsomal enzyme systems and increase plasma concentrations of the TCA. This can translate into conduction abnormalities due to toxic levels of TCA. The combination of SSRIs and monoamine oxidase (MAO) inhibitors has resulted in serious reactions such as hyperthermia, rigidity, and autonomic dysregulation that can be fatal, if developed into 5-HT syndrome. SSRIs are generally well tolerated, inexpensive, and associated with less toxicity than TCAs, which partially explains why the SSRIs and serotonin–norepinephrine reuptake inhibitors (SNRIs)

have largely supplanted the TCAs as first-line options. See the chapter on depression.

Serotonin–Norepinephrine Reuptake Inhibitors

Members of this class inhibit the reuptake of 5-HT and NE, though the selectivity and balance with respect to the extent of inhibition are variable among the SNRIs. **Venlafaxine** XR 75 mg to 225 mg (Effexor XR) daily consistently demonstrated superior efficacy compared to placebo in improving anxious symptom. The additional benefit of venlafaxine's efficacy in treating anxious symptoms in patients with comorbid depression as well as in pure GAD has made it a commonly prescribed first-line drug. The comorbidity of nonspecific somatic pain complaints is common in patients with GAD, which negatively impacts quality of life, worsens outcomes, hampers achievement of remission, and increases the risk of relapse. Response rates for treatment with venlafaxine approach 70%, and remission rates are as high as 43% acutely and as high as 61% long term.

Duloxetine's (Cymbalta) inhibition of 5-HT and NE is more balanced as opposed to venlafaxine, which is more serotonergic at lower dose and more noradrenergic at higher doses. Its dual impact on anxious symptoms and somatic pain has resulted in 53% to 61% of treated patients achieving symptomatic remission and an approximate 47% achieving functional remission.

Adverse Effects

Adverse effects are similar in scope and magnitude to those of the SSRI class; however, the risk of clinically meaningful increases in blood pressure has also been documented, particularly with venlafaxine.

Tricyclic Antidepressants

TCAs are effective in GAD and PD. **Imipramine** (Tofranil) is the only TCA with an indication for the treatment of GAD and has proven effective in controlling panic attacks in patients with PD and GAD. TCAs are typically most useful in attenuating the psychological symptoms of GAD as opposed to the somatic symptoms. TCAs have largely been supplanted by SSRIs and SNRIs as first-line therapy for the treatment of anxiety disorders.

Mechanism of Action

TCA inhibition of 5-HT and NE reuptake are thought to produce anxiolytic and antidepressant effects. Imipramine does not have any direct effects on anticipatory anxiety or phobic avoidance behavior. The response is gradual, over a period of weeks.

Adverse Events

TCAs cause anticholinergic adverse effects such as dryness of the mouth and other mucosal surfaces, blurred vision, tachycardia, constipation, and urinary hesitancy. Other adverse effects are postural hypotension, carbohydrate craving, weight gain, and sexual dysfunction. They lower the seizure threshold and are a relative contraindication in patients with seizure disorders. These drugs are contraindicated in patients with narrow-angle glaucoma, urinary hesitancy, benign prostatic hyperplasia, and heart conduction abnormalities. TCAs enhance the CNS effects of alcohol. Plasma measurements of TCAs should be done in selected situations as needed. The profound risk of toxicity in overdose coupled with these undesired effects has resulted in TCAs being replaced by newer, more tolerable, possibly more effective drugs that are less toxic in overdose. See the chapter on depression.

Benzodiazepines

BZDs are important and widely prescribed sedative–hypnotics. Their pharmacologic properties include reduction of anxiety, sedation, muscle relaxation, anticonvulsant, and amnestic effects. Among the prominent BZDs are **alprazolam** (Xanax), **clonazepam** (Klonopin), **diazepam** (Valium), **lorazepam** (Ativan), and **oxazepam** (Serax). They are best utilized in patients with acute anxiety to a time-limited stressor.

Mechanism of Action

BZDs exert a therapeutic effect by binding to GABA-A receptors in the brain. They cause the GABA-A receptors to increase the opening of chloride channels along the cell membrane, leading to increased response to endogenous GABA, the main inhibitory neurotransmitter. Other neurotransmitters, such as 5-HT and NE, may play a role in the therapeutic effect of BZDs. The exact mechanism of BZDs' antianxiety effect is not yet fully understood. Most of the drugs in this class possess anxiolytic, sedative–hypnotic, and anticonvulsant properties.

BZDs can be used for treating GAD and PD. Approximately 75% of patients with GAD respond moderately or better to BZDs. BZDs are indicated for the short-term management of the acute phase of anxiety (first 2–4 weeks) as well as any subsequent exacerbations of anxiety during stable treatment with an antidepressant. Their rapid onset and tolerability allow them to ease anxious symptoms when immediate anxiolytic effects are necessary. Although more marked improvement is realized in the first 2 weeks of treatment with BZDs, antidepressants consistently achieve the efficacy of BZDs or even surpass it after 6 to 12 weeks of treatment, particularly in alleviating psychic symptoms. Though still a common practice, the utilization of BZDs long term or as monotherapy is not recommended and is inconsistent with evidence-based guidelines. BZDs are most adept at alleviating somatic symptoms but have no effect to a somewhat detrimental effect on the psychic symptoms of GAD. At this time, there is no evidence that one BZD is superior to another for this disorder. The high-potency BZDs, such as **alprazolam**, **clonazepam**, and **lorazepam**, have been effective in controlling panic attacks and anticipatory anxiety in panic attacks. The clinical indications for a specific BZD are not absolute, and

considerable overlap in their use exists. Not only are they effective in pathologic anxiety but also their calming effect is useful in nonpathologic anxiety states (temporary episodes of anxiety due to fear). BZDs have a wider therapeutic window than most other CNS depressants and are associated with fewer side effects.

The various BZDs differ little in their pharmacologic properties, but they differ significantly in their potency, their ability to cross the blood–brain barrier, and their half-lives. High-potency BZDs, such as **alprazolam**, **clonazepam**, and **lorazepam**, have a great affinity for the BZD receptor. The onset and intensity of action of an oral dose of a BZD is determined by the rate of absorption from the GI tract. BZDs are highly bound to plasma proteins (70%–90%) and are highly lipid soluble. The duration of action is related to their lipid solubility as well as hepatic biotransformation to active metabolites. **Oxazepam** and **lorazepam** are metabolized to inactive compounds and therefore have shorter half-lives and durations of activity than other BZDs. This one-step inactivation to an inactive compound makes them the preferred drugs for the treatment of anxiety in elderly patients and patients with liver disease.

Accumulation of BZDs with a long half-life (long-acting BZDs) occurs from one dose to another. Long-acting BZDs (e.g., diazepam, clonazepam, clorazepate) take a longer time to reach steady-state levels, are removed more slowly, and cause more pronounced side effects (e.g., sedation). However, use of these preparations reduces the likelihood and intensity of withdrawal symptoms when discontinued. High lipid solubility results in faster absorption, greater distribution in tissues, and faster entrance and exit from brain sites. Diazepam is a BZD with high lipid solubility used for anxiety (see **Table 40.3** for more information).

On discontinuation of BZD therapy, relapse may occur. Longer-acting drugs, such as clonazepam, can minimize dose-rebound anxiety. Similarly, rapid-onset agents, such as diazepam or alprazolam, can provide acute anxiolysis, whereas short-acting agents such as lorazepam can minimize accumulation and oversedation. In the elderly, use of long-acting BZDs is discouraged because the active metabolites have a tendency to accumulate.

Tolerance and Dependence Issues

Tolerance to the sedative (but not anxiolytic) effects of BZDs develops at moderate doses. BZDs can cause dependence if used continuously for more than several weeks. If the patient's anxiety is episodic, episodic use of BZDs may control symptoms. If anxiety is prolonged, BZDs may control the anxiety, but this therapeutic benefit must be weighed against their capacity to cause dependence. Abuse potential does not appear to be a problem in people who do not abuse alcohol or other substances. See "Monitoring Patient Response" for information on tapering technique and withdrawal issues.

TABLE 40.3

Overview of Selected Drugs Used to Treat Generalized Anxiety Disorder

Generic Name	Trade Name	Usual Adult Dosage Range (mg/d)	Oral Peak (h)	Half-Life (h) Parent + Active Metabolite	Metabolite Activity	Contraindications
Alprazolam	Xanax	0.75–4	1–2	6–20	Inactive	Hypersensitivity to alprazolam or any component of the formulation (cross-sensitivity with other benzodiazepines may also exist), narrow-angle glaucoma, concurrent use of ketoconazole or itraconazole
Chlordiazepoxide	Librium	15–40	0.5–4	30–100	Active	Hypersensitivity to chlordiazepoxide or any component of the formulation (cross-sensitivity with other benzodiazepines may also exist)
Clonazepam	Klonopin	0.5–3	1–2	18–50	Inactive	Hypersensitivity to clonazepam or any component of the formulation (cross-sensitivity with other benzodiazepines may also exist), narrow-angle glaucoma
Clorazepate	Tranxene	7.5–30	1–2	30–100	Active	Hypersensitivity to clorazepate or any component of the formulation (cross-sensitivity with other benzodiazepines may also exist), narrow-angle glaucoma
Diazepam	Valium	6–40	0.5–1	30–100	Active	Hypersensitivity to diazepam or any component of the formulation (cross-sensitivity with other benzodiazepines may also exist), myasthenia gravis, severe respiratory insufficiency syndrome, severe hepatic insufficiency syndrome, sleep apnea syndrome, narrow-angle glaucoma
Lorazepam	Ativan	1–6	2–4	10–20	Inactive	Hypersensitivity to lorazepam or any component of the formulation (cross-sensitivity with other benzodiazepines may also exist), severe respiratory insufficiency syndrome (except during mechanical ventilation), sleep apnea syndrome (parenteral), narrow-angle glaucoma
Oxazepam	Serax	15–120	2–4	8–12	Inactive	Hypersensitivity to oxazepam or any component of the formulation (cross-sensitivity with other benzodiazepines may also exist), narrow-angle glaucoma
Buspirone	BuSpar	15–60	—	2–3	Active	Hypersensitivity to buspirone or any component of the formulation
Hydroxyzine HCl Hydroxyzine pamoate	Atarax Vistaril	75–150	2–4	3	Inactive	Hypersensitivity to hydroxyzine or any component of the formulation
Propranolol	Inderal	10–20	1–4	6–10	Active	Hypersensitivity to propranolol, beta-blockers, or any component of the formulation; uncompensated heart failure; cardiogenic shock; severe sinus bradycardia; sick sinus syndrome; heart block greater than first degree (except in patients with a functioning artificial pacemaker); or bronchial asthma

(Continued)

TABLE 40.3

Overview of Selected Drugs Used to Treat Generalized Anxiety Disorder (*Continued*)

Generic Name	Trade Name	Usual Adult Dosage Range (mg/d)	Oral Peak (h)	Half-Life (h) Parent + Active Metabolite	Metabolite Activity	Contraindications
Clonidine	Catapres, Kapvay	0.3–1.2	1–3	12–16	Inactive	Hypersensitivity to clonidine or any component of the formulation
Mirtazapine	Remeron	15–45	2	20–40	Active	Hypersensitivity to mirtazapine or any component of the formulation; use of MAO inhibitors intended to treat psychiatric disorders (concurrently or within 14 days of discontinuing either mirtazapine or the MAO inhibitor); initiation of mirtazapine in a patient receiving linezolid or intravenous methylene blue

MAO, monoamine oxidase.
Adapted from the following references: Arana, G. W., & Jerrold, R. (2000). *Handbook of psychiatric drug therapy* (4th ed., p. 176). Philadelphia, PA: Lippincott Williams & Wilkins; Schatzberg, A. F., Cole, J. O., & DeBattista, C. (2010). *Manual of clinical psychopharmacology* (7th ed., pp. 382–384). Washington, DC: American Psychiatric Publishing.

Adverse Events

The major adverse events of BZDs are drowsiness and psychomotor impairment. Mild, transitory cognitive and memory impairments are seen occasionally. This is more significant in elderly people and those with high sensitivity to these drugs. Reactions of rage, excitement, and hostility, although rare, have been reported in children, the elderly, and brain-injured patients. Other reported side effects include increased depression, confusion, headache, GI disturbances, menstrual irregularities, and changes in libido. Urticaria may occur in people with drug hypersensitivity, and drug interactions may occur with a variety of medications (**Table 40.4**).

Treatment of Benzodiazepine Overdose

Flumazenil (Mazicon) is a competitive BZD receptor antagonist that reverses the sedative effects of BZDs. Antagonism of BZD-induced respiratory depression is less predictable. Flumazenil is the only BZD receptor antagonist available for clinical use. It blocks many of the actions of BZDs but does not antagonize the CNS effects of other sedative–hypnotics such as ethanol, opioids, or general anesthetics. It is used for BZD overdose and after the use of drugs in anesthetic and diagnostic procedures. When given intravenously, it acts rapidly and has a short half-life (0.7–1.3 hours). Because all BZDs have a longer duration of action than flumazenil, sedation commonly recurs and repeated doses of flumazenil may be needed. Caution should be used to avoid inducing seizures from BZD withdrawal. Other adverse effects of flumazenil include confusion, agitation, dizziness, and nausea/vomiting.

Azapirones

Buspirone is a partial agonist at the 5-HT$_{1A}$ receptors and a full agonist at the presynaptic serotonergic autoreceptors. Though buspirone's effectiveness in treating GAD has been demonstrated inconsistently in several studies, its delayed onset of action, tolerability, and relative lack of efficacy with respect to most comorbid conditions (with the exception of MDD) has resulted in buspirone being used primarily as adjunctive therapy. It has comparable but slightly weaker efficacy compared to diazepam, clorazepate, lorazepam, and alprazolam but has a clearly slower onset of action. Buspirone's utility is mainly associated with its propensity to relieve the cognitive aspects, but it lacks long-term efficacy, particularly in managing the behavioral and somatic manifestations. It is rapidly absorbed from the intestinal tract but undergoes extensive first-pass metabolism. People with liver dysfunction have a decreased clearance of buspirone. Buspirone has no hypnotic, anticonvulsant, or muscle relaxant properties. Patients taking buspirone do not acquire a cross tolerance for alcohol or BZDs. It is generally well tolerated, with only a few patients experiencing adverse effects. When adverse effects do occur, they include nausea, dizziness, and headache (see **Table 40.3**). Doses over 70 mg have caused jitteriness and dysphoria.

In contrast to BZDs, buspirone's therapeutic effect may take 2 to 3 weeks. Because of its delayed effects, this drug is not useful in patients who need immediate relief from anxiety, and patient education is needed to enhance compliance with the medication regimen.

Novel Drugs

Recently, a number of novel entities and also existing medications not initially labeled for use in GAD have been evaluated. **Pregabalin** (Lyrica) has shown some promise in clinical trials, but does not have an indication for the treatment of any anxiety disorder. Two similarly designed randomized, placebo and active comparator-controlled double-blinded studies

TABLE 40.4

Benzodiazepine Drug Interactions

Drug	Interaction	Description	Management
Alcohol/CNS depressants	↑ BZD levels	Increased CNS effects (sedation, psychomotor impairment).	Avoid combination.
Antacids	↓ BZD levels	Antacids alter the rate but not the extent of GI absorption.	Stagger administration times to avoid possible interaction.
Azole antifungals (itraconazole, ketoconazole, voriconazole)	↑ BZD levels	Azole antifungals decrease the metabolism of BZDs, leading into increased CNS depression and sedation.	Alprazolam is contraindicated with itraconazole and ketoconazole.
Carbamazepine	↓ BZD levels	May increase hepatic metabolism and result in decreased pharmacologic effects.	Consider increasing the BZD dose.
Carisoprodol	↑ BZD levels	Increased depressant effects.	Strong association between illicit use of carisoprodol, alprazolam, and oxycodone. Be vigilant for legitimacy of the prescriptions.
Clozapine	↑ BZD levels	Increased risk of respiratory suppression, delirium, and ataxia.	Do not start simultaneously. It may be better to add clozapine to an established BZD routine.
Contraceptives, oral	The clearance rate of BZDs that undergo glucuronidation may be increased (lorazepam and oxazepam). May see decreased clearance and increased free concentrations of chlordiazepoxide, diazepam, and alprazolam, e.g., BZDs that undergo oxidative metabolism		Monitor clinical effects.
CYP3A4 inhibitors (cimetidine, diltiazem, disulfiram, isoniazid, omeprazole, macrolide antibiotics, metoprolol, propranolol, valproic acid)	↑ BZD levels	The elimination of BZDs that undergo oxidative hepatic metabolism (alprazolam, chlordiazepoxide, clonazepam, diazepam) may be decreased by the following drugs due to inhibition of hepatic metabolism.	May need dosage reduction.
Digoxin		Digoxin serum concentrations may be increased.	Monitor digoxin levels.
Hydantoins (e.g., phenytoin)	↓ BZD levels	Serum concentrations of BZDs may be decreased due to induction of hepatic metabolism by hydantoins. Pharmacologic effects of hydantoins may be increased by BZDs.	Monitor clinical effects carefully—consider monitoring serum levels of phenytoin.
Probenecid	↑ BZD levels	Probenecid may interfere with BZD conjugation in the liver, resulting in prolonged effect.	Consider decreasing BZD dose.
Protease inhibitors (e.g., ritonavir, nelfinavir)	↑ BZD levels	May decrease the oxidative metabolism of BZDs leading to severe sedation and respiratory depression.	Decrease BZD dose.

(Continued)

TABLE 40.4

Benzodiazepine Drug Interactions (*Continued*)

Drug	Interaction	Description	Management
Ranitidine	↓ Diazepam	Ranitidine may reduce the GI absorption of diazepam.	Stagger doses.
Rifampin	↓ BZD levels	The oxidative metabolism may be increased due to enzyme induction. Pharmacologic effects of BZDs may be decreased.	Monitor clinically.
Sodium oxybate	↑ BZD levels	Concurrent use may result in an increase in sleep duration and CNS depression.	Avoid combination.
Theophylline	↓ BZD levels.	Theophylline may antagonize the sedative effects of BZDs.	

BZD, benzodiazepine; CNS, central nervous system; GI, gastrointestinal.

evaluated the efficacy of pregabalin versus lorazepam for the treatment of GAD. The pregabalin groups and the lorazepam group all experienced improvements by week 4 as compared to placebo, with no observed statistically significant differences among the active groups. Pregabalin at its highest study dose (600 mg) produced statistically superior reductions in the psychic and somatic symptoms compared to placebo, whereas the lorazepam group only reached statistical significance versus placebo with respect to the somatic symptoms. The relative efficacy and early onset of effect of pregabalin versus commonly used BZDs have been established, and this may represent a new therapeutic intervention for GAD as both a monotherapy (after failure of an initial monotherapy) and an augmentation strategy.

Monoamine Oxidase Inhibitors

MAO inhibitors are effective in controlling panic attacks in most patients with PD. Their effectiveness in GAD has not been explored because of the necessary dietary restrictions and dangerous drug interactions that make their use cumbersome.

Mechanism of Action

MAO inhibitors inhibit the breakdown of 5-HT and NE in the synaptic cleft. The most commonly used MAO inhibitor is **phenelzine** (Nardil), which is typically started at 15 mg once or twice daily, and then increased to a total dose of 60 to 90 mg/day based on response. A response is expected within 4 to 6 weeks, and longer for maximal response to be attained.

Adverse Events

MAO inhibitors have an extensive anticholinergic side-effect profile, including blurred vision, dry mouth and other mucosal surfaces, constipation, urinary hesitancy, and tachycardia. Weight gain, insomnia, and sexual dysfunction frequently occur. These side effects may contribute to overall poor patient tolerability. Hypotension that is aggravated by postural changes may develop, but it usually diminishes in a few weeks.

Palliative measures such as increased fluid intake, salt tablets, and low-dose fludrocortisone (Florinef) can be used to manage hypotension. The greatest danger with MAO inhibitors is hypertensive crisis, which can be caused by food or drug interaction and can result in cerebral hemorrhage and death. MAO inhibitors prevent the breakdown of monoamines, so the patient taking an MAO inhibitor must avoid sympathomimetic substances and foods that contain tyramine, such as cheese, liver, yogurt, yeast, soy sauce, red wine, and beer. See the chapter on depression.

Other Antianxiety Medications

Hydroxyzines are sometimes used to relieve anxiety and tension associated with an anxiety state or as an adjunct in organic disease states with anxiety.

The use of hydroxyzine for long-term treatment of anxiety (>4 months) has not been assessed. **Hydroxyzine hydrochloride** (Atarax) and **hydroxyzine pamoate** (Vistaril) are drugs more commonly used for sedating patients before and after surgery and for managing pruritus, chronic urticaria, and atopic contact dermatitis. See **Table 40.3** for doses and adverse events.

Propranolol has also been used to treat or alleviate the symptoms of anxiety, including PDs, posttraumatic stress disorder, and performance anxiety. Propranolol is a lipophilic nonselective beta-adrenoreceptor blocker. Traditionally used in cardiac populations, its mechanism to blunt sympathomimetic activation also acts as an anxiolytic by dampening symptoms such as tachycardia and diaphoresis. However, no randomized controlled trials have studied these benefits. A 2016 meta-analysis was not able to find a statistically significant difference between the effects of propranolol and BZDs and therefore concluded that use for or against propranolol could not be recommended.

Similar to propranolol's mechanism of action, clonidine is usually used as an antihypertensive that was found to have anxiolytic and sedating effects. It acts as an alpha$_2$-adrenergic agonist, which decreases postsynaptic alpha$_1$-adrenergic receptor activation and inhibits release of catecholamines (e.g., epinephrine, NE). Several small-scale uncontrolled studies have demonstrated clonidine's anxiolytic effects; however, larger studies are still needed to further investigate clonidine's place in therapy.

Lastly, mirtazapine is a TCA with mixed serotonergic and noradrenergic agent that helps increase NE release and 5-HT$_{1A}$ serotonergic neurotransmission. Several studies have compared mirtazapine against placebo and other psychotherapeutic agents that have shown successful results in treatment of anxiety and PDs. Furthermore, its rapid onset of action and low side-effect profile makes mirtazapine a viable adjunct for the treatment of anxiety disorders.

Atypical Antipsychotics

The AAPs have been evaluated mostly for purposes of adjunctive therapy when patients do not respond to, are intolerant of, or do not fully remit with conventional therapies. None of the AAPs have labeled indications for any anxiety disorder, though some do as adjunctive treatments for MDD. Of the eight available AAPs, there are studies evaluating the benefit of five of them in GAD (**aripiprazole**, **quetiapine**, **risperidone**, **ziprasidone**, and **olanzapine**). AAPs have mostly been studied in short-term trials as adjunctive therapies in treatment-resistant GAD. New literature also suggests that AAPs may result in a shorter response rate than in placebo when both were given with SSRIs for GAD in patients with comorbid schizophrenia, bipolar disorder, and MDD. However, the unfavorable side-effect profiles limit their use as first-line long-term drug of choice.

Selecting the Most Appropriate Agent

General Anxiety Disorder

First-Line Therapy

SSRIs and SNRIs are considered drugs of choice for GAD. No evidence exists to support the superiority of any of these drugs individually; however, there are significant differences in adverse effects and drug interactions. Patients may have to try several SSRIs or SNRIs prior to realizing a therapeutic benefit balanced with appropriate tolerability.

Antidepressants all require several weeks to become effective, so BZDs may be given along with an antidepressant until it begins to work. Once this occurs, the patient is slowly tapered off the BZD. BZDs also have a role chronically for purposes of treating exacerbations of anxiety when quick relief is desired. BZDs are considered first-line therapy only for acute anxiety related to a time-limited stressor. The BZDs used most frequently are alprazolam, clonazepam, and diazepam. There is no evidence that one BZD is superior to another in this disorder. When choosing the specific BZD for treatment, the practitioner must consider the drug's onset of action and its half-life and the patient's metabolism (**Figure 40.1** and **Table 40.5**).

Second-Line Therapy

After confirmed failure or intolerance to multiple members of the SSRI and SNRI classes at appropriate doses for an appropriate period of time (i.e., 2–4 weeks), imipramine or buspirone may be considered.

Buspirone may be more appropriate if sedation or psychomotor impairment would be dangerous. Buspirone differs from the SSRIs in its efficacy spectrum and side-effect profile and has fewer adverse effects compared to BZDs and minimal abuse potential. However, the therapeutic effect of the drug may take 1 to 4 weeks. Buspirone may be the most appropriate drug for patients with a history of substance abuse, personality disorder, or sleep apnea.

Third-Line Therapy

Third-line therapy consists of a TCA alone or buspirone.

Fourth-Line Therapy

After the SSRIs, SNRIs, buspirone, and imipramine are exhausted, combination or adjunctive therapy may be considered. Practitioners may even consider combination or adjunctive therapy prior to attempting buspirone or imipramine (third line). Generally, buspirone, pregabalin (not approved for this indication in the United States), or an AAP (not approved for this indication in the United States) could be added to standard therapy in the event that a therapeutic effect is not realized with monotherapy. An SSRI or SNRI plus an AAP, an SSRI or SNRI plus an antihistamine (hydroxyzine), a combination of an SSRI and imipramine, or a combination of an SSRI and a BZD are all reasonable strategies.

Panic Disorder

First-Line Therapy

Nonpharmacologic therapy is especially critical in the treatment of PD. Patients need to be educated on the avoidance of substances that can precipitate panic attacks; these include caffeine, drugs of abuse, and nonprescription stimulants. CBT is associated with short-term improvement in symptoms.

PD is episodic, and patients with PD frequently do well with SSRIs or venlafaxine. Alprazolam (Xanax) is the only BZD that is approved by the FDA for PD, but clonazepam or lorazepam can also be used. These drugs are used along with an SSRI if rapid relief from anxiety is needed and there is no history of substance abuse. The practitioner needs to monitor symptoms, assess for side effects, and gradually increase the dosages of SSRIs, venlafaxine, alprazolam, lorazepam, or clonazepam if needed (**Figure 40.2**).

Second-Line Therapy

Patients who do not respond to SSRIs may be changed to another SSRI or venlafaxine and monitored for effectiveness in decreasing panic attacks and controlling the severity of anxiety or panic symptoms while causing tolerable adverse events.

Third-Line Therapy

Patients who do not respond to venlafaxine or several SSRIs may be switched to yet another SSRI, imipramine, or an MAO

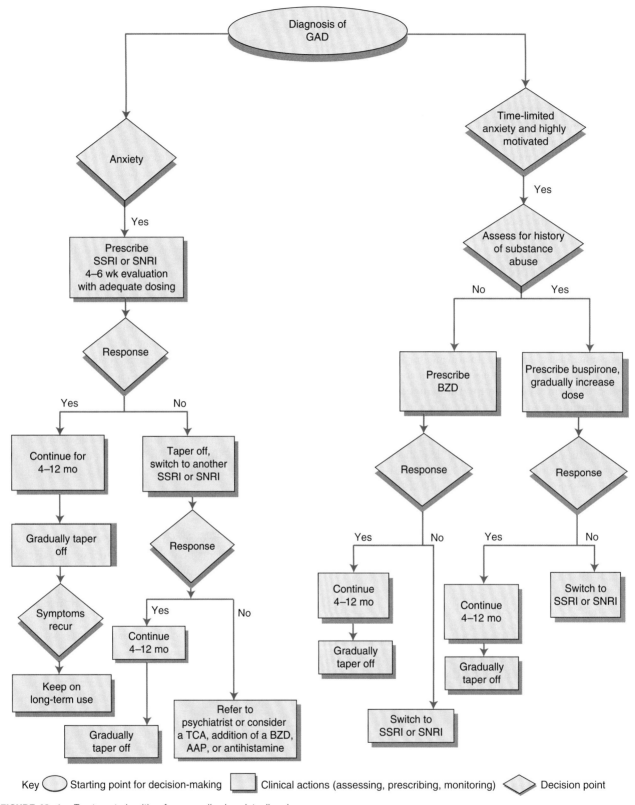

FIGURE 40–1   Treatment algorithm for generalized anxiety disorder.

AAP, atypical antipsychotic; BZD, benzodiazepine; GAD, generalized anxiety disorder; SNRI, serotonin–norepinephrine reuptake inhibitors; SSRI, selective serotonin reuptake inhibitor; TCA, tricyclic antidepressant.

TABLE 40.5

Recommended Order of Long-Term Treatment for Generalized Anxiety Disorder

Order	Agents	Comments
First line	SSRI or SNRI	Useful for anxiety disorder as well as a coexisting comorbidity.
Second line	Buspirone or imipramine	Takes 1–2 weeks for effect.
Third line	Adjunctive therapy with pregabalin, buspirone	Select agent based on drug onset, half-life, and patient metabolism. Do not use if the patient is alcohol or drug dependent. May be first-line drug in motivated patients with acute anxiety to a time-limited stress.

SNRI, serotonin–norepinephrine reuptake inhibitor; SSRI, selective serotonin reuptake inhibitor.

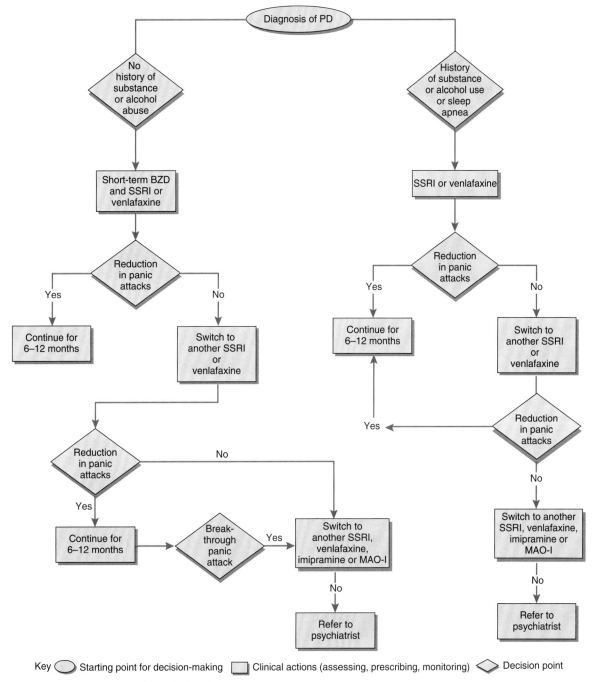

FIGURE 40–2 Treatment algorithm for panic disorder.

BZD, benzodiazepine; MAO-I, monoamine oxidase inhibitors; PD, panic disorder; SSRI, selective serotonin reuptake inhibitor.

inhibitor. MAO inhibitors can be very effective in controlling panic attacks. Before the patient begins therapy, however, the practitioner must assess his or her willingness to avoid the many tyramine-containing sympathomimetic drugs and foods, which can interact with MAO inhibitors to precipitate serious, life-threatening reactions. Washout periods are critical before beginning an MAO inhibitor due to the risk of 5-HT syndrome. In addition, the patient should be referred to a psychiatrist for intensive therapy, particularly if combination therapy is required. When a TCA is given for PD, approximately 33% of patients feel overstimulated when treatment begins. To reduce this problem, the patient may need to start with a lower dose and gradually increase the dose until a therapeutic dose response occurs. BZDs can be used on a short-term basis to lessen these initial symptoms. Because PD is episodic, it is considered a chronic condition that requires long-term management with TCAs. However, approximately 33% of patients on TCAs discontinue their treatment because they cannot tolerate the side effects of the drugs.

Social Anxiety Disorder

SAD or social phobia is characterized by an intense, irrational fear of scrutiny or negative evaluation of others in social situations. In generalized SAD, fear and avoidance extend to various social situations, but can also be confined to only one or two specific situations, such as performing in public. Symptoms most commonly experienced include blushing, shaking, sweating, and heart palpitations.

First-Line Therapy

Generally, the SSRIs and venlafaxine are considered first-line therapies for SAD. CBT is also a potential initial therapy along with a medication or as monotherapy.

Second-Line Therapy

After failure of CBT and an adequate trial of either an SSRI or venlafaxine, the MAO-I phenelzine can be attempted in selected patients (see **Figure 40.3**). Given the adverse effect profile, toxicity in overdose, and drug and food interaction potential, phenelzine should be reserved for refractory cases. **Table 40.6** summarizes drug therapy for GAD, PD, and SAD.

Special-Population Considerations

Patients who have previously been treated for an anxiety disorder may have had drug treatment or psychotherapy that they found unsatisfactory. The practitioner should review with them what the treatments were, what adverse reactions they had, and the number of previous health care providers who treated them. Check with them for any history of drug withdrawal symptoms. If they report that a drug or treatment was unacceptable, plan a different but effective treatment. Assess for adverse effects to the new program. Also assess for drug-seeking behavior to rule out BZD dependence. Sometimes, patients "shop around" for new health care providers when their previous provider has advised withdrawing from BZDs.

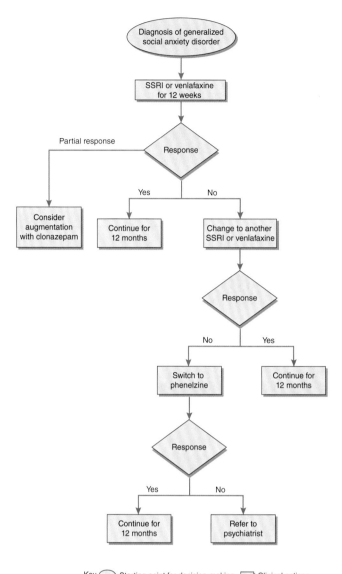

FIGURE 40–3   Treatment algorithm for social anxiety disorder.

SSRI, selective serotonin reuptake inhibitor.

Source: Bandelow, B., Zohar, J., Hollander, E., et al. (2008). World Federation of Societies of Biological Psychiatry (WFSBP) guidelines for the pharmacological treatment of anxiety, obsessive-compulsive and post-traumatic stress disorders—First revision. *World Journal of Biological Psychiatry, 9*(4), 248–312.

TABLE 40.6

Pharmacotherapy for Selected Anxiety Disorders

	SSRIs	TCAs	Buspirone	BZDs	MAOIs	CBT
GAD	+	+	+/−	+	+	+
PD	+	+/−	+	+	+	+
SAD	+	−	+/−	+	+	+

BZDs, benzodiazepines; CBT, cognitive–behavioral therapy; GAD, generalized anxiety disorder; MAOIs, monoamine oxidase inhibitors; PD, panic disorder; SAD, social anxiety disorder; SSRIs, selective serotonin reuptake inhibitors; TCAs, tricyclic antidepressants.

Patients with a history of prescription medication abuse and substance or alcohol abuse can become drug dependent. Buspirone, a nonaddictive drug, is a choice for their treatment regimen.

Pediatric

Similar to adults, the first-line treatment for GAD in children are SSRI antidepressants. SNRI and TCA agents have also shown efficacy in the treatment of pediatric anxiety disorders but, due to their side-effect profiles, are less easily tolerated. A meta-analysis of 16 randomized trials found a number of SSRI and SNRI antidepressants superior to placebo in the treatment of pediatric anxiety (Uthman & Abdulmalik, 2010). The risks associated with SSRIs/SNRI antidepressants for pediatric anxiety should be carefully weighed against their potential benefits whenever their use is considered. Four BZDs—clorazepate, chlordiazepoxide, diazepam, and alprazolam—have been approved by the FDA for use in children. Doses vary according to the child's age and weight. Risks and benefits should be discussed with both the parent and the child before beginning treatment. The FDA recommends close monitoring of the child's clinical status during the early weeks of antidepressant treatment and limiting the duration of their use.

Geriatric

Elderly patients may have decreased liver and renal function and metabolize and excrete drugs more slowly. They also may have neurologic disorders, cardiac disease, hypertension, hypotension, and glaucoma and may be taking drugs for these conditions. Elderly patients may be started on low doses of shorter-acting BZDs, TCAs, SSRIs, and buspirone, and the dosage may be gradually increased. Elderly patients may also experience paradoxical reactions to drugs (see **Tables 40.3** and **40.4**).

Women

Women are more likely than men to seek treatment for anxiety and depression. Women who are taking oral contraceptive drugs may have adverse drug interactions with BZDs (see **Table 40.4**). The practitioner needs to be alert for signs of anxiety disorders in men because they are not as likely as women to report these symptoms. Rather, men are likely to report physical signs of anxiety and not identify the problem as emotional in origin.

Pregnancy

Treatment considerations (to use or not to use antidepressants) during pregnancy *may* pose both maternal and fetal risks: risk of untreated depression or anxiety in the mother and the risk of teratogenicity, malformations, and low birth weight in the fetus, respectively. All antidepressants cross the placenta; however, this does not consistently equate with a risk of teratogenicity. Though somewhat contradictory and arguably not completely clear, some studies have found a modestly increased risk of fetal cardiovascular malformations in fetuses exposed to SSRIs in utero. Other studies have failed to demonstrate this increased risk and suggest that the risk of the aforementioned issues is consistent with that of the general, unexposed population. Thus far, SSRIs have not been associated with maternal complications with the exception of postpartum hemorrhage. The newest evidence, resulting from a large-scale meta-analysis, reveals that fluoxetine may cause fetal heart wall defects and craniosynostosis, and paroxetine may cause fetal heart defects, anencephaly, and abdominal wall defects (Reefhuis et al., 2015). The SNRIs, trazodone, bupropion, and the TCAs are also not generally associated with teratogenicity. The observed cases of fetal defects seem to be dependent on the trimester; therefore, the potential risks associated with antidepressant use during pregnancy vary over the course of the pregnancy. All of the antidepressants discussed in this chapter are pregnancy category C, with the exception of bupropion, which is category B, and paroxetine, which is category D.

The risks of not treating depression in pregnant patients include premature delivery, low birth weight, miscarriage, preeclampsia, and gestational hypertension. Unfortunately, pregnant patients sometimes self-discontinue their antidepressants due to a fear of harming their baby. This can lead to withdrawal in some cases and rebound or worsened anxious symptoms. Fetal organs begin developing early in pregnancy, and therefore a conversation as early as possible is recommended. The patient and practitioner need to design a plan that is acceptable for all parties and will minimize risks to the fetus as well as the patient.

Ethnicity

Understanding a patient's cultural orientation or ethnic background is necessary for making a correct diagnosis and establishing an appropriate treatment plan. What we view as a problem such as anxiety or depression is not always perceived the same way by patients from other cultures. Complaints of anxiety or depression may not be reported by some patients because this is considered to be a mental disorder that is to be kept secret from people outside the family.

Research findings indicate that people from various racial or ethnic groups may metabolize some drugs differently because of their genetic makeup. An example of a drug that is metabolized differently is the antitubercular drug isoniazid (Laniazid). Researchers are beginning to examine other drug classifications for variations. Practitioners need to keep current with research that examines genetic differences in the metabolism of drugs (see Chapters 2 and 3).

Monitoring Patient Response

Patients need to be monitored for self-reports of decreased anxiety symptoms. The practitioner should monitor patients closely for compliance with the medication regimen as well as side effects.

Most side effects from SSRIs are transient. Dose-related sexual effects, such as decreased libido or delayed ejaculation in men and anorgasmia in women, are common and typically do not resolve without intervention. Management of treatment-related sexual dysfunction includes reducing the SSRI dosage reduction and adding or switching to an antidepressant not associated with sexual dysfunction, such as bupropion (Wellbutrin, Wellbutrin SR), nefazodone, or mirtazapine (Remeron). Another strategy includes the use of sildenafil (Viagra) or buspirone.

A non-life-threatening discontinuation syndrome of flu-like symptoms may occur after abrupt cessation of an SSRI. This syndrome can be minimized by gradually tapering the dose. Tapering doses of SSRIs may be a highly individualized process based on patient tolerability and drug agent itself that is being tapered. In general, tapering may take approximately 2 to 4 weeks.

An overdose of TCAs can lead to anticholinergic delirium, ventricular arrhythmias, significant hypotension, seizures, and death. A TCA overdose is a medical emergency and requires close clinical and cardiac monitoring.

Many patients do not like buspirone because it takes 1 to 4 weeks to take effect. Frequently, patients stop taking this medication because they think it is not helping their symptoms. Patient education and monitoring for compliance must be ongoing.

There have been no well-documented fatal overdoses of BZDs, but deaths have resulted from the ingestion of multiple drugs and overdoses of BZDs and other drugs. Prolonged use of BZDs can lead to dependence and withdrawal on discontinuation. Although the duration of therapy is not standardized, most clinicians prescribe the medication for 4 to 6 months and then try decreasing the dosage; however, the relapse rate of anxiety is approximately 60% to 80% within the first year that the patient is off the medication.

There are three components of a withdrawal syndrome: relapse is the return of the original symptoms of anxiety, rebound is a return of symptoms at greater severity than originally experienced, and withdrawal is the appearance of new symptoms.

When a BZD is discontinued, the severity of the withdrawal syndrome depends on how rapidly the drug is tapered, the half-life of the drug, and the duration of therapy. The withdrawal syndrome increases in severity with increased dosage and duration of use: for instance, more patients experience withdrawal symptoms after taking a BZD for 8 months than those taking it for less than 3 months. Withdrawal is relatively infrequent with short-term use, but it can occur with therapy as brief as 2 weeks. Abrupt discontinuation is frequently associated with withdrawal, usually of greater severity. Therefore, the rate of discontinuation should be slowed to moderate the symptoms. The three basic approaches to discontinuation include (1) using the same agent, (2) switching to an agent with a longer half-life, or (3) using adjuvant medications to reduce withdrawal symptoms. Options for adjunctive therapy includes carbamazepine, imipramine, divalproex, and trazodone. Although there is no gold standard for tapering BZD, the tapering period should be at least 4 weeks, and the rate of tapering should be approximately a 10% dosage decrease every 3 to 4 days. **Box 40.5** lists BZD withdrawal symptoms.

| **BOX 40.5** | **Symptoms of Benzodiazepine Withdrawal** |

Frequent
Anxiety
Insomnia
Irritability
Muscle problems

Common
Nausea
Depression
Ataxia
Hyperreflexia
Blurred vision
Fatigue

Rare
Psychosis
Seizures
Delirium
Confusion

Adapted with permission from Schweizer, E., & Rickels, K. (1998). Benzodiazepine dependence and withdrawal: A review of the syndrome and its clinical management. *Acta Psychiatrica Scandinavica, Supplementum, 393*, 95–101. Copyright © John Wiley & Sons.

Patients on long-term (>4 months) BZD therapy need periodic blood counts and liver and thyroid function testing. BZDs can cause elevations in lactate dehydrogenase, alkaline phosphatase, alanine aminotransferase, and aspartate aminotransferase levels. Use of BZDs may cause leukopenia, blood dyscrasias, anemia, thrombocytopenia, eosinophilia, and decreased uptake of I^{125} and I^{131} sodium iodide. (See **Table 40.3**; see the chapter on depression for a discussion of monitoring concerns related to antidepressant medications.)

PATIENT EDUCATION

Drug Information

The patient should know the name of the drug prescribed, dose, frequency of administration, expected outcome of therapy, drug interactions, adverse events, and the amount of time it will take for the drug to take effect. The patient should also know how to report adverse events to the primary caregiver. The patient should be taught to take the drug as ordered and not to increase the dose or stop the drug without first contacting the primary care provider.

The patient should know that the therapeutic effect of the drug needs to be monitored and that the dosage may need to be increased or another drug may be more helpful. If laboratory tests are needed, the patient should know the name of the laboratory test, what the test is, and the frequency of monitoring. The patient also needs to tell all health care providers what medications he or she is taking.

The National Institutes of Health's Web site (www.nih.gov/medlineplus/anxiety.html) provides useful patient information, as does the Anxiety Disorder Association of America's Web site (www.adaa.org).

Lifestyle Information

The patient should know that the physical symptoms of anxiety (e.g., increased heart rate, palpitations, pupillary dilatation, trembling, increased perspiration, muscle tension, and sleep disturbances) are not life threatening. The practitioner should instruct the patient about how combination treatment consisting of medications, psychotherapy, and relaxation therapy can control anxiety. Instruction on performing relaxation exercises is helpful. The practitioner should describe the various psychotherapeutic modalities so that the patient may select the one thought to be most appropriate. If the patient does not seek psychotherapy, the primary caregiver may need to provide emotional support. The patient who does not respond well to drug and relaxation therapy must be referred to a psychiatric specialist.

Providing written instructions is important because the patient may have trouble concentrating on or fully comprehending verbal instructions. After providing all instructions and materials, the practitioner should review the patient's comprehension of the instructions and willingness to comply with the medication regimen. This review should be part of each patient visit.

CASE STUDY 1

A.L. is a 34-year-old female who presents to her primary care physician. She states that over the past 10 months, she has felt more "restless" and "on edge" than usual but also finds herself fatigued by midday. She reports usually having unsatisfying sleep, which she has experienced her "whole life." A.L. works as an attorney at a large law firm, usually requiring 60 to 80 hours of work each week. She does not smoke butdrinks alcohol every one to two days (2glasses of wine). She reports no illicit substance use. She exercises three times a week and generally keeps to a balanced diet. On physical exam, A.L. appears welldeveloped and well-nourished. Her lab work and vital signs are within normal limits. The only medication she takes is oral contraceptive pills, which she has taken for 8 years without any adverse effects, and multivitamins. Upon further questioning, A.L. reveals that she has been under more pressure at work due to higher work volume and her bid to become a partner in her law firm. She feels that she is not performing as well as she should be because of her symptoms and endorses finding it difficult to concentrate, which leads to increased worry (Learning Objectives 2 and 3).

DIAGNOSIS: GENERALIZED ANXIETY DISORDER

1. What first-line therapy would you prescribe for A.L.?
2. Describe specific patient monitoring based on the prescribed therapy.
3. After 3 months, the patient still endorses symptoms. What second-line agent would you start?

Bibliography

*Starred references are cited in the text.

*American Psychiatric Association. (2013). *Diagnostic and statistical manual of mental health disorders: DSM-5* (5th ed.). Washington, DC: American Psychiatric Publishing.

Anttila, S. A., & Leinonen, E. V. (2001). A review of the pharmacological and clinical profile of mirtazapine. *CNS Drug Reviews, 7*(3), 249–264.

Baldwin, D. S., Anderson, I. M., Nutt, D. J., et al. (2014). Evidence-based pharmacological treatment of anxiety disorders, posttraumatic stress disorder and obsessive–compulsive disorder: A revision of the 2005 guidelines from the British Association for Psychopharmacology. *Journal of Psychopharmacology, 28*(5), 403–439.

Bandelow, B., Boerner, J. R., Kasper, S., et al. (2013). The diagnosis and treatment of generalized anxiety disorder. *Deutsches Ärzteblatt International, 110*(17), 300–309.

Bandelow, B., Sher, L., Bunevicius, R., et al. (2012). Guidelines for the pharmacological treatment of anxiety disorders, obsessive-compulsive disorder and posttraumatic stress disorder in primary care. *International Journal of Psychiatry in Clinical Practice, 16*(2), 77–84.

Bandelow, B., Zohar, J., Hollander, E., et al. (2008). World Federation of Societies of Biological Psychiatry (WFSBP) guidelines for the pharmacological treatment of anxiety, obsessive-compulsive and post-traumatic stress disorders—First revision. *World Journal of Biological Psychiatry, 9*(4), 248–312.

Carleton, R. N. (2012). The intolerance of uncertainty construct in the context of anxiety disorders: Theoretical and practical perspectives. *Expert Review of Neurotherapeutics, 12*(8), 937–947.

Combs, H., & Markman, J. (2014). Anxiety disorders in primary care. *The Medical Clinics of North America, 98*(5), 1007–1023.

Dunsmoor, J. E., & Paz, R. (2015). Fear generalization and anxiety: Behavioral and neural mechanisms. *Biological Psychiatry, 78*(5), 336–343. doi: 10.1016/j.biopsych.2015.04.010

Duval, E. R., Javanbakht, A., & Liberzon, I. (2015). Neural circuits in anxiety and stress disorders: A focused review. *Therapeutics and Clinical Risk Management, 11*, 115–126.

Fava, G. A., Gatti, A., Belaise, C., et al. (2015). Withdrawal symptoms after selective serotonin reuptake inhibitor discontinuation: A systematic review. *Psychotherapy and Psychosomatics, 84*(2), 72–81.

Gadot, Y., & Koren, G. (2015). The use of antidepressants in pregnancy: Focus on maternal risks. *Journal of Obstetrics and Gynaecology Canada, 37*(1), 56–63.

Katzman, M. A. (2009). Current considerations in the treatment of generalized anxiety disorder. *CNS Drugs, 23*(2), 103–120.

Khan, A., Joyce, M., Atkinson, S., et al. (2011). A randomized, double-blind study of once-daily extended release quetiapine fumarate (quetiapine XR) monotherapy in patients with generalized anxiety disorder. *Journal of Clinical Psychopharmacology, 31*(4), 418–428.

Martin, E. I., Ressler, K. J., Binder, E., et al. (2009). The neurobiology of anxiety disorders: Brain imaging, genetics, and psychoneuroendocrinology. *The Psychiatric Clinics of North America, 32*(3), 549–575.

Nardi, A. E., Freire, R. C., Mochcovitch, M. D., et al. (2012). A randomized, naturalistic, parallel-group study for the long-term treatment of panic disorder with clonazepam or paroxetine. *Journal of Clinical Psychopharmacology, 32*(1), 120–126.

*Reefhuis, J., Devine, O., Friedman, J. M., et al. (2015). Specific SSRIs and birth defects: Bayesian analysis to interpret new data in the context of previous reports. *British Medical Journal, 351*, h3190.

Reinhold, J. A., Mandos, L. A., Rickels, K., et al. (2011). Pharmacological treatment of generalized anxiety disorder. *Expert Opinion on Pharmacotherapy, 12*(16), 2457–2467.

Rickels, K., Etemad, B., Khalid-Khan, S., et al. (2010). Time to relapse after 6 and 12 months' treatment of generalized anxiety disorder with venlafaxine extended release. *Archives of General Psychiatry, 67*(12), 1274–1281.

Rickels, K., Etemad, B., Rynn, M. A., et al. (2013). Remission of generalized anxiety disorder after 6 months of open label treatment with venlafaxine XR. *Psychotherapy and Psychosomatics, 82*, 363–371.

Rickels, K., Shiovitz, T. M., Ramey, T. S., et al. (2012). Adjunctive therapy with pregabalin in generalized anxiety disorder patients with partial response to SSRI or SNRI treatment. *International Clinical Psychopharmacology, 27*(3), 142–150.

Robinson, G. (2015). Controversies about the use of antidepressants in pregnancy. *Journal of Nervous and Mental Disease, 203*(3), 159–163.

Schweizer, E., & Rickels, K. (1998). Benzodiazepine dependence and withdrawal: A review of the syndrome and its clinical management. *Acta Psychiatrica Scandinavica Supplementum, 393*, 95–101.

Silverstone, P. H., & Salinas, E. (2001). Efficacy of venlafaxine extended release in patients with major depressive disorder and comorbid generalized anxiety disorder. *Journal of Clinical Psychiatry, 62*(7), 523–529.

Steenen, S. A., van Wijk, A. J., van der Heijden, G. J., et al. (2016). Propranolol for the treatment of anxiety disorders: Systematic review and meta-analysis. *Journal of Psychopharmacology, 30*(2), 128–139.

Stein, D. J., Bandelow, B., Merideth, C., et al. (2011). Efficacy and tolerability of extended release quetiapine fumarate (quetiapine XR) monotherapy in patients with generalised anxiety disorder: An analysis of pooled data from three 8-week placebo-controlled studies. *Human Psychopharmacology, 26*(8), 614–628.

Thase, M. E., Chen, D., Edwards, J., et al. (2014). Efficacy of vilazodone on anxiety symptoms in patients with major depressive disorder. *International Clinical Psychopharmacology, 29*(6), 351–356.

*Uthman, O. A., & Abdulmalik, J. (2010). Comparative efficacy and acceptability of pharmacotherapeutic agents for anxiety disorders in children and adolescents: A mixed treatment comparison meta-analysis. *Current Medical Research and Opinion, 26*(1), 53–59.

Varia, I., & Rauscher, F. (2002). Treatment of generalized anxiety disorder with citalopram. *International Clinical Psychopharmacology, 17*(3), 103–107.

Yee, A., Ng, C. G., & Seng, L. H. (2018). Vortioxetine treatment for anxiety disorder: A meta-analysis study. *Current Drug Targets, 19*(12), 1412–1423.

41 Sleep Disorders

Veronica F. Wilbur

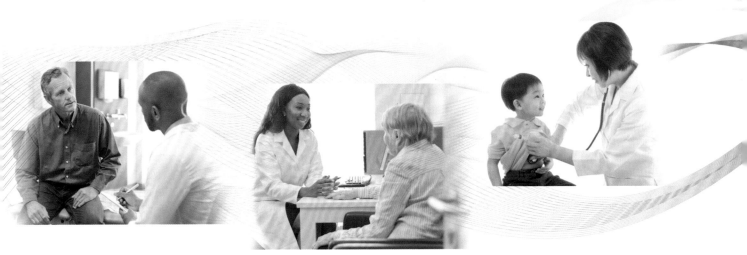

Learning Objectives

1. Identify the scope of the problem for insomnia, restless leg syndrome, and narcolepsy.
2. Differentiate the pharmacology options available to treat patients diagnosed with insomnia.
3. Examine the appropriate pharmacotherapeutics used to treat Willis–Ekbom disease.
4. Describe the evolving pharmacology treatments for narcolepsy.

INTRODUCTION

Sleep, a naturally recurring state of restfulness for the body, is a necessary element of our daily life and occurs in a daily rhythmic pattern. Sleep disorders can affect the quality of sleep and, therefore, how individuals function daily. Poor sleep can often be a symptom of other underlying physical or psychiatric problems. Sleep disorders include insomnia, snoring, and sleep apnea; narcolepsy; and chronic sleep deprivation. Pharmacologic therapy is not appropriate for snoring and sleep apnea but has a role in managing the other diagnoses. The key to a proper treatment plan is to recognize the type of sleep disorder.

INSOMNIA

Although most people occasionally have problems falling or staying asleep, insomnia can be defined as persistent trouble sleeping. However, some experts argue that any sleeping issues may be referred to as *insomnia*; the condition is defined as loss of sleep for a short period. The loss of sleep may be due to physiologic causes such as restless leg syndrome, gastroesophageal reflux, fibromyalgia, or sleep loss due to ignoring sleep cues. Rest that is not refreshing also can be classified as insomnia.

As cited by the Office of Disease Prevention and Health Promotion in Healthy People 2030 (August 2020), the Centers for Disease Control (2019) analysis shows that 1 in 3 adults and adolescents lack sleep greater than 7 hours nightly. Insomnia can have social and economic consequences, as measured through direct and indirect costs. Hafner et al. (2017), as part of the Rand Corporation report, found worldwide that the economic losses by the United States were up to $411 billion annually. More recently, in the managed care environment, the lack of sleep accounts for an aggregate total of $100 million per year in direct and indirect effects (Taddei-Allen, 2020). A Consumer Reports survey of 1767 individuals found that 31% self-medicate for sleep and use over-the-counter (OTC) sleep medication (Carr, 2018). The nonprescription sleeping marker is valued at $576 million and growing. As reported by marketing research by LaRosa 2018, sleeping pills, either nonprescription or OTC pills in the market, valued at $576 million, are growing faster than prescribed sleeping aids. This data illustrates the impact of sleep on health and wellness.

Causes

Insomnia can be of physiologic or psychological origin, and before labeling insomnia as psychological, it is essential to rule out physical causes (**Box 41.1**). Changes in a patient's biological clock can contribute to insomnia (e.g., hyperarousal states, time zone, and schedule changes), as can the sleep environment. Estimates are that up to half of all cases of insomnia are psychological in origin. The *International Classification of*

BOX 41.1 Causes of Insomnia

MEDICAL

- Cardiac problems (e.g., ischemia and congestive heart failure)
- Endocrine problems (e.g., hypothyroidism, hyperthyroidism, degenerative disease)
- Neurologic problems (e.g., stroke, degenerative conditions, dementia, peripheral nerve damage, myoclonic jerks, restless leg syndrome [Willis–Ekbom disease], hypnic jerk, and central sleep apnea)
- Pulmonary problems (e.g., COPD, obstructive sleep apnea)
- Renal problems (e.g., urinary frequency)
- Pain

PSYCHIATRIC

- Anxiety
- Excess stress
- Major depression
- Maladaptive sleep habits
- Sleep performance anxiety

DRUG AND ALCOHOL ABUSE

- Sedatives and stimulants

PRIMARY SLEEP DISORDERS

- Excessive arousal and wakefulness
- Poor sleep hygiene: related to lifestyle
- Sleep state misperception: achievement of adequate sleep but not perceived by patient

---

BOX 41.2 Stages of Sleep

STAGE I

Light NREM: dreamlike state and lasts a few minutes

STAGE II

Relatively light NREM: fragmented thoughts and lasts 15 to 20 min

STAGES III–IV

Deep NREM: lowering of blood pressure, cerebral glucose metabolism, heart rate, and respiratory rate, starts 35 to 40 min after falling asleep, and lasts 40 to 70 min

REM SLEEP

Starts after 90 min of sleep and lengthens toward the end of the night

This cycle alternates throughout the night at intervals of 90 to 100 min, four to six times per night.

Sleep Disorders (ICSD), third edition (2014), defines insomnia categories as *chronic insomnia disorder, short-term insomnia disorder,* and *other insomnia disorders.* In general, insomnia is a serious problem that can adversely impact comorbid conditions. ICSD third edition standardizes the diagnostic criteria for all types of insomnia and does not differentiate between pediatric, adult, and geriatric populations.

Chronic Insomnia

The prevalence of chronic insomnia in the general population is between 10% and 35% and affects more women than men (ICSD, 2014). Previously classified as primary, secondary, or comorbid insomnia, chronic insomnia is a more accurate terminology due to difficulties with overlapping symptoms and features. Specific criteria assist the provider in diagnosing chronic insomnia (see **Box 41.2**). While all requirements are important for diagnosis, the essential element is frequent and

persistent difficulty with initiating sleep and general sleep dissatisfaction (ISCD, 2014).

Characteristics of chronic insomnia include somatized tension and acquired habits that prevent either the initiation or maintenance of sleep. Life stresses such as shift work, a family tragedy, or physical pain can exacerbate chronic insomnia. Neurobiological research about insomnia points to a dysregulation of the brain's neurotransmitters that regulate wakefulness. Non–rapid eye movement (NREM) and REM sleep also contribute to chronic insomnia. Insomnia can start with an initial stressful event, but the hyperarousal state of chronic insomniacs extends well beyond the heightened levels of stress.

Short-Term Insomnia Disorder

The prevalence among adults is 15% to 20% of the general population, more often in women than men and older. Previous classifications of short-term insomnia were acute or adjustment insomnia. Diagnosis is like chronic insomnia but with fewer question categories, see **Box 41.3**. The essential feature here is short-term difficulty initiating or maintaining sleep with general sleep dissatisfaction. Short-term insomnia can be in isolation or comorbid with mental disorders, medical conditions, or substance abuse (ICSD, 2014). Short-term insomnia is often related to environmental factors, such as sleeping in an unfamiliar place or excessive heat, noise, light, or bed partner movement.

Additionally, short-term insomnia can be related to stress, either positive or negative. Many features of short-term insomnia are shared with chronic insomnia with the primary difference of duration. Circadian rhythm disorders, jet lag, and rotating shift work should be considered in the differential.

- What kind of work does the patient do? Is there shift work involved, and which shift?
- What time does the patient go to bed?
- What kind of bed partner does the patient have (restless, still, wakeful sleeper), if any?
- Does the patient regularly take any prescription or OTC drugs?
- How many times during the night does the patient awaken?
- What does the patient do if they cannot go to sleep?
- Does the patient take daytime naps?

Other Insomnia Disorders

The use of *other insomnia disorders* is reserved for those who have difficulty with initiating and maintaining sleep but do not meet the full criteria for either chronic or short-term insomnia. Other sleep disorders, such as restless leg syndrome (RLS) (Willis–Ekbom disease [WED]) and obstructive sleep apnea, should be considered for patients within this category.

Pathophysiology

Understanding insomnia necessitates knowing the physiologic process of sleep. The brain seeks to balance alertness and sleepiness on a continuum between sleep debt, biological alerting, and environmental stimulation. Sleepiness is a function of the brain fighting to get enough sleep to cover the debt. The sleep debt system versus sleep arousal is intricately linked to circadian rhythms and exposure to light. Additionally, various internally regulated biologic systems govern the circadian pattern of the sleep–wake cycle. These biologic systems' interaction includes changes in body temperature, cardiac and renal functions, and hormone secretion throughout the day. The term *circadian* means "approximately one day" and refers to the fact that endogenous rhythms last approximately 24 hours.

Regular sleep is divided into REM sleep and NREM sleep. During the REM stage, which accounts for approximately 20% of the sleep cycle, the brain is active, and most dreaming occurs. NREM, which constitutes about 80% of the sleep cycle, is a phase of deep rest in which pulse, respiration, and brain activity are all slow. NREM sleep can be divided into four phases. Stages I and II are called light NREM sleep. Stage I is the lightest sleep, and fleeting dreams often occur during the transition between the awake state and Stage I. Stage II, which accounts for 50% of NREM sleep, lasts approximately 15 to 20 minutes and is characterized by fragmented thoughts with distinctive EEG changes. Hypnotics commonly increase Stage II. Stages III and IV are called delta or deep NREM sleep. This stage begins after approximately 30 to 45 minutes and lasts 40 to 70 minutes. During Stages III and IV, blood pressure, cerebral glucose metabolism, and heart and respiratory rates are

the lowest in the circadian cycle. The total sleep pattern begins with light NREM, by deep NREM, and then by REM. This cycle lasts approximately 90 to 100 minutes and occurs four to six times per night. **Box 42.2** summarizes the sleep stages.

Required amounts of sleep and NREM sleep vary with age. Newborns sleep approximately 17 to 18 hours each day but have only two phases of sleep: NREM and REM. These two phases cycle every 60 minutes instead of every 90 minutes like adults. Children require 10 hours of sleep. In the early adult years, the total amount of sleep decreases to around 8 hours, which is typical for older adults and younger adults, with some variation among individuals. The total amount of REM sleep stays more constant at 15% to 20% throughout an adult's lifetime. Deep NREM sleep constitutes approximately 20% to 30% of total sleep in young children (Li et al., 2018).

Insomnia is seen more often in people over age 65. The stages and architecture of sleep change, resulting in lighter Stage II and decreases in Stages III and IV sleep. The difference in the earlier stages of sleep results in a decrease in deep NREM sleep. The circadian clock also becomes advanced, causing early morning awakening in the older adults.

Light cues are essential in the process of sleep. The absence of light signals tends to promote longer sleep–wake cycles. Two peaks in the daily need for sleep have been identified: the first at bedtime and the second in midafternoon. Study over the years has linked insomnia and higher hyperarousal states (Pillai et al., 2016; Vargas et al., 2020).

Diagnostic Criteria

Typical complaints of insomnia are malaise, fatigue, and too little sleep. However, since these are self-reported, the patient's subjective report may be unreliable (Alameddine et al., 2015). The problem of insomnia can lead to mild or moderate impairment in concentration and psychomotor abilities. The diagnosis is based on the patient's history, although a complete workup includes evaluating all potential medical and psychological causes. The practitioner must determine the onset and duration of symptoms, the patient's regular sleeping schedule, and general sleep quality. Interviewing other family members and significant others regarding any psychiatric or substance abuse problems can be helpful. If the patient does not sleep alone, the practitioner should elicit information also from the bed partner. Questions about sleep also should be included in the review of systems; **Box 41.4** lists suggested to queries.

A complete physical examination is vital to rule out medical causes of insomnia. Insomnia can be drug related (e.g., stimulating medications or alcohol). Finally, the practitioner should investigate psychiatric causes of insomnia.

The use of sleep questionnaires or diaries and screening tools for depression and anxiety can add to insomnia evaluation (see **Box 41.5**). Sleep patterns may be measured using a special wristwatch that calculates wrist movements, a process called *actigraphy*. In humans, the wrist movement throughout the night is much less frequent than during the day, enabling the practitioner to estimate the patient's sleep and wake

BOX 41.4   Sleep Websites

- National Center on Sleep Disorders Research (NCSDR): http://www.nhlbi.nih.gov/about/ncsdr
- National Heart, Lung, and Blood Institute (NHLBI) Health Information Network: http://www.nhlbi.nih.gov
- Restless Legs Syndrome Foundation: https://www.rls.org/
- Sleep Foundation: http://sleepfoundation.org
- National Institute of Neurological Disorders and Stroke: http://www.ninds.nih.gov/disorders/narcolepsy/narcolepsy.htm
- Healthy Sleep Med Harvard: http://healthysleep.med.harvard.edu/narcolepsy/what-is-narcolepsy/understanding
- Narcolepsy Link: https://www.narcolepsylink.com/
- Know Narcolepsy: https://www.narcolepsylink.com/

BOX 41.5   Patient Screening Sleep Questionnaires—select

- Mini Sleep Questionnaire
- Pittsburgh Sleep Quality Index
- Epworth Sleepiness Scale
- Insomnia Severity Index

times. This tool, however, is not very accurate in assessing the total sleep time of insomniacs. Polysomnography (all-night monitoring of EEG, respiration, muscle activity, and other physiologic parameters) may reveal shallow sleep that is fragmented by multiple arousals. If the patient is depressed, the polysomnogram manifests changes in the REM latency stage. Polysomnograms are indicated when the primary suspected cause of insomnia is sleep apnea. However, the American Sleep Disorders Association does not recommend polysomnography's routine use because a patient may not usually sleep at a sleep disorder center. As technology has advanced, patients can monitor sleep in their homes by purchasing watches and movement devices such as FitBit™ and Apple™ watches.

Initiating Drug Therapy

In combination with behavioral management, the practitioner can consider using specific pharmacologic agents, but only with caution. According to the most recent clinical guidelines for evaluating and managing sleep (Satei et al., 2017), there is weak evidence to use hypnotics and for the lowest dose for the shortest time. There is a potential for the drugs that treat insomnia to be habit-forming.

A wide range of therapies may be necessary to treat insomnia because multiple causes are the rule rather than the exception. Nonpharmacologic treatment includes evaluating the fundamental causes and treating the appropriate intervention first: counseling, behavioral management, and lifestyle alterations for psychiatric problems. Patients with insomnia often have major depression, anxiety, obsessive disorders, dysthymic disorders, and psychotherapy to focus on the specific psychiatric disorder.

Adjunctive to drug therapy, reviewing proper sleep hygiene can enhance the patient's sleep pattern. A thorough examination of sleep hygiene issues can help identify essential lifestyle changes that may improve sleep, and its importance should not be underestimated. The practitioner should implement only one or two behavioral changes at a time. Additional measures, such as exposure to bright light, may help those with circadian rhythm disturbances. Light therapy can retrain the light pacemaker and may be useful for night-shift workers, travelers, and those with delayed or advanced sleep phase disorders.

Goals of Drug Therapy

There are two goals of pharmacotherapy. The first goal is to improve sleep quality and quantity, and the second goal is to improve insomnia-related daytime impairment. The selection of drugs is based on matching the onset and duration to the sleep defect. If given in adequate doses, all hypnotics promote sleep, and the key is to determine the *minimal* amount that will provide efficacy with few or no side effects. Factors in selecting a pharmacologic agent should be directed by (1) symptom pattern, (2) treatment goals, (3) past treatment responses, (4) patient preference, (5) cost, (6) medication interactions, and (7) side effects. Providers need to be aware that there must be a favorable balance between therapeutic effects and potential side effects when treating insomnia with pharmacologic agents.

Hypnotics are the primary drugs used for insomnia, including benzodiazepines and benzodiazepine receptor agonists (BZRA). Other medications utilized to treat insomnia are orexin receptor agonists, melatonin receptor agonists, and first-generation antihistamines. Some sedating antidepressants are useful if the patient has comorbid depression. The practitioner should carefully consider selecting a hypnotic and prescribe use for as short a time as possible. Short-term use is defined as no more than 2 to 3 weeks combined with behavioral interventions; however, specific patients require occasional chronic hypnotic therapy. They may need to use a hypnotic agent two or three times a week over more extended periods than 2 to 3 weeks. Further, it is important to wean patients off hypnotics when not needed due to rebound effects. Careless use of sedative-hypnotics can be dangerous in patients with sleep apnea or a history of substance abuse.

Benzodiazepines

Benzodiazepines are synthetically produced sedative-hypnotics. This group of structurally related chemicals selectively acts on polysynaptic neuronal pathways throughout the central nervous system (CNS). Benzodiazepines appear to enhance gamma-aminobutyric acid (GABA) effects in the ascending reticular activating system, which increases inhibition and blocks thalamic, hypothalamic, and limbic arousal.

When choosing a benzodiazepine (BZD), the practitioner should select an agent with an onset of action that matches the patient's complaint, which has a short duration of effect, lacks rebound insomnia, and causes few or no cognitive problems (e.g., hangover, lack of motor coordination, or memory disturbance) (see **Table 41.1**). The prescriber should also consider the patient's metabolic requirements. Benzodiazepines can be categorized as short acting, intermediate acting, and long acting due to each class's pharmacokinetics. The most used short-acting agent was triazolam, but now, it is not commonly used due to the high incidence of rebound insomnia even after using only a short time and neuropsychiatric adverse effects. Temazepam and lorazepam are examples of intermediate-acting agents, and flurazepam is a long-acting category. When a drug has a longer half-life, there is greater potential for untoward effects such as excessive residual sedation or dizziness. Agents with short-term effects and rapid onset are best for patients who have difficulty falling asleep. Agents with an intermediate onset usually have longer half-lives, useful for patients with sleep maintenance issues. These include temazepam (Restoril) and estazolam. Two agents with a rapid onset of action, flurazepam, and quazepam assist with falling asleep and have a longer duration of action, assisting in maintaining sleep.

Adverse Events

Benzodiazepines have various actions, depending on their half-lives and affinity for the receptor. This class's drugs can produce drowsiness and impaired motor function, which may be persistent due to metabolites and subsequent hepatic and renal accumulation. Other side effects can include short-term memory loss, confusion, and shakiness. Prolonged use of benzodiazepines can lead to physical dependency; abrupt discontinuance can trigger withdrawal symptoms. Drugs in this category are all classified as controlled substances. With this category of medication, there is potential for addiction in addition to physical dependence. The newer agents in the class have fewer side effects, but caution should still be exercised when prescribing. For optimal therapy, the drug selected should address the patient's specific sleep problem.

Interactions

Patients taking benzodiazepines must be cautious with the concomitant use of alcohol. The use of low-dose contraceptives may slightly decrease the clearance of lorazepam and temazepam; the patient may need to alter the dosage or switch to oxazepam. The use of erythromycin (E-mycin) can decrease triazolam clearance by 50%; thus, prescribers must consider reducing the dosage of triazolam in patients taking both drugs.

Benzodiazepine Receptor Agonists

This class of hypnotics was developed to improve the safety profile of the barbiturate-type and longer-acting benzodiazepine compounds. BZRA pharmacologically are like benzodiazepines but instead mimic GABA action, an inhibitory transmitter, which induces sleepiness. The difference between BZD and BZRA is which GABA-A receptor subunits are affected. BZDs act on the subunit of alpha-1, alpha-2, and alpha-3, while BZRAs are selective for alpha-1, which induces sleepiness but not anxiolysis or muscle relaxation. Initially, BZRA were thought to have one of the safest profiles with little or no long-term side effects; however, this proved not to be so with more experience. There is some evidence that long-term use of these drugs can alter sleep microstructure but not sleep architecture (Manconi et al., 2017) and worsen dementia (He et al., 2019). Another issue with the BZRAs is complex sleep-related behaviors. These are defined as completing activities in an altered state of consciousness and also have been reported with the BZRAs. These activities include sleepwalking or sleep-eating and sleep-driving a car. This class's other side effects include decreased motor coordination, confusion, and anterograde amnesia, which were all thought to be less than BZDs.

Eszopiclone

Eszopiclone (Lunesta) is a BZRA indicated for the treatment of insomnia.

Mechanism of Action

The exact mechanism of action is unknown, but eszopiclone is thought to work by interacting with GABA receptors located near benzodiazepine receptors and shares some of the same pharmacologic properties. It is classified as a Schedule IV–controlled substance.

Dosage

For non–older adults, eszopiclone should be started at 2 mg immediately before retiring for bed. The dose may be started or increased to 3 mg to aid in sleep maintenance. For older adult patients, begin at 1 mg to help patients fall asleep and 2 mg if sleep maintenance is the issue. Limited use of the 3-mg dose is recommended due to impairment of driving ability, coordination, and memory for over 11 hours, even if patients do not realize it (PL-Detail Document, 2014).

Time Frame for Response

The onset of action is rapid, with a peak plasma concentration occurring within 1 hour of dosing. This peak concentration is delayed if eszopiclone is taken with or shortly after a high-fat meal.

Contraindications

There are no known contraindications to eszopiclone. However, patients should be cautioned against alcohol's concomitant use due to the sedative effects and the potential for enhancing anterograde amnesia.

Adverse Events

Headache, dry mouth, dizziness, respiratory system infections, and unpleasant taste have occurred in patients taking 2- to 3-mg doses of eszopiclone.

TABLE 41.1

Overview of Selected Drugs Used to Treat Insomnia

Generic (Trade) Name and Dosage	Selected Adverse Events	Contraindications	Special Considerations
Benzodiazepines			
Alprazolam (Xanax) tablets 0.25, 0.5, 1, 2 mg Start: 0.25–0.5 mg PO TID; maximum 4 mg/d in divided doses Range: 0.25–2 mg TID–daily	*CNS:* transient mild drowsiness, sedation, depression, lethargy, apathy, fatigue, light-headedness, disorientation, headache, mild paradoxical excitatory reaction in first 2 wk *GI:* constipation, diarrhea, dry mouth, nausea	Hypersensitivity to benzodiazepines, acute narrow-angle glaucoma, pregnancy, lactation	Use cautiously with impaired liver or kidney function debilitation. Drug dependence and withdrawal result when abruptly discontinued, especially when used for longer than 4 mo. Use cautiously with older adult patients and gradually increase as tolerated.
Estazolam (only available as generic) tablets 1, 2 mg Start: 0.5–1 mg QHS Range: 0.5–2 mg QHS	*CNS:* transient mild drowsiness, sedation lethargy, apathy, fatigue, light-headedness, asthenia, mild paradoxical excitatory reaction in first 2 wk *GI:* constipation, diarrhea, dyspepsia *CV:* bradycardia, tachycardia *GU:* incontinence, urinary retention, changes in libido	Same as above	In addition to above, drug–drug interactions: increased CNS depression with ethanol, omeprazole; increased effects of estazolam with cimetidine, increased sedative effects of estazolam with theophylline. Drug dependence, withdrawal syndrome.
Flurazepam (Dalmane) 15–30 mg PO QHS Start: 15 mg PO QHS Range: 15–30 mg PO QHS	*CNS:* transient mild drowsiness, sedation lethargy, apathy, fatigue, light-headedness, asthenia *GI:* constipation, diarrhea, dyspepsia *CV:* bradycardia, tachycardia *GU:* incontinence, urinary retention, changes in libido	Same as above	Same as above Has a long half-life
Lorazepam (Ativan) 2–4 mg PO QHS	*CNS:* transient mild drowsiness, sedation, depression, lethargy, apathy, fatigue, light-headedness, disorientation, headache, mild paradoxical excitatory reaction in first 2 wk *GI:* constipation, diarrhea, dry mouth, nausea	Same as above	Use cautiously with patients with impaired liver or kidney function Debilitation, drug dependence, and withdrawal result when abruptly discontinued, especially when used for more than 4 mo. Use cautiously with older patients and gradually increase as tolerated.
Quazepam (Doral) 7.5–15 mg PO QHS	*CNS:* transient mild drowsiness, sedation, depression, lethargy, apathy, fatigue, light-headedness, disorientation, restlessness, confusion *GI:* constipation, diarrhea *CV:* bradycardia, tachycardia *GU:* incontinence, urinary retention, changes in libido	Same as above	Drug–drug interactions: increased CNS depression with ethanol, quazepam; increased effects of cimetidine, disulfiram, oral contraceptives; increased sedative effects with theophylline. Half-life of 39 h
Temazepam (Restoril) Start: 15 mg PO QHS Range: 15–30 mg PO QHS	Same as above	Same as above	Drug–drug interactions: increased CNS depression; increased sedative effects with theophylline
Triazolam (Halcion) Start: 0.125 mg PO QHS Range: 0.125–0.5 mg PO QHS Older adults: 0.125–0.25 mg PO QHS	Same as above	Hypersensitivity to benzodiazepines, acute narrow-angle glaucoma, pregnancy, lactation	Same as above

TABLE 41.1

Overview of Selected Drugs Used to Treat Insomnia (Continued)

Generic (Trade) Name and Dosage	Selected Adverse Events	Contraindications	Special Considerations
Benzodiazepine Receptor Agonist			
Eszopiclone (Lunesta) Start: 1–2 mg PO QHS Range: 1–3 mg Older adults: start at 1 mg	*CNS:* morning drowsiness, headache, dizziness *GI:* nausea	Hypersensitivity to eszopiclone	Caution in patients taking strong inhibitors or inducers of CYP3A4. Consider alternative during pregnancy, esp. during 3rd trimester; no known risk of teratogenicity, though risk of neonatal respiratory depression when given near term based on limited human data.
Zolpidem (Ambien, Ambien CR) Ambien Start: 10 mg PO QHS Range: 5–10 mg PO QHS Ambien CR *Female:* 6.25 mg PO QHS; max 12.5 mg *Male:* 6.25–12.5 mg PO QHS Zolpidem tartrate (Intermezzo) Starting: 3.75 mg SL Older adults: 1.75 mg SL	*CNS:* morning drowsiness, hangover, headache, dizziness, suppression of REM sleep *GI:* nausea	Hypersensitivity to drug lass	Use cautiously in patients with acute intermittent porphyria, in patients with impaired hepatic or renal function, in addiction-prone patients, and in pregnancy and lactation. Useful for patients with problems falling asleep and middle-night awakening. Used for middle-night awakening but must have more than 4 h to sleep. Caution with older adults and hepatic impairment. Consider alternative during pregnancy, esp. during 3rd trimester; no known risk of teratogenicity, though risk of neonatal respiratory depression when given near term based on limited human data.
Zaleplon (Sonata) Start: 10 mg PO QHS Range: 5–20 mg PO QHS	*General:* back pain, chest pain *CV:* migraine *GI:* constipation, dry mouth *MS:* arthritis *CNS:* depression, hypertonia, nervousness *Derm:* rash, pruritus	Pregnancy, lactation	Consider alternative during pregnancy, esp. during 3rd trimester; no known risk of teratogenicity, though risk of neonatal respiratory depression when given near term based on limited human data. Patient must use just before bedtime because of quick onset.
Orexin Receptor Antagonist			
Suvorexant (Belsomra) Start: 10 mg PO within 30 min of bed Maximum: 20 mg	Most common side effects were somnolence, headache, dizziness.	Obese women have increased side effects Care with patients with respiratory compromise	Risk of impaired alertness and motor coordination. Must have 7 h to sleep. Reevaluate for persistent insomnia after 7–10 d treatment. Caution with depression. Consider alternative during pregnancy; inadequate human data available to assess risk; possible risk of decreased fetal weight based on conflicting animal data.
Lemborexant (Dayvigo) Start 5 mg PO QHS Maximum 10 mg daily Use lowest effective dose and give immediately before bedtime.	Same as above	Same as above	Same as above Reassess if no response after 7–10 d. Give without food for faster onset.

CNS, central nervous system; CV, cardiovascular; GI, gastrointestinal; GU, genitourinary; REM, rapid eye movement.

Interactions

Eszopiclone is metabolized by the cytochrome P (CYP) 3A4 enzyme system. Therefore, agents that inhibit (e.g., ketoconazole) or induce (e.g., rifampin) this system will affect eszopiclone metabolism.

Zolpidem

Zolpidem tartrate (Ambien), extended-release zolpidem tartrate (Ambien CR), sublingual zolpidem tartrate (Intermezzo), and zolpidem tartrate oral solution (Zolpimist) are also BZRA products.

Mechanism of Action

Zolpidem is also thought to modulate the GABA-A receptors. It appears that zolpidem also modulates the chloride channel macromolecular complex that is responsible for sedative, anticonvulsant, anxiolytic, and myorelaxant properties, therefore, causing sedation and relaxation. Zolpidem has a robust hypnotic component and improves sleep quality while producing less daytime impairment than other hypnotics. The onset of action of zolpidem is rapid; however, regular-release zolpidem peaks quickly, while extended-release zolpidem has a biphasic release assisting with sleep onset and sleep maintenance. Zolpidem has no anxiolytic effects, which makes it less desirable for patients with concomitant anxiety. These drugs are also controlled substances (class IV) due to the potential for abuse.

Dosage

Starting doses of zolpidem are lower for females than males. Zolpidem is started at 5 mg for females and 10 mg for males, while extended-release zolpidem starts at 6.25 mg for females and 12.5 mg for males. Dosing can be increased, but with the understanding, this increases the potential for side effects. Dosing should be altered for patients with hepatic impairment but is not necessary for those with renal impairment.

Time Frame for Response

The onset of action for zolpidem is 10 to 15 minutes of administration and lasts for 2 to 3 hours. Extended-release zolpidem has the same onset, but 60% is initially released, with the remaining drug over the next 6 to 8 hours. The sublingual and oral solution products are taken immediately before bedtime as their onset of action is rapid.

Contraindications

Contraindications to zolpidem include anaphylactic reactions and angioedema. The Food and Drug Administration (FDA; October 1, 2013) also put forth a safety communication bulletin to caution patients about the possibility of complex behaviors that include sleep-driving and other activities.

Adverse Events

The most common adverse events for both drugs are drowsiness, headache, and dizziness. The incidence of complex sleep behaviors can affect up to 15% of those taking zolpidem.

Interactions

Care should be exercised when prescribing zolpidem with other CNS drugs that have depressive effects. Other drugs that inhibit the CYP3A4 isoenzymes may increase the exposure to zolpidem.

Zaleplon

Another BZRA is zaleplon (Sonata). This drug is chemically unrelated to benzodiazepines, barbiturates, and other medications with hypnotic properties.

Mechanism of Action

Zaleplon interacts with the GABA-BZ omega-1 receptor, causing sedation. The drug does not have any myorelaxant, anxiolytic, or anticonvulsant properties. Zaleplon works well for patients who have difficulty falling asleep. It may not be the agent of choice for patients who have difficulty maintaining sleep because of its short elimination half-life. However, provided that at least 4 hours of sleep remain, this drug can be dosed a second time when patients have a nighttime awakening.

Dosage

The dose of zaleplon should be individualized and can range from 5 to 20 mg. The risk of adverse effects is dose dependent.

Time Frame for Response

The onset of action is rapid, within 1 hour after oral administration, but the medication has a short half-life of 1 hour. Zaleplon can be taken as little as 5 hours before the scheduled wake-up time, with no lingering daytime sedation effects.

Contraindications

Hypersensitivity and severe hepatic impairment are contraindications to the use of zaleplon. Dose adjustment is not necessary for renal impairment.

Adverse Events

Headache is the most reported adverse event, followed by dizziness, nausea, and abdominal pain. Postmarketing reports include anaphylaxis and nightmares. Other adverse effects include depression, amnesia, and sleep-related activities.

Interactions

Zaleplon is contraindicated in concomitant use with sodium oxybate (Xyrem) and any type of fentanyl or valerian. Close monitoring is required to use other drugs that are metabolized by the CYP3A4 isoenzyme of the cytochrome P450 system.

Orexin Receptor Antagonists

Orexin receptor antagonists are a new class in the treatment of insomnia. There are two agents in the class, suvorexant (Belsomra) and Lemborexant (Dayvigo).

Mechanism of Action

In 1998, the discovery of the hypothalamic neuropeptide orexin system revealed another influence on the sleep–wake cycle (De Lecea et al., 1998; Sakurai et al., 1998). These neuropeptides (orexin-A and orexin-B) are found in the hypothalamus and other brain areas. The orexin system has a role in the sleep–wake cycle, appetite, metabolism, reward, stress, and autonomic function (Dubey et al., 2015). Early study of the orexin system discovered that blockage resulted in severe sleepiness, which established the role of orexin in wakefulness. Suvorexant and lemborexant are selective dual orexin receptor agonists (DORA) with a binding mechanism to both orexin receptors. The inhibitory action facilitates sleep induction and maintenance.

Dosage

The starting dose for suvorexant is 10 mg and increased to a maximum of 20 mg. For patients taking other drugs that inhibit the CYP3A4 isoenzyme, suvorexant should start at 5 mg and go no higher than 10 mg. The administration should occur within 30 minutes of bedtime, and patients need to have at least 7 hours of planned sleep due to potential complex sleep behaviors. There are no dose adjustments for patients with moderate hepatic impairment, or renal impairment is not required.

Lemborexant starts at 5 mg, and the maximal dose is 10 mg. It can be taken immediately before going to bed; however, sleep time needs to be at least 7 hours. Meals can delay the time of onset. A dose adjustment of no more than 5 mg is required for moderate hepatic impairment and not recommended for severe liver dysfunction.

Time Frame for Response

The onset of action for suvorexant occurs within 30 minutes of administration with peak concentrations in 2 hours. Suvorexant can last up to 6 hours, and the half-life is 12 hours.

Lemborexant has onset with 15 minutes of administration and a peak concentration within 1 to 2 hours and lasts up to 6 hours. The 5-mg dose has a half-life of 17 hours, and the 10 mg dose is 19 hours.

Contraindications

Both suvorexant and lemborexant are contraindicated with narcolepsy, alcohol use, and hypersensitivity to the class. Lemborexant also has precautions for sleep paralysis, hypnagogic/hypnopompic hallucinations, and cataplexy-like symptoms. Use caution with female patients with obesity, depression, concomitant use of other CNS depressants, and impaired respiratory function. Neither drug is recommended for patients who have severe liver disorders.

Adverse Events

The most common adverse reactions to both orexin receptor antagonists include headache, somnolence, dizziness, and abnormal dreams.

Interactions

Drugs that are CYP3A inhibitors such as ketoconazole and clarithromycin are not recommended for concomitant use. Additionally, drugs that are CPY3A inducers, carbamazepine, and phenytoin may reduce the efficacy of the orexin antagonist class. Finally, drugs that are metabolized by the CYP2B6 substrates, such as bupropion or methadone, may need to have the dosage increased when using either suvorexant or lemborexant.

Melatonin Receptor Agonists

There are two approved melatonin receptor agonists approved for use in the United States but for different sleep indications. Ramelteon (Rozerem) was introduced in 2005 as an option to treat insomnia. The other is tasimelteon (Hetlioz) that is only approved for the treatment of circadian rhythm disorder or to shift the sleep–wake cycles of those who are blind. While tasimelteon has shown some promise for insomnia, more research needs to be completed regarding its efficacy (Lankford, 2011). Both drugs have no potential for abuse and are the only agents not classified as schedule medications.

Mechanism of Action

Endogenous melatonin is secreted from the pineal gland and regulates the circadian sleep cycle found in the hypothalamus's suprachiasmatic nucleus (SCN). Secretion of melatonin signals the timing of darkness via specific receptors (MT_1 and MT_2) and decreases neural firing to the SCN. Ramelteon is a synthetic derivative with high selectivity and affinity for the MT_1 and MT_2 receptors, which block the receptors and shorten sleep onset latency. It does not affect other sleep neurotransmitters such as GABA, dopamine, or serotonin.

Dosage

The dose for ramelteon is 8 mg and should be administered within 30 minutes before going to bed. Avoid administration with a high-fat meal.

Time Frame for Response

The onset of action for ramelteon is within 45 minutes, and the half-life is 1 to 2.6 hours. There are no accumulating effects with repeated use of ramelteon due to the short half-life. Administration with a high-fat meal can increase the area under the curve (total exposure).

Contraindications

Ramelteon is contraindicated for patients with hypersensitivity to the class, severe sleep apnea, severe hepatic impairment, and angioedema. Exercise caution prescribing for patients with mild-to-moderate hepatic impairment, depression, and severe chronic obstructive pulmonary disease.

Adverse Events

The most common adverse reactions include somnolence, dizziness, fatigue, nausea, and exacerbated insomnia.

Interactions

Ramelteon interacts with rifampin, ketoconazole, fluconazole, donepezil, doxepin, and alcohol.

Antihistamines

Antihistamines are one of the most used classes of OTC sleep-inducing agents. These drugs often come in combination with analgesics such as acetaminophen and ibuprofen. One of the most used agents is diphenhydramine (Benadryl). The primary mechanism of diphenhydramine is to inhibit histamine at the H1 receptor competitively. It has powerful sedative and anticholinergic effects. No scientific evidence exists in the literature supporting the use of diphenhydramine to relieve insomnia or prolong sleep.

The side effects of diphenhydramine include excessive daytime drowsiness, impaired psychomotor function, and increasing tolerance to the drug. A better approach may be to use a sedating antidepressant before using a trial of diphenhydramine. If a patient takes diphenhydramine while driving under antihistamines' influence (DUI), they can be charged with DUI in many states.

Another first-generation antihistamine agent used for insomnia is doxylamine succinate (Unisom). The mechanism of action is the same as diphenhydramine but stronger and has the addition of anticholinergic effects. Unisom SleepTabs is the only OTC formulation that contains doxylamine succinate. All other oral delivery methods of Unisom, gel caps, minis, liquid, and analgesic combination do not have doxylamine succinate, only diphenhydramine. Precautions for this medication include excessive drowsiness that can affect coordination, therefore, impairing psychomotor coordination.

Antidepressants

Sedating antidepressants may also be used to treat insomnia, but only for patients with comorbid depression. The most used antidepressants in this category are mirtazapine (Remeron), trazodone, and doxepin (Silenor). If the patient has comorbid panic or anxiety, some antidepressant agents can assist with sleep, such as trazodone, which also has some sedating and antianxiety effects (see Chapter 40).

Selecting the Most Appropriate Agent

As previously discussed, therapy aims to improve sleep quality and quantity and improve insomnia-related daytime impairments. Additionally, the appropriate agent's selection is directed by symptom pattern, treatment goals, past treatment responses, patient preference, cost, availability of other treatments, comorbid conditions, contraindications, concurrent medication interactions, and side effects. For short-term insomnia treatment, hypnotic use's suggested duration is 10 to 14 days, but some patients may need a longer course. Practitioners should schedule follow-up visits to monitor the effectiveness of therapy. The time between follow-up visits can vary, but in general, they should fall between every 1 and 2 weeks. Starting the medication at the lowest possible dosage is always a good practice and should minimize side effects. The practitioner should ask the patient about the impact the drug is having on sleep and daytime functioning. Changes may exist with dreaming, learning, memory, and adaptation to stress. Having the patient complete and bring in a sleep log for review can help pinpoint initial management needs and continue to evaluate signs of improvement (**Table 41.2** and **Figure 41.1**). Pharmacologic therapy should be associated with patient education and cognitive therapy (Qaseem et al., 2016; Sateia et al., 2017).

TABLE 41.2

Recommended Order of Treatment for Insomnia

Order	Agents	Comments
First line	Benzodiazepine (e.g., alprazolam, lorazepam, temazepam), BZRAs (zolpidem, zaleplon, escitalopram), or ramelteon First-generation antihistamine—doxylamine succinate	Agent selected should match the sleep deficit. Approved for pregnancy.
Second line	Alternating short-acting BZRAs (zaleplon, eszopiclone) with ramelteon Sedating antidepressants (trazodone, amitriptyline, doxepin, mirtazapine)	Consider short-acting agents, especially with patients who have renal or hepatic problems. Consider antidepressant with comorbid depression.
Third line	Sedating antiepilepsy agents (gabapentin) or atypical antipsychotics (quetiapine, olanzapine) Orexin receptor antagonist (suvorexant, lemborexant)	Do not prescribe anti-psychotics routinely.

BZRAs, benzodiazepine receptor agonists.

First-Line Therapy

As stated previously, the key to pharmacologic therapy is identifying the sleep defect. The practitioner should match the patient's need for an agent to classify insomnia and the altered aspect of sleep. The recommended first-line therapy for short-term insomnia is from any class of BZRA classes or ramelteon. Examples of these medications include zolpidem, eszopiclone, zaleplon, and temazepam.

Doxylamine succinate is the only agent approved to treat any sleep defect in pregnant women. The practitioner must assess the potential side effects and benefits for both the fetus and mother before instituting therapy.

Second-Line Therapy

If therapy is unsuccessful, as evidenced by a lack of improvement in the achievement of treatment goals, alternate short-acting BZRAs or ramelteon. For patients with comorbid conditions such as depression, consider sedating antidepressants such as trazodone, amitriptyline, doxepin, and mirtazapine. These agents may be helpful, especially with patients who have anxiety. The prescriber must also consider the kind of sleep defect being treated and select a drug with the appropriate onset and half-life.

Third-Line Therapy

Various combinations of therapy can be considered for the third line based on lack of goal achievement. The practitioner

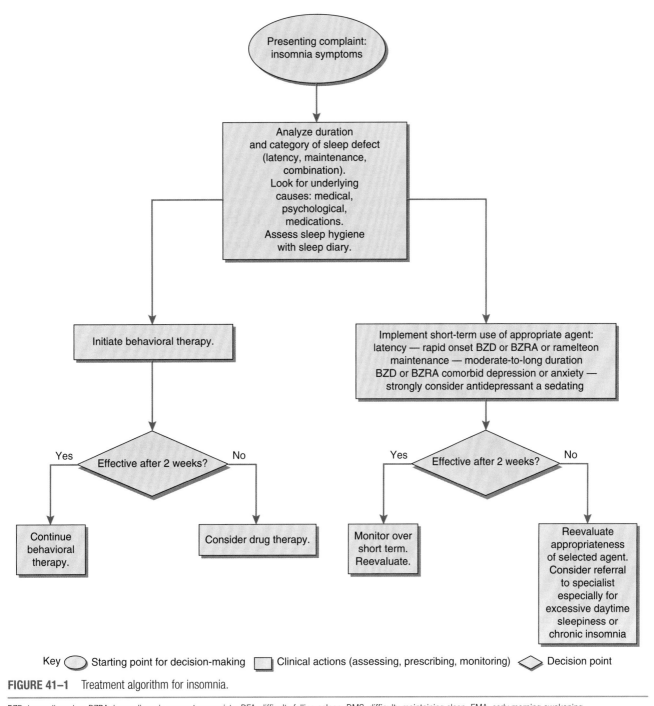

FIGURE 41–1   Treatment algorithm for insomnia.

BZD, benzodiazepine; BZRA, benzodiazepine receptor agonists; DFA, difficulty falling asleep; DMS, difficulty maintaining sleep; EMA, early morning awakening.

should reassess the insomnia situation for patients who fail to respond to both first- and second-line therapies. For chronic insomnia, continual evaluation and behavioral therapy are cornerstones to treatment. Other sedating agents may be used from the antiepilepsy class and atypical antipsychotics. Examples of these drugs include gabapentin, quetiapine, and olanzapine. For discussion of these agents, see Chapters 39 and 40.

Suvorexant and lemborexant are the newest class of hypnotic agents with a unique mechanism of action, different from other known agents already on the market. The cost of either suvorexant or lemobrexant should be a consideration with prescribing.

Special Population Considerations
Pediatric

The use of barbiturates in the pediatric population is usually limited to those who have seizure disorders. In general, benzodiazepines are not indicated for children younger than age 15.

Controlled studies of pharmacologic treatment in this population are lacking, and the use of many drugs is off-label. The provider must be aware when using antihistamines with very young patients; there is a potential for delirium or paradoxical excitation. Melatonin continues to have the best evidence for use in children as a treatment for insomnia (Buscemi et al., 2004; McDonagh et al., 2019; Shamseer & Vohra, 2009).

Geriatric

Older adults may report early morning awakening or general sleep disturbances. The CNS changes potentially affect the sleep of the older adults. Frequent nighttime awakenings may result from secondary changes in circadian rhythms and loss of effective circadian regulation of sleep. Such changes can affect the quality of life. Many older adult patients exhibit daytime sleepiness, which shows that age does not diminish the need for sleep but reduces sleeping ability.

It is essential to evaluate the geriatric patient for underlying comorbidities that contribute to insomnia. Treating the underlying illnesses may assist with reestablishing good sleeping patterns. Extreme caution is necessary when prescribing hypnotic medications to older adult patients because these drugs can increase the potential for delirium and subsequent falls. According to Beers Criteria (American Geriatrics Society, 2019), avoid first-generation antihistamines and short- and intermediate-acting benzodiazepines. Prescribing must consider the pharmacokinetic and pharmacodynamic changes in drug metabolism with the aging process. There is also an increase in falls associated with short- and long-term benzodiazepines (Fixen, 2019, p. 49).

Consistent monitoring of the older adult patient can be vital, mostly with prescribing a long-acting hypnotic due to accumulation in the renal or hepatic system depending on the drug used. Antihistamines can cause delirium or paradoxical excitation.

Women

Pharmacokinetic differences have been noted when select BZRA agents are prescribed for women. Guidance from the FDA in 2013 lowered the dose of zolpidem to 5 mg and, in 2014, eszopiclone to no more than 2 mg. Caution is essential when prescribing all drugs to lactating women and women of childbearing age. Prescribed pharmacologic agents that treat sleep vary in pregnancy restrictions. As a sleep agent, doxylamine succinate has approval for unrestricted use in pregnancy.

Monitoring Patient Response

Sleep can be a reliable predictor of psychological and physical health. Differences in monitoring are related to whether insomnia is an acute or chronic problem. Brief episodes of acute insomnia can warrant treatment to prevent it from progressing and becoming established. A short course (up to 4 weeks) of sedative-hypnotic therapy is the current treatment of choice. The inclusion of cognitive therapy for insomnia improves the chance of an optimal response.

When insomnia becomes a chronic problem, consistent interaction between the patient and health care provider is essential, as is behavioral techniques. With chronic insomnia, there is potential for drug tolerance and rebound insomnia.

Patient Education

Patient education plays a vital role in the treatment of insomnia. Most hypnotic agents can result in excessive drowsiness or hangover from the medication. The clinician must alert the patient to this possibility and monitor the side effects of each agent prescribed (see **Tables 41.1** and **41.2**).

Patient-Oriented Information Sources

Major sleep centers across the country have websites that are useful resources for patients and health care providers. These sites can provide information about the diagnosis of sleep disorders and current research and therapies (**Box 42.4**).

Nutrition/Lifestyle Changes

Good sleep habits include setting a routine bedtime, getting regular exercise, using the bed only for sleeping, and getting in bed only when ready for sleep. Instruct patients to avoid stimulants such as caffeine, alcohol, and excess fluids before bedtime.

Complementary and Alternative Medications

Herbs and botanicals are often used as a "natural" way of promoting sleep. However, this is not without danger, especially if these treatments are taken in conjunction with prescription drugs. According to an analysis by Clarke et al. (2015) of the National Health Statistics in 2012, 32% of adults between 18 and 44 years use some alternative therapy/drugs, while 31% of adults over 65 years of age are likely to use CAM.

Common nonvitamin agents for sleep are melatonin, an endogenous hormone synthesized by the pineal gland from tryptophan. It is mainly secreted at night and its level peaks during regular sleep hours. In 1997, Lavie discovered that endogenous melatonin opens the nocturnal sleep gate and increases nocturnal melatonin secretion. Melatonin does not induce sleep but acts as a gatekeeper in the cascade of events that enables the CNS to favor sleep over wakefulness. Most studies have examined melatonin use to treat sleep disorders resulting from jet lag (Choy & Salbu, 2011; Cingi et al., 2018), but few have looked at melatonin use in short-term insomnia until now. A further meta-analysis of 19 studies showed that melatonin OTC reduced sleep onset time and increased sleep efficiency, total sleep duration, and overall sleep quality (Ferracioli-Oda et al., 2013; Xie et al., 2017).

Valerian is a traditional sleep remedy that is derived from the perennial herb *Valeriana officinalis*. The direct physiologic activity is mediated by the active sesquiterpene components of the volatile oil. This mediation creates a synergistic effect with neurotransmitters such as GABA and produces a direct sedative effect. An effective dosage ranges from 300 to 600 mg of the valerian root; 2 to 3 g of the dried root is soaked in a hot water cup for 10 to 15 minutes, and the patient then drinks the tea. Administration can occur 30 minutes to 2 hours before bedtime. As the U. S. FDA, the German Commission E has not reported significant herb or drug interactions.

As with melatonin, few studies exist regarding the safety and efficacy of valerian. A meta-analysis of those studies found more subjective sleep quality than objective measures (Fernandez-San-Martin et al., 2010). Overall, the clinical guidelines do not support herbal or nutritional substance use due to the lack of efficacy and safety data (Kim et al., 2018).

RESTLESS LEG SYNDROME/WILLIS–EKBOM DISEASE AND PERIODIC LIMB MOVEMENT DISORDER

Restless leg syndrome, also known as Willis–Ekbom disease, is characterized by an intense need to move the legs and affects the arms and trunk. It may also be accompanied by paresthesias and dysesthesias that usually worsen in the evening. Sometimes, the sensations can occur in other large muscle groups, but the legs are often involved. Moving around relieves the feeling, but only for a short time, as the sensation soon returns. Periodic limb movement disorder (PLMD) is another neurologic disorder representing repetitive movements and may or may not associate with RLS/WED. These sensations interfere with sleep. PLMD is characterized by episodes of highly repetitive and stereotyped limb movements only during sleep. Individuals can have both RLS/WED and PLMD.

Both disorders can interfere with sleep and contribute to sleep deprivation and decreased alertness, and daytime function. Population studies worldwide indicate that 5% to 10% of European and North American adults experience symptoms and, of these, 2% to 3% are severe. In the United States, the projection ranges from 2.4% to 10.6% (Piccheietti et al., 2017). PLMD is more common in adults over 60 years of age and is rare in children. Additionally, while 80% to 90% of RLS/WED patients have PLMD, only 30% of PLMD have RLS (Natarajan, 2010).

Causes

Generally, RLS/WED is an idiopathic disorder classified as a central neurologic disorder that causes pain and discomfort in the legs. Secondary causes of RLS/WED can include end-stage renal disease and hemodialysis, specific medication, alcohol use, nicotine and caffeine, neuropathy, and pregnancy. It can also be hereditary or drug induced. There is a definite link between iron deficits and RLS/WED.

Pathophysiology

RLS/WED and PLMD are chronic sensory–motor disorders that are not fully understood. However, recent advances show strong evidence linking RLS/WED to low iron/transferrin,

dopaminergic abnormalities, and excessive glutamate. Primary RLS/WED has a strong hereditary component, with 40% to 60% of patients having a familial association. Genome studies have linked evidence of this familial trait to six different distinct genes for RLS/WED. The onset of RLS/WED before age 45 is consistent with a familial link. Secondary RLS/WED can be associated with neuropathies from changes in axonal and small-fiber neural pathways. Patients with rheumatoid arthritis and diabetes have shown a greater RLS/WED prevalence, again presumably from changes due to neuropathy. Parkinson's disease is frequently associated with RLS/WED, pointing to a commonality in reduced dopaminergic functioning (Peeraully & Tan, 2012). There is also increasing data that supports a link between RLS/WED with obstructive sleep apnea.

The pathophysiology of PLMD is also uncertain, but the theory is there are changes in the descending inhibitory pathways with neuronal hyperexcitability. Dopamine transmission is also decreased, which supports dopaminergic therapy (Earley et al., 2011). Recently, iron deficiency has been implicated in the pathological aspects of RLS/WED and PLMD. According to the International Restless Legs Syndrome Study Group (IRLSSG), every patient should be evaluated for low iron stores (Allen et al., 2017).

Diagnostic Criteria

RLS/WED is diagnosed primarily through the patient history. Clinical criteria have been established by the IRLSSG (**Box 41.6**).

PLMD is associated more with stereotypical repetitive movements of limbs (legs alone or legs more than arms) that occur only during sleep. PLMD is generally diagnosed only through a sleep test.

The physical examination for RLS/WED and PLMD should include a full neurologic examination emphasizing the spinal cord and peripheral nerve function. The vascular examination is also necessary to rule out vascular disorders. Secondary causes of RLS/WED should be evaluated by a serum

---

BOX 41.6 Diagnostic Criteria for Restless Leg Syndrome

1. A compelling urge to move limbs associated with paresthesias/dysesthesias
2. Motor restlessness as evidenced by the following:
   - Floor pacing
   - Tossing and turning in bed
   - Rubbing legs
3. Symptoms worse or exclusively present at rest with variable and temporary relief by activity
4. Symptoms worse in the evening and at night

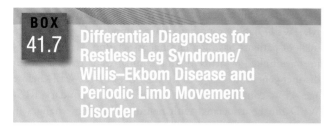

BOX 41.7 Differential Diagnoses for Restless Leg Syndrome/Willis–Ekbom Disease and Periodic Limb Movement Disorder

1. Nocturnal leg cramps
   - Painful, palpable involuntary muscle contractions
   - Focal with sudden onset
   - Unilateral
2. Akathisia
   - Excessive movement without accompanying sensory complaints
3. Peripheral neuropathy
   - Usually tingling, numbness, or pain sensations
   - Not associated with motor restlessness
   - Not helped by movement
   - Evening or nighttime worsening

ferritin level and serum chemistry to rule out uremia and diabetes. Polysomnography is not routinely indicated for RLS/WED but can be helpful to establish the diagnosis. **Box 41.7** lists other possible diagnoses.

Initiating Drug Therapy

Tailor the pharmacotherapy for each patient. Patients with relatively mild symptoms may not need medications. Nonpharmacologic therapy should be instituted, including mental alerting activities and cessation of alcohol, nicotine, and caffeine. Any medications that may precipitate or worsen RLS/WED symptoms, such as antidepressants and dopamine antagonists, should be avoided. Correction of underlying serum iron deficits may be helpful. Short-term studies have shown that drug therapy has significant benefits, but little is known about long-term treatment. There is a concern about long-term treatment due to the dopamine agonists' augmentation effects and should be used more in the short term (Allen et al., 2014; Geyer & Bogan, 2017).

Goals of Drug Therapy

Drug therapy aims to calm the restless legs or periodic limb movements, but there is no cure for the symptoms. For intermittent RLS/WED, treatment with medication should be deferred if possible due to medication and augmentation's potential side effects. Some patients can be refractory to pharmacologic treatment but still achieve partial relief of their symptoms. Pharmacologic agents for RLS/WED include dopaminergic agents, dopamine agonists, opioids, benzodiazepines, anticonvulsants, iron, and gabapentin enacarbil and ferrous iron (see **Table 41.3**). Other than dopamine agonists, many of these drugs are being used in an "off-label" manner.

Dopaminergic Agents

This drug class is approved for RLS/WED that includes the non-ergot dopamine agonist such as pramipexole (Mirapex) and rotigotine (Neupro). Levodopa with dopa decarboxylase inhibitor (carbidopa) is also used when the other dopamine agonist is not working, but this is off-label. See Chapter 38 for a full discussion of these agents.

Adverse Events

The carbidopa–levodopa agents may worsen RLS/WED symptoms in up to 80% of patients. The therapeutic effect may be reduced if taken with high-protein food. Insomnia, sleepiness, and gastrointestinal problems are other adverse events of pramipexole or rotigotine.

Dopamine Agonists

The initial dopamine agonists used for RLS/WED were bromocriptine and pergolide, but both have been discontinued due to the side effects. The newer dopamine agonists replace these drugs. These agents include pramipexole and rotigotine, which are not ergot-based and have fewer side effects. The newer agents' side effects include initial nausea and lightheadedness, nasal stuffiness, edema, and rarely daytime sleepiness. Slowly increasing the dose will help to mitigate these side effects. See Chapter 38 for a full discussion of these agents.

Opioids

Research is limited with using opioids in RLS/WED or PLMD and is reserved for the most severe refractory cases to other therapies. The theory is the same neural pathways are involved for pain and leg movements. Trenkwalder et al. (2013) led a randomized placebo-controlled trial of refractory RLS/WED patients who were treated with combination prolonged-release oxycodone–naloxone. The results show improvement of the quality-of-life indicators, including reducing sensory, restlessness, pain, and sleep. However, according to a review by de Oliveira et al. (2016), the evidence is limited for the use of opioids with RLS/WED. Practitioners need to be judicious in the selection of patients in whom to prescribe potent narcotics. Revised guidelines for RLS/WED treatment support careful opioid usage with careful monitoring (Silber et al., 2013). See Chapter 9 for pain management.

Benzodiazepines

Benzodiazepines (see **Table 42.1**) are only used concomitantly with a dopamine agonist when the use of a sole agent has failed. The most used are clonazepam and temazepam. The expectation is to help the patient sleep through the symptoms, not to stop the restless feeling. However, there is weak evidence, and the potential side effects may negate the benefits. Caution is necessary when using these agents in the older adults, and they can cause daytime sleepiness and cognitive impairment.

Anticonvulsants

Anticonvulsants are considered when dopamine agonists have failed and in patients who describe the RLS/WED discomfort as pain. Gabapentin is helpful in patients with RLS/WED and

TABLE 41.3

Overview of Selected Drugs Used to Treat Willis–Ekbom Disease/Restless Leg Syndrome

Generic (Trade) Name and Dosage	Selected Adverse Events	Contraindications	Special Considerations
Dopaminergic Agents			
Pramipexole (Mirapex) Start: 0.125 mg/d Range: 0.125–0.5 mg Max: 0.5 mg	Common side effects include nausea, somnolence, abdominal pain, dizziness, orthostatic hypotension.	Hypersensitivity to class, caution with alcohol use, concomitant CNS depressant, renal and liver impairment	Start with lower dose for CrCl 20–60 and increase only every 14 d. Augmentation is common with this class.
Rotigotine transdermal (Neupro) Start: 1 mg/24 h patch q24h Range: 1–3 mg/24 h Max: 3 mg/24 h	Same as above	Same as above	Same as above
Anticonvulsants: Alpha-2-Delta Ligands			
Gabapentin enacarbil (Horizant) 600 mg once daily taken at about 5 PM.	Common side effects include somnolence, dizziness, headache, and nausea.	There are no contraindications to using Horizant. Caution with driving and using complex machinery until the effects of Horizant are known. As with any other antiepileptic drug, there is a potential to increase risk of suicidal ideation and depression.	Horizant is not interchangeable with other gabapentin products and there is no generic. Monitor for baseline creatinine, depression, and suicidal ideation. Only approved anticonvulsant drug for RLS/WED. If dose is missed, take the next day.
Iron			
Ferrous Sulfate 150–300 mg/d PO divided BID–QID for 3–6 mo	Common side effects include constipation, black stools, dyspepsia, nausea and vomiting, diarrhea.	Hypersensitivity to drug/class/ components Hemochromatosis, primary, anemia, hemolytic, hemosiderosis, PUD, ulcerative colitis.	Different preparation of FeSO4 contains a variety of equivalent levels of drug. Due to the constipation, side effect prescribe a stool softener in conjunction with iron supplementation.

CNS, central nervous system; PUD, peptic ulcer disease; RLS, Restless Leg Syndrome; WED, Willis–Ekbom Disease.

peripheral neuropathy but is considered "off label". As with the dopamine agonists, lower dosages of gabapentin (100–600 mg one to three times daily) can be successful. The side effect of hypersomnia often limits the dosage. Other side effects can include nausea, sedation, and dizziness. Gabapentin enacarbil is a prodrug of gabapentin and is the only anticonvulsant drug approved for RLS/WED. The starting and continuing dose is 600 mg daily. Adverse effects of the drug are the same as gabapentin (see **Table 42.2**). See Chapter 36 for further discussion of other anticonvulsants.

Ferrous Sulfate

To consider prescribing ferrous sulfate, morning, fasting iron, ferritin, total iron binding capacity (TIBC), and % transferrin saturation guide therapy. When the transferrin saturation is greater than 45%, prescribe ferrous sulfate 325 mg (65 mg elemental iron) twice daily. Accompany the iron with vitamin C 100 mg also twice daily. Intravenous iron can also be considered.

Adverse Effects

The most common reaction to iron replacement is constipation and dark stools. Additionally, there can be nausea, vomiting, and dyspepsia.

Selecting the Most Appropriate Agent

For treatment purposes, the classification of RLS/WED is _intermittent_ (not often enough to require drug therapy), _daily_ (troublesome sufficient to require drug therapy), and _refractory_ (not adequately treated by a dopamine agonist). The ideal agent will minimize or decrease the symptoms of RLS/WED. No one pharmacologic agent appears to be efficacious in all patients, and often, a combination of medications is needed. The severity of RLS/WED can vary, and pharmacologic treatment needs to be individualized. See **Box 41.8** for considerations when selecting a pharmacologic agent (**Figure 41.2**).

Considerations in Pharmacologic Agent Selection in Restless Leg Syndrome/Willis–Ekbom Disease

Age of patient	Benzodiazepines can cause cognitive impairment in older adults.
Severity of symptoms	Mild symptoms: no medication or levodopa or dopamine agonist Severe symptoms: strong opioid
Frequency/ regularity of symptoms	Patients with infrequent symptoms may benefit from PRN medication.
Presence of pregnancy	No safety and efficacy clinical trials on treatment of RLS/WED with medications in pregnancy
Renal failure	Need to decrease dosage if drugs are renally excreted

First-Line Therapy

Dopaminergic antagonists such as low-dose carbidopa–levodopa should be reserved for patients with intermittent RLS/WED. The first choice of therapy for daily RLS/WED is one of the dopamine agonists. Comparative analysis of all dopamine agonists (pramipexole and rotigotine) showed clinically significant improvement in RLS/WED symptomatology. Nausea, dizziness, dyskinesia, and somnolence are potential side effects of both dopaminergic antagonists and agonists. One problem with the dopaminergic antagonists is augmentation (worsening of RLS/WED symptoms), which can occur as early as 10 weeks of therapy.

A prodrug of gabapentin was approved in 2015 for use with RLS/WED. Gabapentin encarbil (Horizant) can be used for first-line treatment. It is the only drug in the anticonvulsant category specifically approved for RLS/WED. Along with other first-line therapies, consider an iron replacement.

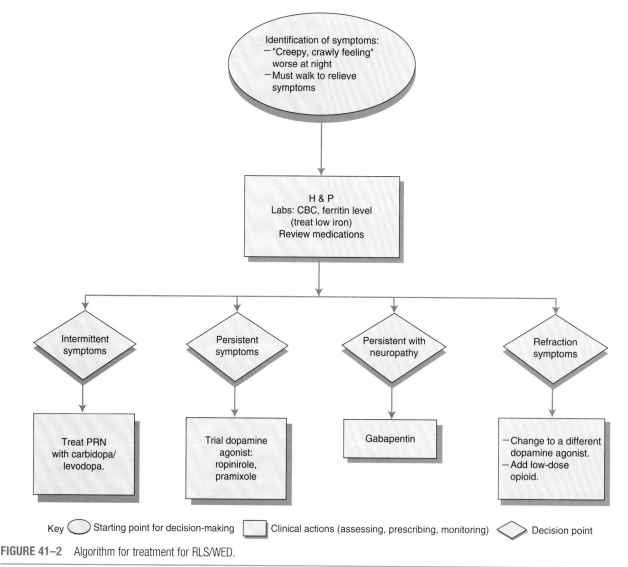

FIGURE 41–2 Algorithm for treatment for RLS/WED.

CBC, complete blood count; RLS, Restless Leg Syndrome; WED, Willis–Ekbom Disease.

Second-Line Therapy

Pharmacologic agents approved for neuropathic pain such as gabapentin (Neurontin) or pregabalin (Lyrica) can be used alone or in conjunction with other agents, but they are also off-label. It is beneficial for patients who describe RLS/WED symptoms as painful. Other anticonvulsant agents such as carbamazepine (Tegretol) can be considered, but the older agents carry an increased risk of adverse effects such as dizziness, drowsiness, and lack of coordination. Patients also may experience nausea with these older agents. An opioid or opioid receptor agonist, tramadol (Ultram), may be added or used alone at low doses. If either the anticonvulsant or opioid fails, a repeat trial of dopamine agonists should be attempted (Silber et al., 2013).

Third-Line Therapy

Patients who continue to have symptoms may be refractory to treatment. Therapeutic doses may not have been obtained, or the patients could not tolerate the side effects of the medications. Consider substituting different medicines in the dopamine agonist class or adding higher-potency opioids. Consider consultation with a sleep specialist for additional therapies.

Monitoring Patient Response

Most patients will have remittance of symptoms with the first therapeutic dose of medication, supporting the theory that dopaminergic abnormality is a cause of this disorder. Another indicator of improvement is a decrease in excessive daytime sleepiness (EDS) from lack of REM sleep. Patients need to be monitored for side effects of the pharmacologic agents. The long-term efficacy of these pharmacologic agents is uncertain, and monitoring for relapse of symptoms is essential. It is also important to monitor for dependence with the use of benzodiazepines or opioids.

Patient Education

Many patients who have RLS/WED use OTC sleep medications, and poor sleep hygiene may contribute to the lack of sleep in RLS/WED sufferers. Implementing cognitive sleep hygiene techniques may provide a modest improvement in short-term sleep symptoms (Edinger, 2003). Patients should inform all their health care providers about their RLS/WED diagnosis, and health care providers should be aware that the patient's inability to keep their limbs still is not due to lack of cooperation. Improper restraint of patients with this syndrome has resulted in mortality and morbidity.

Drug Information

The body of knowledge about medications and RLS/WED is continuing to grow through research. The center for restless legs syndrome at Johns Hopkins (https://www.hopkinsmedicine.org/neurology_neurosurgery/centers_clinics/restless-legs-syndrome/) provides patients and providers with comprehensive information.

Patient-Oriented Information Sources

The Willis–Ekbom Disease Foundation supports research and provides information for patients and health care providers. Extensive international research is also being conducted on this serious sleep problem (see **Box 42.4**).

NARCOLEPSY

Narcolepsy is a sleep disorder caused by deficits in the hypocretin signaling in the brain, leading to poor sleep–wake cycles that can greatly impact those affected daily activities. Individuals with narcolepsy sleep the same amount as the average person but cannot control their sleep timing. The other features of narcolepsy can include EDS, cataplexy (attacks of muscle weakness), sleep paralysis, and hypnagogic hallucinations. Narcolepsy is the second leading cause of EDS and has an overall incidence in the world of 0.2 to 1.6 per thousand individuals (Leschziner, 2014). Narcolepsy can have a dramatic impact on virtually all areas of life. Unfortunately, the diagnosis of narcolepsy is often mislabeled as other chronic sleep disorders, especially if cataplexy is absent.

Causes

Narcolepsy currently lacks distinct etiology and usually starts in the second or third decade of life; however, it has been identified in children as young as 3 years old. EDS or cataplexy may be the first symptom, but most often, cataplexy is delayed 2 to 3 years or can be absent. The precipitation of cataplexy attacks occurs due to specific situations or triggers of strong emotions. Hypnagogic hallucinations can be present but are rarely the first manifestation of narcolepsy. Other possible predisposing factors related to narcolepsy include obesity, head trauma, sleep deprivation, changes in sleep–wake patterns, and viral illnesses (Kornum, et al., 2017).

Pathophysiology

The pathophysiology of narcolepsy is not well understood but is evolving. Current research has focused on the loss of hypocretinergic neurons in the lateral hypothalamus. These neurons stimulate various histaminergic neurons in the basal forebrain, which increase the arousal state and involve activation of the cerebral cortex. This loss creates an unstable neuronal network responsible for maintaining wakefulness and preventing REM sleep (Leschziner, 2014). There is also increasing knowledge about the role of genetics in narcolepsy. A strong genetic component is demonstrated through the human leukocyte antigen (HLA), especially when a first-degree relative has narcolepsy and cataplexy.

Diagnostic Criteria

Patient presentations include complaints of EDS, cataplexy, and sleep-related hallucinations, along with sleep paralysis. These criteria are commonly known as the narcoleptic triad.

BOX 41.9 Diagnostic Criteria for Narcolepsy

Type 1 N

Required:
Hypersomnolence daily × 3 mo
Low CSF hypocretin levels (≤110 pg/mL) OR cataplexy
Short sleep latency (≤8 min)
Two or more sleep-onset rapid eye movement REM episodes on the multiple sleep latency test (MSLT)
Subtype
Type 1 due to a medical condition
Narcolepsy without cataplexy but low hypocretin

Type 2

Required:
Hypersomnolence daily × 3 mo
Hypocretin not measured OR ≥110 pg/mL
Absence of cataplexy
Short sleep latency (≤8 min)
Two or more sleep-onset REM episodes on the MSLT
Subtype
Type 2 due to a medical condition

The International Classification of Sleep Disorders (ICSD), third edition (2014), now classifies narcolepsy as type 1 or type 2 with subtypes. Diagnosis is based on the presence of EDS, levels of hypocretin in the cerebral spinal fluid, and multi latency sleep test (MLST) (**Box 42.9**).

Initiating Drug Therapy

There is no cure for narcolepsy, and pharmacologic therapy must be initiated to control the attacks (**Table 41.4**). Evaluation for cataplexy, sleep-related hallucinations, and sleep paralysis is important to identify the best treatment agent. Most often, antidepressants are used to block the REM paralysis of cataplexy. The mainstay of pharmacologic therapy has been amphetamines and amphetamine-like drugs such as methylphenidate (Ritalin). However, now there are newer drugs on the market that focus on treating the symptoms and the neurobiological deficit. Pharmacologic agents used in treating narcolepsy can be classified into psychostimulants (wake-promoting agents), amphetamines, sodium oxybate, and antidepressants. Recently two additional categories, histamine H3 antagonist/inverse agonist and dopamine–norepinephrine reuptake inhibitors (DNRI), have been added to treatment options.

Goals of Drug Therapy

Pharmacologic therapy should be titrated to promote the optimal dose of stimulation. The provider needs to work with the patient to identify personal treatment goals such as staying awake in a classroom or social situation or driving. The main goal is to experience life as normal as possible, staying awake in typical daily living situations.

Psychostimulants (Wake-Promoting Agents)

Modafinil and armodafinil (the R-enantiomer of modafinil) are psychostimulants with unique properties to promote wakefulness. The potential for these agents' abuse is much lower than with other stimulants, although it still needs to be monitored. The mechanism of action of modafinil and armodafinil is not well understood, but it appears to attenuate the central alpha-1 adrenergic system. The primary sites

of action are the hippocampus's subregions, the centrolateral nucleus of the thalamus, and the amygdala's central nucleus. Modafinil can produce euphoria and psychoactive effects like other CNS stimulants. The drug's absorption occurs rapidly, with peak plasma concentration in 2 to 4 hours and a half-life of 15 hours. The distribution of the drug is throughout the tissues, and it is moderately bound to plasma proteins. The drug is metabolized in the liver and excreted in the urine (see **Table 42.4**).

Amphetamines

Various amphetamine drugs are used to promote wakefulness in narcolepsy. The most used agent is methylphenidate (Ritalin), which is approved for use in narcolepsy. The mechanism of action is generally unknown but thought to stimulate CNS activity and block the reuptake while increasing the release of norepinephrine with dopamine. This agent is metabolized in the liver but not through the CYP450 system. The average half-life of methylphenidate is 3.5 hours, and administration can be adjusted to daily activities.

Sodium Oxybate

Sodium oxybate (Xyrem) is approved to treat two common narcolepsy symptoms: EDS and cataplexy. The active ingredient of sodium oxybate is gamma-hydroxybutyrate (GHB), which can depress the CNS. Another agent with sodium oxybate combined with calcium, magnesium, and potassium (Xywav) is an oral solution. This drug is thought to mediate the GABAb with the noradrenergic and dopaminergic neurons and the thalamocortical neurons. Each drug is only distributed through the manufacturer in a restricted risk evaluation and mitigation strategy (REMS) distribution program due to abuse potential. While the primary care provider may not be the prescriber of this medication, it is important to know about the drugs (Table 42.4).

Antidepressants

Venlafaxine (Effexor) and duloxetine (Cymbalta) act on the serotonergic and noradrenergic systems and may be useful when cataplexy is present (see Chapter 42).

TABLE 41.4

Overview of Selected Drugs Used to Treat Narcolepsy

Generic (Trade) Name and Dosage	Selected Adverse Events	Contraindications	Special Considerations
Psychostimulants			
Armodafinil (Nuvigil) Start: 150–250 mg QAM	*Serious:* arrhythmias, syncope, visual changes, abuse/dependency *Common:* headache, nausea/vomiting, rhinitis, diarrhea	Hypersensitivity to modafinil and armodafinil	Reduce dose in patients with severe hepatic dysfunction. Consider low doses in older adults.
Modafinil (Provigil) Start: 200 mg QAM; maximum 400 mg daily	Same as above	Sensitivity to class, caution with coronary artery disease, mitral valve prolapse, impaired liver failure	Start at 100 mg daily in older adults.
Sodium oxybate (Xyrem) Start: dose 1–2.25 g at HS. Dose 2–2.25 g 2.5–4 h later Increase dose by interval 1.5 g nightly. Range: 6–9 g nightly	*Serious:* CNS and respiratory depression, abuse/dependency, depression, suicidal ideation, psychosis, paranoia, hallucinations, apnea *Common:* nausea, dizziness, vomiting, somnolence enuresis	Sensitivity to class; caution with CNS depressant use; alcohol intake; hepatic, renal, pulmonary, cardiac impairment; psychiatric disorders; drug abuse history	Black box warning for appropriate use—only distributed through Xyrem Success Program and centralized pharmacy Abuse potential due to relation to GHB
Calcium, magnesium, potassium, and sodium oxybates (Xywav) oral solution Initiate dosage at 4.5 g per night orally, divided into two doses Titrate to effect in increments of up to 1.5 g per night per week. Recommended dosage range: 6 g to 9 g per night PO Pediatric dose is by weight based on table in product insert	Same as above	Same as above	Same as above
Histamine H3 Antagonist/Inverse Agonist			
Pitolisant (Wakix) Recommended dosage range is 17.8 to 35.6 mg daily. Titrate dosage weekly from starting dose of 8.9 mg up to 35.6 mg	The most common adverse reactions (≥5% and twice placebo) for Wakik were insomnia, nausea, and anxiety.	Known hypersensitivity to the components of pitolisant Severe hepatic impairment Use caution with drugs that prolong QT_c	Administer once daily in the morning upon wakening. Hepatic & renal impairment dose range is 8.9 mg up to 17.8 mg. Poor metabolizers of CYP2D6: Maximum recommended dosage is 17.8 mg once daily. Only non-schedule narcolepsy medication.
Dopamine–Norepinephrine Reuptake Inhibitors (DNRI)			
Solriamfetol (Sunosi) Starting dose for patients with narcolepsy: 75 mg once daily. Maximum dose is 150 mg once daily.	Most common adverse reactions (≥ 5% and greater than placebo): headache, nausea, decreased appetite, insomnia, and anxiety.	Concurrent treatment with an MAOI or use of an MAOI within the preceding 14 d. Avoid use in patients with unstable cardiovascular disease, serious heart arrhythmias, or other serious heart problems. ESRD: Not recommended.	Take once daily upon awakening. Avoid administration within 9 h of planned bedtime because of the potential to interfere with sleep. Adjust dosing for moderate and severe renal impairment— moderate: start at 37.5 and increase only to 75 mg; severe: start at 37.5 mg with no increase in dose. Schedule IV—No REMS required.

CNS, central nervous system; ESRD, end-stage renal disease; GHB, gamma-hydroxybutyrate; MAOI, monoamine oxidase inhibitor; REMS, risk evaluation and mitigation strategy.

Histamine H3 Antagonist/Inverse Agonist

Pitolisant (Wakix) is the first of the class to treat EDS or cataplexy in adult patients with narcolepsy. It is the first drug for narcolepsy that is not a scheduled medication. A fundamental significance is the lack of REMS measures associated with this medication.

Mechanism of Action

The mechanism of action is unknown but thought to be mediated through its activity as an antagonist/inverse agonist at histamine-3 (H3) receptors, which has a part in the synthesis of wake-promoting excitatory neurotransmitters. In animal models, pitolisant induced central histaminergic and adrenergic transmissions, thereby increasing wakefulness and decreasing REM sleep episodes.

Dosage

The recommended dosage range for pitolisant is 17.8 to 35.6 mg administered orally once daily in the morning upon wakening. Dosage is titrated over 3 weeks, starting with 8.9 mg and doubling until 35.6 mg. Administration in the morning is important not to interrupt sleep.

Time Frame for Response

The half-life of pitolisant is 10 to 12 hours to promote wakefulness. A steady state can be achieved in 5 to 6 days; however, it may take up to 8 weeks to achieve clinical response.

Contraindications

The liver extensively metabolizes pitolisant, and the only absolute contraindication is for severe liver disease. Also, avoid the use of pitolisant in patients with a history of cardiac arrhythmias due to the prolongation of the QTc, which increases the risk of torsade de pointes or sudden death.

Adverse Events

Compared to placebo, the most common side effect is abdominal pain, sleep disturbance, and decreased appetite. Additional side effects can include anxiety and nausea.

Interactions

Pitolisant has different interactions with drugs in the CYP2D6 and histamine-1 systems, for medications are strong CYP2D6 inhibitors that increase pitolisant exposure by 2.2-fold. Examples of these drugs are paroxetine, fluoxetine, and bupropion. In this case, the dose of pitolisant needs to be decreased by 50%. Other strong CYP3A4 inducers, such as rifampin, carbamazepine, and phenytoin, require the pitolisant dose's doubling.

Also, avoid centrally acting H1 receptor antagonists such as pheniramine maleate, diphenhydramine, promethazine (antihistamines), imipramine, clomipramine, and mirtazapine (tri or tetracyclic) antidepressants. Pitolisant functions by increasing the histamine levels in the brain; however, the H1 receptor antagonists cross the blood–brain barrier and reduce the effectiveness of the pitolisant.

Dopamine–Norepinephrine Reuptake Inhibitors

Sunosi (solriamfetol) is a new agent with indications for EDS and narcolepsy. As with other drugs for narcolepsy, it is classified as a Schedule IV drug due to abuse potential. Solriamfetol also does not require participation in REMS.

Mechanism of Action

Solriamfetol's mechanism of wake-promoting action is unclear. Still, the theory is it may be mediated through its activity by selectively binding to DNRI. The liver does not metabolize this drug, nor is it a significant inhibitor in the CYP enzyme system or renal transporters; therefore, it has minimal metabolism. It is excreted unchanged in the urine.

Dosage

For narcolepsy, the starting dose is 75 mg daily to a maximum of 150 mg. Dosages above 150 mg daily do not confer increased effectiveness sufficient to outweigh dose-related adverse reactions. Adjustment in dose is necessary for moderate renal impairment with a maximum of 75 mg and severe impairment of 37.5 mg daily.

Time Frame for Response

The onset of response is within 1 hour, and peak plasma concentration in 2 hours. The half-life of solriamfetol is approximately 7 hours.

Contraindications

Solriamfetol is contraindication when monoamine oxidase (MAO) inhibitors have been administered in the past 14 days. Caution is advised when prescribing for patients with known cardiovascular and cerebrovascular disease. Solriamfetol has not been studied in patients who have a history of psychosis or bipolar disorders.

Adverse Events

The most common adverse reactions are dose dependent and reported as headache, nausea, decreased appetite, anxiety, and insomnia. There have been reports of worsening anxiety and irritability.

Interactions

Concomitant use with MAO inhibitors or noradrenergic drugs increases the risk of hypertensive reaction. Exercise caution with other medications that increase blood pressure, heart rate, or dopamine levels.

Selecting the Most Appropriate Agent

For treatment purposes, narcolepsy classifications include *type 1N* or *type 2* (**Box 42.8**). The ideal agent will minimize the triad of symptoms associated with the disease. As with insomnia and RLS/WED, no one pharmacologic agent appears to help all patients, and often, a combination of medications is needed. Individualizing therapy is also important with narcolepsy. The primary care provider most likely will not prescribe these drugs initially but will continue to be part of the health care team and need knowledge about the disease and treatment.

Special Populations

Pediatrics

Narcolepsy is rare and difficult to diagnose in children. There are limited drug choices, but drugs used in ADHD may be useful (see Chapter 43). Psychostimulating agents, histamine H3 antagonist/inverse agonist, and DNRI have not been studied in children and are not appropriate to prescribe. The sodium oxybates have been evaluated in children and have indications for 7 years and older.

Geriatrics

Due to natural aging changes of the liver and kidneys, there is a potential for decreased metabolism and excretion. There is limited evidence for most drugs for the treatment of narcolepsy in the older adult population. Most studies have an insufficient enrollment of subjects that are 65 years old or greater. A general guideline is to use the medication usually lower doses first and increase slowly.

Women

Modafinil and armodafinil have other risks, including pregnancy in women on hormonal birth control. Most drugs lack adequate data on the developing fetus and lactation.

Monitoring Patient Response

Narcolepsy is a lifelong disease process, and patients must use the medications for their entire lives. Outcome measures include reduction of EDS and adverse effects. Monitoring the patient response is through the lack of side effects from medications and improvement in disease severity symptoms. Achieving the goals identified by the patient can help to improve compliance.

Patient Education

Narcolepsy is a lifelong disease, and patients with their families need to be aware of all available options to treat narcolepsy. Counseling about behavioral treatment such as naps during the day can be beneficial to decrease EDS. Psychological distress is a consequence, not the cause, of the disease due to the impact on lifestyle, including discussion about career limitations such as shift work and jobs that can be hazardous. Information about medication side effects and potential drug interactions is critical to reducing the possibility of suicide, unwanted pregnancy, and addiction.

Drug Information

The Merck Manual—the professional online version–is a good source for treating patients with narcolepsy. Addition resources include Narcolepsy Link https://www.narcolepsylink.com/

Patient-Oriented Sources

Patients can find information about narcolepsy from a variety of sources. Online support groups exist (see **Box 42.4**).

CASE STUDY 1

S.H., ages 47, reports difficulty falling asleep and staying asleep. These problems have been ongoing for many years, but she has never mentioned them to her health care provider. She has generally "lived with it" and self-treated the problem with over-the-counter (OTC) Tylenol PM. Currently, she is also experiencing perimenopausal symptoms of night sweats and mood swings. Current medical problems include hypertension controlled with medications. Past medical history includes childhood illnesses of measles, chickenpox, and mumps. Family history is positive for diabetes on the maternal side and hypertension on the paternal side. Her only medication is an angiotensin-converting enzyme inhibitor and diuretic combination for hypertension control. She generally does not like taking medication and does not take any other OTC products.

DIAGNOSIS: INSOMNIA

1. List specific goals of therapy for S.H.
2. What drug therapy would you prescribe? Why?
3. What are the parameters for monitoring the success of the therapy?
4. Discuss specific patient education based on the prescribed therapy.
5. List one or two adverse reactions for the selected agent that would cause you to change therapy.
6. What would be the choice for second-line therapy?
7. What OTC and/or alternative medicines might be appropriate for this patient?
8. What dietary and lifestyle changes might you recommend?
9. Describe one or two drug–drug or drug–food interactions for the selected agent.

Bibliography

Starred references are cited in the text.

Abad, V. C. (2021). Profile of solriamfetol in the management of excessive daytime sleepiness associated with narcolepsy or obstructive sleep apnea: Focus on patient selection and perspectives. *Nature and Science of Sleep, 13*, 75–91. doi: 10.2147/nss.s245020

*Alameddine, Y., Ellenbogen, J. M., & Bianchi, M. T. (2015). Sleep-Wake time perception varies by direct or indirect query. *Journal of Clinical Sleep Medicine, 11*(2), 123–129. doi: 10.5664/jcsm.4456

*Allen, R. P., Armstrong, M. J., Trenkwalder, C., Zee, P. C., & Winkelman, J. W. (2017). Author response: Practice guideline summary: Treatment of restless legs syndrome in adults: Report of the Guideline Development, Dissemination, and Implementation Subcommittee of the American Academy of Neurology. *Neurology, 88*(24), 2337-2338. https://doi.org/10.1212/wnl.0000000000004047

Allen, R. P., Auerbach, S., Bahrain, H., et al. (2013a). The prevalence of impact of restless legs syndrome on patients with iron deficiency anemia. *American Journal of Hematology, 88*(4), 261–264.

Allen, R. P., Barker, P., Horska, A., et al. (2013b). Thalamic glutamate/glutamine in restless legs syndrome: Increase and related to disturbed sleep. *Neurology, 80*(22), 2028–2034. doi: 10.1212.WNL.0b013e31294b3f6

*Allen, R. P., Chen, C., Garcia-Borreguero, D., et al. (2014). Comparison of pregabalin with pramipexole for restless legs syndrome. *New England Journal of Medicine, 370*, 621–631.

Allison, M. (2012). Evaluation of insomnia in the adult client. *Journal for Nurse Practitioners, 8*(4), 330–331. doi: 10.1016/j.nurpra.2012.02.009

Alshaikh, M. K., Tricco, A. C., Tashkandi, M., et al. (2012). Sodium oxybate for narcolepsy with cataplexy: Systematic review and meta-analysis. *Journal of Clinical Sleep Medicine, 8*(4), 451–458. doi: 10.5664/jcsm.2048

*American Geriatrics Society 2019 updated AGS Beers Criteria® for potentially inappropriate medication use in older adults. (2019). *Journal of the American Geriatrics Society, 67*(4), 674–694. doi: 10.1111/jgs.15767

American Psychiatric Association. (2013). *Diagnostic and Statistical Manual of Mental Disorders* (5th ed., pp. 410–413). Arlington, VA: American Psychiatric Association.

Amos, L., Grekowicz, M., Kuhn, E., et al. (2014). Treatment of pediatric restless leg syndrome. *Clinical Pediatrics, 53*(4), 331–336. doi: 10.1177/0009922813507997

Atkin, T., Comai, S., & Gobbi, G. (2018). Drugs for insomnia beyond benzodiazepines: Pharmacology, clinical applications, and discovery. *Pharmacological Reviews, 70*(2), 197–245. doi: 10.1124/pr.117.014381

Aurora, R. N., Kristo, D. A., Bista, S. R., et al. (2012). The treatment of restless legs syndrome and periodic limb movement disorder in adults—An update for 2012: Practice parameters with evidence-based systematic review and meta-analyses. *Sleep, 35*(8), 1039–1062.

Baglioni, C., Spiegelhalder, K., Lombardo, C., et al. (2011). Sleep and emotions: A focus of insomnia. *Sleep Medicine Reviews, 14*(4), 227–238. doi: 10.1016/j.smrv.2009.10.007

Baldwin, D. S., Aitchison, K., Bateson, A., et al. (2013). Benzodiazepines: Risks and benefits. A reconsideration. *Journal of Psychopharmacology, 27*(11), 967–971. doi: 10.1177/0269881113503509

Bateson, A. (2004). The benzodiazepine site of the GABA$_A$ receptor: An old target with new potential? *Sleep Medicine, 5*(Suppl. 1), S9–S15.

Bent, S., Paudal, A., & Moore, D. (2006). Valerian for sleep: A systematic review and meta-analysis. *American Journal of Medicine, 119*(12), 1005–1012.

Billioti de Gage, S., Ducruet, T., Kurth, T., et al. (2014). Benzodiazepine use and risk of Alzheimer's disease: Case-control study. *BMJ, 349*, g520s.

Bjorøy, I., Jørgensen, V. A., Pallesen, S., & Bjorvatn, B. (2020). The prevalence of insomnia subtypes in relation to demographic characteristics, anxiety, depression, alcohol consumption and use of hypnotics. *Frontiers in Psychology, 11*, 1. doi: 10.3389/fpsyg.2020.00527

Bonnet, M. H., & Arand, D. L. (2010). Hyperarousal and insomnia: State of the science. *Sleep Medicine Reviews, 14*(1), 9–15. doi: 10.1016/j.smrv.2009.05.002

Bozorg, A. (2014). Restless legs syndrome. *EMedicine Drugs & Disease.* Retrieved from http://emedicine.medscape.com/article/1188327-overview on July 8, 2015.

Bozorg, A. (2015). Narcolepsy treatment and management. *EMedicine Drugs & Disease.* Retrieved from http://emedicine.medscape.com/article/1188433overview on August 24, 2015.

Bozorg, J., & Benbadis, S. (2014). Restless legs syndrome clinical presentation. *Medscape: Drugs & Diseases.* Retrieved from http://emedicine.medscape.com/article/1188327-clinica on July 11, 2015.

Brezinski, A., Vangel, M. G., Wurtman, R. J., et al. (2005). Effects of exogenous melatonin on sleep: A meta-analysis. *Sleep Medicine Reviews, 9*(1), 41–50.

Brostrom, A., Stromberg, A., Dahlstrom, U., et al. (2004). Sleep difficulties, daytime sleepiness, and health-related quality of life in patients with chronic heart failure. *Journal of Cardiovascular Nursing, 19*(4), 234–242.

Burbank, F., Buchfuhrer, M., & Kopjar, B. (2013a). Improving sleep for patients with restless legs syndrome. Part II: Meta-analysis of vibration therapy and drugs approved by the FDA for treatment of restless legs syndrome. *Journal of Parkinsonism and Restless Legs Syndrome, 3*, 11–22. doi: 10.2147/JPRLS.S40356

Burbank, F., Buchfuhrer, M., & Kopjar, B. (2013b). Sleep improvement for restless legs syndrome patients. Part I: Pooled analysis of two prospective, double-blind, sham-controlled, multi-center, randomized clinical studies of the effects of vibrating pads on RLS symptoms. *Journal of Parkinsonism and Restless Legs Syndrome, 3*, 1–10. doi: 10.2147/JPRLS.S40354

*Buscemi, N., Vandermeer, B., Randya, R., et al. (2004). Melatonin for treatment of sleep disorders. Evidence Report/Technology Assessment, No. 108. Bethesda, MD: AHRQ Publication No. 05-E002-2.

Buyssee, D. (2004). Insomnia, depression, and aging: Assessing sleep and mood interactions in older adults. *Geriatrics, 59*(2), 47–51.

Buysse, D., Cheng, Y., Germain, A., et al. (2011a). Night-to-night sleep variability in older adults with and without chronic insomnia. *Sleep Medicine, 11*(1), 56. doi: 10.1016/j.sleep.2009.02.010

Buysse, D., Germain, A., Hall, M., et al. (2011b). A neurobiological model of insomnia. *Drug Discovery Today. Disease Models, 8*(4), 129–137. doi: 10.1016/j.ddmopd.2011.07.002

Carden, K. A. (2020). Sleep is essential: A new strategic plan for the American Academy of Sleep Medicine. *Journal of Clinical Sleep Medicine, 16*(1), 1–2. doi: 10.5664/jcsm.8156

*Carr, T. (2018, December 12). The problem with sleeping pills the benefits might be smaller, and the risks greater, than you expect. *Consumer Reports.* https://www.consumerreports.org/drugs/the-problem-with-sleeping-pills/

*Centers for Disease Control. (2019). Short Sleep Duration Among US Adults. Https://Www.Cdc.Gov/Sleep/Data_statistics.Html. https://www.cdc.gov/sleep/data_statistics.html

*Cingi, C., Emre, I. E., & Muluk, N. B. (2018). Jetlag related sleep problems and their management: A review. *Travel Medicine and Infectious Disease, 24*, 59–64. https://doi.org/10.1016/j.tmaid.2018.05.008

Chawla, J. (2014). Insomnia. *EMedicine Drugs & Disease.* Retrieved from http://emedicine.medscape.com/article/1187829-overview on June 30, 2015.

*Choy, M., & Salbu, R. (2011). Jet lag: Current and potential therapies. *P & T, 36*(4), 221–231.

*Clarke, T. C., Black, L. I., Stussman, B. J., et al. (2015). Trends in the use of complementary health approaches among adults: United States, 2002–2012. National health statistics reports; no 79. Hyattsville, MD: National Center for Health Statistics.

Cohen, E. M., Dossett, M. L., Mehta, D. H., Davis, R. B., & Lee, Y. C. (2018). Factors associated with insomnia and complementary medicine use in children: Results of a national survey. *Sleep Medicine, 44*, 82–88. doi: 10.1016/j.sleep.2018.01.007

De la Herran-Arita, A. K., & Garcia-Garcia, F. (2013). Current and emerging options for the drug treatment of narcolepsy. *Drugs, 73*, 1771–1781. doi: 10.1007/s40265-013-0127-y

*De Lecea, L., Kilduff, T. S., Peyron, C., et al. (1998). The hypocretins: Hypothalamus-specific peptides with neuroexcitatory activity. *Proceedings of the National Academy of Sciences of the USA, 95*(1), 322–327.

*de Oliveira, C. O., Carvalho LBC, L. B. C., Carlos, K., Conti, C., de Oliveira, M. M., Prado, L. B. F., & Prado, G. F. (2016). Opioids for restless leg syndrome. *Cochrane Database of Systematic Reviews* , 6, 1. https://doi.org/10.1002/14651858.CD006941.pub2

*Dubey, A. K., Handu, S. S., & Mediratta, P. K. (2015). Suvorexant: The first orexin receptor antagonist to treat insomnia. *Journal of Pharmacology and Pharmacotherapeutics*, 6(2), 118–121. doi: 10.4103/0976-500X.155496

*Earley, D., Kuwabara, H., Wong, D., et al. (2011). The dopamine transporter is decreased in the striatum of subjects with restless legs syndrome. *Sleep*, 34(3), 341–347.

Ebrahim, I. O., Howard, R. S., Kopelman, M. D., et al. (2002). The hypocretin/orexin system. *Journal of the Royal Society of Medicine*, 95(5), 227–230.

*Edinger, J. (2003). Cognitive and behavioral anomalies among insomnia patients with mixed restless legs and periodic limb movement disorder. *Behavioral Sleep Medicine*, 1(1), 37–53.

Edinger, J. D., Arnedt, J. T., Bertisch, S. M., et al. (2021). Behavioral and psychological treatments for chronic insomnia disorder in adults: An American Academy of Sleep Medicine clinical practice guideline. *Journal of Clinical Sleep Medicine*, 17(2), 255–262. doi: 10.5664/jcsm.8986

FDA News Release. (2014). FDA approves new type of sleep drug, Belsomra.

Fernandez-Mendoza, J., Calhoun, S., Bixler, E., et al. (2011). Sleep misperception and chronic insomnia in the general population: The role of objective sleep duration and psychological profiles. *Psychosomatic Medicine*, 73(1), 88–97. doi: 10.1097/PSY.0b013e3181fe365a

*Fernandez-San-Martin, M. I., Masa-Font, R., Palacious-Soler, L., et al. (2010). Effectiveness of valerian on insomnia: A meta-analysis randomized placebo-controlled trials. *Sleep Medicine*, 11(6), 505–511.

*Ferracioli-Oda, E., Qawasmi, A., & Bloch, M. H. (2013). Meta-analysis: Melatonin for the treatment of primary sleep disorders. *PLoS One*, 8(5), E63773. doi: 10.137/journal.pone.0063773

*Fixen, D. R. (2019). 2019 AGS Beers Criteria for older adults. *Pharmacy Today*, 25(11), 42–54. doi: 10.1016/j.ptdy.2019.10.022

Freeman, A. A., & Rye, D. B. (2013). The molecular basis of restless legs syndrome. *Current Opinion in Neurobiology*, 23, 895–900.

Garcia-Borreguero, D., Paul Stillman, P., Benes, H., et al. (2011). Algorithms for the diagnosis and treatment of restless legs syndrome in primary care. *BMC Neurology*, 11, 28. Retrieved from http://www.biomedcentral.com/1471-2377/11/28 on June 8, 2015.

Gentili, A. (2014). Geriatric sleep disorder. *EMedicine Drugs & Disease*. Retrieved from http://emedicine.medscape.com/article/292498-overview on June 21, 2015.

*Geyer, J., & Bogan, R. (2017). Identification and treatment of augmentation in patients with restless legs syndrome: Practical recommendations. *Postgraduate Medicine*, 129(7), 667–675. https://doi.org/10.1080/00325481.2017.1360747

Gibson, M., & Shrader, J. (2018). Time use and labor productivity: The returns to sleep. *The Review of Economics and Statistics*, 100(5), 783–798. doi: 10.1162/rest_a_00746

Goodhines, P. A., Gellis, L. A., Kim, J., Fucito, L. M., & Park, A. (2017). Self-Medication for sleep in college students: Concurrent and prospective associations with sleep and alcohol behavior. *Behavioral Sleep Medicine*, 17(3), 327–341. doi: 10.1080/15402002.2017.1357119

Gulyani, S., Salas, R., & Gamaldo, C. (2012). Sleep medicine pharmacotherapeutics overview today, tomorrow, and the future (Part 1: Insomnia and circadian rhythm disorders). *Chest*, 142(6), 1659–1668. doi: 10.1378/chest.12-0465

*Hafner, M., Troxel, W. M., Stepanek, M., Taylor, J., & Van Stolk, C. (2017). Why sleep matters: The macroeconomic costs of insufficient sleep. *Sleep*, 40(suppl_1), A297. doi: 10.1093/sleepj/zsx050.802

Halloran, L. (2013). Can't sleep? Insomnia treatment. *Journal for Nurse Practitioners*, 9(1), 68–69. doi: 10.1016/j.nurpra.2012.11.007

Hara, C., Stewart, R., Lima-Costa, M. F., et al. (2011). Insomnia subtypes and their relationship to excessive daytime sleepiness in Brazilian community-dwelling older adults. *Sleep*, 34(8), 1111–1117.

Harleen, K., Spurling, B. C., & Pradeep, B. (2020). Chronic insomnia. *StatPearls*, 1. https://www.ncbi.nlm.nih.gov/books/NBK526136/#_NBK526136_pubdet_

Harwell, V., & Fasinu, P. (2020). Pitolisant and other histamine-3 receptor Antagonists—An update on therapeutic potentials and clinical prospects. *Medicines*, 7(9), 55. doi: 10.3390/medicines7090055

*He, Q., Chen, X., Wu, T., Li, L., & Fei, X. (2019). Risk of dementia in Long-Term benzodiazepine users: Evidence from a Meta-Analysis of observational studies. *Journal of Clinical Neurology*, 15(1), 9. https://doi.org/10.3988/jcn.2019.15.1.9

Herring, W. J., Ceesay, P., Snyder, E., et al. (2020). Polysomnographic assessment of suvorexant in patients with probable Alzheimer's disease dementia and insomnia: A randomized trial. *Alzheimer's & Dementia*, 16(3), 541–551. doi: 10.1002/alz.12035

Hirshkowitz, M., Dautovich, N., Hillygus, S., et al. (2014). 2014 Sleep Health Index. Retrieved from http://sleepfoundation.org/sleep-health-index on June 19, 2015.

Ibáñez, V., Silva, J., & Cauli, O. (2018). A survey on sleep assessment methods. *PeerJ*, 6, e4849. https://doi.org/10.7717/peerj.4849

*International Classification of Sleep Disorders (ICSD) (3rd ed.). (2014). *Darien, IL*: American Academy of Sleep Medicine.

Jacobs, L. G. (2019). For older adults, medications are common: An updated AGS Beers Criteria® aims to ensure they Are appropriate, too. *Journal of Gerontological Nursing*, 45(5), 47–48. doi: 10.3928/00989134-20190319-01

Jasvinder, C., Youngsook, P., & Erasmo, A. P. (2018, September 11). *What is the role of ramelteon (Rozerem) in the treatment of insomnia?* https://www.medscape.com/answers/1187829-70581/what-is-the-role-of-ramelteon-rozerem-in-the-treatment-of-insomnia

Jeffrey, S. (2014, May 30). FDA okays first device for restless legs syndrome. Retrieved from http://www.medscape.com/viewarticle/825971 on July 2, 2015.

John Hopkins Medicine. (2015). Center for restless leg syndrome. Retrieved from http://www.hopkinsmedicine.org/neurology_neurosurgery/centers_clinics/restless-legs-syndrome/ on July 11, 2015.

Johnson, D. A., Jackson, C. L., Williams, N., & Alcántara, C. (2019). Are sleep patterns influenced by race/ethnicity: A marker of relative advantage or disadvantage? Evidence to date. *Nature and Science of Sleep*, 11, 79–95. doi: 10.2147/nss.s169312

Joo, E. Y., Seo, D. W., Tae, W. S., et al. (2008). Effect of modafinil on cerebral blood flow in narcolepsy patients. *Sleep*, 31(6), 868–873.

Kalmbach, D., Cuamatzi-Castelan, A., Tonnu, C., et al. (2018). Hyperarousal and sleep reactivity in insomnia: Current insights. *Nature and Science of Sleep*, 10, 193–201. doi: 10.2147/nss.s138823

Kelso, C. (2014). Primary insomnia. *EMedicine Drugs & Disease*. Retrieved from http://emedicine.medscape.com/article/291573-overview on June 30, 2015.

*Kim, J., Lee, S. L., Kang, I., Song, Y. A., Ma, J., Hong, Y. S., Park, S., Moon, S. I., Kim, S., Jeong, S., & Kim, J. E. (2018). Natural products from single plants as sleep aids: A systematic review. *Journal of Medicinal Food*, 21(5), 433–444. https://doi.org/10.1089/jmf.2017.4064

Kitajima, T. (2019). New subtyping of insomnia disorder. *The Lancet Psychiatry*, 6(2), 86–88. https://doi.org/10.1016/s2215-0366(18)30513-3

Klingelhoefer, L., Cova, A., Gupta, B., et al. (2014). A review of current treatment strategies for restless legs syndrome (Willis–Ekbom disease). *Clinical Medicine*, 14(5), 520–524. Retrieved from www.clinmed.rcpjournal.org/content/14/5/520.full.pdf on July 8, 2015.

Krahn, L. E., Hershner, S., Loeding, L. D., et al. (2015). Quality measures for the care of patients with narcolepsy. *Journal of Clinical Sleep Medicine*, 11(03), 335–355. https://doi.org/10.5664/jcsm.4554

*Kornum, B. R., Knudsen, S., Ollila, H. M., Pizza, F., Jennum, P. J., Dauvilliers, Y., & Overeem, S. (2017). Narcolepsy. *Nature Reviews Disease Primers*, 3(1). https://doi.org/10.1038/nrdp.2016.100

Kume, A. (2014). Gabapentin enacarbil for the treatment of moderate to severe primary restless legs syndrome (Willis-Ekbom disease): 600 or 1,200 dose? *Neuropsychiatric Disease and Treatment*, 10, 249–262. doi: 10.2147/NDT.S30160

Lagmaoui, R., Begaud, B., Moore, N., et al. (2002). Benzodiazepine use and risk of dementia: A nested case–control study. *Journal of Clinical Epidemiology*, 55(3), 314–318. doi: 10.1016/s0895-4356(01)00453-x

*Lankford, D. A. (2011). Tasimelteon for insomnia. *Expert Opinion on Investigational Drugs*, *20*(7), 987–993. doi: 10.1517/13543784.2011.583235

*LaRosa, J. (2018, April 25). *Top 6 things to know about the $28 billion sleep market*. Market Research. https://blog.marketresearch.com/top-6-things-to-know-about-the-28-billion-sleep-market

Laudon, M., & Frydman-Marom, A. (2014). Therapeutic effects of melatonin receptor agonists on sleep and comorbid disorders. *International Journal of Molecular Sciences*, *15*(9), 15924–15950. doi: 10.3390/ijms150915924

*Lavie, P. (1997). Melatonin: Role in gating nocturnal rise in sleep propensity. *Journal of Biological Rhythms*, *12*, 657–668.

*Leschziner, G. (2014). Narcolepsy: A clinical review. *Practical Neurology*, *14*, 323–331. doi: 10.1136/practneurol-2014-000837

Levenson, J. C., Kay, D. B., & Buysse, D. J. (2015). The pathophysiology of insomnia. *Chest*, *147*(4), 1179–1192. doi: 10.1378/chest.14-1617

*Li, J., Vitiello, M. V., & Gooneratne, N. S. (2018). Sleep in normal aging. *Sleep Medicine Clinics*, *13*(1), 1–11. doi: 10.1016/j.jsmc.2017.09.001

Lubit, R. (2019, August 21). *Sleep-Wake disorders medication*. https://emedicine.medscape.com/article/287104-medication#3

Maheswaran, M., & Kushida, C. (2006). Restless legs syndrome in children. *Medscape General Medicine*, *8*(2), 79–79. Retrieved from http://www.ncbi.nlm.nih.gov/pmc/articles/PMC1785221/?report=printable on June 30, 2015.

*Manconi, M., Ferri, R., Miano, S., et al. (2017). Sleep architecture in insomniacs with severe benzodiazepine abuse. *Clinical Neurophysiology*, *128*(6), 875–881. doi: 10.1016/j.clinph.2017.03.009

Mazza, M., Losurdo, A., Testani, E., et al. (2014). Polysomnographic fidings in a cohort of chronic insomnia patients with benzodiazepines abuse. *European Psychiatry*, *29*(Suppl. 1), 1.

*McDonagh, M. S., Holmes, R., & Hsu, F. (2019). Pharmacologic treatments for sleep disorders in children: A systematic review. *Journal of Child Neurology*, *34*(5), 237–247. doi: 10.1177/0883073818821030

Michelson, D., Snyder, E., Paradis, E., et al. (2014). Safety and efficacy of suvorexant during 1-year treatment of insomnia with subsequent abrupt treatment discontinuation: A phase 3 randomised, double-blind, placebo-controlled trial. *Lancet Neurology*, *13*(5), 461–471. doi: 10.1016/S1474-4422(14)70053-3

Miller, M. A., Mehta, N., Clark-Bilodeau, C., & Bourjeily, G. (2020). Sleep pharmacotherapy for common sleep disorders in pregnancy and lactation. *Chest*, *157*(1), 184–197. doi: 10.1016/j.chest.2019.09.026

Morin, C., & Benca, R. (2012). Chronic insomnia. *Lancet*, *379*, 1129–1141. doi: 10.1016/S0140-6736(11)60750-2

Morrish, E., King, M., Smith, I., et al. (2004). Factors associated with a delay in the diagnosis of narcolepsy. *Sleep Medicine*, *5*, 37–41.

Narcolepsy. (2015). Medications for treating daytime sleepiness in narcolepsy. Retrieved from http://healthysleep.med.harvard.edu/narcolepsy on August 23, 2015.

*Natarajan, R. (2010). Review of periodic limb movement and restless leg syndrome. *Journal of Postgraduate Medicine*, *56*, 157–162. doi: 10.4103/0022-3859.65284

National Sleep Foundation. (2015). *Melatonin: The basic facts*. Available online at http://sleepfoundation.org/sleep-topics/melatonin-and-sleep

Neubauer, D. N., Pandi-Perumal, S. R., Spence, D. W., Buttoo, K., & Monti, J. M. (2018). Pharmacotherapy of insomnia. *Journal of Central Nervous System Disease*, *10*, 117957351877067. doi: 10.1177/1179573518770672

*Office of Disease Prevention and Health Promotion. (2020, August). *Healthy People 2030: Sleep*. https://health.gov/healthypeople/objectives-and-data/browse-objectives/sleep

Ogilvie, R. P., & Patel, S. R. (2017). The epidemiology of sleep and obesity. *Sleep Health*, *3*(5), 383–388. doi: 10.1016/j.sleh.2017.07.013

Pearson, N. J., Johnson, L. L., & Nahin, R. L. (2006). Insomnia, trouble sleeping, and complementary and alternative medicine: Analysis of the 2002 national health interview survey data. *Archives of Internal Medicine*, *166*(16), 1775–1782.

*Peeraully, T., & Tan, E.-K. (2012). Linking restless legs syndrome with Parkinson disease: Clinical, imaging, and genetic evidence. *Translational Neurodegeneration*, *1*(6). Retrieved from http://www.translationalneurodegeneration.com/content/1/1/6 on August 24, 2015.

Perusse, A., Turcotte, I., St-Jean, G., et al. (2013). Types of primary insomnia: Is hyperarousal also present during napping? *Journal of Clinical Sleep Medicine*, *9*(12), 1273–1280. doi: 10.5664/jcsm.3268

*Picchietti, D. L., Van Den Eeden, S. K., Inoue, Y., & Berger, K. (2017). Achievements, challenges, and future perspectives of epidemiologic research in restless legs syndrome (RLS). *Sleep Medicine, 31*, 3–9. https://doi.org/10.1016/j.sleep.2016.06.007

*Pillai, V., Cheng, P., Kalmbach, D. A., et al. (2016). Prevalence and predictors of prescription sleep aid use among individuals with DSM-5 insomnia: The role of hyperarousal. *Sleep*, *39*(4), 825–832. doi: 10.5665/sleep.5636

*PL-Detail Document. (2014). Comparison of insomnia treatments. *Pharmacist's Letter/Prescriber's Letter*.

*Qaseem, A., Kansagara, D., Forciea, M. A., Cooke, M., & Denberg, T. D. (2016). Management of chronic insomnia disorder in adults: A clinical practice guideline from the American college of physicians. *Annals of Internal Medicine*, *165*(2), 125. doi: 10.7326/m15-2175

Restless legs syndrome fact sheet | national institute of neurological disorders and stroke. (2020, March 17). Https://Www.Ninds.Nih.Gov/Disorders/Patient-Caregiver-Education/Fact-Sheets/Restless-Legs-Syndrome-Fact-Sheet. https://www.ninds.nih.gov/Disorders/Patient-Caregiver-Education/Fact-Sheets/Restless-Legs-Syndrome-Fact-Sheet

Reuben, C. (2019). QuickStats: Percentage* of adults aged ≥18 years who took medication to help fall or stay asleep four or more times in the past week,† by sex and age group—National health interview survey, United States, 2017–2018§. *MMWR. Morbidity and Mortality Weekly Report*, *68*(49), 1150. https://doi.org/10.15585/mmwr.mm6849a5

Richards, K., Shue, V., Beck, C., et al. (2010). Restless legs syndrome risk factors, behaviors, and diagnoses in persons with early to moderate dementia and sleep disturbance. *Behavioral Sleep Medicine*, *8*(1), 48–61. doi: 10.1080/15402000903425769

Romero, K., Goparaju, B., Russo, K., Westover, M. B., & Bianchi, M. (2017). Alternative remedies for insomnia: A proposed method for personalized therapeutic trials. *Nature and Science of Sleep*, *9*, 97–108. doi: 10.2147/nss.s128095

Rosekind, M. R. (2015). Awakening a nation: A call to action. *Sleep Health*, *1*(1), 9–10. doi: 10.1016/j.sleh.2014.12.005

Rosenberg, R., Murphy, P., Zammit, G., et al. (2019). Comparison of lemborexant with placebo and zolpidem tartrate extended release for the treatment of older adults with insomnia disorder. *JAMA Network Open*, *2*(12), e1918254. doi: 10.1001/jamanetworkopen.2019.18254

Ruoff, C., & Black, J. (2014, January). The psychiatric dimensions of narcolepsy. *Psychiatric Times*. Retrieved from http://www.psychiatrictimes.com/sleep-disorders/psychiatric-dimensions-narcolepsy/page/0/1 on August 26, 2015.

*Sakurai, T., Amemiya, A., Matsuzaki, I., et al. (1998). Orexins and orexin receptors: A family of hypothalamic neuropeptides and G protein-coupled receptors that regulate feeding behavior. *Cell*, *92*(4), 573–585. doi: 10.1016/S0092-8674(00)80949-6

*Sateia, M. J., Buysse, D. J., Krystal, A. D., Neubauer, D. N., & Heald, J. L. (2017). Clinical practice guideline for the pharmacologic treatment of chronic insomnia in adults: An American Academy of Sleep Medicine clinical practice guideline. *Journal of Clinical Sleep Medicine*, *13*(2), 307–349. doi: 10.5664/jcsm.6470

Schwartz, J., Feldman, N., Fry, J., et al. (2003). Efficacy of modafinil for improving daytime wakefulness in patients treated previously with psychostimulants. *Sleep Medicine*, *4*, 43–49.

Shahid, A., Chung, S., Phillipson, R., et al. (2012). An approach to long-term sedative-hypnotic use [Dove Press, open access]. *Journal of Nature and Science of Sleep*, *4*, 53–61.

*Shamseer, L., & Vohra, S. (2009). Complementary, holistic, and integrative medicine: Melatonin. *Pediatrics in Review*, *30*(6), 223–228. doi: 10.1542/pir.30-6-223

*Silber, M., Becker, P., Earley, C., et al. (2013). Willis-Ekbom disease foundation revised consensus statement on the management of restless legs

syndrome. *Mayo Clinic Proceedings*, 88(9), 977–986. doi: 10.1016/j.mayocp.2013.06.016

Stevens, M. S. (2013). Normal sleep, sleep physiology, and sleep deprivation. Retrieved from http://emedicine.medscape.com/article/1188226-overview#a3 on July 15, 2015.

*Taddei-Allen, P. (2020). Economic burden and managed care considerations for the treatment of insomnia. *The American Journal of Managed Care*, 26(Suppl 4), S91–S96. doi: 10.37765/ajmc.2020.43008

The National Sleep Foundation. (2014). *2014 Sleep Health Index*. Arlington, VA: Author.

Toro, B. (2014). New treatment options for the management of restless leg syndrome. *Journal of Neuroscience Nursing*, 46(4), 227–232. doi: 10.1097/JNN.0000000000000068

Treatment for restless legs syndrome: Research focus for clinicians. (2013). Minnesota Evidence-based Practice Center under Contract No. 290-2007-10064-I, Review No. 86. Retrieved from www.effectivehealthcare.ahrq.gov/restless-legs.cfm on July 7, 2015.

*Trenkwalder, C., Benes, H., Grote, L., et al. (2013). Prolonged release oxycodone-naloxone for treatment of severe restless legs syndrome after failure of previous treatment: A double-blind, randomised, placebo-controlled trial with an open-label extension. *Lancet Neurology*, 12(12), 1133.

Trevena, L. (2004). Practice corner: Sleepless in Sydney—Is valerian an effective alternative to benzodiazepines in the treatment of insomnia? *ACP Journal Club*, 141(1), 14.

Tsujinom, N., & Sakurai, T. (2009). Orexin/hypocretin: A neuropeptide at the interface of sleep, energy homeostasis, and reward system. *Pharmacological Reviews*, 61(2), 162–176. doi: 10.1124/pr.109.001321

*Vargas, I., Nguyen, A. M., Muench, A., et al. (2020). Acute and chronic insomnia: What has time and/or hyperarousal got to do with it? *Brain Sciences*, 10(2), 71. doi: 10.3390/brainsci10020071

Walters, A., Gabelia, D., & Frauscher, B. (2013). Restless legs syndrome (Willis–Ekbom disease) and growing pains: Are they the same thing? A side-by-side comparison of the diagnostic criteria for both and recommendations for future research. *Sleep Medicine*, 14, 1247–1252. doi: 10.1016/j.sleep.2013.07.013

Wang, X., Li, P., Pan, C., et al. (2019). The effect of Mind-Body therapies on insomnia: A systematic review and Meta-Analysis. *Evidence-Based Complementary and Alternative Medicine*, 2019, 1–17. doi: 10.1155/2019/9359807

Watson, N. F., Badr, M. S., Belenky, G., et al. (2015). Recommended amount of sleep for a healthy adult: A joint consensus statement of the American Academy of Sleep Medicine and Sleep research society. *SLEEP*, 1. https://doi.org/10.5665/sleep.4716

Williams, W. P. T., McLin, D. E., Dressman, M. A., & Neubauer, D. N. (2016). Comparative review of approved melatonin agonists for the treatment of circadian rhythm Sleep-Wake disorders. *Pharmacotherapy: The Journal of Human Pharmacology and Drug Therapy*, 36(9), 1028–1041. doi: 10.1002/phar.1822

Won, C., Mahmoudi, M., Qin, L., et al. (2014). The impact of gender on timeliness of narcolepsy diagnosis. *Journal of Clinical Sleep Medicine*, 10(1), 89–95. doi: 10.5664/jcsm.3370

Wong, E., & Nguyen, T. (2014). Zolpidem use in the elderly and recent safety data. *Journal for Nurse Practitioners*, 10(2), 140–141. doi: 10.1016/j.nurpra.2013.09.012

*Xie, Z., Chen, F., Li, W. A., Geng, X., Li, C., Meng, X., Feng, Y., Liu, W., & Yu, F. (2017). A review of sleep disorders and melatonin. *Neurological Research*, 39(6), 559–565. https://doi.org/10.1080/01616412.2017.1315864

Zee, P. C., Wang-Weigan, S., Wright, K. P., et al. (2011). Effects of ramelteon on insomnia symptoms induced by rapid, eastward travel. *Sleep Medicine*, 11, 525–533.

Zhdanova, I. V., Wurtman, R. J., Regan, M., et al. (2001). Melatonin treatment for age-related insomnia. *Journal of Clinical Endocrinology and Metabolism*, 86(10), 4727–4730.

42 Attention Deficit Hyperactivity Disorder

Kristen M. Audley

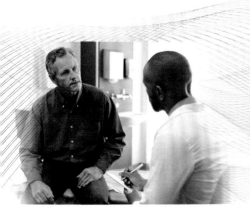 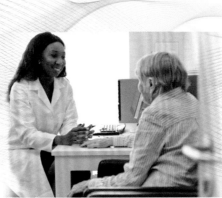 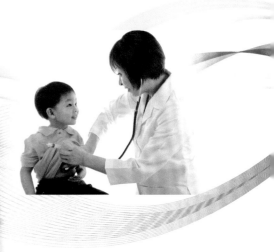

Learning Objectives

1. Understand the causes and pathophysiology of attention deficit hyperactivity disorder (ADHD).
2. Identify the diagnostic criteria used in pediatric, adolescent, and adult patients.
3. Recommend appropriate behavioral interventions and medication management for patients with ADHD.
4. Compare the various medication classes used to treat ADHD and describe their place in therapy.
5. Recommend patient-specific medication formulations (immediate vs. extended release), doses, titrations, and monitoring schedules for stimulants, atomoxetine, and alpha-adrenergic agonists.

INTRODUCTION

Attention deficit hyperactivity disorder (ADHD) is defined as a cluster of characteristics or behaviors that are related to several heterogeneous biopsychosocial behaviors and neurodevelopmental processes, which ultimately negatively influence one's social, occupational, or academic function (Feifel & MacDonald, 2008; Goodman et al., 2012). In children, the clinical presentation typically includes a combination of inattention, impulsivity, and/or hyperactivity. This population tends to endorse symptoms of difficulty concentrating, failure to follow through, forgetfulness, and distractibility, the hallmarks of the inattentive symptom's domain. Many patients also endorse symptoms related to the inability to remain seated, fidgetiness, excessive running or climbing in inappropriate situations, trouble awaiting turn, and propensity to interrupt,

the hallmarks of hyperactivity and impulsivity. The inherent heterogeneity of this disorder complicates the diagnosis and contributes to the lack of uniformly recognized criteria in all populations.

In adults, clinical presentation and functional impacts can vary greatly from their child and adolescent counterparts (Montano & Young, 2012). In addition to the heterogeneity with which ADHD presents, the core symptoms are arguably "normal" depending upon the age of the patient, environmental and social demands, and the extent to which they occur. It is when the symptoms occur more frequently than is considered normal and to an extent that causes functional impairment and are inconsistent with developmental level that a diagnosis of ADHD is made. For example, poor concentration in an academic setting could be considered normal in a child who is under the age of 5, particularly when the poor attention occurs sporadically. If an intervention from a parent or a teacher resolves this issue, then this would not be considered ADHD. If, however, a child of a similar age consistently does not pay attention and does so in the context of parental or teacher intervention and disciplinary action, then this may be considered maladaptive and inconsistent with developmental level.

ADHD is one of the most common neurodevelopmental disorders diagnosed in childhood and often lasts into adulthood. In 2016, the National Survey of Children's Health (NSCH) estimated that approximately 9.4% of children 2 to 17 years of age, or 6.1 million children in the United States, are diagnosed with ADHD (Danielson et al., 2017). The NSCH reported that boys are more than twice as likely as girls to be diagnosed with ADHD, and ADHD is thought to be under-recognized in girls and women. Among those with current ADHD, roughly two thirds were taking medication, and approximately half had received behavioral treatment of ADHD in the past year. Clinically meaningful symptoms persist into adulthood in up to 80% of patients, which suggests that ADHD is not exclusively a condition of childhood that resolves spontaneously but rather is a chronic illness.

CAUSES

A multitude of potential underlying causes of ADHD have been suggested, but none has yet to be fully validated. Secondary to the vast and diverse clinical manifestations, it is likely that the causes are multifactorial. Genetics play an important role in the etiology of ADHD and its comorbidity with other disorders (Faraone et al., 2019). Biologic parents and siblings of children with ADHD have a two to eight times greater chance of being diagnosed with ADHD due to its high heritability. Studies have shown that deoxyribonucleic acid variants in genes or regulatory regions increase the risk for ADHD. ADHD has been associated with the dopamine transporter gene (DAT1, SLC6A3) and the dopamine 4 (D4) receptor gene (DRD4) (Franke et al., 2012). Possible nongenetic causes are neurobiological, such as perinatal stress, low birth weight, traumatic brain injury, maternal smoking during pregnancy, and severe early deprivation. Other theories involve dietary intake of certain chemicals and sugars, but the evidence is inconsistent.

PATHOPHYSIOLOGY

The pathophysiology that underlies the clinical manifestations of ADHD involves reduced volume and function of the prefrontal cortex (PFC), caudate, and cerebellum. These brain regions are primarily responsible for regulating attention, behavior, emotion, distraction inhibition, and executive functioning. Reduced volume or impaired function may manifest as deficits in cognition, attention, motor planning, processing speed, and the complex behavioral complications that are consistent with ADHD. The communication among these areas is regulated by dopamine and norepinephrine and the complex interactions among their multiple receptor subtypes. Dopamine governs reward, motivation, attention, and emotion, and when the available concentrations of dopamine are appropriate, there is sustained focus and on-task behavior and cognition. Norepinephrine, at appropriate levels, improves executive functioning and increases inhibition of thoughts and behavior. Functionally, norepinephrine enhances relevant signals, while dopamine suppresses irrelevant signals. Therefore, a relative balance between the two is critical for optimal function.

Both a hypoactive and a hyperactive norepinephrine and dopamine theory have been proposed, but an integration of the two may be the most realistic theory. The concentrations of available dopamine and norepinephrine relative to one another and the functionality of their receptors influence the expression of ADHD symptoms. The PFC functions optimally under conditions of moderate catecholamine release. Overstimulation or under-stimulation of the PFC can result in impaired cognition. Acquired damage to the previously mentioned brain regions produces behavioral disinhibition, distractibility, impulsivity, organizational deficits, and loss of working memory.

The symptom clusters that tend to emerge in a patient with ADHD include behavioral, cognitive, social–emotional and deficits in executive function. The behavioral symptoms may include hyperactivity, impulsivity, disinhibition, novelty seeking, risk behaviors, and reward dependence. The cognitive features may include organizational issues, poor planning and execution skills, slower or impaired information processing, and deficits in time management. The social–emotional component may include emotional impulsivity, dysphoria, anger, anxiety, emotional lability, trouble reading social cues, and issues with making or keeping friends. Executive functioning refers to a wide range of central control processes that evolve during the process of aging and maturation. Executive function includes self-regulation, sequencing behaviors, planning and organization, working memory, and internalized speech.

Adult patients previously diagnosed and those with undiagnosed ADHD may develop and depend on compensatory mechanisms in order to overcome some of the functional impairments associated with this diagnosis (Santosh et al., 2011). Particularly, patients who are highly functioning professionals with higher-than-average intelligence quotients will tend to develop useful coping mechanisms to overcome symptoms or to hide them from others. Some patients become compulsive list makers or develop a highly structured daily routine in order to minimize forgetting details, completing tasks, or losing belongings. They may unknowingly rely on coworkers or family members to an inappropriate extent for purposes of reminders or assistance in completing tasks or fulfilling responsibilities. Though compensatory mechanisms are generally therapeutic for the patient, they may cloud the clinical picture, particularly in cases where the patient does not self-suspect ADHD but rather a family member or the practitioner suspects ADHD. In any case, the use of appropriate compensatory mechanisms should also be taken into consideration when determining if a drug therapy is indicated. Some patients can adequately manage their symptoms without clinically significant functional impact by relying on compensatory mechanisms and are able to avoid drug therapy.

As patients mature and roles and responsibilities evolve, the functional impairments and symptom presentation evolve in response, thereby presenting a barrier to fulfilling diagnostic criteria (Montano & Young, 2012). Adults are exposed to a variety of social and professional situations, which may provide an opportunity for previously unnoticed symptoms to manifest (Taylor et al., 2011). Inattentive symptoms may manifest as difficulty completing tasks, poor time management, difficulty sustaining attention in work-related activities, distractibility and forgetfulness, and poor concentration. Occupational performance and professional interpersonal relationships may suffer and may ultimately result in frequent job changes, unemployment, failure to live up to one's occupational potential, and lower salaries. Perhaps the most significant evolution of symptoms occurs in the hyperactivity–impulsivity domain. It is often assumed that these symptoms fade or resolve entirely in adults. However, in adults, these symptoms manifest as interrupting conversations, frequent job changes, irritability, quick to anger, relationship discord, dangerous driving habits, and a low frustration tolerance. Maturation results in a shift in this symptom cluster, and it evolves from behavioral to cognitive; patients will feel restless as opposed to running around and leaving their seat (Santosh et al., 2011). Symptoms of inattention may be present in 90% of adult patients.

DIAGNOSTIC CRITERIA

Health care providers use the American Psychiatric Association's *Diagnostic and Statistical Manual of Mental Health Disorders, Fifth Edition* (*DSM-5*) to diagnose ADHD (**Box 42.1**). To make a diagnosis of ADHD, *DSM-5* criteria must be met, including documentation of symptoms and impairment in the social, academic, or occupational setting. The *DSM-5* criteria assess for three kinds of presentations, including the predominantly inattentive presentation, the hyperactivity–impulsivity presentation, or the combined presentation (American Psychiatric Association, 2019). To diagnose ADHD in patients 17 years or older, only five symptoms are needed instead of the six needed for younger children. All iterations of the *DSM*

BOX 42.1 *Diagnostic and Statistical Manual of Mental Health Disorders, Fifth Edition, Criteria for Attention Deficit Hyperactivity Disorder*

A. A persistent pattern of inattention and/or hyperactivity–impulsivity that interferes with functioning or development, as characterized by (1) and/or (2):
1. **Inattention**: Six (6) or more of the following symptoms have persisted for at least 6 months to a degree that is inconsistent with developmental level and that negatively impacts directly on social and academic/occupational activities.
   Note: The symptoms are not solely a manifestation of oppositional behavior, defiance, hostility, or failure to understand tasks or instructions. For older adolescents and adults (age 17 and older), at least five symptoms are required.
   a. Often fails to give close attention to details or makes careless mistakes in schoolwork, work, or during other activities (e.g., overlooks or misses details, work is inaccurate)
   b. Often has difficulty sustaining attention in tasks or play activities (e.g., has difficulty remaining focused during lectures, conversations, or lengthy reading)
   c. Often does not seem to listen when spoken to directly (e.g., mind seems elsewhere, even in the absence of any obvious distraction)
   d. Often does not follow through on instructions and fails to finish schoolwork, chores, or duties in the workplace (e.g., starts tasks but quickly loses focus and is easily sidetracked)
   e. Often has difficulty organizing tasks and activities (e.g., difficulty managing sequential tasks; difficulty keeping materials and belongings in order; messy, disorganized work; has poor time management; fails to meet deadlines)

   f. Often avoids or is reluctant to engage in tasks that require sustained mental effort (e.g., schoolwork or homework; for older adolescents and adults, preparing reports, completing forms, reviewing lengthy papers)
   g. Often loses things necessary for tasks or activities (e.g., school materials, pencils, books, tools, wallets, keys, paperwork, eyeglasses, mobile telephones)
   h. Is often easily distracted by extraneous stimuli (e.g., for older adolescents and adults, may include unrelated thoughts)
   i. Is often forgetful in daily activities (e.g., doing chores, running errands; for older adolescents and adults, returning calls, paying bills, keeping appointments)
2. **Hyperactivity and impulsivity**: Six (or more) of the following symptoms have persisted for at least 6 months to a degree that is inconsistent with developmental level and that negatively impacts directly on social and academic/occupational activities.
   Note: The symptoms are not solely a manifestation of oppositional behavior, defiance, hostility, or failure to understand tasks or instructions. For older adolescents and adults (age 17 and older), at least five symptoms are required.
   a. Often fidgets with or taps hands or squirms in seat
   b. Often leaves seat in situations when remaining seated is expected (e.g., leaves his or her place in the classroom, in the office or other workplace, or in other situations that require remaining in place)

(Continued)

c. Often runs about or climbs in situations where it is inappropriate (e.g., in adolescents or adults, may be limited to feeling restless)

d. Often unable to play or engage in leisure activities quietly

e. Is often "on the go" acting as if "driven by a motor" (e.g., is unable to be or uncomfortable being still for extended time, as in restaurants, meetings; may be experienced by others as being restless or difficult to keep up with)

f. Often talks excessively

g. Often blurts out answers before questions have been completed (e.g., completes people's sentences; cannot wait for turn in conversation)

h. Often has difficulty awaiting turn (e.g., while waiting in line)

i. Often interrupts or intrudes on others (e.g., butts into conversations, games, or activities; may start using other people's things without asking or receiving permission; for adolescents and adults, may intrude into or take over what others are doing)

B. Several inattentive or hyperactive–impulsive symptoms were present prior to age 12 years.

C. Several inattentive or hyperactive–impulsive symptoms are present in two or more settings (e.g., at home, school, or work; with friends or relatives; in other activities).

D. There is clear evidence that the symptoms interfere with, or reduce the quality of, social, academic, or occupational functioning.

E. The symptoms do not occur exclusively during the course of schizophrenia or another psychotic disorder and are not better explained by another mental disorder (e.g., mood disorder, anxiety disorder, dissociative disorder, personality disorder, substance intoxication or withdrawal).

criteria have failed to be validated in the adult population, and therefore up until the release of the *DSM-5* in May of 2013, there was very little consideration for the assessment of adult patients. The *DSM-5* has adapted the previous set of diagnostic criteria such that they are more accurately applied to adults and adult symptom presentation. The verbiage related to the criteria and the descriptors thereof have been changed to reflect more adult-specific situations, though the use of these criteria in adults has been widely criticized. Even considering the newest iteration of the criteria, practitioners are still in a position of having to make a retrospective evaluation of the presence of ADHD in childhood in order to establish a diagnosis in adulthood. This was cited as one of the most problematic components of the criteria as many patients either could not recall the childhood symptoms or could not produce documentation that would substantiate a childhood diagnosis. As ADHD is considered a developmental disorder, the presence of current symptoms as well as a history of previous symptoms (in childhood) needs to be established. Patients with ADHD, by nature of the illness, have impaired short- and long-term memory capabilities, and therefore recall bias may impact the accuracy of assessments (Taylor et al., 2011). The practitioner is also faced with the challenge of determining if this was an established childhood diagnosis, a missed diagnosis in childhood, or a late-onset adult ADHD.

A specialist psychiatrist, pediatrician, or another qualified health care professional should only make a diagnosis of ADHD. This evaluation may include standardized behavioral rating scales or observational data, although each has inherent limitations and should not be considered diagnostic alone. The Adult Self-Report Scale (ASRS) is an 18-item screening tool that is based on the *DSM-IV* criteria. The ASRS has patients rate the items based on the frequency and degree to which they occur. The Conners' Self-Report Scale is a multidimensional assessment scale that both the patient and an observer complete. The long version of this scale is a 66-item tool that assesses symptoms consistent with inattention and memory deficits, impulsivity and emotional lability, hyperactivity and restlessness, and problems with self-conceptualization. Having multiple perspectives is ideal in that the observer may contribute critical data that the patient may either be unaware of or not be willing to disclose. It is also essential for the clinician to interview one or more sources who know the person well.

Another challenge in the evaluation of patients is the degree of *symptom overlap* between ADHD and several other psychiatric diagnoses, namely, mood and anxiety disorders. Patients tend to associate poor concentration with ADHD alone and typically would not consider that an untreated or undiagnosed anxiety disorder can produce similar levels of concentration impairment. It is recommended that practitioners include an assessment for mood and anxiety disorders in their initial evaluations of these patients in order to rule out the presence of an additional psychiatric disorder.

In addition to symptom overlap with other psychiatric illnesses, ADHD is frequently *comorbid* with other psychiatric conditions. Research has shown that more than two thirds of people with ADHD have one or more coexisting conditions.

A determination of whether ADHD is present alone or whether it is present in addition to another psychiatric diagnosis is critical, as mood or anxiety disorders may be the sole diagnosis, which is producing ADHD-like symptoms. Patients with ADHD tend to have high rates of comorbidity with anxiety, depression, learning disabilities, and substance abuse disorders with prevalence rates that are more than double those observed in patients without ADHD. Recent research has established that girls with ADHD are more likely than boys to have a comorbid internalizing condition like anxiety or depression. Substance use disorders (SUDs) are more common in patients with ADHD, and the clinical course of ADHD tends to be more challenging in this patient population. The Society for Developmental and Behavioral Pediatrics is developing guidelines for the diagnosis and treatment of "complex ADHD," including ADHD with comorbid developmental and/or mental health conditions.

INITIATING DRUG THERAPY

Current guidelines and practice advocate for a multimodal treatment plan, which accounts for variations in response. The Multimodal Treatment Study reported that children receiving intensive behavioral management combined with medication fared better than those receiving intensive behavioral management alone (Arnold et al., 1997). The core symptom clusters of ADHD (inattention, hyperactivity, and impulsivity) respond to medication, with or without the behavioral intervention. Behavioral symptoms seem to respond to environmental modification, while skills in sports, academics, and social situations may not respond to medication or behavior modification. Relationship problems usually can be treated through psychotherapy.

Nonpharmacologic aspects of a multimodal treatment plan consist of behavior modification, parent training, family therapy, social skills training, academic skills training, individual psychotherapy, cognitive behavior modification, and therapeutic recreation. These are discussed further in the section titled Nutrition/Lifestyle Changes later in this chapter.

The American Association of Pediatrics (AAP) has an established guideline for the treatment of ADHD, most recently published in 2019 (Wolraich et al., 2019). There is no domestic guideline that governs the treatment of ADHD in adults currently; however, the National Institute for Health and Clinical Excellence (NICE) guideline from the British Psychological Society and the Royal College of Psychiatrists (2018) does include adult guidance (NCCMH, 2018). The NICE guideline for adults parallels the AAP guideline for children, and clinical practice for adult patients in the United States generally aligns with the pediatric/adolescent guidelines and the European guidelines. The AAP guidelines (children 4–18 years old) recommend initiating behavioral therapy in children 4 to 5 years old and only initiating medication, that is, methylphenidate, if the symptoms are severe. In children older than 5 years (and up to 18 years), the initiation of a stimulant medication ± behavioral interventions is considered

first-line therapy. Preference is not given to one stimulant over another except in the case of children less than 6 years of age, in which methylphenidate is recommended (due to increased availability of evidence in this age group). Second-line therapy includes nonstimulant medications with preference given to atomoxetine, then guanfacine, and then clonidine.

The NICE guidelines include recommendations for pediatric patients, adolescents, and adults. Only in cases of significant impairment in at least one domain should drug therapy be initiated in children or adolescent patients per the NICE guidelines. The guidelines recommend obtaining two specialist opinions before initiating therapy in children less than 5 years of age. Methylphenidate is recommended as initial therapy over the other available stimulants in patients over 5 years of age. Amphetamine salts are considered second-line therapies in situations where children or adolescents do not respond to or are intolerant of methylphenidate. Atomoxetine or guanfacine is considered a third-line agent. In adults, drug therapy with amphetamine salts or methylphenidate is considered first line after environmental modifications. Therapy (drug and/or nondrug) should continue for as long as it remains clinically effective.

In practice, practitioners tend to initiate intermediate- to long-acting stimulant medications in children, adolescents, and adults. Medication products that have an extended duration of action tend to have a positive influence on tolerability, provide convenience, and improve compliance. It is also reasonable to start therapy with a short-acting medication product to establish an effective dose and then transition to a longer-acting version of the same drug, if available. The 2018 NICE guidelines recommend using immediate- and modified-release preparations of stimulants to optimize the duration and effectiveness. The prescriber determines which product to initiate based upon experience, patient preference, and other patient-specific factors. A comprehensive list of the currently available, U.S. Food and Drug Administration (FDA)–approved medications for ADHD is available at www.ADHDMedicationGuide.com.

Goals of Drug Therapy

Upon initiation of drug therapy with or without nondrug therapy, the expectation is that the core symptoms of ADHD will abate and the patient will no longer experience functional deficits in social, occupational, or academic domains. This result tends to emerge relatively quickly, particularly after the initiation of medication therapy. It is not uncommon to realize this therapeutic success after the first attempt at drug therapy, and it is also not uncommon to utilize several pharmacotherapeutic modalities before the patient is adequately controlled (**Table 42.1**). There is a careful balance between resolving the core symptoms of ADHD and minimizing the risk of transient or serious adverse effects.

Stimulant Medications

Psychostimulants remain the drug class of choice in treating adults and children with ADHD. Most product formulations

TABLE 42.1

Recommended Order of Treatment for Attention Deficit Hyperactivity Disorder (All Ages)

Order	Agents	Comments
First line	Stimulants	Methylphenidate (Ritalin) or amphetamine works quickly with first dose, is available in extended release formulation, and is easy to titrate. If treatment with one member of the class is unsuccessful, attempt subsequent drugs from this class before initiating second-line therapy.
Second line	Nonstimulants	Atomoxetine (Strattera) should be the next drug utilized in patients who have failed stimulants; this is also appropriate for patients who have contraindications to stimulants. Guanfacine or clonidine has less impressive efficacy but can be added on to existing stimulant or atomoxetine therapy if monotherapy is insufficient. (This could also occur in third-line treatment.)
Third line	Bupropion (Wellbutrin)	Takes a few weeks to have a therapeutic effect. May worsen anxiety and lower seizure threshold.

TABLE 42.2

Neurotransmitters Affected by Pharmacotherapy

	NE	DA	Comments
Methylphenidate	↑	↑	Blocks reuptake
Amphetamine	↑↑	↑	Blocks reuptake
			Causes release of NE
Atomoxetine	↑		Blocks reuptake of NE
Clonidine			Stimulates alpha₂ adrenoceptors
Guanfacine			Stimulates alpha₂ adrenoceptors
Bupropion	↑	↑	Weak blocker of NE, DA reuptake

DA, dopamine; NE, norepinephrine

available are derived from one of two parent molecules: methylphenidate or amphetamine (see **Tables 42.2** and **42.3**). The subtype of ADHD does not appear to be a predictor of response to a specific agent, with about 40% of patients responding to both methylphenidate and amphetamine and 40% of patients responding to only one.

Mechanism of Action

Pharmacologically, the stimulants inhibit the reuptake of dopamine and norepinephrine, thereby increasing concentrations in the presynaptic cleft (Hodgkins et al., 2012). Amphetamines also directly stimulate the release of dopamine and norepinephrine. There are various products currently available in the U.S. market, some of which are immediate-release formulations and some of which are extended-release variations.

Stimulant medications mitigate the traditional ADHD symptoms and have demonstrated utility in improving interpersonal relationships, self-esteem, cognition, and symptoms of comorbid anxiety disorders (Minzenberg, 2012). Prescribing stimulant medications to adults has been a clinical controversy in primary care as well as in psychiatry. This class is arguably the most efficacious in resolving symptoms of ADHD and comorbid psychopathology; however, the risk of adverse effects and abuse potential may impact the rates at which these drugs are prescribed in the adult population.

Though none of the medications within the stimulant class have demonstrated superiority over another member of the class, there are some within-class pharmacokinetic differences that may impact product selection. The immediate-release products generally have a faster onset of action and a more abrupt cessation of effect (both of which can also be observed by the patient). This may be advantageous for patients who only have a discrete period during which they require medication action (e.g., during the school day). It can also be problematic for patients who cannot tolerate the abrupt start and stop of drug action.

The intermediate- and long-acting products have a less pronounced (and therefore less abrupt) onset and offset of therapeutic effect. Extended-release products are formulated to release defined amounts of drug over a 24-hour period. Ritalin LA = (methylphenidate long-acting) releases 50% of the dose in two bursts, whereas Concerta releases 22% immediately and 78% later and Metadate CD releases 30% immediately and 70% later. In addition to their more innocuous presentation, the extended-release products also afford patients a convenience factor, with patients only having to dose once or twice daily (as compared to multiple daily doses with some immediate-acting products). Lisdexamfetamine (Vyvanse) has a 10- to 12-hour duration of action, which necessitates once-daily dosing. In addition to the convenience factor, this drug product is formulated as a prodrug that requires enzymatic degradation in the gastrointestinal (GI) tract to become active. As a result, Vyvanse is far more difficult to abuse or misuse.

The risk of abuse or misuse of stimulants is a legitimate concern, which may ultimately impact treatment. SUDs occur comorbidly with ADHD at an odds ratio of 1.5 to 7.9 (Simon et al., 2015). Utilization of extended-release products minimizes—but does not completely negate—the risk of abuse.

Dosage

It is generally recommended that drug therapy, particularly in adults, consist of an extended-release product in order to maximize compliance and minimize the risk of abuse. In children, many practitioners may decide to begin with a short-acting product in order to gauge response and tolerability and then switch to

TABLE 42.3

Overview of Agents Used to Treat Attention Deficit Hyperactivity Disorder

Generic (Trade) Name and Dosage	Selected Adverse Events	Contraindications	Special Considerations
Atomoxetine (Strattera) Children and adolescents <70 kg: 0.5 mg/kg/d for 3 days, then 1.2 mg/kg/d Patients >70 kg: 40 mg/d; then 80 mg/d after 3 days	Increased heart rate and blood pressure, abdominal pain, decreased appetite, nausea, sedation Urinary retention in adults	Patients on MAO inhibitors, patients with narrow-angle	Atomoxetine does not appear to promote the development of new tics and therefore may be a good choice for patients unable to take stimulant medications due to preexisting tics.
Bupropion (Wellbutrin) Children and adolescents >6 years: 3 mg/kg/d in 2–3 divided doses (maximum 150 mg/d) Adults: 12-hour extended-release: 100 mg QAM; increase in 100 mg/d increments q3–4wk (maximum 200 mg BID) 24-hour extended-release: 150 mg QAM for 1 week, then 300 mg daily for 3 weeks (maximum 450 mg daily)	Insomnia, anorexia, dizziness, anxiety, confusion, xerostomia, constipation, nausea, agitation, fever, headache, vomiting, seizures	Seizure disorders, bulimia, anorexia nervosa Within 14 d of MAO inhibitors	Monitor weight
Clonidine (Catapres) Children: <45 kg: 0.05 mg HS, then titrate in 0.05-mg increments BID >45 kg: 0.1 mg HS, then titrate in 0.1-mg increments BID to QID Range: 27–40.5 kg: 0.05–0.2 mg; 40.5–45 kg: 0.05–0.3 mg; >45 kg: 0.05–0.4 mg Adults: 0.1 mg BID; maximum 2.4 mg	Dizziness, drowsiness, anxiety, confusion, xerostomia, constipation, impotence, nausea, hypotension	Hypersensitivity to clonidine	Monitor blood pressure (standing and supine), respiratory rate and depth, and heart rate.
Long acting: Dexmethylphenidate (Focalin XR 5-, 10-, 15-, 20-, 30-, 40-mg capsule) 10 mg/d; maximum 40 mg/d Dextroamphetamine (Dexedrine Spansule 5-, 10-, 15-mg capsule) 5 mg/d, titrate 5 mg/d weekly; maximum 40 mg/d Dextroamphetamine/amphetamine (Adderall XR 5-, 10-, 15-, 20-, 25-, 30-mg capsule) 10 mg/d; maximum 60 mg/d Lisdexamfetamine (Vyvanse 20-, 30-, 40-, 50-, 60-, 70-mg capsule) 30 mg daily; maximum 70 mg/d Methylphenidate; maximum 60 mg/d: Concerta (18-, 27-, 36-, 54-mg capsule) 18 mg/d; titrate 18 mg/d weekly Daytrana (10, 15, 20, 30 mg/9 h patch) 10 mg patch Metadate CD (10-, 20-, 30-, 40-, 50-, 60-mg capsule) 20 mg QAM Ritalin LA (10-, 20-, 30-, 40-mg capsule) 20 mg QAM	Nervousness, insomnia, arrhythmias, dry mouth, anorexia	Cardiovascular disease, hypertension, arteriosclerosis, hyperthyroidism, glaucoma, alcohol or drug abuse	Monitor growth and CNS activity; high abuse potential; not recommended for children <3 y; avoid late evening dosing.

(Continued)

TABLE 42.3

Overview of Agents Used to Treat Attention Deficit Hyperactivity Disorder (*Continued*)

Generic (Trade) Name and Dosage	Selected Adverse Events	Contraindications	Special Considerations
Short acting: Dexmethylphenidate (Focalin 2.5, 5, 10 mg) 2.5 mg BID; maximum 20 mg/d Dextroamphetamine (Dexedrine 5-, 10-, 15-mg capsule) 5 mg/d, titrate 5 mg/d weekly; maximum 40 mg/d Dextroamphetamine/amphetamine (Adderall 5-, 7.5-, 10-, 12.5-, 15-, 20-, 30-mg tablet) 5 mg daily to BID; maximum 40 mg/d Methylphenidate; >6 y: 5 mg BID (before breakfast and lunch), titrate 5–10 mg/d weekly; maximum 60 mg/d 　　Methylphenidate (5-, 10-mg tablet) 　　Methylin (5-, 10-, 20-mg tablet) 　　Ritalin (5-, 10-, 30-mg tablet)	Tachycardia, nervousness, insomnia, anorexia, dizziness, drowsiness	Marked anxiety, tension, or agitation Glaucoma History of tics or Tourette syndrome in patient or family	Monitor blood pressure, weight, height, heart rate, tics, sleep habits; may potentiate effects of anticoagulants and anticonvulsants; abuse potential; not recommended for children <6 y.
Intermediate acting: Methylphenidate; maximum 60 mg/d 　　Methylphenidate CR (10-, 20-mg tablet) 10 mg QAM 　　Metadate ER (20-mg tablet) 10 mg QAM 　　Methylin ER (10-, 20-mg capsule) 10 mg QAM 　　Ritalin SR (20-mg tablet) 20–60 mg q8h	Same as those for short acting	Same as those for short acting	Same as those for short acting

CBC, comprehensive metabolic panel; CNS, central nervous system; CR, controlled release; ER, extended release; MAO, monoamine oxidase.

a longer-acting product. Initiation of drug therapy, irrespective of the nature of the release of the product, begins at the lowest dose (or the labeled starting dose) and is gradually titrated upward until the benefit is maximized and the patient is without adverse effects.

Time Frame for Response

Most patients taking a therapeutic dose of any stimulant medication will experience an effect on the day of the first dose and certainly within the first few days. If there is no appreciable improvement, then the dose should be increased, if it was well tolerated. As the recommended or maximum dose of the selected drug is approached and there is still an absence of effect, then either (1) the medication should be changed or (2) the diagnosis of ADHD should be reevaluated.

Contraindications

The stimulants are contraindicated in children with certain comorbid disorders. Practitioners should not prescribe methylphenidate to patients with marked anxiety, tension, or agitation; glaucoma; or a history of tics or Tourette syndrome. Stimulants are contraindicated in patients who have existing cardiovascular disease, moderate to severe hypertension, hyperthyroidism, or history of substance abuse. In practice, the presence of a history of substance abuse may be overlooked if the risk of recurrence is determined to be low and the benefit of treatment is determined to be reasonably high.

Adverse Events

The most common adverse events related to stimulant therapy tend to be cardiovascular, GI, or neurologic in nature. Common, transient adverse effects include sleep disturbance, appetite suppression and associated weight loss, agitation, and nervousness. These are typically minimized by taking the drugs with food and using an extended-release formulation. Serious concerns exist related to the potential cardiotoxicity associated with the stimulants. Patients may experience palpitations, tachycardia, and elevations in blood pressure. Critical cardiovascular adverse effects include rhythm disturbances and cardiomyopathy, which precludes use in patients who have an existing cardiovascular abnormality.

Generally, the cardiovascular adverse effects include palpitations, tachycardia, elevated blood pressure, and potentially but uncommonly arrhythmias. Changes in appetite, nausea, vomiting, and other GI disturbances may occur, particularly at the onset of therapy or upon a dosage increase. The neurologic adverse events range from headache and insomnia to seizure activity, particularly in patients predisposed to seizures.

In general, adverse events are manageable, results are quick and predictable with the first dose, and the medications are easy to titrate. The adverse effects of the stimulants, such as headaches, dizziness, appetite suppression, tics, dyskinesias, sleep disturbances, abuse potential, and in particular growth retardation (below height or weight on normal growth charts), may be of concern. Diminished growth may be more common among children on higher and more consistently administered doses of stimulants (Wolraich et al., 2019). Determining the long-term effect of stimulants on children and adults is challenging. To minimize these effects, it is reasonable for the patient to take drug-free periods, usually over the summer. These periods also allow for reassessment of ADHD. Because children frequently seem to show symptoms in structured settings such as school, weekend "drug holidays" are also reasonable, permitting dosage adjustments and disease assessment. Rebound hyperactivity may be more prominent.

Nonstimulant Medications

Owing to their less impressive efficacy rates as compared to those of the stimulants, the nonstimulant medications tend to be prescribed less frequently among all age groups. Generally, practitioners do not initiate drug therapy with a nonstimulant unless the patient has a contraindication to stimulants (cardiac abnormalities, previous or current substance abuse) or is intolerant to or has failed the stimulant class. Currently, the nonstimulant therapeutic class includes atomoxetine (Strattera), immediate- and extended-release guanfacine (Tenex and Intuniv, respectively), clonidine and extended-release clonidine (Catapres and Kapvay, respectively), bupropion (Wellbutrin), and the tricyclic antidepressants.

Atomoxetine

Atomoxetine (Strattera) is the first nonstimulant approved by the FDA for treating ADHD. It is not a controlled substance, and existing data suggest no real potential for abuse or diversion. While stimulants have greater treatment effect than atomoxetine, there are fewer adverse effects on appetite and sleep when compared to stimulants. However, there is more nausea and sedation, and it may be considered first-line therapy for ADHD treatment if the patient has an active substance abuse problem, comorbid anxiety, tics, or severe side effects to stimulants.

Atomoxetine's efficacy and safety have been demonstrated in adults and children; however, its associated rates of response are less impressive than those of the stimulants. In most clinical trails and meta analyses, atomoxetine has improved the core symptoms of ADHD; however, the clinical relevance of the improvements is debatable. It remains an appropriate option in patients who have contraindications to stimulants or who have a comorbid anxiety disorder, as anecdotal evidence suggests some level of anxiolytic activity.

Mechanism of Action

Atomoxetine selectively inhibits the reuptake of norepinephrine by inhibiting the presynaptic norepinephrine transporter. This translates into improved function in the PFC.

Dosage

The medication is available in 10-, 18-, 25-, 40-, 60-, 80-, and 100-mg capsules. For adolescents and adults over 70 kg, the starting dose is 40 mg; the dose is increased to an 80-mg target dose after a minimum of 3 days. The maximum recommended dose is 1.4 mg/kg/d for children and 100 mg for adolescents and adults; dosages should be adjusted only after 2 to 4 weeks of treatment at the lower dose. Since this agent undergoes significant metabolism via the CYP2D6 system, in slow metabolizers or patients taking agents with strong CYP2D6 effects (e.g., paroxetine, fluoxetine), the starting dose should be maintained for up to 4 weeks before dose adjustments are made. Patients with significant hepatic impairment should be started on a dose 50% of the usual starting dose. There are no renal dose adjustments for this medication.

Time Frame for Response

Atomoxetine is rapidly absorbed from the GI tract, leading to 63% bioavailability in extensive metabolizers and 94% bioavailability in poor metabolizers. The onset of action is quick, and dose adjustments are made in the first week. Despite the short half-life in extensive metabolizers, the duration of activity remains consistent throughout the day.

Contraindications

Atomoxetine should not be taken with monoamine oxidase (MAO) inhibitors because it increases synaptic norepinephrine concentrations. Further, due to the risk of angle closure, this agent should not be administered to patients with narrow-angle glaucoma.

Adverse Events

The increase in norepinephrine leads to an increase in blood pressure and heart rate; therefore, atomoxetine should be used cautiously in hypertensive patients or those with underlying cardiovascular disorders. Atomoxetine, like stimulants, should not be administered to patients with uncontrolled hypertension, structural cardiac abnormalities, cardiomyopathy, and abnormalities of the heart rhythm. In adults, there was a 3% rate of urinary retention or hesitation (STRATTERA®, n.d.). Patients may experience initial somnolence and GI tract symptoms, particularly if the dosage is increased too rapidly, and decreased appetite. Other common adverse effects include abdominal pain, vomiting, decreases in appetite, headache, irritability, and dermatitis. Atomoxetine does not appear to promote the development of new tics and therefore may be a good choice for patients who cannot take stimulant medications due to preexisting tics. Boxed warnings regarding rare hepatotoxicity and suicidal ideation in children and adolescents were issued by the FDA in 2005.

Interactions

Atomoxetine is a substrate of the CYP2D6 isoenzyme, and levels of this drug can be increased when CYP2D6 inhibitors are administered.

Alpha Agonists: Guanfacine and Clonidine

The alpha agonists, a decades-old drug class, are traditionally used for the treatment of hypertension. For many years, they have been used off label, particularly in children, for the adjunctive management of ADHD. Their purpose is largely limited to the treatment of behavioral manifestations, aggression, insomnia, and tics and not for the core inattentive symptoms of ADHD. Both guanfacine and clonidine now are available in extended-release dosage forms, which are approved for the treatment of ADHD (Intuniv and Kapvay, respectively). Drugs in this therapeutic class are considered inferior to the stimulants with regard to efficacy and tolerability.

Mechanism of Action

Both guanfacine and clonidine act as postsynaptic alpha$_2$ agonists, which are proposed to regulate subcortical activity in the PFC, the area of the brain responsible for emotions, attention, and behaviors. In some patients, this translates into reduced hyperactivity, impulsivity, and distractibility. Guanfacine demonstrates greater selectivity for the postsynaptic alpha$_2$ receptor, which may confer improved efficacy and tolerability as compared to clonidine. Guanfacine also has a longer half-life, which is associated with less sedation and dizziness as compared to clonidine.

Dosage

Clonidine is dosed at 0.1 mg at bedtime, with a 0.1-mg increase every 7 days until a therapeutic effect is realized (maximum of 0.4 mg daily; ideally, dosed twice daily). Guanfacine is dosed at 1 mg daily with a weekly increase of 1 mg until clinical response is achieved (7 mg maximum daily dose). Dose adjustment for guanfacine may be necessary when administered concomitantly with strong CYP3A4 inhibitors or inducers.

Time Frame for Response

Generally, any therapeutic effects would be realized after approximately 4 weeks of treatment but possibly after several months.

Contraindications

There are no absolute contraindications aside from hypersensitivity to the drug or any other component in the product.

Adverse Events

The adverse effects are generally mild and include fatigue, drowsiness, bradycardia, constipation, dizziness, hypotension, and headache. A gradual upward titration may minimize the emergence of these effects. It is also recommended that a downward taper be employed when discontinuing these medications, as abrupt discontinuation may potentiate a rebound hypertension. For the aforementioned reasons, it is important to educate the patient and/or caregiver about the importance of adherence.

Interactions

Given the central nervous system (CNS) depressant action of clonidine and guanfacine, other concomitant CNS depressants should be avoided.

Bupropion

Bupropion (Wellbutrin) has been evaluated in a small number of studies involving children, adolescents, and adults, in which its efficacy compared to placebo or to an active stimulant comparator has been established. This is not an approved indication for bupropion in any age group, and it is not recommended in the NICE or AAP guidelines discussed previously. Bupropion may be a therapeutic alternative in adults who have contraindications or are intolerant to stimulant medications or in patients who have a comorbid depressive illness.

Mechanism of Action

Bupropion is an aminoketone antidepressant, which is commonly used for the treatment of depressive disorders as well as smoking cessation. It inhibits the reuptake of norepinephrine and dopamine (like the stimulants) but does so less intensely via a mechanism that is not fully understood. Bupropion is not associated with dependence, abuse, or misuse, which provides a therapeutic advantage in patients who have substance abuse issues.

Dosage

An appropriate dose for the treatment of ADHD has not been established, as the treatment of ADHD is an off-label use. In practice, the antidepressant dose (150–450 mg daily) is generally used, though rarely titrated upward to the maximum dose. Bupropion is available as an immediate-release tablet, sustained-release tablet (SR), and extended-release tablet (XL). The XL tablets are dosed once daily, and the SR and immediate-release tablets are both dosed twice daily.

Time Frame for Response

The onset of response is not well documented, but it is considered to be more rapid than the alpha$_2$ agonists (weeks to months) but less rapid than stimulants (same day or a few days).

Contraindications

Bupropion may lower the seizure threshold in predisposed individuals. Therefore, patients with a known seizure disorder or patients taking a medication that has additive effects on the seizure threshold (benzodiazepines, alcohol) should avoid bupropion. This would also include patients who are abruptly discontinuing alcohol or other drugs. Bupropion's labeling includes a boxed warning regarding the risk of suicidal thinking or behavior that is associated with the antidepressant drugs. Bupropion is also contraindicated with the use of MAO inhibitors within the past 14 days.

Adverse Effects

Common adverse effects include dry mouth, nausea, insomnia, dizziness, anxiety, dyspepsia, sinusitis, and tremor. Bupropion may increase the risk of seizures, particularly with higher doses and shorter-acting formulations. Consideration should be given to patients who have a comorbid anxiety disorder, as bupropion has the potential to worsen anxiety.

Interactions

Bupropion is a major substrate and strong inhibitor of CYP2D6, and therefore concurrent use of strong CYP2D6 substrates, inhibitors, or inducers is discouraged. Secondary to its impacts on metabolism, bupropion should not be used concomitantly with vortioxetine or the tricyclic antidepressants.

SELECTING THE MOST APPROPRIATE DRUG

Because of the number of therapeutic options available, this section suggests only a general outline to follow. Nonpharmacologic therapy differs for children and adults and may not always be included in the treatment plan (see **Table 42.1**). **Figure 42.1** outlines the therapeutic treatment algorithm for patients with ADHD.

Medication therapy is indicated in all patients who fulfill the diagnostic criteria and do not have contraindications to the selected medications.

First-Line Therapy

Stimulant medications are considered first-line therapy in children, adolescents, and adults without contraindications. There is no preference given to methylphenidate-type versus amphetamine-type stimulants, though methylphenidate appears to be favored in young children. There is no established difference in efficacy or tolerability among the

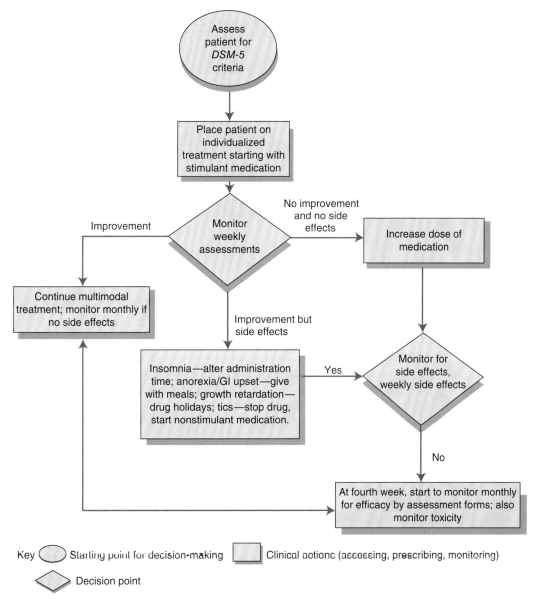

FIGURE 42–1   Treatment algorithm for attention deficit hyperactivity disorder.

DSM-5, Diagnostic and Statistical Manual of Mental Health Disorder, Fifth Edition; GI, gastrointestinal.

members of this class. Product selection tends to be driven by duration of action and individual patient response (efficacy and tolerability). The longer-acting products confer improved convenience, owing to their less complex dosing regimens and possible improved compliance. Lisdexamfetamine (Vyvanse) boasts the longest duration of action and the least abuse potential secondary to its prodrug status, which requires enzymatic activation in the GI tract.

Failure of, or intolerance to, one stimulant does not necessarily mean that the entire therapeutic class is exhausted. In the event that a patient does not realize improvement or is unable to tolerate the initial drug, a different stimulant should be initiated (either from within the subclass of amphetamine-type or methylphenidate-type or from the other subclass).

Second-Line Therapy

Upon clinical failure or intolerance of the stimulants as a therapeutic class, atomoxetine is generally considered second-line therapy. Some practitioners may elect to initiate an alpha$_2$ agonist at this time; however, guidelines generally recommend atomoxetine first.

Third-Line Therapy

Bupropion or the alpha$_2$ agonists may be attempted after failure of, or intolerance to, the stimulants and atomoxetine. At this point, these drugs may also be considered as adjunctive therapy to a partially successfully stimulant or atomoxetine. In the past, the tricyclic antidepressants were also considered third- or fourth-line therapy, but they are generally no longer used for this purpose.

After the failure of several drugs (even if only the stimulants have been attempted), the diagnosis of ADHD should be reevaluated. The response rates for stimulants exceed 90%, and therefore a lack of efficacy is suspicious and may suggest an alternate diagnosis.

MONITORING PATIENT RESPONSE

To determine the efficacy of the drugs used to treat ADHD, practitioners must use the rating scales mentioned previously; no laboratory values or diagnostic tests can determine the patient's improvement. Usually, follow-up visits are scheduled monthly after initiation of a medication and until the patients have achieved a response. When the medication regimen is stable and tolerated, the follow-up visits tend to occur at longer intervals but at least every 6 to 12 months.

Treatment is indicated for as long as the patient is showing core symptoms of ADHD. Practitioners can best determine the need to continue treatment by considering the patient's response during the "drug holidays." If symptoms are no longer present, treatment may not be needed. Continued assessment of the patient even when he or she is not using medication is essential. Medication should be given at the lowest effective dosage.

Studies show that the general side effects of stimulants, namely, insomnia, decreased appetite, dizziness, stomachache, and headache, are usually mild and do not necessitate discontinuation of the drug. Sleep difficulties may actually be related to the ADHD, which causes symptoms that prevent the child from sleeping. Because sleep disturbances cannot be generalized, it is reasonable to assess the patient and determine whether altered bedtimes or altered medication times are appropriate interventions.

In reviewing the complication of tics and dyskinesias, one study determined that transient tics develop in approximately 9% of children. The development of tics does not depend on prior personal or family history. Even though this study showed that tics or dyskinesias are not a contraindication, most health care professionals use stimulants cautiously in patients with prior histories.

Most of the other adverse events have been discussed earlier. If any adverse event occurs that is disturbing to the patient, reasonable alternatives are to lower the dose or discontinue the medication. If the patient is using a stimulant and the outcome is poor, substituting another stimulant is reasonable before trying another medication class.

PATIENT EDUCATION

Medications prescribed for ADHD must be taken exactly as prescribed to get the full benefit. If any adverse events occur that are disturbing, the patient should contact the health care provider immediately. Parents and adult patients should be aware of adverse events to watch for, as previously discussed. Patients need to be evaluated on a regular basis to determine their treatment needs.

Drug Information

The FDA's Web site (www.fda.gov) is a good source of initial prescribing information. Sources such as Micromedex and Lexicomp can also provide information about the use of these agents.

Patient-Oriented Information Sources

The National Institute of Mental Health has an excellent Web site related to ADHD (http://www.nimh.nih.gov/health/topics/attention-deficit-hyperactivity-disorder-adhd/index.shtml). This site provides access to booklets describing strategies for dealing with ADHD directed at parents of young children as well as adolescents. There are also links to local providers, clinical research trials, and other resources. Children and Adults with Attention Deficit Disorder, at www.chadd.org, is a great source of information and support for parents and patients with ADHD.

Nutrition/Lifestyle Changes

Dietary additives and supplements, such as dyes and preservatives, have long been implicated as a cause of ADHD symptoms. The literature is equivocal regarding whether or not removal of these from the diet in certain children is helpful. The 2018 NICE guidelines do not advise elimination of artificial coloring and additives from the diet as a generally applicable treatment for children and young people with ADHD.

Parent training involves teaching parents to recognize situations in which their child could learn or improve social skills. Parents must actively participate in the child's social life, using punishment effectively by clear instruction, positively reinforcing good behavior, ignoring some behaviors, and using negative reinforcement, such as time-out, to decrease the child's stimulation. This method has been shown useful for the short term and is an alternative for parents who do not want to proceed directly to medication therapy.

As mentioned previously, parents also may have ADHD. Family therapy can help teach all members how to negotiate and solve problems together as a unit. Because family therapy may be expensive, parent support groups can promote effective problem-solving techniques and unity.

Social skill training is based on the patient's deficits. Studies show that group training is more effective than individual training because self-observation usually is impossible for this patient population—both children and adults. Academic skills training helps to refine a child's ability to organize, take notes, improve study habits, and prioritize activities. This methodology has not been tested, but in clinical practice, it has been found useful if academic deficiencies are present. Adult patients may also benefit from reappraising their own social, academic, and occupational skill sets. Developing and adhering to a schedule, making commitments to observe deadlines, and accepting consequences when tasks or responsibilities are not successfully completed or maintained will assist in reinforcing good behaviors and minimizing bad behaviors. Adult patients may delay diagnosis by developing compensatory mechanisms and/or relying on others; actively avoiding compensatory mechanisms and not utilizing friends, family, or coworkers as a pathologic support system may also provide a therapeutic benefit.

Psychotherapy is not useful in the treatment of ADHD but can help patients with moralization, self-esteem, and compliance problems. It may also be useful for patients with comorbid illnesses such as anxiety and depression. Psychotherapy may be needed only as difficulties arise.

Cognitive behavior modification teaches stepwise problem solving and self-monitoring by using the reinforcement techniques of rewarding good behavior and removing rewards for unwanted behavior. Although initially believed to be a good strategy, cognitive behavior modification was later found not to improve outcomes when added to medication therapy.

All these techniques offer different benefits, so individual assessment and reassessment are important to determine which techniques (if any) are making a difference for the patient. Some parents may want to try one or more of these methods before trying medication, and practitioners should permit the parents to try whatever methods they feel will be best for their child.

As with children, nonpharmacologic treatment also is beneficial for adults. "Coaching" involves daily encouragement to progress toward set goals. Educational programs help adults to identify their problem, understand it, and not blame themselves for it. Cognitive remediation also is used to teach attention enhancement, memory, problem solving, family relationships, time management, organization skills, and anger control. Medication should not be used as a substitute for treating behaviors with behavior modification. Each patient's therapeutic plan should be assessed and reassessed for success and usefulness.

Complementary and Alternative Medications

There are several herbal medications that may have an impact on a person with ADHD. Ginkgo biloba, a plant-derived medication, has shown some efficacy in improving memory and improving concentration when added to stimulant therapy in children and adolescents (Shakibaei et al., 2015). Supplementation with polyunsaturated acids has also been evaluated as a possible natural adjunctive therapy, but its efficacy has yet to be established.

CASE STUDY 1

S.B., age 8, is always interrupting his teacher, jumping out of his seat in class, fidgeting relentlessly, and butting into other children's games. At home, he runs around recklessly and is uncontrollable. His mother comes to you and wonders why he will not listen. She is concerned because his grades at school are worsening and he has had disciplinary issues with his teachers. After medical evaluation, you find nothing wrong with S.B. physically, and he is taking no other medications. Through questioning, you determine that he has trouble concentrating on his homework, often forgets he has homework, does not complete assignments when he remembers them, loses pieces of games frequently, and hates to sit and read. His mother is unsure of the time frame over which these behaviors developed, but she thinks it has been since her second child was born 4 years ago. While in your office, S.B. did not seem to be hyperactive or inattentive, but you notice he is easily distracted by people passing in the hallway because the door is slightly ajar.

DIAGNOSIS: ATTENTION DEFICIT HYPERACTIVITY DISORDER

1. List specific goals of treatment for S.B.
2. What would be the first-line drug therapy for S.B.? Why?
3. What monitoring parameters would you institute?

4. Discuss specific patient education you would provide to S.B.'s parents based on the prescribed therapy.

5. Describe one or two drug–drug or drug–food interactions that you would be wary of when prescribing this agent.

6. List one or two adverse reactions to the agent you selected that would cause you to change therapy.

7. If the adverse reactions you described previously occurred, what would be your second-line therapy for S.B.? Why?

8. What over-the-counter and/or alternative medications would be appropriate for S.B.?

9. What dietary and lifestyle changes would you recommend to S.B.'s parents?

Bibliography

Starred references are cited in the text.

Adamo, N., Seth, S., & Coghill, D. (2015). Pharmacological treatment of attention-deficit/hyperactivity disorder: Assessing outcomes. *Expert Review of Clinical Pharmacology, 8*(4), 383–397.

*American Psychiatric Association. (2013). *Diagnostic and statistical manual of mental health disorders: DSM-5* (5th ed.). Washington, DC: American Psychiatric Publishing.

*Arnold, L. E., Abikoff, H. B., Cantwell, D. P., et al. (1997). NIMH collaborative multimodal treatment study of children with ADHD (MTA): Design, methodology, and protocol evolution. *Journal of Attention Disorders, 2*(3), 141–158.

Bloch, M. H., & Mulqueen, J. (2014). Nutritional supplements for the treatment of ADHD. *Child and Adolescent Psychiatric Clinics of North America, 23*(4), 883–897.

Brikell, I., Kuja-Halkola, R., & Larsson, H. (2015). Heritability of attention-deficit hyperactivity disorder in adults. *American Journal of Medical Genetics Part B: Neuropsychiatric Genetics, 168*(6), 406–413. doi: 10.1002/ajmg.b.32335

Chen, L. Y., Crum, R. M., Strain, E. C., et al. (2015). Patterns of concurrent substance use among adolescent nonmedical ADHD stimulant users. *Addictive Behaviors, 49*, 1–6.

Danielson, M. L., Bitsko, R. H., Ghandour, R. M., et al. (2018). Prevalence of parent-reported ADHD diagnosis and associated treatment among US children and adolescents, 2016. *Journal of Clinical Child & Adolescent Psychology, 47*(2), 199–212.

Estévez, N., Dey, M., Eich-Höchli, D., et al. (2015). Adult attention-deficit/hyperactivity disorder and its association with substance use and substance use disorders in young men. *Epidemiology and Psychiatric Sciences, 20*, 1–12.

*Faraone, S. V., & Larsson, H. (2019). Genetics of attention deficit hyperactivity disorder. *Molecular Psychiatry, 24*(4), 562–575.

*Feifel, D., & MacDonald, K. (2008). Attention-deficit/hyperactivity disorder in adults: Recognition and diagnosis of this often-overlooked condition. *Postgraduate Medicine, 120*(3), 39–47.

*Franke, B., Faraone, S. V., Asherson, P., et al. (2012). The genetics of attention deficit/hyperactivity disorder in adults, a review. *Molecular Psychiatry, 17*(10), 960–987.

*Goodman, D. W., Surman, C. B., Scherer, P. B., et al. (2012). Assessment of physician practices in adult attention-deficit/hyperactivity disorder. *The Primary Care Companion for CNS Disorders, 14*(4).

*Hodgkins, P., Shaw, M., Coghill, D., et al. (2012). Amfetamine and methylphenidate medications for attention-deficit/hyperactivity disorder: Complementary treatment options. *European Child and Adolescent Psychiatry, 21*(9), 477–492.

Hurt, E. A., & Arnold, L. E. (2014). An integrated dietary/nutritional approach to ADHD. *Child and Adolescent Psychiatric Clinics of North America, 23*(4), 955–964.

Jarrett, M. A. (2015). Attention-deficit/hyperactivity disorder (ADHD) symptoms, anxiety symptoms, and executive functioning in emerging adults. *Psychological Assessment 28*(2), 245 [Epub ahead of print].

*Minzenberg, M. J. (2012). Pharmacotherapy for attention-deficit/hyperactivity disorder: From cells to circuits. *Neurotherapeutics, 9*(3), 610–621.

*Modesto-Lowe, V., Meyer, A., & Soovajian, V. (2012). A clinician's guide to adult attention-deficit hyperactivity disorder. *Connecticut Medicine, 76*(9), 517–523.

*Montano, C. B., & Young, J. (2012). Discontinuity in the transition from pediatric to adult health care for patients with attention-deficit/hyperactivity disorder. *Postgraduate Medicine, 124*(5), 23–32.

*National Collaborating Centre for Mental Health (UK). (2018). Attention deficit hyperactivity disorder: Diagnosis and management of ADHD in children, young people and adults. British Psychological Society.

*NSDUH. (2013). Substance abuse and mental health services administration, results from the 2012 National Survey on Drug Use and Health: Summary of National Findings, NSDUH Series H-46, HHS Publication No. (SMA) 13-4795. Rockville, MD: Substance Abuse and Mental Health Services Administration.

Richardson, M., Moore, D. A., Gwernan-Jones, R., et al. (2015). Non-pharmacological interventions for attention-deficit/hyperactivity disorder (ADHD) delivered in school settings: Systematic reviews of quantitative and qualitative research. *Health Technology Assessment, 19*(45), 1–470.

*Santosh, P. J., Sattar, S., & Canagaratnam, M. (2011). Efficacy and tolerability of pharmacotherapies for attention-deficit hyperactivity disorder in adults. *CNS Drugs, 25*(9), 737–763.

*Shakibaei, F., Radmanesh, M., Salari, E., et al. (2015). Ginkgo biloba in the treatment of attention-deficit/hyperactivity disorder in children and adolescents: A randomized, placebo-controlled, trial. *Complementary Therapies in Clinical Practice, 21*(2), 61–67.

*Simon, N., Rolland, B., & Karila, L. (2015). Methylphenidate in adults with attention deficit hyperactivity disorder and substance use disorders. *Current Pharmaceutical Design, 21*(23), 3359–3366.

*Smith, A. K., Mick, E., & Faraone, S. V. (2009). Advances in genetic studies of attention-deficit/hyperactivity disorder. *Current Psychiatry Reports, 11*(2), 143–148.

STRATTERA* (atomoxetine HCl). (n.d.). Retrieved from https://www.accessdata.fda.gov/drugsatfda_docs/label/2007/021411s004s012s013s015s021lbl.pdf

*Taylor, A., Deb, S., & Unwin, G. (2011). Scales for the identification of adults with attention deficit hyperactivity disorder (ADHD): A systematic review. *Research in Developmental Disabilities, 32*(3), 924–938.

*Wolraich, M. L., Hagan, J. F., Allan, C., et al. (2019). Clinical practice guideline for the diagnosis, evaluation, and treatment of attention-deficit/hyperactivity disorder in children and adolescents. *Pediatrics, 144*(4), e20192528.

43 Substance Use Disorders

Andrew M. Peterson

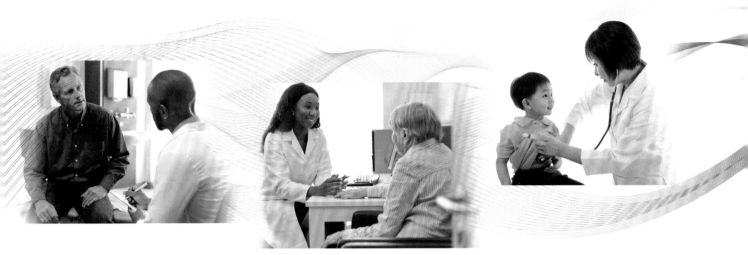

Learning Objectives

1. Use the *Diagnostic and Statistical Manual of Mental Disorders, Fifth Edition* criteria to determine if a patient has a substance use disorder.
2. Select the first-line medication treatment for patients with alcohol and opioid use disorder based on patient-specific clinical data.
3. Describe the common side effects of drugs used to treat alcohol and opioid use disorder.
4. Discuss the signs and symptoms of withdrawal from alcohol and opioids.

INTRODUCTION

Substance use disorders (SUDs) occur when the recurrent use of alcohol and/or drugs causes "clinically significant impairment, including health problems, disability, and failure to meet major responsibilities at work, school, or home" (SAMHSA-a, 2020). The range of substance use/misuse can be considered on a continuum from abstinence to full-blown addiction. Addiction, the severest form of SUD, is a chronic brain disease that is "characterized by impaired control over use of substance, compulsive use, and continued use despite harm and cravings" (Addictionary, 2019). SUDs have impact not only on the individual with the disorder, but the family, employer, and society. For the year 2017, the Centers for Disease Control and Prevention (CDC) reported that 53.9% of adults 35 years and older used alcohol in the past month and 5.6% reported heavy alcohol use (NSDUH, 2018). Nearly 8% of the same population misused prescription or used illicit drugs in the same time frame and more than 70,000 people died of an opioid drug overdose (CDC, 2018). Further, researchers have noted that excessive alcohol use costs the healthcare system more than $28 million, and employers experienced more than $170 million loss in productivity.

In 2013, the Substance Abuse and Mental Health Services Administration (SAMHSA) reported approximately 20.2 million adults aged 18 or older had a past year SUD. Of these adults, 16.3 million had an alcohol use disorder (AUD) and 6.2 million had an illicit drug use disorder. In the same year, 2.5 million adults (~1% of the total adult population) received treatment at a specialty facility. Unfortunately, this translates only into 7.5% of those with an SUD receiving substance use treatment (NSDUH, 2018).

As such, SUD is a large public health problem that is undertreated and requires increased attention by healthcare professionals. In particular, healthcare professionals need to learn to recognize patients potentially experiencing SUD, determine appropriate pharmacotherapeutic and non-pharmacotherapeutic treatment approaches, and support those patients in a long-term recovery program. This chapter will provide a high-level overview of the approaches to two major SUDs—AUD and opioid use disorder (OUD). For nicotine use disorder, see Chapter 52—Smoking Cessation.

CAUSES

The cause of SUD is still unknown, but it is thought that genetics play a significant role. In 2000, Ma and colleagues (2000) reported that race may play a role but more recently, the issue of health disparity among the races might be the more relevant issue (Volkow, 2019). Cotto (2010) showed that gender may also be an influencer, with AUD more prevalent in women and OUD more prevalent in men. Age at first exposure may also play a role, as evidenced by Compton's findings showing use in early teen years leads to an increase in later teen and adult years of a use disorder (Compton, 2019). Repeated use of the substance may lead to an increase in an individual's tolerance of the "feel good" effects, which may progress later on to drug-seeking behavior and SUD/addiction. There may also be some comorbid conditions with an SUD, such as anxiety, depression or bipolar disorder, which may lead some individuals to use substances to combat the ill feelings, or even delay treatment for an SUD due to the mixed diagnoses.

PATHOPHYSIOLOGY

SUD is a brain disease, based on the principle of neurophysiologic reinforcement (NIDA, 2003). The "reward pathway" most commonly invoked to describe the use-addiction cycle

is in the mesolimbic system in the brain where dopaminergic neurons lead to the nucleus accumbens (NAc). These neurons originate in the ventral tegmental area (VTA) and are typically controlled by gamma-aminobutyric acid (GABA). Once the GABA control is removed, dopamine is released and provides a pleasure response to the NAc (**Figure 43.1**).

When GABA is released in the synaptic cleft, it binds to postsynaptic GABA receptor and opens chloride channels; this, in turn, hyperpolarizes the membranes, thereby lowering cell excitability. Alcohol, benzodiazepines (BZ), and barbiturates are believed to enhance GABA control of the postsynaptic neuron—BZ and barbiturates also affect the chloride channel via their own receptor while alcohol just interacts with the GABA-A receptor complex.

Stimulants elevate the synaptic levels of monoamine neurotransmitters such as dopamine, norepinephrine, and serotonin. Cocaine accomplishes this through inhibition of the reuptake mechanism while amphetamines increase the release of dopamine and norepinephrine and block their reuptake.

In contrast to the stimulants and sedatives just discussed, opioids have their own receptors in the brain which are activated by a family of endogenous peptides including endorphins

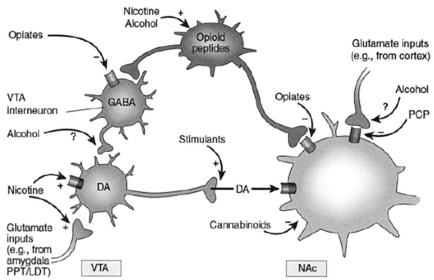

FIGURE 43–1 Simplified schematic of converging acute actions of drugs of abuse on the VTA–NAc pathway. Stimulants directly increase dopaminergic transmission in the nucleus accumbens (NAc). Opiates indirectly increase dopaminergic transmission in the NAc by inhibiting GABAergic interneurons in the ventral tegmental area (VTA), which disinhibits VTA dopamine (DA) neurons. Opiates also act directly on μ-opioid receptors on NAc neurons. μ-Opioid receptors, like D2 dopamine receptors, signal via the inhibitory G-protein Gαi; hence, the two mechanisms converge within some NAc neurons. The actions of other drugs of abuse remain more conjectural. Nicotine seems to activate VTA dopamine neurons directly via stimulation of nicotinic cholinergic receptors on those neurons and indirectly via stimulation of its receptors on glutamatergic nerve terminals that innervate the dopamine cells. Alcohol promotes GABA-A receptor function, which may inhibit GABAergic terminals in the VTA and hence disinhibit VTA dopamine neurons. It may similarly inhibit glutamatergic terminals that innervate NAc neurons. Many additional mechanisms (not shown) are proposed for alcohol. Cannabinoid mechanisms are complex and involve activation of CB1 receptors (which, like D2 and μ-opioid receptors, are Gαi linked) on glutamatergic and GABAergic nerve terminals in the NAc, and on NAc neurons themselves. Phencyclidine (PCP) may act by inhibiting postsynaptic NMDA glutamate receptors in the NAc. Finally, there is some evidence that nicotine and alcohol may activate endogenous opioid pathways and that these and other drugs of abuse (such as opiates) may activate endogenous cannabinoid pathways (not shown). (Used with permission from Nestler, E. J. (2014). Epigenetic mechanisms of drug addiction. *Neuropharmacology, 76*, 259–268.)

GABA, gamma-aminobutyric acid; PPT/LDT, peduncular pontine tegmentum/lateral dorsal tegmentum.

and enkephalins. While widely distributed throughout the brain, opioid receptors are primarily found in the cortex, limbic system, and brain stem. The primary receptor linked to addiction (and pain relief) is the *mu (μ)* opioid receptor. This receptor can also be activated exogenously by agents, such as morphine or fentanyl, and is found largely in the amygdala part of the limbic system.

DIAGNOSTIC CRITERIA

SUD are diagnosed based on the *Diagnostic and Statistical Manual of Mental Disorders, Fifth Edition (DSM-5)* criteria. There are 11 criteria, and a diagnosis requires at least 2 of these criteria to be present, with mild SUD represented by the patient exhibiting two to three criteria, moderate severity being four to five criteria, and severe disorder in patients exhibiting six or more (Hasin, 2013). Many substances cause a SUD and a diagnosis will follow the same pattern. That is, to diagnose an alcohol or other SUD, the same criteria would apply. The most common drugs associated with SUD are listed in **Box 43.1**.

Screening, Brief Intervention, and Referral to Treatment

Screening, Brief Intervention, and Referral to Treatment (SBIRT) is an evidence-based practice that has been endorsed as a viable public health approach to reduce the prevalence of SUD, particularly AUD. The application of SBIRT works best when coupled with strategies for ensuring patients who are identified as likely having an SUD are linked with viable treatment resources. **Screening(s)** helps assess the severity of

substance use and aids to objectively identify a level of treatment for each patient. Screening is the universal use of validated screening instruments to quickly assess a patient's substance use, assess consequences of substance use, and identify the appropriate level of intervention (**Box 43.2**). Using one of these tools allows for the healthcare professional to screen for patterns of substance use and the resulting score informs the professional of the appropriate intervention. **Brief intervention (BI)** centers on behavioral changes by increasing awareness to the problem at hand. It uses the techniques of motivational interviewing to aid in providing motivation to the patient to engage in a behavioral change. **Referral to treatment (RT)** provides patients the opportunity for an evaluation by trained personnel and referral to appropriate level of treatment. **SBIRT** is a key element in the diagnosis and treatment of patients with SUD.

INITIATING DRUG THERAPY

Treatment for SUD can be behavioral and/or medication based, depending on the condition. However, before actual treatment can occur, the patient needs to be detoxified from the substance causing the problem. Detoxification can be dangerous, even deadly, thus it is recommended that it be managed medically to reduce withdrawal symptoms and ensure the patient's safety during the process. However, detoxification is only the first step—it does not result in long-term changes in drug use behavior or impart sobriety. Treatment after detoxification can occur in a variety of settings, such as a rehabilitation center, a hospital, or an intensive outpatient treatment center. An underlying principle is that treatment should be provided in the least restrictive setting and the patient be continually assessed for eligibility to move to the next least restrictive setting. Drug therapy can be initiated in the inpatient or outpatient settings, depending on the substance, the severity of the addiction, and the patient's ability to manage the treatment.

Goals of Drug Therapy

Treatment programs for all substance abuse have three generalized goals:

- Reducing substance abuse or achieving a substance-free life
- Maximizing multiple aspects of life functioning
- Preventing or reducing the frequency and severity of relapse

The specific patient goals are typically based on these and include achieving and maintaining a level of abstinence from the substance being abused which may or may not include a similar substance designed to support abstinence from the offending substance (e.g., methadone for OUD, naltrexone for AUD). Attaining this goal may take numerous attempts and failures and the treatment program tries to minimize the effects of continued use through harm-reduction strategies, education, counseling, and self-help groups that stress reducing risky behavior. These strategies may include assistance in the patient building new relationships with drug-free friends

---

BOX 43.1 **Drugs with Potential for Substance Use Disorder**

Alcohol
- Barbiturates—pentobarbital, phenobarbital, and others
- Benzodiazepines—alprazolam, diazepam, lorazepam, and others
- Cannabinoids—marijuana, tetrahydrocannabinol (THC), and THC derivatives
- Hallucinogens—Lysergic acid diethylamide (LSD), 3,4-Methylenedioxy methamphetamine (MDMA) (e.g., Ecstasy), and mescaline
- Nicotine—cigarettes, vapor cigarettes, cigars, chewing tobacco, and snuff
- Opioids—fentanyl, heroin, hydrocodone, methadone, morphine, oxycodone, and others
- Stimulants—amphetamine, atomoxetine, cocaine, methamphetamine, and methylphenidate (e.g., Ritalin)

BOX 43.2   Example Screening Tools

Tool	Scoring
ASSIST—**A**lcohol, **S**moking, and **S**ubstance **I**nvolvement **S**creening **T**est	0–3—low risk/no intervention 4–26—moderate risk/brief Intervention ≥27—high risk/treatment
AUDIT—**A**lcohol **U**se **D**isorder **I**dentification **T**est	1–7—low risk 8–14—hazardous consumption ≥15—alcohol use disorder likely
CAGE—**C**ut Down; **A**nnoyed; **G**uilty; **E**ye-opener	2 or more positive answers—clinically significant for alcohol misuse
COMM—**C**urrent **O**pioid **M**isuse **M**easure	Score of 9 or greater—high risk for misusing opioids
DAST-10—**D**rug **A**buse **S**creening **T**est—10-question version	0—No risk 1–2—low level risk—continue to monitor 3–5—moderate risk—brief intervention ≥6—Substantial/severe risk—treatment

through 12-step or other recovery programs, changing recreational activities and lifestyle patterns, substituting substances used with less risky ones, with a goal of convincing the patient of their individual responsibility for becoming abstinent (American Psychiatric Association, 1995). Total abstinence is strongly associated with a positive long-term prognosis.

Alcohol Use Disorder

Alcohol is the most common substance that Americans use to alter their state of mind, with more than half of Americans reporting alcohol use in the past month. However, one must note that only approximately 10% of those aged 18 to 25 and approximately 5% aged 26 and older use alcohol in a way that meets the *DSM* criteria of AUD.

The media and scientific outlets typically tout the beneficial effects of alcohol use, including lowering cholesterol levels or reducing the risk of heart disease. However, the overall benefit of alcohol on these conditions does not warrant starting an alcohol regimen to achieve these benefits. In fact, too much alcohol may increase the risk of certain conditions: heavy drinkers see an increase in stroke, hypertension, depression, esophageal cancer, and of course, cirrhosis of the liver. Women who drink 1 drink per day and men who drink 2 drinks per day are considered moderate drinkers. Heavy drinking is more than 4 drinks on any day for men or more than 3 drinks per day for women. A drink can be a glass of wine, a single beer, or one shot of distilled spirits (see **Box 43.3** for alcohol equivalents).

Alcohol Withdrawal

Continued, persistent alcohol use can lead to a tolerance and potentially a physical dependence. Once at this state, reduced alcohol consumption can lead to symptoms of alcohol withdrawal. Symptoms of withdrawal from alcohol range from mild to life-threatening. Withdrawal symptoms may appear 6 to 12 hours after discontinuation of alcohol but can start 1 to 3 days later and may last up to a week (Manasco, 2012). Mild symptoms include anxiety, sweating, restlessness, and insomnia, while moderate symptoms include the mild symptoms plus increased blood pressure or heart rate, confusion, and mild hyperthermia. Severe symptoms include moderate symptoms plus hallucinations, impaired attention, seizures, and delirium tremens (DT) (**Box 43.4**). Patients with mild symptoms can be managed in the ambulatory setting provided they have no prior history of DT or seizures. However, patients with moderate or severe symptoms need closer monitoring, since some people can progress rapidly. Pharmacologic treatment of alcohol withdrawal is typically with BZ. See **Table 43.1** for BZ commonly used in alcohol withdrawal.

Pharmacotherapy

Treatment of AUD includes the management of acute withdrawal episodes, if they occur, and the long-term maintenance of a goal-oriented program designed to minimize the consequences of excessive alcohol use. Clinicians and patients still debate whether the goal is total abstinence from alcohol or just reducing harm by reducing alcohol use (Swift & Aston, 2015). While abstinence is associated with better long-term outcomes, both approaches have merit. The aim of pharmacotherapy for the treatment of AUD is to achieve whichever goal is most important to the patient and the practitioner. See Table 43.2 for drugs used in the treatment of Alcohol Use Disorder.

Acamprosate

Acamprosate is an oral drug indicated for the post-withdrawal maintenance of abstinence from alcohol. Taken consistently, it has the potential to increase the number of days

BOX 43.3 Drink Equivalents

What is a Standard Drink?

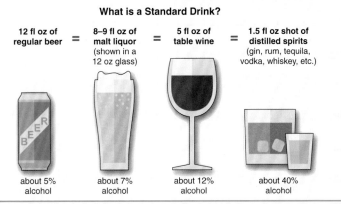

| 12 fl oz of regular beer | = | 8–9 fl oz of malt liquor (shown in a 12 oz glass) | = | 5 fl oz of table wine | = | 1.5 fl oz shot of distilled spirits (gin, rum, tequila, vodka, whiskey, etc.) |

about 5% alcohol   about 7% alcohol   about 12% alcohol   about 40% alcohol

Each beverage portrayed above represents one standard drink (or one alcohol drink equivalent), defined in the United States as any beverage containing .6 fl oz or 14 grams of pure alcohol. The percentage of pure alcohol, expressed here as alcohol by volume (alc/vol), varies within and across beverage types. Although the standard drink amounts are helpful for following health guidelines, they may not reflect customary serving sizes.

BOX 43.4 Delirium Tremens (DT)

DT is characterized by a rapid onset of psychological and neurological changes such as confusion, hallucinations, and sympathetic overdrive. This sympathetic overdrive can lead to seizures and/or cardiovascular collapse. About 33% of those experiencing seizures progress on to the most severe form of alcohol withdrawal, DT. A patient who meets the criteria for alcohol withdrawal plus the following are considered to have DT.

- Decreased attention and awareness
- Disturbance in attention, awareness, memory, orientation, language, visuospatial ability, perception, or all of these abilities that is a change from the normal level and fluctuates in severity during the day
- Disturbances in memory, orientation, language, visuospatial ability, or perception
- No evidence of coma or other evolving neurocognitive disorders

DT occur in less than 5% of those undergoing medical alcohol detoxification and 7% to 20% of those undergoing non-supervised alcohol detoxification. The DT may occur within 24 to 72 hours after cessation of alcohol consumption. DT can be fatal in 5% to 25% of patients and is considered a medical emergency. Treatment of DT involves lab work, frequent vital sign checks, serial mental status evaluation, IV fluids, adequate nutrition, and potential treatment with agents such as BZ to control seizures.

without alcohol and the number of people who do not drink alcohol at all.

Mechanism of Action

Acamprosate may influence GABA transmission via inhibition of presynaptic GABA receptors and may also decrease brain glutamate and increase beta-endorphins. In a dose-dependent manner, acamprosate reduces alcohol intake which in turns helps maintain abstinence in patients with AUD.

Dosage

Acamprosate is available as Campral, a 333 mg tablet. The recommended dosage of acamprosate for maintenance of abstinence from alcohol in adults with normal renal function is 666 mg (2 tablets) thrice daily. For patients with a creatinine clearance (CrCl) between 30 and 50 mL/min, the dose should be reduced to one tablet thrice daily. Acamprosate is not recommended for patients with a CrCl less than 30 mL/min (Table 43.2).

Time Frame for Response

Acamprosate has a bioavailability of about 11% and peak concentrations occur in 3 to 8 hours after oral administration. It has an elimination half-life of approximately 20 hours and does not undergo hepatic metabolism and is primarily excreted via the kidneys.

Contraindications

Due to its renal elimination, it is not recommended for use in patients with CrCl less than 30 mL/min. Since the formulation contains sodium sulfite, patients with severe sulfite sensitivities should not take acamprosate.

TABLE 43.1

Benzodiazepine Use in the Treatment of Alcohol Withdrawal Syndrome

Drug	Advantages/Disadvantages	Dose Equivalents
Chlordiazepoxide	Long half-life does not require tapering upon discontinuation; oral and IV dosage forms; drug accumulation may occur in patients with severe liver dysfunction.	25 mg
Diazepam	Long half-life does not require tapering upon discontinuation; oral and IV dosage forms; drug accumulation may occur in patients with severe liver dysfunction.	5 mg
Lorazepam	Shorter half-life; oral and IV dosage forms; no active metabolites but must be tapered before being discontinued.	1 mg
Oxazepam	Shorter half-life; only available orally; no active metabolites but must be tapered before being discontinued.	15 mg

IV, intravenous.

TABLE 43.2

Medications Used in Alcohol Use Disorder

Medication Generic (Brand)	Contraindications	Adverse Effects	Special Considerations
Acamprosate (Campral) 666 mg PO TID	Hypersensitivity Severe renal impairment (CrCl ≤ 30 mL/min).	GI disturbances	Maintenance of abstinence from alcohol in patients with alcohol use disorder
Disulfiram (Antabuse) 500 mg PO daily	Hypersensitivity Severe cardiovascular, respiratory, or renal disease Severe hepatic dysfunction (i.e., transaminase levels > 3 times upper limit of normal or abnormal bilirubin) Severe psychiatric disorders, especially psychotic and cognitive disorders and suicidal ideation Poor impulse control Metronidazole or ketoconazole therapy which already induces a similar reaction to alcohol	Drowsiness, headache, metallic taste	Management of alcohol use disorder
Naltrexone 50 mg PO daily (ReVia) 380 mg as a once-monthly injection (Vivitrol)	Hypersensitivity Receiving opioid agonists or history of opioid dependence with use within past 7 days Acute opioid withdrawal Failed naloxone challenge test Positive urine opioid screen Acute hepatitis or liver failure	Exacerbation of withdrawal, nausea, headache, injection site reactions	Alcohol dependence and prevention of relapse after opioid detoxification

GI, gastrointestinal.

Adverse Events

Diarrhea (>10%), insomnia (7%), nausea (>5%), pruritus (>4%), and asthenia are common in patients taking acamprosate. Psychological adverse effects include anxiety and depression. Cardiovascular effects may include hypertension, palpitations, vasodilation, syncope, and peripheral edema, which have been reported in about 1% of patients.

Interactions

There are no reported relevant pharmacokinetic interactions with acamprosate.

Disulfiram

Disulfiram, trade name Antabuse, is used to aid in the treatment of AUD. The agent is designed as a deterrent—producing unpleasant effects when alcohol is consumed concomitantly. These reactions are commonly called "disulfiram-like" reactions. It is not used in the acute phase of alcohol detoxification and should only be used when the patient is alcohol free.

Mechanism of Action

Alcohol, or more specifically ethanol, is metabolized by the liver enzyme, ethanol dehydrogenase producing acetaldehyde.

Acetaldehyde is then metabolized by aldehyde dehydrogenase to acetate which is then excreted. Disulfiram is an irreversible aldehyde dehydrogenase inhibitor, thus increasing the level of acetaldehyde in the body. Acetaldehyde causes damage at the cellular level and is often considered the culprit in "hangovers." Thus, when taken concomitantly with alcohol, there is an increase in serum acetaldehyde providing a negative feedback to the patient, deterring further consumption of alcohol. This is often referred to as the "disulfiram-like" reaction.

Dosage

The usual initial oral dose is 500 mg once daily for 1 to 2 weeks then decreased to 250 mg daily as maintenance. Patients may take 125 to 500 mg daily, with a maximum of 500 mg/d. If the patient experiences sedation, the dose may be administered in the evening.

Time Frame for Response

The peak plasma concentration occurs in 1 to 2 hours after ingestion and 80% to 90% of the agent is absorbed. The elimination half-life is 12 hours.

Contraindications

The "disulfiram-like" reaction can occur with small amounts of alcohol. This reaction is characterized by flushing, throbbing headache, respiratory difficulty, nausea and vomiting, and sweating. The patient may also experience chest pain or palpitations, along with respiratory symptoms such as dyspnea and hyperventilation. Severe reactions may include respiratory depression, cardiovascular collapse, arrhythmias, and even myocardial infarction. The intensity of the reaction can vary and is typically dependent on the amounts of disulfiram and alcohol ingested. Mild reactions may occur in the sensitive individual when the blood alcohol concentration is as little as 0.05% to 0.1%. Therefore, the patient should be cautioned about drinking alcohol, and even consuming alcohol from non-liquor–based sources such as mouthwash, cough syrups, and even sauces.

Disulfiram is also contraindicated in patients with significant coronary artery disease or heart failure as heart failure and related deaths have occurred. Disulfiram is contraindicated in patients with underlying psychoses as it may worsen the patient's condition.

Adverse Events

Common adverse reactions to disulfiram include drowsiness, fatigue, and headache. Serious side effects such as hepatic dysfunction and optic and peripheral neuritis as well as peripheral neuropathy have been reported to occur. The neurological adverse effects may occur as early as 10 days after initiation. A metallic or garlic-like taste may occur, as well as a rash/acne.

Interactions

In addition to the inhibition of acetaldehyde dehydrogenase, disulfiram inhibits the cytochrome CYP2C9 activity and has been shown to increase levels of tricyclic antidepressants and BZ.

Naltrexone

Naltrexone, brand names ReVia and Vivitrol, is an opioid antagonist indicated for the treatment of alcohol dependence in patients who are already abstinent from alcohol use. It is also indicated for the prevention of relapse to opioid dependence, following opioid detoxification. It is available as a 50 mg tablet and as a 380 mg intramuscular (IM) injection, as an extended-release polymer formulation.

Mechanism of Action

Naltrexone is an opioid antagonist with high affinity for the *mu* opioid receptor. Occupation of opioid receptors by naltrexone may block the effects of endogenous opioid peptides and thus in turn may be the means by which this agent acts to reduce alcohol consumption, but the exact mechanism of action is not fully known. It is thought that naltrexone decreases craving in people who are alcohol dependent.

Dosage

For AUD, patients start at 50 mg orally daily and the dosage may be increased to 100 mg daily. Alternatively, 150 mg every 3 days may be administered. The extended-release IM form is administered at 380 mg once every 4 weeks in the gluteal muscle.

Time Frame for Response

Naltrexone extended-release injection peaks in about 2 hours after deep IM injection followed by a second peak 2 to 3 days later. Seven days after dosing, plasma concentrations decline with a therapeutic level maintained for about 4 weeks after dosing. Extended-release naltrexone has a half-life of 5 to 10 days due to the polymer degradation. Oral naltrexone is nearly completely absorbed in the gastrointestinal tract and is metabolized almost exclusively by the liver to the primary active metabolite, 6-beta-naltrexol. Peak naltrexone plasma concentrations are reached within 1 hour of dosing. The half-life of the non-polymeric drug is about 4 hours and the half-life of the active metabolite 6-beta-naltrexol is about 13 hours. Over 70% of the dose is excreted in urine.

Contraindications

Naltrexone is contraindicated in patients taking opioid medications, in active withdrawal or actively drinking. Further, patients with hypersensitivity to the drug, or the polymers polylactide-*co*-glycolide, carboxymethylcellulose, should not receive injectable naltrexone.

Adverse Events

For the most part, naltrexone is generally well tolerated. Injection site reactions and pain at the site are the most common reactions for the injectable form, thus making this formulation subject to a Food and Drug Administration (FDA) Risk Evaluation and Mitigation Strategy (REMS). The purpose of this REMS is to inform the patient and healthcare provider about the risk of injection site reactions and strategies to mitigate those reactions. Other adverse effects of naltrexone include headache and nausea. Hepatic toxicity may be seen more frequently in alcohol-dependent patients. Cardiovascular effects such as syncope may occur but are less common.

Interactions

Since the primary action of naltrexone is to block the opioid receptors, there will be a decrease in the efficacy of opioid drugs used to treat pain efficacy of opioids used as antitussives or antidiarrheals. Due to the half-life, the oral formulation should be discontinued 72 hours before surgery and the injectable at least 30 days.

Selecting the Most Appropriate Drug

Long-term pharmacotherapy, if needed, should be planned/started concurrently with any acute withdrawal management program, so long as the patient is cognitively capable of understanding the treatment regimen. At a minimum, clinicians should be sure to put a "warm-handoff" in place, connect the AUD patient to the appropriate level treatment service, and aid in their transition to recovery providers (**Figure 43.2**).

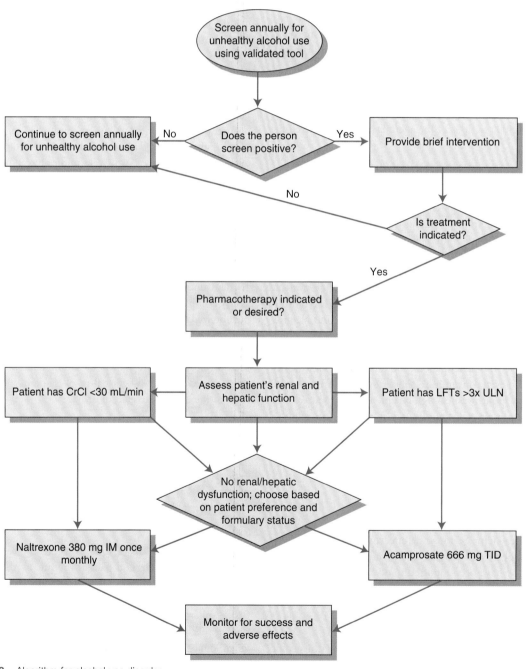

FIGURE 43–2 Algorithm for alcohol use disorder.

CrCl, creatinine clearance; IM, intramuscular; LFT, liver function tests; ULN, Upper limit of normal.

First-Line Therapy

First-line chronic therapy for patients with moderate-to-severe AUD can begin with either naltrexone or acamprosate. The choice of agent depends on various patient factors including renal and hepatic function, side effects and concomitant medications, as well as formulary status and availability of the various dosage forms. Acamprosate should not be used first if the patient has renal dysfunction; if patient has hepatic dysfunction, the patient should not be started on naltrexone.

Second-Line Therapy

Patients who were not successful or intolerant to both naltrexone and acamprosate can be given a trial of disulfiram. To be started on this agent, careful counseling must be provided so that the patient has a good understanding of the risks of alcohol consumption while taking disulfiram.

Opioid Use Disorder

Like AUD, OUD is a specific SUD that is diagnosed using the *DSM-5* criteria. Opioids are a specific type of drug that include prescription medications (morphine, Percocet) typically used to treat pain as well as illicit substances like heroin. As discussed earlier, their action on the *mu* (and *kappa*) receptors reduces pain but also produce a pleasure response. Unfortunately, too, overuse of these medications can lead to respiratory depression and/or arrest and ultimately death. Data from the CDC (CDC/NCHS, 2018) indicate that 128 persons die daily from opioid overdoses. This public health crisis is not new, but recent increase in deaths has been fueled by the increased availability of illicitly manufactured fentanyl and its analogs.

The treatment of OUD requires both acute management of withdrawal as well as long-term, chronic care. Acute care treatment for withdrawal (**Box 43.5**) is typically an inpatient, medically supervised event and must be coupled with a long-term aftercare plan. Recent evidence shows that using medications for OUD for as long as they continue to provide benefit to the patient provides the best chance for maintenance.

Buprenorphine, methadone, and naltrexone are FDA approved for the treatment of OUD. In addition to the three FDA-approved medications for OUD, naloxone, an opioid antagonist, is often used to reverse the effects of an opioid-related overdose. See **Box 43.6** for a brief overview of naloxone use in preventing opioid overdose death. Lofexidine (Lucemyra) is indicated for the management of symptoms associated with opioid withdrawal (See **Table 43.3**).

Buprenorphine

Buprenorphine is the first medication approved by the FDA to treat OUD outside of an opioid treatment program (OTP). Along with methadone, buprenorphine is a first-line treatment option for medication-assisted treatment (MAT) in patients with OUD. Buprenorphine is available in a variety of dosage forms, including buccal, transdermal, oral, injectable, and subdermal implant.

To prescribe buprenorphine for the treatment of OUD, practitioners must apply for and be approved as a qualified practitioner under the Drug Addiction Treatment Act of 2000 (SAMHSA-c, 2020). This act allows clinicians to dispense or prescribe medications such as buprenorphine in settings other than an OTP. Physicians, physician assistants, nurse practitioners, and other healthcare providers can apply for and obtain a "Data-waiver." See SAMHSA (www.samhsa.gov) for information on how to become a buprenorphine-waivered practitioner.

BOX 43.5   Opioid Withdrawal

Withdrawal from opioids such as heroin, opium, morphine, codeine, and methadone can be very uncomfortable and difficult for the patient. Unlike alcohol withdrawal, opioid withdrawal is not usually life-threatening. However, withdrawal from opioids should not be allowed in pregnant women, as this can cause miscarriage or premature delivery. The recommended treatment approach for pregnant, opioid dependent women is methadone maintenance treatment.

Withdrawal from short-acting opioids (e.g., heroin) can be seen in 8 to 24 hours after the last use and may last 4 to 10 days. For long-acting opioids such as methadone, the onset can be as soon as 12 to 24 hours and last upwards of 10 to 20 days due to the long half-life.

Symptoms of withdrawal include GI disturbances like nausea, vomiting and diarrhea, physical changes such as hot/cold flashes, sweating, muscle cramps, and watery discharge from nose/eyes. Further, headaches, anxiety, and insomnia frequently occur.

Patients experiencing withdrawal should be monitored 3 to 4 times daily for symptoms and complications. The Short Opioid Withdrawal Scale (SOWS) is a useful tool for monitoring withdrawal. It should be administered 1 to 2 times daily. The results of the SOWS assessment can help guide management. For mild withdrawal (scores ≤10), symptomatic treatment is indicated. This includes hydration, vitamin B and C supplements and symptomatic treatment for GI effects, sleep disturbances, and headaches/pain.

For moderate withdrawal (scores 10 to 20), symptomatic management and potentially opioid medication (e.g., methadone/buprenorphine) may be indicated. For scores above 20 (severe withdrawal), treatment with opioid medication is indicated in addition to the symptomatic treatment used in mild withdrawal.

BOX 43.6   Naloxone for Overdose Reversal

Naloxone is an opioid antagonist used to block the untoward effects of opioids such as heroin and morphine. Specifically, it reverses the life-threatening depression of the central nervous and respiratory systems acting as a competitive antagonist to the *mu, kappa,* and other opiate receptors in the CNS, with the highest affinity for the *mu* receptor. The onset of action is within 2 minutes when administered IV and 5 minutes for IM or intranasally. The effects of naloxone can last 30 to 60 minutes. If the person does not respond after 5 minutes, the naloxone dose can be repeated.

The IV/IM dosing for adults is 0.4 to 2 mg every 2 to 3 minutes as needed up to a total dose of 10 mg. The nasal spray dosing is 4 mg intranasally and repeat every 2 to 3 minutes in alternating nostrils as needed. If used in the field, the patient should be monitored closely until emergency medical personnel arrive and for at least 24 hours after administration. For patients with chronic opioid addiction, titrate slowly to minimize cardiovascular adverse effects and withdrawal symptoms.

Although traditionally administered in a hospital setting or in the field by emergency response personnel, the advent of the nasal formulation allows for non-healthcare personnel to more readily administer it in an overdose situation. This makes it ideal for treating overdose in people who have been prescribed opioid pain medication and in people who use heroin and other opioids.

Mechanism of Action

Buprenorphine is a mixed agonist/antagonist at the *mu* and *kappa* receptors. This mixed action results in analgesic effects similar to full *mu* agonists yet creates a ceiling effect at the *kappa* receptor which decreases the euphoric and respiratory depression effects.

Dosage

The dosage varies depending on the route of administration. Table 43.3 shows the specific dosage forms and doses. In general, to start buprenorphine treatment (induction therapy), the OUD patient must not have taken opioids for 12 to 24 hours because the agent induces an acute withdrawal due to its antagonistic properties. Further, the patient should be showing signs of early withdrawal. Following the induction phase, the dose of buprenorphine is gradually increased according to the patient's physical and psychological needs but should not exceed a maximum of 24 mg in one day, with typical doses in the range of 8 to 12 mg/d. Maintenance dosing can be achieved typically in 2 to 4 days. The dose of the agent can be reduced after the patient is no longer experiencing cravings and discontinued, or has at least reduced, their opioid use.

Time Frame for Response

The onset of action for the sublingual formulation is about 30 to 60 minutes with a peak clinical effect in about 1 to 4 hours. The effect may last for 6 to 12 hours at low dose (<4 mg) and 24 to 72 hours at higher dose (>16 mg). Patients may be on buprenorphine for months or even years, and treatment can be for life.

Contraindications

The contraindications to buprenorphine treatment are related to its mechanism of action. Patients actively using opioids should not take buprenorphine. Patients with significant respiratory depression, a known or suspected gastrointestinal obstruction, or hypersensitivity to buprenorphine should not take buprenorphine.

Adverse Events

As with the contraindications, the adverse effects associated with buprenorphine primarily relate to its action on the opioid receptors. These include nausea, vomiting, drowsiness, dizziness, headache, memory loss, sweating, dry mouth, and urinary retention. Further, buprenorphine can exert some anticholinergic-like effects and may cause central nervous system (CNS) depression. Other side effects of buprenorphine include nausea, vomiting, drowsiness, dizziness, headache, memory loss, sweating, dry mouth, and urinary retention.

Interactions

Buprenorphine is metabolized by the CYP3A4 enzyme to an active metabolite, nor-buprenorphine. Drugs that inhibit this enzyme (e.g., ketoconazole, erythromycin) may result in increases in buprenorphine and concomitant use may require a reduction in the buprenorphine dose. Drugs that induce CYP3A4 (e.g., phenytoin, phenobarbital, carbamazepine) may result in reduced buprenorphine concentrations.

Lofexidine

Lofexidine is a new, non-opioid adrenergic agonist medication indicated for the mitigation of opioid withdrawal symptoms in adults.

Mechanism of Action

Lofexidine inhibits the release of norepinephrine centrally and peripherally and it is this inhibition that mitigates the symptoms caused by the rebound hyperactivity of epinephrine suppressed by opioids.

Dosage

Lofexidine is dosed at three 0.18 mg tablets (0.54 mg) orally four times daily during the period of peak withdrawal symptoms. Doses should be spaced about 5 to 6 hours apart with the total daily dosage not exceeding 2.88 mg (16 tablets). No single dose should exceed 0.72 mg (4 tablets). Lofexidine may be continued for up to 14 days, depending on symptoms. To discontinue lofexidine, the dose should be gradually reduced

TABLE 43.3

Medications Used in Opioid Use Disorder

Medication	Contraindications	Adverse Effects	Special Considerations
Buprenorphine Sublingual tablet average daily dose: 16 mg/d; (Max daily dose: 32 mg but doses over 24 mg do not seem to provide a clinical advantage) Sublingual tablet/film (with naloxone) average daily dose: 11.4/2.9 mg or 16/4 mg/d depending on product (Max daily dose: 17.2/4.2 mg or 24/6 mg depending on product) Buccal tablet (with naloxone) average daily dose: 8.4/1.4 mg/d (Max daily dose: 12.6/2.1 mg) Extended-release subcutaneous injection average dose: 100 mg monthly (Max monthly dose: 300 mg) Subdermal implant: 4 implants are inserted for 6 month duration; Each implant contains 74.2 mg of buprenorphine, equivalent to 80 mg of buprenorphine hydrochloride	Hypertension Fatigue Headache Dizziness Opioid withdrawal syndrome Anemia Constipation Skin rashes Specific to Implant: Local pruritus, local edema, local hemorrhage Injection: pain at injection site, bruising at injection site, induration at injection site, swelling at injection site, erythema at injection site	Hypersensitivity (e.g., anaphylaxis) to buprenorphine or any component of the formulation Significant respiratory depression. GI obstruction. Extended-release injection is not recommended in patients with moderate-to-severe hepatic impairment.	Discontinuation of therapy: When discontinuing sublingual buprenorphine for long-term treatment of opioid use disorder, use a gradual downward titration of the dose to prevent withdrawal; do not abruptly discontinue. Prescribing for opioid dependence is limited to physicians who have met the qualification criteria and have received a DEA number specific to prescribing this product. Older patients are more sensitive to the CNS depressant effects of opioid analgesic; therefore, use agents with caution. Monitor older patients for sedation and respiratory depression, particularly when initiating therapy. Extended-release injection: indicated for the treatment of moderate-to-severe opioid use disorder in patients who have initiated treatment with a transmucosal buprenorphine-containing product, followed by dose adjustment for a minimum of 7 days. Subdermal implant is indicated for maintenance treatment of opioid dependence in patients who have achieved and sustained prolonged clinical stability on low-to-moderate doses of a transmucosal buprenorphine-containing product (i.e., doses of no more than 8 mg/d of Subutex or Suboxone sublingual tablet or generic equivalent). Neonatal abstinence syndrome is an expected and treatable outcome of use of buprenorphine during pregnancy. Neonatal abstinence syndrome may be life-threatening if not recognized and treated in the neonate.
Methadone Oral: Initial: 20 to 30 mg (as a single dose) Maximum initial dose: 30 mg. Lower doses (5–10 mg) and much slower titration should be considered in patients with no or low tolerance at initiation. Patients should be monitored for oversedation and withdrawal symptoms for 2 to 4 hours after initial dose. An additional 5 to 10 mg may be provided if withdrawal symptoms have not been suppressed or if symptoms reappear after 2 to 4 hours. Total daily dose on the first day should not exceed 40 mg.	Hypotension EKG changes Torsades de pointes Syncope Tachycardia Sedation Nausea Respiratory depression Constipation	Hypersensitivity to methadone or any component.	Older adults: Decrease initial dose and monitor closely when initiating and titrating. Monitor closely due to an increased potential for risks, including certain risks such as falls/fracture, cognitive impairment, and constipation. Clearance may also be reduced in older adults, increasing the risk for respiratory depression or overdose. Neonatal opioid withdrawal syndrome is an expected and treatable outcome of use of methadone during pregnancy. Neonatal opioid withdrawal syndrome may be life-threatening if not recognized and treated in the neonate. Signs and symptoms include irritability, hyperactivity and abnormal sleep pattern, high-pitched cry, tremor, vomiting, diarrhea, and failure to gain weight. Onset, duration, and severity depend on the drug used, duration of use, maternal dose, and rate of drug elimination by the newborn. Incomplete cross-tolerance: Use caution in converting patients from other opioids to methadone. Follow appropriate conversion recommendations. Patients tolerant to other *mu* opioid agonists may not be tolerant to methadone and at risk for severe respiratory depression when converted to methadone.

(Continued)

TABLE 43.3

Medications Used in Opioid Use Disorder (*Continued*)

Medication	Contraindications	Adverse Effects	Special Considerations
Maintenance: Titrate to a dosage that prevents opioid withdrawal symptoms for 24 hours, prevents craving, attenuates euphoric effect of self-administered opioids, and provides tolerance to sedative effects of methadone. Usual range: 80 to 120 mg/d (titration should occur cautiously).			Opioid use disorder: When switching patients from methadone to buprenorphine, patients should preferably be on low doses of oral methadone (<30–40 mg/d) prior to the switch to lessen discomfort. Patients switching from methadone to naltrexone (oral or extended-release IM) require complete withdrawal from methadone or other opioids before naltrexone initiation (typically achieved in 7 days but up to 14 days may be necessary).
Lofexidine (Lucemyra)			
Three 0.18 mg tablets (0.54 mg) PO QID during the period of peak withdrawal symptoms. Doses should be spaced about 5 to 6 hours apart with the total daily dosage not exceeding 2.88 mg (16 tablets). No single dose should exceed 0.72 mg (4 tablets).	No contraindications	Insomnia, sedation and somnolence. Dizziness, hypotension, orthostatic hypotension, and bradycardia. Dry mouth and tinnitus. Prolongation of QTc interval.	To discontinue lofexidine, the dose should be gradually reduced over a 2–4-day period reducing the dose by 1 tablet per dose every 1–2 days.

CNS, central nervous system; DEA, drug enforcement agency; EKG, electrocardiogram; GI, gastrointestinal; IM, intramuscular.

over a 2 to 4 day period, reducing the dose by 1 tablet per dose every 1 to 2 days.

For patients with a CrCl of 30mL/min to 90mL/min, the dose is reduced to 2 tablets four times daily (total dose = 1.44 mg/d) and for patients with a CrCl less than 30mL/min, the dose is 1 tablet four times daily (0.72 mg/d). For those patients with mild and moderate hepatic impairment, the dose is 2.16 mg and 1.44 mg daily, respectively. For those with severe hepatic impairment, the dose is 0.72 mg/d.

Time Frame for Response
Lofexidine is well absorbed orally with a peak plasma concentration occurring in 3 to 5 hours after administration of a single dose.

Contraindications
There are no specific contraindications to lofexidine.

Adverse Events
Insomnia occurs in more than 50% of patients but sedation and somnolence may occur in about 11% to 13% of patients. Dizziness, hypotension, orthostatic hypotension, and bradycardia have been reported in more than 20% of patients. Dry mouth and tinnitus have also been reported.

Interactions
Concurrent use with methadone can cause a prolonged QT interval and, therefore, cardiac monitoring is indicated.

Methadone

Methadone, a Schedule II controlled substance, is effective in treating OUD by reducing cravings and minimizing the euphoric effects of other opioid agonists. Methadone is also used for the treatment of pain, but when being used for OUD, it is only available through federally regulated OTP—often referred to as methadone clinics. At these facilities, the liquid formulation is usually dispensed, and doses are provided daily under supervision of clinic personnel to avoid diversion.

Mechanism of Action
Methadone is a synthetic opioid with full *mu*-agonist activity, similar to morphine. Because of its antagonistic effects at the N-methyl-D-aspartate (NMDA) receptor, it is thought to be less likely to produce tolerance.

Dosage
The initial dose of methadone for OUD is 20 to 30 mg (as a single dose), with careful titration up using 5 to 10 mg increments if withdrawal symptoms have not been suppressed or if symptoms reappear after 2 to 4 hours. Total daily dose on the first day should not exceed 40 mg. Maintenance dosage is one in which opioid withdrawal symptoms such as craving are prevented and the euphoric effect of self-administered opioids are attenuated. Usual range of maintenance is 80 to 120 mg/d.

Time Frame for Response

Methadone has a wide oral bioavailability, ranging from 36% to 100% and peak plasma concentrations are achieved between 1 and 7.5 hours. Methadone's half-life can range between 8 and 59 hours with a duration of effect lasting approximately 30 hours.

Contraindications

Methadone is contraindicated in patients with a known hypersensitivity to the agent, those with a paralytic ileus and any patient in whom opioids are contraindicated, such as those with respiratory depression or acute asthma.

Adverse Events

There is an FDA black box warning emphasizing the potential for respiratory depression and risk of abuse/dependence. There is no ceiling effect and therefore carries a greater risk of respiratory depression if dosed inappropriately. Respiratory rate should be monitored during initiation and titration of methadone doses and extra care is warranted in patients taking other medications that may cause CNS or respiratory depression. Methadone also carries a risk of torsades de pointes. Other adverse events include lightheadedness, dizziness, sedation, nausea, vomiting, and sweating.

Interactions

Methadone is primarily metabolized by CYP2B6, CYP2D6, and CYP3A4 enzyme systems and, therefore, patients taking drugs that inhibit or induce these enzymes will change the pharmacokinetics of the drugs.

Naltrexone

Naltrexone blocks the effects of opioids by competitive binding at opioid receptors. Long-acting injectable is administered once monthly and has shown evidence to decrease heroin use compared to placebo. Its benefits compared to methadone and buprenorphine primarily reside in the fact prescribers do not have to have specialized trainer and obtain a waiver to prescribe it nor must it be dispensed via an OTP. It may decrease cravings for opioids after a number of weeks, and decreases the risk of overdose (see **Table 43.2**).

Selecting the Most Appropriate Drug

Like treatment for AUD, long-term pharmacotherapy for OUD should be considered simultaneously with the detoxification process. All of the FDA-approved medications for OUD are safe and effective and any can be used for most patients. Pharmacotherapy should not be withheld from a patient due to their lack of participation in structured behavioral treatment and all OUD patients and family/support system members should be offered access to naloxone in case of an opioid overdose in the future (**Figure 43.3**). See **Table 43.3** for specifics on each drug.

First-Line Therapy

Buprenorphine or buprenorphine/naloxone is the preferred treatment in primary care because of its efficacy in maintaining reduced opioid use or abstinence and a reduction in opioid overdose deaths. Because it may induce withdrawal, clinicians should verify that the patient is already experiencing signs and symptoms of opioid withdrawal before starting treatment.

Second-Line Therapy

Since methadone and buprenorphine are, at evidence-based recommended doses, equally effective (Mattick et al., 2014), accessing methadone via on OTP makes this agent a second-line drug. Further, the stigma associated with methadone, along with the potential for side effects, further differentiates this drug from buprenorphine. However, if a patient prefers methadone, or has difficulty in accessing buprenorphine, or if the patient has continued cravings (or withdrawal) while on buprenorphine, methadone is a very suitable alternative.

Third-Line Therapy

Oral naltrexone is no better than placebo in the treatment of OUD; therefore, only the injectable formulation is used as primary pharmacotherapy. The primary reason for the lack of success for the oral formulation is attributed to poor medication adherence. To that end, while the injectable formulation is administered once monthly, adherence to continued treatment is essential for success. The clinicians should assure that the patient no longer has opioids in their system by having at least 7 to 10 days of verified abstinence or administer a naloxone challenge before administering naltrexone. This will minimize the potential for a withdrawal reaction from injectable naltrexone.

Special Considerations

Pediatric

It is well accepted that adolescents appear to be disproportionately at risk from the rest of the population, and that initiation of substance misuse during the early teen years places an individual at higher risk for developing an SUD later on in life (Compton, 2019). Further, individuals who have been exposed to childhood trauma are also at an increased risk of developing an alcohol or SUD (Fellitti, 1998) and this risk increases with the increased number of traumas (e.g., physical, mental, sexual).

Geriatric

As the percentage of the population over the age 65 continues to increase, the number of older adults experiencing an SUD also increases. Further, the baby boomer segment of the population, which grew up in the 1960s and 1970s, has a more lenient attitude toward drug and alcohol use. Thus, the perception of misuse among these individuals may be different. Nonetheless, while there is an increasing prevalence of illicit (opioid and cannabis) misuse in this population, alcohol remains the most common substance used by this population.

As discussed in Chapter 5, older adults typically metabolize substances more slowly and their body may be more sensitive

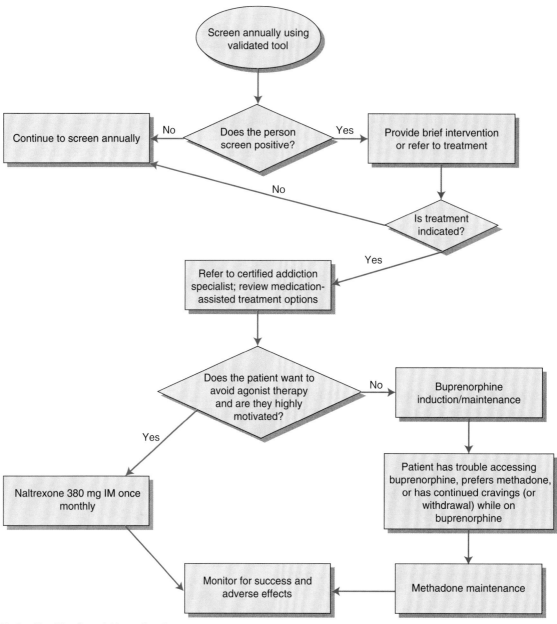

FIGURE 43–3 Algorithm for opioid use disorder.

IM, intramuscular.

to drug effects than younger patients. Changes in reaction time and coordination and impaired judgment from substances can lead to more falls and accidents in this population, which in turn pose a greater risk for other health complications.

Women

While men are more likely than women to misuse drugs, women are just as likely to develop an SUD as men (NIDA, 2020). Further there may be social and environmental factors which can influence drug use/misuse among women, and women who have been subjected to domestic violence and/or sexual trauma or abuse are at increased risk of an SUD. Further, data do suggest that women may have more drug cravings than

men and may be more likely to have a recurrence of use. The clinician should also consider the pregnant patient with an SUD, as it places both the mother and the unborn child at risk. Regular use of drugs during pregnancy can lead to neonatal abstinence syndrome—a condition in which the baby goes through withdrawal—or even still birth.

MONITORING PATIENT RESPONSE

Prior to the initiation of pharmacotherapy for either AUD or OUD, baseline labs including renal and hepatic function need to be obtained. This will help in identifying potential dosage adjustments and will serve as a baseline for monitoring adverse effects and return to normal values (e.g., liver function tests in AUD patient). These laboratory values should be repeated at 6- and 12-month intervals, or more frequently should adverse effects appear or inefficacy of treatment. Patient should be monitored for recurrence of use and/or withdrawal symptoms.

PATIENT EDUCATION

Patients should be educated on the effects and adverse effects of the medication they are taking. With all of these medications, and particularly naltrexone, medication compliance is key to success and the patient needs to be counseled on the importance of taking the medication as prescribed. Further, because of the potential for CNS depression with some of the medications used to treat SUD, patients need to be advised against self-medicating with agents that may affect alertness and cognition.

One of the components of patient education is a discussion of long-term sobriety and recovery in general. SAMHSA defines recovery as "a process of change through which individuals improve their health and wellness, live self-directed lives, and strive to reach their full potential." (SAMHSA-b, 2020), Most research indicates that individuals cannot maintain recovery without a support system. Recovery support systems, designed to prevent a recurrence of harmful use, range from self-help groups to sober living homes. Self-help groups (i.e., Alcoholics Anonymous, Narcotics Anonymous or SMART recovery) are often the mainstay of support groups, but other recovery-oriented care and support systems such as recovery community centers (RCC) exist to help people maintain wellness. A RCC is a peer-operated centered that serves as a local resource for advocacy training and recovery information along with access to self-help groups. These services are provided by trained peers, community allies, or faith-based organizations. Individuals do not live at a RCC, like they do in a sober home, but rather access these services as needed.

Drug Information

There are a variety of sources of information related to SUD, particularly related to pharmacotherapy. In response to the opioid epidemic, SAMHSA has created a website, Providers Clinical Support System, dedicated to the education of medical professionals on the subject of SUD, with a focus on OUD and MAT. Topics include buprenorphine induction, transitioning patients from methadone to buprenorphine, drug–drug interactions, and regulatory issues, including information on how to obtain a DATA waiver to prescribe buprenorphine. The current website is www.pcssnow.org

The National Institute for Drug Abuse (NIDA) also has a host of resources, categorized by professional discipline and specialty. Information and continuing education is available

for dentists, nurse practitioners, physicians, physician assistants, pharmacists, as well as other healthcare professionals. Access to the current, validated screening tools is also available on this site with a comparative chart on which tools are best for which substance, population, and patient age. The current website for this resource is https://www.drugabuse.gov/nidamed-medical-health-professionals

Patient-Oriented Information Sources

The American Society for Addiction Medicine has several resources for patients to access. The information contained therein has information for the patient, the patient's families and friends, along with information on accessing providers specializing in alcohol treatment or those with the ability to prescribe buprenorphine for OUD patients. As noted above, NIDA also has information for clinicians to access to provide to patients including easy-to-read drug facts and information in Spanish.

Nutrition/Lifestyle Changes

Recovering from an SUD involves a life-style change. Nutrition support for patients with an SUD varies by drug and is complicated by other factors including the patient's potential co-occurring mental health disorders, socioeconomic situation, and lack of peer/family support. Both primary malnutrition, which occurs when the substance replaces other dietary nutrients, and secondary malnutrition can occur in patients with misusing any substance.

One of the primary nutritional concerns in patients with AUD is *metabolic syndrome*. This syndrome, characterized by increased abdominal obesity, hyperglycemia, high cholesterol, and high blood pressure, is exacerbated by the cell damage and higher caloric intake seen in patients consuming alcohol in large quantities. Thiamine deficiency may also occur in the AUD patient due to decreased absorption. Thiamine plays a role in metabolizing glucose to produce energy for the brain. Wernicke's encephalopathy, an acute life-threatening neurological condition characterized by the triad of nystagmus, ataxia, and confusion, can result from the administration of glucose in the absence of thiamine. Therefore, in any heavy alcohol user, thiamine needs to be administered prior to initiation of any nutritional intervention.

Complementary and Alternative Medications

Complementary and alternative medicine practices can improve chances of recovery from SUDs, especially when used in addition to traditional SUD treatments. These practices are not designed to replace behavioral and/or pharmacotherapeutic treatments, but to complement them instead. These include meditation, yoga, massage, guided imagery, music therapy, and biofeedback/acupuncture. These can be offered/provided to patients individually or in a group setting.

CASE STUDY 1

Mr. Brightside is a 48-year-old white male. One week ago, his wife, also a patient of yours, started to talk about Mr. B. She related that at times, she has noted Mr. B slurring his words during dinner, only after 1 to 2 glasses of wine; and that on weekends, he sits in front of the TV drinking, mostly beer. About three months ago, Mr. B was stopped while driving and received a Driving Under the Influence (DUI), his second in the past 5 years. She thinks he has a drinking problem. You agreed to talk to Mr. B at his next visit.

1. How would you approach the patient?
2. Which screening test will you use to assess if Mr. B needs a brief intervention or referral to treatment?

3. After further inquiry and investigation, you find it is clear that there is significant clinical impairment in his functioning as a result of his alcohol use. You decide he should be referred to a substance abuse treatment provider for further evaluation and treatment. What medication would you recommend he be started on and why?

BIBLIOGRAPHY

*Starred references are cited in the text.

*Addictionary. (2019). https://www.recoveryanswers.org/addiction-ary/

Anthony, J. C., Warner, L. A., & Kessler, R. C. (1994). Comparative epidemiology of dependence on tobacco, alcohol, controlled substances, and inhalants: Basic findings from the National Comorbidity Survey. *Experimental and Clinical Psychopharmacology, 2*(3), 244–268. doi: 10.1037/1064-1297.2.3.244

*CDC/NCHS. (2018). National Vital Statistics System, Mortality. CDC WONDER, Atlanta, GA: US Department of Health and Human Services, CDC. https://wonder.cdc.gov

Center for Behavioral Health Statistics and Quality. (2016). Key substance use and mental health indicators in the United States: Results from the 2015 National Survey on Drug Use and Health (HHS Publication No. SMA 16-4984, NSDUH Series H-51). Retrieved from https://www.samhsa.gov/data/

*Centers for Disease Control and Prevention (CDC). (2018). 2018 Annual Surveillance Report of Drug-Related Risks and Outcomes—United States. Surveillance Special Report. Centers for Disease Control and Prevention, U.S. Department of Health and Human Services. Published August 31, 2018. https://www.cdc.gov/drugoverdose/pdf/pubs/2018-cdc-drug-surveillance-report.pdf

*Compton, W. M., Jones, C. M., Baldwin, G. T., et al. (2019). Targeting youth to prevent later substance use disorder: an underutilized response to the US opioid crisis. *Am J Public Health. 109*(S3):S185–S189.

*Cotto, J. H., Davis, E., Dowling, G. J., Elcano, J. C., Staton, A. B., & Weiss, S. R. (2010). Gender effects on drug use, abuse, and dependence: A special analysis of results from the National Survey on Drug Use and Health. *Gend Med. 7*(5):402-413.

*Hasin, D. S., O'Brien C. P., Auriacombe, M., et al. (2013). DSM-5 criteria for substance use disorders: Recommendations and rationale. *Am J Psychiatry. 170*(8):834–851.

*Ma, G. X., & Shive, S. (2000). A comparative analysis of perceived risks and substance abuse among ethnic groups. *Addict Behav. 25*(3):361-371.

*Manasco, A., Chang, S., Larriviere, J., Hamm, L. L., & Glass, M. (2012). Alcohol withdrawal. *South Med J. 105*(11), 607–612.

*Mattick, R. P., Breen, C., Kimber, J., et al. (2014). Methadone maintenance therapy versus no opioid replacement therapy for opioid dependence. *Cochrane Database of Systematic Reviews,* (3), CD002209. doi: 10.1002/14651858.CD002209.pub2

*National Survey on Drug Use and Health (NSDUH). (2018). Substance Abuse and Mental Health Services Administration, Center for Behavioral Health Statistics and Quality, National Survey on Drug Use and Health. https://www.cdc.gov/nchs/data/hus/2018/020.pdf. Accessed on November 10, 2020.

*NIDA. (2003, January 1). Diagnosis and Treatment of Drug Abuse in Family Practice—American Family Physician Monograph. Retrieved from https://archives.drugabuse.gov/publications/diagnosis-treatment-drug-abuse-in-family-practice-american-family-physician-monograph on November 10, 2020.

*NIDA. (2020, May 28). Sex and gender differences in substance use. Retrieved from https://www.drugabuse.gov/publications/research-reports/substance-use-in-women/sex-gender-differences-in-substance-use on November 17, 2020.

*Substance Abuse and Mental Health Administration (SAMHSA-a). (2020). Mental health and substance use disorders. https://www.samhsa.gov/find-help/recovery. Accessed on March 14, 2021.

*Substance Abuse and Mental Health Administration (SAMHSA-b). (2020). Mental health and substance use disorders. https://www.samhsa.gov/brss-tacs/recovery-support-tools-resources. Accessed on November 10, 2020.

*Substance Abuse and Mental Health Administration (SAMHSA-c). (2020). Become a Buprenorphine Waivered Practitioner. https://www.samhsa.gov/medication-assisted-treatment/become-buprenorphine-waivered-practitioner. Accessed March 14, 2021.

*Swift, R. M., & Aston, E. R. (2015). Pharmacotherapy for alcohol use disorder: Current and emerging therapies. *Harvard Review of Psychiatry, 23*(2), 122–133. https://doi.org/10.1097/HRP.0000000000000079

*Volkow, N. (2019). Access to addiction services differs by race and gender. https://www.drugabuse.gov/about-nida/noras-blog/2019/07/access-to-addiction-services-differs-by-race-gender. Accessed on November 2020.

UNIT
12

Pharmacotherapy
for Endocrine Disorders

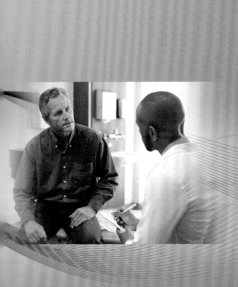

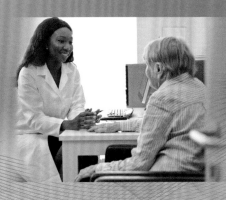

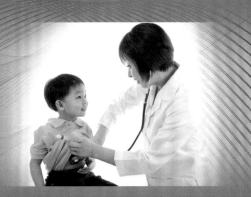

Diabetes Mellitus

Angela Thompson and Lorraine Nowakowski-Grier

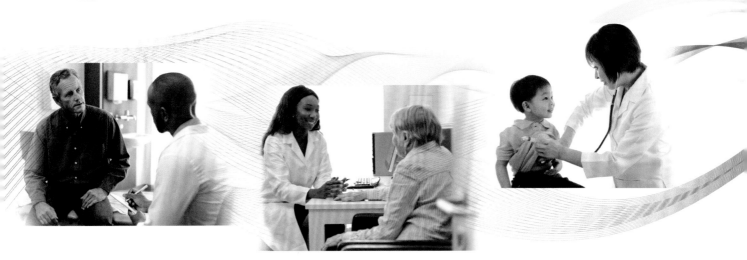

Learning Objectives

1. Identify the various pharmacological approaches to glycemic management in diabetes.
2. Discuss drug- and patient-specific factors to consider when selecting anti-hyperglycemic therapies.
3. Discuss the selection and initiation of insulin therapy.

INTRODUCTION

Diabetes mellitus is the term used to represent a clinically and genetically heterogeneous group of disorders characterized by abnormally high blood glucose levels (hyperglycemia) as a result of either absolute insulin deficiency or a combination of relative insulin deficiency with cellular resistance to the action of insulin. Four major classifications of diabetes have been identified: type 1 diabetes mellitus (formerly known as *insulin-dependent diabetes mellitus*), type 2 diabetes mellitus (formerly known as *non–insulin-dependent diabetes mellitus*), gestational diabetes mellitus, and specific types of diabetes due to other conditions (e.g., drug or chemically induced, diseases of the exocrine pancreas, and monogenic forms).

According to the Centers for Disease Control and Prevention (CDC, 2017a), there are more than 30.3 million people with diabetes in the United States. Among them, 90% to 95% have type 2 diabetes. Additionally, there are another 84.1 million who have a condition called *prediabetes*, which is a high risk condition for the development of diabetes (CDC, 2017a). Diabetes is the seventh leading cause of death in the United States and overall, the risk of death among people with diabetes is approximately twice that of people without diabetes. The annual medical costs for diabetes in the United States in 2017 was 327 billion in direct and indirect costs (CDC, 2017a).

CAUSES

Type 1 diabetes is thought to be an autoimmune disease in which pancreatic beta cells are destroyed. The beta cells are responsible for secreting insulin, a major hormone that promotes cellular uptake and use of glucose and maintains metabolic functions throughout the body. When the beta cells are destroyed, the pancreas produces no insulin, causing glucose levels in the blood to rise dramatically. Onset can occur at any time, but most patients are younger than age 30.

The underlying pathophysiology of type 1 diabetes includes the genetic predisposition for beta cell destruction and environmental factors. The environmental factors that contribute to type 1 diabetes are not as well defined. Viral agents have long been suspected as an environmental trigger in the pathogenesis of type 1 diabetes. Viral illness such as mumps, rubella, varicella, measles, influenza, coxsackievirus, cytomegalovirus, and viral pneumonia have been reported to precede the onset of type 1 diabetes. Furthermore, the incidence increases in the United States during the fall and winter, when viral infections are prevalent. Autoimmunity is evident because 80% of patients with type 1 diabetes test positive for specific human leukocyte antigen. It is likely that a combination of these factors contributes to the destruction of beta cells and the subsequent absence of insulin.

- Family history of diabetes (i.e., parents or siblings with diabetes)
- Obesity (i.e., 20% over desired body weight or body mass index >27 kg/m^2; for Asian Americans, it is >23 kg/m^2)
- Race/ethnicity (e.g., African Americans, Hispanic Americans, Native Americans, Asian Americans, Pacific Islanders have increased risk)
- Age older than 45 years
- Previously identified as having IFG
- Hypertension
- HDL cholesterol level less than 35 mg/dL or triglyceride level greater than 250 mg/dL
- History of gestational diabetes mellitus or delivery of babies weighing greater than 9 lb
- Sedentary lifestyle

In type 2 diabetes, adipose and muscle cells become less sensitive to the actions of insulin and the pancreas produces less insulin than the body needs. As a result, glucose levels in the blood escalate. The highest incidence of type 2 diabetes occurs in those individuals over the age of 30; however, type 2 diabetes can occur at any age. **Box 44.1** lists risk factors for type 2 diabetes; the major risk factors are obesity and family history. Both beta cell defects and insulin resistance are found in patients with type 2 diabetes.

In gestational diabetes, pregnancy causes the woman to become intolerant to glucose. The causes are not fully clear, but they appear to be related to the anti-insulin effects created by progesterone, cortisol, and human placental lactogen. Usually, once the woman has delivered her infant, blood glucose levels return to normal; however, women who have had gestational diabetes have a 20% to 50% chance of developing diabetes in the next 5 to 10 years.

There are other types of diabetes that can occur due to other causes, and they include monogenic forms of diabetes, diabetes from pancreatic exocrine dysfunction, and drug or chemical induction diabetes. These forms of diabetes represent less than 5% of those diagnosed with diabetes (ADA, 2020). Insulin deficiency is the primary defect seen in these secondary forms of diabetes but the offending agent(s) vary.

Cystic fibrosis-related diabetes (CFRD) is one of the most common comorbidities of cystic fibrosis with over 50% propensity (ADA, 2020). Screening for CFRD should be performed using the oral glucose tolerance test (OGTT) within 5 years of initial diagnosis.

Posttransplant diabetes is another less common form of diabetes mellitus. Immunosuppressant agents are considered the primary contributing factor.

Monogenic forms of diabetes are related to autosomal dominant defect. There are over 13 different genets identified to date but maturity-onset diabetes of the young (MODY) is the most common form of monogenic diabetes. MODY is characterized by young age of onset and successive generations of diabetes.

PATHOPHYSIOLOGY

In type 1 diabetes, the pancreatic beta cells are destroyed, causing a subsequent absence of insulin. In genetically susceptible people, an autoimmune attack occurs in which monocytes/macrophages and activated cytotoxic T cells infiltrate the islets. Multiple antibodies against beta cell antigens develop in the blood, and insulin reserve steadily decreases until the amount is insufficient to maintain a normal blood glucose level.

The pathogenesis of type 2 diabetes involves insulin resistance, impaired insulin secretion, and elevated glucose production by the liver. With insulin resistance, circulating insulin concentrations increase as compensation. Researchers have hypothesized that in type 2 diabetes, the ability of insulin to inhibit hepatic glucose production and to stimulate its uptake and use by adipose and muscle cells is diminished. In lean patients with type 2 diabetes, the primary defect appears to occur in the beta cells. In overweight patients, who represent most patients with type 2 diabetes, the most likely primary defect is impairment of the target cells. Although abnormal hepatic glucose metabolism plays an important role in maintaining the diabetic state, it is probably not the earliest development and most likely follows impaired insulin sensitivity in the muscle.

Insulin affects many body systems, and chronic hyperinsulinemia contributes to the pathogenesis and worsening of hypertension, dyslipidemia, and coronary heart disease. Hypertension, high plasma triglyceride levels, and low high-density lipoprotein (HDL) plasma levels correlate with hyperinsulinemia secondary to insulin resistance and a worsened cardiovascular risk profile. This collection of clinical markers or indicators associated with insulin resistance is referred to as *metabolic syndrome*.

Epidemiologic and interventional studies consistently point to the relationship between good glycemic control and the prevention or slowing of the progression of long-term complications of diabetes. The Diabetes Control and Complications Trial Research Group (1993) (DCCT) presented definitive evidence to support the hypothesis that diabetic complications are related to the degree of hyperglycemia. In this landmark study, patients with type 1 diabetes were randomized to two groups and followed for an average of 6.5 years. One group received conventional therapy (one or two daily insulin injections, daily self-monitoring of glucose, and diabetes education) to normalize blood glucose levels; the other group received intensive therapy (three or more daily administrations of insulin and glucose monitoring four times daily). The incidence of microvascular complications was 60% lower in the group that received intensive therapy compared with the group that received conventional therapy. Hence, intensive therapy delayed the onset of complications and slowed their progression. The UK Prospective Diabetes Study Group (1998a, 1998b) (UKPDS) Group answered the question as to whether the DCCT results could be extrapolated to include type 2 diabetes. In the UKPDS, patients with type 2 diabetes were randomized to intensive or conventional therapy and followed over a 10-year period. As in the DCCT, there was a significant (25%) risk reduction in microvascular end points with tight control.

DIAGNOSTIC CRITERIA

Many patients with marked hyperglycemia present with the classic symptoms of polyuria (excessive urination), polydipsia (increased thirst), weight loss, polyphagia (increased hunger and caloric intake), and blurred vision. In type 1 diabetes, the onset of these symptoms usually is more rapid and often preceded by ketoacidosis. In contrast, the course of development for type 2 diabetes can be more gradual, insidious, and frequently undiagnosed for years. The onset and sometimes the presence of symptoms often go unnoticed. Therefore, screening for diabetes as part of a routine medical examination is appropriate if a patient has one or more risk factors (see **Box 44.1**). The more risk factors that the individual has, the greater the chances are that the individual develops diabetes. Because early detection and prompt treatment may reduce the impact of diabetes and its complications, screening is recommended for those at risk.

The new consensus for diagnosis and screening includes use of hemoglobin A1c (A1c). Fasting plasma glucose (FPG) can also be used; less often, the OGTT is employed. FPG and now the A1c are generally the easiest and least expensive diagnostic tests. Fasting is defined as no intake of food or beverage other than water for at least 8 hours before testing. The OGTT is still the preferred screening test for the diagnoses of gestational diabetes in pregnant women. It can be performed in either a one-step or a two-step method and is usually administered between 28 to 30 weeks gestation.

Normal glucose is defined as an FPG level of less than 100 mg/dL and a 2-hour post load glucose (PG) value in the OGTT of less than 140 mg/dL. A normal A1c is less than 5.7 and can be obtained regardless of the last oral intake. Those who test higher than or equal to 6.5% should have repeat testing to confirm the diagnosis. An FPG level of 126 mg/dL or more or a 2-hour PG value in the OGTT of 200 mg/dL or more warrants repeat testing on a different day to confirm the diagnosis. Patients with an FPG of at least 100 mg/dL but less than 126 mg/dL have impaired fasting glucose (IFG). Patients with a 2-hour PG value of at least 140 mg/dL but less than 200 mg/dL in the OGTT are considered as having impaired glucose tolerance (IGT). Patients with IFG or IGT are now referred to as having *prediabetes*, indicating the relatively high risk of developing diabetes. Diagnostic criteria are presented in **Table 44.1**.

TABLE 44.1

Criteria for the Diagnosis of Diabetes Mellitus

Normoglycemia	Impaired Glucose Metabolism (Prediabetes)	Diabetes Mellitus
A1c 4%–5.6%	5.7%–6.4%	A1c ≥ 6.5%
FPG < 100 mg/dL	FPG 100–125 mg/dL (IFG)	FPG ≥ 126 mg/dL
OGTT PG < 140 mg/dL	OGTT 140–199 mg/dL (IGT)	≥200 mg/dL
Random plasma glucose ≥200 mg/dL and symptoms of diabetes mellitus		>200 mg/dL

FPG, fasting plasma glucose; IFG, impaired fasting glucose; IGT, impaired glucose tolerance; OGTT, oral glucose tolerance test; PG, plasma glucose.

Plasma glucose levels can be obtained from patients regardless of the time the patients last ate. Such levels are referred to as random plasma glucose levels. Any random plasma glucose level of 200 mg/dL or more is considered positive for diabetes and warrants additional testing, preferably on another day.

Many medications have an adverse effect on glucose metabolism. While medications are not usually a true etiologic factor for diabetes, they can unmask less obvious glucose intolerance that had not yet been detected. These medications include glucocorticoids, certain antipsychotics, thiazide diuretics, and some HIV medications and immunosuppressant agents.

INITIATING DRUG THERAPY

Effective treatment programs for diabetes mellitus require comprehensive training in self-management, ongoing support from the clinical care team, and, for many, intensive pharmacologic regimens. These programs must be individualized according to each patient's needs and should include the following features:

- Self-monitoring of blood glucose (SMBG)
- Medical nutrition therapy
- Regular exercise or physical activity
- Drug therapy individualized for each patient
- Instruction in the prevention and treatment of acute and chronic complications, including hypoglycemia
- Continuing patient education and support
- Periodic assessment of treatment goals

There are four critical times to evaluate for the appropriateness of diabetes self-management education: at diagnosis, when transitions in care occur, when complicating factors arise (new health conditions, physical limitations, etc.), and annually (ADA, 2020).

The cornerstone of treatment for all patients with diabetes is lifestyle interventions that combine medication nutrition therapy with routine or regular physical activity. The goals of therapy require individualization and often differ between types of diabetes, developmental age, and whether comorbidities and complications of diabetes exist. For those patients who are at their ideal body weight, the lifestyle interventions would be more directed toward regulation of caloric intake to maintain weight and glucose control, whereas those patients above their ideal body weight would have interventions directed to achieving weight loss. Weight loss leads to improved glucose tolerance by enhancing the sensitivity of peripheral glucose receptors. Physical activity and exercise have been shown to be of equal importance in both prevention and in the treatment of type 2 diabetes. Regular physical activity can prevent or delay the onset of type 2 diabetes and its complications. The Diabetes Prevention Program (DPP) was a landmark randomized clinical trial of 3,234 overweight individuals with prediabetes in the United States (DPP, 2002). The DPP found lifestyle intervention to be more effective than metformin in preventing type 2 diabetes. The trial reported that intensive lifestyle intervention decreased the incidence of type 2 diabetes by 58%, compared with 31% in the group taking metformin.

If these interventions fail to achieve desirable glycemic control, practitioners should then consider pharmacological approaches.

Goals of Drug Therapy

The major goals of drug therapy in diabetes mellitus have been established by the ADA and the American Association of Clinical Endocrinology (AACE), and while they are similar, there is some variance, as discussed in the following section.

GLYCEMIC CONTROL

American Diabetes Association

- **A1c** <7.0%. Individualized based on the patient considerations of duration of disease; age/life expectancy; comorbid conditions, known cardiovascular disease (CVD) or advanced microvascular complications; risks for hypoglycemia; resources; and support system, in addition to patient preference.
- More (6.5%) or less (8.0%) stringent glycemic goals may be appropriate based on the previously mentioned criteria.

American Association of Clinical Endocrinologist

- **A1c** 6.5% or less. Individualized based on age, comorbidities, duration of disease
- Closer to normal for healthy
- Less stringent for "less healthy"

American Diabetes Association (ADA) Daily Glucose Goals

- Preprandial glucose 80 to 130 mg/dL
- Postprandial glucose less than 180 mg/dL

American Association of Clinical Endocrinology Daily Glucose Goals

- Preprandial glucose goals less than 110 mg/dL
- Postprandial glucose less than 140 mg/dL

BLOOD PRESSURE

- Less than 140/90 mm Hg in patients with less than 15% 10-year atherosclerotic cardiovascular disease (ASCVD) risk
- 130/80 mm Hg in patients with more than 15% 10-year ASCVD risk of established CVD
- 125/75 in patients with proteinuria

LIPIDS-GOAL IS TO REDUCED LOW-DENSITY LIPOPROTEIN BY 50%

Primary Prevention

Age 20 to 39 years with ASCVD risk factors: Consider initiating statin.

Age 40 to 74 years without ASCVD: Consider moderate intensity statin.

Age 40 to 74 with multiple risk factors for ASCVD: Consider high-intensity statin.

Secondary Prevention

For all ages with established ASCVD, initiate high dose statin.

Consider adding PCSL9 inhibitor or ezetimibe if low-density lipoprotein (LDL) more than 70 despite lifestyle and maximally tolerated statin.

There is less evidence to support treatment of other lipoprotein abnormalities such as hypertriglyceridemia for the primary prevention of ASCVD. In patients with established ASCVD and hypertriglyceridemia between 135 to 499 mg/dL, icosapent ethyl has shown promise for primary prevention (ADA, 2010).

For the primary prevention of hypertriglyceridemia, lifestyle interventions should be employed in addition to the investigation of secondary causes (uncontrolled diabetes, nephrotic syndrome, and liver disease). Pharmacological interventions such as fibric acid derivatives or fish oil can be considered if fasting triglycerides are more than 500 mg/dL for the prevention of pancreatitis.

MICROALBUMIN: RANDOM COLLECTION

The criterion is less than 30 mcg/mL creatinine. In type 1 diabetes, insulin is the mainstay of pharmacological therapy. Lifestyle interventions in addition to metformin are the recommended initial treatment for type 2 diabetes. For individuals with an intolerance to metformin or contraindication, another pharmacological class should be considered. The ADA suggests that pharmacologic therapy be selected with consideration to the following factors:

- Efficacy
- Risk for hypoglycemia
- Impact on weight
- Patient preference
- Cardiovascular (CV) and renal comorbidities
- Cost
- Side effects and adverse reactions

Sulfonylureas

Sulfonylureas are a major group of oral hypoglycemic agents used to treat adults with type 2 diabetes (see **Table 44.2**). They are not approved for use in children with type 2 diabetes.

Mechanism of Action

Sulfonylureas bind to specific receptors on beta cells, causing adenosine triphosphate (ATP)–dependent potassium channels to close. The calcium channels subsequently open, leading to increased cytoplasmic calcium, which stimulates the release of insulin. Theorists have hypothesized that these drugs also have

TABLE 44.2

Overview of Oral Antidiabetic Agents

Generic (Trade) Name and Dosage	Selected Adverse Events	Contraindications	Special Considerations
Sulfonylureas			
SECOND GENERATION			
Glyburide (DiaBeta, Micronase)	Hypoglycemia	Hypersensitivity to sulfonamides and Type 1 Diabetes	Onset occurs within 1.5 h, lasts 18–24 h.
Initially 2.5–5 mg daily; increase by 2.5 mg/wk until desired blood glucose			Same as above.
Older adults start at 1.25 mg/day			
Maximum dose 20 mg/day			
Glyburide, micronized (Glynase) Initially 1.5–3 mg daily; 0.75 mg in older adults	Same as above	Same as above	Onset occurs within 1.5 h, lasts 18–24 h. Same as above.
Maximum dose 12 mg/day			
Glipizide (Glucotrol) Initially 5 mg daily (2.5 mg in older adults); increase weekly to a maximum of 40 mg/day to desired blood glucose	Same as above	Same as above	Patients should take medication 30 min before a meal. Onset occurs within 1 h, lasts for 10–24 h. Same as above.
Glimepiride (Amaryl) Initially 1–2 mg with breakfast; increase by 2 mg/wk until desired blood glucose	Same as above	Same as above	Onset occurs within 2–4 h, lasts 24 h. Same as above.
Maximum dose 8 mg/day			
BIGUANIDE			
Metformin (Glucophage) Initially 500 mg BID; increase by 500 mg/wk until desired blood glucose	GI distress: diarrhea, nausea, bloating, flatulence Rare lactic acidosis	Renal dysfunction, CHF, metabolic acidosis, ketoacidosis, impaired hepatic function, excess alcohol consumption, pregnancy	Patients should take with meals to minimize GI side effects. Medication must be temporarily held when the patient is undergoing IV iodinated contrast study.
Maximum dose 2,550 mg/day in divided doses			Modest synergistic effect may occur when given with sulfonylurea. Medication should be held for patients undergoing surgery.

(Continued)

TABLE 44.2

Overview of Oral Antidiabetic Agents (*Continued*)

Generic (Trade) Name and Dosage	Selected Adverse Events	Contraindications	Special Considerations
Thiazolidinediones			
Rosiglitazone (Avandia) Initially 4 mg/day in single dose; if response is inadequate after 12 wk, increase to 8 mg/day in single dose	Anemia, edema, headache, reversible increase in ALT	Children, ketoacidosis	Monitor ALT at baseline, every 2 mo for the first 12 mo and periodically thereafter. Discontinue medication if ALT is greater than three times the upper limit of normal or if jaundice occurs. Medications may increase plasma volume; caution is necessary for patients with New York Heart Association class III and IV heart failure. Monitor for increased risk of myocardial infarction. Resumption of premenopausal ovulation may occur in anovulatory women. Unintended pregnancy may result. Use restricted for patients unable to take pioglitazone or to manage their blood sugar.
Pioglitazone (Actos) 15–30 mg/day Maximum 45 mg/day as monotherapy and 30 mg/day as combined therapy	Same as above	Same as above	Same as above.
Alpha-Glucosidase Inhibitors			
Acarbose (Precose) Initially 25 mg TID with the first bite of a meal; increase by 25 mg at 4- to 8-wk intervals to a maximum of 300 mg in three divided doses (150 mg if weight <60 kg)	Flatulence, diarrhea, abdominal pain/distention	Renal dysfunction, ketoacidosis, inflammatory bowel disease, colonic ulceration; predisposition to intestinal obstruction; disorders of digestion	Patient should take with first bite of each meal.
Miglitol (Glyset): Same as above	Same as above	Same as above	Same as above.
Meglitinide Analogs			
Repaglinide (Prandin) Initially 0.5 mg with two to four meals daily if the patient has never received other treatment for diabetes; if previous treatment, 1–2 mg with two to four meals daily Double dose weekly to a maximum of 16 mg/day	Hyperglycemia, upper respiratory tract infection, headache, diarrhea, constipation, arthralgia, back or chest pain	Type 1 diabetes, ketoacidosis	To be taken within 30 min of a meal. Patient should skip a dose if he or she skips a meal and add a dose if he or she adds a meal.
Nateglinide (Starlix) Initially 120 mg before each meal to a maximum dose of 360 mg/day	Same as above	Same as above	Same as above.

TABLE 44.2

Overview of Oral Antidiabetic Agents (*Continued*)

Generic (Trade) Name and Dosage	Selected Adverse Events	Contraindications	Special Considerations
Dipeptidyl Peptidase-4 Inhibitors			
Sitagliptin (Januvia) 100 mg PO or 50 mg PO	Common to both acute upper respiratory infection, urinary tract infection, headache Must adjust dosage to mild renal insufficiency Increases tendency toward hypoglycemia when combined with sulfonylureas	Type 1 diabetes	
Saxagliptin (Onglyza) 2.5 or 5 mg daily	Potential for acute pancreatitis, hypersensitivity to medication	History of pancreatitis	
Alogliptin (Nesina) 6.25 mg, 12.5 mg, or 25 mg daily	Same as above		
Linagliptin (Tradjenta) 2.5 or 5 mg daily	Same as above		
Oral Glucagon-Like Peptide Receptor Agonists			
Semaglutide (Rybelsus). Available in 7 or 14 mg tablet	Nausea, vomiting, and diarrhea	GI disorders, family history or personal history of medullary thyroid cancer or MET2, or acute pancreatitis	Dose in the morning 30 min apart from food or medications. Advanced after 1 month to 7 mg dose. If goals not met can advance to 14 mg dose.
Sodium–Glucose Cotransporter 2 Inhibitors			
Canagliflozin (Invokana) 100 or 300 mg daily dapagliflozin (Farxiga) 5 or 10 mg daily empagliflozin (Jardiance) 10 or 25 mg daily Ertugliflozin (Steglatro) 5 mg or 15 mg daily	Hyperkalemia mycotic infections, urinary tract infections, and renal insufficiency, hypotension	Type 1 diabetes or DKA, severe kidney disease (eGFR 30 mL/ min/1.73), or on hemodialysis	Monitor potassium and LDL cholesterol. Check blood pressure and symptoms of mycotic infections.

ALT, alanine aminotransferase; CHF, congestive heart failure; DKA, diabetes ketoacidosis; eGFR, estimated glomerular filtration rate; GI, gastrointestinal; IV, intravenous; LDL, low-density lipoprotein.

extra pancreatic effects involving the liver, muscle, and adipose cells, but because these agents are ineffective in patients with type 1 diabetes, it appears that their predominant hypoglycemic action is on the beta cells. When used alone, these agents have the most significant effect on blood sugar, especially in patients who are lean and insulinopenic or who have monogenic forms of diabetes.

Dosage

Sulfonylureas are divided into first- and second-generation agents. First-generation sulfonylureas include chloropropamide (Diabinese) and tolzamide (Tolinase).

Second-generation drugs are more potent and have less toxicity used than first-generation agents and are therefore more widely prescribed. Second-generation drugs consist of glimepiride (Amaryl), glipizide (Glucotrol and Glucotrol XL), and glyburide (Diabeta, Micronase, Glynase Prestabs). Medications in this class should be started at the lowest dose and titrated as needed to reach target blood glucose levels.

Approximately one third of patients with type 2 diabetes fail to respond adequately to sulfonylureas, most often because of markedly impaired beta cell function, not adhering to diet, or stressful events such as infection. After 10 years of therapy, only 50% of initial responders have adequate glycemic control.

For optimal response, careful patient selection should include the following criteria: duration of disease less than 5 years, no history of prior insulin therapy or good glycemic control on less than 40 units/day of insulin, close to normal body weight, and FPG less than 180 mg/dL.

Adverse Events

The most important consideration for use of sulfonylureas is hypoglycemia. The greatest risk for hypoglycemia is in the older adult population and in people with compromised renal function. The risk for hypoglycemia can be increased with alcohol abuse or overexertion. Most sulfonylureas are classified to use with caution in pregnancy apart from glyburide, which may be used in pregnancy. Prospective studies on rats and rabbits revealed no harm to the fetus, and retrospective human data suggest that glyburide may be a suitable option for pregnant women unable or unwilling to use insulin. The safety and efficacy of sulfonylureas have not been established in children or in the nursing female.

Patient education must include recognition in symptoms of hypoglycemia as well as prevention and treatment plans. Sulfonylureas can cause weight gain of about 2 to 3 kg. They cannot be used in patients with sulfa allergies. Baseline renal and hepatic function levels should be documented prior to starting sulfonylurea therapy.

Interactions

Patients taking sulfonylureas may have enhanced sensitivity to sunlight, so patients should be advised to use appropriate sun protection. Certain drugs may increase the effectiveness of sulfonylureas, resulting in hypoglycemia; a select list of commonly prescribed drugs includes ciprofloxacin (especially with glyburide), clofibrate, gemfibrozil, H_2 antagonists, probenaid, sulfonamides, and tricyclic antidepressants. Drugs that may decrease the effectiveness of the sulfonylureas, resulting in hyperglycemia, include the following: beta blockers, calcium channel blockers, cholestyramine, corticosteroids, diazoxide, estrogens, hydantoins, isoniazid, nicotinic acid, oral contraceptives, phenothiazines, rifampin, sympathomimetics, thiazide diuretics, thyroid medications, and urinary alkalinizers.

Biguanides

Biguanides can be used in conjunction with diet as first-line monotherapy or in combination with other classes of diabetic drugs, including insulin, to treat type 2 diabetes and prediabetes (see **Table 44.2**). Their mechanisms of action and side effect profiles differ from those of sulfonylureas, offering notable advantages. Biguanides do not cause hypoglycemia (when used as monotherapy) and do not promote hyperinsulinemia or weight gain.

Mechanism of Action

This class inhibits hepatic glucose production and moderately improves peripheral sensitivity to insulin. Gluconeogenesis and glycogenolysis are inhibited in the liver. Glycemic control is achieved without stimulating insulin secretion, so hypoglycemia does not develop. Metformin can also decrease intestinal absorption of glucose and improve insulin sensitivity in skeletal muscle. The oral bioavailability is 50% to 60%, and food decreases the bioavailability with a slight delay in the absorption of metformin. Metformin does not bind to liver or plasma proteins and is primarily excreted by the kidneys. Other advantages of biguanides over sulfonylureas include their tendency to induce weight loss and promote favorable effects on lipid profiles. In addition, biguanides can be combined effectively with multiple antidiabetic medications classes. Metformin is available in over 100 combinations with other oral agents from sulfonylureas, thiazolidinediones (TZDs), dipeptidyl peptidase-4 inhibitors (DPP-4i), and sodium–glucose cotransporter 2 (SGLT-2) inhibitors.

Dosage

The dose of metformin is started low and increased weekly as needed to the maximum. The immediate release (IR) form is usually taken before meals in the morning and evening. The extended release (ER) form is usually taken once a day with the evening meal or at bedtime. With metformin IR, the starting dose is 500 or 850 mg daily or twice daily, with increases every 1 to 2 weeks to a maximum of 2,550 mg/day. Peak action is within 2 to 2.5 hours, and the effects last for 10 to 16 hours. Steady-state levels of the drug are achieved in 24 to 48 hours. Metformin ER formula is started at 500 mg daily and increased to a maximum of 2,000 mg daily.

Contraindications

Metformin is contraindicated in the following situations: severe renal impairment as defined by estimated glomerular filtration rate (eGFR) below 30 mL/min/1.73 m^2, chronic alcohol abuse or binge drinking, hepatic disease or impairment, and heart failure. This class also is contraindicated in children under the age of 10. Metformin may be used in pregnancy with low teratogenicity based on human data. It is not known whether metformin is excreted in human milk. Breast-feeding women should discontinue nursing to avoid hypoglycemia in breast-feeding infants. Patients are advised to stop metformin the day of any scheduled radiological study that includes iodinated contrast. Metformin can be restarted 1-2 days postprocedure once the iodinated contrast has been fully excreted through the renal system. Patients should also stop taking metformin when experiencing metabolic acidosis and before surgery until they resume normal oral intake. Metformin may restore ovulation in women, who were anovulatory due to insulin resistance.

Adverse Events

The most common side effect of metformin therapy is gastrointestinal (GI) upset, which includes diarrhea, nausea, vomiting, abdominal bloating, flatulence, anorexia, and a metallic taste in the mouth. Such problems occur in approximately 30% of patients during the initiation of therapy and usually resolve with continued treatment. To minimize these adverse effects, treatment is started with a low dose and increased slowly at no less than weekly intervals. Instruct patients to take metformin with meals to reduce GI side effects.

Because GI upset is rare and late in therapy, any sudden onset of severe vomiting or diarrhea at that time should alert providers to the possibility of lactic acidosis, a rare but potentially fatal complication of metformin therapy. In such cases, patients should discontinue metformin immediately until they can be evaluated and stabilized. From the data collected in Europe for over 20 years, the reported worldwide incidence of metformin-induced lactic acidosis is 0.03 cases/1,000 patient-years. The risk of lactic acidosis increases with advancing age and worsening renal function. Therefore, metformin is contraindicated in patients with renal disease or dysfunction and acute or chronic metabolic acidosis. These conditions predispose patients to impaired perfusion of tissues and decreased elimination of lactate and are therefore contraindications to the use of metformin. In addition, patients should temporarily discontinue metformin during any situation in which an acute decline in renal function may occur (e.g., aggressive diuresis, dehydration from gastroenteritis, surgery).

Some clinical trials have demonstrated an association between metformin and vitamin B_{12} deficiency, which is reversible with discontinuation. It is recommended that B_{12} levels be assessed periodically, especially in those with underlying anemia or peripheral neuropathy (ADA, 2020).

The concomitant use of metformin with cimetidine increases the risk of hypoglycemia. The concomitant use of metformin with alcohol increases the risk of lactic acidosis.

Interactions

While metformin itself does not cause hypoglycemia, combination therapy with sulfonylureas, meglitinides, or insulin can be associated with hypoglycemia.

Thiazolidinediones

This class of antidiabetic agents (**Table 44.2**) reduces insulin resistance at sites of insulin action. They are approved for use in adults with type 2 diabetes. They are not approved for use in children.

Mechanism of Action

TZDs bind to the nuclear steroid hormone receptor peroxisome proliferator–activated receptor gamma, thereby increasing the insulin sensitivity in the skeletal muscle, adipose tissue, and liver cells. Clinically, they decrease peripheral insulin resistance and at higher doses may decrease hepatic glucose production. Like biguanides, they improve the action of insulin without directly stimulating insulin secretion from the pancreatic beta cells. There is an improvement of endothelial function, preservation of beta cell function, and a decrease in albumin excretion.

Dosage

Therapy is usually started at the lowest dose, with gradual increases to reach plasma glucose goals. Dosage varies with the agent chosen.

For use during pregnancy, the prescriber must weigh the risks versus benefits of TZDs; while there are no human data available, there is possible risk of fetal harm based on animal data. This category is not indicated for breast-feeding women or children. In addition, increased risk for fracture in women and macular edema has also been observed with TZD therapy.

A concern specific to pioglitazone is the possible increased risk of bladder cancer. Interim results reported an increased risk of bladder cancer with increasing cumulative dose and duration of therapy. Based on these and other data, pioglitazone was withdrawn from use in France in 2011, and no new prescriptions are authorized for patients in Germany. The studies done in the United States have not been able to reproduce this statistical significance; therefore, it is considered safe to use in the United States.

In 2011, access to rosiglitazone was restricted by the FDA due to a meta-analysis from the RECORD trial findings, which suggested that rosiglitazone may increase the relative risk of myocardial infarction. Later in 2014, the FDA reevaluated the data, determining that an increased risk of myocardial infarction could not be attributed specifically to the use of rosiglitazone; therefore, restricted distribution was removed. Currently, rosiglitazone is available alone and in combination with metformin in the United States.

Adverse Events

Pioglitazone may cause reduced concentrations of combined oral contraceptives; therefore, patients using oral contraceptives should consider alternative contraception methods.

In premenopausal anovulatory women with insulin resistance, ovulation may resume when drugs of this class are used. Thus, the patient may be at risk of unintended pregnancy, and contraception should be considered. Because of increased plasma volume from this class of drugs, TZDs are not recommended for patients with New York Heart Association class III or class IV heart failure. Another contraindication is active liver disease. TZDs can stimulate weight gain from plasma volume expansion and generation and redistribution of fats into the subcutaneous compartments.

Adverse Effects

Serum transaminase levels (Aspartate aminotransaminase [AST] and Alanine aminotransaminase [ALT]) should be monitored prior to initiating therapy and periodically thereafter per the clinical judgment of the health care provider. Liver function studies should also be obtained in the presence of hepatic dysfunction symptoms, such as abdominal pain, fatigue nausea, vomiting, or dark urine. TZD therapy should be discontinued in the presence of jaundice. Edema, shortness of breath, rapid weight gain, and other signs and symptoms of heart failure should be included in assessing TZD therapy. Hypoglycemia may develop in patients taking this class of drug with insulin or sulfonylureas because TZDs are potent sensitizers of insulin. If this occurs, the dose of insulin or sulfonylurea should be reduced. TZDs require several weeks to achieve the maximum benefit from a dosage level. Patients experiencing edema/swelling, shortness of breath, or muscle aches should contact their health care provider.

Interactions

As a class, TZDs are affected by other drugs that are strong CYP2C8 inhibitors, such as gemfibrozil, and other drugs that induce CYP2C8, such as rifampin. Other drugs to be used with caution include digoxin, fexofenadine, midazolam, nifedipine, and warfarin.

Alpha-Glucosidase Inhibitors

This class of drug is approved for use in adults with type 2 diabetes. They are not approved for use in children.

Mechanism of Action

The enzyme alpha-glucosidase, found on the brush border of the intestine, is necessary for the absorption of starch and disaccharides. This class of drugs (**Table 44.2**) acts by slowing the absorption of carbohydrates from the intestines, minimizing the postprandial rise in blood sugar. The result of this delay is decreased levels of postprandial glucose. The alpha-glucosidase inhibitors are most useful in patients with postprandial hyperglycemia. Due to the limited ability of these drugs to lower A1c and their side effect profile, they are not commonly used as monotherapy but as adjuncts to existing therapy.

Dosage

Agents from this class—acarbose (Precose) and miglitol (Glyset)—can be prescribed alone or with a sulfonylurea. Patients should take each dose with the first bite of each meal. Dosages are increased gradually (at 4- to 8-week intervals) to avoid GI side effects. The starting dose is 25 mg thrice daily at the start of each meal. This regimen lasts for 4 to 8 weeks; then, the dose may be increased to 50 mg thrice daily. After 3 months at 50 mg, the dose can be increased to 100 mg thrice daily. Peak concentration occurs in 2 to 3 hours. Patients using alpha-glucosidase inhibitors should be encouraged to maintain physical movement, especially after a meal to limit the buildup of GI tract gas.

Contraindications

Patients with inflammatory bowel disease, colonic ulceration, obstructive bowel disorders, or chronic intestinal disorders of digestion or absorption should not use these agents. Acarbose is contraindicated in patients with cirrhosis of the liver and not recommended in patients with serum creatinine levels of greater than 2.0 mg/dL or a creatinine clearance (CrCl) of less than 25 mL/min. Alpha-glucosidase inhibitors are classified as to be used with caution during pregnancy; there are inadequate human data but there is no known risk. These drugs should not be administered to breast-feeding women. Elevation of serum transaminases (AST or ALT) has been observed in clinical trials in patients taking acarbose at a dose of 200 to 300 mg daily. Liver function should be monitored during the first year of therapy and periodically thereafter to assess for liver toxicity.

Adverse Events

The most common side effects involve the GI tract. Increased fermentation secondary to the delay in carbohydrate absorption increases intestinal gas, causing flatulence, diarrhea, and abdominal distention.

Interactions

Intestinal adsorbents such as charcoal antagonize this class of drugs. The alpha-glucosidase inhibitors may decrease the levels of propranolol and ranitidine.

Meglitinide Analogs

This class is approved for the treatment of adults with type 2 diabetes. They are not approved in children.

Mechanism of Action

Meglitinide analogs are rapid-acting insulin secretagogues that stimulate the release of insulin from the pancreas in response to a meal (see **Table 44.2**). The binding of these agents at characterized sites closes the ATP-dependent potassium channels in the membranes of the beta cells, causing a depolarization of the beta cells and subsequent opening of calcium channels. The resulting increased influx of calcium causes insulin secretion.

Meglitinide analogs are effective in patients who become hypoglycemic while taking sulfonylureas or in those patients with FPG readings in goal range but persistently high postprandial glucose levels. They also are effective for patients with irregular meal schedules because patients take them at meals. Repaglinide (Prandin) and nateglinide (Starlix) are the two drugs available in this class. They lower postprandial blood glucose concentrations without any significant effects on FPG level.

Dosage

Meglitinide analogs can be used as monotherapy or in combination with other oral agents. The starting dose of repaglinide is 0.5 mg before meals if the A1c level is less than 8.0. If the A1c concentration is greater than 8.0, the starting dose is 1 to 2 mg, taken 15 minutes (but no longer than 30 minutes before each meal). Patients must add a dose if they add another meal or skip a dose if they skip a meal. The dose may be doubled to 4 mg before meals to a maximum of 16 mg a day. Nateglinide is similarly administered with a starting dose of 60 to 120 mg before meals.

The peak level is achieved in 1 hour. In 96 hours, the body excretes 90% of the medication. Meglitinide analogs are contraindicated in patients with diabetic ketoacidosis.

Contraindications

Diabetes ketoacidosis (DKA), severe infection, surgery, trauma, or other severe stressors are contraindications. For use during pregnancy, the prescriber must weigh the risks versus benefits of alpha-glucosidase inhibitors; while there are no human data available, there is possible risk of fetal harm based on animal data. This category is not indicated for breast-feeding women or children.

Adverse Events

Adverse events include hypoglycemia, GI disturbances, upper respiratory infections, headache, diarrhea, constipation, arthralgias, and back or chest pain.

Interactions

Concomitant use with beta blockers or alcohol increases the risk of hypoglycemia. Ketoconazole, miconazole, erythromycin, and other cytochrome P-450 (CYP450) 3A4 inhibitors may potentiate the drug, as may nonsteroidal antiinflammatory drugs, aspirin, sulfonamides, and warfarin. Drugs such as rifampin, barbiturates, thiazides, phenothiazines, phenytoin, sympathomimetics, calcium channel blockers, and isoniazid may antagonize it.

Dipeptidyl Peptidase-4 Inhibitors

This class is approved for the treatment of adults with type 2 diabetes. They are not approved for use in children.

Mechanism of Action

Insulinotropic polypeptide and glucagon-like peptide 1 (GLP-1) are two incretin hormones that are released from the distal bowel in response to a glucose load. These hormones account for up to 50% of the response to postprandial glucose. However, dipeptidyl peptidase-4 (DPP-4), which is a surface enzyme, inactivates GLP-1, therefore decreasing the levels of circulating GLP-1 and glucoregulatory functions. The class of agents called DPP-4 inhibitors acts to block the effect against GLP-1 and ultimately increases the amount of native active circulating incretins (see **Table 44.2**).

Currently, there are four DPP-4 inhibitors (DPP-4i) approved in the United States: sitagliptin (Januvia) and saxagliptin (Onglyza), linagliptin (Tradjenta), and alogliptin (Nesina). These medications are indicated for daily administration and coadministration with other oral antidiabetic agents and insulin. Prescribed as monotherapy, these agents do not cause increased risk for hypoglycemia.

Dosage

DPP-4i drugs are administered once daily. Sitagliptin has one starting dose of 100 mg daily. Dosage should be decreased to 50 mg daily for patients with moderate renal insufficiency, defined by CrCl greater than 30 mL/min but less than 50 mL/min. Dosage is further decreased to 25 mg daily if patients on dialysis or those with CrCl less than 30 mL/min.

Saxagliptin has two doses—2.5 or 5 mg—also prescribed daily. The dose of 2.5 mg is used for patients with moderate or severe renal insufficiency. Saxagliptin is a strong CYP3A4/5 inhibitor, which interacts with other drugs that use that pathway. Like sitagliptin, it is approved for combination therapy with sulfonylureas and TZDs but not insulin.

The starting dose of alogliptin in patients with normal kidney function or with mild renal dysfunction is 25 mg daily. In those with moderate renal dysfunction (CrCl 30 mL/min–50 mL/min), a dose of 12.5 mg is advised, with a dose reduction to 6.25 if CrCl is less than 30 mL/min.

Linagliptin does not require renal dosing adjustments.

Contraindications

The contraindications for all medications include hypersensitivity to the agent. Caution for use in pregnancy is advised for all the DPP-4i inhibitors. Consider an alternative in patients who are breast-feeding.

Adverse Events

The most common adverse effects are the same for all the DPP-4i and include upper respiratory infection, urinary tract infection, and headaches. This class also has the potential for hypoglycemia when prescribed in combination therapy with sulfonylureas or insulin.

Additional postmarketing reports include hypersensitivity reactions, bullous phemphigoid, anaphylaxis, angioedema, disabling arthralgias, exfoliative skin conditions including Stevens-Johnson syndrome; hepatic enzyme elevations; and potentially fatal pancreatitis. Additionally, both saxagliptin and alogliptin have been associated with potential increased risk of heart failure.

Interactions

This drug class has no specific pharmacokinetic drug–drug interactions; however, as a potent CYP3A4/5 inhibitor, they can interact with drugs such as ketoconazole, erythromycin, and diltiazem. Additionally, when DPP-4i drugs are used on combination with sulfonylureas, doses of the sulfonylureas may be reduced to avoid hypoglycemia.

Glucagon-Like Peptide Receptor Agonist

This class is approved for treatment of type 2 diabetes in adults. Liraglutide has the indication for treatment of adolescents over the age of 10 (see **Table 44.2** and **44.3**).

Mechanism of Action

The mechanism of action is to stimulate glucose-dependent secretion of insulin from pancreatic beta cells while suppressing the inappropriate release of glucagon from alpha cells, thereby reducing both fasting and postprandial glucose levels. Incretins also slows gastric emptying, thereby increasing satiety. There are presently six glucagon-like peptide receptor agonists (GLP1-RAs) available by injection: exenatide (Byetta, Bydureon), liraglutide (Victoza), lixisenatide (Adlyxin), semaglutide injectable (Ozempic), oral semaglutode (Rrybelsus), and dulaglutide (Trulicity). Albiglutide (Tanzeum) was discontinued by the manufacturer in 2018 due to declining sales.

Three of the GLP1-RAs have demonstrated favorable effects on cardiovascular risk reduction. Liraglutide (Victoza) and dulaglutide (Trulicity) have received FDA approval to reduce the risk of cardiovascular mortality and nonfatal

TABLE 44.3

Comparison of Basal Insulin

Insulin	NPH	Detemir	Glargine	Glargine U300	Degludec
Risk of hypoglycemia	Present	Low	Low	Least	Least
Risk of nocturnal hypoglycemia	Present	Low	Low	Least	Least
Risk of severe hypoglycemia	Present	Low	Low	Least	Least
Weight gain	Present	Low	Low	Low	Low

NPH, neutral protamine hagedorn.

cardiovascular events (myocardial infarction and stroke). Semaglutide (Ozempic) has been shown to reduce the risk of cardiovascular death. The other GLP-1RA agents on the market have not demonstrated superiority over placebo in ASCVD risk reduction. Similarly, three of the GLP1-RAs have shown renal protective effects. Liraglutide (Victoza), semaglutide (Ozempic), and dulaglitide (Trulicity) have demonstrated reduction in new or worsening albuminuria in addition to reduction in new onset of nephropathy (Kristensen, 2019). ASCVD risk reduction may not necessarily be a class effect. Neither exenatide nor lixisenatide have demonstrated ASCVD risk reduction.

Dosage

Exenatide (Byetta) is only available as an injectable and can be used as monotherapy or in conjunction with other oral agents, metformin, sulfonylureas, TZDs, and insulin. The starting dose is 5 mcg, administered within the 60 minutes before morning and evening meals or prior to the largest meals of the day and spaced more than 6 hours apart. Based on response, in 1 month, the dose can be increased to 10 mcg twice a day. If a dose is missed, the treatment should be restarted at the next scheduled dose time.

Liraglutide may be administered once daily at any time. The initial dose of 0.6 mg/day is not effective for glycemic control but should be administered for 1 week to reduce GI symptoms; once initial dose is tolerated, it should be increased to 1.2 mg daily. If glycemic goals are not met after 2 to 4 weeks, the dose may be increased to the maximum of 1.8 mg/day.

Lixisenatide is administered once a day within 1 hour of the first meal of the day. The initial starting dose is 10 mg, which can be increased after 2 weeks to 20 mg.

The ER of exenatide (Bydureon) is dosed once weekly, and timing of the injection may be performed without regard to meals. This injectable is available in a suspension powder for reconstitution or a single-dose auto-injector pen with a hidden needle.

Dulaglutide (Trulicity) may be administered once weekly at any time of the day. This injectable is available in a single dose auto-injector pen with a hidden needle. It is available in 0.75 or 1.5 mg dose.

Semaglutide is available in a multi-dose pen administered once a week (Ozempic) or as an oral tablet (Rybelsus) administered once daily in the morning, at least 30 minutes apart from food and other medications. Semaglutide (Ozempic) is available in a 0.5- or 1-mg dose. Semaglutide is initiated at 0.25 mg and advanced to 0.5 mg after 2 to 4 weeks. If treatment goals are not achieved after 4 weeks at the 0.5-mg weekly dose, patients can be advanced to 1 mg. Semaglutide (Rybelsus) is available in a 7- or 14-mg tablet. Semaglutide (Rybelsus) is initiated at 3 mg daily for the first 30 days and then advanced to a 7-mg daily dose. If treatment goals are not met after 30 days of the 7-mg dose, patients can be advanced to the 14-mg daily dose.

When used with a hypoglycemic agent, GLP1-RAs may cause hypoglycemia; therefore, patients should be cautioned to monitor blood glucose levels carefully.

Contraindications

Contraindications to GLP1-RAs include ketoacidosis and allergy. GLP1-RAs should be avoided in patients with severe GI disorders, including gastroparesis and acute gallbladder disease. GLP1-RAs have not been studied in pregnancy. Breast-feeding women should either discontinue the drug or discontinue nursing. Both exenatide and liraglutide may delay and reduce the peak concentration of digoxin, lisinopril, lovastatin, and acetaminophen.

All GLP1-RAs carry a warning about the possible increased risk of thyroid C-cell tumors. Liraglutide was demonstrated in clinical trials to cause thyroid C-cell tumors in rodents.

Patients with a personal or family history of medullary thyroid carcinoma or multiple endocrine neoplasia syndrome type 2 should not be prescribed GLP1-RAs.

Another precaution is the possible association between acute pancreatitis and GLP1-RAs. It is advised that patients be observed for signs and symptoms of pancreatitis throughout treatment.

Adverse Events

The most common adverse reactions to exenatide are GI related, including nausea, vomiting, diarrhea, and dyspepsia.

Interactions

Due to the decrease in gastric emptying, GLP1-RAs should not be administered close to drugs that have a narrow therapeutic window. Caution should be exercised when patients are taking warfarin, and the international normalized ratio should be monitored closely with drug initiation and dose changes. Exenatide can possibly decrease in the ethinyl estradiol component of oral contraceptives; therefore, exenatide and oral contraceptives should not be administered within 1 hour of each other.

Dopamine Receptor Agonists

Dopamine receptor agonists are used as monotherapy in type 2 diabetes or secondary diabetes with substantial capacity for insulin production. The mechanism by which dopamine receptor agonists improve glycemic control is unknown, but they are theorized to be related to improved insulin sensitivity. Following morning administration of bromocriptine mesylate (Cycloset), postprandial glucose levels are improved without increasing plasma insulin concentrations.

Dosage

The dose of bromocriptine mesylate is 0.8 mg taken 2 hours after waking with the first meal of the day. The dose may be increased by 0.8 mg each week until the maximal tolerated daily dose of 1.6 to 4.8 mg is achieved.

Contraindications

Caution is advised with the use of bromocriptine mesylate in pregnancy. It also inhibits lactation and should not be administered to breast-feeding women. Exacerbation of psychotic disorders or reduction in the effectiveness of drugs that treat psychosis may occur when bromocriptine is coadministered.

Concomitant use of bromocriptine mesylate with other dopamine receptor agonists indicated for the treatment of Parkinson's disease, restless leg syndrome, acromegaly, and other disorders is not recommended.

Adverse Events

The most common side effects include orthostatic hypotension, somnolence, nausea, fatigue, dizziness, vomiting, and headache.

Interactions

Bromocriptine mesylate is highly bound to serum proteins and may increase the unbound fraction of other highly protein-bound drugs (e.g., salicylates, sulfonamides, chloramphenicol, and probenecid), resulting in altered effectiveness and increased risk for side effects.

Bile Acid Sequestrant

This class of medications binds to bile acids in the intestine, thus preventing reabsorption. As the bile acid pool is reduced, hepatic enzymes convert circulating cholesterol to bile acids, thereby upregulating hepatic LDL receptors and clearance of LDL-C from circulation. The glucose-lowering mechanism of action is not well understood but is postulated to be associated the reduced absorption of glucose in the gut. There are three different bile acid sequestrants but only colesevelam is FDA approved as an adjunct to diet and exercise in adults with type 2 diabetes. Colesevelam has not been studied in children for use as a glucose-lowering agent but is approved for the treatment of heterozygous familial hypercholesterolemia in adolescents age 10 and older.

Dosage

Colesevelam is available in 625-mg tablets and 3.75-g suspensions. The recommended dose for the tablets is 6 tablets daily or 3 tablets twice daily. The recommended dose of the oral suspension is 3.75 g packets daily or 1.875 g twice daily. The suspension should be mixed with at least 4 oz of liquid and should not be taken with a meal. Colesevelam should be taken at least 4 hours apart from other medications to prevent interference with drug absorption. Dosing adjustment is not required for hepatic or renal impairment.

Contraindications

Contraindications include a history of bowel obstruction, motility disorders such as gastroparesis, history of major GI surgery, triglyceride levels over 500 mg/dL, and a history of triglyceride-induced pancreatitis. Caution is advised for use of colesevelam during pregnancy and breast-feeding, especially with prolonged use due to a potential alteration of fat-soluble vitamin deficiency.

Adverse Events

The most common adverse reactions with colesevelem are constipation, dyspepsia, and nausea. Additionally, postmarketing reports of bowel obstruction, esophageal obstruction, fecal impactions, dysphagia, and increased transaminases are available.

Interactions

Colesevelam can reduce the absorption of fat-soluble vitamins. Use with caution in patients at risk for or history of fat-soluble vitamin deficiencies. Colesevelam can also interfere with absorption of some medications. Postmarketing reports of increased seizures have occurred with the concomitant administration with phenytoin. Suboptimal levels of warfarin, levothyroxine, ethinyl estradiol, and norethindrone have been reported with the concomitant of colesevelam.

Colesevelam can also raise triglycerides when prescribed in combination with sulfonylureas.

Amylin Analog

A recombinant form of amylin is pramlintide (Symlin). This is an injectable agent that is a synthetic of the pancreatic neurohormone amylin, which is cosecreted with insulin from beta cells in response to food. Pramlintide has three actions as an amylinomimetic agent. First, it helps to delay gastric emptying into the small intestine, which delays the rise in postprandial glucose release. This effect lasts for approximately 3 hours and does not alter nutrient absorption. Second, pramlintide alters the release of additional inappropriate glucagon by pancreatic alpha cells. Finally, there is an increase in satiety, which decreases the total calorie intake and promotes weight loss. Pramlintide is approved for use in adults with type 1 or type 2 diabetes. It is also approved for use with insulin.

Dosage

Pramlintide is available in a multi-dose injector pen. The initiation and dosage of pramlintide differs for type 1 and type 2 diabetes; however, the management of changes in dosage, side effects, and monitoring blood sugar levels is the same for both. The starting dose for those with type 1 diabetes is 15 mcg just prior to any major meal. If tolerated, pramlintide is titrated by 15-mcg increments to a total dose of 30 to 60 mcg. Patients with type 2 diabetes also administer pramlintide just prior to any major meal at 60 mcg per injection. The dose is increased to 120 mcg in 3 to 7 days if there is no nausea. It is recommended that patients started on pramlintide reduce their current insulin regimen by 50%. The ongoing titration of pramlintide is based on blood glucose levels and the presence or absence of nausea. Close monitoring of blood glucose levels is very important to detect hypoglycemia. If significant nausea occurs, the dosage should be decreased until the drug is tolerated. If nausea persists even at the lowest dose, pramlintide should be discontinued.

Contraindications

Few contraindications exist for pramlintide; however, it is critical to select appropriate patients. Those with poor adherence to diabetic care regimens, those with A1c greater than 9%, and those taking drugs that increase gastric motility gastroparesis should not take pramlintide. Additional precaution is needed for anyone with known hypersensitivity to the product. Studies have shown no effects on the drug in those with renal or liver disease and are approved as safe. The safety of pramlintide in pregnancy is unknown; therefore, caution is advised. Alternatives should be considered for breast-feeding women.

Adverse Events

Nausea is the most common side effect. Gradual titration to the recommended dose reduces this reaction. Other side effects include nausea, vomiting, headache, and anorexia.

Interactions

Pramlintide has the potential to delay the absorption of concomitantly administered oral medications such as analgesics, antibiotics, and oral contraceptives. Patients who are taking drugs that alter gastric motility such as anticholinergics should not take pramlintide.

Sodium-Glucose Co-Transporter 2 Inhibitors

This class of medications is approved for use in adults with type 2 diabetes. The safety of this class has not been studied in adolescents. The sodium-glucose co-transporter 2 inhibitors (SGLT-2is) include empagliflozin (Jardiance), canagliflozin (Invokana), dapagliflozin (Farxiga), and ertugliflozin (Steglatro).

The FDA has recently expanded the use of three out of four agents in this class. Canagliflozin has been shown to reduce the progression of diabetic kidney disease and hospitalizations for heart failure in type 2 diabetes with albuminuria more than 300 mg/day. Empagliflozin is approved to reduce the risk for cardiovascular death in adults with type 2 diabetes and established ASCVD. And dapagliflozin has the indication to reduce the risk of hospitalization for heart failure in patients with established ASCVD or multiple ASCVD risk factors and without or without type 2 diabetes mellitus.

Mechanism of Action

This category of medications functions to induce glycosuria through the kidneys by inhibiting the SGLT-2 system in the proximal tubules of the glomerulus, resulting in increased excretion of glucose in the urine and lower excess calorie intake. Normally, 90% of filtered glucose is reabsorbed through SGLT-2 transport system in the proximal tubule of the kidney. A normal glucose load in the tubules is approximately 120 mg/min, and due to reabsorption, there is minimal glucose excretion in the urine. To promote blood sugar control, SGLT-2is will cause an approximately 60% excretion of glucose in the urine. The degree of urinary glucose excretion in SGLT-2is occurs in an insulin-independent fashion, lowering the risk for hypoglycemia and allowing for its use across the spectrum of patients irrespective of the severity or duration of diabetes.

Dosage

Empagliflozin is started at 10 mg orally in the morning and can be titrated up to 25 mg. The medication should be discontinued for persistent eGFR less than 45. Canagliflozin is initiated at 100 mg before the first meal for the day. The dose can be increased to 300 mg daily in patients with normal kidney function, defined as eGFR greater than 60 mL/min/1.73 m. The dose should remain at 100 mg daily for patients with impaired kidney function (eGFR between 30 and 60 mL/min/1.73 m). The initial dose for dapagliflozin is 5 mg with or without food. The dose can be increased to 10 mg. Do not initiate or discontinue dapagliflozin if eGFR is less than 45 mL/min/1.73 m. The recommended starting dose of ertugliflozin is 5 mg once daily in the morning. The dose can be increased to 15 mg daily if needed to gain control of diabetes. Continued use of ertugliflozin is not recommended if the eGFR is persistently between 30 and 60 mL/min/1.73 m.

Contraindications

SGLT-2is should not be used to treat DKA. Patients with severe kidney disease (eGFR, 30 mL/min/1.73) or on hemodialysis should not use SGLT-2is.

Adverse Events

This class of drug can cause hyperkalemia, mycotic infections, urinary tract infections, necrotizing fasciitis of the perineum, and renal insufficiency. Alternatives for any SGLT-2i should be considered in the first trimester and avoided in the 2nd and 3rd trimester. This drug class has not been studied in women who are breastfeeding. Consider an alternate therapy for treatment and the drug class is not approved for use in children. Risk of hypotension may be increased in patients with low volume status, which can be found in patients taking diuretics, angiotensin-converting enzyme inhibitors, or angiotensin receptor blockers. These patients should be carefully monitored and have fluid status corrected before starting an SGLT-2i. The increased glucose excretion is associated with increased urinary frequency. The high urinary glucose concentration also predisposes patients to genital mycotic infections and urinary tract infections. SGLT-2is may cause hyperkalemia, especially in patients with decreased kidney function; therefore, careful monitoring of potassium is indicated. Increases in LDL cholesterol have also been observed. Routine A1c monitoring should be accompanied by potassium and LDL cholesterol monitoring. Check blood pressure and symptoms of mycotic infections.

Interactions

Concomitant use of this class with insulin and sulfonylureas can increase the risk for hypoglycemia.

Combination Oral Medication for Type 2 Diabetes

There are many fixed-dose combination products of two or three different drug classes available to treat type 2 diabetes. Many patients find it easier to take a single medication as opposed to two separate medications, thereby improving overall drug adherence. Fixed-dose combinations are generally tried after a patient has failed to reach reduction of his or her hyperglycemic goals based on one drug alone. The drawback of using these combination medications is the cost. In some cases, the combinations cost more than each drug separately. In addition, starting combination therapy in drug-naive patients can create problems determining the specific cause of drug-induced side effects or allergic reactions.

Insulin

Insulin is the only drug therapy of choice for patients with type 1 diabetes and for those patients with type 2 diabetes who cannot control their condition with diet and exercise alone or in whom combination therapy has failed. Other clinical situations in which insulin therapy is appropriate include newly diagnosed cases of type 2 diabetes presenting with severe, symptomatic hyperglycemia, pregnancy, and surgery.

Just like the insulin normally produced by the pancreas, insulin as drug therapy regulates glucose metabolism in the muscle and other tissues (except the brain). It causes the rapid transport of glucose and amino acids intracellularly, promotes anabolism, and inhibits protein catabolism. In the liver, it promotes the uptake and storage of glucose in the form of glycogen, inhibits gluconeogenesis, and promotes the conversion of excess glucose into fat.

The major characteristics of insulin preparations are onset of action and duration of action (**Tables 44.4** and **44.5**). Semisynthetic insulin, which is produced by recombinant deoxyribonucleic acid technology, has the identical amino acid composition as human endogenous insulin and is therefore referred to as *human insulin*. Human insulin preparations lower the risk of local reactions. An insulin analog, lispro insulin, is a two-amino-acid modification of regular human insulin. Aggregates do not form when lispro insulin is injected subcutaneously, allowing for a more rapid onset and shorter duration than regular insulin and minimizing the postprandial rise in blood sugar and the risk of late hypoglycemia. Another human insulin analog is insulin glargine.

Insulins are categorized as basal (neutral protamine hagedorn [NPH], glargine, detemir, and degludec) or bolus/

TABLE 44.4		
Recommended Order of Treatment for Type 1 Diabetes Mellitus		
Order	**Agents**	**Comments**
First line	Four-injection regimen, a long-acting insulin such as insulin glargine once a day and a rapid-acting or short-acting insulin administered at mealtimes or a combination of intermediate and short acting; dose is 0.4–0.5 units/kg/day	Several schedules are used to administer insulin (see **Table 44.5**). The most used regimen is four injections a day. This regimen best duplicates normal physiologic insulin. The second regimen would be two injections a day, one in the morning and one in the evening. This promotes glycemic control both during the day and while sleeping.
		The insulin dose required is divided into two thirds of the dose in the morning and one third of the dose in the evening. The morning dose is divided into two thirds intermediate insulin and one third short- or rapid-acting insulin. The evening dose is half intermediate insulin and half short- or rapid-acting insulin.
Second line	Insulin dose is gradually increased	Adjustments are made at 1 to 2 units at a time or 10% to 20% twice a week
		Adjustments are based on SMBG records.

SMBG, self-monitoring of blood glucose.

TABLE 44.5

Glucose-Lowering Medication in Type 2 Diabetes: Overall Approach

Initial or First-Line Treatment: Metformin and Lifestyle Therapy (Physical Activity, Portion Control, and Weight Management)							
High-risk ASCVD, or established ASCVD, CKD, HF Independently of A1c		If A1c above target and goal to reduce risk for hypoglycemia				Need to minimize weight gain or promote weight loss		Cost is factor	
SGLT21	GLP-1RA	DPP-4i	GLP-1RA	SGLT-2i	TZD	GLP-1RA	SGLT2-i	SU	TZD
If A1c > target, consider adding		If A1c above target				If A1c above target		If A1c above target	
GLP-1RA	SGLT-2i	SGLT-2i or TZD	SGLT-2i or TZD	GLP-1RA or DPP-4i, or TZD	SGLT-2i or DPP-4i or GLP-1RA	SGLT2i	GLP-1RA	Add TZD	Add SU
Avoid TZD and Saxagliptin if HF		If A1c above target, consider above additions				If A1c above goal		If A1c above target	
In preexisting HF- Consider use of DPP-4i, basal insulin, or SU if A1c remains above target		Add basal insulin or SU with lower risk for hypoglycemia if A1c continues to stay above target				Use regimen with the lowest risk for weight gain		Add basal insulin with lowest cost or consider DPP-4i or SGLT-2i at lowest cost	

ASCVD, atherosclerotic cardiovascular disease; CKD, chronic kidney disease; DDP-4i, Dipeptidyl Peptidase-4 inhibitors; DPP-4i, dipeptidyl peptidase-4 inhibitors; GLP-1RA, glucagon-like peptide receptor agonist; HF; SGLT-2i, sodium-glucose co-transporter 2 inhibitors; SU, Sulfonylurea; TZD, thiazolidinediones.

Source: Adapted from American Diabetes Association. (2020). Standards of Medical Care in Diabetes. *Diabetes Care, 41*(Suppl. 1), S103.

prandial (regular, lispro, glusiline, and aspart). Initial insulin doses should be individualized in patients previously untreated with insulin. The preferred method of insulin therapy administration is through a basal insulin plus a bolus insulin 15 minutes before the start of each meal.

Insulin harvested from animal sources is no longer manufactured. Human insulin is less antigenic than beef insulin and slightly less antigenic than pork insulin. Insulin analogs and U-500 insulin all require a prescription.

The concentrations of insulin currently available in the United States are U-100, U200, U300, and U-500, indicating 100 units/mL, 200 units/mL, 300 units/mL, or 500 units/mL respectively. U-500 insulin is available for patients with extreme insulin resistance classified by needing greater than 200 units total daily dose (TDD). A goal of insulin therapy is to mimic, as nearly as possible, the physiologic profile of insulin secretion (basal/bolus). The evolution of insulin management has moved from a single daily injection therapy to multiple injections with multiple insulin products. This pattern allows the opportunity to adjust the prandial or bolus insulin (rapid-acting or regular) doses based on the results of the blood glucose checks and food quantity consumed while targeting specific glucose levels.

When initiating insulin therapy, it is important to mimic normal physiologic insulin secretion as close as possible. This requires a combination of basal and bolus insulin through multiple daily injections or a combination of inhaled prandial insulin with injectable basal insulin. If an insulin pump delivery device is prescribed, the pump can provide continuous insulin subcutaneously as an infusion to cover both basal insulin and boluses needs utilizing rapid or short-acting insulin only. In the past, multiple daily doses of intermediate insulin, NPH, were prescribed to meet basal insulin needs. And while NPH can still be prescribed as a basal insulin, the ease of the new Peakless basal insulins has led to best practice and predominance of usage.

Premixed insulins that contain both basal and prandial (biphasic) insulins are commercially available as 70/30, 50/50, or 75/25. This insulin regimen may be appropriate for patients who have difficulty mixing their own insulins or for those in whom these ratios are effective. However, for intensive insulin regimens, these insulins are usually not recommended.

Dosage

Insulin is available in an injectable multi-dose vial, injectable multi-dose pen, or inhaled form. The starting dose of insulin injectable is usually based on weight. The recommended starting dose for those with type 1 diabetes is 0.4 to 0.5 units/kg/day with 40% to 50% of the TDD in the form of basal insulin. For example, total daily insulin dose = 0.50 × 70 kg = 35 units of insulin/day, with 14 to 17 units in the form of basal with the remaining amount (14–17 units) divided as a set dose at meals, that is, 3 to 5 units at each meal. Insulin doses can be adjusted up or down by 2 to 4 units every few days until target glucose levels are obtained. See **Table 44.6** on how to determine adjustments.

In type 2 diabetes, basal insulin may be used as a supplement to a regimen that includes one or more oral agents rather than total physiological replacement. In this scenario, it is suggested that basal insulin be estimated utilizing 0.1 to

TABLE 44.6									
Drug-Specific and Patient Factors to Consider When Selecting Antihyperglycemic Treatment in Adults with Type 2 Diabetes									
	Met	**SU/Mel**	**TZD**	**DPP-4i**	**Bromo**	**SGLT-2i**	**AGE**	**Bile Acid**	**GLP-1RA**
Efficacy A1c Change	High (1.5–2)	High (1–2)	Moderate (0.5–1.8)	Moderate (0.5–0.8)	Mild (0.2–0.6)	High (0.8–1)	Moderate (0.5–0.8)	Mild (0.4–0.6)	High (0.8–1.6)
Hypoglycemia	No	High	No	No	No	No	No	No	No
Weight	Neutral	Gain	Gain	Neutral	Neutral	Loss	Gain	Neutral	Loss
CVD Benefit	Moderate	Neutral	Potential (Actos)	Moderate	Neutral	High (empagliflozin, canagliflozin, dapagliflozin)	Neutral	Neutral	High (liraglutide, dulaglutide, semaglutide)
Cost	Low	Low	Low	High	High	High	Low	High	High
Renal Benefits	Neutral	Neutral	Neutral	Renal dose adjustment required for all except linagliptin	Neutral	High	Neutral	Neutral	High (liraglutide, semaglutide) Renal dose adjustments needed for lixisenatide and exenatide

CVD, cardiovascular disease; DPP-4i, dipeptidyl peptidase-4 inhibitors; GLP-1RA, glucagon-like peptide receptor agonist; SGLT-2i, sodium-glucose co-transporter 2 inhibitors; SU, Sulfonylureas; TZD, thiazolidinediones.

Source: Adapted from American Diabetes Association. (2020). Standards of Medical Care in Diabetes. *Diabetes Care, 41*(Suppl. 1), S101.

0.2 unit/kg/day, or a starting dose of 10 units a day. Doses are titrated by 2 units every 3 days until Fasting blood glucose (FBS) is at goal without hypoglycemia. Once the basal dose reaches 0.5 units/kg/day if the A1c is still above target, it is suggested that bolus or prandial insulin be initiated at 4 units a meal or 10% of the basal dose. Titration of prandial insulin can be made every 3 to 4 days by 1 to 2 units or 10% to 15% until goal glucose levels are achieved or hypoglycemia occurs.

Insulin doses should be individualized and closely monitored. The following guidelines can be used to estimate total daily dosage for varying scenarios:

- Children and adults: 0.4 to 1 units/kg/day
- Adolescents during a growth spurt: 1.2 to 1.5 units/kg/day
- Pregnancy: 0.7 to 2 units/kg/day

Insulins mixed with long-acting or intermediate-acting insulin, or premixed formulations (i.e., mixtures such as Humalog Mix 75/25 or NovoLog Mix 70/30), are usually dosed twice a day rather than 3 to 4 times a day, as with basal/bolus regimens. Typically, one injection is given before breakfast and the other injection before dinner. It is recommended that two thirds of the TDD be given in the morning with a 2:1 ratio of intermediate-to short-acting insulin and one third of the TDD be given before dinner with a 1:1 ratio of short-acting insulin and intermediate-acting insulin.

Table 44.7 provides some suggestions on when dosages need adjusting. Insulin glargine, detemir, and degludec cannot

be mixed with other insulins. The advantage of using the basal insulins includes the following:

- Provides a smooth basal effect compared with patterns using multiple injections for intermediate insulin
- Provides moderate flexibility in timing of meals
- Very effective in mimicking normal physiologic acting patterns
- Very effective in controlling the fasting glucose without increasing nocturnal hypoglycemia
- Less weight gain than NPH-based regimens

The 1800 rule is a mathematical algorithm that clinicians can use to provide a means of correcting elevated glucose levels above target by calculating how sensitive the patient is to insulin in a numerical form. This factor, called sensitivity factor (SF), is determined by dividing 1,800 by the TDD of insulin. The SF is the change in blood glucose anticipated by injecting 1 unit of insulin. The formula is as follows: SF = 1,800/TDD. For example, if the patient takes 50 units of insulin in 24 hours, the SF is 1,800/50 = 36.

Therefore, each unit of insulin lowers the blood glucose level by 36 mg/dL. If the SMBG at noon is 170, an addition of 1 unit in the morning should lower the blood glucose level to 134 mg/dL.

Adverse Events

Hypoglycemia, hypokalemia, lipodystrophy, and local or systemic allergic reactions can occur with insulin. The dawn

TABLE 44.7

Recommendations for Initiating Injectable Therapy in Type 2 Diabetes

If A1c above goal and injectable needed

Consider GLP-1RA in most patients and gradually increase to maximum tolerable dose.
Add basal insulin if already on GLP-1RA, GLP-1RA not tolerated, or insulin preferred.

If A1c above target

Add basal insulin or NPH starting dose 0.1 to 0.2 units/kg/day.

Titrate to FBS goal by 2 units every 3 days.

If A1c still above target after basal dose 0.5 units/kg/day

Add prandial insulin at 4 units per meal or 10% of basal dose or if on NPH consider premix split dosing or self-mixed NPH with short/rapid-acting insulin.

Prandial Insulin	Premix Insulin	NPH and short/rapid-acting insulin
Adjust by 1–2 units or 10%–20% twice a week until premeal goals reached. Basal insulin dose may need to be lowered by 4 units or 10% if A1c <8% at initiation.	Usually a 1 unit per 1 unit conversion with two thirds given at breakfast and half give at dinner. Titrate based on individual needs. Consider adjusting by 1 to 2 units or 10% to 20% twice a week until premeal goals reached.	Adjust the dose of the NPH separate from the rapid-acting insulin Consider: Reduce current NPH dose by 20% Add two thirds of calculated dose at breakfast Add one third of calculated dose at dinner Add 4 units or 10% of NPH dose of rapid/short-acting insulin at each NPH injection or BID. Titrate based on individual needs.

FBS, fasting blood glucose; GLP-1RA, glucagon-like peptide receptor agonist; NPH, neutral protamine hagedorn.

phenomenon, so called for worsening hyperglycemia that occurs in the early morning hours, is caused by growth hormone surges that occur during sleep. The Somogyi effect, which also may be mistaken for inadequate control, is a rebound of hyperglycemia that occurs after an early morning episode of insulin-induced hypoglycemia. The hypoglycemia goes unnoticed because it happens while the patient is sleeping. Signs and symptoms include night sweats, nightmares, sleep disturbances, and early morning headaches. Monitoring of blood glucose when hypoglycemia is thought to be occurring helps make the diagnosis.

Interactions

There are many drugs that can decrease or increase the blood glucose effect in a person taking insulin. The following drugs increase the risk of hypoglycemia when used in combination with insulin: angiotensin II receptor blocking agents, disopyramide, fibrates, fluoxetine, monoamine oxidase inhibitors, pentoxifylline, pramlintide, propoxyphene, salicylates, and sulfonamide antibiotics. Drugs that may decrease the blood glucose–lowering effect of insulin are antipsychotics, corticosteroids, diuretics, estrogens, niacin, thyroid hormones, sympathomimetic agents, protease inhibitors, somatropin, and oral contraceptives.

Beta-blockers, clonidine, and resperine have all been shown to blunt the signs and symptoms of hypoglycemia.

Inhaled Rapid-Acting Insulin

Inhaled rapid-acting insulin is approved for the treatment of adults with type 1 and type 2 diabetes. The only available inhaled insulin on the market is Afrezza. Onset of action varies with the dose from 12 to 90 minutes. The peak effect is 35 to 45 minutes and the duration of action is 90 to 180 minutes.

Dosage

Afrezza is dosed at the beginning of each meal and is available in 4-unit, 8-unit, and 12-unit cartridges using the Afrezza inhaler. The recommended initial starting dose is 4 units for the insulin-naive patient or the equivalent amount in patients currently injecting subcutaneous insulin at meals.

Contraindications

Afrezza is contraindicated in patients with chronic lung diseases such as asthma and Chronic Obstructive Pulmonary Disorder (COPD) and in smokers. Lung function studies via spirometry (FEV1) are advised prior to implementation, after 6 months of therapy, and annually thereafter. Lung function studies are also advised if pulmonary symptoms develop such as wheezing, reccurring cough, or shortness of breath.

Adverse Events

The most common side effect is cough, bronchospasm, throat pain or irritation, and bronchitis. Drug interactions are similar with inhaled rapid-acting insulin and other insulin preparations. There is insufficient data to support the safety of rapid-acting inhaled insulin in lactation.

Combination Insulin/Glucagon-Like Peptide Receptor Agonist Injectables

There are two different once-a-day combinations of fixed dose basal insulin and GLP-1RA: lixizenatide/glargine (Soliqua) and liraglutide/degludec (Xiltophy). The starting and maximum doses for each are listed in **Table 44.10**. Titration is similar to basal insulin adjustments.

Continuous Glucose Monitoring

Glucose monitoring has come a long way, from dipstick measurements of urine glucose to glucose meters and strips, to the present era in continuous glucose monitoring (CGM). CGM uses a disposable sensor that measures interstitial glucose every few minutes, 24 hours a day. The patient inserts the sensor subcutaneously just underneath the skin, replacing it every 7 to 14 days. The sensor transmits glucose readings to a separate receiver, insulin pump, or a smartphone. These glucose readings can provide both the patient and the clinician a "video" perspective on the overall glucose patterns throughout the day and the night. The blood sugars can then be correlated with factors such as food intake or activity and can assist with achieving glycemic control. Indications for CGM include frequent hypoglycemia, hypoglycemia unawareness, and elevated A1c despite multiple adjustments in treat plan.

Special Considerations

Pediatric/Adolescent

Until the mid-1990s, type 1 diabetes was the prevalent type of diabetes in children and adolescents. Type 2 diabetes for children is on the rise worldwide, and the mean age is approximately 13.5 years (Rosenbloom et al., 2009). The greatest risk factors are childhood obesity and inactivity. Diabetes is often discovered with glycosuria on a random urinalysis. A red flag for type 2 diabetes in adolescents is acanthosis nigricans, dark pigmentation in skin creases and flexural area. This is a sign of insulin resistance and is present in 60% to 90% of adolescents with type 2 diabetes. It is often easier to see on a physical exam of non-Caucasians, because of more skin pigmentation. Hypertension is present in 20% to 30% of adolescents with type 2 diabetes. In type 1 diabetes, children present with inappropriate polyuria, dehydration, poor weight gain, and ketonuria.

Treatment for type 2 diabetes is weight loss, medical nutritional therapy, exercise, and, in many cases, medication. The only drugs approved for adolescents with type 2 diabetes are insulin, metformin, and liraglutide.

Geriatric

Diabetes in older adults is often complicated by coexisting conditions. Complications develop at an accelerated rate probably because poor glycemic control has been long-standing. Also, older adults usually have a decrease in renal function. Exercise programs for older adults have to be started carefully with comorbid conditions in mind.

Pregnancy

There are two types of diabetes that occur during pregnancy. One is pre-gestational diabetes, as that seen in a woman with type 1 diabetes or type 2 diabetes. This is treated by a specialist and is considered very high risk. The second type is gestational diabetes, which is a form of glucose intolerance detected during pregnancy and associated with resolution after pregnancy.

During pregnancy, human placental lactogen plays a pivotal role in triggering glucose intolerance. It has an antiinsulin and lipolytic effect. Specifically, the peripheral insulin sensitivity decrease as much as 50% from the first trimester to the third trimester while basal hepatic glucose output increases by 30% or more.

Screening for gestational diabetes is recommended between 24 and 28 weeks. There are two choices for screening. Women can have a two-step test, with a 50-g, 1-hour glucose load, followed by a 3-hour glucose tolerance test if necessary. A second alternative is a one-step test, with a 75-g, 2-hour test.

In the gestational diabetic, multiple daily SMBG is required, and it can often be controlled by diet and medical nutritional therapy. If this does not control glucose levels, insulin is required.

Potential neonatal complications include shoulder dystocia, hypoglycemia, polycythemia, and respiratory distress.

Selecting the Most Appropriate Agent

Insulin is necessary in all cases of type 1 diabetes. In patients with type 2 diabetes, a variety of oral agents can be prescribed as monotherapy or in combination. **Table 44.8** lists the potential decrease in A1c with each agent and drug-specific or patient factors to consider for prescribing. The ultimate goal of controlling glycemia is to avoid hyperosmotic symptoms of hyperglycemia, instability of blood sugar over time, minimize hypoglycemia, and prevent or delay complications from diabetes.

First-Line Therapy

In type 1 diabetes, insulin is the only first-line therapy due to absolute insulin deficiency. There are several schedules that can be used for administering acting insulin. The most common regimen is a program that provides basal insulin coverage, using a peakless basal insulin and a rapid-acting insulin before breakfast, lunch, and dinner. The total daily dose requirements typically range from 0.4 to 0.5 units/kg/day with approximately 40% to 50% of the total in the form of basal insulin and the remaining 50% to 60% in the form of Premeal (prandial) insulin (rapid acting or regular insulin) divided into the respective meals. A second regimen is a combination of intermediate- and short-acting insulin. This consists of two injections a day, one in the morning and one in the evening (see **Tables 44.7 and 44.8**).

First-line therapy for type 2 diabetes is monotherapy with metformin if not contraindicated and tolerated. The goal is to achieve or maintain a targeted A1c of less than 7.0% in most patients. If the A1c is above 10%, consider starting insulin therapy or if the A1c is above 9% and symptoms of hyperglycemia are present. See **Tables 44.1 and 44.7**.

Second-Line Therapy

Failure to achieve optimal blood glucose levels in type 2 diabetes after 3 months of monotherapy necessitates the addition of

TABLE 44.8

Comparison of Insulin

Preparation	Brand	Onset (h)	Peak (h)	Duration (h)
Very Rapid-Acting Insulin Analogs				
Aspart	Fiasp	<2.5 min	1–2	3–6
Lispro	Lyumjev	<1 min	1–2	3–5
Rapid-Acting Insulin Analogs				
Lispro	Humalog	<0.5	0.5–3	3–5
Aspart	NovoLog	<0.5	1–3	3–5
Glulisine	Apidra	<0.5	1–2	3–4
Lispro (biosimilar)	Admelog	<0.5	0.5–3	3–5
Short-Acting Insulin				
Regular human insulin	Humulin R	0.5	2–4	6–8
Regular human insulin	Novolin R	Same	Same	Same
Concentrated Regular Insulin				
U500 regular insulin	Humulin R U500	30–45 min	4–8 hours	10–16 hours
Intermediate-Acting Insulin				
NPH	Humulin N	1–4	4–12	14–26
	Novolin N			
Long Acting-Insulin Analogs				
Glargine	Lantus	1–2	None	24
Glargine (biosimilar)	Basaglar	1–2	None	24
Glargine (biosimilar)	Semglee	1–2	None	24
Detemir	Levemir	1	None	14–24 (varies with dose)
Ultra Long-Acting Insulin Analogs				
Glargine	Toujo U300	3–4	None	36 hours
Degludec	Tresiba U100 & U200	30–90 min	None	42 hours
Combination Insulin				
Fixed combination	70/30 (NPH/regular ratio)	30–60 min	Dual	10–16 h
	50/50 (NPL/Lispro ratio)	5–15 min	Dual	10–16 h
	75/25 (NPL/lispro ratio)	5–15 min	Dual	10–16 h
	70/30 (NPA/aspart ratio)	5–15 min	Dual	10–16 h

NPH, neutral protamine hagedorn.

a second oral agent. The choice of the 2nd agent for the treatment of type 2 diabetes should be individualized and based on compelling clinical characteristics, including the need to minimize weight gain or promote weight loss; risk for hypoglycemia; cost; and high risk for or established diagnosis of ASCVD, Heart Failure (HF) or Chronic Kidney Disease (CKD).

GLP-1 RA and SGLT-2i are the choice of therapy for those with indications of HF, ASCVD, or CKD. DPP-4i, GLP-1RA, SGLT-2i, or TZD are appropriate for individuals with higher risk for hypoglycemia. If there is a compelling need to minimize weight gain, then GLP1-RA or SGLT2i is the best choice. Alternately, if cost is a major issue, then sulfonylureas or TZDs

are an appropriate addition to metformin (see **Table 44.9** for an overall approach to pharmacological treatment).

Third-Line Therapy

If the A1c is still above target on a 2nd agent, then consideration for intensification with a third agent should be employed; if the presenting A1c is greater than 9.0 with no symptoms, a third agent can be added. If the goal of decreasing the A1c is not achieved after 3 months, insulin therapy is suggested. An intermediate or basal insulin at bedtime added to the daytime oral regimen can be very effective in treating those with type 2 diabetes.

TABLE 44.9

Comparison of Injectable Glucagon-Like Peptide Receptor Agonist

Short-acting		Administration	Dosing	Comments
Exenatide	Byetta	BID	5 or 10 mcg multi-dose pen	Requires separate pen needle prescription
Liraglutide	Victoza	Daily at any time	1.2 or 1.8 mcg multi-dose pen	Requires separate pen needle prescription
Lixisenatide	Adlyxin	Daily at first meal		Requires separate pen needle prescription
Long-acting				
Extended release Exenatide	Bydureon	Weekly	2 mg single use pen	Pen needle included
Dulaglutide	Trulicity	Weekly	0.75 or 1.5 single use pen	Pen needle included
Semaglutide	Ozempic	Weekly	0.5 mg or 1 mg multi-dose pen	Requires separate pen needle prescription

TABLE 44.10

Glucagon-Like Peptide Receptor Agonist/Basal Insulin Combinations

Name	Strength	Indications/Dosing
Degludec/liraglutide combination (Xultophy)	100/3.6 Maximum daily dose: 50 units	• For use if basal insulin <50 units daily or liraglutide <1.8 mg daily • Administered daily/same time • Starting dose 16 units/0.58 mg (each 1 unit increment = 0.4 mg)
Glargine/lixisenatide combination (Soliqua)	100/33 Maximum daily dose: 60 units	• Administer daily 1 hour before first meal of day • Starting dose 15 units/5 mg if taking glargine <30 units (1 unit = 0.4 mg) • Starting dose 30 units/10 mg if taking 30–60 units of glargine
Dose Adjustment		
FBS above target: +2 to 4 units every weekly	FBS at target: No change in dose	FBS below target: −2 to 4 units weekly

Combination Therapy

Many combination products of two different drug classes are available to treat type 2 diabetes. The following are some of the most common combinations:

- **A sulfonylurea and a biguanide** combination produce mealtime stimulation of endogenous insulin with the sulfonylurea and gluconeogenesis with the biguanide.
- **A biguanide and a TZD** combination provides a synergistic effect on glycemic reduction through insulin sensitization.
- **A DPP-4i and a SGLT-2i** combination reduces insulin resistance, lowers postprandial blood sugars, and can help facilitate weight loss.
- **A biguanide and a SGLT-2i** combination reduces insulin resistance, lowers postprandial glucose levels, and facilitates weight loss.
- **A DPP-4i, SGLT-2i, and biguanide** combination reduces insulin resistance, lowers postprandial glucose levels, and facilitates weight loss.
- **A GLP-1RA and basal insulin** combination reduces fasting and postprandial glucose levels in one convenient daily injection (see **Table 44.10**).

The provider must weigh the risks and benefits of using combinations medications. In some cases, the combination products cost more.

MONITORING PATIENT RESPONSE

Prolonged hyperglycemia of diabetes gives rise to long-term complications that involve lesions of the small (microvascular) and large (macrovascular) blood vessels. Microvascular complications include retinopathy, nephropathy, and neuropathy.

Control is measured using the patient's levels of blood glucose and A1c. Patients use SMBG to keep a daily record of blood glucose. A1c measures blood glucose over 3 months. **Table 44.11** lists the desired levels and levels that require changes in drug regimen.

PATIENT EDUCATION

Drug Information

Education is a hallmark of diabetes therapy. SMBG is essential for monitoring therapeutic response. Practitioners must always educate patients about the signs and symptoms of hypoglycemia and instruct them to carry a source of glucose with them. Possible sources are hard candy (not sugarless) or 4 oz. of juice. All patients with diabetes should have medical identification in the form of a medical alert bracelet or necklace.

TABLE 44.11
Measures of Control of Blood Glucose

Measure of Glucose	Goal	Levels When Adjustment to Regimen Is Indicated
Fasting glucose	80–130 mg/dL	<80 or >140 mg/dL
Random glucose	80–180 mg/dL	<80 or >180 mg/dL
Bedtime glucose	110–150 mg/dL	<110 or >160 mg/dL
A1c	<7	≥7

TABLE 44.12
Estimated Average Glucose

A1c (%)	mg/dL
5	97
6	126
7	154
8	183
9	212
10	240
11	269
12	298

Here are some patient-oriented sources for information and apps that can be downloaded to a smartphone:

- www.diabetes.org is the site from the ADA with information for managing the diabetic's life.
- www.niddk.nih.gov/health/diabetes.htm is a site from the National Institutes of Health that serves as an information clearinghouse.

1. CDC's national website for diabetes:

Diabetes apps

- Glucose Buddy
- mySugr Diabetes Tracker
- DiabetesPal
- Calorie King Food Search
- My Fitness Pal
- One Drop Diabetes Management

Nutritional and Lifestyle Changes

Diabetes management includes medical nutrition therapy, exercise, and, in most cases, drug therapy. Foods high in processed sugar and fat are to be avoided, as is alcohol. Regular daily exercise helps to control blood sugar levels.

Patients with diabetes must follow "sick day guidelines" for the treatment of their condition when dealing with other illnesses. In general, practitioners should instruct people with diabetes not to stop their medication when they are ill. Infection, stress, and other variables increase plasma glucose levels, even though oral intake may be reduced. Practitioners should instruct patients to increase their fluid intake to approximately

8 oz. of water or sugar-free beverage every hour, especially if they have a fever. Patients should monitor blood glucose levels at home more frequently, as often as every 2 to 4 hours. Urine also requires testing for ketones. If the blood glucose concentration is greater than 300 mg/dL on two consecutive readings, fever is persistently high, and symptoms of severe dehydration and ketonuria develop, the patient requires formal evaluation. Sick day plans should be developed with patients before illness occurs (**Table 44.12**).

Complementary and Alternative Medicine

Many people with diabetes combine alternative and traditional medicine. Some of the most common forms of alternative dietary supplements is cinnamon. The use of cinnamon is a popular dietary supplement. Cinnamon is thought to enhance insulin sensitivity and reduce postprandial glucose levels. In a recent study conducted at the U.S. Department of Agriculture, cinnamon reduced serum glucose levels and improved lipid profiles in patients with type 2 diabetes. Patients were randomized into six groups that received 1, 2, or 3 g of cinnamon or a placebo. All groups receiving cinnamon had a decrease of 18% to 30% in fasting serum glucose values, a decrease of 23% to 30% in triglycerides, and a decrease of 7% to 27% in LDL levels. Total cholesterol level declined from 12% to 26%. Doses ranged from 1 to 6 g. Overall cinnamon used as a food is safe. Cinnamon is not currently approved for the treatment of diabetes.

CASE STUDY 1

R.S. is a 55-year-old moderately obese Hispanic woman (body mass index is 29). She was referred to you when her gynecologist noted glucose on a routine urinalysis. She subsequently was tested and found to have a fasting plasma glucose (FPG) of 190 and 200 mg/dL on two separate occasions. She is thirstier than usual and has more frequent

urination. She also complains of decreased energy over the past several months and numbness and tingling in her left lower extremity.

- **Family history:** sister, mother, and maternal grandmother have diabetes

- **Social history:** nonsmoker, drinks alcohol socially (1 drink about 3 times a month), and does not exercise
- **Review of systems:** 20 lb weight gain over the past 2 years, has some blurred vision, has had two urinary tract infections in the past year, and has frequent vaginal yeast infections
  - Gestational diabetes in last two pregnancies
- **Physical exam:** unremarkable except blood pressure of 150/90
  - **Height:** 5.2 in.
  - **Weight:** 200 lb
- **Laboratory results:** FPG, 200 mg/dL; A1c, 10%; low-density lipoprotein, 160 mg/dL; high-density lipoprotein, 35 mg/dL; triglycerides, 266 mg/dL.

DIAGNOSIS: TYPE 2 DIABETES MELLITUS

1. List specific goals for the treatment for R.S.
2. What dietary and lifestyle changes would you recommend for R.S.?
3. What drug therapy would you prescribe? Why?
4. What is the goal for the FPG? Postprandial glucose? A1c?
5. Discuss specific education for R.S. based on the prescribed therapy.
6. List one or two adverse reactions for the therapy selected that would cause you to change the therapy.
7. If the A1c after 3 months on the prescribed therapy is 8.8%, what would be the next line of therapy?

Bibliography

Starred references are cited in the text.

AAC. (2018). Expert consensus decision pathway on novel therapies for cardiovascular risk reduction in patients with type 2 diabetes & atherosclerotic cardiovascular disease. *Journal of American College of Cardiology, 72*(24), 3200–3223. doi: 10.1016/j.jacc.2018.09.020

AACE. (2019). Comprehensive type 2 diabetes management algorithm: Executive summary. Retrieved from https://www.aace.com/pdfs/diabetes/AACE_2019_Diabetes_Algorithm_FINAL_ES.pdf

Abd El Aziz, M. S., Meier, J. J., & Nauck, M. A. (2017). A meta-analysis comparing clinical effects of short- or long-acting GLP-1 receptor agonists versus insulin treatment from head-to-head studies in type 2 diabetes. *Diabetes Obesity Metabolism, 19*, 216–227.

*ADA. (2020). American Diabetes Association Standards of Medical Care in Diabetes. *Diabetes Care, 43*(Suppl. 1), S1–S212.

Adler, A. I., Stratton, I. M., Neil, H. A., et al. (2000). Association of systolic blood pressure with macrovascular and microvascular complications of type 2 diabetes (UKPDS 36): Prospective observational study. *British Medical Journal, 321*, 412–419.

ALLHAT Study Group. (2002). Major outcomes in high-risk hypertensive patients randomized to angiotensin-converting enzyme inhibitor or calcium channel blocker vs. diuretic: The Antihypertensive and Lipid-Lowering Treatment to Prevent Heart Attack Trial (ALLHAT). *Journal of the American Medical Association, 288*, 2981–2997.

American Association of Clinical End (AACE). (2015). American Association of Clinical Endocrinologist and American College of Endocrinology clinical practice guidelines for developing a diabetes mellitus comprehensive care plan. *Endocrine Practice, 21*(Suppl 1), 1–87.

Arslanian, S., Bacha, F., Grey, M., et al. (2018). Evaluation and management of youth-onset type 2 diabetes: A position statement by the American Diabetes Association. *Diabetes Care, 41*, 2648–2668.

*CDC. (2017a). *Diabetes and prediabetes: Fast facts*. Atlanta, GA: U.S. Department of Health and Human Services. Retrieved from https://www.cdc.gov/chronicdisease/resources/publications/factsheets/diabetes-prediabetes.htm

*CDC. (2017b). Number of deaths for the leading causes of death. Retrieved from https://www.cdc.gov/nchs/fastats/leading-causes-of-death.htm

Cefalu, W., Stenlöf, K., Leiter, L., et al. (2015). Effects of canagliflozin on body weight and relationship to A1C and blood pressure changes in patients with type 2 diabetes. *Diabetologia, 58*, 1183–1187. doi: 10.1007/s00125-015-3547-2

Chiang, J. L., Maahs, D. M., Garvey, K. C., et al. (2018). Type 1 diabetes I children and adolescents: A position statement by the American Diabetes Association. *Diabetes Care, 41*, 2026–2044.

Cornell, S., Halstenson, C., & Miller, D. (2019). *The art & science of diabetes self-management education desk reference* (4th ed.). Chicago, IL: American Association of Diabetes Educators.

Davis, M., D'Alessio, D. A., Fradkin, J., et al. (2018). Management of hyperglycemia in type 2 diabetes 2018: A consensus report from the American Diabetes Association and European Association for the Study of Diabetes. *Diabetes Care, 41*(12), 2669–2701. doi: 10.2337/dci18-0033

DCCT/EDIC Research Group. (2000). Retinopathy and nephropathy in patients with type 1 diabetes four years after a trial of intensive therapy. *New England Journal of Medicine, 342*, 381–389.

Diabetes Control and Complications Trial Research Group. (1993). The effect of intensive treatment of diabetes on the development and progression of long-term complications in insulin-dependent diabetes mellitus. *New England Journal of Medicine, 329*, 977–986.

*Diabetes Prevention Program Research Group. (2002). Reduction in the incidence of type 2 diabetes with lifestyle intervention or metformin. *New England Journal of Medicine, 346*, 393–403.

The Diabetes Prevention Program (DPP) Research Group. (2002). The Diabetes Prevention Program (DPP): Description of lifestyle intervention. *Diabetes Care, 25*(12), 2165–2171.

FDA. (2011). FDA drug safety communication: Avandia (rosiglitazone) labels now contain updated information about cardiovascular risks and use in certain patients. Retrieved from http://www.fda.gov/Drugs/DrugSafety/ucm241411.htm

FDA. (2013). FDA drug safety communication: FDA requires removal of some prescribing and dispensing restrictions for rosiglitazone-containing diabetes medicines. http://www.fda.gov/Drugs/DrugSafety/ucm376389.htm

Fitchett, D., Butler, J., van de Borne, P., et al. (2018). EMPA-REG Outcome trial investigators. Effects of empagliflozin on risk for cardiovascular death and heart failure hospitalization across the spectrum of heart failure risk in the EMPA-REG OUTCOME trial. *European Heart Journal, 39*, 363–370.

Gerstein, H. C., Colhoun, H. M., Dagenais, G. R., et al. (2019). REWIND Investigators. Dulaglutide and cardiovascular outcomes in patients with type 2 diabetes (REWIND): A double-blind, randomized placebo-controlled trial. *Lancet, 394*, 121–130.

Hieronymus, L., & Griffin, S. (2015). Role of amylin in type 1 and type 2 diabetes. *Diabetes Educator, 41*(suppl 1), S47–S56. doi: 10.1177/0145721715607642

Ismail-Beigi, F., Craven, T., Banerji, M. A., et al. (2010). Effect of intensive treatment of hyperglycaemia on microvascular outcomes in type 2 diabetes: An analysis of the ACCORD randomised trial. *Lancet (London, England)*, *376*(9739), 419–430. doi: 10.1016/S0140-6736(10)60576-4

James, M. T., Grams, M. E., Woodward, M., et al. (2015). CKD Prognosis Consortium. A meta-analysis of the association of estimated GFR, albuminuria, diabetes mellitus, and hypertension with acute kidney injury. *American Journal of Kidney Disease*, *66*, 602–612.

Kang, H., Lobo, J. M., & Sohn. M. W. (2018). Cost-related medication nonadherence among U.S. adults with diabetes. *Diabetes Research & Clinical Practice*, *143*, 24–33.

Kirkman, M., Rowan-Martin, M. T., Levin, R., et al. (2015). Determinants of adherence to diabetes medications: Findings from a large pharmacy claims database. *Diabetes Care*, *38*(4), 604–609. doi: 10.2337/dc14-2098

*Kristensen, S. L., Rørth, R., Jhund, P. S., et al. (2019). Renal, heart failure, and mortality outcomes with GLP-1 receptor agonists in patients with Type 2 Diabetes: A systematic review and meta-analysis of cardiovascular outcome trials. *Lancet Diabetes Endocrinol*, *7*, 776–785.

Low Wang, C. C., & Shah, A. C. (2017). *Medical management of type 1 diabetes*. Arlington, VA: American Diabetes Association.

Maiorino, M. I., Chiodini, P., Bellastella, G., et al. (2017). Insulin and glucagon like peptide 1 receptor agonist combination therapy in type 2 diabetes: A systematic review meta-analysis of randomized-control trials. *Diabetes Care*, *40*, 614–624.

Marso, S. P. (2016). LEADER steering committee; LEADER trial investigators. Liraglutide and cardiovascular outcomes in type 2 diabetes. *New England Journal of Medicine*, *375*, 311–322.

Marso, S. P., Bain, S. C., Consoli, A., et al. (2016). SUSTAIN-6 Investigators. Semaglutide and cardiovascular outcomes in patients with type 2 diabetes. *New England Journal of Medicine*, *375*, 1834–1844.

Maruther, N. M., Tseng, E., Hutfless, S., et al. (2016). Diabetes medications as monotherapy or metformin-based combination therapy for type 2 diabetes: A systemic review and meta-analysis. *Annals Internal Medicine*, *164*, 740–751.

Neuen, B. L., Ohkuma, T., Neal, B., et al. (2018). Cardiovascular and renal outcomes with canagliflozin according to baseline kidney function: Data from the CANVAS program. *Circulation*, *138*, 1537–1550.

Petrenchik, L., & Loh, F. E. (2017). Factors affecting noninsulin antidiabetic drug adherence in patients with type 2 diabetes. *Diabetes Spectrum*, *67*(1). doi: 10.2337/db18-806-P

Uccellatorre, A., Genovese, S., Dicembrini, I., et al. (2015). Comparison review of short-acting and long-acting glucagon like peptide 1 receptor agonists. *Diabetes Therapeutics*, *6*(3), 239–256.

UK Prospective Diabetes Study Group. (1998a). Effect of intensive blood-glucose control with metformin on complications in overweight patients with type 2 diabetes (UKPDS 34). *Lancet*, *352*, 854–865.

UK Prospective Diabetes Study Group. (1998b). Intensive blood-glucose control with sulfonylureas or insulin compared with conventional treatment and risk of complications in patients with type 2 diabetes (UKPDS 33). *Lancet*, *352*, 837–853.

U.S. Food and Drug Administration. (2019). FDA revises warning regarding use of the diabetes medication metformin in certain patients with reduced kidney function. Retrieved from https://www.fda.gov/drugs/drug-safety-and-availability/fda-drug-safety-communication-fda-revises-warnings-regarding-use-diabetes-medicine-metformin-certain

Vallon, V., & Thomson. S. C. (2017). Targeting renal glucose reabsorption to treat hyperglycaemia: The pleiotropic effects of SGLT2 inhibition. *Diabetologia*, *60*(2), 215–225.

Whittemore, R., Melkus, G., Wagner, J., et al. (2009). Translating the diabetes prevention program to primary care: A pilot study. *Nursing Research*, *58*(1), 2–12. doi: 10.1097/NNR.0b013e31818fcef3

Wilding, J., Rejeev, S., & DeFronzo, R. A. (2016). Positioning SGLT2 inhibitors/incretin-based therapies in the treatment algorithm. *Diabetes Care*, *39*(Suppl. 2), S154–S164.

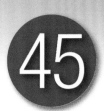

45 Thyroid and Parathyroid Disorders

Alice (Lim) Scaletta and Louis R. Petrone

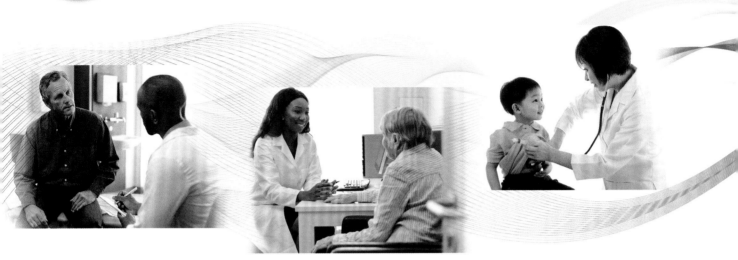

Learning Objectives

1. Explain the role and function of the thyroid and parathyroid and their respective hormones.
2. Compare and contrast the signs and symptoms of hypothyroidism and hyperthyroidism.
3. Based on patient preference, patient presentation, adverse-effect profile, contraindications, and drug interactions, choose appropriate pharmacologic and nonpharmacologic treatment for thyroid and parathyroid disorders.
4. Counsel a patient on administration, adverse effects, and monitoring parameters for medications used to treat thyroid and parathyroid disorders.

INTRODUCTION

The thyroid is the body's largest endocrine gland and is located in the neck anterior to the trachea. It produces two biologically important hormones essential for the metabolic processes of nearly every organ in the body: thyroxine (T_4) and triiodothyronine (T_3). These hormones are vital for fetal growth and central nervous system development. After birth, thyroid hormones are responsible for maintaining tissue thermogenesis, basal metabolic rate, and cardiac functioning.

Reporting epidemiology of thyroid disorders is challenging since prevalence varies across different parts of the world. Factors such as differences in diagnostic standards, assay sensitivities, and availability of iodine nutrition can impact reporting. Iodine-deficient regions include Southeast Asia, South America, and Central Africa, which represents over a billion people worldwide. In these areas, nodular thyroid diseases are most common. Conversely, in iodine-rich countries such as the United States, the most common cause of thyroid disorders is due to autoimmune thyroid disease. Women are disproportionately affected with thyroid disorders compared to men. The older adults are also more susceptible to thyroid disorders.

In iodine-sufficient parts of the world, the prevalence of hypothyroidism is 1% to 2%, and in the United States, it is about 0.3% to 3.7% (Chaker et al., 2017; Taylor et al., 2018). A higher percentage, about 4% to 20%, has mild or subclinical hypothyroidism (Azim & Nasr, 2019). The prevalence of overt hyperthyroidism is 0.2% to 1.3% in iodine-sufficient parts of the world. About 1.3% of the general population has subclinical hyperthyroidism (Taylor et al., 2018; Vanderpump, 2019).

The rate of thyroid cancer diagnosis has increased faster than any other kind of cancer in the United States, occurring at an incidence of 15 cases per 100,000 in a year. However, overdiagnosis may be contributing to these high rates. Thyroid cancer remains one of the least deadly cancers, with 0.4 deaths per 100,000 person-years in the United States (Roman et al., 2017).

Iodine is an essential building block of thyroid hormones. Taken in through the diet, iodine is reduced to iodide in the gastrointestinal tract. It is then transported into the thyroid follicular cells where it is oxidized by thyroid peroxidase. This allows iodide to bind to tyrosine residues found in thyroglobulin, which is a glycoprotein found within the thyroid. Iodide binds to these tyrosine residues to form monoiodotyrosine (MIT), where one iodine is attached, and diiodotyrosine

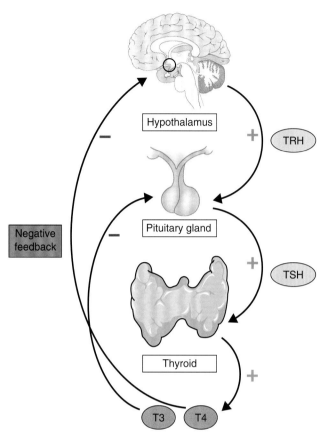

FIGURE 45–1   Hypothalamic-pituitary-thyroid axis (hand-drawn draft).

T₃, triiodothyronine; T₄, thyroxine; TRH, thyroid releasing hormone; TSH, thyroid-stimulating hormone.

(DIT), which has two iodine attached. Once these are formed, they can couple with each other to form T_4 (DIT + DIT) and T_3 (MIT + DIT).

Thyroid hormone synthesis is under the control of the hypothalamic-pituitary-thyroid axis (**Figure 45.1**). In order to detect and respond to the metabolic needs of the body, and because of the potent effects of even small amounts of thyroid hormone, the hypothalamus and pituitary gland serve as a check and balance system to regulate the synthesis and release of thyroid hormones. When the hypothalamus recognizes there is an inadequate supply of thyroid hormone, it releases thyroid releasing hormone (TRH), which stimulates the anterior pituitary to release thyroid-stimulating hormone (TSH). TSH in return stimulates the thyroid to synthesize and release thyroid hormone. When thyroid hormone supplies are adequate, a built in negative feedback system prevents the overproduction of thyroid hormone. Circulating T_3 and T_4 signal the hypothalamus to decrease release of TRH and the anterior pituitary to decrease the release of TSH, thus preventing the overproduction of thyroid hormones.

Thyroid hormones are stored within the thyroglobulin of the thyroid. Once released, over 99% of thyroid hormone is protein bound when traveling throughout the body in the

bloodstream. Protein binding allows for a longer half-life of 7 to 10 days for T_4 and 24 hours for T_3. However, only the unbound or free thyroid hormone is able to exert biological activity. Less than 1% of the total thyroid hormone in the body is responsible for the metabolic processes of virtually the entire body, which highlights the potency of these hormones.

Eighty percent of thyroid hormone made in the thyroid is T_4. While T_3 makes up only 20% of the hormones made by the thyroid, T_3 is more potent than T_4 and is responsible for most of the metabolic activity in the body. The peripheral tissue is able to convert T_4 to T_3 through tissue deiodinases. This ability allows individual organs to dictate the amount of thyroid hormone activity based on its individual metabolic needs. Therefore, T_4 can be seen as a prohormone to T_3.

Serum TSH is the most sensitive and useful marker of thyroid function. It is highly responsive to even subtle changes in circulating thyroid hormones. Thus, it is helpful for initial screening and diagnosis of thyroid dysfunction, even in asymptomatic or subclinical disease. What is considered to be normal serum TSH levels has been highly debated. While most young, healthy euthyroid individuals have TSH levels between 0.5 and 2.5 mIU/L, normal levels increase with age, and the older euthyroid patient can have a serum TSH up to 4.5 mIU/L.

Serum T_3 and T_4 levels are yet more tools to assess thyroid function. Available laboratory testing can measure total thyroid hormone levels (total T_3 or T_4) or unbound thyroid hormone levels (free T_3 and T_4). Because many factors can alter protein binding and because biologic action results from the free form of thyroid hormone, free T_3 and T_4 testing is more sensitive in detecting thyroid dysfunction.

Because thyroid disorders often result from autoimmune disease, detection of various antibodies can help to clarify etiologies and prognoses of thyroid disorders. Thyroid peroxidase antibodies (TPOAb) and thyroglobulin antibodies (TgAb) are often found in autoimmune causes of hypothyroidism, while presence of TSH receptor antibodies (TRAb) often signifies an autoimmune cause for hyperthyroidism. For those with subclinical disease, the presence of antibodies can predict progression to overt disease.

The parathyroid is made up of four pea-sized glands that sit adjacent to the thyroid, and is the smallest endocrine gland in the body (**Figure 45.2**). Despite their close proximity to each other, the thyroid and parathyroid are unrelated and have different functions. The parathyroid gland's primary role is regulating calcium and phosphorus levels in the body through the actions of parathyroid hormone (PTH). Adequate serum calcium is essential for bone, heart, muscular, and nerve health. If serum calcium levels are deficient, PTH stimulates various organs to help raise serum calcium levels. It causes the kidney to increase reabsorption of calcium and stimulates the conversion of vitamin D to its active form 1,25-dihydroxyvitamin D_3 in the kidney. Active vitamin D in return increases the absorption of ingested calcium from the

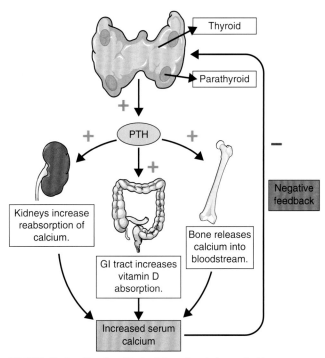

FIGURE 45–2   Parathyroid physiology (hand-drawn draft).

GI, gastrointestinal; PTH, parathyroid hormone.

intestines. PTH also encourages resorption of calcium from the bones into the bloodstream. Similar to thyroid hormones, calcium acts as its own mediator of negative feedback; when calcium binds to receptors on the parathyroid, it signals the parathyroid to decrease the production and release of PTH. Primary hyperparathyroidism is the third most common endocrine disorder and is one of the most common causes of hypercalcemia (Rao, 2018).

HYPOTHYROIDISM

In general, hypothyroidism is a deficiency of thyroid hormones, and it is the most common thyroid disorder. The incidence is higher in women and older adults (Azim & Nasr, 2019). Patients can either present with overt disease or a milder form known as subclinical hypothyroidism.

Causes

Worldwide, the most common cause of hypothyroidism is iodine deficiency. In the United States where iodine is readily available in food and fortified salt, the most common cause is autoimmune thyroiditis, also known as Hashimoto's thyroiditis (Jonklaas et al., 2014; Taylor et al., 2018).

Less commonly, hypothyroidism can result iatrogenically, either from radiation or surgery in the head and neck area, or drugs (amiodarone, lithium, tyrosine kinase inhibitors). When radiation or thyroid surgery is used to treat

hyperthyroidism, hypothyroidism in an expected effect and patients will need to be treated with thyroid replacement therapy. Patients typically become hypothyroid 3 to 12 months after radioactive iodine (RAI), and within 1 month after total thyroidectomy.

Transient hypothyroidism may result from subacute thyroiditis and silent thyroiditis such as postpartum thyroiditis. Because the thyroid is controlled by the actions of both the hypothalamus and pituitary gland, problems with either can lead to secondary hypothyroidism, albeit they occur rarely. Hypothalamic or pituitary failure results in insufficient TSH, which signals the thyroid to decrease production of thyroid hormones.

Pathophysiology

The deficit of thyroid hormone seen in hypothyroidism is due to decreased production and release of thyroid hormones. This most commonly results from a lack of iodine needed to synthesize thyroid hormone, or from Hashimoto's disease, where autoantibodies work against thyroid tissue and thyroid peroxidase.

Long-term sequelae of hypothyroidism include hypercholesterolemia and increased systemic vascular resistance, both of which in turn potentiate cardiovascular disease. Additionally, neuropsychiatric effects like a dementia-like state can occur in the older adults (Barbesino, 2019; Calsolaro et al., 2018; Cappola et al., 2015).

Diagnostic Criteria

Signs and symptoms of hypothyroidism are listed in **Box 45.1**. Symptoms can present very subtly or not at all, especially in subclinical disease. Additionally, many of the classic signs and symptoms of hypothyroidism may progress so gradually or may not immediately be associated with thyroid dysfunction and thus disease may persist for a long time before a diagnosis can be made. Patients with overt disease are more likely to present with symptoms. In long-standing untreated disease, myxedema and delayed deep tendon reflexes can be seen.

Laboratory findings for hypothyroidism are presented in **Table 45.1**. Serum TSH is the primary screening tool for decreased thyroid function. The lack of circulating thyroid hormones causes the anterior pituitary to respond by increasing TSH. In overt hypothyroidism, serum TSH is elevated over 10 mIU/L. Additionally, serum-free T_4 will be low.

TSH is so sensitive to changes in thyroid homeostasis that changes in serum TSH are seen before thyroid hormone levels even become abnormal, which is why it is a more useful biomarker in detecting mild or subclinical disease. Serum TSH is mildly elevated at more than 4.5 to 10 mIU/L, while free T_4 levels will be normal. Oftentimes, patients with subclinical disease may progress to overt disease, especially in those with detectable TPOAb or TgAb titers.

Fatigue
Lethargy
Mental impairment
Depression
Cold sensitivity
Dry skin
Goiter
Hair loss
Decreased perspiration
Decreased appetite
Weight gain
Voice changes
Constipation
Menstrual disturbances
Arthralgia
Paresthesia
Slow movements
Decreased reflexes
Slow speech
Nonpitting edema (myxedema)
Bradycardia
Infertility
Hyperlipidemia

In secondary hypothyroidism where the etiology is due to deficiencies with either the pituitary gland or hypothalamus, TSH would actually be low along with free T_4.

Initiating Drug Therapy

Patients with serum TSH level more than 10 mIU/L should be initiated on thyroid hormone replacement therapy. Treating those with subclinical elevations of TSH between 4.5 and 10 mIU/L is more controversial. There have been no studies to show definitive benefit in treating these patients. Still, the decision should be individualized to the patient, since subclinical

TABLE 45.1
Laboratory Findings in Hypothyroidism

	Serum TSH	Free T_4
Overt hypothyroidism	Elevated (>10 mIU/L)	Low (<0.7 ng/dL)
Mild or subclinical hypothyroidism	Mildly elevated (>4.5–10 mIU/L)	Normal (0.7–1.9 ng/dL)

T_4, thyroxine; TSH, thyroid-stimulating hormone.

hypothyroidism poses many of the same risks of overt disease (Azim & Nasr, 2019; Blum et al., 2015). Consider treating patients without symptoms if they have underlying cardiovascular disease, have high risk for cardiovascular disease, have a goiter, have positive TPOAb titers, have infertility, or are pregnant. The mainstay of treatment will be thyroid hormone replacement therapy.

Goals of Drug Therapy

1. Restore thyroid hormones to normal levels.
2. Relieve signs and symptoms of hypothyroidism.
3. Prevent complications and long-term sequelae of hypothyroidism.
4. Prevent neurological and developmental deficits in newborns and children.

Thyroid Hormone

Synthetic and natural thyroid hormone replacement products are listed in **Table 45.2**. While several products are available, there is no evidence to support the use of any product over the standard of therapy, which is synthetic levothyroxine (LT_4). There is no added benefit to administering exogenous T_3 since peripheral tissue would still be able to convert T_4 to T_3 as needed based on its individual metabolic needs (Kang et al., 2013; Wiersinga, 2019). Therefore, providing LT_4 solely still mimics normal physiologic functioning. Additionally, LT_4's long half-life of 7 to 10 days allows for a steady dose response. The higher cost of the other drugs also limits their use.

Liothyronine is synthetic T_3. Because of its increased potency compared to LT_4, there is an increased risk for toxicity. Peripheral tissues are also unable to control local T_3 activity, unlike with LT_4, which they can convert to T_3 when needed. Its short half-life also necessitates multiple day dosing and leads to more significant peaks and troughs of drug levels.

Desiccated thyroid is derived from cow and pig thyroid and thus has varying and unpredictable T_4 and T_3 hormone content. Occasionally, patients may experience an allergic reaction to these products. Liotrix is a synthetic combination product with a fixed LT_4 to T_3 ratio of 4:1. These combination products tout the ability to mirror thyroid functioning by providing both T_4 and T_3. However, there has been no evidence to show benefit of these therapies over LT_4. Additionally, these products contain a higher amount of T_3 in relation to T_4 than seen in normal thyroid functioning in humans and thus can pose a higher risk for thyrotoxicosis.

Mechanism of Action

Exogenous thyroid hormone, whether synthetic or animal derived, has the same action as endogenous thyroid hormone. It binds to thyroid receptors on cell nuclei to exert metabolic effect in tissues.

Dosage and Administration

The daily dose necessary to achieve a euthyroid state is individual to each patient and can be impacted by age, sex, and weight. The average therapeutic dose of LT_4 is 1.6 mcg/kg/d (using

TABLE 45.2			
Thyroid Replacement Therapies for the Treatment of Hypothyroidism			
Generic (Trade) Name and Dosage	**Selected Adverse Events**	**Contraindications**	**Special Considerations**
Desiccated thyroid (Armour Thyroid) Start: 30–32.5 mg/d Maintenance: 60–130 mg/d	Occurs with excessive dosing: symptoms of hyperthyroidism (palpitations, nervousness, tremor, weight loss, arrhythmias)	Hypersensitivity, untreated thyrotoxicosis, uncorrected adrenal cortical insufficiency	Second-line therapy; contains desiccated pork or beef thyroid glands containing T_4 and T_3
Levothyroxine (Synthroid, Levoxyl, Unithroid) Start: 12.5–100 mcg/d Maintenance: average 1.6 mcg/kg	Same as mentioned earlier	Same as mentioned earlier	First-line therapy; contains synthetic T_4
Liothyronine (Cytomel) Start: 25 mcg/d Maintenance: 25–75 mcg/d	Same as mentioned earlier	Same as mentioned earlier	Second-line therapy; contains synthetic T_3
Liotrix (Thyrolar) Start: levothyroxine 25 mcg/d + liothyronine 6.25 mcg/d Maintenance: levothyroxine 50–100 mcg/d + liothyronine 12.5–25 mcg/d	Same as mentioned earlier	Same as mentioned earlier	Second-line therapy; contains synthetic T_4 and T_3 in combination tablet

T_3, triiodothyronine; T_4, thyroxine.

ideal body weight in obese patients). In young patients without cardiovascular disease, the full therapeutic dose can be started and titrated as needed based on TSH monitoring and symptom improvement. In patients aged 75 and older, starting with a low dose of 25 to 50 mcg/d is appropriate since they generally need less hormone to experience therapeutic effects. Patients with ischemic heart disease are at risk for the cardiovascular risks of overtreatment with LT_4, which can lead to myocardial ischemia and angina. Therefore, these patients should be started on 12.5 to 25 mcg/d.

When treating patients with mild or subclinical disease, the full therapeutic dose is usually not needed. Instead, they can be started on LT_4 25 to 50 mcg/d and titrated up as necessary.

Approximately 70% of the drug is absorbed orally. Therefore, intravenous administration requires a dose decrease to 50% to 70% of the oral dose.

Serum TSH should be checked in 6 to 8 weeks after initiating thyroid replacement therapy. The dose should be titrated based on the TSH level. If a dose change is needed, a slow titration of a 10% to 20% change in dose is recommended. Repeat serum TSH in 6 to 8 weeks after any dosage adjustments and continue to adjust the dose until TSH reaches target range.

Though the Food and Drug Administration rates all brand and generic LT_4 products as bioequivalent, it is widely accepted that they are not therapeutically interchangeable. Because even small differences in thyroid hormone can result in significant physiologic changes, variability in these products, whether in how they are manufactured and what inactive ingredients are present, can lead to differences in bioavailability in an individual. Therefore, patients should avoid switching preparations, either between brand and generic formulations or between different manufacturers of generic LT_4

(Benvenga & Carlé, 2019). If a switch must be made due to insurance or cost, monitoring TSH and adjusting the dosage as necessary is advised.

Time Frame for Response

Patients typically start to feel better after about a week of taking thyroid hormone therapy; however, they may have to wait several weeks for full symptom resolution. It will also take 6 to 8 weeks before TSH and serum thyroid hormone levels to reach normal range. It will take even longer if dose adjustments need to be made.

Contraindications

Thyroid hormone replacement is contraindicated in untreated adrenal insufficiency or thyrotoxicosis, as these agents can aggravate the symptoms of these conditions.

Adverse Drug Reactions

Adverse effects of thyroid hormone replacement occur with overtreatment and present similarly to the symptoms of hyperthyroidism. Patients who are overtreated chronically can develop atrial fibrillation, mental status changes, or fractures in the older adults. Postmenopausal women are also more likely to experience accelerated bone loss and osteoporosis.

Interactions

Several factors influence absorption and therefore dose requirements of LT_4 (**Table 45.3**) (Skelin et al., 2017). For maximal absorption, it should be taken on an empty stomach either 1 hour before the first meal of the day, or at least 4 hours after the last meal of the day. If patients are unable to adhere to this schedule, they should at minimum avoid too much variability in the timing of the medication in respect to food in order to maintain a steady concentration of LT_4.

TABLE 45.3
Drug Interactions of Levothyroxine

Impact of Interaction on LT$_4$	Interacting Medications
Decreased absorption	Metals (calcium, iron, aluminum)
	Bile acid sequestrants (e.g., cholestyramine)
	Sucralfate
	Phosphate binders
	Fiber supplements
	Proton pump inhibitors
Increased clearance	Rifampin
	Carbamazepine
	Phenytoin
	Phenobarbital
Impaired deiodination of T$_4$ to T$_3$	Amiodarone
Unknown mechanism for decreased LT$_4$ effect	Selective serotonin reuptake inhibitors
	Lovastatin

LT$_4$, levothyroxine; T$_3$, triiodothyronine; T$_4$, thyroxine.

In particular, foods containing calcium can significantly decrease absorption of LT$_4$ and thus the medication should be separated from these foods.

Similarly, many drugs can impact absorption or clearance of LT$_4$, as listed in **Table 45.3**. It is recommended to separate administration of these drugs by taking LT$_4$ at least 2 hours before or 6 hours after the interacting medications.

LT$_4$ requires an acidic gastric environment to be absorbed; consequently, it is thought that acid-reducing agents like proton pump inhibitors or histamine-2 receptor antagonists can interact with LT$_4$. However, recent studies have shown conflicting data on whether or not these interactions are clinically significant. Antacids, on the other hand, are known to interact with LT$_4$ absorption due to their calcium or aluminum content.

Thyroid replacement can impact the effects of other medications. In hypothyroidism, there is a decrease in metabolism of vitamin K clotting factors. Therefore, when thyroid hormones are restored, clotting factors may decrease and cause bleeding. Therefore, those taking warfarin should be monitored closely if they initiate or change thyroid hormone therapy.

Selecting the Most Appropriate Drug
First-Line Therapy
For the reasons stated earlier, LT$_4$ remains the gold standard of therapy to treat hypothyroidism. It provides steady reliable dosing, is effective, and is relatively inexpensive.

Second-Line Therapy
Other thyroid hormone replacement therapies contain synthetic or naturally derived T$_3$; however, this does not typically result in better outcomes when compared to LT$_4$ therapy alone. Thus, these agents are considered second-line options

for hypothyroidism. The exception where administering T$_3$ may be beneficial is in the rare case of a patient who has diminished ability to convert T$_4$ to T$_3$.

Special Considerations
Myxedema Coma
When left untreated chronically, hypothyroidism can advance to a decompensated condition known as myxedema coma, in which patients experience hypothermia, central nervous system depression, respiratory depression, cardiovascular instability, electrolyte imbalances, delirium, and even coma. It is a life-threatening condition that carries a mortality rate as high as 30% to 60% (Bridwell et al., 2020) and thus must be treated immediately and aggressively. Management includes a large bolus dose of thyroid hormone replacement with intravenous (IV) LT$_4$ 300 to 500 mcg, followed by a maintenance dose of 75 to 100 mcg IV. Because adrenal suppression often accompanies myxedema coma, IV hydrocortisone is often given in conjunction.

Pediatric
All newborns are screened for congenital hypothyroidism with a TSH level. If it is confirmed, the child must be treated with LT$_4$ indefinitely. Because thyroid hormones are vital during childhood when growth and development is highest, children require more aggressive thyroid hormone replacement compared to adults (Wassner, 2017). The newborn dose is 10 to 17 mcg/kg/d with a goal of achieving T$_4$ concentrations at 10 mcg/dL. Despite potential interactions, it can be crushed and mixed with breast milk or formula for ease of administration. The dose is reduced as the child ages; at 6 months of age, 5 to 7 mcg/kg/d. At ages 1 to 10 years, the dose is 3 to 6 mcg/kg/d. The adult dosage can be given at 12 years and beyond.

Geriatric
Older adults are more prone to hypothyroidism compared to younger individuals (Barbesino, 2019; Calsolaro et al., 2018; Cappola et al., 2015). They are also more susceptible to the adverse effects of thyroid replacement therapies and thus should be started on a low dose and titrated up as needed depending on their symptom improvement and TSH monitoring. Aiming for a TSH goal at the high end of normal range is appropriate, as older patients usually experience resolution of symptoms at a higher TSH compared to younger patients, and this practice helps to minimize the risk of overtreatment.

Pregnancy
During pregnancy, beta-human chorionic gonadotropin (β-hCG) increases and acts like a TSH receptor agonist, which in turn increases the thyroid hormones so important for fetal development. Untreated hypothyroidism during pregnancy can lead to miscarriage, preterm delivery, maternal hypertension, preeclampsia, low birth weight, and stillbirth. The child is also at risk for impaired intellectual development. For this reason, all women should have TSH measured as soon as pregnancy is confirmed (Alexander et al., 2017; Springer et al., 2017).

If a woman is already being treated for hypothyroidism before pregnancy, her dose of LT_4 will need to be increased by 20% to 50% in order to maintain a TSH level in normal range, ideally less than 2.5 mIU/L. TSH should be monitored every 4 weeks during the first half of pregnancy, then once between weeks 26 and 32 of gestation. Typically, patients can return to their prepregnancy dose of LT_4 after delivery.

Women should be counseled to separate administration of LT_4 by 2 hours before or 6 hours after prenatal vitamins, as they contain high levels of calcium and iron.

Monitoring Patient Response

Anytime a thyroid hormone replacement therapy is initiated, the dose is changed, or the formulation is switched, serum TSH should be measured 6 to 8 weeks afterwards. The dose should then be gradually adjusted based on the TSH. Once a stable dose is established, serum TSH can be measured less often at every 6 to 12 months. Additionally, dosing requirements decrease with age. As patients age, the picture of their chronic conditions and medications will change, which may also impact LT_4 levels in the body (Duntas & Jonklaas, 2019). Therefore, periodic monitoring of TSH is recommended to detect when dose adjustments are necessary. The TSH can be checked sooner in the case of any clinical changes such as in weight, interacting medications stopped/started, and pregnancy as that may require a dose adjustment. The goal is to achieve a serum TSH within normal range; however, as emphasized earlier, the range is large, and the TSH level that leads to symptomatic improvement may vary with individuals. Because TSH is a more sensitive marker for therapeutic effect, monitoring free T_4 or total T_3 levels is usually not necessary. The exception is with secondary hypothyroidism, where TSH will not be helpful in guiding therapy. Instead, free T_4 should be measured in these cases.

Patient Education

Drug Information

The most common reason for suboptimal therapy with LT_4 is due to nonadherence (Zsolt et al., 2018). Therefore, patients should be counseled on the importance of adherence in preventing symptoms and complications of hypothyroidism. Patients should also be given instructions on how to best ensure maximal absorption of LT_4. For example, they should take it on an empty stomach, separate from food and other medications. They should also avoid switching formulations.

At times, patients have been known to take excessive thyroid hormone in order to potentiate weight loss. This should be discouraged, as overtreatment with LT_4 can lead to untoward side effects consistent with symptoms seen in hyperthyroidism, including cardiac and bone problems.

Complementary and Alternative Medications

Over-the-counter supplements claim the ability to support thyroid functioning by boosting thyroid hormone with natural ingredients. Some common ingredients include kelp (contains iodine), ashwagandha (a traditional Ayurvedic herb), and various vitamins and minerals. There is a lack of data to support these products. One study conducted in 50 patients in India suggests a possible benefit of ashwagandha compared to placebo, but the small sample size limits the generalizability of these results (Sharma et al., 2018). Additionally, another study revealed that 10 commercially available thyroid supplements were laced with T_3 and T_4. Should patients take these supplements along with prescription thyroid hormone, they may risk toxic effects of overtreatment. Therefore, patients should be encouraged to exercise caution before choosing these supplements.

HYPERTHYROIDISM

Thyrotoxicosis occurs when tissues are exposed to excessive thyroid hormone. Hyperthyroidism is one cause, though there exist non-hyperthyroid causes of thyrotoxicosis. As with hypothyroidism, patients can present with either overt or subclinical disease. One-half percent of the population is affected with overt hyperthyroidism, with higher incidences in women and in those over the age of 80 (De Leo et al., 2016; Taylor et al., 2018; Vanderpump, 2019).

Causes and Pathophysiology

Causes of thyrotoxicosis are listed in **Table 45.4**. The most common cause of hyperthyroidism in the United States is Graves' Disease (De Leo et al., 2016; Smith & Hegedus, 2016), an autoimmune disorder in which TRAb mimic TSH and stimulate TSH receptors to cause thyroid hormone synthesis and release. In older adults, however, toxic multinodular goiter is more common (Samuels, 2018; Taylor et al., 2016).

Secondary causes of hyperthyroidism occur when a pathologic event bypasses the negative feedback loop of the hypothalamic-pituitary-thyroid axis and stimulates the otherwise healthy thyroid to oversecrete thyroid hormones. Examples include pituitary tumors that secrete TSH.

Thyrotoxicosis can occur without an overactive thyroid. In these cases, excessive thyroid hormone is released from its stores due to direct insult to the thyroid. Examples include injury from drugs and inflammation in the thyroid, or thyroiditis.

Complications

Untreated thyrotoxicosis can result in atrial fibrillation, congestive heart failure, embolic events, and osteoporosis (Ross et al., 2016). Those with subclinical disease are at risk for developing these complications. It is recommended for older patients with hyperthyroidism to undergo cardiac evaluation since they are more susceptible to the cardiac effects of thyrotoxicosis. Postmenopausal women should also be considered for anti-osteoporosis agents.

In patients with Graves' disease, autoimmune processes lead to inflammation of the eyes. Known as Graves' ophthalmopathy (GO), symptoms can include eye discomfort,

TABLE 45.4
Causes of Thyrotoxicosis

Causes	Examples
Primary hyperthyroidism	Graves' disease Toxic multinodular goiter Toxic adenoma Thyroid cancer Excessive iodine
Secondary hyperthyroidism	TSH-secreting pituitary tumors Trophoblastic (hCG-secreting) tumors Gestational thyrotoxicosis
Thyrotoxicosis without hyperthyroidism	Subacute thyroiditis Silent (painless) thyroiditis Excessive thyroid hormone intake Drug induced (amiodarone, cytokine or tyrosine kinase inhibitors, interferon, iodine, lithium)

hCG, human chorionic gonadotropin; TSH, thyroid-stimulating hormone.

BOX 45.2   Signs and Symptoms of Hyperthyroidism

Nervousness
Fatigue
Irritability
Hyperactivity
Weakness
Increased perspiration
Heat sensitivity
Palpitations
Tremor
Increased appetite
Decreased weight
Menstrual disturbances
Infertility
Goiter
Increase in frequency of bowel movements
Tachycardia
Atrial fibrillation (especially in older adults)
Hyperreflexia
Tremor in protruded tongue and outstretched hands
Warm, smooth, moist skin
Goiter
Ophthalmopathy and dermopathy in Graves' disease

excessive tearing, sensitivity to light, exophthalmos (bulging, swollen eyes), eyelid retraction, lid lag (lagging of upper lid when looking down), and periorbital edema. The annual incidence of GO is 16 cases per 100,000 women and 3 cases per 100,000 men, affecting 30% of patients with Graves' disease (Kotwal & Stan, 2018; Smith & Hegedus, 2016). Severe cases can lead to excessive pressure on the optic nerve, causing permanent vision loss. The autoimmune effects of Graves' disease can also lead to dermopathy in 1% to 4% of patients (Smith & Hegedus, 2016), including peripheral edema and pretibial myxedema.

Diagnostic Criteria

Clinical presentation of hyperthyroidism is shown in **Box 45.2**. Many may have symptoms for a long time before a diagnosis is made because the progression of disease is gradual and difficult to notice. Often, the signs and symptoms are directly opposite from those seen in hypothyroidism with a few notable exceptions. For example, while constipation is seen in hypothyroidism, diarrhea is not necessarily a symptom of hyperthyroidism. Rather, patients may present with a higher frequency of bowel movements instead. Additionally, patients with either hypo- or hyperthyroidism can both experience fatigue and weakness. Importantly, signs and symptoms of hyperthyroidism can be nonspecific and progress very gradually, especially with mild or subclinical disease. Patients with Graves' disease may also present with an enlarged thyroid, ophthalmopathy, and skin changes. Symptom severity does not seem to correlate with thyroid hormone levels.

Table 45.5 shows laboratory findings for hyperthyroidism. The excessive circulating hormone in thyrotoxicosis creates a negative feedback loop that signals the pituitary to stop releasing TSH. Patients therefore will have low-to-undetectable TSH levels in hyperthyroidism. Identifying the etiology of hyperthyroidism is crucial in determining the most appropriate treatment approach. If the etiology cannot be ascertained from TSH/T_4 testing and clinical presentation alone, further testing is needed. The detection of TRAb can indicate Graves' disease. Radioactive iodine uptake (RAIU) can be used to discern between thyroid hyperactivity versus thyroid injury leading to increased thyroid hormone levels. RAIU measures the amount of radioactivity that penetrates the thyroid tissue after the patient ingests RAI. High uptake into the thyroid is indicative of Graves' disease or toxic nodular goiter since the thyroid is actively taking up iodine in order to form more thyroid hormone. Low uptake on the other hand is indicative of thyroid injury or inflammation causing the thyroid to leak thyroid hormones into the circulation. RAIU testing is contraindicated during pregnancy.

Initiating Drug Therapy

The main choices in therapy include antithyroid drugs (ATD), RAI therapy, or surgery (**Table 45.6**). There is no evidence to show that one treatment modality is better than the other, and the choice should depend on patient preference, tolerability, cost, and existence of contraindications (Ross et al., 2016).

TABLE 45.5

Laboratory Findings in Hyperthyroidism

	Serum TSH	Free T$_4$
Overt hyperthyroidism	Low or undetectable (<0.5 mIU/L)	Elevated (>1.9 ng/dL)
Mild or subclinical hyperthyroidism	Low or undetectable (<0.5 mIU/L)	Normal (0.7–1.9 ng/dL)

T$_4$, thyroxine; TSH, thyroid-stimulating hormone.

Often ATD is considered as a first choice for therapy due to its oral formulation and ability to salvage the thyroid. The goal of treatment is remission of disease, but relapse is common after discontinuation of therapy. ATDs are favored in those who have a high likelihood of remission, including women, those with small goiters, those with mild hyperthyroidism, and those with negative titers for TRAb. Additionally, ATDs are more appropriate for those who have high risk for complications from surgery or radiation, such as older adults and pregnant women.

If patients fail or cannot tolerate ATD therapy, or would prefer more definitive therapy with little risk of relapse, the only remaining option is thyroid ablation. Destroying thyroid tissue would accomplish the goal of abolishing hyperthyroidism, but the consequence is induced hypothyroidism. While replacing one disease state with another may seem counterproductive,

treatment for hypothyroidism is more manageable, tolerable, and predictable than treatment for hyperthyroidism. Thyroid ablation can be accomplished with either RAI therapy or thyroidectomy.

RAI is dosed at 10 to 15 mCi as a single application. The thyroid takes up the RAI, which works to destroy the thyroid tissue. After 6 weeks, 40% to 70% of patients will be euthyroid, and 80% of patients will be cured (Ross et al., 2016). RAI is preferred in those who wish to avoid surgery but should be avoided in pregnancy, lactation, and thyroid cancer. RAI can also worsen GO, so patients with severe eye disease should either avoid RAI or be pretreated with prednisone. Notably, there is no evidence that demonstrates an increased risk of cancer from RAI therapy.

Surgery is favored in those with large goiters and thyroid cancer. Complications of thyroidectomy include hypoparathyroidism, laryngeal nerve injury, and bleeding. It is contraindicated in those with significant comorbid conditions and limited life expectancy. Subtotal thyroidectomy has the least risk of postoperative hypothyroidism; however, this is counterbalanced with a higher risk of recurrence of hyperthyroidism. Total and near total thyroidectomy leads to an almost 100% efficacy rate but will require lifelong thyroid hormone replacement therapy to treat induced hypothyroidism (Ross et al., 2016).

While patients await thyroid ablation with either RAI or thyroidectomy, they can use adjunctive therapies to help control the uncomfortable effects of hyperthyroidism in the meantime. For those with severe hyperthyroidism, patients

TABLE 45.6

Overview of Drug Treatment Options for Hyperthyroidism

Generic (Trade) Name and Dosage	Selected Adverse Events	Contraindications	Special Considerations
Antithyroid Drugs Methimazole (Tapazole) Start: 5–40 mg/d Maintenance: 5–10 mg/d Propylthiouracil (Propyl-Thyracil) Start: 300 mg/d Maintenance: 100–150 mg/d	Common: rash, urticaria, arthralgia, fever Serious: hepatotoxicity (more with propylthiouracil), bone marrow suppression including agranulocytosis	Hypersensitivity	In pregnancy, propylthiouracil preferred in 1st trimester, methimazole preferred in 2nd to 3rd trimester; monitor for agranulocytosis (fever, sore throat, CBC).
Beta-blockers Nadolol (Corgard) Dose: 40–160 mg/d Propranolol (Inderal) Dose: 30–160 mg/d	Bradycardia, fatigue, drowsiness, mood changes, dizziness	Hypersensitivity, uncompensated heart failure, severe sinus bradycardia, sick sinus syndrome, heart block greater than first degree, uncontrolled asthma	Use for symptom control only
Iodine solutions Potassium iodide (SSKI) Dose: 1–2 drops TID Potassium iodide and iodine (Lugol's solution) Dose: 4–8 drops TID	Rash, abdominal discomfort, iodism with prolonged use (burning in mouth, sore teeth/gums, headache, metallic taste, eye swelling, increased salivation, skin lesions)	Hypersensitivity, active tuberculosis, nodular thyroid condition with heart disease	SSKI contains ~38 iodide/drop. Lugol's solution contains ~6.3 mg iodine/iodide/drop.

CBC, complete blood count; SSKI, saturated solution of potassium iodide.

TABLE 45.7

Perioperative Symptom Management for Hyperthyroidism

Procedure	Symptom Management before Procedure	Symptom Management after Procedure
Radioactive iodine therapy	Beta-blocker to control adrenergic symptoms. Methimazole to achieve euthyroid state and control symptoms. Must be stopped 2–3 days before RAI, as it can interfere with efficacy. No role for iodine solutions, as they diminish the effect of RAI.	Beta-blocker to control adrenergic symptoms. Taper as symptoms improve. Resume methimazole 3–7 days after RAI. Taper as symptoms improve.
Thyroidectomy	Beta-blocker to control adrenergic symptoms. Methimazole 6–8 weeks before procedure to achieve euthyroid state and control symptoms. Follow this with iodine solution for 10–14 days to decrease vascularity of thyroid.	Beta-blocker to control adrenergic symptoms. Taper as symptoms improve.

Beta-blocker, beta-adrenergic blocker; RAI, radioactive iodine.

may be pretreated to achieve a euthyroid state in order to prevent complications from RAI or surgery. Additionally, since it takes several weeks for patients to fully experience symptom resolution after thyroid ablation, patients may continue on these therapies after the procedure and taper off as symptoms improve. Adjunctive treatments for perioperative symptom management are presented in **Table 45.7**.

Patients with subclinical hyperthyroidism are at risk for developing cardiovascular and bone effects seen in overt disease. Some patients may even progress to overt disease. Thus, treatment should be considered in those aged 65 or older with TSH less than 0.1 mIU/L. Postmenopausal women, and/or patients with underlying cardiovascular disease, may also be considered for therapy.

Goals of Drug Therapy

1. Reduce thyroid hormone to normal levels to achieve euthyroid state.
2. Relieve signs and symptoms of hyperthyroidism.
3. Prevent long-term complications of hyperthyroidism.

Antithyroid Drugs

Two ATD are available in the United States: methimazole (MMI) and propylthiouracil (PTU). They are most commonly used as first-line therapy for hyperthyroidism of Graves' disease. Thyroid hormones will usually drop after 2 to 3 weeks of therapy, and most patients will be euthyroid by 6 weeks. Forty percent to 60% of patients will achieve remission of Graves' disease after 1 to 2 years of ATD treatment. Relapse can occur in anyone, but the risk is higher in those who maintain positive titers of TRAb after treatment is complete. If relapse occurs, it typically happens within 3 to 6 months after stopping an ATD. At this point, patients may choose to undergo definitive therapy with RAI or surgery.

Mechanism of Action

ATDs inhibit thyroid peroxidase, which is the enzyme needed for iodination of tyrosine in the thyroglobulin. They also prevent the coupling of MIT and DIT. They are known to have immunosuppressant effects in Graves' disease. PTU also has the unique ability to inhibit the conversion of T_4 to T_3 in the peripheral tissues.

Dosage

MMI should be started at 10 to 30 mg/d. Once a euthyroid state is achieved, the dose can be titrated down to a maintenance level of 5 to 15 mg daily. Since PTU has a shorter duration of action, it must be given multiple times daily. The starting dose is 50 to 150 mg three times daily, with reduction to a maintenance dose of 50 mg two to three times daily once a euthyroid state is achieved.

To induce long-term remission, the maintenance therapy should be continued for at least 12 to 18 months (De Leo et al., 2016). The ATD can be tapered off afterwards.

Time Frame for Response

A euthyroid state is usually achieved by 4 to 8 weeks of therapy, at which point patients will start to notice symptom improvement. To help with controlling intolerable symptoms in the meantime, patients may take adjunctive therapies as discussed in the following section.

Contraindications

Both MMI and PTU are contraindicated in known hypersensitivity to antithyroid medications.

Adverse Events

Minor adverse effects include pruritus, rash, and transient elevations in liver enzymes. These can usually be managed by antihistamine therapy in order to prevent the need to stop therapy (Ross et al., 2016). More serious adverse drug reactions include hepatic damage, vasculitis, and agranulocytosis. With PTU, a transient rise in aminotransferases is common. Less frequently, ATDs can cause serious hepatotoxicity, with PTU carrying a higher risk than MMI. PTU carries a black box warning for hepatotoxicity, since it can lead to fulminant hepatotoxicity and death. PTU also has a higher risk of antineutrophil cytoplasmic antibody vasculitis. For these reasons, MMI should be chosen over PTU for nearly every patient (Ross et al., 2016). The exceptions are during the first trimester of pregnancy (during which MMI can be teratogenic), treatment during thyroid storm (due to the quicker action of PTU), and those who cannot tolerate MMI.

Agranulocytosis (absolute neutrophil count <1000 mm^3) is a serious, life-threatening condition that can result from ATD use, with equal risk between PTU and MMI. It occurs in 0.3% of patients, typically within the first 3 months of therapy. The onset is sudden and progresses quickly, so patients must be educated on how to recognize and detect symptoms. Patients should seek immediate medical attention in the case of fever, malaise, and sore throat. Patients may also present with pruritic rash, jaundice, dark urine, arthralgias, abdominal pain, or nausea. To address agranulocytosis, the offending ATD must be stopped, and broad-spectrum antibiotics must be started immediately if the patient is febrile. Granulocyte colony-stimulating factor may also be administered to aid white blood cell count recovery.

Interactions

ATD are sometimes used to achieve a euthyroid state in preparation for RAI therapy. However, ATDs can actually decrease the efficacy of RAI by preventing its full uptake into the thyroid. Therefore, ATDs should be held a few days before the procedure and then restarted 3 to 7 days afterwards.

Adjunctive Agents to Manage Hyperthyroidism

Adjunctive agents can be useful in providing quick relief of symptoms for patients with hyperthyroidism, since ATDs and RAI therapy can take weeks before patients will notice a meaningful effect. Adjunctive agents are also used as pretreatment before surgery and RAI therapy to help with symptoms as they are waiting for the procedure and because patients with severe hyperthyroidism must be euthyroid before undergoing either procedure.

Beta-Blockers

Though beta-adrenergic blockers have no impact on thyroid functioning, they have been shown to quickly reduce the bothersome symptoms of hyperthyroidism such as palpitations, tremor, and anxiety (De Leo et al., 2016; Ross et al., 2016). They can be helpful in controlling the uncomfortable effects of hyperthyroidism while patients wait for other therapies like ATDs to exert their effects. Beta-blockers are recommended in all cases of symptomatic hyperthyroidism, but especially in older adults, those with heart rate more than 90 bpm, and those with cardiovascular disease. Nonselective agents like propranolol are preferred over selective agents due to their ability to hinder the conversion of T$_4$ to the more potent T$_3$. However, nonselective beta-blockers should be avoided in asthma and uncontrolled heart failure. If there exists a contraindication to beta-blockers, a non-dihydropyridine calcium channel blocker (verapamil or diltiazem) or clonidine may be used instead. Because they have no effect on the thyroid, beta-blockers should not be used alone to achieve euthyroid state in a patient scheduled for RAI or surgery.

Iodine Compounds

Large doses of iodine can overwhelm thyroid hormone production and release and cause a rapid and temporary reprieve from hyperthyroidism. Iodine compounds like saturated solution of potassium iodide (38 mg iodide/drop) and Lugol's solution (6.3 mg iodide/drop) offer reduction of serum T$_4$ levels within 24 hours, which can last up to 2 to 3 weeks. They are most commonly used to resolve thyroid storm or to quickly reach euthyroid state prior to thyroid surgery. Iodine solution should not be given before RAI treatment since it will diminish its effect. Adverse effects seen with iodine therapy include hypersensitivity reactions, gynecomastia, and a syndrome known as "iodism," which includes palpitations, mood changes, weight loss, and pustular skin rash.

Treatment of Ophthalmopathy of Graves' Disease

All patients with Graves' disease should be under the care of an ophthalmologist (Kotwal & Stan, 2018; Ross et al., 2016). Although steroids can be used to temporarily calm symptoms, there are no reliable definitive treatments available. Therefore, prevention and risk mitigation are vital. Risk factors for worsening ophthalmopathy include smoking, RAI, and untreated hyperthyroidism. Patients with moderate-to-severe ophthalmopathy should not be considered for RAI.

Special Considerations
Thyroid Storm

Thyroid storm is a life-threatening condition that results from severe thyrotoxicosis (Idrose, 2015). Triggers include infection, trauma, thyroidectomy, RAI treatment, and abrupt discontinuation of anti-thyroid medications. The clinical presentation of thyroid storm includes signs and symptoms seen in hyperthyroidism but intensified and can include high fever, tachycardia, atrial fibrillation, tachypnea, agitation, delirium, gastrointestinal (GI) disturbances, and even seizure or coma. Treatment is aggressive and requires admission to the intensive care unit. Rapid symptom resolution is accomplished with IV beta-blockers, large doses of ATD, iodine solution, corticosteroids, acetaminophen, cooling blankets, fluids, nutritional support, and respiratory care.

Pregnancy

Because fetal development is so dependent on thyroid hormone, an increase in thyroid activity is expected and desired during pregnancy. However, in underlying Graves' disease, pregnant patients may become thyrotoxic, especially due to the TSH mimicking effects of β-hCG. When left untreated, gestational hyperthyroidism can lead to low birth weight, miscarriage, premature delivery, and preeclampsia (De Leo et al., 2016; Illouz et al., 2018). Treatment is usually with ATD, and PTU is preferred in the first trimester due to the teratogenic effect of MMI. PTU may be continued through the rest of the pregnancy or may be switched to MMI in the second or third trimester to avoid possible hepatotoxicity.

Monitoring Patient Response

With ATD therapy, thyroid function tests should be completed every 4 to 6 weeks until the patient is stable, at which point the patient may begin maintenance dosing (Ross et al., 2016). Once maintenance therapy starts, monitor every 4 to 6 weeks and make adjustments to maintain euthyroid levels at the lowest dose. Once this dose is determined, thyroid function can be monitored every 2 to 3 months, then every 6 months during long-term therapy. ATD therapy should be gradually reduced at a rate that maintains euthyroid state, and eventually discontinued. After this, thyroid function should be checked every 6 to 12 months to monitor for possible relapse. Serum TSH will remain suppressed for several months and thus it is not a useful monitoring tool early in therapy.

Patient Education

ATD, RAI therapy, and thyroidectomy are all viable treatment options to treat hyperthyroidism with different risks and benefits that may steer a patient's decision for treatment. Patients should be educated about the advantages and disadvantages to each treatment modality. For ATD therapy, patients should know the goal is remission and not definitive resolution of disease. They should be counseled on the serious side effects of hepatotoxicity and agranulocytosis that can occur, and how to self-monitor for symptoms of each. Patients should also understand that an expected consequence of RAI and surgery is induced hypothyroidism, which will likely need to be treated with thyroid replacement therapy indefinitely. Individual patient preferences should be considered when a decision for therapy is being made.

Complementary and Alternative Medicine

A number of herbals and supplements are used for the treatment of hyperthyroid symptoms, though none have been rigorously studied for safety or efficacy. Examples include L-carnitine, bugleweed, and lemon balm. There is some data to support the use of selenium in controlling GO (Negro et al., 2019; Nordio, 2017), although recommending supplementation has yet to become a standard practice.

HYPERPARATHYROIDISM

Hyperparathyroidism presents as hypercalcemia as a result of overproduction of PTH. Incidence is estimated at 20 cases per 100,000 people every year (Rao, 2018). Resulting complications include decreased bone density and fractures, and kidney stones.

Causes

Primary hyperparathyroidism occurs when there is a pathophysiologic process with the parathyroid gland itself. It is most caused by a single benign adenoma on one of the parathyroid glands which leads the gland to become overactive and overproduce PTH. Fifteen percent to 20% of patients have multiglandular hyperplasia (Bilezikian et al., 2018) in which all four glands are enlarged and overactive. Rarely, overproduction of PTH can result from parathyroid carcinoma. Risk factors for primary hyperparathyroidism are those who received neck radiation and older age. Women are also disproportionately affected at twice the rate of men.

Secondary hyperparathyroidism results from problems that manifest outside of the parathyroid. The most common cause is chronic kidney disease (CKD), which triggers the parathyroid to respond with overproduction of PTH. Since vitamin D is essential for absorption of calcium, another secondary cause is vitamin D deficiency, either from inadequate dietary intake, lack of sun exposure, malabsorption, or liver dysfunction.

Pathophysiology

In primary hyperparathyroidism, the overactive parathyroid produces excessive amounts of PTH that is not under the control of negative feedback from serum calcium levels. As a result, serum calcium levels continue to rise inappropriately. PTH causes bones to release calcium, resulting in weakened bones that increase the risk for osteoporosis and fractures. The kidneys increase reabsorption of calcium, which can give rise to kidney stones.

Because calcium homeostasis is important in heart conduction, heart disease and high blood pressure can result from excessive calcium. Rarely, cognitive and neuromuscular symptoms can occur.

In CKD, a couple pathophysiologic processes lead to secondary hyperparathyroidism. The kidneys have a decreased ability to absorb and activate vitamin D, which is essential for aiding calcium absorption. The kidneys also are unable to maintain phosphorus secretion, and this results in hyperphosphatemia. Phosphorus binds to calcium, creating an insoluble complex. Forming this complex not only lowers the amount of available calcium from the bloodstream, it can also lead to calcification in the heart and consequent cardiovascular disease. The decrease in serum calcium signals the parathyroid to release PTH, and the bones respond by releasing their calcium stores into the bloodstream.

Diagnostic Criteria

In primary hyperparathyroidism, most patients are asymptomatic, but some may present with symptoms of hypercalcemia (**Box 45.3**). Because of the high frequency of electrolyte monitoring in the general population, hypercalcemia is often detected incidentally before patients develop symptoms or complications. Other times, patients may be diagnosed after presentation of symptoms or complications, such as kidney stones or bone fracture.

Diagnosis is confirmed when serum calcium is elevated and intact parathyroid hormone (iPTH) is either normal or elevated (**Table 45.8**). Vitamin D levels may be monitored, since patients with primary hyperparathyroidism often present with low vitamin D levels.

BOX 45.3   Signs and Symptoms of Hypercalcemia

Dyspnea
Angina
Palpitations
Nausea or vomiting
Constipation
Anorexia
Fatigue
Lethargy
Confusion
Anxiety
Depression
Polydipsia
Polyuria
Arthralgia
Fractures
Muscle weakness
Kidney stones

TABLE 45.8   Diagnostic Criteria for Parathyroid Disorders

Disorder	Serum Calcium	Intact Parathyroid Hormone Level
Primary hyperparathyroidism	High	Normal or high
Secondary hyperparathyroidism	Low	High
Hypoparathyroidism	Low	Low

Conversely, hyperparathyroidism as a result of CKD or vitamin D deficiency will show low calcium levels coupled with high iPTH.

Initiating Drug Therapy

While surgery remains the mainstay of therapy for primary hyperparathyroidism, drug therapy with a calcimimetic is available as an option for those who are not candidates for surgery (Bilezikian et al., 2018; Khan et al., 2017).

A full discussion on the pharmacologic management for secondary hyperparathyroidism of CKD is beyond the scope of this chapter. In these cases, there is no pathology associated with the parathyroid gland itself, and therefore treatment is centered around management of the underlying problem.

Goals of Therapy

The goals of therapy in managing primary hyperparathyroidism are as follows:

1. Restore calcium levels to normal range.
2. Resolve symptoms of hypercalcemia.
3. Prevent complications of bone disease and nephrolithiasis.

Calcimimetic Therapy

Cinacalcet (Sensipar) is a calcimimetic that decreases iPTH and helps lower calcium to normal levels in 70% to 80% of patients. Currently, it is the only calcimimetic available and approved for primary hyperparathyroidism. Etelcalcetide (Parsabiv) is an injectable calcimimetic that is only approved for the management of secondary hyperparathyroidism.

Mechanism of Action

Cinacalcet increases the sensitivity of the calcium receptors on the parathyroid gland, thus enhancing the negative feedback mechanism to signal the gland to decrease PTH release. This results in a decrease in calcium levels. However, this decrease in serum calcium does not improve bone density or reduce the risk of kidney stones.

Dosage

Initial dosing of cinacalcet is 30 mg twice daily, and this can be increased every 2 to 4 weeks until serum calcium reaches normal range. It should be given with food for maximal absorption.

Adverse Events

Cinacalcet has many adverse effects which may limit its use in patients who are unable to tolerate the medication. The most common are listed in **Table 45.9**. Less commonly, cinacalcet can increase the risk of more serious adverse effects, including QT prolongation, GI bleeding, seizures, and severe hypocalcemia that can be life-threatening. Patients are at higher risk if they have underlying risk factors for any of the adverse effects mentioned earlier. Constant monitoring of serum calcium and iPTH is essential to prevent overtreatment and consequently serious adverse effects. The risk of overtreatment increases with hepatic impairment, since cinacalcet is primarily metabolized by the liver.

Interactions

Cinacalcet is a minor substrate of several cytochrome P450 enzymes: CYP3A4, CYP2D6, and CYP1A2. Serum calcium and iPTH should be monitored closely if any drugs that use, inhibit, or enhance these metabolic pathways are started or stopped.

Selecting the Most Appropriate Drug

First-Line Therapy

Surgery to remove the overactive parathyroid gland(s) remains the only therapy to cure primary hyperparathyroidism (Wilhelm et al., 2016). Consider surgery in asymptomatic primary hyperparathyroidism if they have any of the following: age younger than 50, serum calcium more than 1.0 mg/dL above the upper limit of normal, creatinine clearance less than 60 mL/min or calcium more than 400 mg/dL in 24-hour urine test, or low-energy fracture or osteoporosis (bone mineral density T-score ≤−2.5 at hip, spine, or wrist). Even if patients

TABLE 45.9

Most Common Adverse Effects of Cinacalcet (occurring >10% of patients)

Organ System	Adverse Effects
Cardiovascular	Hypotension
Central nervous system	Paresthesia, headache, fatigue, depression
Endocrine	Hypocalcemia, dehydration, hypercalcemia, hypoparathyroidism
Gastrointestinal	Nausea, vomiting, constipation, diarrhea, anorexia, abdominal pain
Hematologic	Anemia
Musculoskeletal	Bone fracture, muscle spasms, arthralgia, weakness, myalgia, back pain
Respiratory	Dyspnea, cough, upper respiratory tract infection

do not meet the earlier mentioned criteria, they can still be considered for parathyroidectomy since this is the only known cure for primary hyperparathyroidism.

Second-Line Therapy

If a patient is not a candidate for parathyroidectomy due to comorbid conditions where the risk of surgery would outweigh the benefits, or if the patient refuses surgery, calcimimetic therapy with cinacalcet can be used to reduce calcium and iPTH.

Adjunctively, patients can start bisphosphonate therapy if they have a low-energy fracture or T-score of 2.5 or less in the spine, hip, or wrist. Often, vitamin D supplementation is warranted, since low vitamin D is often seen in primary hyperparathyroidism (Bilezikian et al., 2018; Khan et al., 2017).

Special Considerations

Pregnancy

Primary hyperparathyroidism in pregnancy, though rare, is associated maternal and fetal risk that is proportional to the severity of hypercalcemia (McCarthy et al., 2019; Vera et al., 2016). Maternally, elevated calcium can cause nephrolithiasis, pancreatitis, preeclampsia, and hyperemesis gravidarum. Fetal risks include preterm delivery and miscarriage. Parathyroidectomy is recommended with persistent serum calcium levels above 11 mg/dL (2.75 mmol/L) or if the risk of maternal or fetal complications is high. If surgery is pursued, it should be done during the second trimester (McCarthy et al., 2019). The use of cinacalcet in pregnancy is inadequately studied and poorly understood. Therefore, it should only be reserved in cases where surgery cannot be performed.

Monitoring Patient Response

Serum calcium and iPTH should be monitored continually to guide dose adjustment of cinacalcet as needed until a maintenance dose can be established. Calcium is 40% protein bound, and most of it is bound to albumin. Therefore, when interpreting calcium levels, the albumin-adjusted number should be used.

To check for complications of hyperparathyroidism, three-site bone density should be measured every 1 to 2 years. Serum creatinine should be checked at least annually.

Patient Education

Patients should be counseled on the many adverse effects that are associated with cinacalcet to help inform their decision, especially if surgery remains a viable option. Nonpharmacologically, patients should be encouraged to drink water to avoid dehydration and engage in regular exercise to help strengthen bones. Patients do not need to avoid calcium in the diet.

HYPOPARATHYROIDISM

Characterized by underproduction of PTH and subsequently low circulating calcium, hypoparathyroidism is a relatively rare disorder, affecting 37 per 100,000 person-years in the United States (Clarke, 2018; Rao, 2018). The most common cause is iatrogenic as a result of parathyroidectomy or parathyroid injury during neck surgery. Risks associated include kidney stones, renal insufficiency, cataracts, increased risk for seizure, and neuromuscular effects like tingling and muscle cramps. It does not seem to negatively impact mortality.

Initiating Drug Therapy

Traditionally, calcium and vitamin D supplementation is used to help restore calcium levels. Calcium carbonate is the most commonly employed calcium salt, dosed at 1 to 2 g or more daily, divided into at least 2 doses. It is best absorbed in an acidic environment. Calcitriol dosed at 0.5 to 2 mcg daily is the gold-standard therapy for vitamin D supplementation. Patients should be educated to have a diet rich in calcium (>1 g daily).

More recently, PTH supplementation has become available and has some data to support its use in hypoparathyroidism (Tecilazich et al., 2018). Teriparatide (Forteo) contains only the first 34 amino acids of the PTH molecule, which is the active portion of the hormone. Its approved use is for osteoporosis though, and currently there is not enough robust data to suggest safety or efficacy when used to treat hypoparathyroidism. Recombinant human PTH 1-84, on the other hand, contains the full amino-acid sequence of endogenous PTH and is emerging as a treatment option for hypoparathyroidism. There have been randomized controlled studies and long-term observational studies that show efficacy of PTH 1-84 for patients inadequately controlled on conventional therapy with calcium and vitamin D. The most commonly reported side effects are headache, nausea, hypocalcemia, muscle spasm, and paresthesia.

CASE STUDY 1

Marcy is a 30-year-old White female who presents to the endocrinology clinic after a referral from her primary care provider last week. She reports a notable increase in diaphoresis, fatigue, palpitations, and weight loss despite being hungry and eating several meals a day. She thought these symptoms were due to pregnancy, since she and her husband are trying to get pregnant. But when her home pregnancy test was negative, she decided to see her primary care provider about her symptoms. It was at this appointment that she obtained labs and was diagnosed with Graves' disease. Her lab work from last week is as follows: Thyroid stimulating hormone (TSH) = 0.2 mIU/L, Free T_4 = 2.2 ng/dL, and positive TSH receptor antibodies. She

has no signs of ophthalmopathy. During today's visit, her heart rate is 105 bpm. She has no other significant past medical history (Learning Objective 3).

1. What are the potential risks and benefits of antithyroid medications that should be considered when helping Marcy choose the best option for her?
2. What are the potential risks and benefits for the available options for thyroid ablation that should be considered when helping Marcy choose the best option for her?
3. What adjunctive therapies would be appropriate for Marcy?

Bibliography

*Starred references are cited in the text.

*Alexander, E. K., Pearce, E. N., Brent, G. A., et al. (2017). Guidelines of the American Thyroid Association for the diagnosis and management of thyroid disease during pregnancy and the postpartum. *Thyroid, 27*(3), 315–389.

*Azim, S., & Nasr, C. (2019). Subclinical hypothyroidism: When to treat. *Cleveland Clinic Journal of Medicine, 86*(2), 101–110.

*Barbesino, G. (2019). Thyroid function changes in the elderly and their relationship to cardiovascular health: A mini-review. *Gerontology, 65*(1), 1–8.

Baumgartner, C., Da Costa, B. R., Collet, T. H., et al. (2017). Thyroid function within the normal range, subclinical hypothyroidism, and the risk of atrial fibrillation. *Circulation, 136*(22), 2100–2116.

*Benvenga, S., & Carlé, A. (2019). Levothyroxine formulations: Pharmacological and clinical implications of generic substitution. *Advances in Therapy, 36*(Suppl 2), 59–71.

*Bilezikian, J. P., Bandeira, L., Khan, A., et al. (2018). Hyperparathyroidism. *Lancet, 391*(10116), 168–178.

Biondi, B., & Cooper, D. S. (2018). Subclinical hyperthyroidism. *New England Journal of Medicine, 378*(25), 2411–2419.

*Blum, M. R., Bauer, D. C., Collet, T. H., et al. (2015). Subclinical thyroid dysfunction and fracture risk: A meta-analysis. *The Journal of the American Medical Association, 313*(20), 2055–2065.

*Bridwell, R. E., Willis, G. C., Gottlieb, M., et al. (2020). Decompensated hypothyroidism: A review for the emergency clinician. *American Journal of Emergency Medicine, 39*(1), 207–212.

*Calsolaro, V., Niccolai, F., Pasqualetti, G., et al. (2018). Hypothyroidism in the elderly: Who should be treated and how? *Journal of the Endocrine Society, 3*(1), 146–158.

*Cappola, A. R., Arnold, A. M., Wulczyn, K., et al. (2015). Thyroid function in the euthyroid range and adverse outcomes in older adults. *Journal of Clinical Endocrinology and Metabolism, 100*, 1088–1096.

*Chaker, L., Bianco, A. C., Jonklass, J., et al. (2017). Hypothyroidism. *Lancet, 390*(10101), 1550–1562.

Cianferotti, L., Marcucci, G., & Brandi, M. L. (2018). Causes and pathophysiology of hypoparathyroidism. *Clinical Endocrinology & Metabolism, 32*(6), 909–925.

*Clarke, B. L. (2018). Epidemiology and complications of hypoparathyroidism. *Endocrinology and Metabolism Clinics of North America, 47*(4), 771–782.

*De Leo, S., Lee, S. Y., & Braverman, P. L. (2016). Hyperthyroidism. *Lancet, 388*(10047), 906–918.

Donangelo, I., & Suh, S. Y. (2017). Subclinical hyperthyroidism: When to consider treatment. *American Family Physician, 95*(11), 710–716.

*Duntas, L. H., & Jonklaas, J. (2019). Levothyroxine dose adjustment to optimise therapy throughout a patient's lifetime. *Advances in Therapy, 36*(Suppl 2), 30–46.

Geer, M., Potter, D. M., & Ulrich, H. (2015). Alternative schedules of levothyroxine administration. *American Journal of Health-System Pharmacy, 72*(5), 373–377.

Hennessey, J. V. (2017). The emergence of levothyroxine as a treatment for hypothyroidism. *Endocrine, 55*(1), 6–18.

*Idrose, A. M. (2015). Acute and emergency care for thyrotoxicosis and thyroid storm. *Acute Medicine & Surgery, 2*(3), 147–157.

*Illouz, F., Luton, D., Polak, M., et al. (2018). Graves' disease and pregnancy. *Annals of Endocrinology (Paris), 79*(6), 636–646.

*Jonklaas, J., Bianco, A. C., Bauer, A. J., et al. (2014). Guidelines for the treatment of hypothyroidism. *Thyroid, 24*(12), 1670–1751.

*Kang, G. Y., Parks, J. R., Fileta, B., et al. (2013). Thyroxine and triiodothyronine content in commercially available thyroid health supplements. *Thyroid, 23*(10), 1233–1237.

*Khan, A. A., Hanley, D. A., Rizzoli, R., et al. (2017). Primary hyperparathyroidism: Review and recommendations on evaluation, diagnosis, and management: A Canadian and international consensus. *Osteoporosis International, 28*(1), 1–19.

*Kotwal, A., & Stan, M. (2018). Current and future treatments for Graves' disease and Graves' ophthalmopathy. *Hormone and Metabolic Research, 50*(12), 871–886.

Leung, A. M. (2016). Thyroid emergencies. *Journal of Infusion Nursing, 39*(5), 281–286.

*McCarthy, A., Howarth, S., Khoo, S., et al. (2019). Management of primary hyperparathyroidism in pregnancy: A case series. *Endocrinology, Diabetes & Metabolism Case Reports, 2019*, 19-0039.

*Negro, R., Hegedüs, L., Attanasio, R., et al. (2019). A 2018 European Thyroid Association Survey on the use of selenium supplementation in Graves' hyperthyroidism and Graves' orbitopathy. *European Thyroid Journal, 8*(1), 7–15.

*Nordio, M. (2017). A novel treatment for subclinical hyperthyroidism: A pilot study on the beneficial effects of l-carnitine and selenium. *European Review for Medical and Pharmacological Sciences, 21*(9), 2268–2273.

*Rao, S. D. (2018). Epidemiology of parathyroid disorders. *Clinical Endocrinology & Metabolism, 32*(6), 773–780.

*Roman, B. R., Morris, L. G., & Davies, L. (2017). The thyroid cancer epidemic, 2017 perspective. *Current Opinions in Endocrinology, Diabetes, and Obesity, 24*(5), 332–336.

*Ross, D. S., Burch, H. B., Cooper, D. S., et al. (2016). American Thyroid Association Guidelines for the diagnosis and management of hyperthyroidism and other causes of thyrotoxicosis. *Thyroid*, *26*(10), 1343–1421.

*Samuels, M. H. (2018). Hyperthyroidism in aging. In K. R. Feingold, B. Anawalt, A. Boyce, et al. (Eds.), Endotext. MDText.com, Inc.

*Sharma, A. K., Basu, I., & Singh, S. (2018). Efficacy and safety of ashwagandha root extract in subclinical hypothyroid patients: A double-blind, randomized placebo-controlled trial. *Journal of Alternative and Complementary Medicine*, *24*(3), 243–248.

*Skelin, M., Lucijanić, T., Amidžić Klarić, D., et al. (2017). Factors affecting gastrointestinal absorption of levothyroxine: A review. *Clinical Therapeutics*, *39*(2), 378–403.

*Smith, T. J., & Hegedus, L. (2016). Graves' disease. *New England Journal of Medicine*, *375*(16), 1552–1565.

*Springer, D., Jiskra, J., Limanova, Z., et al. (2017). Thyroid in pregnancy: From physiology to screening. *Critical Reviews in Clinical Laboratory Sciences*, *54*(2), 102–116.

*Taylor, P. N., Albrecht, D., Scholz, A., et al. (2018). Global epidemiology of hyperthyroidism and hypothyroidism. *Nature Reviews Endocrinology*, *14*(5), 301–316.

*Tecilazich, F., Formenti, A. M., Frara, S., et al. (2018). Treatment of hypoparathyroidism. *Clinical Endocrinology & Metabolism*, *32*(6), 955–964.

Trifirò, G., Parrino, F., Sultana, J., et al. (2015). Drug interactions with levothyroxine therapy in patients with hypothyroidism: Observational study in general practice. *Clinical Drug Investigation*, *35*(3), 187–195.

*Vanderpump, M. P. J. (2019). Epidemiology of thyroid disorders. In M. Luster, L. Duntas, & L. Wartofsky (Eds.), *The thyroid and its diseases*. Cham, Switzerland: Springer.

*Vera, L., Oddo, S., Di Iorgi, N., et al. (2016). Primary hyperparathyroidism in pregnancy treated with cinacalcet: A case report and review of the literature. *Journal of Medical Case Reports*, *10*(1), 361.

*Wassner, A. J. (2017). Pediatric hypothyroidism: Diagnosis and treatment. *Paediatric Drugs*, *19*(4), 291–301.

*Wiersinga, W. M. (2019). T$_4$ + T$_3$ combination therapy: Any progress? *Endocrine*, *66*(1), 70–78. doi: 10.1007/s12020-019-02052-2

*Wilhelm, S. M., Wang, T. S., Ruan, D. T., et al. (2016). The American Association of Endocrine Surgeons Guidelines for definitive management of primary hyperparathyroidism. *The Journal of the American Medical Association Surgery*, *151*(10), 959–968.

*Zsolt, H., Lage, M. J., Espaillat, R., et al. (2018). The association between adherence to levothyroxine and economic and clinical outcomes in patients with hypothyroidism in the US. *Journal of Medical Economics*, *21*(9), 912–919.

Pharmacotherapy for Immunology

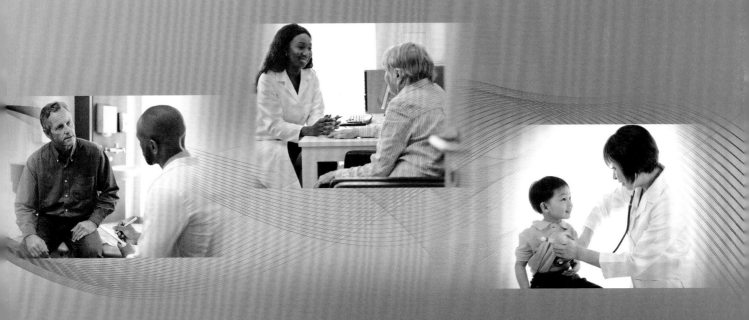

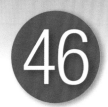

46 Allergies and Allergic Reactions

Lauren M. Czosnowski

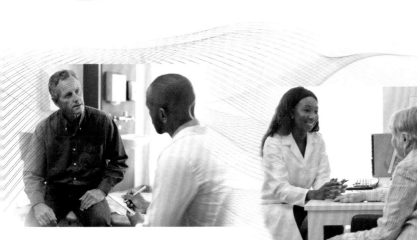

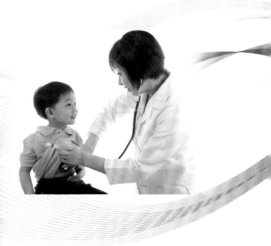

Learning Objectives

1. Discuss the four types of allergic reactions.
2. Differentiate between seasonal and perennial allergic rhinitis.
3. Select an appropriate antihistamine product for a patient experiencing seasonal rhinitis.
4. Determine when an antihistamine, a decongestant, or an intranasal corticosteroid product is needed.
5. Identify and manage the adverse effects associated with treatments for allergic rhinitis.

INTRODUCTION

The term *allergy* is derived from the Greek words *allos* (differing from the normal or usual) and *ergon* (work or energy). To describe it in simple, nonclinical terms, allergy is an abnormal release of energy in the body. In clinical or physiologic terms, allergy is an exaggerated immune response resulting from an antibody–antigen reaction.

Antibodies are soluble protein molecules made by B lymphocytes in response to foreign substances. Antibodies, also referred to as *immunoglobulins*, are tailored specifically and uniquely to bind to each foreign substance and remove it from the circulation. Invasion or contact with a foreign substance results in the production and secretion of antibodies. Therefore, the foreign substance is an *anti*body *generator*—hence the term *antigen*. Antigens are also referred to as *allergens*; the terms are interchangeable.

All people come in contact with the same antigens, yet not all people display allergic symptoms. Allergy symptoms appear when the immune response is exaggerated or inappropriate, causing inflammation and tissue damage. This exaggerated response to an antigen is referred to as *hypersensitivity*. Hypersensitivity is a characteristic of an individual. It is manifested on the second or a subsequent contact with a particular antigen.

Allergens can be food based, chemical, or environmental. Typical food allergens include milk or egg protein, peanut, shellfish, and wheat or soy. Parabens and lanolin, commonly found in makeup and sunscreens; thimerosal, a preservative found in contact lens solutions; and fragrance enhancers found in perfumes are common chemical allergens. Drugs, such as the local anesthetics lidocaine and benzocaine, are also chemical allergens. Environmental allergens include mold, pollen, and dust.

In contrast to allergy, *anergy* is the term used to describe the unexpected failure of the immune system to respond to the challenge of a foreign substance (antigen or allergen). Several skin test antigens may be applied to the skin (an anergy panel) to determine the status of the immune system. The antigens selected are those to which a majority of the population would exhibit a reaction. Examples of these include *Candida* species and histoplasmin. If the characteristic wheals do not appear in the prescribed period, it can be interpreted that the patient has not had prior exposure to the antigen or potentially has a compromised immune system.

CLASSIFICATION OF ALLERGIC REACTIONS

The medical literature describes four types of hypersensitivity reactions (Coombs and Gell classification), which are listed and described in **Box 46.1** (Nairn & Helbert, 2007). There are four

- Type 1 (immediate hypersensitivity)—Immunoglobulin (Ig) E attached to mast cells binds with an antigen, inducing degranulation and release of histamine and other mediators of inflammation. (Asthma and allergic rhinitis are examples of type 1 hypersensitivity.)
- Type 2—IgG attached to a T lymphocyte killer cell is directed against antigens on target cell. This leads to direct cytotoxic action or complement-mediated lysis.
- Type 3—Immune complexes of antibody and antigen are deposited in the tissue. Complement is activated, and polymorphonuclear leukocytes are attracted to the site of the complex. Local tissue damage occurs. (Autoimmune disease is an example of type 3 hypersensitivity.)
- Type 4 (delayed hypersensitivity)—Antigen-sensitized T cells release inflammatory substances after a second contact with the same antigen. (Contact dermatitis, such as poison ivy, and the tuberculin skin test are examples of delayed hypersensitivity.)

types of reactions under this classification system. Type 1 reactions involve the interaction between an antigen and a specific immunoglobulin (Ig) E antibody. These antibodies are bound to member receptors on mast cells and basophils. When an antigen binds to these antibodies, the cell releases histamine, leukotrienes, and prostaglandins. These vasoactive substances produce vasodilation and increase capillary permeability, both of which allow for eosinophils and other inflammatory cells to infiltrate tissues, furthering the allergic response. The first contact results in the formation of the antibody. Subsequent contact with the same antigen results in the antibody–antigen reaction, resulting in this type 1 hypersensitivity reaction. The antibody–antigen reaction triggers the immune response, which results in allergic symptoms (**Figure 46.1**). Allergies can affect the airways, eyes, skin, or the entire body. Type 1 reactions are typically anaphylactic in nature and can be life-threatening.

Type 2 reactions, also known as *cytotoxic reactions*, occur when an antibody reacts with an antigenic component of a cell.

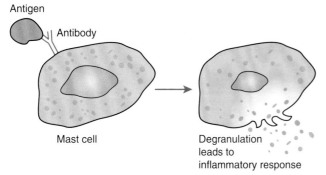

FIGURE 46–1 Antibody–antigen reaction.

This antibody–antigen reaction in turn activates killer T cells or macrophages to aid in the destruction of the antigenic cell. Complement activation is also involved in this process, furthering the cytotoxic process leading to tissue destruction. Transfusion reactions are typically type 2 allergic reactions.

Type 3 reactions result from immune complexes that activate the complement system. Activating this system promotes the migration and release of cells such as polymorphonuclear cells that can release proteolytic enzymes and factors that promote tissue permeability. Systemic lupus erythematosus is a form of a type 3 allergic reaction.

Type 4 reactions are also called *delayed hypersensitivity reactions*. These cell-mediated reactions are the result of sensitized T lymphocytes coming into contact with a specific antigen. The delay typically takes 2 to 3 days or up to a week. Allergic dermatitis is an example of a type 4 reaction.

Immunologic versus Nonimmunologic Reactions

Some cutaneous reactions, such as contact dermatitis, may appear to be allergic reactions, but they do not involve the immune system. Irritant contact dermatitis is the most common cutaneous reaction and is often caused by skin irritants such as powders or chemicals found in gloves.

Contact dermatitis differs from allergic dermatitis in that there is direct tissue insult from the skin irritant that causes the release of inflammatory mediators from skin cells. A common example of irritant contact dermatitis is a reaction to repeated handwashing with soap or other cleaners. In some instances, the cracked, dry skin occurring with contact dermatitis no longer can prevent allergens from entering the systemic circulation. With latex allergies, for example, the powder already present in the glove can give rise to a contact dermatitis, thus allowing for the latex antigens to enter the circulation. This in turn increases the likelihood of an allergic reaction, resulting in allergic contact dermatitis. Because of this phenomenon, it is often difficult to distinguish allergic from nonallergic contact dermatitis. See Chapter 12 for more details on dermatitis.

General Treatment Overview of Allergic Reactions

The first step in treating an allergic reaction is to remove the allergen, if possible. This may involve removing the person from the environment causing the allergy, stopping the offending drug, or washing off the offending chemical. Most allergic reactions clear up within a few days of removing the cause. Symptomatic cutaneous reactions, such as pruritic rash, urticaria, or morbilliform eruptions as well as reactions involving multiple organs, should be treated.

Cutaneous Reactions

Cutaneous reactions such as urticaria, pruritus, and hives are often secondary to the release of histamine, making antihistamine therapy the mainstay of treatment. There are two types of antihistamines used in the general treatment of allergic reactions: first generation and second generation. The first-generation antihistamines include diphenhydramine, hydroxyzine, and chlorpheniramine, among others. These agents are typically very effective, but they may also be very sedating. The second-generation agents, such as loratadine and fexofenadine, are non-sedating antihistamines (NSAs), which work fairly well at controlling mild to moderate symptoms of cutaneous reactions. However, if the symptoms persist for more than a few days, or are not well controlled, a first-generation antihistamine may be substituted for, or added to, the NSA. Close communication with the patient regarding resolution of the symptoms is necessary, along with balancing quality-of-life issues related to side effects, such as sedation, dry mouth, and urinary retention. If the reaction is moderate to severe or if there is no relief from antihistamine therapy, systemic glucocorticoids may be used. Short courses of treatment with oral prednisone or methylprednisolone are usually used. See Chapter 12 for more information on the use of oral steroids for treating cutaneous reactions.

Anaphylaxis and Anaphylactoid Reactions

Anaphylaxis is a type 1 hypersensitivity reaction involving IgE-mediated release of histamine, leukotrienes, and other mediators from already sensitized mast cells and basophils. The release of these mediators initiates a systemic chain of events that includes symptoms such as angioedema, flushing, pruritus, urticaria, nausea, vomiting, and wheezing. The onset of the reaction is quick, generally within 1 to 30 minutes. The histamine release causes a smooth muscle contraction and vasodilation. The wheezing resulting from smooth muscle contraction in the lungs decreases oxygenation, whereas vasodilation results in a release of fluids into the tissues, thus causing a lower effective plasma volume, leading to shock. Prolonged vasodilation, coupled with decreased oxygenation, can lead to arrhythmias, convulsions, and death.

Anaphylactoid reactions are similar in appearance to anaphylaxis but may occur after the *first* injection of certain drugs and contrast media. They are non-IgE mediated, and the agent causes a direct release of histamine and other inflammatory toxins. They have a dose-related, idiosyncratic mechanism rather than an immunologically mediated one. A classic example of an anaphylactoid reaction is the "red man syndrome" associated with vancomycin. Patients may experience itching, redness, and hives with rapid infusion of vancomycin due to histamine release; slowing the infusion rate usually improves the reaction.

Treatment

Immediate treatment with epinephrine is imperative. Epinephrine effectively increases the blood pressure and is an antagonist to the effects of histamine on smooth muscle and other tissues.

At the onset of anaphylactic symptoms, such as generalized pruritus, urticaria, angioedema, or wheezing, 0.01 mL/kg aqueous epinephrine 1:1,000 (1 mg/mL) subcutaneously or intramuscularly (IM; usual dose, 0.2–0.5 mL in adults; 0.3 mL maximum for children) should be given. This dose may be repeated every 5 to 15 minutes as necessary to control symptoms, and a continuous intravenous (IV) infusion could be necessary for patients without an adequate response to IM injection plus fluid resuscitation. IM injection into the lateral thigh muscle results in a shorter time to peak concentrations of epinephrine in the blood, compared to subcutaneous injection or IM injection into the deltoid muscle. An injectable antihistamine such as diphenhydramine (usual dose for adults, 25–50 mg; children, 1 mg/kg) may also be given in addition to epinephrine to treat symptoms related to anaphylaxis, such as itching and hives. Nebulized albuterol at a dose of 2.5 to 5 mg may be considered for airway obstruction. These agents alone do not treat airway obstruction, hypotension, or shock.

If the reaction does involve the cardiovascular system, then IV fluids should be rapidly infused to maintain volume. Hypovolemia is usually the major cause of the hypotension due to fluid moving out of the intravascular space. Colloid plasma expanders such as dextran are rarely necessary. Normal saline is an appropriate choice for most patients, and 1 to 2 L should be given as an initial bolus. Fluids may be continued as necessary to maintain hemodynamic stability. If fluid replacement is ineffective at restoring blood pressure, then dopamine or norepinephrine may be *cautiously* introduced. Alternatively, if the patient is experiencing bradycardia, atropine may be used to increase heart rate. Patients with severe reactions should be observed in the hospital for 24 hours after recovery in case of relapse.

Systemic corticosteroids may help prevent late-phase reactions in some cases of anaphylaxis, although they will not have an effect for 4 to 6 hours. Typically, methylprednisolone 1 to 2 mg/kg/d divided every 6 to 8 hours for adults and 1 to 2 mg/kg/d divided every 8 to 12 hours for children is needed to prevent the onset of late-phase reactions. For milder attacks, oral prednisone dosed at 0.5 mg/kg/d may be administered, although there are not strong data to support in administering glucocorticoids.

Prophylaxis

The primary means of preventing an allergic reaction is avoidance. However, when this is not feasible or practical, immunotherapy is an effective means of preventing reactions, particularly anaphylactic reactions from insect bites. This form of "desensitization" is only effective when a specific allergen can be identified. Some ragweed and pollen allergies respond well to immunotherapy, though it may take several months before immunity is conferred.

Desensitization may be rapidly achieved in patients requiring drug therapy to which they have an established allergy. For example, patients with anaphylactic reactions to penicillin may be desensitized by administering increasing concentrations of penicillin every 15 minutes. To ensure patient safety, desensitization is best done under constant supervision and in consultation with an experienced allergist. There are numerous protocols for penicillin desensitization

Step	Administered dose (mg)	Cumulative dose (mg)
1	0.05	0.05
2	0.125	0.175
3	0.25	0.425
4	0.5	0.925
5	1.25	2.175
6	2.5	4.675
7	5	9.675
8	10	19.675
9	25	44.675
10	50	94.675
11	100	194.675
12	805.325	1,000

FIGURE 46–2   Example IV cephalosporin desensitization protocol.

and an increasing number for patients who are allergic to sulfa drugs. For one such example, see **Figure 46.2**. Each dose through step 11 is administered over 15 minutes, and then step 12 is administered over 60 minutes, which completes the total dose of the drug.

In January 2020, the U.S. Food and Drug Administration (FDA) approved the first oral immunotherapy agent to mitigate allergic reactions in children with peanut allergies. This peanut allergen powder, brand-named Palforzia, must be combined with a continued avoidance of peanuts in the diet but can help decrease the severity of allergic reactions, including anaphylaxis. This drug works similarly to a desensitization protocol for drug allergies but consists of increasing oral doses over several months. The very first dose and the first doses of any dose increase are administered in a health care setting due to the risk of anaphylaxis, and patients need to be observed for at least one hour. Due to the risk of anaphylaxis, Palforzia may only be prescribed through a risk evaluation and mitigation strategy program, in which the prescriber, pharmacy, and patient must all be enrolled. Other adverse reactions include vomiting, nausea, itching, cough, sneezing, and dyspnea; patients with uncontrolled asthma should not initiate Palforzia, and it should be withheld if the patient experiences an asthma exacerbation.

ALLERGIC RHINITIS: HAY FEVER OR POLLEN ALLERGY

Allergic rhinitis is an *airway allergy*. Asthma, also an airway allergy, is discussed in Chapter 24. Many people have hay fever. The National Institute of Allergy and Infectious Diseases

TABLE 46.1

Seasonal versus Perennial Allergies

Causes of Seasonal Allergies	Causes of Perennial Allergies
Tree pollen (spring)	Mold (indoor)
Grass pollen (spring through fall)	Dust (dust mites)
Weeds (late summer)	Animal dander (skin flakes)
Leaf mold (early spring and late summer)	Animal fur Foods (nuts, shellfish, milk, eggs)

(NIAID) states that pollen allergy may affect approximately 7% of adults and 9% of children in the United States (NIAID, 2015).

Causes

Common inhaled allergens that cause allergic rhinitis in sensitized people include pollen (grass, trees, weeds), dust mites, mold spores, enzymes (in detergents), and insect body parts. The two most common types of allergic rhinitis are seasonal and perennial (**Table 46.1**). The incidence of seasonal rhinitis is approximately 10 times greater than that of perennial rhinitis.

In seasonal allergic rhinitis, symptoms correspond with seasonal peaks in tree, grass, and weed pollens. During the spring, tree pollens such as alder, birch, and oak cause problems for many people. In the summer, grass pollens, such as timothy grass, can cause allergies. Weeds, such as mugwort and ragweed, pollinate in late summer and autumn. Pollens usually are wind-borne, and patients with seasonal allergic rhinitis often are said to have *hay fever*. The most common cause of seasonal allergic rhinitis is ragweed pollen.

Patients with perennial allergic rhinitis have symptoms throughout the year, instead of only during certain months. They usually require chronic treatment. The most common causes of perennial rhinitis are animal dander and dust mites. In many cases, causative agents are difficult for patients to avoid because many such agents are indoor allergens. Perennial rhinitis may worsen when patients are exposed to nonnatural irritants such as paint, cleaners, or tobacco smoke.

Genetic predisposition plays a major role in the development of allergic rhinitis. The genetically determined tendency to produce increased quantities of IgE expresses itself after prolonged exposure to an allergen. Consequently, allergic rhinitis is uncommon before age 3. Those in later childhood or young adulthood are at greatest risk for development of new symptoms. In general, neither sex exhibits more of a predilection for allergic rhinitis; however, some sources indicate that the perennial form is more common in women.

Patients with a family history of asthma or eczema are more likely to have an allergic basis for rhinitis. The incidence of allergic rhinitis increases by approximately 20% to 30% when one parent has a history and is even higher when both parents have allergic disorders. Studies of pediatric populations have uncovered certain factors that may increase the expression of allergy: maternal smoking, especially during pregnancy, female gender, and exposure to air pollution (Corren et al., 2014).

Pathophysiology

Initial exposure to the antigen/allergen stimulates the B lymphocytes (plasma cells) to produce an antigen-specific antibody (IgE) that binds to mast cell membranes (tissue-fixed antibody). The person is now sensitized to that specific antigen and susceptible to allergic reactions when reexposed to it. On subsequent exposure, the antigen binds to the tissue-fixed IgE antibody and triggers breakdown of the mast cells (degranulation) and release of mediators (histamine, prostaglandins, leukotrienes, kinins, thromboxanes, and serotonin). Histamine, which is stored primarily in mast cells and basophils, is believed to be the mediator most responsible for the clinical signs and symptoms of allergic rhinitis.

Common symptoms in patients with allergic rhinitis are ocular pruritus (itching of the eyes) and conjunctival inflammation (inflammation of the membrane lining the eyelids). Other symptoms of allergic rhinitis are irritability, lethargy, fatigue, and loss of appetite. Once released into the nasal mucosa, the mediators cause vasodilation, increased capillary permeability, increased mucus production, and stimulation of nerve endings. The resulting symptoms are rhinorrhea (profuse, watery nasal discharge), nasal congestion (obstruction by mucus), and nasal pruritus. The most severe symptoms include violent episodes of sneezing (often a dozen or more times in a row) and total obstruction of nasal airflow resulting from copious amounts of mucus (**Figure 46.3**).

The specific IgE antibody made in response to the allergen also may attach to eosinophils. Antigen-provoked degranulation of eosinophils also causes allergic symptoms. The symptoms associated with eosinophils are related to a late-phase allergic response, occurring hours to days after the initial reaction.

Diagnostic Criteria

The diagnosis of allergic rhinitis begins with a thorough history determining the presence of classic signs and symptoms and the time, place, and circumstances under which they occur. A family history is also important because it may establish the familial predisposition to allergy.

Physical examination of the patient with suspected allergic rhinitis begins with assessment of facial appearance, which often includes teary eyes and a red, swollen nose with scaling and crusting from frequent blowing and rubbing with facial tissues. There also may be dark circles under the eyes (allergic shiners), pinched nostrils, and a gaping mouth (from mouth breathing). The nasal mucous membranes are typically pale, swollen, and coated with a clear, watery secretion. Some erythema and bleeding may be noted. Swelling, streaks of erythema, and mucus may be present in the posterior pharynx. Other positive physical findings include swelling around and watery discharge from the eyes.

Nasal Smears

Practitioners may use the Wright stain for nasal secretions to detect eosinophils. Although eosinophilia suggests an allergic etiology for rhinitis symptoms (in infectious rhinitis, neutrophils predominate), it is not diagnostic. Conversely, an absence of eosinophilia does not rule out allergy. Eosinophilia may be absent in patients who have superimposed infections or have not had a recent exposure to allergens.

Skin Testing

Skin testing with extracts of suspected allergens usually provides the most effective means of identifying specific sensitivities in patients with allergic rhinitis. In this test, a superficial scratch or prick is made in the skin and a diluted extract of antigen is applied. If the patient has allergen-specific IgE antibodies bound to tissue mast cells, a classic wheal-and-flare

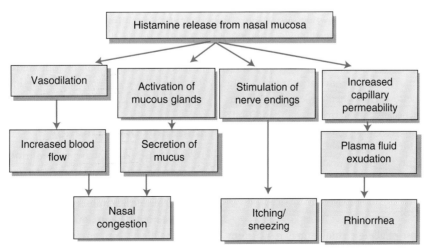

FIGURE 46–3 Results of histamine release in the nasal mucosa.

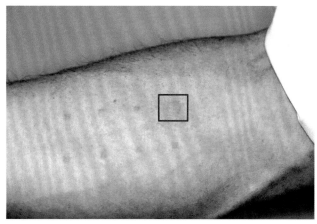

FIGURE 46–4 Skin wheal-and-flare reaction from a positive control (**upper right**) using Histamine base 6 mg/mL. Other sites are negative. (Used with permission from Johnson, J. [2013]. *Bailey's head and neck surgery* [5th ed.]. Philadelphia, PA: Wolters Kluwer.)

TABLE 46.2

Symptoms of Seasonal Allergies versus Respiratory Infections

Symptoms	Seasonal Allergy (Hay Fever)	Upper Respiratory Infection
Head congestion/ runny nose	Yes	Yes
Sneezing	Yes	Sometimes
Itchy, watery eyes	Yes	No
Cough	Usually dry	Dry or productive
Predictable seasonal patterns	Yes	Uncommon
Fever	No	Yes
Short duration (3–7 days)	No	Yes
Long duration (weeks)	Yes	No
Productive cough	Uncommon (except in asthma)	Yes

reaction appears over the next 15 to 30 minutes (**Figure 46.4**). To avoid false-negative results, patients should discontinue the use of antihistamines before they undergo skin testing. Clinicians should individualize this time frame based on the pharmacokinetics of the specific antihistamine that the patient is taking. In most cases, it is adequate to stop taking antihistamines 48 to 72 hours before testing. If patients do not stop taking antihistamines before skin testing, practitioners may mistakenly exclude a diagnosis of allergic rhinitis and subject patients to unnecessary further evaluations.

If the results of the scratch test are negative or unclear, practitioners may administer a more dilute extract of antigen intradermally. Clinicians should not use the intradermal test in patients with a positive response to scratch testing because of the risk of significant allergic reaction, including anaphylaxis.

Radioallergosorbent Testing

Radioallergosorbent testing (RAST) permits in vitro detection of serum IgE antibodies to allergens. Because only 1% of IgE molecules circulate in the blood (the remainder are bound to tissue), RAST results may not reflect the biologic situation. Although RAST is more specific, skin testing is less costly, more sensitive, and simpler to perform. Despite these shortcomings, RAST is helpful when the results of skin testing are unclear. The test is likewise useful when patients are unable to undergo skin testing because of dermatologic conditions or a history of anaphylactic reaction to the suspected allergen. RAST is also indicated for evaluating children younger than age 2 as well as for patients unable to discontinue using antihistamines, as required before skin testing.

Differential Diagnosis

Symptoms similar to those of allergic rhinitis may result from *mechanical nasal obstruction* (foreign body or anatomic factors), as a *side effect of medications* (oral contraceptives, hormone

replacement therapy, tricyclic antidepressants, propranolol [Inderal], reserpine [Serpasil], methyldopa [Aldomet], and aspirin-containing compounds) or from *medical conditions associated with increased vasodilation* (e.g., hypothyroidism, cystic fibrosis, tumors, alcoholism, or pregnancy). **Table 46.2** compares the symptoms of seasonal rhinitis with common cold symptoms to illustrate the similarities and differences between these conditions.

Although seasonal rhinitis usually is relatively easy to diagnose, identification of perennial rhinitis may be more elusive. Other nonallergic conditions could cause similar symptoms. *Vasomotor rhinitis* (congestion of the nasal mucosa without infection or allergy) could be difficult to differentiate from perennial rhinitis. In vasomotor rhinitis, however, irritants (e.g., fumes, cold air, high humidity, alcoholic beverages, or emotional stress) rather than allergens usually trigger symptoms. Moreover, vasomotor rhinitis is associated with an absence of nasal, palatal, or conjunctival pruritus. In *nonallergic rhinitis with eosinophilia*, testing likewise fails to indicate a specific allergen.

Initiating Drug Therapy

Allergic rhinitis may be treated through avoidance of the allergen, pharmacologic agents, and immunotherapy. The basic approach to pharmacologic management of allergic rhinitis is the use of antihistamines, nasal decongestants, and intranasal corticosteroids (**Figure 46.5**).

The ideal treatment for allergic rhinitis is avoidance of the offending allergen. Complete avoidance often is not feasible, but most patients usually can reduce exposure. Basic strategies

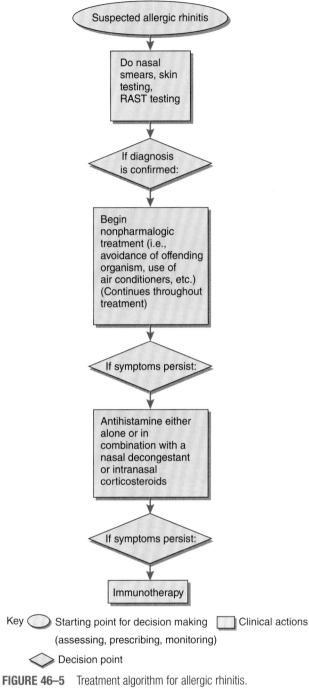

Key ⬭ Starting point for decision making   ▢ Clinical actions
(assessing, prescribing, monitoring)

◇ Decision point

FIGURE 46–5   Treatment algorithm for allergic rhinitis.

RAST, radioallergosorbent testing.

include the use of air conditioners in homes and automobiles to lessen exposure to pollen by keeping windows closed and use of dehumidifiers to discourage the growth of molds and mites. If possible, humidity should be maintained at 30% to 40% throughout the year. Patients can lessen exposure to mites by encasing mattresses in plastic, washing all bedding in very hot water every week, and removing carpeting and upholstered furniture. They can use high-efficiency particulate air cleaners to help filter out dust molds and pollen. Ideally, pets should be removed from the home; however, many patients

and their families find doing so unacceptable. At a minimum, families should keep pets out of the allergic person's bedroom, as well as away from heating and cooling systems.

Immunotherapy, also known as *desensitization, hyposensitization,* or *allergy shots,* has been used for decades for the treatment of allergic rhinitis and asthma. It consists of repeated subcutaneous injections of gradually increasing concentrations of the allergens considered to be specifically responsible for the patient's allergy symptoms. However, patients must have documented IgE antibodies to these allergens. The injections are purified extracts of the "trigger" substances such as ragweed, grass, dust mite, and animal dander. Clinical benefits are related to the administration of high doses of allergens weekly or every other week. The duration of treatment is typically 3 to 5 years, but if there is no improvement after first year, consider discontinuing immunotherapy. Treatment is discontinued based on minimal symptoms over two consecutive seasons of exposure. The benefit is derived from a reduction in the percentage of histamine released after immunotherapy compared with before treatment. The result is milder or no symptoms of allergy. Immunotherapy is not the first-line treatment. It is usually initiated when avoidance of the triggers and drug therapy fail to control the symptoms of hay fever and other allergies.

Goals of Drug Therapy

The goal of drug therapy for patients with allergies is to alleviate the symptoms with a little to no adverse effects from medications. This is accomplished primarily through decreasing the release or inhibiting the effect of histamine release and other mediators of inflammation from mast cells. Mast cells are distributed throughout the body; however, the greatest concentration of histamine occurs in the skin, respiratory system, and gastrointestinal (GI) mucosa. Relief of symptoms with minimal drug side effects should lead to an improved quality of life.

Histamine released in the GI tract does not cause allergic symptoms. It may result in hyperacidity by stimulating histamine type 2 (H_2) receptors and lead to peptic ulcer disease or gastroesophageal reflux disease. Treatment of these conditions is with H_2 blockers. It is the histamine released in the skin and respiratory tract (H_1 receptors) that causes classic allergic symptoms. The medications used to treat these symptoms are antihistamines (H_1 blockers), nasal decongestants, intranasal corticosteroids, and intranasal cromolyn. Suggestions for their selection are outlined in the following sections. The decision to treat with medications will depend on the severity of symptoms and patient tolerance of symptoms, as well as the balance of symptoms versus medication side effects. If drug treatment is chosen by the patient, it will be required as long as exposure to the triggers continues or until the patient becomes desensitized to the trigger, either naturally ("outgrowing the allergy") or through immunotherapy (described earlier).

Antihistamines

Antihistamines are classified according to their sedative effects or as first generation (older) and second generation (newer) depending on when they were marketed. The older antihistamines cross the blood–brain barrier, causing the greatest degree of sedation as well as other central nervous system (CNS) effects. These agents can be subclassified on the basis of chemical structure. The main groupings include the ethanolamines, alkylamines, phenothiazines, piperazines, and piperidines.

Mechanism of Action

Antihistamines are drugs that exert their effect in the body primarily by blocking the actions of histamine at receptor sites. They are classified as pharmacologic antagonists of histamine. They do not prevent histamine release but act by competitive inhibition. Most antihistamines can be classified as either H_1-receptor blockers, which block the smooth muscle response, or H_2-receptor blockers, which block the histaminic stimulation of gastric acid. In general, H_2-receptor blockers are not used for patients with allergies. If the concentration of antihistamine drug at the receptor site exceeds the concentration of histamine, then the effects of histamine are blocked. Antihistamines usually ameliorate itching, sneezing, ocular symptoms, and nasal discharge but do not always reduce nasal congestion.

First-Generation Antihistamines

The first-generation antihistamines, such as diphenhydramine, chlorpheniramine, and brompheniramine, are the older antihistamines. As noted earlier, these tend to be more sedating than newer, second-generation agents such as loratadine or cetirizine.

Dosage

The dosage varies depending on the age and weight of the patient. The frequency of dosing is typically every 4 to 6 hours as needed but can be upward of every 12 hours depending on the half-life of the drug and the formulation. For example, diphenhydramine (Benadryl) is given every 4 to 6 hours, but brompheniramine is dosed every 12 to 24 hours. These are often over-the-counter (OTC) agents and are supplied as tablets, capsules, elixirs, or suspensions. Furthermore, these formulations come in a variety of flavors, and some are even free of dye.

Time Frame for Response

The onset of action of these agents typically ranges from 15 to 30 minutes and lasts nearly as long as the dosing interval. Those agents with a longer half-life will take longer to get to steady state, but the initial effect is often seen fairly rapidly.

Some regular users of antihistamines find that tolerance, or drug failure, develops after several weeks or months. One reason for this decreased effectiveness is that some antihistamines are capable of hepatic enzyme induction, resulting in increased metabolism in the liver. Essentially, the antihistamine drug hastens its own destruction and removal from circulation. The various antihistamine classes differ in their capacity to induce hepatic enzymes. Some practitioners have found that if tolerance develops, patients may benefit by switching to another antihistamine in a different chemical category. The effectiveness of this technique has not been evaluated by controlled studies.

Contraindications

First-generation antihistamine therapy is contraindicated in lactating mothers. Additionally, the anticholinergic side effects of the first-generation antihistamines put patients with narrow-angle glaucoma at risk for an increase in intraocular pressure. Similarly, men with benign prostatic hyperplasia (BPH) should avoid these agents due to the drug's ability to decrease urine flow. The sedating effects of these agents should also be considered when patients are required to perform hazardous tasks or drive. Because of the sedating and anticholinergic properties, first-generation antihistamines are on the Beers list, a list of drugs that should be avoided or used with extreme caution in elderly patients (American Geriatrics Society [AGS], 2019). Antihistamines are recommended for the treatment of itching and rhinitis in pregnant women; diphenhydramine is considered acceptable and may also be used as adjunctive treatment for nausea and vomiting during pregnancy.

Adverse Events

Knowledge of the chemical category to which an antihistamine belongs can help determine the relative degree of sedation and anticholinergic effects associated with the particular agent. In general, the ethanolamine derivatives, such as diphenhydramine, and the phenothiazine derivatives, such as promethazine (Phenergan), cause the greatest degree of sedation and anticholinergic effects. The most problematic anticholinergic effects are dry mouth, blurred vision, urinary hesitancy, constipation, confusion, and mental cloudiness.

The sedative effects of the older antihistamines vary among patients and may not cause problems for some. Tolerance to the sedative effect develops, and many patients find that sedation either disappears or becomes less bothersome after several days of continued use. Nonetheless, sedation may affect the patient's acceptance of the older antihistamine drugs.

Less-Sedating Antihistamines

More recently, antihistamines have been developed that do not cross the blood–brain barrier to the extent exhibited by the older agents. These newer antihistamines, commonly referred to as *NSAs*, are considered to act peripherally and do not produce sedation or cause clinically important changes in mental status. In general, the anticholinergic effects of these agents are also minimal. Cetirizine, a metabolite of the antipruritic hydroxyzine (Atarax), is not always accepted as an NSA because it is reported to have a higher incidence of sedation than the other newer antihistamines. It is generally classified as a peripherally acting antihistamine and is often still listed in the same category. Nonetheless, it is an effective antihistamine approved by the FDA for seasonal and perennial rhinitis. The NSAs are listed and compared in **Table 46.3**.

TABLE 46.3

Overview of Selected Antihistamines and Decongestants

Generic (Trade) Name and Dosage	Selected Adverse Events	Contraindications	Special Considerations
Non-sedating Antihistamines			
Cetirizine (Zyrtec) 10 mg PO daily Children 2–6 years: 2.5 mg daily 6–11 years: 5–10 mg daily	Somnolence, dry mouth, pharyngitis, dizziness	Known hypersensitivity to cetirizine or hydroxyzine	Renal or hepatic impairment: Adults: 5 mg daily; Children: not recommended with CrCl < 10 mL/min
Desloratadine (Clarinex) 5 mg PO daily Children 2–5 years: 1.25 mg daily 6–11 years: 2.5 mg daily	Same as loratadine	Known hypersensitivity to any ingredients or loratadine	Give same dose every other day in renal or hepatic impairment.
Fexofenadine (Allegra) 60 mg PO BID 180 mg tablet PO daily Children 2–11 years: 30 mg BID	Viral infection (cold, influenza), nausea, headache, drowsiness, dyspepsia, fatigue	Known hypersensitivity to any of its ingredients	Erythromycin and ketoconazole may increase plasma levels of fexofenadine. Dose adjustment in renal disease
Levocetirizine (Xyzal) 2.5–5 mg PO daily Children 2–5 years: 1.25 mg daily 6–11 years: 2.5 mg PO daily	Same as cetirizine	Known hypersensitivity to levocetirizine or cetirizine, end-stage renal disease, hemodialysis, renal impairment in children	Use with caution in patients with renal impairment.
Loratadine (Claritin) 10 mg PO daily Children 2–5 years: 5 mg daily	Headache, somnolence, fatigue, dry mouth	Known hypersensitivity to any of its ingredients	Give same dose every other day in renal or hepatic impairment.
Intranasal Antihistamines			
Azelastine (Astelin or Astepro nasal spray) 1–2 sprays in each nostril BID; 100 doses per bottle Children 2–13 years: 1 spray in each nostril BID	Bitter taste, headache, somnolence, nasal burning, pharyngitis, dry mouth, paroxysmal sneezing, nausea, rhinitis, fatigue, dizziness	Known hypersensitivity	Amount of drug per spray: 137 mcg (Astelin), 205.5 mcg (Astepro) Astepro may be dosed two sprays once daily rather than BID.
Olopatadine (Patanase) two sprays per nostril BID Children 6–11 years: one spray per nostril BID	Headache, somnolence, cough, epistaxis, throat irritation, bitter taste, dry mouth	None	Amount of drug per actuation (spray): 127 mcg
Oral Nasal Decongestants			
Phenylephrine 10–20 mg q4h Children 6–12 years: 10 mg q4h	Same as pseudoephedrine	Same as pseudoephedrine	Pregnancy: Not preferred
Pseudoephedrine 60 mg q6h (240 mg); extended release, 120 mg q12h; controlled release 240 mg q24h Children 6–12 years: 30 mg q6h (120 mg) Children 4–6 years: 15 mg q6h (60 mg)	Headache, insomnia, dry mouth, somnolence, nervousness, dizziness, fatigue, dyspepsia, nausea, pharyngitis, anorexia, thirst	Hypersensitivity to drug or its components Use within 14 days of an MAO inhibitor.	Extended release should not be recommended for children <12 years. Pregnancy: Not recommended; avoid in first trimester
Intranasal Cromolyn			
Cromolyn (Nasalcrom nasal solution) Patients ≥2 years: one spray in each nostril three to six times daily until symptom relief, then q8–12h	Common: burning, stinging, or irritation inside nose, increase in sneezing Rare: cough, headache, unpleasant taste, bloody nose	Hypersensitivity to cromolyn or the formula; acute asthma attacks	Comes in 13 mL bottles and 26 mL bottles; 13 mL bottle = 100 sprays, 26 mL bottle = 200 sprays Not recommended in children <2 years

MAO, monoamine oxidase.

Dosage

Loratadine (Claritin) is dosed as 10 mg once daily for adults and children aged 6 and older. For children aged 2 to 5, the dose is 5 mg once daily. Cetirizine (Zyrtec) is given 5 to 10 mg once daily for children older than age 6 and adults. The lower dosage can be used for younger children or for patients with less severe symptoms. Children aged 2 to 5 should be started on 2.5 mg once daily. Levocetirizine and desloratadine are generally half the dose of cetirizine and loratadine. Fexofenadine (Allegra) doses are for adults and children aged 12 and older. The starting dose is 60 mg twice daily or 180 mg once daily for the extended-release formulation. Children aged 6 to 11 should start at 30 mg twice daily. These agents are available over the counter for both children and adults.

Time Frame for Response

This class of agents has a rapid onset of action, with a time to maximum effect ranging from 1 to 2.5 hours. The half-life of these drugs is 8 to 28 hours, leading to a 1- to 3-day delay in reaching a steady state. Food can delay the time to peak of cetirizine and loratadine, but not fexofenadine.

Contraindications

The lower propensity for anticholinergic effects allows for wider use of NSAs in older adults, patients with glaucoma, and men with BPH because they do not share the same contraindications. NSAs are contraindicated in patients with previous hypersensitivity to these drugs and are not recommended in lactating mothers. Using antihistamines is generally considered safe during pregnancy; preference may be given to cetirizine or loratadine, as these agents have more data in pregnancy compared to the other agents in this category.

Adverse Events

Overall, this class of drugs is well tolerated in patients. Common adverse events include headache, dry mouth, dyspepsia, nausea, and fatigue. See **Table 46.3** for specific agents. It is important to note that cetirizine and levocetirizine are known to be more sedating than the other drugs in this class. More serious but rare side effects include dizziness, myalgia, somnolence, and dysmenorrhea.

Interactions

While loratadine and desloratadine do not have any significant drug interactions, fexofenadine does have some interactions that should be clinically considered. Fexofenadine concentrations may be increased by azole antifungals and erythromycin. Antacids and grapefruit juice administered with fexofenadine may decrease the absorption of fexofenadine. There is also a remote possibility that fexofenadine may prolong the QT interval on an electrocardiogram when administered with other drugs that concurrently prolong the QT interval. Cetirizine or levocetirizine administered with sedating drugs may increase sedation.

Intranasal Antihistamines

Azelastine (Astelin) and olopatadine (Patanase) intranasal antihistamines are also available to treat allergic rhinitis. In placebo-controlled trials, they significantly improved the symptoms of rhinorrhea, sneezing, and nasal pruritus. The adverse events that occurred more frequently than in the patients treated with placebos were bitter taste (19.7% vs. 0.6% for placebo) and somnolence (11.5% vs. 5.4%) (Astelin Package Insert, 2014). These agents still have some systemic absorption, so it is important to remember that they may cause side effects and interact with allergy skin tests. Intranasal prescribing information is noted in **Table 46.3**.

Nasal Decongestants

Mechanism of Action

Nasal decongestants are sympathomimetic amines chemically related to norepinephrine, a major neurotransmitter of the sympathetic nervous system. These drugs are vasoconstrictors. They offer relief from nasal congestion by constricting the blood vessels of the nasal mucosa that have been dilated by histamine and are available in either oral or topical nasal formulations. The results are a shrinking of swollen nasal passages and more air movement to make breathing easier. However, just as norepinephrine is a CNS stimulant, so are the synthetic oral and topical (nasal) decongestants, which is an important clinical consideration.

Dosage

Dosing for common nasal decongestant products is noted in **Table 46.3**. Many decongestants are available in combination with antihistamines. Fixed combination products containing antihistamines and sympathomimetic amines are convenient, but the effective dose of oral decongestants varies among patients. If use of a fixed combination causes side effects or does not relieve symptoms, then clinicians should titrate with single agents to achieve the required dosage.

Because these agents are available OTC, counsel patients to read all labels carefully in order to select a product with only the components that they need to treat symptoms. Many of these combination products may also contain pain relievers or caffeine in addition to antihistamines and decongestants. If patients are also taking separate doses of pain relievers, they could be in danger of overdose.

Since September 2006, the sale of OTC pseudoephedrine has been restricted to "behind-the-counter" status, which means that customers may not directly access any products containing this drug. This could be behind the pharmacy counter or in a locked cabinet. This change was the result of the "Combat Methamphetamine Epidemic Act of 2005," which sought to deter citizens from synthesizing illicit methamphetamine from pseudoephedrine-containing products. Purchasers are not required to have a prescription but must present photo identification. The seller must keep a record of the purchaser's name and information, along with the quantity purchased. The quantity limits may vary per state, but most states have a maximum of 3.6 g that may be purchased in a 24-hour period; many states set a limit of 9 g in a 30-day period (U.S. Food and Drug Administration, 2014). Some states have also imposed a minimum age for purchasing pseudoephedrine (e.g., 18 years and older).

Time Frame for Response

The onset of action for these agents, in immediate-release form, is typically 15 to 30 minutes with a peak response within 30 to 60 minutes. The half-life of pseudoephedrine is 9 to 16 hours, but the effect of the decongestant activity wears off within 4 to 6 hours after administration.

Contraindications

Caution should be used when recommending OTC oral decongestants. Patients with high blood pressure, heart disease, hyperthyroidism, narrow-angle glaucoma, seizure disorders, and BPH may see exacerbation of their disease. In addition, use of oral decongestants is contraindicated in patients taking monoamine oxidase (MAO) inhibitors within 14 days of the administration of pseudoephedrine. Pseudoephedrine and phenylephrine cause the release of norepinephrine into the synapse, and MAO inhibitors inhibit the enzymatic degradation of norepinephrine. As such, the concomitant use of these agents increases the sympathetic activity of the nervous system and can lead to hypertensive crisis. Nasal decongestants are not recommended during pregnancy, and pseudoephedrine should be avoided during the first trimester of pregnancy.

Adverse Events

Oral decongestants constrict blood vessels throughout the body and also act as CNS stimulants, thus increasing blood pressure and heart rate and causing palpitations. Stimulation of the CNS can lead to insomnia, irritability, restlessness, and headache. Many patients find that they can use oral decongestants only during the daytime because the stimulatory effects of these drugs can cause nervousness, agitation, and insomnia.

Topical (Intranasal) Decongestants

Intranasal application (sprays or drops) of sympathomimetic amines provides a prompt and dramatic decrease of nasal congestion. A rebound phenomenon (rhinitis medicamentosa), however, often follows topical application of these drugs. In this scenario, the nasal mucous membrane becomes even more congested and edematous as the drug's vasoconstrictor effect wears off. This secondary congestion is believed to result from ischemia caused by the drug's intensive local vasoconstriction and local irritation of the agent itself. If the use of a topical decongestant is limited to 3 or 4 days, rebound congestion is minimal. With chronic use or overuse of these drugs, rebound nasal stuffiness may become quite pronounced. This phenomenon may begin a vicious cycle, leading to more frequent use of the drug that causes the problem. Should this occur, patients should discontinue topical decongestant therapy. They may use an oral decongestant, isotonic saline drops or spray, or both instead (**Table 46.4**). Side effects from topically administered agents include local irritation and rebound congestion.

Intranasal Corticosteroids

Nasal-inhaled corticosteroids are the most effective forms of therapy for allergic rhinitis. They help to relieve congestion and rhinorrhea by limiting the late-phase response and reducing inflammation. Corticosteroids have a wide range of inhibitory activities against multiple cell types (e.g., mast cells, eosinophils, neutrophils, macrophages, and lymphocytes) and mediators of inflammation (e.g., histamine, eicosanoids, leukotrienes, and cytokines).

Mechanism of Action

Corticosteroids exert their antiinflammatory effect by disabling the cells that present antigen to antibody. Interfering with the antigen–antibody reaction reduces the stimulus for mast cell degranulation. With reduced mast cell degranulation, secretion of cytokines is diminished. The result is a weaker inflammatory reaction with milder or no symptoms of runny nose, nasal congestion, itching, and sneezing.

TABLE 46.4						
Topical Nasal Decongestants						
			Patient Age			
Generic	**Trade**	**Concentration (%)**	**>6 mo**	**2–6 y**	**6–12 y**	**>12 y**
Oxymetazoline	Afrin	0.05	No	No	Yes	Yes
Phenylephrine	Neo-Synephrine	0.125	Yes	Yes	Yes	Yes
	Neo-Synephrine	0.25	No	No	Yes	Yes
	Neo-Synephrine	0.5	No	No	No	Yes
Tetrahydrozoline	Tyzine Pediatric	0.05	No	Yes	Yes	Yes
	Tyzine	0.1	No	No	Yes	Yes
Xylometazoline	Triaminic Nasal and Sinus Congestion	0.05 0.1	No	Yes	Yes	Yes

Dosage

The dosage of the individual intranasal steroids is listed in **Table 46.5**. In general, mometasone furoate, fluticasone propionate, and budesonide have been rated as most potent in vitro. However, these differences have not been shown to translate into meaningful clinical differences in patients. Intranasal corticosteroids must be primed before initial use. Clinicians should counsel patients to squeeze the pump a few times until a fine spray appears. If patients do not use the pump for more than 1 week, they should reprime it.

Time Frame for Response

The therapeutic effects of intranasal corticosteroids are not immediate but will begin working within 3 to 12 hours. Clinicians must counsel patients that they may not experience maximal effects for 1 to 2 weeks if they are using intranasal steroids continuously. Although continuous use is more efficacious, as-needed dosing has also been shown to be useful in patients with seasonal allergic rhinitis. Intranasal corticosteroids should be initiated 2 to 4 weeks before the start of allergy season in patients with recurrent seasonal allergic rhinitis for maximal benefit.

If nasal blockage is severe, patients should use a topical nasal decongestant for the first 2 to 3 days to reduce the swelling and increase the delivery of corticosteroid to the nasal mucosa. Use of nasal corticosteroids should not continue beyond 3 weeks in the absence of significant symptomatic improvement, according to the manufacturers' professional product information.

Contraindications

Intranasal corticosteroids are generally considered to be acceptable treatment for allergic rhinitis in patients who are pregnant, especially if the patient was already maintained on one prior to conception. If an intranasal steroid is to be initiated during pregnancy, agents such as fluticasone and mometasone may be preferred due to lower systemic absorption and more long-term safety data.

Adverse Events

These agents are supplied as aqueous solutions in manually activated metered-dose nasal spray pumps, with separate patient instructions for use with every package. Some of these formulations have a flowery odor, which some patients may find annoying. Local side effects such as irritation, bleeding, and septal perforation may occur but are rare; ensure that patients are using these products correctly in order to minimize these side effects.

Overall, intranasal steroids do not achieve significant systemic concentrations, although the effects of long-term systemic absorption could be concerning. Probably, the most concerning adverse effects of intranasal steroids are the possibility of decreasing the rate of growth and suppressing the

TABLE 46.5

Intranasal Corticosteroid Prescribing Information

Drug	Brand Name (Manufacturer)	Amount of Drug per Spray/Doses per Bottle	How Supplied	Suggested Dose Adult	Pediatric (6–12 y)
Beclomethasone	Beconase AQ (GlaxoSmithKline)	42 mcg/200	25 g amber glass bottle with spray pump	One or two sprays in each nostril BID spray pump	Same as adult
Budesonide	Rhinocort Allergy (Astra)	32 mcg/120	8.6 g bottle with spray pump, available OTC	One to four sprays in each nostril daily	Same as adult
Ciclesonide	Omnaris (Covis)	50 mcg/120	12.5 g bottle with spray pump	Two sprays in each nostril daily	One to two sprays per nostril daily
Flunisolide	N/A	25 mcg/200	25 mL bottle with spray pump	Two sprays in each nostril BID	Same as adult
Fluticasone	Flonase (GlaxoSmithKline)	50 mcg/120	16 g bottle with spray pump, available OTC	Two sprays in each nostril daily	One spray in each nostril daily
	Xhance (Optinose)	93 mcg/120	16 mL bottle with spray pump, fragrance and alcohol free	One to two sprays in each nostril BID	Approved for >18 y
Mometasone	Nasonex (Merck)	50 mcg/120	17 g bottle with spray pump	Two sprays in each nostril daily	One spray in each nostril daily
Triamcinolone	Nasacort Allergy (Aventis)	55 mcg/60	10.8 mL bottle, available OTC	Two sprays in each nostril daily	One to two sprays in each nostril daily

OTC, over the counter.

hypothalamic–pituitary–adrenal axis. Transient effects on growth in children have been noted, but the studies looking at this end point have varied widely. At normal recommended doses, fluticasone, mometasone, and budesonide have not shown growth suppression. The only study to show growth suppression used higher than recommended doses for long periods, so this should not be a serious concern in clinical practice.

All aqueous preparations contain preservatives. Benzalkonium chloride, which may cause ciliary dysfunction, is the preservative in the beclomethasone, flunisolide, fluticasone, mometasone, and triamcinolone products, whereas budesonide contains potassium sorbate as the preservative.

Interactions

Interactions with other drugs are generally not a concern due to low systemic absorption of intranasal corticosteroids.

Intranasal Cromolyn

Cromolyn is classified as a mast cell stabilizer. It prevents antigen-induced degranulation, thereby inhibiting the release of histamine and other cytokines that mediate inflammatory cell function. Cromolyn is of no value in treating acute allergic rhinitis. It is helpful only in preventing the nasal symptoms of allergic rhinitis. Treatment is more effective if it begins 2 to 4 weeks before exposure and continues throughout the exposure period. Intranasal cromolyn is available to patients as Nasalcrom 4% Nasal Solution. It does not require a prescription. Patient use information is noted in **Table 46.3**.

Selecting the Most Appropriate Agent

Nasal symptoms of allergic rhinitis include watery rhinorrhea (runny nose), paroxysmal sneezing (sudden fits of sneezing), nasal congestion (stuffy nose, sinus headache, or both), and postnasal drip that may cause coughing. Allergic rhinitis also may involve the conjunctiva (allergic conjunctivitis). The resulting symptoms are ocular pruritus (itching eyes), lacrimation (watery eyes), conjunctival hyperemia (bloodshot eyes), and chemosis (swollen eyelids). Drug treatment must be tailored to address the most bothersome symptoms. See **Box 46.2** and **Figure 46.5** for a stepwise approach to treating allergic rhinitis. **Table 46.6** lists the recommended treatment order for allergies.

First-Line Therapy

Intranasal corticosteroids are the most potent agents available for the relief of *established* seasonal or perennial rhinitis. They provide efficacy with substantially reduced side effects compared with oral corticosteroids (Dykewicz et al., 2017). Selection of the best agent mostly depends on the patient's insurance formulary; patients may also choose a product that is available OTC, depending on cost.

However, due to the long time frame for response and that they may not be as effective for systemic symptoms, these

---

BOX 46.2   A Stepwise Approach Is Used to Manage the Symptoms of Allergic Rhinitis

1. Identify the offending allergens by history with confirmation of the allergy by skin test.
2. Teach the patient to avoid the offending allergens.
3. For mild symptoms, prophylactic treatment with cromolyn nasal spray (Nasalcrom) or treatment with an antihistamine/decongestant combination may be necessary.
4. For prominent symptoms, begin with topical corticosteroid nasal spray.
5. For treatment failures despite avoidance and pharmacotherapy, progress to immunotherapy.

TABLE 46.6   Recommended Order of Treatment for Allergies

Order	Agents	Comments
First line	Intranasal corticosteroids	Intranasal corticosteroids are the most potent agents available for relief of established seasonal or perennial rhinitis
Second line	Antihistamines/nasal decongestants	Either first- or second-generation agent can be used
		Product selection is based on dosing frequency, potential for adverse effects, and cost
		Second-generation antihistamines may be given only once or BID, and they are relatively non-sedating. First-generation antihistamines are given TID to QID. Pseudoephedrine and phenylephrine are the most popular oral nasal decongestants
Third line	Intranasal cromolyn	Must be used prophylactically

---

agents are often given in combination with antihistamines. First-generation antihistamines were considered first-line agents for the prevention and treatment of allergic symptoms. However, the sedative side effects of the traditional antihistamines limit their usefulness in patients who must remain awake and alert. Fortunately, NSAs cause minimal sedation because they do not cross the blood–brain barrier into the CNS.

The various first- and second-generation antihistamines are equally effective in treating symptoms of allergic rhinitis. Product selection is based on dosing frequency (i.e., duration of action), potential for adverse effects, and cost. Second-generation antihistamines may be given only once or twice daily, and they are relatively non-sedating. First-generation antihistamines are given three to four times daily. Some products are available in long-acting dosage forms that may be given only twice daily. While more sedating, first-generation antihistamines are also significantly less expensive than the second-generation drugs. These agents have the best results when patients take them before exposure to a known allergen. During seasonal attack, patients may need to take antihistamines around the clock for maximal effectiveness.

Second-Line Therapy

Because antihistamines do not reduce nasal congestion, they are often used in combination with nasal decongestants. Pseudoephedrine and phenylephrine are the most popular oral nasal decongestants. Nasal decongestants are α-adrenergic receptor agonists. As such, they stimulate α-adrenergic receptors, causing vasoconstriction in the nasal mucosa, decreasing congestion, and opening nasal passages. Side effects include CNS and cardiovascular stimulation. Elevation in blood pressure may also occur. Many prescription and nonprescription drugs contain a combined antihistamine and nasal decongestant. Some examples are given in **Table 46.3**.

Topical (intranasal) decongestants avoid systemic adverse effects. Prolonged use leads to rebound nasal congestion, however, so they are impractical for seasonal or perennial allergies. Their use should be limited to short periods (a few days).

Third-Line Therapy

Cromolyn, in the form of a metered-dose nasal spray, could be considered a first-line treatment for allergic rhinitis, but it is a prophylactic measure only. It is classified as a mast cell stabilizer in that it prevents or attenuates the allergen activation of nasal mast cells. To be efficacious, cromolyn must be administered continuously (usually four times daily) during seasonal allergen exposure or immediately before an anticipated exposure such as animal dander.

Intranasal cromolyn is an alternative to antihistamines and nasal decongestants for allergic rhinitis. It generally is considered less effective than intranasal corticosteroids, but it is virtually free of side effects.

SPECIAL POPULATION CONSIDERATIONS

Pediatric

If one parent has allergies, the child has a 50% chance of having allergies. Allergies may also be more common in children who were formula-fed, of low birth weight, or exposed to tobacco smoke early in life. In childhood, more boys have allergic rhinitis than do girls, but this difference begins to disappear after adolescence. No sex differences are found in adults.

To determine the dose of allergy medication for a child, practitioners should use weight if possible. Otherwise, they may base according to age. The official product literature usually provides child dosage recommendations by age and weight. Parents should also be counseled to look at package labeling carefully and use dose recommendations for their child's weight if the directions specify. Also, parents should use appropriate teaspoon or tablespoon measurements rather than kitchen utensils. Counsel patients to ask the pharmacist at their local pharmacy if they are not sure if they have an accurate measuring tool.

In determining the dose of medication for a child, practitioners must recognize that infants and small children are not merely "scaled-down" adults. Organs such as the GI tract, liver, and kidneys are not developed enough in children for them to handle medications. Estimating a child's dose based on the adult dose is not always safe. Most pharmaceutical manufacturers do not provide such comprehensive pediatric dosing guidelines. Usually, an age range for children's doses is stated in the official package insert or on the commercial package. If not, prescribers should contact the manufacturer or consult with a specialist who is experienced with the treatment.

As noted earlier, a major consideration in prescribing intranasal steroids in children is the impact on growth. The FDA has approved the use of mometasone and fluticasone furoate for children older than age 2; fluticasone propionate for children older than age 4; and ciclesonide, budesonide, and flunisolide for children aged 6 and older. The other agents are approved for use in children older than age 6.

Geriatric

Although few factors provoke rhinitis in older adults, treatments need to be more tailored because of slower metabolism and the potential for side effects, especially in the CNS. Also, this population is more likely to be taking multiple medications and therefore runs a greater risk of drug interactions than most other patients.

Women

In women, allergic rhinitis symptoms may worsen during pregnancy. The antihistamines diphenhydramine, loratadine, and cetirizine are considered to be acceptable and preferred for use during pregnancy, whereas desloratadine and fexofenadine are less desirable due to lack of data. All intranasal steroids are generally considered to be acceptable due to low likelihood of systemic absorption, but the clinician should consider trying a more preferred agent first if initiating therapy during pregnancy.

MONITORING PATIENT RESPONSE

Assessing the efficacy of treatment requires monitoring the patient's adherence to the drug therapy plan, quality of life, and degree of satisfaction with the care provided. **Box 46.3** could be a useful office tool for this purpose.

> **BOX 46.3   Questions to Ask the Allergic Patient at Every Office Visit**
>
> ### MONITORING SIGNS, SYMPTOMS, AND FUNCTIONAL STATUS
>
> - Has your allergy been better or worse since your last visit?
> - In the past 2 weeks, how many days have you had? (*Ask the patient to tell you how symptoms developed, what they were like, and how long they lasted.*)
>   A runny, stuffy, or itchy nose?
>   Any wheezing or coughing?
>   Any hives or swelling?
>   Eczema or other skin rashes?
>   Reactions to foods?
>   Reactions to insects?
> - Since your last visit, how many days has your allergy caused you to
>   miss work or school?
>   reduce your activities? or
>   (for caregivers) change your activity because of your child's allergies?
> - Since your last visit, have you had any unscheduled or emergency department visits or hospital stays?
> - Since your last visit, have you had any times when your allergy symptoms were a lot worse than usual?
>   If yes, what do you think caused the symptoms to get worse?
>   If yes, what did you do to control the symptoms?
> - Have there been any changes in your home, school, or work environment (e.g., new smokers or pets)? Any new hobbies or recreational activities?
> - Has there been difficulty sleeping at night due to symptoms of allergy?
>
> ### MONITORING PHARMACOTHERAPY
>
> - What medications are you taking?
> - How often do you take each medication? How much do you take each time?
>
> - Have you had any unusual reactions to your medications?
> - Have you missed or stopped taking any regular doses of your medications for any reason?
> - Have you had trouble filling your prescriptions (e.g., for financial reasons, not on formulary)?
> - Have you tried any other medications?
> - Has your allergy medicine caused you any problems (e.g., sleepiness, bad taste, sore throat)?
> - Have you had any nighttime awakenings?
>
> ### MONITORING PATIENT–PROVIDER COMMUNICATION AND PATIENT SATISFACTION
>
> - What questions do you have about your allergy management?
> - What problems have you had in following your allergy management plan, such as taking your medications or reducing your exposure to allergens?
> - Has anything prevented you from getting the treatment you need for your allergies?
> - Have the costs of your allergy treatment interfered with your ability to get appropriate care?
> - How can we improve your allergy care?
>
> This information is provided by the AAFA as part of its educational outreach to patients and their caregivers. The information was adapted from the 2007 National Asthma Education and Prevention Program's Guidelines for the Diagnosis and Treatment of Asthma published by the National Heart, Lung, and Blood Institute.

AAFA, Asthma and Allergy Foundation of America.

PATIENT EDUCATION

Patient education is extremely important in the prevention and management of allergy symptoms. Teaching each patient about the causes of allergic reactions, how triggers evoke symptoms, the various medications available and their use, when to self-treat and when to seek medical help, and how to assess whether treatment is working is highly desirable and appropriate during an office visit. But comprehensive teaching may not be practical because of time constraints. It may be more efficient to determine what

the patient *does not* understand and fill in the gaps at that time. For example, at the end of the visit, practitioners could ask the patient three very basic questions about treatment:

- What is the name of the medication you are taking for allergy symptoms?
- What beneficial effects do you expect, and what side effects may occur?
- How do you take the medication (i.e., dose, time of day, with meals, and what to avoid taking with it)?

If the patient can articulate the correct answers to these questions, little more needs to be discussed about treatment. Practitioners could provide verbally or in writing those things that the patient does not know or understand. Also, they should encourage patients to accept written materials that pharmacists provide when they fill prescriptions and to question any ambiguous or contradictory information.

Drug Information

A variety of sources provide information regarding the treatment of allergic rhinitis. The American Association of Allergies, Asthma, and Immunology provides practice parameters for the treatment of allergic rhinitis (www.aaaai.org). Furthermore, the FDA provides drug information specific to the product, particularly in relation to children or pregnant women.

Patient-Oriented Information Sources

The American Association of Allergies, Asthma, and Immunology provides patient-directed information (http://www.aaaai.org/patients/resources/fastfacts/rhinitis.stm). Similarly, the FDA has information regarding medications in an easy-to-use format for patients.

Complementary and Alternative Medications

There is some suggestion that acupuncture and biofeedback may be effective means of treating allergic rhinitis. However, controlled studies evaluating the effectiveness of these treatment modalities are lacking.

ALLERGIC CONJUNCTIVITIS

The signs and symptoms of allergic conjunctivitis result from the same allergens that cause allergic rhinitis. Mast cells are abundant in the eyelid and conjunctiva but are infrequently found in the eye. This limits allergic ocular inflammation to the lining of the eyelid and the ocular surface (the conjunctiva).

Histamine and arachidonic acid derivatives are the mediators that probably cause most ocular signs and symptoms. Mast cell activation, however, also leads to recruitment of eosinophils, which can be found in the conjunctiva 3 to 5 hours after mast cell degranulation.

Many patients experience ocular symptoms only when allergens directly contact the eyes. For example, patients with sensitivity to cat dander may not have reactions in a room with cats but experience symptoms if they bring their hands to their face. Patients who have symptoms even without direct contact need to be particularly rigorous in their efforts to eliminate or avoid allergens in their homes, workplaces, or schools. Eye rubbing not only introduces allergens into the eye but also may degranulate mast cells mechanically.

Practitioners should encourage patients to apply cool compresses to their eyelids rather than rubbing their eyes to alleviate symptoms. Artificial tears also may reduce symptoms and wash away allergens and inflammatory mediators from the conjunctiva. Often, however, these approaches are inadequate. In such cases, patients require pharmacologic intervention. The types of eye drop medications used to treat allergic conjunctivitis are corticosteroids, antihistamines, vasoconstrictor/antihistamine combinations, mast cell stabilizers, and nonsteroidal antiinflammatory drugs (NSAIDs).

First-generation oral antihistamines, which can help reduce ocular itching, may cause more problems by decreasing tear production due to anticholinergic effects. NSAIDs provide temporary relief of ocular itching due to seasonal allergic conjunctivitis. They work by inhibiting biosynthesis of prostaglandin, a mediator of pain and inflammation. See Chapter 16 for more information on treating allergic conjunctivitis.

CASE STUDY 1

G.B. is a 21-year-old college student who recently moved away from home for the first time. She has been at college since the beginning of the fall semester, approximately 2 weeks. She presents today with a chief complaint of fits of sneezing (sometimes 10 in a row); a runny, itchy, stuffy nose; and red, tearing eyes. Her temperature is 99°F; blood pressure is 118/78. She denies cough and headache. Her chest is clear. Her past medical history is unremarkable, except she states that her mother told her she had *hay fever* when she was younger, which she "outgrew" during high school. These symptoms are the same. She is having difficulty studying because of the sneezing and itching nose, and she is embarrassed to be in class with these symptoms. She picked up diphenhydramine recently and has been taking it once or twice daily as needed, but she says that it makes her too sleepy to study or concentrate. GB is supporting herself through college, so she is concerned about costs of treatment (Learning Objectives 3 and 5).

DIAGNOSIS: ALLERGIC RHINITIS/CONJUNCTIVITIS

1. List specific goals for treatment for G.B.
2. What drug therapy would you recommend? Why?
3. What are the parameters for monitoring success of the therapy?
4. Discuss specific patient education based on the prescribed therapy.

Bibliography

Starred references are cited in the text.

*The American Geriatrics Society (AGS) 2019 Beers Criteria Update Expert Panel. (2019). American Geriatrics Society updated Beers Criteria for potentially inappropriate medication use in older adults. *Journal of American Geriatrics Society, 67,* 674–694.

Bland, C. M., & Jones, B. M. (2020). Drug allergy. In *Pharmacotherapy: A pathophysiologic approach* (11 ed.), New York: McGraw-Hill. http://accesspharmacy.mhmedical.com.ezproxy.butler.edu/content.aspx?bookid=2577&sectionid=240763240.

Choo, K. J., Simons, F. E., & Sheikh, A. (2012). Glucocorticoids for the treatment of anaphylaxis. *Cochrane Database of Systematic Reviews, 4,* CD007596.

*Corren, J., Baroody, F. M., & Pawankar, R. (2014). Allergic and nonallergic rhinitis. In *Middleton's allergy: Principles and practice* (8th ed.). St. Louis, MO: Elsevier.

*Dykewicz, M. S., Wallace, D. V., Baroody, F., et al. (2017). Treatment of seasonal allergic rhinitis: An evidence-based focused 2017 guideline update. *Annals of Allergy, Asthma & Immunology,* 1–23.

Gendo, K., & Larson, E. B. (2004). Evidence-based diagnostic strategies for evaluating suspected allergic rhinitis. *Annals of Internal Medicine, 140,* 278–289.

Lichtenstein, L., & Fauci, A. (1996). *Current therapy in allergy, immunology, and rheumatology* (5th ed.). St. Louis, MO: Mosby-Year Book.

Lieberman, P., Nicklas, R. A., Randolph, C., et al. (2015). Anaphylaxis: A practice parameter update 2015. *Annals of Allergy, Asthma & Immunology, 115,* 341–384.

Middleton, E., Reed, C., Ellis, E., et al. (Eds.). (1998). *Allergy: Principles and practice* (5th ed., Vols. I and II). St. Louis, MO: Mosby-Year Book.

*Nairn, R., & Helbert, M. (2007). Hypersensitivity reactions. In R. Nairn & M. Helbert (Eds.), *Immunology for medical students.* St. Louis, MO: Elsevier.

National Institute of Allergy and Infectious Disease. (1997). *Disease state management sourcebook.* New York, NY: Faulkner and Gray.

*National Institute of Allergy and Infectious Disease. (2015). Pollen allergy fact sheet. Retrieved from http://www.niaid.nih.gov/topics/allergicDiseases/Documents/PollenAllergyFactSheet.pdf on July 2015.

Patterson, R., Grammar, L., & Greenberg, P. (1997). *Allergic diseases: Diagnosis and management* (5th ed.). Philadelphia, PA: Lippincott-Raven.

Solensky, R., & Khan, D. A. (2010). Drug allergy: An updated Practice Parameter. *Annals of Allergy and Clinical Immunology, 105,* 259–273.

*U.S. Food and Drug Administration. (2014). Legal requirements for the sale and purchase of drug products containing pseudoephedrine, ephedrine, and phenylpropanolamine. Retrieved from http://www.fda.gov/Drugs/DrugSafety/InformationbyDrugClass/ucm072423.htm on August, 2015.

Wheatley, L. M., & Togias, A. (2015). Allergic rhinitis. *New England Journal of Medicine, 372*(5), 456–463.

Wingard, L., Brody, T., Larner, J., et al. (1991). *Human pharmacology: Molecular to clinical.* St. Louis, MO: Mosby-Year Book.

Yanez, A., & Rodrigo, G. J. (2002). Intranasal corticosteroids versus topical H_1 receptor antagonists for the treatment of allergic rhinitis: A systematic review with meta-analysis. *Annals of Allergy, Asthma & Immunology, 89,* 479–484.

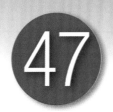

47 Human Immunodeficiency Virus

Linda M. Spooner

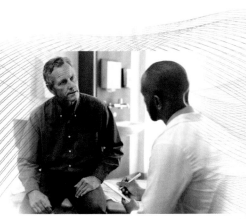
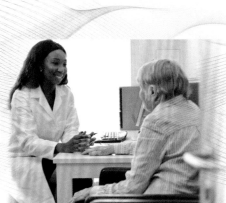
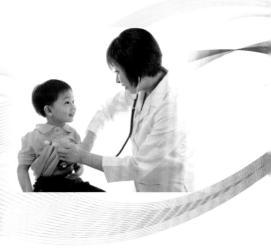

Learning Objectives

1. Discuss the epidemiology and pathophysiology of human immunodeficiency virus (HIV) infection.
2. Describe the features of antiretroviral therapy that must be considered when selecting initial treatment and providing education to people living with HIV, including those in selected populations.
3. Review strategies for pre- and post-exposure prophylaxis for HIV infection.

INTRODUCTION

The first known case of human immunodeficiency virus (HIV) infection was documented in 1959 in a man from Kinshasa, Congo. How he became infected with the virus is unknown. Furthermore, how the disease grew to epidemic proportions also is unclear. In the United States, HIV infection was first recognized in 1981, after it was discovered that young homosexual men were contracting unusual cases of pneumonia and rare cancers that typically were not seen in immunocompetent patients.

HIV is the virus that causes acquired immunodeficiency syndrome (AIDS). A diagnosis of AIDS is based on the presence of an AIDS-defining condition (**Box 47.1**) or a CD4+ T-cell count of less than 200/mm³ (Centers for Disease Control and Prevention [CDC], 2014). Although rates of progression from HIV infection to AIDS vary greatly among individuals, the median is approximately 10 years in patients not receiving antiretroviral medications.

The two types of HIV that have been identified are HIV-1 and HIV-2. HIV-1 accounts for the majority of cases

worldwide, including in the United States, whereas HIV-2 is primarily found in West Africa. HIV-2 is less efficiently transmitted and results in a slower disease progression than HIV-1. Unfortunately, since there are no randomized clinical trials that have assessed the efficacy of antiretroviral medications for the treatment of HIV-2 infection, the ideal initial treatment regimen is unknown. It is recommended to use two nucleoside reverse transcriptase inhibitors plus an integrase inhibitor as preferred initial management of HIV-2 infection (Panel on Antiretroviral Guidelines, 2019).

Over the past three decades, HIV infection has reached epidemic proportions. The World Health Organization (WHO) estimates that approximately 37.9 million people worldwide are infected with HIV, with more than two thirds of cases occurring in Africa (WHO, 2018). Of these, 1.7 million children younger than age 15 are infected. In 2018, 1.7 million people were newly infected with HIV, and there were 770,000 deaths attributed to HIV throughout the world. Explanations for these overwhelming numbers include limited access to health care and antiretroviral medications as well as lack of education about prevention and transmission of HIV. It is exciting to note that these numbers have declined over recent years, largely due to global progress made in efforts to treat more people and to prevent more cases of mother-to-child transmission.

According to the most recent estimates, 1.1 million individuals were living with HIV in the United States at the end of 2015 (CDC, 2017). The number of new infections occurring annually has remained stable at approximately 40,000 per year.

The management of patients infected with HIV is challenging for several reasons. First, the selection of antiretroviral therapy (ART) regimens can be complex, requiring the practitioner to individualize treatment selection based upon genotypic resistance testing results, comorbidities, concomitant

BOX 47.1   Acquired Immunodeficiency Syndrome-Defining Conditions

Candidiasis, pulmonary or esophageal
Cervical cancer, invasive
Coccidioidomycosis, disseminated or extrapulmonary
Cryptococcosis, extrapulmonary
Cryptosporidiosis, chronic intestinal
Cytomegalovirus disease
Herpes simplex virus, chronic ulcers, pulmonary, or esophageal
Histoplasmosis, disseminated or extrapulmonary
HIV-related encephalopathy
HIV-associated wasting
Isosporiasis
Kaposi sarcoma
Lymphoma
Mycobacterium avium complex or *Mycobacterium kansasii* infection
Pneumocystis jiroveci pneumonia
Other pneumonias, recurrent
Progressive multifocal leukoencephalopathy
Salmonella septicemia, recurrent
Toxoplasmosis
Tuberculosis

HIV, human immunodeficiency virus.

medications, and patient preferences. Second, adverse effects of the medications may affect a patient's ability to tolerate and comply with therapy. Third, nonadherence to ART results in treatment failure as well as the development of resistance due to suboptimal serum concentrations of antiretroviral drugs. The health care practitioner should collaborate with the individual patient to select a regimen that the patient can take successfully and still manage potential adverse effects and drug interactions.

CAUSES

HIV is transmitted through four types of contact: sexual intercourse, blood-borne contact, perinatal transmission, and breast-feeding. *Prevention is the key to avoiding transmission* (**Box 47.2**). The most common route of transmission worldwide is through sexual contact with an infected person's genital fluids. The virus is also transmitted via intravenous (IV) transfer of infected blood through transfusions, IV drug use and needle sharing, or occupational exposure. An infected mother may transmit the virus to her baby prior to or during birth as well as during breast-feeding. It is important to note that HIV is *not* transmitted through casual contact (e.g., contact with tears, saliva, toilet facilities).

Effective treatment with ART reduces the risk of transmission to sexual partners, as lower concentrations of HIV

BOX 47.2   Preventing Human Immunodeficiency Virus Transmission

PREVENTING SEXUAL TRANSMISSION

Abstinence, safer sexual practices, use of latex condoms, risk factor modification, notification of sexual partners, education (especially to adolescents), treating sexually transmitted infections, pre-exposure prophylaxis, and consistent and effective use of ART may be used to prevent sexual transmission of HIV. The use of ART to prevent HIV transmission to sexual partners is known as TasP, also known as Undetectable = Untransmittable (U = U).

PREVENTING BLOOD EXPOSURE TRANSMISSION

Since 1985, all donated blood is tested for the presence of HIV. Implementation of universal precaution training programs has decreased transmission among health care workers. Needle exchange and drug treatment programs are available throughout the United States.

PREVENTING PERINATAL TRANSMISSION

Universal prenatal HIV counseling and testing, lowering antepartum viral load to undetectable in the mother with combination ART, appropriate pre- and post-exposure prophylaxis of the infant with ART, and avoidance of breast-feeding by women living with HIV.

ART, antiretroviral therapy; HIV, human immunodeficiency virus; TasP, treatment as prevention.

ribonucleic acid (RNA) in plasma are associated with decreased levels of HIV in genital secretions. Therefore, consistent use of ART leading to sustained reductions in HIV viral loads should be combined with safer sexual and drug use practices to prevent HIV transmission. Pre-exposure prophylaxis (PrEP) with ART is also used to reduce the risk of acquiring HIV infection in high-risk individuals.

PATHOPHYSIOLOGY

HIV is a retrovirus; each viral particle contains two single-stranded molecules of RNA rather than deoxyribonucleic acid (DNA). Following infection of host cells, the viral enzyme reverse transcriptase allows the synthesis of a DNA molecule that is then inserted into the DNA of the host cell, allowing the virus to replicate. In the case of HIV, the host cells are CD4[+] T lymphocytes, white blood cells involved in cell-mediated immunity. As the virus replicates, it destroys the CD4[+] T lymphocytes, thereby leading to immune deficiency.

HIV incorporates itself into the host cell through a number of steps. A viral envelope surrounding the HIV RNA contains proteins on its outer surface that react specifically with the CD4$^+$ receptor on the T lymphocyte (CD4$^+$ T cell). Additionally, the viral membrane uses coreceptors (CCR5 or CXCR4) to attach to the CD4$^+$ T cell. Once this is completed, the viral envelope fuses to the host cell and allows the HIV RNA to enter the host cell. Next, reverse transcriptase catalyzes the formation of a single-stranded DNA intermediate from the viral RNA. This step is followed by duplication of the single-stranded DNA to form a double-stranded DNA. Catalyzed by the enzyme integrase, viral DNA is integrated into the host cell's nucleus. After the DNA is transcribed and translated back to RNA, the virus then makes long chains of polyproteins that are split by the enzyme protease to form new copies of HIV RNA. To protect the viral RNA, a protective core protein called a *capsid* surrounds the genetic material. This process is rapidly repeated, producing an estimated 10 billion new particles each day. The average half-life of a viral particle is 6 hours. The largest concentration of viral particles is found in lymph node tissue and genital secretions.

DIAGNOSTIC CRITERIA

The signs and symptoms of HIV disease vary among patients. The acute retroviral syndrome occurs 2 to 3 weeks following exposure to the virus. During this time, the number of CD4$^+$ T lymphocytes (CD4$^+$ count) declines dramatically, and the number of HIV RNA particles in the plasma (viral load) increases greatly. Clinically, the patient may experience fever, swollen lymph nodes, sore throat, skin rash, muscle soreness, headache, nausea, vomiting, and diarrhea. The specific symptoms and their duration vary among patients, and their presence alone does not constitute a diagnosis; most patients have nonspecific and mild to moderate symptoms. Diagnosis of HIV is based on the presence of HIV RNA or p24 antigen in the plasma or serum, often with a negative or indeterminate HIV antibody test (Panel on Antiretroviral Guidelines, 2019).

The currently used method for diagnosing HIV-1 infection is a combination immunoassay, also known as a fourth-generation assay, which detects circulating antibodies to the HIV-1, HIV-2, and HIV p24 antigen. This assay is highly sensitive and specific for established infection (99% sensitivity and specificity), but false-positive results may rarely occur in patients with autoimmune disorders. If the result of the test is positive, a confirmatory test known as an HIV-1/HIV-2 antibody differentiation assay is performed. If the result of this assay is negative, an HIV RNA or nucleic acid test is performed to determine if virus is present.

Laboratory Parameters

Once the diagnosis of HIV has been confirmed using the above tests, initiation of therapy should be guided by the patient's clinical status as well as two main laboratory parameters, including the CD4$^+$ T-cell count, the plasma HIV RNA

(viral load), and viral resistance testing. Determination of these results allows the clinician to understand the patient's risk of opportunistic infections and risk for disease progression and to monitor response to the selected drug therapy.

CD4$^+$ T-Cell Count

The CD4$^+$ T-cell count indicates the extent to which HIV has damaged the immune system. Normally, the CD4$^+$ T-cell count ranges between 500 and 1,600/mm^3. As the viral infection progresses, the CD4$^+$ count declines, correlating with increasing immunosuppression. Its value is especially important *before* initiating ART. CD4$^+$ T-cell counts of less than 200/mm^3 are associated with an increased risk of AIDS malignancies, such as Kaposi sarcoma, and opportunistic infections, such as *Pneumocystis jiroveci* pneumonia, toxoplasmosis, and cytomegalovirus infection.

Plasma Human Immunodeficiency Virus Ribonucleic Acid: Viral Load

Quantification of HIV replication is determined by measuring the viral load in number of copies per milliliter of plasma. The primary assay used is the HIV-1 reverse transcriptase–polymerase chain reaction assay, which has a lower limit of detection of 20 to 75 copies/mL. Clinical trials demonstrate that viral loads that are undetectable (e.g., <20–75 copies/mL) are associated with a longer duration of suppression of viral replication as compared with detectable levels. The viral load is a useful tool to monitor a patient's virologic status, disease progression, and ART regimen.

Human Immunodeficiency Virus Drug Resistance Testing

Because of the significant association between the presence of drug-resistant HIV and failure of antiretroviral treatment regimens, HIV resistance assays have become useful mechanisms for guiding the selection of appropriate therapy. When used in combination with medication histories and patient counseling, these assays have assisted in the attainment of more efficient and sustained viral suppression. Drug resistance testing is recommended for all patients in the initial laboratory testing they receive as they enter into care.

The two methods used to assess resistance include genotypic and phenotypic assays. Genotypic assays detect genetic mutations that may confer viral resistance. Interpretation of these genotypes requires an understanding of the mutations and their correlation with resistance to specific classes of antiretroviral medications. Results are typically available within 1 to 2 weeks. Treatment should not be delayed while waiting for the results. Phenotypic assays calculate the concentrations of antiretroviral drugs required to inhibit HIV replication by 50%. This value is known as the *median inhibitory concentration* and is abbreviated as IC$_{50}$. The ratio of the IC$_{50}$ of the patient's and reference virus is noted as the fold increase in IC$_{50}$ for a variety of antiretroviral medications. Results of phenotypic assays are available within 2 to 3 weeks due to automation techniques, but they are more expensive to perform than genotypic assays and more complicated to interpret. Thus, genotypic assays are preferred. Both assays may be unsuccessful in patients with low viral loads (<500–1,000 copies/mL) due to the inadequate presence of the virus.

Several limitations exist with HIV drug resistance testing. First, there is no standardized method for quality assurance for the available genotypic and phenotypic assays. Second, they are expensive to perform. Lastly, if a drug-resistant virus comprises less than 10% to 20% of a patient's total virus population, the assays will not detect the resistant virus. Overall, these assays provide a method for making decisions on initiating ART, changing ART in patients experiencing virologic failure or suboptimal response, and selecting ART in pregnant women.

INITIATING DRUG THERAPY

When considering treatment of patients with HIV infection, it is important to note that all patients, regardless of CD4+ count, should be offered treatment as soon as possible with ART (Panel on Antiretroviral Guidelines, 2019). Additionally, regardless of CD4+ count, effective ART reduces the risk of sexual transmission of HIV infection. Urgent initiation of ART is especially important for any individual with AIDS-defining conditions, pregnancy, and early or recent HIV infection since delayed treatment in these situations has been linked to increased morbidity, mortality, and transmission of HIV.

Before therapy is started for any patient, a thorough history and physical examination should be performed, in addition to a complete blood count, basic chemistry profile, liver function tests, fasting lipid profile and glucose, urinalysis, CD4+ T-cell count, viral load, genotypic resistance testing, and additional evaluation of various serologies (e.g., hepatitis B and C).

Goals of Therapy

Because currently available antiretroviral regimens cannot eradicate HIV, goals of therapy primarily focus on the sustained suppression of viral replication to undetectable levels. There are five main goals of ART (Panel on Antiretroviral Guidelines, 2019). These include maximal and sustained suppression of viral load, restoration and preservation of immune system function, enhancement of quality and duration of life, reduction in morbidity and mortality from HIV-related complications, and prevention of HIV transmission. Patients' responses to ART are variable, although successful regimens initiated in treatment-naive patients can decrease viral loads to undetectable levels within 12 to 24 weeks. Virologic success is improved with high-potency ART, excellent treatment adherence, low baseline viral load, and regimen tolerability and convenience.

To maximize the benefits of ART, it is important to select drug regimens carefully based on drug resistance testing, pretreatment viral load (e.g., greater than or less than 100,000 copies/mL), adverse effects, convenience, patient preference, drug interaction profile, pregnancy or pregnancy potential, comorbidities, and cost. There are several recommended regimens that may be used as initial therapy for HIV infection, as they have potent efficacy in suppressing viral replication. These primarily include integrase strand transfer inhibitor (INSTI)-based regimens. Additionally, boosted protease inhibitor (PI)-based regimens and nonnucleoside reverse transcriptase inhibitor-based regimens may be used as initial therapy in certain clinical situations. **Table 47.1** lists the characteristics of all of the currently available antiretroviral medications.

Reverse Transcriptase Inhibitors

There are two subclasses of reverse transcriptase inhibitors (RTIs): the nucleoside reverse transcriptase inhibitors (NRTIs) and the nonnucleoside reverse transcriptase inhibitors (NNRTIs).

Nucleoside Reverse Transcriptase Inhibitors

There are six NRTIs marketed in the United States. These include abacavir (Ziagen), didanosine (Videx), emtricitabine (Emtriva), lamivudine (Epivir), stavudine (Zerit), and zidovudine (Retrovir). There is one nucleotide RTI, tenofovir, available as tenofovir disoproxil fumarate (TDF, Viread) and tenofovir alafenamide (TAF, Vemlidy), which is similar in the mechanism of action but is slightly different in structure than the nucleoside analogs. In addition, several combination products are available for dosing convenience; these are listed in **Table 47.1**.

Mechanism of Action
The NRTIs must be phosphorylated in the target cells before becoming active. This intracellular phosphorylation results in an active triphosphorylated form that interferes with the transcription of viral RNA to DNA. This interference can occur through two mechanisms: chain termination and competitive inhibition.

The *chain termination* process results in the reverse transcriptase enzyme adding the NRTI to the growing chain of HIV viral DNA instead of the needed DNA nucleoside. The NRTI acts as a nucleoside analog in DNA production, and its addition is relatively simple. Once this is accomplished, no more DNA nucleosides can be added to the chain, thus terminating its growth and halting the production of viral DNA.

Competitive inhibition occurs when the active (phosphorylated) NRTI competes with the cell's own nucleoside building block. By competing for the cell's building block, these agents also halt the production of viral DNA.

Dosing
With the exception of abacavir, all NRTIs require elimination by the kidneys and, therefore, must be dose adjusted for patients with renal insufficiency. This is an important concept because it helps to minimize the incidence of adverse effects.

The first NRTI that received U.S. Food and Drug Administration (FDA) approval in the United States was zidovudine. It has been studied extensively as a component of ART and has proven to be effective in delaying the progression of the disease, reducing the incidence of opportunistic infections, and

TABLE 47.1			
Overview of Drugs Used to Treat Human Immunodeficiency Virus Infection			
Generic (Trade) Name and Adult Dosage	**Selected Adverse Effects**	**Contraindications**	**Special Considerations**
NRTIs			
Abacavir (Ziagen) 300 mg PO BID or 600 mg PO daily	Hypersensitivity reaction (fever, rash, malaise, fatigue, nausea, vomiting, respiratory symptoms), possible increased risk of myocardial infarction	Hypersensitivity to any component Moderate-to-severe hepatic impairment Rechallenge following the hypersensitivity reaction	Take without regard to meals. Hypersensitivity reaction can be fatal (black box warning) Discontinue immediately. Do not rechallenge Requires HLA-B*5701 screening prior to use Available in combination with lamivudine (Epzicom), zidovudine + lamivudine (Trizivir), and lamivudine + dolutegravir (Triumeq)
Didanosine (Videx EC) ≥60 kg: 400 mg PO daily; with TDF, 250 mg PO daily <60 kg: 250 mg PO daily; with tenofovir, 200 mg PO daily	Pancreatitis, peripheral neuropathy, optic neuritis, lactic acidosis with hepatic steatosis, noncirrhotic portal hypertension	Concomitant use of allopurinol or ribavirin	Take 30 minutes before or 2 hours after a meal Dose adjustment is required for renal insufficiency
Emtricitabine (Emtriva) 200 mg PO daily	Skin hyperpigmentation, severe acute exacerbation of hepatitis B in coinfected patients who discontinue treatment	Hypersensitivity to any component	Take without regard to meals. Dose adjustment is required for renal insufficiency Available in combination with TDF (Truvada), TAF (Descovy), TDF + efavirenz (Atripla), TDF + rilpivirine (Complera), TAF + rilpivirine (Odefsey), TDF + elvitegravir/ cobicistat (Stribild), TAF + elvitegravir/cobicistat (Genvoya), TAF + bictegravir (Biktarvy), and TAF + darunavir/cobicistat (Symtuza)
Lamivudine (Epivir) 150 mg PO BID or 300 mg PO daily	Severe acute exacerbation of hepatitis B in coinfected patients who discontinue treatment	Hypersensitivity to any component	Take without regard to meals Dose adjustment is required for renal insufficiency Available in combination with zidovudine (Combivir), abacavir (Epzicom), TDF (Cimduo), dolutegravir (Dovato), zidovudine + abacavir (Trizivir), abacavir + dolutegravir (Triumeq), TDF + doravirine (Delstrigo), TDF + efavirenz (Symfi, Symfi Lo)
Stavudine (Zerit) ≥60 kg: 40 mg PO BID <60 kg: 30 mg PO BID	Peripheral neuropathy, pancreatitis, lactic acidosis with hepatic steatosis, lipoatrophy, hyperlipidemia	Hypersensitivity to any component	Take without regard to meals Do not use with zidovudine Dose adjustment is required for renal insufficiency

(Continued)

TABLE 47.1

Overview of Drugs Used to Treat Human Immunodeficiency Virus Infection (*Continued*)

Generic (Trade) Name and Adult Dosage	Selected Adverse Effects	Contraindications	Special Considerations
TAF (Vemlidy)	Nausea, diarrhea, headache, possible weight gain when used with INSTIs, severe acute exacerbation of hepatitis B in coinfected patients who discontinue treatment Less likely to result in renal insufficiency or decreased bone mineral density than TDF	Hypersensitivity to any component	Take without regard to meals Not recommended for patients with creatinine clearance less than 30 mL/min Available in combination with emtricitabine (Descovy), emtricitabine + bictegravir (Biktarvy), emtricitabine + elvitegravir/cobicistat (Genvoya), emtricitabine + rilpivirine (Odefsey), emtricitabine + darunavir/cobicistat (Symtuza)
TDF (Viread) 300 mg PO daily	Nausea, vomiting, diarrhea, headache, asthenia, renal insufficiency, decreased BMD, severe acute exacerbation of hepatitis B in coinfected patients who discontinue treatment	Hypersensitivity to any component	Take without regard to meals Dose adjustment is required for renal insufficiency Available in combination with emtricitabine (Truvada), lamivudine (Cimduo), emtricitabine + efavirenz (Atripla), emtricitabine + rilpivirine (Complera), lamivudine + doravirine (Delstrigo), lamivudine + efavirenz (Symfi and Symfi Lo), and emtricitabine + elvitegravir/cobicistat (Stribild)
Zidovudine (Retrovir) 200 mg PO TID or 300 mg PO BID	Nausea, headache, malaise, bone marrow suppression, lactic acidosis with hepatic steatosis, nail pigmentation	Hypersensitivity to any component	Take without regard to meals Dose adjustment is required for renal insufficiency Available in combination with lamivudine (Combivir) and lamivudine + abacavir (Trizivir)
NNRTIs			
Doravirine (Pilfeltro) 100 mg PO daily	Nausea, dizziness, fatigue, increased bilirubin, increased serum creatinine	Concomitant administration of strong cytochrome P450 inducers	Take without regard to meals Available in combination with TDF + emtricitabine (Delstrigo)
Efavirenz (Sustiva) 600 mg PO bedtime	Neuropsychiatric symptoms (hallucinations, abnormal dreams, suicidality, dizziness, impaired concentration, euphoria, confusion), rash, elevated liver function tests, hyperlipidemia, false-positive cannabinoid and benzodiazepine screening tests, late-onset neurotoxicity (including ataxia and encephalopathy)	Hypersensitivity to any component Numerous drug interactions; see **Table 47.2** for contraindicated combinations	Take on an empty stomach at bedtime Available in combination with emtricitabine + TDF (Atripla), lamivudine + TDF (Symfi: 600 mg efavirenz; Symfi Lo: 400 mg efavirenz)
Etravirine (Intelence) 200 mg PO BID	Rash (including Stevens–Johnson syndrome), hypersensitivity reactions, nausea	Hypersensitivity to any component	Take following a meal

TABLE 47.1

Overview of Drugs Used to Treat Human Immunodeficiency Virus Infection (*Continued*)

Generic (Trade) Name and Adult Dosage	Selected Adverse Effects	Contraindications	Special Considerations
Nevirapine (Viramune, Viramune XR) 200 mg PO daily for 14 days, followed by 200 mg PO BID or XR tablet 400 mg PO daily	Rash (including Stevens–Johnson syndrome), symptomatic hepatitis, including fatal hepatic necrosis (significantly higher risk in treatment-naive women with CD4$^+$ count > 250 and men CD4$^+$ count > 400)	Moderate–severe hepatic impairment	Take without regard to meals. Lead-in period can be extended in patients who develop a rash without constitutional symptoms but should not exceed 28 days
Rilpivirine (Edurant) 25 mg PO daily	Rash, depression, headache, insomnia, hepatotoxicity, QT interval prolongation	Coadministration of anticonvulsants (phenytoin, phenobarbital, carbamazepine, oxcarbazepine), rifampin, St. John's wort, proton pump inhibitors Numerous drug interactions; see **Table 47.2** for contraindicated combinations	Take with a meal Available in combination with dolutegravir (Juluca), TDF + emtricitabine (Complera), and TAF + emtricitabine (Odefsey)
Protease Inhibitors			
	Class adverse effects: lipodystrophy, GI intolerance, hepatotoxicity, hyperlipidemia, hyperglycemia	Numerous drug interactions; see **Table 47.2** for contraindicated combinations	
Atazanavir (Reyataz) 300 mg PO daily plus ritonavir 100 mg PO daily OR 300 mg PO daily plus cobicistat 150 mg PO daily	Prolonged PR interval with first-degree AV block, indirect hyperbilirubinemia, nephrolithiasis, cholelithiasis, rash, increase in serum creatinine when administered with cobicistat	Hypersensitivity to any component	Take with food Use caution when dosing with acid-reducing agents Available coformulated with cobicistat (Evotaz) Dose adjustment is required in hepatic insufficiency
Darunavir (Prezista) 800 mg PO daily plus ritonavir 100 mg PO daily OR 800 mg PO daily plus cobicistat 150 mg PO daily	Rash (Stevens–Johnson syndrome and erythema multiforme reported), headache, increase in serum creatinine when administered with cobicistat	Same as above	Take with food. Available coformulated with cobicistat (Prezcobix) and with TAF + emtricitabine + cobicistat (Symtuza)
Fosamprenavir (Lexiva) 1,400 mg PO BID **or** 1,400 mg PO daily plus ritonavir 100–200 mg PO daily **or** 700 mg PO BID plus ritonavir 100 mg PO BID	Rash, headache, nephrolithiasis	Same as above	Take with a meal if boosted with ritonavir. Dose adjustment is required for hepatic insufficiency
Indinavir (Crixivan) 800 mg PO q8h or 800 mg PO BID plus ritonavir 100–200 mg PO BID	Nephrolithiasis, hyperbilirubinemia, headache, dizziness, metallic taste, rash	Same as above	Should be taken 1 hour before or 2 hours after meals when unboosted. Take without regard to meals when boosted with ritonavir Drink 1.5 L fluid daily to avoid renal stones Dose adjustment is required for hepatic insufficiency

TABLE 47.1

Overview of Drugs Used to Treat Human Immunodeficiency Virus Infection (*Continued*)

Generic (Trade) Name and Adult Dosage	Selected Adverse Effects	Contraindications	Special Considerations
Lopinavir/ritonavir (Kaletra) 400/100 mg PO BID or 800/200 mg PO daily	Prolonged PR interval or QT interval, asthenia	Same as above	Take without regard to meals Alternative dosing is required in patients taking concomitant efavirenz or nevirapine
Nelfinavir (Viracept) 1,250 mg PO BID or 750 mg PO TID	Diarrhea	Same as above	Take with food
Ritonavir (Norvir) Use only as a pharmacokinetic enhancer (booster) with other PIs; 100–400 mg PO daily in 1–2 divided doses	Circumoral and peripheral paresthesias, taste perversion, asthenia	Same as above	Take with food
Saquinavir (Invirase) 1,000 mg PO BID plus ritonavir 100 mg PO BID	Prolonged PR interval, prolonged QT interval, headache	Same as above, plus severe hepatic impairment	Take within 2 hours of a large meal Avoid use in patients with pretreatment QT interval >450 msec
Tipranavir (Aptivus) 500 mg PO BID plus ritonavir 200 mg PO BID	Hepatotoxicity (including hepatic decompensation and fatal hepatitis) rash, fatal and nonfatal intracranial hemorrhage	Same as above, plus moderate-to-severe hepatic impairment	Take with food Must be boosted with ritonavir
Fusion Inhibitors			
Enfuvirtide (Fuzeon) 90 mg subcutaneously BID	Local injection site reactions (almost 100% of patients), increased rate of bacterial pneumonias, hypersensitivity reaction (<1%)	Hypersensitivity to any component	Store reconstituted solution in refrigerator and use within 24 hour
Integrase Inhibitors			
Bictegravir (only available coformulated with other ART) 50 mg PO daily	Diarrhea, nausea, headache	Coadministration with dofetilide or rifampin	Take without regard to meals Available coformulated with TAF + emtricitabine (Biktarvy)
Dolutegravir (Tivicay) 50 mg PO once daily or 50 mg PO BID	Hypersensitivity reactions, insomnia, headache, weight gain, increased risk of neural tube defects when taken at the time of conception	Hypersensitivity to any component Concomitant use with dofetilide	Take without regard to meals Alternative agent for women trying to conceive Twice-daily dosing used when coadministered with efavirenz, fosamprenavir/ritonavir, tipranavir/ritonavir, rifampin. Also used for treatment-experienced patients with resistance mutations Available coformulated with lamivudine (Dovato), rilpivirine (Juluca), and abacavir + lamivudine (Triumeq)
Elvitegravir (only available coformulated with other ART) 150 mg PO daily	Nausea, diarrhea, depression, and suicidal ideation (rare)	Hypersensitivity to any component	Available coformulated with TDF + emtricitabine + cobicistat (Stribild) and TAF + emtricitabine + cobicistat (Genvoya) Numerous drug interactions and renal considerations due to cobicistat component

TABLE 47.1

Overview of Drugs Used to Treat Human Immunodeficiency Virus Infection (*Continued*)

Generic (Trade) Name and Adult Dosage	Selected Adverse Effects	Contraindications	Special Considerations
Raltegravir (Isentress, Isentress HD) 400 mg PO BID or 1200 mg PO daily (Isentress HD)	Nausea, diarrhea, headache, creatine kinase elevation, muscle weakness, fever, depression, and suicidal ideation (rare)	Hypersensitivity to any component	Take without regard to meals When dosed with rifampin, administer raltegravir 800 mg PO BID (Isentress HD not recommended) Use caution with concomitant agents that cause myopathy
CCR5 Antagonists			
Maraviroc (Selzentry) 150 mg PO BID with strong CYP450 3A inhibitors (including PIs other than tipranavir/ritonavir); 300 mg PO BID with nonstrong CYP450 3A inhibitors or inducers; 600 mg PO BID with CYP450 3A inducers (efavirenz, etravirine)	Hepatotoxicity, cough, dizziness, rash, orthostatic hypotension	Severe renal impairment or end-stage renal disease with concomitant use of potent CYP450 3A inhibitors or inducers Numerous drug interactions; see **Table 47.2** for contraindicated combinations	Take without regard to meals
CD4 Post-attachment Inhibitors			
Ibalizumab (Trogarzo) 200 mg IV loading dose, followed by maintenance dose of 800 mg IV q14d	Dizziness, nausea, diarrhea, rash	None listed	Dosing in renal and hepatic impairment not studied Contains polysorbate 80, which may cause delayed hypersensitivity reactions Administer as IV infusion over at least 30 minutes (loading dose) or 15 minutes (maintenance dose)
Fostemsavir (Rukobia) 600 mg PO BID	Nausea, QT prolongation, increased liver function tests (especially in patients with concomitant hepatitis B or C infection)	Hypersensitivity to any component Concomitant use of CYP450 3A4 inducers (consult product labeling for detailed list)	Not for use in treatment-naïve patients Take without regard to meals Use with caution in patients with history of QT prolongation or those taking medications that prolong the QT interval

ART, antiretroviral therapy; AV, atrioventricular node; BMD, bone mineral density; GI, gastrointestinal; HLA, human leukocyte antigen; HD, hemodialysis; INSTI, integrase strand transfer inhibitor; IV, intravenous; NRTIs, nucleoside reverse transcriptase inhibitors; NNRTI, nonnucleoside reverse transcriptase inhibitors; PI, protease inhibitor; TAF, tenofovir alafenamide; TDF, tenofovir disoproxil fumarate.

prolonging survival. Significant adverse effects of zidovudine include bone marrow suppression, which can lead to clinically significant anemia and neutropenia, gastrointestinal (GI) toxicity, fatigue, and lactic acidosis with hepatic steatosis. Thus, it is not recommended as a component of initial treatment.

Lamivudine is one of the better-tolerated NRTIs and was the second NRTI to receive FDA approval. Other NRTIs have been available for many years, including didanosine and stavudine. The bioavailability of didanosine is decreased in the presence of gastric acidity. Therefore, it is formulated as an enteric-coated capsule or as a solution that is reconstituted with liquid antacid to allow for improved absorption. Dosing of didanosine and stavudine should be based on weight (see **Table 47.1**). Both of these NRTIs have similar toxicities, including pancreatitis, peripheral neuropathy, and

GI disturbances. Didanosine also has been associated with noncirrhotic portal hypertension. Neither of these agents is recommended as part of initial treatment for treatment-naive patients.

In contrast, TAF, TDF, and emtricitabine are the most commonly used NRTIs in clinical practice due to their excellent tolerability and dosing convenience. The two forms of tenofovir are available coformulated with emtricitabine and within a number of single-tablet regimens (see **Table 47.1**).

Contraindications

Abacavir is an effective component of ART. Patients who initiate treatment with this agent must be cautioned about the hypersensitivity reaction that occurs in 2.5% to 8% of patients. Symptoms of the hypersensitivity reaction include fever, rash,

GI disturbances, lethargy, and malaise. These can occur at any time after initiating therapy (median, 9 days), although the majority of reactions occur within the first 6 weeks of therapy. Symptoms resolve after discontinuation of the drug but may recur and result in death if abacavir is restarted. The risk of this reaction is correlated with the presence of the human leukocyte antigen (HLA)-B*5701 allele. As a result, pretreatment screening for this allele must be performed before initiating therapy. Abacavir should not be used in those individuals who test positive for the HLA-B*5701 allele on the screening test, and they should be considered allergic to abacavir. Patients who test negative for the allele should still be counseled about the signs and symptoms of the hypersensitivity reaction. Additionally, there is controversy over an association between abacavir and cardiovascular disease, as some analyses have demonstrated an increased risk of myocardial infarction, while others have not. At this time, it is recommended to use caution when considering the initiation of abacavir in patients with risk factors for cardiovascular disease.

Tenofovir and emtricitabine are the two newest NRTIs available for use as a part of an ART regimen. Both are well tolerated, are dosed once daily, and can be taken without regard to meals. TDF (more so than TAF) may cause renal insufficiency, with a higher risk in patients with advanced HIV infection, long treatment duration, low body weight, and pre-existing renal impairment. Baseline and periodic assessment of serum creatinine and phosphorous, along with urinary glucose and protein, should be performed. Also, since both forms of tenofovir and emtricitabine exhibit activity against hepatitis B virus, they are the agents of choice for the management of patients who are coinfected with HIV and hepatitis B.

Dual NRTIs are used as part of ART in combination with a boosted PI, an NNRTI, or an integrase inhibitor. Recommended dual NRTIs include TDF/emtricitabine (coformulated as Truvada), TAF/emtricitabine (coformulated as Descovy), and abacavir/lamivudine (coformulated as Epzicom). Triple NRTI regimens are less effective than PI- or NNRTI-based regimens; therefore, they should not be used in routine clinical practice.

Adverse Effects

A class adverse effect observed with all NRTIs includes lactic acidosis with hepatic steatosis. Although this adverse effect is rare, especially with newer NRTIs, it results in a high risk of death. This may be due to mitochondrial dysfunction that occurs on the administration of NRTIs. The clinical presentation of lactic acidosis varies greatly among patients but often includes nonspecific GI symptoms (nausea, vomiting, abdominal pain) as well as generalized weakness, myalgias, and paresthesias that can progress to tachycardia, tachypnea, mental status changes, and multiorgan failure. Hepatic steatosis may manifest as an enlarged fatty liver on computed tomography scan as well as increased liver transaminases.

Risk factors for the development of this syndrome include female gender, pregnancy, obesity, regimen components (stavudine, didanosine, zidovudine), and prolonged use of NRTIs. If this syndrome develops, the NRTIs should be discontinued immediately, and supportive care should be initiated. Because

other clinical interventions such as administration of thiamine, riboflavin, and levocarnitine have not been adequately assessed in clinical trials, their efficacy cannot be determined at this time. Patients taking NRTIs should be cautioned about the signs and symptoms of lactic acidosis, and if these are observed, the patient should notify the practitioner immediately. It is optimal to use NRTIs with less risk of mitochondrial toxicity, such as TAF, TDF, emtricitabine, lamivudine, or abacavir, instead.

Additionally, all NRTIs can decrease bone mineral density (BMD). The risk is greater with regimens containing TDF. BMD assessment can be considered for individuals with a history of fractures or other risk factors for osteoporosis or BMD loss. Calcium and vitamin D supplementation can also be considered.

Nonnucleoside Reverse Transcriptase Inhibitors
Mechanism of Action and Clinical Use

By binding to reverse transcriptase, NNRTIs also interfere with the conversion of RNA to DNA. The available NNRTIs are delavirdine (Rescriptor), doravirine (Pilfeltro), efavirenz (Sustiva), etravirine (Intelence), nevirapine (Viramune), and rilpivirine (Edurant). Delavirdine is the least potent NNRTI and, therefore, is not recommended as part of initial ART. Nevirapine has a higher incidence of rash and hepatotoxicity than efavirenz; thus, it is no longer recommended for initial treatment. It can be continued in patients who are stabilized on the drug already. Etravirine has primarily been studied in treatment-experienced patients with prior virologic failure, and its use is reserved for this purpose. Trials have shown that efavirenz-based regimens have similar virologic efficacy as compared with PI- and integrase inhibitor-based regimens, although some studies show that other regimens are superior to efavirenz because of fewer discontinuations due to central nervous system side effects and possible association with suicidality. Thus, the Department of Health and Human Services (DHHS) Panel considers efavirenz as recommended in certain clinical situations. Rilpivirine is also an alternative NNRTI since it was shown to be noninferior to efavirenz overall. However, its use should be restricted to individuals with a pretreatment viral load of less than 100,000 copies/mL and CD4+ count above 200 cells/mm^3. This is because comparative clinical trials with rilpivirine and efavirenz showed a higher rate of virologic failure with rilpivirine in patients with very high viral loads or low CD4+ counts, due to the development of resistance mutations. Both efavirenz and rilpivirine are available in coformulations with tenofovir and emtricitabine to reduce pill burden. Doravirine is the newest NNRTI, and it is available coformulated with TDF and emtricitabine as a single-tablet regimen (Delstrigo) which can be used as initial treatment in certain clinical situations (e.g., where an INSTI cannot be used).

Adverse Effects

The most frequently reported adverse effects of NNRTIs include GI disturbances, rash, and elevations in hepatic transaminases. Efavirenz commonly causes central nervous system adverse effects, including dizziness, impaired concentration, abnormal dreams, and hallucinations. These events occur within the first few days of initiating therapy but resolve over

2 to 4 weeks with continued treatment. Dosing at bedtime is helpful in minimizing these adverse effects. More recently, efavirenz has been linked to late-onset neurotoxicity, including ataxia and encephalopathy. This can appear months to years following initiation of treatment.

Nevirapine has been associated with severe, life-threatening hepatotoxicity, including hepatic necrosis and hepatic failure, primarily occurring within the first few weeks of initiation. This may also occur along with a hypersensitivity reaction that includes rash and fever. A black box warning in the nevirapine labeling notes that women with CD4$^+$ counts greater than 250 cells/mm^3 and men with CD4$^+$ counts greater than 400 cells/mm^3 have a considerably higher risk of hepatotoxicity. Therefore, all patients who initiate therapy with nevirapine should initiate dosing once daily for 14 days followed by twice daily, and they should receive close monitoring of liver function tests and clinical symptoms throughout the treatment course. If hepatotoxicity occurs, nevirapine should be discontinued permanently.

Etravirine demonstrates activity against some HIV viruses that express mutations conferring resistance to the other four NNRTIs and is reserved for treatment-experienced patients. Its adverse effects include nausea, rash, and hypersensitivity reactions associated with organ dysfunction.

Rilpivirine causes fewer central nervous system adverse effects than efavirenz. Its side effects include depression, headache, insomnia, and rash. Doravirine may cause dizziness, fatigue, and increased serum creatinine.

Drug Interactions

All of the NNRTIs are metabolized by the cytochrome P-450 (CYP450) 3A4 isoenzyme system in the liver. Each NNRTI also has variable effects on inhibiting or inducing this enzyme system. Therefore, caution should be used when administering NNRTIs with drugs dependent on CYP450 3A4 for metabolism, including PIs, phenytoin, phenobarbital, and clarithromycin. Concomitant use of rifampin with etravirine or rilpivirine is contraindicated because of the increased metabolism of etravirine that results in reduced serum concentrations and reduced efficacy. Rifampin may be used with caution with nevirapine. Rifampin must be used with an increased dose of efavirenz (800 mg daily). Concomitant use of St. John's wort is contraindicated with all NNRTIs due to the risk of virologic failure secondary to the resulting suboptimal NNRTI concentrations. Use of rilpivirine with proton pump inhibitors is contraindicated due to reduced absorption and subsequent decreased concentrations of rilpivirine. Additional contraindicated concomitant medications can be found in **Table 47.2**.

Protease Inhibitors

Mechanism of Action

Introduced in the mid-1990s, PIs have demonstrated potent virologic efficacy, durable effects, and high barriers to resistance. They act near the final stage of HIV viral replication by inhibiting the protease-mediated cleavage of the polyproteins. These polyproteins are responsible for creating new HIV RNA copies. Inhibiting this final stage by the use of PIs decreases the production of HIV RNA copies.

Nine PIs are available: atazanavir (Reyataz), darunavir (Prezista), fosamprenavir (Lexiva), indinavir (Crixivan), lopinavir/ritonavir (Kaletra), nelfinavir (Viracept), ritonavir (Norvir), saquinavir (Invirase), and tipranavir (Aptivus). These agents vary greatly in terms of their potency, adverse effects, and pharmacokinetic characteristics.

Dosing

PI-based regimens provide excellent efficacy in virologic suppression. Either ritonavir or cobicistat, potent CYP450 3A4 isoenzyme inhibitors, can be used to increase the concentrations of other PIs, allowing greater exposure of the virus to the PI. These "boosted" regimens demonstrate more potent virologic activity while reducing pill burden and adverse effects. However, it is important to note that there are numerous drug–drug interactions that result from the presence of these pharmacokinetic enhancing agents in a regimen. Despite this, boosting regimens with low-dose ritonavir or cobicistat is the standard of care in PI-based ART regimens, as this results in a high genetic barrier for resistance.

The pharmacokinetic characteristics of the PIs vary greatly across the class. Food affects the bioavailability of many of the PIs (see **Table 47.1**). For example, administration of atazanavir with food increases its bioavailability substantially and therefore should be administered with a meal. In contrast, concentrations of indinavir decrease by 77% with food, resulting in the requirement that this drug be taken on an empty stomach or with a small, low-fat snack (e.g., pretzels) when used without ritonavir booster doses.

Adverse Effects

The adverse effects of all PIs include GI disturbances, such as nausea, vomiting, and diarrhea, occurring upon treatment initiation. All PIs can cause increases in the levels of hepatic transaminases. Clinical hepatitis and hepatic decompensation are more common in patients receiving regimens containing tipranavir/ritonavir. Risk factors for hepatotoxicity with PIs include hepatitis B or C coinfection, alcohol abuse, underlying liver disease, and concomitant use of hepatotoxic agents. This should be monitored carefully.

A class effect of the PIs includes fat maldistribution, also known as *lipodystrophy*. This results in the accumulation of fat in the abdomen, breasts, and dorsocervical fat pad (*buffalo hump*). This occurs in a large percentage of patients receiving ART, depending upon the regimen used and the duration of treatment. Fat maldistribution may be accompanied by metabolic abnormalities such as hyperlipidemia and hyperglycemia. Management of lipodystrophy includes the use of diet and exercise as well as administration of tesamorelin, a growth hormone-releasing factor. Improvements have been demonstrated in clinical trials of patients changed from lopinavir/ritonavir to atazanavir.

All of the PIs, with the exception of unboosted atazanavir, have been associated with hyperlipidemia, including increased levels of triglycerides, total serum cholesterol, and low-density

TABLE 47.2

Nonantiretroviral Medications That Are Contraindicated for Concomitant Use with Nonnucleoside Reverse Transcriptase Inhibitors, Protease Inhibitors, Integrase Strand Transfer Inhibitors, or Tenofovir Alafenamide

Class/Drug	Contraindicated Medications and/or Classes	Comments
All NNRTIs	St. John's wort, enzalutamide, mitotane	Results in virologic failure
	Rifapentine (except efavirenz)	Results in tuberculosis treatment failure
	Simeprevir, dasabuvir, ombitasvir, paritaprevir	Results in concomitant medication toxicity
Efavirenz	Bedaquiline, cisapride, pimozide, midazolam, triazolam	Results in concomitant medication toxicity
Etravirine	Bedaquiline, rifampin, carbamazepine, phenytoin, phenobarbital	Results in decreased etravirine concentrations
Rilpivirine	Proton pump inhibitors, rifampin	Results in virologic failure
	Rifampin, carbamazepine, oxcarbazepine, phenytoin, phenobarbital, >1 dose dexamethasone	Results in decreased rilpivirine concentrations
All PIs	Simvastatin, lovastatin	Results in increased risk of rhabdomyolysis
	Amiodarone, dronedarone, flecainide, propafenone, quinidine, eplerenone, ranolazine, rivaroxaban, cisapride, pimozide, midazolam, triazolam, lurasidone, ergot alkaloids, alfuzosin, salmeterol, fluticasone, salmeterol, elbasvir/grazoprevir, sofosbuvir/velpatasvir/voxilaprevir, glecaprevir/pibrentasvir sildenafil (when used for pulmonary arterial hypertension), silodosin	Results in concomitant medication toxicity
	Rifampin, carbamazepine, oxcarbazepine, phenytoin, phenobarbital	Results in virologic failure
	Rifapentine	Results in tuberculosis treatment failure
	St. John's wort	Results in virologic failure
Atazanavir	Proton pump inhibitors	When used with unboosted atazanavir, results in decreased atazanavir concentrations
All INSTIs	Dofetilide (except raltegravir)	Results in concomitant medication toxicity
	Carbamazepine, oxcarbazepine, phenytoin, phenobarbital, St. John's wort	Results in virologic failure
Elvitegravir/ cobicistat	Apixaban, rivaroxaban, cisapride, pimozide, ranolazine, midazolam, triazolam, lurasidone, ergot alkaloids, alfuzosin, salmeterol, fluticasone, elbasvir/ grazoprevir, sofosbuvir/velpatasvir/voxilaprevir, glecaprevir/pibrentasvir, silodosin, lovastatin, simvastatin, sildenafil (when used for pulmonary arterial hypertension)	Results in concomitant medication toxicity
TAF	Rifampin, rifabutin, rifapentine, St. John's wort, tipranavir/ritonavir	Results in virologic failure

INSTIs, integrase strand transfer inhibitors; NNRTIs, nonnucleoside reverse transcriptase inhibitors; PIs, protease inhibitors; TAF, tenofovir alafenamide.

lipoproteins. Lopinavir/ritonavir and fosamprenavir/ritonavir cause a substantial increase in triglycerides when compared to atazanavir/ritonavir or darunavir/ritonavir. These lipid abnormalities may be associated with accelerated coronary artery disease in HIV patients. Management includes dietary modifications, exercise, smoking cessation, and changing to agents with a lower likelihood of lipid abnormalities, as well as the addition of lipid-lowering treatments, such as 3-hydroxy-3-methylglutaryl-coenzyme A reductase inhibitors (statins). However, it is important to note that most statins cause drug interactions with the PIs, and some are contraindicated (**Table 47.2**). Therefore, pravastatin is a preferred agent because it does not have as many interaction concerns.

Another class effect of PIs includes hyperglycemia, which may lead to new-onset diabetes mellitus as a result of insulin resistance in approximately 3% to 5% of patients. Patients should be cautioned about warning signs of hyperglycemia, including polydipsia, polyphagia, and polyuria. Management of hyperglycemia includes lifestyle modifications (diet and exercise), consideration of NNRTI or integrase inhibitor use as an alternative, and pharmacologic management according to the American Diabetes Association.

Clinical Use

Based upon virologic efficacy and durability data, dosing convenience and low pill burden, and good tolerability, the guidelines published by the Panel on Antiretroviral Guidelines (2019) list darunavir/ritonavir as the recommended component of an initial PI-based regimen, stating that its use is preferred over boosted atazanavir (**Table 47.3**). Clinical trials comparing

TABLE 47.3

Recommended Initial Treatment Regimens for Most People with Human Immunodeficiency Virus

Bictegravir/TAF/emtricitabine#

or

Dolutegravir + abacavir‡/lamivudine*

or

Dolutegravir + TDF or TAF/emtricitabine*

or

Raltegravir + TDF or TAF/emtricitabine*

or

Dolutegravir/lamivudine^

---

*May substitute lamivudine for emtricitabine or vice versa.

‡Do not use abacavir in patients who are HLA-B*5701 positive.

#Do not initiate if creatinine clearance less than 30 mL/min.

^Do not initiate if pre-treatment human immunodeficiency virus ribonucleic acid (HIV RNA) > 500,000 copies/mL, active co-infection with hepatitis B virus, or if antiretroviral therapy (ART) initiation occurs before receipt of results of genotyping and hepatitis B screening.

TAF, tenofovir alafenamide; TDF, tenofovir disoproxil fumarate.

darunavir/ritonavir to lopinavir/ritonavir demonstrated superior virologic efficacy with darunavir/ritonavir after 96 weeks of treatment. Darunavir contains a sulfa moiety and, therefore, can cause a rash. The rash is typically mild to moderate in severity and self-limited. However, the agent should be discontinued if the rash is severe or in the presence of fever or elevated liver function tests. Atazanavir/ritonavir has fewer adverse effects on lipids when compared to other PI-based regimens, but it has a higher rate of discontinuation due to adverse effects when compared to darunavir/ritonavir or raltegravir. The primary adverse effect of atazanavir is hyperbilirubinemia with or without jaundice or icteric sclerae. It may also cause nephrolithiasis, nephrotoxicity, and cholelithiasis. Since it requires an acidic GI environment for dissolution, acid-reducing agents such as antacids, histamine$_2$ receptor antagonists, and proton pump inhibitors may inhibit the absorption of atazanavir, requiring staggered dosing and limitations on the use of these agents.

Drug Interactions

All PIs are metabolized by the CYP450 3A4 isoenzyme system in the liver. Each of the PIs has a different effect on inducing or inhibiting the efficiency of this isoenzyme system. Therefore, caution must be used when combining PIs with any medications that are metabolized by CYP450 3A4 or that induce or inhibit this system. Concurrent use of PIs with ergot alkaloids, simvastatin, lovastatin, rifampin, and St. John's wort is contraindicated. A summary of these contraindicated medications is provided in **Table 47.2**.

Fusion Inhibitors

Enfuvirtide (Fuzeon) is the only available agent in this class of antiretroviral drugs. It inhibits the fusion of the virus to the cell membrane of the CD4+ T cell, thereby preventing HIV from entering the cell. Because its mechanism of action is distinct from the intracellular agents previously discussed, it may be useful for highly treatment-experienced patients with the virus that is resistant to other currently available antiretroviral agents.

Enfuvirtide must be injected subcutaneously twice daily. Adverse effects include local injection site reactions, such as erythema, induration, and pain, which occur in almost all patients. Less than 1% of patients experience hypersensitivity reactions, including rash and fever. Enfuvirtide significantly increases tipranavir/ritonavir concentrations, resulting in an increased risk of adverse effects.

Integrase Inhibitors

Three INSTIs are available for the treatment of HIV infection. These include bictegravir, dolutegravir, elvitegravir, and raltegravir. They prevent the integration of viral DNA into the host cell's genome. With the exception of elvitegravir, each of these agents is recommended for use with a dual NRTI backbone as initial therapy in treatment-naive individuals, per the Panel's guidelines (2019), as they have similar virologic efficacy as other recommended regimens and are well tolerated.

Raltegravir was the first INSTI approved, and it is metabolized via UDP glucuronosyltransferase family 1 member A1 (UGT1A1)-mediated glucuronidation and therefore exhibits minimal drug–drug interaction risk. This agent can cause elevations in creatine kinase with possible rhabdomyolysis and should be used with caution in patients receiving concomitant medications that have similar adverse effects. Rare cases of hypersensitivity reactions have been documented in postmarketing surveillance.

Elvitegravir is only available coformulated with the booster agent cobicistat, emtricitabine, and TDF or TAF (Stribild or Genvoya), which permits the product to be dosed once daily but results in numerous drug interactions. The most common adverse effects of elvitegravir include nausea, headache, and diarrhea. Additionally, because cobicistat inhibits the active renal tubular secretion of creatinine, increases in serum creatinine and decreases in creatinine clearance occur without reducing renal function. This combination product is not recommended for use in individuals with a baseline creatinine clearance of less than 70 mL/min, and it should be discontinued if creatinine clearance decreases to less than 50 during treatment.

Dolutegravir and bictegravir are considered second-generation INSTIs, in that they have a higher genetic barrier to resistance. The dosing of dolutegravir is once daily for treatment-naive patients and twice daily in treatment-experienced patients. It is available as a single agent or coformulated with abacavir and lamivudine (Triumeq). Bictegravir is only available coformulated with TAF/emtricitabine as Biktarvy. Both dolutegravir and bictegravir are well tolerated, causing insomnia or headache in rare cases. Because their absorption is affected by agents containing polyvalent cations (e.g., calcium supplements, antacids, iron supplements), their dosing should be 2 hours before or 6 hours after the administration of these products.

CCR5 Antagonist

Maraviroc (Selzentry) is the only available agent in this class of antiretrovirals. It blocks the CCR5 receptor on the membrane of CD4$^+$ T cells, preventing entry of the HIV. Prior to use, a coreceptor tropism assay (e.g., Trofile) must be performed to determine if the patient's virus utilizes the CCR5 receptor since not all HIV strains do. Maraviroc has a black box warning in its package insert describing hepatotoxicity that may be preceded by a systemic allergic reaction. This agent may also cause cough, orthostatic hypotension, rash, and fever. It also has a multitude of drug–drug interactions associated with its use, requiring dose adjustment. The Panel (2019) does not recommend maraviroc-based regimens as initial therapy for treatment-naive patients; rather, its utility is for highly treatment-experienced patients who have failed other treatment regimens.

CD4 Post-attachment Inhibitor

Ibalizumab (Trogarzo) is a humanized monoclonal antibody that binds to domain 2 of the CD4 receptor on the surface of the cell, thereby preventing the entry of the HIV virus into the host cells via interference with the required post-attachment steps. The drug does not interfere with CD4 activity and therefore does not cause immunosuppression. Its utility is as an addition to an optimized background ART regimen in patients who have multi-drug resistant virus and experienced virologic failure. It is administered as an IV infusion every 2 weeks.

gp120-directed Attachment Inhibitor

Fostemsavir (Rukobia) is a prodrug that is hydrolyzed to temsavir, an active drug that serves as a gp120-directed attachment inhibitor. This results in prevention of attachment by the virus to CD4+ cell receptors. Fostemsavir is a gp120-directed attachment inhibitor that is only indicated for use in heavily treatment-experienced adults with multidrug-resistant HIV infection who are failing their current ART regimen.

Selecting the Most Appropriate Regimen

Although guidelines exist for the combinations of agents to be used in ART, each patient must have a highly individualized regimen. Although current regimens are effective at keeping the viral load at undetectable levels, eradication of the virus is not yet attainable. This is due to the early development of latently infected CD4$^+$ T cells with a long half-life that, even with prolonged therapy, persist.

Previously Untreated Patients

One of the most important therapeutic interventions in the care of a patient with HIV infection is the initial treatment regimen (**Tables 47.1** and **47.3**). It is essential to select the most potent and appropriate therapy possible, keeping in mind adverse effects and adherence issues. Discontinuing recommended therapy due to nonadherence increases the risk of drug resistance and failure with alternate regimens.

"Recommended initial regimens for most people with HIV" have been selected by the DHHS Panel based on optimal efficacy and durability demonstrated in clinical trials as well as tolerability and convenience of use. "Recommended initial regimens in certain clinical situations" are also provided by the DHHS Panel for situations where alternatives may be preferred.

Recommended initial therapy is comprised of two NRTIs (also known as the dual nucleoside "backbone") plus a third drug: an INSTI (for most people) or either an NNRTI or a PI (in certain clinical situations) (**Table 47.3**). Recommended dual NRTI backbones include either TDF or TAF/emtricitabine or abacavir/lamivudine. Since they are each available as coformulated tablets with once-daily dosing, selection depends upon consideration of clinical data, adverse effects, and comorbidities. Since TDF can cause nephrotoxicity and decreased BMD, use of TAF/emtricitabine or abacavir/lamivudine can be considered in patients at increased risk of these adverse effects. Prior to initiation of abacavir, testing for the HLA B*5701 allele to determine the risk of hypersensitivity must be performed. If a patient is coinfected with HIV and hepatitis B, tenofovir/emtricitabine is the preferred backbone due to its activity against the hepatitis B virus.

Selection of the third drug in the regimen depends upon clinical data, adverse effects, dosing convenience, genetic barrier to resistance, comorbid conditions, and drug interaction potential. The INSTI-based regimens of raltegravir, bictegravir, or dolutegravir plus a dual NRTI backbone are recommended as initial regimens for most treatment-naive patients. Their advantages include comparable virologic efficacy to other regimens with fewer adverse effects and lipid abnormalities. They also have fewer drug interactions than PI- or NNRTI-based regimens. Raltegravir may have a lower genetic barrier to resistance as compared with the other INSTIs. Bictegravir has been shown to be similar to dolutegravir in terms of safety, efficacy, and tolerability. Dolutegravir was shown to be superior to darunavir/ritonavir and efavirenz in virologic efficacy, primarily due to fewer discontinuations for side effects. Due to preliminary data that show an increased risk of neural tube defects in pregnant women taking dolutegravir at the time of conception, the risks and benefits of this medication should be discussed with women who plan to become pregnant or who are not using effective contraception.

Recently, the option of use of a single NRTI (lamivudine) with an INSTI (dolutegravir) was added to the list of recommended regimens for most people with HIV. This combination is available as a single tablet known by the brand name Dovato. Dovato should be avoided in people with pre-treatment HIV viral loads of more than 500,000 copies/mL, those who have active co-infection with hepatitis B virus, and those who will initiate ART in advance of receiving results of genotype resistance testing or hepatitis B screening.

Treatment-Experienced Patients

When antiretroviral treatment failure occurs, it is necessary to assess why this occurred to determine the appropriate therapy change. Virologic failure is a term that encompasses all potential reasons for suboptimal response to therapy that must be assessed, including patient factors (e.g., incomplete medication adherence, psychiatric illness, presence of resistant virus, interruption of access to ART, high pill burden and/or dosing frequency) and drug-related factors (e.g., suboptimal pharmacokinetics, drug interactions, medication errors, and HIV-related factors, such as the presence of resistance or prior treatment failure) (Panel on Antiretroviral Guidelines, 2019). *Virologic failure* is defined as the failure to achieve or maintain HIV RNA plasma levels less than 200 copies/mL. An *incomplete virologic response* results when two consecutive viral loads are above 200 copies/mL after 24 weeks on ART in a patient who has not been previously suppressed on the regimen. *Virologic rebound* occurs when the viral load increases to 200 copies/mL or higher after virologic suppression has been achieved. It is also important to note that virologic blips can occur, where an isolated occurrence of the detectable virus happens but is followed by a return to undetectable concentrations. Blips are not typically associated with virologic failure.

After the practitioner considers the causes and types of treatment failure, the drug regimen should be changed accordingly. The patient's previous treatment experience and current drug resistance pattern must be considered because there may be cross-resistance between agents within the same therapeutic class. In addition, if an adverse effect or unacceptable toxicity caused a cessation of therapy, the practitioner should avoid alternative agents likely to cause that adverse effect. Furthermore, agents with complicated dosing schedules and strict food and timing requirements should be avoided if that is what caused the first treatment failure. Selecting agents that are free of side effects and strict food or timing requirements may not be easy, but each patient must be given the regimen to which he or she will most likely adhere.

When changing therapy, one or more of the agents in the regimen may need to be replaced so that the regimen contains at least two (preferably three) fully active drugs based upon resistance testing, treatment history, and mechanism of action. This will vary depending on the individual patient's situation. Expert advice from an HIV clinician is crucial to selecting the most appropriate option and performing proper monitoring and follow-up.

Special Population Considerations

Pediatric

Guidelines exist for treating HIV infection in the pediatric patient (Panel on Antiretroviral Therapy and Medical Management of Children Living with HIV, 2020). Although the principles remain the same in all HIV-infected individuals, unique considerations in subsets of the pediatric population need brief discussion. These include diagnosis of disease, differences in CD4$^+$ T-cell counts and viral loads, changes in pharmacokinetic parameters, and adherence issues.

Diagnostic testing for suspected HIV-infected infants can be performed as early as at birth and by age 2 weeks in almost all infants. Testing in high-risk infants should occur within the first 48 hours of life because in 20% to 30% of infected infants, the diagnosis can be made within this time frame. If the initial test is negative, repeat testing should be performed at age 1 to 2 months and age 4 to 6 months. Detailed testing schedules for low- and high-risk infants are found in the guidelines. HIV DNA polymerase chain reaction assays or RNA assays, collectively known as nucleic acid tests, are the preferred virologic methods for diagnosing HIV in infants. Antibody testing is not accurate due to the transfer of maternal HIV antibodies to the infant.

The CD4$^+$ T-cell counts in children younger than age 5 are typically higher than adult counts. Pediatric patients with a positive virologic test should have CD4$^+$ T-cell counts and viral loads monitored every 3 to 4 months if not on ART, or more frequently in those initiating or changing ART. CD4$^+$ counts can be monitored every 6 to 12 months in children who have demonstrated treatment adherence, sustained virologic suppression, stable clinical status, and high CD4$^+$ counts for at least 2 to 3 years. Similarly, because of immunologic differences, particularly in those patients acquiring the disease perinatally, viral loads may be difficult to interpret during the first year of life. Using CD4$^+$ T-cell count and viral load together can more accurately predict prognosis and survival.

Pharmacokinetic variables, particularly volume of distribution and clearance, change as a person ages. These changes should be considered when designing drug therapy regimens for children and adolescents. Similarly, the issue of medication adherence in this population is crucial, and concerns vary across the span of childhood through adolescence. Some of the solution formulations for these agents may be unpalatable, depending on the child's preferences. Also, absorption of drugs can be affected by food, and the timing of drug administration around food schedules can be extremely difficult. Mixing medications in bottles with formula may increase palatability but may create compatibility issues. Additionally, children depend upon their caregivers to administer ART; therefore, the complexity and convenience of the regimen must be considered. It is preferable for an HIV expert to manage these patients to select optimal treatment and monitor short- and long-term adverse effects and quality of life.

Women/Pregnancy

Thresholds for the initiation of ART in HIV-infected women are the same as those for HIV-infected men. Selection of antiretrovirals in women of childbearing potential should reflect regimen efficacy as well as its potential for teratogenicity if the woman becomes pregnant. For example, dolutegravir is an alternative agent for women trying to conceive but is a preferred agent throughout pregnancy. It is also important to note that the efficacy of many oral contraceptives is reduced by ART.

When considering the use of ART in pregnant women with HIV infection, practitioners must consider two main issues: ART of HIV in the mother and prophylaxis to reduce the risk of perinatal HIV infection (Panel on Treatment of HIV-Infected Pregnant Women and Prevention of Perinatal Transmission, 2020). The safety and efficacy of ART regimens must be assessed prior to initiating therapy in a pregnant patient as well as special considerations for dosing, adverse effects, and other medication counseling points.

The acquisition of disease through exposure in utero is a major source of HIV infection in infants. Therefore, early identification of HIV-infected women is crucial before or during pregnancy. Preconception HIV prevention counseling and testing for all pregnant women have been advocated by national organizations, including the American College of Obstetricians and Gynecologists and the CDC. All pregnant women should be tested for HIV infection as early as possible, and repeat testing should be performed in those at high risk of acquiring the infection.

One of the more remarkable aspects of zidovudine therapy was the discovery that this agent reduced the maternal–fetal transmission of HIV. The pivotal study by Connor and colleagues showed a maternal–fetal transmission rate of 8.3% with zidovudine versus 25.5% with placebo in expectant mothers between 14 and 34 weeks of gestation (Connor et al., 1994). Therefore, antiretroviral chemoprophylaxis with IV zidovudine during labor is recommended for all pregnant women with viral loads greater than 1,000 copies/mL or unknown viral loads at the time of delivery. This is not required for women adherent to ART whose viral loads have remained consistently below 1,000 copies/mL during late pregnancy and delivery. Postnatally, the infant should receive oral chemoprophylaxis in an effort to reduce perinatal transmission. Additionally, breast-feeding is not recommended for any HIV-positive woman in the United States, regardless of ART regimen.

Health Care Workers/Occupational Exposure

The primary means of transmission of HIV in the health care worker population is through an accidental needlestick. However, transmission can occur through the exposure of HIV-infected blood or other infected body fluids to a health care worker's nonintact skin or mucous membranes. The risk of HIV transmission after a percutaneous exposure to infected blood is approximately 0.3%; the risk decreases to approximately 0.09% for a mucous membrane exposure.

In theory, initiation of antiretroviral postexposure prophylaxis (PEP) within 1 to 2 hours after exposure may prevent or inhibit systemic infection by limiting the replication of the virus in the lymphocytes and lymph nodes. As such, the U.S. Public Health Service has published recommendations regarding the initiation and continuation of PEP in health care personnel (Kuhar et al., 2013). The primary role of PEP is to prevent HIV infection after accidental occupational exposure.

Current guidelines recommend a preferred PEP regimen of TDF/emtricitabine plus raltegravir, due to its potency, tolerability, dosing convenience, and minimal drug interactions. Alternative regimens are listed in **Table 47.4**; these can be considered if there are contraindications, cost concerns, or intolerability with the preferred regimen. PEP should be initiated as soon as possible after exposure while awaiting results of source identification, resistance profile, or both. Therapy should be continued for 28 days and should only be discontinued early if the source patient is proven to be HIV negative, if the exposed health care worker is shown to be HIV positive, if the adverse

TABLE 47.4	
Alternative Human Immunodeficiency Virus Postexposure Prophylaxis for Occupational Exposure	
Column A	**Column B**
Atazanavir 300 mg PO daily + ritonavir 100 mg PO daily	TDF/emtricitabine tablet PO daily
Darunavir 800 mg PO daily + ritonavir 100 mg PO daily	TDF 300 mg PO daily + lamivudine 300 mg PO daily
Etravirine 200 mg PO BID	Zidovudine/lamivudine tablet PO BID
Lopinavir/ritonavir 2 tablets PO BID	Zidovudine 300 mg PO BID + emtricitabine 200 mg PO daily
Raltegravir 400 mg PO BID	
Rilpivirine 25 mg PO daily	

Preferred regimen: Tenofovir/emtricitabine tablet PO daily PLUS raltegravir 400 mg PO BID.

Alternative regimen: Choose one drug or drug pair from Column A and one drug or drug pair from Column B. May also use elvitegravir/cobicistat/tenofovir/emtricitabine (Stribild) PO daily.

Adapted from Kuhar, D. T., Henderson, D. K., Struble, K. A., et al. (2013). Updated U.S. public health service guidelines for the management of occupational exposures to HIV and recommendations for postexposure prophylaxis. *Infection Control and Hospital Epidemiology, 34,* 875–892. Courtesy of JSTOR. Retrieved from http://nccc.ucsf.edu/wp-content/uploads/2014/03/Updated_USPHS_Guidelines_Mgmt_Occupational_Exposures_HIV_Recommendations_PEP.pdf

TDF, tenofovir disoproxil fumarate.

effects of PEP are intolerable and there is no other alternative available, or if the exposed health care worker decides to discontinue treatment based on risks and benefits. HIV antibody testing should be performed at baseline, 6 weeks, 12 weeks, and 6 months after exposure. If a fourth-generation combination HIV antigen/antibody test is used, the final test can be completed at 4 months. Extended follow-up (e.g., at 12 months) is recommended for health care workers who become infected with hepatitis C virus following exposure to a coinfected patient.

Nonoccupational Postexposure Prophylaxis

Use of ART within 72 hours of exposure to HIV outside of the workplace, such as through sexual assault, unprotected sexual intercourse, and sharing needles during injection drug use, is a method that has never been studied in clinical trials but is employed to prevent HIV infection. Each case should be considered individually, to assess if the source is HIV negative (nonoccupational postexposure prophylaxis [nPEP] not recommended), unknown (consider nPEP), or HIV positive (nPEP recommended). As with occupational PEP, the preferred regimen is TDF/emtricitabine plus raltegravir or dolutegravir for 28 days. Use of dolutegravir as a component of nPEP should be avoided in non-pregnant women of child-bearing potential who have been sexually active or assaulted and are not utilizing an effective method of contraception as well as women in early pregnancy, due to the risk of development of neural tube defects in the unborn infant.

Preexposure Prophylaxis

Use of daily PrEP with tenofovir/emtricitabine in sexually active adults at risk of becoming infected with HIV has helped to decrease transmission. One of the largest clinical trials assessing the efficacy of this approach, known as the Preexposure Prophylaxis Initiative (iPrEX) study, demonstrated a 44% relative risk reduction in HIV infection incidence in HIV-negative men who have sex with men (Grant et al., 2010). Studies in heterosexual populations also show that this strategy is effective in reducing the incidence of HIV infection. The decision to use PrEP must be considered carefully. Since the effectiveness of the regimen is linked with adherence, it is crucial to emphasize the importance of taking the regimen every day, not just on days when sexual intercourse would occur. Intermittent regimens are being studied but are not currently recommended in the guidelines. Per recommendations from the U.S. Public Health Service, individuals must test negative for HIV infection within 1 week of PrEP initiation and every 3 months during treatment, to prevent the development of resistance in the presence of HIV infection (U.S. Public Health Service, 2017). Additionally, patients should receive safer sexual practice counseling at each visit, to further reduce the risk of transmission. No more than a 90-day supply of PrEP should be prescribed, and patients should be seen every 3 months for lab work and adherence assessments. The current guidelines only recommend TDF/emtricitabine (Truvada) for use as PrEP; however, TAF/emtricitabine (Descovy) received FDA approval for this indication in late 2019, with the exception of use in receptive vaginal intercourse.

MONITORING PATIENT RESPONSE

The CD4$^+$ T-cell counts are important not only because they indicate the risk of development of opportunistic infections before treatment but also because they help the health care provider initiate or discontinue opportunistic infection prophylaxis during ART. Once ART is started, a CD4$^+$ count should be checked at baseline and after 3 months to assess reconstitution of the immune system. It is important to check CD4$^+$ counts every 3 to 6 months to assess response to ART during the first 2 years of treatment and to determine the necessity of opportunistic infection prophylaxis. CD4$^+$ counts may be obtained once yearly in those individuals who are receiving suppressive ART and have CD4$^+$ counts well above the threshold for risk of opportunistic infections, consistently ranging between 300 and 500 cells/mL. More frequent monitoring would be required in patients with changes in clinical status, those who are unable to achieve virologic suppression on ART, or in those initiating treatment with interferon, steroids, or cancer chemotherapeutic agents. CD4$^+$ count monitoring is optional for those patients with CD4$^+$ counts above 500 cells/mm^3 after 2 years on suppressive ART.

Viral load indicates both initial and sustained responses to treatment with ART, and decreases in viral load correlate with decreased risk of progression to AIDS and death. Viral load should be measured at baseline for all patients, to permit appropriate ART selection. Once therapy has been initiated or changed,

viral load should be assessed immediately before treatment and again 2 to 8 weeks later. The viral load should be repeated every 4 to 8 weeks until it is less than 200 copies/mL. Subsequent testing should reveal an undetectable viral load by 8 to 12 weeks in those patients adherent to ART. At that point, viral load testing should be repeated every 3 to 4 months to determine continuing effectiveness of the regimen. This duration can be extended to 6 months in those patients who are immunologically stable and have fully suppressed viral loads for at least 2 years. If a patient exhibits a suboptimal response, it is important to review medication adherence, drug interactions, and resistance mutations to permit consideration of regimen changes.

Genotypic resistance testing is recommended for all patients at baseline, regardless of when treatment is initiated, to optimize regimen selection by determining which drugs still retain activity. It is also useful for patients with suboptimal viral load reduction and virologic failure. Resistance testing is not recommended for patients with viral loads of fewer than 500 copies/mL because the assays cannot consistently determine resistance patterns with such low-level viremia. Recommendations for genotypic resistance testing in pregnant patients include baseline testing prior to therapy as well as testing those with detectable viral loads while taking ART.

PATIENT EDUCATION

To minimize the likelihood of treatment regimen failure and development of drug resistance, the health care professional must be aware of who is at high risk for adherence issues as well as the most common reasons for poor adherence. Risk factors for poor adherence to antiretroviral regimens include active substance abuse, active mental illness, lack of disease and medication education, low levels of literacy, and stigma. Several treatment factors affect adherence, such as pill burden, frequency of dosing, food requirements, adverse effects, and treatment fatigue.

Strategies the practitioner can use to minimize the risk of failure due to nonadherence include encouraging the patient to develop a strong relationship with the health care team, taking an active role in his or her therapy, and involving the patient's family, friends, and peers in the therapy. In addition, counseling on HIV and the goals of achieving viral suppression (e.g., reduction in HIV-related morbidity and mortality, prevention of sexual transmission) may encourage an otherwise indifferent patient to adhere to a regimen.

Another strategy the practitioner should use to promote drug adherence is preparing the patient for adverse events. The patient needs to know which adverse events are likely to occur, how to minimize the risk of experiencing adverse events, and which adverse events demand discontinuation of therapy. The patient also needs to understand the importance of following the dosing schedule in addition to the food requirements for each agent (Panel, 2019). **Table 47.1** provides information on dosing, diet, and fluid requirements of each agent.

Developing a plan for scheduling medications and carefully explaining to the patient how the medication should be taken is imperative. This plan should focus on daily pill taking as well as future events in a patient's life that threaten to interrupt the established schedule (e.g., holidays or vacations). This plan must consider lifestyle factors such as work schedule and privacy issues (e.g., taking medication at work or storage of medication at work). Regardless of how much or little assistance the patient needs in developing strategies for ensuring adherence, success is often determined by the patient's outlook. If the patient perceives that therapy will lead to an improved quality of life or increased length of life, chances for adherence are greater (Reynolds, 1998). Therefore, before attacking the logistics of a medication schedule, the health care provider must convince the patient of the benefits of continuing therapy.

Once the daily plan is developed, it should evolve into a long-term plan that allows the patient to adhere to therapy and allows the health care provider to monitor adherence. Aids for adherence include pill boxes that separate doses per day, alarms to remind patients of their doses, or something as simple as a calendar that lists dosing schedules. Whatever method is used, the patient must remain adherent and be checked for adherence. The simplest way to check for adherence is to ask the patient. However, a patient may not confess to missed doses or may not be aware of missed doses. Pill counting is another option, but patients may remove missed doses to appear adherent. Testing the viral load may reveal adherence information, but if levels increase because of resistance, not nonadherence, the results will be misleading. Adherence counseling and effective engagement and retention in care are all closely linked to improving treatment success.

CASE STUDY 1

Anna is a 36-year-old woman who was diagnosed with human immunodeficiency virus (HIV) infection 2 days ago at a community outreach clinic. She has been feeling well for the past 2 years, and she maintains a healthy, active lifestyle by exercising three to four times a week and eating a balanced diet. Her medications include a multivitamin and occasional antacids for heartburn, and she does not consistently use birth control methods. She has never received antiretroviral therapy (ART). She comes to your office for an initial physical exam and blood work in preparation for treatment initiation. The physical examination is unremarkable, and the laboratory results are as follows:

Electrolytes, serum creatinine, liver function tests: within normal limits.

Complete blood count with differential: within normal limits.

CD4$^+$ T-cell count: 400 cells/mm^3.

Viral load: 110,000 copies/mL.

Genotype: no resistance mutations detected.

(Learning Objective 2)

1. List specific goals for treatment for this patient.
2. Describe the rationale behind the drug therapy would you prescribe for Anna.
3. What are the parameters for monitoring safety and effectiveness of Anna's ART?

Bibliography

Starred references are cited in the text.

*Centers for Disease Control and Prevention. (2014). Revised surveillance case definition for HIV infection- United States, 2014. *Morbidity and Mortality Weekly Report, 63*(3), 1–10.

*Centers for Disease Control and Prevention. (2017). Diagnoses of HIV infection in the United States and dependent areas. 2016 *HIV Surveillance Report, 28.* [Online]. Retrieved from https://www.cdc.gov/hiv/pdf/library/reports/surveillance/cdc-hiv-surveillance-report-2016-vol-28.pdf

*Connor, E. M., Sperling, R. S., Gelber, R., et al. (1994). Reduction of maternal-infant transmission of human immunodeficiency virus type 1 with zidovudine treatment: Pediatric AIDS Clinical Trials Group Protocol 076 Study Group. *New England Journal of Medicine, 331*, 1173–1180.

*Grant, R. M., Lama, J. R., Anderson, P. L., et al. (2010). Preexposure chemoprophylaxis for HIV prevention in men who have sex with men. *New England Journal of Medicine, 363*, 2587–2599.

*Kuhar, D. T., Henderson, D. K., Struble, K. A., et al. (2013). Updated U.S. public health service guidelines for the management of occupational exposures to HIV and recommendations for postexposure prophylaxis. *Infection Control and Hospital Epidemiology, 34*, 875–892.

Lacy, C. F., Armstrong, L. L., Goldman, M. P., et al. (2020). *Adult drug information handbook* (29th ed.). Hudson, OH: Lexi-Comp.

Olin, J. L., Klibanov, O., Chan, A., et al. (2019). Managing pharmacotherapy in people living with HIV and concomitant malignancy. *Annals of Pharmacotherapy, 53*, 812–832.

*Panel on Antiretroviral Guidelines for Adults and Adolescents. (2019). Guidelines for the use of antiretroviral agents in adults and adolescents with HIV. Department of Health and Human Services [Online]. Retrieved from http://www.aidsinfo.nih.gov/ContentFiles/AdultandAdolescentGL.pdf

*Panel on Antiretroviral Therapy and Medical Management of Children Living with HIV. (2020). Guidelines for the use of antiretroviral agents in pediatric HIV infection. HHS Panel on Antiretroviral Therapy and Medical Management of Children Living with HIV—A Working Group of the Office of AIDS Research Advisory Council (OARAC). Retrieved from http://aidsinfo.nih.gov/contentfiles/lvguidelines/pediatricguidelines.pdf

*Panel on Treatment of Pregnant Women with HIV Infection and Prevention of Perinatal Transmission. (2020). Recommendations for use of antiretroviral drugs in pregnant women with HIV infection and interventions to reduce perinatal HIV transmission in the United States. [Online]. Retrieved from http://www.aidsinfo.nih.gov/ContentFiles/lvguidelines/PerinatalGL.pdf

*Reynolds, N. R. (1998). Initiatives to get HIV-infected patients to adhere to their treatment regimens. *Drug Benefit, 10*(11), 23–25, 29–30, 32.

Saag, M. S., Gandhi, R. T., Hoy, J. F., et al. (2020). Antiretroviral drugs for treatment and prevention of HIV infection in adults: 2020 Recommendations of the International Antiviral Society–USA Panel. *Journal of the American Medical Association, 324*(16), 1651–1669.

*U.S. Public Health Service. (2017). *Preexposure prophylaxis for the prevention of HIV infection in the United States–2017 Update.* [Online]. Retrieved from http://www.cdc.gov/hiv/pdf/risk/prep/cdc-hiv-prep-guidelines-2017.pdf

*World Health Organization (WHO). (2018). *HIV/AIDS: Data and statistics* [Online]. Retrieved from http://www.who.int/hiv/data/en

48

Organ Transplantation

David M. Salerno

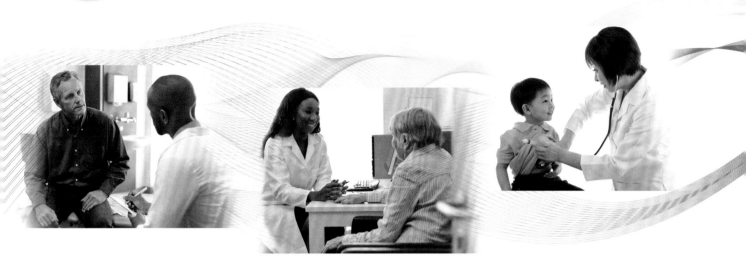

Learning Objectives

1. Describe the immune response in organ transplantation and the specific targeted pathways for T-cell inhibition.
2. Identify the role of induction and maintenance therapy in solid organ transplantation.
3. List drug interactions and side effects associated with immunosuppressive medications.

INTRODUCTION

Organ transplantation is a life-saving intervention for patients with end-stage organ disease. Each year, there are more than 100,000 patients in the United States who are in need of an organ transplant. According to the United Network for Organ Sharing, there were fewer than 40,000 solid organ transplants performed in 2018, primarily due to shortage of deceased donor organs (OPTN/SRTR, 2020). Currently, patients can receive various types of solid organ transplants, including kidney, pancreas, liver, intestine, heart, lung or vascular allografts, or a combination of multiple-organ transplants. Transplanted organs between genetically diverse individuals of the same species are referred to as *allogenic grafts* or *allografts*. Immunosuppressive medications are required to maintain long-term allografts and patient survival to combat the fundamental function of the immune system of distinguishing self from nonself.

PATHOPHYSIOLOGY

The immune system is primarily responsible for defense against infections and cancer. The immune response to an organ allograft can be divided into three phases: recognition of foreign antigens, activation of antigen-specific lymphocytes, and the effector phase of graft rejection.

Recognition of Foreign Antigens

The ability of the immune system to reject an allograft is derived from genes located on chromosome 6, termed the *major histocompatibility complex* (MHC). The MHC encodes a group of diverse cell surface proteins commonly referred to as *antigens*. The initiation of organ transplant rejection is due to MHC and peptide complexes from the donor being recognized by T-cell receptor (TCR) present on the recipient T cells. In humans, the MHC genes are called *human leukocyte antigen* (HLA). HLA is divided into two different types: class I and class II genes, which are the basis for the formation of antigens. HLA loci are highly polymorphic, which allows for T cells to easily distinguish self from nonself. The degree of HLA matching between a donor allograft and a recipient is a risk factor for rejection; the magnitude is determined based upon the organ allograft being transplanted. The relative immunogenicity, or ability of an allograft to induce an immune response, also varies per organ.

Activation of Antigen-Specific Lymphocytes

Recipient T cells are able to recognize an allograft in two distinct manners: through direct or indirect antigen presentation. Direct antigen presentation is a response of recipient T cells to donor-derived antigen-presenting cells (APC) that are from an allograft. In this case, the recipient T cells can detect allogenic MHC molecules on the surface of the APCs and become activated. Conversely, for indirect antigen presentation, recipient T cells recognize allopeptides that are derived from the donor but are presented from recipient APCs. The mechanism

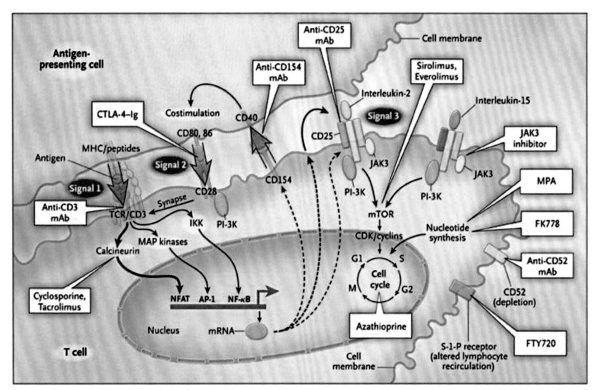

FIGURE 48-1   Mechanisms of T-cell activation. Note, Anti-CD154 antibody, FTY720, and FK778 have been withdrawn from clinical trials. (Used with permission from Danovitch, G. M. [2017]. *Handbook of kidney transplantation* [6th ed.]. Philadelphia, PA: Wolters Kluwer.)

MAP, Mitogen-activated protein kinase; MHC, major histocompatibility complex; MPA, mycophenolic acid; mTOR, mammalian target of rapamycin; NFAT, nuclear factor of activated T cells; TCR, T-cell receptor.

by which APCs can activate T cells has been described in the three-signal model of T-cell activation and proliferation by Halloran (2004) (**Figure 48.1**).

Briefly, signal 1 involves APCs recognizing a foreign substance and presenting the peptide on its MHC for a T cell to recognize with a TCR. This binding of the MHC/peptide to the TCR causes an influx of calcium and activates calcineurin as part of a complex to dephosphorylate nuclear factor of activated T cells (NFAT), which can translocate to the nucleus and act as a transcription factor to promote the production of interleukin-2 (IL-2). Signal 2 is termed a *costimulation event.* The goal of this pathway is to enhance signal 1. The CD80/86 receptor on the APC binds to the T cell at CD28 receptor, and this causes an upregulation of signal 1 to promote IL-2 formation. IL-2 is utilized to upregulate and directly activate neighboring T cells through the CD25 receptor, which is signal 3. Signal 3 works through the mammalian target of the rapamycin (mTOR) pathway to cause T-cell proliferation through the cell cycle. The three-signal model is the basis for understanding the specific targets of each class of immunosuppressive agents.

Effector Phase of Graft Rejection

Once a T cell becomes activated through either direct or indirect antigen recognition, it can cause direct destruction to the allograft either by release of cytotoxic factors or by potentiating

a cascade for cell death. T cells can also activate B cells, which proliferate and differentiate into plasma cells. Plasma cells release antibodies that can cause additional cell damage by fixing complement to cause destruction.

DIAGNOSTIC CRITERIA

Symptoms of Rejection

Symptoms of organ transplant rejection vary by organ. Kidney and liver transplant recipients may not experience any symptoms at all other than derangements in serum creatinine or liver function tests, respectively. In some cases, patients may experience pain over the graft site. For patients with heart or lung transplantation, symptoms of rejection might manifest as symptoms of end-stage organ dysfunction, such as swelling, trouble breathing, hypoxemia, and shock.

Biopsy is the gold standard for each organ discipline to make a diagnosis of rejection. Biopsy findings are beyond the scope and focus of this chapter, but the classification can range from mild to moderate to severe cases of rejection. Each transplant center develops protocols that specify either protocol-based biopsies at specific milestones post-transplant versus only biopsying patients who are experiencing signs and symptoms of rejection.

INITIATING DRUG THERAPY

Goals of Drug Therapy

The goals of immunosuppressive therapy are to mitigate the risk of rejection while balancing the risks of infection and adverse drug events. Many transplant centers utilize specific protocols for immunosuppression in the perioperative and postoperative periods; however, immunosuppression goals need to be patient specific. To prevent allograft rejection, immunosuppressive medications are divided into induction therapy and maintenance therapy. Induction therapy is potent immunosuppression utilized within the perioperative period (in the operating room and for the first several days thereafter) to prevent early acute T-cell-mediated rejection of the allograft. Maintenance therapy is the lifelong immunosuppression provided to the patient to prevent long-term rejection of the organ. Patients must stay on immunosuppressive medications lifelong to prevent rejection.

Drug Class: Lymphocyte-Depleting Agents

Lymphocyte-depleting therapy consists of either monoclonal or polyclonal antibodies that are targeted for a variety of T-cell surface receptors. Antibody-dependent lysis of the T cell ensues upon binding causing destruction of the T cell.

Rabbit-Derived Anti-thymocyte Globulin

Anti-thymocyte globulin is derived from immunizing either horses or rabbits with human lymphoid tissue and then filtering the sera to obtain concentrated gammaglobulin. The efficacy and safety of rabbit anti-thymocyte globulin versus horse anti-thymocyte globulin was compared by Alloway et al. (2019). In kidney transplant recipients, rabbit anti-thymocyte preparation significantly reduced the rate of rejection at one year and increased allograft survival when compared to the horse-derived product. Additionally, there is a risk of allergic reaction to either preparation, but the risk is significantly higher with the horse-derived product. As such, rabbit-anti-thymocyte globulin (rATG) is the preferred product. Patients receiving rATG for the first time should be screened for rabbit protein allergies prior to the administration of the first dose.

Mechanism of Action

Cytotoxic antibodies directed against T-cell markers cause a depletion of peripheral blood lymphocytes through lysis and disposal through the reticuloendothelial system.

Dosage

The usual dose for induction immunosuppressive therapy is 1.5 mg/kg given via intravenous infusion over 6 to 10 hours for 4 to 7 days in duration. The dose is rounded to the nearest 25 mg, per vial size. The maximum daily dose is 150 mg/d. Typically, the first dose is given intraoperatively. To avoid thrombophlebitis, anti-thymocyte globulin can be given through a central vein or through a peripheral vein with the addition of hydrocortisone sodium succinate 20 mg and heparin 1,000 units to the infusion solution. For patients with a history of heparin-induced thrombocytopenia, heparin can be removed from the bag without resultant adverse drug sequelae. Premedications with acetaminophen 650 mg IV/PO, diphenhydramine 25 to 50 mg IV/PO, and methylprednisolone 1 mg/kg or equivalent should be given 30 minutes prior to infusion. As needed, medications including supplemental doses of acetaminophen and diphenhydramine should be made available. Vital signs should be monitored every 15 minutes during the first hour of infusion and then hourly until the infusion is complete.

Time Frame for Response

Anti-thymocyte globulin depletes peripheral lymphocytes immediately. Prolonged lymphopenia may last between 6 and 12 months.

Contraindications

rATG is contraindicated in patients with severe rabbit protein allergy.

Adverse Events

Fever, chills, and arthralgias are the most common reactions seen with the administration of thymoglobulin, necessitating the use of premedications. The infusion rate should be slowed in patients who have these symptoms or develop tachycardia during the infusion. Infrequently, flash pulmonary edema and serum sickness have been reported. Thymogloblin is associated with thrombocytopenia and leukopenia. The dose of thymoglobulin should be decreased by 50% in patients with a platelet count of 50,000 to 100,000 cells/mL or a white blood cell count of 2,000 to 3,000 cells/mL. Administration of thymoglobulin should be discontinued in patients with a platelet count of less than 50,000 cells/mL or white blood cell count of less than 2,000 cells/mL.

Interactions

No specific pharmacokinetic drug interactions are known.

Alemtuzumab

Alemtuzumab is a recombinant deoxyribonucleic acid (DNA)–derived humanized anti-CD52 monoclonal antibody. It has been used as an induction agent and for the treatment of organ transplant rejection although it does not have an Food and Drug Administration (FDA)–labeled indication for use. It has not undergone extensive comparison with thymoglobulin.

Mechanism of Action

Alemtuzumab is an antibody directed against the glycoprotein CD52. CD52 is highly expressed on peripheral T and B cells.

Dosage

The dose is 30 mg as either an intravenous infusion over 6 hours or subcutaneous administration. Premedications with acetaminophen 650 mg IV/PO, diphenhydramine 25 to 50 mg IV/PO, and methylprednisolone 1 mg/kg or equivalent should be given 30 minutes prior to administration.

Time Frame for Response

Peripheral lymphocytes undergo lysis within 1 hour of administration. Although the half-life of this monoclonal antibody is 12 days, the therapeutic effect of T-cell depletion can last for months to years.

Contraindications

No contraindications are listed in the product labeling.

Adverse Events

Alemtuzumab can cause infusion reactions including fever, chills, and hypotension. The use of premedications is necessary to mitigate this risk. Additionally, alemtuzumab is associated with neutropenia and thrombocytopenia. Secondary to the profound and prolonged depletion of lymphocytes, patients are also at risk for viral infections including cytomegalovirus and herpes viruses as well as other infections.

Interactions

No drug interactions are listed in the product labeling.

Drug Class: Non-lymphocyte-Depleting Basiliximab

Basiliximab is a monoclonal antibody that is directed against the IL-2 receptor, also known as CD25. CD25 is found on the surface of activated T cells. Basiliximab is approved for use in kidney transplant recipients as induction therapy. It is routinely used off-label as induction therapy in liver, heart, and lung transplant recipients. Non-lymphocyte-depleting agents are generally considered to be less immunosuppressive than lymphocyte-depleting agents. In patients at high risk for rejection, lymphocyte-depleting agents are preferred to decrease the risk of rejection and graft loss but careful attention must be paid to balance the lower risk of rejection but higher risk of infection.

Mechanism of Action

Basiliximab binds the IL-2 receptor decreasing the affinity of IL-2 to its receptor. This competitive inhibition leads to blocking signal 3 of the T-cell activation pathway. Through this mechanism, it does not cause T-cell lysis.

Dosage

Basiliximab is given as a 20 mg infusion over 30 minutes on postoperative day 0 and postoperative day 4.

Time Frame for Response

The half-life is 7 days, and the therapeutic effect on the IL-2 receptor persists for up to 3 to 4 weeks.

Contraindications

Basiliximab is contraindicated in patients with known hypersensitivity to basiliximab or any other component of the formulation.

Adverse Events

Randomized clinical trials showed no difference in the reported side effects between basiliximab and placebo.

Interactions

No drug interactions are listed in the product labeling.

Drug Class: Calcineurin Inhibitors

Calcineurin inhibitors (CNI), cyclosporine and tacrolimus, have been considered the backbone of maintenance immunosuppressive regimens for the last several decades. Calcineurin is a calcium-dependent protein phosphatase that forms a complex with several other proteins in response to an APC binding to a T cell. This complex dephosphorylates the transcription factor, NFAT, which upregulates key mediators involved in T-cell activation. Although both agents act by inhibiting calcineurin and ultimately the expression of several cytokine genes that promote T-cell activation, each agent is biochemically different and achieves the inhibition of the calcineurin complex in two distinct manners. The nuances between the agents are discussed in **Table 48.1**, which also explains the differences in side effect profiles.

Cyclosporine

Cyclosporine is a lipophilic polypeptide that was isolated from the fungus *Tolypocladium inflatum* and approved for use in organ transplant recipients in 1978. Cyclosporine changed the field of organ transplantation since it was responsible for significant improvements in allograft survival.

Mechanism of Action

Cyclosporine achieves signal 1 inhibition by binding to cyclophilin, preventing the formation of the calcineurin complex. This inhibition of calcineurin prevents T-cell proliferation.

Dosage

Cyclosporine is available in two distinct formulations: non-modified and modified cyclosporine. The initial non-modified version is available as Sandimmune®, which is poorly absorbed and requires the presence of bile for absorption. Neoral® is a micro-emulsified capsule that has significantly improved bioavailability. This modified version is the preferred product for patients newly started on cyclosporine. Typical starting doses of cyclosporine range from 3 to 6 mg/kg/day in divided doses every 12 hours. Dosing is then titrated to maintain serum trough concentrations between 200 and 350 ng/mL, contingent upon the duration from transplant.

Time Frame for Response

Non-modified cyclosporine has a peak serum concentration in 2 to 6 hours after administration and modified cyclosporine peaks in 1.5 to 2 hours after oral administration.

Contraindications

Intravenous cyclosporine is contraindicated in patients with a hypersensitivity to polyoxyethylated castor oil (Cremophor EL).

TABLE 48.1

Comparison of Cyclosporine and Tacrolimus

Feature	Cyclosporine	Tacrolimus
Mechanism to inhibit calcineurin	Inhibition of cyclophilin	Inhibition of FK-binding protein
Daily oral maintenance dose	3–6 mg/kg	0.1 mg/kg
IV: PO conversion ratio	1:3	1:5
Routes of administration	PO and IV	PO, sublingual, and IV
Metabolism	CYP3A4/5	CYP3A4/5
Interactions	Inhibits CYP 2C9 (weak), CYP 3A4 (weak), P-glycoprotein	Inhibits P-glycoprotein
Side effects		
Alopecia	N/A	+
Gingival hyperplasia	+	N/A
Hirsutism	+	N/A
Hyperglycemia/new-onset diabetes after transplant	+	++
Hyperkalemia	+	+
Hyperlipidemia	++	+
Hypomagnesemia	+	+
Hypertension	++	+
Hyperuricemia	++	+
Nephrotoxicity	+	+
Neurotoxicity	+	++

+, Known effect.

++, Effect more pronounced.

Adapted from Danovitch, G. M. (2009). *Handbook of kidney transplantation* (5th ed.). Philadelphia, PA: Lippincott Williams & Wilkins.

Adverse Events

Side effects of cyclosporine include nephrotoxicity, neurotoxicity, hypertension, hyperlipidemia, gingival hyperplasia, and hirsutism (**Table 48.1**). The mechanism of CNI-induced nephrotoxicity includes both an acute and chronic component. CNIs cause a reversible afferent arterial vasoconstriction as well as activation of the renin-angiotensin system. The chronic form of CNI nephrotoxicity includes hyaline thickening in the afferent arterioles as well as interstitial fibrosis. Nephrotoxicity can be treated with either a dose reduction or discontinuation of the CNI. Neurotoxicity from CNIs can range on a spectrum from headaches, tremors, confusion, agitation, dysarthria, seizures, and posterior reversible encephalopathy syndrome. Neurotoxicity is more frequent with tacrolimus compared to cyclosporine. Symptoms can often be improved with a dose reduction or dose discontinuation. Other potential side effects include new-onset diabetes after transplant, hypertension, hyperlipidemia, and hyperkalemia.

Interactions

Cyclosporine is a substrate of cytochrome P450 3A4 and a P-glycoprotein. Medications that inhibit cytochrome P450 and therefore raise the serum concentration of cyclosporine include azole antifungals such as fluconazole and voriconazole, macrolides such as erythromycin and clarithromycin, calcium channel blockers such as diltiazem and verapamil, and protease inhibitors for both human immunodeficiency virus and hepatitis C virus such as ritonavir. In addition, several foods including grapefruit, pomegranate, and star fruit should be avoided in patients receiving cyclosporine due to enzyme inhibition.

Conversely, medications that induce cytochrome P450 enzymes and therefore decrease the serum concentration of cyclosporine include antituberculosis medications rifampin and rifabutin, antiepileptic medications including phenobarbital and phenytoin. A more complete list of drug interactions is listed in **Box 48.1**. Additionally, cyclosporine is a moderate inhibitor of cytochrome P450 3A4 and can be considered both the perpetrator and victim drug in an interaction. Care should be taken when introducing a new drug onto the medication profile for an organ transplant recipient. Patients should be counseled to call their transplant team when starting any new prescription or over-the-counter medications to mitigate unknown drug interactions in patients seeing multiple providers.

Additionally, there are several pharmacodynamic interactions that should be avoided. Non-steroid antiinflammatory drugs have similar adverse effects on the kidney including afferent arteriole vasoconstriction and should not be used concomitantly with CNIs. Conversely, angiotensin-converting enzyme inhibitors (ACEi) dilate the efferent arteriole, which, in combination with afferent arteriole vasoconstriction from CNIs, can cause acute kidney injury. Furthermore, medications that

BOX 48.1   Inducers and Inhibitors of Cytochrome P450 3A4

STRONG INDUCERS

Carbamazepine
Phenobarbital
Phenytoin
Primidone
Rifampin
St. John's Wort

MODERATE INHIBITORS

Clotrimazole
Diltiazem
Erythromycin
Fluconazole
Verapamil

STRONG INHIBITORS

Atazanavir
Clarithromycin
Cobicistat
Darunavir
Fosamprenavir
Indinavir
Itraconazole
Letermovir
Lopinavir
Nelfinavir
Posaconazole
Ritonavir
Saquinavir
Tipranavir
Voriconazole

are associated with hyperkalemia (ACEi, angiotensin II receptor blockers, spironolactone) may compound toxicity and should be avoided.

Tacrolimus

Tacrolimus is a macrolide that was isolated from the bacterium *Streptomyces tsukubaensis*. The efficacy and safety of tacrolimus was demonstrated in a 1994 landmark trial, which compared the outcomes in patients receiving tacrolimus versus cyclosporine in liver transplant recipients. Although graft and patient survival were similar between the two groups, tacrolimus was associated with significantly fewer episodes of acute cellular rejection. Tacrolimus has become the backbone of the immunosuppressive regimen in all disciplines of solid organ transplant.

Mechanism of Action

Tacrolimus prevents signal 1 of the three-signal model for T-cell activation. It interferes with FK506-binding protein, which prevents the formation of the calcineurin complex. This decreases the production of IL-2 and subsequently prevents T-cell proliferation.

Dosage

Tacrolimus is 40 to 50 times more potent than cyclosporine. The starting dose is 0.05 to 0.1 mg/kg by mouth divided twice a day. Tacrolimus dose is titrated to maintain serum trough concentrations between 8 and 15 ng/mL within the first three months after transplant. Trough concentration targets vary based on the organ transplanted as well as the individual patient goals. Trough concentrations should be checked after the patient has reached steady state pharmacokinetics, which requires the same dose for 3 to 5 half-lives. Trough concentrations are checked 30 minutes prior to the next dose after the patient has received 3 to 5 doses spaced 12 hours apart.

Two once-daily formulations of tacrolimus are approved for use in organ transplantation. Astagraf XL® was approved in 2014 and is indicated for prophylaxis of organ rejection in kidney transplant recipients. This extended-release version is not interchangeable with immediate-release tacrolimus due to its significantly different pharmacokinetic profile, although the conversion ratio is 1:1 of the total daily dose of tacrolimus. This formulation contains the addition of ethylcellulose to decrease the diffusion rate and prolong the release of tacrolimus. Use of Astagraf XL® has been slow secondary to an FDA-boxed warning citing increased mortality in female liver transplant recipients. Envarsus® utilizes a proprietary technology to improve the solubility of tacrolimus by dispersing tacrolimus in a polymeric matrix. This increases the bioavailability of the product. Envarsus® is not interchangeable with immediate-release tacrolimus. The conversion ratio is 1:0.7 (1 mg of immediate-release tacrolimus to 0.7 mg of Envarsus®). Advantages of Envarsus® include an overall lower peak or maximum concentration while maintaining a similar drug exposure. This results in less neurological toxicity including tremors and headache.

Time Frame for Response

The time to peak drug concentration is 2 to 6 hours post dose.

Contraindications

There are no contraindications to use of tacrolimus other than any known serious hypersensitivity reaction.

Adverse Events

Adverse effects are similar to cyclosporine and are shown in **Table 48.1**. Tacrolimus is more frequently associated with neurotoxicity and new-onset diabetes after transplant when compared to cyclosporine.

Interactions

Tacrolimus is a substrate for cytochrome P450 3A4 and therefore is subject to similar drug interactions as cyclosporine and those listed in **Box 48.1**.

Drug Class: Antimetabolites

Antimetabolites are considered adjunctive therapy in immunosuppressive maintenance regimens and are rarely used alone for maintenance immunosuppression. While azathioprine has been used for nearly 50 years, the advent of mycophenolic acid (MPA) derivatives has continued to decrease the post-transplant rejection rates and is now considered the standard of care in maintenance immunosuppressive regimens when paired with a CNI.

Mycophenolate

Mycophenolate mofetil (MMF) (Cellcept®) and the enteric-coated mycophenolate sodium (Myfortic®) are both esters that are hydrolyzed to the active form MPA.

Mechanism of Action

MPA blocks de novo purine synthesis (guanosine monophosphate) by inhibiting the enzyme inosine monophosphate dehydrogenase (IMPDH). This halts the cell cycle in the S phase specifically in B and T lymphocytes, contributing to overall immunosuppression. Although IMPDH is present in other cell lines, most other cells contain a salvage pathway that has the ability to produce guanosine monophosphate using the enzyme hypoxanthine-guanine phosphoribosyltransferase; thus, the cell cycle is not halted in these cells.

Dosage

MMF is dosed 1 to 3 g by mouth in divided doses twice daily. Mycophenolate sodium is dosed 720 to 2,160 mg in divided doses twice daily.

Time Frame for Response

Peak plasma concentrations of MPA from MMF occur in 1 to 1.5 hours post-administration and 1.5 to 2.75 hours for mycophenolate sodium.

Contraindications

MPA is contraindicated in patients with hypersensitivity to mycophenolate or its derivatives. Cellcept® IV is also contraindicated in patients who are allergic to polysorbate 80 (Tween).

Adverse Events

Gastrointestinal disturbances including nausea, vomiting, diarrhea, abdominal pain, and heartburn are the most common side effects from MPA. Typically, these side effects are dose related and can be reversed by either a dose reduction or giving the same total daily dose divided three or four times daily. If symptoms persist, the patient may be converted to the other formulation. Neutropenia is also a common side effect from MPA. Neutropenia can be treated by either a dose reduction and/or treatment with filgrastim (or equivalent). Mycophenolate products are subject to the FDA Risk Evaluation and Mitigation Strategy program that recommends discontinuing mycophenolate in females at least 6 weeks before pregnancy is attempted. MPA use during pregnancy is associated with a risk of first-trimester pregnancy loss and congenital malformations. Patients who become pregnant while on MPA must be immediately converted to another agent. Women of childbearing age must receive contraceptive counseling and use effective contraception while taking MPA.

Interactions

MPA undergoes metabolism through glucuronidation in the liver to MPA glucuronide, which is an inactive metabolite that is subject to enterohepatic recirculation. Administration of MPA with cyclosporine inhibits enterohepatic recirculation and reduces total MPA exposure. MPA should not be administered with cholestyramine as this can inhibit the absorption of MPA. A theoretical drug interaction with ferrous sulfate exists by blocking the absorption of MPA; however, this has not been shown to be clinically relevant.

Azathioprine

Azathioprine (Imuran®) has been used in organ transplant for over 60 years. It is used as a second-line agent.

Mechanism of Action

Azathioprine is a prodrug that is converted to the active form 6-mercaptopurine. 6-Mercaptopurine decreases the metabolism of purines and produces metabolite nucleotides that are incorporated into DNA chain elongation to arrest the cell cycle in B and T lymphocytes.

Dosage

Starting doses of azathioprine range from 1 to 2 mg/kg given daily by mouth.

Time Frame for Response

Although the time to peak drug concentration is 1 to 2 hours, the time to peak therapeutic effect in T cells is generally considered to take 1 to 3 months.

Contraindications

Azathioprine is contraindicated in patients with hypersensitivity to azathioprine or any component of the formulation.

Adverse Events

Myelosuppression and other cytopenias are the most common side effects of azathioprine in a dose-dependent fashion. Gastrointestinal disturbances, including nausea and vomiting, are also common side effects of azathioprine.

Interactions

Allopurinol inhibits the metabolism of 6-mercaptopurine by inhibiting the enzyme xanthine oxidase. Concomitant therapy of allopurinol with azathioprine requires a 75% reduction in azathioprine daily dosage or should be avoided.

Drug Class: Mammalian Target of Rapamycin Inhibitors

The mTOR pathway is involved in cellular homeostasis, regulating the intracellular and extracellular environment. mTOR coordinates cellular growth and proliferation. Most notably in organ transplantation, mTOR is responsible for the transition of the cell cycle from G1 to S phase in lymphocytes. mTOR inhibitors can be utilized as either adjunctive or the backbone immunosuppressive agent in a maintenance regimen. The specific niche of mTOR inhibitors in organ transplantation is to avoid CNI-induced nephrotoxicity or neurotoxicity, prevent post-transplant cancer recurrence, and potentially reduce chronic conditions related to graft loss in lung and heart transplantation. Given their mechanism of action of inhibition of signal 3, mTOR inhibitors are considered less immunosuppressive than CNIs and are associated with higher rates of organ transplant rejection within the first year after the transplant.

Sirolimus

Sirolimus is a macrolide derived from the bacterium *Streptomyces hygroscopicus*. It is FDA approved only to prevent organ transplant rejection in kidney transplant recipients.

Mechanism of Action

Sirolimus binds with the same immunophillin FKBP-12 as tacrolimus, but this complex instead inhibits mTOR, preventing the progression of the cell cycle from G1 to S phase. Sirolimus is a signal 3 inhibitor, as this pathway is downstream of IL-2 binding of the CD25 receptor described previously.

Dosage

Starting doses of sirolimus are 1 to 2 mg by mouth daily. Doses are titrated to obtain serum trough concentrations between 4 and 10 ng/mL when used alone or 3 to 7 ng/mL in combination with CNIs. Sirolimus has a half-life of 63 hours; therefore, dose adjustments and trough monitoring should occur on weekly basis. Loading doses of mTOR inhibitors are no longer recommended secondary to wound-healing complications, including higher rates of incisional hernia and lymphocele.

Time Frame for Response

Sirolimus achieves peak plasma concentration between 1 and 6 hours after administration. With a long half-life, it takes several days to weeks to achieve therapeutic trough concentrations that have been associated with a reduction in organ transplant rejection.

Contraindications

Sirolimus is contraindicated in patients with hypersensitivity to sirolimus or any component of the formulation.

Adverse Events

Adverse events of mTOR inhibitors are similar and summarized in **Box 48.2**. Hyperlipidemia and hypertriglyceridemia are commonly reported adverse events for patients on mTOR inhibitors. A baseline cholesterol and lipid panel should be obtained prior to the start of mTOR inhibitors. Additionally, patients should not be started on mTOR inhibitors if their serum triglycerides are greater than 350 mg/dL at baseline. Both statin therapy and agents to lower triglycerides may be needed concomitantly with mTOR inhibitors to maintain acceptable lipid concentrations within reference ranges. mTOR inhibitors are also associated with impaired wound healing and

> **BOX 48.2 Side Effects of Mammalian Target of Rapamycin Inhibitors**
>
> Anemia
> Hypercholesterolemia
> Hypertriglyceridemia
> Impaired wound healing
> Leukopenia
> Lymphocele
> Mouth ulcers
> Peripheral edema
> Pneumonitis
> Proteinuria

should be discontinued 2 weeks prior to elective surgeries and should not be started within 4 weeks after surgery including index transplantation. mTOR inhibitors can cause proteinuria through an unknown mechanism. Patients need to be screened for proteinuria through either a 24-hour urine collection or a spot urine protein/creatinine ratio prior to initiation of mTOR inhibitors. Additionally, patients should be monitored every few months for new-onset proteinuria when using mTOR inhibitors. Sirolimus has an FDA–boxed warning regarding hepatic artery thrombosis with use early after liver transplantation; as such, use within the first 4 weeks post-transplant is generally avoided.

Interactions

Sirolimus is a substrate of cytochrome P450 3A4 and is therefore subject to similar drug interactions listed for CNIs and those medications listed in **Table 48.2**.

Everolimus

Everolimus is structurally similar to sirolimus and is a macrolide.

Mechanism of Action

The mechanism of action is similar to sirolimus.

Dosage

Starting doses of everolimus are typically 1 to 2 mg given by mouth in divided doses twice daily. Doses are titrated to achieve a serum trough concentration between 3 and 8 ng/mL. Everolimus can be used in addition to or in place of CNIs. The half-life of everolimus is 32 hours; therefore, serum trough concentrations should be checked 5 to 7 days after a dose adjustment.

Time Frame for Response

Time to peak plasma concentration of everolimus is 1 to 2 hours.

Contraindications

Everolimus is contraindicated in patients with clinically significant hypersensitivity to everolimus. Everolimus does have several FDA-boxed warnings including increased risk of kidney arterial and venous thrombosis when used within 30 days

TABLE 48.2

Table of Induction Agents

Generic (Trade) Name and Dosage	Selected Adverse Effects	Contraindications	Special Considerations
Rabbit-anti-thymocyte globulin 1.5 mg/kg per dose	Flash pulmonary edema, respiratory distress, leukopenia, thrombocytopenia, fever, chills, thrombophlebitis	Hypersensitivity (allergy or anaphylaxis) to rabbit proteins or any component of the formulation; active infections	Dose is rounded to the nearest vial size of 25 mg; maximum daily dose is 150 mg.
Alemtuzumab (Lemtrada) 30 mg given IV over 6 hours or SQ	Flash pulmonary edema, respiratory distress, leukopenia, thrombocytopenia, fever, chills, thrombophlebitis	Hypersensitivity or anaphylactic reactions to alemtuzumab or any component of the formulation; active infections; underlying immunodeficiency; active secondary malignancies; current or history of progressive multifocal leukoencephalopathy	Restricted distribution; Participation in FDA REMS program required
Basiliximab (Simulect) 20 mg IV on postoperative day 0 (intraoperatively) and postoperative day 4	Similar side effect profile comparable to placebo	Known hypersensitivity to basiliximab or any component of the formulation	N/A

FDA, Food and Drug Administration; REMS, Risk Evaluation Mitigation Strategy.

post transplant, increased nephrotoxicity when used in combination with cyclosporine, and increased mortality often associated with infection in heart transplant recipients.

Adverse Events

Adverse effects of everolimus are similar to those of sirolimus and are listed in **Box 48.2**.

Interactions

Everolimus is a substrate of cytochrome P450 3A4 and is therefore subject to similar drug interactions listed for CNIs and those medications listed in **Box 48.1**.

Drug Class: Corticosteroids

Corticosteroids are used both as induction and maintenance therapy. During induction, methylprednisolone IV is utilized, whereas patients are converted to oral prednisone for slow tapering over time. Each solid organ transplant discipline differs in the amount and duration of steroid use. Recently, many centers for kidney transplantation are moving toward steroid withdrawal protocols, which eliminate the use of chronic steroids to minimize long-term side effects.

Mechanism of Action

It is unknown which of the three signals of T-cell proliferation are inhibited by corticosteroids. Steroids have several immunomodulatory mechanisms including inhibition of the production of cytokines and decreasing lymphocyte production and trafficking.

Dosage

Induction doses are typically between 250 and 1,000 mg given IV as methylprednisolone. Maintenance doses of oral

prednisone typically range from 5 to 20 mg by mouth daily. Steroids can be tapered rapidly if used for a short duration of time or more slowly over a period of several months.

Time Frame for Response

Steroids are rapidly effective and work within 30 minutes to 1 hour.

Contraindications

Steroids are contraindicated in uncontrolled active infections.

Adverse Events

Corticosteroids are associated with both short- and long-term side effects as well as dose-related toxicities. Acute side effects of steroids include elevations in blood glucose, hypertension, anxiety, trouble sleeping, confusion, hallucinations, and fluid retention. Long-term side effects include metabolic complications such as diabetes and fat redistribution such as central obesity, "moon" face, and "buffalo hump." Other long-term side effects include osteoporosis and osteopenia leading to bone fractures; ophthalmic changes such as cataracts; and glaucoma and skin changes including acne, bruising, and impaired wound healing.

Interactions

Limited drug interactions exist.

Drug Class: Costimulation Blockade— Belatacept

In order to achieve sustained T-cell response after antigen recognition in signal 1, there needs to be co-stimulatory signals delivered through accessory T-cell surface molecules from signal 2. Costimulation blockade, using belatacept (Nulojix®), is achieved by blockage of the CD28 and B7 interaction to

TABLE 48.3

Table of Maintenance Agents

Generic (Trade) Name and Dosage	Selected Adverse Effects	Contraindications	Special Considerations
Azathioprine (various) 1–2 mg/Kg PO daily	Leukopenia, gastrointestinal disturbances, hepatotoxicity	Hypersensitivity to azathioprine or any component of the formulation; pregnancy	TPMT genotyping or phenotyping may assist in identifying patients at risk for or with abnormally low CBC unresponsive to dose reduction
Belatacept (Nulojix) 10 mg/kg during initiation phase 5 mg/kg maintenance phase	Post-transplant lymphoproliferative disorder, infections	Transplant patients who are EBV seronegative or with unknown EBV serostatus due to increased risk for PTLD	Therapy is not recommended in liver transplant patients due to increased risk of graft loss and death.
Cyclosporine (Sandimmune, Neoral) 6 mg/kg per day in two divided doses given PO	Monitor serum trough concentration; therapeutic concentrations range from 200 to 400 ng/mL Monitor for side effects including nephrotoxicity, neurotoxicity, hypertension, hyperglycemia, and hyperkalemia.	Hypersensitivity to cyclosporine or any component of the formulation; contraindicated in hypersensitivity to polyoxyethylated castor oil (Cremophor EL)	Avoid grapefruit and pomegranate juice, fruit, seeds, and extract; cyclosporine concentrations may be falsely elevated if sample is drawn from the same central venous line through which dose was administered.
Everolimus (Afinitor) 1–2 mg PO BID	Monitor serum trough concentration; therapeutic concentrations range from 3 to 8 ng/mL Monitor for side effects including proteinuria, hypercholesterolemia, hypertriglyceridemia, anemia, and fatigue	Hypersensitivity to everolimus or any component of the formulation	May be associated with wound dehiscence and impaired healing; discontinuation several weeks before a planned operation or for several weeks after surgery is recommended.
Mycophenolic acid Mycophenolate mofetil (CellCept, Myfortic): 500–1,500 mg PO BID Mycophenolate sodium: 360–1080 mg PO BID	Leukopenia, gastrointestinal disturbances	Hypersensitivity to mycophenolate mofetil, mycophenolic acid, mycophenolate sodium, or any component of the formulation; intravenous formulation is also contraindicated in patients who are allergic to polysorbate 80 (Tween).	Use during pregnancy is associated with increased risks of first trimester pregnancy loss and congenital malformations. Females of reproductive potential must be counseled regarding pregnancy prevention and planning. Participation in FDA REMS program required
Sirolimus (Rapamune) 1–2 mg PO daily	Monitor serum trough concentration; therapeutic concentrations range from 3 to 10 ng/mL Monitor for side effects including proteinuria, hypercholesterolemia, hypertriglyceridemia, anemia, and fatigue	Hypersensitivity to sirolimus or any component of the formulation	May be associated with wound dehiscence and impaired healing; discontinuation several weeks before a planned operation or for several weeks after surgery is recommended.
Tacrolimus (Astagraf, Protopic) 0.1 mg/kg/d in two divided doses given PO	Monitor serum trough concentration; therapeutic concentrations range from 8 to 15 ng/mL. Monitor for side effects including nephrotoxicity, neurotoxicity, hypertension, hyperglycemia, and hyperkalemia	Hypersensitivity to tacrolimus, polyoxyl HCO-60, or any other component of the formulation	Avoid grapefruit and pomegranate juice, fruit, seeds, and extract

CBC, complete blood count; EBV, Epstein-Barr virus; FDA, Food and Drug Administration; HCO-60, 60 hydrogenated castor oil; PTLD, post-transplant lymphoproliferative disorder; REMS, Risk Evaluation Mitigation Strategy; TPMT, Thiopurine S-methyltransferase.

mitigate organ rejection. Belatacept is used alone or in combination with CNIs as the backbone agent in a maintenance immunosuppression regimen, specifically in kidney transplantation. The use of belatacept in other organ disciplines to prevent rejection either has not been studied sufficiently or is associated with graft loss and mortality.

Mechanism of Action

Belatacept is a fusion protein that causes selective T-cell costimulation inhibition by binding to CD80 and CD86 receptors on APCs, blocking the interaction between these receptors and CD28 receptors on T cells. This results in a decreased production of cytokines and less proliferation of T cells.

Dosage

Belatacept dosing is divided into an initial phase and a maintenance phase. In the de novo initial phase, belatacept is given as 10 mg/kg IV on days 1, 5, 14, 28, 56, and 96 following kidney transplant. The maintenance phase is 5 mg/kg every 4 weeks thereafter. Belatacept is dosed based on actual body weight, and each dose should be administered within 3 days of the scheduled date.

Time Frame for Response

Although the onset of action is immediate, clinical trials have shown an increased risk of acute cellular rejection within the first year when compared to CNIs.

Contraindications

Owing to a higher risk of post-transplant lymphoproliferative disorder, transplant recipients who are Epstein-Barr virus (EBV) seronegative or with unknown EBV serostatus should not receive belatacept.

Adverse Events

Adverse events to belatacept are generally considered mild and may be more associated with other agents as part of a combination regimen.

Interactions

No known drug interactions exist at this time.

Selecting the Most Appropriate Drug

First-Line Therapy

Both induction and maintenance strategies in organ transplantation are patient specific and vary based on the organ transplanted to balance the risks of rejection, infection, and drug toxicity. There are several factors that must be weighed by the treating clinician when determining what induction strategy to be utilized including immunogenicity of the organ, number of HLA mismatches, risk factors for rejection in each specific patient, risk of toxicity, and the results of crossmatch testing performed at the time of transplant. Immunogenicity, or the ability of an antigen to provoke an immune response, varies with each organ transplanted. This follows the percentage

of patients who typically receive induction therapy with T-cell-depleting agents: pancreas 80%, kidney 75%, lung 69%, intestine 64%, heart 52%, and liver 30%. Thymoglobulin is the most commonly used T-cell-depleting therapy, and basiliximab is the most common non-T-cell-depleting therapy utilized for induction in organ transplantation.

Maintenance immunosuppression is typically comprised of either two or three drug regimens to achieve sufficient immunosuppression to prevent rejection while balancing the risks of infection and toxicity. The most commonly used regimen is tacrolimus, MMF and prednisone, utilized after organ transplantation with nearly 60% of kidney and liver transplant recipients receiving this combination. Over the last decade, the percentage of patients receiving maintenance corticosteroids has been decreasing, as more centers move toward a steroid-sparring protocol using the combination of tacrolimus and MMF.

Second-Line Therapy

For those patients who are not able to tolerate tacrolimus, cyclosporine can be used instead. Common reasons for needing to switch to cyclosporine include tacrolimus-associated neurotoxicity or nephrotoxicity. Similarly, patients unable to tolerate MMF can be switched to an alternative antimetabolite such as azathioprine.

Belatacept use in kidney transplant recipients in the United States has been increasing in the last decade. While there is a higher risk of rejection within the first year after kidney transplant, its popularity has increased secondary to its relatively mild adverse effect profile and ability to maintain superior kidney function compared to cyclosporine. Belatacept use does not impact any of the major risk factors for cardiovascular death, whereas CNIs can cause nephrotoxicity, hypertension, hyperlipidemia, and new-onset diabetes after transplant. Cardiovascular mortality remains the leading cause of death for kidney transplant recipients within 10 years after transplant with a functioning graft. The use of belatacept will continue to increase in selected patient populations as clinicians develop strategies to mitigate the higher risk of rejection within the first year after transplantation, and additional data are available for comparing belatacept to tacrolimus-based maintenance regimens.

Third-Line Therapy

Currently, mTOR inhibitors are not considered the standard of care after organ transplantation. They are typically reserved for specific situations in which patients are unable to tolerate CNIs due to toxicity. Additionally, mTOR inhibitors are utilized for their presumed anti-tumor properties.

Special Considerations

Geriatric

Older patients generally have less risk of rejection than younger patients. Immunosuppressive regimens in older patients may therefore have lower immunosuppressive goals, and providers are more sensitive to lower immunosuppression in the setting of infections.

Ethnic

African-American patients have a higher risk for acute rejection. As such, some center-specific protocols have empiric dose increases in MMF to 1,500 mg by mouth twice daily to mitigate the increased risk. Conversely, Asian patients may be at higher risk of infection, and some protocols call for a reduced dose of MMF 500 mg by mouth twice daily to prevent increased infections.

Genomics

Gain-of-function mutations in CYP P450 3A4/5 have been described and play a role in the maintenance dose of CNIs. Currently, genomic alterations in cytochrome P450 enzymes are not utilized routinely for empiric dosing and are still considered for research purposes only.

MONITORING PATIENT RESPONSE

While much of the decision-making in immunosuppressive therapy is protocol based, health care providers are encouraged to monitor patients for signs and symptoms of rejection, infection, and medication-related toxicities. Many patients need to have their immunosuppression medications adjusted to increase or decrease the level of immunosuppression for these reasons. Overtime, the patient's risk for rejection will decrease and providers are able to lower the amount of immunosuppression.

PATIENT EDUCATION

Drug Information

Patients should be counseled to call their transplant team when starting any new prescription or over-the-counter medications to mitigate the risk of new drug–drug interactions. As many patients will begin several new medicines post-transplant, it is important to review the indication, dose, duration, route, schedule, frequency, and side effects of each medicine with patients and their primary caregivers. Adherence to medication is a significant predictor of long-term allograft survival, and each episode of rejection should prompt the clinician to discuss barriers to medication adherence with patients. Strategies to promote medication adherence including use of a pillbox, medication schedule, timers, digital applications, and routines should be reviewed with the patients before discharge.

Nutrition/Lifestyle Changes

Patients require extensive education to mitigate side effects and infections post-transplant as they will be on lifelong immunosuppression. To prevent infection, patients should be counseled to thoroughly cook meat to appropriate temperatures and wash vegetables. Patients should avoid raw foods such as sushi to prevent infection. Some patients may experience hyperkalemia from CNIs and therefore may need to follow a potassium-restricted diet for the first few months post-transplant.

Patients should be counseled to avoid grapefruit, pomegranate, and star fruit when prescribed CNIs or mTOR inhibitors. Each of these fruits can cause cytochrome P450 3A4 enzyme inhibition that can raise serum drug concentrations to toxic ranges.

Complementary and Alternative Medications

Patients should be counseled to avoid dietary and herbal supplements as it is not currently known how these supplements might interaction with immunosuppressive medications. Additionally, probiotics should be avoided in patients on active immunosuppression secondary to the risk of infection/fungemia.

CASE STUDY 1

I.G. underwent a deceased-donor kidney transplant and is now receiving postoperative day 1 dose 2 of 4 of anti-thymocyte globulin for induction immunosuppression. One hour into the infusion, the nurse calls to report a change in the patient's vital signs, including a blood pressure of 95/65, new tachycardia of 115 beats per minute, and a fever of 101°F. Other medications on the profile at the time are tacrolimus 2 mg twice daily, mycophenolate mofetil 500 mg twice daily, and prednisone 5 mg daily.

1. Which medication is causing these adverse drug reactions?
   a. Anti-thymocyte globulin
   b. Mycophenolate mofetil
   c. Prednisone
   d. Tacrolimus

2. What changes in therapy are necessary to treat this patient's new symptoms?
   a. Discontinue anti-thymocyte globulin.
   b. Discontinue maintenance therapy until the conclusion of the induction therapy.
   c. Slow down the infusion rate of the anti-thymocyte globulin and give acetaminophen 650 mg orally for fever.
   d. Give the patient an additional dose of prednisone 20 mg.

3. The following day, I.G.'s complete blood count reports a white blood cell count of 2.3 cells/mcL, a hemoglobin count of 10.3 mg/dL, and a platelet count of 76,000 cells/mcL. What should the dose of anti-thymocyte globulin be for today?

a. 1.5 mg/kg; not to exceed 150 mg
b. 0.75 mg/kg; not to exceed 150 mg
c. 1.5 mg/kg; no dose maximum
d. 0.75 mg/kg; no dose maximum

Bibliography

*Starred references are cited in the text.

*Alloway, R. R., Woodle, E. S., Abramowicz, D., et al. (2019). Rabbit anti-thymocyte globulin for the prevention of acute rejection in kidney transplantation. *American Journal of Transplantation*, 19(8), 2252–2261. doi: 10.1111/ajt.15342

Atreya, I., & Neurath, M. F. (2009). Understanding the delayed onset of action of azathioprine in IBD: Are we there yet? *Gut*, 58(3), 325–326. doi: 10.1136/gut.2008.163485

Awan, A. A., Niu, J., Pan, J. S., et al. (2018). Trends in the causes of death among kidney transplant recipients in the United States (1996–2014). *American Journal of Nephrology*, 48(6), 472–481. doi: 10.1159/000495081

Ben-Horin, S., Goldstein, I., Fudim, E., et al. (2009). Early preservation of effector functions followed by eventual T-cell memory depletion: A model for the delayed onset of the effect of thiopurines. *Gut*, 58(3), 396–403. doi: 10.1136/gut.2008.157339

Busuttil, R. W., & Klintmalm, G. B. (2015). *Transplantation of the liver.* Maarssen, Netherlands: Elsevier Gezondheidszorg.

Campath® [Package insert]. (2019). Cambridge, MA: Genzyme Corporation.

Cellcept® [Package insert]. (2019). South San Francisco, CA: Genentech USA, Inc.

Colvin, M., Smith, J. M., Hadley, N., et al. (2020). OPTN/SRTR 2018 annual data report: Heart. *American Journal of Transplantation*, 20(Suppl s1), 340–426. doi: 10.1111/ajt.15676

Danovitch, G. M. (2009). *Handbook of kidney transplantation* (Lippincott Williams & Wilkins Handbook Series) (5th ed.). Philadelphia, PA: Lippincott Williams & Wilkins.

Durrbach, A., Pestana, J. M., Pearson, T., et al. (2010a). A phase III study of belatacept versus cyclosporine in kidney transplants from extended criteria donors (BENEFIT-EXT study). *American Journal of Transplantation*, 10(3), 547–557. doi: 10.1111/j.1600-6143.2010.03016.x

Geissler, E. K., Schnitzbauer, A. A., Zülke, C., et al. (2016). Sirolimus use in liver transplant recipients with hepatocellular carcinoma: A randomized, multicenter, open-label phase 3 trial. *Transplantation*, 100(1), 116–125. doi: 10.1097/TP.0000000000000965

Gelone, D. K., Park, J. M., & Lake, K. D. (2007). Lack of an effect of oral iron administration on mycophenolic acid pharmacokinetics in stable renal transplant recipients. *Pharmacotherapy*, 27(9), 1272–1278. doi: 10.1592/phco.27.9.1272

*Halloran, P. F. (2004). Immunosuppressive drugs for kidney transplantation. *The New England Journal of Medicine*, 351, 2715–2729.

Hart, A., Smith, J. M., Skeans, M. A., et al. (2020). OPTN/SRTR 2018 annual data report: Kidney. *American Journal of Transplantation*, 20(Suppl s1), 20–130. doi: 10.1111/ajt.15672

Imuran® [Package insert]. (2018). Roswell, GA: Sebela Pharmaceuticals Inc.

Kandaswamy, R., Stock, P. G., Gustafson, S. K., et al. (2019). OPTN/SRTR 2017 annual data report: Pancreas. *American Journal of Transplantation*, 19(Suppl 2), 124–183. doi: 10.1111/ajt.15275

Klintmalm, G. (1994). The U.S. multicenter FK506 liver study group: A comparison of tacrolimus (FK 506) and cyclosporine for immunosuppression in liver transplantation. *The New England Journal of Medicine*, 331, 1110–1115.

Klintmalm, G. B., Feng, S., Lake, J. R., et al. (2014). Belatacept-based immunosuppression in de novo liver transplant recipients: 1-year experience from a phase II randomized study. *American Journal of Transplantation*, 14(8), 1817–1827. doi: 10.1111/ajt.12810

Kwong, A., Kim, W. R., Lake, J. R., et al. (2020). OPTN/SRTR 2018 annual data report: Liver. *American Journal of Transplantation*, 20(Suppl s1), 193–299. doi: 10.1111/ajt.15674

Lorenz, M., Wolzt, M., Weigel, G., et al. (2004). Ferrous sulfate does not affect mycophenolic acid pharmacokinetics in kidney transplant patients. *American Journal of Kidney Diseases*, 43(6), 1098–1103. doi: 10.1053/j.ajkd.2004.03.021

Myfortic® [Package insert]. (2020). East Hanover, NJ: Novartis Pharmaceuticals Corporation.

Neoral® [Package insert]. (2015). East Hanover, NJ: Novartis Pharmaceuticals Corporation.

Nulojix® [Package insert]. (2014). Princeton, NJ: Bristol-Myers Squibb.

*OPTN/SRTR 2018 Annual Data Report: Introduction. (2020). *American Journal of Transplantation*, 20(Suppl s1), 11–19. doi: 10.1111/ajt.15671

Phan, K., Moloney, F. J., Hogarty, D. T., et al. (2019). Mammalian target of rapamycin (mTOR) inhibitors and skin cancer risk in nonrenal solid organ transplant recipients: Systematic review and meta-analysis. *International Journal of Dermatology*. doi: 10.1111/ijd.14549

Prograf® [Package insert]. (2018). Northbrook, IL: Astellas Pharma US, Inc.

Rapamune® [Package insert]. (2019). Philadelphia, PA: Wyeth Pharmaceuticals, LLC.

Simulect® [Package insert]. (2003). East Hanover, NJ: Novartis Pharmaceuticals Corporation.

Smith, J. M., Weaver, T., Skeans, M. A., et al. (2020). OPTN/SRTR 2018 annual data report: Intestine. *American Journal of Transplantation*, 20(Suppl s1), 300–339. doi: 10.1111/ajt.15675

Tremblay, S., Nigro, V., Weinberg, J., et al. (2017). A Steady-State Head-to-Head Pharmacokinetic Comparison of All FK-506 (Tacrolimus) Formulations (ASTCOFF): An open-label, prospective, randomized, two-arm, three-period crossover study. *American Journal of Transplantation*, 17(2), 432–442. doi: 10.1111/ajt.13935

U.S. Multicenter FK506 Liver Study Group. (1994). A comparison of tacrolimus (FK 506) and cyclosporine for immunosuppression in liver transplantation. *The New England Journal of Medicine*, 331(17), 1110–1115. doi: 10.1056/NEJM199410273311702

Ventura, C., Guarnieri, C., Stefanelli, C., et al. (1991). Comparison between alpha-adrenergic- and K-opioidergic-mediated inositol (1,4,5)P3/inositol (1,3,4,5) P4 formation in adult cultured rat ventricular cardiomyocytes. *Biochemical and Biophysical Research Communications*, 179(2), 972–978. doi: 10.1016/0006-291x(91)91913-w

Vincenti, F., Charpentier, B., Vanrenterghem, Y., et al. (2010). A phase III study of belatacept-based immunosuppression regimens versus cyclosporine in renal transplant recipients (BENEFIT study). *American Journal of Transplantation*, 10(3), 535–546. doi: 10.1111/j.1600-6143.2009.03005.x

Yarbrough, G. G., & Singh, D. K. (1978). Intravenous thyrotropin releasing hormone (TRH) enhances the excitatory actions of acetylcholine (ACh) on rat cortical neurons. *Experientia*, 34(3), 390. doi: 10.1007/BF01923054

Zortress® [Package insert]. (2018). East Hanover, NJ: Novartis Pharmaceuticals Corporation.

Pharmacotherapy for Thromboembolic Disorders

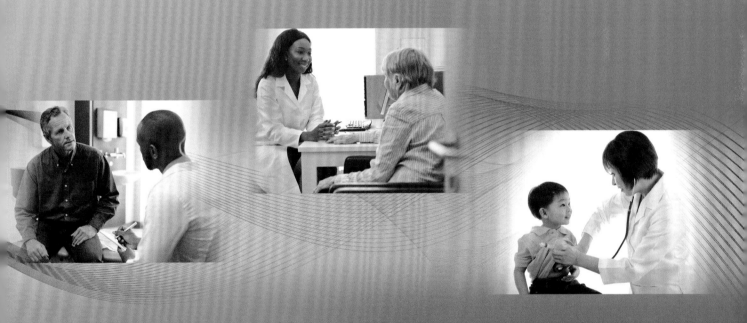

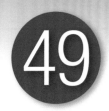

49 Thromboembolic Disorders

Sarah A. Spinler and Lyndsay Carlson

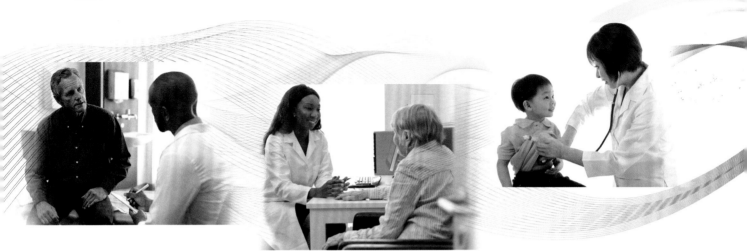

Learning Objectives

1. Describe the epidemiology and pathophysiology of thromboembolism responsible for stroke, deep vein thrombosis (DVT) and pulmonary embolism (PE).
2. List the signs, symptoms, risk stratification scoring, and testing used in the diagnosis of ischemic stroke, DVT, and PE.
3. Select appropriate parenteral anticoagulation, oral anticoagulation, and antiplatelet therapy for prevention of ischemic stroke in patients with prosthetic heart valves and/or atrial fibrillation, acute treatment of DVT and PE, and secondary prevention of DVT and PE based on patient's thrombosis and bleeding risk, diet, drug interactions, and renal function.
4. Transition patients from warfarin to a direct-acting oral anticoagulant (DOAC) or from a DOAC to warfarin.
5. Monitor for and manage a patient who experiences anticoagulation-associated major bleeding.

INTRODUCTION

Thromboembolic disease and patients with risk factors for thromboembolic disease and patients with risk factors for thromboemboli are frequently encountered in the ambulatory population, and an understanding of the pathogenesis of these conditions and underlying patient risk factors, along with the clotting cascade, is essential for determining appropriate treatment. The indications for anticoagulation (AC) continue to expand, and treatment for some conditions has now shifted to the outpatient setting. Several disorders warrant anticoagulant therapy, including venous thromboembolism (VTE) prevention and treatment, stroke prevention in atrial fibrillation (SPAF), ischemic stroke, prosthetic cardiac valves, coronary and peripheral arterial disease (PAD), and hypercoagulable conditions. Recognizing when prophylaxis for clotting events is appropriate is also important, including during orthopedic surgery and during hospitalization in patients with multiple risk factors for VTE. AC practices are an important component of quality metrics and patient safety practices for hospitalized patients. AC management strategies for the prevention and treatment of VTE and SPAF and the prevention of systemic thromboembolism in patients with prosthetic heart valves are discussed in this chapter.

DISORDERS REQUIRING ANTICOAGULATION AND THEIR CAUSES

Venous Thromboembolism

VTE is a thromboembolic event occurring in the venous system, and it is manifested as either deep vein thrombosis (DVT) or pulmonary embolism (PE). VTE contributes significantly to patient morbidity and mortality and is considered a major global disease burden (Raskob et al., 2014). Venous thrombus formation occurs in the setting of venous stasis (sluggish blood flow), vascular endothelial wall injury, and hypercoagulability (propensity for increased blood clotting); these three features are classically referred to as *Virchow's triad* (Merli, 2008).

The components of Virchow's triad can assist with categorizing the most common causes and risk factors for VTE. Venous stasis, which results in pooling of blood in the lower extremity veins, is precipitated by prolonged immobility occurring during hospitalization, surgery, spinal cord injury, or paralyzing stroke, in conditions that increase venous pressure, including varicose veins or venous insufficiency from the postthrombotic syndrome, or, less frequently, in obesity or pregnancy. Vascular intimal injury is often related to recent surgery, especially abdominal and orthopedic surgery, recent trauma or fracture to the pelvis or lower extremities, childbirth, and previous venous thrombosis. Imbalances between the body's regulatory mechanisms of procoagulant and anticoagulant proteins can result in hypercoagulable conditions. Hypercoagulability may be present secondary to inherited abnormalities of coagulation (thrombophilia), malignancy, oral contraceptive use, and estrogen therapy (Heit et al., 2016). In addition, central venous catheters and age older than 40 years also increase the risk of venous thromboembolic disease (Heit et al., 2016). The incidence of VTE is approximately from 0.75 to 2.69 per 1,000 individuals in the general population and is increased to between 2 and 7 per 1,000 among those age ≥70 years and to 1 in 200 in patients with active cancer (Easaw et al., 2015; Raskob et al., 2014). Risk factors for VTE should be identified and corrected, if possible. Inherited thrombophilia is the most common risk factor in patients presenting with VTE under the age of 50 years (Heit et al., 2016). See **Box 49.1** for more information on predisposing risk factors for VTE.

BOX 49.1 Risk Factors for Deep Vein Thrombosis and Pulmonary Embolism

REVERSIBLE

Trauma, surgery, pregnancy, estrogen therapy, chemotherapy, prolonged or transient immobility, fractures, central venous catheters, obesity, long-haul air travel

ACQUIRED

Increasing age >40 years, malignancy, previous VTE, hematologic disease, HF, stroke, inflammatory bowel disease, nephrotic syndrome, spinal cord injury, varicose veins, superficial vein thrombosis, aPL antibodies, LA

INHERITED DISORDERS

Activated protein C resistance, antithrombin III deficiency, protein C deficiency, protein S deficiency, anticardiolipin antibodies, factor V Leiden, prothrombin gene mutation

---

HF, heart failure; LA, lupus anticoagulant; VTE, venous thromboembolism.
Data adapted from Geerts, W. H., Bergqvist, D., Pineo, G. F., et al. (2008). Prevention of venous thromboembolism: American College of Chest Physicians evidence-based clinical practice guidelines (8th ed.). *Chest, 133*(6 Suppl.), 381S–453S; Osinbowale, O., Ali, L., & Chi, Y. W. (2010). Venous thromboembolism: A clinical review. *Postgraduate Medicine, 122*(2), 54–65.

In DVT, the characteristic symptom of lower extremity swelling is due to the thrombus partially or completely occluding the vein. Proximal DVT develops in the popliteal, femoral, or iliac veins above the knee, while calf vein DVT is isolated below the knee. Calf vein DVT may extend proximally in 40% to 50% of patients without AC.

The major complication of proximal DVT is thrombus dislodgment and extension into the pulmonary circulation. PE is a life-threatening emergency, with an associated mortality rate of 25%. Lower extremity DVTs are the source of 90% of PEs (Piazza & Goldhaber, 2006). Distal DVT isolated to the calf veins has a lower risk of long-term complications. In hospitalized patients, proximal DVT accounts for 80% of cases, with distal DVT comprising 20% (Righini & Bounameaux, 2008).

Nearly 50% of patients experiencing DVT develop chronic venous insufficiency or postthrombotic syndrome. The acute thrombus and accompanying inflammation lead to valvular incompetence and venous stasis, with resultant chronic lower extremity edema, ulceration, and chronic pain (Makedonov et al., 2020). These symptoms are frequently debilitating to the patient's quality of life. The lower extremities should be assessed for edema, skin pigmentation changes, spider veins, varicosities, and scarring from previous ulcers to assist with recognizing chronic venous insufficiency and implementing preventive measures, if possible (Makedonov et al., 2020).

Patients with a proximal DVT have a higher risk of recurrence than those with a distal DVT, and patients with PE have a higher recurrent VTE risk than those with isolated DVT. Patients presenting with provoked VTE have a lower risk of recurrence than those with idiopathic (unprovoked VTE). Other risk factors for recurrent VTE include malignancy (recurrence rates exceed 20% at 1 year), antiphospholipid (aPL) antibody syndrome, male sex, persistent positive D-dimer (checked 3 weeks to 2 months following cessation of AC), and residual thrombosis. Several web-based risk prediction models are available to estimate a patient's risk of recurrent VTE (Fahrni et al., 2015) (see **Box 49.2**).

Atrial Fibrillation

Atrial fibrillation (AF) is a cardiac arrhythmia characterized by loss of coordination of electrical and mechanical activity in the atria. Thrombi can form in the left atrial appendage due to impaired ventricular filling and incomplete emptying of the atria. AF may initially present with the embolic complication of stroke, when atrial thrombi dislodge and travel through the bloodstream to the brain. AF is responsible for up to 12% of ischemic strokes nationwide (Ahmad & Wilt, 2016). Other major complications of AF include heart failure (HF), dementia, and death (January et al., 2014). Patients with mitral stenosis (any cause), rheumatic mitral valve disease, or prosthetic heart valves (mechanical or bioprosthetic) and AF have a 17-fold increased risk systemic embolization/stroke compared to those in sinus rhythm (Ahmad & Wilt, 2016). Patients with AF but without valvular heart disease or a prosthetic heart valve have a fivefold increased risk of ischemic stroke compared to those in sinus rhythm (January et al., 2014).

BOX 49.2 Helpful Online Resources

Calculator	Purpose	URL
AnticoagEvaluator	An app from the ACC that may be used to select guideline recommended anticoagulation therapy	https://www.acc.org/anticoagevaluator
CHA$_2$DS$_2$-VASc	Estimates annual risk of ischemic stroke in patients with AF	https://www.mdcalc.com/cha2ds2-vasc-score-atrial-fibrillation-stroke-risk
DASH Prediction Score	Estimates risk of recurrent VTE to evaluate risk–benefit of continuing anticoagulation	https://www.mdcalc.com/dash-prediction-score-recurrent-vte
Dynamic Vienna Prediction Model	Estimates risk of recurrent VTE	http://www.meduniwien.ac.at/user/georg.heinze/dvpm/
FDA drug interactions checker	Identifies drug and herbal supplement interactions with warfarin and DOACs	https://www.drugs.com/drug_interactions.html
Geneva Score (Revised)	Estimates risk of PE	https://www.mdcalc.com/geneva-score-revised-pulmonary-embolism
Global RPh Warfarin Maintenance Dose Consult Tool	Assists in making inpatient and outpatient warfarin dose changes	https://globalrph.com/medcalcs/warfarin-maintenance-dose-consult-tool/
HAS-BLED Score	Estimates the risk of oral anticoagulant major bleeding in a patient with AF	https://www.mdcalc.com/has-bled-score-major-bleeding-risk
HERDOO2 Prediction Rule	Estimates risk of recurrent VTE to evaluate risk–benefit of discontinuing anticoagulation	https://www.mdcalc.com/herdoo2-rule-discontinuing-anticoagulation-unprovoked-vte
PERC Rule	Rules out PE if no criteria are present and low pretest probability of PE	https://www.mdcalc.com/perc-rule-pulmonary-embolism
Simplified Pulmonary Embolism Severity Index	Predicts 30-day outcome of patients with PE	https://www.mdcalc.com/simplified-pesi-pulmonary-embolism-severity-index
University of Washington Warfarin maintenance dose nomogram	Assists in making outpatient warfarin maintenance dose changes based on INR	https://globalrph.com/medcalcs/warfarin-maintenance-dose-consult-tool/, https://www.soapnote.org/blood-lymph/coumadin-calculator/
VTE-BLEED Score	Identifies patients with VTE at either low or high risk of major bleeding on oral anticoagulation	https://practical-haemostasis.com/Clinical%20Prediction%20Scores/Formulae%20code%20and%20formulae/Formulae/VTED_bleedng/vte_bleed_score.html
Warfarin dose adjustment calculator	Assists in making warfarin dose changes	https://www.soapnote.org/blood-lymph/coumadin-calculator/
Wells Criteria	Uses presenting signs and symptoms to estimate the risk of PE	https://www.mdcalc.com/wells-criteria-pulmonary-embolism

ACC, American College of Cardiology; AF, atrial fibrillation; DOAC, direct-acting oral anticoagulant; FDA, Food and Drug Administration; INR, international normalized ratio; PE, pulmonary embolism; PERC, Pulmonary Embolism Rule-out Criteria; VTE, venous thromboembolism.

AF is the most common cardiac rhythm disturbance seen in clinical practice. Hospitalization for this arrhythmia is increasing, accounted for by the aging of the population and an increased incidence of chronic heart disease (Chung et al., 2020). The incidence increases with advancing age and is highest in those older than age 65 or in younger patients with comorbidities of hypertension (HTN) or underlying heart disease. Other risk factors associated with the development of AF include HTN, prior myocardial infarction (MI), HF, and valvular heart disease. Additional cardiac causes include atrial enlargement, atrial septal defect, and coronary artery bypass graft surgery. Noncardiac etiologies include diabetes mellitus, sleep apnea, thyrotoxicosis, chronic pulmonary disease, electrolyte disorders, PE, alcohol intoxication, obesity, and genetic predisposition (Chung et al., 2020).

The three key components to managing AF include preventing transient ischemic attack (TIA) and ischemic stroke with oral anticoagulant (OAC) drugs, restoring and maintaining sinus rhythm in selected patients, and controlling the ventricular heart rate. The patient's risk of stroke determines the need for AC. Patients with a history of stroke or TIA have the highest risk of a recurrent event. Other independent risk factors for stroke in AF are increasing age, HTN, congestive HF (either symptomatic HF with reduced or preserved systolic function), and diabetes mellitus. Female gender is considered a "risk modifier" where excess risk is evident only in the presence of other non-sex-related stroke risk factors (Ding et al., 2020). Patients older than age 75 comprise over half of AF-associated strokes; thus, the older adults represent a population in which stroke prophylaxis is essential. AC therapy is the cornerstone for SPAF.

Prosthetic Valvular Heart Disease

Prosthetic heart valves confer a high risk of systemic embolism, and antithrombotic therapy, antiplatelet therapy, AC, or a combination of antiplatelet and AC is warranted in most patients. Valvular heart disease is most commonly caused by degenerative valve disease due to increasing life spans and rheumatic heart disease. Indications for prosthetic heart valve replacement include mitral stenosis, mitral regurgitation, aortic stenosis, and aortic regurgitation, as progressive deterioration of the native valve can lead to syncope, dyspnea, angina, and HF. There are two main types of prosthetic heart valves: mechanical, made from synthetic materials, or bioprosthetic, of porcine or bovine origin. Mechanical prosthetic valves are more thrombogenic than bioprosthetic valves and require lifelong AC, but they are more durable. Factors contributing to thrombus formation with mechanical valve replacement include disruption of the vessel wall during surgery, leading to altered blood flow and activation of hemostasis, or exposure of circulating blood to the artificial surfaces of the valve prosthesis (Sun et al., 2010).

Prosthetic valves in the mitral position are more thrombogenic than those in the aortic position. In the mitral position, shear stress is low, blood flow is stagnant, and stasis occurs. In the aortic position, blood flow is rapid and shear stress is high, which causes red blood cell hemolysis and activation of platelets and coagulation factors (Sun et al., 2010).

The risk of thromboembolism in native valvular heart disease is influenced by the position of the valve, for example, mitral versus aortic, heart chamber dimension, ventricular performance, and concomitant risk factors such as prior thromboembolism and AF. In native valvular disease, individuals with rheumatic mitral valve disease have the greatest incidence of systemic embolism. Thromboembolism in aortic valve disease has been noted but is uncommon. Without the coexistence of mitral valve disease or AF, AC is not indicated in these patients (Nishimura et al., 2017).

PATHOPHYSIOLOGY OF COAGULATION AND CLOTTING DISORDERS

Disrupting the body's normal system of checks and balances for hemostasis will lead to either excessive bleeding or inappropriate clotting. The three major components of the coagulation system—endothelial cells, platelets, and coagulation proteins—preserve hemostasis by promoting clot formation in response to vascular injury. The intact vessel wall of the vascular endothelium maintains blood fluidity by inhibiting blood coagulation and platelet aggregation while promoting fibrinolysis. When the vessel wall is injured, substances in the endothelial cell lining stimulate the formation of a hemostatic plug by promoting platelet adhesion and aggregation and by activating blood coagulation, resulting in a fibrin clot (Colman et al., 2006).

Role of Clotting Cascade

In response to tissue injury, a series of complex enzymatic reactions (the clotting cascade, **Figure 49.1**) is initiated that leads to the formation of a stable fibrin clot. Circulating inactive coagulation factors are sequentially converted into activated coagulation factor complexes. The final step in the cascade is the formation of thrombin (factor IIa), which leads to the conversion of fibrinogen to fibrin and the formation of a fibrin clot (Colman et al., 2006).

Platelets also participate in repairing tissue injury by adhering to the site of injured blood vessels, attracting other platelets to the site, and forming large platelet aggregates that help stabilize the platelet–fibrin clot. When platelets are activated, receptors for clotting factors are exposed. This also provides a stable environment for the initiation of the clotting cascade (Colman et al., 2006).

The coagulation system is traditionally divided into the intrinsic and extrinsic pathways. Activity through the extrinsic pathway is initiated by components from the blood and vasculature, with factor VII as the major initiating factor. Activation occurs when procoagulant components migrate to sites of vascular damage or when blood is exposed to substances released as a result of vascular wall damage. In contrast, activity through the intrinsic coagulation pathway is initiated by activation of factor XII when blood comes in contact with a foreign surface (such as a prosthetic device) or damaged endothelial blood vessels. Once factor X is activated in either the extrinsic or intrinsic pathways, the two pathways merge to form a final common pathway for clot formation by converting prothrombin to thrombin (Colman et al., 2006) (see **Figure 49.1**).

Several inhibitory processes limit the clotting process. One of the main regulatory proteins of the clotting cascade is antithrombin III, which inhibits the activated clotting factors Xa, VIIa, IXa, XIa, XIIa, and IIa (thrombin). Three other regulatory proteins, proteins C, S, and Z, must be present in sufficient amounts because they prevent excessive clot formation by inactivating factors Va and VIIIa (activated protein C

COAGULATION PATHWAY

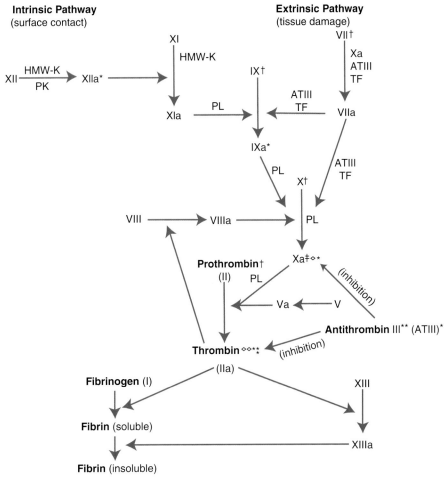

* Major site of activity for unfractionated heparin
† Site of activity for warfarin
‡ Major site of activity for low molecular weight heparin, apixaban rivaroxaban and edoxaban
⁑ Site of activity for low molecular weight heparin
◊◊ Major site of activity for dabigatran

FIGURE 49–1   The coagulation system.

ATIII, antithrombin III; HMW-K, high-molecular-weight kininogen; PK, prekallikrein; PL, phospholipids from activated platelets; TF, tissue factor.

with its cofactor protein S) and preventing the degradation of factor Xa (protein Z). Deficiency in any of these proteins creates a predisposition to pathologic thrombosis (Colman et al., 2006).

Thrombotic Process

Thrombi can form in any part of the cardiovascular (CV) system—the veins and arteries (including those of the brain) as well as the heart. Thrombi can cause local complications by obstructing vessels or by breaking off and traveling to a distant site (embolization). Arterial thrombi often form in the setting of preexisting atherosclerosis or other vascular diseases, especially at the sites of ruptured atherosclerotic plaques.

In the heart, thrombi can develop on damaged cardiac valves, in a dilated or dyskinetic heart chamber, or on prosthetic valves. Although most intracardiac thrombi cause no symptoms, serious consequences can arise if the thrombi migrate to the systemic circulation, especially the brain. In the venous system, thrombi usually occur in the lower extremities as DVT or in the pulmonary circulation as PE. Venous thrombi form in areas of sluggish blood flow (venous stasis) and contain primarily red cells held together with fibrin, with only small amounts of platelets. In contrast, arterial thrombi form in areas of high blood flow and are composed primarily of platelets bound with fibrin strands (Colman et al., 2006). The type of thrombus will dictate whether treatment is most appropriate with anticoagulant drugs or antiplatelet drugs.

Hypercoagulable States

Patients with thrombophilia, or hypercoagulable conditions, have an increased tendency to develop thrombosis, most often venous thrombosis. Hypercoagulability may be inherited or acquired. Genetic risk factors for VTE fall into two categories: loss of function and gain of function mutations. The two most common genetic risk factors for VTE are the gain of function mutations, factor V Leiden mutation and the prothrombin G20210A mutation. The aPL antibody syndrome is the most common nongenetically acquired thrombophilia. While heritable thrombophilia increases the risk of VTE, it does not influence the initiation of OAC, intensity of AC or for a first episode of VTE, often the duration of OAC (Hotoleanu, 2017).

A mutation in coagulation factor V, one of the key proteins in the coagulation cascade, occurs with factor V Leiden. Normally, activated protein C and S will inactivate factor V; in individuals with factor V Leiden, activated factor V is not degraded as efficiently, resulting in increased coagulability (Varga, 2008). Factor V Leiden occurs in 1% to 15% of Caucasians in the United States and increases the risk of VTE tenfold in heterozygotes and 30- to 140-fold in homozygotes (Hotoleanu, 2017).

Another genetic mutation that causes an increased risk of thrombosis is prothrombin G20210A. Some patients will have increased prothrombin activity, which is thought to contribute to thrombosis. The incidence in the general population is 1% to 4% and its presence increases the risk of VTE fivefold. Both the factor V Leiden and prothrombin gene mutation are uncommon in Blacks and Asians (Hotoleanu, 2017).

Loss of function mutations causing deficiencies in antithrombin III, activated protein C, and activated protein S (natural anticoagulants), although very rare, will also induce a prothrombotic state, corresponding to a five- to tenfold increase in VTE risk (Hotoleanu, 2017).

Homocysteine is an amino acid formed when the essential amino acid methionine is metabolized. Genetic defects (polymorphism) in the enzymes that regulate homocysteine metabolism can lead to elevated levels (hyperhomocysteinemia), but the exact association between this defect and resultant VTE is still uncertain. Hyperhomocysteinemia has been linked to an increased risk of stroke. Hyperhomocysteinemia is likely due to genetic and acquired causes (e.g., dietary deficiencies of folate, vitamin B_6, or vitamin B_{12}) (Hotoleanu, 2017).

The presence of a genetic risk factor superimposed with an acquired risk factor significantly increases the risk of VTE (Coppola et al., 2009). Clues that a patient with VTE has an underlying inherited hypercoagulable condition include thrombosis in patients younger than age 50, a positive family history of VTE, idiopathic or unprovoked thrombosis, recurrent thrombosis, and thrombosis in unusual locations, such as the adrenal glands, renal veins, or upper extremities (Merli, 2008).

A wide spectrum of acquired hypercoagulable states exist, including aPL antibody syndrome, malignancy, hematologic disorders, and nephrotic syndrome. For the purposes of this chapter, only aPL antibody syndrome will be discussed. aPLs are autoantibodies that bind to membrane phospholipid proteins, which are thought to cause the proteins to be antigenic and initiate thrombosis. Several aPLs have been identified, but the most significant are lupus anticoagulant (LA), IgG and IgM anticardiolipin antibodies (aCL) and anti-b2-glycoprotein I. aPLs are a strong predictor of thrombotic risk for arterial and venous thrombosis, and patients who have all three ("triple positive") are at the highest risk for thrombosis. LA is often found in patients with systemic lupus erythematosus but can occur in other diseases, including syphilis. The hallmark characteristics of aPL antibody syndrome are recurrent arterial or venous thrombosis, unexplained fetal loss, and thrombocytopenia with the presence of circulating aPLs. Ischemic stroke is a well-established criterion for the diagnosis of aPL antibody syndrome (Hotoleanu, 2017).

A workup for thrombophilia is usually deferred until after the acute thrombosis phase because diagnosis does not impact treatment as current thromboprophylaxis is not recommended for asymptomatic patients, including those who are triple positive (Arachchillage & Laffan, 2020; Hotoleanu, 2017). Widespread screening for inherited disorders is not recommended unless it is expected to change clinical management. A hematologist referral is required to determine what, if any, laboratory testing is required and whether wider testing of family members is warranted. The presence of certain anticoagulant drugs, in particular, warfarin and direct-acting oral anticoagulants (DOACs), will dictate the best timing for laboratory testing because they interfere with aPL testing (Flieder et al., 2018).

Although inherited thrombophilia increases the risk of VTE, prophylaxis with long-term AC is not necessary because the risk of bleeding, including fatal bleeding, outweighs the benefits of prophylaxis. However, in the setting of a potential triggering risk factor (e.g., surgery), AC prophylaxis is beneficial during the period of exposure (Coppola et al., 2009). Current guidelines on aPL-positive patients recommend lowdose aspirin for primary prevention in aPL-positive patients (Tektonidou et al., 2019). Warfarin (international normalized ratio [INR] 2.0–3.0) is the preferred OAC for secondary prevention of a first-time unprovoked VTE and warfarin (either INR 2.0–3.0 or 3.0–4.0) is recommended for first-time arterial thromboembolism (Tektonidou et al., 2019). The data with DOACs are limited (Arachchillage & Laffan, 2020).

DIAGNOSTIC CRITERIA

Venous Thromboembolism

Unilateral erythema, pain, swelling, venous distention, and warmth in the affected leg are common presenting symptoms of DVT. Other conditions, such as muscle strain, cellulitis, and postphlebitic syndrome, may mimic symptoms of DVT. Approximately 50% of patients with DVT have no symptoms.

Diagnosing VTE based on clinical factors is often unreliable because only 20% of patients who present with suspected VTE actually have a thrombosis. Therefore, objective of the use of pretest probability (PTP) plus a confirmatory D-dimer laboratory test is required (Lim et al., 2018).

Clinical prediction models that divide patients into low-, intermediate-, or high-risk categories for DVT/PE have been validated. For a first-time DVT, the Wells score may be calculated to determine the PTP of DVT and PE, and either the Wells score for PE or modified GENEVA score to determine the PTP of PE (Lim et al., 2018) (see **Box 49.2**). For patients with suspected DVT and low-calculated PTP, guidelines recommend measuring the laboratory blood test D-dimer to exclude the diagnosis of DVT (Lim et al., 2018). D-dimer is the major degradation product released into the circulation when cross-linked fibrin undergoes fibrinolysis. Levels of a highly sensitive D-dimer are elevated (>500 ng/mL) in most patients with ongoing thrombosis. Current assays for D-dimer are over 95% sensitive but not specific. Therefore, a negative highly sensitive D-dimer (<500 ng/mL) test helps to rule out DVT or PE and no further testing or AC is required. Patients with intermediate or high PTP for DVT and those with low PTP but a positive highly sensitive D-dimer should proceed to diagnostic testing with proximal or whole-leg ultrasound (Lim et al., 2018).

The most common method used for detecting DVT is compression ultrasonography (CUS) with Doppler. CUS measures the rate and direction of blood flow and can visualize clot formation in the proximal leg veins. CUS is the diagnostic method of choice because it is noninvasive, can be conducted at the bedside, and is relatively easy to perform. In CUS, DVT is diagnosed if the common femoral or popliteal veins cannot be compressed. For CUS, the sensitivity is 95% and specificity is 96% with a first episode of symptomatic proximal DVT (Merli, 2008).

PE is the most serious complication of DVT. The PE mortality rate is related to the size of the thrombus. A massive PE obstructs 50% of the pulmonary vasculature. The term *submassive* is used when less than 50% of the pulmonary circulation is affected. Death occurs from acute right-sided HF in untreated patients. The diagnosis of PE is difficult when based on symptoms because presenting symptoms are not specific. For patients presenting with PE, shortness of breath with or without leg pain may be the first symptom. Other physical findings include sudden onset of dyspnea, pleuritic chest pain, cough, tachycardia, tachypnea, and pre-syncope or syncope; these symptoms may also occur in HF, interstitial lung disease, and pneumonia, so thorough examination and further testing is important (Konstantinides et al., 2019). Suspicion of PE is based on symptoms along with such risk factors as immobility, recent trauma or surgery, underlying malignancy, and oral contraceptive use. Baseline tests for evaluating PE include a chest radiograph, an electrocardiogram (ECG) to differentiate between PE and MI, and arterial blood gas evaluations (to assess the severity of hypoxemia). The chest radiograph is often normal, so it is most useful in excluding the diagnosis of other conditions with similar symptoms of PE, including pneumothorax. The PTP using the Wells score is estimated as low, intermediate, or high. For patients with suspected PE and low or intermediate calculated PTP, guidelines recommend measuring the laboratory blood test D-dimer to exclude the diagnosis of PE (Lim et al., 2018). For patients with low PTP, some clinicians also apply the Pulmonary Embolism Rule-out Criteria (PERC) rule (see **Box 49.2**). If all eight criteria of the PERC rule are present (age < 50 years, heart rate < 100 bpm, oxyhemoglobin saturation ≥95%, no hemoptysis, no estrogen use, no prior DVT or PE, no unilateral leg swelling, and no surgery/trauma requiring hospitalization within the prior 4 weeks), the likelihood of PE is low and no further testing or no AC is required (Konstantinides et al., 2019; Lim et al., 2018).

For PE, planar ventilation–perfusion (VQ) lung scan or computed tomography pulmonary angiography (CTPA) is used to diagnose PE (Lim et al., 2018). A VQ scan measures the distribution of blood and air flow in the lungs. The results are reported as high, intermediate, or low probability or normal. A normal scan excludes clinically important PE and is sufficient evidence to withhold anticoagulant therapy. An abnormal scan, even though it might suggest PE, can result from other disease states. Both a VQ scan and a CTPA have high specificity (>95%) but a CTPA has higher sensitivity compared to a VQ scan. For patients with high PTP of PE, the guidelines recommend a CTPA as the initial diagnostic test. For patients with intermediate PTP of PE, the guidelines recommend a VQ scan as the initial diagnostic test. Disadvantages to CTPA include radiation exposure and the need for injected contrast agent and subsequent risk of renal impairment. A VQ scan is also preferred in patients who are at risk of contrast nephropathy such as those with preexisting kidney disease or hypotension. Both CTPA and VQ lung scanning can reliably exclude the diagnosis of PE. For patients with low PTP of PE, the guidelines recommend evaluating the results of a highly sensitive D-dimer test. If positive, diagnostic testing should proceed with a VQ scan (Lim et al., 2018).

Atrial Fibrillation

Symptoms associated with AF include palpitations, chest discomfort, shortness of breath, fatigue, hypotension, dizziness, and syncope. Clinical signs of AF include acute HF, pulmonary edema, exertional dyspnea, and possibly hemodynamic instability (Kirchhof et al., 2016). On physical examination, findings of an irregular pulse, irregular jugular venous pulsations, variations in the intensity of the first heart sound (S_1), or signs of associated valvular heart disease can guide the practitioner in suspecting AF. The ECG is used to confirm the diagnosis; an irregularly irregular rhythm is the hallmark of AF. Other ECG characteristics include the absence of P waves and ventricular response rates of 100 to 180 bpm. A thorough history and physical examination is needed to rule out underlying causes of AF. Other baseline assessments include evaluation of electrolytes, thyroid function tests, complete blood count (CBC), and chest radiograph. A sleep study is warranted if sleep apnea is suspected. The diagnostic workup also includes a transthoracic echocardiogram, which can detect left ventricular dysfunction, left ventricular hypertrophy, valvular heart disease, and atrial enlargement. In some cases, a stress test is ordered to rule out the presence of ischemic heart disease. Transesophageal echocardiography is frequently used to identify left atrial thrombi in preparation for electrical cardioversion, which attempts to restore normal sinus rhythm (January et al., 2014).

Nurses and physician assistants can assist with the initial management of AF by remembering the mnemonic *SALTE*—stabilize (monitor heart rate, blood pressure, respiratory status, and medication), assess (fluid and electrolyte status, medication management, risk factor identification, and modification), label/treat (arrhythmia management, reducing anxiety, and AC management), and educate (disease process, AC teaching, and prescribed medications) (McCabe, 2005). Patients with stroke, TIA or risk factors for stroke should be taught the acronym FAST, a mnemonic that stands for facial drooping, arm weakness, speech difficulty, and time to call 911 (Powers et al., 2018).

Ischemic Stroke

Ischemic stroke is characterized by a sudden or progressive onset of focal neurologic signs due to an inadequate blood supply to the brain. The resulting neurologic deficits depend on the location of cerebral infarction. Most often, the deficits are confined to one side of the body, right or left. The most common presenting stroke symptom is tingling, numbness, and weakness or paralysis on one side of the body. Ataxia, aphasia, dysarthria, visual field loss, and sensory loss also can occur. Other manifestations include changes in mental status or loss of consciousness. The time of onset of symptoms is a key piece of historical information to determine from the patient or family members because it will dictate treatment. Neurologic signs or symptoms may progress in approximately 25% of patients in the first 24 to 48 hours. Approximately 50% of patients are left with a permanent disability (Hankey, 2017).

The physical examination may show signs of trauma or seizures (e.g., contusions, tongue lacerations) or carotid disease (bruits). A comprehensive neurological exam is necessary to determine the extent of neurological deficit, identify the possible location of the thrombus, and help determine the most appropriate intervention (Hankey, 2017).

All patients presenting with suspected ischemic stroke require several diagnostic tests, including blood glucose, electrolytes, CBC with platelets, 12-lead ECG, troponin, prothrombin time (PT), INR, activated partial thromboplastin time (aPTT), and oxygen saturation (Hankey, 2017; Powers et al., 2018). Only blood glucose and assessment of INR in patients receiving warfarin should precede the administration of alteplase in candidates eligible for fibrinolysis (Powers et al., 2018).

Brain imaging studies, including noncontrast computerized tomography scan and magnetic resonance imaging, are used to detect the presence, extent, and progression of a cerebral infarction and if there is intracranial bleeding. Several tests can help detect the source of a presumed thromboembolic ischemic stroke. Noninvasive carotid ultrasound will show occlusion or stenosis. An ECG differentiates between AF and MI. Transthoracic and transesophageal echocardiograms visualize cardiac function and the presence of an atrial thrombus. Carotid cerebral angiography can be performed to examine the arteries and veins of the brain and neck. This provides the most accurate visualization to detect abnormalities such as stenosis or occlusion that may have caused the ischemic event (Powers et al., 2019).

Native and Prosthetic Valvular Heart Disease

Signs and symptoms of valvular heart disease vary depending on the valve that is affected. In aortic stenosis, the cardinal symptoms are dyspnea, angina, syncope, and HF. Aortic regurgitation is often asymptomatic. Dyspnea is the hallmark symptom of mitral stenosis, although this usually is present with exertion and has a gradual onset over approximately 20 years. Mitral regurgitation also progresses slowly and may be asymptomatic for many years. The initial symptoms may be fatigue, dyspnea on exertion, and palpitations that, in severe cases, may lead to pulmonary edema. Each valvular disorder is associated with a characteristic murmur, but the intensity of the murmur does not always correlate with the severity of the valvular disorder (Maganti et al., 2010).

Findings on physical examination also vary with the severity of the valve calcification, severity of stenosis, and left ventricular dysfunction. The chest radiograph will show cardiomegaly, which can occur with aortic stenosis. A 12-lead ECG is used to determine the possible cardiac effects of valve incompetence or stenosis such as left ventricular hypertrophy in mitral and aortic regurgitation. Confirmation of the diagnosis of valvular disease is best accomplished by an echocardiogram, which will also give an estimate of disease severity. Cardiac catheterization and angiography are used when noninvasive tests are inconclusive. When physical symptoms of valvular disease lead to limitations in daily activities or if cardiac decompensation occurs despite medical treatment, surgical intervention either with surgical repair, surgical valve replacement, or minimally invasive transcatheter aortic valve replacement (TAVR) is recommended (Maganti et al., 2010).

INITIATING DRUG THERAPY

AC is the cornerstone of stroke prevention in AF as well as acute treatment and secondary prevention of DVT/PE. Antiplatelet therapy is indicated for prevention of DVT/PE in patients undergoing orthopedic surgery as well as secondary prevention of stroke. An overview of drugs used in thromboembolic disorders is presented in **Table 49.1**.

TABLE 49.1

Overview of Drugs Used in Thromboembolic Disorders

Generic (Trade) Name	Dosage	Selected Adverse Effects	Contraindications[1]	Special Considerations[2]
Unfractionated heparin	Initial IV bolus and continuous infusion; Varies based on indication and dose adjusted via nomogram	Bleeding, HIT	Active bleeding, recent history of HIT	Dose adjusted to aPTT or anti-Xa level via a nomogram
Enoxaparin (Lovenox)	For VTE: 1 mg/kg subcutaneous BID	Bleeding, HIT	Active bleeding, recent history of HIT	Dose adjustment in renal disease required
Dalteparin (Fragmin)	For VTE treatment: 200 IU/kg subcutaneous every 24 h or 100 IU/kg subcutaneous BID	Bleeding, HIT	Active bleeding, recent history of HIT	
Fondaparinux	For VTE treatment: Body weight > 100 kg: 10 mg subcutaneously once daily; body weight 50–100 kg: 7.5 mg subcutaneous once daily; body weight < 50 kg: 5 mg subcutaneous once daily	Bleeding	Active bleeding, CrCl < 30 mL/min	
Warfarin (Coumadin) (Jantoven)	Typical initial dose 5 mg PO daily but varies by patient characteristics (see WARFARINDOSING.org), dose adjusted based on INR	Bleeding	Active bleeding, pregnancy	Numerous drug–food, drug–drug, and drug–herbal interactions; narrow therapeutic index drug
Apixaban (Eliquis)	For AF: 5 mg PO BID For VTE treatment: Initial therapy: 10 mg PO BID for 7 days followed by 5 mg PO BID For secondary prevention of VTE following initial treatment: Either 5 mg PO BID or 2.5 mg PO BID	Bleeding	Active bleeding Avoid use with drugs that are combined P-gp and strong CYP3A4 inducers	For AF: Dose adjusted for 2 of the following: SCr ≥ 1.5 mg/dL, age ≥ 80 years, or body weight ≤ 60 kg Reduce dose or avoid use with combined P-gp and strong CYP3A4 inhibitors
Dabigatran (Pradaxa)	150 mg PO BID	Bleeding, dyspepsia, gastritis-like symptoms	Active bleeding	Dose adjustment in renal disease and certain P-gp inhibitors required
Edoxaban (Savaysa)	60 mg PO daily	Bleeding	Active bleeding For AF: CrCl > 95 mL/min	Dose adjustment in renal disease and with certain P-gp inhibitors required
Rivaroxaban (Xarelto)	For AF: 20 mg PO daily For initial VTE treatment: 15 mg PO BID for 21 days followed by 20 mg PO daily For secondary prevention of VTE following initial treatment: Either 20 mg PO daily or 10 mg PO daily	Bleeding	Active bleeding Avoid use with drugs that are combined P-gp and CYP3A4 inducers Avoid use with certain combined P-gp and strong CYP3A4 inhibitors	Dose adjustment in renal disease required in AF Doses larger than 10 mg must be taken with a meal
Aspirin	Low-dose aspirin: 81 mg PO daily	Bleeding	Active bleeding	Initial dose for acute ischemic stroke is 325 mg
Clopidogrel	For secondary prevention of ischemic stroke and TIA: 75 mg PO daily For secondary prevention of minor stroke or high-risk TIA: initial dose 300 mg followed by 75 mg daily on days 2 to 21 with aspirin 81 mg PO daily	Bleeding, rash, TTP (rare)	Active bleeding	

(Continued)

TABLE 49.1

Overview of Drugs Used in Thromboembolic Disorders (Continued)

Generic (Trade) Name	Dosage	Selected Adverse Effects	Contraindications[1]	Special Considerations[2]
Ticagrelor	For secondary prevention of ischemic stroke and TIA: 180 mg PO loading dose followed by 90 mg PO BID on days 2 to 30 with aspirin 81 mg PO daily	Bleeding, rash, dyspnea	Active bleeding	
Aspirin/Extended-release Dipyridamole (Aggrenox)	For secondary prevention of ischemic stroke: 1 capsule (25 mg aspirin and 200 mg extended-release dipyridamole) BID	Headache, dizziness, GI intolerance, flushing, rash, pruritus, bleeding	Active bleeding	

[1]See text for additional contraindications.

[2]See text for discussion regarding use of anticoagulants in patients receiving neuraxial anesthesia.

AF, atrial fibrillation; aPTT, activated partial thromboplastin time; CrCl, creatinine clearance; GI, gastrointestinal; HIT, heparin-induced thrombocytopenia; INR, international normalized ratio; IV, intravenous; P-gp, P-glycoprotein; TIA, transient ischemic attack; TTP, thrombotic thrombocytopenic purpura; VTE, venous thromboembolism.

Goals of Drug Therapy

Preventing the development of an ischemic stroke is the primary goal of antithrombotic therapy in patients with AF and prosthetic heart valves and in those with a history of cardioembolic stroke. AC treatment in patients with existing DVT/PE is initiated to prevent extension of the thrombus; thromboembolic complications, including postthrombotic syndrome; and development of a new thrombus. Aspirin may be used for secondary prevention of DVT/PE in selected patients after initial AC therapy for at least 6 months (Witt et al., 2018). Antithrombotic prophylaxis after orthopedic surgery is initiated with aspirin or AC to decrease the risk of DVT or PE (Anderson et al., 2019). Aspirin is used for primary prevention of ischemic stroke in patients with a 10-year atherosclerotic cardiovascular disease (ASCVD) risk score of at least 20% (Arnett et al., 2019). For patients presenting with minor stroke or TIA and without AF, dual antiplatelet therapy (DAPT) with aspirin and clopidogrel is recommended for 21 days with aspirin continued thereafter indefinitely (Campbell et al., 2019). Clopidogrel may also be used as single antiplatelet therapy for secondary prevention of ischemic stroke in patients without AF (Campbell et al., 2019). Aspirin is no longer recommended as stroke prevention in patients with AF (January et al., 2019). Other indications for antiplatelet therapy for primary or secondary prevention of cardiovascular disease events will not be discussed in this chapter.

Anticoagulants

Anticoagulants include the injectable agents unfractionated heparin (UFH) and low-molecular-weight heparins (LMWHs) (e.g., enoxaparin), oral vitamin K antagonist (VKA) warfarin,

and the DOACs dabigatran etexilate (a direct thrombin inhibitors), and oral factor Xa inhibitors (rivaroxaban, apixaban, edoxaban, and betrixaban) (see **Figure 49.1**).

A valid indication for AC is essential before starting anticoagulant therapy. UFH and LMWHs are used for treatment and secondary prevention of VTE and treatment of acute coronary syndromes. In addition, UFH is used in hospitalized patients undergoing procedures such as cardiothoracic surgery, electrophysiology arrhythmia catheter ablation, cardioversion for AF, and percutaneous coronary intervention as well as in patients undergoing hemodialysis. Warfarin is used in the prevention of valve thrombosis in patients with mechanical heart valves as well as for SPAF, prevention of VTE in patients undergoing orthopedic surgery, and treatment and secondary prevention of VTE. Food and Drug Administration (FDA)–approved indications for DOACs are described in **Table 49.2**.

Contraindications to Anticoagulation

Absolute contraindications to AC are active major bleeding, recent intracranial hemorrhage (ICH), intracranial mass with a high bleeding risk, end-stage liver disease, severe thrombocytopenia, recent trauma or traumatic surgery, the immediate postoperative period after central nervous system (CNS) or ocular surgery, or the presence of spinal catheters and aneurysms (Steinberg et al., 2015). Warfarin is contraindicated in pregnancy, and there are no data with DOACs in pregnancy. Therefore, UFH or LMWH, which does not cross the placenta, is preferred. Active or a recent (within 100 days) history of heparin-induced thrombocytopenia (HIT) is a contraindication to UFH and LMWHs. Neuraxial anesthesia with spinal or epidural catheter placement or removal poses a risk of

TABLE 49.2

Food and Drug Administration–Approved Indications for Direct-Acting Oral Anticoagulants

Drug	Dabigatran	Rivaroxaban	Apixaban	Edoxaban
Stroke and systemic thromboembolism prevention in NVAF	X	X	X	X
Prophylaxis of DVT (which may lead to PE) following hip and knee orthopedic surgery	X	X	X	
For prophylaxis of VTE in acutely ill medical patients		X		
Treatment of DVT and PE	X[1]	X	X	X[1]
To reduce risk of recurrence of DVT and PE in patients previously treated	X	X	X	
To reduce the risk of MACE in patients with chronic CAD and/or PAD		X		

[1]In patients who have been treated with a parenteral anticoagulant for 5–10 days.

CAD, coronary artery disease; DVT, deep vein thrombosis; MACE, major adverse cardiac events; NVAF, nonvalvular atrial fibrillation; PAD, peripheral arterial disease; PE, pulmonary embolism; VTE, venous thromboembolism.

spinal hematoma in the anticoagulated patient. Therefore, the American Society of Regional Anesthesia and Pain Medicine released guidelines regarding timing for neuraxial needle placement and removal relative to UFH, LMWH, and DOAC dose were published (Narouze et al., 2018).

Anticoagulants: Considerations Before Starting Therapy

In addition to a valid indication, several patient factors also warrant consideration to determine if the risk of major hemorrhage outweighs the benefit of therapy.

Baseline laboratory values including PT, INR, aPTT, urinalysis, CBC (with platelet count), and a liver profile are recommended before initiating AC. In women of childbearing age, laboratory testing for β-human chorionic gonadotropin is strongly encouraged to rule out pregnancy. Obtaining the patient's telephone number and an alternative contact, such as a responsible family member or neighbor (obtain consent to contact others per the Health Insurance Portability and Accountability Act rules), is also advised. In addition, rule out any active major bleeding from the CNS or gastrointestinal (GI) tract. A digital rectal examination or guaiac test to detect blood in the stool is recommended. A detailed medical, surgical, and medication history, including over-the-counter (OTC) medications and dietary supplements, is needed to assess the patient's risk of bleeding events or inadequate AC. It is also important to document the indication for AC, which determines the duration of therapy, and, if warfarin is selected, to define the corresponding target INR, which defines the intensity of AC. When all these issues are addressed, AC is initiated (Witt, 2010). For patients receiving an LMWH or DOAC, body weight (kg), serum creatinine, and estimation of renal function creatinine clearance (CrCl) should be calculated. For patient receiving UFH, body weight (kg) should also be obtained. Although not currently recommended as a routine practice, a bleeding risk estimate for patients with AF may be obtained from calculating the HAS-BLED score and is discussed later in this chapter (see **Box 49.2**).

Parenteral Anticoagulants: Unfractionated Heparin and Low-Molecular-Weight Heparin

UFH and LMWH are used for the treatment of acute venous or arterial thrombosis and prophylaxis of DVT/PE.

Unfractionated Heparin

Mechanism of Action.   UFH inhibits reactions that lead to clotting, but it does not alter the concentration of the normal clotting factors of the blood. When UFH binds to antithrombin III, the shape of the structure changes, which increases the inactivation rate of the intrinsic clotting cascade pathway, including activated clotting factors XII, XI, X, and IX and thrombin (factor II). Once active thrombosis has developed, UFH inhibits further coagulation by inactivating thrombin and preventing the conversion of fibrinogen to fibrin. UFH is a very large molecule (i.e., it has an average molecular weight of 15,000 Da with chains of 18 to 50 saccharide units), but only a small portion of the entire structure is necessary for binding with antithrombin III. Because the structure is so large, UFH can bind to both factors Xa and thrombin. Heparin derivatives with smaller structures cannot bind to thrombin but can bind to and inhibit factor Xa (Hirsh et al., 2008). One disadvantage of heparin's large size is that it cannot inactivate clot-bound thrombin or activated factor X that is bound to platelets. Clot-bound thrombin can continue to generate more thrombin, activate platelets, and convert fibrinogen into fibrin, promoting clotting. In contrast to UFH, direct thrombin inhibitors do not activate platelets (Spyropoulos, 2008).

Heparin is not absorbed from the GI tract, so it must be administered parenterally. UFH has an immediate onset of action and is administered by intravenous (IV) infusion when rapid AC is needed, as in acute DVT, PE, or acute coronary syndromes. UFH may also be administered subcutaneously with peak levels occurring at 2 to 4 hours after administration, depending on the dose. Subcutaneous dosing must be at a sufficient amount to overcome the lower bioavailability, approximately 30%, associated with this route of administration. The duration of action and half-life are dose dependent. The average half-life is 30 to 180 minutes, which may be significantly prolonged at high doses. UFH is metabolized by liver heparinase and the reticuloendothelial system and possibly secondarily in the kidneys. It is then excreted in urine as unchanged drug.

Limitations of UFH include variability in its size, anticoagulant activity, and pharmacokinetic profile. UFH can range in size from 5,000 to 30,000 Da. Agents with higher molecular weights are cleared from the circulation more rapidly than agents with lower molecular weights. UFH is highly bound to plasma proteins and cellular components, including endothelial cells and macrophages, which reduces its therapeutic effect and increases the incidence of immunologic reactions (e.g., HIT). Furthermore, some patients exhibit heparin resistance. This is characterized by no measurable change in anticoagulant effect despite receiving large doses (35,000 units) of heparin daily. UFH also has a nonlinear dose response, so that small changes in dosage can result in large changes in anticoagulant effect (Hirsh et al., 2008).

Dosage and Monitoring Patient Response. Before initiating UFH therapy, define the target aPTT, establish the frequency of aPTT monitoring, and determine the duration of therapy. UFH treatment dosing is based on weight. Initial dosing for treatment of VTE is 80 units/kg as an IV bolus and then 18 units/kg/hour as a continuous IV infusion. UFH's effect is monitored by aPTT or anti-Xa level. Dosage changes should be made based on aPTT levels monitored every 6 hours until the patient is stable and then every 12 to 24 hours. Each individual hospital defines a reagent-specific aPTT therapeutic range depending upon an antifactor Xa concentration—aPTT curve. Hospitals construct a dosing algorithm for dose adjustment depending on the resultant aPTT or utilize heparin anti-Xa activity measures directly. One popular method is the weight-based nomogram (Hirsh et al., 2008) shown in **Table 49.3**.

TABLE 49.3

Weight-Based Heparin Dosing Nomogram

Activated Partial Thromboplastin Time	Rate Change
Initial dose	80 units/kg bolus, then 18 units/kg/h
<35 s	80 units/kg bolus, then increase infusion by 4 units/kg/h
35–45 s	40 units/kg/h bolus, then increase infusion by 2 units/kg/h
46–70 s	No change (Therapeutic range determined by anti-Xa calibration curve 0.3–0.7 IU/mL)
71–90 s	Decrease infusion rate by 2 units/kg/h
>90 s	Hold infusion for 1 h; then decrease infusion rate by 3 units/kg/h

AC may be subtherapeutic or supratherapeutic despite the use of validated dosing protocols. UFH in a fixed low dose of 5,000 units subcutaneously every 8 to 12 hours is used for VTE prophylaxis. This regimen may be used in postoperative patients and acutely ill medical patients (Anderson et al., 2019; Schünemann et al., 2018).

Low-Molecular-Weight Heparins and Fondaparinux

Mechanism of Action. LMWHs are fragments of UFH, prepared by the depolymerization of porcine heparin. Like UFH, LMWHs produce their major anticoagulant effect via thrombin and factor Xa. Fondaparinux is a synthetic specific inhibitor of factor Xa. LMWHs are used for prophylaxis of VTE in patients after orthopedic and abdominal surgery, in acutely ill medical patients with decreased mobility or increased risk of VTE, and for treatment of DVT/PE. Fondaparinux (Arixtra) is used for VTE prophylaxis in surgical patients and in treatment of VTE. As with UFH, most patients need subsequent treatment with warfarin or a DOAC, depending on the indication for AC. Other uses that will not be discussed in this chapter include the treatment of acute coronary syndromes. Two LMWHs are available in the United States: dalteparin (Fragmin) and enoxaparin (Lovenox).

LMWH bind to antithrombin III and preferentially inhibit activated factor Xa with minimal effects of thrombin (factor IIa) because of their size. The average molecular weight of LMWHs ranges from 4,000 to 6,500 Da with 13 to 22 saccharide units. (UFH has a mean molecular weight of 12,000 to 15,000 Da with 18 to 50 saccharide units.) Only the LMWHs with saccharide chains having 18 or more units can bind to and inhibit thrombin. UFH has a ratio of anti-Xa to anti-IIa activity of 1:1, and the anti-Xa to anti-IIa activity of LMWHs ranges from 2:1 to 4:1 (Hirsh et al., 2008).

LMWHs given by the subcutaneous route have a bioavailability of greater than 90% of the given dose. In contrast to UFH, LMWHs have minimal binding to cells or plasma proteins, which results in the persistence of free drug in the circulation and a longer half-life of activity. The half-lives of LMWHs range from 108 to 252 minutes. Dosing is fixed in prophylaxis but is based on weight for treatment. The peak effect occurs at approximately 4 hours following a subcutaneous dose.

Dosage and Monitoring Patient Response. As previously noted, the major antithrombotic and bleeding effects of LMWHs arise through their ability to inactivate factor Xa. UFH is monitored using aPTT, which primarily reflects anti-activated factor II (IIa) activity, but LMWHs have minimal effects on the aPTT. Theoretically, LMWHs may be monitored by anti-Xa activity, with a target range for treatment regimens of a chromogenic anti-Xa peak of 0.5 to 1.2 units/mL measured 3 to 4 hours after a subcutaneous dose. Studies have demonstrated that the anti-Xa effect of LMWHs is linearly related to the dose administered. Therefore, plasma levels are predictable, and anti-Xa activity monitoring is not routinely performed. Monitoring may be considered in selected patients, such as those with renal dysfunction because LMWHs are cleared primarily by the renal route, morbidly obese patients (>150 kg) because weight-adjusted dosing has not been evaluated in patients with severe obesity, and pregnant patients because their weight changes, volume shifts occur, and clearance changes as pregnancy progresses. However, the American Society of Hematology (ASH) recommends against such monitoring for LMWHs because of concerns related to anti-Xa assay standardization and variability and a lack of evidence that correlates levels with bleeding events (Witt et al., 2018). Therefore, obese patients should be dosed based upon total body weight, and usual manufacturer recommendations regarding dosing in kidney disease should be followed. Because of a lack of data in patients with end-stage kidney disease (CrCl < 15 mL/min), most clinicians avoid preferring using UFH over LMWH in those patients.

Each LMWH has a unique dosing regimen because of its unique chemical properties and the relative proportions of anti-Xa to anti-IIa activity. Because of differences in the manufacturing process, molecular weight, half-life, ratio of anti-Xa to anti-IIa activity, and dose, the FDA does not consider these agents therapeutically interchangeable (Hirsh et al., 2008). Enoxaparin at 30 mg every 12 hours or 40 mg daily is currently approved for prophylaxis in medical inpatients and patients after hip, knee, and abdominal surgery. Dalteparin at 2,500 international units every 12 hours or 5,000 units daily is approved for prophylaxis in patients after hip and abdominal surgery. For VTE treatment, current FDA-approved dosing for enoxaparin is 1 mg/kg subcutaneous every 12 hours or 1.5 mg/kg daily subcutaneous for inpatients with acute DVT with and without PE when administered in conjunction with warfarin and for outpatients with acute DVT without PE when administered in conjunction with warfarin. Dosing adjustment is required for enoxaparin in patients with CrCl less than 30 mL/min. Dalteparin is dosed at 100 international units/kg subcutaneous every 12 hours or 200 international units/kg every 24 hours for patients with acute DVT with or without PE. Fondaparinux has a longer half-life than LMWHs and is administered as a once-daily dose for VTE prophylaxis (2.5 mg/d) and treatment (5 mg/d for patients weighing <50 kg, 7.5 mg/d for patients weighing 50 to 100 kg, and 10 mg/d for patients weighing >100 kg). Fondaparinux is contraindicated for VTE prophylaxis in patients weighing less than 50 kg due to increased bleeding risk and as well as patients with CrCl less than 30 mL/min for all indications (see **Table 49.1**). The use of UFH, fondaparinux, and LMWH for acute coronary syndromes will not be discussed in this chapter.

Selection Considerations Between Low-Molecular-Weight Heparins and Unfractionated Heparin

Advantages of LMWHs and fondaparinux over UFH include greater bioavailability with subcutaneous administration; longer duration of anticoagulant effect, allowing for once-daily or twice-daily dosing; high degree of correlation between anti-Xa

and body weight, allowing for fixed dosing; less intensive nursing care; and less intensive laboratory monitoring and more predictable anticoagulant response, permitting use in the outpatient setting (Hull & Pineo, 2004).

Adverse Effects

Patients are carefully assessed for bleeding including hematuria and GI bleeding/blood in stools or hemoptysis. Reversal of AC is discussed later in this chapter.

Platelet counts should be closely monitored during UFH and LMWH therapy because a drop in platelet count below 150×10^9/L or greater than 50% of baseline necessitates an evaluation for heparin-induced thrombocytopenia (HIT), antibody-mediated prothrombotic reaction. This immune-mediated thrombocytopenia, HIT, has been reported in less than 1% of patients. The incidence of thrombocytopenia is lower with LMWH than with UFH. Clinical effects of HIT can result in DVT, PE, MI, limb ischemia, gangrene requiring limb amputation, cerebral thrombosis, and death. Suspected HIT should be evaluated using the "4Ts" score: Thrombocytopenia, Timing, Thrombosis, and oTher. Patients with a low-probability score of 3 or less can continue UFH/LMWH. In patients with an intermediate or high score of 4 or more, all sources of UFH or LMWH (such as heparin flushes and heparin-coated catheters, infusions, and subcutaneous injections) should be discontinued, a functional diagnostic test, such as the enzyme-linked immunosorbent assay (ELISA) antibody test, performed, and therapeutic AC with a nonheparin alternative anticoagulant started. The 2018 ASH guidelines recommend bivalirudin or argatroban as well as fondaparinux and DOACs. If the ELISA test is negative, UFH/LMWH can be resumed as the test has high sensitivity. However, if positive, alternate AC is continued and a more specific diagnostic test, a serotonin-release assay (SRA), is performed. Both ELISA and SRA tests may take several days for results to be available. Most clinicians use bivalirudin and argatroban for the acute phase of HIT, especially if there is thrombosis, until the platelet count normalizes (>150×10^9/L). After the platelet count is normal, therapeutic AC is typically continued out to 6 weeks using less expensive, but less studied, fondaparinux or a DOAC (Cuker et al., 2018).

Vitamin K Antagonist (Warfarin)
Mechanism of Action

Warfarin inhibits activation of the clotting factors in the liver that depend on vitamin K for synthesis—factors II, VII, IX, and X and the coagulation inhibitor proteins C, Z, and S. Warfarin interferes with the conversion of vitamin K from its inactive form to active vitamin K. Vitamin K is depleted, and the rate of clotting factor formation is decreased, which ultimately prevents clot formation and extension. Warfarin does not affect the function of existing clotting factors and has no effect on an existing thrombus (Ansell et al., 2008).

Time Frame for Response

A significant limitation to warfarin is its long onset of effect. The half-lives of clotting factors range from 6 hours (factor VII) to 60 hours (factor II) (Tran & Ginsberg, 2006).

The average half-life of warfarin is 36 to 42 hours. The onset of anticoagulant effect depends on both the half-life of warfarin and the time required to deplete the vitamin K–dependent clotting factors.

Dosage and Monitoring Patient Response

Because of its long half-life, warfarin is administered once daily. Warfarin is completely absorbed after oral administration and is metabolized to inactive metabolites by the liver. Warfarin has a narrow therapeutic window; therefore, the dose needed to exert clinical efficacy is similar to the dose that causes adverse effects. Individual patients vary widely in their ability to absorb and eliminate warfarin (pharmacokinetic variations) and in their rate of clinical response and dosage requirements (pharmacodynamic variations). Patient variability in the dose response to warfarin is not related to weight or sex but is influenced by age, comorbid disease states, concomitant medications, and one's genetically predetermined rate of metabolism (Ageno et al., 2012).

The anticoagulant effect of warfarin is monitored with the INR, which is derived from the PT (**Table 49.4** and **Box 49.3**). The INR will show an initial prolongation 1 to 3 days after warfarin is first administered, which is due to the rapid depletion of factor VII. However, the full antithrombotic effect of warfarin will not be seen for 8 to 14 days, when factor II (prothrombin) is depleted. In cases of acute DVT or PE, UFH or LMWHs is often given with warfarin when rapid AC is needed or in hypercoagulable patients (protein C or S deficiency). Warfarin causes a quick fall in protein C (half-life of 8 to 10 hours), which can induce a temporary hypercoagulable state, putting patients at risk for thrombosis. The injectable anticoagulant is continued along with warfarin for at least 5 days until the INR is stable for at least 2 days, which allows for additional reductions in the levels of factors X and II (Ageno et al., 2012). During therapy in hospitalized patients, daily CBCs and platelet counts are usually obtained and daily INRs with warfarin to determine the dose.

If the patient receives a prescription for warfarin, the prescriber needs to choose among nine different dosage strengths and colors (e.g., a 1-mg tablet is pink, whereas a 5-mg tablet

---

TABLE 49.4

Relationship between the Prothrombin Time Ratio and the International Normalized Ratio for Thromboplastins with Varying International Sensitivity Index Values

Hospital	ISI	Control PT (s)	PT (s)	PT ratio	INR
A	1.3	14.8	33.9	2.3	2.9
B	2.3	11.4	18.2	1.6	2.9

Note: The INR takes into account the differences in thromboplastin sensitivity, thus giving a more accurate reflection of the level of anticoagulation.

PT, prothrombin time; PT ratio, observed PT divided by control PT; ISI, International Sensitivity Index; INR, international normalized ratio (INR = PT ratio^{ISI}).

BOX 49.3 International Normalized Ratio: Test for Warfarin Monitoring

The INR is the universally accepted laboratory test for monitoring anticoagulation therapy with the VKAs (e.g., warfarin). PT is the time in seconds for a blood sample to clot after the addition of laboratory reagents, including specific plasma proteins (tissue thromboplastins) that aid in coagulation. PT measures the reduction in three of the four vitamin K–dependent clotting factors (II, VII, and X) of the extrinsic coagulation cascade. The PT ratio is simply the patient's individual PT divided by a laboratory's control PT. A change in the tissue thromboplastin source from human brain to rabbit brain 40 years ago resulted in a reduced sensitivity in the PT test, leading to lower PT values, and accordingly higher PT ratio goals, with subsequent increased bleeding risk. The International Sensitivity Index (ISI) was developed by the World Health Organization (WHO) as a reference standard to correct this problem.

Mathematically, the INR is the PT ratio raised to the power of the ISI, or INR = PT ratio^{ISI}. The ISI for commercially available tissue thromboplastins varies between individual lots and manufacturers. The WHO reference standard was assigned an ISI of 1.0, although most commercial laboratories use tissue thromboplastins with ISIs ranging from 1.0 to 2.88. The ISI for a particular reagent is identified in the package insert. The INR can be determined using a calculator, if needed.

Most laboratories commonly report PT and INR. However, only the INR should be used for warfarin dosing changes. Relying on the INR minimizes variability in reported results if different laboratories, with different thromboplastin preparations, are used. The INR represents the best method for standardizing results from different thromboplastin reagents. The American College of Chest Physicians has standardized the desired target INR goal for anticoagulation therapy for each clinical indication. Current guidelines recommend an INR range of 2 to 3 for most indications of anticoagulation. INRs of 2.5 to 3.5 are reserved for patients with certain prosthetic heart valves. The PT and INR may be elevated in the presence of certain DOACs, for example, dabigatran and rivaroxaban, but should not be used for dosage adjustments.

Data adapted from Ansell, J., Hirsh, J., Hylek, E., et al. (2008). Pharmacology and management of the VKAs: American College of Chest Physicians evidence-based clinical practice guidelines (8th ed.). *Chest, 133*(6 Suppl.), 160S–198S.

is peach). For safety's sake and to avoid confusing the patient, prescribe only one warfarin tablet strength (e.g., 2.5- or 5-mg tablets, but not both) where possible. Patients also need to be taught to remember the tablet color, shape, and tablet strength with each new prescription and refill.

The goal INR for various indications is described in **Box 49.4**. It is difficult to predict an individual's warfarin requirement needed to reach the INR range that is considered therapeutic for the disease state. The initial dose of warfarin is typically 5 to 10 mg/d orally administered for 1 to 3 days. Certain patient populations, such as the older adults, patients experiencing malnutrition, those with congestive

HF, underlying malignancy, with severely impaired renal or hepatic function, or those taking interacting drugs that increase warfarin's effect, are at high risk for bleeding, and lower initial starting doses (≤5 mg) are appropriate. Larger starting doses, such as 7.5 to 10 mg, may be used in younger patients without comorbid conditions if rapid effect is urgently needed, but this is unnecessary for most patients. During the initial titration phase, daily dosage increases or decreases are commonly made in 2- to 2.5-mg increments based on INR values. Administering warfarin at the same time daily is recommended to reduce variability in effects. Warfarin is overlapped with an injectable anticoagulant in patients with acute VTE and in patients with AF at high risk of stroke or those with AF who were recently cardioverted. This overlap process is referred to as "bridging" to therapeutic AC (Ageno et al., 2012).

The relationship between the warfarin dose and the INR is not linear. Therefore, minor changes in dose can result in greater than expected changes in the INR. The maintenance warfarin dose varies widely among individuals. Questions to ask to help determine the cause of an out-of-range INR in a patient previously stabilized on warfarin are described in **Box 49.5**.

BOX 49.4 Target International Normalized Ratios for Thrombosis Prevention with Vitamin K Antagonists

INR GOAL 1.5 TO 2.0

Mechanical On-X aortic valve in patients without other risk factors for stroke (e.g., AF)

INR GOAL 2.0 TO 2.5

Patients with a disease-specific AC goal of 2.0 to 3.0 (see in the following point, excluding valves) who also are taking DAPT with both aspirin and a P2Y12 inhibitor

INR GOAL 2.0 TO 3.0

Prophylaxis of VTE
Treatment of DVT
Treatment of PE
Stroke prevention in AF
Tissue (bioprosthetic) heart valves with other risk factors for stroke
Mechanical prosthetic heart valves (bileaflet valves or single-valve tilting disk; e.g., St. Jude Medical, Medtronic Hall) in the aortic position with no additional risk factors for stroke (e.g., AF)
For 3 to 6 months following bioprosthetic aortic or mitral valve surgery in patients at low risk of bleeding
Hypercoagulable conditions (aPL antibodies with LA)— certain patients with thromboembolism

INR GOAL 2.5 TO 3.5

Mechanical prosthetic heart valves (caged ball, tilting disk) in the mitral position or in the aortic position for patients with additional stroke risk factors (e.g., AF)
Hypercoagulable conditions (aPL antibodies with LA)— if a history of thromboembolic events with INR of 2 to 3

AC, anticoagulant; AF, atrial fibrillation; aPL, antiphospholiid; DAPT, dual antiplatelet therapy; DVT, deep vein thrombosis; international normalized ratio; LA, lupus anticoagulant; PE, pulmonary embolism; VTE, venous thromboembolism.

BOX 49.5 Questions to Ask When International Normalized Ratio Results Are Unexpected

- Have any warfarin doses been missed in the past 7 to 10 days? May decrease INR.
- Have extra warfarin tablets been ingested? May increase INR.
- Is the patient taking a warfarin regimen other than prescribed?
- Is the patient experiencing bleeding problems?
- Is the patient experiencing thromboembolic complications?
- Have any new medications (prescription, OTC, herbal) been started, deleted, or changed from the patient's medication regimen?
- Has the patient's underlying condition changed, as in acute HF exacerbation or worsening renal or hepatic impairment? May increase INR.
- Has the patient had a recent acute febrile or GI illness with diarrhea? May increase INR.
- Has thyroid status changed? Hyperthyroidism may increase INR and new hypothyroidism may decrease the INR.
- Has a malignancy been diagnosed? Patient is at increased risk of thromboembolism and bleeding. INRs may be fluctuating and difficult to maintain in the therapeutic range.

GI, gastrointestinal; INR, international normalized ratio; OTC, over the counter.

For maintenance therapy changes, calculating the total weekly warfarin dose and then increasing or decreasing the weekly regimen by only 10% to 20%, spread over the course of the week, can cause measurable changes in the INR. Some clinicians advocate administering the same dosage daily, whereas others agree that giving varying doses on alternate days is rational. Patients with low educational levels and cognitive impairments or those receiving several other medications may benefit from a simple dosing schedule. If an alternating-day regimen is chosen, defining the actual dosage for each day of the week is recommended (e.g., 5 mg administered on Tuesdays, Thursdays, Saturdays, and Sundays and 7.5 mg on Mondays, Wednesday, and Fridays, rather than 5 mg alternating with 7.5 mg every other day). This helps to reduce patient's confusion and avoid fluctuations in the INR. Sensitive patients with reduced requirements should receive warfarin daily rather than alternating between drug and drug-free days, for example, 1.5 mg given every day, rather than 2 mg alternating with 1 mg every other day (Ansell et al., 2008). Once a patient has reached a therapeutic INR with a consistent warfarin dose, INR monitoring should continue at least every 4 weeks. Patients with a stable INR, defined as no dosing adjustments needed to maintain the INR in the therapeutic range for 3 or more consecutive months, may be monitored up to every 6 to 12 weeks (Witt et al., 2018).

Warfarin dose initiation was described earlier. Several dosing nomograms and calculators are also available to assist in making maintenance dose changes (see **Box 49.2**). It is important to note that these nomograms were developed in patients who were not taking interacting medications. The addition or subtraction of an interacting medication requires more frequent INR monitoring. If possible, patients taking warfarin should be managed by specialized AC clinics as the clinic-reported patient time spent in the therapeutic INR range is higher than "usual" care and bleeding events lower (Garcia et al., 2008).

When transitioning a patient from a DOAC to warfarin, the prescribing information for each specific DOAC should be consulted. Because the AC response to warfarin is delayed, the DOAC and warfarin should be overlapped for several days if the DOAC is initiated with the INR is therapeutic. The DOAC may also affect coagulation tests, including the INR and therefore one recommended approach is switching to a parenteral anticoagulant, such an LMWH at the time the dose of the DOAC is due and starting warfarin. The LMWH would be discontinued when the INR is in the therapeutic range ("bridging" to warfarin).

Adverse Effects

Patients are carefully assessed for bleeding including hematuria and GI bleeding/blood in stools or hemoptysis. Reversal of AC is discussed later in this chapter.

Interactions

S-Warfarin (the more potent enantiomer) is metabolized by the liver isoenzymes CYP2C9 with minor contribution of CYP3A4. *R*-warfarin (the less potent enantiomer) is primarily metabolized by CYP1A2 with less contribution of CYP3A4 and CYP2C19. Medications that inhibit or are substrates for these isoenzymes may decrease warfarin metabolism and increase the INR. Medications that induce these isoenzymes increase the clearance of warfarin and decrease the INR. The most clinically significant interactions are with fluconazole, amiodarone, sulfamethoxazole–trimethoprim, and metronidazole where single doses result in an immediate increase in INR (Vazquez, 2018). For patients where an interacting drug is clinically indicated, a therapeutic alternative should be considered. If an inducer is coprescribed, monitor the INR within 5 days of adding and consider aggressive warfarin dose increases until a therapeutic INR is achieved. If an inhibitor is coprescribed, monitor the INR within 3 to 5 days and anticipate a 20% to 50% decrease in warfarin dose (Vazquez, 2018). A switch to a noninteracting appropriate DOAC should also be considered. Herbal and nutritional product interactions are described later in this chapter.

Selection Considerations Between Warfarin and Direct-Acting Oral Anticoagulants

While the number of prescriptions of DOACs is rapidly increasing in the United States, about half of all patients requiring chronic AC are still prescribed warfarin (Barnes et al., 2015). However, it has numerous drug–drug interactions (**Table 49.5**), has a very narrow therapeutic index, and requires routine laboratory monitoring of the INR at least every 4 to 12 weeks. Warfarin is appropriate for patients with end-stage kidney disease because information on DOAC safety from clinical trials of DOACs is limited.

Direct-Acting Oral Anticoagulants

Dabigatran etexilate (Pradaxa), rivaroxaban (Xarelto), apixaban (Eliquis), and edoxaban (Savaysa) are DOACs. FDA-approved indications of DOACs are described in **Table 49.2**.

Mechanism of Action

Dabigatran etexilate is a prodrug that is metabolized by blood esterases to dabigatran, which binds to and inhibits thrombin that prevents the conversion of fibrinogen to fibrin. Thrombin is also the most potent stimulator of platelet aggregation (see **Figure 49.1**). Blocking thrombin is an effective method of inhibiting coagulation since thrombin is needed for fibrin formation and to activate factors V, VII, VIII, IX, and XIII. Dabigatran directly inhibits free and clot-bound thrombin. The direct-acting agents, rivaroxaban, apixaban, and edoxaban bind directly to factor Xa and do not require antithrombin like LMWHs do. IV direct thrombin inhibitors are available (e.g., bivalirudin, and argatroban) and are administered via infusion in the hospital and used primarily for percutaneous coronary intervention (bivalirudin) or treatment of HIT (argatroban and bivalirudin).

Dosage and Monitoring Patient Response

One of the most important advantages of the DOACs over warfarin is that the DOACs have a faster onset of action. The time to anticoagulant effect of a DOAC depends on the time

TABLE 49.5

Common Warfarin Drug Interactions

Increase the INR	Decrease the INR
Acetaminophen	Adalimumab
Amiodarone	Carbamazepine
Atazanavir	Cholestyramine
Cannabinoid-containing products	Darunavir
Cimetidine	Eslicarbazepine
Ciprofloxacin	Lopinavir
Clarithromycin	Nafcillin
Cyclosporine	Methimazole
Efavirenz	Phenobarbital
Erythromycin	Phenytoin
Esomeprazole	Rifampin
Fenofibric acid derivatives	Rifamycin
Fluconazole	Ritonavir
Fluorouracil	Vitamin K
Fluvastatin	
Fluoxetine	
Fluvoxamine	
Itraconazole	
Ketoconazole	
Letermovir	
Levofloxacin	
Lovastatin	
Metronidazole	
Methylphenidate	
Miconazole	
Omeprazole	
Phenytoin	
Prednisone	
Rosuvastatin	
Saquinavir	
Simvastatin	
Sulfamethoxazole	
Tamoxifen	
Tezacaftor and ivacaftor (Symdeko)	
Tramadol	
Vemurafenib	
Venetoclax	

to maximum plasma concentration, which typically occurs within 2 to 4 hours of first dose administration. Therefore, bridging between an injectable anticoagulant and a DOAC is not necessary.

The dosing of rivaroxaban and apixaban for the treatment of SPAF and VTE differs (**Tables 49.6–49.8**). Apixaban has the least dependency on renal clearance, and edoxaban has the fewest labeled drug–drug interactions (**Table 49.9**). Edoxaban has a black box warning for SPAF to avoid use in patients with CrCl greater than 95 mL/min due to reduced efficacy for ischemic stroke. Reduced efficacy was not proportional to CrCl and was not apparent in the primary endpoint of stroke or systemic thromboembolism. Dabigatran should be avoided for treatment of VTE in patients taking

P-gp inhibitors (**Table 49.9**) with CrCl < 50 mL/min but not for SPAF. Dosing for patients with renal insufficiency and end-stage kidney disease on hemodialysis are inconsistent for rivaroxaban based on indication.

Determining a patient's past history of medication adherence is also recommended because dabigatran and apixaban require twice-daily dosing, and anticoagulant efficacy will be decreased if a patient misses one dose. Dabigatran cannot be crushed or put in weekly pillboxes to help with compliance because it is packaged in moisture-proof containers. Rivaroxaban doses greater than 10 mg, as well as betrixaban should be taken with a meal.

In a patient transitioning from warfarin to a DOAC, warfarin should be discontinued and the DOAC should be started when the INR is at the lower end of the warfarin therapeutic range. In a patient transitioning from UFH to a DOAC, discontinue UFH at the time that the DOAC is administered. In a patient transitioning from LMWH to a DOAC, discontinue the LMWH and administer the DOAC at the time of the next scheduled LMWH dose. When switching between DOACs, give the first dose of the new DOAC at the time the previous DOAC scheduled dose was due.

Adverse Effects

Patients are carefully assessed for bleeding including hematuria and GI bleeding/blood in stools or hemoptysis. Reversal of AC is discussed later in this chapter. Other than bleeding, DOACs are well tolerated. Notably, as many as 30% of patients taking dabigatran may experience GI upset which may lead to discontinuation (Chan et al., 2016). Taking dabigatran with food may or may not alleviate the GI upset.

Interactions

The DOACs have fewer drug–drug interactions compared to warfarin (**Table 49.9**). However, unlike warfarin where you can increase the frequency of INR monitoring to accommodate the drug interaction, drug interactions with DOACs require either a dose reduction or avoidance with a switch to warfarin. Dabigatran requires dose reduction (or avoid use) with certain P-gp inhibitors. Inducers of P-glycoprotein (P-gp) (e.g., rifampin, carbamazepine, phenytoin, St. John's wort) should be avoided with all DOACs. Apixaban and rivaroxaban should be avoided with a drug that is a combined P-gp inhibitor and a strong CYP3A4 inhibitor (e.g., ketoconazole and ritonavir), especially in patients with renal dysfunction. Although clarithromycin is a combined P-gp and strong CYP3A4 inhibitor, it does not require dose adjustment for apixaban and rivaroxaban. When combined with a P-gp inhibitor, the dose of dabigatran should be reduced if the patient's CrCl is 30 to 50 mL/min or avoided if the CrCl is < 30 mL/min.

Selection Considerations Between Direct-Acting Oral Anticoagulants and Warfarin

Disadvantages of DOACs compared to warfarin include lack of a specific antidote for reversal of edoxaban, a higher acquisition cost, and potentially a faster offset of action so that adherence is key to a sustained effect.

TABLE 49.6

Dosing and Renal Adjustment for Direct-Acting Oral Anticoagulants for Stroke and Systemic Thromboembolism Prevention in Atrial Fibrillation

	Dabigatran	Rivaroxaban	Apixaban	Edoxaban
SPAF	150 mg BID	20 mg once daily taken with a meal	5 mg BID	60 mg once daily if CrCl is 51–95 mL/min
Renal adjustment	75 mg BID if CrCl is 15–30 mL/min No dosing recommendation if CrCl < 15 mL/min	15 mg daily take with a meal if CrCl ≤ 50[1]	2.5 mg BID if 2 of the following 3 are present: SCr ≥ 1.5 mg/dL, age ≥80 years, or weight ≤ 60 kg No dose adjustment for patients with CrCl < 15 mL/min recommended[1]	Do not use if CrCl > 95 mL/min 30 mg once daily if CrCl is 15–50 mL/min Not recommended in patients with CrCl < 15 mL/min

[1]Dosing for patients with CrCl < 15 mL/min was not studied in clinical trials; therefore, dosing recommendations are based on single-dose pharmacokinetic and pharmacodynamic data in subjects with end-stage kidney disease maintained on hemodialysis.

CrCl, creatinine clearance; SPAF, Stroke Prevention in Atrial Fibrillation.

Source: Pradaxa (dabigatran etexilate mesylate) [prescribing information]. Ridgefield, CT: Boehringer Ingelheim Pharmaceuticals Inc.; 11/2019. Xarelto (rivaroxaban) [prescribing information]. Titusville, NJ: Janssen Pharmaceuticals, Inc.; 03/2020. Eliquis (apixaban) [prescribing information]. Princeton, NJ: Bristol-Myers Squibb Company; 11/2019. Savaysa (edoxaban) [prescribing information]. Parsippany, NJ: Daiichi Sankyo, Inc; 08/2019.

TABLE 49.7

Dosing and Renal Adjustment for Direct-Acting Oral Anticoagulants for Venous Thromboembolism Treatment and Secondary Prevention of Venous Thromboembolism

	Dabigatran	Rivaroxaban	Apixaban	Edoxaban
VTE Treatment				
VTE	Following 5–10 days of parenteral therapy, 150 mg BID	15 mg BID with a meal for 21 days, then 20 mg daily with a meal for the remaining treatment period	10 mg BID for 7 days, then 5 mg BID	Following 5–10 days of parenteral therapy, 50 mg once daily when weight > 60 kg; 30 mg once daily if ≤60 kg
Renal Adjustment	No dosage recommendation if CrCl ≤ 30 mL/min	Avoid use if CrCl < 15 mL/min	No adjustment required[1]	30 mg once daily if CrCl ≤ 15–50 mL/min
VTE Secondary Prevention				
Long-Term Secondary Prevention	150 mg BID	10 mg daily after at least 6 months of standard treatment (as described above)	2.5 mg BID	Not approved for this indication
Renal Adjustment	No dosage recommendations for CrCl ≤ 30 mL/min	Avoid use if CrCl < 15 mL/min	No adjustment required[1]	Not approved for this indication

Note: See Table 49.9 for important drug interactions that affect dosing.

[1]Dosing for patients with CrCl < 30 mL/min was not studied in clinical trials; therefore, dosing recommendations are based on single-dose pharmacokinetic and pharmacodynamic data in subjects with end-stage kidney disease maintained on hemodialysis.

CrCl, creatinine clearance; VTE, venous thromboembolism.

Source: Pradaxa (dabigatran etexilate mesylate) [prescribing information]. Ridgefield, CT: Boehringer Ingelheim Pharmaceuticals Inc.; 11/2019. Xarelto (rivaroxaban) [prescribing information]. Titusville, NJ: Janssen Pharmaceuticals, Inc.; 03/2020. Eliquis (apixaban) [prescribing information]. Princeton, NJ: Bristol-Myers Squibb Company; 11/2019. Savaysa (edoxaban) [prescribing information]. Parsippany, NJ: Daiichi Sankyo, Inc; 08/2019.

TABLE 49.8

Treatment Options for Venous Thromboembolism

Agent	Initial Dosing or Lead In	Maintenance Dosing
Preferred for Hospitalized Inpatients with Renal Insufficiency (<30 mL/min)		
UFH[1]	Weight-based bolus (80 units/kg) followed by weight-based continuous infusion (18 units/kg/h) adjusted to a hospital-specific aPTT or anti-Xa level[2]	
Other Options for VTE Treatment in Hospitalized or Ambulatory Outpatients		
LMWH[3]	**Dalteparin:** 200 IU/kg subcutaneous every 24 h or 100 IU/kg subcutaneous BID	
	Enoxaparin: 1 mg/kg subcutaneous BID or 1.5 mg/kg subcutaneous every 24 h (CrCl ≥ 30 mL/min) 1 mg/kg subcutaneous once daily (CrCl < 30 mL/min)	
Fondaparinux[3]	Body weight (CrCl < 30 mL/min) <50 kg: 5 mg subcutaneous once daily 50–100 kg: 7.5 mg subcutaneous once daily >100 kg: 10 mg subcutaneous once daily	
Warfarin[4]	Bridge with LMWH or UFH ≥ 5 d 0.5–10 mg/d	• 5 mg/d for most patients (lower for older adults or those taking interacting drugs,[4] which reduce warfarin clearance and increase the INR, e.g., 2 mg/d; higher doses for young patients without interacting drugs, e.g., 7.5–10 mg/d) individualized to INR 2.0–3.0
Apixaban[5]	10 mg BID for 7 d followed by 5 mg BID	• Either continue 5 mg BID or reduce dose to 2.5 mg
Dabigatran[5]	5–10 days parenteral anticoagulant	• 150 mg BID (CrCl > 30 mL/min)
Edoxaban[5]	5–10 days parenteral anticoagulant	• 60 mg/d (CrCl > 50 mL/min) • 30 mg/d (CrCl 15–50 mL/min, ≤60 kg, or with some P-gp inhibitors[5])
Rivaroxaban[5]	15 mg BID for 21 days with a meal followed by 20 mg/d with a meal (CrCl ≥ 15 mL/min)	• CrCl ≥ 15 mL/min: 10 mg/d with or without meals

[1]Bridged to a DOAC or warfarin.

[2]See Table 49.3 for an example weight-based dosing nomogram.

[3]Bridged to DOAC or warfarin or may be continued in a patient with active cancer.

[4]See Table 49.4 for interacting drugs.

[5]See Table 49.9 for interacting drugs.

Source: Pradaxa (dabigatran etexilate mesylate) [prescribing information]. Ridgefield, CT: Boehringer Ingelheim Pharmaceuticals Inc.; 11/2019. Xarelto (rivaroxaban) [prescribing information]. Titusville, NJ: Janssen Pharmaceuticals, Inc.; 03/2020. Eliquis (apixaban) [prescribing information]. Princeton, NJ: Bristol-Myers Squibb Company; 11/2019. Savaysa (edoxaban) [prescribing information]. Parsippany, NJ: Daiichi Sankyo, Inc; 08/2019. Arixtra (fondaparinux sodium injection) [prescribing information]. Canonsburg, PA: Mylan Pharmaceuticals, Inc.; 08/2017. Lovenox (enoxaparin sodium injection) [prescribing information]. Bridgewater, NJ: Sanofi Aventis US, LLC; 12/2018. Coumadin (warfarin sodium) [prescribing information]. Princeton, NJ: Bristol-Myers Squibb Company; 12/2019.

Managing Anticoagulation-Related Bleeding

Bleeding is the most worrisome adverse event associated with antithrombotic therapy. In patients with AF, DOACs reduce the risk of major bleeding compared to warfarin. The annual risk of major bleeding is approximately 2% to 3% with DOACs and 3% to 4% with warfarin with fatal bleeding occurring in up to 0.5% (Garg et al., 2016; Kovacs et al., 2015; Werth et al., 2015). In patients with VTE, the annual risk of major bleeding for warfarin and DOACs is approximately 1% to 2% (Werth et al., 2015). The highest risk of bleeding with warfarin, especially ICH, occurs when the INR exceeds a 4 to 5 range. The frequency of major bleeding in patients with a target INR of 2 to 3 is half of that seen in patients with a target INR above 3 (Holbrook et al., 2012). One of the greatest advantages of DOACs over warfarin for SPAF is that they reduce the risk of ICH by more than 50% (Wolfe et al., 2018).

In addition to the intensity of AC, the other major factors that determine bleeding risk include individual patient characteristics such as older age, chronic kidney disease, liver disease, a prior history of stroke (for patients with AF), a labile INR (for patient taking warfarin), anemia, active cancer, uncontrolled HTN, ethanol use, concomitant antiplatelets (such as aspirin, other nonsteroidal anti-inflammatory drugs [NSAIDs], P2Y12 inhibitors such as clopidogrel, prasugrel, and ticagrelor) and concomitant use of selective serotonin

TABLE 49.9

Direct-Acting Oral Anticoagulant Drug Interactions

Anticoagulant	Property of Interacting Drug			
	P-gp Inhibitor Alone	**P-gp Inducer Alone**	**Combined P-gp Inhibitor and Strong CYP3A4 Inhibitor**	**Combined P-gp Inhibitor and Moderate CYP3A4 Inhibitor**
Apixaban and Rivaroxaban	No interaction	Avoid use with carbamazepine, phenytoin, rifampin, and St. John's wort	Avoid—except clarithromycin (e.g., ketoconazole, ritonavir)	Rivaroxaban: For CrCl 15–79 mL/min: Use only if the potential benefit outweigh the potential risk (e.g., erythromycin, dronedarone, verapamil)
Edoxaban	No labeled interaction in SPAF; For VTE treatment: Verapamil, quinidine, azithromycin, clarithromycin, oral erythromycin, oral itraconazole, oral ketoconazole; reduce dose to 30 mg/d	Avoid use with rifampin	No interaction for SPAF For VTE treatment: See P-gp inhibitor alone	No interaction
Dabigatran	Not recommended if CrCl < 30 mL/min; Reduce dose to 75 mg BID or avoid with CrCl 30–50 mL/min	Avoid	See P-gp inhibitors	
Pharmacodynamic (increased risk of bleeding)	Aspirin NSAIDs P2Y12 inhibitors Other antiplatelets (e.g., cilostazol, vorapaxar, dipyridamole) Other anticoagulants Thrombolytics			

CrCl, creatinine clearance; NSAIDs, nonsteroidal anti-inflammatory drugs; P-gp, P-glycoprotein; SPAF, stroke prevention in atrial fibrillation; VTE, venous thromboembolism.

reuptake inhibitors (SSRIs) (such as sertraline, fluoxetine, and citalopram), ethanol intake, as well as a longer duration of therapy (Schulman et al., 2008). The greatest risk of bleeding occurs within the first months of OAC therapy (Ansell et al., 2008). Coadministration of aspirin plus an anticoagulant increases a patient's bleed risk by about 50% and, therefore, indications for concomitant antiplatelet therapy should be scrutinized carefully (Schaefer et al., 2019). While patients with AF who are at high risk of major bleeding can be identified using the HAS-BLED score (see **Box 49.2**). Currently there is no cut-point above which AC is contraindicated as risks for ischemic stroke are also increased in patients with higher HAS-BLED score. Rather, the HAS-BLED score is used to identify modifiable risk factors for bleeding such as uncontrolled HTN or concomitant antiplatelets (Lip et al., 2018). In patients with VTE, the VTE-Bleed Score can be calculated and potentially be used to determine a duration of VTE treatment (Nishimoto et al., 2020) (see **Box 49.2**). In patients with a higher bleeding risk (VTE-Bleed Score ≥ 2), a lower dose/intensity DOAC or possibly aspirin may be used for secondary prevention following an initial 6 months of higher dose therapy (**Table 49.8**).

Minor bleeding is defined as that which is self-terminating and does not require hospitalization or an office visit or treatment by a health care provider. Clinically relevant non-major bleeding is defined as overt bleeding that does not meet the criteria for major bleeding but does require either hospitalization and prompt physician-guided medical or surgical care or change in antithrombotic therapy. Major bleeding involves bleeding into a major organ, intracranial or epidural bleeding, and pericardial, intraocular, retroperitoneal, intra-articular, or intramuscular with compartment syndrome bleeding. Bleeding that is overt with a 2 g/dL drop in hemoglobin, or requires transfusion of at least 2 units, or requires surgical correction or administration of IV vasoactive agents, is also described as major bleeding (Kovacs et al., 2015).

Common locations of antithrombotic bleeding include the oral or nasal mucosa, urine, stool, or soft tissues. Bleeding complications in order of frequency are epistaxis, purpura, hematuria, GI bleeding, and hemoptysis (Jacobs, 2008). Women are more likely to experience minor bleeding than men (Schulman et al., 2008). Minor bleeding is usually managed by temporarily discontinuing 1 to 2 doses of OAC therapy (Tomaselli et al., 2020).

Management of Warfarin-Associated Bleeding

When the INR is elevated, management depends on the patient's potential risk of bleeding, whether the patient is actively bleeding, and the INR level. Treatment options include simply omitting one or more warfarin doses with more frequent INR testing or administering vitamin K.

In the inpatient setting, management of major bleeding focuses on reversing the AC effects of warfarin which includes administration of either IV or oral vitamin K with or without clotting factor replacement. Four-factor prothrombin complex concentrates (4F-PCCs) contain purified vitamin K–dependent clotting factors, II, IV, IX, X, as well as the endogenous inhibitor proteins C and S. The 2012 American College of Chest Physicians Guidelines and the 2016 AC Forum Guidelines for VKA reversal according to INR and presence or absence of bleeding are described in **Box 49.6** (Holbrook et al., 2012; Witt et al., 2016). Currently, administration of 4F-PCCs is recommended over fresh frozen plasma for warfarin reversal because of a more rapid and complete effect with similar incidence of thromboembolic events (Witt et al., 2018). Any bleeding event should be adequately investigated because an underlying comorbidity, such as malignancy, may be contributory.

Management of Direct-Acting Oral Anticoagulant–Associated Bleeding

Currently, there are no available antidotes for edoxaban-associated bleeding. Idarucizumab, a humanized monoclonal antibody fragment, binds to dabigatran with a higher affinity than thrombin thus neutralizing dabigatran's anticoagulant effect. The half-life of idarucizumab is 45 to 70 minutes. It may be administered to treat major bleeding or to reverse anticoagulant effects for surgery or medical procedures. Andexanet alpha is a modified factor Xa decoy protein that binds to factor Xa with a higher affinity than factor Xa inhibitors (Dobesh et al., 2019). While activity has been shown with reversing the anticoagulant activity of apixaban, edoxaban, rivaroxaban, betrixaban, and LMWHs, currently, only reversal of apixaban- and rivaroxaban-associated major bleeding is FDA approved.

For minor bleeding, the bleeding site should be manually compressed. Rarely, should a DOAC dose be held given the short half-life and risk of thromboembolic event. The situations should be evaluated to determine whether or not the DOAC should be continued, dose adjusted, or changed to a different DOAC or warfarin (Tomaselli et al., 2020).

For major and life-threatening bleeding, such as ICH, other CNS bleed, pericardial tamponade, airway, hemothorax, or other critical access bleeds, the DOAC should be discontinued and manual or mechanical compression of the bleeding site

---

BOX 49.6 Guidelines for Reversing the Anticoagulant Effects of Warfarin

The reason for bleeding should be evaluated. Consider discontinuing or holding 1–2 doses of VKA. Stop concomitant medications that predispose to bleeding as appropriate (e.g., aspirin). Consider restarting with a lower maintenance dose and monitor the INR more frequently.

INRs 4.5 TO 10 AND NO EVIDENCE OF BLEEDING

In addition to omitting the next one or two doses of warfarin and monitoring the INR more frequently, apply either one of two strategies: (1) Do not administer vitamin K or (2) Consider administering 1.25 to 2.5 mg of oral vitamin K. Depending on cause of elevated INR, considering resuming therapy at a lower dose is one approach.

INRs > 10 AND NO EVIDENCE OF BLEEDING

In addition to omitting the next one or two doses of warfarin and monitoring the INR more frequently, administer one dose of oral vitamin K (2.5 or 5 mg). The INR will fall substantially in 24 to 48 hours. Frequent INR checks are necessary, and additional doses of oral vitamin K can be given if the INR is still elevated. Once the INR falls within the target range, warfarin can be resumed at a lower dose.

SIGNIFICANT BLEEDING

Patients experiencing major, life-threatening bleeding, regardless of what the INR is (even if elevated compared to normal value 1.0, but within the therapeutic range), need immediate reversal of the INR and should have their warfarin temporarily discontinued; 4F-PCCs should be administered (e.g., Kcentra; see dosing information based on INR at Kcentra.com), as well as IV vitamin K 5 to 10 mg should be administered via slow IV infusion over 1 hour. Depending on the INR, repeat doses of vitamin K can be given every 12 hours.

Recommendations from Holbrook, A., Schulman, S., Witt, D. M., et al. (2012). Evidence-based management of anticoagulant therapy: Antithrombotic therapy and prevention of thrombosis: American College of Chest Physicians Evidence-Based Clinical Practice Guidelines (9th ed.) *Chest, 141*(2 Suppl.), e152S–e184S; Witt, D. M., Clark, N. P., Kaatz, S., et al. (2016). Guidance for the practical management of warfarin therapy in the treatment of venous thromboembolism. *Journal of Thrombosis and Thrombolysis, 41*(1), 187–205.

4F-PCCs, 4-factor prothrombin complex concentrates; INR, international normalized ratio; IV, intravenous; VKA, vitamin K antagonist.

should be performed if possible. If the last administered dose was within 2 to 3 hours, administer activated charcoal. The 2020 ACC Expert Consensus Decision Pathway on Management of Bleeding in Patients Receiving Oral Anticoagulants recommends idarucizumab for reversal of major bleeding with dabigatran and andexanet for reversal of major bleeding with factor Xa inhibitors (betrixaban, apixaban, rivaroxaban and edoxaban). If those antidotes are not available, administration of 4F-PCCs is recommended (Tomaselli et al., 2020). For dabigatran, administer idarucizumab 5 g by rapid IV bolus or infusion. Andexanet is administered as an IV bolus and a 2-hour infusion as either a low or high dose determined by the apixaban or rivaroxaban dose and estimated time since last DOAC dose. Hemostatic efficacy may be seen within minutes after idarucizumab or andexanet alpha administration. In patients with chronic kidney disease or acute kidney injury, the DOAC half-life may be prolonged and the patient should be monitored for a longer period of time.

Management of Unfractionated Heparin-Associated Bleeding

Excessive AC with UFH can be reversed with IV protamine sulfate, which is high in arginine and is cationic binding tightly to heparin, which is highly anionic, thus reversing the anticoagulant effect (Nutescu et al., 2016). Unfortunately, protamine has other undesirable effects in some patients, including immediate and delayed allergic response.

Management of Low-Molecular-Weight Heparin–Associated Bleeding

There is no proven method for reversing excessive AC occurring with LMWHs, although consensus guidelines provide dosing recommendations for using protamine and it has been found useful in some, but not all, coagulopathic patients (Witt et al., 2018). Preliminary data suggests that andexanet alpha may reverse enoxaparin coagulopathy (Dobesh et al., 2019).

Antiplatelet Agents

Antiplatelet agents that have been used in the prevention and treatment of ischemic stroke are aspirin, aspirin/dipyridamole (Aggrenox), and the P2Y12 inhibitor clopidogrel (Plavix). Aspirin has been studied in primary and secondary prevention of VTE. Aspirin has been studied as a sole therapy for stroke prevention in patients with bioprosthetic heart valves and as add-on therapy to warfarin for stroke prevention in patients with mechanical heart valves. Aspirin has been shown to be inferior to warfarin and apixaban for SPAF. Two other P2Y12 inhibitors, prasugrel (Effient) and ticagrelor (Brilinta), as well as clopidogrel are used to prevent CV death, MI, or stroke following acute coronary syndrome and to prevent stent thrombosis following percutaneous coronary intervention. The use of P2Y12 inhibitors for secondary coronary heart disease indications will not be discussed in this chapter.

Aspirin

Mechanism of Action

Aspirin prevents prostaglandin synthesis in platelets and other tissues by irreversibly modifying and inhibiting the enzyme cyclooxygenase (COX), which catalyzes the conversion of arachidonic acid to thromboxane A_2, a prostaglandin derivative, which is a potent vasoconstrictor and promoter of platelet aggregation. The onset of antiplatelet effects is within 5 minutes of oral administration. After discontinuing aspirin, platelets are impaired for their normal life span of 7 to 10 days because of the irreversible inhibition of COX. Every 24 hours, 10% of platelets are replaced; 5 to 6 days after aspirin ingestion, approximately 50% of platelets function normally (Patrono et al., 2008).

Dosage

The optimal aspirin dosage for thrombotic disorders is still controversial because doses ranging from 30 to 1,500 mg/d are effective (Adams et al., 2008; Albers et al., 2008). Randomized trials have found lower aspirin doses ranging between 50 and 100 mg/d effective as an antithrombotic agent (Patrono et al., 2008). There is no benefit to higher doses over low-dose aspirin for ASCVD prevention. Because higher doses may be associated with increased risk for GI bleeding, a lower dose, such as 81 mg orally daily, is preferred (Abdelaziz et al., 2019). However, doses as high as 300 mg/d as single antiplatelet therapy are recommended for up to 2 weeks during hospitalization for secondary prevention of noncardioembolic ischemic stroke in the 2019 National Institute for Health and Care Excellence stroke guidelines (National Institute for Health and Care Excellence, 2019).

Aspirin's contraindications are active GI bleeding (unless a recent coronary stent has been placed) or aspirin allergy or hypersensitivity. The most common adverse effects of aspirin are GI upset, such as nausea, dyspepsia, heartburn, epigastric discomfort, anorexia, and bleeding. These effects are dose related and are more likely to occur at doses greater than 325 mg/d. Although lower aspirin doses cause fewer GI symptoms, they still can cause significant GI bleeding. Aspirin may also potentiate peptic ulcer disease. Caution should be exercised when using aspirin with other drugs that affect platelet function (e.g., NSAIDs, P2Y12 inhibitors, and SSRI antidepressants) or anticoagulants because the bleeding potential will be increased.

Aspirin/Extended-Release Dipyridamole

A combination product containing 25-mg aspirin and 200-mg extended-release dipyridamole (Aggrenox) administered twice daily is available for preventing stroke in patients who have experienced a TIA or previous ischemic stroke. Dipyridamole inhibits, the uptake of adenosine, increasing local adenosine concentrations, which stimulates platelet adenosine cyclase resulting in increased cyclic adenosine monophosphate, which inhibits platelet aggregation, and causes arteriolar vasodilation. The most common adverse effects include GI complaints, diarrhea, and headache. Elevations in hepatic enzymes have also been reported. Capsules should not be chewed. Contraindications are similar to those for aspirin alone.

Clopidogrel

Clopidogrel is a thienopyridine P2Y12 inhibitor that irreversibly inhibits adenosine diphosphate-mediated platelet aggregation. Dose-dependent inhibition of platelet aggregation is seen 2 hours after a single oral dose with a peak effect about 6 hours after the dose, and platelet aggregation and bleeding time return to baseline approximately 5 to 7 days after discontinuing clopidogrel.

Clopidogrel is a prodrug and must be activated (bio-transformed) to inhibit platelet aggregation. Clopidogrel is extensively metabolized by the liver primarily by CYP2C19. Strong CYP2C19 inhibitors (e.g., fluconazole, fluvoxamine, and fluoxetine) may decrease the antiplatelet effect of clopidogrel and should be avoided. Although patients who are poor metabolizers of CYP2C19 will have a poor antiplatelet effect as measured by tests such as VerifyNow P2Y12 assay, no current clinical practice guidelines recommend pharmacogenetic testing prior to clopidogrel initiation. If a patient is a known poor metabolizer of CYP2C19, an alternative antiplatelet agent should be selected (Zeb et al., 2018).

Contraindications to clopidogrel are active major bleeding, including from peptic ulcer or ICH. Bruising and bleeding are the primary risks of clopidogrel therapy, and the risk is increased in the setting of DAPT with aspirin. Diarrhea is relatively common, occurring in approximately 5%. A pruritic, macular, erythematous rash starting on the trunk or face and spreading to the extremities occurs in about 1% with an onset within the first week of therapy. Rarely clopidogrel causes life-threatening thrombocytopenic purpura (Lokhandwala et al., 2011).

Selecting the Most Appropriate Agent
Treatment of Deep Vein Thrombosis or Pulmonary Embolism

Anticoagulant treatment options for VTE are shown in **Table 49.9**. Guidance for treating VTE in patients without cancer is provided by the ASH and European Society of Cardiology (ESC) (Konstantinidis et al., 2019; Ortel et al., 2020). Patients without cancer with uncomplicated DVT may be treated at home. Patients presenting with PE without cancer may be stratified by the simplified pulmonary embolism severity index score to identify patients at low risk for death, recurrent VTE and bleeding, after the diagnosis of PE has been made (see **Box 49.2**). A patient with a score of 0 is identified as low risk and could be treated at home provided appropriate support services available. Some hemodynamically unstable patients with acute PE may require treatment with alteplase. For initial management in hemodynamically stable patients, DOACs are preferred over warfarin because they have similar efficacy, but lower bleeding risk compared to warfarin. Treatment duration is determined by the presence or absence of chronic risk factors for recurrence balanced by the risk of bleeding. For patients without cancer and either unprovoked VTE or with chronic risk factors, indefinite AC should be considered (longer than 6 months) balanced by the patient's risk for bleeding. For patients with a time-limited risk factor, short-term (3–6 months) AC is recommended. Validated risk scores for identifying patients with low risk of recurrence, in whom AC may be stopped after 6 months of treatment, are available but with limited validation (e.g., Vienna Prediction Model, DASH Prediction Score, and HERDOO2 (see **Box 49.2**). Lower doses of rivaroxaban and apixaban can be considered for secondary prevention following the first 6 months of higher-intensity AC. While aspirin following initial 3 to 6 months

of AC treatment has been shown to be more effective than placebo for preventing VTE recurrence, it is less effective with similar bleeding to lower-intensity DOACs and therefore DOACs are preferred for secondary prevention.

For patients with cancer, guidelines for VTE treatment are available from ESC, the American Society of Clinical Oncology and the National Comprehensive Cancer Network (NCCN) (NCCN Guidelines Version 1.2020. Cancer Associated Venous Thromboembolic Disease) (Key et al., 2019; Konstantinidis et al., 2019). Guidelines differ with respect to preference of LMWH (preferred over UFH) versus a DOAC. DOACs should be avoided and LMWH used in patients with gastric or gastroesophageal lesions as there is an increased risk of bleeding. LMWH is also preferred for patients with CrCl <25 mL/min. For long-term AC, either LMWH, edoxaban, or rivaroxaban is recommended because they are superior to warfarin and have fewer drug interactions with chemotherapy. LMWH is preferred in the NCCN guidelines for patients with GI malignancies secondary to increased bleeding risk with DOACs. For noncatheter-associated VTE, treatment should continue indefinitely while cancer is active, under treatment, or if risk factors for recurrence exist. For central venous catheter–associated VTE, treatment should continue for as long as the catheter is in place (NCCN Guidelines Version 1.2020. Cancer Associated Venous Thromboembolic Disease).

Prophylaxis of Deep Vein Thrombosis and Pulmonary Embolism

Patients undergoing total hip replacement (THR), total knee replacement (TKR), or hip fracture surgery should receive AC prophylaxis to reduce the high risk of DVT or PE. Several studies have found the prevalence of total DVT at 7 to 14 days after THR, TKR, and hip fracture surgery to be approximately 50% to 60% in patients not receiving antithrombotic therapy. The incidence of PE is less certain, but in studies in which a VQ scan was performed, about 7% to 11% of THR and TKR patients had a high probability scan within 7 to 14 days after surgery. It has also been found that total DVT rate is greater in TKR than THR. Overall, the data suggest that asymptomatic VTE is common after orthopedic surgery and, in the absence of prophylaxis, will affect at least half of these patients (Geerts et al., 2008).

Numerous pharmacologic and nonpharmacologic agents have been used in the postoperative setting to decrease the risk of DVT or PE. According to the ASH 2019 guidelines for VTE prophylaxis in surgical patients, effective drugs for prophylaxis of VTE following orthopedic surgery include aspirin, LMWHs (e.g., enoxaparin 40 mg subcutaneous daily), apixaban (2.5 mg PO twice daily), rivaroxaban (10 mg PO daily), dabigatran (110 mg subcutaneous day 1 followed by 220 mg subcutaneously daily). The guidelines note that the data indicate with low certainty that there may be no difference in mortality between anticoagulants and aspirin and no difference in symptomatic PE (Anderson et al., 2019).

For the hospitalized medical patient, LMWH (e.g., enoxaparin 40 mg subcutaneously once daily) is recommended over both UFH and DOACs (rivaroxaban and betrixaban)

(Anderson et al., 2019). LMWHs had similar mortality (low certainty data), were cost-effective, and have fewer injections per day compared to UFH. DOACs have a higher risk of major bleeding compared to enoxaparin.

Secondary Prevention of Noncardioembolic Ischemic Stroke and Transient Ischemic Attack

The choice of either aspirin, clopidogrel, or aspirin/dipyridamole for long-term secondary prevention of stroke is based on contraindications, patient tolerance, availability, and cost (Powers et al., 2019). Pharmacotherapy for secondary prevention of stroke/TIA is described in the 2014 American Heart Association (AHA)/ American Stroke Association (ASA) guidelines (Kernan et al., 2014). Antiplatelet therapy reduces the relative risk of death, MI, or recurrent stroke by 22% (Kernan et al., 2014). These guidelines recommend treatment with either aspirin (50–325 mg/d), aspirin plus dipyridamole (25/200 mg twice daily), or clopidogrel monotherapy (75 mg daily). A head-to-head trial comparing clopidogrel monotherapy and aspirin/dipyridamole in patients with TIA or ischemic stroke in more than 20,000 patients found similar rates of recurrent stroke but a higher dropout rate with aspirin/dipyridamole than clopidogrel mostly due to headache (Sacco et al., 2008). A large individual patient data network meta-analysis of 6 randomized controlled trials (approximately 43,000 patients) from the Cerebrovascular Antiplatelet Trialists' Collaborative Group found similar efficacy between clopidogrel monotherapy and aspirin/ dipyridamole and both more effective compared to aspirin alone with similar major bleeding with clopidogrel and aspirin/dipyridamole for secondary stroke/TIA prevention (Greving et al., 2019).

Compared to aspirin alone, clopidogrel plus aspirin has similar efficacy but increases bleeding events in major stroke. In minor stroke [National Institutes of Health Stroke Scale (NIHSS) score ≤ 3], the AHA stroke guidelines recommend the combination of low-dose aspirin (e.g., 81 mg/d) and clopidogrel 75 mg/d for 21 days followed by aspirin or clopidogrel alone upon a reduction in 30-day recurrent stroke risk at a cost of a slightly higher increased major bleeding risk (Powers et al., 2019). Either aspirin or clopidogrel or aspirin/dipyridamole are guideline-recommended for long-term secondary prevention of noncardioembolic stroke (Kernan et al., 2014; Powers et al., 2019). Recently, low-dose aspirin plus ticagrelor administered as a 180 mg loading dose followed by 90 mg twice daily for 30 days was approved by the FDA for secondary stroke prevention in patients with minor stroke (NIHSS score ≤ 5) or high-risk TIA (Johnston et al., 2020). For patients experiencing recurrent noncardioembolic stroke while taking low-dose aspirin, another antiplatelet agent or increased dose of aspirin should be used (Powers et al., 2019).

Stroke Prevention in Atrial Fibrillation

Antithrombotic therapy selection for the prevention of stroke is based upon a discussion with the patient about the risk of stroke and the benefits/risks of antithrombotic therapy. Patients with valvular heart disease (mitral stenosis, rheumatic mitral valve disease, or prosthetic heart valves) and AF are at high risk of stroke. For patients without valvular heart disease, an annual risk of stroke is estimated using the $CHAS_2DS_2$-VASc Score

(or via a mobile phone app AnticoagEvaluator) (see **Box 49.2**). Risk factors included in this estimate are age, female gender, HF, HTN, prior history of stroke or TIA, diabetes mellitus, and presence of concomitant vascular disease, such as MI, PAD, or aortic plaque (January et al., 2014).

Antithrombotic therapy for stroke prevention in AF in patients without mechanical heart valves or mitral stenosis is outlined in the 2019 AHA/ American College of Cardiology/ Heart Rhythm Association (HRS) guidelines (January et al., 2019). No antithrombotic prophylaxis is needed for patients with a CHA_2DS_2-Vasc score of 0 as stroke risk is less than 0.2% per year. OAC is recommended for men with a CHA_2DS_2-Vasc score of 2 or more and 3 or more in women. DOACs are recommended over warfarin except in patients with mechanical heart valves where warfarin is recommended. Warfarin can be considered instead of a DOAC in patients with CrCl <15 mL/ min or who are on dialysis where there are sparse data on patient outcomes. For patients with end-state kidney disease, the recommended DOACs are rivaroxaban and apixaban (FDA approved for use in this patient group). If warfarin is used, the INR should be measured monthly and the target range is 2.0 to 3.0. Aspirin should not be used for stroke thromboprophylaxis in AF.

OAC may be considered in men with a CHA_2DS_2-Vasc score of 1 in men and 1 or 2 in women for patients with certain high risk for stroke features and a low major bleeding risk as assessed by the HAS-BLED score (see **Box 49.2**). This personalized approach, as recommended by the ESC, includes such individual risk factors as age >65 years, type 2 diabetes, permanent/persistent AF (Sulzgruber et al., 2019).

DOACs have been found to have superior or similar efficacy to warfarin for the prevention of stroke or systemic thromboembolism with similar or lower major bleeding and an approximate 50% reduction in ICH (Chan et al., 2014; Ruff et al., 2014). Drug selection is often made by patient preference based upon cost (insurance copay) or convenience (dosing frequency, lack of INR monitoring).

Prophylaxis Against Systemic Embolism in Patients with Prosthetic Heart Valves

Anticoagulant therapy for thromboprophylaxis with warfarin is recommended in all patients having prosthetic valve replacement. The rate of embolism reported with mechanical valves (St. Jude bileaflet valve) when antithrombotic prophylaxis was not administered ranged from 12% per year with aortic valves to 22% per year with mitral valves (Salem et al., 2008). Bioprosthetic tissue valves present a much lower risk of thromboembolism, averaging 1% per year; the risk of thromboembolic events is highest in the first 3 months following surgery, after which anticoagulant therapy is usually discontinued (Nishimura et al., 2017).

Patients with mechanical valves in the (1) mitral position or (2) patients with aortic valves with additional risk factors such as AF, previous thromboembolism, left ventricular ejection fraction less than 40%, as well as those with older caged ball valves require lifelong therapy with warfarin maintained at a target INR of 2.5 to 3.5 (target INR 3.0). A lower INR of 2 to 3 (target 2.5) is recommended for patients with mechanical bileaflet or single-tilting disk (e.g., Medtronic Hall) valves in the aortic position because studies show there is not an increased risk of thromboembolism and the bleeding risk is lower than with a higher target INR (Nishimura et al., 2017). The On-X aortic valve is a newer heart valve that requires less intense AC with warfarin compared to other valve types (INR 1.5–2.0) and is taken with low-dose aspirin (Otto et al., 2021).

Previously, low-dose aspirin was recommended to be added to warfarin to further reduce thromboembolism risk. However, with newer generation mechanical heart valves, the risk of thromboembolism in patients treated with therapeutic warfarin is approximately 0.5% to 0.7% per year. Therefore, routinely adding low-dose aspirin to warfarin therapy is no longer recommended. Aspirin is indicated for patients at higher thromboembolic risk (for example, prior thromboembolism on therapeutic AC) or for other indications such as ASCVD (Otto et al., 2021).

Warfarin is recommended with an INR of 2 to 3 (target 2.5) for at least 3 months and up to 6 months following surgery for aortic and mitral bioprosthetic tissue valves (e.g., porcine heart valves) in patients at low risk of bleeding (Otto et al., 2021). Aspirin monotherapy 75 to 100 mg/d is then recommended lifelong after the first 3 months regardless of the valve position (Otto et al., 2021).

Patients with mechanical heart valves can experience thromboembolic events even if antithrombotic therapy is administered appropriately. Options in these cases from expert consensus are to increase the target INR for patients on warfarin, to add aspirin to patients not already receiving warfarin, or to add warfarin if the patient is receiving aspirin (Otto et al., 2021).

TAVR for aortic stenosis is associated with a lower stroke than bioprosthetic or mechanical valve replacement. While a short 3- to 6-month course of DAPT with low-dose aspirin and clopidogrel followed by life-long aspirin is common, recent data and current guidelines suggest that a regimen of aspirin alone may have similar thromboembolic outcomes and a lower bleeding risk (Otto et al., 2021; Saito et al., 2020). Use of a lower-intensity DOAC, for example either rivaroxaban or apixaban, in the absence of another indication (such as SPAF) has been associated with an increased mortality, thromboembolism, and bleeding risk and is not recommended (Dangas et al., 2020; Otto et al., 2021). For patients with a long-term indication for AC, such as AF, patients undergoing TAVR should be maintained on the OAC regimen used for SPAF prior to the surgery, either a direct-acting oral anticoagulant (DOAC) or warfarin, without the addition of short-term concomitant antiplatelet therapy (clopidogrel) as the combination is associated with significantly higher risk of major bleeding without reducing the risk of ischemic events (Nijenhuis et al., 2020). It should be noted, however, that all DOACs carry a warning to avoid use in patients with prosthetic heart valves.

Special Considerations
Genomics
Gene variants have been identified affecting CYP2C9 (warfarin metabolism) as well as vitamin K epoxide reductase complex 1 (VKORC1) (an enzyme involved in the conversion of vitamin K from active to inactive forms affecting the body's sensitivity to warfarin). The prescribing information contains recommended initial doses of warfarin for warfarin-naive patients based upon selected genotypes combinations of CYP2C9 and VKORC1. Genetic-guided initial warfarin dosing has been shown to shorten the time to a stable INR but has not been found to consistently reduce bleeding because additional factors besides genotype influence warfarin clearance and thus dose (Johnson et al., 2017). Warfarin initiation should not be delayed to await the results of pharmacogenetic testing. An algorithm for warfarin dosing for less experienced clinicians is available from WARFARINDOSING.org (WARFARINDOSING. org, 2016). In addition to genotype, other factors such as patient age, sex, race, height, weight, smoking status, interacting drugs, and target INR are included. Lower warfarin initiation doses are used for the older adults, patients with hepatic dysfunction including those with hepatic congestion secondary to symptomatic HF and those who take concomitant interacting drugs such as amiodarone. Currently, measurement of pharmacogenetic testing for these genetic variants prior to starting warfarin is currently not recommended by any professional organization (Witt et al., 2016).

NONDRUG THERAPY

Nondrug therapies help prevent or treat the complications of DVT, including venous stasis ulcers and the postthrombotic syndrome. Mechanical measures, including intermittent pneumatic compression (IPC) devices and graduated compression stockings, offer the advantage of carrying no risk of bleeding compared to anticoagulants. IPC sleeves applied to the lower extremities periodically inflate and deflate, to squeeze the calf and prevent venous stasis and pooling of blood in the leg veins. Use of IPC alone is recommended in patients with a high risk of bleeding following general orthopedic or general surgery, until the bleeding risk resolves (Geerts et al., 2008). IPC may be combined with pharmacologic prophylaxis in orthopedic surgical patients and high-risk medical patients (e.g., critically ill) to reduce the risk of VTE (Anderson et al., 2018, 2019).

Although there is little evidence for effectiveness, routine use of compression stockings should be considered following DVT (Ortel et al., 2020). Routine use of inferior vena cava (IVC) filters to prevent distal emboli from reaching the lungs to prevent PE is not recommended but may be considered for patients with absolute contraindications to AC or recurrent PE despite therapeutic AC (Konstantinidis et al., 2019). Complications of IVC filters include thrombosis, migration of the filter (rarely to the heart), and obstruction of the vena cava.

In patients with AF who have an indication for AC but have an unacceptable high risk for bleeding while taking an anticoagulant, placement of a left atrial appendage occlusion device reduces the risk of ischemic stroke (Essa et al., 2020).

PATIENT EDUCATION

Oral Anticoagulant Patient Education

Drug Information

Patient education is essential because patients must comply with laboratory follow-up and accurately follow dosing instructions. An assessment of any contraindications to therapy, including active bleeding and pregnancy, is necessary before starting therapy. The risk of bleeding may exceed the benefits in patients with a previous history of medication nonadherence, significant alcohol consumption, memory impairment, and lack of adequate support from family members or caregivers. Patients and caregivers must agree with the decision

to initiate therapy (Witt, 2010). Common elements of AC patient education are described in **Box 49.7**.

When LMWHs are used in the outpatient setting, patient education regarding subcutaneous injection is necessary. Establish that the patient or their caregiver can reliably and accurately administer the subcutaneous injection, or consider arranging for home health care visits. An instructional video for patient self-injection is available on the Lovenox website (Lovenox enoxaparin sodium injection).

Nutrition Education for Warfarin

Education concerning food restrictions for patients taking warfarin is essential. Vitamin K_1 (phylloquinone), the antidote to warfarin, is naturally found in several plant foods. In contrast,

---

BOX 49.7 **Elements of Anticoagulation Patient Education**

Indicate the reason for initiating AC therapy (e.g., stroke prevention or prevention of VTE) and how it relates to clot formation.

Review the name of anticoagulant drug(s) (generic and trade) and discuss how they work to reduce the risk of clotting complications.

Discuss the potential duration of therapy.

Describe the common signs/symptoms of bleeding and what to do if they occur.

Describe the common signs/symptoms of clotting (e.g., leg pain/swelling for DVT or sudden acute shortness of breath for PE or F.A.S.T signs and symptoms for stroke) complications and what to do if they occur.

Outline precautionary measures to minimize the risk of trauma or bleeding.

Discuss potential drug interactions (prescription and, in addition for warfarin, OTC, herbal) and what to do when normal medication regimens change.

Clarify whether or not the patient may take concomitant low-dose aspirin and other NSAIDs.

Discuss the need to avoid or limit alcohol consumption.

Explain the need for birth control measures for women of childbearing age.

Review the importance of notifying all health care providers (e.g., physicians, dentist) of the use of AC therapy.

Review the importance of notifying the AC provider when dental, surgical, or invasive procedures and hospitalization are scheduled.

Explain when to take anticoagulant mediations and what to do if a dose is missed.

Discuss the importance of carrying identification (ID card, medical alert bracelet/necklace).

Document in the patient's medical record that the patient education session has occurred.

In addition, for warfarin only:

Discuss the delayed onset of effect and the need for the use of warfarin with a parenteral anticoagulant for 5 to 10 days of treatment.

Explain the meaning and significance of the INR.

Explain the need for frequent INR testing and target INR values appropriate for the patient's treatment.

Identify the laboratory location where the patient will go for the INR test and the date and time of the next test.

Identify the prescriber who will interpret the INR and the method of communicating those changes to the patient.

Discuss the narrow therapeutic index of warfarin and emphasize the importance of regular monitoring as a way to minimize the risk of bleeding/thrombosis.

Discuss the influence of dietary vitamin K use on the effects of the INR.

In addition, for rivaroxaban, apixaban, and edoxaban only:

Explain the importance of periodic serum creatinine laboratory tests to monitor renal function.

Identify the prescriber or their designee as the individual to contact regarding questions, bleeding, and refills.

Review the date, time, and location of the patient's next follow-up appointment.

In addition, for rivaroxaban only:

Explain that doses greater than 10 mg should be taken with a large meal.

For dabigatran only:

Explain that the capsule cannot be crushed and cannot be removed from the original packaging.

AC, anticoagulant; DVT, deep vein thrombosis; F.A.S.T., facial drooping, arm weakness, speech difficulty, time to call 911; ID, identification; INR, international normalized ratio; NSAIDs, nonsteroidal anti-inflammatory drugs; OTC, over-the-counter; PE, pulmonary embolism.

Adapted from Garcia, D. A., Witt, D. M., Hylek, E., et al. (2008). Delivery of optimized anticoagulant therapy: Consensus statement from the anticoagulation forum. *Annals of Pharmacotherapy, 42*, 979–988.

vitamin K_2 (menaquinones) is primarily synthesized by normal intestinal flora. The estimated adequate intake of vitamin K_1 for adults is 120 mcg/d for men and 90 mcg/d for women older than age 19. In the United States, typical American dietary vitamin K_1 intake is 122 mcg/d for women and 138 mcg/d for men (National Institutes of Health Vitamin K Fact Sheet for Health Professionals). Excessive amounts of dietary vitamin K_1 may antagonize warfarin's clinical effect and decrease the INR. Khan and coworkers (2004) found that for every 100-mcg increase in vitamin K_1 intake in the 4 days before an INR measurement, the INR fell by 0.2. In another study, it was found that higher warfarin doses at 5.7 ± 1.7 mg/d were needed by those consuming 250 mcg or more of vitamin K daily compared to that of 3.5 ± 1.0 mg/d by those consuming less than 250 mcg of vitamin K daily (Khan et al., 2004).

Dark green leafy vegetables (spinach and turnip, collard, and mustard greens), broccoli, Brussels sprouts, and cabbage are the primary sources of vitamin K and contain high amounts, greater than 100 mg/100 g serving. Herbal and green teas may also contain large quantities of vitamin K_1 (1,400 mg/100 g), and high levels of vitamin K_1 (50 mg/100 g) are found in soybean and soy products and olive oils, whereas peanut and corn oils contain minimal amounts. Vitamin K is also found in certain plant oils and prepared foods containing these oils, such as baked goods, margarine, and salad dressings.

Food preparation with oils rich in vitamin K may also contribute to total vitamin K intake and affect warfarin action. The *Coumadin Cookbook* (available from amazon.com) is a great resource for patients taking warfarin because it provides tips for monitoring and maintaining a consistent vitamin K intake and provides many recipes with a low vitamin K content. Patients should be encouraged to eat a healthy diet, maintain consistency in their choice of foods, and avoid large fluctuations in dietary vitamin K_1 intake. Instructing patients to maintain a consistent intake of vitamin K–containing foods, rather than trying to eliminate all sources of dietary vitamin K_1, is essential. Patients must also be educated on portion sizes and their vitamin K content so that they are not only consistent with the frequency of intake of vitamin K foods but also consistent with the number of servings of vitamin K they consume. Fad diets, such as the "cabbage soup" diet, are discouraged, and if diets such as the Atkins diet or low-carbohydrate diets are to be started, the patient must notify the practitioner so that INRs can be monitored more often. These diets, when strictly followed, frequently lead to a change in the intake amount of vitamin K foods. **Table 49.10** lists examples of vitamin K food content and serving sizes. A complete listing of the vitamin K content of foods (from highest to lowest content) is available from the United States Department of Agriculture (USDA National Nutrient Database for Standard

TABLE 49.10
Vitamin K Content of Common Foods

Description	Weight (g)	Common Measure	Vitamin K per Measure (mcg)
Asparagus, frozen, cooked, boiled, drained, without salt	180	1 cup	144
Beans, snap, green, canned, regular pack, drained solids	135	1 cup	53
Beet greens, cooked, boiled, drained, without salt	144	1 cup	697
Broccoli, cooked, boiled, drained, without salt	156	1 cup	220
Broccoli, raw	88	1 cup	89
Broccoli, cooked, boiled, drained, without salt	37	1 spear	52
Broccoli, frozen, chopped, cooked, boiled, drained, without salt	184	1 cup	162
Brussels sprouts, frozen, cooked, boiled, drained, without salt	155	1 cup	300
Brussels sprouts, cooked, boiled, drained, without salt	156	1 cup	219
Cabbage, raw	70	1 cup	53
Cabbage, cooked, boiled, drained, without salt	150	1 cup	163
Cabbage, Chinese (pak choi), cooked, boiled, drained, without salt	170	1 cup	58
Celery, cooked, boiled, drained, without salt	150	1 cup	57
Collards, frozen, chopped, cooked, boiled, drained, without salt	170	1 cup	1,059
Collards, cooked, boiled, drained, without salt	190	1 cup	836
Cowpeas (blackeyes), immature seeds, frozen, cooked, boiled, drained, without salt	170	1 cup	63
Cucumber, with peel, raw	301	1 large	49
Dandelion greens, cooked, boiled, drained, without salt	105	1 cup	579
Endive, raw	50	1 cup	116

(Continued)

TABLE 49.10

Vitamin K Content of Common Foods (Continued)

Description	Weight (g)	Common Measure	Vitamin K per Measure (mcg)
Kale, frozen, cooked, boiled, drained, without salt	130	1 cup	1,147
Kale, cooked, boiled, drained, without salt	130	1 cup	1,062
Lettuce, iceberg (includes crisphead types), raw	539	1 head	130
Lettuce, green leaf, raw	56	1 cup	71
Lettuce, cos or romaine, raw	56	1 cup	57
Lettuce, butterhead (includes boston and bibb types), raw	163	1 head	167
Mustard greens, cooked, boiled, drained, without salt	140	1 cup	419
Onions, spring or scallions (includes tops and bulb), raw	100	1 cup	207
Okra, cooked, boiled, drained, without salt	160	1 cup	64
Okra, frozen, cooked, boiled, drained, without salt	184	1 cup	88
Parsley, fresh	10	10 sprigs	164
Peas, green (includes baby and lesuer types), canned, drained solids, unprepared	170	1 cup	63
Peas, edible podded, frozen, cooked, boiled, drained, without salt	160	1 cup	48
Plums, dried (prunes), stewed, without added sugar	248	1 cup	65
Rhubarb, frozen, cooked, with sugar	240	1 cup	51
Spinach, frozen, chopped or leaf, cooked, boiled, drained, without salt	190	1 cup	1,027
Spinach, canned, regular pack, drained solids	214	1 cup	988
Spinach, cooked, boiled, drained, without salt	180	1 cup	888
Spinach souffle	136	1 cup	172
Spinach, raw	30	1 cup	145
Turnip greens, frozen, cooked, boiled, drained, without salt	164	1 cup	851
Turnip greens, cooked, boiled, drained, without salt	144	1 cup	529
Pie crust, cookie type, prepared from recipe, graham cracker, baked	239	1 pie shell	59
Noodles, egg, spinach, cooked, enriched	160	1 cup	162
Fast foods, coleslaw	99	¾ cup	70
Bread crumbs, dry, grated, seasoned	120	1 cup	55

Source: USDA National Nutrient Database—Vitamin K. Available from: https://www.nal.usda.gov/sites/www.nal.usda.gov/files/vitamin_k.pdf

Reference Release 28). The vitamin K content of individual foods may be searched at the U.S. Department of Agriculture Food Central (USDA FoodData Central). A helpful patient information sheet listing foods high, moderate, and low or with no vitamin K content is available from the Department of Veterans Affairs Food Services (Veterans Affairs [VA] Food Services Vitamin K Content of Foods).

Hidden sources of excess vitamin K include enteral supplements, which can cause resistance to warfarin. Checking the amount of vitamin K in any nutritional supplement is advised because several of these preparations are now marketed directly to patients through the lay press. In addition, many OTC vitamin preparations contain vitamin K, and patients should be counseled to read the label or bring in all medication bottles to the practitioner. For example, one Viactiv calcium chew

contains 40 mcg of vitamin K; this translates to 80 mcg of vitamin K daily if the recommended dose of two chews is ingested. Questioning patients regarding any changes in dietary habits may provide clues when the INR varies.

Several herbal and nutritional products can potentially interfere with the anticoagulant effect of warfarin. Although stringently performed clinical trials are lacking, feverfew, garlic, cranberry, ginger, fish oil, and turmeric may increase INR and/or an enhance the bleeding risk when used with warfarin. Herbal and natural products that can decrease the effect of warfarin include ginseng, coenzyme Q, and green tea (due to its vitamin K content) (Di Minno et al., 2017).

Consumer and professional information on herbal supplement drug interactions with supporting literature can be accessed on an FDA drug interactions checker (see **Box 49.2**).

Case: Transitioning a patient from a direct-acting oral anti-coagulant (DOAC) to warfarin

C.F. is a 76-year-old woman (80 kg, 5 ft. 5 in.) who presents to a follow-up visit with her primary care provider stating she can no longer afford her Eliquis prescription. She was started on Eliquis last month after an ischemic stroke and new diagnosis of atrial fibrillation. Other past history includes prior myocardial infarction, diabetes, and hypertension. C.F. was given a coupon for a free 30-day supply of Eliquis which is just about gone. When she went to the pharmacy to pick up her next fill, they informed her that her copay would be $100 per month. She feels she cannot afford this copay and is requesting a less expensive option. The office has already contacted C.F.'s insurance company and none of the other DOACs are covered by her plan. Her provider wishes to switch her to warfarin, for which she will have $5 per month copay. She has no past history of bleeding. (Learning objective: Transition patients from warfarin to a DOAC or from a DOAC to warfarin.)

Pertinent laboratory values include the following: hemoglobin 13.2, hematocrit 39.1%, platelet count 157,000/mcL, serum creatinine 1.0 mg/dL.

1. What is C.F.'s CHA_2DS_2-VASc Score?
2. What are some important points you should review with patient prior to making the decision to switch from Eliquis to warfarin?
3. C.F. would like to proceed with the switch from Eliquis to warfarin. What instructions should she be given?
4. What are important points for patient education regarding anticoagulation and stroke prevention in atrial fibrillation?

Bibliography

Starred references are cited in the text.

*Abdelaziz, H. K., Saad, M., Pothineni, N. V. K., et al. (2019). Aspirin for primary prevention of cardiovascular events. *Journal of the American College of Cardiology, 73*(23), 2915–2929.

*Adams, R. J., Albers, G., Alberts, M. J., et al. (2008). Update to the AHA/ASA recommendations for prevention of stroke in patients with ischemic stroke or transient ischemic attack. *Stroke, 39,* 1647–1652.

*Ageno, W., Gallus, A. S., Wittkowsky, A., et al. (2012). Oral anticoagulant therapy: Antithrombotic therapy and prevention of thrombosis, 9th ed: American College of Chest Physicians evidence-based clinical practice guidelines. *Chest, 141*(2 Suppl), e44S–e88S.

*Ahmad, S., & Wilt, H. (2016). Stroke prevention in atrial fibrillation and valvular heart disease. *Open Cardiovascular Medicine Journal, 10,* 110–116.

*Albers, G. W., Amarenco, P., Easton, J. D., et al. (2008). Antithrombotic and thrombolytic therapy for ischemic stroke: American College of Chest Physicians evidence-based clinical practice guidelines (8th ed.). *Chest, 133*(6 Suppl.), 630S–669S.

*Anderson, D. R., Morgano, G. P., Bennett, C., et al. (2019). American Society of Hematology 2019 guidelines for management of venous thromboembolism: Prevention of venous thromboembolism in surgical hospitalized patients. *Blood Advances, 3*(23), 3898–3944.

*Ansell, J., Hirsh, J., Hylek, E., et al. (2008). Pharmacology and management of the vitamin K antagonists: American College of Chest Physicians evidence-based clinical practice guidelines (8th ed.). *Chest, 133*(6 Suppl.), 160S–198S.

*Arachchillage, D. R. J., & Laffan, M. (2020). What is the appropriate anticoagulation strategy for thrombotic antiphospholipid syndrome? *British Journal of Haematology, 189*(2), 216–227. doi: 10.1111/bjh.16431.

*Arnett, D. K., Blumenthal, R. S., Albert, M. A., et al. (2019). 2019 ACC/AHA Guideline on the primary prevention of cardiovascular disease: Executive summary: A report of the American College of Cardiology/American Heart Association Task Force on Clinical Practice Guidelines. *Journal of the American College of Cardiology, 74*(10), 1376–1414.

*Barnes, G. D., Lucas, E., Alexander, G. C., et al. (2015). National trends in ambulatory oral anticoagulant use. *American Journal of Medicine, 128*(12), 1300–1305.

*Campbell, B. C. V., De Silva, D. A., Macleod, M. R., et al. (2019). Ischemic stroke. *Nature Review Disease Primers, 5*(1), 70.

*Chan, N. C., Paikin, J. S., Hirsh, J., et al. (2014). New oral anticoagulants for stroke prevention in atrial fibrillation: Impact of study design, double counting and unexpected findings on interpretation of study results and conclusions. *Thrombosis and Haemostasis, 111*(5), 798–807.

*Chan, P. H., Hai, J. J., Huang, D., et al. (2016). Burden of upper gastrointestinal symptoms in patients prescribed dabigatran for stroke prevention. *SAGE Open Medicine, 4,* 2050312116662414.

*Chung, M. K., Refaat, M., Shen, W. K., et al. (2020). Atrial fibrillation: JACC Council perspectives. *Journal of the American College of Cardiology, 75*(14), 1689–1713.

*Colman, R. W., Clowes, A. W., George, J. N., et al. (2006). Overview of hemostasis. In R. W. Colman (Ed.), *Hemostasis and thrombosis: Basic principles and clinical practice* (5th ed., pp. 13–17). J. B. Lippincott.

*Coppola, A., Tufano, A., Cerbone, A. M., et al. (2009). Inherited thrombophilia: Implications for prevention and treatment of venous thromboembolism. *Seminars in Thrombosis and Hemostasis, 35,* 683–694.

*Cuker, A., Arepally, G. M., Chong, B. H., et al. (2018). American Society of Hematology 2018 guidelines for management of venous thromboembolism: Heparin-induced thrombocytopenia. *Blood Advances, 2*(22), 3360–3392.

*Dangas, G. D., Tijssen, J. G. P., Wöhrle, J., et al. (2020). A controlled trial of rivaroxaban after transcatheter aortic-valve replacement. *New England Journal of Medicine, 382*(2), 120–129.

*Di Minno, A., Frigerio, B., Spadarella, G., et al. (2017). Old and new oral anticoagulants: Food, herbal medicines and drug interactions. *Blood Reviews, 31*(4), 193–203.

*Ding, W. Y., Harrison, S., Gupta, D., et al. (2020). Stroke and bleeding risk assessments in patients with atrial fibrillation: Concepts and controversies. *Frontiers in Medicine* (Lausanne), 7, 54.

*Dobesh, P. P., Bhatt, S. H., Trujillo, T. C., et al. (2019). Antidotes for reversal of direct oral anticoagulants. *Pharmacology and Therapeutics, 204,* 107405.

*Easaw, J. C., Shea-Budgell, M. A., Wu, C. M. J., et al. (2015). Canadian consensus recommendations on the management of venous thromboembolism in patients with cancer. Part 1: Prophylaxis. *Current Oncology, 22,* 133–143.

*Essa, H., Hill, A. M., & Lip, G. Y. H. (2020). Atrial fibrillation and stroke. *Cardiac Electrophysiology Clinics, 13,* 243–255.

*Fahrni, J., Husmann, M., Gretener, S. B., & Keo, H. H. (2015). Assessing the risk of recurrent venous thromboembolism – A practical approach. *Vascular Health and Risk Management, 11,* 451–459.

*Flieder, T., Weiser, M., Eller, T., et al. (2018). Interference of DOACs in different DRVVT assays for diagnosis of lupus anticoagulants. *Thrombosis Research, 165*, 101–106.

*Garcia, D. A, Witt, D. M., Hylek, E., et al. (2008). Delivery of optimized anticoagulant therapy: Consensus statement from the anticoagulation forum. *Annals of Pharmacotherapy, 42*(9), 79–88.

*Garg, J., Chaudhary, R., Krishnamoorthy, P., et al. (2016). Safety and efficacy of oral factor-Xa inhibitors versus Vitamin K antagonist in patients with non-valvular atrial fibrillation: Meta-analysis of phase II and III randomized controlled trials. *International Journal of Cardiology, 218*, 235–239.

*Geerts, W. H., Bergqvist, D., Pineo, G. F., et al. (2008). Prevention of venous thromboembolism: American College of Chest Physicians evidence-based clinical practice guidelines (8th ed.). *Chest, 133*(6 Suppl.), 381S–453S.

*Greving, J. P., Diener, H. C., Reitsma, J. B., et al. (2019). Antiplatelet therapy after noncardioembolic stroke. *Stroke, 50*(7), 1812–1818.

*Hankey, G. J. (2017). Stroke. *Lancet, 389*(10069), 641–654.

*Heit, J. A., Spencer, F. A., & White, R. H. (2016). The epidemiology of venous thromboembolism. *Journal of Thrombosis and Thrombolysis, 41*(1), 3–14.

*Hirsh, J., Bauer, K. A., Donati, M. B., et al. (2008). Parenteral anticoagulants: American College of Chest Physicians evidence-based clinical practical guidelines (8th ed.). *Chest, 133*(6 Suppl.), 141S–159S.

*Holbrook, A., Schulman, S., Witt, D. M., et al. (2012). Evidence-based management of anticoagulant therapy: Antithrombotic therapy and prevention of thrombosis. American College of Chest Physicians Evidence-Based Clinical Practice Guidelines (9th ed.). *Chest, 141*(2 Suppl.), e152S–e184S.

*Hotoleanu, C. (2017). Genetic risk factors in venous thromboembolism. *Advances in Experimental Medicine and Biology, 906*, 253–272.

*Hull, R. D., & Pineo, G. (2004). Heparin and low molecular-weight heparin therapy for venous thromboembolism: Will unfractionated heparin survive? *Seminars in Thrombosis and Hemostasis, 30*(Suppl. 1), 11–23.

*Jacobs, L. G. (2008). Warfarin pharmacology, clinical management, and evaluation of hemorrhagic risk for the elderly. *Cardiology Clinics, 26*, 157–167.

*January, C. T., Wann, L. S., Alpert, J. S., et al. (2014). 2014 AHA/ACC/HRS guideline for the management of patients with atrial fibrillation: A report of the American College of Cardiology/American Heart Association task force on practice guidelines and the heart rhythm society. *Journal of the American College of Cardiology, 64*, e1–e76.

*January, C. T., Wann, L. S., Calkins, H., et al. (2019). 2019 AHA/ACC/HRS focused update of the 2014 AHA/ACC/HRS guideline for the management of patients with atrial fibrillation: A report of the American College of Cardiology/American Heart Association Task Force on Clinical Practice Guidelines and the Heart Rhythm Society in collaboration with the Society of Thoracic Surgeons. *Circulation, 140*(2), e125–e151.

*Johnson, J. A., Caudle, K. E., Gong, L., et al. (2017). Clinical Pharmacogenetics Implementation Consortium (CPIC) guideline for pharmacogenetics-guided warfarin dosing: 2017 update. *Clinical Pharmacology and Therapeutics, 102*(3), 397–404.

Johnston, S. C., Amarenco, P., Denison, H., et al. (2020). Ticagrelor and aspirin or aspirin alone in acute ischemic stroke or TIA. *New England Journal of Medicine, 383*(3), 207–217.

*Kernan, W. N., Pvbiagele, B., Black, H. R., et al. (2014). Guidelines for the prevention of stroke in patients with stroke and transient ischemic attack: A guideline for healthcare professionals from the American Heart Association/American Stroke Association. *Stroke, 45*(7), 2160–2236.

*Key, N. S., Bohlke, K., & Falanga, A. (2019). Venous thromboembolism prophylaxis and treatment in patients with cancer: ASCO clinical practice guideline update summary. *Journal of Oncology Practice, 15*(12), 661–664.

*Khan, T., Wynne, H., Wood, P., et al. (2004). Dietary vitamin K influences intra-individual variability in anticoagulant response to warfarin. *British Journal of Haematology, 124*(3), 348–354.

*Kirchhof, P., Benussi, S., Kotecha, D., et al. (2016). ESC Scientific Document Group: 2016 ESC Guidelines for the management of atrial fibrillation developed in collaboration with EACTS. *European Heart Journal, 37*(38), 2893–2962.

*Konstantinides, S. V., Myer, G., Becattini, C., et al. (2019). The 2019 ESC guidelines on the diagnosis and management of acute pulmonary embolism. *European Heart Journal, 40*(42), 3453–3455.

*Kovacs, R. J., Flaker, G. C., Saxsonhouse, S. J., et al. (2015). Practical management of anticoagulation in patients with atrial fibrillation. *Journal of the American College of Cardiology, 65*(13), 1340–1360.

*Lim, W., Le Gal, G., Bates, S. M., et al. (2018). American Society of Hematology 2018 guidelines for management of venous thromboembolism: Diagnosis of venous thromboembolism. *Blood Advances, 2*(22), 3226–3256.

*Lip, G. Y. H., Banerjee, A., Boriani, G., et al. (2018). Antithrombotic Therapy for Atrial Fibrillation: CHEST Guideline and Expert Panel Report. *Chest, 154*(5), 1121–1201.

*Lokhandwala, J., Best, P. J. M., Henry, Y., et al. (2011). Allergic reactions to clopidogrel and cross-reactivity to other agents. *Current Allergy and Asthma Reports, 11*, 52–57.

*Lovenox (enoxaparin sodium injection) prescribing information. Available from: https://www.lovenox.com/patient-self-injection-video. Viewed February 16, 2021.

*Maganti, K., Rigolin, V. H., Enriquez Sarano, M., et al. (2010). Valvular heart disease: Diagnosis and management. *Mayo Clinic Proceedings, 85*, 483–500.

*Makedonov, I., Kahn, S. R., & Galanaud, J. P. (2020). Prevention and management of the post-thrombotic syndrome. *Journal of Clinical Medicine, 9*(4), 923.

*McCabe, P. J. (2005). Spheres of clinical nurse specialist practice influence evidence-based care for patients with atrial fibrillation. *Clinical Nurse Specialist, 19*(6), 308–317.

*Merli, G. J. (2008). Pathophysiology of venous thrombosis and the diagnosis of deep venous thrombosis-pulmonary embolism in the elderly. *Cardiology Clinics, 26*, 203–219.

*Narouze, S., Benzon, H. T., Provenzano, D., et al. (2018). Interventional spine and pain procedures in patients on antiplatelet and anticoagulant medications (second edition): Guidelines from the American Society of Regional Anesthesia and Pain Medicine, the European Society of Regional Anaesthesia and Pain Therapy, the American Academy of Pain Medicine, the International Neuromodulation Society, the North American Neuromodulation Society, and the World Institute of Pain. *Regional Anesthesia and Pain Anesthesia Pain Medicine, 43*(3), 225–262.

*National Comprehensive Cancer Network Guidelines Version 1.2020. Cancer Associated Venous Thromboembolic Disease. Available from: https://www.nccn.org/professionals/physician_gls/pdf/vte.pdf. Viewed May 8, 2020.

National Institute for Health and Care Excellence. (2019): Stroke and transient ischaemic attack in over 16s: Diagnosis and initial management. Available from: https://www.nice.org.uk/guidance/ng128/resources/stroke-and-transient-ischaemic-attack-in-over-16s-diagnosis-and-initial-management-pdf-66141665603269. Viewed May 14, 2020.

*National Institutes of Health. Vitamin K: Fact Sheet for Health Professionals. Available from: https://ods.od.nih.gov/factsheets/vitaminK-HealthProfessional/. Accessed February 4, 2021.

*Nijenhuis, V. J., Brouwer, J., Delewi, R., et al. (2020). Anticoagulation with or without clopidogrel after transcatheter aortic-valve implantation. *New England Journal of Medicine, 382*(18), 1696–1707.

*Nishimoto, Y., Yamashita, Y., Morimoto, T., et al. (2020). Validation of the VTE-BLEED score's long-term performance for major bleeding in patients with venous thromboembolisms: From the COMMAND VTE registry. *Journal of Thrombosis and Haemostasis, 18*(3), 624–632.

*Nishimura, R. A., Otto, C. M., Bonow, R. O., et al. (2017). 2017 AHA/ACC focused update of the 2014 AHA/ACC Guideline for the management of patients with valvular heart disease: A report of the American College of Cardiology/American Heart Association Task Force on Clinical Practice Guidelines. *Journal of the American College of Cardiology, 70*(2), 252–289.

*Nutescu, E. A., Burnett, A., Fanikos, J., et al. (2016). Pharmacology of anticoagulants used in the treatment of venous thromboembolism. *Journal of Thrombosis and Thrombolysis, 41*, 15–31.

*Ortel, T. L., Neumann, I., Ageno, W., et al. (2020). American Society of Hematology 2020 guidelines for management of venous thromboembolism: Treatment of deep vein thrombosis and pulmonary embolism. *Blood Advances, 4*(19), 4693–4738.

Otto, C. M., Nishimura, R. A., Bonow, R. O., et al. (2021). 2020 ACC/AHA guideline for the management of patients with valvular heart disease: A report of the American College of Cardiology/American Heart Association Joint Committee on Clinical Practice Guidelines. *Circulation, 143*(5), e72–e227.

*Patrono, C., Baigent, C., Hirsh, J., et al. (2008). Antiplatelet drugs: American College of Chest Physicians Evidence-Based clinical practice guidelines (8th ed.). *Chest, 133*(6 Suppl.), 199S–233S.

*Piazza, G., & Goldhaber, S. Z. (2006). Acute pulmonary embolism. Part 1: Epidemiology and diagnosis. *Circulation, 114,* e28–e32.

*Powers, W. J., Rabinstein, A. A., Ackerson, T., et al. (2018). American Heart Association Stroke Council. 2018 guidelines for the early management of patients with acute ischemic stroke: A guideline for healthcare professionals from the American Heart Association/American Stroke Association. *Stroke, 49*(3), e46–e110.

*Powers, W. J., Rabinstein, A. A., Ackerson, T., et al. (2019). Guidelines for the early management of patients with acute ischemic stroke: 2019 update to the 2018 guidelines for the early management of acute ischemic stroke: A guideline for healthcare professionals from the American Heart Association/American Stroke Association. *Stroke, 50*(12), e344–e418.

*Raskob, G. E., Angchaisuksiri, P., Blanco, A. N., et al. (2014). Thrombosis: A major contributor to global disease burden. *Thrombosis Research, 134,* 931–938.

*Righini, M., & Bounameaux, H. (2008). Clinical relevance of distal deep vein thrombosis. *Current Opinion in Pulmonary Medicine, 14,* 408–413.

*Ruff, C. T., Giugliano, R. P., Braunwald, E., et al. (2014). Comparison of the efficacy and safety of new oral anticoagulants with warfarin in patients with atrial fibrillation: A meta-analysis of randomised trials. *Lancet, 383*(9921), 955–982.

*Sacco, R. L., Diener, H. C., Yusuf, S., et al. (2008). Aspirin and extended-release dipyridamole versus clopidogrel for recurrent stroke. *New England Journal of Medicine, 359*(12), 1238–1251.

*Saito, Y., Nazif, T., Baumbach, A., et al. (2020). Adjunctive antithrombotic therapy for patients with aortic stenosis undergoing transcatheter aortic valve replacement. *JAMA Cardiology, 5*(1), 92–101.

*Salem, D. V., O'Gara, P. T., Madias, C., et al. (2008). Valvular and structural heart disease: American College of Chest Physicians Evidence-Based Clinical Practice Guidelines (8th ed.). *Chest, 133*(6 Suppl.), 593S–626S.

*Schaefer, J. K., Li, Y., Gu, X., et al. (2019). Association of adding aspirin to warfarin therapy without an apparent indication with bleeding and other adverse events. *JAMA Internal Medicine, 179*(4), 533–541.

*Schulman, S., Beyth, R. J., Kearon, C., et al. (2008). Hemorrhagic complications of anticoagulant and thrombolytic treatment: American College of Chest Physicians Evidence-Based Clinical Practice Guidelines (8th ed.). *Chest, 133*(6 Suppl.), 257S–298S.

*Schünemann, H. J., Cushman, M., Burnett, A. E., et al. (2018). American Society of Hematology 2018 guidelines for management of venous thromboembolism: Prophylaxis for hospitalized and nonhospitalized medical patients. *Blood Advances, 2*(22), 3198–3225.

*Spyropoulos, A. C. (2008). Brave new world: The current and future use of novel anticoagulants. *Thrombosis Research, 123,* S29–S35.

*Steinberg, B. A., Greiner, M. A., Hammill, B. G., et al. (2015). Contraindications to anticoagulation therapy and eligibility for novel anticoagulants in older patients with atrial fibrillation. *Cardiovascular Therapeutics, 33*(4), 177–183.

*Sulzgruber, P., Wassmann, S., Semb, A. G., et al. (2019). Oral anticoagulation in patients with non-valvular atrial fibrillation and a CHA2DS2-VASc score of 1. *European Heart Journal, 40*(36), 3010–3012.

*Sun, J. C., Davidson, M. J., Lamy, A., et al. (2010). Antithrombotic management of patients with prosthetic heart valves: Current evidence and future trends. *Lancet, 374,* 565–576.

*Tektonidou, M. G., Andreoli, L., Limper, M., et al. (2019). EULAR recommendations for the management of antiphospholipid syndrome in adults. *Annals of Rheumatic Disease, 78*(10), 1296–1304.

*Tomaselli, G. F., Mahaffey, K. W., Cuker, A., et al. (2020). 2020 Expert Consensus decision pathway on the management of bleeding in patients on oral anticoagulants. *Journal of the American College of Cardiology, 76*(5), 594–622.

*Tran, H. A., & Ginsberg, J. S. (2006). Anticoagulant therapy for major arterial and venous thromboembolism. In R. W. Colman (Ed.), *Hemostasis and thrombosis: Basic principles and clinical practice* (5th ed., pp. 1676–1680). Philadelphia, PA: J. B. Lippincott.

*United States Department of Agriculture FoodData Central. Available from: https://fdc.nal.usda.gov/. Viewed February 16, 2021.

*United States Department of Agriculture USDA National Nutrient Database for Standard Reference Release 28. Available from: https://ods.od.nih.gov/pubs/usdandb/VitK-Phylloquinone-Content.pdf. Viewed February 4, 2021.

*Varga, E. A. (2008). Genetics in the context of thrombophilia. *Journal of Thrombosis and Thrombolysis, 25,* 2–5.

*Vazquez, S. R. (2018). Drug-drug interactions in an era of multiple anticoagulants: A focus on clinically relevant drug interactions. *Blood, 132*(21), 2230–2239.

Veteran's Affairs Nutrition and Food Services Vitamin K Content. Available from: https://www.nutrition.va.gov/docs/UpdatedPatientEd/VitaminKContentofFoods-nationalboard03-2011.pdf. Viewed February 16, 2021.

WARFARINDOSING.org. Available from: http://warfarindosing.org/Source/Home.aspx. Viewed February 16, 2021.

*Werth, S., Breslin, T., NiAinle, F., et al. (2015). Bleeding risk, management and outcome in patients receiving non-VKA oral anticoagulants (NOACs). *American Journal of Cardiovascular Drugs, 15*(4), 235–242.

*Witt, D. M. (2010). Optimizing use of current anticoagulants. *Hematology Oncology Clinics of North America, 24,* 717–726.

*Witt, D. M., Clark, N. P., Kaatz, S., et al. (2016). Guidance for the practical management of warfarin therapy in the treatment of venous thromboembolism. *Journal of Thrombosis and Thrombolysis, 41*(1), 187–205.

*Witt, D. M., Nieuwlaat, R., Clark, N. P., et al. (2018). American Society of Hematology 2018 guidelines for management of venous thromboembolism: Optimal management of anticoagulation therapy. *Blood Advances, 2*(22), 3257–3291.

*Wolfe, Z., Khan, S. U., Nasir, F., et al. (2018). A systematic review and Bayesian network meta-analysis of risk of intracranial hemorrhage with direct oral anticoagulants. *Journal of Thrombosis and Haemostasis, 16*(7), 1296–1306.

*Zeb, I., Krim, N., & Bella, J. (2018). Role of CYP2C19 genotype testing in clinical use of clopidogrel: Is it really useful? *Expert Review of Cardiovascular Therapy, 16*(5), 369–377.

50 Anemias

Caroline Attia and Kelly Barranger

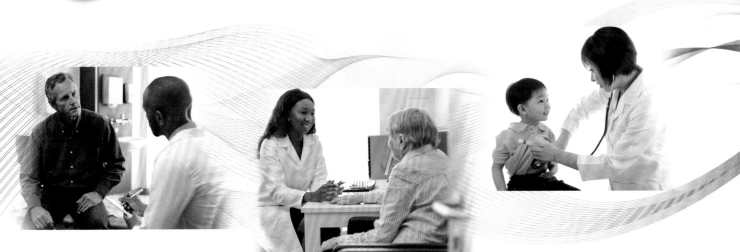

Learning Objectives

1. Discuss the pathophysiology, evaluation, and treatment of the various types of anemia.
2. Interpret laboratory tests in patients with anemia.
3. Select the appropriate pharmacologic agents for treatment of anemias.
4. Formulate appropriate monitoring plans for patients with various types of anemias.

INTRODUCTION

Anemia is a condition in which there is a decrease in the number of red blood cells (RBCs) or hemoglobin in the blood. Anemia can also be defined as a reduced ability to carry oxygen to meet physiologic needs, which varies by age, sex, altitude, and pregnancy status. There is no one set of "normal ranges" for hemoglobin, hematocrit, and RBCs. In general, anemia can be defined as values that are more than 2 standard deviations below the mean. The World Health Organization (WHO) criteria for anemia in men and women are less than 13.0 and less than 12.0 g/dL, respectively (**Table 50.1**). These values are also supported by the second National Health and Nutrition Examination Survey (Centers for Disease Control and Prevention, 2012).

CAUSES

Anemia may develop through blood loss, nutritional deficiency, or malabsorption syndromes; develop concurrently with inflammation or malignancy; or be inherited, as in sickle cell disease (SCD), thalassemia, or hemoglobinopathy. Anemia may also occur from the treatment of diseases such as cancer, HIV/AIDS, or hepatitis C.

PATHOPHYSIOLOGY

RBCs, also known as *erythrocytes*, are formed in the marrow of the ribs, sternum, clavicle, vertebrae, pelvis, and proximal epiphyses of the humerus and femur. RBCs play a vital role in the support of metabolism by transporting oxygen to and removing carbon dioxide from tissue. To maintain proper tissue oxygenation and sustain a normal acid–base balance, an adequate number of RBCs must be available, and they must be in specific shape and size. The average adult blood cell concentration for mean corpuscular volume (MCV) is 80 to 96 fL. These values may vary slightly from laboratory to laboratory.

RBCs develop from a pluripotent cell, which differentiates into an erythroid precursor. The cells shed their nuclei and obtain hemoglobin. The production of RBCs is initiated by the hormone erythropoietin (EPO), which is produced by the kidneys in response to a decrease in tissue oxygen concentration. Decreased tissue oxygen then signals the kidneys to increase production and release EPO. This EPO stimulates the stem cell to differentiate into proerythroblasts. EPO also increases the rate of mitosis and increases the release of reticulocytes from the marrow and induces hemoglobin formation. When hemoglobin synthesis is accelerated, the critical hemoglobin concentration necessary for maturity is reached more rapidly, causing an earlier release of reticulocytes. The appearance of reticulocytes in peripheral circulation indicates that RBC production is being stimulated. The maturation process takes about 1 week. Several days are then required for the reticulocyte to become an erythrocyte (**Figure 50.1**). The normal RBC survival time is 120 days; the survival time can be decreased to 18

TABLE 50.1

Hemoglobin Thresholds

Age or Gender Group	Hemoglobin Thresholds (g/dL)
Children (0.5–4.99 y)	11.0
Children (5.00–11.99 y)	11.5
Children (12.0–14.99 y)	12.0
Nonpregnant women (15.00 y)	12.0
Pregnant women	11.0
Men (15.00 y)	13.0

to 20 days before occurrence of an anemia if the bone marrow functions at maximal capacity. When hemolytic destruction of RBCs exceeds marrow production, anemia will develop, causing the hemoglobin value to decrease.

DIAGNOSTIC CRITERIA

Anemia is a reduction in the number of circulating RBCs (the hemoglobin concentration) or the volume of packed RBCs (hematocrit) in the blood. Anemias are classified according to their pathophysiologic basis and occur due to decreased production or increased destruction of RBCs. They are also classified according to cell size using the MCV (**Figure 50.2**). Microcytic anemias are those anemias due to RBCs with a lower than normal size. These include iron deficiency anemia, thalassemia, and anemia of chronic disease, infection, inflammation, or malignancy. In contrast, macrocytic anemia may be megaloblastic, such as folate or vitamin B_{12} deficiency, or due to nonmegaloblastic causes, such as myelodysplasia, liver disease, or reticulocytosis (**Box 50.1**).

The signs and symptoms of anemia depend on the rate of development, age, and cardiovascular status of the patient. Rapid onset of anemia is most likely to present with cardiorespiratory symptoms (tachycardia, light-headedness, breathlessness). Anemia of a chronic nature may present with vague symptoms, including fatigue, weakness, headache, vertigo, faintness, sensitivity to cold, pallor, and loss of skin tone.

Normal ranges may not be appropriate for all populations. Patients living at high altitude have values higher than those living at sea level. Smokers or those who have a significant exposure to secondary smoke have higher than normal levels. African Americans of both sexes have lower values compared to the Caucasian population.

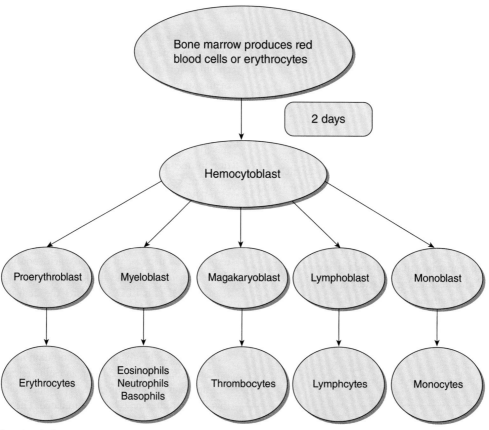

FIGURE 50–1   Hematopoiesis.

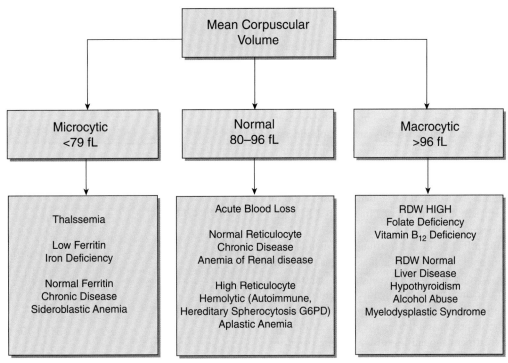

FIGURE 50–2   Anemias classified by mean corpuscular volume.

RDW, red cell distribution width.

**BOX
50.1   Classification of Anemias
by Pathophysiology**

Increased destruction
    Blood loss
    Hemolysis
    SCD
    G6PD deficiency
    Thrombotic thrombocytopenic purpura
    Hemolytic–uremic syndrome
    Clostridial infection
    Hypersplenism
Decreased production
    Iron deficiency
    Thalassemia
    Anemia of chronic disease
    Aplastic anemia
    Myeloproliferative leukemia
G6PD, glucose-6-phosphate dehydrogenase

EVALUATION

Anemia is never normal. A history, physical examination, and simple laboratory testing are useful in evaluating patients with anemia. The first thing to consider in evaluating anemia is the stability of the patient. Second, consider whether it is recent or lifelong. Recent anemia is almost always acquired, whereas lifelong

anemia is likely inherited (hemoglobinopathies, thalassemia, hereditary spherocytosis). Next, obtain a thorough history including recent and past infections, malignancy, renal disease, and a history of autoimmune disease. The review of systems should include weight loss or weight gain, fever, chills or night sweats, change in bowel habits, and black tarry stools.

The goal of the physical examination is to assess the patient's condition and to find signs of organ or multisystem involvement. During the physical examination, note the presence or absence of tachycardia, dyspnea, fever, or postural hypotension. Also, note the presence or absence of lymphadenopathy, hepatosplenomegaly, and bone tenderness, especially over the sternum (chronic myeloid leukemia) or lytic lesion (multiple myeloma or metastatic cancer). Assess the skin for signs of petechiae due to thrombocytopenia, ecchymosis, or coagulation abnormalities. During the physical examination, a stool examination for occult blood should be performed.

Laboratory evaluation should be performed and include a complete blood count (CBC), including differential and reticulocytes.

A low white blood cell (WBC) count (leukopenia) may be associated with hypersplenism, cobalamin deficiencies, or bone marrow suppression or replacement, whereas high WBC count may be associated with a primary hematologic malignancy, inflammation, or infection.

The WBC differential, in conjunction with the total WBC count, may show the absolute number of various cell types:

• Absolute neutrophil count may be elevated due to infection and may be decreased after having chemotherapy.
• Absolute monocyte count may be elevated in myelodysplasia.

- Absolute eosinophil count may be elevated in certain infections.
- Absolute lymphocyte count may be decreased in HIV infection or following treatment with glucocorticoids.

Pancytopenia is the combination of anemia, thrombocytopenia, and neutropenia. Mild pancytopenia is seen in patients with splenomegaly and splenic trapping. The presence of severe pancytopenia is associated with disorders such as aplastic anemia, folate or cobalamin deficiency, hematologic malignancy, and marrow ablation from chemotherapy or radiation.

Hemolysis should be considered in patients with a rapid fall in hemoglobin concentration, reticulocytosis, and/or abnormally shaped RBC (spherocytes or fragmented RBC) in the absence of blood loss.

An important principle in the treatment of anemia is to initiate treatment only when a specific diagnosis is made. In the acute setting, anemia may be severe, and a red cell transfusion is required, but this is rare. Frequently, the cause of anemia is multifactorial. In most cases, it is important to evaluate a patient's iron status before and during the treatment for anemia. Moreover, treatment modalities for anemia are based on the underlying cause and are discussed separately further in the chapter.

ANEMIAS CAUSED BY INCREASED DESTRUCTION

Acute Posthemorrhagic Anemia/Chronic Blood Loss

Posthemorrhagic anemia results from massive hemorrhage associated with spontaneous or traumatic rupture or incision of a large blood vessel. It can also be from an erosion of an artery by a lesion (peptic ulcer, neoplasm) or failure to maintain normal hemostasis. The sudden loss of one third of blood volume may be fatal, whereas a two-thirds loss of blood volume slowly over 24 hours is without immediate risk. During and immediately after hemorrhage, the RBC count, hemoglobin value, and hematocrit may be high due to vasoconstriction. Fluid from tissue enters the circulation within a few hours, resulting in hemodilution, causing a drop in the RBC count and hemoglobin value. This result is proportional to the severity of bleeding. Signs of vascular instability (hypotension and decreased organ perfusion) appear with acute losses of 10% to 15% of the total blood volume. When more than 30% of blood volume is lost suddenly, hypotension and tachycardia occur. When more than 40% of blood volume is lost, signs of hypovolemic shock (confusion, dyspnea, diaphoresis, hypotension, and tachycardia) appear.

Diagnostic Criteria

Initial evaluation of anemia includes a careful history and physical examination. Laboratory evaluation includes CBC, reticulocyte index, iron studies, examination of the peripheral blood smear, and a stool sample for occult blood (**Table 50.2**).

TABLE 50.2	
Laboratory Values for Anemia	
	Reference Range*
Hemoglobin	
Adult male	13.3–16.2 g/dL
Adult female	12.0–15.8 g/dL
Hematocrit	
Adult male	38.8%–46.4%
Adult female	35.4%–44.4%
Reticulocyte count	
Adult male	0.8%–2.3% RBCs
Adult female	0.8%–2.0% RBCs
WBC (leukocyte)	3.54–9.06 L
MCH	26.7–31.9 pg
MCV	79–93 fL
MPV	9.0–12.95 fL
MCHC	32.3–35.9 g/dL
Platelet	165–415 mn
Ferritin	
Adult male	15–400 ng/mL
Adult female	10–200 ng/mL
Vitamin B$_{12}$	200–600 pg/mL
Folate	3–16 ng/mL

*These values may vary from laboratory to laboratory.

MCH, mean corpuscular hemoglobin; MCHC, mean corpuscular hemoglobin concentration; MCV, mean corpuscular volume; MPV, mean platelet volume; WBC, white blood cell.

Further studies are indicated based on the results of the preliminary evaluation.

Initiating Therapy

Immediate therapy consists of hemostasis, restoration of blood volume, and treatment of shock. In many cases, the blood lost needs to be replaced promptly. Blood transfusion is the only means of rapidly restoring blood volume.

Sickle Cell Anemia

Sickle cell anemia is an autosomal recessive disorder in which abnormal hemoglobin leads to chronic hemolytic anemia with numerous clinical consequences. SCD affects approximately 100,000 Americans (Data & Statistics, 2019). The disease affects predominately African Americans and to a lesser number Hispanic Americans.

Pathophysiology

Patients with SCD predominantly make hemoglobin S, which is present in RBCs. Normal adult hemoglobin is made up of hemoglobin A. When the erythrocyte in patient with SCD becomes stressed, the erythrocyte loses its oxygen, causing the cell integrity to be lost. These cells form long, stiff rod-like structures that bend the erythrocyte into a sickle shape. This causes the cells to get stuck in the blood vessels and cut off blood supply to organs. This vaso-occlusion and blockage of microvasculature causes significant damage to the endothelium of the arterial and venous circulation, which leads to a sickle cell crisis. Crisis occurs when patients are physically stressed (e.g., from strenuous exercise), are exposed to high altitude or cold temperatures, or have a high fever or infection. The underlying cause includes hypoxia, dehydration, and acidosis. Sickle cell crises last about a week but may not resolve for several weeks to months. Pain typically occurs in the back, ribs, and limbs. Patients with sickle cell anemia are susceptible to infection, particularly *Streptococcus pneumoniae* and *Haemophilus influenzae*, and are prone to gallstones and renal failure. Other complications include chronic leg ulcer, priapism, aseptic necrosis of the humoral and femoral heads, and chronic osteomyelitis. Long-term effects include stroke, heart failure, and death. Patients should be screened for renal disease, pulmonary hypertension, hypertension, retinopathy, risk of stroke, and pulmonary disease and should receive reproductive and contraception counseling.

Therapeutic transfusion therapy is reserved for individuals with acute stroke, acute chest syndrome, acute multiorgan failure, and acute symptomatic anemia. A lifelong cure for SCD is available through an human leukocyte antigens (HLA)-matched sibling donor hematopoietic stem cell transplant. In the past, this treatment was limited to individuals who are younger than age 16 due to toxicities and adverse outcomes, including stroke, acute chest syndrome, osteonecrosis, and osteomyelitis and a mortality rate of 10% (Bernaudin et al., 1997). However, more recently, older adolescents and adults with severe SCD have been included in treatment protocols (Nickel & Kamani, 2018).

Diagnostic Criteria

Examination of peripheral blood smears for sickling and checking a reticulocyte count can provide supportive data for the diagnosis of SCD. Hemoglobin electrophoresis or a sickle cell preparation can also be useful in the diagnosis of SCD. Laboratory findings also show reduced hemoglobin and an RBC count between 2 and 3 million/mcL.

For those at risk, techniques such as chorionic biopsy have been used during early gestation (6–8 weeks of pregnancy) to identify SCD. Genetic counseling and education must also be offered. Risk of the procedure to mother and fetus, risks of false-positive and false-negative results, and the acceptability of therapeutic abortion should also be discussed.

Initiating Drug Therapy

The management of SCD focuses on primary prevention and treatment of the complication as well as a potential cure. Children with SCD should be immunized against S.

pneumoniae, *H. influenzae* type B, hepatitis B virus, and influenza. All individuals should be immunized as recommended by the Advisory Committee on Immunization Practices. The immunization schedule can be found online through the Centers for Disease Control and Prevention (n.d.) and is updated on a continual basis. Infants are at increased risk for pneumococcal disease and should receive 13-valent conjugate pneumococcal vaccine shortly after birth and 23-valent pneumococcal polysaccharide vaccine at 2 years of age. A second dose should be given at 5 years of age. Other immunizations include hepatitis B and meningococcal vaccine.

Additionally, patients are maintained on folic acid supplementation of 1 mg/day. There is a folate deficiency and supplementation will have an effect on hemoglobin concentration, growth, infection and episodes of pain; however, while the evidence is weak, harm was not found (Dixit et al., 2018).

Hydroxyurea

In selected patients, hydroxyurea is used for prophylaxis treatment to reduce the number of crises (acute chest syndrome or greater than three crises per year) in adults and children. The effects of hydroxyurea on RBCs include increasing hemoglobin F levels, increasing water content of RBCs, increasing deformability of sickled cells, and altering the adhesion of RBCs to endothelium. Evidence suggests that hydroxyurea reduces the number of chest syndromes and transfusions and may reverse organ dysfunction (Wong et al., 2014).

The starting dose of hydroxyurea for adults is 15 mg/kg/d (round up to the nearest 500 mg). For patients with chronic kidney disease (CKD), the dose is adjusted to 5 to 10 mg/kg/day. The starting dosage for infants and children is 20 mg/kg/day. While adjusting the dose of hydroxyurea, a CBC with differential and reticulocyte count should be done every 4 weeks. The goal of therapy is for an absolute neutrophil count 2,000/mcL or more and a platelet count 80,000/mcL or more. In younger patients, an absolute neutrophil count down to 1,250/mcL may be safely tolerated. If neutropenia or thrombocytopenia occurs, hydroxyurea should be held and a CBC with differential should be performed weekly. Once blood counts have recovered, reinstitute hydroxyurea at a dose 5 mg/kg/day lower than the dose given before onset of cytopenias.

The dose of hydroxyurea should be increased by 5 mg/kg/day every 8 weeks until mild myelosuppression (absolute neutrophil count 2,000–4,000/mcL) is achieved, up to a maximum of 35 mg/kg/day. Laboratory studies including a CBC with differential, reticulocyte count, and platelet count should be performed every 2 to 3 months. The effectiveness of hydroxyurea depends on adherence, and patients should be counseled not to miss a dose and not to double up on doses. Keep in mind that it may take 3 to 6 months of treatment with hydroxyurea to see a clinical response. Patients should be maintained on a maximum tolerated dose for 6 months before discontinuation or treatment failure is considered. During hospitalizations, patients should be continued on hydroxyurea (National Heart, Lung, and Blood Institute, 2014).

Hydroxyurea should not be used in patients likely to become pregnant or those unwilling or unable to follow instructions regarding treatment. Patients should be monitored for myelotoxicity. Serious adverse reactions include myelosuppression and the risk of cancer. Side effects include cutaneous hyperpigmentation, alopecia, xerosis, nail pigmentation, and leg ulcers.

Oxbryta (Voxelotor)

Voxelotor is an Hb S polymerization inhibitor indicated for the treatment of SCD in adults and children 12 years of age and older. Accelerated approval on November 2019 was based on an increase in Hb in a phase III randomized, double-blind, placebo-controlled multicenter trial (HOPE trial). The response rate was defined as an increase in Hb of more than 1 g/dL from baseline at week 24 and was described as 51.1% (46/90) compared to 6.5% (6/92) in the placebo group (p, 0.001) (Ballas, 2020).

The dose of voxelotor is 1,500 mg orally once daily and can be taken with or without food. The dose is 1,000 mg orally once daily in the presence of severe hepatic impairment. If taken concomitantly with CYP3A4 inhibitors or fluconazole, the dose should be decreased to 1,000 mg once daily. If taken in the presence of strong or moderate CYP3A4 inducers, the dose should be increased to 2,500 mg once daily.

Pain Management

Management of acute painful episodes consists of exclusion of causes (infection), hydration by oral or intravenous (IV) fluid resuscitation, and aggressive pain relief, including analgesics and opiates. Acetaminophen has analgesic and antipyretic effects. The 24-hour maximum daily dose of acetaminophen in four divided doses should not exceed 4 g for healthy individuals and 3 g in individuals with liver disease or who are pregnant. High dosages of acetaminophen can damage the liver and could be fatal (Han, 2017).

Nonsteroidal antiinflammatory agents (NSAIDs) have antiinflammatory effects in addition to pain and antipyretic proprieties. NSAIDs have potentially serious adverse effects, including gastritis and gastrointestinal (GI) bleeding, which may result in anemia. NSAIDs are contraindicated in patients with a history of GI bleed and renal disease (Han, 2017). The management of acute painful crisis includes aggressive narcotic analgesia, such as morphine or hydromorphone (see Chapter 19). Adverse effects of opioid analgesics include severe sedation and respiratory depression. Side effects include itching, nausea, and vomiting. Opioid analgesics should be used carefully in patients with asthma, impaired ventilation, liver failure, renal failure, and increased intracranial pressure.

Meperidine should not be utilized as a first-line medication and should be used with caution in the treatment of acute SCD because multiple doses are associated with the accumulation of its major metabolite, normeperidine, and central toxicity, including twitching, multifocal clonus, and seizures. Coadministration with antipsychotics may cause neuromuscular disorders, including dystonia, tardive dyskinesia, akathisia, and neuroleptic malignant syndrome. Meperidine in combination with monoamine oxidase inhibitors may cause severe adverse reactions, including excitation, hyperpyrexia, convulsions, and death.

Patients with chronic sickle cell pain are managed with long-acting opioids and short-acting opioids for breakthrough pain, according to the National Heart, Lung, and Blood Institute's guidelines.

ANEMIAS CAUSED BY DIMINISHED PRODUCTION OF RED BLOOD CELLS

Iron Deficiency Anemia

Iron deficiency anemia is the most common nutritional deficiency worldwide. The diagnosis of iron deficiency anemia is made by low hemoglobin and iron stores, whereas iron deficiency is made by low iron stores without anemia. According to WHO, iron deficiency is most prevalent in young children and women of childbearing age. The goal of treatment is to identify the underlying causes and administer the appropriate therapy (Benoist, 2008).

Causes

The cause of iron deficiency is related to insufficient iron intake, inadequate absorption from the GI tract, and increased iron demands. It is also exacerbated by chronic intestinal blood loss due to parasitic and malarial infections.

Insufficient Iron Intake and Inadequate Absorption

One of the main causes for the insufficient iron intake is a vegetarian diet or a diet low in the consumption of animal proteins that contain iron. Inadequate absorption from the GI tract is usually related to various malabsorption syndromes such as celiac disease, Whipple disease, and bacterial overgrowth. Surgical procedures also may contribute to poor iron absorption include post-gastrectomy and gastric bypass because iron is absorbed in the duodenum. Other factors that can affect iron absorption is the presence of certain foods (dietary fiber, coffee, tea, eggs, or milk) or drugs (quinolones, tetracycline, histamine-2 [H_2] blockers, proton pump inhibitors, calcium supplements) or unrelenting diarrhea.

Increased Iron Demands

Iron demands are increased in menstrual blood loss, pregnancy, and lactation. Iron requirements are highest during infancy and pregnancy. Iron deficiency in pregnancy has been implicated as a cause of perinatal complications such as low birth weight and premature delivery in affected mothers. In children, long-term findings include increased susceptibility to infection, poor growth, developmental and behavioral delays, and low mental and motor test scores. Pregnant women should routinely receive iron supplementation and continue into postpartum.

BOX 50.2   Causes of Iron Deficiency

Deficient diet
Decreased absorption
Increased requirements
    Pregnancy
    Lactation
Blood loss
    GI
    Menstrual
    Blood donation
Hemoglobinuria
Iron sequestration

Chronic alcoholism, food faddism, prolonged illness with anorexia, or poor nutrition also contribute to iron deficiency (**Box 50.2**). Interventions such as foods fortified with iron and iron supplementation are in place to prevent and correct iron deficiency.

Pathophysiology

The predominant use of iron is for the creation of heme groups that are incorporated into hemoglobin and myoglobin. Additionally, iron is involved in the production of cytochromes and other enzymes. Immediately bioavailable, iron is bound in the bloodstream to a specific carrier protein, transferrin. Excess of immediate iron needs is stored in the liver, spleen, and bone marrow as ferritin. Patients with iron deficiency anemia may be asymptomatic or have vague symptoms. Other manifestations include koilonychia (spoon nail), angular stomatitis, glossitis, and pica (eating dirt, paint, clay, ice, or cornstarch).

Diagnostic Criteria

Laboratory findings are critical for the diagnosis. The classic criteria for iron deficiency anemia include low serum iron and ferritin concentrations and a high total iron-binding capacity (TIBC). In mild iron deficiency, the hemoglobin, hematocrit, and RBC indices remain normal. In the later stages, the hemoglobin and hematocrit levels fall below normal values (**Table 50.2**).

A low concentration of ferritin (<0–120 ng/L) is the earliest and most sensitive indication of iron deficiency. However, patients with renal or liver disease, malignancies, or infectious or inflammatory processes may have elevated ferritin levels that may not correlate with iron stores in the bone marrow. Transferrin saturation (serum iron divided by TIBC) is also used to assess iron deficiency anemia. Low values (<15%) indicate iron deficiency anemia, although low serum transferrin saturation values may also be present in inflammatory disorders. In this case, TIBC helps to

differentiate the diagnosis. A TIBC over 400 mcg/dL suggests iron deficiency anemia, whereas values below 200 mcg/dL usually represent inflammatory disease. Free erythrocyte protoporphyrin (FEP) can also be used to distinguish between iron deficiency anemia and thalassemia minor. Iron binds with protoporphyrin to form heme. The serum concentration of protoporphyrin not bound to iron is elevated when iron levels are low. Thus, FEP is elevated in patients with iron deficiency anemia, inflammatory disorders, and lead poisoning. Rarely, a bone marrow examination is performed to assess iron stores.

Initiating Drug Therapy

The successful treatment of iron deficiency anemia depends on identifying the underlying cause. The treatment of iron deficiency anemia consists of dietary supplementation and iron preparations (**Table 50.3**). Oral iron is inexpensive and effective in the treatment of anemia. Iron is best absorbed from red meat, fish, and poultry. Plant-based foods are good sources of iron, although they are less easily absorbed. Whole-grain or iron-fortified cereals, breads, and pastas are among the best. Beverages such as tea or milk will reduce the absorption of iron and should be consumed in moderation between meals. Medications such as antacids, proton pump inhibitors, and H_2 antagonists reduce absorption and should be avoided if possible. Vitamin C (500 mg daily), as well as orange juice, increases the absorption of iron due to increased stomach acidity. They should be given together and are recommended with meals. Transfusion should be considered for patients with iron deficiency anemia complaining of fatigue or dyspnea on exertion.

Indications for the use of IV iron include chronic bleeding, intestinal malabsorption, intolerance to oral iron, nonadherence, or hemoglobin of less than 6 g/dL with signs of poor perfusion.

Goals of Drug Therapy

The goal of therapy is based on how the anemia affects the patient's quality of life, activities of daily living, and general well-being. Treatment with oral iron may take 6 to 8 weeks for the hemoglobin to improve and as long as 6 months to replete iron stores. Minimization of the impact chronic iron deficiency anemia has on adequate iron replacement has typically occurred when the serum ferritin level reaches 500 ng/L

TABLE 50.3

Elemental Iron Content of Various Iron Salts

Iron Salt	Percentage Iron
Ferrous fumarate	33
Ferrous gluconate	11.6
Ferrous sulfate	20
Ferrous sulfate, anhydrous	30

and when the hemoglobin and hematocrit have returned to normal levels.

Iron Replacement Therapy

Dosage

Treatment of iron deficiency anemia in adults should start with 100 to 200 mg of elementary iron (Adamson, 2012). For children, treatment is 3 to 6 mg/kg. Supplemental iron should be administered in divided doses without food. The addition of vitamin C may improve absorption.

Non–enteric-coated ferrous salts containing ferrous sulfate are the least expensive and provide adequate elemental iron. Typically, a dose of 325 mg ferrous sulfate three times daily provides sufficient iron replacement (195-mg elemental iron or about 2.7 mg/kg for a 70-kg adult). Slow-release or sustained-release iron preparations do not dissolve until reaching the small intestines, significantly reducing iron absorption.

Iron dextran is administered intravenously in one large dose of 200 to 500 mg. Safer alternatives include sodium ferric gluconate and iron sucrose. Sodium ferric gluconate is administered intravenously in eight weekly 125-mg doses for a total of 1,000 mg, and iron sucrose is administered intravenously five times over 2 weeks in 200-mg doses. Side effects of IV iron supplementation include nausea, vomiting, pruritus, headache, and flushing. Myalgia, arthralgia, and back and chest pain usually resolve in 48 hours.

Blood transfusion should be reserved for those patients who are hemodynamically unstable or show signs of end-organ ischemia from acute GI bleeding.

Time Frame for Response

Therapeutic doses of iron should increase hemoglobin value by 0.7 to 1 g/wk. Reticulocytosis occurs within 7 to 10 days after initiation of iron therapy. Iron therapy should be continued for at least 3 to 6 months. Common causes of treatment failure include noncompliance with therapy, malabsorption, and blood loss equal to the rate of production. Malabsorption can be ruled out by the iron test, which is rarely used, in which plasma iron levels are measured 1 to 2 hours afterward. Refractory responses to treatment may be due to a patient with *Helicobacter pylori* infection or celiac disease. Eradicating *H. pylori* or following a gluten-free diet may eliminate the need for iron supplementation.

Adverse Events

Adverse reactions to oral iron are primarily GI difficulties, consisting of discolored feces, anorexia, constipation or diarrhea, nausea, and vomiting. To minimize the GI side effects, iron supplements should be taken with food. However, the impact of this on bioavailability of agents may be as high as a 66% decrease in iron absorption. Changing to a different iron salt or to a controlled-release preparation may reduce side effects.

A major adverse reaction of iron dextran is the risk of anaphylaxis, which can be fatal. Delayed reactions include myalgias, headache, and arthralgias.

Interactions

There is a host of drug–drug interactions with iron preparations. Many antibiotics, such as tetracyclines and fluoroquinolones, cause a decrease in absorption due to the formation of a chelation product with the ferrous ions. The absorption of iron may be decreased when it is given with products containing aluminum, calcium, or magnesium. This effect may be as much as 30% to 40% reduction in absorption. The theory is that the reduced stomach acidity secondary to the antacid-like properties of products reduces the iron absorption. Similarly, patients taking proton pump inhibitors or H_2 antagonists may also have decreased iron absorption due to the lowered stomach acid. If the patient is taking both medications, space them at least 1 to 2 hours apart. In contrast, acidifying agents such as ascorbic acid (vitamin C) may enhance the absorption of iron-containing salts.

ANEMIA OF CHRONIC RENAL FAILURE

Anemia is a common complication of chronic renal failure and is primarily due to reduced EPO production by the kidney. Anemia occurs when the glomerular filtration rate (GFR) declines below 60 mL/min. Stages of CKD are defined according to the estimated GFR (**Table 50.4**) based on National Kidney Foundation guidelines (Kidney Dialysis Outcomes Quality Initiative [KDOQI, 2007]). Risk factors that increase the risk of CKD include hypertension, diabetes mellitus, autoimmune disease, older age, African ancestry, a family history of renal disease, a previous episode of acute renal failure, and the presence of proteinuria, abnormal urinary sediment, or structural abnormalities of the urinary tract. Measurement of albuminuria is a good test for early detection of renal disease; a 24-hour urine collection is the gold standard. A first-morning urine sample is often more practical and correlates well but not perfectly. Persistence in the urine of greater than 17 mg of albumin per gram of creatinine in adult males and 25 mg of albumin per gram of creatinine in adult females usually signifies chronic renal damage.

TABLE 50.4	
Classification of Chronic Kidney Disease	
Stage	**GFR, mL/min/1.73 m²**
0	>90*
1	>90†
2	60–89
3	30–59
4	15–29
5	<15

*With risk factors for CKD.

†With demonstrated kidney damage (e.g., persistent proteinuria, abnormal urine sediments, abnormal blood and urine chemistry, and abnormal imaging studies).

CKD, chronic kidney disease; GFR, glomerular filtration rate.

Progressive renal impairment is associated with worsening systemic inflammation, as seen with elevated levels of C-reactive protein, which contributes to the acceleration of vascular disease and comorbidities associated with advanced renal disease. As renal impairment advances, metabolic and endocrine functions are impaired and result in anemia, malnutrition, and abnormal metabolism of carbohydrates, fats, and proteins. Plasma levels of hormones, including parathyroid hormone (PTH), insulin, glucagon, sex hormones, and prolactin, change with renal failure because of urinary retention, decreased degradation, and abnormal regulation. Calciphylaxis is a devastating condition seen in patients with advanced kidney disease. It is heralded by livedo reticularis and advances to patches of ischemic necrosis, especially on the legs, thighs, abdomen, and breasts.

Pathophysiology

CKD is characterized by the progressive loss of functioning nephrons. With a reduction in nephron mass, renal vasodilation occurs and leads to hypoperfusion of the remaining glomeruli. Nephrons exposed to prolonged hyperperfusion begin to leak protein, become sclerotic, and eventually are destroyed. Substances that are filtered that are neither secreted nor resorbed by the tubule, such as urea, begin to rise early in the course of renal impairment.

Serum concentration of phosphorus, which is under the influence of PTH, is kept within the normal range until more than 80% of real function is lost. This is because increased PTH reduces the amount of phosphorus resorbed by the tubule. Failure of the kidney to fulfill its excretory, endocrine, and metabolic function results in inadequate quantities of EPO and 1,25-dihydroxy-vitamin D_3. Other hormones, such as PTH, insulin, and prolactin, are present in excess. The primary cause of anemia in patients with CKD is insufficient EPO production by the diseased kidneys. The mechanisms impairing renal EPO production are not well understood.

Initiating Drug Therapy

Patients should be placed on a multivitamin to replace the vitamins lacking in restrictive diets. Adequate bone marrow iron stores should be available before EPO treatment is initiated. Iron supplementation is usually essential to ensure an adequate response to EPO because the demand for iron by the marrow frequently exceeds the amount of iron immediately available for erythropoiesis (measured by percentage of transferring saturation) as well as the amount of iron stores (measured by serum ferritin). Current practice is to target a hemoglobin concentration of 10 to 12 g/dL.

The treatment of anemia caused by chronic renal failure begins with treating reversible causes of deteriorating renal function. Poor metabolism of minerals including calcium and are common in CKD. Oral phosphorus-binding agents, calcium carbonate, and calcium acetate are used to treat hyperphosphatemia. Phosphorus-binding agents that do not contain calcium are sevelamer and lanthanum. Vitamin D or vitamin D analogs (calcitriol, paricalcitol) are given to treat secondary hyperparathyroidism.

Many of the immunologically mediated renal diseases (e.g., membranous nephropathy, Wegener disease, Goodpasture syndrome, lupus nephritis) respond to treatment with corticosteroids, cytotoxic agents, or plasmapheresis. This will not be discussed here. These patients should be under the care of a rheumatologist and/or a nephrologist.

When renal disease is associated with a metabolic disorder such as diabetes (Chapter 45) or gout (not discussed here), the treatment is directed at metabolic control to slow the course of renal deterioration.

When a drug (methicillin, indomethacin, NSAID, metformin, meperidine, and oral hypoglycemics) or other toxic substance is identified as the cause of renal failure, the offending agent should be withheld or avoided. Many antibiotics, antihypertensives, and antiarrhythmics require a reduced dosage or a change in the dose interval in patients with kidney disease.

The Kidney Disease: Improving Global Outcomes (KDIGO) 2012 recommendations for erythropoiesis-stimulating agents (ESA) therapy in patients on non-dialysis and dialysis follow the recommendation from the FDA (Kliger et al., 2013). That is, a hemoglobin target range of 10 to 12 g/dL should be replaced by using the lowest possible dose of ESA to prevent transfusion. The concern is that increased blood transfusions will expose eligible kidney transplant recipients to allosensitizing effects of blood transfusions. Furthermore, the ESA dose should be reduced or interrupted if the hemoglobin exceeds 11 g/dL. The ESA dosing strategy should be individualized for each patient considering the risks and benefits. KDIGO guidelines add an additional goal to avoid hemoglobin levels of less than 9 g/dL. The Normal Hematocrit Study reported worse outcomes in patients with hemoglobin 13 to 15 g/dL compared to 9 to 11 g/dL. While the FDA removed quality-of-life benefits in the use of ESA, the KDIGO recommendation is that it is still reasonable to start ESA in some patients with a hemoglobin level above 10 g/dL. The disagreement falls in interpreting quality of life.

For the naive pediatric patient with anemia, not on iron or ESA, the KDIGO recommendation is for oral iron when the transferrin is less than 20% and ferritin is less than 100 ng/mL. For pediatric patients on dialysis, oral or IV iron is recommended.

Goals of Drug Therapy

The goals of therapy are to (1) treat the underlying renal disease; (2) slow the progression of renal deterioration by modifying the known or suspected factors that are thought to aggravate the primary process and avoid factors that may aggravate existing renal failure; and (3) treat the specific complications of renal disease and prevent long-term complications of uremia. Correction of anemia decreases morbidity and reduces hospitalization and mortality among patients with CKD.

The benefits of correcting anemia include improvements in quality of life, exercise capacity, cognitive function, and sexual function.

Epoetin and Darbepoetin

The KDOQI anemia guidelines 2007 recommend individualizing the risks and benefits of ESA therapy. The goal is to avoid transfusion for a hemoglobin target of 11.0 to 12.0 g/dL and should not be above 13.0 g/dL. Recombinant EPO (epoetin, Epogen, Procrit) is indicated for the treatment of anemia due to chronic renal failure, zidovudine administration (in HIV-infected patients), and chemotherapy administration. Other indications include a reduction in blood transfusions in anemic patients undergoing elective, noncardiac, nonvascular surgery. Similarly, darbepoetin is indicated for patients with chronic renal failure and patients receiving chemotherapy. Recombinant EPO is indicated in chronic renal failure to elevate the hemoglobin when the hemoglobin is less than 10.0 g/dL and to decrease the need for transfusion. Epogen should be avoided for a hemoglobin greater than 12.0 g/dL.

Mechanism of Action

Epoetin and darbepoetin are recombinant hormones that stimulate the production of RBCs from the erythroid tissues in the bone marrow. Epoetin also stimulates the division and differentiation of erythroid progenitors in bone marrow. Darbepoetin is a longer-acting erythropoietic agent than epoetin (serum half-life of 25 vs. 8.5 hours).

Dosage

The starting dose of epoetin is 50 to 100 units/kg given subcutaneously three times a week for a hemoglobin less than 10 g/dL for anemia due to CKD. For patients on dialysis, this should be administered intravenously. Dosing should be individualized and the lowest dose used to reduce the need for transfusion. The dose should be reduced or interrupted for a hemoglobin greater than 10 g/dL or if the hemoglobin rises greater than 1 g/dL in a 2-week period. In the latter case, the dose should be reduced by 25% or more.

The recommended starting dose for darbepoetin is 0.45 mcg/kg body weight, administered as a single IV or subcutaneous injection once weekly (Amgen, 2013). Dosing is the same whether it is given subcutaneously or intravenously. Treat to a target hemoglobin concentration of 10 to 11 g/dL. After initiating therapy, the hemoglobin level should be monitored weekly for at least 4 weeks until the hemoglobin value has stabilized.

All patients receiving erythropoietic stimulation should receive iron supplementation unless iron stores are already in excess. Iron supplementation should be initiated no later than the beginning of treatment and continue throughout the course of therapy. Oral therapy with ferrous sulfate 325 mg once to thrice daily is adequate. Monitor the patient's hematocrit, ferritin, transferrin, vitamin B_{12} and folate levels, blood pressure, clotting times, platelet counts, blood urea nitrogen level, and serum creatinine concentration.

Time Frame for Response

Two to 6 weeks may be required to evaluate the effectiveness of epoetin. If the response is not satisfactory in terms of reduced transfusion requirements or increased hematocrit after 8 weeks of therapy, the dose may be increased up to 300 units/kg three times a week. If patients do not respond, it is unlikely that they will respond to higher doses. Maintenance doses are individualized for each patient.

With once-weekly dosing, steady-state serum levels are achieved within 4 weeks with darbepoetin. Dose adjustment should not be increased more frequently than once a month. If the hemoglobin is increasing and approaching 11 g/dL, the dose should be reduced by 25%. If the hemoglobin continues to increase, the dose is withheld temporarily until the hemoglobin begins to stabilize.

Contraindications

Epoetin and darbepoetin are contraindicated in patients with uncontrolled hypertension or hypersensitivity to mammalian cell–derived products or human albumin. In 2011, the Food and Drug Administration (FDA) revised the labeling of ESA, warning that the risks may outweigh the benefits in patients who have current malignancy and had previous stoke. The KDIGO 2012 guidelines agree about using caution when using ESA. ESA is not intended for patients with chronic renal failure who require correction of severe anemia or in patients with iron folate deficiencies or GI bleeding.

Adverse Events

Epoetin and darbepoetin are generally well tolerated. Adverse reactions may include hypertension, headache, seizure, arthralgia, nausea, edema, fatigue, diarrhea, vomiting, chest pain, asthenia, and dizziness. Other adverse reactions include infection, hypertension, hypotension, and myalgia. Serious adverse reactions include vascular access thrombosis, heart failure, sepsis, and cardiac arrhythmia. There are no significant drug interactions.

ANEMIA OF CHRONIC DISEASE

Anemia of chronic disease is a hypoproliferative anemia and is associated with infection, organ failure, trauma, inflammation, and neoplasia (**Box 50.3**).

Pathophysiology

Anemia of chronic disease typically occurs despite adequate reticuloendothelial iron stores and is characterized by reduced concentrations of serum iron, transferrin, and TIBC; normal or raised ferritin levels; and high erythrocyte sedimentation rate. RBCs are often normochromic and normocytic. In patients with rheumatoid arthritis and Crohn disease, RBCs are similar to those effects of iron deficiency, with hypochromic and microcytic indices.

Causes of Anemia of Chronic Disease

COMMON CAUSES

Chronic infections
  Tuberculosis
  Subacute bacterial endocarditis
  Osteomyelitis
Chronic inflammation
  Rheumatoid arthritis and inflammatory osteoarthritis
  Systemic lupus erythematosus
  Collagen vascular diseases
  Gout
Malignancies

LESS COMMON CAUSES

Alcoholic liver disease
Heart failure
Thrombophlebitis
Chronic obstructive lung disease
Ischemic heart disease

Diagnostic Criteria

In anemia of chronic disease, hematocrit rarely falls below 60% of baseline. The MCV is usually normal or slightly reduced. Serum iron values may be unmeasurable, and transferrin saturation may be extremely low. Serum ferritin values should be normal or increased. A serum ferritin value lower than 300 ng/L suggests coexistent iron deficiency.

Initiating Drug Therapy

Treatment is directed at the underlying cause and at eliminating exacerbating factors such as nutritional deficiencies and marrow-suppressive drugs. Other causes of anemia should be treated before initiating therapy.

Doses of recombinant epoetin are higher for anemia of chronic disease than those in renal anemia. Epoetin is administered subcutaneously, and doses may vary from 150 to 1,500 units/kg/wk.

Goals of Drug Therapy

A good response is likely if, after 2 weeks of therapy, the hemoglobin increases more than 0.5 g/dL. If no response has been observed at 900 units/kg/wk, further escalation is unlikely to be effective. Iron supplements are required to ensure an adequate epoetin response.

THALASSEMIA

Thalassemia is a hereditary disorder of hemoglobin synthesis, which is considered among the hypoproliferative anemias. The alpha-thalassemia syndromes are seen primarily in persons from India and China and are less commonly seen in African Americans. The beta-thalassemia syndrome affects primarily persons of Mediterranean origin (Italian, Greek). Every year, more than 200,000 babies are born with thalassemia major. They have a life expectancy of less than 30 years and are dependent on blood transfusions. Repeated transfusions result in cirrhosis of the liver, cardiomyopathy, endocrinopathies, and death due to hemosiderosis (Savulescu, 2004).

Pathophysiology

Normal adult hemoglobin is primarily hemoglobin A. Hemoglobin A consists of equal quantities of alpha- and beta-globin chains. Thalassemia is present when a hemoglobinopathy is associated with a decreased production of either the alpha- or the beta-globins or a structurally abnormal globin chain. In alpha-thalassemia, the production of alpha-globin chains is controlled by four genes. Mutation of all four genes is incompatible with life (hydrops fetalis). Mutation of only one of the four is considered a silent carrier. Mutations of two of the four genes result in both microcytosis and mild anemia. Mutations of three of the four genes allow excess beta-chains to form tetramers (hemoglobin H) and result in severe anemia in addition to microcytosis. Physical examination will reveal pallor and splenomegaly. Beta-thalassemia is commonly classified by the severity of anemia; many genotypes exist for each phenotype. In beta-thalassemia, the beta-globin chain is controlled by two genes. Mutations of one of two genes results in beta-thalassemia trait (beta-thalassemia minor). Thalassemia intermedia is associated with dysfunction of both beta-globin genes. Clinical severity is intermediate (hemoglobin level of 7–10 g/dL), and patients are usually not dependent on transfusions. Thalassemia major (Cooley anemia) results from mutations of both genes and reveals a majority of hemoglobin F, which results in severe anemia, and RBC transfusions are required to sustain life. Clinical problems include growth failure, bony deformities (abnormal facial structure, pathologic fractures), hepatosplenomegaly, jaundice, leg ulcers, and cholelithiasis. As a result of transfusion dependency, iron overload results because of the body's inability to excrete iron from the transfused RBCs. This results in hemochromatosis, heart failure, cirrhosis, and endocrinopathies typically after more than 100 units.

Diagnostic Criteria

Alpha-Thalassemia Trait

Patients with mild anemia have a hematocrit between 28% and 40%. The MCV is low despite modest anemia, and the RBC bound is normal or increased. Blood smear shows microcytic, hypochromia, target cell and acanthocytes (cell with irregularly spaced bulbous projections). The reticulocyte and iron parameters are normal.

Hemoglobin H

Patients have marked hemolytic anemia with a hematocrit between 22% and 32%. The MCV is low. The peripheral blood smear reveals hypochromia, microcytosis, target cells, and poikilocytosis. The reticulocyte count is elevated. A peripheral blood smear demonstrates the presence of hemoglobin.

Beta-Thalassemia Minor

Patients have modest anemia with a hematocrit between 28% and 40%. The MCV ranges from 50 to 75 fL, and the RBC count is normal or increased. The peripheral blood smear reveals hypochromia, microcytosis, and target cells, and basophilic stippling may be present. The reticulocyte count is normal or slightly elevated.

Beta-Thalassemia Major

Patients have severe anemia, and the hematocrit may fall to less than 10%. The peripheral blood smear is bizarre, revealing severe poikilocytosis, hypochromia, microcytosis, target cells, basophilic stippling, and nucleated RBCs.

Initiating Drug Therapy

Patients with mild thalassemia (alpha-thalassemia trait or beta-thalassemia minor) require no treatment. Patients should be identified so that they will not be subjected to repeated evaluation and treatment for iron deficiency. Patients with hemoglobin H should take folate supplements and avoid iron and oxidative drugs such as sulfonamides. Patients with severe thalassemia are maintained on a regular transfusion schedule and receive folate supplementation. Iron chelation therapy with deferoxamine mesylate may be used when transfusions result in tissue iron overload. Deferoxamine is administered by continuous subcutaneous infusion for 10 to 24 hours/day. Adverse reactions include local irritation at the injection site, pruritus, hypotension, tachycardia, abdominal discomfort, diarrhea, nausea, and vomiting. Ocular and auditory disturbances may occur, and patients should have baseline and annual vision and hearing examinations.

VITAMIN B$_{12}$ DEFICIENCY

Vitamin B$_{12}$ (cyanocobalamin) deficiency, or pernicious anemia, is a disorder of impaired deoxyribonucleic acid synthesis. Vitamin B$_{12}$ deficiency is considered a macrocytic anemia and may arise because of genetic or acquired abnormalities. Special populations, such as older adults, alcoholics, patients with malnutrition, strict vegans, and patients who had weight loss surgery, namely, Roux-en-Y anastomosis, are at high risk for developing vitamin B$_{12}$ deficiency. Vitamin B$_{12}$ is essential to maintaining the integrity of the neurologic system.

Pathophysiology

Vitamin B$_{12}$ deficiency has several causes, including lack of intrinsic factor, inadequate intake, decreased absorption, and inadequate utilization. Other causes include fish tapeworm infestation, *H. pylori* infection, malignancy, pancreatitis,

---

BOX 50.4 Causes of Vitamin B$_{12}$ Deficiency

Dietary deficiency
Decreased production of intrinsic factor
    Pernicious anemia
    Gastrectomy
H. pylori infection
Fish tapeworm
Pancreatic insufficiency
Surgical resection of ileum
Crohn disease

---

gluten enteropathy, sprue, and small bowel bacterial overgrowth (**Box 50.4**). More recently, the increased incidence of obesity and the option of gastric bypass surgery raise greater concerns about vitamin B$_{12}$ deficiency. Vitamin B$_{12}$ is water soluble and obtained by ingestion of fish, meat (beef, pork, organ meat), and dairy products. Its absorption occurs in the terminal ileum and requires intrinsic factor (found in gastric mucosa) for transport across the intestinal mucosa. Ileal absorptive sites may be congenitally absent or destroyed by inflammation or surgical resection. Other causes of decreased absorption include chronic pancreatitis, malabsorption syndromes, and drugs (oral calcium-chelating drugs, aminosalicylic acid, and biguanides).

Vitamin B$_{12}$ deficiency can present with gastric mucosal atrophy, neuropsychiatric abnormalities (paranoia, delirium, confusion, irritability, dementia), and yellow-blue color blindness. GI manifestations include anorexia, intermittent constipation and diarrhea, and poorly localized abdominal pain. An early symptom may be glossitis or weight loss. In the early stages, neurologic symptoms include peripheral loss of position and vibratory sensation in the extremities, weakness, and loss of reflexes. Later stages include spasticity, Babinski responses, and ataxia. Early diagnosis is important because neurologic defects, if left untreated, are irreversible.

Diagnostic Criteria

Serum vitamin B$_{12}$ assay is the most used method for establishing B$_{12}$ deficiency. There is variability between laboratories as to what is a low normal vitamin B$_{12}$ level. This ranges from 150 to 200 pg/mL. Serum concentrations of homocysteine as well as serum and urinary concentrations of methylmalonic acid can aid in the detection of vitamin B$_{12}$ deficiency. These levels are elevated in vitamin B$_{12}$ deficiency due to a decreased metabolism rate. If an intrinsic factor deficiency is suspected, a serum level of the intrinsic factor deficiency antibody can be obtained.

Initiating Drug Therapy

Pernicious anemia, malabsorption syndromes, weight loss surgery, or surgical removal of the stomach causes absence of intrinsic factor. Therefore, dietary vitamin B_{12} cannot be absorbed. In this case, therapy consists of parenteral administration of vitamin B_{12}. In the case of inadequate intake, dietary allowance and supplementation can be recommended.

Goals of Drug Therapy

Clinical improvement is evidenced by increased alertness, appetite, and cooperation. Reticulocytosis occurs within 2 to 3 days and peaks within 5 to 8 days. The hematocrit begins to rise within 2 weeks and reaches normal values within 2 months. The MCV will increase initially due to increased reticulocytes and then will gradually decrease to normal.

Vitamin B_{12} (Cyanocobalamin)

Pernicious anemia is typically treated with parenteral (i.e., intramuscular or deep subcutaneous) cyanocobalamin in a dose of 1,000 mcg (1,000 mcg, 1 mg) every day for 1 week followed by 1 mg every week for 4 weeks. Then, if the underlying disorder persists (e.g., pernicious anemia, surgical removal of the terminal ileum), 1 mg is administered every month for the remainder of the patient's life. Oral vitamin B_{12} 1,000 mcg daily can be an adequate substitution for the parenteral injection.

Due to the lack of intrinsic factor, the original premise was therapy had to be injectable; however, a more recent study (Chan et al., 2016) found that oral therapy has efficacy and can be substituted for the injection.

For dietary insufficiency, the recommended daily doses of vitamin B_{12} are 0.4 mcg for patients ages 0 to 6 months; 0.5 mcg, ages 7 to 12 months; 0.9 mcg, ages 1 to 3; 1.2 mcg, ages 4 to 8; 1.8 mcg, ages 9 to 13; 2.4 mcg, ages 14 and older; 2.6 mcg in pregnant patients; and 2.8 mcg in breast-feeding women.

FOLATE DEFICIENCY

Pathophysiology

Folic acid is necessary to produce nucleic proteins, amino acids, purines, and thymine. Humans are unable to synthesize total daily folate requirements and depend on a dietary source. Major sources of folate include fresh vegetables and fruits, yeast, mushrooms, and animal organs such as liver and kidney. The minimum daily requirement is 50 to 100 mcg. Folic acid deficiency results in the development of large functionally immature erythrocytes (megaloblasts). Major causes of folic acid deficiency include inadequate intake, inadequate absorption, inadequate utilization, increased requirement (pregnancy, lactation, infancy, malignancy, increased metabolism), and increased excretion (renal dialysis, **Box 50.5**). Folic acid deficiency is associated with poor eating habits as seen in older adults, alcoholics, food faddists, and those who are chronically ill. It is also seen in patients with malabsorption syndromes, Crohn disease, and celiac disease. Drugs reported to cause folic

---

BOX 50.5 Causes of Folate Deficiency

Dietary deficiency
Decreased absorption due to
    Phenytoin
    Sulfasalazine
    Trimethoprim–sulfamethoxazole
Increased requirements
    Chronic hemolytic anemia
    Pregnancy
    Exfoliative skin disease

---

acid deficiency include co-trimoxazole, primidone, phenytoin, and phenobarbital.

Symptoms associated with folate deficiency are similar to those in patients with vitamin B_{12} deficiency. Symptoms include weakness, fatigue, difficulty concentrating, irritability headache, shortness of breath, and palpitations. However, the major difference is the absence of neurologic manifestations.

Diagnostic Criteria

Laboratory assessment of folate status includes a serum folic acid level. Serum folic acid levels less than 4 ng/mL suggest deficiency. A low RBC folate level identifies tissue deficiency; however, the values depend on the laboratory method used. Serum homocysteine measurement provides the best evidence of tissue deficiency. Both methylmalonic acid and homocysteine must be measured because B_{12} uses the same pathway. A normal methylmalonic acid level with an elevated homocysteine level confirms the diagnosis of folate deficiency.

Initiating Drug Therapy

A serum folate level less than 4 ng/mL indicates deficiency. Folic acid 1 mg daily is started to replenish the vitamin deficiency. A serum folate level can be followed to evaluate adequate folate stores.

Goals of Drug Therapy

The evaluation of symptomatic improvement is the same as those with vitamin B_{12} deficiency.

Folate Replacement

Folic acid is present in most fruits and vegetables (citrus fruits and green leafy vegetables). The recommended dietary allowances for adult men and women are 0.15 to 0.2 mg and 0.15 to 0.18 mg, respectively. Total body stores are approximately 5 mg and supply requirements for up to 2 to 3 months. Folate deficiency is treated by oral replacement therapy. The usual dose of folate is 1 mg daily. Higher doses up to 5 mg daily may be required for folate deficiency due to malabsorption. The duration of therapy depends on the cause of deficiency. Patients with hemolytic anemia or those with malabsorption or chronic malnutrition should receive oral folic acid indefinitely. Side effects include erythema, skin rash, nausea, abdominal distention, altered sleep patterns, irritability, mental depression, confusion, and impaired judgment.

APLASTIC ANEMIA

Aplastic anemia is a condition of bone marrow failure that can be hereditary or arise from injury to or abnormal expression of the stem cell. Aplastic anemia is defined as pancytopenia with a hypocellular bone marrow in the absence of an abnormal infiltrate and with no increase in reticulin (Marsh et al., 2009). There are several causes of aplastic anemia (**Box 50.6**). One cause is direct stem cell injury from radiation, chemotherapy (alkylating agents), antimetabolites, antimitotics, toxins (benzenes), or pharmacologic agents (**Box 50.7**).

Pathophysiology

Erythrocytes, granulocytes, and platelets, which are normally produced in the bone narrow, decrease to dangerously low levels. The bone marrow becomes hypoplastic with replacement of normal marrow hematopoietic cells by fat cells, and pancytopenia develops. This results in bleeding and increased risk of infection. Patients most commonly present with fatigue, dyspnea, weakness, and skin or mucosal hemorrhage or visual disturbance due to retinal hemorrhage. Physical examination may reveal signs of pallor, purpura, and petechiae.

Diagnostic Criteria

A CBC typically shows pancytopenia. In most cases, the hemoglobin level and neutrophil, reticulocyte, and platelet counts are depressed with a preserved lymphocyte count. The bone marrow aspirate and bone marrow biopsy appear hypocellular

---

BOX 50.6 Causes of Aplastic Anemia

Congenital
Idiopathic/autoimmune
Systemic lupus erythematosus
Chemotherapy
Radiation therapy
Toxins
    Benzene, toluene, insecticides
Heavy metals
    Gold, arsenic, bismuth, mercury
Drugs
Pregnancy

BOX 50.7 Drugs Associated with Aplastic Anemia

Antiprotozoals (quinacrine and chloroquine, mepacrine)
NSAIDs (phenylbutazone, indomethacin, ibuprofen, sulindac, aspirin)
Anticonvulsants (hydantoins, carbamazepine, phenacemide, felbamate)
Sulfonamides
    Antithyroid drugs (methimazole, methylthiouracil, propylthiouracil)
    Antidiabetic drugs (tolbutamide, chlorpropamide)
    Carbonic anhydrase inhibitors (acetazolamide, methazolamide)
Antihistamines (cimetidine, chlorpheniramine)
D-penicillamine
Estrogens
Sedatives and tranquilizers (chlorpromazine, prochlorperazine, piperacetazine, chlordiazepoxide, meprobamate, methyprylon)
Allopurinol
Methyldopa
Quinidine
Lithium
Guanidine
Potassium perchlorate
Thiocyanate
Carbimazole

---

with scant amounts of normal hematopoietic progenitors. Magnetic resonance imaging of the vertebrae shows uniform replacement of marrow with fat.

Initiating Drug Therapy

Mild cases of aplastic anemia may be treated with supportive care. Foremost, RBC transfusions and platelets are given for bleeding, and antibiotics are given for infections (Marsh et al., 2009). Antifungals are given prophylactically for a low neutrophil count. Treatment for severe acquired aplastic anemia includes hematopoietic stem cell transplantation and immunosuppression therapy. When the cause of aplastic anemia is related to drugs or chemicals, these should be discontinued. Patients presenting with aplastic anemia should be referred to a hematologist/oncologist.

SPECIAL POPULATION CONSIDERATIONS

Pediatric

The American Academy of Pediatrics recommends hemoglobin screening and risk evaluation for iron deficiency anemia in all children at 1 year of age. The Centers for Disease Control and Prevention recommends screening for low-income or newly immigrated families to begin at 9 to 12 months of age and for low-birth-weight infants before 6 months of age if they are not fed iron-fortified formula. Iron deficiency anemia significantly impairs mental and psychomotor development in infants and children. Iron deficiency can be reversed with treatment; however, the reversibility of the mental and psychomotor effects is unclear. Furthermore, iron deficiency increases a child's susceptibility to lead toxicity as lead replaces iron in the absorptive pathway when iron is unavailable.

Young children are at greatest risk for iron deficiency anemia due to rapid growth, increased iron requirements, and lack of iron in the diet. Poverty, abuse, and living in a home with poor household conditions also place children at risk for iron deficiency anemia. Iron deficiency anemia is seen most commonly in children ages 6 months to 3 years. Those at highest risk are low-birth-weight infants after age 2 months, breast-fed term infants who receive no iron-fortified food or supplemental iron after age 4 months, and formula-fed term infants who are not consuming iron-fortified formula. During the first months of life, the newborn rapidly uses iron stores due to an accelerated growth rate and increased blood volume. Maternally derived iron stores are generally sufficient for the first 4 to 6 months; however, sustained growth demands an increased iron supply. By the end of the second year of life, the growth rate decreases and accompanying iron needs level off. During adolescence, growth accelerates and iron needs increase. Adolescent girls are at increased risk and need additional iron to compensate for menstrual loss. Patients with iron deficiency who are responding poorly to the usual dietary supplementation regimens should be screened for lead poisoning. Heavy metal poisoning, as with lead and bismuth, is often overlooked.

Geriatric

Anemia should not be accepted as an inevitable consequence of aging. Mild anemia, less than 10 g/dL as defined by the WHO criteria, is associated with significant negative outcomes, including decreased physical performance, increased number of falls, increased frailty, decreased cognition, increased dementia, increased hospitalization, and increased mortality.

Anemia in older adults is a risk factor of adverse outcomes, including hospitalization, morbidity, and mortality. The prevalence of anemia increases after 50 years of age and exceeds 20% of those 85 years and older (Goodnough & Schrier, 2014). There is no specific recommended hemoglobin threshold, but it is prudent to maintain a hemoglobin level of 9 to 10 g/dL unless otherwise indicated. The most common causes of anemia in older patients are chronic disease (CKD, infections, malignancies, and inflammatory disorders), iron deficiency, and nutritional and metabolic disorders. Anemia resulting from blood loss due to surgery, injury, and GI and genitourinary bleeding is more common in hospitalized patients.

Women

Pregnant women and women who are 4- to 6-week postpartum are at risk for asymptomatic iron deficiency anemia. As such,

the American Academy of Family Physicians, U.S. Preventive Services Task Force, and the Centers for Disease Control and Prevention recommend routine screening. Pregnant women who are iron deficient are at increased risk for a preterm delivery and delivering a low-birth-weight baby. Two to three times more iron is required in pregnancy and in childhood. In pregnant women who had a previous pregnancy with a fetus or infant with a neural tube defect, the recommended dose of folate is 5 mg daily. Also, women who may become pregnant and have seizure disorders should take folate supplementation.

MONITORING PATIENT RESPONSE

In almost all cases of anemia, evaluation should proceed in an orderly manner and therapy be withheld until a specific diagnosis can be made. Patients with significant cardiopulmonary disease, who may be compromised by a decreased oxygen capacity, require immediate correction for anemia. This may require inpatient evaluation and consideration of transfusion therapy when they are experiencing dyspnea, angina, or marked fatigue related to anemia. Once treatment has been initiated, patient response should be evaluated on at least a monthly basis. Correction of anemia decreases morbidity and reduces hospitalization and mortality among patients with CKD. Benefits of correcting anemia include improvements in the patient's quality of life, exercise capacity, cognitive function, and sexual function.

PATIENT EDUCATION

Patients need to be told to what extent the anemia accounts for symptoms, what the possible causes are, and what the appropriate workup will be. Patient education and the importance of adherence to therapy are integral to successful management. Because some patients with anemia require the need for medication, the patient needs to be informed about possible side effects and when to report dangerous side effects.

Nutrition

All patients are encouraged to limit the use of alcohol, to avoid tobacco, to exercise, and to consume a diet of meat, poultry, fish, and fresh fruits and vegetables. To prevent deficiency, all patients are encouraged to eat fortified foods (fortified cereals, dairy products) or take supplements as prescribed by their physician. Patients with specific problems, such as pica, may need additional counseling.

Complementary and Alternative Medications

Patients should be educated that herbs are not regulated by the U.S. FDA and may interact with prescription medications. Patients must also understand that they should report any adverse reactions and stop the herbal medication immediately.

CASE STUDY 1

M.W. is a 69-year-old African-American man and was referred to clinic for evaluation of increasing shortness of breath.

Past medical history
  Chronic renal insufficiency
  Hypertension
  Congestive heart failure
  Diabetes mellitus type 2, poor control
  Deep vein thrombosis
  Alcohol abuse
  Chronic obstructive pulmonary disease with respiratory
    failure
Family history
  Noncontributory
Physical examination
  Height 69 in., weight 205 lb
  Blood pressure: 138/88
  Pulse 86 beats/min, regular
  Lungs clear, neck supple negative for jugular venous
    distention
  Lower extremities +1 edema
Laboratory findings
  Scr = 2.8 K$^+$ = 5.1
  BUN = 56 Na$^+$ = 147

WBC = 5.0 Hb = 8.2
Hct = 24.6
Serum ferritin 189 mg/dL
Social history
  Tobacco: 52 pack-years
  Alcohol: distant past

DIAGNOSIS: ANEMIA OF CKD

1. List specific goals of treatment for M.W.
2. What drug therapy would you prescribe? Why?
3. What are the parameters for monitoring success of therapy?
4. Discuss specific patient education based on the prescribed therapy.
5. List one or two adverse reactions for the selected agent that would cause you to change therapy.
6. What would be the choice for second-line therapy?
7. What over-the-counter and/or alternative medications would be appropriate for M.W.?
8. What dietary and lifestyle changes would you recommend for M.W.?
9. Describe one or two drug–drug or drug–food interactions for the selected agent.

Bibliography

Starred references are cited in the text.

Abramson, J., Jurkovitz, C., Vaccarino, V., et al. (2003). Chronic kidney disease, anemia, and incident stroke in a middle-aged, community-based population: The ARIC study. *Kidney International, 64,* 610–615.

*Adamson, J. (2012). Iron deficiency and other hypoproliferative anemias. In D. Longo, A. Fauci, D. Kasper, et al., (Eds.), *Harrison's principles of internal medicine* (pp. 448–457). New York, NY: McGraw-Hill.

Aigner, E., Feldman, A., & Datz, C. (2014). Obesity as an emerging risk factor for iron deficiency. *Nutrients, 6,* 3587–3600.

Alleyne, M., Horne, M., & Miller, J. (2008). Individualized treatment for iron-deficiency anemia in adults. *The American Journal of Medicine, 121,* 943–948.

*Amgen. (2013). ARANESP (darbepoetin alfa) package insert. Thousand Oaks, CA: Amgen.

Andrews, N. (2008). Forging a field: The golden age of iron biology. *Blood, 112,* 219–230.

Angerio, A., & Lee, N. (2003). Sickle cell crisis and endothelin antagonists. *Critical Care Nursing Quarterly, 26,* 225–229.

Bacigalupo, A. (2008). Treatment strategies for patients with severe aplastic anemia. *Bone Marrow Transplantation, 42,* S42–S44.

Ballas, S. (2005). Pain management of sickle cell disease. *Hematology/Oncology Clinics of North America, 19,* 785–802.

*Ballas, S. K. (2020). The evolving pharmacotherapeutic landscape for the treatment of sickle cell disease. *Mediterranean Journal of Hematology and Infectious Diseases, 12*(1), e2020010. doi: 10.4084/MJHID.2020.010

*Benoist, B., McLean, E., Egli, I., et al. (2008). *Worldwide prevalence of anaemia 1993–2005: WHO global database on anaemia.* Geneva, Switzerland: World Health Organization.

*Bernaudin, F., Souillet, G., Vannier, J., et al. (1997). Report of the French experience concerning 26 children transplanted for severe sickle cell disease. *Bone Marrow Transplantation, 19,* S112–S115.

Borgna-Pignatti, C. (2009). Modern treatment of thalassaemia intermedia. *British Journal of Haematology, 138,* 291–304.

Brawley, O., Cornelius, L., Edwards, L., et al. (2008). National Institutes of Health Consensus Development Conference statement: Hydroxyurea treatment for sickle cell disease. *Annals of Internal Medicine, 148,* 932–938.

Butler, C., Vidal-Alaball, J., Cannings-John, R., et al. (2006). Oral vitamin B$_{12}$ versus intramuscular vitamin B$_{12}$ for vitamin B$_{12}$ deficiency: A systematic review of randomized controlled trails. *Family Practice, 23,* 279–285.

Camaschella, C. (2015). Iron-deficiency anemia. *New England Journal of Medicine, 372,* 1832–1843.

Cao, A., & Galanello, R. (2002). Effect of consanguinity on screening for thalassemia. *New England Journal of Medicine, 347,* 1200–1202.

*Centers for Disease Control and Prevention. (n.d.). ACIP Vaccine Recommendations | CDC. ACIP Vaccine Recommendations and Guidelines. https://www.cdc.gov/vaccines/hcp/acip-recs/index.html

*Centers for Disease Control and Prevention. (2012). National health and nutrition examination survey. Retrieved from http://www.cdc.gov/nchs/nhanes/nhanesii.htm

*Centers for Disease Control and Prevention, Sickle Cell Disease (SCD), Data & Statistics on Sickle Cell Disease | CDC, Accessed December 2019.

*Chan, C. Q. H., Low, L. L., & Lee, K. H. (2016). Oral vitamin B$_{12}$ replacement for the treatment of pernicious anemia. *Frontiers in Medicine, 3*, 1. doi: 10.3389/fmed.2016.00038

Cravens, D., Nasheisky, J., & Oh, R. (2007). Clinical inquiries. How do we evaluate a marginally low B$_{12}$ level? *Journal of Family Practice, 56*, 62–63.

*Dixit, R., Nettem, S., Madan, S. S., et al. (2018). Folate supplementation in people with sickle cell disease. *SSRN Electronic Journal, 1*. doi: 10.2139/ssrn.3297902

Global Blood Therapeutics. (2019). Oxbryta package insert. San Francisco, CA: Global Blood Therapeutics.

*Goodnough, L., & Schrier, S. (2014). Evaluation and management of anemia in the elderly. *American Journal of Hematology, 89*, 88–96.

Guidi, G., & Santonastaso, C. (2010). Advancements in anemias related to chronic conditions. *Clinical Chemistry & Laboratory Medicine, 48*, 1217–1226.

Gurusamy, K., Nagendran, M., Broadhurst, J., et al. (2014). Iron therapy in anaemic adults without chronic kidney disease. *Cochrane Database System Review, 12*, 1–132.

*Han, J., Saraf, S. L., Lash, J. P., et al. (2017). Use of anti-inflammatory analgesics in sickle-cell disease. *Journal of Clinical Pharmacy and Therapeutics, 42*(5), 656–660. doi: 10.1111/jcpt.12592

Inker, L., Astor, B., Fox, C., et al. (2014). KDOQI US commentary on the 2012 KDIGO clinical practice guideline for the evaluation and management of CKD. *American Journal of Kidney Disease, 63*, 713–735.

Killip, S., Bennett, J., & Chambers, M. (2007). Iron deficiency anemia. *American Family Physician, 75*, 671–678.

*Kliger, A., Foley, R., Goldfarb, D. S., et al. (2013). KDOQI US commentary on the 2012 KDIGO clinical practice guideline for anemia in CKD. *American Journal of Kidney Disease, 62*(5), 849–859.

Lanzkron, S., Strouse, J., Wilson, R., et al. (2008). Systematic review: Hydroxyurea for the treatment of adults with sickle cell disease. *Annals of Internal Medicine, 12*, 939–950.

Liu, K., & Kaffes, A. (2011). Iron deficiency anaemia: A review of diagnosis, investigation and management. *European Journal of Gastroenterology & Hepatology, 24*, 109–116.

*Marsh, J., Ball, S., Cavenagh, J., et al. (2009). Guidelines for the diagnosis and management of aplastic anaemia. *British Journal of Haematology, 147*, 43–70.

Miller, H., Hu, J., Valentine, J., et al. (2010). Efficacy and tolerability of intravenous ferric gluconate in the treatment of iron deficiency anemia in patients without kidney disease. *Archives of Internal Medicine, 167*, 1327–1328.

*National Kidney Foundation. (2007). KDOQI clinical practice guideline and clinical practice recommendations for anemia in chronic kidney disease: 2007 update of hemoglobin target. Retrieved from http://www2.kidney.org/professionals/KDOQI/guidelines_anemiaUP/guide1.htm

*Nickel, R. S., & Kamani, N. R. (2018). Ethical challenges in hematopoietic cell transplantation for sickle cell disease. *Biology of Blood and Marrow Transplantation, 24*(2), 219–227. doi: 10.1016/j.bbmt.2017.08.034

Poskitt, E. (2003). Early history of iron deficiency. *British Journal of Haematology, 122*, 504–562.

Robinson, A., & Mladenovic, J. (2001). Lack of clinical utility of folate levels in the evaluation of macrocytosis or anemia. *American Journal of Medicine, 110*, 88–90.

*Savulescu, J. (2004). Thalassaemia major: The murky story of deferiprone. *British Medical Journal, 328*, 358–359.

Short, M., & Domagalski, J. (2013). Iron deficiency anemia: Evaluation and management. *American Family Physician, 87*, 98–104.

Simon, E., Long, B., & Koyfman, A. (2016). Emergency medicine management of sickle cell disease complications: An evidence-based update. *The Journal of Emergency Medicine, 51*(4), 370–381. doi: 10.1016/j.jemermed.2016.05.042

Tefferi, A. (2003). Anemia in adults: A contemporary approach to diagnosis. *Mayo Clinic Proceedings, 78*, 1274–1280.

*U.S. Department of Health and Human Services. National Heart, Lung, and Blood Institute. (2014). Evidence-based management of sickle cell disease. Retrieved from http://www.nhlbi.nih.gov/health-pro/guidelines/sickle-cell-disease-guidelines

U.S. Renal Data System. (2001). USRDS 2001 annual data report. Bethesda, MD: National Institute of Diabetes and Digestive and Kidney Diseases, National Institutes of Health.

Vajpayee, N., Graham, S., & Bem, S. (2011). Basic examination of blood and bone marrow. In R. A. McPherson & M. R. Pincus (Eds.), *Henry's clinical diagnosis and management by laboratory methods* (22nd ed.). Philadelphia, PA: Elsevier/Saunders.

*Wong, T., Brandow, A., Lim, W., et al. (2014). Update on the use of hydroxyurea therapy in sickle cell disease. *Blood, 24*, 3850–3857.

Yawn, B., Buchana, G., Afenyi-Annan, A., et al. (2014). Management of sickle cell disease. Summary of the 2014 evidence-based report by expert panel members. *Journal of American Medical Association, 312*, 1033–1048.

Yen, P. (2000). Nutritional anemia. *Geriatric Nursing, 21*, 111–112.

Young, N. (2002). Acquired aplastic anemia. *Annals of Internal Medicine, 136*, 534–546.

Pharmacotherapy for Health Promotion

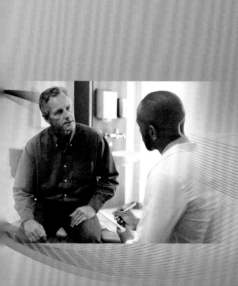
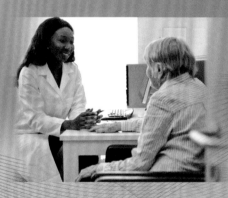
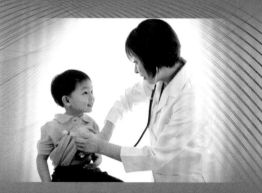

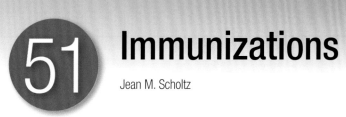

51 Immunizations

Jean M. Scholtz

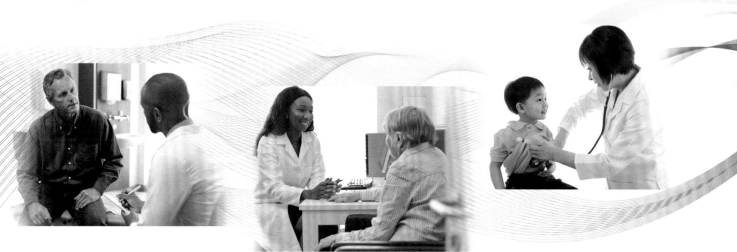

Learning Objectives

1. Understand the need for immunizations.
2. Know the immunization schedule for children and adults.
3. Understand the special circumstances for immunizations.

INTRODUCTION

The use of immunizations is described as one of the 10 greatest public health achievements. Immunization rates in the United States are at their highest with more than 90% of children 3 years of age receiving all required vaccines (Hill et al., 2015). In the 2018-to-2019 school year, coverage for state-required doses of measles, mumps, rubella diphtheria, tetanus, and pertussis was around 95% (Seither et al., 2019). As a result, cases of diphtheria, polio, rubella, mumps, measles, and *Haemophilus influenzae* type b (Hib) are at record low levels. Immunization prophylaxis is important for all age groups—infants through older adults. Unfortunately, immunization rates in adolescents and adults are not as high as those in preschool-age children. Immunization rates in persons 18 to 64 years of age against influenza and pneumococcus range from 33% to 70%, with pneumonia and influenza the eighth leading cause of death in the United States (Williams et al., 2017). There are even lower immunization rates in the socioeconomically disadvantaged and various ethnicities. In addition, there are individuals who continue to be antivaccinators due to the fear of autism. In 2019, the World Health Organization named vaccine hesitancy as one of the ten threats to global health (Geoghegan

et al., 2020). Practitioners need to develop a system that facilitates review of immunization status at all health care visits so that no opportunity is missed to educate and update immunizations for those who are not adequately vaccinated and thus inadequately protected against preventable diseases.

Immunization prophylaxis offers an opportunity to prevent disease, improve clinical outcomes for those at high risk, and realize significant savings to the person in terms of cost, time, and resources. Healthy People 2020 continues to promote the movement throughout the United States to increase immunization rates and reduce preventable infectious diseases. They continue to have a significant impact on preventing communicable diseases, reducing preventable complications, and improving clinical outcomes. However, adult vaccination coverage remains low for most routinely recommended vaccines and below the Healthy People 2020 target (Williams et al., 2017). Plans are underway for the creation of Healthy People 2030 goals to continue this charge.

However, because these diseases persist in other countries, immunization prophylaxis needs to be continued. Recommendations for immunization prophylaxis come from multiple sources, and useful resources are listed in **Box 51.1**. The Centers for Disease Control and Prevention (CDC) is responsible for providing vaccine management, technical assistance, information, epidemiology, and assessment. In February of each year, the immunization schedule is reviewed and revised as indicated.

CHARACTERISTICS OF IMMUNIZATIONS

Many infectious diseases can be prevented by immunoprophylaxis, which is accomplished either through active or passive immunization. Active immunization involves giving a person

Advisory Committee on Immunization Practices (ACIP): http://www.cdc.gov/vaccines/acip/

American Academy of Pediatrics (AAP): http://aap.org

American Academy of Family Physicians: http://www.aafp.org/online/en/home.html

Centers for Disease Control General Best Practice Guidelines for Immunization: http://www.cdc.gov/vaccines/ed/general-recs/index.html

Children's Hospital of Philadelphia Vaccine Education Center: http://www.vaccine.chop.edu

Epidemiology and Prevention of Vaccine-Preventable Diseases—The Pink Book, 13th Edition (2015): http://www.cdc.gov/vaccines/pubs/pinkbook/index.html

U.S. Preventive Task Force and the Centers for Disease Control and Prevention (CDC):http://www.cdc.gov/vaccines/

Vaccine-Preventable Adult Diseases: http://www.cdc.gov/vaccines/adults/vpd.html

Immunization Action Coalition: http://www.immunize.org

Infectious Disease Society of America: http://www.idsociety.org/

Morbidity & Mortality Weekly Report: www.cdc.gov/mmwr

National Network for Immunization Information: www.immunizationinfo.org

Directory of Immunization Coalitions: http://www.izcoalitions.org/

The Vaccine Handbook: A Practical Guide for Clinicians, 6th edition: https://www.immunize.org/va/va53_vaccine-handbook.pdf

The Yellow Book: CDC Health Information for International Travel 2020: http://wwwnc.cdc.gov/travel/page/yellow-book-home)

either live or attenuated (live but killed; inactivated) vaccine to stimulate the development of immune system defenses against future natural exposure.

Active immunization involves administration of all or part of a microorganism or a modified product of that microorganism (e.g., toxoid, a purified antigen, or an antigen produced by genetic engineering) to evoke an immune response that mimics the response of the body to natural infection but that usually presents little or no risk to the recipient. Protection may be afforded for a limited time or for a lifetime. If protection is for a limited time, the vaccine must be readministered at specified intervals.

Passive immunization is used for those people who have already been exposed or who have the potential to be exposed to certain infectious agents. Passive immunization involves the administration of a preformed antibody when the recipient has a congenitally acquired defect or immunodeficiency, when exposure is likely to result in high-risk complications, or when time does not permit adequate protection by active immunization (e.g., immunizations against rabies or hepatitis B). In addition, passive immunity can be used therapeutically during active disease states to help suppress the effects of a toxin or the inflammatory response.

VACCINES

Vaccines are the pharmacologic substances used to provide or boost immunity to disease. The major constituents of vaccines include active immunizing antigens (toxoid, live virus, or killed bacteria), suspending fluid, preservatives, stabilizers, antibiotics, and adjuvants. The differences depend on the manufacturer, and the person prescribing or administering the vaccine should

check the package insert for the active and inert ingredients for each product. Potential allergic reactions may result from one or more of the preservatives, stabilizers, adjuvants, or antibiotics in the vaccine, and the recipient's sensitivity to one or more of the additives should be anticipated as a hypersensitivity. Current vaccines licensed in the United States are identified in **Box 51.2**.

The recommended immunization schedule for persons aged 0 through 18 years in the United States is listed in **Figure 51.1**. The schedules have columns added at 4 to 6 years and 11 to 12 years of age to highlight school entry and adolescent age group vaccine recommendations. Footnotes are listed for each vaccine and contain the recommendations for routine vaccination, catchup, and vaccination to individuals with high-risk conditions or special circumstances. **Figure 51.2** presents the recommended immunizations for persons aged 4 months through 18 years who are behind in immunizations.

Recommendations for hepatitis B; rotavirus (RV1/RV5); diphtheria, tetanus, and acellular pertussis (DTaP); tetanus, diphtheria, and pertussis (Tdap); *H. influenzae* type b (Hib); pneumococcus; poliomyelitis; influenza; measles, mumps, and rubella (MMR); varicella; hepatitis A; human papillomavirus (HPV); and meningococcus are included from birth to age 18.

Combination vaccines are available that assist in reducing the number of injections a child must receive at any one time. In addition, recommended acceptable ranges for administration provide some flexibility regarding the number of injections administered at any one time as recommendations for catch-up vaccinations. A consideration for flexible scheduling should include parental or guardian compliance with appointments as well as office follow-up methods used for those patients who do not keep scheduled appointments for immunizations.

Adenovirus types 4 and 7
Anthrax
Bacillus Calmette-Guerin (BCG)
Diphtheria and tetanus toxoid adsorbed
Diphtheria and tetanus toxoids and acellular pertussis vaccine adsorbed
Diphtheria and tetanus toxoids and acellular pertussis vaccine adsorbed and inactivated polio
Diphtheria and tetanus toxoids and acellular pertussis adsorbed, inactivated polio, and *H. influenzae* B conjugate
H. influenzae B conjugate
H. influenzae B conjugate and hepatitis B
Hepatitis A
Hepatitis B
Hepatitis A and hepatitis B
Human papillomavirus 9-valent
Influenza A (H1N1)
Influenza (H5N1)
Influenza virus (trivalent, types A and B)
Influenza vaccine (quadrivalent, types A and B, intranasal, live)
Influenza vaccine (quadrivalent, types A and B, injectable)
Japanese encephalitis
Measles and mumps (live)
Measles, mumps, and rubella (live)
Measles, mumps, rubella, and varicella (live)
Meningococcal (groups A, C, Y, and W-135) oligosaccharide diphtheria CRM197 conjugate

Meningococcal polysaccharide (serogroups A, C, Y, and W-135) diphtheria toxoid conjugate
Meningococcal polysaccharide groups A, C, Y, and W-135 combined
Meningococcal (groups C and Y) and *Haemophilus* b tetanus toxoid conjugate and W-135
Meningococcal (groups A, C, Y, and W-135) polysaccharide diphtheria toxoid conjugate
Meningococcal group B
Plague
Pneumococcal polyvalent
Pneumococcal 13-valent conjugate
Poliovirus, inactivated
Rabies
Rotavirus (live, oral)
Smallpox (live)
Tetanus and diphtheria toxoids adsorbed for adults
Tetanus toxoid adsorbed
Tetanus toxoid, reduced diphtheria toxoid, and acellular pertussis, adsorbed
Typhoid (live, oral)
Typhoid Vi polysaccharide
Varicella virus (live)
Yellow fever
Zoster (live)
Zoster (recombinant)

Special Circumstances

Preterm infants and children who are immunocompromised, infected with human immunodeficiency virus (HIV), lack a spleen, or have a personal or family history of seizures require special consideration when immunization prophylaxis is reviewed and administered.

Preterm Infants

Preterm (<37 weeks' gestation) and low-birth-weight (<2,500 g) infants are at high risk for vaccine-preventable deaths due to an immature immune system and possible decreased maternal antibody levels. Preterm infants born to mothers who are hepatitis B surface antigen (HBsAg) negative should receive their first hepatitis B immunization at 1 month of age or at hospital discharge.

Preterm infants born to mothers who test positive for HBsAg should receive hepatitis B immune globulin within 12 hours of birth and concurrent hepatitis B vaccine (in the appropriate dose per package insert) at a different site. If the maternal HBsAg status is unknown, the vaccine should be given at 1, 2, and 6 months

of age. In addition, all preterm infants should receive the influenza vaccine annually in the fall beginning at age 6 months.

Immunosuppressed Children

Children who are immunosuppressed or immunodeficient are at risk for actually contracting the disease or experiencing serious adverse effects from live bacteria or live virus vaccines. Live vaccines are therefore contraindicated. In general, experience with vaccine administration to an immunosuppressed or immunodeficient child is limited. Efficacy is suboptimal because their ability to develop immunogenicity to a specific agent is altered owing to a depressed immune system. Theoretical considerations are the only guide because experiential data are lacking or adverse consequences have not been reported.

Children with a deficiency in antibody-synthesizing capacity cannot respond to vaccines. These children should receive regular doses of immune globulin, usually intravenous (IV) immune globulin, which provides passive protection against many infectious diseases. Specific immune globulins (e.g., varicella-zoster immune globulin) are available for postexposure prophylaxis for some infections. An exception appears to be the judicious use of

Recommended Child and Adolescent Immunization Schedule for ages 18 years or younger
UNITED STATES 2020

Vaccines in the Child and Adolescent Immunization Schedule*

Vaccines	Abbreviations	Trade names
Diphtheria, tetanus, and acellular pertussis vaccine	DTaP	Daptacel® Infanrix®
Diphtheria, tetanus vaccine	DT	No trade name
Haemophilus influenzae type b vaccine	Hib (PRP-T) Hib (PRP-OMP)	ActHIB® Hiberix® PedvaxHIB®
Hepatitis A vaccine	HepA	Havrix® Vaqta®
Hepatitis B vaccine	HepB	Engerix-B® Recombivax HB®
Human papillomavirus vaccine	HPV	Gardasil 9®
Influenza vaccine (inactivated)	IIV	Multiple
Influenza vaccine (live, attenuated)	LAIV	FluMist® Quadrivalent
Measles, mumps, and rubella vaccine	MMR	M-M-R® II
Meningococcal serogroups A, C, W, Y vaccine	MenACWY-D MenACWY-CRM	Menactra® Menveo®
Meningococcal serogroup B vaccine	MenB-4C MenB-FHbp	Bexsero® Trumenba®
Pneumococcal 13-valent conjugate vaccine	PCV13	Prevnar 13®
Pneumococcal 23-valent polysaccharide vaccine	PPSV23	Pneumovax® 23
Poliovirus vaccine (inactivated)	IPV	IPOL®
Rotavirus vaccine	RV1 RV5	Rotarix® RotaTeq®
Tetanus, diphtheria, and acellular pertussis vaccine	Tdap	Adacel® Boostrix®
Tetanus and diphtheria vaccine	Td	Tenivac® Tdvax™
Varicella vaccine	VAR	Varivax®
Combination vaccines (*use combination vaccines instead of separate injections when appropriate*)		
DTaP, hepatitis B, and inactivated poliovirus vaccine	DTaP-HepB-IPV	Pediarix®
DTaP, inactivated poliovirus, and *Haemophilus influenzae* type b vaccine	DTaP-IPV/Hib	Pentacel®
DTaP and inactivated poliovirus vaccine	DTaP-IPV	Kinrix® Quadracel®
Measles, mumps, rubella, and varicella vaccine	MMRV	ProQuad®

*Administer recommended vaccines if immunization history is incomplete or unknown. Do not restart or add doses to vaccine series for extended intervals between doses. When a vaccine is not administered at the recommended age, administer at a subsequent visit. The use of trade names is for identification purposes only and does not imply endorsement by the ACIP or CDC.

How to use the child/adolescent immunization schedule

1 Determine recommended vaccine by age (Table 1)

2 Determine recommended interval for catch-up vaccination (Table 2)

3 Assess need for additional recommended vaccines by medical condition and other indications (Table 3)

4 Review vaccine types, frequencies, intervals, and considerations for special situations (Notes)

Recommended by the Advisory Committee on Immunization Practices (www.cdc.gov/vaccines/acip) and approved by the Centers for Disease Control and Prevention (www.cdc.gov), American Academy of Pediatrics (www.aap.org), American Academy of Family Physicians (www.aafp.org), American College of Obstetricians and Gynecologists (www.acog.org), and American College of Nurse-Midwives (www.midwife.org).

Report
• Suspected cases of reportable vaccine-preventable diseases or outbreaks to your state or local health department
• Clinically significant adverse events to the Vaccine Adverse Event Reporting System (VAERS) at www.vaers.hhs.gov or 800-822-7967

 Download the CDC Vaccine Schedules App for providers at www.cdc.gov/vaccines/schedules/hcp/schedule-app.html.

Helpful information
• Complete ACIP recommendations: www.cdc.gov/vaccines/hcp/acip-recs/index.html
• General Best Practice Guidelines for Immunization: www.cdc.gov/vaccines/hcp/acip-recs/general-recs/index.html
• Outbreak information (including case identification and outbreak response), see Manual for the Surveillance of Vaccine-Preventable Diseases: www.cdc.gov/vaccines/pubs/surv-manual

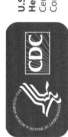

U.S. Department of Health and Human Services
Centers for Disease Control and Prevention

FIGURE 51–1 Recommended child and adolescent immunization schedule for ages 18 years or younger, United States, 2020. (From Centers for Disease Control and Prevention, 2020a.)

The figure below provides catch-up schedules and minimum intervals between doses for children whose vaccinations have been delayed. A vaccine series does not need to be restarted, regardless of the time that has elapsed between doses. Use the section appropriate for the child's age. Always use this table in conjunction with Figure 52.1 and the footnotes that follow.

Vaccine	Minimum Age for Dose 1	Dose 1 to Dose 2	Dose 2 to Dose 3	Dose 3 to Dose 4	Dose 4 to Dose 5
Children age 4 months through 6 years			Minimum Interval Between Doses		
Hepatitis B[1]	Birth	4 weeks	8 weeks *and* at least 16 weeks after first dose. Minimum age for the final dose is 24 weeks.		
Rotavirus[2]	6 weeks	4 weeks	4 weeks[2]		
Diphtheria, tetanus, and acellular pertussis[3]	6 weeks	4 weeks	4 weeks	6 months	6 months[3]
Haemophilus influenzae type b[4]	6 weeks	4 weeks if first dose was administered before the 1st birthday. 8 weeks (as final dose) if first dose was administered at age 12 through 14 months. No further doses needed if first dose was administered at age 15 months or older.	4 weeks if current age is younger than 12 months **and** first dose was administered at younger than age 7 months, **and** at least 1 previous dose was PRP-T (ActHib, Pentacel) or unknown. 8 weeks *and* age 12 through 59 months (as final dose)[4] • if current age is younger than 12 months **and** first dose was administered at age 7 through 11 months (wait until at least 12 months old); OR • if current age is 12 through 59 months **and** first dose was administered before the 1st birthday, and second dose administered at younger than 15 months; OR • if both doses were PRP-OMP (PedvaxHIB; Comvax) **and** were administered before the 1st birthday (wait until at least 12 months old). No further doses needed if previous dose was administered at age 15 months or older.	8 weeks (as final dose) This dose only necessary for children age 12 through 59 months who received 3 doses before the 1st birthday.	
Pneumococcal[4]	6 weeks	4 weeks if first dose administered before the 1st birthday. 8 weeks (as final dose for healthy children) if first dose was administered at the 1st birthday or after. No further doses needed for healthy children if first dose administered at age 24 months or older.	4 weeks if current age is younger than 12 months and previous dose given at <7months old. 8 weeks (as final dose for healthy children) if previous dose given between 7-11 months (wait until at least 12 months old); OR if current age is 12 months or older and at least 1 dose was given before age 12 months. No further doses needed for healthy children if previous dose administered at age 24 months or older.	8 weeks (as final dose) This dose only necessary for children aged 12 through 59 months who received 3 doses before age 12 months or for children at high risk who received 3 doses at any age.	
Inactivated poliovirus[6]	6 weeks	4 weeks[6]	4 weeks	6 months[6] (minimum age 4 years for final dose).	
Measles, mumps, rubella[8]	12 months	4 weeks			
Varicella[9]	12 months	3 months			
Hepatitis A[10]	12 months	6 months			
Meningococcal[11] (Hib-MenCY ≥ 6 weeks; MenACWY-D ≥ 9 mos; MenACWY-CRM ≥ 2 mos)	6 weeks	8 weeks[11]	See footnote 11	See footnote 11	
Children and adolescents age 7 through 18 years					
Meningococcal[11] (Hib-MenCY ≥ 6 weeks; MenACWY-D ≥ 9 mos; MenACWY-CRM ≥ 2 mos)	Not Applicable (N/A)	8 weeks[11]			
Tetanus, diphtheria, tetanus, diphtheria, and acellular pertussis[12]	7 years[12]	4 weeks if first dose of DTaP/DT was administered before the 1st birthday. 6 months (as final dose) if first dose of DTaP/DT or Tdap/Td was administered at or after the 1st birthday.	4 weeks	6 months if first dose of DTaP/DT was administered before the 1st birthday.	
Human papillomavirus[12]	9 years	Routine dosing intervals are recommended[12]			
Hepatitis A[10]	N/A	6 months			
Hepatitis B[1]	N/A	4 weeks	8 weeks and at least 16 weeks after first dose.		
Inactivated poliovirus[6]	N/A	4 weeks	4 weeks[6]	6 months[6]	
Measles, mumps, rubella[8]	N/A	4 weeks			
Varicella[9]	N/A	3 months if younger than age 13 years. 4 weeks if age 13 years or older.			

NOTE: The above recommendations must be read along with the footnotes of this schedule.

FIGURE 51–2 Recommended catch-up immunization schedule for children and adolescents who start late or who are more than 1 month behind, United States, 2020. (From Centers for Disease Control and Prevention, 2020a.)

live virus varicella vaccine in children with acute lymphocytic leukemia in remission in whom the risk of natural varicella outweighs the risk from the attenuated vaccine virus. This vaccine may be obtained from the manufacturer on a compassionate use protocol for patients aged 12 months to 17 years who have acute lymphocytic leukemia in remission for at least 1 year.

Children with Transplants

Transplant recipients (e.g., bone marrow transplant recipients) should also be viewed in a special light. Some experts elect to reimmunize all children without serologic evaluation, and others, because of the limited amount of data, recommend that immunization protocols be developed for these children in conjunction with experts in the fields of infectious disease and immunology. Information about the use of live virus vaccines in organ transplant recipients is also limited. Only inactivated poliovirus vaccine should be given to transplant recipients and their household contacts.

Children Taking Corticosteroids

Children receiving corticosteroids also need careful consideration and thorough review of their medical history, including a review of the underlying disease, the specific dose and schedule of corticosteroids prescribed, and the current immunization status, which includes an evaluation of risk factors relative to infectious disease. In general, children who have a disease (which suppresses the immune response) and who are receiving either systemic or locally administered corticosteroids (which also suppress the immune response) should not be given live virus vaccines except in special circumstances. The guidelines for administering a live virus vaccine to patients receiving corticosteroid therapy are based on the dosage in relation to the child's weight in kilograms and the duration of corticosteroid therapy. The following treatments do not contraindicate administration:

1. Topical, inhaled, and compartmental depot injection of corticosteroids
2. Physiologic maintenance doses of corticosteroids
3. Systemic corticosteroids of less than 2 mg/kg/d of prednisone or its equivalent or less than 20 mg/d or on alternate days if greater than 10 kg

Special consideration should be given if high-dose corticosteroids are prescribed. Administration of high-dose corticosteroids ($\geq$2 mg/kg/d of prednisone or its equivalent or $\geq$20 mg/d if the child weighs >10 kg) given daily or on alternate days for 14 days or less preempts the administration of live virus vaccines until the treatment is discontinued. Some experts recommend delaying immunization until 4 weeks after discontinuation of therapy (Marshall, 2019).

Patients who receive high doses of systemic corticosteroids—daily or on alternate days for 14 days or more—should not receive live virus vaccines until steroid therapy has been discontinued for at least 1 month. In addition, if clinical or laboratory evidence of systemic immunosuppression results from prolonged application, live virus vaccines should not be administered until corticosteroid therapy has been discontinued for at least 1 month.

Children with Seizures

Infants and children with a personal or family history of seizures are at increased risk for having a convulsion after receiving either pertussis (as DTaP) or measles (as MMR) vaccine. Seizures are usually brief, self-limited, and generalized and occur in conjunction with fever (Pickering et al., 2009). However, in the case of DTaP vaccine administered during infancy, administration may coincide with or hasten the inevitable recognition of a seizure-related disorder such as infantile spasms or epilepsy. This causes confusion about the role of the pertussis vaccine, and in this instance, pertussis immunization should be deferred until a progressive neurologic disorder is excluded or the cause of the seizure diagnosed.

Measles immunization, however, is usually given at an age when the cause and nature of the seizure activity have been established. Therefore, measles immunization should not be deferred in children with a history of one or more seizures.

Adolescents

Adolescents continue to be adversely affected by vaccine-preventable diseases, including varicella, hepatitis B, measles, meningococcus, HPV, and rubella. Recommendations for adolescents at ages 11 and 12 aim to improve the vaccine coverage and to establish routine visits to health care providers. These strategies reflect the recommendations (see **Box 51.1**) of the Advisory Committee on Immunization Practices (ACIP), American Academy of Pediatrics (AAP), American Academy of Family Physicians, and American Medical Association. In addition to providing an opportunity for administering needed vaccines, such as hepatitis B, varicella, second dose of MMR, tetanus and diphtheria booster, and HPV, this visit provides an opportunity to render other recommended preventive services, including health behavior guidance; screening for biomedical, behavioral, and emotional conditions; and delivery of other health services. For more information, see **Figure 51.1** and **Box 51.1**.

IMMUNIZATION RECOMMENDATIONS FOR ADULTS

Immunization prophylaxis is as important for adults as it is for children. However, the practice of assessing the vaccination status of adults at their routine health visits remains an issue.

As a result, many adults continue to be affected adversely by vaccine-preventable diseases such as varicella, pertussis, measles, and rubella. The guidelines are updated yearly in February, and all schedules are published in *Morbidity and Mortality Weekly Report* (http://www.cdc.gov/mmwr/index.html) and may be found at http://www.cdc.gov/vaccines/schedules/index.html. The ACIP recommendations are available at http://www.cdc.gov/vaccines/hcp/acip-recs/. Each patient's immunization records should be reviewed at each patient visit and determined if any vaccines are required. For more information, see **Figure 51.3** and **Box 51.1**.

Recommended Adult Immunization Schedule
for ages 19 years or older

UNITED STATES

2020

How to use the adult immunization schedule

1 Determine recommended vaccinations by age **(Table 1)**

2 Assess need for additional recommended vaccinations by medical condition and other indications **(Table 2)**

3 Review vaccine types, frequencies, and intervals and considerations for special situations **(Notes)**

Recommended by the Advisory Committee on Immunization Practices (www.cdc.gov/vaccines/acip) and approved by the Centers for Disease Control and Prevention (www.cdc.gov), American College of Physicians (www.acponline.org), American Academy of Family Physicians (www.aafp.org), American College of Obstetricians and Gynecologists (www.acog.org), and American College of Nurse-Midwives (www.midwife.org).

Report
- Suspected cases of reportable vaccine-preventable diseases or outbreaks to the local or state health department
- Clinically significant postvaccination reactions to the Vaccine Adverse Event Reporting System at www.vaers.hhs.gov or 800-822-7967

Injury claims
All vaccines included in the adult immunization schedule except pneumococcal 23-valent polysaccharide (PPSV23) and zoster (RZV, ZVL) vaccines are covered by the Vaccine Injury Compensation Program. Information on how to file a vaccine injury claim is available at www.hrsa.gov/vaccinecompensation.

Questions or comments
Contact www.cdc.gov/cdc-info or 800-CDC-INFO (800-232-4636), in English or Spanish, 8 a.m.–8 p.m. ET, Monday through Friday, excluding holidays.

 Download the CDC Vaccine Schedules App for providers at www.cdc.gov/vaccines/schedules/hcp/schedule-app.html.

Helpful information
- Complete ACIP recommendations: www.cdc.gov/vaccines/hcp/acip-recs/index.html
- General Best Practice Guidelines for Immunization (including contraindications and precautions): www.cdc.gov/vaccines/hcp/acip-recs/general-recs/index.html
- Vaccine information statements: www.cdc.gov/vaccines/hcp/vis/index.html
- Manual for the Surveillance of Vaccine-Preventable Diseases (including case identification and outbreak response): www.cdc.gov/vaccines/pubs/surv-manual
- Travel vaccine recommendations: www.cdc.gov/travel
- Recommended Child and Adolescent Immunization Schedule, United States, 2020: www.cdc.gov/vaccines/schedules/hcp/child-adolescent.html

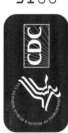

U.S. Department of Health and Human Services
Centers for Disease Control and Prevention

Vaccines in the Adult Immunization Schedule*

Vaccines	Abbreviations	Trade names
Haemophilus influenzae type b vaccine	Hib	ActHIB® Hiberix® PedvaxHIB®
Hepatitis A vaccine	HepA	Havrix® Vaqta®
Hepatitis A and hepatitis B vaccine	HepA-HepB	Twinrix®
Hepatitis B vaccine	HepB	Engerix-B® Recombivax HB® Heplisav-B®
Human papillomavirus vaccine	HPV vaccine	Gardasil 9®
Influenza vaccine (inactivated)	IIV	Many brands
Influenza vaccine (live, attenuated)	LAIV	FluMist® Quadrivalent
Influenza vaccine (recombinant)	RIV	Flublok® Quadrivalent
Measles, mumps, and rubella vaccine	MMR	M-M-R® II
Meningococcal serogroups A, C, W, Y vaccine	MenACWY	Menactra® Menveo®
Meningococcal serogroup B vaccine	MenB-4C MenB-FHbp	Bexsero® Trumenba®
Pneumococcal 13-valent conjugate vaccine	PCV13	Prevnar 13®
Pneumococcal 23-valent polysaccharide vaccine	PPSV23	Pneumovax® 23
Tetanus and diphtheria toxoids	Td	Tenivac® Tdvax™
Tetanus and diphtheria toxoids and acellular pertussis vaccine	Tdap	Adacel® Boostrix®
Varicella vaccine	VAR	Varivax®
Zoster vaccine, recombinant	RZV	Shingrix
Zoster vaccine live	ZVL	Zostavax®

*Administer recommended vaccines if vaccination history is incomplete or unknown. Do not restart or add doses to vaccine series if there are extended intervals between doses. The use of trade names is for identification purposes only and does not imply endorsement by the ACIP or CDC.

FIGURE 51-3 Recommended adult immunization schedule for ages 19 years or older, United States, 2020. (From Centers for Disease Control and Prevention, 2020b.)

DISEASE-SPECIFIC VACCINE RECOMMENDATIONS

Pneumococcal Vaccine 23-Valent

Pneumococcal infection causes an estimated 5,000 deaths annually in the United States, accounting for more deaths than any other vaccine-preventable bacterial disease. *Streptococcus pneumoniae* colonizes the upper respiratory tract and can cause disseminated invasive infections including bacteremia and meningitis, pneumonia and other lower respiratory tract infections, and upper respiratory tract infections including otitis media and sinusitis. The pneumococcal vaccine protects against invasive bacteremic disease, although existing data suggest that it is less effective in protecting against other types of pneumococcal infections.

The ACIP recommends giving one dose of pneumococcal vaccine to older patients (65 years or older), with an additional dose given earlier to identified high-risk populations (**Box 51.3**). Two available vaccines include a 13-valent

pneumococcal conjugate and a 23-valent purified capsular polysaccharide antigens of *S. pneumoniae*. If an older patient's vaccination status is unknown, he or she should receive one dose of the vaccine. There are no data to support revaccination beyond two doses.

Response to Vaccine

Antibodies develop within 2 to 3 weeks in healthy young adults; immune responses are not consistent among all 23 serotypes in the vaccine. Antibody concentrations and responses to individual antigens tend to be lower in the following populations:

- People aged 65 years or older
- People with alcoholic cirrhosis, chronic obstructive pulmonary disease, type 1 diabetes mellitus, Hodgkin's disease, or asthma
- People who smoke
- People with chronic renal failure requiring dialysis, renal transplantation, or nephrotic syndrome
- People with acquired immunodeficiency syndrome (AIDS) or HIV infection

Special Circumstances

Antibody response is diminished or absent in people who are immunocompromised or who have leukemia, lymphoma, or multiple myeloma. The antibody levels to most pneumococcal vaccine antigens remain elevated for at least 5 years in healthy adults.

A more rapid decline (within 3–5 years) occurs in certain children who have undergone splenectomy after trauma and in those who have sickle cell disease. Antibody concentrations also decline after 5 to 10 years in older people, those who have undergone splenectomy, patients with renal disease requiring dialysis, and people who have received transplants. A lower antibody response or rapid decline in antibody levels is also noted in patients with Hodgkin's disease and multiple myeloma. At least 2 weeks should elapse between immunization and the initiation of chemotherapy or immunosuppressive therapy.

Revaccination is recommended once for patients who are aged 2 or older, who are at highest risk for serious pneumococcal infection, and who are likely to have a rapid decline in antibody levels provided that 5 years have elapsed since receiving the first dose of vaccine.

Pneumococcal Conjugate Vaccine

In February 2010, the U.S. Food and Drug Administration (FDA) licensed a 13-valent pneumococcal conjugate vaccine, PCV-13 (Prevnar-13). This vaccine is recommended for universal use in children aged 23 months and younger. The number of doses for the primary series varies with the age of the child at the first dose.

Children aged 24 to 59 months who are at high risk for invasive pneumococcal infection and who have not been

---

BOX 51.3 Recommendations for the Use of Pneumococcal Vaccine

GROUPS FOR WHICH VACCINATION IS RECOMMENDED

People aged 65 years or older

People aged 2 to 64 years with chronic cardiovascular disease including congestive heart failure and cardiomyopathies; chronic pulmonary disease including chronic obstructive lung disease, emphysema, and asthma; sickle cell disease; diabetes mellitus; and people who smoke

People aged 2 to 64 years with alcoholism, chronic liver disease including cirrhosis, cochlear implants, or cerebrospinal fluid leaks

People aged 2 to 64 years with functional or anatomic asplenia

People aged 2 to 64 years living in nursing homes or other long-term care facilities

IMMUNOCOMPROMISED PEOPLE

Immunocompromised people aged 2 years or older, including those with HIV infection, leukemia, lymphoma, Hodgkin's disease, multiple myeloma, generalized malignancy, chronic renal failure, or nephrotic syndrome; those receiving immunosuppressive chemotherapy (including corticosteroids); and those who have received an organ or bone marrow transplant

HIV, human immunodeficiency virus.

previously immunized should also receive 23-valent vaccine to expand the serotype coverage. In June 2012, the ACIP recommended routine use of the PCV-13 for adults with immunocompromising conditions. It should be administered in addition to the pneumococcal vaccine 23-valent (PPSV-23) to all eligible adults. In June 2019, ACIP recommended PCV-13, based on shared clinical decision-making, for adults aged 65 years or older who do not have an immunocompromising condition, cerebrospinal fluid leak, or cochlear implant and who have not previously received PCV-13. All adults aged 65 years or older should receive a dose of PPSV-23 (Matanock et al., 2019).

Influenza Vaccine

Influenza and pneumonia are the eighth leading causes of death in the United States and fifth in older adults. Fatalities from influenza begin to rise in midlife and are highest in persons with chronic disease. Measures available to reduce the incidence of influenza include immunoprophylaxis with inactivated (killed virus) vaccine and chemoprophylaxis. Before the influenza season gets under way, vaccination of people at risk and those likely to transmit influenza to at-risk populations is the most effective measure. The vaccine is associated with a decrease in influenza-related respiratory illness in all age groups, decreased hospitalization and death in people at high risk, decreased incidence of otitis media in children, and decreased work and school absenteeism. Influenza vaccine is recommended for anyone aged 6 months or older.

Two types of influenza vaccine are available—inactivated influenza vaccine (IIV) and live attenuated influenza vaccine (LAIV in the form of nasal spray). LAIV was not recommended to be used from 2015 to 2018 due to its low efficacy. It is now recommended for those aged 2 to 49 years and is contraindicated in patients who are immunocompromised and require a protected environment, health care workers, and household members who are in close contact with the immunocompromised individual. If a live virus is given, the patient should not have contact with those who are immunocompromised for 7 days. The antigenic composition of the influenza vaccine changes each year; thus, this vaccine must be administered every year. It provides protection against influenza A and B and is available as either a trivalent inactivated influenza vaccine (IIV3) or a quadrivalent live (LAIV4) or inactivated vaccine (IIV4). The IIV3 vaccine is available in a high-dose formulation for patients aged 65 years or older, and there is an intradermal IIV4 formulation approved for patients aged 18 to 64 years. Children aged 6 months through 8 years require two doses of influenza vaccine (administered ≥4 weeks apart) during their first season of vaccination to optimize response. Recombinant (RIV3) and cell-cultured (ccIIV3) influenza vaccines should be utilized in patients with severe allergic and anaphylactic reactions to various influenza vaccine components (Centers for Disease Control and Prevention, 2020a, 2020b, 2020d; Grohskopf et al., 2019). There is no preference for any particular version of IIV in any target group, and there is no preference between LAIV and IIV for healthy persons 2 to 49 years of age.

Groups at Risk

People at increased risk for influenza-related complications include the following:

1. Adults aged 65 years or older
2. Children younger than 2 years old
3. Pregnant women and women up to 2 weeks after the end of pregnancy
4. American Indians and Alaska Natives
5. People who live in nursing homes and other long-term care facilities
6. Although all children younger than 5 years old are considered at high risk for serious flu complications, the highest risk is for those younger than 2 years old, with the highest hospitalization and death rates among infants younger than 6 months old.
7. People with asthma
8. People with neurologic and neurodevelopment conditions
9. People with blood disorders (such as sickle cell disease)
10. People with chronic lung disease (such as chronic obstructive pulmonary disease and cystic fibrosis)
11. People with endocrine disorders (such as diabetes mellitus)
12. People with heart disease (such as congenital heart disease, congestive heart failure and coronary artery disease)
13. People with kidney disorders
14. People with liver disorders
15. People with metabolic disorders (such as inherited metabolic disorders and mitochondrial disorders)
16. People who are obese with a body mass index of 40 or higher
17. People younger than 19 years of age on long-term aspirin- or salicylate-containing medications.
18. People with a weakened immune system due to disease (such as people with HIV or AIDS, or some cancers such as leukemia) or medications (such as those receiving chemotherapy or radiation treatment for cancer, or persons with chronic conditions requiring chronic corticosteroids or other drugs that suppress the immune system)

Transmission of Influenza

Just as immunizing people in groups at high risk for flu and its complications is important, so too is immunizing those who are most likely to transmit the disease. Groups that can transmit influenza to people at high risk include health care workers (in hospital and outpatient settings and in emergency response service), employees of nursing homes and chronic care facilities who have contact with patients or residents, employees of assisted living and other residences for people in high-risk groups, providers of home care to people at high risk (e.g., visiting nurses, volunteers), household contacts of high-risk individuals, and providers of essential community services. Additional populations for consideration include people with HIV infection, breast-feeding mothers, people traveling to foreign countries, students or other people in institutional settings, and the general populace who want to reduce the likelihood of contracting influenza.

The current 2- to 3-month time frame over which patients are traditionally immunized is too short to fully implement immunization recommendations and inconsistent with the duration of influenza activity. Health care providers and patients should reevaluate their approach to influenza vaccination and recognize the need to extend the immunization time period into January and beyond. To increase influenza immunization rates, the CDC and other professional societies recommend an expanded immunization season with vaccination offered at every opportunity between October and May.

Antibody development after vaccination can take as long as 2 weeks in healthy adults and as long as 6 weeks in children—or 2 weeks after the second dose. Most persons recommended for influenza vaccination should receive a single dose each year. The exception is children aged 6 months to 9 years who are receiving an influenza vaccine for the first time. They should receive 2 doses administered at least 1 month apart. No influenza vaccine is currently approved for children aged 6 months and younger; these vulnerable infants should be protected indirectly through the vaccination of close contacts.

Chemoprophylaxis with antiviral agents, Oseltamivir (Tamiflu), zanamivir (Relenza), or peramivir (Rapivab), is recommended. When administered within 48 hours of the onset of illness, they can reduce the severity and shorten the duration of illness in otherwise healthy people. To be effective as chemoprophylaxis, the antiviral must be taken each day for the duration of potential exposure to a person with influenza and continued for 7 days after the last known exposure. Amantadine (Symmetrel) and rimantadine (Flumadine) are no longer recommended due to the high rate of resistance.

Meningococcal Vaccine

Approximately 3,000 cases of invasive meningococcal diseases (IMD) occur in the United States each year. The overall case-fatality rate for IMD is 10% but is higher in adolescents (20%) than in young children (5%) despite antibiotic therapy early in the illness. The three serogroups of meningococcal disease that are most commonly seen in the United States are serogroups B, C, and Y. Two kinds of meningococcal vaccines are now available. Two single-component meningococcal conjugate vaccines (Menactra [MenACWY-D] and Menveo [MenACWY-CRM]) and two recombinant serogroup B meningococcal (MenB-FHbp [Trumenba] and MenB-4C [Bexsero]) are licensed in the United States.

Meningococcal conjugate (MenACWY) provides coverage against types A, C, Y, and W. The recently released serogroup B meningococcal (MenB) vaccines provide short-term protection against most strains of serogroup B meningococcal disease. The ACIP recommends routine vaccination of all adolescents aged 11 to 18 years with the quadrivalent meningococcal conjugate vaccine (MenACWY). A single dose should be administered at age 11 or 12 years with a booster dose at age 16 years for persons who receive the first dose before age 16 years. The MenB vaccine series should be administered to persons aged 16 to 23 years (preferred age 16 to 18 years) with routine vaccination of certain persons at increased risk for meningococcal disease with MenACWY and serogroup B meningococcal (MenB) vaccine. Both meningococcal vaccines (MenACWY and MenB) are recommended for high-risk patients (e.g., sickle cell disease, anatomic or functional asplenia, complement deficient) beginning at 2 months and 10 years of age respectively.

Pertussis Vaccine

Pertussis continues to be poorly controlled in the United States despite high compliance with childhood pertussis vaccination. In 2009, 16,858 pertussis cases and 12 infant deaths were reported. This continued to increase with 18,975 cases in 2017 and 15,609 cases in 2018.

In October 2010, the ACIP expanded the use of tetanus toxoid and reduced diphtheria toxoid and acellular pertussis (Tdap) for adolescents and adults to improve immunity against pertussis. Adolescents aged 11 through 18 years who have completed the recommended childhood diphtheria and tetanus toxoids and pertussis/diphtheria and tetanus toxoids and acellular pertussis (DTaP) vaccination series and any adults greater than 19 years should receive a single dose of Tdap. Pregnant women should receive one dose of Tdap during each pregnancy at 27 to 36 weeks' gestation. ACIP recommendations have been updated to allow either tetanus and diphtheria toxoids (Td) vaccine or Tdap to be used for the decennial Td booster, tetanus prophylaxis for wound management, and for additional required doses in the catch-up immunization schedule if a person has received at least 1 Tdap dose (Havers et al., 2020).

Human Papillomavirus Vaccine

Three HPV vaccines, bivalent (2vHPV), quadrivalent (4vHPV), and 9-valent (9vHPV), are licensed, but since the end of 2016, only 9vHPV vaccine has been distributed in the United States. All three vaccines target HPV types 6 and 11, which are most commonly associated with clinical diseases and cause over 95% of genital warts. Types 16 and 18, believed to be responsible for approximately 66% of cases of cervical cancer, are contained in the quadrivalent and 9-valent vaccines. The 9-valent product provides additional protection against HPV 31, 33, 45, 52, and 58, which account for 14% females and 4% males of HPV-associated cancers. The ACIP (Robinson et al., 2020) recommends routine HPV vaccination at age 11 or 12 years; vaccination can be given starting at age 9 years. ACIP also recommends catch-up vaccination for persons through age 26 years who are not adequately vaccinated. ACIP recommends HPV vaccination based on shared clinical decision-making for individuals aged 27 through 45 years who are not adequately vaccinated. HPV vaccines are not licensed for use in adults older than age 45 years. Ideally, the vaccine should be administered before potential exposure to HPV through sexual contact. The vaccine is a series of three doses. The second dose is administered 1 to 2 months after the first dose, and the third dose is administered

6 months after the first dose. It can be given to immunocompromised women, but the immune response may be reduced. Pregnant women should not receive the HPV vaccine, even if the series has been started before pregnancy. It can be administered to lactating women (Petrosky et al., 2015).

Rotavirus Vaccine

Rotavirus is the most common cause of severe gastroenteritis in children younger than age 5.

Before rotavirus vaccines were available in the United States, more than 200,000 children younger than age 5 received care in hospital emergency departments for rotavirus disease each year, and 55,000 to 70,000 young children were hospitalized. Two years after the introduction of the vaccine in 2006, a significant reduction in rotavirus hospitalization rates ($P < 0.001$) was observed among all age groups (87% reduction in 6 to less than 12 months old, 96% reduction in 12 to less than 24 months old, and 92% reduction in 24 to less than 36 months old). Multiple studies have continued to show that the U.S. rotavirus season has become less pronounced and shorter since the utilization of the vaccine (Payne et al., 2011b).

Rotavirus is very contagious. People who get a rotavirus infection shed large amounts of the virus in their feces. The disease spreads when infants or young children get rotavirus in their mouth. This happens through contact with the hands of other people or objects (such as toys) that have been contaminated with small amounts of rotavirus.

The first dose of the rotavirus vaccine can be given as early as age 6 weeks and needs to be given before an infant is of age 15 weeks. Children should receive all doses of rotavirus vaccine before they are of age 8 months.

Haemophilus Influenzae Type b Vaccine

Hib vaccine prevents meningitis and pneumonia caused by Hib. It is given to all infants at 2, 4, and 6 months for a total of two- to three-dose primary series (depending on brand) and a booster dose at age 12 to 15 months. More than 95% of infants will develop protective antibody levels after a primary series with clinical efficacy estimated at 95% to 100%. Invasive Hib disease in a completely vaccinated infant is very uncommon. Unimmunized older children, adolescents, and adults with certain specified medical conditions (anatomic or functional splenectomy, HIV infection, sickle cell disease, immunoglobulin or complement deficiency, chemotherapy recipients, hematopoietic stem cell transplant) should receive additional doses of Hib vaccine as they have an increased risk for invasive Hib disease.

Hepatitis A Vaccine

Hepatitis A is a serious liver disease caused by hepatitis A virus (HAV) and transmitted by hand-to-mouth contact through eating and drinking. Proper sanitation and good personal hygiene can help prevent its spread. It is typically self-limiting but may lead to jaundice and, if severe, death (about 3–6 deaths per 1,000 cases) (Hamborsky et al., 2015). In 2006, the hepatitis A

vaccine became available for the long-term protection of HAV infections. A two-dose series should be routinely administered to children beginning at 12 months of age. This vaccine should also be given to individuals traveling to countries with an intermediate to high prevalence of hepatitis A, men who have sex with men, drug abusers, chronic liver disease, or those treated with clotting factors.

Hepatitis B Vaccine

Hepatitis B is a serious disease caused by hepatitis B virus (HBV) that attacks the liver. The virus is very resilient and is viable outside the body for up to 7 days. It can cause life-long infection, cirrhosis (scarring) of the liver, liver cancer, liver failure, and death. It is spread through person-to-person contact through blood, semen, or other body fluids. All children should get their first dose of hepatitis B vaccine at birth and complete the vaccine series by 6 to 18 months of age. Children and adolescents younger than 19 years of age who have not yet gotten the vaccine and adults with risk factors (e.g., men who have sex with men, IV drug users, health care and public safety personnel, persons with chronic liver disease, persons with HIV, persons undergoing renal dialysis, those residing in correctional facilities, and travelers to endemic regions) should also be vaccinated. A series of 3 or 4 shots should be given over a 6-month period. The hepatitis B vaccine provides greater than 90% protection to infants, children, and adults if they are immunized prior to being exposed to HBV.

Inactivated Poliovirus

Polio is an infectious disease caused by *Enterovirus*. A polio outbreak in the United States in 1952 resulted in over 21,000 cases of paralysis. The incidence fell rapidly following introduction of effective vaccines. The inactivated polio vaccine (IPV) is the only polio vaccine available in the United States. Children should receive a total of 4 doses of IPV beginning at 2, 4, 6 to 18 months and a booster dose at 4 to 6 years. The last case of wild-virus polio reported in the United States was in 1979, and global polio eradication may be achieved within the next decade.

Measles, Mumps, and Rubella Vaccine

The MMR vaccine provides protection against three diseases and has been administered since 1967. Two doses of MMR provide complete protection. Children should be given the first dose of MMR vaccine at 12 to 15 months of age. The second dose can be given 4 weeks later but is usually given before the start of kindergarten at 4 to 6 years of age. Measles and mumps are contagious diseases transmitted by contact with an infected person through coughing and sneezing, and both spread very easily. The measles consists of an erythematous, maculopapular, pruritic, splotchy rash, which lasts about 5 days and is preceded with a several-day prodrome of malaise, fever, coryza, and conjunctivitis. It may result in encephalitis (permanent brain damage) or death in 1 to 2 of every 1,000 cases (Marshall, 2020). The mumps consists of fever, headache, malaise, myalgias, and bilateral swelling of the parotid glands (parotitis).

Testicular swelling and tenderness (orchitis) and aseptic meningitis may occur in 30% and 10% of patients, respectively. Patients with rubella (also called *German measles* or *3-day measles*) exhibit a transient, erythematous, and sometimes pruritic rash, with about 60% of postpubertal women developing arthritis. If a woman in her first trimester of pregnancy contracts rubella, fetal damage is almost 100%. If contracted in second or third trimester, babies are born with congenital rubella syndrome (CRS) at birth. CRS will result in deafness, cataracts, cardiac defects, and central nervous system abnormalities.

By 2001, administration of the MMR vaccine eradicated measles from the United States, decreased the incidence of mumps by 99%, and provided lifelong protection against rubella. However, due to parents' concern of the MMR vaccine causing autism, mumps and measles cases have increased over the last several years. In 2010, there were 2,600 cases of the mumps, which decreased to 229 in 2012. In 2014, there were over 600 cases of measles reported, which decreased to 189 cases in the United States from January to September 2015 (Hamborsky et al., 2015; Perry et al., 2015). During January 1 to October 1, 2019, a total of 1,249 measles cases and 22 measles outbreaks were reported in the United States. This represents the most U.S. cases reported in a single year since 1992 and the second highest number of reported outbreaks annually since measles was declared eliminated in the United States in 2000 (Patel et al., 2019).

Between January 2016 and June 2017, 9,200 mump cases were reported. Health departments reported 150 outbreaks (9,200 cases), with the largest outbreak involving nearly 3,000 cases. In 2018, a third dose of mumps-containing vaccine was recommended for persons at increased risk during outbreaks (Marin et al., 2018).

Varicella Vaccine

Chickenpox is a highly contagious disease caused by the varicella-zoster virus (VZV). In an unvaccinated child, it appears as an itchy, uncomfortable rash with blisters and vesicles. Before the chickenpox vaccine was widely used, nearly 11,000 people were hospitalized each year and about 50 children and 50 adults died every year from chickenpox. A live varicella vaccine was licensed for use in the United States in 1995, and since then, the number of hospitalizations and deaths due to chickenpox has decreased by more than 90% (Hamborsky et al., 2015). Two doses of the chickenpox vaccine are recommended, with the first dose given at age 12 to 15 months old and the second at age 4 through 6 years.

Zoster Vaccine

Herpes zoster, or shingles, occurs when latent VZV reactivates and causes recurrent disease. Patients contracting zoster experience a painful, vesicular eruption unilaterally along a sensory nerve. The patient may experience pain and paresthesias a few days prior to the rash. Shingles is typically associated with aging and immunosuppression. A complication that may result after the lesions have resolved is postherpetic neuralgia or pain in the area of the occurrence. About 30% of Americans will develop herpes zoster each year, and the risk of the disease increases with increasing age with more than half the cases occurring in people aged 60 years or older. In May 2006, the FDA approved herpes zoster vaccine (ZVL, Zostavax) for use in persons 60 years of age or older. It is a live vaccine with 64% efficacy in people aged 60 through 69 years versus about 18% efficacy in people aged 80 years or older. Recombinant zoster vaccine (RZV, Shingrix) for the prevention of herpes zoster in adults aged 50 years or older is a recombinant nonlive vaccine that contains an immune-response boosting adjuvant. Based on studies showing greater efficacy and longer duration of protection, the ACIP recommends RZV for healthy adults aged 50 years or older to prevent herpes zoster infection and its related complications, as well as for adults who previously received Zostavax, stating that RZV is the preferred vaccine for herpes zoster prevention and its complications.

ADVERSE EVENTS ASSOCIATED WITH VACCINES

Risks of vaccination vary from inconvenient to severe and life threatening. Common vaccine side effects (e.g., fever and local irritation to DTaP vaccine) are usually mild to moderate in severity and without permanent consequences. However, serious side effects and adverse reactions are possible, although the occurrence of an adverse event does not prove causation by the vaccine (i.e., the adverse event may be caused by factors other than the vaccine).

Reporting of adverse events is important because it may provide clues to unanticipated adverse reactions. It is important to interview the patient or guardian regarding any side effects after past immunizations. Any unexpected, reported, and observed event that required medical attention soon after the administration should be described in detail in the patient's medical record and reported using the Vaccine Adverse Events Reporting System (VAERS) (accessible online, https://vaers.hhs.gov/esub/index).

The VAERS is a result of the National Childhood Injury Act of 1986, which made provisions for health care providers to report occurrences of certain adverse events and to maintain permanent immunization records. Pertinent information to be reported includes a detailed description of the event (signs and symptoms reported and observed) and the time from administration of vaccine to presentation of signs and symptoms.

Pertinent patient history information should be noted regarding any existing physician-diagnosed allergies, medical conditions, and birth defects as well as any illness at the time of vaccine administration. In addition, information about the vaccine must be included. Documentation should identify the type of vaccine; the manufacturer, lot number, site, and route of administration; and any previous doses received.

Staff members from the VAERS contact the provider (reporter) to follow up about the patient's condition at 60 days and at 1 year after the initial reporting of adverse events. **Figure 51.4** contains the VAERS form.

VAERS Vaccine Adverse Event Reporting System
www.vaers.hhs.gov

Adverse events are possible reactions or problems that occur during or after vaccination. Items **2, 3, 4, 5, 6, 17, 18** and **21** are **ESSENTIAL** and should be completed. Patient identity is kept confidential. Instructions are provided on the last two pages.

INFORMATION ABOUT THE PATIENT WHO RECEIVED THE VACCINE (Use Continuation Page if needed)

1. Patient name: (first) _____ (last) _____

Street address: _____

City: _____ State: _____ County: _____

ZIP code: _____ Phone: ( ) _____ Email: _____

2. Date of birth: (mm/dd/yyyy) _____ 📅 3. Sex: ☐ Male ☐ Female ☐ Unknown

4. Date and time of vaccination: (mm/dd/yyyy) _____ 📅 Time: hh:mm ☐AM ☐PM

5. Date and time adverse event started: (mm/dd/yyyy) _____ 📅 Time: hh:mm ☐AM ☐PM

6. Age at vaccination: _____ Years _____ Months 7. Today's date: (mm/dd/yyyy) _____ 📅

8. Pregnant at time of vaccination?: ☐ Yes ☐ No ☐ Unknown
(If yes, describe the event, any pregnancy complications, and estimated due date if known in item 18)

9. Prescriptions, over-the-counter medications, dietary supplements, or herbal remedies being taken at the time of vaccination:

10. Allergies to medications, food, or other products:

11. Other illnesses at the time of vaccination and up to one month prior:

12. Chronic or long-standing health conditions:

INFORMATION ABOUT THE PERSON COMPLETING THIS FORM

13. Form completed by: (name) _____

Relation to patient: ☐ Healthcare professional/staff ☐ Patient (yourself)
☐ Parent/guardian/caregiver ☐ Other: _____

Street address: _____ ☐ Check if same as item 1

City: _____ State: _____ ZIP code: _____

Phone: ( ) _____ Email: _____

14. Best doctor/healthcare professional to contact about the adverse event: Name: _____ Phone: ( ) _____ Ext: _____

INFORMATION ABOUT THE FACILITY WHERE VACCINE WAS GIVEN

15. Facility/clinic name: _____

Fax: ( ) _____

Street address: _____ ☐ Check if same as item 13

City: _____

State: _____ ZIP code: _____

Phone: ( ) _____

16. Type of facility: (Check one)
☐ Doctor's office, urgent care, or hospital
☐ Pharmacy or store
☐ Workplace clinic
☐ Public health clinic
☐ Nursing home or senior living facility
☐ School or student health clinic
☐ Other: _____
☐ Unknown

WHICH VACCINES WERE GIVEN? WHAT HAPPENED TO THE PATIENT?

17. Enter all vaccines given on the date listed in item 4: (Route is HOW vaccine was given, Body site is WHERE vaccine was given) Use **Continuation Page** if needed

Vaccine (type and brand name)	Manufacturer	Lot number	Route	Body site	Dose number in series
select			select	select	select
select			select	select	select
select			select	select	select
select			select	select	select

18. Describe the adverse event(s), treatment, and outcome(s), if any: (symptoms, signs, time course, etc.)

Use **Continuation Page** if needed

19. Medical tests and laboratory results related to the adverse event(s): (include dates)

Use **Continuation Page** if needed

20. Has the patient recovered from the adverse event(s)?: ☐ Yes ☐ No ☐ Unknown

21. Result or outcome of adverse event(s): (Check all that apply)
☐ Doctor or other healthcare professional office/clinic visit
☐ Emergency room/department or urgent care
☐ Hospitalization: Number of days (if known) _____
Hospital name: _____
City: _____ State: _____
☐ Prolongation of existing hospitalization (vaccine received during existing hospitalization)
☐ Life threatening illness (immediate risk of death from the event)
☐ Disability or permanent damage
☐ Patient died – Date of death: (mm/dd/yyyy) _____ 📅
☐ Congenital anomaly or birth defect
☐ None of the above

ADDITIONAL INFORMATION

22. Any other vaccines received within one month prior to the date listed in item 4: Use **Continuation Page** if needed

Vaccine (type and brand name)	Manufacturer	Lot number	Route	Body site	Dose number in series	Date Given
select			select	select	select	
select			select	select	select	

23. Has the patient ever had an adverse event following any previous vaccine?: (If yes, describe adverse event, patient age at vaccination, vaccination dates, vaccine type, and brand name)
☐ Yes _____ ☐ No ☐ Unknown

24. Patient's race: ☐ American Indian or Alaska Native ☐ Asian ☐ Black or African American ☐ Native Hawaiian or Other Pacific Islander
(Check all that apply) ☐ White ☐ Unknown ☐ Other: _____

25. Patient's ethnicity: ☐ Hispanic or Latino ☐ Not Hispanic or Latino ☐ Unknown   26. Immuniz. proj. report number: (Health Dept use only)

COMPLETE ONLY FOR U.S. MILITARY/DEPARTMENT OF DEFENSE (DoD) RELATED REPORTS

27. Status at vaccination: ☐ Active duty ☐ Reserve ☐ National Guard ☐ Beneficiary ☐ Other: _____   28. Vaccinated at Military/DoD site: ☐ Yes ☐ No

FORM FDA VAERS 2.0 (02/20)

[SAVE]

FIGURE 51–4 Vaccine adverse event reporting system form (https://vaers.hhs.gov/)

VAERS **CONTINUATION PAGE** (Use only if you need more space from the front page)

17. Enter all vaccines given on the date listed in item 4 (continued):					Dose number
Vaccine (type and brand name)	Manufacturer	Lot number	Route	Body site	in series
select			select	select	select
select			select	select	select
select			select	select	select
select			select	select	select

22. Any other vaccines received within one month prior to the date listed in item 4 (continued):					Dose number	Date
Vaccine (type and brand name)	Manufacturer	Lot number	Route	Body site	in series	Given
select			select	select	select	
select			select	select	select	
select			select	select	select	
select			select	select	select	
select			select	select	select	
select			select	select	select	

Use the space below to provide any additional information (indicate item number):

FORM FDA VAERS 2.0 (02/20) SAVE

FIGURE 51–4 *(Continued)*

COMPLETING THE VACCINE ADVERSE EVENT REPORTING SYSTEM (VAERS) FORM

GENERAL INSTRUCTIONS

- Submit this form electronically using the Internet. For instructions, visit www.vaers.hhs.gov/uploadfile/.

- If you are unable to submit this form electronically, you may fax it to VAERS at 1-877-721-0366.

- If you need additional help submitting a report you may call the VAERS toll-free information line at 1-800-822-7967, or send an email to info@vaers.org.

- Fill out the VAERS form as completely as possible and use the **Continuation Page** if needed. Use a separate VAERS form for each individual patient.

- If you do not know exact numbers, dates, or times, please provide your best guess. You may leave these spaces blank if you are not comfortable guessing.

- You can get specific information on the vaccine and vaccine lot number by contacting the facility or clinic where the vaccine was administered.

- Please report all significant adverse events that occur after vaccination of adults and children, even if you are not sure whether the vaccine caused the adverse event.

- Healthcare professionals should refer to the VAERS Table of Reportable Events at www.vaers.hhs.gov/reportable.html for the list of adverse events that must be reported by law (42 USC 300aa-25).

- Healthcare professionals treating a patient for a suspected vaccine adverse event may need to contact the person who administered the vaccine in order to exchange information and decide how best to complete and submit the VAERS form.

SPECIFIC INSTRUCTIONS

Items 2, 3, 4, 5, 6, 17, 18 and 21 are **ESSENTIAL** and should be completed.

- **Items 4 and 5:** Provide dates and times as specifically as you can and enter as much information as possible (e.g., enter the month and year even if you don't know the day). If you do not know the exact time, but know it was in the morning ("AM") or afternoon or evening ("PM"), please provide that information.

- **Item 6:** If you fill in the form by hand, provide age in years. If a child is less than 1 year old, provide months of age. If a child is more than 1 year old but less than 2 years old, provide year and months (e.g., 1 year and 6 months). If a child is less than 1 month of age when vaccinated (e.g., a birth dose of hepatitis B vaccine) then answer 0 years and 0 months, but be sure to include the patient's date of birth (item 2) and date and time of vaccination (item 4).

- **Item 8:** If the patient who received the vaccine was pregnant at time of vaccination, select "Yes" and describe the event, any pregnancy complications, and estimated due date if known in item 18. Otherwise, select "No" or "Unknown."

- **Item 9:** List any prescriptions, over-the-counter medications, dietary supplements, herbal remedies, or other non-traditional/alternative medicines being taken by the patient when the vaccine(s) was given.

- **Item 10:** List any allergies the patient has to medications, foods, or other products.

- **Item 11:** List any short-term or acute illnesses the patient had on the date of vaccination AND up to one month prior to this date (e.g., cold, stomach flu, ear infection, etc.). This does **NOT** include the adverse event you are reporting.

- **Item 12:** List any chronic or long-standing health conditions the patient has (e.g., asthma, diabetes, heart disease).

- **Item 13:** List the name of the person who is completing the form. Select the "Check if same as item 1" box if you are the patient or if you live at the same address as the patient. The contact information you provided in item 1 will be automatically entered for you. Otherwise, please provide new contact information.

- **Item 14:** List the doctor or other healthcare professional who is the best person to contact to discuss the clinical details of the adverse event.

- **Item 15:** Select the "Check if same as item 13" box if the person completing the form works at the facility that administered the vaccine(s). The contact information provided in item 13 will be automatically entered for you. Otherwise, provide new contact information.

- **Item 16:** Select the option that best describes the type of facility where the vaccine(s) was given.

FIGURE 51–4 (*Continued*)

RETURN TO PAGE 1

- **Item 17:** Include only vaccines given on the date provided in item 4. The vaccine route options include:

  - Injection/shot (intramuscular, subcutaneous, intradermal, jet injection, and unknown)
  - By mouth/oral
  - In nose/intranasal
  - Other (specify)
  - Unknown

  For body site, the options include:

  - Right arm
  - Left arm
  - Arm (side unknown)
  - Right thigh
  - Left thigh
  - Thigh (side unknown)
  - Nose
  - Mouth
  - Other (specify)
  - Unknown

  For vaccines given as a series (i.e., 2 or more doses of the same vaccine given to complete a series), list the dose number for the vaccine in the last column named "Dose number in series."

- **Item 18:** Describe the adverse event(s), treatment, and outcome(s). Include signs and symptoms, when the symptoms occurred, diagnosis, and treatment. Provide specific information if you can (e.g., if patient had a fever, provide the temperature).

- **Item 19:** List any medical tests and laboratory results related to the adverse event(s). Include abnormal findings as well as normal or negative findings.

- **Item 20:** Select "Yes" if the patient's health is the same as it was prior to the vaccination or "No" if the patient has not returned to the same state of health prior to the vaccination, and provide details in item 18. Select "Unknown" if the patient's present condition is not known.

- **Item 21:** Select the result(s) or outcome(s) for the patient. If the patient did not have any of the outcomes listed, select "None of the above." Prolongation of existing hospitalization means the patient received a vaccine during a hospital stay and an adverse event following vaccination occurred that resulted in the patient spending extra time in the hospital. Life threatening illness means you believe this adverse event could have resulted in the death of the patient.

- **Item 22:** List any other vaccines the patient received within one month prior to the vaccination date listed in item 4.

- **Item 23:** Describe the adverse event(s) following any previous vaccine(s). Include patient age at vaccination, dates of vaccination, vaccine type, and brand name.

- **Item 24:** Check all races that apply.

- **Item 25:** Check the single best answer for ethnicity.

- **Item 26:** For health department use only.

- **Items 27 and 28:** Complete only for U.S. Military or Department of Defense related reports. In addition to active duty service members, Reserve and National Guard members, beneficiaries include: retirees, their families, survivors, certain former spouses, and others who are registered in the Defense Enrollment Eligibility Reporting System (DEERS).

GENERAL INFORMATION

- VAERS (www.vaers.hhs.gov) is a national vaccine safety monitoring system that collects information about adverse events (possible reactions or problems) that occur during or after administration of vaccines licensed in the United States.

- VAERS protects patient identity and keeps patient identifying information confidential.

- The Health Insurance Portability and Accountability Act (HIPAA) Privacy Rule permits reporting of protected health information to public health authorities including the Centers for Disease Control and Prevention (CDC) and U.S. Food and Drug Administration (FDA) (45 CFR § 164.512(b)).

- VAERS accepts all reports without judging the importance of the adverse event or whether a vaccine caused the adverse event.

- Acceptance of a VAERS report by CDC and FDA does not constitute admission that the vaccine or healthcare personnel caused or contributed to the reported event.

- The National Vaccine Injury Compensation Program (VICP) is administered by the Health Resources and Services Administration (HRSA). The VICP is separate from the VAERS program and reporting an event to VAERS does not constitute filing a claim for compensation to the VICP (see www.hrsa.gov/vaccinecompensation/index.html).

- Knowingly filing a false VAERS report with the intent to mislead the Department of Health and Human Services is a violation of Federal law (18 U.S. Code § 1001) punishable by fine and imprisonment.

FIGURE 51–4 *(Continued)*

CONTRAINDICATIONS TO VACCINATIONS

The primary contraindications to vaccine administration are acute febrile illness, allergy to a vaccine component, or history of hypersensitivity/anaphylactic reaction to vaccine constituents. **Table 51.1** includes a detailed listing of contraindications by vaccine. The four main types of hypersensitivity reactions include the following:

1. Allergic reactions to egg-related antigens (e.g., yellow fever, influenza)
2. Mercury sensitivity in some recipients of vaccines or immune globulin
3. Antibiotic-induced allergic reactions (e.g., inactivated poliovirus vaccine—trace streptomycin, neomycin, and polymyxin B; MMR, including single or combined with varicella—trace neomycin; varicella and herpes zoster vaccines-neomycin)
4. Hypersensitivity to other vaccine components, including the infectious agent (e.g., gelatin: shingles vaccine)

Acute febrile illness suggesting a moderate to severe illness is sufficient reason to defer vaccination until the person recovers. Guidelines in this instance are based on the provider's assessment of the illness and the vaccines scheduled for administration. The rationale for withholding vaccination in moderate to severe illness, with or without fever, is that evolving signs and symptoms associated with the illness may be difficult to distinguish from the reaction to the vaccine. Minor illness (minor respiratory, gastrointestinal, or other illness) and low-grade fevers are not contraindications to immunization.

TABLE 51.1

Guide to Contraindications and Precautions to Commonly Used Vaccines in Adults

Vaccine	Contraindications	Precautions
IIV	Severe allergic reaction (e.g., anaphylaxis) to any component of the vaccine (except egg) or to a previous dose of influenza vaccine	Moderate or severe acute illness with or without fever History of Guillain-Barré syndrome within 6 weeks of previous influenza vaccination Egg allergy other than hives (e.g., angioedema, respiratory distress, lightheadedness, or recurrent emesis) or required epinephrine or another emergency medical intervention (IIV may be administered in a medical setting under the supervision of a health care provider who is able to recognize and manage severe allergic conditions)
RIV	Severe allergic reaction (e.g., anaphylaxis) to any vaccine component or to a previous dose of influenza vaccine	Moderate or severe acute illness with or without fever History of Guillain-Barré syndrome within 6 weeks of previous influenza vaccination
LAIV	Severe allergic reaction (e.g., anaphylaxis) after a previous dose or to any component of the vaccine Pregnant women Immunocompromised due to any cause Close contacts and caregivers of severely immunosuppressed persons Adults who have taken influenza antiviral medications within the previous 48 hours	Moderate or severe acute illness with or without fever History of Guillain-Barré syndrome within 6 weeks of previous influenza vaccination Asthma Other chronic medical conditions, for example, other chronic lung diseases, chronic cardiovascular disease (excluding isolated hypertension), diabetes, chronic renal or hepatic disease, hematologic disease, neurologic disease, and metabolic disorders
Tdap;Td	Severe allergic reaction (e.g., anaphylaxis) after a previous dose or to a vaccine component For pertussis-containing vaccines: encephalopathy (e.g., coma, decreased level of consciousness, or prolonged seizures) not attributable to another identifiable cause occurring within 7 days of administration of a previous dose of Tdap or diphtheria and tetanus toxoids and acellular pertussis (DTaP) vaccine	Moderate or severe acute illness with or without fever History of Guillain-Barré syndrome within 6 weeks after a previous dose of vaccine containing tetanus toxoid component History of Arthus-type hypersensitivity reactions after a previous dose of tetanus or diphtheria toxoid–containing vaccine; defer at least 10 years since the last tetanus toxoid–containing vaccine For pertussis-containing vaccines: progressive or unstable neurologic disorder, uncontrolled seizures, or progressive encephalopathy until condition has stabilized

(Continued)

TABLE 51.1

Guide to Contraindications and Precautions to Commonly Used Vaccines in Adults (*Continued*)

Vaccine	Contraindications	Precautions
Varicella	Severe allergic reaction (e.g., anaphylaxis) after a previous dose or to a vaccine component Severe immunodeficiency (e.g., ematologic and solid tumors, chemotherapy, congenital immunodeficiency, or long-term immunosuppressive therapy) or persons with HIV infection who are severely immunocompromised Family history of congenital or hereditary immunodeficiency in first-degree relatives (i.e., parents and siblings) unless the immune competence of the potential vaccine recipient has been substantiated clinically or verified by a laboratory test Pregnancy	Recent (within 31 months) receipt of antibody-containing blood products (specific interval dependent on the products) Moderate or severe acute illness with or without fever Receipt of specific antivirals (i.e., acyclovir, famciclovir, or valacyclovir) 24 hours before vaccination; avoid these for 14 days after vaccination Use of aspirin or aspirin-containing products For MMRV only: family history of seizures
HPV	Severe allergic reaction (e.g., anaphylaxis) after a previous dose or to a vaccine component	Moderate or severe acute illness with or without fever Pregnancy
RZV	Severe allergic reaction (e.g., anaphylaxis) to a vaccine component Known severe immunodeficiency Pregnancy	Receipt of specific antivirals (i.e., acyclovir, famciclovir, or valacyclovir) 24 hours before vaccination; avoid these for 14 days after vaccination Moderate or severe acute illness with or without fever
MMR	Severe allergic reaction (e.g., anaphylaxis) after a previous dose or to a vaccine component Severe immunodeficiency Pregnancy	Recent (within 3–11 months) receipt of antibody-containing blood products (specific interval dependent on the products) Moderate or severe acute illness with or without fever
PCV-13	Severe allergic reaction (e.g., anaphylaxis) after a previous dose or to a vaccine component, including any vaccine containing diphtheria toxoid	Moderate or severe acute illness with or without fever
PPSV-23	Severe allergic reaction (e.g., anaphylaxis) after a previous dose or to a vaccine component	Moderate or severe acute illness with or without fever
MenACWY; serogroup B meningococcal (MenB)	Severe allergic reaction (e.g., anaphylaxis) after a previous dose or to a vaccine component	Moderate or severe acute illness with or without fever
Hepatitis A	Severe allergic reaction (e.g., anaphylaxis) after a previous dose or to a vaccine component	Moderate or severe acute illness with or without fever
Hepatitis B	Severe allergic reaction (e.g., anaphylaxis) after a previous dose or to a vaccine component	Moderate or severe acute illness with or without fever
Hib	Severe allergic reaction (e.g., anaphylaxis) after a previous dose or to a vaccine component	Moderate or severe acute illness with or without fever

DTaP, diphtheria, tetanus, and acellular pertussis; Hib, *Haemophilus influenzae* type b; HIV, human immunodeficiency virus; HPV, human papillomavirus; IIV, inactivated influenza vaccine; LAIV, live attenuated influenza vaccine; MenACWY, meningococcal conjugate A, C, W, and Y; MMR, measles, mumps, rubella; MMRV, measles, mumps, rubella vaccine; PCV-13, pneumococcal conjugate vaccine 13-valent; PPSV-23, pneumococcal polysaccharide vaccine 23-valent; RIV, recombinant influenza vaccine; RZV, recombinant zoster vaccine; Td, diphtheria toxoids; Tdap, diphtheria toxoid and acellular pertussis.

Source: Centers for Disease Control and Prevention (2014). Use of MenACWY-CRM vaccine in children aged 2 to 23 months at increased risk for meningococcal disease. *Morbidity and Mortality Weekly Report, 63*(24), 527–530.

The benefit of the immunization at the recommended age, regardless of the presence of mild illness, outweighs the risk of vaccine failure (Pickering et al., 2009).

One needs to use special attention to contraindications when administering live vaccines. Contraindications for all live vaccines include pregnancy and known severe immunodeficiency (e.g., from hematologic and solid tumors, receipt of chemotherapy, congenital immunodeficiency, or long-term immunosuppressive therapy, or patients with HIV infection who are severely immunocompromised) (see the preceding discussions on immunocompromised children).

PATIENT AND PROVIDER EDUCATION AND ISSUES

Patient and health care provider/practitioner education, updates on immunization protocols, and established office systems with designated areas of responsibility are significant factors in improving immunization rates. Office routines and systems should incorporate pediatric immunization standards (**Box 51.4**) and facilitate the use of all possible opportunities to review and update the immunization status of each patient (National Vaccine Advisory Committee, 2003). Tickler systems, chart reminders, and flow sheets that identify needed immunizations clearly and visibly are useful adjuncts to patient care.

A team approach to staff involvement also helps to enhance vaccination rates. Support staff should be aware of immunization needs when scheduling return or preventive visits as well as visits for illness or minor health problems. Visual reminders on the patient's chart or visit encounter form can be used to alert the practitioner to review specific vaccine needs or requests. **Box 51.5** presents recommendations related to the immunization schedule, and **Box 51.6** offers answers to frequently asked questions about immunization.

Vaccines should be stored in the office in sufficient amounts to meet the needs of the patients. Staff should have specific assignments to monitor stock levels, lot numbers, and expiration dates. Vaccines should be stored according to the manufacturer's recommendations with a backup system to address times when power outages may have affected vaccines, particularly during nonbusiness hours. Methods can range from plugging in a digital clock in the same outlet to use of alarm systems on the freezer or refrigerator. An inexpensive method of detecting a power outage uses a cup of ice with a penny or other coins placed on top of the ice. The length of a power outage may be judged by how far the coin sinks in the previously completely frozen ice. If power outages occur, the pharmaceutical manufacturer should be contacted for information about vaccine use, revised

---

BOX 51.4 Standards for Pediatric Immunization Practices

Standard 1: Immunization services are readily available.

Standard 2: No barriers or unnecessary prerequisites to the receipt of vaccines exist.

Standard 3: Immunization services are available free or for a minimal fee.

Standard 4: Providers use all clinical encounters to screen and, when indicated, immunize children.

Standard 5: Providers educate parents and guardians about immunization in general terms.

Standard 6: Providers question parents or guardians about contraindications and, before immunizing a child, inform them in specific terms about the risks and benefits of the immunizations their child is to receive.

Standard 7: Providers follow only true contraindications.

Standard 8: Providers administer simultaneously all vaccine doses for which a child is eligible at the time of each visit.

Standard 9: Providers use accurate and complete recording procedures.

Standard 10: Providers co-schedule immunization appointments in conjunction with appointments for other child health services.

Standard 11: Providers report adverse events after immunization promptly, accurately, and completely.

Standard 12: Providers operate a tracking system.

Standard 13: Providers adhere to appropriate procedures for vaccine management.

Standard 14: Providers conduct semiannual audits to assess immunization coverage levels and to review immunization records in the patient populations they serve.

Standard 15: Providers maintain up-to-date, easily retrievable medical protocols at all locations where vaccines are administered.

Standard 16: Providers operate with patient-oriented and community-based approaches.

Standard 17: Vaccines are administered by properly trained individuals.

Standard 18: Providers receive ongoing education and training on current immunization recommendations.

From Centers for Disease Control and Prevention (1993). Standard for pediatric immunization practices—recommended by National Vaccine Advisory Committee (ACIP). *Morbidity and Mortality Weekly Report, 42*(RR-5), 1–13.

RESTARTING VACCINE SERIES

With the exception of oral typhoid vaccine, it never is necessary to restart a vaccine series because the interval has been prolonged—yet every effort should be made to adhere to the recommended schedule.

VACCINES GIVEN TOO SOON

These will not be accepted at school entry and revaccination will be recommended.

LACK OF WRITTEN VACCINATION RECORD

An attempt should be made to verify vaccination status. If no record can be verified, the child should be considered unimmunized and should be revaccinated as appropriate for age.

HEPATITIS B

In the case of an *interrupted* or *incomplete* series, resume the series; do not repeat or restart. Dose should be appropriate in accord with the manufacturer's instructions. The *third dose* should be given at least 2 months after the second dose and at least 4 months after the first dose but not before 6 months of age.

PPD/MEASLES, MUMPS, RUBELLA

PPD can be done before or at the same time as the measles vaccine is administered. Give PPD 4 to 6 weeks after measles vaccine, if measles is given first, because measles can reduce

the reactivity of PPD. This reduction in reactivity is due to mild suppression of cell-mediated immunity, which can lead to false-negative test results.

DIPHTHERIA, TETANUS, AND PERTUSSIS

The fourth dose can be given if a child is more than or equal to 12 months of age and 6 months have elapsed since DTaP dose 3 (especially if the child is unlikely to return at 15–18 months of age). The fifth dose should be given at 4 to 6 years. Children should not receive more than six doses of diphtheria or tetanus-containing toxoid before their seventh birthday. No pertussis-containing vaccines are licensed for use in people more than or equal to 7 years of age.

HAEMOPHILUS INFLUENZAE TYPE B

No Hib vaccine should be given to infants younger than 6 weeks of age, and it is not recommended after 5 years of age. Minimum age for last Hib is 12 months if at least 2 months has passed since the previous dose. DTaP/Hib combination products should not be used for primary series (2, 4, 6 months of age).

VARICELLA

Dosage for people aged 12 months or older: single 0.5 mL dose subcutaneously suffices for protection for 12 months to 12 years. People aged 13 years of age or older should receive two 0.5 mL doses at least 4 weeks apart.

DTaP, diphtheria, tetanus, and acellular pertussis; Hib, *Haemophilus influenzae* type b; MMR, measles, mumps, rubella; PPD, purified protein derivative skin test.

---

expiration dates, or unusable vaccine. Staff members should not automatically assume that vaccine should be discarded.

A central log book, including date and time and lot numbers and expiration dates of the vaccines, is recommended. Used with patient schedule information and chart documentation, the log book helps identify patients should a pharmaceutical company notify the office of a vaccine recall or a need to reimmunize patients receiving a specific lot of vaccine. Immunization screening processes are necessary for all populations to determine if an individual can receive the required vaccines. The screening questions, asked prior to vaccination, should be as follows:

1. Is the patient sick today?
2. Does the patient have any severe allergies to drugs, foods, vaccine components, or latex?
3. Has the patient had any serious reactions to previous vaccinations?

4. Is the patient on long-term aspirin?
5. Has the patient or close family member had seizures or a brain or neurologic problem?
6. Does the patient have a history of bowel obstruction?
7. Does the patient have asthma or another chronic medical condition (e.g., lung, heart, kidney, or metabolic)?
8. If the patient is a child between 2 and 4 years, has a health care provider diagnosed wheezing or asthma in the past year?
9. Does the patient have cancer, leukemia, a blood disorder, HIV infection, AIDS, tuberculosis, or any problem with the immune system?
10. In the past 3 months, has the patient received any treatment that might weaken their immune system, such as steroids, cancer chemotherapy, or radiation?
11. Are there any family members who have problems with their immune system?
12. Has the patient received blood transfusions or immune globulin in the past year?

BOX 51.6 Questions and Answers about Immunization

Question 1: How long should the vaccination needle be?

a. Subcutaneous injections for children and adults: ⅝ to ¾ in., 23- to 25-gauge needle.

Intramuscular injections for infants and children: minimum needle length of ⅞ in. for anterolateral thigh and minimum of ⅝ in. for deltoid injection; for adults: 1 to 1½ in. needle (Marshall, 2012).

Question 2: What are the immunization recommendations for children of parents or household residents who were never vaccinated for polio?

a. If the unvaccinated or inadequately vaccinated person resides in the household, an IPV schedule is recommended for the child. Parents and household contacts may receive IPV too.

Question 3: Which Hib vaccines are the best?

a. Products of different manufacturers are considered interchangeable for the primary series and the booster. However, no Hib vaccine is recommended for infants younger than 6 weeks of age. If it is given, it may make the child incapable of responding to subsequent doses.

Question 4: What are some special concerns related to pregnancy?

a. There are no contraindications to immunization of a household member if another household member is pregnant. However, if a woman in the household wants to become pregnant and also wants to be vaccinated, she should wait to become pregnant at least 1 month after receiving mumps, measles, varicella and 3 months after receiving rubella.

Question 5: What happens if someone has an extra vaccination?

a. Extra doses of live vaccine do not appear to have adverse consequences, and they may boost immunity. Extra doses of inactivated vaccines can induce very high antibody titers. If these people are revaccinated, large local inflammatory reactions may ensue.

Question 6: Is it harmful to receive vaccines simultaneously?

a. No evidence exists that simultaneous administration of vaccines reduces vaccine effectiveness or increases adverse events.

Question 7: What are the implications of an error, such as previous administration of a vaccine at the wrong site, in a wrong dose, by a wrong route?

a. Unfortunately, they do not count. Only full doses in acceptable sites should be counted. Revaccinate according to age. The exception to the rule is live vaccines (MMR, varicella), which are recommended to be administered subcutaneously—intramuscular administration of these vaccines is not likely to decrease immunogenicity. *Note:* Reducing or dividing doses of any vaccine including those to preterm or low-birth-weight infants is not indicated.

Question 8: What is the recommended way to administer multiple injections to infants?

a. The recommended approach is to place the vaccine most likely to cause a local adverse reaction (e.g., DTaP) in one leg and the two less reactive in different sites in the other leg.

Question 9: How effective is the varicella vaccine?

a. Effectiveness is 70% to 90% protection against infection with 95% protection against severe disease. Protection persists at least 7 to 10 years. The risk of transmission appears low but somewhat higher if the vaccine develops a varicella-like rash after vaccination. Recommend that immunocompromised people avoid contact with patients who develop a varicella-like rash.

Question 10: Why is the MMR vaccine given twice?

a. The second dose is given because 2% to 5% of people do not develop immunity after the first dose, and 95% of the people who did not respond to the first dose respond to the second.

Note: Birth before 1957 is generally considered evidence of rubella immunity; laboratory evidence of immunity is recommended. Combined MMR vaccine is the drug of choice if vaccination is needed.

Question 11: What is the standard dosing schedule for hepatitis B vaccine?

a. There is no standard dose. That is why it is so important to read the package insert for hepatitis B vaccine carefully. The formulations vary, and the appropriate microgram dose must be selected.

DTaP, diphtheria, tetanus, and acellular pertussis; Hib, *Haemophilus influenzae* type b; IPV, inactivated polio vaccine; MMR, measles, mumps, rubella.

---

13. Is the patient pregnant or is there a chance she could become pregnant in the next 3 months?
14. Has the patient received any other vaccines in the last 4 weeks?

Focusing on adolescent and adult populations as well as infants and children is critical. Current recommendations include routine screening at ages 11, 12, and 50. An interim process for high-risk people in combination with aforementioned recommended screenings provides the best mechanism for implementing a comprehensive immunization program.

It is extremely important to keep updated and be familiar with Web sites and organizations that provide vaccine information to be aware of changes that occur.

CASE STUDY 1

E.S. is a 66-year-old male with no food or drug allergies. He presents to your clinic on December 10 as a follow-up visit for pneumonia one month ago. His history is significant for the following:

- Type 2 diabetes mellitus controlled with diet and exercise
- Newborn grandson
- Vaccination history: oral polio vaccine 1964; diphtheria toxoids 2010; physician-confirmed chicken pox, mumps, and measles as a child

   1. You assess that E.S. requires several vaccines. Which of the screening questions should you ask to determine if he can be immunized today?

2. You determine that E.S. can be immunized today and needs to be immunized against pneumococcal infection. Which of the vaccines should E.S. receive today?

3. What additional vaccines does E.S. require at this time? Should all of these be given today?

4. E.S. asks you if he really needs all of these vaccines and if there are any side effects. How should you respond?

Bibliography

Starred references are cited in the text.

American Academy of Pediatrics, Committee on Infectious Diseases. (1999). Poliomyelitis prevention: Revised recommendations for use of inactivated and live oral poliovirus vaccines. *Pediatrics, 103,* 171–172.

Anon. (2020). Antiviral drugs for influenza. *Medical Letter on Drugs and Therapeutics, 62*(1589), 1–4.

Centers for Disease Control and Prevention. (1993). Standards for pediatric immunization practices. *Morbidity and Mortality Weekly Report, 42* (RR-5), 1–13.

Centers for Disease Control and Prevention. (2010a). Updated recommendations for prevention of invasive pneumococcal disease among adults using the 23-valent pneumococcal polysaccharide vaccine. *Morbidity and Mortality Weekly Report, 59*(34), 1102–1106.

Centers for Disease Control and Prevention. (2010b). Prevention of pneumococcal disease among infants and children—Use of 13-valent pneumococcal conjugate vaccine and 23-valent pneumococcal polysaccharide vaccine. *Morbidity and Mortality Weekly Report, 59*(RR11), 1–18.

Centers for Disease Control and Prevention. (2011). Updated recommendations for use of tetanus toxoid, reduced diphtheria toxoid and acellular pertussis (Tdap) vaccine from the Advisory Committee on Immunization Practices, 2010. *Morbidity and Mortality Weekly Report, 60*(1), 13–15.

Centers for Disease Control and Prevention. (2012). Use of 13-valent pneumococcal conjugate vaccine and 23-valent pneumococcal polysaccharide vaccine for adults with immunocompromising conditions. *Morbidity and Mortality Weekly Report, 6*(40), 816–819.

Centers for Disease Control and Prevention. (2013). Prevention and control of meningococcal disease. *Morbidity and Mortality Weekly Report, 62*(RR02), 1–22.

*Centers for Disease Control and Prevention. (2014). Use of MenACWY-CRM vaccine in children aged 2 through 23 months at increased risk for meningococcal disease. *Morbidity and Mortality Weekly Report, 63*(24), 527–530.

Centers for Disease Control and Prevention. (2015). Use of serogroup B meningococcal vaccines in persons aged >10 years at increased risk for serogroup B meningococcal disease. *Morbidity and Mortality Weekly Report, 64*(22), 608–612.

Centers for Disease Control and Prevention. (2016). Barriers and strategies to improving influenza vaccination among health care personnel. Retrieved from http://www.cdc.gov/flu/toolkit/long-term-care/strategies.htm on January 15, 2020.

*Centers for Disease Control and Prevention. (2020a). Immunization schedules: Recommended Child and Adolescent Immunization Schedule for ages 18 years or younger, United States, 2020. Retrieved from http://www.cdc.gov/vaccines/schedules/hcp/child-adolescent.html on February 2, 2020.

*Centers for Disease Control and Prevention. (2020b). Immunization schedules. Retrieved from http://www.cdc.gov/vaccines/schedules/hcp/adult.html on February 2, 2020.

Centers for Disease Control and Prevention. (2020c). ACIP vaccine recommendations and guidelines: Advisory Committee on Immunization Practices (ACIP). Retrieved from http://www.cdc.gov/vaccines/hcp/acip-recs/index.html on February 2, 2020.

*Centers for Disease Control and Prevention. (2020d). Information for Health Care Professionals: Influenza (Flu). Retrieved from https://www.cdc.gov/flu/professionals/index.htm on January 5, 2021.

Dooling, K. L., Guo, A., Patel, M., et al. (2018). Recommendations of the advisory committee on immunization practices for use of herpes zoster vaccines. *Morbidity and Mortality Weekly Report, 67,* 103–108.

Eliscu, A. (2017). Human papillomavirus and HPV vaccines. *Pediatrics in Review, 38*(9), 443–445.

Freedman, M. S., Hunter, P., Ault, K., et al. (2020). Advisory committee on immunization practices recommended immunization schedule for adults aged 19 years or older—United States, 2020. *Morbidity and Mortality Weekly Report, 69,* 133–135.

*Geoghegan, S., O'Callaghan, K. P., & Offit, P. A. (2020). Vaccine safety: Myths and misinformation. *Frontiers in Microbiology, 11,* 372.

*Grohskopf, L. A., Alyanak, E., Broder, K. R., et al. (2019). Prevention and control of seasonal influenza with vaccines: Recommendations of the Advisory Committee on Immunization Practices—United States, 2019–20 Influenza Season. *MMWR Recommendations and Reports, 68*(3), 1–21.

*Hamborsky, J., Kroger, A., & Wolfe, C. (Eds.). (2015). *Epidemiology and prevention of vaccine-preventable diseases (The Pink Book)* (13th ed.). Washington, DC: Public Health Foundation. Retrieved from http://www.cdc.gov/vaccines/pubs/pinkbook/index.html on January 15, 2020.

*Havers, F. P., Moro, P. L., Hunter, P., et al. (2020). Use of tetanus toxoid, reduced diphtheria toxoid, and acellular pertussis vaccines: Updated recommendations of the Advisory Committee on Immunization Practices—United States, 2019. *Morbidity and Mortality Weekly Report, 69,* 77–83.

Heron, M. (2019). Deaths: Leading causes for 2017. *National vital statistics reports, 68*(6). Hyattsville, MD: National Center for Health Statistics.

*Hill, H. A., Elam-Evans, L. D., Yankey, D., et al. (2015). National, state, and selected local area vaccination coverage among children aged 19–35 months—United States, 2014. *Morbidity and Mortality Weekly Report, 64*(33), 889–896.

Hughes, M. M., Reed, C., Flannery, B., et al. (2019). Projected population benefit of increased effectiveness and coverage of influenza vaccination on influenza burden—United States. *Clinical Infectious Diseases, 10,* 1093–2000.

Hussain, A., Ali, S., Ahmed, M., et al. (2018). The anti-vaccination movement: A regression in modern medicine. *Cureus, 10*(7), e2919.

Kobayashi, M., Bennett, N. M., Gierke, R., et al. (2015). Intervals between PCV13 and PPSV23 vaccines: Recommendations of the Advisory Committee on Immunization Practices (ACIP). *Morbidity and Mortality Weekly Report, 64*(34), 944–947.

Kroger, A. T., Duchin, J., & Vázquez, M. (2017). General best practice guidelines for immunization: Best practices guidance of the Advisory Committee on Immunization Practices (ACIP). Retrieved from https://www.cdc.gov/vaccines/hcp/acip-recs/general-recs/index.html on March 15, 2020.

Lindley, M. C., Kahn, K. E., Bardenheier, B. H., et al. (2019). Burden and prevention of influenza and pertussis among pregnant women and infants—United States. *Morbidity and Mortality Weekly Report, 68,* 885–892.

*Marin, M., Marlow, M., Moore, K. L., et al. (2018). Recommendation of the advisory committee on immunization practices for use of a third dose of mumps virus–containing vaccine in persons at increased risk for mumps during an outbreak. *Morbidity and Mortality Weekly Report, 67,* 33–38.

Marshall, G. (2020). *The vaccine handbook: A practical guide for clinicians* (9th ed.). West Islip, NY: Professional Communications, Inc.

*Matanock, A., Lee, G., Gierke, R., et al. (2019). Use of 13-valent pneumococcal conjugate vaccine and 23-valent pneumococcal polysaccharide vaccine among adults aged ≥65 years: Updated recommendations of the advisory committee on immunization practices. *Morbidity and Mortality Weekly Report, 68,* 1069–1075.

*National Vaccine Advisory Committee. (2003). Standards for child and adolescent immunization practices. *Pediatrics, 112,* 958–963.

National Vaccine Advisory Committee. (2014). Recommendations from the national vaccine advisory committee standards for adult immunization practice. *Public Health Reports, 129,* 115–123.

National Vaccine Advisory Committee. (2020). 2020 National Vaccine Plan Development: Recommendations from the national vaccine advisory committee. *Public Health Reports, 135*(2), 181–188.

Opel, D. J., & Omer, S. B. (2015). Measles, mandates, and making vaccination the default option. *JAMA Pediatrics, 169*(4), 303–304.

*Patel, M., Lee, A. D., Clemmons, N. S., et al. (2019). National update on measles cases and outbreaks—United States, January 1–October 1, 2019. *Morbidity and Mortality Weekly Report, 68,* 893–896.

*Payne, D. C., Staat, M. A., Edwards, K. M., et al. (2011a). Direct and indirect effects of rotavirus vaccination upon childhood hospitalizations in 3 US counties, 2006–2009. *Clinical Infectious Diseases, 53*(3), 245–253.

Payne, D. C., Wikswo, M., & Parashar, U. M. (2011b). Chapter 13: Rotavirus. In *Manual for the surveillance of vaccine-preventable diseases.* VPD Surveillance Manual (5th ed.). Atlanta, GA: Centers for Disease Control and Prevention.

*Perry, R. T., Murray, J. S., Gacic-Dobo, M., et al. (2015). Progress toward regional measles elimination—Worldwide, 2000–2014. *Morbidity and Mortality Weekly Report, 64*(44), 1246–1251.

*Petrosky, E., Bocchini, J. A., Hariri, S., et al. (2015). Use of 9-valent human papillomavirus (HPV) vaccine: Updated HPV vaccination recommendations of the Advisory Committee on Immunization Practices. *Morbidity and Mortality Weekly Report, 64*(11), 300–304.

*Pickering, L., Baker, C., Kimberlin, D., et al. (Eds.). (2009). *The 2009 red book: Report of the committee on infectious diseases* (26th ed.). Elk Grove Village, IL: American Academy of Pediatrics.

Poland, G., & Johnson, D. (2008). Increasing influenza vaccination rates: The need to vaccinate throughout the entire influenza season. *American Journal of Medicine, 121*(7 Suppl. 2), S3–S10.

Ranee, S., Calhoun, K., Knighton, C. L., et al. (2015). Vaccination coverage among children in kindergarten—United States, 2014–15 school year. *Morbidity and Mortality Weekly Report, 64*(33), 897–904.

*Robinson, C. L., Bernstein, H., Poehling, K., et al. (2020). Advisory committee on immunization practices recommended immunization schedule for children and adolescents aged 18 years or younger—United States, 2020. *Morbidity and Mortality Weekly Report, 69,* 130–132.

*Seither, R., Loretan, C., Driver, K., et al. (2019). Vaccination coverage with selected vaccines and exemption rates among children in kindergarten—United States, 2018–19 school year. *Morbidity and Mortality Weekly Report, 68,* 905–912.

Trimble, C., & Frazer, I. (2009). Development of therapeutic HPV vaccines. *The Lancet Oncology, 10*(10), 975–980.

*Williams, W. W., Lu, P., O'Halloran, A., et al. (2017). Surveillance of vaccination coverage among adult populations—United States, 2015. *MMWR Surveillance Summaries, 66*(No. SS-11), 1–28.

Xu, J. Q., Murphy, S. L., Kochanek, K. D., et al. (2020). Mortality in the United States, 2018. *NCHS Data Brief, no. 355.* Hyattsville, MD: National Center for Health Statistics.

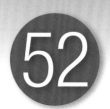

52 Smoking Cessation

Tyan F. Thomas

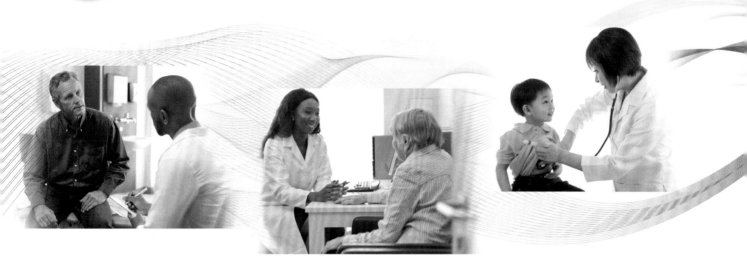

Learning Objectives

1. Describe the various nicotine-containing products available for purchase in the United States.
2. Identify the medical conditions associated with tobacco use.
3. Define nicotine addiction and tobacco use disorder.
4. Describe the course of nicotine addiction and tobacco use disorder.
5. List steps in the stages of change model to assess a person's readiness to quit nicotine-containing products.
6. Outline the goals of therapy of nicotine cessation.
7. Recite nondrug therapies used to help people stop smoking.
8. List the medications used to treat nicotine addiction and tobacco use disorder.
9. Describe the place in therapy of the various medications used to treat nicotine addiction and tobacco use disorder.
10. Identify adverse events associated with medications used to help people stop using nicotine-containing products.

INTRODUCTION

Nicotine is the addictive substance contained in the tobacco plant. A traditional cigarette is one of many nicotine-containing products, and smoking of a traditional cigarette is one of many methods to consume nicotine. Nicotine-containing products include cigarettes, cigars, smokeless tobacco, hookah tobacco, and electronic cigarettes (e-cigarettes). Electronic nicotine delivery systems (ENDS), also called *e-cigarettes*, do not contain tobacco but deliver nicotine by vaporizing nicotine-containing liquids. **Table 52.1** provides a list of forms of tobacco and nicotine delivery devices available in the United States (Food and Drug Administration [FDA], 2020a, 2020b). Because the majority of adult nicotine users smoke traditional cigarettes, this chapter will focus on evidence-based interventions used for cessation of cigarette smoking (Creamer et al., 2019).

Cigarette smoking is a chronic condition. Like sufferers of other chronic conditions, many cigarette smokers cycle through periods of remission (i.e., periods of abstinence from cigarette use) and relapse (i.e., periods of active cigarette use). Similar to other chronic conditions, cigarette smoking contributes to morbidity and mortality and is the leading cause of preventable morbidity and mortality in the United States (U.S. Department of Health and Human Services [USDHHS], 2014, 2020).

The USDHHS estimates that in the United States, cigarette smoking and secondhand exposure to cigarette smoke result in at least 480,000 premature deaths annually. Lung cancer, coronary heart disease (CHD), and chronic obstructive pulmonary disease (COPD) are the three leading causes of smoking-related deaths (USDHHS, 2014, 2020). Smoking accounts for a little over 80% of all lung cancer deaths and is attributable to deaths caused by 11 non-lung-related cancers, including oral–pharyngeal and stomach cancers (Siegel et al., 2015). Life expectancy is estimated to be 10 years shorter for smokers compared to lifelong nonsmokers (Jha et al., 2013; USDHHS, 2020).

In addition to the variety of cancers, smoking is a major risk factor for cardiovascular diseases, such as CHD and aortic aneurysm, cerebrovascular disease, and peripheral arterial disease. It is estimated that each year, as many as 24% of all

TABLE 52.1

Tobacco and Nicotine Delivery Products Available in the United States

Combustible tobacco products	Traditional cigarettes: tobacco and other chemical additives rolled in a paper wrapper and contains a filter
	Bidis: tobacco rolled in a tendu or temburni leaf (plants native to Asia)
	Cigars
	Pipes
Chewable tobacco	Tobacco leaf
	Cured tobacco plug
	Tobacco leaf roll
Ground tobacco (snuff)	Dry
	Moist
	U.S. snus (moist snuff packaged in ready-to-use pouches resembling tea bags)
Dissolvable tobacco	Lozenges
	Orbs
	Sticks
	Strips
Electronic Nicotine Delivery Products	e-cigarettes
	e-hookahs
	e-pipes
	Vape pens

deaths related to CHD in American adults 35 years of age and older may be attributable to cigarette smoking (USDHHS, 2014) and that smoking doubles the risk of ischemic stroke (Boehme et al., 2017; Meschia et al., 2014). Furthermore, smoking increases the risk of acute respiratory infections. It is also a major risk factor for the development of COPD and is estimated to account for nearly 80% of COPD-related deaths (USDHHS, 2014).

In the United States, the annual costs for medical expenditures for care of smoking-related illnesses are estimated to be at least $196 billion, and annual costs related to lost earnings and loss of productivity are estimated to be at least $190 billion (USDHHS, 2014, 2020).

Adverse health effects associated with smoking seem to lessen with smoking cessation. Jha and colleagues found that adult smokers who quit at younger ages gained years of life compared to adults who continued smoking: adults who quit when aged 25 to 34 years gained 10 years of life compared to 9 years of life gained when quitting from ages 35 to 44 years and 6 years gained when quitting from ages 45 to 55 years. In fact, adults who quit smoking between 25 and 34 years of age had survival curves similar to adults who never smoked (Jha et al., 2013).

The CDC estimates that in 2018, approximately 13.7% (34.2 million) of adults in the United States smoked cigarettes, which is down from 17.8% (42.1 million) in 2013 (Creamer et al., 2019; Jamal et al., 2014) and 42.4% in 1964, when the first surgeon general's report on smoking was published

(Li et al., 2020). According to the CDC, more men than women in the United States smoke cigarettes (15.6% of adult males compared to 12.0% of adult females) (Creamer et al., 2019). Among racial and ethnic populations in the United States, Asians have the lowest rates of cigarette use (7.1%), while American Indians/Alaska natives had the highest rates (22.6%) (Creamer et al., 2019). Smoking rates vary by age group as well, with the lowest rates among those older than age 65 years (8.4%) and higher rates among adults aged 25 to 64 years (16.4%) (Creamer et al., 2019). While cigarette smoking rates have significantly declined since 1964, the current smoking rate is still above the goal rate of less than 12%, as set by the U.S. Healthy People 2020 initiative.

In 2019, an estimated 31.2% (4.7 million) of U.S. high school students and 12.5% (1.5 million) of middle school students reported current use of nicotine-containing products (including e-cigarettes, hookah, traditional cigarettes, and other tobacco products) on the National Youth Tobacco Survey (Wang et al., 2019). Use of e-cigarettes was most common, with cigars and traditional cigarettes rounding out the top three most commonly used nicotine-containing products by youth completing this survey (Wang et al., 2019). While use of cigarettes has decreased in this age group, this decrease is offset by the increased use of other forms of nicotine-containing products (Arrazola et al., 2015; Wang et al. 2019).

Although nearly 70% of adult cigarette smokers report that they would like to quit, only 55.4% will make a quit attempt during any given year, and less than 10% are likely to be successful; however, many who attempt to quit smoking do not use recommended cessation methods, and most relapse within the first week of quitting (Fiore et al., 2008; Malarcher et al., 2011; USDHHS, 2020). Fortunately, most cigarette smokers make multiple attempts, and nearly half of users will eventually abstain (American Psychiatric Association [APA], 2013).

The U.S. Preventive Services Task Force (USPSTF) recommends that all health care professionals, including physicians, nurses, and pharmacists, ask about and document their patients' smoking status, advise patients to quit, and refer them to initiate evidence-based interventions (Siu, 2015). In addition, experts urge clinicians to treat tobacco use disorder as a chronic disease similar in many respects to other diseases such as hypertension, diabetes mellitus, and hyperlipidemia and to provide patients with appropriate advice and pharmacotherapy (Fiore et al., 2008).

PATHOPHYSIOLOGY

Nicotine, the addictive substance in tobacco and nontobacco nicotine-containing products, is absorbed and distributed to most tissues of the body, where it binds with nicotinic receptors to produce its physiologic effects on the heart, brain, and other organ systems. Nicotine is a ganglionic cholinergic receptor agonist whose pharmacologic effects are highly dose dependent. At blood concentrations achieved by recreational nicotine use, effects include central and peripheral nervous system stimulation; respiratory stimulation; skeletal muscle relaxation; epinephrine release by the adrenal medulla; peripheral vasoconstriction; and increased blood pressure, heart rate, cardiac output, and oxygen consumption (Hibbs & Zambon, 2018). In addition, nicotine increases dopamine levels in the central nervous system, thus stimulating the reward system and reinforcement of its use (Hibbs & Zambon, 2018; Prochaska & Benowitz, 2016). Activation of nicotine receptors in the brain produces relaxation, decreases stress and anxiety, and improves concentration and reaction times (Benowitz, 2010). Cessation of smoking leads to depressed mood, irritability, difficulty concentrating, and anxiety. Smokers use nicotine to experience the rewarding effects and to avoid the unpleasant effects of nicotine withdrawal.

OTHER PHYSIOLOGIC EFFECTS

A common endocrine and metabolic effect of nicotine is weight loss. Smokers tend to weigh 2.4 to 4.5 kg less than nonsmokers (Audrain-McGovern & Benowitz, 2011; Molarius et al., 1997). Additional endocrine effects include increased risk of osteoporosis and earlier menopause (Mishra et al., 2019; National Institute of Arthritis and Musculoskeletal and Skin Diseases, 2018).

Finally, smoking alters the liver's metabolic effects by inducing hepatic (cytochrome P-450) enzymes. These effects on hepatic enzymes result in the increased metabolism of certain medications, such as theophylline and acetaminophen, and substances such as caffeine.

DIAGNOSTIC CRITERIA

Chronic nicotine ingestion may lead to physical and physiologic dependence and tolerance to some of its pharmacologic effects. The American Psychiatric Association (APA) labels nicotine addiction as tobacco use disorder and defines it as a form of substance abuse that can lead to clinically important impairment or distress (2013). The key features required for the diagnosis of this disorder are continued use despite wanting to quit; prior attempts at quitting; and persistent use despite the presence of physical illness, tolerance, and presence of withdrawal symptoms (APA, 2013). **Box 52.1** highlights the APA criteria for tobacco use disorder and tobacco withdrawal. Another clinical assessment tool for tobacco/nicotine dependence is the Fagerstrom Test for Nicotine Dependence, which assesses a patient's level of nicotine dependence, in part, by determining the time to first cigarette (TTFC) of the day (Heatherton et al., 1991). Nicotine has a relatively short half-life, and nicotine-dependent cigarette users may experience significant discomfort on waking unless they quickly have their first cigarette (Mallin, 2002). The number of cigarettes smoked per day and the TTFC both have been shown to correlate with the degree of

nicotine dependence. Therefore, the Fagerstrom test may be used (**Box 52.2**) in addition to the APA criteria for diagnosis of tobacco use disorder among smokers.

Development and Course of Tobacco Use Disorder and Nicotine Dependence

Many teenagers experiment with use of tobacco and nicotine products, and by age 18, 20% use these products at least monthly; many of these individuals will become daily users (APA, 2013). Commencement of tobacco use after the age of 21 is rare (APA, 2013). Individuals may have some of the APA-defined criteria of tobacco use disorder soon after beginning use of nicotine-containing products, and many individuals will have a pattern of use that meets the APA's definition of tobacco use disorder by late adolescence (APA, 2013).

Patients who are addicted to nicotine may experience withdrawal symptoms. Onset of these symptoms usually occurs within 24 hours and may last for days, weeks, or longer (APA, 2013; Henningfield et al., 2009). Nicotine withdrawal is associated with a well-described syndrome characterized by irritability, awakening from sleep, anxiety, impaired concentration, impaired reaction time, restlessness, drowsiness, confusion, increased appetite, and weight gain (Henningfield et al., 2009; O'Brien, 2018; Shiffman, et al., 2004).

Initiating Drug and Nondrug Therapy

The DHHS/Public Health Service (PHS) (Fiore et al., 2008) and the USPSTF (Siu, 2015) provide recommendations on treatment approaches to help adults stop smoking. While there are many different ways to consume nicotine, these guidelines mainly focus on recommendations for cessation of cigarette smoking.

Before exploring drug and nondrug therapy interventions, it is essential for the reader to recognize the importance of identifying current nicotine product users. Both guidelines recommend that health care providers complete the Five A's: ask every patient about nicotine product use, advise all nicotine users to quit, assess the users' willingness to make a quit attempt, assist users with their quit attempt, and arrange follow-up (**Box 52.3**).

After the Five A's have been performed, the patient may be categorized as unwilling to quit, willing to quit, and recently quit. Health care providers may utilize motivational interviewing techniques to encourage the unwilling patient to quit. Motivational interviewing may include the 5R's: relevance, risks, rewards, roadblocks, and repetition (Fiore et al., 2008) (**Box 52.4**). It is also helpful to determine the patient's readiness to change (Fiore et al., 2008). The five-step transtheoretical stages of change (SOC) model is useful for assessing the patient's readiness to quit. The SOC model identifies behavioral change as a process involving movement through a series of five motivational stages (Mallin, 2002; Prochaska & Velicer, 1997):

- **Stage 1**—Precontemplation: the patient has no intention to quit smoking/using nicotine-containing products.
- **Stage 2**—Contemplation: a smoker/nicotine user is interested in quitting but has no definite plans.

BOX
52.1   APA Criteria for Tobacco Use Disorder and Tobacco Withdrawal

TOBACCO USE DISORDER

Tobacco use disorder is defined as a problematic pattern of use of tobacco that leads to clinically important impairment or distress, as demonstrated by the presence of two or more of the following, occurring within a 12-month period:

1. Tobacco is taken in larger amounts over a longer period of time than was intended.
2. There exists a persistent desire to cut down or control tobacco use, or unsuccessful efforts are made to cut down or control tobacco use.
3. A significant amount of time is spent in activities necessary to obtain or use tobacco.
4. Craving, or a strong desire or urge to use tobacco, exists.
5. Recurrent tobacco use results in a failure to fulfill important obligations or responsibilities at work, school, or home.
6. Tobacco use continues despite its contribution to persistent or recurrent social or interpersonal problems (e.g., tobacco use causes or contributes to arguments with others).
7. Tobacco use results in the individual giving up important social, occupational, or recreational activities.
8. Tobacco use recurs in situations that are physically hazardous (e.g., smoking in bed).
9. Persistent tobacco use despite knowledge of having chronic tobacco-related physical or psychosocial problems
10. Tolerance to tobacco exists, with tolerance being defined as either one of the following: (1) the need for a markedly increased amount of tobacco to produce the intended effect or (2) a markedly diminished effect with the continued use of the same amount of tobacco.
11. Withdrawal occurs. Withdrawal is manifested by either one of the following: (1) presence of characteristic co-relate withdrawal symptoms; (2) tobacco, or other nicotine containing products, is taken to relieve or avoid withdrawal symptoms.

WITHDRAWAL

Withdrawal symptoms may be initiated and characterized by the following:

1. Daily use of tobacco for at least several weeks
2. Abrupt cessation of nicotine use, or reduction in the amount of nicotine used, followed within 24 hours by four or more of the following:
   a. Irritability, frustration, or anger
   b. Anxiety
   c. Difficulty concentrating
   d. Increased appetite
   e. Restlessness
   f. Depressed mood
   g. Insomnia
3. The signs and symptoms outlined in item 2 cause clinically significant distress or impairment in social, occupational, or other important areas of functioning.
4. The signs or symptoms are not due to a different medical condition and are not better accounted for by another mental disorder, including intoxication or withdrawal from another substance.

- **Stage 3**—Preparation: a smoker/nicotine user in this stage is planning to quit within the next month and often has made a failed attempt to quit during the previous year.
- **Stage 4**—Action: a smoker/nicotine user makes a serious effort to quit by modifying his or her behavior and environment. During this stage, the patient has abstained anywhere from 1 day to 6 months. After 6 months of abstinence, the patient enters the final stage.
- **Stage 5**—Maintenance: at this stage a smoker/nicotine user is now a former smoker/nicotine user who works to prevent relapse into active smoking/nicotine use.

Patients willing to quit should be encouraged to identify a target quit date; otherwise, the patient may never actually make the attempt. Next, they should be offered support, which may include behavioral therapy and drug therapy. Patients who have recently quit may need both behavioral and drug therapy interventions to prevent relapse. Quit rates are improved with use of behavioral counseling alone and drug therapy alone when compared to unaided smoking cessation, commonly called *quitting cold turkey*. However, the combination of behavioral counseling and drug therapy further improves a patient's chances of a successful quit attempt than use of behavioral counseling or drug therapy alone.

NONDRUG THERAPY

Nondrug therapy consists of behavioral interventions. Both the DHHS/PHS and the USPSTF categorize behavioral interventions by the method of delivery: in-person counseling, telephonic counseling, and self-help materials. In addition to method of delivery, behavioral interventions are also described by level of intensity, with *minimal* defined as one encounter lasting fewer than 20 minutes and *intensive* defined as one encounter lasting 20 minutes or more plus more than one follow-up encounter (Siu, 2015). Minimal and intensive

Fagerstom Tolerance Test for Nicotine Dependence

Write the number of the answer that is most applicable on the line to the left of the question.

_____1. How soon after you awake do you smoke your first cigarette?
   3 points: Within 5 minutes
   2 points: 6 to 30 minutes
   1 point: 31 to 60 minutes
   0 points: After 60 minutes

_____2. Do you find it difficult to refrain from smoking in places where it is forbidden such as the library, theater, or doctor's office?
   1 point: Yes
   0 points: No

_____3. Which cigarette would you hate most to give up?
   1 point: The first one in the morning
   0 points: Any other cigarette

_____4. How many cigarettes a day do you smoke?
   0 points: 10 or less
   1 points: 11 to 20
   2 point: 21 to 30
   3 points: 31 or more

_____5. Do you smoke more frequently during the first hours after waking than during the rest of the day?
   1 point: Yes
   0 points: No

_____6. Do you smoke when you are so ill that you are in bed most of the day?
   1 point: Yes
   0 points: No

Scoring Instructions: Add up your responses to all the items. Total scores should range from 0 to 10, where a score of 6 to 7 suggests a high level of physical dependence to nicotine and a score of 8 to 10 suggests a very high level of physical dependence to nicotine.

TOTAL SCORE:_____

Source: Heatherton, T. F., Kozlowski, L. T., Frecker, R. C., et al. (1991). The Fagerstrom Test for nicotine dependence: A revision of the Fagerstrom Tolerance Questionnaire. _British Journal of Addictions, 86,_ 1119–1127.

The Five A's Model for Treating Tobacco Use and Dependence

Ask every patient about tobacco use and record information in patient's medical record at every visit.
Strongly **_advise_** every tobacco user to quit, using a personalized approach.
Assess the patient's willingness to make an attempt to quit.
Assist the patient who is willing to make an attempt to quit by offering medication and providing or referring for smoking cessation counseling.
Arrange for follow-up contact within the first week after the quit date. For patients unwilling to make a quit attempt, address willingness to quit at next visit.

Source: U.S. Department of Health and Human Services, Public Health Service, Agency for Health Care Policy and Research. (2008). Treating tobacco use and dependence: 2008 update. Rockville, MD: Author.

brief interventions, but even a short discussion of fewer than 3 minutes may have an impact.

When in-person counseling is an option, the DHHS/PHS guideline recommends a minimum of four sessions. There is no guidance about the duration of each session, but data suggest no additional benefit after a total of 90 minutes of counseling time. These in-person sessions may be delivered by different health care providers, including physicians, nurses, and psychologists. In-person counseling may be delivered one-on-one or in a group. These sessions should provide support and help patients to develop a plan to avoid smoking triggers and overcome barriers to quitting.

Telephone counseling is effective in increasing cessation rates as well. The DHHS/PHS guideline recommends at least 3 telephone calls be provided. These calls may be done by counselors and health care providers who have received training to offer counseling via phone.

Finally, self-help materials tailored to an individual's needs are effective in improving chances of a smoking cessation. It is important to note that these materials should go beyond simply describing the health effects of smoking. In addition to printed self-help materials, evidence is emerging about the potential benefits of computer-based programs and mobile phone applications. A 2019 Cochrane review found automated text messaging to be more effective than minimal cessation support, and the combined use of automated text messaging with other smoking cessation interventions was more effective than other smoking cessation interventions alone (Whitaker et al., 2019). The CDC has a free mobile application called quitSTART, which provides tips to help patients manage cravings and provide support if a patient slips and smokes during the quit attempt. All nicotine users, including pregnant women and adolescents, should be encouraged to quit use, and all should be offered behavioral interventions to help them in their quit attempts.

behavioral interventions increase the proportion of adults who successfully quit smoking cigarettes and remained smoke-free for at least 6 months. Longer sessions and more sessions have been linked with higher cessation rates; this is called a _dose–response relationship_. However, even brief interventions lasting fewer than 3 minutes have increased cessation rates in some studies (Siu, 2015). In other words, intensive interventions increase cessation rates to a greater degree than

BOX 52.4 Tobacco Users Unwilling to Quit: The Five R's

RELEVANCE

Encourage patient to discuss why quitting is personally relevant to him or her. Motivational information has the highest impact when it is relevant to a patient's disease status or risk, family or social situation (e.g., having children in the home), health concerns, and other patient factors (e.g., prior quitting experience, personal barriers to cessation).

RISKS

The clinician should ask the patient to identify potential negative consequences of tobacco use. The clinician may suggest and highlight the negative consequence that seems most relevant to the patient. The clinician should also emphasize that smoking low-tar/low-nicotine cigarettes or use of other forms of tobacco (e.g., smokeless tobacco, cigars, and pipes) will not eliminate these risks.

REWARDS

The clinician should ask the patient to identify potential benefits of stopping tobacco use. The clinicians may suggest and

highlight the benefits that seem most relevant to the patient. Examples of rewards include improved health; greater ability to taste food; improved sense of smell; saving money; less smoke-related odors in home, car, and clothing; feeling better physically; and improved appearance (less wrinkling/aging of skin and whiter teeth).

ROADBLOCKS

The clinician should ask the patient to identify barriers or impediments to quitting and provide treatment (e.g., problem-solving counseling, medication) that could address barriers. Typical barriers may include withdrawal symptoms, fear of weight gain, lack of support, depression, and being around other tobacco users.

REPETITION

The motivational intervention should be repeated every time an unmotivated patient is encountered in a clinical setting. Tobacco users who have failed previous quit attempts should be encouraged by telling them that most people make repeated quit attempts before they are successful.

Source: U.S. Department of Health and Human Services, Public Health Service, Agency for Health Care Policy and Research. (2008). Treating tobacco use and dependence: 2008 update. Rockville, MD: Author.

Self-Management

Self-management techniques are commonly used to make patients more aware of their smoking habits and cues. By becoming more familiar with the environment and events that precede smoking a cigarette, patients may be able to interrupt these patterns by avoiding certain situations. If a relapse occurs, the patient should determine what may have triggered the failed attempt and eliminate those factors. Some nondrug methods to enhance smoking cessation and prevent relapse include getting rid of ashtrays, drinking water and breathing deeply between sips, avoiding places with smoke-filled air, making a dental appointment to get teeth cleaned, exercising, calling on friends or family for support and encouragement, eating a balanced diet, chewing gum or a toothpick, and avoiding the routine that causes craving a cigarette, such as drinking coffee every morning with a cigarette (Mallin, 2002). An analysis of self-help programs showed these programs to be relatively ineffective compared to individual, group, or proactive telephone counseling.

Nicotine Fading

Nicotine fading consists of a slow decrease in the intake of nicotine without use of pharmacologic therapy during the

cut down period (compared to the *cut down to quit* method described in the next section). This can be accomplished by decreasing the number of puffs taken or the number of cigarettes smoked per day or by switching to a brand of cigarettes that contains less nicotine. However, the success rate of this technique may be limited because the patient can compensate by inhaling more deeply or for longer periods. Lindson and colleagues (2019) did not find a significant difference between quit rates of study participants who were asked to reduce nicotine intake before quitting compared to participants who were asked to completely stop smoking on a specific date. This method is not discussed in the 2008 or 2015 smoking cessation recommendations; however, based on the findings of Lindson and colleagues (2019), this option may be acceptable for the patient who wishes to use it, as it does not seem to reduce the chances for a successful quit rate.

Cut Down to Quit Method in Combination with Pharmacologic Therapies

This method requires the smoker to reduce the number of cigarettes smoked per day in combination with use of a fast-acting nicotine replacement product or varenicline. Lindson and colleagues (2019) found in their review that cutting down cigarette consumption supplemented by use of a fast-acting nicotine product or varenicline may increase chances of a successful quit attempt compared to the nicotine fading method (i.e., cutting down cigarette consumption without use of supplemental pharmacologic therapy). No studies comparing the cutting down of nicotine consumption in combination with pharmacologic therapy and abrupt cessation prior to use of pharmacologic agents were included in Lindon and colleagues' analysis. This method is not endorsed at this time by any U.S. smoking cessation treatment guideline, and no nicotine replacement product currently has the U.S. FDA (2013) approval for this use. This method may be an option for a person who has failed prior quit attempts when abruptly stopping smoking cessation before using pharmacologic therapy.

Aversion Therapy

Finally, aversion techniques have been used to make smoking less desirable to the patient. The first method, satiation, requires the patient to smoke double or triple the usual amount in a short time. In the second method, rapid smoking, the patient must inhale rapidly every 6 to 8 seconds until the cigarette is finished or the patient is nauseated. The use of these methods is limited because of possible health problems and compliance issues. Aversive smoking procedures (e.g., rapid smoking, puffing) have been shown to be more effective than providing no counseling, but this method is not recommended by the DHHS/PHS or the USPSTF.

Goals of Drug Therapy

All nonpregnant adults attempting to quit should be encouraged to use effective pharmacotherapies for smoking cessation to aid in their quit efforts. Use of pharmacotherapy in pregnant patients requires a shared decision-making process between the patient and her health care providers. Long-term smoking cessation pharmacotherapy should be considered as a strategy to reduce the likelihood of relapse (Fiore et al., 2008; Siu 2015). Smoking cessation requires repeated intervention and multiple quit attempts (Fiore et al., 2008). The most effective treatment of tobacco dependence requires the use of multiple treatment modalities (Fiore et al., 2008; Sui, 2015). Long-term abstinence is the ultimate goal of treatment of smoking cessation. In patients unwilling to quit, initial goals include moving them from precontemplating to contemplating quitting.

DRUG THERAPY

Overview

Bupropion SR (sustained release), varenicline, and nicotine replacement therapy (NRT) are the only FDA-approved drugs currently on the market to help with smoking cessation. Two second-line medications (clonidine and nortriptyline) were identified for smoking cessation in previous guidelines (Fiore et al., 2008). The USPSTF recommendations do not mention these second-line therapies. These agents are not FDA-approved for smoking cessation, and they are not commonly prescribed for this indication.

Nicotine Replacement Therapy

NRT, the most commonly used pharmacotherapy for smoking cessation, aims to control nicotine levels in the bloodstream so that withdrawal does not occur while the patient is adjusting to life without cigarette smoking. The goal of therapy is to maintain the cessation of smoking for a period that allows the patient to develop preventive strategies to avoid relapse.

The primary mechanism of action by which NRT enhances smoking cessation is to obtain plasma levels of nicotine that can relieve or prevent withdrawal symptoms. The pharmacokinetic effects underlie the concept of nicotine replacement as an aid to smoking cessation, providing that steady-state levels of nicotine can prevent a smoker from experiencing intense withdrawal while not providing the reinforcing peaks achieved from smoking (Le Houezec, 2003). **Figure 52.1** shows the pharmacokinetic profiles of currently available NRT products. Smokers can, therefore, achieve abstinence by dealing with the various behavioral aspects of smoking. Once abstinence is achieved, the smoker can taper of the nicotine by gradual reduction (Le Houezec, 2003). While patients are exposed to nicotine when using NRT, they are not being exposed to the carcinogens and other toxins in cigarette smoke. **Table 52.2** provides an overview of selected NRT products currently available in the United States.

The USPSTF expert panel found in research studies that the abstinence rate with NRT was higher than with no drug therapy at 6 months after quit attempt (10% in group with no drug therapy and 17% in patients using any form of NRT) (Siu, 2015). There appears to be no difference in abstinence rates among the different NRT. However, combined use of NRT, compared to use of one product, increases the chance for continued abstinence from smoking after 6 months (Patnode et al., 2015; Siu 2015). Neither guideline endorses the use of any one NRT over another because of similar effectiveness demonstrated with all products. Patient preference will help guide the clinician's treatment decisions. Some clinicians recommend use of a transdermal patch for continuous nicotine delivery and use of gum, lozenges, or some other fast-acting nicotine delivery for acute cravings.

Nicotine Transdermal Patches

Currently, there are two nicotine transdermal systems on the market, and both products are available without a prescription (**Table 52.2**): Nicoderm CQ and Habitrol are available as brand-name products and as various generic nicotine transdermal patch products.

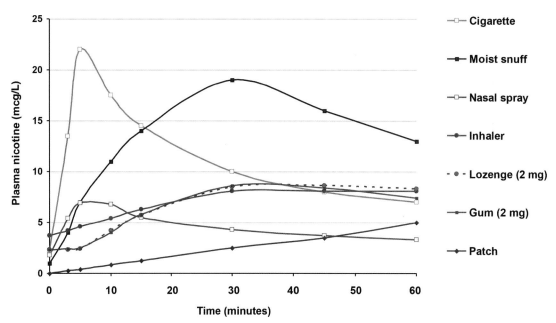

FIGURE 52–1 Pharmacokinetics of nicotine replacement products. (Reprinted with permission from *Rx for Change: Clinician-Assisted Tobacco Cessation* program. Copyright © 1999–2020 The Regents of the University of California. All rights reserved.)

Nicoderm CQ varies slightly from other available products in its weaning regimen. The recommended dosing regimen for Nicoderm CQ patches for patients who smoke more than 10 cigarettes daily is 21 mg for 6 weeks, 14 mg for 2 weeks, and 7 mg for 2 weeks. The recommended dosing regimens for Habitrol, for other generic patch products, and for patients who smoke more than 10 cigarettes daily are 21 mg for 4 weeks, 14 mg for 2 weeks, and 7 mg for 2 weeks. For all available products, it is recommended that patients who smoke 10 cigarettes or less per day start at a 14-mg patch for 6 weeks and then decrease to a 7-mg patch for 2 weeks. Patients may continue using the patch for longer periods of time, after discussing with a clinician, if they feel they may relapse upon stopping.

All available transdermal products may be worn for 16 to 24 hours and should be applied at the same time each day. Patients who experience nightmares or other sleep disturbances when wearing the patch for 24 hours may be counseled to wear it for 16 hours and to remove the patch prior to falling asleep. Persistence of sleep disturbances despite removing patch before sleeping may signal the presence of nicotine withdrawal. A new patch should then be applied on waking, and only one patch should be applied at a time.

The most common side effects of the transdermal patches include a mild skin reaction with pruritus, burning, and erythema. The skin reactions are usually mild and self-limiting, resolving within 24 hours of removing the patch. Rotating application sites, changing brands, and applying nonprescription strength hydrocortisone cream may reduce the incidence and severity of these events. Transdermal patches should not be used on patients with systemic eczema, atopic dermatitis, or psoriasis because these patients are more likely to develop skin reactions.

The initial patch should be applied immediately on awakening on the patient's targeted quit date. The application site should be clean and dry before applying the patch. The patient should press the patch onto a hairless portion of the upper outer arms or upper chest and hold it for approximately 10 seconds. To decrease irritation that may occur with the patches, the patient should rotate application sites with each new patch. It is common to experience mild tingling, itching, or burning sensations for the first minute after application. If these symptoms persist for more than 4 days, however, the prescriber should be notified and an alternative method should be used.

If the patch gets wet or if it falls off, a new patch should be applied to a different site and then removed at the original time the first patch would have been removed. Proper disposal of the patch is important. After the patch is removed, it should be placed in the wrapper from the newly applied patch and discarded responsibly—out of the reach of children and pets.

It is ideal, but unnecessary, that the patient stops smoking completely before initiating treatment. The FDA has found that overlapping use of NRT with an occasional cigarette poses no significant health risks; this may be communicated to patients who "slip" with use of a cigarette while using NRT (FDA, 2013). It is important to remind patients that nicotine in the skin will continue to enter the bloodstream for several hours after the patch is removed.

Nicotine Gum

Nicotine polacrilex gum (Nicorette) was the first NRT to be approved and is available without a prescription. The patient

TABLE 52.2

Overview of Selected Agents Used in Smoking Cessation

Generic (Trade) Name and Dosage	Selected Adverse Events	Contraindications	Special Considerations
Nicotine Products			
Nicotine patch (Habitrol and various generic products) ≥10 cigarettes/d: 21 mg for 4 wk, then 14 mg for 2 wk, then 7 mg for 2 wk <10 cigarettes/d: 14 mg for 6 wk, then 7 mg for 2 wk	Cutaneous irritation, GI disturbances, dizziness, headaches	None noted	Available without a prescription People under 18 years of age, pregnant and breast-feeding women should use under guidance of a health care provider. Patch worn for 16–24 h/d
Nicotine patch (Nicoderm CQ) ≥10 cigarettes/d: 21 mg for 6 wk, then 14 mg for 2 wk, then 7 mg for 2 wk <10 cigarettes/d: 14 mg for 6 wk, then 7 mg for 2 wk	Same as nicotine patch	Same as nicotine patch	Same as nicotine patch
Nicotine polacrilex gum (Nicorette) Start: 2 mg q1–2 h for 6 wk 2 mg q2–4 h for 2 wk 2 mg q4–8 h for 2 wk Range: 1–24 pieces per day	Sore throat, hiccups, undesirable taste	None	Available without a prescription People under 18 years of age, pregnant and breast-feeding women should use under guidance of a health care provider. Gum should be chewed until patient feels a tingling sensation and then "parked" between cheek and gum. Repeat chewing every 15–30 min. Consider an alternative if patient wears dentures or has temporomandibular joint disease When given as monotherapy, patient should chew at least nine pieces each day during the first 6 wk. Patient should take no more than 24 pieces in a 24-hour period.
Nicotine nasal spray (Nicotrol NS) Start: 1–2 sprays in each nasal hourly (one spray = 0.5 mg) Range: 1–40 sprays per day	Nasal irritation, sore throat, dizziness, headache	Hypersensitivity to preservatives contained in spray	Prescription required for this product No more than five sprays per hour When given as monotherapy, patient should use at least eight doses each day. Patients with rhinitis may have a reduced peak in nicotine plasma concentrations and a delayed time in achieving peak plasma nicotine concentrations. Use of nasal decongestants may prolong the time to achieve peak plasma nicotine concentrations.
Nicotine inhaler (Nicotrol inhaler) Start: six cartridges per day; self-titrated to avoid withdrawal Range: 6–16 cartridges per day	Throat irritation, dizziness, headache, cough, dependence	Hypersensitivity to menthol	Prescription required for this product A minimum of six cartridges must be used for 3–6 wk. Do not use for >6 mo. Product may cause airway irritation—use with caution in people with airway disease.
Nicotine lozenge (Commit) First cigarette within 30 min of waking: 4 mg First cigarette >30 min after waking: 2 mg One lozenge q1–2h for first 6 wk, then one q2–4h for 2 wk, and one lozenge q4–8h for 2 wk	Hiccups, dyspepsia, dry mouth, and irritation/soreness of the mouth	None	Available without a prescription People under 18 years of age, pregnant and breast-feeding women should use under guidance of a health care provider. Lozenge should be placed in mouth and allowed to dissolve for about 20–30 min. Do not swallow or chew the lozenge. Occasionally, move the lozenge from one side of the mouth to other until completely dissolved. Patient should not use more than five lozenges in 6 hours and no more than 20 per day. When given as monotherapy, patient should chew at least nine pieces each day during the first 6 wk.

(Continued)

TABLE 52.2

Overview of Selected Agents Used in Smoking Cessation (*Continued*)

Generic (Trade) Name and Dosage	Selected Adverse Events	Contraindications	Special Considerations
Non-nicotine Products			
Bupropion (Zyban) Start: 150 mg PO once daily for 3 d, then increase to 150 mg PO BID for 7–12 wk Range: 150–300 mg/d	Headache, dry mouth, insomnia	History of seizures, eating disorders Do not use in people undergoing abrupt discontinuation of alcohol, benzodiazepine, barbiturate, or antiepileptic medication (use in this setting may further increase seizure risk).	Patient must set a target quit date the second week of therapy. May be a good agent for initial therapy in smokers with concomitant depression
Varenicline (Chantix) Start: 0.5 mg PO once daily for 3 d, then increase to 0.5 mg PO BID for 4 d, then increase to 1 mg PO BID for 12–24 wk	Neuropsychiatric disturbances such as mood changes, anxiety, suicidal ideation	History of anaphylaxis or skin reactions to varenicline	Do not start in patients with preexisting psychiatric illness. Patient should set quit date for eighth day of therapy.

GI, gastrointestinal.

should chew the gum slowly until he or she senses a peppery, citrus, or minty taste or tingling. Then, the gum should be "parked" between the cheek and the gingiva to increase absorption. This cycle should be repeated with the same piece of gum approximately every minute for 15 to 30 minutes. The gum is more effective if used on a fixed schedule as opposed to an "as-needed" basis (APA, 1996). This may be explained in part by the fact that one piece of gum stays in the bloodstream for 2 to 3 hours. Therefore, a fixed schedule will help to ensure consistent nicotine levels in the blood, and the patient should be advised to chew one piece of gum every 1 to 2 hours (Hukkanen et al., 2005). Chewing at least nine pieces a day during the first 6 weeks of attempting to quit has been shown to increase the patient's chance of success. Most patients should use a 2-mg dose, but a 4-mg dose is also available and may be used as the initial dose in the following:

- Patients with a history of severe withdrawal symptoms
- Patients who smoke their first cigarette within 30 minutes of awakening
- Patients for whom the 2-mg gum failed
- Patients who request it

The TTFC method is used to determine the initial gum strength to be used. Those who smoke their first cigarette within 30 minutes of awakening are advised to use 4-mg strength. It is hypothesized that the TTFC is a better method than number of cigarettes smoked per day as a way of identifying patients who are highly nicotine dependent. This is because some patients may not smoke often each day but are physiologically dependent on nicotine since they develop withdrawal symptoms during prolonged periods without smoking (i.e., upon awakening after no cigarette use while sleeping) (Shiffman et al., 2002).

The initial duration of therapy is 6 weeks regardless of what strength is used. After the first 6 weeks, the patient should be slowly weaned off the gum to avoid withdrawal symptoms. The manufacturer of Nicorette gum recommends that the patient chew a piece of gum every 1 to 2 hours during the first 6 weeks of therapy, then decrease to one piece of gum every 2 to 4 hours during weeks 7 and 8, and then one piece of gum every 4 to 8 hours during weeks 8 to 12. The maximum dose is 24 pieces per day (see **Table 52.2**). Patients may continue using nicotine gum for longer periods of time, after discussing with a clinician, if they feel they may relapse upon stopping.

It is ideal, but unnecessary, that the patient stops smoking completely before initiating treatment. The FDA has found that overlapping use of NRT with an occasional cigarette poses no significant health risks; this may be communicated to patients who "slip" with use of a cigarette while using NRT (FDA, 2013). In addition, food and drink should not be taken for at least 15 minutes before and after chewing the gum because certain foods (e.g., coffee, tea, carbonated beverages) cause the saliva to become more acidic, consequently decreasing the absorption of the gum. Patients should dispose of the gum and wrapper properly to avoid ingestion by small children and pets.

Common adverse effects of nicotine gum use include jaw muscle aches and fatigue, oral sores, hiccups, belching, throat irritation, and nausea. Some of these events (i.e., hiccups, throat irritation, nausea) result from rapid chewing, leading to excessive nicotine release and absorption. Patient education on the proper use of the gum decreases the incidence of these events. Gum may stick to dentures. If this is a concern, the clinician may suggest use of nicotine lozenge, which is also available without a prescription.

Nicotine Lozenge

The newest formulation of NRT is the nicotine lozenge (formerly Commit, now Nicorette), which was approved by the FDA in October 2002 and is available without a prescription. The nicotine lozenge is available in 2-mg and 4-mg strengths. One study found that treatment with the nicotine lozenge results in significantly greater 28-day abstinence at 6 weeks for the 2-mg (46.0% vs. 29.7%; $p < 0.001$) and the 4-mg lozenges compared with a placebo (48.7% vs. 20.8%; $p < 0.001$) (Shiffman et al., 2002). Similar treatments were maintained for a full year. Use of more lozenges also resulted in reducing cravings and withdrawal (Shiffman et al., 2002).

Similar to nicotine gum, nicotine lozenge helps control cravings by delivering craving-fighting medicine quickly. The lozenge strength, like nicotine gum, depends on the smoker's TTFC. Those who smoke their first cigarette within 30 minutes of waking are directed to use the 4-mg strength, whereas those who smoke their first cigarette after 30 minutes of waking are directed to use the 2-mg strength (Shiffman et al., 2002). It is recommended that during the first 6 weeks, an individual should take one lozenge every 1 to 2 hours and should use at least nine lozenges per day during this time when using as monotherapy. This dosage is then reduced to one lozenge every 2 to 4 hours in weeks 7 to 9 and every 4 to 8 hours in weeks 10 to 12. The recommended length of treatment of therapy for the nicotine lozenge is 12 weeks; however, a patient may discuss with his or her clinician to extend use of the product if he or she fears relapse upon discontinuation after 12 weeks. Because it delivers 25% more nicotine per dose, the lozenge may be an alternative for patients who report the presence of withdrawal symptoms with the gum (Shiffman et al., 2002).

The patient should be advised not to eat or drink for 15 minutes before using the nicotine lozenge. The lozenge should be placed in the mouth and sucked on for 20 to 30 minutes to allow the lozenge to slowly dissolve. The lozenge should not be swallowed or chewed. The patient will feel a warm or tingly sensation. Occasionally, the lozenge should be moved from one side of the mouth to the other until it is completely dissolved. Only one lozenge should be used at a time, and patients should not use more than five lozenges in 6 hours or more than 20 per day. The lozenge may be a good option for patients who are concerned about a gum product sticking to dentures. Lozenges, similar to nicotine gum, are available for purchase without a prescription. Other fast-acting replacement therapies such as nicotine nasal spray and nicotine inhaler require a prescription.

The most common side effects of the nicotine lozenge are hiccups, dyspepsia, dry mouth, nausea, and irritation/soreness in the mouth and throat (Shiffman et al., 2002). These effects mainly occurred in patients who chewed or swallowed the lozenge. Patient education on how to properly administer the lozenge can help decrease these incidences. Finally, because the lozenge looks similar to hard candy, it should be stored and disposed properly to avoid access to children.

Nicotine Nasal Spray

The nicotine nasal spray is a prescription product and is marketed under the brand name Nicotrol NS. Compared to other NRT products, nicotine nasal spray has the fastest rate of absorption and thus is the most similar to the onset of the effect that occurs with cigarette smoking (Hukkanen et al., 2005). This formulation may have a role for patients who fail to quit smoking by using the gum or patch or who are highly dependent smokers who require nicotine replacement at a quicker rate than the gum and patch can provide.

Each spray contains 0.5 mg of nicotine, and the minimum dose is 1 mg—delivered as one 0.5-mg spray in each nostril. The recommended initial dosage of the nasal spray is 1 mg (i.e., one spray in each nostril) or 2 mg (two sprays in each nostril) per hour. The dosage may be increased as needed to prevent withdrawal symptoms. The maximum dose is five doses (i.e., 5 mg) per hour or 40 sprays per day. A minimum of eight doses should be used each day to increase the chance of success. After the initial 6 to 8 weeks of treatment, the dosage should be slowly tapered over the next 4 to 6 weeks. No one titration schedule has proven superior; some health care providers may recommend that the patient taper by inhaling half of the dose while maintaining the same dosing frequency used during the initial 8 weeks of therapy or extending the dosing interval (i.e., skipping doses) while maintaining the same dose. Using the nasal spray for longer than 6 months is not recommended because there is no greater efficacy, and the safety of use beyond 6 months has not been well studied.

Before administering the first dose, the patient must prime the pump. This is accomplished by pumping the medication into a tissue six to eight times until a fine spray appears. If the spray is not used for 24 hours or more, the pump must be primed again. Once the pump is ready for use, the patient must follow the manufacturer's directions. The difference between the nicotine nasal spray and other nasal sprays is that the patient must remember not to sniff or inhale while administering Nicotrol NS. If the spray comes in contact with the mouth, eyes, or skin, the patient should rinse the area immediately with cold water to prevent toxicity. The patient must be aware that it takes approximately 1 week to adjust to the side effects.

Common side effects of the nicotine nasal spray include dependence, nose and throat irritation, rhinitis, sneezing, coughing, and watery eyes. Other side effects were transient changes in sense of taste or smell, nasal congestion, and transient epistaxis. These events can occur in more than 75% of patients. Nicotine spray has a higher abuse potential compared to other NRT because of its short onset of action. Nearly a third of spray users in clinical trials reported feelings of dependency. The clinician should monitor for this side effect.

Nicotine Inhaler

The nicotine inhaler is available in the United States as a prescription drug for smoking cessation. The inhaler is thought to improve smoking cessation through two mechanisms: when it is used, it mimics the hand-to-mouth ritual that occurs when smoking a cigarette, and it produces a sensation of inhaled smoke on the back of the throat. However, because of the limited evidence, the inhaler is often reserved for patients who have failed initial treatment with other products (see **Table 52.2**).

The inhaler consists of a mouthpiece and a cartridge. These two separate pieces are pressed together to break the seal on the cartridge. Once the seal is broken, the nicotine-filled air is inhaled into the mouth as a cigarette would be inhaled. The best results have been found when the patient takes shallow, frequent puffs over 20 minutes.

The recommended dose is 6 to 16 cartridges per day. A minimum of six cartridges must be used during the first 3 to 6 weeks of therapy, and therapy should be continued for at least 3 months. After 3 months, the dose should be tapered over the next 6 to 12 weeks. No standard tapering schedule exists; patient and health care provider may devise a patient-specific tapering schedule. Use of the Nicotrol inhaler should not exceed 6 months. Like the nasal spray, the inhaler must be used regularly for 1 week before the patient adjusts to the side effects. Finally, because the cartridges contain high concentrations of nicotine, they should be stored and disposed of in a place that cannot be accessed by children and pets.

The nicotine inhaler is associated with dyspepsia, throat or mouth irritation, oral burning, rhinitis, and cough after inhalation. Patients should adjust to side effects after the first week of continued inhaler use.

NON-NICOTINE THERAPIES

Bupropion

Bupropion is the first non-nicotine product approved for smoking cessation. The drug has been commonly used as an antidepressant under the brand name Wellbutrin SR. It is available by prescription as an aid to smoking cessation under the brand name Zyban. The exact mechanism of action is unknown; however, it is believed to be related to dopaminergic or noradrenergic properties. Patnode and colleagues' review of the literature found 6-month abstinence rates of 19.7% in bupropion groups compared to 11.5% in placebo groups.

The initial dose of bupropion SR is 150 mg/d for 3 days to decrease the incidence of insomnia. After 3 days, the dose can be increased to 150 mg twice daily for 7 to 12 weeks. Dosages higher than 300 mg/d are not recommended because of the increased risk of seizures. Unlike NRT, bupropion SR therapy should be initiated while the patient is still smoking because the drug takes approximately 1 week to reach steady-state plasma concentrations. The patient should set a target quit date during week 2 of therapy. If the patient has not made significant improvements by week 7 of treatment, the attempt is unlikely to be successful and the medication should be discontinued. Additionally, a patient who successfully quits after 7 to 12 weeks of treatment should be considered for continuation of bupropion SR therapy. Tapering the dose is not required when stopping the medication.

The most common side effects of bupropion SR are dry mouth and insomnia. Insomnia may be reduced by avoiding bedtime administration, but the patient must be counseled to allow 8 hours between the two daily doses. Other adverse events that can occur include nervousness or difficulty concentrating, rash, and constipation. Seizures have also occurred but are very rare at doses used for smoking cessation (ScieGen Pharmaceuticals, 2019).

It is important that patients taking bupropion SR participate in behavioral therapy programs that include counseling both during and after therapy. Patients need to be informed not to use Wellbutrin, Wellbutrin SR, or Wellbutrin XL while taking Zyban because these medications all contain bupropion. In addition, monoamine oxidase inhibitors should not be used during or within 14 days of bupropion SR treatment. The interaction between these agents increases bupropion toxicity (i.e., seizures, psychotic changes). Zyban SR should not be chewed or crushed because it will damage the SR formulation, which may increase the risk of overdose and adverse events.

Varenicline

Varenicline is the newest approved agent on the market to aid in smoking cessation. It is available in the United States with a prescription under the brand name Chantix. It aids in smoking cessation by binding to a subunit of the nicotinic acetylcholine receptor. When attached to this subunit, varenicline blocks nicotine's binding to the same subunit and blocks nicotine's effects in the brain (i.e., reward, stimulant, depressant affects). Varenicline is also a partial agonist of the nicotine acetylcholine receptor, so it alleviates withdrawal symptoms produced with smoking cessation. In short, varenicline provides patients attempting to quit some of the rewarding effects felt with smoking while blocking the reinforcement effects of continued nicotine use. Patnode and colleagues' review found an estimated abstinence rates of 28% and 12% in patients taking varenicline and placebo, respectively.

To reduce the risk of nausea, varenicline should be titrated over a 1-week period to its effective dose of 1 mg twice daily. The starting dose is 0.5 mg once daily for days 1 to 3, which is then increased to 0.5 mg twice daily for days 4 to 7 and finally increased to the target dose of 1 mg twice daily on day 8. Patients who develop intolerable nausea when taking 1 mg twice daily may have the dose reduced to 1 mg once daily, but a dose titration to 1 mg twice daily should be attempted at a later time. For people with severe renal impairment (creatinine clearance less than 30 mL/min), the starting dose is 0.5 mg once daily, which may be titrated to a target dose of 0.5 mg twice daily. Varenicline should be started 1 week before the patient's set quit date. As with other smoking cessation treatments, varenicline should be given along with behavioral counseling.

The most commonly reported adverse events are nausea, constipation, and abnormal dreams. Other side effects are headaches, difficulty concentrating, somnolence, somnambulism (i.e., performing tasks while sleeping), and visual disturbances. There have been several reports of accidents and near-miss accidents while driving or operating heavy machinery in people taking varenicline, which may have been a result of somnolence and visual disturbances. Patients should be counseled not to drive or operate heavy machinery until they know how varenicline will affect them.

Varenicline use has been reported to cause neuropsychiatric symptoms (e.g., mood changes, psychosis, hallucinations, suicidal ideation, suicide attempts, and completed suicides). Because of this effect, varenicline should be prescribed with careful observation and monitoring to patients with preexisting psychiatric conditions, and patients who experience any changes in mood or behavior or develop suicidal ideation should immediately stop varenicline and contact their health care provider immediately (Pfizer Pharmaceuticals, 2019).

Uses of Electronic Nicotine Delivery Systems to Aid in Smoking Cessation

No ENDS (e-cigarettes) manufacturer has applied for or has received FDA approval for smoking cessation to date. However, approximately two-thirds of physicians reported that they believed e-cigarettes were helpful for smoking cessation; 35% recommended ENDS use to their patients (Siu 2015). Patients also use them to aid in their smoking cessation efforts. In a recent survey of e-cigarette users, 56% reported using them to help them to quit smoking cigarettes; 26% of those surveyed reported using them to smoke in places where cigarette smoking was banned. Patnode and colleagues reviewed two studies of e-cigarettes for smoking cessation. One study found no statistical difference in 6-month smoking cessation rates in patients randomized to use an e-cigarette (7.3%), nicotine patch (5.8%), and placebo e-cigarettes (4.1%). In the second study, investigators observed that more patients randomized to an ENDS product had stopped smoking one year after trial enrollment (11% vs. 4%, $p = 0.04$). Because e-cigarettes are not regulated by the FDA, ingredients in various products may be unknown. According to the American Cancer Society (2020), some e-cigarettes may contain formaldehyde and other compounds linked to adverse health effects. Use of e-cigarettes should not be recommended to aid in smoking cessation efforts because of unconfirmed effectiveness and potential safety concerns (Siu 2015). FDA-regulated NRT may be considered for the patient who finds appealing the hand-to-mouth ritual associated with the use of e-cigarettes.

Comparison of Pharmacotherapy Agents

• NRT compared to bupropion: There were no statistically significant differences in smoking cessation rates between these single-agent NRT and bupropion based on the results

of two reviews of multiple head-to-head trials (Patnode et al., 2015). A pooled analysis of two studies found that patients taking nicotine patch and nicotine lozenges had a slightly higher abstinence rate compared to bupropion alone.
• NRT compared to varenicline: No differences in smoking cessation rates were observed in two head-to-head trials (Patnode et al., 2015).
• Bupropion compared to varenicline: Four head-to-head studies showed higher quit rates with varenicline compared with bupropion therapy; however, some of these differences in quit rates were not statistically different.

Combination Drug Therapy

Although most of the drugs included in this chapter have only been approved as single pharmacologic agents, combined treatment may be appropriate for smokers who are unable to quit with monotherapy.

Combined Nicotine Replacement Therapy Products

Nicotine patch is often combined with short-acting nicotine delivery products such as gum or lozenges. The patch gives a consistent level of nicotine in the body, and the short-acting product provides additional relief for cravings. Three combinations of nicotine replacement have shown to be safe and effective in smoking cessation and are recommended by the DHHS/PHS expert panel: long-term (greater than 14 weeks) nicotine patch + other NRT (gum or spray) and nicotine patch + nicotine inhaler (Fiore et al., 2008). A 2012 review of many NRT studies found that study participants taking a combination of NRT products had, on average, a 20.6% abstinence rate compared to 15.6% in participants taking only one NRT product (Siu, 2015). In addition, a pooled analysis of two studies showed nicotine patch and nicotine lozenge combination therapy to yield slightly higher quit rates than bupropion alone (Patnode et al., 2015).

Combined Nicotine Replacement Therapy and Bupropion

In a pooled analysis of 12 studies, Patnode and colleagues did not find a benefit with combined use of NRT and bupropion when compared to NRT alone. Conversely, in a pooled analysis of four studies, Patnode and colleagues found a small but significant favorable effect of NRT and bupropion combination, compared to bupropion alone.

Nicotine Replacement Therapy and Varenicline

Koegelenberg and colleagues published study results showing the combination of varenicline and nicotine transdermal patch to have higher abstinence rates at 12 weeks compared to varenicline monotherapy (Koegelenberg et al., 2014). This placebo-controlled study included 446 participants and was conducted in South Africa. The continuous abstinence rates at 12 weeks were 55.4% versus 40.9% (OR 1.85; 95% CI: 1.19–2.89; $p = 0.007$) in the combination and varenicline monotherapy groups, respectively. Continuous cessation rates were also higher in the combination group at 6 months: 49% versus 32.6% (OR 1.98; 95% CI: 1.25–3.14; p = 0.004). There were more reports of nausea, sleep disturbances, depression, and skin reactions in the combination group; however, skin reactions were the only adverse effect that was statistically higher than the monotherapy group (14.9% vs. 7.8%; p = 0.03). While these results are promising, more studies are needed, and more information about the adverse effect profile with this combination are needed before being routinely prescribed.

Bupropion and Varenicline Combination

Ebbert and colleagues observed statistically significant differences in long-term smoking cessation (defined as no smoking from 2 weeks after quit date) at 12 and 26 weeks for patients taking the combination of the two medications compared to those participants taking varenicline monotherapy (Ebbert et al., 2014). More

patients in the combination group had maintained smoking cessation at 52 weeks, but the difference was not statistically significant. The potential benefit of higher quit rates was offset by increased reports of anxiety and depressive symptoms with combination therapy. Rose and Bhem studied the benefit of combined use of varenicline and bupropion in participants who did not respond to nicotine patch therapy. They found no difference in abstinence rates between varenicline + bupropion and varenicline only at 8 to 11 weeks. At this time, combination therapy with bupropion and varenicline should not be recommended.

Selecting the Most Appropriate Agent

Which therapeutic agent is most effective depends on the patient and the patient's smoking history, among other factors. For a review of the recommended treatments and the clinical guidelines for prescribing pharmacotherapy for smoking cessation, see **Tables 52.3** and **52.4** and **Figure 52.2**.

TABLE 52.3

Summary of Treatment Recommendations for Smoking Cessation in Nonpregnant Adults, Pregnant Adults, and Nonpregnant Adolescents

Intervention	Nonpregnant Adults	Pregnant Adults	Nonpregnant Adolescents*
Behavioral therapy	Recommended by USPSTF	Recommended by USPSTF Recommended by ACOG	Recommended by AAP
Nicotine replacement therapy	Recommended by USPSTF	Inadequate evidences to recommend, according to USPSTF ACOG recommends use of NRT only after a detailed discussion with the patient about risks and benefits and the need for medical supervision	Recommended by AAP
Bupropion	Recommended by USPSTF	Inadequate evidence to recommend according to USPSTF May be used after discussing the risks and benefits, according to ACOG	No recommendation provided by USPSTF or AAP
Varenicline	Recommended by USPSTF	Inadequate evidence to recommend according to USPSTF May be used after discussing the risks and benefits, according to ACOG	No recommendation provided by USPSTF or AAP
Combination of FDA-approved therapies^	Recommended Consider using combinations with favorable effect compared to monotherapy	Inadequate evidence to recommend, according to USPSTF	No recommendation provided by USPSTF or AAP
ENDS	Inadequate evidence to recommend, according to USPSTF	Inadequate evidence to recommend according to USPSTF According to ACOG, ENDS appear to affect fetal lung development. No recommendation provided by ACOG. Ill-advised due to limited evidence of effectiveness in this population.	No recommendation provided by USPSTF or AAP Ill-advised due to limited evidence of effectiveness Unclear role of ENDS, as many adolescents may use ENDS as primary means of nicotine delivery

*Source document does not distinguish between pregnant and nonpregnant adolescents.

^ Does *not* include use of ENDS.

AAP, American Academy of Pediatrics; ACOG, American College of Obstetrics and Gynecology; ENDS, electronic nicotine delivery systems; FDA, Food and Drug Administration; USPSTF, U.S. Preventive Services Task Force.

Sources: American College of Obstetrics and Gynecologists. (2017). Tobacco and nicotine cessation during pregnancy. Committee Opinion No. 807. *Obstetrics and Gynecology, 135*(5), e221–e229; American Academy of Pediatrics. (2020, May 14). Counseling about smoking cessation. https://www.aap.org/en-us/advocacy-and-policy/aap-health-initiatives/Richmond-Center/Pages/Counseling-About-Smoking-Cessation.aspx; Siu, A. L. (2015). Behavioral and pharmacotherapy interventions for tobacco smoking cessation in adults, including pregnant women: U.S. Preventive Services Task Force recommendation statement. *Annals of Internal Medicine, 163*, 622–634.

TABLE 52.4

Clinical Guidelines for Prescribing Pharmacotherapy for Smoking Cessation

Who should receive pharmacotherapy for smoking cessation?	All nonpregnant, adult smokers and nonpregnant adolescent smokers trying to quit. Special consideration should be given before using pharmacotherapy with selected populations: those with medical contraindications, those smoking fewer than 10 cigarettes/d, breast-feeding women May be considered in pregnant adults based on shared decision-making between prescriber and patient.
What intervention should pregnant women receive?	Pregnant women should always be offered behavioral interventions. Pregnant women may be offered NRT, bupropion, or varenecline after discussing risks and benefits with their obstetrician or obstetrics care provider.
What interventions should an adolescent receive?	The USPSTF recommendations do not discuss smoking cessation tools in adolescents. The American Academy of Pediatrics recommend nicotine replacement therapy. Use of all nicotine replacement therapy products in people under 18 years of age requires a prescription.
What first-line pharmacotherapies are recommended?	All seven of the FDA-approved pharmacotherapies for smoking cessation are recommended, including bupropion SR, nicotine gum, nicotine inhaler, nicotine lozenge, nicotine nasal spray, nicotine patch, and varenicline. The clinician should consider the first-line medication regimens that have been shown to be more effective than the nicotine patch alone—varenicline 2 mg/d or the combination of nicotine patch and as-needed use of nicotine gum or nicotine nasal spray.
What factors should a clinician consider when choosing among the seven first-line pharmacotherapies?	Because of the lack of sufficient data to rank-order these seven medications, choice of a specific pharmacotherapy, factors such as clinician familiarity with the medications, contraindications for selected patients, patient preference, previous patient experience with a specific pharmacotherapy (positive or negative), and patient characteristics (e.g., history of depression, concerns about weight gain) should guide decisions.
Are pharmacotherapeutic treatments appropriate for lighter smokers (e.g., 10–15 cigarettes/d)?	If pharmacotherapy is used with lighter smokers, clinicians should consider reducing the dose of first-line NRT pharmacotherapies. No adjustments are necessary when using bupropion SR or varenicline.
Which pharmacotherapies should be considered with patients particularly concerned about weight gain?	Bupropion SR and nicotine replacement therapies, in particular nicotine gum and nicotine lozenge, have been shown to delay, but not prevent, weight gain.
Are there pharmacotherapies that should be especially considered in patients with a history of depression?	Bupropion SR may be considered given its dual indication for smoking cessation and depression. NRT also provides some help, but varenicline should be used with caution in this population because of its association with neuropsychiatric adverse effects.
Should nicotine replacement therapies be avoided in patients with a history of cardiovascular disease?	No. The nicotine patch in particular is safe and has been shown not to cause adverse cardiovascular effects.
May tobacco dependence pharmacotherapies be used long term (e.g., 6 mo or more)?	Yes. This approach may be helpful with smokers who report persistent withdrawal symptoms during the course of pharmacotherapy, who have relapsed in the past after stopping therapy, or who desire long-term therapy. A minority of individuals who successfully quit smoking use ad libitum NRT (gum, nasal spray, inhaler) long term. The use of these medications long term does not present a known health risk.
May pharmacotherapies ever be combined?	Yes. There is evidence that combining the nicotine patch with either nicotine gum or nicotine nasal spray, nicotine patch with nicotine inhaler, and nicotine patch with bupropion increases long-term abstinence rates over a placebo. The use of nicotine patch with either nicotine gum or nicotine nasal spray increases long-term abstinence over the use of a single nicotine replacement product.

FDA, Food and Drug Administration; NRT, nicotine replacement therapy; SR, sustained release; USPSTF, U.S. Preventive Services Task Force.

Source: U.S. Preventive Service Task Force. (2015). Behavioral and pharmacotherapy interventions for tobacco smoking cessation in adults, including pregnant women: U.S. Preventive Services Task Force recommendation statement. Rockville, MD: Author. U.S. Department of Health and Human Services, Public Health Service, Agency for Health Care Policy and Research. (2008). Treating tobacco use and dependence: 2008 update. Rockville, MD: American College of Obstetrics and Gynecologists. (2017). Tobacco and nicotine cessation during pregnancy. Committee Opinion No. 807. *Obstetrics and Gynecology*, 135(5), e221 – e229.

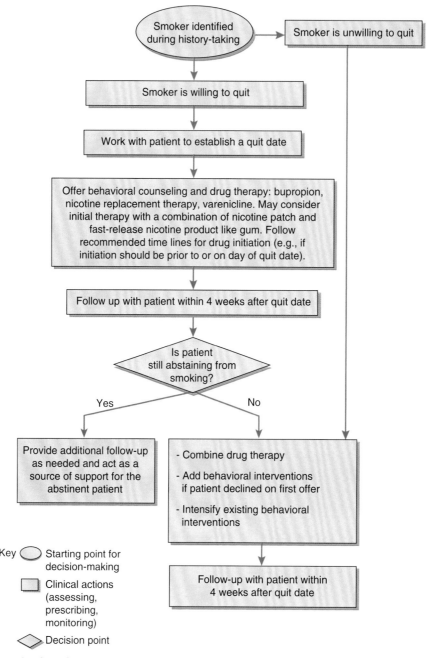

FIGURE 52–2 Treatment algorithm for smoking cessation.

SPECIAL POPULATION CONSIDERATIONS

Pregnant Women

The USPSTF does not recommend use of pharmacotherapy because of limited study data to determine the risks and benefits. Data are limited because many studies of NRT have been stopped early because of failure to show effectiveness or adverse pregnancy effects (American College of Obstetricians and Gynecologists [ACOG], 2017). The ACOG, however, recommends behavioral interventions and consideration of the use of FDA-approved therapies, such as NRT, varenicline,

or bupropion (ACOG, 2017). If the clinician is considering use of medication therapy for a pregnant smoker, the clinician must provide in-depth education about side effect profiles, including any potential risk to fetus, of medications. The nicotine gum and lozenge are classified as pregnancy category C (risk cannot be excluded: animal studies have shown an adverse effect on the fetus, but there are no adequate, well-controlled studies in pregnant women), and the patches, nasal spray, and inhaler are classified as category D (positive evidence of risk: studies in humans or postmarketing have demonstrated a risk to the fetus). Bupropion and varenicline also are classified as category C. A systematic review of 18 studies of bupropion and varenicline use in pregnancy did not find an increased risk of fetal anomalies, low birth weight, or preterm birth.

Breast-Feeding Women

Nicotine is distributed into milk, but use of NRT is expected to produce lower nicotine levels in breast milk than smoking because NRT yields lower nicotine blood levels (AHFS, 2020). Safety of NRT in breast-fed infants has not been evaluated. Use of NRT should be considered only if the benefit to the mother outweighs possible harm to the breast-fed infant.

Varenicline has not been evaluated in nursing women, so it is unknown if the product is excreted in breast milk; however, it has been shown to be excreted in milk of lactating animals. For these reasons, the manufacturer recommends to avoid varenicline use in breast-feeding women, unless the benefit to the mother outweighs possible harm to the breast-fed infant. ACOG also recommends use of a different agent in breast-feeding women because of lack of published data regarding varenicline use in breast-feeding women. Daily doses of bupropion up to 300 mg are associated with low levels of drug in breastmilk that are unlikely to cause adverse effects in infants (ACOG, 2017).

Cardiovascular Disease

NRT should be used with caution in those patients with cardiovascular disease because it can cause tachydysrhythmia and worsen angina. However, the risks are small compared with the cardiovascular effects of smoking. Nicotine concentrations are higher and delivered more rapidly from cigarettes compared with NRT products.

Adolescents

As previously described in this chapter, many adult nicotine users start during adolescence. Health care providers must ask adolescents about nicotine use at every encounter. The USPSTF does not offer guidance for smoking cessation in adolescents. The American Academy of Pediatrics (2020) recommends use of NRT if pharmacotherapy is needed. It does not offer recommendations for use of bupropion or varenicline. Behavioral therapy is an important component and should be provided as well. ENDS should not be used due to potential harms of impurities in the liquid and a lack of data demonstrating effectiveness. Moreover, it is important to note that an adolescent may be using ENDS for nicotine delivery—another reason why ENDS use for smoking cessation may be less favorable in this population.

Monitoring Patient Response

Smoking status must be assessed and monitored in all patients. As mentioned, patients starting NRT should be advised to stop smoking completely before initiating treatment to avoid nicotine toxicity. Common signs of nicotine toxicity include nausea, vomiting, diarrhea, hypersalivation, abdominal pain, perspiration, dizziness, headache, hearing and visual disturbances, confusion, and weakness. On the other hand, patients beginning treatment with Zyban SR or varenicline must set a quit date after the medication has been taken for at least 1 week (1 week for varenicline and 1 to 2 weeks for bupropion SR).

A follow-up telephone call from the practitioner should occur within 1 week after the patient's scheduled quit date. If the patient is aware of the future call, compliance may be improved. In addition, the follow-up call may help detect ineffective use or adverse events early in the course of treatment. Additional follow-up contacts should occur as needed. If the patient has been successful at the time of the call, the clinician should offer congratulations and additional support. However, if the patient has relapsed, it is important to reassure the patient that it is not indicative of ultimate failure. Many smokers attempt to quit several times before achieving their goal. The reasons for failure should be identified and eliminated for the next attempt, and the patient should be encouraged to try again. Intensification of behavioral counseling may also be warranted. Drug therapy may be prolonged beyond 3 months if the patient develops cravings or feels he or she may relapse upon discontinuation (Prochaska & Benowitz, 2016).

Patient Education

The occurrence of adverse events with any medication has a definite correlation with patient compliance. Therefore, it is important that both the practitioner and patient be aware of the common side effects that may occur when using smoking cessation products. In addition, the patient needs to be informed that tolerance to the adverse effects associated with NRT usually occurs.

Weight gain is a common outcome of smoking cessation, and many patients are hesitant to quit for this reason. Many former smokers gain 4 to 5 kg, but as many as 13% gain 11 kg or more (Pisinger & Jorgensen, 2007). The mechanism for this is thought to be a slowing of metabolism. As mentioned earlier, the average smoker weighs 2.4 to 3.0 kg less than the average nonsmoker (Audrain-McGovern & Benowitz, 2011; Molarius et al., 1997). Therefore, with the cessation of smoking, the average former smoker should weigh approximately the same as the average nonsmoker. Patients must be informed that weight gain is possible but not significant. In addition, the health risk of increased weight is small compared with continued smoking. The increase in weight can be addressed after the patient has achieved complete abstinence. If weight gain is a major deterrent to treatment, nicotine replacement therapies, particularly nicotine gum and nicotine lozenge, and bupropion may be used since these agents may delay the weight gain.

Furthermore, patient counseling on the proper use of nicotine products including dose and administration can improve efficacy and safety of the medications. Finally, patient should be reminded of the beneficial health effects and other benefits of smoking cessation.

CASE STUDY 1

A.P., a 55-year-old man, has been smoking one pack of cigarettes per day for the last 38 years. He has a very stressful job as an executive of a large marketing company. A.P. and his coworkers frequently go to happy hour at the local bar after a long day at work. When he is at home, A.P. has a sedentary lifestyle that consists of lounging by the pool or watching television. He tried to quit smoking cold turkey 2 years ago and remained abstinent for approximately 6 months but has never tried any pharmacologic smoking cessation aids. During his previous attempt to quit, he became very anxious, irritable, and depressed and had trouble sleeping and concentrating at work. He has a medical history of hypertension for the last 10 years and a bout of successfully treated depression 5 years ago after the death of his mother. His family has been encouraging him to stop smoking for years. He is currently at the doctor's office for his blood pressure checkup and inquires about smoking cessation options; he doesn't have a definitive timeline for a quit date.

He smokes one pack per day and describes craving his first cigarette of the day about 10 to 15 minutes after awakening. He has observed that smoking with his morning coffee, smoking when drinking at the bar with his friends, and smoking after meals are triggers that led to his relapse with his prior smoking cessation efforts. He would like to try something to help with acute cravings.

1. What symptoms experienced by this patient during his previous attempt to quit smoking are consistent with withdrawal from tobacco/nicotine?
2. What motivational level (stage of change) is this patient in?
3. When A.P. reaches the action stage, what pharmacologic options are available for him?
4. Which smoking cessation aid would you recommend starting in this patient? Why?
5. How would your recommendation for smoking cessation aids change if patient reported smoking his first cigarette more than 30 minutes upon awakening?
6. What adverse events may the patient experience with the product that you chose in the previous question?
7. What are some nondrug methods that may enhance smoking cessation in this patient?

Bibliography

*Starred references are cited in the text.

*American Academy of Pediatrics. (2020, May 14). Counseling about smoking cessation. https://www.aap.org/en-us/advocacy-and-policy/aap-health-initiatives/Richmond-Center/Pages/Counseling-About-Smoking-Cessation.aspx

*American Cancer Society. (2020, June 12). What do we know about e-cigarettes? https://www.cancer.org/cancer/cancer-causes/tobacco-and-cancer/e-cigarettes.html

*American College of Obstetricians and Gynecologists. (2017). Tobacco and nicotine cessation during pregnancy. Committee Opinion No. 807. *Obstetrics and Gynecology, 135*(5), e221–e229.

*American Psychiatric Association. (1996). Practice guideline for the treatment of patients with nicotine dependence. *American Journal of Psychiatry, 153*(Suppl. 10), 1–31.

*American Psychiatric Association. (2013). Substance-related and addictive disorders. In *Diagnostic and Statistical Manual of Mental Disorders* (5th ed.). doi: 10.1176/appi.books.9780890425596.dsm16

Anthenelli, R. M., Morris, C., Ramey, T. S., et al. (2013) Effects of varenicline on smoking cessation in adults with stably treated current or past major depression. *Annals of Internal Medicine, 159*, 390–400.

*Arrazola, R. A., Singh, T. S., Corey, C. G., et al. (2015). Tobacco use among middle and high school students–United States, 2011–2014. *Morbidity and Mortality Weekly Report, 64*(14), 381–385.

*Audrain-McGovern, J., & Benowitz, N. L. (2011). Cigarette smoking, nicotine, and body weight. *Clinical Pharmacology and Therapeutics, 9*(1), 164–168. doi: 10.1038/clpt.2011.105

*Benowitz, N. L. (2010). Nicotine addiction. *New England Journal of Medicine, 362*(24), 2295–2303.

*Boehme, A. K., Esenwa, C., & Elkind, M. S. (2017). Stroke risk factors, genetics, and prevention. *Circulation Research, 120*(3), 472–495. doi: 10.1161/CIRCRESAHA.116.308398

*Creamer M. R., Wang, T. W., Babb, S., et al. (2019). Tobacco use and cessation indicators among adults – United States, 2018. *Morbidity and Mortality Weekly Report, 68*(45), 1013–1019.

*Ebbert, J. O., Hatsukam, D. K., Croghan, I. T., et al. (2014) Combination varenicline and bupropion SR for tobacco-dependence treatment in cigarette smokers. *Journal of the American Medical Association, 311*(2), 155–163.

Final National Pollutant Discharge Elimination System and Storm Water Multi-Sector General Permit for Industrial Activities, Part XIV (Notice). Modifications to the labeling of nicotine replacement therapy products for over-the-counter human use. *Federal Register, 78*(63), 19718–19721.

*Fiore, M. C., Jaen, C. R., Baker T. B., et al. (2008). Treating tobacco use and dependence: 2008 update. *Clinical Practice Guideline*. Rockville, MD: U.S. Department of Health and Human Services, Public Health Service.

Glover, E. D., Glover, P. N., Franzon, M., et al. (2002). A comparison of a nicotine sublingual tablet and placebo for smoking cessation. *Nicotine and Tobacco Research, 4*, 441–450.

*Heatherton, T. F., Kozlowski, L. T., Frecker, R. C., et al. (1991). The Fagerstrom Test for nicotine dependence: A revision of the Fagerstrom Tolerance Questionnaire. *British Journal on Addiction, 86*(9), 1119–1127.

*Henningfield, J. E., Shiffman, S., Ferguson, S. G., et al. (2009). Tobacco dependence and withdrawal: Science base, challenges and opportunities for pharmacotherapy. *Pharmacology and Therapeutics, 123*(1), 1–16.

*Hibbs, R. E., & Zambon A. C. (2018). Chapter 11. Nicotine and agents acting at the neuromuscular junction and autonomic ganglia. In L. L. Burton, R. Hilal-Dandan, & B. C. Knollmann (Eds.), *Goodman & Gilman's: The pharmacological basis of therapeutics* (13th ed.) Retrieved from https://accessmedicine-mhmedical-com.db.usciences.edu/content.aspx?bookid=2189&sectionid=167889972. Accessed on May 27, 2020.

*Hukkanen, J., Jacob III, P., & Benowitz, N. L. (2005). Metabolism and disposition kinetics of nicotine. *Pharmacological Reviews, 57*, 79–115.

Hurt, R. D., Sachs, D. P. L., Glover, E. D., et al. (1997). A comparison of sustained-release bupropion and placebo for smoking cessation. *New England Journal of Medicine, 337*, 1195–1202.

*Jamal, A., Agaku, I. T., O'Conner, E., et al. (2014). Current cigarette smoking among adults—United States, 2005–2013. *Morbidity and Mortality Weekly Report, 63*(47), 1108–1112.

*Jha, P., Ramasundarahettige, C., Landsman, V., et al. (2013). 21st century hazards of smoking and benefits of smoking cessation in the United States. *New England Journal of Medicine, 368*(4), 341–350.

*Koegelenberg, C. F. N., Noor, F., Bateman, E. D., et al. (2014). Efficacy of varenicline combined with nicotine replacement therapy vs varenicline alone for smoking cessation: A randomized clinical trial. *JAMA, 312*(2), 155–161.

*Le Houezec, J. (2003). Nicotine pharmacokinetics in nicotine addiction and nicotine replacement: A review. *International Journal of Tuberculosis and Lung Disease, 7*(9), 809–810.

*Li, R. M., Dupree, L., & Doering, P. (2020). Substance-related disorders II: alcohol, nicotine, and caffeine. In J. T. DiPiro, G. C. Yee, M. Posey, S. T. Haines, T. D. Nolin, & V. Ellingrod (Eds.), *Pharmacotherapy, a pathophysiologic approach.* McGraw-Hill. https://accesspharmacy-mhmedical-com.db.usciences.edu/content.aspx?bookid=2577&sectionid=223397102. Accessed on June 11, 2020.

*Lindson N., Klemperer E., Hong B., et al. (2019). Smoking reduction interventions for smoking cessation (Review). *Cochrane Database of Systematic Reviews, 2019*(9), 1–187. doi: 10.1002/14651858.CD013183.pub2

*Malarcher, A., Dube, S., Shaw, L., et al. (2010). Quitting smoking among adults–United States, 2001–2010. *Morbidity and Mortality Weekly Report, 60*(44), 1513–1519.

*Mallin, R. (2002). Smoking cessation integration of behavioral and drug therapies. *American Family Physician, 65*(16), 1107–1114.

*Meschia, J. F., Bushnell, C., Boden-Abala, B., et al. (2014). Guidelines for the primary prevention of stroke: A statement for health care professionals from the American Heart Association and the American Stroke Association. *Stroke, 45*(12), 3754–3832.

*Mishra, G. D., Chung, H., Cano, A., et al. (2019). EMAS position statement: Predictors of premature and early natural menopause. *Maturitas, 123*, 82–88. doi: 10.1016/j.maturitas.2019.03.008

*Molarius, A., Seidell, J. C., Kuulasmaa, K., et al. (1997). Smoking and relative body weight: An international perspective from the WHO MONICA project. *Journal of Epidemiology and Community Health, 51*, 252–260.

*National Institute of Arthritis and Musculoskeletal and Skin Diseases. (2018). Smoking and bone health. Retrieved from https://www.bones.nih.gov/health-info/bone/osteoporosis/conditions-behaviors/bone-smoking#b. Accessed on May 27, 2020.

*Nicotine. AHFS Drug Information (Adult and Pediatric). AHFS Clinical Drug Information. American Society of Health-System Pharmacists, Bethesda, MD. Updated March 3, 2020. http://online.lexi.com.db.usciences.edu/lco/action/home. Accessed on May 16, 2020.

*O'Brien, C. P. (2018). Drug use disorders and addiction. In L. L. Brunton, R. Hilal-Dandan, & B. C. Knollmann (Eds.), *Goodman & Gilman's the pharmacologic basis of therapeutics* (13th ed.). McGraw-Hill. Retrieved from https://accessmedicine-mhmedical-com.db.usciences.edu/book.aspx?bookid=2189. Accessed on June 11, 2020.

*Patnode, C. P., Henderson, J. T., Thompson, J. H., Senger, C. A., Fortmann, S. P., & Whitlock, E. P. (2015). Behavioral counseling and pharmacotherapy interventions for tobacco cessation in adults, including pregnant women: A review of reviews for the U.S. Preventive Services Task Force. Evidence Synthesis No. 134. AHRQ Publication No. 14-05200-EF-1. Agency for Healthcare Research and Quality, Rockville, MD.

*Pfizer Pharmaceuticals. (2019). Chantix (Varenicline) tablets: Highlights of prescribing information. Retrieved from https://dailymed.nlm.nih.gov/dailymed/drugInfo.cfm?setid=d52bc40b-db7b-4243-888c-9ee95bbc6545

*Pisinger, C., & Jorgensen, T. (2007). Weight concerns and smoking in a general population: The Inter99 study. *Preventive Medicine, 44*, 283–289.

*Prochaska, J. J., & Benowitz, N. L. (2016). The past, present, and future of nicotine addiction therapy. *Annual Review of Medicine, 67*, 467–486. doi: 10.1146/annurev-med-111314-033712

*Prochaska, J. O., & Velicer, W. F. (1997). The transtheoretical model of health behavior change. *American Journal of Health Promotion, 12*(1), 38–48.

*ScieGen Pharmaceuticals, Inc. (2019). Bupropion hydrochloride extended-release tablets (SR): Highlights of prescribing information. Retrieved from https://dailymed.nlm.nih.gov/dailymed/drugInfo.cfm?setid=8069c521-c49a-4b6d-baa8-4b0be897d585

*Shiffman, S., Dresler, C. M., Hajek, P., et al. (2002). Efficacy of a nicotine lozenge for smoking cessation. *Archives of Internal Medicine, 162*(22), 2632–2633.

*Shiffman, S., Dresler, C. M., Rohay, J. M., et al. (2004). Successful treatment with a nicotine lozenge of smokers with prior failure in pharmacological therapy. *Addiction, 99*(1), 83–92.

Shiffman, S., West, R. J., & Gilbert, D. G. (2004). Recommendation for the assessment of tobacco craving and withdrawal in smoking cessation trials. *Nicotine and Tobacco Research, 6*(4), 599–614.

*Siegel, R., Jacobs, E. J., Newton, C. C., et al. (2015). Deaths due to cigarette smoking for 12 smoking-related cancers in the United States. *Journal of the American Medical Association: Internal Medicine, 175*(9), 1574–1576. doi: 10.1001/jamainternmed.2015.2398

*Siu, A. L. (2015). Behavioral and pharmacotherapy interventions for tobacco smoking cessation in adults, including pregnant women: U.S. Preventive Services Task Force recommendation statement. *Annals of Internal Medicine, 163*, 622–634.

*U.S. Department of Health and Human Services. (2014). The health consequences of smoking—50 years of progress. A report of the surgeon general. U.S. Department of Health and Human Services, Centers for Disease Control and Prevention, National Center for Chronic Disease Prevention and Health Promotion, Office on Smoking and Health, Atlanta, GA. https://www.ncbi.nlm.nih.gov/books/NBK179276/pdf/Bookshelf_NBK179276.pdf. Accessed on January 24, 2021.

*U.S. Department of Health and Human Services. (2020). Smoking cessation: A report of the surgeon general. https://www.hhs.gov/sites/default/files/2020-cessation-sgr-full-report.pdf

*U.S. Food and Drug Administration. (2013). Modifications to the labeling of nicotine replacement therapy products for over-the-counter human use. *Federal Register, 78*(63), 19718–19721.

*U.S. Food and Drug Administration. (2020a). Vaporizers, e-cigarettes, and other electronic nicotine delivery systems (ENDS). https://www.fda.gov/tobacco-products/products-ingredients-components/vaporizers-e-cigarettes-and-other-electronic-nicotine-delivery-systems-ends

*U.S. Food and Drug Administration. (2020b). Recognize tobacco in its many forms. https://www.fda.gov/consumers/consumer-updates/recognize-tobacco-its-many-forms

*Wang, T. W., Gentzke, A. S., Creamer, M. R., et al. (2019). Tobacco product use and associated factors among middle and high school students – United States, 2019. *Morbidity and Mortality Weekly Report Surveillance Summary, 68*(12), 1–22.

*Whitaker, R., McRobbie, H., Bullen, C., Rodgers, A., Gu, Y., & Dobson, R. (2019). Mobile phone text messaging and app-based interventions for smoking cessation. *Cochrane Database of Systematic Reviews, 2019*(4), 1–83. doi: 10.1002/14651858.CD006611.pub5

53 Weight Loss

Amy M. Egras

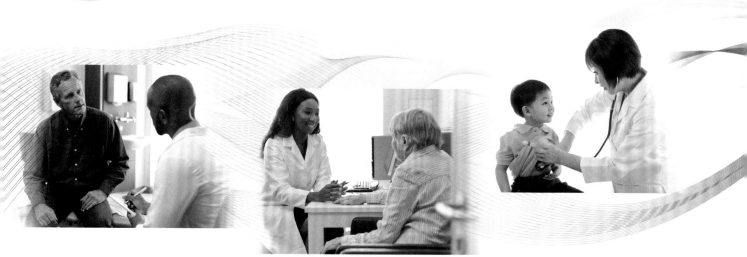

Learning Objectives

1. Identify factors involved in obesity.
2. Differentiate available treatments.
3. Formulate an individual treatment plan.

INTRODUCTION

Obesity has reached epidemic proportions, affecting more than 650 million adults worldwide. According to the most recent National Health and Nutrition Examination Survey for 2017 to 2018, 42.4% of U.S. adults are obese (body mass index [BMI] ≥ 30 kg/m²) and 9.2% have severe obesity, with a BMI of 40 kg/m² or higher. These numbers have increased from 30.5% and 4.7%, respectively, compared with data for the period 1999 to 2000.

Additionally, childhood obesity is on the rise. The prevalence of obesity among U.S. youth aged 2 to 19 years in 2015 to 2016 was 18.5%. This is approximately 13.7 million children and adolescents.

CAUSES OF OBESITY

Obesity is determined by overall body energy stores and the energy balance. When the calories consumed exceed the calories burned, the result is an increase in body fat storage and ultimately obesity. However, we are learning that the etiology of obesity is very complex. It is influenced by genetic, physiologic, psychological, environmental, social, and economic factors. Researchers link obesity to the development of chronic debilitating disease states such as cardiovascular disease, type 2 diabetes mellitus, cancer, nonalcoholic fatty liver disease, obstructive sleep apnea, and mental illness. Additionally, obesity is resulting in a large economic burden. Overall, the medical burden of obesity is costing the United States as much as $147 billion per year (in 2008 dollars).

Genetic Factors

It is clear that genetics may predispose people to be obese. Although estimates vary, it is shown that heritability of BMI is 40% to 70%. In fact, there are now 11 monogenic forms of obesity identified. These include things such as a deficiency of leptin and melatonin-4 receptors, which are expressed in the hypothalamus and involved in regulating energy homeostasis. Additionally, over 300 loci have been identified in genome-wide association studies. Continuation of whole-exome and whole-genome sequencing potentially can lead to the possibility of identifying new molecular targets and risk-predication markers that could help with tackling the obesity epidemic.

Environmental Factors

While we know that genetics likely play a role in the development of obesity, the environment has also shifted in a way that promotes overeating and less physical activity. In the United States, high-calorie, high-fat foods are easily accessible and inexpensive (e.g., processed food, fast-food restaurants). In addition to this, these convenient, easy-to-prepare foods are often available in large portion sizes, which has also contributed to the increase in obesity. Americans are eating more calories than they were 30 to 40 years ago.

On top of the increased consumption of calories is the decrease in energy expenditure. Some contributors to this include less access to physical activity (e.g., sidewalks), less physical education in schools, and advancements in technology. Advancements in technology, such as the Internet and video games, have led to more sedentary behaviors.

Psychological Factors

Psychological factors may also influence eating habits. Mood disorders and obesity frequently occur together. In fact, the relationship between depression and obesity is bidirectional. Some eating behaviors associated with obesity may include heightened food responsiveness and enjoyment of eating, eating in the absence of hunger, eating disinhibition, impulsive eating, and eating during stressful times.

Other Causes

Some illnesses can also contribute to obesity. These include hypothyroidism, Cushing syndrome, depression, and some neurologic problems. Certain drugs, such as steroids and some antidepressants, may cause excessive weight gain. There are also data to show a link between sleep debt and increased body weight. Sleep deprivation has shown to increase hunger and appetite.

PATHOPHYSIOLOGY

The adipocyte is the cellular basis for obesity. Adipocytes are metabolically active cells. These cells secrete adipocytokines, which are proinflammatory (e.g., tumor necrosis factor, interleukin-6), or may play a role in blood coagulation (e.g., plasminogen activator inhibitor-1, prostaglandins), insulin sensitivity (e.g., adiponectin), and appetite regulation (e.g., leptin). Obesity is more than just a disorder of body weight regulation. If this were the case, it would be easy for people to lose weight. However, losing weight is difficult. This is due to some biological adaptive responses to weight loss. Some of these changes are due to dysfunctional hormonal systems.

In addition, hormones also have a big role in appetite regulation. Signals from the gut, adipose tissue, liver, and pancreas to the hypothalamus and brain stem control appetite. While ghrelin is an appetite stimulant, neuropeptide YY (PYY) and cholecystokinin in the gastrointestinal (GI) tract, and gastric inhibitory polypeptide and glucagon-like peptide-1 (GLP-1), which are secreted in response to glucose, and leptin all signal satiety. Leptin deficiency, dysfunction, and resistance are all potentially related to the pathophysiology of obesity. Overall, a disruption of this hormonal system is believed to play a role in the pathophysiology of obesity.

Diagnostic Criteria

The best way to classify obesity would be the quantitative measurement of body fat. However, methods such as underwater weighing, dual-energy X-ray absorptiometry scanning, computed tomography, and magnetic resonance imaging are not practical for everyday clinical practice. The more commonly used measurement of obesity in the clinical setting is the BMI.

Body Mass Index

The BMI is the measurement of choice for clinicians and researchers studying obesity. Besides its simplicity, associations have been demonstrated between increased BMI and increased morbidity and mortality.

The BMI takes into account both a person's height and weight (BMI, kg/m^2). **Table 53.1** shows the mathematics and metric conversions. To use the table, find the appropriate height in the left-hand column and then move across the row to the given weight. The number at the top of the column is the BMI for that height and weight. **Table 53.2** gives the current guidelines for classification of obesity based on BMI. A limitation of BMI is that it does not distinguish excess fat from muscle, similar to the weight-for-height tables. Therefore, people with increased lean weight due to intense exercise or resistance training may be mistakenly classified as obese using BMI alone. In addition, BMI does not take body fat distribution into account, which is an independent predictor of health risk.

Waist Circumference

Waist circumference is a marker of abdominal fat and indicative of increased cardiometabolic risk. Waist circumference is found by measuring the circumference around the waist at the level of the iliac crest (just above the hip bone). A waist circumference exceeding 40 in. (102 cm) in men and 35 in. (88 cm) in women signifies increased health risk.

INITIATING DRUG THERAPY

Weight loss for those who are overweight and obese can provide many benefits, such as prevention of disease and improvements in emotions and function. In fact, even modest weight loss, 5% to 10%, has been shown to significantly improve many health conditions. According to the 2013 American Heart Association (AHA)/American College of Cardiology (ACC)/the Obesity Society (TOS) Guidelines for the Management of Overweight and Obesity in Adults, those with a BMI of 30 kg/m^2 or more or a BMI of 25 to 29.9 kg/m^2 with additional cardiovascular disease (CVD) risk factors (e.g., diabetes, prediabetes, hypertension, dyslipidemia, elevated waist circumference) should try to lose weight.

Weight loss requires creating an energy deficit by reducing calorie intake, increased physical activity, and behavioral therapy. All patients recommended to lose weight should be offered a comprehensive lifestyle intervention that involves trained professionals (e.g., registered dietician). A comprehensive lifestyle intervention results in greater weight loss initially

TABLE 53.1

Body Mass Index Conversion Chart

Body Mass Index (kg/m²)

19	20	21	22	23	24	25	26	27	28	29	30	35	40	45
Height (in.) and Body Weight (lbs)														
58	91	96	100	105	110	115	119	124	129	134	138	143	167	191
59	94	99	104	109	114	119	124	128	133	138	143	148	173	198
60	97	102	107	112	118	123	128	133	138	143	148	153	179	204
61	100	106	111	116	122	127	132	137	143	148	153	158	185	211
62	104	109	115	120	126	131	136	142	147	153	158	164	191	218
63	107	113	118	124	130	135	141	146	152	158	163	169	197	225
64	110	116	122	128	134	140	145	151	157	163	169	174	204	232
65	114	120	126	132	138	144	150	156	162	168	174	180	210	240
66	118	124	130	136	142	148	155	161	167	173	179	186	216	247
67	121	127	134	140	146	153	159	166	172	178	185	191	223	255
68	125	131	138	144	151	158	164	171	177	184	190	197	230	262
69	128	135	142	149	155	162	169	176	182	189	196	203	236	270
70	132	137	146	153	160	167	174	181	188	195	202	207	243	278
71	136	143	150	157	165	172	179	186	193	200	208	215	250	286
72	140	147	154	162	169	177	184	191	199	206	213	221	258	294
73	144	151	159	166	174	182	189	197	204	212	219	227	265	302
74	148	155	163	171	179	186	194	202	210	218	225	233	272	311
75	152	160	168	176	184	192	200	208	216	224	232	240	279	319
76	156	164	172	180	189	197	205	213	221	230	238	246	287	328

Note: Each entry gives the body weight in pounds for a person of a given height and body mass index. Pounds have been rounded off. To use the table, find the appropriate height in the left-hand column. Move across the row to a given weight. The number at the top of the column is the body mass index for the height and weight.

From *Understanding adult obesity*. National Institute of Diabetes and Digestive and Kidney Diseases, U.S. Department of Health and Human Services, http://win.niddk.nih.gov/publications/understanding.htm

TABLE 53.2

Classification of Obesity by Body Mass Index

	BMI (kg/m²)
Underweight	<18.5
Normal	18.5–24.9
Overweight	25.0–29.9
Obesity, class	
I	30.0–34.9
II	35.0–39.9
III (extreme)	≥40

BMI, body mass index.

and, over the long term, helps minimize weight regain. The lifestyle intervention should include the following:

- **Reduced calorie diet:** Decrease calorie intake by 500 kcal/d or more; this is typically prescribed as 1,200 to 1,500 kcal/d for women or 1,500 to 1,800 kcal/d for men.
- **Increased physical activity:** Increased aerobic physical activity for 150 min/wk or more (approximately ≥30 min/d, most days of the week).
- **Behavior therapy:** A behavior change program that may include self-monitoring of food intake, physical activity, and weight.

Adjunctive therapy with pharmacotherapy is recommended for patients with a BMI of more than 30 kg/m² or a BMI of 27 kg/m^2 or higher with comorbidity (e.g., type 2 diabetes, hypertension, dyslipidemia, CVD, nonalcoholic fatty liver disease, osteoarthritis, major depression, sleep apnea) who are unable to successfully lose weight or sustain weight loss (**Table 53.3**). Furthermore, patients with a BMI of 40 kg/m^2 or higher or a BMI of 35 kg/m^2 or higher with a comorbidity who have not been able to successfully lose weight with behavioral therapy (with or without pharmacotherapy) may be candidates for bariatric surgery.

Goals of Drug Therapy

The goals of therapy are to reduce body weight and maintain a lower body weight for the long term. A weight loss program that consists of diet, physical activity, and behavior therapy interventions typically results in a 5% to 10% weight loss in the first 6 months. However, it is important to note that sustained weight loss of even 3% to 5% can lead to beneficial effects, such as reductions in triglycerides, blood glucose, hemoglobin A1c, and the risk of developing type 2 diabetes. Greater weight loss results in even greater benefits.

In order to achieve weight loss, it is recommended that patients initiate a comprehensive lifestyle intervention that includes dietary, physical activity, and behavioral therapy. However, weight loss is difficult for most patients. The addition of weight loss medications may actually help with adherence to behavior change by helping to create the negative energy balance needed for weight loss. Weight loss medications should be used in combination to lifestyle changes. It should also be noted that medications do not change the underlying physiology of weight regulation. Therefore, gradual weight gain typically occurs when the medications are stopped. Keeping this in mind, it is important to note that, previously, most weight loss medications were only approved for short-term use. Currently, there are several medications approved for long-term weight management.

Appetite Suppressants

Appetite suppressants are noradrenergic medications used for weight loss. These medications are also referred to as *anorexiants*. Medications in this class (see **Table 53.3**) include benzphetamine, diethylpropion extended release (ER) or immediate release, phendimetrazine ER or immediate release, and phentermine (Adipex-P, Lomaira). They are considered adjuncts to a comprehensive weight management program. In addition, tolerance to the anoretic effects can occur after a few weeks of use. Because of tolerance and the lack of long-term data, these agents are only approved for short-term use: 12 weeks or fewer.

Mechanism of Action

The mechanism of action of appetite suppressants is to decrease appetite by stimulating the hypothalamus to release norepinephrine. The immediate release formulations are short-acting agents

---

TABLE 53.3

Overview of Agents Prescribed for Weight Loss

Generic (Trade) Name and Dosage	Selected Adverse Events	Contraindications	Special Considerations
Appetite Suppressants			
Benzphetamine Start 25–50 mg PO daily (may increase to 25–50 mg 1–3 times daily)	Increased heart rate, increased blood pressure, insomnia, tremor, and headache	Coronary artery disease, arrhythmias, heart failure, stroke, uncontrolled hypertension, hyperthyroidism, glaucoma, pregnancy, breast-feeding Approved for those aged ≥12 years old	Schedule C-III drug
Diethylpropion Start 25 mg PO TID or QID (immediate release) or 75 mg daily (controlled release)	Same as above	Same as above Approved for those aged >16 years old	Schedule C-IV drug
Phendimetrazine Tablet: 17.5–35 mg PO BID or TID, 1 hour before meals (maximum 70 mg TID) Capsule: 105 mg PO 30–60 minutes before morning meal	Same as above	Same as above Approved for those aged ≥17 years old	Schedule C-III drug
Phentermine (Adipex-P, Lomaira) Capsule/tablet (excluding Lomaira): 15–37.5 mg PO daily in 1–2 divided doses Tablet (Lomaira only): 8 mg PO TID	Same as above	Same as above Approved for those aged >16 years old	Schedule C-IV drug

TABLE 53.3

Overview of Agents Prescribed for Weight Loss (Continued)

Generic (Trade) Name and Dosage	Selected Adverse Events	Contraindications	Special Considerations
Lipase Inhibitor			
Orlistat (Xenical, Alli) Rx: 120 mg TID with meals OTC: 60 mg TID with meals	Oily spotting, flatus with discharge, fecal urgency, and fatty/oily stool	Chronic malabsorption syndrome, cholestasis, pregnancy Xenical approved for those ≥12 years old	May decrease absorption of fat-soluble vitamins (A, D, E, K)
Glucagon-Like Peptide-1 Receptor Agonist			
Liraglutide (Saxenda) Start 0.6 mg subcutaneously once daily; titrate up weekly to target dose of 3 mg subcutaneously daily	Nausea, vomiting, diarrhea, constipation, and pancreatitis	Medullary thyroid cancer, multiple endocrine neoplasia type 2, pregnancy	
Combination			
Phentermine ER/topiramate Start phentermine ER 3.75 mg/topiramate 23 mg PO once daily (maximum phentermine ER 15 mg/topiramate 92 mg once daily)	Increased heart rate, insomnia, dry mouth, constipation, paresthesia, dizziness, and dysgeusia	MAOIs, hyperthyroidism, and glaucoma	Schedule C-IV drug
Naltrexone/bupropion Start naltrexone 8 mg/bupropion 90 mg PO once daily (maximum naltrexone 32 mg/ bupropion 360 mg once daily)	Increased heart rate, increased blood pressure, nausea, constipation, headache, vomiting, and dizziness	MAOIs, uncontrolled hypertension, seizure disorders, bulimia or anorexia nervosa, and drug or alcohol withdrawal	Boxed warning: suicidal ideation and serious neuropsychiatric events

ER, extended release; MAOI, monoamine oxidase inhibitor; OTC, over-the-counter.

and usually dosed twice or thrice daily. For ER formulations, these are usually dosed once daily. The dosing varies by individual response, but it is recommended to start at the lowest dose and increase based on weight loss and tolerance of adverse events.

Contraindications

All of these medications are classified as Schedule 3 (C-III) or 4 (C-IV) drugs and have abuse potential. Caution should be used when prescribing these agents in patients with a history of substance abuse.

Because they lead to increased levels of norepinephrine, these agents can result in elevations of blood pressure and heart rate. Therefore, they are contraindicated in patients with a history of cardiovascular disease such as coronary artery disease, arrhythmias, heart failure, stroke, and uncontrolled hypertension, as well as hyperthyroidism and glaucoma. In addition, patients taking monoamine oxidase (MAO) inhibitors should not take these medications due to the potential increase in blood pressure, which could lead to hypertensive crisis. They are also contraindicated in pregnancy and breast-feeding.

Adverse Events

Adverse events include central nervous system stimulation such as insomnia, restlessness, dizziness, and headache. Overstimulation may result in an impairment of ability to perform activities requiring mental alertness (e.g., driving or operating

heavy machinery). Occasionally, xerostomia, constipation, and changes in libido may occur.

Serious adverse events that may occur are cardiovascular effects such as increases in blood pressure and tachycardia. For this reason, blood pressure and heart rate should be monitored on a regular basis, even more frequently in patients with preexisting hypertension.

Lipase Inhibitor: Orlistat

Orlistat (Xenical, Alli) differs from other available weight loss medications as it works nonsystemically, acting locally in the GI tract. Orlistat is a GI pancreatic lipase inhibitor that aids weight loss by lowering the absorption of dietary fat, on average by 30%. In clinical trials, orlistat users also saw improvements in total cholesterol, low-density lipoprotein, blood pressure, and blood glucose levels.

Dosage

Orlistat is available as a prescription or an over-the-counter (OTC) medication. Prescription orlistat (Xenical) should be administered at a dose of 120 mg thrice daily (maximum dose: 360 mg/d), while OTC orlistat (Alli) should be administered at a dose of 60 mg thrice daily (maximum dose: 180 mg/d). The doses should be taken during or up to 1 hour after a meal containing fat. The meal should contain less than 30% fat, and orlistat should be omitted if the meal contains no fat or if a meal is missed. Orlistat has the potential to decrease the absorption of the fat-soluble vitamins A, D, E, and K. Multivitamins should be taken by all patients taking orlistat, and these should be separated from the orlistat dose by 2 or more hours to ensure vitamin absorption.

Contraindications and Precautions

Orlistat is contraindicated in patients with chronic malabsorption syndrome, cholestasis, and pregnancy. In addition, orlistat is not indicated in patients younger than age 12.

Adverse Events

Because orlistat works locally in the GI tract, the primary side effects of orlistat include frequent bowel movements, bowel urgency, fatty stools, and flatulence with discharge. Patients should be counseled on these adverse events given the fact that fatty stools may appear as an oily leakage, particularly after flatus, and may intolerable for some patients. Nausea and abdominal pain may also occur. Because the GI effects associated with orlistat worsen with the more fat the patient eats, it is recommended that daily fat intake be distributed over 3 meals and that a single meal contain less than 30% fat. However, data suggest that concomitant administration of natural fiber (e.g., psyllium) may reduce the self-reported frequency and severity of GI side effects associated with orlistat use.

Caution should be used in patients taking oral warfarin (Coumadin) because orlistat may inhibit the absorption of vitamin K, resulting in an increased international normalized ratio. In addition, orlistat may decrease the serum concentration of the following medications: cyclosporine, levothyroxine, amiodarone, and anticonvulsants. Cyclosporine should be dosed 3 hours after orlistat; and levothyroxine and orlistat should be dosed at least 4 hours apart from orlistat. For amiodarone and anticonvulsants, it is unclear if separating the doses will reduce this interaction; patients on these therapies who are also taking orlistat should be monitored more closely.

Rarely, orlistat can result in hepatotoxicity. Patients should be advised to stop using orlistat and contact their health care provider if they experience any signs or symptoms of liver injury, such as anorexia, pruritis, jaundice, dark urine, light-colored stools, and/or right upper quadrant pain. In addition, although not common, orlistat can potentially cause an increase in urinary oxalate, which could potentially lead to oxalate nephrolithiasis and oxalate nephropathy with renal failure. It is recommended to monitor renal function in those patients at risk for renal impairment.

Glucagon-Like Peptide-1 Receptor Agonist: Liraglutide

Liraglutide is a GLP-1 receptor agonist, which is a medication approved for obesity as the trade name Saxenda and is also indicated for type 2 diabetes as the trade name Victoza. In regards to obesity, it is approved for weight loss in conjunction with comprehensive lifestyle changes at target doses of 3 mg subcutaneously daily versus a target dose of 1.8 mg subcutaneously daily for type 2 diabetes. Liraglutide is considered a preferred pharmacological for obese or overweight patients who also have type 2 diabetes and especially those with atherosclerotic cardiovascular disease (ASCVD).

Mechanism of Action

Liraglutide influences diabetes by stimulating glucose-dependent insulin secretion, decreases glucagon secretion, and slows gastric emptying. As it relates to weight loss, liraglutide also activates the proopiomelancortin (POMC) neurons, which results in the feeling of satiety and decreased food intake.

Dosage

Liraglutide should be titrated up over the course of 5 weeks to help minimize GI side effects. Liraglutide is dosed at 0.6 mg subcutaneously once daily for a week; then, the dose is increased by 0.6 mg subcutaneously daily at weekly intervals until the target dose of 3 mg subcutaneously daily is achieved. Although efficacy has not been established at doses of less than 3 mg, some experts will continue the medication if goal weight loss has been achieved.

Contraindications and Precautions

Liraglutide has a boxed warning for the potential of medullary thyroid cancer and multiple endocrine neoplasia type 2. Both of these conditions were observed in animal studies. However, patients with a history of either of these conditions should not use liraglutide. It is also contraindicated in pregnancy.

Adverse Events

The most common side effects experienced with liraglutide are nausea, vomiting, diarrhea, and/or constipation. The dose is titrated up at weekly intervals to help minimize these GI side effects. In addition to these side effects, patients have reported headache and increased heart rate. Liraglutide has also been associated with pancreatitis, and patients should be monitored for associated signs and symptoms.

Combination Medications

Phentermine Extended Release/Topiramate

Phentermine ER/topiramate (Qsymia) is a medication that is a combination of low-dose phentermine ER, an anorexiant medication, and topiramate, an anticonvulsant medication that is also indicated for use in migraine prevention. This medication is approved for weight loss in conjunction with comprehensive lifestyle changes. A risk evaluation and mitigation strategy is in place for Qsymia. This drug safety program was issued to inform prescribers and female patients about the increased risk for congenital malformations seen in infants exposed to Qsymia during the first trimester of pregnancy. While the drug is still available, providers must go through special training to prescribe the drug.

Mechanism of Action

As mentioned previously, the mechanism of action of phentermine works to decrease appetite by stimulating the hypothalamus to release norepinephrine. While the mechanism of action in regard to weight loss for topiramate is not fully understood, it is believed to be due to the enhancement of gamma-aminobutyric acid, the inhibition of carbonic anhydrase, and antagonism of glutamate, which results in reduced food intake.

Dosage

Phentermine ER/topiramate should be titrated up over several weeks. The starting dose is phentermine ER 3.75 mg/topiramate 23 mg once daily for 2 weeks. If the patient is tolerating this dose, then it can be increased to phentermine ER 7.5 mg/topiramate 46 mg once daily for 12 weeks; weight loss can be evaluated thereafter. If after 12 weeks 3% of baseline body weight has not been lost then the medication can be increased to phentermine ER 11.25 mg/topiramate 69 mg once daily for 2 weeks and then to phentermine ER 15 mg/topiramate 92 mg once daily.

Contraindications and Precautions

Phentermine ER/topiramate is contraindicated in patients with hyperthyroidism and glaucoma. In addition, patients taking MAO inhibitors should not take these medications due to the potential increase in blood pressure that could lead to hypertensive crisis. Due to the potential risk of orofacial clefts, women who are taking Qsymia and become pregnant must immediately stop the drug. It should not be used while breast-feeding. Although low, phentermine ER/topiramate does have a potential for abuse and as such is classified as a Schedule 4 (C-4) drug.

Adverse Events

The most common side effects experienced with phentermine ER/topiramate are increased heart rate, insomnia, dry mouth, constipation, paresthesia, dizziness, and dysgeusia. Due to the carbonic anhydrase inhibition of this medication, electrolytes should be monitored for hypokalemia and metabolic acidosis, and patients should be cautioned to monitor closely during strenuous exercise or extreme heat for signs of hyperthermia. In addition, be aware of any changes in behavior that may indicate any cognitive dysfunction or psychiatric disturbances. Due to the topiramate component, this medication should be withdrawn gradually as there is an increased risk of seizures with abrupt discontinuation.

Naltrexone Sustained Release/Bupropion

Naltrexone sustained release/bupropion (Contrave) is a medication that is a combination of naltrexone, an opioid antagonist, and bupropion, a dopamine/norepinephrine reuptake inhibitor. Bupropion as monotherapy is indicated for use in depression and smoking cessation. This medication is used for weight loss in conjunction with comprehensive lifestyle changes.

Mechanism of Action

Together, naltrexone and bupropion target two areas of the brain that are involved in the regulation of food intake. They work on the arcuate nucleus of the hypothalamus, which is involved in appetite regulation; they also work on the mesolimbic dopamine reward circuit, which stimulates the POMC neurons, which lead to appetite suppression.

Dosage

Naltrexone/bupropion should be titrated up over several weeks. The starting dose is naltrexone 8 mg/bupropion 90 mg taken 1 tablet by mouth in the morning for 1 week. Starting week 2, the dose should be increased to 1 tablet by mouth in the morning and 1 tablet by mouth with dinner. At week 3, the dose should be increased to 2 tablets by mouth in the morning and 1 tablet by mouth with dinner. At week 4, the dose should be increased to 2 tablets by mouth in the morning and 2 tablets by mouth with dinner. The final target dose should be naltrexone 16 mg/bupropion 180 mg by mouth twice daily. If a patient is taking a medication that is a CYP2B6 inhibitor, such as ticlopidine or clopidogrel, then the maximum dose should be naltrexone 8 mg/bupropion 90 mg by mouth twice daily.

Contraindications and Precautions

Naltrexone/bupropion is contraindicated in patients with uncontrolled hypertension, seizure disorders, bulimia or anorexia nervosa, and drug or alcohol withdrawal. In opioid-dependent patients, naltrexone/bupropion may precipitate acute withdrawal; patients should be opioid free for 7 to 10 days before starting naltrexone/bupropion. In addition, patients taking MAO inhibitors should not take these medications due to the potential increase in blood pressure, which could lead to hypertensive crisis; do not start naltrexone/bupropion in a patient receiving linezolid or intravenous methylene blue. It should not be used during pregnancy or breast-feeding.

Naltrexone/bupropion has a boxed warning for potential suicidal ideation and serious neuropsychiatric events. Patients should be monitored for severe psychiatric changes, such as depression or mania, psychosis, hallucinations, hostility, anxiety, and suicidal ideation or attempt.

Adverse Events

The most common side effects experienced with naltrexone/bupropion are nausea, constipation, headache, vomiting, and dizziness. In addition, use caution in patients with cardiovascular disease, due to the potential increase in heart rate and blood pressure.

Other Medications

Some antidepressant, antiseizure, and diabetes medications have been studied for use in weight loss. The use of these medications for weight loss is considered an *off-label* use.

Anticonvulsant medications: Zonisamide (Zonegran) is an anticonvulsant medication that has resulted in weight loss for binge eating disorder. However, adverse effects of the medication seem to be limiting its use.

Diabetes medications: Metformin (Glucophage) has demonstrated the ability to help people with type 2 diabetes and obesity lose weight. In addition, GLP-1 receptor agonists such as semaglutide and exenatide, sodium-glucose-linked transporter-2 inhibitors (SGLT2i) such as canagliflozin and empagliflozin, and pramlintide (Symlin), an amylin analog, have also demonstrated weight loss.

Alternative Medications

There are many OTC weight loss products on the market. The only nonprescription product, which is reviewed and approved by the Food and Drug Administration (FDA), is orlistat (Alli), which was discussed previously. All other weight loss products on the market are dietary supplements. Dietary supplements are not medications and not intended to treat, diagnosis, mitigate, prevent, or cure diseases. In addition, because they require premarket review or approval by the FDA, the manufacturer is responsible for making sure their product is safe. It has been reported that approximately 15% of U.S. adults have used a weight loss dietary supplement at some point in their lives (Blanck et al., 2007). Due to their perceived safety and efficacy, and easy availability, these are often an attractive choice for people. However, many of the weight loss supplements on the market do not have much evidence to support their claim of weight loss. See **Table 53.4** for a summary of

some of the most common dietary supplements available on the market.

Drugs That Cause Weight Gain

In addition to considering whether or not overweight or obese patients should be started on weight loss medication, it is also important to assess their current medication profile to see if they are taking any medications that may be associated with weight gain. Whenever possible, it is recommended to use an alternative medication that may not be associated with weight gain. However, if there is no acceptable therapeutic alternative, it is advised to try and use the lowest dose to achieve the desired clinical outcome. See **Table 53.5** for a list of drugs that may cause weight gain and potential alternatives.

TABLE 53.4

Dietary Supplements for Weight Loss

Name	Selected Adverse Events
Bitter orange	Increased heart rate and blood pressure
Chitosan	Well tolerated: gastrointestinal side effects
Chromium	Well tolerated: gastrointestinal side effects
Coleus forskohlii	Unknown
Conjugate linoleic acid	Dyspepsia, constipation, diarrhea
Garcinia cambogia	Hepatotoxicity
Green tea extract	Insomnia, agitation, nausea, vomiting, bloating, diarrhea
Guar gum	Abdominal pain, gas, bloating
Hoodia	Headache, dizziness, nausea, vomiting
Raspberry ketone	Unknown

TABLE 53.5

Drugs That May Cause Weight Gain

Medical Condition	Drug Class or Name	Alternative Medications
Type 2 diabetes	Insulin Sulfonylureas Meglitinides Thiazolidinediones	Metformin (Glucophage) Pramlintide (Symlin) GLP-1 receptor agonists SGLT2 inhibitors
Hypertension	Beta-adrenergic blockers	ACE inhibitors ARBs Calcium channel blockers
Depression	Paroxetine (Paxil) Amitriptyline Mirtazapine (Remeron) Venlaflaxine (Effexor)	Fluoxetine (Prozac) Sertraline (Zoloft) Citalopram (Celexa) Escitalopram (Lexapro) Bupropion (Wellbutrin)
Psychiatric disorders	Clozapine Olanzapine (Zyprexa) Quetiapine (Seroquel) Risperidone (Risperdal)	Ziprasidone (Geodon) Aripiprazole (Abilify)
Seizures	Carbamazepine (Tegretol) Gabapentin (Neurontin) Valproate (Depakote) Pregabalin (Lyrica)	Topiramate (Topamax) Lamotrigine (Lamictal) Zonisamide (Zonegran)
Chronic inflammatory diseases (e.g., rheumatoid arthritis)	Corticosteroids	Nonsteroidal anti-inflammatory drugs Disease-modifying antirheumatic drugs

ACE, angiotensin-converting enzyme; ARB, angiotensin receptor blocker; GLP-1, glucagon-like peptide-1; SGLT2, sodium-glucose-linked transporter-2.

Selecting the Most Appropriate Agent

The selection of the most appropriate agent for treating an obese patient depends on a number of factors. In particular, the provider should use a patient-centered approach to determine which medication would be best for a patient. The provider should assess the patient's other health conditions and consider both potential contraindications and benefits of certain medications as they pertain to weight loss. For example, a patient with underlying cardiovascular disease or uncontrolled hypertension would not be a good candidate for any medication that increases heart rate or blood pressure, such as phentermine, phentermine ER/topiramate, or naltrexone/bupropion. On the other hand, a patient with uncontrolled type 2 diabetes may benefit from the addition of liraglutide as it may help with blood glucose control in addition to weight loss.

Finally, as mentioned previously, all pharmacotherapeutic treatments should be coupled with comprehensive lifestyle intervention that involves calorie restriction, physical activity, and behavior modification.

Special Population Considerations

Pregnancy and Breast-Feeding

All of the weight loss medications are contraindicated in pregnancy and breast-feeding. Women who are pregnant or breast-feeding and concerned with their weight should discuss this with their provider and be monitored closely.

Pediatrics

Overweight and obesity are on the rise among the youth in the United States. For people aged 2 to 19 years old, 18.5% are considered to be obese. Young children aged 2 to 5 years old have lower rates of obesity: 13.9%. However, among children aged 6 to 11 years old, 18.4% are obese, and in adolescents aged 12 to 19, the prevalence of obesity is 20.6%. Obesity in childhood affects both physical and psychosocial health. Like treatment for adults, childhood obesity should be addressed with a comprehensive lifestyle intervention that targets healthy eating, physical activity, and behavioral therapy. This is the cornerstone, and pharmacotherapy is not routinely recommended. With regard to pharmacotherapy, however, only a few of the aforementioned medications are approved for use in children or adolescents (see **Table 53.3**). Childhood obesity is complex and should be facilitated by the child's primary care provider and parents/legal guardians.

Diabetes

Caution should also be used when any of these weight loss agents are prescribed for patients with diabetes. The decrease in caloric intake may decrease a patient's blood glucose level, requiring adjustment of insulin or oral hypoglycemic agents. Liraglutide is the preferred medication for those who are overweight or obese with type 2 diabetes, especially those with ASCVD.

Smokers

Smoking in itself is a risk factor for cardiovascular disease. The additional burden of obesity places the obese smoker in a much higher risk category for long-term cardiovascular effects. Nicotine has some thermogenic and metabolic effects, which are known to decrease appetite and often associated with a lower BMI. Quitting smoking is associated with a decreased resting metabolic rate and alterations in hormones, which results in weight gain. Therefore, the obese patient who then quits smoking runs the risk of gaining weight or thwarting efforts at weight loss. These patients may benefit from the use of naltrexone/bupropion given that bupropion is also indicated for smoking cessation.

MONITORING PATIENT RESPONSE

The patient should be monitored for weight loss, decreases in BMI, and changes in waist circumference. A comprehensive lifestyle intervention is key; patients who have a high-intensity intervention (≥14 sessions in 6 months) have the greatest weight loss. However, even low to moderate interventions result in more weight loss than usual care, defined as limited advice or educational materials on weight loss.

For patients taking weight loss medications, it is recommended that efficacy and safety are monitored monthly for the first 3 months and then at least every 3 months thereafter. If a patient loses 5% or more of his or her body weight at 3 months and the medication is deemed safe, then the medication can be continued. However, if a patient loses less than 5% of his or her body weight at 3 months or if there are any issues with safety or tolerability, then the medication should be discontinued.

PATIENT EDUCATION

Patients should be educated that obesity is more than just a cosmetic problem. Patients should be educated on the fact that obesity has been linked to several serious medical conditions, such as diabetes, heart disease, high blood pressure, and stroke. It is also associated with higher rates of certain types of cancer. A patient-centered approach for weight loss is essential. The provider and the patient should determine an appropriate weight loss strategy, keeping in mind health goals using a comprehensive lifestyle intervention together as a team. In addition to the weight loss strategies, the provider–patient team must also acknowledge and address the fact that weight loss maintenance is a lifelong challenge and address the challenges as they arise.

CASE STUDY 1

A.P. is a 34-year-old woman who comes into your clinic looking for a medication to help her lose weight. She states that she has tried several times to lose weight but seems to gain it back within months after stopping her dieting.

Your workup reveals a normal, young, well-developed woman in no acute distress. She is 66 in. tall and weighs 200 lbs. Pertinent labs include A1c 5.9%. Her blood pressure is 128/88 and heart rate is 80. She has a history of monthly migraine headaches, for which she takes sumatriptan 50 mg PO PRN; she may repeat the dose in 2 hours if there is no relief; she also has hypothyroidism, for which she take levothyroxine 112 mcg PO daily. She does not smoke or drink alcohol. She works as a secretary in an office. She has a body mass index of 32.3 kg/m².

1. What drug therapy would you prescribe? Why?
2. Discuss specific patient education based on the prescribed therapy.
3. Suppose A.P. experiences an increase in blood pressure and heart rate while on the current therapy. What would be an alternative therapy you could recommend?

Bibliography

Barrea, L., Altieri, B., Polese, B., et al. (2019). Nutritionist and obesity: Brief overview on efficacy, safety, and drug interactions of the main weight-loss dietary supplements. *International Journal of Obesity Supplements, 9*(1), 32–49.

Bays, H. E., McCarthy, W., Christensen, S., et al. (2020). Obesity algorithm slides, presented by the Obesity Medicine Association. www.obesityalgorithm.org. https://obesitymedicine.org/obesity-algorithmpowerpoint/. Accessed on April 17, 2020.

Blanck, H. M., Serdula, S. K., Gillespie, C., et al. (2007). Use of nonprescription dietary supplements for weight loss is common among Americans. *Journal of the American Dietetic Association, 107*(3), 441–447.

Budd, G. M., & Peterson, J. A. (2014). The obesity epidemic. Part 1: Understanding the origins: A review of underlying physical, psychological, and social factors. *American Journal of Nursing, 114*(12), 40–46.

Centers for Disease Control and Prevention. (2020). Adult obesity causes and consequences. Retrieved from https://www.cdc.gov/obesity/adult/causes.html on April 17, 2020.

Domecq, J. P., Prutsky, G., Leppin, A., et al. (2015). Drugs commonly associated with weight change: A systemic review and meta-analysis. *The Journal of Clinical Endocrinology and Metabolism, 100*(2), 363–370.

Farrington, R., Musgrave, I. F., & Byard, R. W. (2019). Evidence for the efficacy and safety of herbal weight loss preparations. *Journal of Integrative Medicine, 17*(2), 87–92.

Filozof, C., Fernandez Pinilla, M. C., & Fernandez-Cruz, A. (2004). Smoking cessation and weight gain. *Obesity Reviews, 5*(2), 25–103.

Gadde, K. M., Apolzan, J. W., & Berthoud, H. R. (2018). Pharmacotherapy for patients with obesity. *Clinical Chemistry, 64*(1), 118–129.

Hales, C. M., Carroll, M. D., Fryar, C. D., et al. (2017). Prevalence of obesity among adults and youth: United States, 2015–2016. NCHS data brief, no 288. Hyattsville, MD: National Center for Health Statistics.

Hales, C. M., Carroll, M. D., Fryar, C. D., et al. (2020). Prevalence of obesity and severe obesity among adults: United States, 2017–2018. NCHS Data Brief, no 360. Hyattsville, MD: National Center for Health Statistics.

Hamdy, O., Uwaifo, G. I., & Oral, E. A. (2020). Obesity. [Updated February 14, 2020]. In R. Khardori, & F. Talavera (Eds.), Medscape [Internet].

Heymsfield, S. B., & Wadden, T. A. (2017). Mechanisms, pathophysiology, and management of obesity. *The New England Journal of Medicine, 376*, 254–266.

Jensen, M. D., Ryan, D. H., Apovian, C. M., et al. (2013). AHA/ACC/TOS Guideline for the management of overweight and obesity in adults: A report of the American College of Cardiology/American Heart Association Task Force on Practice Guidelines and The Obesity Society. *Circulation.* Published online November 12, 2013.

Kumar, S., & Kelly, A. S. (2017). Review of childhood obesity: From epidemiology, etiology, and comorbidities to clinical assessment and treatment. *Mayo Clinic Proceedings, 92*(2), 251–265.

Kushner, R. F. (2014). Weight loss strategies for treatment of obesity. *Cardiovascular Diseases, 56*, 465–472.

Lexi-Comp Online™, Lexi-Drugs Online™, Hudson, Ohio: Lexi-Comp, Inc.; 2020; April 17, 2020.

Maunder, A., Bessell, E., Lauche, R., et al. (2020). Effectiveness of herbal medicines for weight loss: A systematic review and meta-analysis of randomized controlled trials. *Diabetes, Obesity and Metabolism*, Published online January 27, 2020.

May, M., Schindler, C., & Engeli, S. (2020). Modern pharmacological treatment of obese patients. *Therapeutic Advances in Endocrinology and Metabolism, 11*. Published online January 22, 2020.

Parto, P., & Lavie, C. J. (2017). Obesity and cardiovascular diseases. *Current Problems in Cardiology, 42*(11), 376–394.

Purnell, J. Q. (2018). Definitions, classification, and epidemiology of obesity. [Updated April 12, 2018]. In K. R. Feingold, B. Anawalt, A. Boyce et al. (Eds.), Endotext [Internet]. South Dartmouth, MA: MDText.com, Inc.

Saunders, K. H., Umashanker, D., Igel, L. I., et al. (2018). Obesity pharmacotherapy. *Medical Clinics of North America, 120*(1), 135–148.

Sharma, A., & Kushner, R. (2009). A proposed clinical staging system for obesity. *International Journal of Obesity, 33*, 289–295.

Velazquez, A., & Apovian, C. M. (2018). Updates on obesity pharmacotherapy. *Annals of the New York Academy of Sciences, 1411*(1), 106–119.

Wasim, M., Awan, F. R., Najam, S. S., et al. (2016). Role of leptin deficiency, inefficiency, and leptin receptors in obesity. *Biochemical Genetics, 54*, 565–572.

Wharton, S., Raiber, L., Serodio, K. J., et al. (2018). Medications that cause weight gain and alternatives in Canada: A narrative review. *Diabetes, Metabolic Syndrome and Obesity, 11*, 427–438.

World Health Organization. (2020). *Obesity and overweigh.* Retrieved from https://www.who.int/en/news-room/fact-sheets/detail/obesity-and-overweight on April 17, 2020.

Wright, S. M., & Aronne, L. J. (2012). Causes of obesity. *Abdominal Radiology, 37*, 730–732.

Pharmacotherapy for Women's Health

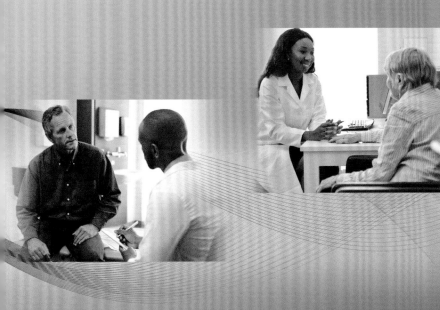

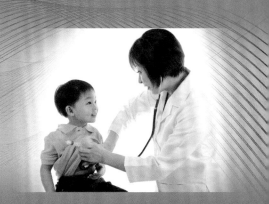

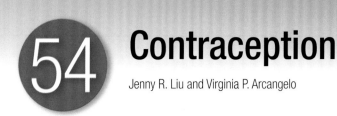

54 Contraception

Jenny R. Liu and Virginia P. Arcangelo

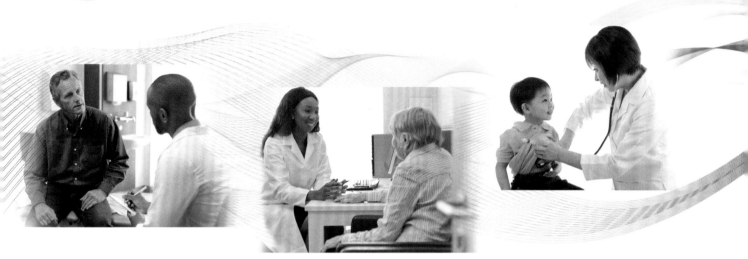

Learning Objectives

1. Understand the methods of action of contraceptive options.
2. Compare and contrast the available methods of contraception.
3. Formulate an individualized contraceptive treatment plan.

INTRODUCTION

Contraception is the inhibition of pregnancy by a process, device, or method. The U.S. Food and Drug Administration (FDA) first approved oral contraception (OC), the use of hormones to prevent pregnancy, in the 1960s, and the last law prohibiting its use in the United States was overturned in 1973 (Speroff & Darney, 2000). Regardless of the type used, one of the major benefits of contraception is its potential impact on the rate of unplanned pregnancies. In 2008, women reported that more than half of all pregnancies (51%) were unintended. By 2011, the percentage of unintended pregnancies declined to 45% (Finer & Zolna, 2016).

Most recently published statistics from 2014 indicate there are 13 abortions per 1,000 women of reproductive age in the United States (Singh et al., 2018). Unintended pregnancies that continue, including both unwanted and mistimed pregnancies, are positively associated with late-entry prenatal care, low birth weight, child abuse or neglect, and behavioral problems in children. One way to decrease unintended pregnancies is through increased awareness of contraception and the various available options. The widespread use of contraception in health care in the United States has expanded opportunities for women. Its use has allowed women to take on roles beyond (or in addition to) motherhood. Contraception has increased women's ability to decide when pregnancy and subsequent child-rearing will occur.

Age and desire for future pregnancy greatly influence a woman's method of choice. Reversible forms of contraception are the regimens of choice among most women planning future pregnancies. Oral, transdermal, and vaginal hormonal contraception are a first choice because return of fertility after discontinuing use is expected. Data from the 2015–2017 National Survey of Family Growth showed that in the United States, among women aged 15 to 49 years who use contraception, the most common contraceptive methods used were female sterilization (18.6%), oral contraceptive pills (12.6%), long-acting reversible contraceptives (10.3%), and male condoms (8.7%) (Daniels & Abma, 2019).

Oregon became the first state in passing a landmark law in 2016 that allows pharmacists to prescribe contraceptives to women aged 18 years or older. As of April 2019, pharmacists in 13 states legally can prescribe and directly dispense some types of hormonal contraception: California, Colorado, District of Columbia, Hawaii, Idaho, Maryland, New Mexico, New Hampshire, Oregon, Tennessee, Utah, Washington, and West Virginia (Free the Pill, 2019).

PHYSIOLOGY

A woman's ability to reproduce begins after she has completed the developmental stage of puberty. The average age of the onset of puberty is 11.2 years, whereas the length of time for the completion of this process is 4 years. Menarche, the last step in the pubertal process, is when menses commences. The average age for menarche is 12.7 years.

The cause or trigger for the onset of puberty is not completely understood. It is thought that a decreased sensitivity of the hypothalamus and pituitary glands to already circulating sex hormones results in an increased production of luteinizing hormone (LH) and follicle-stimulating hormone (FSH). Increased LH and FSH further stimulate the gonadal response of increased secretion of estrogen, progesterone, and testosterone. LH subsequently surges, inciting the release of ova. In the absence of fertilization, menses ensues.

A woman's menstrual cycle can be described in terms of either the follicular or luteal phase. In addition, in each of these phases, endometrial, ovarian, and pituitary hormone-secreting changes occur. These two major phases and the physiologic changes occurring in each are illustrated in **Figure 54.1**.

The endometrial changes can be subdivided. Menstruation, occurring on days 1 to 4 of the menstrual cycle, is the shedding of the endometrial lining. The next three phases are the proliferative phase (day 4 or 5 through ovulation), the secretory phase (immediately after ovulation), and the implantation phase (~21–27 days). During these phases, the endometrial lining is prepared for implantation of a fertilized ovum. In the event that an ovum does not implant, the next phase, endometrial breakdown, begins once again.

Relative to the ovarian changes that occur during the menstrual cycle, three major subdivisions can be identified: the follicular, ovulatory, and luteal phases. During the follicular phase, a dominant follicle is produced that will be released and await possible fertilization. The regulatory hormone largely responsible for this portion of the ovarian phase of the menstrual cycle is FSH. FSH stimulates the conversion of androgens to estrogen in the granulosa cells of the ovaries. Stimulation by FSH contributes to the development of a dominant follicle that produces further estrogen. The overall increase in estrogen production stimulates development of the glandular epithelium of the uterine lining, increases cervical mucus production and reduces the viscosity of this mucus, and increases vaginal pH.

Opposing the normal negative feedback mode of the menstrual cycle, in which high concentrations of estrogen inhibit the release of FSH and LH, the eventual peak in estrogen in this late follicular phase stimulates a surge in LH. The LH surge is subsequently responsible for the final maturation, release, and rupture of the dominant follicle. Follicular rupture and ovulation occur approximately 24 to 36 hours after the beginning of the LH surge and encompass the ovulatory phase of the menstrual cycle.

After the ovulatory phase, the luteal phase of the menstrual cycle enables the implantation of a fertilized ovum and maintenance of the uterine lining. The corpus luteum that remains after the follicle ruptures, releasing the ovum, secretes progesterone and 17-beta-estradiol. The secretion of these hormones increases the secretory activity of the endometrial glands. Cervical mucus also increases in viscosity. In the event that pregnancy occurs, the life of the corpus luteum is extended

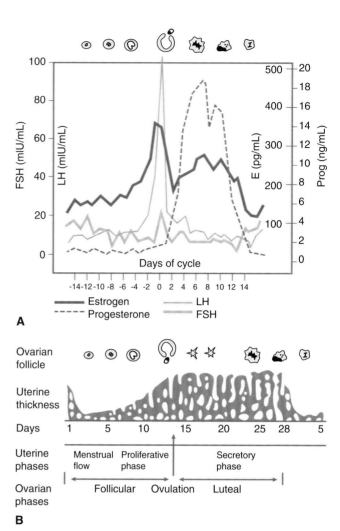

FIGURE 54–1   Comparison of the phases of the reproductive cycle. **A.** Plasma hormone concentrations in the normal female reproductive cycle. **B.** Ovarian events and uterine changes during the menstrual cycle. (Reprinted from Bullock, B. A., & Henze, R. L. [2000]. *Focus on pathophysiology* [p. 1100]. Philadelphia, PA: Lippincott Williams & Wilkins, with permission.)

FSH, follicle-stimulating hormone; LH, luteinizing hormone.

to continue production of these hormones. In the absence of pregnancy, the corpus luteum dies, estrogen and progesterone levels decline, and menstruation occurs.

INITIATING DRUG THERAPY

Given the normal menstrual cycle, pregnancy can be inhibited by preventing fertilization, manipulating hormones of the menstrual cycle such that ovulation never occurs, or interfering with implantation. Contraceptive options may be nonpharmacologic or pharmacologic. **Figure 54.2** identifies these options and the failure rates of each.

Nonpharmacologic options include the rhythm method, barrier devices, and intrauterine devices (IUDs) and intrauterine systems (IUSs). The rhythm method, also called the *calendar*

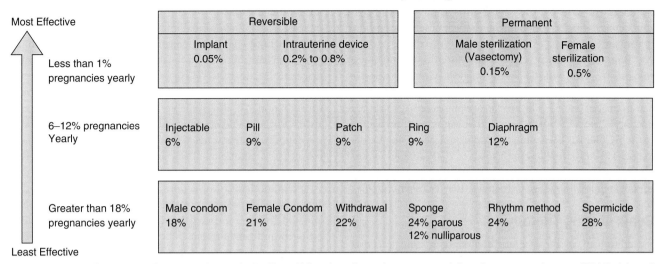

FIGURE 54–2 Effectiveness of contraceptive methods. (From U.S. selected practice recommendations for contraceptive use. [2013]. Adapted from the World Health Organization selected practice recommendations for contraceptive use 2nd ed. *Mortality and Morbidity Weekly Report, 62*[RR05], 1–46.)

method, is a form of natural family planning for women who may have a complex medical history or religious reasons that limit traditional birth control options. It can be done by tracking a woman's menstrual cycle, monitoring basal body temperature, and watching for changes to cervical mucus. However, this method is only about 76% effective at preventing pregnancy. Women using the rhythm method monitor their body and analyze their past menstrual cycles to try to determine when their fertile days are. They can then either choose to abstain from intercourse during those days or use a barrier device.

The rhythm method takes into account the viability of sperm in the female reproductive tract, which is up to 6 days after intercourse, and the ovum is available for fertilization for up to 24 hours after being released from the ovaries. It is assumed, therefore, that the period of maximum fertility occurs in the 5 days before ovulation and ends on the day of ovulation. Prediction of ovulation is important in recognizing the dates to avoid sexual intercourse; therefore, this method works best for women whose cycles are consistent. Several methods may be incorporated into the rhythm method to better identify the time of ovulation. Examples include the use of ovulation predictor kits, monitoring of basal body temperature, and testing of cervical mucus. The increase in progesterone concentration just before the LH surge is accompanied by a 0.4°F to 0.8°F increase in basal body temperature. It is recommended that women avoid unprotected intercourse for the 5 days prior to a basal body temperature increase, and they can resume intercourse 24 hours after the spike ("Rhythm Method for Natural Family Planning," 2018). Cervical mucus can also be used as a guide to predict ovulation. Midcycle cervical mucus, just before ovulation, is clear, thin, and stretchy. Peak mucus production occurs on the day of ovulation. It is recommended to avoid unprotected intercourse 2 to 3 days before the first signs of slippery mucus, about 3 days after slippery mucus

peaks, and also during menses. In general, it is safe to have intercourse again after the cervical mucus becomes cloudy and sticky or dry ("What Is the Cervical Mucus Method?" 2020).

Other nonpharmacologic options for the prevention of pregnancy include the use of barrier devices such as condoms, diaphragms, and cervical caps. These options vary not only in their efficacy rates but in their abilities to prevent sexually transmitted infections (STIs). The male latex condom helps to prevent the spread of human papillomavirus and many other STIs. It is the only contraceptive option clinically proven to prevent the spread of the human immunodeficiency virus (HIV). The female condom has been shown to act as a barrier to most STIs. However, limitations include its cost, decrease in spontaneity, and improper placement.

The diaphragm and cervical cap are both devices that require fitting by a health care provider. The woman can insert a diaphragm up to 6 hours before intercourse and must leave it in place for at least 6 hours (but no more than 24 hours) after intercourse. The diaphragm has been shown to reduce the risk of cervical gonorrhea, pelvic inflammatory disease (PID), and tubal infertility secondary to STIs. It is not, however, effective against HIV infection, and urinary tract infections are twice as common in diaphragm users compared with nonusers. Comparably, the cervical cap may be left in place for a total of 48 hours. It must remain in place, however, for at least 8 hours after sexual intercourse. Like the diaphragm, it has not been shown to afford any protection against HIV infection.

The third major type of nonpharmacologic contraception is the IUD/IUS. Although its mechanism of action is not clearly understood, the copper IUD is thought to act as a spermicide by interfering with sperm transport into and within the uterus to prevent pregnancy. The intrauterine environment is rendered unreceptive to sperm or the implantation of a fertilized ovum should fertilization occur. In progesterone-implanted

IUSs, the continued release of progesterone contributes to the contraceptive action of this device through production of viscous cervical mucus, which further impedes the sperm's ability to reach the ovum.

Both the American College of Obstetricians and Gynecologists (ACOG) and the North American Menopause Society recommend that women continue contraceptive use until menopause or ages 50 to 55. The median age of menopause is approximately 51 years in North America but can range from ages 40 to 60. ACOG has been a huge proponent of decreasing barriers to access of contraception. In October of 2019, ACOG released a statement supporting over-the-counter access to hormonal contraception without age restrictions (Isley & Allen, 2019).

Goals of Drug Therapy

In addition to, or in place of, the nonpharmacologic contraceptive options available, pharmacologic options do exist. The primary mechanism by which these agents prevent pregnancy is through manipulation of the normal menstrual cycle, effects on cervical mucus, or both. Estrogen plus progesterone or progesterone alone is used to interfere with the process of ovulation, conception, or both. Optimal contraception features, as defined by the World Health Organization, include the following:

- Safety
- Effectiveness
- Convenience
- Regular bleeding episodes
- Rapid reversibility

Combined (Estrogen and Progestin) Oral, Transdermal, and Vaginal Contraceptives

These prescription methods use a "combination" of two hormones: estrogen and progesterone. All combination methods work primarily by preventing ovulation. They are highly effective when taken every day, with perfect-use failure rates of less than 1%. However, the typical failure rate of combination birth control pills is 3% to 8% and much higher in some populations. They also have several noncontraceptive benefits, including but not limited to a decreased risk of ovarian and endometrial cancers, benign breast disease, ectopic pregnancy, ovarian cysts, endometriosis, ovulation pain, and premenstrual syndrome. They also might improve acne, hirsutism, and other manifestations of polycystic ovary syndrome. The improvement occurs secondary to an increase in the level of sex hormone binding globulin, which reduces circulating free testosterone and ameliorates many androgenic effects. These methods are reversible and can be used by women of all ages.

The combination contraceptive agents contain estrogen, usually in the form of ethinyl estradiol. Doses of estrogen range from 20 to 35 mg; 98% of all prescribed OCs contain less than 35 mg of estrogen, and even OCs with as little as 20 mg of estrogen are considered effective. Pills with low estrogen content are considered safer than higher-dose OCs for certain patients, including perimenopausal women, those with a family history of heart disease, and smokers younger than age 35 (although women who take OCs and smoke remain at an increased risk of myocardial infarction [MI] and stroke due to OC-associated changes in coagulation factors). Progesterone-only birth control comes in the form of desogestrel, ethynodiol diacetate, levonorgestrel (LNg), norethindrone, norethindrone acetate, norgestimate, or norgestrel. A synthetic progesterone (drospirenone) is also available. Drospirenone has additional antiandrogenic and antimineralocorticoid properties and is associated with less water retention than other progesterones, less negative emotional affect, and less appetite increase after 6 months of use.

The mechanism of action of combination contraceptive agents is the suppression of the pituitary gonadotropins FSH and LH by the continued high concentrations of circulating estrogen and progesterone. The suppression of LH, primarily by the progesterone component, inhibits the LH surge responsible for ovulation. Progesterone also increases cervical mucus viscosity, resulting in impaired sperm transport. FSH suppression, largely through estrogen's influence, prevents the selection and emergence of a dominant follicle. Therefore, the combination of estrogen and progesterone inhibits selection of a dominant follicle and ovulation.

In addition to their influence on the reproductive cycle, the hormones used in OC pills (OCPs) exert other actions. All forms of progesterone exhibit some estrogenic, androgenic, or anabolic activity. For example, highly androgenic forms of progesterone affect lipid and carbohydrate metabolism and increase the appearance of acne, weight gain, and hirsutism. As such, practitioners should consider the various progesterone formulations relative to their androgenic effects when choosing an OCP regimen. The least androgenic forms include the newer, third-generation progesterones desogestrel and norgestimate. In addition to their relative lack of androgenic side effects, they are also more potent than the other progesterones norethindrone, ethynodiol diacetate, and LNg. Knowledge of the differences in the progesterone formulations becomes important when managing, or prospectively avoiding, certain side effects of OCPs.

An important consideration to keep in mind is potential drug interactions with OCPs. A recent study showed the drug interactions among ethinyl estradiol/estradiol and valproate (Depacon), oxcarbazepine (Trileptal), and carbamazepine to be among the most prevalent interactions (Bosak et al., 2019). Antibiotics may reduce the efficacy of OCPs when taken concurrently; however, there have been few well-documented reports about OCP failure with antimicrobials. Antibiotics more likely to reduce OCP effectiveness include azithromycin, erythromycin, ketoconazole, penicillin (and derivatives), rifampin, rifabutin, and tetracycline antibiotics (Dickinson et al., 2001). Rifampin, an inducer of enzymes that metabolizes estrogens, is known to decrease the effectiveness of OCPs (Simmons et al., 2018). Although, in literature, the absolute risk of unintended pregnancy is small, the most conservative approach is to advise patients to use a backup method of contraception during times of antibiotic use.

Many options exist when choosing an OC regimen for a patient. In general, combination OCPs are divided into monophasic, biphasic, and triphasic combinations. **Tables 54.1** and **54.2** list the available formulations. Monophasic combinations provide a set amount of estrogen and progesterone daily for 21 days. Placebo or nothing is given on days 22 to 28, the days during which menstruation occurs. The monophasic combinations may be useful in managing adverse effects such as breakthrough vaginal bleeding. Also, women who are sensitive to fluctuations in hormone levels that occur with the biphasic and triphasic OCPs may respond more positively to the monophasic formulations. Side effects, including breast tenderness, nausea, headaches, and bloating, are usually limited to the first 1 to 2 months of use but may discourage continuation. A backup method of birth control, such as condoms, should

TABLE 54.1
Monophasic Contraception

Brand Name	Hormonal Components
Alesse, Aviane, Lessina	20 mcg EE, 0.1 mg levonorgestrel
Brevicon	35 mcg EE, 0.5 mg norethindrone
Apri, Desogen, Ortho-Cept	30 mcg EE, 0.15 mg desogestrel
Kelnor 1/35	35 mcg EE, 1 mg ethynodiol diacetate
Levlen, Nordette, Portia	30 mcg EE, 0.15 mg levonorgestrel
Loestrin 1/20	20 mcg EE, 1.0 mg norethindrone acetate
Loestrin 1.5/30	30 mcg EE, 1.5 mg norethindrone acetate
Lo/Ovral, Cryselle	30 mcg EE, 0.3 mg norgestrel
Norethin 1/35E	35 mcg EE, 1 mg norethindrone
Norinyl 1 + 35	35 mcg EE, 0.5 mg norethindrone
Nortrel 0.5/35	30 mcg EE, 3 mg drospirenone
Ocella, Yasmin	35 mcg EE, 0.25 mg norgestimate
Ortho-Cyclen	35 mcg EE, 1 mg norethindrone
Ortho-Novum 1/35, Nortrel	50 mcg EE, 1 mg norethindrone
Ortho-Novum 1/50, Norinyl 1 + 50	35 mcg EE, 0.4 mg norethindrone
Ovcon 35	50 mcg EE, 1 mg norethindrone
Ovcon 50	50 mcg EE, 0.5 mg norgestrel
Ovral	30 mcg EE, 0.15 mg levonorgestrel
Seasonale	20 mcg EE, 3 mg drospirenone
Yaz	35 mcg EE, 1 mg norethindrone
Extended Cycle	
Jolessa, Seasonale	30 mcg EE, 0.15 mg levonorgestrel
Lybrel	20 mcg EE, 0.09 mg levonorgestrel

EE, ethinyl estradiol.

TABLE 54.2
Biphasic and Triphasic Oral Contraceptive Pills

Brand Name	Hormonal Components
Biphasic Oral Contraceptive Pills	
Kariva, Mircette	20/10 mcg EE, 15 mg desogestrel
Ortho-Novum 10/11	35/35 mcg EE, 0.5/1 mg norethindrone
Triphasic Oral Contraceptive Pills	
Cyclessa, Velivet	25/25/25 30 mcg EE, 0.1/0.125/0.15 mg desogestrel
Estrostep	20/30/35 mcg EE, 1 mg norethindrone acetate
Ortho-Novum 7/7/7, Nortrel 7/7/7	35/35/35 mcg EE, 0.5/0.75/1 mg norethindrone
Ortho Tri-Cyclen, Tri-Previfem, Tri-Sprintec	35/35/35 mcg EE, 0.18/0.215/0.25 mg norgestimate
Tri-Levlen, Triphasil, Enpresse	30/40/30 mcg EE, 0.05/0.075/0.125 mg levonorgestrel
Tri-Norinyl, Aranelle	35/35/35 mcg EE, 0.5/1/0.5 mg norethindrone
Triphasil	30/40/30 mcg EE, 0.05/0.075/0.125 mg levonorgestrel
Extended Cycle	
Seasonique	30/10/30 mcg EE, 0.15 mg levonorgestrel

EE, ethinyl estradiol.

be used for the first week after pills are started. Few clinical differences have been noted among the myriad pill formulations (monophasic, biphasic, triphasic, different generation progestins, and other formulations), so it is reasonable to prescribe a generic monophasic pill containing 30 to 35 mcg of estrogen for most patients.

There is also a variation to the traditional monophasic OCP. This formulation provides a constant amount of estrogen and progesterone daily on days 1 to 21. Placebo tablets are taken on days 22 to 23. Then, on days 24 to 28, a lower dose of estrogen alone is given. The rationale for providing estrogen on days 24 to 28 is to help manage problems in women who may exhibit symptoms of estrogen deficiency, such as rebound headaches, during the traditional week-long placebo period.

The biphasic and triphasic OCP combinations were developed to better mimic the fluctuations in hormones during the menstrual cycle. Changes in the estrogen or progesterone components occur every 7 to 10 days in these products. The phasic OCPs have not been shown to have any proven advantages in efficacy over the monophasic products. The major difference between the biphasic and triphasic regimens and the monophasic regimens is the net amount of progesterone delivered per cycle. The biphasic and triphasic regimens contain, in general, less progesterone (see **Tables 54.1** and **54.2**). Therefore, for women experiencing progesterone-related side effects, such as weight gain, fluid retention, and acne, switching to a regimen containing lower doses of progesterone with less androgenic effects may be beneficial.

Extended-cycle OCPs are also now available. During the standard 7-day hormone-free interval that occurs with the use of low-dose estrogen formulations, the function of the hypothalamic–pituitary–ovarian axis recovers rapidly, and this increases the risk of ovarian follicle development, ovulation with unintended pregnancy, and spotting due to endogenous estradiol production. Fluctuating hormone levels allow endometrial buildup and can exacerbate premenstrual symptoms and menstrual headaches by creating hormone excess and withdrawal states. Extended-cycle OCPs with a shorter or eliminated hormone-free interval reduce the risk of these unwanted effects by preventing endogenous estradiol production while still providing highly effective and safe contraception.

When initiating therapy for patients, a contraceptive regimen is started relative to the woman's menstrual cycle. Initiation can occur with either a day 1 start or a Sunday start regimen. A day 1 regimen has the contraceptive agent begin on the first day menses, regardless of the day of the week. While a Sunday start regimen begins the OCP on the Sunday after the onset of menses. This means that the woman will not menstruate on a weekend, which is desirable to many patients. OCP packs are produced with the Sunday start regimen in mind. In the event that a patient is a day 1 start, the pharmacist places a special label on the pack noting the beginning day of the pack and the end. The situation in which the day 1 versus Sunday start becomes an issue is relative to missed doses, which is discussed later in the chapter.

In reality, combined hormonal contraceptives can be initiated at any time if it is reasonably certain that the woman is not pregnant. If combined hormonal contraceptives are started within the first 5 days since menstrual bleeding began, no additional contraceptive protection is needed. If they are initiated more than 5 days since menstrual bleeding started, abstinence from sexual intercourse or additional contraceptive protection is required for the next 7 days.

Another form of contraception is the transdermal patch containing 75 mcg of ethinyl estradiol and 6 mg of norelgestromin. The patch releases hormones through the skin and can be applied to the abdomen, buttocks, upper outer arm, or upper torso. It is important to counsel the patient that the patch should only be applied on clean, dry, healthy skin free of lotions. However, the patient can bathe, shower, or swim while wearing the patch. A new patch is applied each week, worn for 7 days, and removed and replaced with a new patch. During the fourth week, no patch is worn. The first patch should be applied on the first day of menses and a new one on the same day the next week. Detachment has been shown in only 5% of cases, but if it becomes loose or falls off, it must be replaced with a new patch. If the patch is off for more than 24 hours,

a new cycle is started and backup methods of birth control are used for the next 7 days.

The most frequent complaint from users of the patch is reactions at the application site. With respect to weight, studies showed women who weigh more than 198 lbs experienced a higher failure rate, so these women should consider a different form of contraception.

Combination contraceptive vaginal rings are also available. These come as a small, flexible, plastic ring inserted into the vagina by the patient. It releases 15 mcg of ethinyl estradiol and 120 mcg of etonogestrel daily. It is removed after 3 weeks and a new ring is inserted after 1 week. The vaginal ring contains lower hormonal doses because there is no hepatic or gastrointestinal (GI) interference. It can remain in place during bathing, swimming, and intercourse.

Progestin-Only Hormonal Contraceptives

Progesterone-only contraceptives are available in formulations of oral tablets, intramuscular (IM) injections, subdermal implants, or hormonal IUDs. They are the hormonal contraceptive of choice in women who cannot take or cannot tolerate estrogen-containing formulations. They are a better choice for women with certain comorbidities, such as high blood pressure and history of thrombosis and women who are smokers and aged over 35; they may be negatively impacted by estrogen-containing pills. The progestin-only pill is often recommended for breast-feeding women. In ease of administration, compliance, and efficacy, however, the formulations vary greatly.

The progesterone-only contraceptive pill, commonly referred to as the *minipill*, contains a very low dose of progesterone. **Table 54.3** lists the available formulations and active components of each. The minipills do not consistently suppress the pituitary gonadotropins LH and FSH. Their primary effect is exerted through changing the endometrial and cervical mucus environments. The time from dosing to changes in the cervical mucus is 2 to 4 hours. The impermeability of the mucus declines 22 hours after the dose. Therefore, to help ensure maximum efficacy, it is imperative that the pill is taken at exactly the same time daily. It is recommended that if the dose is more than 3 hours late, a backup form of contraception should be used. When beginning the minipill, it should start on the first day of menses and a backup contraceptive should be used for the first 7 days. The minipill, unlike combination OCPs, does not contain placebo pills, and should be taken daily without a placebo week.

TABLE 54.3	
Progesterone-Only Oral Contraceptive Pills	
Brand Name	**Hormonal Component**
Micronor, Camila, Errin, Nor-QD	0.35 mg norethindrone
Ovrette	0.075 mg norgestrel

The FDA approved the use of depot-medroxyproges-terone acetate (DMPA) in 1992. The dose of DMPA used suppresses ovulation in addition to affecting cervical mucus. DMPA is dosed every 13 weeks and is a good choice for women for whom daily compliance with a combination or progester-one-only OCP is an issue. When beginning DMPA, the recommendation is that it be given within the first 5 days after the onset of menses. It can be given to postpartum women and to those who are breast-feeding. Subsequent doses must be given no later than 13 weeks from the prior dose to ensure efficacy. If a woman presents later than 13 weeks for her next injection, the provider needs to determine that the patient is not pregnant before administering the drug.

DMPA, like other progesterone-only contraceptives, is safe for women with a history of cardiovascular disease, stroke, thromboembolism, or peripheral vascular disease. It is ideal for women with hemoglobinopathies, such as sickle cell disease, because some studies have shown a decrease in hemolytic crises in this patient population.

In addition to the positive compliance effects of this dosage formulation, women wishing future pregnancy also frequently prefer DMPA. On discontinuation of DMPA, 70% of women conceive within the first year and 90% within 24 months. The most common adverse effects of DMPA are weight gain, amenorrhea, and irregular bleeding, with episodes of unpredictable bleeding lasting more than 7 days. The latter problem occurs more commonly in the first few months of therapy. Another important consideration for DMPA is that prolonged use may result in significant loss of bone mineral density; however, this bone loss was reversible with discontinuation of DMPA. Therefore, patients on DMPA should be recommended to increase their intake of calcium and vitamin D as well as to exercise regularly.

The Intrauterine System

Another form of contraception is IUSs, categorized into nonhormonal and hormonal IUDs. These are flexible plastic devices that are inserted into the uterus and cause a sterile inflammatory reaction within the uterus, which interferes with sperm transport into and within the uterine cavity. This is the most effective method of reversible contraception with a failure rate of less than 1% (Daniels & Abma, 2019). There are currently five IUDs approved by the FDA. One is the hormone-free copper-containing IUD (ParaGard®). It is effective for up to 10 years and can be inserted anytime as long as the woman is not pregnant. It can also be inserted within 5 days of the first act of unprotected sexual intercourse as an emergency contraceptive (Espey et al., 2008; see **Table 54.4**).

Another IUS is the hormonal IUD, containing the progestin hormone LNg. There are currently four available in the United States. One releases 20 mcg/d of LNg (Mirena®) and is approved for 5 years of use. Liletta® is approved for 6 years and initially releases 20 mcg/d and then subsequently decreases over 6 years to 8.6 mcg/d. Skyla® is slightly smaller

TABLE 54.4
Intrauterine Systems

Nonhormonal IUD		
Brand Name	**Maximum Duration of Use (Years)**	**Component**
(ParaGard®)	10	Copper-containing
Hormonal (Levonorgestrel) IUD		
Brand Name	**Maximum Duration of Use (Years)**	**Levonorgestrel Dose (mcg/d)**
Mirena®	5	20 (reduced by ~50% after 5 years)
Liletta®	6	20 (declines to ~8.6 mcg/d after 6 years)
Skyla®	3	14 (declines to 5 mcg/d after 3 years)
Kyleena®	5	17.5 (declines to 7.4 mcg/d after 5 years)

IUD, intrauterine device.

than the Mirena®, which may make it a better option for nulliparous women. It releases 14 mcg/d of LNg initially and then decreases to 5 mcg/d after 3 years and is approved for 3 years of use. Kyleena®, the newest IUD approved in 2016, is approved for 5 years of use. It initially releases 17.5 mcg/d of LNg and then subsequently decreases to 7.4 mcg/d after 5 years.

Because the IUS contains no estrogen component, it is appropriate for women in whom estrogen is contraindicated. The IUS has been shown to lessen dysmenorrhea and bleeding, so it may be an effective treatment for women with dysmenorrhea, menorrhagia, and anemia and may serve as an effective transition from contraception to hormone replacement therapy. Insertion can be done in the physician's office, and little maintenance is required. The only maintenance required for the patient is to check the string after each menstrual period to ensure that the IUS is still in place. For women who choose to become pregnant, the device can be removed by the clinician at any time. No waiting period is required before conception, and IUS use is not associated with a decline in fertility.

The only contraindications to the use of this method are suspected pregnancy, uterine abnormalities that cause significant distortion of the uterus, PID, or unexplained vaginal bleeding prior to insertion. Immediate postpartum insertion is appropriate.

Progestin-Only Implants

Nexplanon® is a subdermal rod that releases etonogestrel, which is the same progestin used in the NuvaRing. It is implanted in the upper arm as an office procedure and remains active for 3 years.

Like other progestin-only contraceptives, Nexplanon® works by blocking the LH surge, thereby preventing ovulation. It also thickens the cervical mucus and thins the endometrial lining. Unlike other progestin-only methods, Nexplanon® causes estradiol to gradually increase to normal endogenous levels after an initial decrease. Progestin-only implants are extremely effective in preventing pregnancy and have an efficacy rate similar to that associated with sterilization or use of an IUD. Women experience a quick return to normal cycles after implant removal, and there have been no reports of infertility after removal. Implantation and removal can be performed as simple office procedures.

The main side effects are irregular bleeding (50%), acne (12%), headaches (16%), and weight gain (12%) ("Progesterone Only Contraceptives," 2015). It is important to note that Nexplanon® is contraindicated in women with active liver disease or current or past history of thrombosis. This differs from most other progestin-only methods of contraception that have long been considered safe to use in women with an increased risk of venous thromboembolism (e.g., women who smoke or have hypertension, diabetes mellitus, migraine headaches, or a history of venous thromboembolism).

Emergency Contraception

Two forms of emergency contraceptive pills (ECPs) are currently available in the United States: the Cu-IUD, as described previously, and three options of ECPs (Daniels & Abma, 2019), LNg, ulipristal acetate (UPA), and combined estrogen and progestin (Yuzpe regimen). LNg is given as a single dose of 1.5 mg or as a split dose of 0.75 mg taken 12 hours apart. UPA is a progesterone receptor antagonist and is given as a single dose of 30 mg. It inhibits follicle rupture and is effective even near ovulation. Combined estrogen and progestin, also known as the *Yuzpe method* that was developed in the 1970s, utilizes everyday birth control pills as emergency contraception. It is given in 2 doses, 1 dose of 100 mcg of ethinyl estradiol plus 0.5 mg of LNg followed by the same dose 12 hours later. However, this regimen is less effective than UPA or LNg and is also associated with more frequent occurrence of side effects (nausea and vomiting). All ECPs should be taken as soon as possible within 120 hours (5 days) of unprotected intercourse. Both UPA and LNg have similar effectiveness when taken within 3 days; however, UPA has been shown to be more effective than the LNg formulation 3 to 5 days after unprotected sexual intercourse. LNg has an initial efficacy of 94% with subsequent decrease in effectiveness between 72 and 120 hours. The LNg formulation might also be less effective than UPA among obese women. LNg is available over the counter while UPA requires a prescription (Daniels & Abma, 2019).

The copper IUD is another form of emergency contraception. It is the most effective and can remain in place for continued contraception. See the section on IUS for more information.

Regardless of the regimen chosen, menstruation should occur within 21 days. If menstruation does not occur, a pregnancy test is recommended. Providers should take note to counsel women to wait at least 5 days after taking UPA before starting or continuing their hormonal contraception. If a woman opts for a method that would require an appointment with a physician (e.g., DMPA, implants, IUDs), starting it at the same time as ulipristal is an option. Although this could make ulipristal less effective, it is a risk that should be balanced with the risk of not initiating regular contraception (Croke, 2017).

According to the ACOG and the World Health Organization, there are no absolute medical contraindications to the use of emergency contraception with the exception of pregnancy.

Drug Interactions

Any agent that increases GI motility or causes diarrhea may reduce the plasma concentration of ethinyl estradiol by decreasing its absorption. Agents, such as ascorbic acid, that inhibit sulfation of ethinyl estradiol in the GI tract may increase the bioavailability of ethinyl estradiol and lead to an increase in estrogenic adverse effects.

Ethinyl estradiol is metabolized by the cytochrome P-450 (CYP) 3A4 enzyme pathway. Drugs known to induce CYP3A4 (phenytoin, primidone, barbiturates, carbamazepine, ethosuximide, topiramate, methsuximide, rifampin, and griseofulvin) can lead to decreased plasma ethinyl estradiol levels and may cause failure of emergency contraception. Reports suggest that the enterohepatic circulation of ethinyl estradiol is decreased in women taking antibiotics, which may lead to a decrease in systemic concentrations of ethinyl estradiol. Ethinyl estradiol can inhibit microsomal enzymes, which may slow the metabolism of other drugs (i.e., theophylline), increasing their plasma and tissue concentrations thereby increasing the risk of adverse effects. There is a potential interaction between warfarin and LNg given as an emergency contraceptive. The proposed mechanism is the displacement of warfarin by LNg from the F1S binding site of human alpha$_1$-acid glycoprotein, the main transport protein for drugs in the plasma. This potential interaction should be taken into consideration so the patient's international normalized ratio levels can be monitored carefully.

Selecting the Most Appropriate Agent

Before using any of the hormonal regimens, all sexually active patients should receive a gynecologic examination with the Papanicolaou test to observe cervical cytology. They also should have a pregnancy test and a thorough physical examination before they begin use, including blood pressure, weight, and body mass. This is because obese women require higher doses of estrogen and progesterone for efficacy. A lipid panel, including baseline total cholesterol, high-density lipoprotein cholesterol, and triglyceride levels, may be especially important in women with other risk factors for heart disease. Identification of blood glucose control before and after initiating hormonal contraception is important in women with diabetes mellitus. Before copper or LNg-releasing IUD (Mirena®) insertion, bimanual examination and cervical inspection should be performed to determine uterine size and position, as well as to identify cervical or uterine abnormalities that could be a sign of infection or that could prevent IUD insertion. No examinations or tests are needed before using an implant or initiating depot medroxyprogesterone or progestin-only pills (Croke, 2017).

Most women can tolerate up to 735 mcg of ethinyl estradiol for a 28-day cycle. But a 3-month trial should be done to determine tolerability. Most side effects subside after 3 months.

With the wide variety of forms of hormonal contraception, many questions exist about which agent should be used first and for whom. **Table 54.5** addresses some of these issues and is provided as a guide to the prescription of hormonal contraception.

MONITORING PATIENT RESPONSE

Therapeutic drug monitoring of hormonal contraception includes, primarily, monitoring for adverse effects and preventing complications from their use.

In addition to the initial workup and physical examination, it is also important to maintain a high index of suspicion for adverse effects associated with the use of either the estrogen or progesterone components, or both, in women receiving hormonal contraception. It is estimated that 25% to 50% of women discontinue hormonal contraception within the first 12 months of use because of physical side effects. Therefore, it is important to look for these side effects and know how to manage them. **Box 54.1** identifies side effects related to excess estrogen and progesterone.

TABLE 54.5	
Treatment Order for Available Hormonal Contraceptive Agents	
Clinical Scenario	**Therapeutic Options**
Women wish to use hormonal contraception—adolescents; perimenopausal women; and postpartum, nonlactating women with no other medical risks	Any OCP <50 mcg EE either continuous or cyclic
History of: • Smoking and over age 35 • Uncontrolled hypertension • Undiagnosed abnormal vaginal bleeding • Diabetes with vascular complications or more than 20 years' duration • Deep vein thrombosis or pulmonary embolism or history of ischemic heart disease • Headaches with focal neurological symptoms • Breast cancer • Active viral hepatitis or cirrhosis History of cholestasis with OCP use or pregnancy	Consider progestin-only OCPs, Depo-Provera, Implanon, or IUD
Endometriosis	Monophasic continuous therapy
Postpartum, lactating	Progesterone-only minipill
Noncompliance	Depot medroxyprogesterone acetate *or* levonorgestrel subdermal implants
Breakthrough bleeding—first half of cycle	Change to combination pill with higher estrogen content in first half of cycle.
Breakthrough bleeding—second half of cycle	Change to combination pill with higher progestin content in second half of cycle

Data from Zieman, M., Hatcher, R., Cwiak, C., et al. (2010). *A pocket guide to managing contraception.* Tiger, GA: Bridging the Gap Foundation.

EE, ethinyl estradiol; IUD, intrauterine device; OCP, oral contraception pills.

BOX 54.1 Causes of Side Effects of Hormone Contraception

Too Much Estrogen
Heavy bleeding
Cystic breasts
Breast enlargement
Breast tenderness
Dysmenorrhea
Bloating
Premenstrual edema
Gastrointestinal symptoms
Premenstrual headache
Premenstrual irritability
Cervical exstrophy

Too Little Estrogen
Bleeding (spotting) early in cycle
Too light bleeding
Bleeding throughout the cycle
Amenorrhea

Too Much Progestin
Increased appetite
Candidiasis
Depression
Fatigue
Cervicitis

Too Little Progestin
Bleeding for fewer days
Bleeding (spotting) late in the cycle
Heavy bleeding
Delayed withdrawal bleeding
Bloating
Dysmenorrhea
Premenstrual edema
Gastrointestinal symptoms
Premenstrual headache
Premenstrual irritability

Side effects due to insufficient estrogen and progesterone, such as breakthrough bleeding, also may occur. In the first half of the menstrual cycle, breakthrough bleeding is likely due to insufficient estrogen; in the second half of the cycle, it is likely due to insufficient progesterone. Therefore, practitioners can simplify management by adding supplemental estrogen or progesterone when appropriate or changing to a new regimen with higher estrogen or progesterone as necessary.

If there is breakthrough bleeding early in the cycle, a change to a pill with more estrogen but the same level of progestin is appropriate. Breakthrough bleeding late in the cycle requires a pill with more progestin. Periods with heavy bleeding and bloating indicate a lower dosage of estrogen is needed since increased estrogen causes the uterine lining to thicken which causes heavier bleeding. Elevated blood pressure and depression indicate the need for a lower progestin dose.

PATIENT EDUCATION

Poor outcomes secondary to the use of hormonal contraception may include treatment failures, potentially life-threatening side effects, or side effects beyond those commonly expected. Treatment failures frequently are related to compliance with the regimen. In the case of combination OCs, guidelines exist, which explain what to do in the event of a missed pill (or pills)

TABLE 54.6 Guidelines for Missed Pills

Number of Missed Pills	Recommended Action
One pill	Take missed pill as soon as possible and resume schedule; backup method of contraception is not necessary.
Two 30 to 35 mg pills	Take missed pill as soon as possible and resume schedule; backup method of contraception is not necessary.
Two 20 mg pills	Follow directions for more than two pills.
More than two pills	Take pill and continue taking a pill daily. Use condom or abstinence for 7 days. If missed in week 3, finish active pills in current pack and start a new pack the next day (skip current inactive pills). If missed pills in first week and had sex, use EC and then resume taking pills the next day after EC.

EC, emergency contraception.

to help ensure continued contraceptive efficacy. **Table 54.6** illustrates these guidelines. Another cause of treatment failure includes drug interactions that may affect the efficacy of the hormonal contraceptive. Agents proven to reduce circulating estrogen concentrations, therefore affecting efficacy, include rifampin, phenytoin, and carbamazepine. Recommendations to reduce the risk of treatment failure relative to these agents include the use of higher daily doses of estrogen (50 mg ethinyl estradiol) or use of progesterone-only options.

Patients can best avoid life-threatening side effects of the hormonal contraceptives, especially combination OCs, if they follow the contraindications to their use. **Box 54.2** identifies

BOX 54.2 Absolute Contraindications to the Use of Combination Oral Contraceptive Pills

- Thrombophlebitis, thromboembolic disorders, cerebral vascular disease, coronary occlusion*
- Markedly impaired liver function
- Breast cancer (known or suspected)
- Abnormal vaginal bleeding in the absence of a diagnosed cause
- Pregnancy
- Smokers older than age 35

*Includes a past history or other situations that may put the patient at risk for developing these conditions.

absolute contraindications to the use of combination OCs. In addition, the acronym *ACHES* is useful in teaching patients about the potential severe side effects that may occur with the use of OCPs. Clinicians should instruct patients to call their primary care provider if any of the following occurs:

- Severe **A**bdominal pain (indicative of gallbladder disease)
- **C**hest pain (potentially related to pulmonary embolism or MI)
- **H**eadache (relative to stroke, hypertension, or migraine)
- **E**ye problems (relative to stroke or hypertension)
- **S**evere leg pain (indicative of deep vein thrombosis)

It is crucial to relay this information to the patient. Early recognition and treatment of these adverse events save lives.

Many women are unaware of the health risks and side effects of the various forms of hormonal contraception. Likewise, 25% of women are unaware that the use of combination contraceptive agents imparts benefits in addition to the prevention of pregnancy. Some of these benefits include a 50% to 60% reduction in ovarian cancer risk with 5 years of use. This benefit persists for up to 10 or more years after discontinuation. In addition, 50% to 60% reductions in PID risk and 30% to 50% reductions in the occurrence of menstrual disorders have been observed with combination agents.

Another benefit of OCPs is their use in other indications. For example, 60% to 94% of women with endometriosis who

---

BOX 54.3 Noncontraceptive Benefits of Combined Oral Contraceptives

- Decreased iron deficiency anemia
- Decreased dysmenorrhea
- Decreased dysfunctional uterine bleeding
- Decreased incidence of ovarian cysts
- Improvement in acne
- Decreased incidence of pelvic inflammatory disease
- Decreased risk of osteoporosis
- Decreased incidence of endometrial cancer
- Decreased risk of benign breast disease

Several Web sites contain patient information on contraception: www.contraception.net, http://www.nlm.nih.gov/medlineplus/birthcontrol.html, and www.plannedparenthood.org.

---

are treated with daily monophasic contraceptive agents for 6 to 9 months experience symptomatic improvement. After treatment, a 5% to 10% annual recurrence rate of the disease is noted. Benefits of contraceptive agents are listed in **Box 54.3**.

CASE STUDY 1

R.M. is a 36-year-old woman who comes into the clinic requesting a prescription for oral contraception (OCP). She does not have any medical problems or a family history of venous thromboembolism. However, she reports currently smoking about a pack of cigarettes (20 cigarettes/pack) per day. Previously, R.M. was smoking up to 2 packs of cigarettes daily, but over the past month, she has been chewing approximately 8 pieces of 4-mg nicotine gum per day to help decrease her cigarette smoking.

1. Before prescribing an OCP regimen, what tests or examinations would you like to perform?
2. What is the appropriate OCP recommendation for R.M.?

Bibliography

Starred references are cited in the text.

Ahern, R., Frattarelli, L., Delto, J., et al. (2010). Knowledge and awareness of emergency contraception in adolescents. *Journal of Pediatric and Adolescent Gynecology, 23*(5), 273–278.

Allsworth, J. E., Secura, G. M., Zhao, Q., et al. (2013). The impact of emotional, physical, and sexual abuse on contraceptive method selection and discontinuation. *American Journal of Public Health, 103*(10), 1857–1864.

Bonnema, R., Mcnamara, M., & Spencer, A. (2010). Contraceptive choices in women with underlying medical conditions. *American Family Physician, 82*(6), 621–628.

*Bosak, M., Słowik, A., Iwańska, A., et al. (2019). Co-medication and potential drug interactions among patients with epilepsy. *Seizure, 66*, 47–52.

*Croke, L. M. (2017). CDC updates recommendations for contraceptive use. *American Family Physician.* January 15, 2017. www.aafp.org/afp/2017/0115/p125

Curtis, K. M., Jatlaoui, T. C., Tepper, N. K., et al. (2016). U.S. selected practice recommendations for contraceptive use, 2016. *MMWF Recommendations and Reports, 65*(4), 1–66.

*Daniels, K., & Abma, J. C. (2019). Products – Data Briefs – Number 327 – December 2018. *Centers for Disease Control and Prevention.* February 14, 2019. www.cdc.gov/nchs/products/databriefs/db327.htm

*Dickinson, B. D., Altman, R. D., Nielsen, N. H., et al. (2001). Council on Scientific Affairs, American Medical Association: Drug interactions between oral contraceptives and antibiotics. *Obstetrics & Gynecology, 98*(5 pt 1), 853–860.

*Espey, E., Ogburn, T., & Fotieo, D. (2008). Contraception: What every internist should know. *Medical Clinics of North America, 92*(5), 1037–1058.

*Finer, L. B., & Zolna, M. R. (2016). Declines in unintended pregnancy in the United States, 2008–2011. *The New England Journal of Medicine, 374*(9), 843–652.

*Free the Pill. (2019). *What's the Law in Your State?* Cambridge, MA: Ibis Reproductive Health; 26 June 2019. http://freethepill.org/statepolicies

*Isley, M., & Allen, R. H. (2019). Over-the-counter access to hormonal contraception. *ACOG Committee Opinion*, *134*(4), e96–102.

*Mayo Clinic Staff. (2018). Rhythm Method for Natural Family Planning. *Mayo Clinic*, Mayo Foundation for Medical Education and Research, January 6, 2018, www.mayoclinic.org/tests-procedures/rhythm-method/about/pac-20390918

Mosher, W. D., & Jones, J. (2010). Use of contraception in the United States: 1982–2008. *Vital and Health Statistics*, *29*, 1–44.

*Planned Parenthood. (2020). What is the Cervical Mucus Method?: Cycle, stages & chart. *Planned Parenthood*, www.plannedparenthood.org/learn/birth-control/fertility-awareness/whats-cervical-mucus-method-fams

*Progesterone Only Contraceptives. (2015). *The Oncofertility Consortium*. oncofertility.northwestern.edu/resources/progesterone-only-contraceptives

Secretary's advisory committee on National Health Promotion and Disease Prevention Objectives for 2020. (2010). *Evidence-based clinical and public health: Generating and applying the evidence*. Washington, DC: CDC.

*Simmons, K. B., Haddad, L. B., Nanda, K., et al. (2018). Drug interactions between rifamycin antibiotics and hormonal contraception: A systematic review. *BJOG*, *125*(7), 804–811.

*Singh, S., Remez, L., Sedgh, G., et al. (2018). Abortion worldwide 2017: Uneven progress and unequal access. https://www.guttmacher.org/report/abortion-worldwide-2017

Spencer, A., Bonnema, R., & McNamara, M. (2009). Helping women choose appropriate hormonal contraception: Update on risks, benefits and indications. *American Journal of Medicine*, *122*(6), 497–506.

*Speroff, L., & Darney, P. (2000). *A clinical guide for contraception* (3rd ed.). Philadelphia, PA: Lippincott Williams & Wilkins.

Steinauer, J., & Autry, A. (2007). Extended cycle combined hormonal contraception. *Obstetrics and Gynecology Clinics*, *34*(1), 43–55.

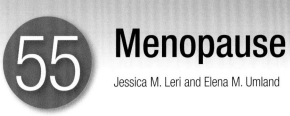

55 Menopause

Jessica M. Leri and Elena M. Umland

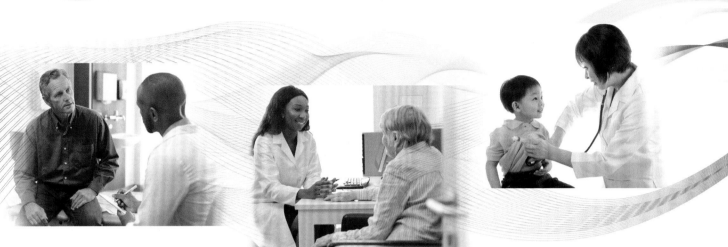

INTRODUCTION

Menopause is the permanent cessation of menstruation resulting from loss of ovarian function. It is an endocrinopathy resulting from failure of the ovary to produce estrogen. Menopause is not an acute condition but rather a gradual transition from perimenopause to menopause and finally postmenopause. The menopausal transition is defined as that period of time from the first changes in the menstrual cycle to the final menstrual period (FMP). The menopausal transition typically begins about 2 years prior to the FMP, however, this time frame varies from woman to woman (Harlow et al., 2012).

Healthy women typically spend one third of their lives in a menopausal state. According to the North American Menopause Society (NAMS), the postwar baby boom of the 1940s and 1950s led to an absolute increase in the over-50 population (NAMS, 2010). Every day, over 6,000 women enter menopause. American women today can expect to live beyond age 80. The mean age of menopause in the United States is 51 years, with a range of 40 to 58 years. Approximately 4% of women experience their FMP before age 40. Overall, women can expect to spend approximately 30 years postmenopause. Factors that contribute to menopause occurring at an earlier-than-average age include a history of irregular menses before the perimenopause, African-American heritage, cigarette smoking, and weight reduction diets and hysterectomy.

The increased incidence of chronic disease in postmenopausal women appears to be influenced by decreased levels of estrogen or progesterone. Following menopause, women can expect to experience an increased probability of developing coronary heart disease (CHD), stroke, hip fracture, breast cancer, colorectal cancer, and endometrial cancer. Furthermore, postmenopausal women have a greater increased risk of Alzheimer disease over men. While efforts in preventing these disease states as well as diagnosing them in a timely manner and effectively managing them are often the focus of health care providers, it is the management of the symptoms associated with menopause directly, namely, vasomotor symptoms (VMS) and urogenital symptoms, that is the focus of this chapter.

PATHOPHYSIOLOGY

Menopause involves an age-related loss of ovarian function and a resulting decrease in estrogen secretion by the ovarian follicular unit. The ovary produces 17-beta-estradiol, the major circulating estrogen. At birth, approximately 1 to 2 million ovarian follicles are present. By age 45, the number drops to approximately 10,000.

During the menopausal transition, the woman herself notices changes in her menstrual pattern. This may include a change in the time span from the first day of one menstrual period to the first day of the next (variable by greater than 7 days from what was previously considered normal for the patient); the amount of menstrual flow and the number of days of bleeding may vary from month to month, increasing or decreasing. It is expected that later in the menopausal transition, cycles become skipped with phases of amenorrhea lasting 60 days or more (Harlow et al., 2012).

Amenorrhea in menopause results from the remaining follicles becoming resistant to the effect of follicle-stimulating hormone (FSH). The ovaries have a large number of follicles. These atrophy during the reproductive years at steady state rate until there are too few to produce significant amounts of estradiol. During perimenopause (the time frame inclusive of the menopause transition and 1 year following the FMP), estradiol and progesterone production declines. The reduction in hormone levels reduces the negative feedback loop of the hypothalamic–pituitary system, which leads to a rise in FSH levels.

Estrogen has an impact on many body tissues and systems: bone, teeth, brain, eyes, vasomotor, heart, colon, and urogenital. Ovarian failure causes changes in many organ systems, but the changes are subtle and usually not distressing to women. The most noticeable change is amenorrhea. This is the change in reproductive function that all women experience. Women are considered postmenopausal following their FMP.

Morbidity in postmenopausal women is largely the result of alterations in hormone production, notably the decline in estradiol production. During the menopause transition and early postmenopause, women seek treatment for the related occurrences of VMS insomnia, mood changes, and urogenital symptoms. The most commonly noted symptoms are the VMS. Risk factors associated with the occurrence and severity of VMS include obesity, cigarette smoking, depression, anxiety, lack of exercise, low socioeconomic status, and race, specifically African-American women (Thurston & Joffe, 2011). The occurrence of VMS is felt to be due to a disruption of the thermoregulatory circuitry that functions under the influence of consistent concentrations of the neurotransmitter's serotonin and norepinephrine. Changes in estradiol levels have been associated with fluctuations in serotonin and norepinephrine, hence the link between declining estradiol concentrations and the presence of VMS (Deecher & Dorries, 2007; Rossaminth & Ruebberdt, 2009). According to the American College of Obstetricians and Gynecologists (ACOG), approximately 87% of women experience these symptoms on a daily basis, occurring in the form of hot flashes or flushes, perspiration, chills, and clamminess (ACOG, 2014). These are transient sensations typically lasting from 1 to 5 minutes. Of women experiencing VMS, approximately 33% experience more than 10 hot flashes per day. They are the most annoying consequences of menopause for many women, often affecting mood and disrupting sleep.

There are also changes in the genitourinary system as a result of menopause. And it is estimated that the symptoms resulting from these changes affect up to 40% of midlife women (ACOG, 2014). The vagina, vulva, urethra, and bladder have a large number of estrogen receptors. As estrogen concentrations decline, the potential for urogenital symptoms increases. The vulva loses collagen, adipose tissue, and the ability to retain water. There is a shortening and narrowing of the vagina; the walls become thin and pale and elasticity decreases. Vaginal secretions decrease, thereby decreasing vaginal lubrication. The urethra may become irritated as well. Vulvovaginal atrophy in addition to other estrogen-deficiency-related changes to the labia, vagina, urethra, and bladder is referred to as the *genitourinary syndrome of menopause* (GSM) (NAMS, 2017). Unlike VMS, which do tend to improve and subside over time, menopause-related genitourinary symptoms such as vaginal dryness, itching and burning, and subsequent dyspareunia tend to be chronic and progressive and are unlikely to resolve over time.

INITIATING DRUG THERAPY

Goals of Drug Therapy

In managing symptoms related to menopause, notably VMS and menopause-related genitourinary symptoms, the goal is reduction in symptom severity and frequency and a subsequent improvement in quality of life (QOL). There are many treatment options available including regimens containing estrogen with or without the addition of a progestin. There are also a variety of nonhormonal options such as the selective serotonin reuptake inhibitors (SSRIs) and gabapentin, to name just two. Newer products such as estrogen agonist/antagonist agents and tissue selective estrogen complexes (TSECs) have also been recently added to the list of options. Regardless of the treatment regimen, the goals remain the same—minimizing menopause symptoms of estrogen deficiency. Contrary to the suggested findings of early observational studies, and subsequent to prospective, randomized trials, it is no longer acceptable to use estrogen with or without the addition of a progestin to prevent long-term chronic conditions, particularly CHD (Moyer, 2013).

Hormone Therapy

Estrogen decreases the frequency of night sweats and periods of wakefulness during the night, reduces sleep latency (time between going to bed and falling asleep), and improves sleep in postmenopausal women with sleeping difficulty. Estrogen regimens reduce frequency and intensity of hot flashes by 75% and 87%, respectively (ACOG, 2014). No other method provides such consistent and significant relief of menopausal symptoms as estrogen. Hormone therapy (HT) generally refers to treatment with estrogen and progestin. In women with a uterus, the combination of estrogen and progestin should be used together. In women without an intact uterus, estrogen is used alone. See **Table 55.1** for a summary overview of select HT and related products to treat menopausal symptoms.

TABLE 55.1

Overview of Available Hormone Therapy and Related Agents to Treat Menopausal Symptoms

Generic (Trade) Name and Dosage	Side Effects	Contraindications	Special Considerations
Oral Menopause Hormone Therapy			
CEE (Premarin) Usual daily dose 0.3–0.65 mg Doses available: 0.3, 0.45, and 0.625 mg	Nausea, vomiting, breakthrough bleeding, edema, weight changes, swollen/tender breasts, hypertension, depression, hair loss, changes in libido, venous thromboembolic events	Estrogen-dependent neoplasia Thrombophlebitis or thromboembolic disorder Pregnancy Undiagnosed vaginal bleeding Uncontrolled hypertension Acute liver disease	May cause GI upset, may take with food Treatment should occur at the lowest effective dose for the shortest duration as needed
Estradiol (Estrace) 1 mg/d	Nausea, vomiting, breakthrough bleeding, edema, weight changes, swollen/tender breasts, hypertension, depression, hair loss, changes in libido, venous thromboembolic events	Estrogen-dependent neoplasia Thrombophlebitis or thromboembolic disorder Pregnancy Undiagnosed vaginal bleeding Uncontrolled hypertension Acute liver disease	May cause GI upset, may take with food Treatment should occur at the lowest effective dose for the shortest duration as needed
Combination Products			
Estradiol/norethindrone acetate (Activella, Amabelz, Mimvey, Lopreeza) Doses: 0.5 mg estrogen/0.1 mg progestogen 1 mg estrogen/0.5 mg progestogen (Mimvey) 1 tablet daily	Nausea, vomiting, breakthrough bleeding, edema, weight changes, swollen/tender breasts, hypertension, depression, hair loss, changes in libido, venous thromboembolic events	Estrogen-dependent neoplasia Thrombophlebitis or thromboembolic disorder Pregnancy Undiagnosed vaginal bleeding Acute liver disease	May cause GI upset, may take with food Treatment should occur at the lowest effective dose for the shortest duration as needed
Estradiol/drospirenone (Angeliq) Doses: 1 mg estrogen/0.5 mg progestogen, 0.5 mg estogren/0.25 mg progestogen 1 tablet daily	Breakthrough bleeding, abdominal pain, gastrointestinal pain, venous thromboembolic events, swollen/tender breasts	Estrogen-dependent neoplasia Thrombophlebitis or thromboembolic disorder Pregnancy Undiagnosed vaginal bleeding Acute liver disease	
Estradiol/levonorgestrel (Climara Pro) Dose: 0.045 mg estrogen/0.015 mg progestogen 1 patch weekly	Vaginal hemorrhage, application site reaction, back pain, swollen/tender breasts	Estrogen-dependent neoplasia Thrombophlebitis or thromboembolic disorder Pregnancy Undiagnosed vaginal bleeding Acute liver disease	Apply to clean, dry area on lower abdomen, hips, or buttocks (not breast or waistline)
Estradiol/norethindrone acetate (CombiPatch) Doses: 0.05 mg estogren/0.14 mg progestogen, 0.05 mg estrogen/0.25 mg progestogen 1 patch twice weekly	Breakthrough bleeding, abdominal pain, gastrointestinal pain, venous thromboembolic events, swollen/tender breasts	Estrogen-dependent neoplasia Thrombophlebitis or thromboembolic disorder Pregnancy Undiagnosed vaginal bleeding Acute liver disease	Apply to clean, dry area on lower abdomen, hips, or buttocks (not breast or waistline)
Ethinyl estradiol/norethindrone acetate (Femhrt, Jinteli, Fyavolv, Jevantique Lo) Doses: 2.5 mcg estrogen/0.5 mg progestogen, 5mcg estrogen/1 mg progestogen 1 tablet daily	Breakthrough bleeding, abdominal pain, gastrointestinal pain, venous thromboembolic events, swollen/tender breasts	Estrogen-dependent neoplasia Thrombophlebitis or thromboembolic disorder Pregnancy Undiagnosed vaginal bleeding Acute liver disease	

(Continued)

TABLE 55.1

Overview of Available Hormone Therapy and Related Agents to Treat Menopausal Symptoms (*Continued*)

Generic (Trade) Name and Dosage	Side Effects	Contraindications	Special Considerations
Conjugated estrogens/ medroxyprogesterone acetate (Premphase) Dose: 0.625 mg estrogen with 5 mg progestogen 0.625 mg/d for 14 days; then 0.625 mg and 5 mg/d for 14 days	Breakthrough bleeding, abdominal pain, gastrointestinal pain, venous thromboembolic events, swollen/tender breasts	Estrogen-dependent neoplasia Thrombophlebitis or thromboembolic disorder Pregnancy Undiagnosed vaginal bleeding Acute liver disease	Women recently menopausal (< 2 years) with a uterus may benefit from cyclic treatment versus continuous. Continuous may increase risk of unscheduled bleeding.
Conjugated estrogens/ medroxyprogesterone acetate (Prempro) Doses: 0.625 mg estrogen with 2.5 or 5 mg progestogen, 0.3 or 0.45 mg estrogen with 1.5 mg progestogen 1 tablet daily	Breakthrough bleeding, abdominal pain, gastrointestinal pain, venous thromboembolic events, swollen/tender breasts	Estrogen-dependent neoplasia Thrombophlebitis or thromboembolic disorder Pregnancy Undiagnosed vaginal bleeding Acute liver disease	Same as above
Conjugated estrogens and bazedoxifene (Duavee) Doses: 0.45 mg/20 mg, 0.625 mg/20 mg	Breakthrough bleeding, abdominal pain, gastrointestinal pain, venous thromboembolic events, swollen/tender breasts	Estrogen-dependent neoplasia Thrombophlebitis or thromboembolic disorder Pregnancy Undiagnosed vaginal bleeding Acute liver disease	Addition of bazedoxifene further minimizes the bone loss observed with estrogen and reduces the risk for developing endometrial hyperplasia
Esterified estrogen 1.25 mg and methyltestosterone 2.5 mg (Estratest) Esterified estrogen 0.625 mg and methyltestosterone 1.25 mg (Estratest H.S.) Taken daily for 3 wk and then 1 wk off	Liver function changes, nausea, breakthrough bleeding, edema, weight gain, hypertension, depression, intolerance to contact lenses, changes in libido, virilization, jaundice, gallbladder disease	Breast or endometrial cancer, undiagnosed genital bleeding, thromboembolic disease, pregnancy, lactation	Report any adverse events immediately May take at bedtime to prevent nausea
Progestins			
Medroxyprogesterone acetate (Amen, Curretab, Cycrin, Provera) Dose: 2.5–10 mg either daily or cyclic	Vision changes, migraine, porphyria, depression, insomnia, jaundice, nausea, thrombophlebitis, pulmonary embolism, increased blood pressure, breakthrough bleeding, breast tenderness, rash, hirsutism, increased weight, decreased glucose tolerance	Thrombophlebitis, hepatic disease, breast cancer, undiagnosed vaginal bleeding, pregnancy, lactation Caution in epilepsy, migraine, asthma, cardiac dysfunction	Report any adverse events immediately May take at bedtime to prevent nausea
Norethindrone acetate (Aygestin) Dose: 2.5 – 10 mg/d	Vision changes, migraine, porphyria, depression, insomnia, jaundice, nausea, thrombophlebitis, pulmonary embolism, increased blood pressure, breakthrough bleeding, breast tenderness, rash, hirsutism, increased weight	Thrombophlebitis, hepatic disease, breast cancer, undiagnosed vaginal bleeding, pregnancy, lactation Caution in epilepsy, migraine, asthma, cardiac dysfunction	Report any adverse events immediately May cause GI upset, may take with food

TABLE 55.1

Overview of Available Hormone Therapy and Related Agents to Treat Menopausal Symptoms (*Continued*)

Generic (Trade) Name and Dosage	Side Effects	Contraindications	Special Considerations
Transdermal Menopause Hormone Therapy			
Estradiol (Alora, Climara, Minivelle, Vivelle Dot, Menostar) Change transdermal patch once a week Climara—0.025, 0.0375, 0.05, 0.06, 0.075, 0.1 Menostar—0.014 Change transdermal patch twice a week Alora— 0.025, 0.05, 0.075, 0.1 mg/d Minivelle—0.025, 0.0375, 0.05, 0.075, 0.1 Vivelle Dot—0.025, 0.0375, 0.05, 0.075, 0.1 mg/d	Irritation at application site, headache, breakthrough bleeding, nausea, abdominal cramps	Undiagnosed abnormal vaginal bleeding, thromboembolic disorder, pregnancy, breast or estrogen-dependent tumor	Apply to clean, dry area on lower abdomen, hips, or buttocks (not breast or waistline) Rotate application sites Use 3 wk on and 1 wk off in patient with intact uterus; continuous in patient without uterus Menostar is only for prevention of postmenopausal osteoporosis
Estradiol transdermal gel (Divigel, Elestrin, EstroGel) Divigel 0.1%—0.25, 0.5, or 1g of gel Elestrin 0.06%—0.87 g/d (1 pump) or 1.7 g/d (2 pumps) Estrogel 0.06%—1.25 g/d (1 pump)	Breakthrough bleeding, abdominal pain, gastrointestinal pain, venous thromboembolic events, swollen/tender breasts, application site reaction	Undiagnosed abnormal vaginal bleeding, thromboembolic disorder, pregnancy, breast or estrogen-dependent tumor	Divigel should be applied to one leg daily, alternating sites each day Elestrin pump must be primed prior to use. Apply to upper arm Estrogel should be applied from wrist to shoulder
Other Related Options			
Ospemifene (Osphena) 60 mg daily	Vaginal discharge, hot flashes, muscle spasms	Undiagnosed, abnormal genital bleeding, known or suspected estrogen-dependent neoplasia, a history of or active thromboembolic disease	As it is an antagonist in breast cancer, it does not have the same risk as estrogen The only product in its class approved in the United States for dyspareunia associated with vulvovaginal atrophy
Vaginal Hormones			
Estradiol 0.01% (Estrace Vaginal Cream) Initially 2–4 g/d for 1–2 wk, then 1–2 g/d for 1–2 wk; maintenance dose: 1 g 1–3 times/wk (3 wk on and 1 wk off)	Uterine bleeding, vaginal candidiasis	Breast or estrogen-dependent cancer, thrombophlebitis, thrombophilic disorders, undiagnosed genital bleeding, pregnancy, lactation, impaired liver function	Need to take progestin if uterus present
Estring (vaginal ring) 2mg ring into the vagina; replaced every 90 d	Headache, leukorrhea, back pain, urinary tract infection, vaginitis, vaginal pain, abdominal pain, bacterial growth	Breast or estrogen-dependent cancer, thrombophlebitis, thrombophilic disorders, undiagnosed genital bleeding, pregnancy, lactation, impaired liver function	Remove while treating vaginitis Re-evaluate every 3–6 mo
Femring 0.05 mg/24hr, 0.1mg/24h	Headache, urinary tract infection, vaginitis, vaginal pain	Breast or estrogen-dependent cancer, thrombophlebitis, thrombophilic disorders, undiagnosed genital bleeding, pregnancy, lactation, impaired liver function	Dose is released daily for 3 months

(Continued)

TABLE 55.1

Overview of Available Hormone Therapy and Related Agents to Treat Menopausal Symptoms (*Continued*)

Generic (Trade) Name and Dosage	Side Effects	Contraindications	Special Considerations
Premarin vaginal cream 0.625 mg/g 0.5–2 g/d	Nausea, vomiting, breakthrough bleeding, edema, weight changes, swollen/tender breasts, hypertension, depression, hair loss, changes in libido	Breast or estrogen-dependent cancer, thrombophlebitis, thrombophilic disorders, undiagnosed genital bleeding, pregnancy, lactation, impaired liver function	Therapeutic regimen consists of 3 wk on therapy and 1 wk off

CEE, conjugated equine estrogen; GI, gastrointestinal.

QOL data have been reported for the estrogen plus progestin arm of the Women's Health Initiative (WHI). Approximately 16,600 women completed surveys at baseline and year 1. About 1,500 women completed surveys at year 3. At year 1, there was statistically significant improvement in sleep disturbance, physical functioning, and bodily pain as compared with the placebo group. However, the differences were so small that there is a question about clinical significance. There was no significant difference at year 3. In women reporting moderate to severe VMS, those taking estrogen plus progestin had significant improvement in the severity of hot flashes and night sweats (WHI, 2002). Furthermore, the Society for Women's Health Research unanimously recommends that significant improvement in health-related QOL and global QOL be provided via HT; the greatest benefits are observed when started in a timely fashion related to the onset of menopausal symptoms (Davies et al., 2013).

In the women's health, osteoporosis, progestin, estrogen trial, healthy postmenopausal women aged 40 to 65 were randomly assigned to treatment with conjugated equine estrogen (CEE) alone (0.625, 0.45, or 0.3 mg daily), CEE plus medroxyprogesterone acetate (MPA) (0.625/2.5, 0.45/2.5, 0.45/1.5, or 0.3/1.5 mg daily), or a placebo. Over 13 cycles, women in all active treatment groups had a significant reduction in VMS. In women taking CEE alone, benefit increased with increased dosage. In women taking CEE plus MPA, the benefit was comparable with all doses (Utian et al., 2001).

If HT is prescribed solely for vaginal symptoms, health care providers are advised to consider the use of topical vaginal products (gel or cream applied locally) secondary to reduced systemic effects as compared to oral or transdermal formulations.

The slight decrease in testosterone production that accompanies menopause can cause a significant decrease or complete loss of libido in some women. For these women, testosterone can be added to HT in doses of 1.25 to 2.5 mg methyltestosterone. The adverse events of testosterone in these doses are hirsutism, voice change, and a decrease in the high-density lipoprotein cholesterol level. Long-term use is associated with the risk of hepatocellular neoplasm, increased edema, and possible elevation of cholesterol level. The only indication for treatment is severe vasomotor disturbances and decreased libido. The most frequent treatment choice is either Estratest,

which is 1.25 mg esterified estrogen and 2.5 mg methyltestosterone, or Estratest H.S., which is 0.625 mg esterified estrogen and 1.25 mg methyltestosterone. Estratest H.S. may be used safely as long as baseline lipid levels are normal. Estratest, with its 1.25 mg esterified estrogen, is a high dose of estrogen and should be used only for short periods.

HT started after age 65 does not improve memory and, in fact, has been observed to increase the risk for developing dementia (Coker et al., 2010). While preliminary data suggest that there may be cognitive benefits when HT is used in younger women, it has not been well studied. The WHI memory study of younger women found no long-term posttreatment effects on cognitive function and no changes in cognitive function when HT was prescribed to women aged 50 to 54 (Espeland et al., 2017).

Mechanism of Action

HT with estrogen minimizes VMS and genitourinary symptoms related to estrogen deficiency. Estrogen assists in temperature control that occurs in the anterior hypothalamus. Furthermore, estrogen receptors are located throughout the entire female genitourinary tract. Increasing the estrogen levels that declined via menopause through estrogen replacement helps to improve the symptoms of deficiency. Progestins are added to systemic estrogen formulations (oral and transdermal) in women who have a uterus. The unopposed use of estrogen in these women can lead to endometrial hyperplasia, increasing the risk for developing endometrial cancer. However, progestins may increase the risk of breast cancer more than that observed with estrogen alone (further discussed under adverse events).

Dosage

Several systemic estrogen and progestin formulations (oral and transdermal) are available, and there is no strong evidence that one formulation is superior to another relative to the impact on VMS or genitourinary symptoms. Hormones delivered via a transdermal patch are associated with a lower risk of venous thromboembolism (VTE) compared to oral formulations. A reasonable starting dose of estrogen for women who are having hot flashes is 0.025 mg of transdermal estradiol, 0.5 mg of oral estradiol, or 0.3 mg of CEE. The transdermal and vaginal routes of administration of estrogen avoid first-pass hepatic metabolism and may be the reason for which reduced thromboembolic risk (VTE and stroke) is observed. In relation, there is not an increase in C-reactive protein (perhaps contributing to this lower risk of VTE) seen with the non-oral products as is observed with oral therapy. However, no randomized controlled trials to support this concept have been published to date.

When considering the use of vaginal estrogen products, especially for the management of genitourinary symptoms, it is important to note that 10% to 15% of systemic estrogen users may not achieve adequate relief of their symptoms such that additional low-dose vaginal products can be added (NAMS, 2013). For genitourinary symptoms including vulvovaginal atrophy, recurrent urinary tract infections, and overactive bladder, low-dose vaginal estrogen is very effective; 80% to 90% efficacy is noted with vaginal products as compared to 75% efficacy with systemic estrogen formulations. Vaginal formulations are available as vaginal rings (7.5 mcg estradiol released daily over 90 days), vaginal tablets, and vaginal creams. The vaginal tablets contain 10 mcg estradiol and should be dosed one tablet daily for 2 weeks and then one tablet twice weekly thereafter. The vaginal creams contain 0.1 mg active estradiol per 1 g dose. The vaginal creams are dosed 2 to 4 g of cream vaginally per day for 1 to 2 weeks followed by 1 g of cream vaginally one to three times per week. Unlike the systemic estrogen products, the vaginal formulations appear safe alone (in the absence of a progestin) relative to endometrial hyperplasia and endometrial cancer risk; however, long-term data are lacking. Overall, the benefits of these products are dose dependent and patient specific.

In addition, and during the menopause transition in particular, low-dose oral contraceptives can be used to prevent and control symptoms until the patient reaches menopause and to ensure prevention of conception because these women are still fertile. To determine when, in fact, the patient taking oral contraceptives is postmenopausal—so that alternative treatment regimens can be considered—FSH levels can be determined on the last hormone-free day of the oral contraceptive package.

The postmenopausal estrogen–progestin intervention (PEPI) trial showed that CEE with cyclic micronized progesterone had the best lipid profile of any of the combined regimens. Micronized progesterone and norethindrone acetate (NETA) have better side effect profiles than MPA and should be considered when choosing a progestin (PEPI Writing Group, 1995).

Time Frame for Response and Treatment Duration

In the past, it was recommended that HT should be used at the lowest effective dose and for the shortest duration possible. The new concept is "appropriate dose, duration, regimen and route of administration" (NAMS, 2017, p. 742). Personal preferences, QOL, benefits, and risks should be considered when determining duration of treatment. Improvement in symptoms may be realized over a short period of time, from days to weeks. Symptom improvement is dose related. Owing to the long-term effects such as increased risk of breast cancer, CHD, and VTE, the duration of HT should be individualized looking at patients' risk, whether it be personal or familial. Women with premature menopause who are candidates for

HT can use this treatment until the median age of menopause, 52 years, with longer treatment considered, if needed, for symptom management (NAMS, 2017). Women 59 years and younger, whose onset of menopause has been within the past 10 years and who have no contraindications for HT use, benefit outweighs the risk for VMS at women at an elevated risk of bone loss or fracture (NAMS, 2017). Women over the age of 60 or those who initiate HT greater than 10 or 20 years after menopause onset have a less favorable benefit–risk ratio. There is a greater absolute risk of CHD, stroke, VTE, and dementia (NAMS, 2017).

Contraindications

The WHI was a large, 8- to 10-year study of healthy, postmenopausal women, with a randomized controlled component of 27,347 postmenopausal women, aged 50 to 79 years (WHI Writing Group, 2002). They were randomized to HT (estrogen alone, estrogen plus progestin) or placebo. The estrogen used was continuous-combined CEE 0.625 mg daily and 2.5 mg MPA daily. The estrogen plus progestin arm was stopped early (after about 5.2 years). This group also had increased risk of coronary events, stroke, pulmonary embolism, and invasive breast cancer. The thought is that because there was an increased incidence of invasive breast cancer, HT promotes the growth of existing breast cancer rather than causing cancer. There was a reduced risk of colorectal cancer and hip fractures. Many of the risks appeared in year 1 (coronary and VTE events) and year 2 (stroke). It was determined based on the data that the risk–benefit profile of estrogen plus progestin was such that its use for primary prevention of chronic conditions was not validated and it should not be prescribed to prevent chronic conditions. The study was stopped in 2002. Poststopping, and representing 13 years of cumulative follow-up for the WHI, there continues to be (1) lack of support for the use of HT for chronic disease prevention and (2) acknowledgment that the lowest risks of long-term negative effects occur in younger women with hysterectomy receiving CEE alone. Additional subanalyses focusing on the younger cohort of the WHI (estrogen alone or HT) have failed to find adverse cardiac outcomes among this subset. In fact, women in their 50s who took estrogen appear to have less coronary artery calcification than controls (Manson et al., 2013).

Box 55.1 identifies specific contraindications to the use of HT in postmenopausal women; in addition, oral contraceptives are contraindicated in smokers older than 35 years of age.

Adverse Events

The routine physical examination for a postmenopausal woman should include the patient's measured height, a gynecologic examination, and clinical breast examination. Investigative studies should include a pregnancy test, mammogram, and Papanicolaou (Pap) smear. Conditions that predispose women to increased risk of endometrial cancer include a lifelong history of irregular menses, polycystic ovary disease, or a recent history of irregular menses occurring closer than 21 days apart or menses lasting longer than 10 days. These

<table>
<tr><td>

BOX 55.1 Contraindications to Hormone Therapy

</td></tr>
</table>

ABSOLUTE CONTRAINDICATIONS

- Known or suspected breast cancer
- Known or suspected endometrial cancer
- Untreated endometrial hyperplasia
- Uncontrolled hypertension
- Acute liver disease
- Active thromboembolic disease or history of thrombo-embolic disease
- Known or suspected pregnancy

RELATIVE CONTRAINDICATIONS

- Chronic, mild liver dysfunction
- Smoking (cigarettes, marijuana)
- Acute intermittent porphyria

women should have an endometrial biopsy before beginning HT. Adverse events include intolerance to contact lenses from steepening of corneal curvature, headache, gallbladder disease, an increase in serum triglycerides, nausea, vomiting, abdominal cramps, increased blood pressure, thromboembolic disease, edema, breast cancer, breast tenderness, and break-through bleeding. **Table 55.1** identifies side effects associated with various elements of HT.

All continuous HT regimens can cause breakthrough bleeding. About 30% of all women who are recently meno-pausal have some breakthrough bleeding; this decreases with women who are more than 3 years postmenopausal. Amenorrhea usually occurs within 1 year of initiating therapy.

Relative to the longer term, more serious adverse events, data from the WHI show that short-term use of combined estrogen and progestin increases the incidence of breast can-cer and abnormal mammograms. Those women in the study taking HT were diagnosed at a more advanced stage of breast cancer. In the WHI, this risk resulted in an additional eight cases of breast cancer per 10,000 women using estrogen plus progestin for 5 or more years.

The results of the WHI showed that for every 10,000 women taking menopausal hormone therapy for 1 year, there was an increase of eight cases of stroke, seven cases of CHD, eight more invasive breast cancers, and eight additional pulmo-nary embolisms (Manson et al., 2013).

Interactions

Drug interactions with CEE include increased effects of cor-ticosteroids and decreased levels of estrogen with barbiturates, phenytoin, and rifampin. Patients taking phenytoin metabolize estrogen more quickly. An increased dose of estrogen may be needed in smokers because only half the serum level achieved in nonsmokers is reached. However, any changes in CEE dose

should be based upon symptom response, not anticipated responses. Alternatively, alcohol increases the circulating levels of estrogen due to the liver's preoccupation with metabolizing the alcohol at the expense of the estrogen.

Additional/Summary Recommendations

The Endocrine Society issued conclusions on the use of HT (Santen, 2010). Select conclusions with "A level" of evidence include the following:

- "Standard-dose" estrogen used with or without a progesto-gen is associated with marked reduction in frequency and severity of hot flashes. For many women, lower doses of estrogen are also effective.
- For symptoms of vaginal atrophy, very low doses of vaginal estradiol are effective.
- Symptoms of overactive bladder may be reduced by estro-gen given vaginally or systemically.
  - Vaginal estrogen is associated with lower rates of recur-rent urinary tract infections.
  - For women in late postmenopause, estrogen given with or without a progestogen is as effective as bisphospho-nate therapy for preventing early postmenopausal bone loss and increasing bone mass.
  - Use of estrogen alone and estrogen plus a progestogen is associated with a lower incidence of hip and vertebral fractures.
  - Use of HT containing estrogen plus a progestogen is linked to a lower risk of colon cancer.
  - Mammographic density is increased in women taking estrogen alone or with a progestogen.
  - Risk for venothrombotic episodes is approximately dou-bled in women using HT, and this risk is multiplicative with baseline risk factors such as age, increased body mass index, thrombophilias, surgery, and immobilization.
  - Although continuous estrogen plus a progestogen does not cause endometrial cancer, estrogen alone without a progestogen is associated with an increased incidence of endometrial cancer.
  - The risk of gallbladder disease is increased in women using estrogen alone or with a progestogen.

Estrogen Agonist/Antagonist

Ospemifene (Osphena), the only agent in this class of drugs approved for postmenopausal symptom management, notably for the treatment of the genitourinary symptom of dyspareunia, is an alternative to HT for this indication. Furthermore, it is recommended by the NAMS as a nonestrogen alternative (NAMS, 2017).

Ospemifene binds to both estrogen receptor alpha and estrogen receptor beta. It acts as an agonist in some tissues and as an antagonist in other tissues. Specifically, it acts sim-ilarly to estrogen in vaginal tissues (i.e., minimizing dyspa-reunia) and has very weak estrogen activity in the uterus (i.e., minimal role in contributing to endometrial hyperplasia). It is a triethylene derivative, similar to tamoxifen, and as such may also have antiestrogenic activity in breast tissue, therefore, lacking the increased risk of breast cancer observed with traditional HT. Similar to HT, it has been shown to reduce bone turnover as measured by biochemical markers of bone turnover.

Dosage

Ospemifene is administered orally at a dose of 60 mg daily. It is recommended that it be taken with food to maximize its absorption from the gut.

Time Frame for Response

Clinical trials evaluating ospemifene have included those of 12 weeks' duration and up to 52 weeks. While a meaningful response was not noted to occur before 2 weeks of treatment, clinical efficacy was realized by 12 weeks and observed to continue through to 52 weeks.

Contraindications

Ospemifene use should be avoided in women with undiagnosed, abnormal vaginal bleeding; women with known or suspected estrogen-dependent neoplasia; and women with a history of or active thromboembolic disease.

Adverse Events

Overall, in studies with ospemifene, 61% of women experienced an adverse event. Among these, the most common were vaginal discharge, muscle spasms, hot flashes, and hyperhidrosis. In particular, the rate of hot flashes observed with ospemifene was more than double than that observed in the placebo groups (8% vs. 3%). To date, there are no studies exceeding 1 year in duration, so any long-term side effects are yet to be identified.

The labeling for ospemifene includes a boxed warning for increased risk of VTE events, cardiovascular disease, and endometrial cancer with its use. And while the U.S. Food and Drug Administration (FDA) currently recommends the concomitant use of a progestin in women receiving ospemifene who have an intact uterus, there is currently no study to evaluate this combination.

Interactions

Ospemifene is metabolized by the cytochrome (CYP) P-450 isoenzyme system and is a highly protein-bound agent. Its concurrent use with other drugs that are inhibited or induced by CYP 3A4, 2C9, or 2C19 or that are greater than 89% protein bound may significantly alter ospemifene's effects. The manufacturer specifically recommends avoiding the concomitant use of fluconazole and rifampin.

Tissue Selective Estrogen Complex

TSEC describes the combination of CEE and bazedoxifene, an estrogen agonist/antagonist. This product is currently marketed under the brand name Duavee and is approved for the treatment of moderate to severe VMS.

Mechanism of Action

Like ospemifene, bazedoxifene acts as an estrogen agonist in some tissues and an antagonist in others. In particular, it acts as an antagonist in uterine tissue, reducing the risk for developing endometrial hyperplasia. Its effect as an estrogen agonist is responsible for its role in minimizing bone loss. When bazedoxifene is combined with CEE, the effects include a further reduction in bone mineral density loss, a reduction in VMS, and no greater increased risk of VTE (compared to the combination of CEE and progestin).

Dosage

The recommended dose following dose-ranging studies and based upon safety and efficacy data is 20 mg bazedoxifene plus 0.45 mg OR 0.625 mg CEE by mouth daily.

Time Frame for Response

A significant 74% to 80% reduction in the severity and frequency of hot flashes (compared to placebo) was observed following 12 weeks of treatment. A secondary outcome of improvement in sleep symptoms was also observed.

Contraindications

Use of the combination of bazedoxifene plus CEE should be avoided in patients with active or past history of VTE disorder, active or past history of an arterial thromboembolic disorder, a history of or current breast cancer, hepatic impairment or disease, and protein C and S or antithrombin deficiency that would predispose a woman to clot formation.

Adverse Events

In clinical trials, the adverse events observed with the combination of bazedoxifene plus CEE were comparable to those observed in the placebo treatment groups.

Interactions

The concomitant use of bazedoxifene and ospemifene is to be avoided. Other interactions with this combination product include those noted with estrogen in the HT treatment section of this chapter.

Selective Serotonin Reuptake Inhibitors and Selective Serotonin–Norepinephrine Reuptake Inhibitors

Agents including paroxetine, sertraline, venlafaxine, desvenlafaxine, citalopram, and escitalopram have been evaluated for their efficacy in reducing VMS associated with menopause. Only paroxetine, marketed as Brisdelle, has received FDA approval for the treatment of moderate to severe VMS.

Mechanism of Action

The preoptic area of the anterior hypothalamus, responsible for temperature regulation, is under the influence of serotonin and norepinephrine. The action of these two neurotransmitters at the hypothalamus is negatively affected by fluctuating estrogen levels. Therefore, the use of the SSRIs and selective serotonin–norepinephrine reuptake inhibitors (SNRIs) reestablishes the neurotransmitters in the thermoregulatory center of the hypothalamus, improving VMS.

Dosage

Recommended starting doses of the abovementioned agents for the management of VMS associated with menopause are citalopram 10 mg by mouth daily, escitalopram 10 mg by mouth daily, venlafaxine 37.5 mg by mouth daily, desvenlafaxine 100 mg by mouth daily, sertraline 50 mg by mouth daily, and paroxetine 7.5 mg by mouth daily. The doses of citalopram, escitalopram, and venlafaxine can be increased to 30, 20, and 75 mg, respectively.

Time Frame for Response

While maximal dose–response effect to HT occurs in approximately 4 weeks, improvement in symptoms may be observed within the first week of treatment. To the contrary, the effects of the SSRIs and SNRIs are typically not realized until several weeks of therapy have been completed. After 4 to 8 weeks of treatment, an overall 30% to 75% reduction in hot flashes compared to placebo has been observed.

Contraindications

The SSRIs and SNRIs are not to be used within 14 days of the use of any of the monoamine oxidase inhibitors because such use may result in the development of serotonin syndrome.

Adverse Events

The most common adverse events observed with the use of the SSRIs and SNRIs include nausea, dizziness, dry mouth, nervousness, constipation, and sexual dysfunction.

Interactions

As noted under contraindications, the concomitant use of this class of drugs and a monoamine oxidase inhibitor may result in the development of the serotonin syndrome. Carbamazepine may increase the metabolism of the SSRIs/SNRIs and, conversely, the SSRIs/SNRIs may reduce carbamazepine metabolism. Cimetidine reduces the metabolism of the SSRIs/SNRIs. The SSRIs/SNRIs enhance the antiplatelet effects of nonsteroidal antiinflammatory agents.

Gabapentin

Mechanism of Action

Gabapentin is an anticonvulsant that has been used to treat VMS associated with tamoxifen treatment in breast cancer patients as well as those associated with menopause. The mechanism of action of gabapentin for these purposes is unknown.

Dosage

Trials of gabapentin in postmenopausal women have utilized starting doses of 600 to 900 mg gabapentin in divided doses daily. Doses have been titrated to effect to a maximum total daily dose of 2.7 g.

Time Frame for Response

While efficacy may be appreciated at approximately 4 to 6 weeks of treatment, full effects may not be observed until as late as 12 weeks. In clinical trials, hot flash frequency was reduced by 45%, and the composite hot flash score (including frequency and severity) was reduced by as much as 54% when compared to placebo (Guttuso et al., 2003).

Contraindications

Gabapentin should not be used in women with a history of hypersensitivity to gabapentin or any of its components.

Adverse Events

Somnolence, fatigue, dizziness, rash, and peripheral edema have been observed in women taking gabapentin for the treatment of VMS.

Interactions

Antacids may significantly reduce the absorption of gabapentin so gabapentin should be dosed 2 hours after any antacids.

Clonidine

Clonidine is a centrally acting α-2 agonist used in the management of hypertension that has also been observed to treat VMS associated with menopause.

Mechanism of Action

The exact mechanism of clonidine in treating VMS is unclear, but it is thought to be related to its central activity and potential impact on the thermoregulatory center in the hypothalamus.

Dosage

The recommended dose of clonidine for postmenopausal VMS is 0.1 mg by mouth daily.

Time Frame for Response

Improvement in VMS may be experienced following 4 to 6 weeks of clonidine treatment. Overall, clinical trial data for clonidine used to minimize VMS are lacking. What is available illustrates that clonidine is more effective than placebo but less effective than HT.

Contraindications

As clonidine is an antihypertensive agent, women with baseline low blood pressure would not be candidates for its use in managing VMS.

Adverse Events

The most common side effects noted with clonidine use include dry mouth, insomnia, drowsiness, and increased risk for hypotension.

Interactions

Clonidine may potentiate the effects of other central nervous system depressants.

SELECTINGP THE MOST APPROPRIATE THERAPY

The options for managing VMS and the GSM are varied, and there is not one regimen that fits all patients. The regimens vary in dosage formulation as well as active drug. In addition, nondrug recommendations should also be considered. Regardless,

a patient-centered approach identifying the potential benefits and risks of each regimen as well as patient preference(s) and potential for regimen adherence for each patient must be considered. The choice of regimen should be arrived at by the "team" of patient and provider.

The Patient-Centered Approach

The decision of how to manage VMS or symptoms of the GSM is one that must be reached by both patient and provider. While HT remains the most effective treatment modality, its duration of use must be limited and many women do not view its benefits to outweigh its risks, so alternative modalities are desired. Any treatment agreed to should be in addition to the lifestyle changes identified later in this chapter. **Figure 55.1** illustrates a decision tree that can be used in determining initial treatment modalities for women presenting with menopause-related symptoms. As noted, and included within the

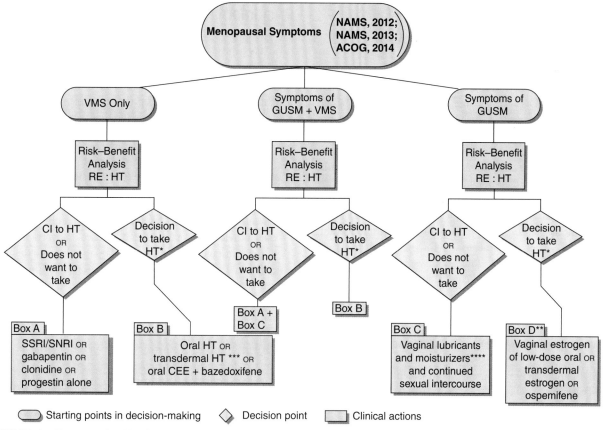

FIGURE 55–1   Treatment algorithm for menopause.

* Systemic estrogen (oral, transdermal) use requires the addition of a progestin in all women with an intact uterus; estrogen + bazedoxifene, however, does not require a progestin.

** Drug choices listed in order of preference/choice dated up clinical trial data and available guidelines.

*** Transdermal preferred for women with hyperlipidemia (esp. triglycerides).

**** Vaginal moisturizers versus lubricants have resulted in the decrease or elimination of symptoms for many women (NAMS, 2013).

ACOG, American College of Obstetricians and Gynecologists; CEE, conjugated equine estrogen; CI, contraindication(s); GUSM, genitourinary syndrome of menopause; HT, hormone therapy, estrogen + progestin; NAMS, North American Menopause Society; SNRI, serotonin–norepinephrine reuptake inhibitor; SSRI, selective serotonin reuptake inhibitor; VMS, vasomotor symptoms.

previous text of this chapter, whether or not a woman has had any history of estrogen-dependent cancer is a factor that contributes to the final management decision. Debate still exists over the short-term use of HT in women following treatment of estrogen-dependent cancers, including breast, ovarian, and endometrial cancers. One retrospective study found that in spite of being treated for an estrogen-dependent cancer, 19.5% of women chose to take estrogen for menopause-related symptoms (primarily VMS) in spite of the contraindications to its use (Sekar et al., 2013). In addition, while there appears little question or controversy surrounding the use of HT in younger women at the time of menopause as having a very positive benefit to risk profile and being the most effective treatment for VMS, the increasing evidence of the risks and benefits of HT beyond the age of 65 years makes HT as an initial treatment choice in this older population a much less clear decision. Alternative treatments to HT should be carefully considered in this population (Davies et al., 2013; Moyer, 2013).

MONITORING PATIENT RESPONSE

The decision to continue HT should be revisited yearly, and therapy should be discontinued when symptoms resolve—usually in 1 to 3 years after menopause. And owing to an increase in breast cancer risk, its use beyond 3 to 5 years is not recommended (NAMS, 2012). The patient should be seen 4 to 8 weeks after starting therapy to evaluate response and make any necessary dosage adjustments and then in 3 to 6 months to monitor continued response to therapy, the need for any further dosage adjustments, and the occurrence of any side effects. After that, annual visits are required.

The health status of a woman on HT must be evaluated annually. Their medical history for the past year should be reviewed, including questions about vaginal bleeding. The woman should have an annual clinical breast examination and mammogram if she is older than age 40. Any woman on continuous-combined HT who has vaginal bleeding beyond the first year of treatment should be evaluated with an endometrial biopsy. The physical examination should include the following:

- Height and weight measurements to screen for osteoporosis and obesity
- Fasting lipid panel according to recommendations
- Blood pressure evaluation to screen for cardiovascular disease
- Clinical breast examination and review of procedures for breast self-examination
- Full pelvic examination, including a Pap smear

Prescriptions for HT should not be renewed without a full annual history and physical. Discontinuing HT should be done gradually as abrupt discontinuation may lead to a rebound of symptoms. This may be done in several ways. The patient may begin to skip more days between doses or the daily dose may be decreased at 4- to 6-week intervals.

PATIENT EDUCATION

Following publication of many prospective, randomized trials in the late 1990s and early 2000s, and the subsequent unbalanced media coverage that ensued, many women abruptly discontinued their HT (resulting in a plethora of women with rebounding symptoms of menopause). This only further illustrated the need for practitioners to remain current with the HT research and be able to put the clinical trial data in a balanced light for their patients. It also illustrated the need for practitioners to be more aware than ever of the alternatives that exist to HT and to effectively communicate this to their patients without overwhelming them. Menopause is a natural part of the aging process and women need to know that their providers realize the gravity of the impact its consequences may have on QOL and trust that their providers will assist them in managing this part of their life.

Drug Information

Several options are available for the postmenopausal woman with VMS. If she decides to begin HT, the decision must be an informed decision. To make an informed decision, the patient must be provided with detailed information on the risks and benefits of therapy and other options available. It is also important to understand the side effects and that there may be monthly bleeding. General key teaching points include the following:

- The patient must be aware that it may take up to 4 weeks or more (depending on treatment option chosen) before symptoms to respond to treatment. Efficacy of the treatment chosen is typically dose dependent.
- Encourage patients to be aware of and communicate with their provider the occurrence of potential adverse events as, in some instances, there may be ways to minimize them. For example, HT can be taken with food or at bedtime to prevent nausea. For other more severe adverse events such as VTE, patients should be educated regarding the signs and symptoms and be encouraged to contact their provider in a very timely manner or seek emergency treatment as needed.
- Patients should be instructed to never, in the event of missed doses, double the next dose.
- Patients should be aware that the management of menopause-related symptoms is at the lowest necessary dose for the shortest duration as is needed, and they should be empowered to follow up with their provider regarding potential discontinuation of treatment in a timely manner.

Patient information sources for menopause include the following:

- The American Congress of Obstetricians and Gynecologists: http://www.acog.org/Patients
- Harvard Health Publications: http://www.health.harvard.edu/topics/womens-health
- The North American Menopause Society: http://www.menopause.org/for-women

TABLE 55.2

Herbal Treatment of Menopausal Symptoms

Menopausal Symptom	Herbal Treatment	Usual Dose	Adverse Events and Contraindications
Hot flashes	Black cohosh (*Cimicifuga*)	40–200 mg/d; not to be taken for >6 mo	Not to be used during pregnancy Potential side effects: GI disturbances, hypotension
	Isoflavones (soy)	20–40 mg/d	Flatulence
Mood swings	St. John wort (*Hypericum*)	300 mg TID	Do not take with any antidepressant. May cause sun sensitivity

GI, gastrointestinal.

Nutrition/Lifestyle Changes

The reduction in intake of refined carbohydrates, caffeine, and alcohol has been reported by women to result in minimizing hot flashes. Wearing only cotton clothing and maintaining low environmental temperatures may also allow women to feel more comfortable during hot flashes. Further recommendations to reduce VMS include dressing in layers, smoking cessation, and weight loss. The latter two suggestions are also beneficial to overall good health.

For genitourinary symptoms associated with menopause, specifically the symptoms of atrophy, regular sexual activity should be encouraged.

Complementary and Alternative Medications

In women not wishing to take pharmacologically active agents to minimize the symptoms of vaginal atrophy, the use of long-acting vaginal moisturizers and lubricants is an option. Such agents may increase the vaginal pH to premenopausal levels, and their use during intercourse may reduce friction-related effects worsened by atrophy.

Women are also turning to other herbs, such as soy or black cohosh, or the phytoestrogens for managing menopausal symptoms, specifically VMS (**Table 55.2**). Phytoestrogens,

estrogens obtained from plant sources, are marketed in oral formulations for the management of VMS. An example of this is the brand-named product Promensil. Phytoestrogens are also found in a number of common foods, including soybeans and soy products, cashews, peanuts, oats, corn, wheat, flaxseeds, and sunflower seeds. While phytoestrogens appear to lack the negative effects of estrogen relative to stimulation of the breast and uterus, they must be used for 4 to 6 weeks before any improvement may be noticed. Soy, chickpeas, and other legumes contain isoflavones, which exhibit estrogenic properties. They can provide some VMS relief, although their effectiveness in menopause is still being investigated.

Another option is vitamin E. While vitamin E has been evaluated, the results have illustrated that the treatment group had minimal to no positive impact on daily hot flashes compared to placebo (Loprinzi et al., 2008). Some clinical trials have shown improvement of hot flashes with soy and black cohosh, and some have shown no improvement (Faure et al., 2002).

And while black cohosh is also used to treat menopause, specifically purportedly inducing vaginal maturation and improving VMS, no long-term scientific data are available, and concern regarding the development of hepatitis and myopathy with long-term use exists.

CASE STUDY 1

D.W. is a 56-year-old woman who has been complaining of amenorrhea for the past 11 months. Her current complaints are vaginal dryness, dyspareunia, and hot flashes. Her surgical history includes a hysterectomy. Of note, her sister has a history of estrogen receptor+ breast cancer (Learning Objectives 1, 2, 3, and 4).

1. What are the presenting signs and symptoms of menopause that are being experienced by D.W.?

2. What drug therapy would you prescribe? Why?
3. What are the parameters for monitoring success of the therapy?
4. Discuss specific patient education based on the prescribed therapy.
5. What lifestyle changes would you recommend for D.W.?

Bibliography

Starred references are cited in the text.

*American College of Obstetricians and Gynecologists. (2014). Practice Bulletin No. 141: Management of menopausal symptoms. *Obstetrics and Gynecology, 123*(1), 202–216.

Barnes, K. N., Pearce, E. F., Yancey, A. M., et al. (2014). Ospemifene in the treatment of vulvovaginal atrophy. *Annals of Pharmacotherapy, 48*(6), 752–757.

Carris, N., Kutner, S., & Reilly-Rogers, S. (2014). New pharmacological therapies for vasomotor symptoms management: Focus on bazedoxifene/conjugated equine estrogens and paroxetine mesylate. *Annals of Pharmacotherapy, 48*(10), 1343–1349.

Carroll, D. G., Lisenby, K. M., & Carter, T. L. (2015). Critical appraisal of paroxetine for the treatment of vasomotor symptoms. *International Journal of Women's Health, 7*, 615–624.

*Coker, L. H., Espeland, M. A., Rapp, S. R., et al. (2010). Postmenopausal hormone therapy and cognitive outcomes: The Women's Health Initiative Memory Study (WHIMS). *The Journal of Steroid Biochemistry and Molecular Biology, 118*(4–5), 304–310.

*Davies, E., Mangongi, N. P., & Carter, C. L. (2013). Is timing everything? A meeting report of the Society for Women's Health Research roundtable on menopausal hormone therapy. *Journal of Women's Health, 22*(4), 303–312.

*Deecher, D. C., & Dorries, K. (2007). Understanding the pathophysiology of vasomotor symptoms (hot flushes and night sweats) that occur in perimenopause, menopause, and postmenopause. *Archives of Women's Mental Health, 10*, 247–257.

Eder, S. E. (2014). Ospemifene: A novel selective estrogen receptor modulator for treatment of dyspareunia. *Women's Health, 10*(5), 499–503.

*Espeland, M. A., Rapp, S. R., Manson, J. E., et al. (2017). Long-Term effects on cognitive trajectories of postmenopausal hormone therapy in two age groups. *The Journal of Gerontology Series A: Biological Sciences Medical Sciences, 72*(6), 838–845. doi: 10.1093/Gerona/glw156

*Faure, E., Chantre, P., & Mares, P. (2002). Effects of a standardized soy extract on hot flushes: A multicenter, double-blind randomized, placebo-controlled study. *Menopause, 9*, 329–334.

*Guttuso, T. Jr., Kurlan, R., McDermott, M. P., et al. (2003). Gabapentin's effects on hot flashes in postmenopausal women: A randomized controlled trial. *Obstetrics and Gynecology, 101*(2), 337–345.

*Harlow, S. D., Gass, M., Hall, J. E., et al. (2012). Executive summary of the stages of reproductive aging workshop +10: Addressing the unfinished agenda of staging reproductive aging. *Menopause, 19*(4), 1–9.

Krause, M. S., & Nakajima, S. T. (2015). Hormonal and nonhormonal treatments of vasomotor symptoms. *Obstetric and Gynecologic Clinics of North America, 42*, 163–179.

*Loprinzi, C. L., Barton, D. L., Sloan, J. A., et al. (2008). Mayo Clinic and North Central Cancer treatment group hot flash studies: A 20-year experience. *Menopause, 15*, 655–660.

*Manson, J. E., Chlebowski, R. T., Stefanick, M. L., et al. (2013). Menopausal hormone therapy and health outcomes during the intervention and extended post stopping phases of the Women's Health Initiative randomized trials. *Journal of the American Medical Association, 310*(13), 1353–1368.

McLendon, A. N., Clinard, V. B., & Woodis, C. B. (2014). Ospemifene for the treatment of vulvovaginal atrophy and dyspareunia in postmenopausal women. *Pharmacotherapy, 34*(10), 1050–1060.

Mirkin, S., Komm, B., & Pickar, J. H. (2014). Conjugated estrogen/bazedoxifene tablets for the treatment of moderate-to-severe vasomotor symptoms associated with menopause. *Women's Health, 10*(2), 135–146.

*Moyer, V. A., on behalf of the U.S. Preventive Services Task Force. (2013). Menopausal hormone therapy for the primary prevention of chronic conditions: U.S. Preventive Services Task Force Recommendation Statement. *Annals of Internal Medicine, 158*(1), 47–54.

*North American Menopause Society. (2010). Overview of menopause. In *Menopause Practice: A Clinician's Guide* (4th ed., Chapter 1). Retrieved from http://menopause.org/publications/other-resources/terms-statistics# on June 19, 2015.

North American Menopause Society. (2011). The role of soy isoflavones in menopausal health: Report of the North American Menopause Society/Wulf H. Utian Translational Science Symposium in Chicago, IL (October 2010). *Menopause, 18*(7), 732–753.

*North American Menopause Society. (2012). The 2012 hormone therapy position statement of the North American Menopause Society. *Menopause, 19*(3), 257–271.

*North American Menopause Society. (2013). Management of symptomatic vulvovaginal atrophy: 2013 position statement of the North American Menopause Society. *Menopause, 20*(9), 888–902.

*North American Menopause Society. (2017). The 2017 hormone therapy position statement of the North American Menopause Society. *Menopause, 24*(7), 728–753.

*Portman, D. J., & Gass, M. L. (2014). Genitourinary syndrome of menopause: New terminology for vulvovaginal atrophy from the International Society for the Study of Women's Sexual Health and the North American Menopause Society. *Menopause, 21*(10), 1–6.

Rao, S., Singh, S., Parker, M., et al. (2008). Health maintenance for postmenopausal women. *American Family Physician, 78*(5), 583–591.

Reed, S., Newton, K., LaCroix, A., et al. (2007). Night sweats, sleep disturbances and depression associated with diminished libido in late menopausal transition and early postmenopause: Baseline data from the Herbal Alternatives for Menopause Trial (HALT). *American Journal of Obstetrics and Gynecology, 196*(6), 1–7.

*Rossaminth, W. G., & Ruebberdt, W. (2009). What causes hot flashes? The neuroendocrine origin of vasomotor symptoms in the menopause. *Gynecological Endocrinology, 25*(5), 303–314.

*Santen, R. J. (2010). Postmenopausal hormone therapy: An Endocrine Society scientific statement. *Journal of Clinical Endocrinology and Metabolism, 7*(Suppl. 1), S1–S66.

*Sekar, H., Singhal, T., Holloway, D., et al. (2013). The use of hormone therapy and its alternatives in women with a history of hormone dependent cancer. *Menopause International, 1*–6. doi: 10.1177/1754045312473874

*Thurston, R. C., & Joffe, H. (2011). Vasomotor symptoms and menopause: Findings from the Study of Women's Health Across the Nation. *Obstetrics and Gynecology, 38*, 489–501.

Umland, E. M., & Falconieri, L. (2012). Treatment options for vasomotor symptoms in menopause: Focus on desvenlafaxine. *International Journal of Women's Health, 4*, 305–319.

*Utian, W. H., Shoupe, D., Bochman, G., et al. (2001). Relief of vasomotor symptoms and vaginal atrophy with lower doses of conjugated equine estrogen and medroxyprogesterone acetate. *Fertility Sterility, 75*, 1065–1079.

Vaughan, L., Espeland, M. A., Snively, B., et al. (2013). The rationale, design, and baseline characteristics of the Women's Health Initiative Memory Study of Younger Women (WHIMS-Y). *Brain Research, 1514*, 3–11.

*Writing Group for the PEPI Trial. (1995). Effects of estrogen or estrogen/progestin on heart disease risk factors in post-menopausal women. *Journal of the American Medical Association, 273*, 199–208.

*Writing Group for the Women's Health Initiative. (2002). Risks and benefits of estrogen plus progestin in healthy postmenopausal women. *Journal of the American Medical Association, 288*, 321–333.

56 Vaginitis

Iman I. Aberra and Virginia P. Arcangelo

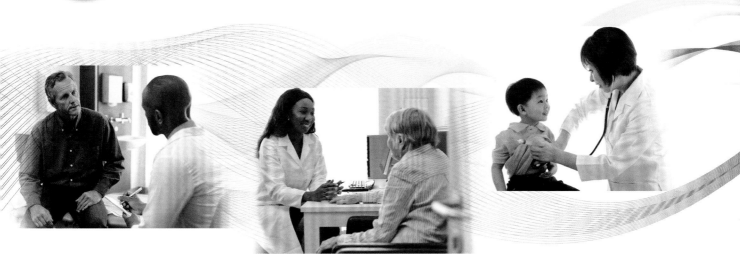

Learning Objectives

1. Understand the causes and risk factors of different forms of vaginitis.
2. Recognize the signs and symptoms of different types of vaginitis and how to confirm the diagnosis.
3. Identify the goals of treatment and compose a patient-specific treatment plan for a patient presenting with vaginitis.

INTRODUCTION

Vaginitis is inflammation or irritation of the vagina or vulva that can be caused by infection, immune-related responses, or physiological changes of the vaginal mucosa. Vaginitis from infection is one of the most common gynecologic complaints. The most common causes of vaginitis are vulvovaginal candidiasis (VVC), bacterial vaginosis (BV), and *Trichomonas vaginalis*. Common symptoms include vaginal or perineal itching, burning, vulvar or vaginal irritation, and abnormal vaginal discharge. Many women may be asymptomatic.

CAUSES

Bacterial Vaginosis

BV is a polymicrobial vaginal infection that occurs when the hydrogen peroxide–producing *Lactobacillus* normally present in the vagina diminish, allowing other bacteria to proliferate. Bacteria, such as *Gardnerella vaginalis*, *Prevotella* species, *Mobiluncus* species, and *Mycoplasma hominis*, are commonly

responsible for BV. Although the cause of BV is not well understood, risk factors include sexual activity with multiple male and female partners, douching, lack of condom use, intrauterine contraceptive devices, and lack of vaginal lactobacilli.

BV is considered the most common form of infectious vaginitis and affects approximately 30% of women. African-American (51%) and Mexican-American (32%) women are affected more than white women. Up to 84% of women with BV are asymptomatic.

Because most women who have BV exhibit no or minor symptoms, there is a tendency to overlook this condition. Sociodemographic factors associated with BV include younger age, being non-Hispanic black or Mexican American, having less than a high school education, and living at or near the federal poverty level. Sexual risk factors, such as being sexually active, age of first sexual intercourse, and having multiple male lifetime sexual partners, particularly multiple over the past year, all are risk factors for BV. In lesbian women, female partners of women who have BV have a higher incidence of BV. Despite the sexual risk factors associated with BV, it is considered sexually associated but not sexually transmitted. While infection is rare in women who have never been sexually active, treatment of male sex partners has not proven to be beneficial in preventing recurrence.

Candidiasis

VVC is the second most common form of infectious vaginitis. Most vaginal yeast infections are caused by *Candida albicans*, although other organisms, such as *Candida tropicalis* and *Candida glabrata*, are seen in recurrent or complicated candidiasis. Symptoms occur when there is an overgrowth of yeast that normally colonizes the vagina. This can be due to recent antibiotic use, pregnancy, steroid use, or an immunocompromised state. Other risk factors include uncontrolled diabetes and increased estrogen levels. Oral contraceptives, use of a diaphragm, spermicide, and the use of an intrauterine device are associated with an increased risk for infection.

Behavioral risk factors, in particular orogenital sex, may contribute to the introduction of microorganisms or cause microtrauma to the vulva and vestibule. While sexual activity can increase the incidence of VVC, it is not a sexually transmitted disease.

Trichomoniasis

T. vaginalis, an anaerobic protozoan, is the most common non-viral sexually transmitted infection. Increased numbers of sexual partners, a recent new sexual partner, or early initiation of sexual activity (younger than age 16) is associated with increased prevalence of infection. It is more common in African-American women than in white women. Up to 86% of trichomoniasis infections may be asymptomatic. Infection can persist for months and sometimes years in asymptomatic patients who are not treated. Males often tend to be asymptomatic and can be a vector of transmission. Trichomonads can live for several hours on moist surfaces and may be transmitted by fomites such as towels or sexual toys.

Allergies and Irritants

Conditions or products that irritate the vulva or vaginal epithelium or local allergic reactions may produce symptoms similar to those of infectious vaginitis. Examples of irritants include vaginal lubricants, condoms, spermicides, and feminine hygiene products. Women who have other atopic skin conditions may experience vaginal and vulvar manifestations as well.

Atrophy

Low levels of estrogen in postmenopausal women may lead to atrophy of the vaginal epithelium and subsequent irritation and inflammation, which may predispose these women to vaginitis.

Inflammatory Vaginitis

The cause of inflammatory vaginitis is thought to be autoimmune related and associated with low estrogen levels. It is also postulated that the inflammation present in the vagina results in an aberration of the normal vaginal flora. The exact cause of this type of vaginitis is unknown.

PATHOPHYSIOLOGY

A review of the normal physiology of the vaginal environment forms the basis for understanding the possible causes and pathophysiology of vaginitis. In postpubertal women, both anaerobic and aerobic bacteria make up the normal vaginal flora. These include potential pathogens, such as *Staphylococcus*, *Streptococcus*,

and *Bacteroides* species, and nonpathogens, such as lactobacilli and diphtheroids. *C. albicans* is a saprophytic fungus that is a normal vaginal inhabitant in 15% to 25% of women.

One of the most important factors in the defense against infection is an acidic vaginal pH of 3.8 to 4.2, which the vaginal flora helps to maintain. An acidic vagina prevents the overgrowth of pathogenic bacteria. In women of reproductive age, estrogen produces glycogen from the vaginal mucosa. Glycogen serves as a nutrient to the vaginal flora and is metabolized to lactic acid, keeping the vagina acidic. Hydrogen peroxide–producing strains of lactobacilli in vaginal secretions have been associated with protection against some vaginal infections as well. Variables that alter the vaginal pH or destroy lactobacilli may predispose a woman to vaginal infection. Among these variables are pregnancy, diabetes, sexual activity, hormonal changes, antibiotic therapy, and the use of feminine hygiene products. The thickness of the vaginal epithelium may also influence antimicrobial defenses.

DIAGNOSTIC CRITERIA

Bacterial Vaginosis

Clinical signs and symptoms of BV include malodorous homogeneous vaginal discharge and vaginal irritation. Routine screening in asymptomatic women is not recommended due to the lack of clear benefit.

Gram staining is considered the gold standard laboratory test in diagnosing BV. It is interpreted using the Nugent score. This standardized scoring system quantifies the organisms seen on the stain. A score of 0 to 3 is given for normal flora, 4 to 6 for mixed flora, and 7 to 10 for BV. This method is time consuming and requires personnel to interpret the Gram stain. This typically cannot be done in an office visit and is often reserved for research purposes.

Other forms of diagnostic testing include Affirm VP (Becton Dickinson, Sparks, Maryland) and OSOM BV Blue Test (Sekisui Diagnostics, Framingham, Massachusetts). The Affirm VPIII is a deoxyribonucleic acid (DNA) hybridization probe for *G. vaginalis*, and the OSOM BV Blue Test detects vaginal sialidase activity. Both tests have high sensitivity and specificity, and results come back within 30 minutes, making them ideal point-of-care tests to use in the office setting. Furthermore, the manufacturer of the Affirm VP assay produced the Affirm VPIII assay (Becton Dickinson, Sparks, Maryland), which is also able to test for *Candida* spp. and *T. vaginalis*.

A clinical diagnosis of BV requires three out of four Amsel criteria and utilizes saline microscopy, which is also known as a wet mount. The Amsel criteria comprise abnormal homogeneous discharge, vaginal pH greater than 4.5, positive amine or "whiff test" ("fishy" odor with potassium hydroxide [KOH] applied to discharge), and positive clue cells (epithelial cells surrounded by adherent coccobacilli) on microscopy (Amsel et al., 1983) (**Box 56.1**). This test can be used in the office setting for quick results.

BOX 56.1   Amsel Criteria

- Thin homogeneous discharge
- Positive whiff test
- Clue cells positive on microscopy
- pH > 4.5

The presence of three of the four criteria above establish a diagnosis for BV (Amsel et al., 1983).

UNCOMPLICATED

Sporadic VVC
and
Mild to moderate VVC
and
Likely to be *Candida albicans*
and
Non-immunocompromised women

COMPLICATED VVC

Recurrent VVC (defined as 4 or more episodes in a year)
or
Severe VVC
or
Nonalbicans candidiasis
or
Immunocompromised women (e.g., HIV infection, on immunosuppressive medication, debilitation) or diabetes (CDC, 2015)

Routine cultures and cervical Papanicolaou (Pap) smears are not helpful in diagnosing BV since it is a polymicrobial infection. Proline aminopeptidase card tests, such as the FemExam test card (CooperSurgical, Shelton, Connecticut) and Pip Activity TestCard (Litmus Concepts, Inc., Santa Clara, California), are no longer recommended because of their low specificity and sensitivity.

Candidiasis: Vulvovaginal Candidiasis

Symptoms of VVC include intense pruritus and erythema, dysuria, and a thick, white, curd-like vaginal discharge that tends to adhere to the vaginal walls. Diagnosis is made on the basis of presenting complaints, physical findings, and observation of pseudohyphae on KOH wet mount slide. Gram stain and culture of the vaginal discharge are other methods that may be employed in the diagnosis of VVC. Vaginal cultures can confirm the diagnosis and identify the species of *Candida* causing infection. Since 10% to 20% of women harbor *Candida* in the vagina, it is not recommended that asymptomatic women be treated. If the vaginal pH is tested, the value should be normal, usually less than 4.5. *Candida* may also be identified on Papanicolaou (Pap) smears of symptomatic or asymptomatic women. VVC may be classified as complicated or uncomplicated (**Box 56.2**).

Trichomoniasis

Patients with vaginitis caused by *Trichomonas* organisms report a profuse, frothy, green-yellowish malodorous vaginal discharge, vaginal and vulvar irritation, dysuria, and dyspareunia. Sometimes, postcoital bleeding can occur. Most patients are asymptomatic and carry the organism, which can be spread to sexual partners.

Under microscope, trichomonads often appear in motion on a vaginal secretion saline wet mount, "swimming" with the flagella in a jerking or tumbling action. It is important that vaginal samples be examined within 10 minutes to best identify the parasite. Saline wet mounts have low sensitivity and are not recommended to diagnose *Trichomonas* vaginitis, although they can be used if there are cost concerns. The Centers for Disease Control and Prevention (CDC) suggests that if nucleic

acid amplification test (NAAT) cannot be utilized as initial diagnostic testing, wet mounts with a negative result be tested using molecular testing to increase sensitivity.

The CDC recommends diagnostic testing by highly specific and sensitive methods, which can be achieved through molecular testing. The APTIMA *T. vaginalis* assay (Hologic Gen-Probe, San Diego, California) and BD Probe Tec TV Qx Amplified DNA Assay (Becton Dickinson, Franklin Lakes, New Jersey) are Food and Drug Administration (FDA)–approved NAATs for the detection of *T. vaginalis* from vaginal, endocervical, and urine samples.

Other point-of-care tests include the OSOM Trichomonas Rapid Test (Sekisui Diagnostics, Framingham, Massachusetts) and the Affirm VPIII test, which was mentioned previously. The OSOM Trichomonas Rapid Test is an antigen detection test that can produce results in about 10 minutes. Both tests are highly sensitive and specific.

Trichomonas organisms may also be identified on a Pap smear. This method is not recommended due to the high rates of false positives and negatives. Culture is very sensitive (95%) and specific (greater than 95%) but delays diagnosis and is not routinely performed.

Allergic Vaginitis

Vaginitis resulting from allergy or irritants may be characterized by vaginal pruritus and burning. The diagnosis often relies on exclusion. Although vaginal discharge may be increased, the secretions, when examined microscopically, do not harbor candidal organisms, trichomonads, or clue cells.

Atrophic Vaginitis

Vaginitis associated with atrophy of the vaginal walls produces pruritus, thin clear discharge, dryness, and dyspareunia. Physical examination reveals thinning of the vaginal walls with a characteristic shiny-smooth appearance. Introduction of the speculum into the vaginal introitus may cause bleeding. Microscopic examination reveals no candida organisms, trichomonads, or clue cells.

Inflammatory Vaginitis

Presentation of inflammatory vaginitis typically includes increased vaginal secretions, dyspareunia, and inflammation of the vagina. Vaginal discharge is homogenous, purulent, and odorless. Diagnosis is made by wet mount microscopic visualization of inflammatory cells such as leukocytes and parabasal epithelial cells and is negative for infectious etiology.

INITIATING DRUG THERAPY

When considering pharmacotherapy for vaginitis, the practitioner explores lifestyle choices that may predispose the patient to infection or inflammation. Questions to ask regard the use of douches or other feminine hygiene products, sexual practices and partners, the possible relationship between sexual activity and appearance of symptoms, and recent antibiotic or oral contraceptive use. The practitioner should perform a thorough assessment to identify other possible irritants or complaints.

Before choosing a plan of therapy, the practitioner and patient also need to consider the issue of recurrent infection. In the case of recurrent VVC (four or more symptomatic episodes annually), the practitioner should be alert to the possibility of diabetes, and the need for screening should be discussed. In the case of recurrent trichomonal infection, sex partners should be examined and treated if they are found to be transmitting the organisms. It is also common for BV to recur.

Goals of Therapy

The primary goal of therapy in treating infectious vaginitis is eradication of the offending organism. The primary goals of therapy for allergic vaginitis and inflammatory vaginitis include avoiding irritants and reducing inflammation, respectively. Addressing the hypoestrogenic state of postmenopausal women with hormone replacement therapy alleviates the symptoms of atrophic vaginitis. A discussion of atrophic vaginitis is available elsewhere in this text book.

Another important goal of therapy is relief of symptoms. Vaginitis can cause considerable discomfort, both physically and emotionally. Women with vaginitis often experience

---

BOX 56.3 | **Self-Diagnosis and Self-Treatment of Vaginitis**

There are multiple studies assessing the accuracy of self-diagnosis of vaginal symptoms, and the incidence of misdiagnosis was found to be high. Ferris et al. (2002) observed women who were self-treating symptoms that they attributed to VVC with OTC antifungals. Of the 95 women studied, only 34% actually had VVC. The authors found that reading the package label or a prior diagnosis of VVC did not significantly increase the chances of a correct self-diagnosis.

Although misuse of these pharmaceuticals rarely causes acute adverse reactions, a delay in diagnosis of infections such as pelvic inflammatory disease, BV, or urinary tract infections could have significant consequences. Furthermore, repeated use of these medications unsuccessfully by women before their visit to the provider can make accurate assessment of the symptoms and physical findings difficult.

---

embarrassment and even fear, particularly of the implications of a sexually transmitted disease. The frustration associated with recurrent infection may lead women to repeated attempts to self-treat, which delays proper evaluation by their primary care provider. For more information on self-treatment, see **Box 56.3**.

In the treatment of BV, additional goals of therapy include reduction of the risk of complications following gynecological procedures (e.g., abortion and hysterectomy) and reduction in the risk of acquiring other sexually transmitted infections. Adverse pregnancy outcomes have been associated with BV and trichomoniasis. The treatment of asymptomatic women with BV is not recommended since there is a paucity of evidence to suggest that treatment prevents any of these complications.

Topical Azole Antifungals

Topical vaginal preparations for treating uncomplicated VVC include the following azoles: clotrimazole, butoconazole, tioconazole, miconazole, and terconazole. Clotrimazole, butoconazole, and tioconazole are available over the counter. All topical antifungals are considered equal for the treatment of uncomplicated VVC. Treatment duration with these agents is 1, 3, 7, or 14 days depending on the product. Types of topical preparations include creams, ointments, and suppositories. These topical azoles are considered to be more effective than the antifungal nystatin (Mycostatin) in uncomplicated VVC. **Table 56.1** lists the azole drugs currently available by prescription or without a prescription. Practitioners should advise women whose symptoms persist or recur within 2 months of treatment to seek medical care. In general, the only

TABLE 56.1

Overview of Antifungal Agents

Generic (Trade) Name and Dosage

OTC Preparations

Clotrimazole 1% cream (Gyne-Lotrimin), 1 application (5 g) intravaginally QHS for 7–14 d

Clotrimazole 2% cream (Gyne-Lotrimin), 1 application (5 g) intravaginally QHS for 3 d

Miconazole 2% cream (Monistat 7), 1 application (5 g) intravaginally QHS for 7 d

Miconazole 4% cream (Monistat 3), 1 application (5 g) intravaginally QHS for 3 d

Miconazole 100-mg suppository (Monistat 7), 1 suppository intravaginally QHS for 7 d

Miconazole 200-mg suppository (Monistat 3), 1 suppository intravaginally QHS for 3 d

Miconazole 1,200-mg suppository (Monistat 1), 1 suppository intravaginally QHS for 1 dose

Tioconazole 6.5% ointment (Monistat 1), 1 application (5 g) intravaginally QHS for 1 dose

Prescription Preparations

Butoconazole 2% cream (Gynazole-1), single dose bioadhesive, 5 g intravaginally for 1 dose

Terconazole 0.4% cream (Terazol 7), 1 application (5 g) intravaginally QHS for 7 d

Terconazole 0.8% cream (Terazol 3), 1 application (5 g) intravaginally QHS for 3 d

Terconazole 80-mg suppositories (Terazol 3), 1 suppository intravaginally QHS for 3 d

Fluconazole 150-mg tablet (Diflucan), 1 tablet PO, single dose

Note: All products can cause vaginal irritation, skin rash, hives. Refer to product labeling for more information.

OTC, over the counter.

Source: Centers for Disease Control and Prevention. (2015). Sexually transmitted treatment guidelines, 2015. *Morbidity and Mortality Weekly Reports, 64*(RR-3), 1–137.

contraindication to the topical antifungals is hypersensitivity to the azole or components of the cream or gel.

Time Frame for Response

The cure rates for topically applied azoles have long been established at between 80% and 90%. It can take a few days to see the effect of the medications.

Adverse Events

Topical azoles seldom cause systemic adverse events, although they may cause local irritation. Unfortunately, these effects may be difficult to distinguish from the conditions for which they are being used. Less common events may include penile irritation of the sex partner, abdominal cramps, or headache.

Interactions

Since these preparations are oil based, they may weaken latex condoms and diaphragms. Patients should be instructed to read condom product labeling for more information.

Oral Azole Antifungal Agents

Fluconazole, the only oral azole to be recommended by the CDC for treating uncomplicated VVC, is available by prescription in a single 150-mg dose. It is as effective as topical azoles. The findings of a study evaluating the acceptance of single-dose oral fluconazole by patients and physicians showed that most participants believed the drug to be effective in relieving or alleviating the symptoms of VVC. Oral weekly fluconazole (100 mg, 150 mg, or 200 mg) maintenance therapy for recurrent VVC should be extended for 6 months. Caution should be used in patients with hepatic and renal impairment since hepatotoxicity may occur, although it is unlikely given the low-dose weekly regimen recommended.

Contraindications

Contraindications to oral azole antifungals include known hypersensitivity to these azoles and the concomitant use of drugs with which they interact.

Time Frame for Response

It may take a few days for symptoms to resolve. Failure to respond necessitates reevaluation.

Adverse Events

The most commonly reported adverse events noted in patients treated with oral fluconazole are headache, nausea, and abdominal pain. Liver enzyme levels may need to be monitored for long-term use in women with a history of hepatic impairment. Adverse effects tend to be dose related. Significant interactions through cytochrome P450 enzymes are unlikely to occur with low doses used for VVC.

Antibiotics

Metronidazole (Flagyl) may be used orally or intravaginally for treating BV. Oral metronidazole 500 mg twice daily for 7 days is the standard treatment for BV, and only the oral form is effective in treating *Trichomonas* infection. Tinidazole can also be used for both trichomoniasis and BV, although it is more expensive than metronidazole. Topical clindamycin cream 2% (Cleocin) should be used in patients with BV who are allergic to metronidazole (see **Table 56.2** for specific dosages). Clindamycin 300 mg twice daily may also be used orally for a 7-day course for BV. It is contraindicated in patients with

TABLE 56.2

Centers for Disease Control and Prevention Recommendations for Treating Bacterial Vaginosis

Generic (Trade) Name and Dosage	Selected Adverse Events	Contraindications	Special Considerations
Recommended Regimens			
Metronidazole 500-mg tablets (Flagyl), 1 tablet PO BID for 7 d	Metallic taste, headache, GI distress	Allergy (no longer contraindicated in pregnancy)	Avoid alcohol during therapy and for 72 hours after stopping (will cause nausea and vomiting) May potentiate the anticoagulant effects of warfarin
Clindamycin 2% cream (Cleocin), 1 applicator intravaginally QHS for 7 d	Vaginal irritation, skin rash, hives	Allergy	Oil based; may weaken latex condoms and diaphragms. Refer to product labeling for more information
Metronidazole gel 0.75% (MetroGel), 1 applicatorful intravaginally daily for 5 d	Vaginal irritation, skin rash, metallic taste, GI distress	Same as above	Although blood levels are lower than with the use of oral metronidazole, alcohol still should be avoided

Note: Centers for Disease Control and Prevention recommendations as of 2015.

GI, gastrointestinal.

hypersensitivity to it or to other preparations containing linco-mycin. Clindamycin ovules intravaginally are also effective if inserted at bedtime for three nights.

Contraindications

The use of metronidazole with disulfiram, a drug used for alcohol abstinence, is contraindicated due to the risk of psychosis from enhancement of metronidazole. It is recommended that these two medications are not administered within 14 days of each other. Metronidazole is no longer thought to be terato-genic, and therefore, it is not contraindicated in the first tri-mester of pregnancy. Tinidazole is contraindicated in the first trimester of pregnancy and breast-feeding since animal studies show potential risk to fetus. Metronidazole and tinidazole are contraindicated in patients with a known hypersensitivity to them or other nitroimidazoles.

Adverse Events

Metallic taste, headache, and gastrointestinal (GI) distress are common side effects of metronidazole, tinidazole, and clin-damycin. They can be given with food to minimize GI side effects. To avoid the disulfiram-like effect of nausea and vomit-ing, patients must not consume alcohol during treatment with metronidazole and tinidazole and for at least 3 days after treat-ment stops.

Interactions

Metronidazole may potentiate the anticoagulant effect of warfarin (Coumadin). Clindamycin ovules and cream are made from an oleaginous base, which might impair the use of rubber or latex products such as condoms and dia-phragms. These products should not be used during or within 3 days following treatment of intravaginal clinda-mycin ovules and within 5 days following treatment with clindamycin vaginal cream.

Estrogens

Treatment of atrophic vaginitis consists of topical estrogen creams administered externally or intravaginally or systemic estrogen replacement therapy. Treatment of atrophic vaginitis is discussed elsewhere in this text book.

Antiinflammatories

Mild topical steroid preparations can be used on a short-term or episodic basis for inflammatory vaginitis. Careful monitor-ing of the patient's response is advised.

Selecting the Most Appropriate Agent

First-Line Therapy: Candidiasis

In an attempt to guide therapeutic options, the CDC classifies VVC as either uncomplicated or complicated (see **Box 56.2**).

Over-the-counter (OTC) topical antifungals are typical first-line therapy of uncomplicated VVC. Appropriate therapy consists of 1 to 14 days of treatment with the topical antifun-gals. Self-treatment with OTC antifungals can be reserved for women who have been previously diagnosed with VVC and who have not experienced a recurrence within 2 months.

Single-dose oral antifungals are an alternative first-line therapy in uncomplicated VVC, especially because of the ease of administration. Fluconazole is the oral azole of choice. For severe VVC, oral fluconazole 150 mg every 72 hours for 2 to 3 doses is recommended. The patient's sex partners do not need treatment because candidiasis is not sexually transmit-ted. See **Figure 56.1** and **Table 56.3** for an overview of VVC treatment.

Second-Line Therapy: Candidiasis

If symptoms persist beyond the recommended course of therapy with first-line agents, second-line therapy involves assessing for

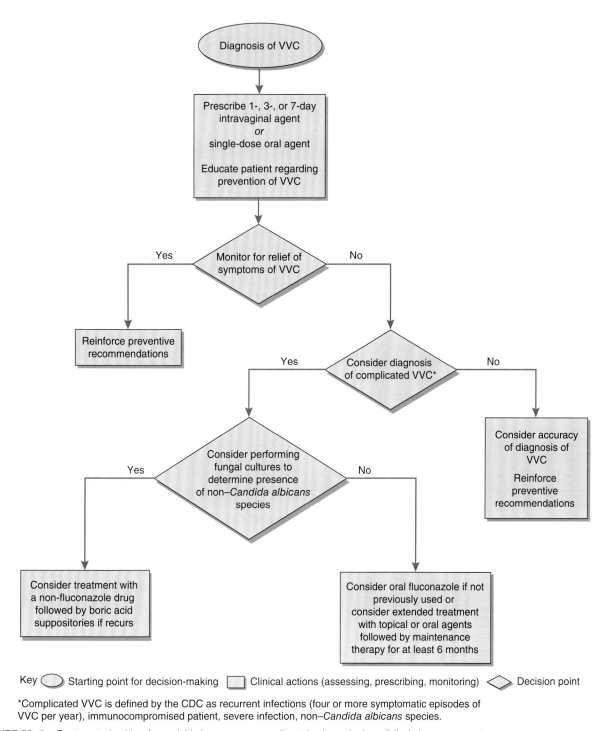

FIGURE 56–1   Treatment algorithm for vaginitis known as uncomplicated vulvovaginal candidiasis in nonpregnant women.

VVC, vulvovaginal candidiasis

possible recurrent VVC or infection with non-*albicans Candida*, such as *C. glabrata*. Vaginal cultures should be obtained to confirm the diagnosis and identify the species of *Candida* involved. If the patient has had three or fewer recurrences of *C. albicans* VVC in a 1-year period, the patient should be treated with longer courses of topical antifungals (7–14 days) or orally with fluconazole 150 mg every 72 hours for 3 doses.

Recurrent VVC, defined as at least four episodes of VVC in a year, occurs in approximately 5% of women. The Infectious Diseases Society of America (IDSA, 2016) recommends 10 to 14 days of induction therapy with either a topical azole or oral fluconazole. Maintenance therapy recommended is oral fluconazole 150 mg once weekly for 6 months. This is well tolerated and convenient. Approximately 90% of patients achieve symptom

TABLE 56.3

Recommended Order of Treatment for Vulvovaginal Candidiasis Caused by *Candida Albanians* in Immunocompetent Women

Order	Agents
First line (uncomplicated VVC)	OTC topical antifungal *or* Oral single-dose fluconazole 150 mg.
Second line (i.e., for recurrence after 2 months of initial presentation and less than 4 times per year)	Same as first line, although longer duration (7–14 days) of topical therapy, *or* 3 doses of oral fluconazole given every 72 hours.
Third line (i.e., recurrent VVC/more than 4 episodes in a year)	Induction therapy for 10–14 days with either a topical azole or an oral fluconazole. Maintenance therapy for 6 months with oral once weekly fluconazole 150 mg.

Note: Refer to text for treatment of immunocompromised or non–*albicans* VVC.

OTC, over the counter; VVC, vulvovaginal candidiasis.

Source: Centers for Disease Control and Prevention. (2015). Sexually transmitted treatment guidelines, 2015. *Morbidity and Mortality Weekly Reports, 64*(RR-3), 1–137.

control with this regimen, and the rate of recurrence is approximately 45% after cessation of maintenance therapy. If symptoms are not resolved while on maintenance therapy, consultation with a specialist is recommended. Topical clotrimazole cream 200 mg intravaginally twice weekly, clotrimazole vaginal suppository 500 mg once weekly, or another intermittent oral or topical antifungal can be used if fluconazole therapy is not possible.

A small number of patients will have VVC caused by non-*albicans Candida*. It is important to exclude all other causes of vaginal symptoms prior to diagnosing a woman with non-*albicans* VVC since it is possible for non-*albicans Candida* to be a colonizer. Most *Candida* species are susceptible to oral fluconazole. *C. krusei* and *C. glabrata* are typically inherently resistant to fluconazole. *C. krusei* infections can be treated successfully with any topical antifungal. *C. glabrata* does not respond to any azole antifungal. Though evidence for treatment of *C. glabrata* VVC is limited, the IDSA (2016) recommends intravaginal boric acid 600 mg vaginal capsules daily for 14 days or nystatin 100,000-unit intravaginal suppositories daily for 14 days. As a weak recommendation, topical flucytosine 17% cream alone or with amphotericin B 3% cream administered vaginally daily for 14 days is an option. These medications are not available commercially and thus a compounding pharmacy will need to make them for the patient. Insurance will typically not cover costs for compounded medications, and this can be expensive as patients will likely need to pay out of pocket. Consultation with a specialist is recommended.

Women who are immunocompromised benefit from prolonged therapy (7–14 days) with either topical agents or oral agents.

First-Line Therapy: Bacterial Vaginosis

Oral metronidazole (500 mg twice daily) 7-day therapy has long been considered standard first-line treatment for BV. However, the CDC (2015) also recommends topical clindamycin cream 2% (intravaginally for 7 days) or metronidazole gel 0.75% (intravaginally for 5 days) as acceptable first-line therapy.

Alternative regimens for first-line therapy include clindamycin 300 mg twice daily orally for a 7-day course or clindamycin ovules 100 mg intravaginally at bedtime for 3 days. Once-daily dosing with metronidazole 750-mg extended-release tablets for 7 days has been approved by the U.S. FDA for the treatment of BV, but data are limited regarding the efficacy of this regimen (CDC, 2015). Treatment of sex partners is not recommended because clinical trials have not shown a relationship between treatment of partners and recurrence of BV. See **Figure 56.2** and **Table 56.4** for an overview of treatment.

Second-Line Therapy: Bacterial Vaginosis

Treatment reduces symptoms, although recurrences are common. Recurrent BV should be treated. Treatment of recurrent BV has not been adequately studied. The CDC (2015) suggests treatment with the same or a different recommended first-line agent. One randomized trial for persistent BV indicated that metronidazole gel 0.75% twice per week for 6 months after completion of a recommended regimen was effective in maintaining a clinical cure for 6 months (Sobel et al., 2006). However, recurrence can result after cessation of the maintenance therapy. Routine treatment of sex partners is not recommended due to lack of evidence of any benefit.

First-Line Therapy: Trichomoniasis

Only one treatment regimen is considered to be clinically efficacious for trichomoniasis: metronidazole or tinidazole given as a single 2-g dose. An alternative regimen is metronidazole 500 mg twice daily for 7 days. Treatment of male sex partners (who are usually asymptomatic) is recommended, and patients and their partners should avoid intercourse until they have completed therapy and are symptom free. Condom use should be encouraged to prevent transmission. Patients should be cautioned to avoid alcohol, as previously described. See **Figure 56.3** and **Table 56.5** for an overview of treatment.

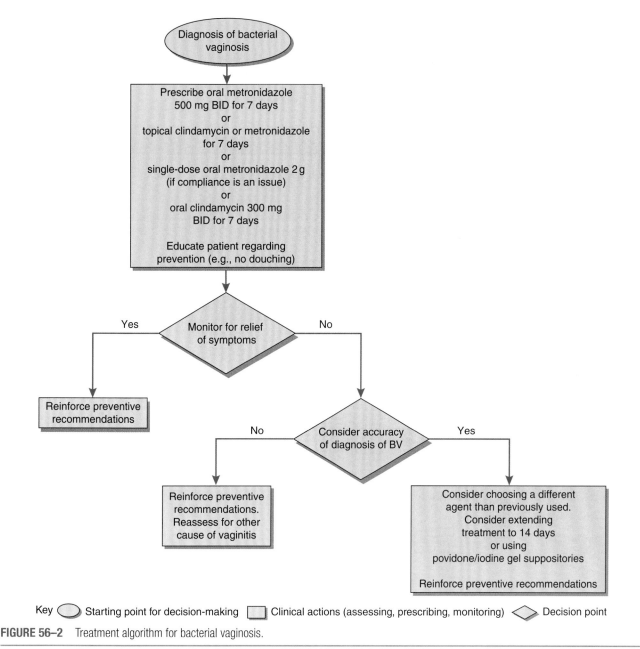

FIGURE 56–2 Treatment algorithm for bacterial vaginosis.

BV, bacterial vaginosis.

Second-Line Therapy: Trichomoniasis

Some strains of *T. vaginalis* can have diminished susceptibility to metronidazole but may respond to tinidazole. Resistance to metronidazole occurs in approximately 4% to 10% of cases while resistance to tinidazole happens in approximately 1% of cases. If first-line treatment fails and reinfection from an untreated partner is excluded, metronidazole 500 mg orally twice daily for 7 days can be used. For patients failing this regimen, tinidazole or metronidazole at 2 g orally for 7 days should be initiated. If this regimen fails multiple times, then susceptibility testing for metronidazole and tinidazole should be obtained for the organism. Consultation of a specialist is recommended since treatment options are limited when metronidazole and tinidazole are resistant. It is always

important to evaluate compliance with medication therapy. If patients are not compliant with their medication regimen, that can likely be the cause of treatment failure. Treatment regimens for sexual partners for patients with recurrent trichomoniasis are not well studied, although the CDC (2015) suggests using the same treatment regimen as the presenting patient and that the sexual partner is evaluated by a health care professional.

Special Population Considerations
Pediatric

Before menarche, when estrogen levels are low, the vaginal epithelium is thin and the vaginal pH tends to be between 6.0 and 7.0. These conditions create a vaginal environment that

TABLE 56.4

Recommended Order of Treatment for Bacterial Vaginosis in Nonpregnant Women

Order	Agents
First-line treatment	Oral metronidazole 500 mg BID for 7 days *or* Clindamycin cream 2% cream, one full applicator (5 g) intravaginally HS for 7 days *or* Metronidazole gel 0.75%, one full applicator (5 g) intravaginally HS for 5 days
First-line alternative therapies	Tinidazole 2 g PO once daily for 2 days *or* Tinidazole 1 g PO for 5 days *or* Clindamycin 300 mg PO BID for 7 days *or* Clindamycin ovules 100 mg intravaginally HS for 3 days
Second-line treatment (i.e., for recurrence)	Choose different agent or same agent
Third-line treatment (i.e., for recurrence)	First-line therapy; then metronidazole 0.75% gel vaginally twice weekly for 4–6 weeks

Source: Centers for Disease Control and Prevention. (2015). Sexually transmitted treatment guidelines, 2015. *Morbidity and Mortality Weekly Reports, 64*(RR-3), 1–137.

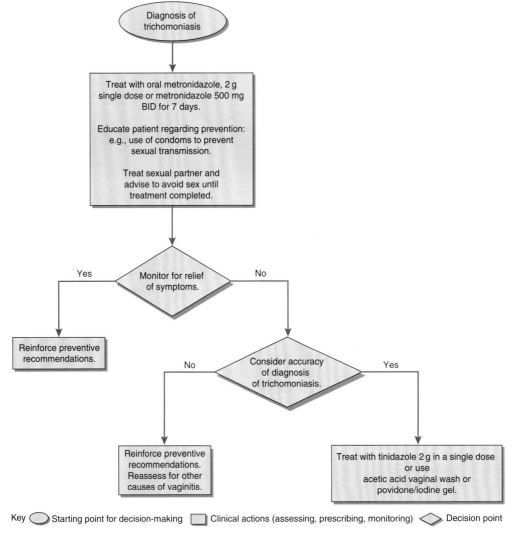

FIGURE 56–3   Treatment algorithm for vaginitis resulting from *Trichomonas* organisms in nonpregnant women.

TABLE 56.5

Recommended Order of Treatment for *Trichomonas* Infection in Nonpregnant Women

Order	Agents
First-line treatment	Metronidazole or tinidazole, single oral dose of 2 g
	Metronidazole 500 mg PO BID for 7 days in women with HIV
Second-line treatment (after treatment failure)	Metronidazole 500 mg PO BID for 7 days
Third-line treatment (after treatment failure)	Metronidazole or tinidazole 2 g PO daily for 7 days

Note: Consultation with a specialist and susceptibility testing for metronidazole and tinidazole should be obtained after several failed third-line treatments.

HIV, human immunodeficiency virus.

Source: Centers for Disease Control and Prevention. (2015). Sexually transmitted treatment guidelines, 2015. *Morbidity and Mortality Weekly Reports, 64*(RR-3), 1–137.

BOX 56.4

Centers for Disease Control and Prevention Recommendations for Treatment of Infectious Vaginitis in Pregnancy

VULVOVAGINAL CANDIDIASIS

Topical azole therapies, *only*, for 7 days

BACTERIAL VAGINOSIS

Same as first-line therapy in nonpregnant women

TRICHOMONIASIS

Metronidazole 2 g PO single dose

Data are current for 2015.

is more susceptible to invading anaerobic bacteria if the child is exposed. Infections may be sexually transmitted or caused by contamination with fecal flora, and the possibility of sexual abuse must be considered. Poor hygiene and the use of vaginal irritants such as bubble baths and other products may also contribute to infections in the prepubertal child. Because of the high vaginal pH of the prepubertal child, candidiasis usually does not occur.

Postmenopausal Women

The decline in estrogen levels that occurs in the postmenopausal woman produces conditions similar to those in prepubertal children, and these conditions predispose the woman to infection and atrophy. As noted previously, the practitioner needs to be aware that atrophic vaginitis is a common cause of vaginal symptoms, and accurate diagnosis is essential.

Pregnant Women

Because vaginitis may occur during pregnancy, therapeutic goals include relieving symptoms and avoiding complications. Depending on the cause of vaginitis, therapy aims to achieve one or both of these goals. Refer to **Box 56.4** for the CDC's recommendations for the treatment of vaginitis in pregnancy.

Physiologic conditions of pregnancy increase the risk of VVC. For treatment of VVC during pregnancy, the CDC recommends that only topical azoles be used for a 7-day course of therapy.

Adverse pregnancy outcomes (premature rupture of membranes, preterm labor, preterm birth, intraamniotic infection, and postpartum endometritis) have been reported in patients with BV, although there is no evidence to suggest that treatment prevents these outcomes. Symptomatic BV in pregnant women should be treated to relieve symptoms. There is lack of evidence suggesting benefit in the treatment of asymptomatic

pregnant women. Oral and topical metronidazole and clindamycin may be used in both groups (see **Table 56.3**). Follow-up of high-risk pregnant women who have been treated for BV is recommended at 1 month after completion of treatment to ensure a successful response.

Trichomonas infections have been associated with preterm delivery, premature ruptures of membranes, and low birth-weight infants. It is not clear if treatment reduces complications. Symptomatic infections during any stage of pregnancy should be treated with oral metronidazole 2 g once. Tinidazole should be avoided due to lack of evidence in pregnant women and potential risk of harm to animal fetuses. Treatment and screening of asymptomatic high-risk pregnant women is inconclusive; the decision to test and treat is at the discretion of the obstetrician (van Schalkwyk et al., 2015). Screening and treatment in all pregnant women with human immunodeficiency virus (HIV) at the first prenatal visit is recommended by the CDC (2015) since infection with *Trichomonas* is a risk factor for vertical transmission of HIV. To confirm eradication, a retest after 3 months should be performed.

Immunocompromised Patients

In women with HIV, metronidazole 500 mg twice daily for 7 days was shown to be more effective than a once dose of metronidazole 2 g in the treatment of trichomoniasis. Screening should be done at diagnosis and yearly thereafter. Patients should be retested 3 months after completing treatment. Trichomoniasis is significantly associated with pelvic inflammatory disease in women with HIV. Treatment reduces genital-tract HIV viral load and viral shedding.

Patients with HIV or other immunocompromising conditions should be treated for BV the same as those without.

Immunocompromised patients presenting with VVC should be treated with longer courses of topical antifungals (7–14 days) or orally with fluconazole 150 mg every 72 hours for 3 doses.

MONITORING PATIENT RESPONSE

Diagnosis and management of vaginitis can be frustrating for both the patient and the practitioner, especially in patients with chronic symptoms and recurrent infections. Symptoms may recur or persist despite adherence to prescribed therapy. The practitioner should consult an expert if the patient fails to respond to current treatment recommendations.

The use of fungal cultures to assess response to therapy and to identify the offending *Candida* species is beneficial in assessing and treating patients with recurrent VVC. Fungal cultures play a role in detecting non-*albicans Candida* infections that may require second-line therapy.

Practitioners need to individualize the plan of care with each patient. They also need to maintain current knowledge of research regarding alternative therapies and to inform patients of findings. In many situations, yogurt and similar products may cause no harm and may provide patients with a perception of control over a frustrating condition.

Because of the increased risk of postoperative gynecologic infectious complications associated with BV, some specialists suggest that before performing surgical abortion or hysterectomy, providers should screen for and treat women with BV in addition to providing routine surgical prophylaxis. However, more evidence is needed in the treatment of asymptomatic BV before procedures. Treatment of sex partners is not routinely recommended because studies have shown that treatment of partners does not reduce the incidence of recurrence or relapse.

PATIENT EDUCATION

Drug Information

Metronidazole and tinidazole can cause nausea and vomiting if alcohol is ingested during therapy and up to 72 hours after therapy stops. Patients should be instructed to be compliant with drug therapy. The practitioner should reinforce the importance of following directions carefully and completing the full course of antibiotic therapy even if symptoms subside early.

Lifestyle Changes

The patient should avoid tight-fitting clothing, should wear undergarments that allow adequate vaginal ventilation, and should avoid douches and other feminine hygiene products that may alter the normal vaginal pH. The possibility that sexual activity may be associated with the onset of symptoms should be discussed, and the patient should be instructed to monitor these patterns. The patient should use condoms to protect against sexually transmitted disease. Because the use of antibiotics and oral contraceptives may be factors that predispose patients to vaginitis, other treatment options should be explored.

Receiving orogenital sex, using any form of contraceptive, having a high body mass index, having impaired glucose tolerance, consuming excessive sweets, and having high stress levels are some risk factors for recurrent VVC.

Complementary and Alternative Medicine

Probiotics are supplements that contain live bacteria. They promote healthy normal flora. The true benefit of supplementation with lactobacilli probiotics, however, as protection against infectious vaginitis has not been established.

CASE STUDY 1

R.S. is a 32-year-old woman who seeks treatment for a vaginal discharge that she has had for the past month. She is sexually active and has had the same partner for the past 6 months. She reports noticing an odor, especially after sexual intercourse. Her history reveals that she has been using a commercial douche on a biweekly basis during the past year for hygienic purposes in an attempt to prevent vaginal infections. She denies any other associated symptoms. The physical examination reveals a white vaginal discharge. Microscopic examination of the vaginal discharge shows clue cells, and the pH is 5.5 (Learning Objectives 1, 2, and 3).

DIAGNOSIS: BACTERIAL VAGINOSIS

1. List the specific goals of treatment for this patient.
2. What are the potential causes and risk factors this patient has?

3. How would you confirm the diagnosis of bacterial vaginosis (BV)?
4. What drug therapy would you prescribe? Why?
5. What are the parameters for monitoring the success of the therapy?
6. Discuss specific patient education based on the prescribed therapy.
7. List one or two adverse reactions for the selected agent that would cause you to change therapy.
8. What over-the-counter or alternative medications would be appropriate for this patient?
9. What dietary or lifestyle changes should be recommended?
10. Describe one or two drug–drug or drug–food interactions for the selected agent.

Bibliography

Starred references are cited in the text.

*Amsel, R., Totten, P. A., Spiegel, C. A., et al. (1983). Nonspecific vaginitis: Diagnostic criteria and microbial and epidemiologic associations. *The American Journal of Medicine, 74*(1), 14–22.

*Centers for Disease Control and Prevention. (2015). Sexually transmitted treatment guidelines, 2015. *Morbidity and Mortality Weekly Reports, 64*(RR-3), 1–137.

Coleman, J. S., & Gaydos, C. A. (2018). Molecular diagnosis of bacterial vaginosis: An update. *Journal of Clinical Microbiology, 56*(9), e00342–18. doi: 10.1128/JCM.00342-18

*Ferris, D. G., Nyirjesy, P., Sobel, J. D., et al. (2002). Over-the-counter antifungal drug misuse associated with patient-diagnosed vulvovaginal candidiasis. *Obstetrics and Gynecology, 99*(3), 419–425.

Hildebrand, J. P., & Kansagor, A. T. Vaginitis. [Updated December 16, 2019]. In: *StatPearls* [Internet]. Treasure Island, FL: StatPearls Publishing; January 2020. https://www.ncbi.nlm.nih.gov/books/NBK470302/

Kaambo, E., Africa, C., Chambuso, R., et al. (2018). Vaginal microbiomes associated with aerobic vaginitis and bacterial vaginosis. *Frontiers in Public Health, 6*, 78. doi: 10.3389/fpubh.2018.0007

Lee, A., Kim, T. H., Lee, H., et al. (2018). Therapeutic approaches to atrophic vaginitis in postmenopausal women: A systematic review with a network meta-analysis of randomized controlled trials. *Journal of Menopausal Medicine, 24*(1), 1–10.

Martin Lopez, J. E. (2015). Candidiasis (vulvovaginal). *BMJ Clinical Evidence, 2015*, 0815.

Paavonen, J., & Brunham, R. C. (2019). Bacterial vaginosis and desquamative inflammatory vaginitis. *The New England Journal of Medicine, 380*(11), 1089.

Paladine, H. L., & Desai, U. A. (2018). Vaginitis: Diagnosis and treatment. *American Family Physician, 97*(5), 321–329.

Pappas, P. G., Kauffman, C. A., Andes, D. R., et al. (2016). Executive summary: Clinical practice guideline for the management of Candidiasis: 2016 Update by the Infectious Diseases Society of America. *Clinical Infectious Diseases: An Official Publication of the Infectious Diseases Society of America, 62*(4), 409–417.

Santoro, N., Epperson, C. N., & Mathews, S. B. (2015). Menopausal symptoms and their management. *Endocrinology and Metabolism Clinics of North America, 44*(3), 497–515.

*Sobel, J. D., Ferris, D., Schwebke, J., et al. (2006). Suppressive antibacterial therapy with 0.75% metronidazole vaginal gel to prevent recurrent bacterial vaginosis. *American Journal of Obstetrics and Gynecology, 194*, 1283–1289.

*van Schalkwyk, J., Yudin, M. H., & Infectious Disease Committee. (2015). Vulvovaginitis: Screening for and management of trichomoniasis, vulvovaginal candidiasis, and bacterial vaginosis. *Journal of Obstetrics and Gynaecology Canada, 37*(3), 266–274.

Wang, Z., He, Y., & Zheng, Y. (2019). Probiotics for the treatment of bacterial vaginosis: A meta-analysis. *International Journal of Environmental Research and Public Health, 16*(20), 3859.

Wolters Kluwer Clinical Drug Information, Inc. (Lexi-Drugs). (2020). Wolters Kluwer Clinical Drug Information, Inc.; February 10, 2020.

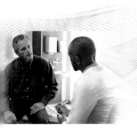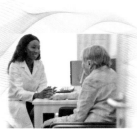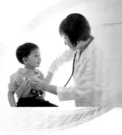

Note: Page numbers followed by "f" denote figures; those followed by "t" denote tables; and those followed by "b" denote boxes.

A

Abacavir, for HIV infection, 851t, 950, 959t
Abatacept
    for psoriasis, 232t
    for rheumatoid arthritis, 684–685
Abreva (docosanol), for viral skin infections, 222, 222t
Abscesses
    causes of, 201
    tubo-ovarian, in pelvic inflammatory disease, 632
Absence (petit mal) seizures, 726–727
Absorbents, for diarrhea, 485
Absorica (isotretinoin)
    for acne, 244t, 246–247, 249
    for rosacea, 252
Absorption, drug, 19–21
    active transport in, 20
    vs. age, 57t
    bioavailability and, 19, 20b
    biologic membranes and, 19–20
    blood flow and, 20–21
    complementary alternative medicine interactions, 44, 44t
    in drug–disease interactions, 46
    in drug–drug interactions, 34, 35t
    drug–food interactions, 41–42, 42b
    enteral, 20
    factors affecting, 19–21
    formulation and, 20
    gastrointestinal motility and, 21
    intramuscular and subcutaneous, 58
    methods of, 19
    mucosal, 59
    in older adults, 72
    oral, 57–58
    parenteral, 21–22
    passive diffusion in, 19–20
    in pediatric patients, 57–59
    percutaneous, 58–59
    pharmaceutical preparation and, 20
    in pregnancy, 57–59, 57t
    pulmonary, 59
    rate of, 34
    solubility and, 19–20
Acacia, complementary alternative medicine interactions, 44
Academic skills training, for ADHD, 867
Acamprosate, for alcohol use disorder, 873–875, 874t
Acarbose, for diabetes mellitus, 892t, 896
Accelerated approval, 4
ACCF/AHA guidelines, for heart failure, 358, 360, 362, 364–366
Accolate (zafirlukast), for asthma and COPD, 429t, 438–439
Accupril (quinapril)
    for chronic stable angina, 334, 335t, 338
    for heart failure, 352, 353t
Accutane (isotretinoin)
    for acne, 244t, 246–247, 249
    for rosacea, 252
Acebutolol
    for chronic stable angina, 340
    for hypertension, 301
Aceon (perindopril)
    for chronic stable angina, 334
    for heart failure, 352

Acetaminophen
    for headache, 696–697, 697t
    metabolism of, 61
    for osteoarthritis, 647–648
    for pain, 81–82, 152, 154, 155
    for pain management in opioid use disorder, 173
    pharmacokinetics and pharmacodynamics of, 156t
Acetylcholinesterase inhibitors, for Alzheimer's disease, 758–759, 760t
Acetylcysteine, for asthma and COPD, 432t, 441–442
Acetylsalicylic acid. *See* Aspirin
ACHES acronym, for hormonal contraceptive side effects, 1099
Achromycin (tetracycline)
    absorption and, 41
    α₁-acid glycoprotein, drug binding to, in older adults, 72
    adsorption and, 34
    for gonorrhea, 624, 625t
    for syphilis, 624, 625t
Acidophilus capsules, for diarrhea, 488
AcipHex (rabeprazole)
    for GERD, 529t, 530t
    for peptic ulcer disease, 529t, 537t
Acitretin (etretinate), for psoriasis, 232t
Aclidinium bromide, for asthma and COPD, 430t, 438
Acne vulgaris, 241–250
    causes of, 241, 242t
    classification of, 242, 242t
    diagnostic criteria of, 242
    drug-induced, 241, 242t
    epidemiology of, 241
    pathophysiology of, 242
    patient education on, 249, 249b
    in pediatric patients, 249
    in pregnancy, 249
    selection of drugs, 247–249, 248f, 248t
    therapeutic monitoring of, 249
    treatment of, 242–249, 243t–244t, 248f, 248t
Acquired immunodeficiency syndrome. *See* Human immunodeficiency virus infection
Actemra, for rheumatoid arthritis, 685
Actigraphy, in sleep disorders, 831
ACTION HF organization guidelines, for heart failure, 363, 367
Action potential, in cardiac function, 371, 372b
Actiq (fentanyl), for pain, 152, 156, 157, 158t, 159–160, 159t
Activated charcoal, constipation and, 469b
Active transport
    in absorption, 20
    in excretion, 39
Actonel (risedronate), for osteoporosis, 667, 668t
Actos (pioglitazone), for diabetes mellitus, 892t, 895
Acular (ketorolac), for conjunctivitis, 263t, 265
Acupuncture, for allergic rhinitis, 944
Acute coronary syndromes, 329–330, 333. *See also* Myocardial infarction (MI)
    treatment selection in, 346
Acute emesis, nausea and vomiting, 463–465, 464b, 465b
Acyclovir
    for herpes simplex virus infections, 628, 629t, 631
    for viral skin infections, 221–222, 222t, 223
Aczone (dapsone), for acne, 243t, 245
Adalat (nifedipine)
    for chronic stable angina, 336t, 341
    for hypertension, 303t, 304

Adalimumab
    for inflammatory bowel disease, 503t, 508
    for psoriasis, 232t, 236
    for rheumatoid arthritis, 680t, 684
Adapalene, for acne, 243t, 244, 247
Adderall (amphetamine and dextroamphetamine), for ADHD, 861t–862t
Addiction
    definition of, 162
    opioids, 161–162, 167–168, 168f
Adefovir, for hepatitis B virus, 557, 558t
Adenine, 122, 122b
Adenocard (adenosine), for arrhythmias, 374t, 385
Adenosine, for arrhythmias, 374t, 385
Adenosine triphosphate-citrate lyase inhibitors, for hyperlipidemia, 324–325
ADHD. *See* Attention-deficit/hyperactivity disorder (ADHD)
Adherence issues, 13–14, 14t
    in older adults, 76–78
Adipex-P (phentermine), for obesity, 1080, 1080t
Adipose tissue. *See* Fat (body)
Adjunctive agents
    for hyperthyroidism, 921
    for spontaneous bacterial peritonitis, 551
Administration routes
    buccal, 21
    inhalation, 21
    intra-arterial, 22
    intramuscular, 58
        drug absorption in, 22
    intravenous, 22
    oral, 21, 57–58, 60, 66
    parenteral, 21–22
        for pediatric patients, 67
    in prescriptions, 12
    rectal, 21, 58, 66–67
    subcutaneous, 22
    sublingual, 21
    topical (*See* Topical administration)
    transdermal, 22
Adolescents
    absorption in, 57t
    acne vulgaris in, 241–250
    depression in, 800
    diabetes mellitus, 905
    distribution in, 57t, 59–60
    elimination in, 57t
    immunization for, 1038
    metabolism in, 57t
    nausea and vomiting in, 468b
Adrenergic agonists, for glaucoma, 274t, 276
ADRs. *See* Adverse drug reactions (ADRs)
Adsorbents, for diarrhea, 485
Adsorption, drug, in drug–drug interactions, 34
Adult education, on side effects, 87
Advair Diskus (fluticasone propionate/salmeterol), for asthma and COPD, 431t
Adverse drug reactions (ADRs), 33–51. *See also specific drugs*
    death rate in, 33
    definition of, 48
    drug interactions (*See* Drug interactions)
    medication errors, 49, 49t, 49f
    in older adults, 76, 77t
    prescription errors causing, 9
    tracking of, 49, 50f
    types of, 49
Advicor (lovastatin/niacin), for hyperlipidemia, 325

Advil (ibuprofen), pharmacokinetic and pharmacodynamic properties of, 152, 156t, 159
Aeromonas species infections, 480b, 482
Aerosol drug delivery, 59
    devices, 67, 68t
Affinity, drug, 18b, 29, 37
Afinitor (everolimus), for organ transplantation, 972–973, 974t
Afrin (oxymetazoline hydrochloride), for upper respiratory infections, 405, 405t, 408, 412
Afrin Children (phenylephrine hydrochloride), for upper respiratory infections, 405, 405t, 408, 412
After-depolarization, in cardiac cells, 372
Age. *See also* Older adults; Pediatric patients
    chronic stable angina and, 330
    pediatric dosage calculated from, 65
    on pharmacokinetics and pharmacodynamics, 31
Agency for Health Care Policy and Research (AHCPR) guidelines, for smoking cessation, 1061–1062, 1071t, 1072f
Aging. *See also* Older adults
    body changes with, 72–74, 74b, 75t
Agonists, receptor interaction with, 30
Agranulocytosis, 921
Agricultural Improvement Act, 181
AHCPR guidelines. *See* Agency for Health Care Policy and Research (AHCPR) guidelines
AIDS. *See* Human immunodeficiency virus Infection
Aimovig, for migraine prevention, 717t, 718–719
Air travel, with sinusitis, 417
Airway
    allergic inflammation of (*See* Allergic rhinitis; Asthma)
    chronic obstruction of (*See* Chronic obstructive pulmonary disease [COPD])
Ajovy, for migraine prevention, 717t, 719
AK-Con (naphazoline), for conjunctivitis, 264t, 265
AK-Dex (dexamethasone), for conjunctivitis, 264t
Akynzeo (netupitant/palonosetron), for nausea and vomiting, 457t
Albumin
    drug binding to, 34, 46
        in older adults, 72
        pregnancy, 59, 62
    hepatorenal syndrome, 552t
Albuterol, for asthma and COPD, 428t, 436
Alcaftadine, for conjunctivitis, 262, 263t
Alclometasone dipropionate, for contact dermatitis, 193t
Alcohol ear drops, for otitis externa, 290
Alcohol intake
    adverse drug reactions and, 76
    drug interactions and, 48
    in heart failure, 369
    moderation of, for hyperlipidemia, 317
    in older adults, 76
Alcohol use disorder (AUD)
    alcohol equivalents, 872, 873b
    algorithm for, 877f
    medications used in, 880t
    treatment for, 872, 873–877
Alcohol withdrawal syndrome, 872–873
    benzodiazepine for, 874t
    delirium tremens, 873, 873b
Aldactone (spironolactone)
    for acne, 244t, 247
    for chronic stable angina, 334, 335t, 338
    for heart failure, 354t, 359
    for hypertension, 300, 300t
Aldara (imiquimod), for human papilloma virus infections, 635–636, 636t
Aldosterone antagonists
    for chronic stable angina, 334, 335t, 338
    for hypertension, 300
Aldosterone, in blood pressure regulation, 295, 296
Alemtuzumab, for organ transplantation, 967–968, 973t

Alendronate, for osteoporosis, 667, 668t
Aleve (naproxen)
    for headache, 697, 698t
    pharmacokinetic and pharmacodynamic properties of, 156t
    for upper respiratory infections, 406t, 409
Alfenta (alfentanil), for pain, 160
Alfentanil, for pain, 160
Alfuzosin, for overactive bladder, 601t, 603t
Algorithms. *See also specific disorders*
    development of, 138
Alirocumab, for hyperlipidemia, 321t, 322
Aliskiren, for hypertension, 303, 303t
Alkalinization, in drug excretion, 39
All-or-none phenomenon, in neurons, 725
Allegra (fexofenadine), for allergic rhinitis, 937t, 938
Alleles, 122b, 123
Allergens, 830b, 830f, 929–930
    in rhinitis, 931, 932t, 933
Allergic conjunctivitis, 261–265, 944
Allergic contact dermatitis (ACD), 191
Allergic rhinitis, 932–944
    algorithm for, 935
    causes of, 932, 932t
    complementary and alternative medicine for, 944
    diagnosis of, 933–934
    differential diagnosis of, 934, 934t
    genetic factors in, 932
    information sources for, 944
    in older adults, 942
    pathophysiology of, 933, 933f
    patient education on, 943–944
    in pediatric patients, 942
    perennial, 932, 932t, 934
    in pregnancy, 942
    seasonal, 932, 932t, 934
    therapeutic monitoring of, 942, 943b
    treatment of, 934–942
    in women, 942
Allergic vaginitis, 1116, 1117–1118
Allergy(ies), 929–944
    definition of, 929
    reactions in
        classification of, 929–930, 930b, 930f
        prevention of, 931
        to vaccines, 1049
Allicin. *See Allium sativum*
Allium sativum, 418
    urinary tract infection, 575
Allogenic grafts, 965
Allografts, 965
Allopurinol, for gout, 654
Allosteric site, definition of, 18b
Allowable substitutions, 12
Allylamine antifungals, 215, 215t–216t, 217
Almotriptan, for migraine headache, 703, 706t, 711
Alocril (nedocromil), for conjunctivitis, 263t, 265
Aloe vera, for psoriasis, 239
Alomide (lodoxamide), for conjunctivitis, 263t, 265
Alosetron, 495
Aloxi (palonosetron), for nausea and vomiting, 460
Alpha-adrenergic antagonists, 601t, 603t, 608
Alpha-adrenergic blockers, for benign prostatic hyperplasia, 584–585, 584t
Alpha-glucosidase inhibitors, 892t, 896
Alphagan (brimonidine), for glaucoma, 274t, 276
5-alpha-reductase inhibitors, for benign prostatic hyperplasia, 583–584, 584t
Alprazolam
    for anxiety disorders, 80, 816, 817t, 819t
    drug interactions of, 41
    for insomnia, 834t
Altace (ramipril)
    for chronic stable angina, 334, 335t, 338
    for heart failure, 352, 353t, 356–357
    for hypertension, 302, 302t
Altered intestinal motility, 481
Alternative medicine. *See also* Complementary and alternative medicine (CAM)

Alzheimer's disease, 755–763
    causes of, 756, 756b
    complementary and alternative medicine for, 762
    diagnosis of, 756–757
    epidemiology of, 755
    information sources for, 758b, 762
    pathophysiology of, 756–757
    patient education on, 762
    support groups for, 758, 758b
    therapeutic monitoring of, 761–762
    treatment of, 757–761, 757b, 758b, 760t, 761t
Amantadine
    for influenza, 1042
    for Parkinson disease, 772
Ambien (zolpidem), for insomnia, 835t, 836
Amcinonide, for contact dermatitis, 193t
Amenorrhea, in menopause, 1102
Amerge (naratriptan), for migraine headache, 705t, 710
American Association of Clinical Endocrinologist (AACE), 890
American Diabetes Association (ADA), 890
American dwarf plant (*Serenoa repens*), 612
American Hospital Formulary Service, 14t, 133
American Psychiatric Association, nicotine dependence test of, 1058, 1060b
American Urological Association Symptom Index Scale of, 582, 582t
Amikacin
    dosages of, 107t
    monitoring of, 108t
    sensitivity of, 97t
Amikin. *See* Amikacin
Amiloride
    for ascites, 547t, 549
    for heart failure, 354t
    for hypertension, 300t
Aminoglycoside antibiotics, for otitis externa, 289
Aminoglycosides, 97t, 107–108, 107t, 118t
Aminopenicillins, 100t. *See also specific drugs*
Aminophylline, for asthma and COPD, 440–441
Aminosalicylates, for inflammatory bowel disease, 502t, 504–505
Amiodarone
    for arrhythmias, 374t, 379b, 381–383
    for heart failure, 366
Amitiza (lubiprostone)
    for constipation, 472t, 475, 476–477
    for irritable bowel syndrome, 493t, 495, 497t
Amitriptyline
    for headache, 697, 699
    for insomnia, 838
    for irritable bowel syndrome, 494, 497t
    for migraine prevention, 716t, 718
    for pain, 162
Amlodipine
    for chronic stable angina, 336t, 341
    for hypertension, 303t, 304, 308
Amoxicillin
    for community-acquired pneumonia, 422, 422t
    for GERD, 529t, 532
    for otitis media, 285, 285t
    for peptic ulcer disease, 529t, 532
    sensitivity of, 95t
    for sinusitis, 413–414
    for urinary tract infections, 569
Amoxicillin–ampicillin, 100t
Amoxicillin–clavulanate
    causing diarrhea, 479
    for community-acquired pneumonia, 422, 422t
    dosages of, 101t
    for otitis media, 284, 285t
    sensitivity of, 95t
    for sinusitis, 407t, 413–414
    for skin infections, 205t, 207
Amoxil (amoxicillin)
    for community-acquired pneumonia, 422, 422t
    for GERD, 529t, 532
    for otitis media, 285, 285t

for peptic ulcer disease, 529t, 532
sensitivity of, 95t
for sinusitis, 413–414
for urinary tract infections, 569
Amphetamine
drug excretion, 39
for narcolepsy, 846
Ampicillin, 100t
sensitivity of, 95t
Ampicillin–sulbactam, 95t, 101t
Amylin analog, for diabetes mellitus, 899–900
Amyloid plaques, in Alzheimer's disease, 756
Anaerobic infections, antimicrobial agents for,
114–115, 115t
Anakinra, for rheumatoid arthritis, 679t
Analgesics, 145, 152
central, 160
for decongestants, 406t, 409
5 A's of, 175, 175b
multiple-mechanism, 160
nonopioid, 155–161
opioid, 156–157, 158t
for osteoarthritis, 648–649
for pain management in opioid use disorder, 173
vs. type of pain, 145, 153–155, 153t, 156t
for urinary tract infections, 569, 571t
Anaphylaxis and anaphylactoid reactions, 931
Ancef (cefazolin), 95t, 102t
for skin infections, 205t, 207
Anectine (succinylcholine), metabolism of, 31
Anemia(s), 1013–1028
aplastic, 116, 1026, 1026b
in blood loss, 1016
causes of, 1013
of chronic disease, 1022–1023
in chronic renal failure, 1020–1022
classification of, 1014, 1015b, 1015f
complementary and alternative medicine for,
1027
Cooley (thalassemia), 1023–1024
diagnosis of, 1014
in folate deficiency, 1025–1026, 1025b
iron deficiency, 1018–1020, 1019b, 1019t, 1027
iron replacement therapy, 1020
macrocytic, 1014, 1024, 1024b
microcytic, 1014, 1023
vs. normal hematologic values, 1014t
nutrition for, 1027
in older adults, 1027
pathophysiology of, 1013–1014, 1015b
patient education on, 1027
in pediatric patients, 1027
pernicious, 1024–1025, 1024b
posthemorrhagic, 1016
sickle cell, 1016–1018
signs and symptoms of, 1016
in thalassemia, 1023–1024
therapeutic monitoring of, 1027
types of, 1013
in vitamin B_{12} deficiency, 1024–1025, 1024b
in women, 1027
Angioedema, from angiotensin-converting enzyme
inhibitors, 357
Angiography
cerebral
in seizures, 728
in stroke, 988
pulmonary, in pulmonary embolism, 987
Angiomax (bivalirudin), for chronic stable angina, 337t
Angiotensin-converting enzyme inhibitors
for chronic stable angina, 334, 335t, 338
drug interactions of, 358, 358t
for heart failure, 352, 353t, 356t, 358t
for hypertension, 302, 302t, 307–308
for older adults, 358, 368
therapeutic monitoring of, 88
Angiotensin II receptor blockers
for chronic stable angina, 334, 335t, 338
for heart failure, 354t, 359–360

for hypertension, 302–303, 302t, 307–308
Angiotensin, in blood pressure regulation, 295
Angiotensin receptor-neprilysin inhibitor, for heart
failure, 354t, 360–361
Anorexiants, 1080, 1080t–1081t
Anoro Ellipta (umeclidinium/vilanterol), for asthma
and COPD, 431t
Antabuse (disulfiram), for alcohol use disorder,
874t, 875
Antacids
constipation and, 469b
drug interactions with, 34, 35t
for GERD, 528, 529t, 530t
for nausea and vomiting, 458t, 462, 467
for peptic ulcer disease, 528, 529t
Antagonist/estrogen agonist, in menopause, 1108–
1109
Antagonists, receptor interaction with, 30
Anterior blepharitis, 257
Anthralin, for psoriasis, 231t, 233
Anti-immunoglobulin E agent, 433t, 442–443
Anti-interleukin-4R agent, 433t, 442–443
Anti-interleukin-5/5R agents, 433t, 442–443
Anti-thymocyte globulin, for organ transplantation,
967, 973t
Antianaerobic agents, 98t, 114–115, 115t
Antiarrhythmic agents
adenosine, 385
for atrial fibrillation/flutter, 374t, 386t, 388–391,
389f, 390f
atropine, 385
for bradycardia, 387t, 395–396
characteristics of, 374t–378t
Class I (sodium channel blockers), 378, 379b
Class IA, 378–379, 379b
Class IB, 379–380, 379b
Class IC, 379b, 380–381
Class II (beta blockers), 379b, 381
Class III (potassium channel blockers), 379b,
381–384
Class IV (calcium channel blockers), 379b, 384
classification of, 374, 378, 379b
digoxin, 385
for geriatrics, 396–397
goals of, 374
information sources for, 397–398
interactions of, with complementary
medicines, 398
monitoring of, 397
for paroxysmal supraventricular tachycardia, 386t,
392–393, 393f
patient education on, 397–398
for pediatric patients, 396
selection of, 385–395, 389f–395f
for ventricular fibrillation, 374t, 387t, 393–394,
395f
for ventricular tachycardia, 374t–378t, 387t,
393–394
Antibody(ies)
in allergic reactions, 930
in allergic rhinitis, 933, 933f
Antibody–antigen reactions, 930, 930f
Anticholinergics
constipation and, 469b
for older adults, 75t
for overactive bladder, 601t, 602, 602t–603t,
604–605, 606t
for Parkinson disease, 767–768
for upper respiratory infections, 406t, 409–410
Anticipatory emesis, nausea and vomiting, 465–466
Anticipatory nausea and vomiting, 451
Anticoagulants, 990. *See also* Heparin; Warfarin
for chronic stable angina, 337t, 342–343
considerations for, 991
contraindications of, 990–991
direct-acting oral, 996–997
fibrinolytic therapy for, 337t, 342–343
invasive procedures and, 1006b
managing, 999–1002

nutrition with, 1008
parenteral, 991–993, 992t, 994b, 994t
patient education on, 1006–1008, 1006b, 1008t
selection of, 1003–1005
therapeutic monitoring of, 992
types of, 990
Anticonvulsants, 728t, 729, 729f, 737b, 739, 740b,
750
for migraine prevention, 714, 715t
for pain, 162–163
for psychiatric disorders, in older adults, 82
for restless legs syndrome, 842–843
Antidepressants, 838, 846
adverse events due to, 788–789, 792
for Alzheimer's disease, 761
for anxiety disorders, 814–821, 814t
atypical, 789t, 795t, 796
classification of, 787–788, 789t
in continuation phase, 787
for depression, 786–800
acute, 787
drug interactions of, 793t
in emergencies, 801, 801b
goals of, 786
herbal, 802
for irritable bowel syndrome, 494–495, 497t
in maintenance phase, 787
mechanism of action of, 787, 787f
metabolism of, genetic variations in, 801
for migraine prevention, 716t, 718
monoamine oxidase inhibitors, 789t, 793t, 794,
795t
neurotransmitters affected by, 789t
for obesity, 1078
in older adults, 80–81, 800
for pain, 162
in pediatric patients, 800
selection of, 798
selective serotonin reuptake inhibitors, 788–789,
790t–791t, 792, 795t
tricyclic, 789t, 790t, 794, 795t
in women, 801
Antidiarrheal agents, 482
atypical, 484
for irritable bowel syndrome, 492t, 494
Antidiuretic drugs, 609
Antiemetics, 713–714. *See also* Nausea and vomiting
Antiepileptic drugs, 727, 730t, 732t, 737b, 739,
740b, 748–750
Antifungals
allylamine, 215, 215t–216t, 217
azole, 215, 215t–217t, 1118–1119, 1119t
for skin infections, 215–218, 215t–217t
systemic azole, 217–218
Antigen-specific lymphocytes, activation of, 965–
966, 966f
Antigens, 965
in allergic reactions, 829–830, 930b, 930f
Antihistamines
for allergic conjunctivitis, 941t, 944
for allergic rhinitis, 936–938, 937t
for conjunctivitis, 262, 263t, 265
constipation and, 469b
for contact dermatitis, 194
for cutaneous allergic reactions, 931
for insomnia, 837–838
nonsedating, 936, 937t
for upper respiratory infections, 406t–407t, 410
Antihistamines-anticholinergics, for nausea and
vomiting, 456t, 458–459, 467
Antiinflammatories, for decongestants, 406t, 409
Antimalarials, for rheumatoid arthritis, 682
Antimetabolites, for organ transplantation, 971
Antimicrobial agents, 93–119. *See also specific drugs*
for acne, 246
aminoglycosides, 97t, 107–108, 107t
antianaerobic, 98t, 114–115, 115t
antibiotics-induced ototoxicity
for asthma and COPD, 444

Antimicrobial agents (*continued*)
  beta-lactam/beta-lactamase inhibitors, 95t, 100–101, 101t
  carbapenems, 96t, 104, 104t
  cephalosporins, 95t–96t, 101–103, 102t
  chloramphenicol, 98t, 115–116, 116t
  for community-acquired pneumonia, 421–423
  for conjunctivitis, 262
  for contact dermatitis, 194
  for empiric therapy, 93, 94t
  fluoroquinolones, 96t, 104–106, 105t
  for GERD, 529t, 531–533
  for inflammatory bowel disease, 503t, 507
  lipopeptides, 98t, 112–113, 112t
  for lower respiratory tract infections, 419
  macrolides, 97t, 106, 106t
  monobactams, 96t, 103, 103t
  oxazolidinones, 98t, 112, 112t, 118t
  parenteral-to-oral switching of, 94
  penicillins (*See* Penicillin(s))
  for peptic ulcer disease, 529t, 531–533, 536t
  pleuromutilins, 98t, 114, 114t
  for prostatitis, 579–580, 579t, 580f
  resistance mechanisms of, 117–118, 118t
  for rhinosinusitis, 413–416
  for rosacea, 250–252, 251t
  selection of, 93–99, 94t–98t
  sensitivity of, 94t–98t
  for sinusitis, 416
  skin infections, 206t, 208, 209t, 210f
  stewardship programs, 118
  streptogramins, 98t, 113–114, 113t
  sulfonamides, 97t, 109–110, 110t
  tetracyclines, 97t, 108–109, 109t
  therapeutic monitoring of, 94
  for urinary tract infections, 569, 570t–571t
Antimicrobial resistance, 283
Antimotility agents, 482–484, 484t
Antimuscarinic drugs, for overactive bladder, 601t, 602, 602t–603t, 604–605, 606t
Antiparasitic agents, for rosacea, 251
Antiphospholipid antibody syndrome, hypercoagulability in, 982
Antiplatelet agents, 1002–1003
  for chronic stable angina, 337t, 341–342
  ischemic stroke, 1002
  precautions with, 1006b
  therapeutic monitoring of, 992
Antipsychotic drugs
  for Alzheimer's disease, 760–761
  constipation and, 469b
  for older adults, 79–80
Antireflux therapy. *See* Gastroesophageal reflux disease (GERD), treatment of
Antiretroviral agents, for HIV infection, 950–963, 951t–954t
Antiseptics, for contact dermatitis, 194
Antispasmodic agents, for irritable bowel syndrome, 492t–493t, 494, 497t
Antispastic agents, for pain, 164
Antithrombin III, 342
  deficiency, hypercoagulability in, 986
Antithrombotic therapy. *See* Anticoagulants; Antiplatelet agents
Antithyroid drugs (ATDs), 919t, 920–921
Antitussin (guaifenesin), for upper respiratory infections, 406t, 408
Antitussives
  for lower respiratory tract infections, 419
  for upper respiratory infections, 406t, 408–409
Antivert (meclizine), for nausea and vomiting, 456t, 459
Antiviral agents
  for lower respiratory tract infections, 419–420, 423
  for viral skin infections, 221–223, 222t
Anusol-HC (hydrocortisone), for inflammatory bowel disease, 502t
Anxiety, definition of, 810

Anxiety disorders, 809–827
  algorithms for, 822f
  antidepressants for, 814–821
  definitions of, 810, 810t
  diagnosis of, 811–812, 812b–813b
  ethnic differences in, 825
  genetic factors in, 811
  information sources for, 826–827
  lifestyle changes for, 827
  in older adults, 825
  pathophysiology of, 811, 811b
  patient education on, 826–827
  in pediatric patients, 825
  therapeutic monitoring of, 825–826, 826b
  treatment of, 813–826
  in women, 825
Anxiolytic drugs, for older adults, 80
Anzemet (dolasetron), for nausea and vomiting, 457t, 460
Aplastic anemia, 116, 1026, 1026b
Apolipoprotein E, in Alzheimer's disease, 756
Apomorphine, for Parkinson disease, 770t, 773
Appetite suppressants, for obesity, 1078, 1080–1081, 1080t–1081t, 1083
Apraclonidine, for glaucoma, 274t, 276
Apremilast, for psoriasis, 231t, 235
Aprepitant, for nausea and vomiting, 457t
Apresoline (hydralazine)
  for heart failure, 355t, 364–365
  for hypertension, 305, 305t
Apriso (mesalamine), for inflammatory bowel disease, 502t, 504–505, 510
Aqueous humor, outflow obstruction of, glaucoma in, 272
Arava (leflunomide), for rheumatoid arthritis, 679t, 683
Arcaptag Neohaler (indacaterol), for asthma and COPD, 430t, 436
Area under the plasma concentration curve, 6
Arformoterol, for asthma and COPD, 430t, 436
Argatroban, 342–343
Aricept (donepezil), for Alzheimer's disease, 758, 760t
Armour Thyroid (desiccated thyroid), 914
  for hypothyroidism, 914, 915t
Arrhythmias, 371–398
  atrial fibrillation/flutter (*See* Atrial fibrillation/flutter)
  atrioventricular nodal, 372
  bradycardia, 387t, 395–396, 396f
  causes of, 371
  complementary and alternative medicine for, 398
  definition of, 371
  diagnosis of, 373
  junctional, 372, 373b
  nonsustained ventricular tachycardia, 387t, 393
  nutrition for, 398
  in older adults, 396–397
  paroxysmal supraventricular tachycardia, 386t, 392–393, 393f
  pathophysiology of, 371–372, 372b
  patient education on, 397–398
  in pediatric patients, 396
  premature ventricular contractions, 373b, 380
  reentry, 372
  supraventricular, 372, 373b
  sustained ventricular tachycardia, 387t, 393–394
  therapeutic monitoring of, 397
  treatment of (*See* Antiarrhythmic agents)
  types of, 372, 373b
  ventricular, 372, 373b
  ventricular fibrillation, 378t, 387t, 393–394, 395f
  ventricular tachycardia, 378t, 387t, 394–395, 395f
ART (antiretroviral therapy), for HIV infection, 947–950, 955
Arthritis
  definition of, 641
  degenerative (*See* Osteoarthritis)
  rheumatoid (*See* Rheumatoid arthritis)

Artificial tears, for keratoconjunctivitis sicca, 269, 270t
Asacol (mesalamine), for inflammatory bowel disease, 502t, 504–505, 510
Ascites, 548–549
  diagnosis of, 548
  diuretic therapy for, 547t
  therapeutic monitoring for, 549
  treatment of, 548–549
Asoconstrictors, for rosacea, 251–252
Aspirin
  for chronic stable angina, 337t, 342–343, 346
  for coagulation disorders, 1000
  for common cold, 409
  contraindications to, 1002
  for headache, 696–697, 697t
  mechanism of action of, 1002
  for migraine headache, 703, 704t
  for pain, 153, 155, 156
  for stroke prevention, 1002
Astagraf (tacrolimus), for organ transplantation, 969t, 970, 974t
Astelin (azelastine), for allergic rhinitis, 937t, 938
Asthma, 425–447
  causes of, 425
  complementary and alternative medicines for, 447
  culturally specific beliefs, 445
  diagnosis of, 427, 427t
  genomics, 445
  guidelines for, 425
  immunizations for, 443
  information sources for, 447
  lifestyle changes in, 447
  nutrition for, 447
  in older adults, 445
  pathophysiology of, 426, 426t–427t
  patient education for, 445–447
  in pediatrics, 444–445
  personalized management for ages 12 years and above, 436t
  personalized management for children 6–11 years, 436t
  in pregnancy, 445
  respiratory drug delivery systems, 445–446, 445t
  risk factor for, 435t
  self-monitoring, 445
  severity, 435t
  spirometry findings of, 427t
  supplemental oxygen for, 443–444
  symptom control for ages 6 and above, 434t
  therapeutic monitoring for, 445
  treatment of, 427–444, 428t–433t
  in women, 445
Asthma Control Test, 434
Atacand (candesartan)
  for chronic stable angina, 334
  for heart failure, 360
  for hypertension, 302t
Atarax (hydroxyzine)
  for anxiety disorders, 817t, 820
  for nausea and vomiting, 456t, 458–459
Atazanavir, for HIV infection, 953t, 957
Atenolol
  for chronic stable angina, 336t, 340
  for hypertension, 300, 301t
Atherosclerosis
  chronic stable angina in, 331
  hypertension and, 331
  pathogenesis of, 314–315, 331–332
Athlete's foot, 214
Ativan (lorazepam)
  for Alzheimer's disease, 761
  for anxiety disorders, 80, 816, 817t
  for insomnia, 833, 834t
  for nausea and vomiting, 456t, 459
  for seizures, 746–747
Atomoxetine, for ADHD, 861t, 863
Atonic seizures, 727

Atopic conjunctivitis, 266–267, 266t
Atopic dermatitis (eczema), 191
Atorvastatin, for hyperlipidemia, 317t, 319
Atrial fibrillation/flutter
    characteristics of, 982
    diagnosis of, 986–988
    embolism in, treatment of, 1003–1004
    treatment of, 374t, 386t, 388–391, 389f, 390f
Atrioventricular nodal arrhythmias, 372
Atrioventricular node, function of, 372
Atrophic vaginitis, 1116, 1118
Atropine, for arrhythmias, 374t, 385
Atrovent (ipratropium bromide)
    for asthma and COPD, 428t, 438
    for upper respiratory infections, 406t, 409–410
Attention-deficit/hyperactivity disorder (ADHD),
        855–868
    in adults, 856
    algorithm for, 865
    causes of, 856
    complementary and alternative medicine for, 867
    diagnosis of, 857–859
    epidemiology of, 855
    information sources for, 866
    lifestyle changes for, 866–867
    nutrition for, 866–867
    pathophysiology of, 856–857
    patient education on, 866–867
    risk factors for, 856
    therapeutic monitoring of, 866
    treatment of, 857t–858t, 859–866, 860t, 865f
Atypical absence seizures, 727
Auditory canal, infections of (otitis externa), 282,
        282t, 287–290, 288t, 289t
Augmentin (amoxicillin–clavulanic acid)
    causing diarrhea, 479
    for community-acquired pneumonia, 422, 422t
    dosages of, 101t
    for otitis media, 284, 285t
    for respiratory infections, 407t
    sensitivity of, 95t
    for sinusitis, 413–414
    for skin infections, 205t, 207
Auranofin, for rheumatoid arthritis, 679t
Aurothioglucose, for rheumatoid arthritis, 679t
Autoimmune thyroiditis, 913
Autoinduction, of enzymes, 39
Automaticity, in cardiac cells, 372
Autonomic nervous system, in blood pressure
        regulation, 296
Autosomal, 122b
Avanafil, for benign prostatic hyperplasia, 590, 590t
Avapro (irbesartan)
    for chronic stable angina, 334
    for heart failure, 360
Avelox (moxifloxacin), 105, 105t
    for community-acquired pneumonia, 423
    sensitivity of, 96t
    for skin infections, 206t, 208
    for upper respiratory infections, 407t, 414–415
Aversion therapy, for smoking cessation, 1063
Avodart (dutasteride), for benign prostatic
        hyperplasia, 583–584, 584t
Avoidance
    in allergic reaction prevention, 931, 934
    in contact dermatitis, 192
Avycaz (ceftazidime–avibactam), 95t, 101t
Axent (almotriptan), for migraine headache, 703,
        706t, 711
Axid (nizatidine)
    for GERD, 529t, 530t
    for peptic ulcer disease, 529t, 537t
Azactam (aztreonam), 96t, 103, 103t
    causing diarrhea, 480
Azapirones, for anxiety disorders, 818
Azathioprine
    for chronic gout, 654–655
    for contact dermatitis, 195

for inflammatory bowel disease, 503t, 506–507,
        514
    for organ transplantation, 971, 974t
    for rheumatoid arthritis, 679t, 682
Azelaic acid, for acne, 243t, 245
Azelastine
    for allergic rhinitis, 937t, 938
    for conjunctivitis, 263t, 265
Azelex (azelaic acid)
    for acne, 243t, 245
    for rosacea, 251
Azithromycin, 106, 106t
    for asthma and COPD, 444
    for bronchitis, 419t, 420
    causing diarrhea, 479, 486
    for Chlamydia trachomatis infections, 616t, 617,
        618t
    for community-acquired pneumonia, 422–423,
        422t
    for conjunctivitis, 265
    for gonorrhea, 621–622, 621t
    for otitis media, 286
    for prostatitis, 580
    sensitivity of, 97t
Azole antifungals, 215, 215t–217t, 217–218,
        1118–1119, 1119t
Azopt (brinzolamide), for glaucoma, 273t, 276
Aztreonam, 96t, 103, 103t
    causing diarrhea, 480
Azulfidine (sulfasalazine), 110
    for inflammatory bowel disease, 502t, 504,
        510, 515
    for rheumatoid arthritis, 678t, 681–682

B
Bacillus cereus infections, 480b, 482
Baclofen, for pain, 164
Bacterial conjunctivitis, 265–267, 266t
Bacterial skin infections. See specific infections
Bacterial vaginosis
    causes of, 1115
    diagnosis of, 1116–1117, 1117b
    pathophysiology of, 1116
    patient education on, 1126
    in pregnancy, 1125, 1125t
    therapeutic monitoring of, 1126
    treatment of, 1116–1117, 1120–1126, 1120t,
        1122t, 1123f
Bacteriuria, asymptomatic, 574
Bactrim (sulfamethoxazole–trimethoprim), 97t,
        109–110, 110t
    for prostatitis, 579, 579t
    for sinusitis, 413
    for skin infections, 206t, 208
    for spontaneous bacterial peritonitis, 550,
        550t, 551
    for urinary tract infections, 569, 570t, 572
Bactroban (mupirocin), for skin infections, 204, 208
Balanitis, 214
Balsalazide, for inflammatory bowel disease,
        502t, 505
Barbita (phenobarbital), for seizures, 728t, 731t,
        738–740
Barbiturates
    for migraine headache, 713
    for seizures, 731t, 739–741
Baroreceptors, in blood pressure regulation, 296
Basiliximab, for organ transplantation, 968, 973t
Baxdela (delafloxacin), 96t, 105, 105t
Bazedoxifene, 1109
Beclomethasone, for allergic rhinitis, 940t, 941
Behavioral therapy. See Cognitive-behavioral therapy
        (CBT)
Belatacept, for organ transplantation, 973, 974t, 975
Belbuca (buprenorphine), 169, 170t–171t, 171–172,
        172t, 174–175
Belladonna alkaloids, for irritable bowel syndrome,
        492t, 494, 497t
Bempedoic acid, for hyperlipidemia, 321t, 324–325

Benadryl (diphenhydramine)
    for allergic rhinitis, 936
    for insomnia, 837–838
    for nausea and vomiting, 456t, 461
    for upper respiratory infections, 406t, 410
Benazepril, for chronic stable angina, 334
Benefiber (wheat dextrin), for constipation, 471,
        471t, 473
Benicar (olmesartan)
    for chronic stable angina, 334
    for heart failure, 360
Benign prostatic hyperplasia (BPH), 581–586
    alternative therapies for, 586, 586t
    causes of, 581
    diagnosis of, 581–582, 582t
    epidemiology of, 581
    hypertension in, 304
    information resources of, 586
    lifestyle changes in, 586
    pathophysiology of, 581
    patient education on, 586, 586t
    therapeutic monitoring of, 586
    treatment of, 582–586, 584t–585t, 585f
Benralizumab, for asthma and COPD, 433t,
        442–443
Bentyl (dicyclomine), for irritable bowel syndrome,
        492t, 494, 497t
BenzaClin Gel (clindamycin–benzoyl peroxide), for
        acne, 247
Benzamycin (erythromycin–benzoyl peroxide), for
        acne, 247
Benzathine penicillin G, for syphilis, 616t, 624, 625t
Benzodiazepine(s)
    for alcohol withdrawal syndrome, 874t
    for Alzheimer's disease, 761
    for anxiety disorders, 80, 816–818, 817t–818t
    for insomnia, 832–833, 838t, 842
    mechanism of action of, 816
    for nausea and vomiting, 456t, 459–460
    overdose of, 818, 826
    for restless legs syndrome, 842
    for seizures, 737b, 745–747
    withdrawal from, 826, 826b
Benzodiazepine receptor agonists, for insomnia,
        833, 835t
Benzonatate, for upper respiratory infections, 406t,
        408–409
Benzoyl peroxide, for acne, 243t, 245, 247, 263
Benzquinamide, for nausea and vomiting, 456t
Benztropine (Cogentin), for Parkinson disease,
        767–768, 769t
Bepotastine, for conjunctivitis, 263t, 265
Bepreve (bepotastine), for conjunctivitis, 263t, 265
Best Pharmaceuticals for Children Act of 2002, 56
Beta-adrenergic blockers
    cardioselective, 300
    for hypertension, 300–302, 301t
    increased sensitivity of, in depression, 784, 784b
Beta-adrenoreceptor agonists, for overactive bladder,
        601t, 603t, 605–607
Beta blockers
    for arrhythmias, 379b, 381
    cardioselective, 340
    for chronic stable angina, 336t, 339–341
    for glaucoma, 272, 273t, 275
    for heart failure, 354t–355t, 362–363
    for hyperthyroidism, 919t, 921
    for migraine prevention, 714, 715t
Beta cells, destruction of, 887
Beta-hydroxy-beta-methylglutaryl coenzyme
        reductase inhibitors (statins), 317t,
        319–320, 320f
Beta-lactams
    beta-lactamase inhibitors, 95t, 100–101, 101t
    for community-acquired pneumonia, 421–422
Beta$_2$-adrenergic agonists (short and long acting),
        428t, 434–438
Betamethasone dipropionate, for contact dermatitis,
        193t

Betamethasone valerate, for contact dermatitis, 193t
Betamol, for migraine prevention, 716t
Betapace (sotalol), for arrhythmias, 377t, 379b, 383–384
Betaxolol, for glaucoma, 273t, 275
Betimol (timolol), for glaucoma, 273t, 275
Betoptic S (betaxolol), for glaucoma, 273t, 275
Bevespi Aerosphere (glycopyrrolate/formoterol fumarate), for asthma and COPD, 430t
Bextra (valdecoxib), 82, 647
Biaxin (clarithromycin), 97t, 106, 106t
    for bronchitis, 419t, 420
    causing diarrhea, 479
    for community-acquired pneumonia, 422–423, 422t
    for GERD, 529t, 532
    for peptic ulcer disease, 529t, 532
    for prostatitis, 580
    sensitivity of, 97t
Bichloracetic acid, for human papilloma virus infections, 616t, 636, 636t
Bicillin (benzathine penicillin G), for syphilis, 616t, 624, 625t
Biguanides, for diabetes mellitus, 891t, 894–895
Bile acid
    resins, for hyperlipidemia, 320f, 321t, 322–323
    sequestrants
        constipation and, 469b
        for diabetes mellitus, 899
Biliary tract, in drug excretion, 40
Bimatoprost, for glaucoma, 274t, 275–276
Binding
    for peptic ulcer disease drug (See Albumin, drug binding to; Protein binding)
    tissue, in pediatric patients, 60
Bioavailability, 18b, 19, 20b
Bioequivalent drugs, 134, 135
Biofeedback, for allergic rhinitis, 944
Biological agents, for inflammatory bowel disease, 507–509, 513
Biomarkers, 122, 122b
    asthma and COPD, 426
Biopsy
    for diagnosis of organ transplant rejection, 966
    in human papilloma virus infections, 635
Biotransformation, definition of, 18b
Bipolar disorder
    causes of, 803
    diagnosis of, 803
    overview of, 802–803
    pathophysiology of, 803
    pharmacotherapy for, 804, 804t–806t
Birth control. See Contraception
Bisacodyl
    for constipation, 472t, 474
    for irritable bowel syndrome, 492t, 493–494, 497t
Bismuth subsalicylate
    for diarrhea, 484, 484t, 485–486
    for GERD, 529t, 533
    for peptic ulcer disease, 529t, 533
Bisoprolol
    for heart failure, 354t, 362
    hypertension, 300, 301t
Bisphosphonates, for osteoporosis, 667, 668t, 670–671
Bivalirudin, for chronic stable angina, 337t
Bivalirudin, 342–343
Black cohosh, 1113, 1113t
Blackheads, 242
Bladder
    control of, prostatic hyperplasia and, 581
    infections of (See Urinary tract infections [UTIs])
Bleeding, from warfarin, 994b, 995
Blepharitis, 257–261
    causes of, 257
    diagnosis of, 258
    pathophysiology of, 257–258

patient education, 260
    treatment of, 258–260, 259t–261t
Blood
    flow, absorption and, 20–21
    loss of, anemia in, 1016
Blood pressure
    classification of, 297, 297t
    elevated (See Hypertension [HTN])
    goals, 298t
    measurement of, 296
    regulation of, 295
Blood transfusion, for blood loss, 1016
Blood volume, in pregnancy, drug distribution and, 59
Body composition, of pediatric patients, 59–60
Body mass index, 1078, 1079t
Boggs Act of 1951, 180
Bone
    loss of (See Osteoporosis)
    remodeling of, in osteoarthritis, 642
Bone marrow, failure of, aplastic anemia in, 1026, 1026b
Bone mineral density, measurement of, in osteoporosis, 665, 673
Bonine (meclizine), for nausea and vomiting, 456t, 459
Bonjesta (doxylamine/pyridoxine), for nausea and vomiting, 458t, 467
Botox (onabotulinumtoxinA)
    for migraine prevention, 716t
    for overactive bladder, 601t, 603t, 607
Botulinum A toxin, 609
Bouchard's nodes, in osteoarthritis, 643
BPH (benign prostatic hyperplasia), 581–586, 582t, 584t–585t, 585f, 586t
Bradycardia, treatment of, 387t, 395–396, 396f
Bradykinin, in pain transduction, 148
Branched-chain amino acids, for hepatic encephalopathy, 554
Brand name drugs vs. generic drugs, 6, 6t
Breakthrough therapy, 4
Breast-feeding
    drug therapy in, 63–64
    drugs used in, prescription considerations for, 11
    in obesity, 1085
    viral hepatitis and, 560
Breast milk, 63–64
Breo Ellipta (fluticasone furoate/vilanterol), for asthma and COPD, 431t
Breviblec (esmolol), for arrhythmias, 376t, 379b
Brief intervention (BI), 871
Brilinta (ticagrelor)
    for chronic stable angina, 337t, 342
    for coagulation disorders, 1002
Brimonidine
    for glaucoma, 274t, 276
    for rosacea, 251–252
Brinzolamide, for glaucoma, 273t, 276
Brivaracetam, for seizures, 735t, 748
Brodalumab, for psoriasis, 232t, 236–237
Bromocriptine, for restless legs syndrome, 842
Bronchitis
    causes of, 418
    chronic, in COPD (See Chronic obstructive pulmonary disease [COPD])
    diagnosis of, 418–419
    in older adults, 82
    pathophysiology of, 418
    patient education, 420
    therapeutic monitoring, 420
    treatment of, 419–420, 419t
Brovana (arformoterol), for asthma and COPD, 430t, 436
Buccal administration, 21
Budesonide
    for allergic rhinitis, 940t, 941
    for inflammatory bowel disease, 503t, 505–506
Bulk-forming laxatives
    for constipation, 161, 471, 471t, 473
    for irritable bowel syndrome, 491, 491t

Bullous impetigo
    causes of, 199, 200t
    diagnosis of, 202
    treatment of, 204, 205t–206t, 207–209, 209t, 210f
Bumetanide
    for heart failure, 354t
    for hypertension, 299, 299t
Bumex (bumetanide)
    for heart failure, 354t
    for hypertension, 299, 299t
Bunavail (buprenorphine/naloxone), 169, 170t–171t, 171–172, 172t, 174–175
Buprenex (buprenorphine), 169, 170t–171t, 171–172, 172t, 174–175
Buprenorphine
    for opioid use disorder, 876–878, 879t
    for pain, 154
    for pain management in opioid use disorder, 169, 170t–171t, 171–172, 172t, 174–175
Bupropion
    for ADHD, 860t, 861t, 864–865
    for depression, 791t, 795t, 796
    for smoking cessation, 1066t, 1068–1070
Burow solution, for contact dermatitis, 192
BuSpar (buspirone)
    for Alzheimer's disease, 761
    for anxiety disorders, 80, 817t, 818
Buspirone
    for Alzheimer's disease, 761
    for anxiety disorders, 80, 817t, 818
Butalbital, in combination product, for headache, 697, 698t
Butoconazole, for candidiasis, 1118, 1119t
Butrans (buprenorphine), 169, 170t–171t, 171–172, 172t, 174–175
Butterbur, for migraine headache, 721
Bystolic (nebivolol), for hypertension, 300, 301t

C
Cafergot (ergotamine/caffeine), for migraine headache, 708t, 713
Caffeine
    in combination product, for headache, 697, 698t, 703, 704t
    drug interactions with, in older adults, 76, 77t
    metabolism of, in pediatric patients, 60
Calan (verapamil)
    for arrhythmias, 378t, 379b, 384
    for chronic stable angina, 337t, 341
    for hypertension, 303t, 304
    for migraine prevention, 716t, 718
Calcimimetic therapy, for hyperparathyroidism, 923
Calcineurin inhibitors (CNIs), for organ transplantation, 968–970, 969t, 970b
Calcipotriene, for psoriasis, 231t, 233
Calcipotriol, for psoriasis, 233
Calcitonin, for osteoporosis, 668t, 671
Calcitriol, for hypoparathyroidism, 924
Calcium carbonate, for hypoparathyroidism, 924
Calcium channel blockers
    for arrhythmias, 379b, 384
    for chronic stable angina, 336t–337t, 341
    grapefruit juice interactions with, 42, 42b
    for heart failure, 358
    for hypertension, 303–304, 303t
    for migraine prevention, 716t, 718
Calcium polycarbophil, for irritable bowel syndrome, 491t
Calcium supplements
    constipation and, 469b
    for osteoporosis, 666, 668t, 672
Caldolor (ibuprofen), pharmacokinetic and pharmacodynamic properties of, 152, 156t, 159
CAM. See Complementary and alternative medicine (CAM)
Campral (acamprosate), for alcohol use disorder, 873–874, 874t

Campylobacter infections, 480, 480b, 481, 482
Canasa (mesalamine), for inflammatory bowel disease, 502t, 504–505, 510
Cancer
  pain in, 148, 155
  prostate, 586–587
  screening and inflammatory bowel disease, 515
  smoking-related, 1057
Candesartan
  for chronic stable angina, 334
  for heart failure, 360
  for hypertension, 302t
Candidiasis
  causes of, 213
  complementary and alternative medicine for, 219
  diagnosis of, 214
  pathophysiology of, 213
  patient education on, 219
  therapeutic response of, 219
  treatment of, 214–215, 215t–217t, 217–219
  vulvovaginal
    algorithm for, 1121f
    causes of, 1115–1116
    classification of, 1117, 1117b
    complementary and alternative medicine for, 1126
    diagnosis of, 1116–1118, 1118b
    pathophysiology of, 1116
    patient education on, 1126
    in pregnancy, 1125, 1125b
    treatment of, 1117, 1120–1126, 1120t, 1121f, 1122t
Cangrelor, for chronic stable angina, 342
Cannabidiol
  for pain, 179, 183t, 185–186, 185t
  for seizures, 735t, 747
Cannabinoids
  for nausea and vomiting, 461–462
  for pain management, 180–181 (*See also specific cannabinoids*)
  use in older adults, 81
Cannabis
  ethnic, 187
  genomics and, 187
  legal status of, 180–181
  as medicine, 180
  for pain, 164
  and pain management, 179–188
    information sources of, 187
    lifestyle changes in, 187
    nutrition for, 187
    in older adults, 187
    patient education for, 187
    in pediatrics, 187
    in pregnancy, 187
    therapeutic monitoring, 187
    in women, 187
  as plant, 179–180, 180f
  terpenes in plants, 186, 186b
Cannabis indica, 179–180, 187
Cannabis ruderalis, 179–180
Cannabis sativa, 179–180, 181, 187
Cannabis use disorder, 187
Capitated pharmacy benefits, 138
Capoten (captopril)
  for chronic stable angina, 334, 335t, 338
  for heart failure, 352, 353t, 356
  for hypertension, 302, 302t
Capsaicin
  for osteoarthritis, 644
  for overactive bladder, 609
Capsid, of HIV, 949
Captopril
  for chronic stable angina, 334, 335t, 338
  for heart failure, 352, 353t, 356
  for hypertension, 302, 302t
Carafate (sucralfate)
  constipation and, 469b

for GERD, 529t, 533
  for peptic ulcer disease, 529t, 533, 537t
Carbamazepine
  for Alzheimer's disease, 761
  in cytochrome P-450 system induction, 39
  for pain, 163
  for psychiatric disorders, in older adults, 82
  for seizures, 728t, 730t, 736–737
  therapeutic monitoring of, 88
Carbapenems, 96t, 104, 104t, 118t
Carbidopa–levodopa, for restless legs syndrome, 842
Carbonic anhydrase inhibitors, for glaucoma, 273t, 276
Carbunculosis
  algorithm for, 210f
  causes of, 200t, 201
  complementary and alternative medicine for, 212
  diagnosis of, 203
  lifestyle changes in, 212
  pathophysiology of, 202, 202b
  patient education on, 211–212
  therapeutic monitoring of, 211
  treatment of, 204, 205t–206t, 207–210, 209t, 210f
Cardiac Arrhythmia Suppression Trial (CAST), 373
Cardiac output, decreased, in heart failure, 350, 350f, 351b
Cardiovascular system, evaluation of, for erectile dysfunction drugs, 591, 591b
Cardioversion
  anticoagulants before, 988
  for atrial fibrillation, 388
Cardizem (diltiazem)
  for arrhythmias, 375t, 379b, 384
  for chronic stable angina, 337t, 341
  hypertension, 303t, 304
Cardura (doxazosin)
  for benign prostatic hyperplasia, 584, 584t
  for hypertension, 304, 304t
  for overactive bladder, 601t, 603t, 608
Carotid sinus massage, for arrhythmias, 388
Carteolol, for glaucoma, 273t, 275
Cartia (diltiazem), for chronic stable angina, 303t, 304
Cartilage, degeneration of
  in osteoarthritis, 642
  in rheumatoid arthritis, 676
Carvedilol
  for heart failure, 355t, 362–363
  for hypertension, 300–301, 301t
  for variceal hemorrhage, 546, 546t
CAST (Cardiac Arrhythmia Suppression Trial), 373
Castor oil, for constipation, 472t, 477
Cataflam (diclofenac), for osteoarthritis, 644, 645t
Cataplexy, in narcolepsy, 845–846
Catapres (clonidine)
  for ADHD, 861t, 863–864
  for hypertension, 304, 305t
Catechol-*O*-methyltransferase Inhibitors, for Parkinson disease, 775
Ceclor (cefaclor), for skin infections, 205t, 207
Cedocard (isosorbide dinitrate), for chronic stable angina, 336t, 338–339
Cefaclor, 102t
  for skin infections, 205t, 207
Cefadroxil, 102t
  sensitivity of, 95t
Cefazolin, 95t, 102t
  for skin infections, 205t, 207
Cefdinir, 102t
  for community-acquired pneumonia, 422
  for otitis media, 285t, 286
Cefepime, 96t, 102t, 103
Cefiderocol, 96t, 102t, 103
Cefixime
  for *Chlamydia trachomatis* infections, 616t
  for gonorrhea, 616t, 621, 621t
  for upper respiratory infections, 407t, 415–416
Cefotaxime, 102t, 103

for gonorrhea, 622
  sensitivity of, 96t
  for spontaneous bacterial peritonitis, 550, 550t
Cefotetan, 95t, 102t, 103
Cefoxitin, 95t, 102t, 103
  for gonorrhea, 616t
Cefpodoxime, 102t
  for community-acquired pneumonia, 422
  for otitis media, 286, 286t
  for respiratory infections, 407t, 415–416
  for skin infections, 205t, 207
Cefprozil, 102t
  for skin infections, 205t, 207
Ceftaroline, 96t, 102t, 103
Ceftazidime, 96t, 102t, 103
  for skin infections, 207
Ceftazidime–avibactam, 95t, 101t
Ceftibuten, 102t
Ceftin (cefuroxime)
  for community-acquired pneumonia, 422
  for otitis media, 286, 286t
  in pregnancy, 61
  for skin infections, 205t, 207
Ceftolozane–tazobactam, 95t, 101t
Ceftriaxone, 96t, 102, 102t, 103
  causing diarrhea, 479
  for conjunctivitis, 265
  for diarrhea, 483t
  for gonorrhea, 621, 621t
  for otitis media, 285t
  for skin infections, 205t, 207
  for spontaneous bacterial peritonitis, 550, 550t
Cefuroxime, 95t, 102t
  for community-acquired pneumonia, 422
  for otitis media, 286, 286t
  in pregnancy, 61
  for skin infections, 205t, 207
Cefzil (cefprozil), 102t
  for skin infections, 205t, 207
Celebrex (celecoxib), 537
  for osteoarthritis, 644, 646t, 647
  for pain, 82, 156
Celecoxib, 537
  for osteoarthritis, 644, 646t, 647
  for pain, 82
Celexa (citalopram), for depression, 81
Cellcept (mycophenolate mofetil), for organ transplantation, 971, 974t
Cellulitis
  causes of, 200–201, 200t, 201t
  complementary and alternative medicine for, 212
  diagnosis of, 202–203
  lifestyle changes for, 212
  pathophysiology of, 202, 202b
  patient education on, 211–212
  therapeutic monitoring of, 211
  treatment of, 204, 205t–206t, 207–209, 209t, 210f
Central alpha-2 receptor agonists, for hypertension, 304–305, 305t
Central sensitization, 150
Cephalexin, 102t
  sensitivity of, 95t
  for skin infections, 205t, 207
Cephalosporins, 95t–96t, 101–103, 102t, 118t. See *also specific drugs*
  for community-acquired pneumonia, 422t
  for diarrhea, 483t
  for otitis media, 284, 286
  for skin infections, 205t, 207–208
  for spontaneous bacterial peritonitis, 550
CeraVe, for psoriasis, 231t
Cerebral angiography, in stroke, 988
Cerebyx (fosphenytoin), for seizures, 730t, 749–750
Certikuzumab
  for inflammatory bowel disease, 503t, 508
  for psoriasis, 232t, 236
Cervical cap, 1091, 1091f

Cervical mucus, in menstrual cycle, 1092
Cervix, dysplasia of, in human papilloma virus infections, 635
Cesamet (nabilone)
  for nausea and vomiting, 462
  for pain, 183t, 184–185
Cetaphil, for psoriasis, 231t
Cetirizine, for allergic rhinitis, 936, 938
Cevimeline, for keratoconjunctivitis sicca, 270t
Chain termination, in retroviral replication, 950
Chancre, in syphilis, 624
Chemical mediators, in pain transmission, 150
Chemoreceptor trigger zone (CTZ), 453
Chemotherapy-induced nausea and vomiting, 462–463
  acute emesis, 463–465, 464b, 465b
  anticipatory emesis, 465–466
  corticosteroids for, 461
  delayed emesis, 465
Chest pain, in ischemic heart disease. *See* Chronic stable angina
Chickenpox. *See* Varicella-zoster virus (VZV)
Child-Turcotte Pugh score, for cirrhosis, 545, 545t
Children. *See also* Pediatric patients
  absorption in, 57t
  definition of, 56t
  dehydration with diarrhea, 487
  distribution in, 57t, 59–60
  elimination in, 57t
  metabolism in, 57t
  nausea and vomiting in, 468b
Chirality, 18b, 29–30
Chlamydia pneumoniae infections, 95t–98t
Chlamydia trachomatis infections, 480b, 617–619
  causes of, 617
  conjunctivitis, 261, 265
  diagnosis of, 617
  gonorrhea with, 620
  pathophysiology of, 617
  in pediatric patients, 617
  pelvic inflammatory disease in, 631–634, 633t, 634f
  in pregnancy, 619
  screening for, 620
  treatment of, options for, 616t
Chlor-Trimeton (chlorpheniramine), for upper respiratory infections, 406t, 410
Chloramphenicol, 98t, 115–116, 116t, 118t
Chlordiazepoxide, for anxiety disorders, 817t
Chloride channel activators
  for constipation, 472t, 475
  for irritable bowel syndrome, 495
Chloroquine and derivatives, in rheumatoid arthritis, 682
Chlorothiazide, for hypertension, 298t
Chlorpheniramine, for upper respiratory infections, 406t, 410
Chlorpromazine, for nausea and vomiting, 456t, 458
Chlorthalidone
  for heart failure, 353t
  for hypertension, 298t, 306, 308
Cholesterol
  in atherosclerosis, 314
  elevated (*See* Hyperlipidemia)
  -lowering therapy, treatment algorithm for, 318f
  physiology of, 314
Cholesterol absorption inhibitors, for hyperlipidemia, 321–322, 321t
Cholestyramine, for hyperlipidemia, 321t, 322–323
Cholinergic agonists
  for glaucoma, 274t, 276
  for keratoconjunctivitis sicca, 269, 270t
Cholinergic blockers. *See* Anticholinergics
Chondroitin, for osteoarthritis, 651
Chromosomes, 122, 122b, 123f
Chronic disease, anemia of, 1022–1023, 1023b
Chronic kidney disease (CKD), 922

Chronic Kidney Disease Epidemiology Collaboration (CKD-EPI), 26–27, 27t
Chronic liver disease (CLD), 543. *See also specific diseases*
Chronic obstructive pulmonary disease (COPD), 425–447
  causes of, 425
  combined assessment to initiate therapy, 437t
  complementary and alternative medicines for, 447
  culturally specific beliefs, 445
  diagnosis of, 427, 427t
  genomics, 445
  guidelines for, 425
  immunizations for, 443
  information sources for, 447
  lifestyle changes in, 447
  nutrition for, 447
  in older adults, 445
  pathophysiology of, 426, 426t–427t
  patient education for, 445–447
  pharmacologic options for, 437b
  in pregnancy, 445
  respiratory drug delivery systems, 445–446, 445t
  self-monitoring, 445
  spirometry findings of, 427t
  supplemental oxygen for, 443–444
  therapeutic monitoring for, 445
  treatment of, 427–444, 428t–433t
  in women, 445
Chronic stable angina, 329–348
  acute, 343, 345
  algorithm for, 344f
  anginal equivalent, 329
  angiotensin-converting enzyme inhibitors for, 334, 338
  anticoagulant and fibrinolytic therapy for, 337t, 342–343
  antiplatelet agents for, 337t, 341–342
  in atherosclerosis, 315
  beta blockers for, 336t, 339–341
  calcium channel blockers for, 336t–337t, 341
  causes of, 330–331, 330b
  classification of, 330–331, 330b
  complementary and alternative medicine for, 347
  in coronary artery vasospasm, 332
  decubitus, 330
  definition of, 329
  diagnosis of, 332–333
  equivalent, 329
  information sources for, 347
  nitrates for, 336t, 338–339
  nocturnal, 330
  pathophysiology of, 331–332
  patient education on, 347
  postinfarction, 330
  prevention of, 345–346, 345t
  risk factors for, 330–331, 330b
  stable, 329, 330b
  symptoms of, 329–330, 330b
  therapeutic monitoring of, 346–347
  treatment of, 333–346, 335t–337t, 344f, 345t
  unstable, 329
  variant (Prinzmetal), 330
Chronulac (lactulose)
  for constipation, 472t, 473–474
  for hepatic encephalopathy, 553–554, 553t
  for irritable bowel syndrome, 491, 491t, 497t
Chylomicrons, 314
Cialis (tadalafil)
  for benign prostatic hyperplasia, 585
  for erectile dysfunction, 589–590, 590t
Ciclopirox, for fungal infections, 215t
Cigarette smoking. *See* Smoking
Cimetidine
  in cytochrome P-450 system inhibition, 37
  for GERD, 529t, 530t, 534
  for peptic ulcer disease, 529t, 534, 537t
Cimzia (certikuzumab)
  for inflammatory bowel disease, 503t, 508

for psoriasis, 232t, 236
Cinacalcet, for hyperparathyroidism, 923, 924t
Cinnamon, for diabetes mellitus, 908
Cinqair (reslizumab), for asthma and COPD, 433t, 442–443
Cipro (ciprofloxacin)
  for diarrhea, 483t, 485
  for inflammatory bowel disease, 503t, 507, 514
  in pediatrics, 64
  for skin infections, 206t, 208
  for urinary tract infections, 570t
Ciprodex (combination product), for otitis externa, 288
Ciprofloxacin, 41, 96t, 105, 105t
  for conjunctivitis, 262
  for diarrhea, 483t, 485
  for inflammatory bowel disease, 503t, 507, 514
  for otitis externa, 288
  in pediatrics, 64
  for skin infections, 206t, 208
  for urinary tract infections, 570t
Circadian rhythm, sleep and, 830
Cirrhosis, 541–554
  acute liver injury, 541
  ascites and, 547t, 548–549
    diagnosis of, 548
    therapeutic monitoring for, 549
    treatment of, 548–549
  causes of, 541–542, 542f, 542t
  complementary and alternative medications for, 554
  diagnosis of, 544–545, 545t
  drug-induced liver injury, 541–542
  hepatic encephalopathy and
    diagnosis of, 552–553
    therapeutic monitoring for, 554
    treatment of, 553–554
  hepatorenal syndrome and
    diagnosis of, 551, 551b
    therapeutic monitoring for, 552
    treatment of, 551–552, 552b
  information resources, 554
  lifestyle changes in, 554
  nutrition for, 554
  pathophysiology of, 542–544, 543f
  patient education on, 554
  portal hypertension and, 545
    gastroesophageal varices, 545–546
    nonselective beta blockers for, 546, 546t
    in older adults, 547
    therapeutic monitoring for, 547
    treatment of, 546–548, 546t–547t
  spontaneous bacterial peritonitis and
    adjunctive therapy for, 551
    diagnosis of, 549, 549b
    prophylaxis, 551, 551b
    therapeutic monitoring for, 551
    treatment of, 549–551, 550t
  variceal hemorrhage and
    diagnosis of, 547
    therapeutic monitoring for, 548
    treatment of, 547–548
Citalopram, for depression, 81
Citroma (magnesium citrate), for irritable bowel syndrome, 492t, 493, 497t
Citrucel (methylcellulose)
  for constipation, 471, 471t, 473
  for irritable bowel syndrome, 491t
Claforan (cefotaxime), 96t, 102t, 103
Clarithromycin, 106, 106t
  for bronchitis, 419t, 420
  causing diarrhea, 479
  for community-acquired pneumonia, 422–423, 422t
  for GERD, 529t, 532
  for peptic ulcer disease, 529t, 532
  for prostatitis, 580
  sensitivity of, 97t
Claritin (loratadine), for allergic rhinitis, 937t, 938

Clear Eyes (naphazoline), for conjunctivitis, 264t, 265
Clearance, 18b, 26–27, 26b, 27t
Clenia (sodium sulfacetamide), for rosacea, 251
Cleocin (clindamycin), 118t
  for acne, 114–115, 115t, 243t
  for bacterial vaginosis, 1119, 1120t, 1122
  sensitivity of, 98t
  for skin infections, 206t, 208
  for upper respiratory infections, 407t, 415
Clidinium, for irritable bowel syndrome, 492t, 494, 497t
Clindagel (clindamycin), for acne, 243t, 245
Clindamycin, 114–115, 115t, 118t
  for acne, 243t, 245
  for bacterial vaginosis, 1119–1120, 1120t, 1122
  for otitis media, 286, 286t
  sensitivity of, 98t
  for skin infections, 206t, 208
  for upper respiratory infections, 407t, 415
Clindamycin–benzoyl peroxide, for acne, 247
Clindamycin/tretinoin, for acne, 243t, 247
Clinical trials, 3–4, 4f
  pediatric patients included in, 56
Clobazam, for seizures, 746
Clobetasol propionate, for contact dermatitis, 193t
Clock-drawing test, for Alzheimer's disease, 757, 757f
Clocortolone pivalate, for contact dermatitis, 193t
Clofibrate, for hyperlipidemia, 323
Clonazepam
  for anxiety disorders, 816, 817t, 819t
  for seizures, 746–747
Clonic seizures, 727
Clonidine
  for ADHD, 861t, 863–864
  constipation and, 469b
  for hypertension, 304, 305t
  menopause systems, 1110–1111
Clopidogrel
  for chronic stable angina, 337t, 342
  for coagulation disorders, 1002–1003
  metabolism and polymorphism of, 124, 124f, 125b
Clostridium difficile infections, 480b
  clindamycin-induced, 115
  diarrhea, 479–480, 480b
Clotrimazole
  for candidiasis, 1118, 1119t, 1122
  for fungal infections, 215t
Clotting cascade, 984–985, 985f
Cloxacillin, 100t
Clue cells, in bacterial vaginosis, 1116
Cluster headaches, 719
Coagulation disorders
  anticoagulants for (See Anticoagulants; specific drugs)
  antiplatelet agents for (See Antiplatelet agents)
  clotting cascade, role of, 984–985, 985f
  diagnosis of, 986–988
  pathophysiology of, 984–986, 985f
  patient education on, 1006–1008, 1006b, 1008t
  in pregnancy, 1006
  therapeutic monitoring in, 992
  thrombotic process, 985
Coal tar, for psoriasis, 231t, 233
Coanalgesics, for pain management in opioid use disorder, 173
Cockcroft and Gault formula, for creatinine clearance, 26–27, 27t, 74
Codeine, for pain, 156, 159, 159t
Cognitive-behavioral therapy (CBT)
  for ADHD, 867
  for anxiety disorders, 813
  for pain, 151, 152b
  for pain management in opioid use disorder, 175
  for weight loss, 1080
Colace (docusate sodium)
  for constipation, 471t, 474–475
  for irritable bowel syndrome, 492t, 494, 497t

Colazide (balsalazide), for inflammatory bowel disease, 502t, 505
Colchicine, 657–658
Cold, common. See Common cold
Cold therapy, for pain, 152
Colesevelam, for hyperlipidemia, 321t, 322–323
Colestid (colestipol), for hyperlipidemia, 322–323
Colestipol, for hyperlipidemia, 322–323
Colitis, ulcerative. See Ulcerative colitis (UC)
Colyte (polyethylene glycol–electrolyte solution), for constipation, 473–474
Combigan (brimonidine and timolol), 275t, 277
Combination immunoassay, in HIV infection, 949
Combination oral medication, for type 2 diabetes, 901
Combivir (combination product), for HIV infection, 951
Comedolytic bactericidals, for acne, 245
Comedolytics, for acne, 242, 244–245
Comedones, 242
Commit (nicotine lozenge), 1065t, 1067
Common cold, 403–412
  algorithm for, 411f
  alternative therapies for, 417–418
  analgesics for, 406t, 409
  anticholinergics for, 406t, 409–410
  antihistamines for, 406t–407t, 410
  antiinflammatory agents for, 406t, 409
  antitussives for, 406t, 408–409
  causes of, 404
  combination products for, 410–411
  complementary and alternative medicine for, 417–418
  decongestants for, 405, 405t, 408
  diagnosis of, 404
  epidemiology of, 403
  expectorants for, 406t, 408
  pathophysiology of, 404
  patient education on, 416–417
  in pediatric patients, 404, 411
  prevention of, 404–405
  therapeutic monitoring of, 412
  treatment of, 404–412, 405t–407t, 411f
Communication, prescription errors and, 9
Community-acquired pneumonia (CAP)
  causes of, 420
  definition of, 421t
  diagnosis of, 421, 421t
  pathophysiology of, 420–421
  therapeutic monitoring, 423
  treatment of, 421–423, 422t
Community drug take-back programs, 7
Compazine (prochlorperazine), for nausea and vomiting, 455, 456t, 458
Competitive inhibition
  of cytochrome P-450 system, 37–38, 37f, 38t
  in retroviral replication, 950
Complementary and alternative medicine (CAM), 6–7, 447. See also Herbal preparations
  absorption and, 44, 44t
  for ADHD, 867
  for allergic rhinitis, 944
  for Alzheimer's disease, 762
  antiarrhythmic agent interactions with, 398
  for asthma and COPD, 447
  for benign prostatic hyperplasia, 586, 586t
  for candidiasis, 219
  for chronic stable angina, 347
  for cirrhosis, 554
  for common cold, 417–418
  for constipation, 479
  for contact dermatitis, 198
  for depression, 802
  for diabetes mellitus, 908
  for diarrhea, 488
  in distribution, 44–45
  for erectile dysfunction, 592
  for GERD, 535
  for gout, 660

  for headache, 721
  for hypertension, 309
  for hyperthyroidism, 922
  for hypothyroidism, 917
  for inflammatory bowel disease, 515–516
  for insomnia, 840
  for menopausal symptoms, 1113, 1113t
  in metabolism, 45–46, 46b
  for migraine headache, 721
  for nausea and vomiting, 468
  for obesity, 1084
  for organ transplantation, 976
  for osteoarthritis, 651
  for otitis externa, 290
  for overactive bladder, 612
  for pain management, 152b, 153
  for Parkinson disease, 779
  for peptic ulcer disease, 538
  pharmacodynamic interactions, 45–46, 46b
  pharmacokinetics, 44–45, 44t, 45t
  for psoriasis, 239
  for rheumatoid arthritis, 689
  for skin disorders, 250
  for skin infections, 212
  for substance use disorders, 884
  target drug, 44b
  for tinea, 219
  for tinea versicolor, 219
  for urinary tract infections, 575
  for vaginitis, 1126
  for viral hepatitis, 562
Complementary medicine. See also Complementary and alternative medicine (CAM)
Complex partial (psychomotor) seizures, 727
Compliance
  with practice guidelines and formularies, 138–139, 138t
  with treatment (See Adherence issues)
Complicated lesions, in atherosclerosis, 332
Compression ultrasonography (CUS), in venous thromboembolism, 868
Computed tomography
  in pulmonary embolism, 987
  in seizures, 727–728
  in stroke, 988
Concentration, drug, 37–38
Concerta (methylphenidate), for ADHD, 860, 861t
Condoms, 1091
Condyloma acuminata. See Human papilloma virus infections
Condylox (podofilox), for human papilloma virus infections, 635, 636t
Congestive heart failure. See Heart failure (HF)
Conjugated equine estrogen, for menopausal symptoms, 1103t, 1106–1108
Conjunctivitis, 261–268
  algorithm for, 267f
  allergic, 261–265, 944
  atopic, 266–267, 266t
  bacterial, 265–267, 266t
  causes of, 261
  diagnosis of, 261–262
  giant papillary, 262, 266t, 267
  hay fever, 261, 265–266
  in keratoconjunctivitis sicca, 268–271, 270t–271t
  pathophysiology of, 261
  patient education on, 268
  pediatric patients, 262
  therapeutic monitoring of, 268
  treatment of, 262–267, 263t–264t, 266t, 267f
  vernal, 266–267, 266t
  viral, 262, 266t, 267
Constilac (lactulose)
  for constipation, 472t, 473–474
  for hepatic encephalopathy, 553–554, 553t
  for irritable bowel syndrome, 491, 491t, 497t
Constipation
  bowel regimen for prevention of, 161
  bulk-forming laxatives for, 471, 471t, 473

Constipation (*continued*)
    causes of, 469
    chloride channel activators for, 472t, 475
    chronic, history and physical examination for, 470b
    complementary and alternative medications for, 479
    defined, 469
    diagnosis of, 470
    disorders associated with, 469b
    guanylate cyclase-C agonist for, 472t, 475
    hyperosmotic laxatives for, 472t, 473–474
    information sources for, 479
    irritable bowel syndrome with, 490b
    lifestyle changes in, 479
    lubricant laxatives for, 471t
    medication associated with, 469b
    nutrition for, 479
    in older adults, 82, 478
    pathophysiology of, 470
    patient education for, 479
    in pediatrics, 477–478
    peripherally acting mu-opioid receptor antagonist for, 472t, 475–476
    in pregnancy, 478–479
    saline laxatives for, 472t, 474
    secretagogues for, 472t, 475
    serotonin-4 (5-HT$_4$) receptor agonist for, 476
    stimulant laxatives for, 472t, 474
    surfactants laxatives for, 471t, 474–475
    therapeutic monitoring of, 479
    treatment of, 470–477, 471t–472t, 477f, 478t
    in women, 478–479
Contact dermatitis (CD), 191–198
    allergic, 191
    causes of, 191
    complementary and alternative medicine for, 198
    definition of, 191
    diagnosis of, 192
    irritant, 191
    in older adults, 197
    pathophysiology of, 191–192, 930
    patient education on, 197–198
    in pediatric patients, 196
    pharmacogenomics, 192
    therapeutic monitoring of, 197
    treatment of, 192–196, 193t, 195t–196t, 196f–197f
    in women, 197
Contact lenses, conjunctivitis with, 261–262, 265, 266t
Contraception combined products, 1090–1097, 1093t
    definition of, 1089
    emergency, 1096
    failure rates of, 1091f
    intrauterine systems for, 1095
    methods for, 1089, 1091f
    nonpharmacologic, 1090, 1091f
    optimal features of, 1092
    oral (*See* Oral contraceptives)
    physiology of, 1089–1090, 1090f
    progestin-only, 1094–1095, 1094t
    reversible forms of, 1089
    usage of, 1089
    vaginal devices for, 1094
Contraception, oral. *See* Oral contraceptives
Contrave (naltrexone/bupropion), in obesity, 1083
Controlled Substances Act of 1970, 4, 5b, 180
Copayment, plans, 139
COPD. *See* Chronic obstructive pulmonary disease (COPD)
Cordarone (amiodarone)
    for arrhythmias, 374t, 379b, 381–383
    for heart failure, 366
Coreg (carvedilol)
    for heart failure, 355t, 362–363
    for hypertension, 300–301, 301t
    for variceal hemorrhage, 546, 546t

Corgard (Nadolol), for hyperthyroidism, 919t
Corlanor (ivabradine), for heart failure, 355t, 365–366
Corn syrup (Karo), for constipation, 478
Coronary artery(ies)
    calcium, 316, 316t
    vasospasm of, 332
Coronary heart disease
    hyperlipidemia and, 315, 315b
    after menopause, 1101
    pathogenesis of, 314–315
    premature, 330
    prevention of, 317
    risk assessment for, 315–317
    risk factors for, 330–331, 330b
Cortenema (hydrocortisone enema), for inflammatory bowel disease, 502t
Corticosteroids
    for allergic conjunctivitis, 944
    for allergic rhinitis, 939–941, 940t
    for anaphylaxis and anaphylactoid reactions, 931
    for asthma and COPD, 429t, 432t, 439–440
    for chemotherapy-induced nausea and vomiting, 461, 468
    for conjunctivitis, 264t, 265
    for contact dermatitis, 193–195, 193t, 195t–196t
    for gout, 656, 657
    immunization and, 1038
    for inflammatory bowel disease, 502t–503t, 505–506, 510, 513, 514
    for keratoconjunctivitis sicca, 269
    for organ transplantation, 973
    for osteoarthritis, 647, 649
    for otitis externa, 288–289
    potency of, 193, 193t
    for psoriasis, 233
    for rheumatoid arthritis, 678
Cortisporin (hydrocortisone)
    for otitis externa, 289, 289t
    for psoriasis, 231t
Corvert (ibutilide), for arrhythmias, 376t, 379b, 384
Coryza. *See* Common cold
Cosentyx (secukinumab), for psoriasis, 232t, 236–237
Cosopt (dorzolamide and timolol), 275t, 277
Cost-effectiveness analysis, for managed care, 132
Cost factors, in adherence, 77
Cost minimization analysis, for managed care, 132
Cost–benefit analysis, for managed care, 132
Costimulation blockade, for organ transplantation, 973, 975
Cost–utility analysis, for managed care, 132
Cough
    from angiotensin-converting enzyme inhibitors, 357–358
    in common cold, 406t, 408, 411
Coumadin. *See* Warfarin
Cozaar (losartan)
    for chronic stable angina, 334, 335t, 338
    for heart failure, 354t, 359–360
    for hypertension, 302, 302t
Cranberry juice, for urinary tract infections, 575
Creatinine
    clearance, 26–27, 26b, 27t
    level of, in older adults, 74, 75t
Crepitus, in osteoarthritis, 643
Crescendo angina, 329
Crestor (rosuvastatin), for hyperlipidemia, 317t, 319
Crisaborole, for contact dermatitis, 194
Crixivan (indinavir), for HIV infection, 953t, 957
Crohn's disease (CD)
    aminosalicylates for, 502t, 504–505
    antibiotics for, 503t, 507, 513
    biological agents for, 507–509, 513
    cancer screening and, 515
    causes of, 499
    complementary and alternative therapies for, 515–516
    corticosteroids for, 502t–503t, 505–506, 510, 513, 514

    definition of, 501t
    diagnosis of, 500
    etiology of, 499
    fulminant, 501t, 509t
    immunosuppressive agents for, 503t, 506–507, 513
    incidence of, 499
    information sources for, 514–515
    nutrition for, 515
    pathophysiology of, 499–500, 500t
    patient education for, 514–516
    in pediatrics, 513
    in pregnancy, 513–514
    preventive care for, 515
    surgical interventions in, 516t
    therapeutic monitoring of, 514
    treatment of, 500–513, 501t, 502t–504t, 509t, 511f
    vs. ulcerative colitis, 500t
    vaccination for, 515
    in women, 513–514
Crolom (cromolyn)
    for allergic rhinitis, 937t, 941
    for conjunctivitis, 263t, 265
Cromolyn
    for allergic rhinitis, 937t, 941
    for conjunctivitis, 263t, 265
Cryptosporidium infections, 480, 480b
Cubicin (daptomycin), 98t, 112–113, 112t, 206t, 208
Cultural factors, in pain management, 152
Culture
    bacterial
        for antimicrobial selection, 93
        in peptic ulcer disease, 527
    fungal, in candidiasis, 1117
    urine
        in prostatitis, 578
        in urinary tract infections, 568
    viral, in herpes simplex virus infections, 628
Cutar (coal tar), for psoriasis, 233
Cutibacterium acnes (*C. acnes*), 242, 245
Cyclobenzaprine
    drug interactions of, 41
    for pain, 163
Cyclooxygenase-2 inhibitors
    for osteoarthritis, 644
    for pain, 82, 155, 156
Cyclooxygenase, in inflammation, 647
Cyclosporine
    for contact dermatitis, 195
    for inflammatory bowel disease, 503t, 506–507, 514
    for keratoconjunctivitis sicca, 269, 270t
    for organ transplantation, 968–970, 969t, 974t
    for psoriasis, 231t, 235
    for rheumatoid arthritis, 680, 688
Cymbalta (duloxetine), for overactive bladder, 601t, 603t, 607–608
CYP enzymes. *See* Cytochrome P-450 system
CYP2D6 genotype, 157
Cystitis. *See* Urinary tract infections (UTIs)
Cytochrome P-450 system
    actions of, 36–39, 36f, 37f, 38t
    description of, 35
    in drug–drug interactions, 792, 793t
    in drug metabolism, 60, 60t
    in drug–food interactions, 42
    genetic differences in, 48
    induction of, 38–39, 38t
    inhibition of, 37–38, 37f, 38t
    in metabolism, 24, 24t
    nomenclature of, 35
Cytomegalovirus, 220
Cytomel (liothyronine), for hypothyroidism, 914, 915t
Cytosine, 122, 122b
Cytotec (misoprostol)
    for GERD, 529t, 532–533

for NSAID-induced ulcers, 647
for peptic ulcer disease, 529t, 532–533, 537t
Cytotoxic reactions, 930, 930b
Cytoxan (cyclophosphamide), for rheumatoid
arthritis, 679t, 680

D

D-dimer assay, in venous thromboembolism, 987
Dalbavancin, 97t, 110–111, 111t, 208
Daliresp (roflumilast), for asthma and COPD, 432t,
440
Dalmane (flurazepam)
for anxiety disorders, 80
for insomnia, 833, 834t
Dalteparin (fragmin), 992, 999t
Dalvance (dalbavancin), 97t, 110–111, 111t
Dapsone, for acne, 243t, 245
Daptomycin, 98t, 112–113, 112t, 206t, 208
Darbepoetin, for anemia, 1022
Darifenacin, for overactive bladder, 601t, 602, 603t,
604, 604t
DAW (dispense as written) code, 135
Dawn phenomenon, in insulin therapy, 903
Decadron (dexamethasone)
for conjunctivitis, 264t
for inflammatory bowel disease, 503t
for nausea and vomiting, 457t, 461
Declomycin (demeclocycline), 109
Decongestants. *See also* Vasoconstrictors
for allergic rhinitis, 937t, 938–939, 939t
for rosacea, 251–252
topical, 939
for upper respiratory infections, 405, 405t, 408
Deep venous thrombosis. *See* Venous
thromboembolism
Deferoxamine, for iron overload, in thalassemia,
1024
Degenerative arthritis. *See* Osteoarthritis
Delafloxacin, 96t, 105, 105t
Delavirdine, for HIV infection, 956
Delayed emesis, nausea and vomiting, 465
Delayed-hypersensitivity reactions, 930, 930b
Delirium tremens (DT), 873, 873b
Delsym (dextromethorphan), for upper respiratory
infections, 406t, 408–409
Delta-9-tetrahydrocannabinol, 81
Deltasone (prednisone), for inflammatory bowel
disease, 502t, 505–506
Delzicol (mesalamine), for inflammatory bowel
disease, 502t, 504–505, 510
Demadex (torsemide), for heart failure, 354t
Demeclocycline, 109
Dementia
Alzheimer's (*See* Alzheimer's disease)
behavioral and psychological symptoms of, 83–84
nonadherence in, 83–84
Denavir (penciclovir), for viral skin infections,
221–222, 222t
Denosumab, for osteoporosis, 669t, 672
Deoxyribonucleic acid (DNA), 121, 122b, 123f
Depakene (valproic acid)
for Alzheimer's disease, 761
for migraine prevention, 714, 715t
for psychiatric disorders, 88
for seizures, 731t, 738–739
therapeutic monitoring, 88
Dependence
on benzodiazepines, 816
on opioids, 161–162
Depot medroxyprogesterone acetate, 1095, 1097t,
1104t, 1106
Depression, 783–802
algorithm for, 799f
antidepressants for (*See* Antidepressants)
causes of, 783
complementary and alternative medicine for, 802
conditions associated with, 786, 786b
definition of, 783
diagnosis of, 784–785, 784b

dysthymia, 785
emergencies in, 801, 801b
epidemiology of, 783
genetic factors in, 801
information sources for, 802
nonpharmacologic treatment of, 785
in older adults, 80–81, 800
pathophysiology of, 784, 784b
patient education on, 801–802
in pediatric patients, 800
postpartum, 785, 801
risk factors for, 741
seasonal affective disorder, 785
severity of, 785, 786
St. John's wort for, 802
suicide in, 801–802, 801b
therapeutic monitoring of, 801, 801b
treatment of, 785–798
types of, 785
Depression and Bipolar Support Alliance, 802
Dermaspray, for wound cleansing, 212
Dermatitis. *See* Contact dermatitis
Dermatophytosis. *See* Tinea
Dermuspray, for wound cleansing, 194
Desensitization, for allergic reactions, 831, 935
Desiccated thyroid, for hypothyroidism, 914, 915t
Desipramine
for irritable bowel syndrome, 494, 497t
for overactive bladder, 601t, 609
for pain, 162
Desonide, for contact dermatitis, 193t
Desoximetasone, for contact dermatitis, 193t
Desyrel (trazodone)
for Alzheimer's disease, 761
for anxiety disorders, 80
for depression, 791t, 793t, 795t, 796
Detrol (tolterodine), 602t
for overactive bladder, 601t, 602, 604–605, 604t
Detrusor overactivity, 595
Dexamethasone
for conjunctivitis, 264t
for contact dermatitis, 193t
for inflammatory bowel disease, 503t
for migraine headache, 709t, 713
for nausea and vomiting, 457t, 461
Dexedrine (dextroamphetamine), for ADHD, 861t
Dexilant (dexlansoprazole)
for GERD, 529t, 530t, 531
for peptic ulcer disease, 529t, 531, 537t
Dexlansoprazole
for GERD, 529t, 530t, 531
for peptic ulcer disease, 529t, 531, 537t
Dextroamphetamine, for ADHD, 861t
Dextromethorphan
as isomer, 30
for upper respiratory infections, 406t, 408–409
Diabetes mellitus, 887–909
biguanides for, 891t, 894–895
causes of, 887–888
chronic stable angina in, 331
classification of, 887
complementary and alternative medicine for, 908
definition of, 887
diagnosis of, 889, 889t
epidemiology of, 887–888
glucosidase inhibitors for, 892t, 896
hypertension in, 302, 308
information sources for, 907–908
insulin for, 901–904, 906t
intensive therapy for, 888–889
lifestyle changes for, 908
meglitinide analogs for, 892t, 896–897
neuropathic pain in, 162
nutrition for, 908
in obesity, 1085
in older adults, 905
pathophysiology of, 888
patient education on, 907–908
in pediatric patients, 905

pre-gestational, 905
in pregnancy, 905
risk factors for, 888b
sulfonylureas for, 891, 891t, 893–894
therapeutic monitoring of, 907
thiazolidinediones for, 892t, 895–896
treatment of, 889–908
type 1
causes of, 887
diagnosis of, 889, 889t
pathophysiology of, 888
in pediatric patients, 905
treatment of, 901–905, 901t, 906t
type 2
causes of, 888
complementary and alternative medicine for,
908
diagnosis of, 889
pathophysiology of, 888
in pediatric patients, 905
risk factors for, 888b
treatment of, 890, 901–905
Diabetic foot infection
causes of, 201
diagnosis of, 203–204, 203t
pathophysiology of, 202, 202b
treatment of, 204, 205t–206t, 207–211, 209t,
210f
Diabinese (chlorpropamide), for diabetes mellitus, 893
*Diagnostic and Statistical Manual of Mental Disorders,
Fifth Edition* (*DSM*-5), 871, 871b
Dialose (docusate potassium), for constipation, 472t
Diaper dermatitis, 214
Diaphragm, as contraceptive method, 1091
Diarrhea
absorbents for, 485
adsorbents for, 485
altered intestinal motility, 481
antidiarrheal agents for, 482
antimotility agents for, 482–484, 484t
atypical antidiarrheals for, 484
causes of, 479
Clostridium difficile, treating, 480t
complementary and alternative medications, 488
diagnosis of, 481–482
disorders and procedures associated with, 480t
exudative (inflammatory) diarrhea, 481
infectious diarrhea, empiric and specific
antimicrobial therapy in, 483t
infective organisms associated with, 480–481, 480t
information sources, 487–488
irritable bowel syndrome with, 490b
lifestyle changes in, 488
medications causing, 479–480, 480t
nutrition for, 488
in older adults, 487
osmotic, 481
pathophysiology of, 481
patient education for, 487, 488t
in pediatrics, 486
in pregnancy, 487
secretory, 481
semisynthetic antibiotic for, 484t, 485
therapeutic monitoring of, 487
travelers', 480–481
treatment for, 482–486, 483t–485t, 486f
in women, 487
Diazepam, 164
for anxiety disorders, 80, 816, 817t, 819t–820t
for nausea and vomiting, 456t, 459
for seizures, 747
Dichlorodiphenyltrichloroethane, drug interactions
in, 48
Diclegis (doxylamine/pyridoxine), for nausea and
vomiting, 458t, 467
Diclofenac
for osteoarthritis, 644, 645t
pharmacokinetic and pharmacodynamic
properties of, 156t

Dicloxacillin, 95t, 100t, 205t, 207
Dicyclomine, for irritable bowel syndrome, 492t, 494, 497t
Didanosine, for HIV infection, 950, 951t, 955
Diet. See Nutrition
Dietary Approaches to Stop Hypertension, 309
Dietary Supplement Health and Education Act of 1994, 7
Dietary supplements. See Complementary and alternative medicine (CAM)
Diethylpropion (tenuate), for obesity, 1080, 1080t
Dieting. See Weight loss
Differin (adapalene gel), for acne, 244
Diffusion, passive, 19–20
Dificid (fidaxomicin), 106
Diflorasone diacetate, for contact dermatitis, 193t
Diflucan (fluconazole), 217t
    for candidiasis, 1119, 1119t
Diflunisal
    for osteoarthritis, 646t, 647
    pharmacokinetic and pharmacodynamic properties of, 156t
Digoxin, 34, 40
    for arrhythmias, 375t, 385
    for heart failure, 355t, 363–364
    metabolism of, 58
    steady state of, 26
    therapeutic monitoring of, 88
Dihydropyridines
    for chronic stable angina, 341
    for hypertension, 303t
Dihydrotestosterone, 612
    in prostate hyperplasia, 581
Diiodohydroxyquin, for diarrhea, 483t
Dilacor (diltiazem), for hypertension, 337t, 341
Dilantin (phenytoin), for seizures, 728, 730t, 736
Dilaudid (hydromorphone), dose-response relationship of, 30
Diloxanide furoate, for diarrhea, 483t
Diltiazem
    for arrhythmias, 375t, 379b, 384
    for chronic stable angina, 337t, 341
    for hypertension, 303t, 304
Dimenhydrinate, for nausea and vomiting, 456t, 459
Diovan (valsartan)
    for chronic stable angina, 334, 335t, 338
    for heart failure, 354t, 360
    for hypertension, 302t
Dipentum (olsalazine), for inflammatory bowel disease, 502t, 505
Dipeptidyl peptidase-4 inhibitors, for diabetes mellitus, 897
Diphenhydramine
    for allergic rhinitis, 936
    for insomnia, 837–838
    for nausea and vomiting, 456t, 461
    for upper respiratory infections, 406t, 410
Diphenoxylate/atropine
    for diarrhea, 482–484, 484t–485t, 486
    for irritable bowel syndrome, 492t, 494, 497t
Dipivefrin, for glaucoma, 276
Direct acting antivirals, for hepatitis C virus, 559–560, 559t, 561
Direct fluorescent antibody test, for syphilis, 624
Disopyramide, for arrhythmias, 375t, 379, 379b
Dispense as written code, 135
Displacement interactions, in drug binding, 36, 36t
Disposal of medications, 7
Distribution, drug, 22–23, 23f, 23b
    complementary alternative medicine interactions, 44–45
    in drug–disease interactions, 46
    in drug–drug interactions, 34, 36, 36t
    in older adults, 72–73
    in pediatric patients, 57t, 59–60
    in pregnancy, 57t, 59–60
Disulfiram, for alcohol use disorder, 874t, 875
Ditropan (oxybutynin)
    constipation due to, 82
    for overactive bladder, 601t, 602, 602t, 604, 604t

Diuretics
    for ascites, 547t
    classes of, 298
    constipation and, 469b
    effect of drugs on, 43–44
    for heart failure, 353t–354t, 358–359
    for hypertension, 298–300, 298t–300t, 308
    loop, 299–300, 299t
    nutrient interactions with, 44
    potassium-sparing, 300, 300t
    thiazide, 298–299, 298t
Diuril (chlorothiazide), for hypertension, 298t
Divalproex, for migraine prevention, 714, 715t
DNA sequence, 122
Dobutamine, for heart failure, 355t, 357
Dobutrex (dobutamine), for heart failure, 355t, 357
Docosanol, for viral skin infections, 222, 222t
Docusate calcium
    for constipation, 472t, 474–475
    for irritable bowel syndrome, 492t, 494, 497t
Docusate potassium, for constipation, 472t
Docusate sodium
    for constipation, 161, 471t, 474–475
    for irritable bowel syndrome, 492t, 494, 497t
Dofetilide, for arrhythmias, 375t, 379b, 384
Dolasetron, for nausea and vomiting, 457t, 460
Dolobid (diflunisal), 646t, 647
    pharmacokinetic and pharmacodynamic properties of, 156t
Donepezil, for Alzheimer's disease, 758–759, 760t, 761
Donnatal (belladonna alkaloids), for irritable bowel syndrome, 492t, 494, 497t
Dopamine
    for anaphylaxis and anaphylactoid reactions, 931
    for bradycardia, 395–396
    deficiency of, in depression, 784, 784b
    heart failure, 359
    for restless legs syndrome, 842
Dopamine receptor agonists, for diabetes mellitus, 899
Dopamine transporter (DAT), for Parkinson disease, 767
Dopamine–norepinephrine reuptake inhibitors, 848
Dopaminergic agents, for restless legs syndrome, 842
Doribax (doripenem), 96t, 104, 104t
Doripenem, 96t, 104, 104t
Doryx (doxycycline), for rosacea, 252
Dorzolamide, for glaucoma, 273t, 276
Dose
    for pediatric patients, 65–66
    in prescriptions, 12
    response relationships with, 30, 30f
    timing of, in breast-feeding, 64
Dovonex (calcipotriene), for psoriasis, 231t, 233
Downregulation, definition of, 18b
Doxazosin
    for benign prostatic hyperplasia, 584, 584t
    for hypertension, 304, 304t
    for overactive bladder, 601t, 603t, 608
Doxycycline, 97t, 108–109, 109t, 206t
    for acne, 246
    for Chlamydia trachomatis infections, 616t, 617, 618t
    for conjunctivitis, 262
    for gonorrhea, 622, 622t
    for lower respiratory tract infections, 419t, 420, 422t
    for pelvic inflammatory disease, 616t, 633t
    for prostatitis, 579t, 580
    for rosacea, 252
    for syphilis, 616t, 624, 625t
    for upper respiratory infections, 407t, 414
Doxylamine/pyridoxine, for nausea and vomiting, 458t, 467
Drainage, of skin infections, 209
Dramamine (dimenhydrinate), for nausea and vomiting, 456t, 459
Dravet syndrome, 185
Dressing, for topical corticosteroids, 194

Drithocreme (anthralin), for psoriasis, 231t, 233
Driving, epilepsy and, 751
Dronabinol
    for nausea and vomiting, 458t, 462
    for pain, 183t, 184, 187
Dronedarone, for arrhythmias, 375t, 379b, 383
Drospirenone, in contraceptives, 1092
Drug abuse, potential for, 4b
Drug interactions, 33–51
    with disease, 46–47, 47t
    with food, 41–44, 42b, 43b, 696b, 796
    in older adult, 76
    P-glycoprotein interactions, 40–41, 41t
    patient factors in, 47–48
    tracking of, 49, 50f
Drug receptors, 27–29
    action of, 27–28, 28f
    affinity of, 29
    for agonists, 30
    for antagonists, 30
    chirality of, 29–30
    definition of, 18b
    dose–response relationships and, 30, 30f
    drug interactions with, 29–30
    G-protein–coupled, 28f, 29
    gated ion channels, 28, 28f
    intracellular, 28f, 29
    in older adults, 74
    transmembranous, 28f, 29
    types of, 28, 28f
Drug–drug interactions, 34–41
    in absorption, 34, 35t
    in adsorption, 34
    cytochrome P-450 system and, 792, 793t
    definition of, 34
    in distribution, 34, 36, 36t
    in excretion, 39–40, 40t
    in metabolism, 36–39, 36f, 37f, 38t
    object drug in, 34, 35t, 36t
    in older adults, 76
    with over-the-counter drugs, 72
    pharmacodynamic, 41
    target drug in, 34, 35t, 36t
Dry eye disease. See Keratoconjunctivitis sicca
Dry eye syndrome. See Keratoconjunctivitis sicca
Dry powder inhalers, 67, 68t
Duac Gel (clindamycin–benzoyl peroxide), for acne, 247
Dual antiplatelet therapy (DAPT), 990
Dulcolax (bisacodyl)
    for constipation, 472t, 474
    for irritable bowel syndrome, 492t, 493–494, 497t
Dulera (mometasone furoate/formoterol fumarate dihydrate), for asthma and COPD, 431t
Duloxetine
    for overactive bladder, 601t, 603t, 607–608
    for pain, 162
Duobrii (halobetasol proprionate and tazarotene lotion), for psoriasis, 231t, 234
Duodenum, peptic ulcers of. See Peptic ulcer disease (PUD)
Duphalac (lactulose)
    for constipation, 472t, 473–474
    for hepatic encephalopathy, 553–554, 553t
    for irritable bowel syndrome, 491, 491t, 497t
Dupilumab, for asthma and COPD, 433t, 442–443
Dupixent (dupilumab), for asthma and COPD, 433t, 442–443
Duragesic (fentanyl), for pain, 152, 156, 157, 158t, 159–160, 159t
Dutasteride, for benign prostatic hyperplasia, 583–584, 584t
Dye staining test, in keratoconjunctivitis sicca, 262
Dynacirc (isradipine), for hypertension, 303t, 304
Dynapen (dicloxacillin), for skin infections, 205t, 207
Dyrenium (triamterene)
    for heart failure, 354t
    for hypertension, 299, 300t

Dyslipidemia. *See* Hyperlipidemia
Dysthymia, 785

E

E-mycin (erythromycin), 97t, 106, 106t
  causing diarrhea, 479
  for rosacea, 252
Ear, infections of
  external (otitis externa), 281–283, 282t, 287–290, 288t–289t
  inner (otitis media), 281–287, 282t, 284t, 285t–286t, 285f
Ear drops, for otitis externa, 288, 288t
Echinacea angustifolia, 417
Echinacea pallida, 417
Echinacea purpurea, 417
Echocardiography
  in atrial fibrillation, 988
  in chronic stable angina, 333
  in valvular heart disease, 988
Economic issues. *See* Pharmacoeconomics
Ecthyma
  algorithm for, 210f
  causes of, 199, 199t
  complementary and alternative medicine for, 212
  diagnosis of, 202
  lifestyle changes for, 212
  pathophysiology of, 202, 202b
  patient education on, 211–212
  therapeutic monitoring of, 211
  treatment of, 204, 205t–206t, 207–209, 209t, 210f
Eczema. *See* Atopic dermatitis
Edecrin (ethacrynic acid)
  for heart failure, 354t
  for hypertension, 299, 299t
Education, patient. *See* Patient education; *specific drugs and diseases*
Efavirenz, for HIV infection, 956, 958t
Effexor (venlafaxine)
  for anxiety disorders, 814t, 815
  for depression, 789t, 791t, 795t, 802
  for headache, 699
  insomnia, 846
  for menopausal symptoms, 1109–1110
  for overactive bladder, 607–608
Effient (prasugrel), for coagulation disorders, 1002
Elavil (amitriptyline)
  for depression, 789t, 790t, 794
  for fibromyalgia, 718
  for headache, 697, 700t
  for irritable bowel syndrome, 494, 497t
  for migraine prevention, 700t, 720
Elbasvir, for hepatitis C virus, 559, 559t
Electrocardiography (ECG)
  in arrhythmias, 373
  in atrial fibrillation, 987–988
  in chronic stable angina, 333
  in heart failure, 351
  in valvular heart disease, 988
Electroencephalography (EEG), in seizures, 749
Electronic health records, 139–140
Electronic prescriptions, 13, 139–140
Elestat (epinastine), for conjunctivitis, 263t, 265
Eletriptan, for migraine headache, 706t, 711
Elimination, drug, 23–27, 24t, 25f–26f, 26b, 27t. *See also* Excretion, drug; Metabolism, drug
  vs. age, 57t
  clearance in, 26–27, 26b, 27t
  half-life and, 25, 25f
  in older adults, 73–74, 74b, 75t
  in pediatrics, 61
  in pregnancy, 67
  steady state and, 26, 26f
Elixophyllin (theophylline), for asthma and COPD, 432t, 440–441
Emadine (emedastine), for conjunctivitis, 262, 263t
Emedastine, for conjunctivitis, 262, 263t
Emend (aprepitant), for nausea and vomiting, 457t
Emergencies, hypertensive, 308

Emergency Use Authorization (EUA), 4
Emesis. *See* Nausea and vomiting
Emete-con (benzquinamide), for nausea and vomiting, 456t
Emetic complex (EC), 453
Emgality, for migraine prevention, 717t, 719
Emollients, for psoriasis, 231t, 233
Emphysema. *See* Chronic obstructive pulmonary disease (COPD)
Empiric antibiotic therapy, 94, 94t
Emtricitabine, for HIV infection, 950, 951t, 956
Emtriva (emtricitabine), for HIV infection, 950, 951t, 956
Enablex (darifenacin), for overactive bladder, 601t, 602, 603t, 604, 604t
Enalapril
  for chronic stable angina, 334, 335t, 338
  for heart failure, 352, 353t
  for hypertension, 302, 302t
Enantiomers, 18b, 29
Enbrel (etanercept), 232t, 236
  for rheumatoid arthritis, 680t, 684
Endocannabinoid system, 179
  and relationship to pain, 181–182
  structure and function of, 182f
Endocytosis, 20
Endometritis, in pelvic inflammatory disease, 632
Endorphins, in pain management, 149
Endoscopy
  in GERD, 525
  in peptic ulcer disease, 527
Endotype, asthma and COPD, 426
Enemas, drug absorption from, 21
Enfuvirtide, for HIV infection, 954t, 959
Enoxaparin, 990, 992, 999t
  for chronic stable angina, 337t, 342
  drug–disease interactions of, 48
Enstilar, for psoriasis, 234
Entamoeba histolytica infections, 480b
Entecavir, for hepatitis B virus, 557, 558t
Enteral absorption, 20
Enterobacter infections, skin, 201t
Enterococcus infections, antimicrobial sensitivity in, 95t–98t
Enterohepatic recirculation, 18b, 25, 25f
Entocort EC (budesonide), for inflammatory bowel disease, 503t, 505–506
Entourage effect, 186
Entresto (sacubitril/valsartan), for heart failure, 354t, 360–361
Entyvio (vedolizumab), for inflammatory bowel disease, 504t, 508
Envarsus (tacrolimus), for organ transplantation, 969t, 970, 974t
Environmental factors
  in keratoconjunctivitis sicca, 268
  migraine headache, 701, 701b
  in obesity, 1077–1078
Enzyme(s). *See also specific enzyme*, e.g., Cytochrome P-450 system induction
  induction, 38
  inhibition, 24
  and metabolism of, 23–24
Eosinophilia, in allergic rhinitis, 933
Epaned (enalapril), for hypertension, 302, 302t
Epidermophyton infections, 213
Epidiolex (cannabidiol), for pain, 179, 183t, 185–186, 185t
Epiduo (adapalene/BPO), for acne, 243t, 247
Epilepsy, 725–752
  algorithm for, 729f, 729t
  causes of, 725–726
  definition of, 725
  diagnosis of, 727–728
  information sources for, 751
  lifestyle changes for, 751
  in older adults, 750
  pathophysiology of, 726–727
  in pediatric patients, 750
  pharmacogenetics, 750

reflex, 725
  seizure classification in, 726–727
  status epilepticus in, 727
  surgery for, 728
  therapeutic monitoring of, 751
  treatment of, 728–750, 728t, 729f, 730t–735t, 736b, 737b, 740b
  in women, 750
Epileptic focus, 726
Epinastine, for conjunctivitis, 263t, 265
Epinephrine, 28
  for anaphylaxis and anaphylactoid reactions, 931
  for glaucoma, 276
  for ventricular fibrillation, 395–396
Epivir (lamivudine), for HIV infection, 950, 951t, 956
Eplerenone
  for ascites, 550
  for chronic stable angina, 334, 335t, 338
  for hypertension, 300, 300t
Epoetin, for anemia, 1022
Epogen (epoetin), for anemia, 1022
Eprosartan
  for chronic stable angina, 334
  for heart failure, 360
Epsom salt (magnesium sulfate), for constipation, 472t, 474
Epstein-Barr virus infection, 220
Eptinezumab-jjmr (Vyepti), for migraine prevention, 717t, 719
Equalactin (calcium polycarbophil), for irritable bowel syndrome, 491t
Eravacycline, 97t, 108, 109t
Erectile dysfunction (ED), 587–592
  algorithm for, 591f
  causes of, 588, 588b
  complementary and alternative medicine for, 592
  diagnosis of, 589
  drug-induced, 791t, 792
  epidemiology of, 587–588
  information sources of, 592
  pathophysiology of, 588–589
  patient education on, 592
  therapeutic monitoring of, 592
  treatment of, 589–592, 590t, 591b, 591f, 592t
Erenumab-aooe (Aimovig), for migraine prevention, 717t, 718–719
Ergostat (ergotamine), for migraine headache, 707t, 713
Ergotamines, for migraine headache, 707t, 713
Errors, in drug prescription, 9
Ertapenem, 96, 104, 104t
Ery-base (erythromycin, base), for lower respiratory tract infections, 419t, 420
Ery-Tab (erythromycin), for rosacea, 252
Erysipelas
  causes of, 200–201, 200t
  complementary and alternative medicine for, 212
  diagnosis of, 202–203
  lifestyle changes for, 212
  pathophysiology of, 202, 202b
  patient education on, 211–212
  therapeutic monitoring of, 211
  treatment of, 204, 205t–206t, 207–209, 209t, 210f
Erythrocytes. *See* Red blood cells
Erythrodermic psoriasis, 230
Erythromycin(s), 34, 106, 106t
  for acne, 243t, 246, 247
  causing diarrhea, 479
  for *Chlamydia trachomatis* infections, 616t, 617, 619
  for conjunctivitis, 262
  for diarrhea, 483t
  for gonorrhea, 623, 623t
  for lower respiratory tract infections, 419t, 420
  for otitis media, 286
  for rosacea, 252
  sensitivity of, 97t
  for skin infections, 243t, 247

Erythropoietin, in red blood cell production, 1013
Escherichia coli infections, 480b, 481
    in cirrhosis, 544
    skin, 201t, 202, 207
    urinary tract, 568, 572, 574
Escitalopram
    for Alzheimer's disease, 761
    for anxiety disorders, 814t, 815
    for depression, 81
Esketamine (Spravato), for depression, 791t,
    797–798
Eslicarbazepine, for seizures, 738
Esmolol, for arrhythmias, 376t, 379b
Esomeprazole
    for GERD, 529t, 530t, 531
    for peptic ulcer disease, 529t, 531, 537t
Esophagogastroduodenoscopy, 545
Esophagus
    candidiasis of (*See* Candidiasis)
    gastric contents reflux into (*See* Gastroesophageal
        reflux disease [GERD])
Estazolam, for insomnia, 833, 834t
Estrace (estrogen), for menopausal symptoms, 1102,
    1103t–1106t
Estraderm (estradiol), for menopausal symptoms,
    1103t, 1105t
Estradiol
    in contraceptives, 1093t, 1094, 1096
    for menopausal symptoms, 1102, 1103t, 1105t
    for overactive bladder, 608
Estratest (combination product), for menopausal
    symptoms, 1104t, 1106
Estring (vaginal ring)
    hormone replacement, 1105t, 1107
    for overactive bladder, 608
Estrogen(s), 608–609
    actions of, 1106
    for Alzheimer's disease, 1101
    contraceptives, 1092–1094, 1093t
    deficiency of, in menopause, 1102
    drug interactions of, 1096
    for menopausal symptoms, 1102, 1103t
    in menstrual cycle, 1090, 1090f
    metabolism of, 1097
    for osteoporosis, 669t, 671
    for overactive bladder, 601t
    replacement of (*See* Hormone replacement
        therapy)
Estrogen agonist/antagonist, in menopause, 1108–
    1109
Estrogen receptor alpha, in menopause, 1108
Estrogen receptor beta, in menopause, 1108
Eszopiclone, for insomnia, 833, 836
Etanercept
    for psoriasis, 232t, 236
    for rheumatoid arthritis, 680t, 684
Etelcalcetide, for hyperparathyroidism, 923
Ethacrynic acid
    for heart failure, 354t
    for hypertension, 299, 299t
Ethical issues, in prescribing drugs, 7–8
Ethinyl estradiol, in contraceptives, 1093t, 1097
Ethnic factors
    in acne medications, 249
    in anxiety disorders, 825
    in pharmacokinetics and pharmacodynamics, 31
Ethosuximide, for seizures, 728t, 739
Ethynodiol diacetate, in contraceptives, 1092, 1093t
Etonogestrel, in contraceptives, 1096
Etretinate, for psoriasis, 232t
Eucerin products, for psoriasis, 231t
Eustachian tube, in otitis media, 282–283
Everolimus, for organ transplantation, 972–973,
    974t
Evista (raloxifene), for osteoporosis, 669t, 671
Evolocumab (repatha), for hyperlipidemia, 321t, 322
Evoxac (cevimeline), for keratoconjunctivitis sicca,
    270t
Excedrin (combination product), for headache, 703,
    704t

Excretion, drug, 24–25, 25f
    in drug–disease interactions, 47
    in drug–drug interactions, 39–40, 40t
    in drug–food interactions, 43
    in pediatric patients, 61
Exelderm (sulconazole), for fungal infections, 215t
Exelon (rivastigmine), for Alzheimer's disease, 758,
    759, 760t
Exercise
    for chronic stable angina, 331
    for coronary heart disease prevention, 331
    for diabetes mellitus, 889, 890
    for heart failure, 352
    for hyperlipidemia, 316
    for hypertension, 296
    lack of, obesity in, 1083
    therapeutic, for pain management in opioid use
        disorder, 175
Exercise tolerance test, in chronic stable angina, 333
Exon, 122b
Expectorants, for respiratory infections, 406t, 408
Extemporaneous formulations, for pediatric patients,
    65
Extensive metabolizers, 124
Extrapyramidal side effects (EPSs), 79
Exudative (inflammatory) diarrhea, 481
Eye, anatomy of, 271f
Eye disorders. *See* Ophthalmic disorders
Eye drops, application of, 265
Eyelid, infections of (blepharitis), 257–260,
    259t–261t
EyeScrub, for blepharitis, 258
Ezetimibe, for hyperlipidemia, 321–322, 321t

F

Factor V Leiden, hypercoagulability and, 982b, 986
Fading, nicotine, 1062
Fagerstrom Test for Nicotine Dependence, 1059,
    1061b
Falls, medication and, in older adults, 79–81, 79t
Famciclovir
    for herpes simplex virus infections, 616t, 628,
        629t, 631
    for viral skin infections, 222, 222t, 223
Familial hypercholesterolemia, homozygous, 325
Family planning. *See* Contraception
Family therapy, for ADHD, 867
Famotidine, 34
    drug interactions of, 34
    for GERD, 529t, 530t, 534
    for peptic ulcer disease, 529t, 537t
Famvir (famciclovir)
    for herpes simplex virus infections, 616t, 628,
        629t, 631
    for viral skin infections, 222, 222t, 223
Fansidar (sulfadoxine), 109
Fasciitis, necrotizing. *See* Necrotizing fasciitis
Fasenra (benralizumab), for asthma and COPD,
    433t, 442–443
Fast track, 4
Fastin (phentermine), for obesity, 1080t, 1082–1083
Fasting plasma glucose test, 889, 889t
Fat (body)
    distribution of, 1078
    in fetus, drug distribution and, 62
    in older adults, 72
    in pregnancy, drug distribution and, 59
Fat (blood), elevated. *See* Hyperlipidemia
Fat (dietary), in hyperlipidemia, 316
Fatty acid supplements, for keratoconjunctivitis
    sicca, 269
Fatty streak, in atherosclerosis pathogenesis,
    315, 332
Fear, normal, 811
Fee-for-service insurance, 131–132
Felbamate, for seizures, 734t, 744
Felodipine
    for chronic stable angina, 341
    for hypertension, 303t, 304
Felon, 199, 201, 203

FemCare (clotrimazole), for candidiasis, 1118, 1119t,
    1122
Femring (vaginal ring), for menopausal symptoms,
    1105t, 1107
Femstat (butoconazole), for candidiasis, 1118, 1119t
Fenofibrate, for hyperlipidemia, 321t, 323–324
Fentanyl, for pain, 152, 156, 157, 158t, 159–160,
    159t
Fentora (fentanyl), for pain, 152, 156, 157, 158t,
    159–160, 159t
Ferritin, deficiency of, in iron deficiency anemia,
    1019
Ferrous salts
    constipation and, 469b
    for iron deficiency anemia, 1020
Ferrous sulfate, for restless legs syndrome, 843
Fesoterodine, for overactive bladder, 601t, 602, 603t,
    604–605, 604t
Fetroja (cefiderocol), 96t, 102t, 103
Fetus, drug transfer to, 61–63, 62t
    metabolism of, 62
    risk categories of, 63t
    teratogenic, 62–63, 63t, 247
Feverfew, for migraine headache, 721
Fexofenadine, for allergic rhinitis, 937t, 938
Fiber-Con (polycarbophil), for diarrhea, 484t, 485
Fiberall (polycarbophil)
    for constipation, 471, 471t, 473
    for diarrhea, 484t, 485
    for irritable bowel syndrome, 491t
Fibric acid derivatives, for hyperlipidemia, 320f,
    321t, 323–324
Fibrous plaque, atherosclerotic, 315, 332
Fick's law of diffusion, 19, 20
Fidaxomicin, 106
Fight-or-flight response, 811, 811b
Filiform warts (verruca filiformis), 221
Finacea (azelaic acid), for rosacea, 251
Finasteride, for benign prostatic hyperplasia,
    583–584, 584t
Fioricet (combination product), for headache, 697,
    698t, 699
Fiorinal (combination product), for headache, 697,
    698t, 713
First-order kinetics, in drug elimination, 25
First-pass effect, 18b, 20b
First-pass metabolism, 541
Fish oil
    for hyperlipidemia, 316
    for psoriasis, 239
Fish tapeworm infections, 1024, 1024b
Five A's, for smoking cessation, 1059, 1061b
Five R's, for smoking cessation, 1059, 1062b
Flagyl (metronidazole), 98t, 115, 115t, 118t
    for bacterial vaginosis, 1119, 1120t
    for GERD, 529t, 532
    for inflammatory bowel disease, 503t, 507, 514
    for peptic ulcer disease, 529t, 532
Flat warts (verruca plana), 221
Flavoxate, for urinary tract infections, 571t, 572
Flecainide, for arrhythmias, 376t, 379b, 380
Flector (diclofenac), pharmacodynamic and
    pharmacologic properties of, 156t
Fleet enemas, for constipation, 472t, 474
Flomax (tamsulosin)
    for benign prostatic hyperplasia, 584–585, 584t
    for overactive bladder, 601t, 603t, 608
Floxin (ofloxacin)
    for *Chlamydia trachomatis* infections, 616t, 617
    for gonorrhea, 618t
    for otitis externa, 288, 288t
Fluconazole
    for candidiasis, 1119, 1119t, 1120
    in cytochrome P-450 system inhibition, 38
    for fungal infections, 217t, 218
Fludrocortisone, for reactions to monoamine oxidase
    inhibitors, 794, 796
Fluid therapy, for upper respiratory infections, 408,
    411
Flumadine (rimantadine), for influenza, 1042

Flumazenil, for benzodiazepine overdose, 818
Fluocinolone acetonide, for contact dermatitis, 193t
Fluorometholone, for conjunctivitis, 264t
Fluoroquinolone, 96t, 104–106, 105t, 118t. *See also specific drugs*
    absorption and, 41
    adsorption and, 34
    for community-acquired pneumonia, 422t, 423
    for otitis externa, 288–289
    for prostatitis, 579t, 580
    for skin infections, 206t, 208
    for spontaneous bacterial peritonitis, 550
Fluoxetine
    for anxiety disorders, 814t, 815, 825
    for depression, 81, 789t, 790t, 795t, 796
    for headache, 699
Fluphenazine, for nausea and vomiting, 456t
Flurandrenolide, for contact dermatitis, 193t
Flurazepam
    anxiety disorders, 80
    for insomnia, 833, 834t
Fluticasone propionate, for contact dermatitis, 193t
Fluvastatin, for hyperlipidemia, 317t, 319
Fluvoxamine, for anxiety disorders, 814t
Foam cells, in atherosclerosis pathogenesis, 315
Folate deficiency, anemia in, 1025–1026, 1025b
Follicle-stimulating hormone, in menstrual cycle, 1090, 1090f
Folliculitis
    causes of, 200t, 201
    complementary and alternative medicine for, 212
    diagnosis of, 203
    lifestyle changes in, 212
    pathophysiology of, 202, 202b
    patient education on, 211–212
    therapeutic monitoring of, 211
    treatment of, 204, 205t–206t, 207–210, 209t, 210f
Fondaparinux (Arixtra), 342–343, 992, 999t
Food. *See also* Nutrition
    additives, ADHD and, 867
    allergens in, 829
    drug interactions with, 31, 41–44, 42b, 43b
    drug interactions with, 796, 796b
Food and Drug Administration, 863
    cannabis drugs approved by, 183, 183t
    clinical trial oversight by, 3–4
    Controlled Substances Act of 1970, 4, 5b
    fast track, 4–5
    generic drug criteria of, 134–135
    herbal preparations and, 7
    Modernization Act of 1997, 56
    pregnancy risk categories of, 62t, 63
    therapeutic equivalence ratings of, 6t
Foot infection, diabetic. *See* Diabetic foot infection
Foreign antigens, recognition of, 965
Foreign body, nasal *vs.* allergic rhinitis, 934
Foreign medications, 7
Formoterol, for asthma and COPD, 430t, 436
Formularies
    advantages of, 133
    closed, 133
    committee for, 137–138
    compliance with, 138–139, 138t
    drug-dispensing limitations, 135–136
    evolution of, 133
    example of, 133, 133t
    functions of, 134–136
    generic substitution in, 134–135
    management of, 137–138, 137b
    medical necessity in, 136
    new agents added to, 137, 137b
    open, 133–134
    patient impact of, 134
    prior authorization in, 136
    restrictive, 135
    structure of, 133–134, 133t
    therapeutic interchange in, 135
    tiered, 134
Formulary medication, 133

Formulations, drug
    absorption and, 20
    for pediatric patients, 65
Fortaz (ceftazidime), 96t, 102t, 103
    for skin infections, 207
Forteo (teriparatide)
    for hypoparathyroidism, 924
    for osteoporosis, 669t, 671
Fosamax (alendronate), for osteoporosis, 667, 668t
Fosamprenavir (Lexiva), for HIV infection, 953t, 954t, 957
Fosfomycin, for urinary tract infections, 569, 570t, 572
Fosinopril
    for chronic stable angina, 335t
    for heart failure, 352, 353t
Fosphenytoin, for seizures, 728–729, 728t, 730t, 736
Fostemsavir (Rukobia), for HIV infection, 955t
Fractures, in osteoporosis, 663
Fragmin (dalteparin), 992, 999t
Free (unbound) drug, definition of, 22–23, 23f
Free erythrocyte production, in iron deficiency anemia, 1019
Fremanezumab-vfrm (Ajovy), for migraine prevention, 717t, 719
Friction acne, 241
Frova (frovatriptan), for migraine headache, 706t, 710, 711
Frovatriptan, for migraine headache, 706t, 710, 711
Functional bowel disorders. *See specific disorders*
Fungal infections, 212–219. *See also* Antifungals
Furosemide
    for ascites, 547t, 548–549
    for heart failure, 354t, 358–359
    hypertension, 299, 299t
Furunculosis
    causes of, 200t, 201
    complementary and alternative medicine for, 212
    diagnosis of, 203
    lifestyle changes in, 212
    pathophysiology of, 202, 202b
    patient education on, 211–212
    treatment of, 204, 205t–206t, 207–210, 209t, 210f
Fusion inhibitors, for HIV infection, 954t, 959
Fuzeon (enfuvirtide), for HIV infection, 954t, 959

G
G-protein–coupled drug receptors, 28f, 29
Gabapentin
    menopause systems, 1110
    for pain, 162
    for restless legs syndrome, 842–843
    for seizures, 728t
Gabitril (tiagabine), for seizures, 733t, 742–743
Galantamine, for Alzheimer's disease, 758–759, 760t
Galcanezumab-gnlm (Emgality), for migraine prevention, 717t, 719
Gamma-aminobutyric acid (GABA), 181
    as drug receptor, 28
Garamycin (gentamicin), 114–115
    dosages of, 107t
    monitoring of, 108t
    sensitivity of, 97t
    for skin infections, 208
Gardnerella vaginalis infections, 1115
GAS infections. *See Streptococcus pyogenes* infections
Gastric emptying time
    in pediatric patients, 57–58
    in pregnancy, 57–58
Gastric pH
    in pediatric patients, 57
    in pregnancy, 57
Gastroesophageal reflux disease (GERD), 523–526
    antacids for, 528, 529t
    antibiotics for, 529t, 531–533
    causes of, 523–524, 524t
    complementary and alternative medicines for, 535
    complications of, 525, 525t

    definition of, 523
    diagnosis of, 525–526, 525t
    epidemiology of, 523
    histamine-2 receptor antagonists for, 528, 529t, 530–531
    in older adults, 534
    pathophysiology of, 524–525, 524f, 525t
    patient education on, 535
    in pediatric patients, 534
    in pregnancy, 535
    proton pump inhibitors for, 529t, 531
    risk factors for, 524, 524t, 525
    symptoms of, 525t
    therapeutic monitoring of, 535
    treatment of, 526, 528–534, 529t, 530t
    in women, 535
Gastroesophageal varices, cirrhosis and, 545–546
Gastrointestinal enzymes
    in pediatric patients, 58
    in pregnancy, 58
Gastrointestinal system
    absorption in, 19, 21, 34, 35t
    in older adults, 82
Gastrointestinal tract, stimulating nausea and vomiting, 453
Gated ion channels, as drug receptors, 28, 28f
Gemfibrozil, for hyperlipidemia, 321t, 323–324
Gemifloxacin, 96t, 105, 105t
    for community-acquired pneumonia, 423
Gender differences. *See also* Women
    in chronic stable angina risk, 330
    in HIV infection, 963
    in pharmacokinetics and pharmacodynamics, 31
Generalized anxiety disorder
    algorithm for, 822f
    definition of, 810t
    diagnosis of, 811–812, 812b, 813b
    epidemiology of, 809
    treatment of, 813–818, 814t, 817t, 818–825, 818t
Generalized (convulsive or nonconvulsive) seizures, 726–727
Generic drugs, substitution with, 134–135
Genes, definitions, 121, 122b
Genetic factors
    in allergic rhinitis, 932
    in Alzheimer's disease, 756
    in antidepressant metabolism, 801
    in anxiety disorders, 811
    in cytochrome P-450 system, 36–37, 48, 801
    in drug interactions, 48
    in gout, 652
    in hypercoagulability, 986
    in hyperlipidemia, 313, 314b
    in obesity, 1077
    in periodic limb movement disorder, 841
    in pharmacokinetics and pharmacodynamics, 31
    in restless legs syndrome, 841
    in rheumatoid arthritis, 975
Genetic Information Nondiscrimination Act (GINA), 127
Genetic testing, for drug efficacy and adverse response, 126
Genital herpes. *See* Herpes simplex virus infections, genital
Genital warts. *See* Human papilloma virus infections
Genome, definitions, 121, 122b
Genotypic assay, in HIV infection, 949
Gentamicin, 114–115
    dosages of, 107t
    monitoring of, 108t
    sensitivity of, 97t
    for skin infections, 208
GERD. *See* Gastroesophageal reflux disease (GERD)
Geriatric population. *See* Older adults
Gestational diabetes, 888, 905
Giant papillary conjunctivitis, 262, 266t, 267
Giardia infections, 480, 480b
Ginger, for nausea and vomiting, 468

Gingko biloba
    for ADHD, 867
    in Alzheimer's disease, 762
Glasgow Coma Scale, 554
Glaucoma, 271–278
    causes of, 272
    diagnosis of, 272
    pathophysiology of, 272
    patient education for, 277
    therapeutic monitoring of, 277
    treatment of, 272–277, 273t–275t, 277t
    types of, 272
Glecaprevir, for hepatitis C virus, 559, 559t
Glibenclamide (glyburide), complementary
    alternative medicine interactions, 46
Glomerular filtration rate, 61
    estimation of, with creatinine clearance, 26
    in older adults, 74, 75t
GLP-1 receptor agonist (glucagon-like peptide-1
    receptor agonist), 1081t, 1082
Glucagon-like peptide receptor agonist
    for diabetes mellitus, 897–899
    for obesity, 1081t, 1082
Glucocorticoids. *See* Corticosteroids
Glucosamine
    for osteoarthritis, 651
    for psoriasis, 239
Glucose, impaired metabolism of. *See* Diabetes
    mellitus
Glucosidase inhibitors, for diabetes mellitus, 892t,
    896
Glutamate, release of, 181
Glycopeptides, 97t, 110–111, 111t, 118t
Glycopyrrolate, for asthma and COPD, 430t, 438
Gold compounds, for rheumatoid arthritis, 679t, 680
Golimumab, for psoriasis, 232t
Gonioscopy, in glaucoma, 272
Gonorrhea, 620–623
    algorithm for, 623f
    causes of, 620
    Chlamydia trachomatis infections with, 620
    diagnosis of, 620
    epidemiology of, 620
    pathophysiology of, 620
    patient education on, 623
    in pediatric patients, 621t, 622–623, 623t
    pelvic inflammatory disease in, 631, 633t, 634f
    in pregnancy, 620
    therapeutic monitoring of, 623
    treatment of, 620–623, 621t, 623f, 623t
Gout
    causes of, 652
    complementary and alternative medicine, 660
    diagnosis of, 653
    information sources, 660
    lifestyle changes, 660
    nutrition for, 660
    pathophysiology, 652–653
    patient education, 660
    therapeutic monitoring of, 659–660
    treatment of, 653–656, 653b, 657t
    xanthine oxidase inhibitors, 653–654
Graft rejection, effector phase of, 966
Gram-negative infections, antimicrobial sensitivity
    in, 95t–98t
Grand mal (tonic-clonic) seizures, 726, 727, 736
Granisetron, for nausea and vomiting, 457t, 460
Granulex, for wound cleansing, 212
Grapefruit juice, drug interactions with, 42–43, 42b
Graves' ophthalmopathy (GO), 917–918, 921
"Gray baby" syndrome, 115
Grazoprevir, for hepatitis C virus, 559, 559t
Griseofulvin, for fungal infections, 215, 216t, 217
Guaifenesin, for upper respiratory infections, 406t,
    408
Guanfacine
    for ADHD, 863–864
    for hypertension, 304, 305t
Guanine, 122, 122b

Guanylate cyclase-C agonist
    for constipation, 472t, 475
    for irritable bowel syndrome, 495
Gum, nicotine, 1064, 1065t, 1066–1067, 1069
Guselkumab, for psoriasis, 232t
Gut microflora, for constipation, 479
Guttate psoriasis, 230
Guzelkumab, for psoriasis, 234
Gyne-Lotrimin (clotrimazole), for candidiasis, 1118,
    1119t, 1122

H
Habitrol (nicotine patch), 1063–1064, 1065t
Haemophilus infections, conjunctivitis, 261, 262
Haemophilus influenzae infections
    otitis media, 282, 284
    sinusitis, 412
    skin, 201t, 207
Halcinonide, for contact dermatitis, 193t
Halcion (triazolam), for insomnia, 833, 834t
Half-life, 18b, 25, 25f
    analgesic, 156t
    clearance and, 26b
    in drug interactions, 37
    enzyme induction, 39
    steady state and, 26, 26f
Halobetasol propionate
    for contact dermatitis, 193t
    and tazarotene, 231t, 234
Haplotype, 122b
Harrison Act, 180
Hashimoto's thyroiditis, 913
Hay fever conjunctivitis, 261, 265–266
Hay fever rhinitis. *See* Allergic rhinitis
Head & Shoulders shampoo, for fungal infections,
    219
Headaches, 693–722
    alarm signs in, 695
    classification of, 693, 694b
    cluster, 693, 719
    complementary and alternative medicine for, 721
    migraine (*See* Migraine headache)
    nutrition for, 721
    in older adults, 720
    patient education on, 721
    in pediatric patients, 720
    in pregnancy, 720–721
    primary, 693
    rebound, 693–696
    secondary, 696
    tension, 694–699, 697t–698t, 700t
    therapeutic monitoring of, 721
    in women, 720–721
Health insurance
    economics of (*See* Pharmacoeconomics)
    electronic prescribing, 139–140
    history of, 131–132
Health Maintenance Organization Act of
    1973, 132
Hearing loss, mitochondrial mutation and, 126
Heart, electrophysiology of, 371–372, 372b
Heart failure (HF), 349–369
    algorithm for, 367f
    angiotensin-converting enzyme inhibitors for,
        352–358, 353t–355t, 356f, 358t
    angiotensin II type 1 receptor blockers for,
        359–360
    angiotensin receptor-neprilysin inhibitor for,
        354t, 360–361
    beta blockers for, 354t–355t, 362–363
    causes of, 349–350
    classification of, 351t
    clinical manifestations of, 351, 351b
    diagnosis of, 351b, 351–352, 351t
    digoxin for, 355t, 363–364
    diuretics for, 353t–354t, 358–359
    drug-induced, 349
    economic impact of, 349
    epidemiology of, 349

hydralazine–isosorbide dinitrate combination for,
    355t, 364–365
    left ventricular, 351, 351b
    lifestyle changes for, 369
    nutrition for, 369
    in older adults, 368
    pathophysiology of, 350, 350f
    patient education on, 368–369
    in pediatric patients, 368
    in pregnancy, 368
    right ventricular, 351, 351b
    therapeutic monitoring of, 368
    treatment of, 352–369
    vicious circle of, 350, 350f
Heart Failure Society of America guidelines, for heart
    failure, 361
Heart transplantation, 965. *See also* Organ
    transplantation
Heat therapy, for pain, 152
Heberden's nodes, in osteoarthritis, 643
Helicobacter pylori infections, in peptic ulcer disease,
    527, 528–533, 535–538, 536t
Hematocrit
    in anemia, 1013
    in thalassemia, 1019, 1023–1024
Hematuria, in urinary tract infections, 569
Hemoglobin A$_{1C}$, in diabetes mellitus therapy, 889,
    889t
Hemoglobin H, in thalassemia, 1023–1024
Hemoglobin, level of, in anemia, 1013, 1014t
Hemoglobin S, in sickle cell disease, 1016
Hemolytic anemia, in thalassemia, 1016, 1023–1024
Hemorrhage, anemia after, 1016
Hemostasis, normal, 984
Heparin
    invasive procedures and, 1006b
    laboratory tests prior to, 991
    low-molecular-weight, 992–993, 996, 999t,
        1001, 1003
    in pregnancy, 1006
    therapeutic monitoring of, 992
    unfractionated, 990–993, 999t
Heparin-induced thrombocytopenia, 343
Hepatic encephalopathy (HE)
    diagnosis of, 552–553
    therapeutic monitoring for, 554
    treatment of, 553–554
Hepatic extraction ratio, 18b
Hepatitis A vaccine, 1036f, 1039f, 1043
Hepatitis B vaccine, 1035, 1036f, 1043, 1053b
Hepatitis B virus (HBV)
    causes of, 554–555
    classification of chronic infection, 556t
    complementary and alternative medications for,
        562
    diagnosis of, 555
    information resources, 561
    lifestyle changes in, 562
    nutrition for, 562
    in older adults, 560
    pathophysiology of, 555
    patient education on, 561
    in pediatrics, 560
    in pregnancy, 560
    serologic markers and interpretation, 556t
    therapeutic monitoring for, 548
    treatment of, 555–559, 556t, 558t
    in women, 560
Hepatitis C virus (HCV)
    causes of, 554–555
    complementary and alternative medications for,
        562
    diagnosis of, 555
    genomics, 560–561, 561t
    information resources, 561
    interpretation of serologic results, 557t
    lifestyle changes in, 562
    nutrition for, 562
    in older adults, 560

pathophysiology of, 555
patient education on, 561
in pediatrics, 560
in pregnancy, 560
therapeutic monitoring for, 548
treatment of, 555, 557, 557t, 559–560, 559t
in women, 560
Hepatorenal syndrome (HRS)
diagnosis of, 551, 551b
therapeutic monitoring for, 552
treatment of, 551–552, 552t
types of, 551
Herbal preparations
for Alzheimer's disease, 762
for anemia, 1027
for depression, 802
menopause, 1113t
Herbal preparations, 7
Heredity. See also Genetic factors
chronic stable angina and, 330
Herpes simplex virus (HSV)
causes of, 220
complementary and alternative medicine for, 225
diagnosis of, 220–221
genital
algorithm for, 630f
diagnosis of, 626
pathophysiology of, 628
patient education on, 631
in pediatric patients, 631
in pregnancy, 631
recurrent, 628, 631
suppression of, 631
syndromes of, 628
treatment of, 628–631, 629t, 630f
lifestyle changes in, 225
pathophysiology of, 220
patient education for, 225
in pregnancy, 225
prevention of, 225
treatment of, 221–224, 222t, 224f
Highly active antiretroviral therapy, for HIV
infection, 947–950
Histamine
in allergic rhinitis, 933, 933f, 935
in pain transduction, 148
Histamine-2 receptor antagonists
for GERD, 528, 529t, 530–531, 530t
for peptic ulcer disease, 528, 529t, 530–531, 537t
Histamine H3/inverse agonist, for narcolepsy, 847t,
848
History, inadequate, prescription errors and, 9
HIV infection. See Human immunodeficiency virus
infection
Hives, 930
HMG-CoA reductase inhibitors, 317t, 319–320,
320f
constipation and, 469b
Homocysteinemia, hypercoagulability in, 986
Homozygous familial hypercholesterolemia, 325
Hormone replacement therapy, for osteoporosis, 668t
Hormone therapy, 1102–1108
for menopausal symptoms
adverse events, 1103t–1106t, 1107–1108
algorithm for, 1111f
clinical studies of, 1102, 1106
contraindications, 1107, 1108b
discontinuation of, 1112
dose–response effect to, 1110
goals of, 1102
patient education on, 1112–1113
products for, 1102, 1103t–1106t, 1106, 1111f
recommendations for, 1107, 1108
risk/benefit of, 1107
selection of, 1111–1112
treatment duration of, 1107
Hot flashes, for menopausal symptoms, 1102, 1105t,
1106, 1108–1110, 1113t
Human chromosomes, 123f

Human genome, 121
Human herpes virus type 6 (HHV-6), 220
Human immunodeficiency virus infection, 947–964
AIDS-defining conditions in, 947, 948b
causes of, 948, 948b
CD4 T lymphocyte count in, 963
diagnosis of, 949–950
drug resistance in, 949–950
epidemiology of, 948
genotypic assay in, 949
in health care workers, 962, 962t
history of, 947
laboratory parameters in, 949
patient education on, 963–964
in pediatric patients, 961
phenotypic assay in, 949
post-exposure prophylaxis of, 962, 962t
in pregnancy, 961–962
prevention of, 947, 948b, 961
previously untreated persons, 959t, 960
signs and symptoms of, 949
syphilis with, 626
therapeutic monitoring in, 963
transmission of, 947, 948b, 962, 1091
treatment-experienced patients, 960–961
treatment of, 950–963, 951t–954t, 958t, 962t
types of, 947
viral load in, 949, 963–964
Human leukocyte antigen (HLA), 965
Human papilloma virus infections
genital, 635–638
algorithm for, 637
causes of, 635
diagnosis of, 635
pathophysiology of, 635
patient education on, 638
in pediatric patients, 637
in pregnancy, 637
therapeutic monitoring of, 638
treatment of, 635–638, 636t, 637f
Human papillomavirus, 220, 225t
Humidifier, for upper respiratory infections, 416
Humira (adalimumab)
for inflammatory bowel disease, 503t, 508
for psoriasis, 232t, 236
for rheumatoid arthritis, 680t, 684
Hydantoins, for seizures, 728, 729, 736
Hydralazine
for heart failure, 355t, 364–365
for hypertension, 305, 305t
Hydrochlorothiazide
for heart failure, 353t
for hypertension, 298t, 299
Hydrocodone, in pain, 156, 158t, 159, 159t
Hydrocortisone
for contact dermatitis, 193t
for inflammatory bowel disease, 502t
for otitis externa, 288t
for psoriasis, 231t
HydroDIURIL (hydrochlorothiazide), for heart
failure, 353t
Hydromorphone, 30, 152, 156, 157, 158t, 159, 159t
Hydrophilic (lipophobic), 18b
Hydrophobic (lipophilic), 18b
Hydroxychloroquine, for rheumatoid arthritis, 679t,
681, 682
Hydroxyurea, for sickle cell anemia, 1017–1018
Hydroxyzine
for anxiety disorders, 817t, 820
for nausea and vomiting, 456t, 458–459
Hygroton (chlorthalidone), for heart failure, 353t
Hyoscyamine sulfate, for irritable bowel syndrome,
493t, 494, 497t
Hyperactivity, in ADHD. See Attention-deficit/
hyperactivity disorder (ADHD)
Hyperarousal state, insomnia and, 831
Hypercalcemia, signs and symptoms of, 923b
Hypercholesterolemia. See Hyperlipidemia
Hypercoagulability. See Venous thromboembolism

Hyperglycemia, in diabetes mellitus, 888, 889t, 891,
892t
Hyperhomocysteinemia, hypercoagulability in, 986
Hypericin, for depression, 802
Hyperinsulinemia, 296
pathophysiology of, 888
Hyperkalemia, in chronic stable angina, 338
Hyperlipidemia, 313–326
in cardiovascular risk assessment, 315–317, 315b,
316f
causes of, 313–314, 314b
cholesterol-lowering therapy, treatment algorithm
for, 318f
chronic stable angina in, 332
coronary artery calcium for, 316
definition of, 313
diet for, 316
epidemiology of, 313
exercise for, 316–317
genetic factors in, 313, 314b
lifestyle changes for, 316–317
in older adults, 325
pathophysiology of, 314–315
patient education on, 326
in pediatric, 325
statin benefit groups, 317–320, 317t
treatment of, 317–325, 318f, 319b, 320f
in women, 325
Hyperosmotic laxatives
for constipation, 472t, 473–474
for irritable bowel syndrome, 491, 491t–492t,
493, 497t
Hyperparathyroidism, 922–924
causes of, 922
diagnosis of, 922–923, 923b, 923t
pathophysiology of, 922
patient education on, 924
in pregnancy, 924
therapeutic monitoring for, 924
treatment of, 923–924, 924t
Hypersensitivity reactions
classification of, 829–830, 930b, 930f
definition of, 829
prevention of, 931
treatment of, 931
to vaccines, 1049
Hypertension (HTN), 295–309
in African-Americans, 307–308
angiotensin-converting enzyme inhibitors for,
302, 302t
angiotensin II receptor blockers for, 302–303,
302t
in benign prostatic hypertrophy, 304
beta-adrenergic blockers for, 300–302, 301t
calcium channel blockers for, 303–304, 303t
as cardiovascular risk factor, 295
causes of, 295–296
central alpha-2 receptor agonists for, 304–305,
305t
in cerebrovascular disease, 305
classification of, 295
complementary and alternative medicine for, 309
coronary heart disease in, 331
definition of, 296, 297t
in diabetes mellitus, 308
diagnosis of, 296–297
diuretics for, 298–300, 298t–300t
epidemiology of, 295
in heart failure, 308
in ischemic heart disease, 298, 306
kidney disease, 295
in left ventricular hypertrophy, 298
lifestyle changes for, 267, 309
malignant, 308
in obesity, 295, 307
in older adults, 307
pathophysiology of, 296
patient education on, 309
in pediatric patients, 307

Hypertension (HTN) (*continued*)
  peripheral alpha-1 receptor blockers for, 304, 304t
  in pregnancy, 307
  racial factors in, 307–308
  rebound, in nitrate discontinuation, 333
  renin inhibitors for, 303, 303t
  therapeutic monitoring of, 308–309
  treatment of, 297–307, 298t–306t, 307f
  vasodilators for, 305, 305t
  white coat, 296
  in women, 307
Hypertension in the Very Elderly Trial (HYVET), 297
Hyperthyroidism, 917–922
  causes of, 917
  complementary and alternative medicine for, 922
  complications of, 917–918, 918t
  diagnosis of, 918, 918b, 919t
  laboratory findings in, 919t
  mild or subclinical, 919t
  overt, 919t
  pathophysiology of, 917
  patient education on, 922
  in pregnancy, 921
  primary, 918t
  secondary, 918t
  signs and symptoms of, 918t
  therapeutic monitoring for, 922
  thyroid storm and, 921
  thyrotoxicosis without, 918t
  treatment of, 918–921, 919t–920t
Hypoglycemia, in diabetes mellitus therapy, 903–904
Hypokalemia, from angiotensin-converting enzyme inhibitors, 357
Hyponatremia, from selective serotonin reuptake inhibitors, 81
Hypoparathyroidism, 924
Hyposensitization, for allergic rhinitis, 935
Hypotension, from angiotensin-converting enzyme inhibitors, 357
Hypothalamic-pituitary-thyroid axis, 912, 912f
Hypothyroidism, 913–917
  causes of, 913
  complementary and alternative medications for, 917
  diagnosis of, 913–914, 914b, 914t
  information sources of, 917
  laboratory findings for, 913, 913t
  in myxedema coma, 916
  in older adults, 916
  overt, 913, 914t
  pathophysiology of, 913
  patient education on, 917
  in pediatrics, 916
  in pregnancy, 916–917
  signs and symptoms of, 913, 913b
  subclinical, 913, 914t
  therapeutic monitoring for, 917
  treatment for, 914–917, 915t, 916t
Hytrin (terazosin)
  for benign prostatic hyperplasia, 584, 584t
  multiple uses of, 86
HYVET (Hypertension in the Very Elderly Trial), 297

I

Ibalizumab (Trogarzo), for HIV infection, 955t
Ibuprofen
  for headache, 697, 698t
  for osteoarthritis, 646t
  for pain, 152, 156t, 159
Ibutilide, for arrhythmias, 376t, 379b, 384
Ilumya (tildrakizumab), for psoriasis, 232t
Imdur (isosorbide mononitrate), for chronic stable angina, 336t, 338, 339
Imipenem, 95t–96t, 104, 104t
Imipenem-cilastatin-relebactam, 95t, 101t, 104

Imipramine
  for irritable bowel syndrome, 494, 497t
  for migraine prevention, 718
  for overactive bladder, 600
Imiquimod, for human papilloma virus infections, 635–636, 636t
Imitrex (sumatriptan), for migraine headache, 704t, 710
Immune complexes, 930, 930b
Immunization
  active, 1034
  adolescent, 1035b, 1036f, 1038
  adverse events in, 1044, 1045f–1048f
  characteristics of, 1033–1034
  contraindications to, 1049, 1049t–1050t, 1051
  hepatitis A, 1036f, 1039f, 1043
  hepatitis B, 1035, 1036f, 1043, 1053b
  human papillomavirus, 1042–1043
  importance of, 1033
  influenza, 1035, 1039f, 1041–1042
  measles, mumps, rubella, 1036f, 1043–1044, 1050t, 1052b–1053b
  meningococcal, 1042
  passive, 1034
  patient education on, 1051–1053, 1051b–1053b
  pediatric, 1035, 1036f, 1037f, 1038, 1039f, 1051b
  pertussis, 1042
  pneumococcal, 1039f, 1040, 1040b
  polio, 912f, 1043
  preterm infants, 1035
  recommendations for
    adult, 1038
    agencies, 1035, 1036f, 1037f
    pediatric, 1035, 1036f, 1037f, 1038, 1039f, 1051b
  rotavirus, 1043
  scheduling of, 1051b
  tetanus, diphtheria, 1039f
  to vaccines, 1033–1054
  vaccines for (*See* Vaccine(s))
  varicella, 1036f, 1038, 1039f, 1044
  zoster, 1044
Immunodeficiency. *See also* Human immunodeficiency virus infection
  immunization in, 1035
Immunoglobulin(s), in allergic reactions, 829, 930b, 930f
Immunomodulators, for rheumatoid arthritis, 685, 688
Immunosuppressive agents, for inflammatory bowel disease, 503t, 506–507, 513
Immunotherapy, for allergic rhinitis, 935
Imodium (loperamide)
  for diarrhea, 482–484, 484t–485t, 485
  for irritable bowel syndrome, 492t, 494, 497t
Impaired fasting glucose, 889, 889t
Impaired glucose tolerance, 889, 889t
Impetigo
  causes of, 199, 200t
  complementary and alternative medicine for, 212
  diagnosis of, 202
  lifestyle changes for, 212
  pathophysiology of, 202, 202b
  patient education on, 211–212
  therapeutic monitoring of, 211
  treatment of, 204, 205t–206t, 207–209, 209f, 210f
Implantable cardioverter-defibrillators, for arrhythmias, 373
Impotence. *See* Erectile dysfunction (ED)
Imuran (azathioprine)
  for inflammatory bowel disease, 503t, 506–507, 514
  for organ transplantation, 971, 974t
  for rheumatoid arthritis, 679t, 682
Inattention. *See* Attention-deficit/hyperactivity disorder (ADHD)

Incruse Ellipta (umeclidinium bromide), for asthma and COPD, 430t, 438
Indacaterol, for asthma and COPD, 430t, 436
Indapamide, for hypertension, 298t
Inderal (propranolol)
  for chronic stable angina, 336t, 340
  for migraine prevention, 714, 715t
Indinavir, for HIV infection, 953t, 957
Indocin (indomethacin), for pain, 156
Indomethacin, for pain, 156
Induction, of cytochrome P-450 system, 38–39, 38t
Infants. *See also* Neonates
  absorption in, 57t
  body composition of, 59–60
  Chlamydia trachomatis infections in, 617–619
  dehydration with diarrhea, 487
  distribution in, 57t, 59–60
  elimination in, 57t, 61
  GERD in, 534
  gonorrhea in, 621t, 622, 623
  intestinal microorganisms in, 58
  kidney function in, 61
  metabolism in, 57t
  nausea and vomiting in, 468b
  oral administration for, 66
  pulmonary absorption in, 59
  weight changes in, 56
Infections. *See also specific infections*
  ear
    external (otitis externa), 281–283, 282t, 287–290, 288t–289t
    inner (otitis media), 281–287, 282t, 284t, 285t–286t, 285f
  eyelid margin, 257–260, 259t–261t
  prostatic, 578–581, 579t, 580f
  respiratory (*See* Bronchitis; Common cold; Pneumonia; Sinusitis; *specific infections*, e.g.)
  sexually transmitted (*See* Sexually transmitted infections)
  urinary tract (*See* Urinary tract infections [UTIs])
Infectious organisms, diarrhea and, 480–481
Inferior vena cava filters, for pulmonary embolism, 1005
Inflammation, joint. *See* Osteoarthritis; Rheumatoid arthritis
Inflammatory bowel disease (IBD), 498–499
  aminosalicylates for, 502t, 504–505
  antibiotics for, 503t, 507, 513
  biological agents for, 507–509, 513
  cancer screening and, 515
  causes of, 499
  complementary and alternative therapies for, 515–516
  corticosteroids for, 502t–503t, 505–506, 510, 513, 514
  Crohn's disease (*See* Crohn's disease [CD])
  diagnosis of, 500
  etiology of, 499
  fulminant, 501t, 509t
  immunosuppressive agents for, 503t, 506–507, 513
  incidence of, 499
  information sources for, 514–515
  nutrition for, 515
  pathophysiology of, 499–500, 500t
  patient education for, 514–516
  in pediatrics, 513
  in pregnancy, 513–514
  preventive care for, 515
  surgical interventions in, 516t
  therapeutic monitoring of, 514
  treatment of, 500–513, 501t, 502t–504t, 509t, 511f–512f
  ulcerative colitis (*See* Ulcerative colitis [UC])
  vaccination for, 515
  in women, 513–514
Inflammatory vaginitis, 1116, 1118

Infliximab
for inflammatory bowel disease, 503t, 508, 509
for psoriasis, 232t, 236
for rheumatoid arthritis, 680t, 684
Influenza
amantadine, 1042
Flumadine (rimantadine), 1042
immunization, 1035, 1039f, 1041–1042
oseltamivir, 1042
Relenza (zanamivir), 1042
Rimantadine, 1042
Symmetrel (amantadine), 1042
Tamiflu (oseltamivir), 1042
Information resources, 14, 14t, 15t
for acne, 249, 249b
for allergic rhinitis, 944
for Alzheimer's disease, 760b, 762
for antiarrhythmic agents, 397–398
for antibiotics, 211
for anxiety disorders, 826–827
for asthma and COPD, 447
for attention-deficit/hyperactivity disorder, 866
for cannabis pain management, 187
for chronic stable angina, 347
for cirrhosis, 554
for constipation, 479
for depression, 802
for diabetes mellitus, 907–908
for diarrhea, 487–488
for epilepsy, 751
for GERD, 535
for gout, 660
for inflammatory bowel disease, 514–515
for irritable bowel syndrome, 498, 498b
for menopause, 1112
for narcolepsy, 845
for nausea and vomiting, 468
for osteoarthritis, 651
for osteoporosis, 673
for otitis externa, 290
for otitis media, 290
for peptic ulcer disease, 538
for psoriasis, 238
for rheumatoid arthritis, 688
for rosacea, 252
for seizures, 751
for sinusitis, 417
for sleep disorders, 832b, 845
for viral hepatitis, 561
Inhalation, of drugs
absorption of, 21, 65
pediatric patients, 65, 67
Inhaler, nicotine, 1065t, 1068
Inhibition
of cytochrome P-450 system, 37–38, 37f, 38t
enzyme, 24
INR (international normalized ratio), 988, 994b,
994t, 995b
Insomnia, 829–840
acute, 830
algorithm for, 839f
in Alzheimer's disease, 762
causes of, 829–830, 830b
chronic or learned, 830
classification of, 829–830
complementary and alternative medicine for,
840–841
definition of, 829
diagnosis of, 831–832, 832b
economic burden of, 829
epidemiology of, 829
information sources for, 840
lifestyle changes for, 840
nutrition for, 840
in older adults, 840
pathophysiology of, 731
patient education on, 840
in pediatric patients, 839–840

therapeutic monitoring of, 840
treatment of, 832–837, 834t–835t, 838t, 839f
in women, 840
Inspra (eplerenone)
for chronic stable angina, 334, 335t, 338
for hypertension, 300, 300t
Institute for Clinical Systems Improvement (ICSI),
for pain management, 151, 153t
Insulin
action of, 888
deficiency of, in type 1 diabetes mellitus, 888
for diabetes mellitus, 901, 906t
inhaled rapid-acting, 904–905
resistance to, in type 2 diabetes mellitus, 888
Insurance health
economics of (See Pharmacoeconomics)
history of, 131–132
Integrase inhibitors, for HIV infection, 959
Interactions, drug. See Drug interactions; Drug–drug
interactions
Interdigital candidiasis, 214
Interferon alfa-2b, for hepatitis B virus, 558t
Interferon(s), for human papilloma virus infections,
637
Interleukin-6 receptor antagonists, for rheumatoid
arthritis, 685
Interleukin-17 inhibitors, for psoriasis, 230, 236–237
Interleukin-23 inhibitors, for psoriasis, 230, 237
Intermediate metabolizers, 124
Intermittent coronary syndrome, 329
International League Against Epilepsy (ILAE), 726
International normalized ratio, 988, 994b, 994t,
995b
Intertrigo, 214
Intestine, microorganisms in, in pediatric patients, 58
Intestine transplantation, 965. See also Organ
transplantation
Intra-arterial administration, 22
Intra-articular therapy, for osteoarthritis, 649
Intracellular drug receptors, 28f, 29
Intramuscular administration
drug absorption in, 22
for pediatric patients, 58
in pregnancy, 58
Intraocular pressure, increased, glaucoma in, 272,
273t–275t, 275–277
Intrauterine contraceptive systems, 1095
Intravenous administration
drug absorption in, 22
for pediatric patients, 66
Intrinsic factor, deficiency of, anemia in, 1024,
1024b
Intrinsic sympathomimetic activity (ISA), 340
of beta blockers, 300–301
Intropin (dopamine), for heart failure, 359
Intuniv (guanfacine), for hypertension, 304, 305t
Invanz (ertapenem), 96t, 104, 104t
Invirase (saquinavir), for HIV infection, 954t, 957
Iodine, 911–912
Iodine solutions, for hyperthyroidism, 919t
Iodism, 921
Ion channels, gated, as drug receptors, 28, 28f
Ionization status, of drug, placental transfer and, 61
Iopidine (apraclonidine), for glaucoma, 274t, 276
Ipratropium bromide
for asthma and COPD, 428t, 438
for upper respiratory infections, 406t, 409–410
Irbesartan
for chronic stable angina, 334
for heart failure, 360
Iron, deficiency of, anemia in, 1016–1017
Irritable bowel syndrome (IBS)
antidepressants for, 494–495
antidiarrheal agents for, 492t, 494
antispasmodic agents for, 492t–493t, 494
bulk-forming laxatives for, 491, 491t
causes of, 488–489
chloride channel activators for, 495

with constipation, 490b
diagnosis of, 489–490, 489b
with diarrhea, 490b
dietary and lifestyle changes, 490, 491b
guanylate cyclase-C agonist for, 495
hyperosmotic laxatives for, 491, 491t–492t, 493
lifestyle changes in, 498
mixed, 490b
nutrition for, 498
in older adults, 498
pathophysiology of, 489
patient education for, 498
patient-oriented information sources, 498, 498b
in pediatrics, 497–498
secretagogues for, 493t, 495
semisynthetic antibiotic for, 493t, 495
serotonin-3 receptor antagonists for, 495
stimulant laxatives for, 492t, 493–494
surfactant laxatives for, 492t, 494
therapeutic monitoring of, 498
treatment of, 490–497, 491t–493t, 496f, 497t
types of, 490, 490b
unclassified, 490b
in women, 498
Irritants
conjunctivitis due to, 261
dermatitis due to, 191
vaginitis due to, 1116
Ischemic stroke, 988
antiplatelet agents, 1002
secondary prevention of, 1004
Ismo (isosorbide mononitrate), for chronic stable
angina, 336t, 338, 339
Isoflavones, for menopausal symptoms, 1113, 1113t
Isomers, 18b, 29
Isoniazid, nutrient interactions with, 43
Isoptin (verapamil), for chronic stable angina, 337t,
341
Isopto Carpine (pilocarpine), for glaucoma, 274t,
276
Isordil (isosorbide dinitrate)
for chronic stable angina, 336t, 338–339
for heart failure, 355t, 364–365
Isosorbide dinitrate
for chronic stable angina, 336t, 338–339
for heart failure, 355t, 364–365
Isosorbide mononitrate, for chronic stable angina,
336t, 338, 339
Isotretinoin
for acne, 244t, 246–247, 249
for rosacea, 252
Isradipine
for chronic stable angina, 341
for hypertension, 303t, 304
Itraconazole, for fungal infections, 216t, 217–218
IUD (intrauterine device), 1091, 1095, 1097t
Ivabradine, for heart failure, 355t, 365–366
Ivermectin, for rosacea, 251
Ixekizumab, for psoriasis, 232t, 236–237

J
Jalyn (dutasteride/tamsulosin), 585
Jarisch-Herxheimer reaction, for syphilis, 626
Jock itch (tinea cruris), 214
Joint(s), inflammation of. See Rheumatoid arthritis
Joint National Committee guidelines, 296, 297t
Juxtapid (lomitapide), 325

K
Kaletra (combination product), for HIV infection,
954t, 957
Kanamycin, 107t, 108t
Kanus kinase inhibitors, for rheumatoid arthritis,
683–684
Kaolin and bismuth salicylate, for diarrhea, 484,
484t, 485
Kaopectate (kaolin and bismuth salicylate), for
diarrhea, 484, 484t, 485

Kaposi sarcoma-associated herpesvirus (HHV-8), 220
Keflex (cephalexin), for skin infections, 205t, 207
Keppra (levetiracetam), for seizures, 733t, 742
Keratinocytes, dysfunction of, in psoriasis, 230
Keratoconjunctivitis sicca, 268–271, 270t–271t
Ketamine, 163
Ketek (telithromycin), 106
Ketoconazole
    drug interactions of, 34, 38
    for fungal infections, 215t, 219
Ketoprofen
    for headache, 697, 698t
    for pain, 156
Ketorolac
    for conjunctivitis, 263t, 265
    pharmacokinetic and pharmacodynamic
        properties of, 156t
Ketotifen, for conjunctivitis, 263t, 265
Kidney
    in blood pressure regulation, 295–296
    clearance in, 26, 26b
    drug excretion from, 24–25, 39–40, 40t, 61
        in drug–disease interactions, 47
        in drug–food interactions, 43
        drug interactions in, 48
        hypertension in, 300
        in older adults, 73–74, 75t
        in pregnancy, 61
    dysfunction or failure of, anemia in,
        1020–1022
    transplantation, 965. *See also* Organ
        transplantation
Kief, in cannabis plant, 179
Kineret (anakinra), for rheumatoid arthritis, 680t
Klebsiella infections, skin, 201t, 202, 207, 208
Klebsiella pneumonia infections, in cirrhosis, 544
Klonopin (clonazepam)
    for anxiety disorders, 816, 817t
    for seizures, 746–747
Koebner's phenomenon, in psoriasis, 229
Konsyl (psyllium), for irritable bowel syndrome, 491,
        491t, 497t
Kynamro (mipomersen), 325
Kytril (granisetron), for nausea and vomiting, 457t,
        460

L
Labetalol, for hypertension, 300, 301t, 307
Lacosamide, for seizures, 733t, 741
Lacrimal system, dysfunction of, keratoconjunctivitis
        sicca in, 268–271, 270t
Lactation. *See also* Breast-feeding
    labeling rule, 63, 63t
LactMed database, 63
Lactobacilli, vaginal, 1116
Lactulose
    for constipation, 472t, 473–474
    for hepatic encephalopathy, 553–554, 553t
    for irritable bowel syndrome, 491, 491t, 497t
Lamictal (lamotrigine), for seizures, 733t, 741
Lamisil (terbinafine), for tinea, 216t, 217, 217t
Lamivudine
    for hepatitis B virus, 557, 558t
    for HIV infection, 951t, 954t, 955
Lamotrigine, for seizures, 733t, 741
Lanoxin (digoxin)
    for arrhythmias, 375t, 385
    for heart failure, 355t, 363–364
    metabolism of, 58
    steady state of, 26
    therapeutic monitoring of, 88
Lansoprazole
    for GERD, 529t, 530t, 531
    for peptic ulcer disease, 529t, 531
Laryngeal papillomatosis, in pediatric patients, 637
Lasix (furosemide)
    for heart failure, 354t, 358–359
    for hypertension, 299, 299t

Lasmiditan (Reyvow), for migraine headache, 707t,
        711–712
Lastacaft (alcaftadine), for conjunctivitis, 262, 263t
Latanoprost, for glaucoma, 274t, 275–276
Latanoprostene bunod, 274t, 276
Ledipasvir, for hepatitis C virus, 559, 559t
Lefamulin, 98t, 114, 114t, 118t
Leflunomide, for rheumatoid arthritis, 679t, 680,
        683
Left ventricular hypertrophy, hypertension in, 298
Leg(s), restless, 841–845, 841b–842b, 844b, 844f
Legionella infections, 95t–98t
Lemtrada (alemtuzumab), for organ transplantation,
        967–968, 973t
Lennox-Gastaut syndrome, 185
Lescol (fluvastatin), for hyperlipidemia, 317t, 319
Leukocyte dipstick test, for urinary tract infections,
        569
Leukotriene modifier drugs, for asthma and COPD,
        429t–430t, 438–439
Levalbuterol tartrate, for asthma and COPD, 428t,
        436
Levaquin (levofloxacin), 105, 105t
    sensitivity of, 96t
    for skin infections, 206t, 208
    for upper respiratory infections, 407t, 414–415
    for urinary tract infections, 571t
Levbid (hyoscyamine sulfate), for irritable bowel
        syndrome, 493t, 494, 497t
Levetiracetam, for seizures, 733t, 742
Levitra (vardenafil), for erectile dysfunction, 590,
        590t
Levo-Dromoran (levorphanol), as isomer, 30
Levobunolol, for glaucoma, 273t, 275
Levodopa
    metabolism of, 43
    for Parkinson disease, 767, 768f, 770t–771t, 774
Levofloxacin, 105, 105t
    for *Chlamydia trachomatis* infections, 616t, 617
    for community-acquired pneumonia, 423
    sensitivity of, 96t
    for skin infections, 206t, 208
    for spontaneous bacterial peritonitis, 550t
    for upper respiratory infections, 407t, 414–415
Levonorgestrel, in contraceptives, 1092, 1093t, 1097t
Levorphanol, as isomer, 30
Levothyroxine, for hypothyroidism, 914, 915t
Levoxyl (levothyroxine), for hypothyroidism, 914,
        915t
Levsin (hyoscyamine sulfate), for irritable bowel
        syndrome, 493t, 494, 497t
Lexapro (escitalopram)
    for anxiety disorders, 814t, 815
    for depression, 81
Lexiva (fosamprenavir), for HIV infection, 953t,
        957, 958
Lialda (mesalamine), for inflammatory bowel disease,
        502t, 504–505, 510
Librax (clidinium), for irritable bowel syndrome,
        492t, 494, 497t
Libritabs (chlordiazepoxide), for anxiety disorders,
        817t, 819t, 825
Librium (chlordiazepoxide), for anxiety, 817t
License number, of prescriber, 12–13, 13f
Licorice, for peptic ulcer disease, 538
Licorice root (glycyrrhizin), 562
Lidocaine, for arrhythmias, 376t, 379–380, 379b
Lifestyle changes
    in adverse drug reactions, in older adults, 76
    in anxiety disorders, 827
    in asthma and COPD, 447
    in attention-deficit/hyperactivity disorder,
        866–867
    in benign prostatic hyperplasia, 586
    in cannabis pain management, 187
    in cirrhosis, 554
    in constipation, 479
    in diarrhea, 488

in epilepsy, 751
in GERD, 535
in gout, 660
in headache, 696
in heart failure, 369
in herpes simplex virus, 225
in hyperlipidemia, 316–317
in hypertension, 267, 309
in insomnia, 832
in irritable bowel syndrome, 498
in menopause, 1113
in nausea and vomiting, 468
in otitis externa, 290
in Parkinson disease, 778–779
in peptic ulcer disease, 538
in psoriasis, 238–239
in rheumatoid arthritis, 688
in seizures, 751
in sinusitis, 417
in skin infections, 212
in urinary tract infections, 574–575
in vaginitis, 1126
in varicella-zoster virus, 225
in viral hepatitis, 562
in warts (verrucae), 225
Lifitegrast, for keratoconjunctivitis sicca, 269, 270t
Ligands, 18b, 27
Light therapy, for insomnia, 832
Limbic system, stimulating nausea and vomiting, 454
Linaclotide
    for constipation, 472t, 475, 476–477
    for irritable bowel syndrome, 495, 497t
Linezolid, 98t, 112, 112t
    for skin infections, 206t, 208
Linzess (linaclotide)
    for constipation, 472t, 475, 476–477
    for irritable bowel syndrome, 495, 497t
Liothyronine, for hypothyroidism, 914, 915t
Liotrix, for hypothyroidism, 914, 915t
Lipase, in pediatric patients, 58
Lipase inhibitor, for obesity, 1081–1082
Lipid bilayer
    absorption through, 19
    receptors on, 29
Lipitor (atorvastatin), for hyperlipidemia, 317t, 319,
        320
Lipopeptides, 98t, 112–113, 112t
Lipophilic drugs, 62, 63–64
    distribution of, in older adults, 72
    metabolism of, 36–39
Lipoprotein(s)
    in atherosclerosis, 314
    in coronary heart disease risk assessment, 313,
        315b
    drug therapy effects on, 317–325, 319f, 320f,
        321t
    elevated (See Hyperlipidemia)
    high-density (good), 314, 321t
    intermediate-density, 314
    low-density (bad), 314, 321t
    physiology of, 314
    smoking effects on, 330
    structures of, 313
    very-low-density, 314, 321t, 322
Liquid paraffin, for constipation, 475
Liraglutide (saxenda), for obesity, 1081t, 1082
Lisinopril
    for chronic stable angina, 334, 335t, 338
    for heart failure, 352, 353t, 356
    for hypertension, 302, 302t
Livalo (pitavastatin), for hyperlipidemia, 317t
Liver
    diseases, 541–562
        chronic, defined, 541
        cirrhosis, 541–554
        laboratory findings in, 542t
        viral hepatitis, 554–562
    drug excretion from, 25, 25f

drug metabolism in, 23–24
    in older adults, 73–74, 74b
    pediatric patients, 60–61, 61t
dysfunction of
    drug interactions in, 48, 49
    drug pharmacokinetics in, 46
fibrosis, 545
first-pass effect in, 18b, 20b
functions of, 542f
Liver transplantation, 965. *See also* Organ transplantation
Loading dose, for steady state, 26
Local anesthetics
    administration, 67, 67t
    for pain, 163
Lodoxamide, for conjunctivitis, 263t, 265
Lofexidine, for opioid use disorder, 880, 880t
Lomaira (phentermine), for obesity, 1080, 1080t
Lomitapide, 325
Lomotil (diphenoxylate/atropine)
    for diarrhea, 482–484, 484t–485t, 486
    for irritable bowel syndrome, 492t, 494, 497t
Long-term care, drugs used in
    for constipation, 82
    falls related to, 79–81, 79t
    for incontinence, 82
    for pain management, 82
Loop diuretics
    for heart failure, 354t
    for hypertension, 299–300, 299t
Loperamide
    for diarrhea, 482–484, 484t–485t, 485
    for irritable bowel syndrome, 492t, 494, 497t
Lopid (gemfibrozil), for hyperlipidemia, 321t, 323–324
Lopinavir, for HIV infection, 954t, 957, 958
Lopressor (metoprolol)
    for arrhythmias, 376t, 379b
    for chronic stable angina, 336t, 340
    for hypertension, 300, 301t
Loprox (ciclopirox), for fungal infections, 215t
Loratadine, for allergic rhinitis, 936, 937t, 938
Lorazepam
    for Alzheimer's disease, 833
    for anxiety disorders, 80, 816, 817t, 819t
    for insomnia, 833, 834t
    for nausea and vomiting, 456t, 459
    for seizures, 746–747
Losartan
    for chronic stable angina, 334, 335t, 338
    for heart failure, 354t, 359–360
    for hypertension, 302, 302t
Lotensin (benazepril), for chronic stable angina, 334
Loteprednol, for conjunctivitis, 263t
Lotrimin (clotrimazole), for fungal infections, 215t
Lovastatin
    for hyperlipidemia, 317t, 319, 320, 324
    and niacin, for hyperlipidemia, 325
Lovenox (enoxaparin), 992, 999t
    for chronic stable angina, 337t, 342
Lozenge, nicotine, 1065t, 1067
Lubiprostone
    for constipation, 472t, 475, 476–477
    for irritable bowel syndrome, 493t, 495, 497t
Lubricant laxatives, for constipation, 471t
Lubricant(s), ocular, for keratoconjunctivitis sicca, 269, 270t
Lubriderm, for psoriasis, 231t
Lucemyra (lofexidine), for opioid use disorder, 880, 880t
Lugol's solution, 921
Lumigan (bimatoprost), for glaucoma, 274t, 275–276
Lung
    scan, in pulmonary embolism, 987
    transplantation, 965. *See also* Organ transplantation
Luvox (fluvoxamine), for anxiety disorders, 814t

Lymphocyte-depleting agents
    for organ transplantation, 967–968
Lyrica, for anxiety disorders, 818, 820

M
Macrobid (nitrofurantoin), for urinary tract infections, 569, 570t, 572
Macrocytic anemias, 1014, 1024, 1024b
Macrodantin (nitrofurantoin), for urinary tract infections, 569, 570t, 572
Macrolides, 97t, 106, 106t, 118t. *See also specific drugs*
    for lower respiratory tract infections, 420, 422–423, 422t
    for otitis media, 286
Macrophages, in atherosclerosis pathogenesis, 314–315
Mafenide, 110
Magnesium citrate
    for constipation, 472t, 474, 477
    for irritable bowel syndrome, 492t, 493, 497t
Magnesium hydroxide
    for constipation, 472t, 474
    for irritable bowel syndrome, 494, 497t
Magnesium sulfate
    for constipation, 472t, 474
Magnetic resonance imaging
    in seizures, 728
    in stroke, 988
Maintenance dose, for steady state, 26
Maintenance medications, in managed care, 134
Major histocompatibility complex (MHC), 965
    molecules, in rheumatoid arthritis, 675
Malabsorption, 1024, 1024b
    drug-induced, 43
Malt soup extract, for constipation, 471, 471t, 473, 478
Maltsupex (malt soup extract), for constipation, 471, 471t, 473, 478
Mammalian target of rapamycin inhibitors (mTOR), for organ transplantation, 971–973, 972b, 973t
Managed care organizations (MCOs)
    compliance issues in, 138–139, 138t
    current issues in, 140–141
    electronic prescribing, 139–140
    formularies used by, 133–136
    medical necessity policy of, 136
    origin of, 131–132
    pharmacoeconomics, 132
    pharmacy and therapeutics committee of, 137–138, 137b
    practice guidelines of, 138–139, 138t
    prior authorization by, 136
    treatment algorithms of, 138
    types of, 131
MAO-B Inhibitors, for Parkinson disease, 772
Marijuana. *See* Cannabis
Marijuana Tax Act of 1937, 180
Marinol (dronabinol)
    for nausea and vomiting, 458t, 462
    for pain, 183t, 184, 187
Massage, for pain, 152b, 153
Mast cell stabilizers, for conjunctivitis, 263t, 265
Mavik (trandolapril), for heart failure, 352, 353t, 356, 357
Maxalt (rizatriptan), for migraine headache, 705t, 710–711
Maxipime (cefepime), 96t, 102t, 103
Mazicon (flumazenil), for benzodiazepine over-dose, 818
Meclizine, for nausea and vomiting, 456t, 459
Medical necessity, 136
Medical Therapy of Prostatic Symptoms trial, 583
Medicare
    health maintenance organization supplements for, 132
    Part D, 77

Medication errors, 49, 49t, 49f
    preventing, 68, 68b
Medrol (methylprednisolone), for inflammatory bowel disease, 502t, 505–506
Medroxyprogesterone acetate, depot, 1095, 1097t
MedWatch program, 49, 49f
Meglitinide analogs, for diabetes mellitus, 892t, 896–897
Meibomian gland dysfunction (MGD blepharitis), 257–258
Melatonin, 832, 840
Melatonin receptor agonists, for insomnia, 837
MELD-Na score, for cirrhosis, 545, 545t
Memantine, for Alzheimer's disease, 759–760, 761t
Membranes, absorption through, 19–20
Meningococcal vaccine, 1042
Menopause, 1101–1113
    age of, 1101
    algorithm for, 111f
    complementary and alternative medicine for, 1113, 1113t
    definition of, 1101
    herbal treatment of, 1113t
    hormone therapy for, 1102–1108, 1103t–1106t, 1108b
    information sources for, 1112
    lifestyle changes for, 1113
    migraine headache in, 721
    monitoring of, 1112
    nonhormonal therapy for, 1102
    pathophysiology of, 1101–1102
    patient education on, 1112–1113
Menstrual cycle
    migraines related to, 721
    physiology of, 1090, 1090f
Menthol, for upper respiratory infections, 405
Meperidine, for pain, 156, 160
Mepolizumab, for asthma and COPD, 433t, 442–443
6-mercaptopurine, for inflammatory bowel disease, 503t, 506–507, 514
Meropenem, 96t, 104, 104t
Meropenem-vaborbactam, 101t
    sensitivity of, 95t
Merrem (meropenem), 96t, 104, 104t
Mesalamine, for inflammatory bowel disease, 502t, 504–505, 510
Metabolic syndrome, 883
    hypertension in, 299
Metabolism, drug, 23–24, 24t
    vs. age, 57t
    complementary alternative medicine interactions, 45–46, 46b
    in drug–disease interactions, 47
    in drug–drug interactions, 33, 36–39, 36f, 37f, 38t
    in drug–food interactions, 42–43, 42b
    in fetus, 62
    first-pass, 541
    in older adults, 73, 74b
    in pediatric patients, 60–61, 61t
    in placenta, 62
    tissues involved in, 24
Metamucil (psyllium)
    for constipation, 471, 471t, 473
    for irritable bowel syndrome, 491, 491t, 497t
Metformin, for diabetes mellitus, 891t, 894–895
Methadone
    clinics, 172
    for opioid use disorder, 879t–880t, 881–882
    for pain, 155, 157, 158t, 160
    for pain management in opioid use disorder, 170t, 172–173, 174–175
Methenamine, for urinary tract infections, 571t, 572
Methicillin-resistant *Staphylococcus aureus* (MRSA), 421
Methimazole, for hyperthyroidism, 919t, 920–921

Methotrexate
    for chronic gout, 655
    for contact dermatitis, 195
    for inflammatory bowel disease, 503t, 506–507, 513
    for psoriasis, 232t, 235
    for rheumatoid arthritis, 678t, 681, 684
Methylcellulose
    for constipation, 471, 471t, 473
    for irritable bowel syndrome, 491t
Methyldopa, for hypertension, 304, 305t
Methylphenidate
    for ADHD, 759, 859, 860t
    for reactions to monoamine oxidase inhibitors, 794
Methylprednisolone
    for anaphylaxis and anaphylactoid reactions, 931
    for inflammatory bowel disease, 502t, 505–506
    for nausea and vomiting, 457t, 461
Methyltestosterone, for menopausal symptoms, 1104t, 1106
Methylxanthines, for asthma and COPD, 432t, 440–441
Metipranolol, for glaucoma, 273t, 275
Metoclopramide
    absorption of, 34
    for migraine headache, 713
    for nausea and vomiting, 458t, 460–461, 467
Metolazone
    for heart failure, 353t, 359
    for hypertension, 298t
Metoprolol
    for arrhythmias, 376t, 379b
    for chronic stable angina, 336t, 340
    for heart failure, 355t, 362
    for hypertension, 300, 301t
Metric units, in prescriptions, 12
MetroGel (metronidazole), for rosacea, 250–251, 251t
Metronidazole, 115, 115t, 118t
    for bacterial vaginosis, 1119–1120, 1120t
    for diarrhea, 483t
    for GERD, 529t, 532
    for hepatic encephalopathy, 554
    for inflammatory bowel disease, 503t, 507, 514
    for peptic ulcer disease, 529t, 532
    for rosacea, 250–251, 251t
    sensitivity of, 98t
    for trichomoniasis, 1122, 1123, 1125t
Mevacor (lovastatin), for hyperlipidemia, 317t, 319, 320, 324
Mexiletine, for arrhythmias, 377t, 379b, 380
Miacalcin (calcitonin), for osteoporosis, 668t, 671
Micanol (anthralin), for psoriasis, 231t, 233
Micardis (telmisartan)
    for chronic stable angina, 334
    for heart failure, 360
Micatin (miconazole), for fungal infections, 215t
Miconazole
    for candidiasis, 1118, 1119t
    for fungal infections, 215t, 219
Microcytic anemias, 1014, 1019t, 1022, 1023b
Micronor (progesterone), 1094–1095, 1094t
Microorganisms
    in pediatric patients, 58
    in pregnancy, 58
Microsporum infections, 213, 218
Microwave thermotherapy, for benign prostatic hyperplasia, 586
Microzide (hydrochlorothiazide), for heart failure, 353t
Midamor (amiloride)
    for heart failure, 354t
    for hypertension, 300t
Midodrine, for hepatorenal syndrome, 552, 552t
Migraine headache, 700–719
    causes of, 700–701, 702b
    classification of, 702b
    complementary and alternative medicine for, 721

diagnosis of, 702, 702b
    nutrition for, 721
    in older adults, 720
    pathophysiology of, 701–702
    patient education on, 721
    in pediatric patients, 720
    in pregnancy, 720–721
    prevention of, 714
    therapeutic monitoring of, 721
    treatment of, 703–721, 704t
    triggers of, 700, 702b
    with or without aura, 702
    in women, 720–721
Migranal (dihydroergotamine), for migraine headache, 708t, 713
Milk thistle (silymarin), 562
Mineral oil, for constipation, 471t, 475
Mini-Mental State Examination, for Alzheimer's disease, 757
Minipress (prazosin)
    for benign prostatic hyperplasia, 584–585
    for hypertension, 304, 304t
Minitran (nitroglycerin), for chronic stable angina, 336t, 338, 339
Minocin (minocycline), 97t, 108–109, 109t
Minocycline, 97t, 108–109, 109t
    for acne, 246
Minoxidil, for hypertension, 305, 305t
Mipomersen, 325
Mirabegron, for overactive bladder, 601t, 603t, 605–607
MiraLAX (polyethylene glycol)
    for constipation, 473–474
    for irritable bowel syndrome, 491
Mirena, as contraceptive device, 1095
Mirtazapine, for depression, 789t, 795t, 796
Mirvaso (brimonidine 0.33% gel), for rosacea, 251–252
Misoprostol
    for GERD, 529t, 532–533
    for NSAID-induced ulcers, 647
    for pain, 156
    for peptic ulcer disease, 529t, 532–533, 537t
Misuse, of drugs
    harm and, prevention of, 4–5
    from lack of knowledge, 9
Mitochondrial mutation, antibiotics-induced ototoxicity, 126
Mitrolan (calcium polycarbophil), for irritable bowel syndrome, 491t
Mobiluncus infections, bacterial vaginosis, 1115
Modafinil, for narcolepsy, 846
Modification of Diet in Renal Disease (MDRD), 26–27, 27t
Moisturel, for psoriasis, 231t
Molecular weight, of drug, placental transfer and, 61, 62t
Mometasone furoate, for contact dermatitis, 193t
Monistat (miconazole)
    for candidiasis, 1119t
    for fungal infections, 215t
Monitoring, therapeutic. *See* Therapeutic monitoring; *specific drugs and disorders*
Monoamine oxidase inhibitors
    adverse reactions to, 790b, 794, 795t, 796
    for anxiety disorders, 814t, 820
    for depression, 794, 795t, 796
    tyramine interactions with, 31, 43, 43b, 46, 794, 796
Monobactams, 96t, 103, 103t, 118t
Monoclonal antibodies, for asthma and COPD, 433t, 442–443
Monodox (doxycycline), for rosacea, 252
Monoket (isosorbide mononitrate), for chronic stable angina, 336t, 338, 339
Monopril (fosinopril)
    for chronic stable angina, 335t
    for heart failure, 352, 353t
Montelukast, for asthma and COPD, 429t, 438–439

Monurol (fosfomycin), for urinary tract infections, 569, 570t, 572
Moraxella catarrhalis infections
    otitis media, 282, 284
    sinusitis, 412
Moraxella infections, conjunctivitis, 261, 262
Moricizine, for arrhythmias, 380
Morning sickness, 466
Morning stiffness, in rheumatoid arthritis, 676
Morphine
    for pain, 152, 153, 157–159, 158t, 159t
    for sickle cell anemia, 1018
Motegrity (prucalopride), for constipation, 476
Motrin (ibuprofen)
    for osteoarthritis, 646t
    pharmacokinetic and pharmacodynamic properties of, 152, 156t, 159
Movantik (naloxegol), for constipation, 472t, 476–477
Moxifloxacin, 105, 105t
    for community-acquired pneumonia, 423
    sensitivity of, 96t
    for skin infections, 206t, 208
    for upper respiratory infections, 407t, 414–415
Mucinex (guaifenesin), for upper respiratory infections, 406t, 408
Mucinex Sinus (oxymetazoline hydrochloride), for upper respiratory infections, 405, 405t, 408, 412
Mucolytics, for asthma and COPD, 432t, 441–442
Mucosal absorption in, 59
Mucus, cervical, in menstrual cycle, 1090
Multaq (dronedarone), for arrhythmias, 375t, 379b, 383
Mupirocin, for skin infections, 204, 208
Murine (tetrahydrozoline), for conjunctivitis, 264t, 265
Muscarinic antagonists (short and long acting), for asthma and COPD, 428t, 430t, 438
Muscle(s)
    drug administration into, 22
    drug administration into
        for pediatric patients, 58
    tension of, headache in, 695
Muscle relaxants, for pain, 163–164
Mycobacterium avium-intracellulare infections, 480b
Mycophenolate, for contact dermatitis, 195
Mycophenolate mofetil, for organ transplantation, 971, 974t
Mycophenolate sodium, for organ transplantation, 971, 974t
Mycoplasma hominis infections, bacterial vaginosis, 1115
Mycostatin (nystatin)
    for candidiasis, 1118
    for fungal infections, 216t, 218
Myfortic (mycophenolate mofetil) for organ transplantation, 971, 974t
Myocardial infarction (MI)
    in atherosclerosis, 332
    chronic stable angina after, 329–330
    hypertension in, 297
    non-ST elevation, 333
    ST elevation, 333
    treatment of, 346, 346t
Myocardial ischemia, activation of, 332
Myochrysine (gold sodium thiomalate), for rheumatoid arthriti, 679t
Myoclonic seizures, 726–727
Myrbetriq (mirabegron), for overactive bladder, 601t, 603t, 605–607
Myrtol, 418
Mysoline (primidone), for seizures, 732t, 740–741
Myxedema coma, hypothyroidism in, 916

N

N-methyl-*D*-aspartate receptor antagonists, 163
Nabilone
    for nausea and vomiting, 462
    for pain, 183t, 184–185

Nabiximols (sativex), for pain, 186t
Nabumetone, for osteoarthritis, 645t
Nadolol
    for hyperthyroidism, 919t
    for variceal hemorrhage, 546–547, 546t
Nafcillin, 95t, 100t, 107
Naftifine, for fungal infections, 215t
Naftin (naftifine), for fungal infections, 215t
Nails, fungal infections of
    diagnosis of, 214
    treatment of, 217–219
Naldemedine, for constipation, 476–477
Naloxegol, 161
    for constipation, 472t, 476–477
Naloxone, for opioid reversal, 160–161
Naltrexone/bupropion (contrave)
    for alcohol use disorder, 874t, 875
    in obesity, 1083
    for opioid use disorder, 879t, 882
    for overdose reversal, 878b
Namenda (memantine), for Alzheimer's disease,
    759–760, 760t
Naphazoline, for conjunctivitis, 264t, 265
Naprosyn (naproxen)
    for headache, 697, 698t
    pharmacokinetic and pharmacodynamic
        properties of, 156t
    for upper respiratory infections, 406t, 409, 412
Naproxen
    for headache, 697, 698t
    pharmacokinetic and pharmacodynamic
        properties of, 156t
    for upper respiratory infections, 406t, 409, 412
Naratriptan, for migraine headache, 703, 705t, 710
Narcan (naloxone), for opioid reversal, 160–161
Narcolepsy, 845–849
Narcotic analgesics, constipation and, 469b
Narcotics Control Act of 1956, 180
Nardil (phenelzine), for anxiety disorders, 814t, 820
Nasal smears, in allergic rhinitis, 933
Nasal spray, nicotine, 1065t, 1067–1068
Nasalcrom Nasal Solution (cromolyn), for allergic
    rhinitis, 937t, 941–942
Natalizumab, for inflammatory bowel disease, 504t,
    508, 509
Nateglinide, for diabetes mellitus, 892t, 896
National Digestive Diseases Information
    Clearinghouse (NDDIC), 479
National Foundation for Depressive Illness Inc., 802
National Institute for Drug Abuse (NIDA), 883
National Institute of Mental Health, depression
    information of, 802
National Plan and Provider Enumeration System
    (NPPES), 5
National Provider Identifier (NPI), 5
Natural endocannabinoids, for pain management,
    150
Nausea and vomiting
    algorithm for, 463f
    antacids for, 458t, 462, 467
    anticipatory, 451
    antiemetics for, 456t–458t, 460–461
    antihistamines-anticholinergics, 456t, 458–459,
        467
    benzodiazepines for, 456t, 459–460
    cannabinoids for, 461–462
    causes of, 451–452
    central nervous system stimulating, 453–454
    complementary and alternative therapies for, 468
    complications of, 455b
    corticosteroids for, 461, 468
    diagnosis of, 454
    etiologies of, 451, 452b
    gastrointestinal tract stimulating, 453
    information sources for, 468
    lifestyle changes in, 468
    limbic system stimulating, 454
    metoclopramide for, 458t, 460–461, 467
    modulation of, 453

NK1 antagonist for, 457t
    nutrition for, 468
    pathophysiology of, 452–454, 453f
    patient education for, 468
    in pediatrics, 466, 468b
    phenothiazines, 455, 456t, 458, 467
    in pregnancy, 466–468
    prevalence of, 452
    serotonin antagonists for, 457t, 460
    stimulatory centers of, 453–454
    therapeutic monitoring of, 468
    treatment of, 454–468, 456t–458t, 463f, 464t
        chemotherapy-induced nausea and vomiting,
            462–466, 464b–465b, 466t, 467f
    in women, 466–468
Nebivolol, for hypertension, 300, 301t
Nebulizers, 67, 68t
Necrotizing fasciitis
    causes of, 201
    complementary and alternative medicine for, 212
    diagnosis of, 204
    lifestyle changes for, 212
    pathophysiology of, 202, 202b
    patient education on, 211–212
    therapeutic monitoring of, 211
    treatment of, 204, 205t–206t, 207–211, 209t,
        210f
    types, 201
Nedocromil, for conjunctivitis, 263t, 265
Nefazodone
    for anxiety disorders, 826
    for depression, 789t, 795t, 796
Nelfinavir, for HIV infection, 954t, 957
Neo-Synephrine (oxymetazoline hydrochloride), for
    upper respiratory infections, 405, 405t,
    408, 412
Neomycin
    for hepatic encephalopathy, 554
    for otitis externa, 288, 288t
Neonatal abstinence syndrome, 174–175
Neonates
    absorption in, 57t
    body composition of, 59–60
    Chlamydia trachomatis infections in, 261, 262,
        265, 617
    definition of, 56t
    distribution in, 57t, 59–60
    drug dosing in, 65–66
    elimination in, 57t, 61
    gastric emptying time in, 58
    gastrointestinal enzymes of, 58
    gonorrhea in, 261, 262, 619
    intramuscular absorption in, 58
    metabolism in, 57t
    percutaneous absorption in, 58–59
    pharmacokinetics in, 56–61
    plasma protein binding in, 60
    vascular perfusion in, 59
Neoral (cyclosporine)
    for inflammatory bowel disease, 503t, 506–507,
        514
    for organ transplantation, 968–970, 969t, 974t
    for rheumatoid arthritis, 679t, 680, 682
Nephrotoxicity, of aminoglycosides, 107–108
Netarsudil, for glaucoma, 275t, 277
Netilmicin, 107t, 108t
Netupitant/palonosetron, for nausea and vomiting,
    457t
Neuritic plaques, in Alzheimer's disease, 756
Neurofibrillary tangles, in Alzheimer's disease, 756
Neurokinin 1 (NK) receptors, 453
Neuron(s)
    abnormal communication between, in seizures,
        725–726
    destruction of, in Alzheimer's disease, 756
Neurontin (gabapentin)
    for restless legs syndrome, 844
    for seizures, 732t
Neuropathic pain, 146, 147b, 162, 181

Neurosyphilis, 624, 626, 628t
Neurotoxicity, of carbapenems, 104
Neurotransmitters
    for ADHD, 860, 860t
    in Alzheimer's disease, 756
    in depression, 784, 784b
    in pain transmission, 148
    peripheral chemical mediators, 150
    in seizures, 726
    in stress, 811, 816
Nevirapine, for HIV infection, 953t, 956
New York Heart Association, heart failure
    classification of, 351, 351t
Newborn, nausea and vomiting in, 468b
Nexium (esomeprazole)
    for GERD, 529t, 530t, 531
    for peptic ulcer disease, 529t, 531, 537t
Nexletol (bempedoic acid), for hyperlipidemia, 321t,
    324–325
Nexterone (amiodarone), for arrhythmias, 374t,
    379b, 381–383
Niacin, for hyperlipidemia, 320f, 321t, 323
Nicardipine
    for chronic stable angina, 341
    for hypertension, 303t, 304
Nicoderm (nicotine patch), 1063–1064, 1065t
Nicomide, 250
Nicorette (nicotine gum), 1064, 1065t, 1066–1067
Nicotinamide, 250
Nicotine. See also Smoking
    aversion to, 1063
    dependence on
        definition of, 1057–1058, 1060b
        diagnosis of, 1059–1060, 1060b, 1061b
        pathophysiology of, 1058–1059
        treatment of (See Smoking, cessation of)
    drug interactions with, in older adults, 76, 77t
    fading process for, 1062
    physiologic effects of, 1059
    in replacement therapy, 1063–1068, 1065t–1066t
        bupropion, 1069–1070
        gum, 1064, 1065t, 1066–1067
        inhaler, 1065t, 1068
        lozenge, 1065t, 1067
        nasal spray, 1065t, 1067–1068
        patches, 1063–1064, 1065t
        for special populations, 1072–1073
        varenicline, 1068–1070
    toxicity of, 1073
    withdrawal from, 1059, 1060b
Nicotinic acetylcholine receptor, 28
Nicotinic acid (niacin), for hyperlipidemia, 321t, 323
Nicotrol (nicotine inhaler), 1065t, 1068
Nicotrol (nicotine patch), 1065t, 1069
Nicotrol NS (nicotine nasal spray), 1065t, 1067–
    1068
Nifedipine
    for chronic stable angina, 336t, 341
    for hypertension, 303t, 304
Nisoldipine, for hypertension, 304
Nitrates
    for chronic stable angina, 336t, 338–339
    tolerance of, 339
Nitric oxide donating prostaglandin analogs, for
    glaucoma, 274t, 276
Nitro-Bid (nitroglycerin), for chronic stable angina,
    336t, 338, 339
Nitro-Dur (nitroglycerin), for chronic stable angina,
    336t, 338, 339
Nitrofurantoin, 98t, 116t, 117, 118t
    for urinary tract infections, 569, 570t, 572
Nitroglycerin, for chronic stable angina, 336t, 338,
    339
Nitrol (nitroglycerin), for chronic stable angina,
    336t, 338, 339
Nitroquick (nitroglycerin), for chronic stable angina,
    336t, 339
Nitrostat (nitroglycerin), for chronic stable angina,
    336t, 339

Nizatidine
    for GERD, 529t, 530t
    for peptic ulcer disease, 529t, 537t
Nizoral (ketoconazole), for fungal infections, 215t, 219
NK1 antagonist, for nausea and vomiting, 457t
Nociception, 167
Nociceptive pain, 146, 147b, 148, 181
Nocturnal chronic stable angina, 330
Nodules, gout, 653
Non-dihydropyridines, for hypertension, 303–304, 303t
Non-lymphocyte-depleting basiliximab, for organ transplantation, 968
Non-nucleoside reverse transcriptase inhibitors, for HIV infection, 951, 956–957
Non-opioid analgesics, for pain management in opioid use disorder, 173
Non-rapid eye movement sleep, 830b, 831
Non-ST elevation MI, 333
Non-statin cholesterol-lowering drugs, for hyperlipidemia, 320–325
Non-stimulants, for ADHD, 863
Nonallergic rhinitis, with eosinophilia, 934
Noncompetitive inhibition, of cytochrome P-450 system, 37–38, 37f
Noncompliance. See Adherence issues
Nondihydropyridines, for chronic stable angina, 341
Nonformulary medications, 133
Nonpharmacologic treatments, for pain management in opioid use disorder, 175, 175b
Nonpreferred drugs, in formularies, 133
Nonprescription drugs, vs. prescription drugs, 5–6
Nonpsychoactive cannabidiol, 81
Nonselective beta blockers, for portal hypertension, 546, 546t
Nonsteroidal anti-inflammatory drugs (NSAIDs), 1018. See also specific drugs, e.g., Aspirin
    for Alzheimer's disease, 759
    for conjunctivitis, 263t, 265
    drug interactions of, 41
    for headache, 697, 698t
    for keratoconjunctivitis sicca, 270t
    mechanism of action of, 644, 647
    for migraine headache, 703, 704t, 713
    for osteoarthritis, 644, 645t–646t, 647
    for pain, 82, 152, 154, 155–156
    for pain management in opioid use disorder, 173
    peptic ulcer disease due to, 527
        pathophysiology of, 524–525
        treatment of, 526, 536–537
    for rheumatoid arthritis, 678
    for upper respiratory infections, 409
Norelgestromin, in contraceptives, 1094
Norepinephrine
    for anaphylaxis and anaphylactoid reactions, 931
    deficiency of, in depression, 784, 784b
    for hepatorenal syndrome, 552, 552t
    in stress, 811, 814t, 815
Norfloxacin, 105t
    for conjunctivitis, 262
    for diarrhea, 483t
    sensitivity of, 96t
    for spontaneous bacterial peritonitis, 551
Noritate (metronidazole), for rosacea, 250–251, 251t
Normeperidine, 156
Norpace (disopyramide), for arrhythmias, 375t, 379
Norpramin (desipramine), for irritable bowel syndrome, 494, 497t
Nortriptyline, for pain, 162
Norvasc (amlodipine), for chronic stable angina, 336t, 341
Norvasc (amlodipine) for hypertension, 303t, 304, 308
Norvir (ritonavir), for HIV infection, 954t, 957–958
Nose, obstruction of vs. allergic rhinitis, 933
NREM (non-rapid eye movement sleep), 830b, 831
NS3/4A Protease Inhibitors, 560, 561t

NS5A Inhibitors, 560, 561t
NS5B Polymerase Inhibitors, 560, 561t
Nucala (mepolizumab), for asthma and COPD, 433t, 442–443
Nucleoside reverse transcriptase inhibitors, for HIV infection, 851, 950, 951t
Nucleotide, 122, 122b
Nulojix (belatacept), for organ transplantation, 973, 974t, 975
Numerical rating scale, for pain assessment, 151, 151f
Nurtec, for migraine headache, 707t
Nutrition
    with anticoagulants, 1008
    for arrhythmias, 398
    for asthma and COPD, 447
    for attention-deficit/hyperactivity disorder, 866–867
    for cannabis pain management, 187
    for cirrhosis, 554
    for constipation, 479
    for diabetes mellitus, 889, 908
    for diarrhea, 488
    drug interactions and, 48
    for folate deficiency, 1026
    for GERD, 535
    for gout, 660
    for headache, 721
    for heart failure, 369
    for hypertension, 309
    for inflammatory bowel disease, 515
    for insomnia, 840
    for iron deficiency anemia, 1018, 1027
    for irritable bowel syndrome, 498
    for menopausal symptoms, 1113
    for nausea and vomiting, 468
    for obesity, 1077
    for osteoarthritis, 651
    for Parkinson disease, 778–779
    for peptic ulcer disease, 538
    in pharmacokinetics and pharmacodynamics, 31
    for rheumatoid arthritis, 688
    for seizures, 751
    for skin infections, 212
    for viral hepatitis, 562
NuvaRing (estrogens), for contraception, 1096
Nuzyra (omadacycline), 97t, 108, 109t
Nystatin, for candidiasis, 216t, 218, 1118

O

Obesity, 1077–1086
    breast-feeding, 1085
    causes of, 1077–1078
    chronic stable angina in, 331
    classification of, 1079t
    complementary and alternative medicine for, 1084
    contrave, 1083
    defined, 66
    diabetes, 1085
    diagnosis of, 1078, 1079t
    environmental factors in, 1077–1078
    epidemiology of, 1077
    genetic factors in, 1077
    gout, 652
    hypertension in, 295, 307
    medical conditions with, 1085
    osteoarthritis in, 641
    pathophysiology of, 1078
    patient education on, 1085
    in pediatrics, 66, 1085
    phentermine extended release/topiramate, 1082–1083
    pregnancy, 1085
    psychological factors in, 1078
    in smokers, 1085
    therapeutic monitoring of, 1085
    treatment of, 1078–1085, 1080t–1081t
Object drug, in interactions, 34, 35t, 36t

Octreotide
    for hepatorenal syndrome, 552, 552t
    for variceal hemorrhage, 548
Ofloxacin, 105t
    for Chlamydia trachomatis infections, 616t, 617, 618t
    for conjunctivitis, 262
    for diarrhea, 483t
    for otitis externa, 288, 288t
    for pelvic inflammatory disease, 616t
    for urinary tract infections, 571t
Olanzapine, for Alzheimer's disease, 761
Older adults, 71–89, 573–574
    absorption in, 72
    adherence issues in, 76–78
    adverse drug interactions in, 76, 77t
    alcohol intake in, 76
    alternatives to medication for, 86
    anemia in, 1027
    angiotensin-converting enzyme inhibitors for, 358
    antiarrhythmic agents for, 396–397
    antibiotics for, 85
    anxiety disorders in, 825
    asthma and COPD in, 445
    benign prostatic hyperplasia in, 581
    body systems in, 72–74, 74b, 75t
    caffeine use in, 76, 77t
    cannabis in, 187
    consequences of longevity, 72
    constipation in, 82, 478
    contact dermatitis in, 197
    dementia and behavioral and psychological symptoms of dementia, 83–84
    depression in, 80–81, 800
    diabetes management in, 85
    diabetes mellitus, 905
    diarrhea in, 487
    distribution in, 72–73
    dosage regimens for, 86–87
    drug interactions in, 76
    drug receptors in, 74
    drugs to avoid in, 87t
    drugs with reduced hepatic metabolism in, 74b
    elimination in, 73–74, 74b, 75t
    environmental changes affecting, 72b
    erectile dysfunction in, 589
    falls in, medication and, 79–81, 79t
    functional deficits in, 78
    GERD in, 534
    guidelines for safe prescribing, 82–88, 83t, 86b, 87t
    headache in, 720
    heart failure in, 368
    Helicobacter pylori infections in, 538
    hyperlipidemia in, 325
    hypertension in, 307
    hypothyroidism in, 916
    insomnia in, 831, 840
    irritable bowel syndrome in, 498
    life expectancy and goals of care, 78
    medication review for, 87–88
    narcolepsy in, 845
    nicotine use in, 76, 77t
    nondrug alternative therapies for, 86
    nonselective beta blockers for, 547
    nutritional support for, 85–86
    organ transplantation in, 975
    osteoarthritis in, 651
    overactive bladder in, 610–611
    pain management in, 81–82, 174
    patient education for, 75
    peptic ulcer disease in, 538
    pharmacodynamics in, 74
    pharmacokinetics in, 72, 74b, 75t
    physical and mental changes, 78
    polypharmacy in, 74–76, 77t
    population of, 71–72
    prescribing for, 9–10, 82–88, 83t, 86b, 87t

prescription considerations for, 11
for rheumatoid arthritis, 688
screening and medication management, 84
seizures in, 750
self-medication in, 78
special considerations in long-term care, 78–82, 79t
substance use disorders in, 882
therapeutic monitoring of, 83b, 88
urinary tract infections in, 573–574
viral hepatitis in, 560
Olmesartan
for chronic stable angina, 334
for heart failure, 360
Olodaterol, for asthma and COPD, 430t, 436
Olopatadine, for conjunctivitis, 263t, 265
Olsalazine, for inflammatory bowel disease, 502t, 505
Omadacycline, 97t, 108, 109t
Omalizumab, for asthma and COPD, 433t, 442–443
Omega-3 fatty acids, for hyperlipidemia, 324
Omeprazole
for GERD, 529t, 530t, 531
for peptic ulcer disease, 529t, 531, 537t
Omnicef (cefdinir), for otitis media, 285t, 286
OnabotulinumtoxinA
for migraine prevention, 716t
for overactive bladder, 601t, 603t, 607
Ondansetron, for nausea and vomiting, 457t, 460, 467
Onychomycosis, 214, 217, 218
Ophthalmic disorders, 257–278
conjunctivitis, 261–268
eyelid margin infections, 257–260, 259t–261t
glaucoma, 271–278
keratoconjunctivitis sicca, 268–271
in neonates (ophthalmia neonatorum)
chlamydial, 617
gonorrheal, 621t, 623
Ophthalmopathy of Graves' disease, 917–918, 921
Opioid receptors, 149
Opioid risk tool, 169, 169b
Opioid use disorder (OUD)
algorithm for, 881f
assessment of, 168–169
buprenorphine for, 169, 170t–171t, 171–172, 172t, 174–175
medications used in, 879t–880t
methadone for, 170t, 172–175
multimodal analgesia for, 173
naloxone for, 169, 171–172
non-opioid analgesics for, 173
nonpharmacologic treatments for, 175, 175b
in older adults, 174
opioid withdrawal, 876, 878b
opioids for, 173
pain management in, 167–176
patient education for, 176
in pregnancy, 174–175
risk assessment and monitoring tools for, 169b
screening of, 168–169
therapeutic monitoring of, 175–176, 175b
treatment for, 169–174, 170t–172t
in women, 174–175
Opioid withdrawal, 876, 878b
Opioids, 156–161. *See also specific drugs*
addiction, 161–162
antagonist, 160–161
dependence on, 161–162
metabolism of, 157
for migraine headache, 708t, 713
for osteoarthritis, 648
for pain management in opioid use disorder, 173
pseudo-addiction, 161–162
receptors for, 159
for restless legs syndrome, 842
safety of, 161
tolerance, 161–162
use in chronic pain, 147–148

Optivar (azelastine), for conjunctivitis, 263t, 265
Oracea (doxycycline)
for lower respiratory tract infections, 419t, 420, 422t
for rosacea, 252
for upper respiratory infections, 407t, 414
Oral administration, 21, 57–58, 66
Oral contraceptives
for acne, 243t–244t, 247
benefits of, 1099, 1099b
biphasic, 1093, 1093t
combined products for, 1092–1094, 1093t
drug interactions with, 1096
emergency, 1096
failure rate of, 1091f
hypertension due to, 307
initiation of, 1094
mini-pills, 1094
missed pill guidelines for, 1098, 1098t
monitoring of, 1097–1098
monophasic, 1093, 1093t
patient education on, 1098–1099, 1098t, 1099b
perimenopause, 1101–1102
progestin-only, 1094–1095, 1094t
selection of, 1096–1097, 1097t
side effects of, 1098–1099, 1098b
triphasic, 1093, 1093t
Oral glucose tolerance test, 888, 889t
Oral hypoglycemic agents
alpha-glucosidase inhibitors, 892t, 896
biguanides, 891t, 894–895
meglitinide analogs, 892t, 896–897
sulfonylureas, 891, 891t, 893–894
thiazolidinediones, 892t, 895–896
Oral rehydration therapy (ORT), 487, 488t
Oral replacement solutions (ORSs), 487
Orasone (prednisone)
for inflammatory bowel disease, 502t, 505–506
Orbactiv (oritavancin), 97t, 110–111, 111t
Orchiectomy, for prostate cancer, 587
Orencia (abatacept)
for psoriasis, 232t
for rheumatoid arthritis, 684–685
Orexin receptor agonists, for insomnia, 836–837
Organ transplantation, 965–977
in African-Americans, 976
antigen-specific lymphocytes, activation of, 965–966, 966f
antimetabolites for, 971
calcineurin inhibitors for, 968–970, 969t, 970b
complementary and alternative medications, 976
corticosteroids for, 973
costimulation blockade, belatacept for, 973, 975
diagnosis of, 966
foreign antigens, recognition of, 965
genomics of, 976
graft rejection, effector phase of, 966
information resources, 976
lifestyle changes in, 976
lymphocyte-depleting agents for, 967–968
mammalian target of rapamycin inhibitors for, 971–973, 972b, 973f
non-lymphocyte-depleting basiliximab for, 968
nutrition for, 976
in older adults, 975
pathophysiology of, 965–966, 966f
patient education on, 976
symptoms of rejection, 966
therapeutic monitoring for, 976
treatment for, 967–975
Oritavancin, 97t, 110–111, 111t, 208
Orlistat, for obesity, 1081–1082, 1081t
Ortho Tri-Cyclen (ethinyl estradiol with norgestimate), for acne, 244t
Orthopedic surgery, anticoagulants for, 1003
Oseltamivir
for bronchitis, 419–420, 419t
for community-acquired pneumonia, 423

for influenza, 1042
Osmotic diarrhea, 481
Ospemifene (osphena), for postmenopausal symptom, 1108
Osphena (ospemifene), for postmenopausal symptom, 1108
Osteoarthritis, 641–652
causes of, 641
complementary and alternative medicine for, 651
diagnosis of, 642–643
epidemiology of, 641
information resources for, 651
joints affected in, 641
in older adults, 651
pathophysiology of, 641–642, 642f
patient education on, 651–652
polypharmacy in, 74
primary (idiopathic), 641
secondary, 641
therapeutic monitoring of, 651
treatment of, 643–649, 643b, 645–646, 651f
in women, 651
Osteophytes, in osteoarthritis, 643
Osteoporosis, 663–673
algorithm for, 667f
bisphosphonates for, 667, 668t
calcitonin for, 668t, 671
calcium supplements for, 666, 668t, 672
causes of, 663, 664b
diagnosis of, 665
information sources for, 673
pathophysiology of, 663–664
postmenopausal, 663, 664b
secondary, 663, 664b
selective estrogen receptor modulators for, 669t, 671
senile, 663, 664b
therapeutic monitoring of, 673
treatment and prevention of, 663–673
types of, 663, 664b
Otezla (apremilast), for psoriasis, 231t, 235
Otitis externa (OE), 281–283, 287–290
causes of, 282
in children, 289
clinical presentation of, 287
complementary and alternative medications for, 290
definition of, 281
diagnosis of, 287
information sources for, 290
lifestyle changes in, 290
malignant, 282, 282t
nutrition for, 290
vs. otitis media, 282t
pathophysiology of, 283
patient education on, 290
prevention of, 289–290
therapeutic monitoring of, 289
treatment of, 287–289, 288t, 289t
Otitis media (OM), 281–287
acute, 282t
algorithm for, 285f
causes of, 282
clinical presentation of, 282–283
definition of, 281
diagnosis of, 283–284, 284t
epidemiology of, 281
information sources for, 290
pathophysiology of, 282–283
prevention of, 287
prophylaxis of, 287
recurrent, 287
therapeutic response of, 287
treatment of, 284–286, 285t–286t, 285f
Ototoxicity
of aminoglycosides, 107–108
antibiotics-induced, 126

Outcomes, in drug prescribing, 11
Ovary
    age-related functional loss of (*See* Menopause)
    physiology of, in menstrual cycle, 1090, 1090f
Over-the-counter (OTC) drugs
    antacid preparations, 462
    older adults using, 78, 87–88
    vs. prescription drugs, 5–6
Overactive bladder (OAB), 595–613
    alpha-adrenergic antagonists for, 601t, 603t, 608
    anticholinergic/antimuscarinic drugs for, 601t,
        602, 602t–603t, 604–605, 606t
    antidiuretic drugs, 609
    behavioral modifications, 602b
    beta-adrenoreceptor agonists for, 601t, 603t,
        605–607
    causes of, 596
    complementary and alternative medications for,
        612
    diagnostic criteria, 598–600, 599b, 600t
    estrogens, 608–609
    evaluation of, 598–600
    information resources, 611–612
    lifestyle changes in, 612
    nutrition for, 612
    in older adults, 610–611
    onabotulinumtoxinA for, 601t, 603t, 607
    pathophysiology, 596–598, 596f, 597f, 598f,
        599b
    patient education on, 611–612
    in pediatrics, 610
    refractory, 610
    serotonin norepinephrine reuptake inhibitors for,
        601t, 603t, 607–608
    therapeutic monitoring, 611
    treatment of, 600–611, 601t–604t, 606t
    in women, 611
Overflow incontinence, 596
Overweight. *See* Obesity
Oxacillin, 99, 100t
Oxazepam
    for anxiety disorders, 80, 816t, 817t
    for insomnia, 833
Oxazolidinones, 98t, 112, 112t, 118t
Oxbryta (Voxelotor), for anemia, 1018
Oxcarbazepine
    for pain, 163
    for seizures, 730t, 737–738, 743
Oxiconazole, for fungal infections, 215t
Oxistat (oxiconazole), for fungal infections, 215t
Oxybutynin
    constipation due to, 82
    for overactive bladder, 601t, 602, 602t, 604, 604t
Oxycodone, for pain, 152, 156, 157, 158t, 159, 159t
Oxymetazoline hydrochloride
    for rosacea, 251–252
    for upper respiratory infections, 405, 405t, 408,
        412
Oxymorphone, for pain, 152, 156, 158t, 159, 159t

P
P-glycoprotein interactions, 40–41, 41t
P2Y12 inhibitors, for chronic stable angina, 342
Pacerone (amiodarone), for arrhythmias, 374t, 379b,
    381–383
Pain. *See also* Headaches
    acute, 146, 154
    and addiction, pathophysiology between, 167–
        168, 168f
    assessment of, 151–152, 151b, 151f, 168
    chronic, 146–147, 154–155, 154b
    definition of, 145
    diagnosis of, 182–183
    endocannabinoid system and relationship to,
        181–182, 182f
    malignant, 148
    mixed, 146, 147b
    modulation of, 149
    neuropathic, 146, 147b, 181

nociception, 167
nociceptive, 146, 147b, 148, 181
nonmalignant, 151
osteoarthritis, 641
on pathophysiology, 181
pathophysiology of, 148–150, 149f
perception of, 148–149
receptors, 150
screening for, 168
in sickle cell disease, 1018
transduction of, 148
treatment of, 183–187, 183t, 185b, 186b
types of, 146–148, 147b
Pain management, 145–164
    acute, 154
    adjunctive options for, 152b
    assessment in, 151–152, 151b, 151f
    breakthrough, 148
    cancer pain, 148, 155
    cannabis, 179–188
        ethnic, 187
        genomics and, 187
        information sources of, 187
        legal status of, 180–181
        lifestyle changes in, 187
        as medicine, 180
        nutrition for, 187
        in older adults, 187
        patient education for, 187
        in pediatrics, 187
        as plant, 179–180, 180f
        in pregnancy, 187
        therapeutic monitoring, 187
        in women, 187
    central sensitization, 150
    chemical mediators in, 150
    chronic, 154–155, 154b
    co-analgesics for, 162–164
    goals of, 152
    malignant, 148
    mild to moderate, 152, 153t, 156t
    moderate to severe, 152, 153t, 156t
    muscle relaxants for, 163–164
    neuropathic, 164
    noncancer pain, 154–155
    nonopioids for, 155–161, 156t
    nonpharmacologic methods for, 152, 152b
    in older adults, 81–82
    in opioid use disorder, 167–176
        assessment of, 168–169
        buprenorphine for, 169, 170t–171t, 171–172,
            172t, 174–175
        methadone for, 170t, 172–175
        multimodal analgesia for, 173
        naloxone for, 169, 171–172
        non-opioid analgesics for, 173
        nonpharmacologic treatments for, 175, 175b
        in older adults, 174
        opioids for, 173
        patient education for, 176
        in pregnancy, 174–175
        risk assessment and monitoring tools
            for, 169b
        screening of, 168–169
        therapeutic monitoring of, 175–176, 175b
        treatment for, 169–174, 170t–172t
        in women, 174–175
    opioids for, 156–161
    pain-modulating receptors for, 149–150
    peripheral sensitization, 150
    severe, 152–153, 153t
    in sickle cell disease, 1018
    vs. type of pain, 153–155, 153t, 154b
Pain-modulating receptors, 149–150
Palonosetron, for nausea and vomiting, 460
Panax ginseng, 417
Panax quinquefolius, 417
Pancreas transplantation, 965. *See also* Organ
    transplantation

Pantoprazole
    for GERD, 529t, 530t
    for peptic ulcer disease, 529t, 537t
Parathyroid hormone (PTH), 912–913
    for osteoporosis, 669t, 671–672
Parenteral absorption, 21–22
Parenteral administration, for pediatric patients, 67
Parkinson disease (PD), 765–779
    causes of, 765–766
    complementary and alternative medications, 779
    definition of, 767
    diagnosis of, 766–767
    information sources, 778
    lifestyle changes for, 778–779
    nutrition for, 778–779
    pathophysiology of, 766
    patient education on, 778–779
    therapeutic monitoring of, 777–778
    treatment of, 765–779, 768f, 769t–771t
Paromomycin, for diarrhea, 483t
Paronychia
    causes of, 200t, 201
    diagnosis of, 203
    treatment of, 210
Paroxetine
    for anxiety disorders, 81
    for depression, 81
    for menopausal symptoms, 1109–1110
Paroxysmal supraventricular tachycardia, 386t,
    392–393, 393f
Parsabiv (etelcalcetide), for hyperparathyroidism, 923
Partial (focal, local) seizures, 726
Passive diffusion, 19–20
Pasteurella infections, skin, 200, 200t
Patanol (olopatadine), for conjunctivitis, 263t, 265
Patch
    contraceptive, 1094
    hormone replacement, 1103t, 1105t, 1106
    nicotine, 1065t, 1069
    nitroglycerin, for chronic stable angina, 336t, 339
Pathophysiology, in pharmacokinetics and
    pharmacodynamics, 30–31
Patient-centered approach, for menopausal
    symptoms, 111–1112, 111f
Patient education, 416–417. *See also specific disorders*
    for irritable bowel syndrome, 498
Patient prescription copayment, 139
Paxil (paroxetine)
    for anxiety disorders, 81, 814t, 815
    for menopausal symptoms, 1109–1110
Pectin, 485
Pediatric patients, 55–63
    absorption in, 57–59, 57t
    acne in, 249
    administration routes for, 57–59, 60
    age groups of, 55, 56t
    allergic rhinitis in, 942
    anemia in, 1026–1027
    antiarrhythmic agents for, 396
    anxiety disorders in, 825
    asthma in, 444–445
    body composition of, 59–60
    cannabis in, 187
    Chlamydia trachomatis infections in, 619, 622–623
    clinical trials including, 56
    common cold in, 404, 411
    constipation in, 477–478
    contact dermatitis in, 196
    depression in, 800
    diabetes mellitus in, 905
    diarrhea in, 486
    distribution in, 57t, 59–60
    dosages for, 65–66
    drug misadventures in, 55
    drug selection for, 64–68, 64f, 67b
    elimination in, 57t, 61
    formulations for, 65
    GERD in, 534
    gonorrhea in, 621t, 622–623, 623t

headache in, 720
heart failure in, 368
Helicobacter pylori infections in, 538
herpes simplex virus infections in, 631
HIV infection in, 961
human papilloma virus infections in, 637
hyperlipidemia in, 325
hypertension in, 307
immunization of, 1035, 1038, 1039f, 1041–1042
inflammatory bowel disease in, 513
insomnia in, 839–840
intramuscular administration, 58
irritable bowel syndrome in, 497–498
long-term effects, 65
metabolism in, 57t, 60–61, 61t
migraine headache in, 720
mucosal absorption in, 59
narcolepsy in, 849
nausea and vomiting in, 466, 468b
obesity in, 66, 1085
oral administration, 57–58, 66
overactive bladder in, 610
pain management in, 146
parenteral administration, 67
peptic ulcer disease in, 538
percutaneous absorption in, 58–59
pharmacokinetics in, 56–61
plasma protein binding in, 60
prescription considerations for, 9, 11
preventing medication errors, 68b
pulmonary absorption in, 59
pulmonary administration in, 67
rectal administration, 58, 66–67
risks and benefits, 64–65
seizures in, 750
sinusitis in, 413–415
sleep requirements of, 831
syphilis in, 625t, 626
tissue-binding characteristics in, 60
topical administration, 67–68
urinary tract infections in, 574
vaccines for, 1034, 1035, 1036f–1037f, 1038
vaginitis in, 1123–1125
viral hepatitis in, 560
Pediatric Research Equity Act of 2003, 56
Pediatrics
hypothyroidism in, 916
substance use disorders in, 882
Peginterferon, for hepatitis B virus, 557, 558t
Pegloticase, 655
Pelargonium sidoides extract, 418
Pelvic inflammatory disease, 616t, 631–634, 633t, 634f
Pelvic pain syndrome, 578
Penciclovir, for viral skin infections, 221–222, 222t
Penicillamine, for rheumatoid arthritis, 679t, 680
Penicillin(s), 99–100, 100t. *See also specific drugs*
for otitis media, 284
resistance of, 118t
resistance to, beta-lactam/beta-lactamase inhibitors for, 95t, 100–101, 101t
sensitivity of, 95t
for skin infections, 205t, 207
for syphilis, 616t, 624–626, 625t
Penicillin G, 100t
sensitivity of, 95t
for syphilis, 616t, 624, 625t, 628t
Penicillin G benzathine, 100t
Penicillin G procaine, 100t
Penicillin V, 95t
Penicillin VK, 100t
Penis, dysfunction of. *See* Erectile dysfunction (ED)
Penlac (ciclopirox), for fungal infections, 215t
Pentasa (mesalamine), for inflammatory bowel disease, 502t, 504–505, 510
Pepcid (famotidine)
for GERD, 529t, 530t
for peptic ulcer disease, 529t, 537t
Peppermint, for GERD, 535

Peptic ulcer disease (PUD), 526–528
antacids for, 528, 529t
antibiotics for, 529t, 531–533
causes of, 526, 526t
complementary and alternative medicines for, 538
diagnosis of, 547–548
epidemiology of, 526
histamine-2 receptor antagonists for, 528, 529t, 530–531
information sources for, 538
nonsteroidal anti-inflammatory drug–induced, 536–537, 537t
NSAID-induced, 645t
in older adults, 538
pathophysiology of, 526–527
patient education on, 538
pediatric patients, 538
proton pump inhibitors for, 529t, 531
risk factors, 526t
therapeutic monitoring of, 538
treatment of, 528–533, 529t, 535–537, 536t–537t
in women, 538
Pepto-Bismol (bismuth subsalicylate)
for diarrhea, 484, 484t, 485–486
for GERD, 529t, 533
for peptic ulcer disease, 529t, 533
Per-member-per-month reports, 138, 138t
Perampanel, for seizures, 733t, 743
Perception, pain, 148–149
Perdiem (psyllium), for irritable bowel syndrome, 491, 491t, 497t
Performist (formoterol), for asthma and COPD, 430t, 436
Pergolide, for restless legs syndrome, 842
Perimenopause, physiology of, 1101–1102
Perindopril
for chronic stable angina, 334
for heart failure, 352
Periodic limb movement disorder, 841–845, 842b, 844b, 844f
Peripheral alpha-1 receptor blockers, for hypertension, 304, 304t
Peripheral sensitization, 150
Peripherally acting mu-opioid receptor antagonist, for constipation, 472t, 475–476
Peritonitis, in pelvic inflammatory disease, 632
Permissive hypothesis, of depression, 784, 784b
Pernicious anemia, 1024–1025, 1024b
Perphenazine, for nausea and vomiting, 456t, 458
Personalized medicine, 127. *See also* Precision medicine
pH
drug absorption and, 21, 34, 35t
gastric contents
in pediatric patients, 57
in pregnancy, 57
urine, drug excretion and, 39, 43
Pharmacist reimbursement, 139
Pharmacodynamics, 27–30
complementary alternative medicine interactions, 45–46, 46b
definition of, 17, 18b
dose–response relationships in, 30, 30f
of drug–disease interactions, 48
of drug–drug interactions, 41
of drug–food interactions, 31, 43, 43b
drug receptors in, 27–29, 28f
factors affecting, 30–31
of nonopioid c analgesics, 156t
pharmacokinetics relationship with, 17, 18f
terminology of, 18b
Pharmacoeconomics, 132
compliance issues, 138–139, 138t
cost–benefit analysis, 132
cost-effectiveness analysis, 132
cost minimization analysis, 132
cost–utility analysis, 132
definition of, 132

and electronic health records, 139–140
electronic prescribing, 139–140
formularies, 133t, 138t
overview of, 132
pharmacy and therapeutics committee, 137–138, 137b
Pharmacogenetics, definitions, 121, 122b
Pharmacogenomics, 10, 121–128
basic concepts, 121–123
definitions, 121, 122b
and precision medicine, 121
single nucleotide polymorphisms, 123
clinical applications of, 123–124
clopidogrel, 124, 124f, 125b
genetic testing for drug efficacy and adverse response, 126
mitochondrial mutation linked to antibiotics-induced ototoxicity, 126
warfarin, 124–126, 125f
clinical pharmacogenomics science, 127
information sources for, 128b
promises, pitfalls, and policy implications, 126–128
Pharmacokinetics, 17–27
bioavailability in, 19, 20b
complementary alternative medicine interactions, 44–45, 44t, 45t
absorption and, 44, 44t
distribution, 44–45
metabolism, 45–46, 46b
definition of, 17, 18b
of drug–disease interactions, 46–47, 47t
of drug–drug interactions, 34–41
absorption, 34, 35t
distribution, 34, 36, 36t
excretion, 39–40, 40t
metabolism, 36–39, 36f, 37f, 38t
P-glycoprotein interactions, 40–41, 41t
of drug–food interactions, 31, 41–44, 42b, 43b
factors affecting, 30–31
of Nonopioid analgesics, 156t
in pediatrics, 56–61
pharmacodynamics relationship with, 17, 18f
in pregnancy, 56–61
purpose of, 17
terminology of, 18b
Pharmacy and therapeutics committee, 137–138, 137b
Pharmacy benefit managers, 131
Phenazopyridine, for urinary tract infections, 571t, 572
Phendimetrazine, for obesity, 1080, 1080t
Phenelzine, for anxiety disorders, 814t, 820, 824
Phenergan (promethazine)
for allergic rhinitis, 936
for nausea and vomiting, 455, 456t
Phenobarbital
in cytochrome P-450 system induction, 39
for seizures, 728t, 731t, 738, 740
Phenothiazines, for nausea and vomiting, 455, 456t, 458, 467
Phenotype, asthma and COPD, 426
Phenotypic assay, in HIV infection, 949
Phentermine (adipex-P), for obesity, 1080, 1080t
Phentermine (lomaira), for obesity, 1080, 1080t
Phentermine extended release/topiramate, in obesity, 1082–1083
Phenylephrine hydrochloride, for upper respiratory infections, 405, 405t, 408, 412
Phenytoin
for arrhythmias, 378, 383
for seizures, 728–729, 728t, 736
therapeutic monitoring of, 88
Phillips' milk of magnesia (magnesium hydroxide)
for constipation, 472t, 474
for irritable bowel syndrome, 494, 497t
Phosphodiesterase 4 inhibitors, for asthma and COPD, 432t, 440

Phosphodiesterase-5 inhibitors, for erectile dysfunction, 589–590, 591b, 592t
Phospholipid(s), in lipoprotein transport, 314
Physical therapy
for osteoarthritis, 643
for rheumatoid arthritis, 676
Physicochemical properties, of drug, 60
Phytoestrogens, 1113, 1113t
Pibrentasvir, for hepatitis C virus, 559, 559t
Pigmentation, loss of, in fungal infections, 212, 213
Pilocarpine
for glaucoma, 274t, 276
for keratoconjunctivitis sicca, 270t
Pimecrolimus, for contact dermatitis, 192–193, 194, 196
Pindolol
for chronic stable angina, 340
for hypertension, 301
Pink eye. See Conjunctivitis
Pioglitazone, for diabetes mellitus, 892t, 895
Piperacillin, 95t, 100t
Piperacillin–tazobactam, 101t
sensitivity of, 95t
Pitavastatin, for hyperlipidemia, 317t
Pitolisant (Wakix), for narcolepsy, 847t, 848
Pityriasis versicolor. See Tinea versicolor
Placebo effect, 8
Placenta, drug transfer across, 61–63
Plantar warts (verruca plantaris), 221
Plaque
atherosclerotic, 315, 332
psoriasis, 230
Plaquenil (hydroxychloroquine)
for rheumatoid arthritis, 679t, 682
Plasma protein binding, in pediatrics, 60
Platelet(s), in clotting cascade, 984, 985f
Plavix (clopidogrel)
for chronic stable angina, 337t, 342
coagulation disorders, 1002–1003
Plazomicin, 107, 107t, 108t
Plecanatide, 475
Plendil (felodipine), for hypertension, 303t, 304
Pleuromutilins, 98t, 114, 114t
Plexion (sodium sulfacetamide), for rosacea, 251
Pneumococcal vaccine, 283, 289–290, 1040, 1040b
Pneumococcus infections, conjunctivitis, 262
Pneumonia, in older adults, 82
Podofilox, for human papilloma virus infections, 616t, 635, 636t
Podophyllin resin, for human papilloma virus infections, 616t, 635, 636t
Poison ivy, 191, 195
Polio vaccine, 1053b
Pollen allergy. See Allergic rhinitis
Polycarbophil
for constipation, 471, 471t, 473
for diarrhea, 484t, 485
Polyethylene glycol, 473–474
for constipation, 161
for constipation, 473–474
for hepatic encephalopathy, 553t, 554
Polygenic disorders, 122
Polymerase chain reaction, 220–221
Polymorphisms, 121, 122b
Polymyxin B, for otitis externa, 288, 288t
Polypharmacy, in older adults, 74–76, 77t
Polysomnography, in sleep disorders, 832
Pomade acne, 241
Poor metabolizers, 124
Portal hypertension (PH), 545
gastroesophageal varices, 545–546
nonselective beta blockers for, 546, 546t
in older adults, 547
therapeutic monitoring for, 547
treatment of, 546–548, 546t–547t
Positron emission tomography, in seizures, 728
Postantibiotic effect, 99b
Posthemorrhagic anemia, 1016
Postinfarction chronic stable angina, 330, 330b

Postmenopausal osteoporosis, 663, 664b
Postoperative nausea and vomiting (PONV), 452
Postpartum depression, 785, 801
Potassium channel blockers, for arrhythmias, 379b, 381–384
Potassium hydroxide test, 214
in candidiasis, 1116
Potassium iodide (SSKI), 921
for hyperthyroidism, 919t
Potassium-sparing diuretics
for heart failure, 354t, 359
for hypertension, 300, 300t
Povidone–iodine suppositories, for bacterial vaginosis, 1122
PQRSTU mnemonic, for pain assessment, 151, 151b
Practice guidelines, 138–139, 138t
Praluent (alirocumab), for hyperlipidemia, 321t, 322
Pramipexole (Mirapex), for restless legs syndrome, 842
Prasugrel (effient)
for chronic stable angina, 337t, 342
for coagulation disorders, 1002
Pravachol (pravastatin), for hyperlipidemia, 317t, 325
Pravastatin, for hyperlipidemia, 317t, 325
Prazosin
for benign prostatic hyperplasia, 584–585
for hypertension, 304, 304t
Precision medicine, 121, 122b
Precose (acarbose), for diabetes mellitus, 892t, 896
Prednicarbate, for contact dermatitis, 193t
Prednisolone, for conjunctivitis, 263t
Prednisone
for asthma and COPD, 432t, 439
for gout, 657
for inflammatory bowel disease, 502t, 505–506
for rheumatoid arthritis, 678
Preferred drugs, in formularies, 133
Preferred provider organizations, 132
Pregabalin (Lyrica)
for anxiety disorders, 818, 820
for pain, 162–163
for seizures, 732t, 741
Pre-gestational diabetes mellitus, 905
Pregnancy
acne in, 249
allergic rhinitis in, 942
anemia in, 1027
asthma and COPD in, 445
cannabis in, 187
Chlamydia trachomatis infections in, 615, 619
constipation in, 478–479
contact dermatitis in, 197
diabetes mellitus in, 889, 905
diarrhea in, 487
drugs in, 55–63
absorption, 57t
distribution, 57t, 59–60
elimination, 57t, 61
fetal physiology, 62
intramuscular administration, 58
labeling rule, 63, 63t
metabolism, 57t
mucosal absorption in, 59
oral administration, 57–58
percutaneous absorption in, 58–59
pharmacokinetics in, 56–61
physiologic changes and, 56
placental and fetal metabolism, 62
placental transfer of medications, 61–62, 62t
pulmonary absorption in, 59
rectal administration, 58
teratogenicity of medications, 62–63
GERD in, 535
gonorrhea in, 623
headache in, 720–721
heart failure in, 368
herpes simplex virus infections in, 631
HIV infection in, 961–962

human papilloma virus infections in, 637
hyperlipidemia in, 325
hyperparathyroidism in, 924
hypertension in, 307
hypothyroidism in, 916–917, 921
immunization during, 1051
inflammatory bowel disease in, 513–514
insomnia in, 840
menopause, 1103t–1106t, 1107, 1108b, 1113t
migraine headache in, 720–721
nausea and vomiting in, 466–468
in obesity, 1085
for osteoarthritis, 651
pain management in opioid use disorder in, 174–175
postpartum depression after, 785, 801
prescription considerations for, 11
rheumatoid arthritis, 688
skin infections in, 211
smoking cessation in, 1072–1073
substance use disorders in, 883
syphilis in, 626
unintended, 1089
urinary tract infections in, 574
vaginitis in, 1125, 1125b
viral hepatitis in, 560
Preinfarction angina, 329
Premarin (conjugated equine estrogen), for menopausal symptoms, 1103t, 1106t
Premature infants
definition of, 56t
gastric emptying time in, 58
gastrointestinal enzymes of, 58
pharmacokinetics in, 56–61
plasma protein binding in, 60
Premature ventricular contractions, treatment of, 373b, 380
Prescribing of drugs
adherence issues in, 13–14, 14b
authority for, 8
errors in, 9
ethical considerations in, 7–8
from formularies (See Formularies)
for older adults, 82–88, 83t, 86b, 87t
patient education in, 8
practical issues in, 7–8
refills, 12
selection in, 7, 8b, 10, 11, 11b
steps of, 10–11, 10f, 11b
writing prescription in, 11–13, 13f
Prescription copayment, patient, 139
Prescription Drug Marketing Act (PDMA), 8–9
Prescription drug monitoring program, 169
Prescription drugs, vs. nonprescription drugs, 5–6
Pressurized metered-dose inhalers, 67, 68t
Preterm infants, immunization of, 1035
Prevacid (lansoprazole)
for GERD, 529t, 530t, 531
for peptic ulcer disease, 529t, 531
Prevalite (cholestyramine), for hyperlipidemia, 321t, 322–323
Prevotella infections, bacterial vaginosis, 1115
Prilosec (Omeprazole)
for GERD, 529t, 530t, 531
for peptic ulcer disease, 529t, 531, 537t
Primary hyperparathyroidism. See Hyperparathyroidism
Primary open-angle glaucoma (POAG). See Glaucoma
Primaxin (imipenem), 95t–96t, 104, 104t
Primidone, for seizures, 732t, 738, 740–741
Prinivil (lisinopril)
for chronic stable angina, 334, 335t, 338
for heart failure, 352, 353t, 356
for hypertension, 302, 302t
Prinzmetal chronic stable angina, 330
Prior authorization, of drugs, 136
Priority review, 4
prn drugs, 12

ProAir (albuterol), for asthma and COPD, 428t, 436
Probenecid, 655
for pelvic inflammatory disease, 616t, 633t
for syphilis, 628t
Probuphine (buprenorphine), 169, 170t–172t, 171–172, 174–175
Procainamide, for arrhythmias, 377t, 379, 379b
Procaine, in ear drops, 284
Procardia (nifedipine)
for chronic stable angina, 336t, 341
for hypertension, 303t, 304
Prochlorperazine
for headache, 713–714
for nausea and vomiting, 455, 456t, 458
Procrit (epoetin), for anemia, 1022
Prodrugs, 18b, 24, 24t
metabolism of, 47
Progesterone
in contraceptives, 1091f, 1092–1094, 1093t, 1094t, 1098
in IUDs, 1090, 1095
for menopausal symptoms, 1104t, 1106
in menstrual cycle, 1090, 1090f
Progestins
in contraceptives, 1092–1095, 1094t
for menopausal symptoms, 1104t, 1106
Prolia (denosumab), for osteoporosis, 669t, 672
Prolixin (fluphenazine), for nausea and vomiting, 456t
Promensil (phytoestrogens), 1113, 1113t
Promethazine
allergic rhinitis in, 936
for nausea and vomiting, 455, 456t
Propafenone, for arrhythmias, 377t, 379b, 380–381
Propionibacterium acnes. See Cutibacterium acnes (C. acnes)
Propofol, 452
Propoxyphene, for pain, 87t
Propranolol
for arrhythmias, 377t, 379b
for chronic stable angina, 336t, 340
for migraine prevention, 714, 715t
for variceal hemorrhage, 546, 546t
Proprotein convertase subtilisin/kexin type 9 (PCSK9) inhibitors, 321t, 322, 325
Propyl-Thyracil (propylthiouracil), for hyperthyroidism, 919t, 920–921
Propylthiouracil, for hyperthyroidism, 919t, 920–921
Proscar (finasteride), for benign prostatic hyperplasia, 583–584, 584t
ProSom (estazolam), for insomnia, 833, 834t
Prostaglandin analogs
for glaucoma, 274t, 275–276
for nitric oxide donating prostaglandin analogs, 274t, 276
Prostaglandins, in pain transduction, 148
Prostate
-specific antigen, in prostate cancer, 582
benign hyperplasia of, 581–586, 582t, 584t–585t, 585f, 586t
cancer of, 586–587
inflammation of (prostatitis), 578–581, 579t, 580f
Prostatectomy, for benign prostatic hyperplasia, 586
Prostatitis, 574, 578–581
acute, 578
algorithm for, 580f
causes of, 578
chronic, 578
diagnosis of, 578
nonbacterial, 578
pathophysiology of, 578
patient education on, 581
therapeutic monitoring of, 580
treatment of, 579–580, 579t, 580f
Prostatodynia, 578
Prosthetic valvular heart disease, 984

Protease inhibitors, for HIV infection, 953t, 957–959
Protein binding
of drugs, 22–23, 23f (See also Albumin, drug binding to)
in pediatric patients, 59
plasma, 60
Protein C deficiency, hypercoagulability in, 982b, 986
Protein S deficiency, hypercoagulability in, 982b, 986
Proteus infections, skin, 207
Prothrombin defects, hypercoagulability in, 986
Prothrombin time, 988, 994b, 994t
Proton pump inhibitors
for GERD, 529t, 530t, 531
for peptic ulcer disease, 529t, 531, 537t
Protonix (pantoprazole)
for GERD, 529t, 530t
for peptic ulcer disease, 529t, 537t
Proventil (albuterol), for asthma and COPD, 428t, 436
Prozac (fluoxetine)
for anxiety disorders, 814t, 815
for depression, 81, 789t, 790t, 798
for headache, 699
for obesity, 1084t
Prucalopride, for constipation, 476
"Pseudo-addictive" behavior, 169
Pseudoephedrine
allergic rhinitis in, 937t, 938
for upper respiratory infections, 405, 405t, 412
Pseudomonas aeruginosa, 421
Pseudomonas infections
antimicrobial sensitivity in, 95t–98t
otitis externa, 282, 282t
prostatitis, 578
skin, 201, 201t, 208, 211
Psoriasis, 229–239
algorithm for, 238f
causes of, 229, 230b
complementary and alternative medicine for, 239
diagnosis of, 230
drugs exacerbating, 229, 230b
epidemiology of, 229
lifestyle changes for, 238–239
pathophysiology of, 229–230
patient education on, 238–239
therapeutic monitoring of, 238
treatment of, 230–237, 231t–232t, 237t, 238f
Psychiatric disorders. See also Anxiety disorders; Depression
in older adults, 78–79
Psychogenic factors, in erectile dysfunction, 589
Psychomotor (complex partial) seizures, 726
Psychostimulants (Wake-promoting agents), for narcolepsy, 846, 847t
Psychotherapy
for ADHD, 867
for anxiety disorders, 827
for depression, 785
Psychotropic agents, for older adults, 79
Psyllium
for constipation, 471, 471t, 473
for irritable bowel syndrome, 491, 491t, 497t
Pulmonary absorption, 59
Pulmonary administration, for pediatric patients, 67
Pulmonary angiography, in pulmonary embolism, 868
Pulmonary embolism
from deep venous thrombosis, 981, 982b
diagnosis of, 987
prevention of, 1003
prophylaxis of, 1003–1004
treatment of, 999t, 1003
Pure Food and Drug Act, 180
Purinethol (6-mercaptopurine), for inflammatory bowel disease, 503t, 506–507, 514
Pustular infections
causes of, 201

complementary and alternative medicine for, 212
diagnosis of, 203
lifestyle changes in, 212
pathophysiology of, 202, 202b
patient education on, 211–212
treatment of, 204, 205t–206t, 207–211, 209t, 210f
Pustular psoriasis, 230
Pyelonephritis, uncomplicated, treatment for, 569, 573, 573t
Pygeum, for benign prostatic hyperplasia, 586, 586t
Pyridium (phenazopyridine), for urinary tract infections, 571t, 572
Pyrithione zinc, for fungal infections, 219

Q
Quality-adjusted life years, in cost–utility analysis, 132
Quality of life
in cost–utility analysis, 132
in heart failure, 352
Quazepam, for insomnia, 833, 834t
Questionnaires, insomnia, 831
Questran (cholestyramine), for hyperlipidemia, 321t, 322–323
Quinacrine, for aplastic anemia, 1026b
Quinaglute (quinidine), arrhythmias, 377t, 378, 379b
Quinapril
for chronic stable angina, 334, 335t, 338
for heart failure, 352, 353t
Quinicine, for diarrhea, 483t
Quinidine, for arrhythmias, 377t, 378, 379b
Quinolone
causing diarrhea, 480
for diarrhea, 483t
Quinupristin–dalfopristin, 98t, 113–114, 113t

R
Rabbit-anti-thymocyte globulin (rATG), for organ transplantation, 967, 973t
Rabeprazole
for GERD, 529t, 530t
for peptic ulcer disease, 529t, 537t
Radioactive iodine therapy, 919, 920t
Radioactive iodine uptake (RAIU), 918
Radioallergosorbent testing, in rhinitis, 934
Radiofrequency catheter ablation, for arrhythmias, 373, 393
Radiography
heart failure, 366
for osteoarthritis, 653
Raloxifene (Evista), for osteoporosis, 669t, 671
Ramipril
for chronic stable angina, 334, 335t, 338
for heart failure, 352, 353t, 356–357
for hypertension, 302, 302t
Randomized Spironolactone Evaluation Study, 300
Ranexa (ranolazine), for chronic stable angina, 337t, 343
Ranitidine, 76t, 77t
for GERD, 529t, 530t
for peptic ulcer disease, 529t, 537t
RANK ligand inhibitor, for osteoporosis, 672
Ranolazine, for chronic stable angina, 337t, 343
Rapaflo (silodosin), for benign prostatic hyperplasia, 584, 584t
Rapamune (sirolimus), for organ transplantation, 972, 974t
Rapid eye movement sleep, 788, 831
Rapid plasma reagin test, for syphilis, 624
RAST (radioallergosorbent testing), in rhinitis, 934
Recarbrio (imipenem-cilastatin-relebactam), 95t, 101t, 104
Recovery community centers, 883
Recreation, therapeutic, for ADHD, 859
Rectal administration, 21, 58, 66–67
Recurrent acute otitis media, 287

Red blood cells
    aplastic anemia, 1026, 1026b
    chronic disease, anemia of, 1022–1023, 1023b
    chronic renal failure, anemia of, 1020–1022,
        1023b
    folate deficiency, 1025–1026, 1025b
    iron deficiency anemia, 1018–1020, 1019b,
        1019t
    vitamin B$_{12}$ deficiency, 1024–1025, 1024b
Referral to treatment (RT), 871
Refills, in prescriptions, 12
Reflex epilepsy, 725
Refractory overactive bladder, 610
Reglan (metoclopramide), for nausea and vomiting,
    458t, 460–461, 467
Reimbursement, pharmacist, 139
Relafen (nabumetone), for osteoarthritis, 645t
Relaxation techniques, for headache, 703
Relenza (zanamivir), for influenza, 1042
Relpax (eletriptan), for migraine headache, 706t, 711
REM (rapid eye movement) sleep, 788, 831
Remeron (mirtazapine), for depression, 818t, 826
Remicade (infliximab), 680t, 684
    for inflammatory bowel disease, 503t, 508, 509
    for psoriasis, 232t, 236
Remodeling, bone, in osteoarthritis, 642, 642f
Renal system, 296
Renin-angiotensin-aldosterone system, 544
        heart failure, 350
        hypertension, 295, 296
Renin inhibitors, for hypertension, 303, 303t
Repaglinide, for diabetes mellitus, 892t, 896
Repatha (evolocumab), for hyperlipidemia, 321t, 322
Rescriptor (delavirdine), for HIV infection, 956
Resiniferatoxin, for overactive bladder, 609
Reslizumab, for asthma and COPD, 433t, 442–443
Respiratory drug delivery systems, for asthma and
    COPD, 445–446, 445t
Respiratory tract infections (RTIs). *See specific
    instructions*
Response, dose relationship with, 30, 30f
Restless leg syndrome, 829, 841–845, 841b–842b
Restoril (temazepam), for insomnia, 833, 834t
Retching, 454
Retin A (retinoic acid), for acne, 242, 243t
Retinoic acid, for acne, 242, 243t
Retinoids, for psoriasis, 234
Retroviruses, mechanism of action of, 948
Revefenacin, for asthma and COPD, 438
Reverse cholesterol transport, 314
Reverse transcriptase, in HIV replication, 948, 949
Reverse transcriptase inhibitors, for HIV infection
    non-nucleoside, 950, 951t, 956–957, 960
    nucleoside, 950, 951t, 956
Reverse transcriptase-polymerase chain reaction, in
    HIV detection, 949
ReVia (naltrexone), for alcohol use disorder, 874t,
    875
Reyataz (atazanavir), for HIV infection, 953t, 957
Reyvow, for migraine headache, 707t, 711–712
Rheumatoid arthritis, 675–689
    causes of, 675
    complementary and alternative medicine for, 689
    corticosteroids for, 678
    definition of, 675
    diagnosis of, 676
    disease-modifying antirheumatic drugs for,
        678–684
    early stages of, 676
    immunomodulators for, 685, 688
    information sources for, 688
    nutrition for, 688
    in older adults, 688
    pathophysiology of, 675–676
    patient education on, 688–689
    in pregnancy, 688
    progression of, 676
    severe, 676

    therapeutic monitoring, 688
    in women, 688
Rheumatoid factor, in rheumatoid arthritis, 676
Rheumatrex (methotrexate)
    for inflammatory bowel disease, 503t, 506–507,
        513
    psoriasis, 232t, 235
    rheumatoid arthritis, 678t, 680
Rhinitis
    allergic, 932–944, 935f
    nonallergic, with eosinophilia, 934
    vasomotor, 934
Rhinitis medicamentosa, 408
Rhinophyma, 250
Rhinosinusitis, 412–418
    algorithm for, 411f
    antibiotics for, 413–416
    causes of, 412–413
    chronic *vs.* acute, 412
    diagnosis of, 413
    information sources for, 417
    lifestyle changes for, 417
    pathophysiology of, 413
    patient education on, 416–417
    in pediatric patients, 413–415
    risk factors for, 412b
    therapeutic monitoring of, 416
    treatment of, 405t–407t, 413–418
Rho Kinase Inhibitors, for glaucoma, 275t, 277
Rhofade (oxyometazoline HCl cream 1%), for
    rosacea, 251–252
Rhopressa (netarsudil), for glaucoma, 275t, 277
Rhythm method, as contraceptive method,
    1090–1091, 1091f
Ribavirin, for hepatitis C virus, 559, 559t
Ribonucleic acid (RNA), 122b
Ridaura (auranofin), for rheumatoid arthritis, 679t
Rifampin, 39, 40, 98t, 116–117, 116t, 118t
Rifaximin
    for diarrhea, 483t, 484t–485t, 485–486
    for hepatic encephalopathy, 553t, 554
    for irritable bowel syndrome, 493t, 495, 497t
Rimantadine, for influenza, 1042
Rimegepant (Nurtec), for migraine headache, 707t
Ring, estradiol, 1105t
Ringworm (tinea corporis), 213
Risarkizymab, for psoriasis, 232t, 234
Risedronate, for osteoporosis, 668t, 670
Risk-benefit, for pediatric patients, 64–65
Risperdal (risperidone), for Alzheimer's disease, 761
Risperidone, for Alzheimer's disease, 761
Ritalin (methylphenidate), 794, 860, 861t
Ritonavir, for HIV infection, 954t, 957, 958, 960
Rituxan, for rheumatoid arthritis, 680t, 685–686
Rituximab (Rituxan), for rheumatoid arthritis, 680t,
    685–686
Rivastigmine, for Alzheimer's disease, 758–759, 760t
Rizatriptan, for migraine headache, 703, 705t,
    710–711
Robitussin (guaifenesin), for upper respiratory
    infections, 406t, 408
Robitussin DM (dextromethorphan), as isomer, 30
Rocephin (ceftriaxone), 96t, 102, 102t, 103
    causing diarrhea, 479
    for ophthalmic disorders, 265
    for otitis media, 285t
    for sexually transmitted infections, 621, 621t,
        625t, 633t
    for skin infections, 205t, 207
Rocklatan (netarsudil and latanoprost), 275t, 277
Rofecoxib, for pain, 82, 596
Roflumilast, for asthma and COPD, 432t, 440
Rosacea, 250–253
    antiparasitics for, 251
    causes of, 250
    decongestants and vasoconstrictors for, 251–252
    diagnosis of, 250
    oral antibiotics for, 252

    pathophysiology of, 250
    patient education, 252
    selection of drugs, 252, 252t, 253f
    therapeutic monitoring of, 252
    topical antibacterials for, 250–251, 250t
    treatment of, 252, 252t, 253f
Rosiglitazone, for diabetes mellitus, 892t, 895
Rosula (sodium sulfacetamide), for rosacea, 251
Rosuvastatin, for hyperlipidemia, 317t, 319, 320
Rowasa (mesalamine), for inflammatory bowel
    disease, 502t, 504–505, 510
Rufinamide, for seizures, 735t, 745
Rukobia, for HIV infection, 955t
Rythmol (propafenone), for arrhythmias, 377t, 379b,
    380–381

S
Sacubatril/valsartan, for heart failure, 354t, 360–361
Safety, drug, 3–7, 5b, 6t, 68
Salagen (pilocarpine), for keratoconjunctivitis sicca,
    270t
Salicylates, nonacetylated, for osteoarthritis, 647,
    647b
Salicylic acid, for viral skin infections, 223
Saline laxatives, for constipation, 472t, 474
Saline nasal flushes, for respiratory infections, 405
Salmeterol, for asthma and COPD, 430t, 436
Salmonella infections, 480, 480b, 481, 482
Salpingitis, in pelvic inflammatory disease, 632
Sampling, drug, 8–9
Sanctura (trospium), for overactive bladder, 601t,
    602t, 604–605, 604t
Sancuso (granisetron), for nausea and vomiting,
    457t, 460
Sandimmune (cyclosporine)
    for inflammatory bowel disease, 503t, 506–507,
        514
    for organ transplantation, 968–970, 969t, 974t
    for psoriasis, 231t, 235
    for rheumatoid arthritis, 679t, 680, 682
Saquinavir, for HIV infection, 954t, 957
Sarecycline, for acne, 243t, 246
Sativex, for pain, 186t
Saw palmetto, 586, 586t, 612
Saxenda (liraglutide), for obesity, 1081t, 1082
Scalded skin syndrome, 207
Scalp, fungal infections of, 213
Scheduled drugs, 4, 5b
Sclerostin inhibitor, for osteoporosis, 672
Scopolamine, for nausea and vomiting, 456t, 459
Screener and Opioid Assessment for Patients with
    Pain-Revised (SOAPP-R), 169, 169b
Screening, Brief Intervention, and Referral to
    Treatment (SBIRT), 871, 872b
Seasonal affective disorder, 785
Seasonal (hay fever) conjunctivitis, 265–266, 266t
Seborrheic blepharitis, 257–258
Second messenger, definition of, 18b
Secondary hyperparathyroidism. *See*
    Hyperparathyroidism
Secretagogues
    for constipation, 472t, 475
    for irritable bowel syndrome, 493t, 495
Secretory diarrhea, 481
Secukinumab, for psoriasis, 232t, 236–237
Seebri (glycopyrrolate), for asthma and COPD,
    430t, 438
Seizures, 725–752
    absence (petit mal), 726–727
    acute, 726
    algorithm for, 729f
    atonic, 727
    atypical absence, 727
    causes of, 725–726
    classification of, 726–727
    clonic, 726–727
    complex partial (psychomotor), 726
    diagnosis of, 727–728

first aid for, 751
generalized (convulsive or nonconvulsive),
726–727
immunization and, 1038
lifestyle changes for, 751
myoclonic, 726–727
in older adults, 750
partial (focal, local), 726
pathophysiology of, 726–727
patient education on, 770
in pediatric patients, 750
persistent (status epilepticus), 727
recurrent (See Epilepsy)
secondary, 726
surgery for, 728
therapeutic monitoring of, 751
tonic, 727
tonic-clonic (grand mal), 726, 727
treatment of, 728–750, 728t, 729f, 730t–735t,
736b, 740b
unknown onset, 727
in women, 750
Selective adhesion molecule inhibitors, 504t, 508
Selective estrogen receptor modulators, for
osteoporosis, 669t, 671
Selective norepinephrine reuptake inhibitors (SNRIs),
for pain, 162
Selective serotonin reuptake inhibitors
adverse reactions to, 788–789, 790t–791t, 792
for anxiety disorders, 80, 814t, 815, 824
for depression, 80, 788–789, 789t, 790t–791t,
792, 795t
for menopausal symptoms, 1102, 1109–1110
response time for, 788
withdrawal from, 825–826
Selegiline, for Alzheimer's disease, 762
Selenium sulfide, for fungal infections, 216t, 218
Self-management techniques, for smoking cessation,
1062
Self-monitoring, of asthma and COPD, 445
Selsun (selenium sulfide), for fungal infections, 216t,
218
Semisynthetic antibiotic
for diarrhea, 484t, 485
for irritable bowel syndrome, 493t, 495
Senile osteoporosis, 663, 664b
Senna
for constipation, 472t, 474
for irritable bowel syndrome, 492t, 493–494,
497t
Senokot (senna)
for constipation, 472t, 474
for irritable bowel syndrome, 492t, 493–494,
497t
Sensipar (cinacalcet), for hyperparathyroidism, 923,
924t
Sensitization, in contact dermatitis, 191, 194
Septra (trimethoprim–sulfamethoxazole)
for prostatitis, 579, 579t
for sinusitis, 413
Serax (oxazepam), for anxiety disorders, 80, 816,
817t
Serevent Diskus (salmeterol), for asthma and COPD,
430t, 436
Serotonin
antagonists of (See Selective serotonin reuptake
inhibitors [SSRIs])
deficiency of, in depression, 784, 784b
in pain transduction, 148
in stress, 815
Serotonin-3 receptor antagonists, for irritable bowel
syndrome, 495
Serotonin-4 (5-HT₄) receptor agonist, for
constipation, 476
Serotonin antagonists, for nausea and vomiting,
457t, 460
Serotonin norepinephrine reuptake inhibitors
adverse events, 1110

menopause systems, 1109–1110
for overactive bladder, 601t, 603t, 607–608
Serotonin reuptake inhibitors, menopause systems,
1109–1110
Sertraline
for Alzheimer's disease, 761
for anxiety disorders, 814t, 815
for depression, 81
Serum-ascites albumin gradient approach, 548
Serzone (nefazodone), depression, 789t, 795t, 796
Sex differences, in pharmacokinetics and
pharmacodynamics, 31
Sexual activity, urinary tract infections in, 568
Sexual dysfunction, after menopause, 1110
Sexually transmitted infections, 615–638
Chlamydia, 616t, 617–619, 618t, 619f
contraceptive methods and, 1091
epidemiology of, 617
gonorrhea, 616t, 620–623, 621t, 623f, 623t
herpes simplex virus, 616t, 626–631, 629t, 630f
human immunodeficiency virus infection,
947–964
human papilloma virus, 616t, 635–638, 636t,
637f
pelvic inflammatory disease, 616t, 631–634,
633t, 634f
syphilis, 616t, 624–626, 625t, 627f
Seysara (sarecycline), for acne, 243t, 246
Shigella infections, 480, 480b, 481, 482
Shingrix vaccine, 225
Sick day guidelines, for diabetes mellitus, 908
Sickle cell anemia, 1016–1018
Side effects. See Adverse drug reactions (ADRs)
education on, 87
nonadherence in, 77
Sildenafil, for erectile dysfunction, 589–590, 590t
Siliq (brodalumab), for psoriasis, 232t, 236–237
Silodosin, for benign prostatic hyperplasia, 584, 584t
Silvadene (silver sulfadiazine), 110
Silver sulfadiazine, 110
Simbrinza (brinzolamide and brimonidine), 275t,
277
Simcor (simvastatin/niacin), for hyperlipidemia, 325
Simponi (golimumab), for psoriasis, 232t
Simulect (basiliximab), for organ transplantation,
968, 973t
Simvastatin/niacin, for hyperlipidemia, 317t, 321,
325
Single-nucleotide polymorphisms (SNPs), 122–123,
122b
Singulair (montelukast), for asthma and COPD,
429t, 438–439
Sinoatrial node, function of, 372
Sinusitis, 412–418. See also Rhinosinusitis
Sirolimus, for organ transplantation, 972, 974t
Sjögren's syndrome, keratoconjunctivitis sicca in, 269
Skin
acne of, 241–253
allergic reactions in, 930
contact dermatitis of, 191–198
drug administration across, 22
drug administration through, 58
drug administration under, 22, 58
fungal infections of, 212–219
in pregnancy, 211
prevention of, 205b
psoriasis manifestations in, 229–239
risk factors for, 202b
rosacea manifestations in, 250–253, 251t, 252t,
253f
Skin testing, in allergic rhinitis, 933–934
Skyrizi (risankizumab), for psoriasis, 232t, 234
Sleep
history of, 831, 831b
importance of, 829
physiology of, 830b, 831
Sleep disorders. See also Insomnia

chronic stable angina and, 330b, 341
narcolepsy, 845–849
periodic limb movement disorder, 841–845,
842b, 844b, 844f
types of, 829
Smoking
cessation of, 1057–1074, 1062b, 1065t–1066t,
1071t
in adolescents, 1073
algorithm for, 1072f
in breast-feeding, 1073
in cardiovascular disease, 1073
in heart failure, 369
in hyperlipidemia, 317
nicotine delivery systems, uses of, 1069
patient education on, 1073
pharmacotherapy agents, comparison
of, 1069
in pregnancy, 1072–1073
relapse in, 1073
therapeutic monitoring in, 1073
treatment recommendations, 1070t
weight gain in, 1085
coronary heart disease and, 330
diagnostic criteria for, 1059–1060, 1060b
drug interactions in, 48, 77t, 79
economic impact of, 1058
epidemiology of, 1057–1058
GERD, 535
health impact of, 1058
pathophysiology of, 1058–1059
peptic ulcer disease and, 538
in pregnancy, 1072–1073
SNRIs (Serotonin–norepinephrine reuptake
inhibitors), 1109–1110
SOAPP-R (Screener and Opioid Assessment for
Patients with Pain-Revised), 169, 169b
Social Anxiety Disorder (SAD), 715
Social phobia. See Social Anxiety Disorder (SAD)
Social skills training, for ADHD, 867
Sodium, dietary restriction of
for heart failure, 369
for hypertension, 309
Sodium biphosphate enema, 474, 477
Sodium channel blockers
for arrhythmias, 378, 379b
for pain, 163
Sodium-glucose co-transporter 2 inhibitors, for
diabetes mellitus, 900–901
Sodium oxybate, for narcolepsy, 846
Sodium phosphate enema, for constipation, 472t,
474
Sodium polystyrene sulfonate, constipation and,
469b
Sodium sulfacetamide, for rosacea, 251
Sofosbuvir, for hepatitis C virus, 559, 559t
Solfoton (phenobarbital), for seizures, 731t
Solifenacin, for overactive bladder, 601t, 602, 602t,
604–605, 604t
Solriamfetol (Sunosi), for narcolepsy, 847t, 848
Solu-Cortef (hydrocortisone), for inflammatory
bowel disease, 502t
Solu-Medrol (methylprednisolone)
for inflammatory bowel disease, 502t
for nausea and vomiting, 457t, 461
Solubility, drug, absorption and, 19–20
Somatic pain, 146
Somogyi effect, 801
Sonata (zaleplon), for insomnia, 835t, 836
Soolontra (ivermectin), for rosacea, 251
Sorbitol
for constipation, 472t, 473–474
for irritable bowel syndrome, 491
Sorbitrate (isosorbide dinitrate), for chronic stable
angina, 336t, 338–339
Soriatane (acitretin), for psoriasis, 234–235
Sotalol, for arrhythmias, 377t, 379b, 383–384
Soy products, for menopausal symptoms, 1113

Spiriva (tiopropium bromide), for asthma and COPD, 430t
Spironolactone
  for acne, 244t, 247
  for ascites, 547t, 548–549
  for chronic stable angina, 334, 335t, 338
  for heart failure, 354t, 359
  for hypertension, 300, 300t
Splanchnic nerves. See Visceral afferent nerves
Spontaneous bacterial peritonitis (SBP)
  adjunctive therapy for, 551
  diagnosis of, 549, 549b
  prophylaxis, 551, 551b
  therapeutic monitoring for, 551
  treatment of, 549–551, 550t
Sporanox (itraconazole), for fungal infections, 216t, 217–218
Spravato, for depression, 791t, 797–798
ST elevation MI, 333
St. John's wort, 802
Stable angina, 329, 330b
Stages of change model, for smoking cessation, 1059
Staphylococcus aureus infections, 480b, 482
  antimicrobial sensitivity in, methicillin, 95t–98t
  contact dermatitis and, 194
  sinusitis, 412
  skin, 199–201, 201t, 207–210
Staphylococcus infections
  antimicrobial sensitivity in, 95t–98t
  blepharitis, 257–258
  conjunctivitis, 261, 262, 265
Starlix (nateglinide), for diabetes mellitus, 892t, 896
Statins, for hyperlipidemia, 317t, 319–320, 320f
Status epilepticus, 727
Stavudine, for HIV infection, 950, 951t
Staxyn (vardenafil), for erectile dysfunction, 590, 590t
Steady state, 26, 26f
Stelara (ustekinumab)
  for inflammatory bowel disease, 504t, 508
  for psoriasis, 232t, 236
Stendra (avanafil), for benign prostatic hyperplasia, 590, 590t
Stereoselectivity, 30
Stewardship programs, antimicrobial, 118
Stigmas, in cannabis plant, 179
Stimulant laxatives
  for ADHD, 859–860, 860t, 862–863
  for constipation, 472t, 474
  for irritable bowel syndrome, 492t, 493–494
Stiolto Respimat (tiotropium bromide/olodaterol), for asthma and COPD, 431t
Stomach
  contents of, pH of, in pediatric patients, 57
  peptic ulcers of (See Peptic ulcer disease [PUD])
Strattera (atomoxetine), for ADHD, 861t, 863
Streptococcus infections
  antimicrobial sensitivity in, 95t–98t
  conjunctivitis, 261, 262, 265
  skin, 199, 201, 201t
Streptococcus pneumonia infections
  in cirrhosis, 544
  conjunctivitis, 261, 265
  otitis media, 284
  sinusitis, 412, 413
  vaccines for, 1040
Streptococcus pyogenes infections, skin, 199, 201
Streptogramins, 98t, 113–114, 113t, 118t
Streptomycin
  dosages of, 107t
  monitoring of, 108t
Stress, response to, 809, 811b
Stress test, in chronic stable angina, 333
Striverdi Respimat (olodaterol), for asthma and COPD, 430t, 436
Stroke
  hypertension in, 298, 306, 307
  ischemic
    characteristics of, 988

diagnosis of, 988
prevention of, 990
treatment of, 1004
Subclinical hypothyroidism, 913, 914t
Subcutaneous administration
  drug absorption in, 22
  for pediatric patients, 58
  for pregnancy, 58
Sublingual administration, 21
Sublocadelate (buprenorphine), 169, 170t–171t, 171–172, 172t, 174–175
Suboxone (buprenorphine/naloxone), 169, 170t–171t, 171–172, 172t, 174–175
Substance use disorders (SUDs), 869–884
  alcohol use disorder, 872, 873b, 873–876, 874t, 877f
  alcohol withdrawal, 872–873, 873b, 874t
  causes of, 869–870
  complementary and alternative medications for, 884
  diagnosis of, 871, 871b, 871t
  Diagnostic and Statistical Manual of Mental Disorders, Fifth Edition for, 871, 871b
  drugs with potential for, 871b
  information resources for, 883
  lifestyle changes in, 883
  nutrition for, 883
  in older adults, 882
  opioid use disorder, 876–882, 878b, 881f, 879f–880b
  pathophysiology of, 870–871, 870f
  patient education on, 883
  in pediatrics, 882
  in pregnancy, 883
  screening, brief intervention, and referral to treatment, 871, 872b
  therapeutic monitoring for, 883
  treatment for, 871–882, 873b, 874t, 877f, 878b, 879t–880t, 881
  in women, 883
Substitutions, allowable, 12
Subutex (buprenorphine), 169, 170t–171t, 171–172, 172t, 174–175
Succinylcholine, metabolism of, genetic factors in, 31
Sucralfate
  constipation and, 469b
  for GERD, 529t, 533
  for peptic ulcer disease, 529t, 533, 537t
Sudafed (pseudoephedrine), for upper respiratory infections, 405, 405t, 408, 412
Sufenta (sufentanil), for pain, 160
Sufentanil, for pain, 160
Suicide, in depression, 801–802, 801b
Sulconazole, for fungal infections, 215t
Sulfacet-R (sodium sulfacetamide), for rosacea, 251
Sulfadiazine, 110t
Sulfadoxine, 109
Sulfamethoxazole, 109. See also Trimethoprim-sulfamethoxazole (TMP-SMZ)
Sulfamethoxazole–trimethoprim
  for prostatitis, 579, 579t
  for sinusitis, 413
  for skin infections, 206t, 208
  for spontaneous bacterial peritonitis, 550, 550t, 551
  for urinary tract infections, 569, 570t, 572
Sulfamylon (mafenide), 110
Sulfasalazine
  for inflammatory bowel disease, 502t, 504, 510, 515
  for rheumatoid arthritis, 681–682
Sulfisoxazole, 110t
Sulfonamides, 97t, 109–110, 110t
Sulfonylureas, for diabetes mellitus, 891, 891t, 893–894
Sumatriptan, for migraine, 703, 704t, 710
Sumycin (tetracycline), 108–109
  dosage of, 109t
  sensitivity of, 97t

Sunosi, for narcolepsy, 847t, 848
Suppositories, absorption of, 21
Supraventricular tachycardia, paroxysmal, 386t, 392–393, 393f
Suprax (cefixime)
  for gonorrhea, 621, 621t
  for upper respiratory infections, 407t, 415–416
Surface area
  in pediatric patients, 57–58
  in pregnancy, 57–58
Surfactant laxatives
  for constipation, 471t, 474–475
  for irritable bowel syndrome, 492t, 494
Surfak (docusate calcium)
  for constipation, 472t, 474–475
  for irritable bowel syndrome, 492t, 494, 497t
Surgery
  for epilepsy, 728
  for necrotizing fasciitis, 211
  orthopedic, anticoagulants for, 990
  for thyroid and parathyroid disorders, 919
Sustained-release dosage, 20
Swimmer's ear. See Otitis externa
Symbicort (budesonide/formoterol), for asthma and COPD, 431t
Symmetrel (amantadine), for influenza, 1042
Symproic (naldemedine), for constipation, 476–477
Synapses, in neurons, 726
Syndros (dronabinol), for pain, 183t, 184, 187
Synercid (quinupristin–dalfopristin), 98t, 113–114, 113t
Synovial fluid
  in gout, 652
  in osteoarthritis, 642
Synovial membrane, proliferation and erosion of, in rheumatoid arthritis, 675
Synthroid (levothyroxine), for hypothyroidism, 914, 915t
Syphilis, 624–626
  algorithm for, 627f
  causes of, 624
  diagnosis of, 624
  pathophysiology of, 624
  patient education on, 626
  in pediatric patients, 626
  in pregnancy, 626
  therapeutic monitoring of, 626, 628t

T
T lymphocytes, CD4, in HIV infection, 961, 963
Taclonex, for psoriasis, 231t, 234
Tacrolimus
  for contact dermatitis, 194, 196
  for organ transplantation, 969t, 970, 974t
Tadalafil
  for benign prostatic hyperplasia, 585
  for erectile dysfunction, 589–590, 590t
Tafluprost, for glaucoma, 274t, 275–276
Tagamet (cimetidine)
  for GERD, 529t, 530t, 531
  for peptic ulcer disease, 529t, 531, 537t
Tai chi, for pain management in opioid use disorder, 175
Taltz (ixekizumab), for psoriasis, 232t, 236–237
Talwin (pentazocine), for pain, 87t
Tamiflu (oseltamivir)
  for bronchitis, 419–420, 419t
  for community-acquired pneumonia, 423
  for influenza, 1042
Tamsulosin
  for benign prostatic hyperplasia, 584–585, 584t
  for overactive bladder, 601t, 603t, 608
Tapazole (methimazole), for hyperthyroidism, 919t, 920–921
Tapentadol, for pain, 158t, 160
Targadox (doxycycline)
  for acne, 246
  for rosacea, 252

Target drug
    complementary alternative medicine interactions,
        44b
    in interactions, 34, 35t, 36t
Tazarotene
    for acne, 244–245, 249
    for psoriasis, 231t, 234
Tazorac (tazarotene)
    for acne, 244–245, 249
    for psoriasis, 231t, 234
Tea tree oil for skin disorders, 250
Tear(s)
    artificial, for keratoconjunctivitis sicca, 269, 270t
    deficiency of, in keratoconjunctivitis sicca,
        268–272
Tear break-up time testing, in keratoconjunctivitis
        sicca, 269
Tedizolid, 98t, 112, 112t, 208
Teflaro (ceftaroline fosamil), 103
Tegretol (carbamazepine)
    for Alzheimer's disease, 761
    psychiatric disorders, 82
    seizures, 730t, 736–737
    therapeutic monitoring of, 88
Telangiectasia, in rosacea, 250
Telavancin, 97t, 110–111, 111t, 208
Telbivudine, 558t, 559
Telehealth, 140
Telemedicine, 140
Telithromycin, 106
Telmisartan
    for chronic stable angina, 334
    for heart failure, 360
Temazepam, for insomnia, 833, 834t, 838t
Temporal lobe (complex partial) seizures, 726
Tenex (guanfacine), for ADHD, 863
Tenofovir, for HIV infection, 951t, 955–956
Tenofovir alamfenamide, for hepatitis B virus, 557,
        558t
Tenofovir disoproxil fumarate, for hepatitis B virus,
        557, 558t
Tenormin (atenolol)
    for chronic stable angina, 336t, 340
    for hypertension, 300, 301t
Tension headache
    causes of, 694–695
    diagnosis of, 695, 695b
    epidemiology of, 693–694
    pathophysiology of, 695
    in pediatric patients, 720
    prevention of, 699, 700t
    prophylaxis of, 697, 699
    treatment of, 703, 704t–709t, 710–714
Tenuate (diethylpropion), for obesity, 1080, 1080t
Teratogenicity, 62–63
    nausea and vomiting in pregnancy, 466
    retinoic acid derivatives, 247
Terazol (terconazole), for candidiasis, 1119t
Terazosin
    for benign prostatic hyperplasia, 584, 584t
    for hypertension, 304, 304t
    multiple uses of, 86
Terbinafine
    for fungal infections, 216t, 217, 217t
Terconazole, for candidiasis, 1118, 1119t
Teriparatide
    for hypoparathyroidism, 924
    for osteoporosis, 669t, 671–672
Terpenes
    in cannabis plant, 179
    in pain management, 186, 186b
Tessalon Perles (benzonatate), for upper respiratory
        infections, 406t, 408–409
Testosterone, for menopausal symptoms, 1104t,
        1106
Tetracycline(s), 108–109, 118t. See also specific drugs
    absorption and, 41
    for acne, 243t, 246, 249
    adsorption and, 34

causing diarrhea, 479–480
    dosage of, 109t
    for GERD, 529t, 532
    for gonorrhea, 620, 622t
    for peptic ulcer disease, 529t, 532
    for rosacea, 252
    sensitivity of, 97t
    for syphilis, 616t, 624, 625t
Tetrahydrocannabinol, 179, 461–462
Tetrahydrozoline, for conjunctivitis, 264t, 265
Teveten (eprosartan)
    for chronic stable angina, 334
    for heart failure, 360
Thalassemia, 1023–1024
Theo-Dur (theophylline)
    for asthma and COPD, 432t, 440–441
    metabolism of, in pediatric patients, 60
    therapeutic monitoring of, 88
Theo24 (theophylline)
    for asthma and COPD, 432t, 440–441
    metabolism of, in pediatric patients, 60
    therapeutic monitoring of, 88
Theophylline
    for asthma and COPD, 432t, 440–441
    metabolism of, in pediatric patients, 60
    therapeutic monitoring of, 88
Therapeutic equivalence ratings, 6t
Therapeutic interchange, of drugs, 135
Therapeutic lifestyle changes diet, for hyperlipidemia,
        316
Therapeutic monitoring. See also specific drugs and
        diseases
    of older adults, 88
Therapeutic threshold, 18, 19f
Therapeutic window, 18–19, 18b, 19f
Theratype, asthma and ADHD, 426
Thiamine deficiency, in alcohol use disorder, 883
Thiazide diuretics
    for heart failure, 358, 364, 367
    for hypertension, 298–299, 298t
Thiazolidinediones, for diabetes mellitus, 892t,
        895–896
Thorazine (chlorpromazine), for nausea and
        vomiting, 456t, 458
Threshold
    definition of, 18b
    therapeutic, 18, 19f
Thrombocytopenia, heparin-induced, 986, 990
Thrombolysis in myocardial infarction, 334, 334b
Thymine, 122, 122b
Thyroid and parathyroid disorders, 911–913, 912f,
        913f
    hyperparathyroidism, 922–924
    hyperthyroidism, 917–922
    hypoparathyroidism, 924
    hypothyroidism, 913–917
Thyroid disorders. See also Hyperthyroidism;
        Hypothyroidism
Thyroid hormones
    deficiency of (See Hypothyroidism)
    excess of (See Hyperthyroidism)
    for hypothyroidism, 914–916, 915t, 916t
Thyroid-stimulating hormone (TSH), 912
Thyroid storm, hyperthyroidism and, 921
Thyroidectomy, 919, 920t
Thyrolar (liotrix), for hypothyroidism, 914, 915t
Thyrotoxicosis, 917
    causes of, 917, 918b
    untreated, 917
Tiagabine, for seizures, 733t, 742–743
Tiazac (diltiazem), for chronic stable angina, 337t,
        341
Ticagrelor
    for chronic stable angina, 337t, 342
    for coagulation disorders, 1002
Tigan (trimethobenzamide), for nausea and
        vomiting, 456t
Tigecycline, 97t, 108–109, 109t
    for skin infections, 206t, 208

Tikosyn (dofetilide), for arrhythmias, 375t, 379b,
        384
Tildrakizumab, for psoriasis, 232t, 234
Timolol (Betamol)
    for glaucoma, 273t, 275
    for migraine prevention, 716t
Timoptic (timolol), for glaucoma, 273t, 275
Tinactin (tolnaftate), for tinea, 164, 216t
Tinea
    causes of, 212, 212b
    complementary and alternative medicine for, 219
    diagnosis of, 213–214
    infections, varieties of, 212b
    pathophysiology of, 213
    patient education on, 219
    therapeutic response of, 219
    treatment of, 214–215, 215t–217t, 217–219
Tinea capitis, 212, 213, 218
Tinea corporis, 212, 213–214, 218
Tinea cruris, 214, 218
Tinea manuum, 214, 218
Tinea pedis, 212, 214, 218
Tinea unguium, 214, 217–218
Tinea versicolor
    causes of, 212–213, 213b
    complementary and alternative medicine
        for, 219
    diagnosis of, 214
    pathophysiology of, 213
    patient education on, 219
    therapeutic response of, 219
    treatment of, 214–215, 215t–217t, 217–219
Tinidazole, for diarrhea, 483t
Tioconazole, for candidiasis, 1118, 1119t
Tiopropium bromide, for asthma and COPD, 430t,
        438
Tissue-binding characteristics in pediatrics, 60
Tissue selective estrogen complex, 1109
Tizanidine, for pain, 163–164
Tobramycin
    dosages of, 107t
    monitoring of, 108t
    sensitivity of, 97t
Tocilizumab (Actemra), for rheumatoid arthritis, 685
Toenails, fungal infections of, 217, 218, 219
Tofacitnib, for psoriasis, 232t
Tofranil (imipramine)
    for anxiety, 814t, 815
    for irritable bowel syndrome, 494, 497t
Tolerance
    of benzodiazepines, 840
    of nitrates, 339
    of opioids, 161–162
Tolnaftate, for tinea, 216t
Tolterodine, for overactive bladder, 601t, 602, 602t,
        604–605, 604t
Tongue, drug administration under, 21
Tonic-clonic (grand mal) seizures, 726, 727
Tonic seizures, 727
Tonometry, in glaucoma, 272
Topamax (topiramate)
    for migraine prevention, 714, 715t
    for seizure, 734t, 743
Topical administration, 22, 67
Topical calcineurin inhibitors, for contact dermatitis,
        194
Topiramate
    for headaches, 714, 715t
    for seizure, 734t, 743
Toprol (metoprolol)
    for chronic stable angina, 336t, 340
    for hypertension, 300, 301t
Toradol (ketorolac), pharmacokinetic and
        pharmacodynamic properties of, 156t
Torsemide
    for heart failure, 354t
    for hypertension, 299, 299t
Toviaz (fesoterodine), for overactive bladder, 601t,
        602, 603t, 604–605, 604t

Toxicity
from antacids, 462
cytochrome P-450 system, 38
above therapeutic window, 18
Toxoplasma gondii infections, in immunodeficiency, 110
Tramadol
osteoarthritis, 648
for pain, 158t, 160
Trandolapril
for heart failure, 352, 353t, 356, 357
for hypertension, 302
Transcutaneous electrical nerve stimulation, for pain, 152–153, 152b
Transderm-Nitro (nitroglycerin), for chronic stable angina, 336t, 338, 339
Transderm Scop (scopolamine), for nausea and vomiting, 456t, 459
Transdermal administration, 22
Transduction, pain, 148
Transfusion, blood, in blood loss, 1016
Transmission, pain, 148
Transurethral resection of prostate, for benign prostatic hyperplasia, 586
Tranxene (clorazepate), for anxiety disorders, 817t, 818
Travatan Z (travoprost), for glaucoma, 274t, 275–276
Travelers' diarrhea (TD), 480–481
Travoprost
for Alzheimer's disease, 761
for anxiety disorders, 80
for depression, 796
for glaucoma, 274t, 275–276
Trelegy Ellipta (fluticasone furoate/umeclidinium/vilanterol), for asthma and COPD, 431t
Tremfya (guselkumab), for psoriasis, 232t, 234
Tretinoin, for acne, 242–244
Tri-Sprintec (ethinyl estradiol with norgestrate), for acne, 244t
Trial of Nonpharmacological Interventions in the Elderly, 307
Triamcinolone acetonide, for contact dermatitis, 193t
Triamterene
for heart failure, 354t
hypertension, 299, 300t
Triazolam, for insomnia, 833, 834t
Trichloroacetic acid (TCA), for human papilloma virus infections, 616t, 636, 636t
Trichomoniasis
algorithm for, 1124f
causes of, 1116
diagnosis of, 1117
pathophysiology of, 1116
patient education on, 1126
in pregnancy, 1125
treatment of, 1118, 1120–1126, 1120t, 1122t, 1123f
Trichophyton infections, 213
TriCor (fenofibrate), for hyperlipidemia, 321t, 323–324
Tricyclic antidepressants
adverse reactions to, 794, 795t
for Alzheimer's disease, 761
for anxiety disorders, 814t, 815–816
constipation and, 469b
for depression, 789t, 790t–791t, 794, 795t
drug interactions with, 794
for migraine prevention, 716t, 718
for pain, 162
therapeutic ranges of, 794
Triglycerides, 321t
dietary, 316
elevated (*See* Hyperlipidemia)
physiology of, 314
Trihexyphenidyl (Artane), for Parkinson disease, 767–768, 769t

Trilafon (perphenazine), for nausea and vomiting, 456t, 458
Trileptal (oxcarbazepine), for seizure, 730t, 737
Trimethobenzamide, for nausea and vomiting, 456t
Trimethoprim, 109–110, 110t
for urinary tract infections, 569, 570t
Trimethoprim-sulfamethoxazole (TMP-SMZ), 38, 109–110, 110t, 118t
diarrhea and, 480, 483t
for prostatitis, 579, 579t
sensitivity of, 97t
for sinusitis, 413
for urinary tract infections, 569, 570t, 572
Trimpex (trimethoprim), for urinary tract infections, 569, 570t
Triptans, for migraine headache, 703, 704t–706t
Trizivir (combination product), for HIV infection, 951t–952t
Trogarzo, for HIV infection, 955t
Tropical ear. *See* Otitis externa
Trospium, for overactive bladder, 601t, 602t, 604–605, 604t
Trulance (plecanatide), 475
Trusopt (dorzolamide), for glaucoma, 273t, 276
Trypsin, for wound cleansing, 212
TSEC (Tissue selective estrogen complex), 1109
Tubo-ovarian abscess, in pelvic inflammatory disease, 632
Tudorza (aclininium bromide), for asthma and COPD, 430t
Tumor necrosis factor
in psoriasis, 230
for rheumatoid arthritis, 684
Tumor necrosis factor inhibitors, 503t, 508
Tygacil (tigecycline), 97t, 108–109, 109t
for skin infections, 206t, 208
Tylenol (acetaminophen)
metabolism of, 61
for pain, 152, 154, 155, 156t
for pain, 81–82
Tympanic membrane, in otitis media, 283–284
Tympanometry, for otitis media, 284
Tyramine, monoamine oxidase inhibitor interactions with, 31, 794, 796, 796b
Tysabri (natalizumab), for inflammatory bowel disease, 504t, 508, 509
Tzanck test, 221

U
Ubrelvy, for migraine headache, 707t
Ubrogepant (Ubrelvy), for migraine headache, 707t
Ulcer(s)
peptic (*See* Peptic ulcer disease[PUD])
in syphilis, 624
Ulcerative colitis (UC)
aminosalicylates for, 502t, 504–505
antibiotics for, 503t, 507, 513
biological agents for, 507–509, 513
cancer screening and, 515
causes of, 499
complementary and alternative therapies for, 515–516
corticosteroids for, 502t–503t, 505–506, 510, 513, 514
criteria for severity of, 501t
Crohn's disease *vs.*, 500t
diagnosis of, 500
etiology of, 499
fulminant, 501t, 509t
immunosuppressive agents for, 503t, 506–507, 513
incidence of, 499
information sources for, 514–515
nutrition for, 515
pathophysiology of, 499–500, 500t
patient education for, 514–516
in pediatrics, 513
in pregnancy, 513–514

preventive care for, 515
surgical interventions in, 516t
therapeutic monitoring of, 514
treatment of, 500–513, 501t, 502t–504t, 509t, 512f
vaccination for, 515
in women, 513–514
Ultra tears (artificial tears), for keratoconjunctivitis sicca, 269, 270t
Ultram (tramadol)
for osteoarthritis, 648
for restless legs syndrome, 845
Ultrarapid metabolizers, 124
Umeclidinium bromide, for asthma and COPD, 430t, 438
Unasyn (ampicillin–sulbactam), 95t, 101t
Unbound (free) drug, definition of, 22–23
Unfractionated heparin, for chronic stable angina, 342
Uni-Tussin (guaifenesin), for upper respiratory infections, 406t, 408
Unipen (nafcillin), 95t, 100t, 107
Uniphyl (theophylline), for asthma and COPD, 432t, 440–441
Unithroid (levothyroxine), for hypothyroidism, 914, 915t
Units, in prescription, 12
Upregulation, definition of, 18b
Urate-lowering therapies (ULT), 603
Ureasetest, in *Helicobacter pylori* infections, 527
Ureidopenicillins, 100t
Urge incontinence, 604, 607–608
Urinary tract infections (UTIs)
algorithm for, 572f
causes of, 568, 568b
complementary and alternative medicine for, 575
complicated, 568
definition of, 568
diagnosis of, 568–569
information sources for, 574
lifestyle changes for, 574–575
older adults, 573–574
pathophysiology of, 567–568
patient education on, 574–575
pediatric patients, 574
pregnancy, 574
risk factors for, 568
therapeutic monitoring of, 574
treatment of, 569–573, 570t–571t, 572f, 573t
uncomplicated, 457
Urine
culture of, 578
pH of, drug excretion and, 24–25, 39
Urised (methenamine), for urinary tract infections, 571t, 572
Urispas (flavoxate), for urinary tract infections, 571t, 572
Uristat (phenazopyridine), for urinary tract infections, 571t, 572
Uroxatral (alfuzosin), for overactive bladder, 601t, 603t
Use of urodynamic testing (UDT), 599–600, 600t
Ustekinumab
for inflammatory bowel disease, 504t, 508
for psoriasis, 232t, 236
Utibron (indacaterol/glycopyrrolate), for asthma and COPD, 431t

V
Vabomere (meropenem-vaborbactam), 101t
Vaccination. *See also* Immunization
for asthma and COPD, 443
for inflammatory bowel disease, 515
pneumococcal immunization, 290
for viral skin infections, 225
Vaccine(s)
administration routes for, 1034
adverse events of, 1044

contraindications to, 1049, 1049t–1050t, 1051
definition of, 1033
diphtheria, tetanus, pertussis, 1034, 1035b
Haemophilus influenzae, 1033, 1035b, 1036f
hepatitis A, 1034, 1035b, 1043
hepatitis B, 1034, 1035, 1035b, 1038, 1043,
    1052b
human papillomavirus, 1042–1043
influenza, 1035, 1039f, 1041–1042
licensed, 1035b
measles, mumps, rubella, 1036f, 1043–1044,
    1050t, 1052b–1053b
patient education on, 1051–1053, 1051b–1053b
for pediatric patients, 1051b
pertussis, 1042
pneumococcal, 1039f, 1040, 1040b
polio, 1037f, 1043
rotavirus, 1043
tetanus, diphtheria, 1035b, 1052b
varicella, 1035, 1036f, 1037f, 1038, 1044
zoster, 1044
Vaccine Adverse Events Reporting System (VAERS),
    1044, 1045f–1048f
Vagifem (estradiol)
for menopausal symptoms, 1102
for overactive bladder, 608
Vagina, contraceptives for, 1102
Vaginitis
algorithm for, 1121f
allergic, 1116, 1117–1118
anti-inflammatories for, 1120
antibiotics for, 1119–1120
antifungal agents for, 1119
atrophic, 1116, 1118
causes of, 1115–1116
complementary and alternative medicine for,
    1126
diagnosis of, 1116–1118, 1118b
estrogens for, 1120
inflammatory, 1116, 1118
lifestyle changes for, 1126
pathophysiology of, 1116
patient education on, 1126
in pediatric patients, 1123–1125
in postmenopausal women, 1125
in pregnancy, 1125
self-diagnosis and self-treatment of, 1118b
therapeutic monitoring of, 1120
treatment of, 1116–1119, 1118b, 1121f, 1122t,
    1123f, 1124f, 1124t, 1125b, 1125t
Vaginosis, bacterial. *See* Bacterial vaginosis
Valacyclovir
for herpes simplex virus infections, 628
for viral skin infections, 222, 222t, 223
Valdecoxib, 82, 647
13-valent pneumococcal conjugate vaccine (PCV-
    13), 443
23-valent pneumococcal polysaccharide vaccine
    (PPSV-23), 443
Valerian, 840–841
Valium (diazepam)
anxiety, 816, 817t, 819t, 820t
for nausea and vomiting, 456t, 459
Valproic acid, 88
headaches, 714, 715t, 716t
seizures, 728t, 731t, 733t, 738–739
Valsartan
for chronic stable angina, 334, 335t, 338
for heart failure, 354t, 360
for hypertension, 302t
Valtrex (valacyclovir), for viral skin infections, 222,
    222t, 223
Valvular heart disease
diagnosis of, 988
embolism in, 373
native and prosthetic, 988
Vancenase (beclomethasone), for allergic rhinitis,
    940t, 941

Vancocin (vancomycin)
causing diarrhea, 479
for skin infections, 206t, 208
Vancomycin, 97t, 110
causing diarrhea, 479
dosage of, 111t
half-life of, 25
for skin infections, 206t, 208
Vanilloid receptors, for overactive bladder, 609
Vantin (cefpodoxime)
for community-acquired pneumonia, 422
for otitis media, 286, 286t
for skin infections, 205t, 207
upper respiratory infections, 407t, 415–416
Vardenafil, for erectile dysfunction, 590, 590t
Varenicline, for smoking cessation, 1068–1070
Variant angina, 330
Variceal hemorrhage
diagnosis of, 547
prophylaxis, 456t
therapeutic monitoring for, 548
treatment of, 547–548
Varicella vaccine, 225
Varicella-zoster virus (VZV)
causes of, 220
complementary and alternative medicine for, 225
diagnosis of, 220–221
lifestyle changes in, 225
pathophysiology of, 220
patient education for, 225
in pregnancy, 225
prevention of, 225
treatment of, 221–224, 222t, 224f
Varicose veins, 982, 982b
Vascular perfusion in neonates, 59
Vasoactive agents, for variceal hemorrhage, 548
Vasoconstrictors, for conjunctivitis, 264t, 265
Vasodilators, for hypertension, 305, 305t
Vasomotor rhinitis, 934
Vasospasm, coronary artery, 332
Vasotec (enalapril)
for chronic stable angina, 334, 335t, 338
for heart failure, 352, 353t
for hypertension, 302, 302t
Vaughn Williams classification, of antiarrhythmic
    agents, 366
Vedolizumab, for inflammatory bowel disease, 504t,
    508
Velpatasvir, for hepatitis C virus, 559, 559t
Veltin (clindamycin/tretinoin), for acne, 243t, 247
Venereal Disease Research Laboratory test (VDRL),
    624
Venlafaxine
headaches, 699
for overactive bladder, 607–608
pain management, 162
Venous thromboembolism
characteristics of, 982
diagnosis of, 986–987
pathophysiology of, 984–986
prevention of, 1004
treatment of, 986–987, 990
Ventilation/perfusion scan, in pulmonary embolism,
    987
Ventolin (albuterol), for asthma and COPD, 428t,
    436
Ventricular fibrillation, 373b, 387t, 393–394, 395f
Ventricular tachycardia, pulseless, 373b, 374t, 387t,
    394–395, 395f
Verapamil
for arrhythmias, 378t, 379b, 384
chronic stable angina, 337t, 341
constipation and, 469b
headaches, 716t, 718
hypertension, 303t, 304
Verbal description scales, for pain assessment, 151,
    151f
Verelan (verapamil), for hypertension, 303t, 304

Vernal conjunctivitis, 266–267, 266t
VESIcare (solifenacin), for overactive bladder, 601t,
    602, 602t, 604–605, 604t
Viagra (sildenafil), for erectile dysfunction, 589–590,
    590t
Vibativ (telavancin), 97t, 110–111, 111t
Vibramycin (doxycycline), 97t, 108–109, 109t
for prostatitis, 579t, 580
for rosacea, 252
for upper respiratory infections, 407t, 414
Vicks Sinex (oxymetazoline hydrochloride), for upper
    respiratory infections, 405, 405t, 408, 412
Videx (didanosine), for HIV infection, 950, 951t
Vigabatrin, for seizures, 735t, 744–745
Vilanterol, for asthma and COPD, 436
Vilazodone, depression, 796–797
Viracept (nelfinavir), for HIV infection, 954t, 957
Viral agents infections, 480b
Viral hepatitis, 554–562
hepatitis B virus
causes of, 554–555
complementary and alternative medications
    for, 562
diagnosis of, 555
information resources, 561
lifestyle changes in, 562
nutrition for, 562
in older adults, 560
pathophysiology of, 555
patient education on, 561
in pediatrics, 560
in pregnancy, 560
therapeutic monitoring for, 548
treatment of, 555–559, 556t, 558t
in women, 560
hepatitis C virus
causes of, 554–555
complementary and alternative medications
    for, 562
diagnosis of, 555
genomics, 560–561, 561t
information resources, 561
lifestyle changes in, 562
nutrition for, 562
in older adults, 560
pathophysiology of, 555
patient education on, 561
in pediatrics, 560
in pregnancy, 560
therapeutic monitoring for, 548
treatment of, 555, 557, 557t, 559–560, 559t
in women, 560
Viral infections. *See also specific infections*
common cold, 403–412
conjunctivitis, 261–268, 266t
skin, 219–225
Viramune (nevirapine), for HIV infection, 953, 956
Virchow's triad, 981–982
Viread (tenofovir), for HIV infection, 852t, 950
Visceral afferent nerves, 453
Visceral pain, 146, 147b
Vistaril (hydroxyzine)
anxiety, 817t, 820
for nausea and vomiting, 456t, 458–459
Visual analog scale, for pain assessment, 151, 151f
Vitamin A derivative. *See* Retinoids
Vitamin B$_1$ (thiamine), for nausea and vomiting, 468
Vitamin C
anemias, 1020
for common cold, 417
Vitamin D analogs, for psoriasis, 231t, 233–234
Vitamin E, Alzheimer's disease, 762
Vitamin K
epoxide reductase complex, subunit 1
    (VKORC1), 124
warfarin interactions with, 993–996
Vivitrol (naltrexone), for alcohol use disorder, 874t,
    875

Voltaren (diclofenac), pharmacokinetic and pharmacodynamic properties of, 156t
Volume of distribution, 23, 23b
  definition of, 18b
Vortioxetine, depression, 797
Voxelotor, for anemia, 1018
Voxilaprevir, for hepatitis C virus, 559, 559t
Vyepti, for migraine prevention, 717t, 719
Vytorin Efficacy International Trial, 321
Vyzulta (latanoprostene bunod), 274t, 276

W
Waist circumference, in obesity, 1078, 1085
Waist-to-hip ratio, in obesity, 1078, 1085
Wakix, for narcolepsy, 847t, 848
Warfarin, 38, 48, 88
  anticoagulation disturbances, 993–996, 997t
  metabolism and polymorphism of, 124–126, 125f
  vitamin K antagonists, 993–996
Warts (verrucae)
  causes of, 220
  diagnosis of, 221
  lifestyle changes in, 225
  pathophysiology of, 220
  patient education for, 225
  treatment of, 221–224, 224f
Water (body), in pediatrics, 56
Weight
  dysfunctional hormonal system, 1078
  pediatric dosage calculated from, 66
Weight-for-height tables, in obesity, 1078, 1079t
Weight gain, in smoking cessation, 1060b, 1062b
Weight loss, 1077–1086
  dietary supplements for, 1084, 1084t
Welchol (colesevelam), for hyperlipidemia, 321t, 322–323
Wellbutrin (bupropion)
  for ADHD, 861t, 863
  smoking cessation, 1068
Wernicke's encephalopathy, 883
Wet-wrap therapy, 193
Wheat dextrin, for constipation, 471, 471t, 473
Whiff test, in bacterial vaginosis, 1116
Whiteheads, 242, 242t
Wild-type allele, 122b
Witch hazel for skin disorders, 250
Withdrawal
  alcohol or sedative drugs, 725
  antidepressants, 579
  antiepileptic drugs (AEDs), 727
Women. See also Pregnancy
  acne vulgaris and rosacea, 249
  allergies and allergic reactions, 942
  anemias, 1027
  anxiety, 825
  asthma and COPD in, 445
  cannabis in, 187
  constipation in, 478–479
  contact dermatitis in, 197
  contraception, 1089–1099
  diarrhea in, 487
  gastroesophageal reflux disease, 535

gout, 652
headaches, 720–721
heart failure, 368
human immunodeficiency virus, 961–962
hyperlipidemia, 325
hypertension, 307
inflammatory bowel disease in, 513–514
insomnia, 840
irritable bowel syndrome in, 498
major depressive disorder, 801
menopause, 1101–1113
nausea and vomiting in, 466–468
osteoarthritis, 651
overactive bladder in, 611
pain management in opioid use disorder in, 174–175
peptic ulcer disease, 538
rheumatoid arthritis, 688
seizure disorders, 750
sexually transmitted infections, 626, 631, 637
sleep disorders, 840
substance use disorders in, 883
viral hepatitis in, 560
Wood's lamp, in tinea detection, 213
World Health Organization (WHO), adverse drug reaction definition of, 48
Writing prescription
  dosage regimen, and route of administration, 12
  drug dose, 12
  electronic prescriptions, 13
  name of drug, 12
  patient details, 12
  practice of, 11
  prescriber details, 12
  signature and license number, 12–13
  substitutions, 12

X
Xalatan (latanoprost), 274t, 275–276
Xanax (alprazolam), insomnia, 834t, 838t
Xeljanz (tofacitnib), for psoriasis, 232t
Xenical (orlistat), for obesity, 1081, 1081t
Xenleta (lefamulin), 98t, 114, 114t, 118t
Xerava (eravacycline), 97t, 108, 109t
Xifaxan (rifaximin)
  for diarrhea, 483t, 484t–485t, 485–486
  for hepatic encephalopathy, 553t, 554
  for irritable bowel syndrome, 493t, 495, 497t
Ximino (minocycline), for acne, 246
Xnthine oxidase inhibitors, in gout, 653–654
Xolair (omalizumab), for asthma and COPD, 433t, 442–443
Xopenex (levalbuterol tartrate), for asthma and COPD, 428t, 436
Xylocaine (lidocaine), antiarrhythmic agents, 376t, 379–380, 379b

Y
Yersinia infections, 480b, 482
Yoga, for pain management in opioid use disorder, 175
Yohimbine, for erectile dysfunction, 592
Yuzpe regimen, for emergency contraception, 1096

Z
Zafirlukast, for asthma and COPD, 429t, 438–439
Zaleplon, for insomnia, 836, 838t
Zanaflex (tizanidine), for pain, 163–164
Zanamivir, for influenza, 1042
Zantac (ranitidine)
  for GERD, 529t, 530t
  for peptic ulcer disease, 529t, 537t
Zarontin (ethosuximide), for seizures, 731t, 739
Zaroxolyn (metolazone), for heart failure, 353t, 359
Zebeta (bisoprolol), for heart failure, 354t, 362
Zegerid (omeprazole-sodium bicarbonate)
  for GERD, 529t, 530t, 531
  for peptic ulcer disease, 529t, 531, 537t
Zemdri (plazomicin), 107, 107t, 108t
Zerbaxa (ceftolozane–tazobactam), 95t, 101t
Zerit (stavudine), for HIV infection, 851t, 950
Zero-order kinetics, in drug elimination, 25
Zestril (lisinopril)
  for chronic stable angina, 334, 335t, 338
  for heart failure, 352, 353t, 356
  for hypertension, 302, 302t
Zetia (ezetimibe), for hyperlipidemia, 321–322, 321t
Ziagen (abacavir), for HIV infection, 950, 951t
Ziana (clindamycin/tretinoin), for acne, 243t, 247
Zidovudine, for HIV infection, 950, 951t–952t, 955
Zileuton, for asthma and COPD, 429t
Zinacef (cefuroxime), for skin infections, 205t, 207
Zinc, 586, 586t
  for common cold, 418
  for skin disorders, 250
Zioptan (tafluprost), for glaucoma, 274t, 275–276
Zithromax (azithromycin), 106, 106t
  for bronchitis, 419t, 420
  causing diarrhea, 479, 486
  for community-acquired pneumonia, 422–423, 422t
  genitourinary tract disorders, 617
  sensitivity of, 97t
Zocor (simvastatin), 317t, 321
Zofran (ondansetron), for nausea and vomiting, 457t, 460, 467
Zolmitriptan, for migraine headache, 705t, 710
Zoloft (sertraline)
  major depressive disorder, 796, 802
  seizure disorders, 747
Zolpidem, for insomnia, 836, 838t
Zomig (zolmitriptan), for migraine headache, 705t, 710
Zonisamide, for seizures, 734t, 744
Zostavax vaccine, 225
Zosyn (piperacillin–tazobactam), 101t
Zovirax (acyclovir), for viral skin infections, 221–222, 222t, 223
Zubsolv (buprenorphine/naloxone), 169, 170t–171t, 171–172, 172t, 174–175
Zyban (bupropion), for smoking cessation, 1066t, 1068
Zyflo (zileuton), for asthma and COPD, 429t
Zyprexa (olanzapine), for Alzheimer's disease, 761
Zyvox (linezolid), 98t, 112, 112t
  for skin infections, 206t, 208